ADOLESCENT HEALTH CARE

A PRACTICAL GUIDE

FIFTH EDITION

ADOLESCENT HEALTH CARE

A PRACTICAL GUIDE

Editor-in-Chief

Lawrence S. Neinstein, MD

Executive Director
USC University Park Health Center
Professor of Pediatrics and Medicine
Chief, Division of College Health
USC Keck School of Medicine
Los Angeles, California

Associate Editors

Catherine M. Gordon, MD, MSc
Debra K. Katzman, MD, FRCP (C)
David S. Rosen, MD, MPH
Elizabeth R. Woods, MD, MPH

Wolters Kluwer | Lippincott Williams & Wilkins
Health
Philadelphia • Baltimore • New York • London
Buenos Aires • Hong Kong • Sydney • Tokyo

Acquisitions Editor: Sonya Seigafuse
Developmental Editor: Nancy Hoffmann
Managing Editor: Ryan Shaw
Project Manager: Rosanne Hallowell
Manufacturing Manager: Kathleen Brown
Marketing Manager: Kimberly Schonberger
Design Coordinator: Stephen Druding
Cover Designer: Larry Didona
Production Services: Laserwords Private Limited, Chennai, India

Fifth Edition
© 2008 by Lippincott Williams & Wilkins, a Wolters Kluwer business
530 Walnut Street
Philadelphia, PA 19106
LWW.com

© 2002 by Lippincott Williams & Wilkins (fourth edition). © 1996 by Williams & Wilkins
(third edition). © 1991 by Urban & Schwarzenberg (second edition). © 1984 by Urban & Schwarzenberg
(first edition).

Printed in the United States

Library of Congress Cataloging-in-Publication Data

Adolescent health care : a practical guide / edited by Lawrence S. Neinstein ; associate
editors, Catherine M. Gordon ... [et al].—5th ed.
   p. ; cm.
  Rev. ed. of: Adolescent health care / Lawrence S. Neinstein. 4th ed. c2002.
  Includes bibliographical references and index.
  ISBN 978-0-7817-9256-1
  1. Adolescent medicine. I. Neinstein, Lawrence S. II. Neinstein, Lawrence S. Adolescent
health care.
  [DNLM: 1. Adolescent Medicine—Handbooks. WS 39 A2384 2007]
  RJ550.N45 2007
  616.00835—dc22

2007035316

Care has been taken to confirm the accuracy of the information presented and to describe generally
accepted practices. However, the authors, editors, and publisher are not responsible for errors or
omissions or for any consequences from application of the information in this book and make no warranty,
expressed or implied, with respect to the currency, completeness, or accuracy of the contents of the
publication. Application of this information in a particular situation remains the professional responsibility
of the practitioner.

The authors, editors, and publisher have exerted every effort to ensure that drug selection and
dosage set forth in this text are in accordance with current recommendations and practice at the time of
publication. However, in view of ongoing research, changes in government regulations, and the constant
flow of information relating to drug therapy and drug reactions, the reader is urged to check the package
insert for each drug for any change in indications and dosage and for added warnings and precautions.
This is particularly important when the recommended agent is a new or infrequently employed drug.

Some drugs and medical devices presented in this publication have Food and Drug Administration
(FDA) clearance for limited use in restricted research settings. It is the responsibility of health care
providers to ascertain the FDA status of each drug or device planned for use in their clinical practice.

The publishers have made every effort to trace copyright holders for borrowed material. If they
have inadvertently overlooked any, they will be pleased to make the necessary arrangements at the first
opportunity.

To purchase additional copies of this book, call our customer service department at (800) 638-3030 or
fax orders to (301) 223-2320. International customers should call (301) 223-2300.
Visit Lippincott Williams & Wilkins on the Internet: at LWW.com. Lippincott Williams & Wilkins
customer service representatives are available from 8:30 am to 6 pm, EST.

10 9 8 7 6 5 4 3 2 1

To my incredible family:
my wife, Debra,
and my children,
Yael and Yossi, Aaron, and David.
In addition, to my parents
Shirley, Roz, and Ben.

And in memory of my father Alvin.

CONTENTS

CONTRIBUTORS

William P. Adelman, MD
Associate Professor
Department of Pediatrics
F. Edward Hebert School of Medicine
Uniformed Services
University of the Health Sciences;
Head
Department of Adolescent Medicine
National Naval Medical Center and Walter Reed Army Medical
    Center
Bethesda, Maryland

Mark E. Alexander, MD
Assistant Professor of Pediatrics
Department of Pediatrics
Harvard University;
Associate in Cardiology
Department of Pediatric Cardiology
Children's Hospital Boston
Boston, Massachusetts

Seth D. Ammerman, MD
Associate Clinical Professor
Department of Pediatrics
Division of Adolescent Medicine
Stanford University
Mountain View, California;
Attending Physician
Department of Pediatrics
Division of Adolescent Medicine
Lucile Packard Children's Hospital
Palo Alto, California

Martin M. Anderson, MD, MPH
Professor of Clinical Pediatrics
Department of Pediatrics
David Geffen School of Medicine at UCLA;
Professor of Clinical Pediatrics
Department of Pediatrics
Mattel Children's Hospital at UCLA
Los Angeles, California

Raquel D. Arias, MD
Associate Dean for Women
USC Keck School of Medicine;
Associate Professor
Department of Obstetrics and Gynecology
LAC-USC Women's and Children's Hospital
Los Angeles, California

Marvin E. Belzer, MD
Associate Professor of Pediatrics and Medicine
Department of Pediatrics
USC Keck School of Medicine;
Associate Director of Research
Division of Adolescent Medicine
Childrens Hospital Los Angeles
Los Angeles, California

Robert J. Bielski, MD
Assistant Professor
Department of Surgery
Division of Orthopaedics
University of Chicago
Comer Children's Hospital
Chicago, Illinois

Margaret J. Blythe, MD
Professor of Pediatrics
Department of Pediatrics
Indiana University School of Medicine;
Director of Adolescent Clinical Services
Associate Medical Director of Indiana University Medical
    Group—Primary Care
Department of Pediatrics
Wishard Hospital
Indianapolis, Indiana

Terrill Bravender, MD, MPH
Associate Professor
Department of Pediatrics, Psychiatry, Family Medicine
Duke University School of Medicine;
Director of Adolescent Medicine
Department of Pediatrics
Duke University Medical Center
Durham, North Carolina

Paula K. Braverman, MD
Professor of Pediatrics
Department of Pediatrics
University of Cincinnati College of Medicine;
Director of Community Programs
Division of Adolescent Medicine
Cincinnati Children's Hospital Medical Center
Cincinnati, Ohio

Cora Collette Breuner, MD, MPH
Associate Professor
Department of Pediatrics
University of Washington;
Director
Adolescent Medicine Clinic
Children's Hospital and Regional Medical Center
Seattle, Washington

Matthew J. Bueche, MD
Clinical Associate Professor
Department of Orthopaedic Surgery and Rehabilitation
Loyola University Chicago
Stritch School of Medicine
Maywood, Illinois;
Attending Physician
Department of Surgery
Edward Hospital
Naperville, Illinois

Gale R. Burstein, MD, MPH, FAAP
Medical Director
Department of Epidemiology and Surveillance and STD and TB
    Control
Erie County Department of Health;
Clinical Assistant Professor
Department of Pediatrics
The Women and Children's Hospital of Buffalo
Buffalo, New York

Jeremi M. Carswell, MD
Instructor
Department of Pediatrics
Division of Endocrinology
Harvard University Medical School;
Clinical Instructor
Division of Endocrinology
Children's Hospital Boston
Boston, Massachusetts

Mariam R. Chacko, MD
Professor
Department of Pediatrics
Section of Adolescent Medicine & Sports Medicine
Texas Children's Hospital
Baylor College of Medicine
Houston, Texas

Heather Champion, PhD
Research Associate
Department of Social Science & Health Policy
Wake Forest University School of Medicine
Winston-Salem, North Carolina

Sonia Chehil, MD, FRCPC
Assistant Professor
Department of Psychiatry
Dalhousie University;
Staff Psychiatrist
Child and Adolescent Psychiatry
IWK Health Centre
Halifax, Nova Scotia

Michael Cirigliano, MD, FACP
Assistant Professor of Medicine
University of Pennsylvania School of Medicine
Philadelphia, Pennsylvania

Susan M. Coupey, MD
Professor of Pediatrics
Department of Pediatrics
Albert Einstein College of Medicine;
Chief
Division of Adolescent Medicine
Children's Hospital at Montefiore
Bronx, New York

Joanne E. Cox, MD
Assistant Professor
Department of Pediatrics
Harvard Medical School;
Associate Chief
Division of General Pediatrics
Department of Medicine
Children's Hospital Boston
Boston, Massachusetts

Lawrence J. D'Angelo, MD, MPH
Professor
Department of Pediatrics, Medicine, Epidemiology, and
    Prevention and Community Health
George Washington University;
Chief
Division of Adolescent and Young Adult Medicine
Goldberg Center for Community Pediatric Health
Children's National Medical Center
Washington, DC

Ralph J. DiClemente, PhD
Charles Howard Candler Professor
Department of Behavioral Sciences & Health Education
Rollins School of Public Health
Emory University
Atlanta, Georgia

Amy D. DiVasta
Instructor of Pediatrics
Department of Pediatrics
Harvard Medical School;
Assistant in Medicine
Department of Medicine
Division of Adolescent Medicine
Children's Hospital Boston
Boston, Massachusetts

Wendi G. Ehrman, MD
Assistant Professor of Pediatrics and Adolescent Medicine
Department of Pediatrics
Medical College of Wisconsin;
Department of Pediatrics
Childrens' Hospital of Wisconsin
Milwaukee, Wisconsin

Lawrence F. Eichenfield, MD
Professor
Department of Pediatrics & Medicine (Dermatology)
University of California, San Diego;
Chief
Department of Pediatric & Adolescent Dermatology
Rady Children's Hospital-San Diego
San Diego, California

Jean S. Emans, MD
Professor
Department of Pediatrics
Harvard Medical School;
Chief
Division of Adolescent/Young Adult Medicine
Children's Hospital Boston
Boston, Massachusetts

Abigail English, JD
Director
Center for Adolescent Health & the Law
Chapel Hill, North Carolina

James A. H. Farrow, MD
Professor
Department of Pediatrics & Medicine;
Director
Department of Tulane Student Health Service
Tulane University
New Orleans, Louisiana

Martin Fisher, MD
Professor
Department of Pediatrics
New York University School of Medicine
New York, New York;
Chief
Department of Pediatrics
Division of Adolescent Medicine
Schneider Children's Hospital
New Hyde Park, New York

Amy Fleischman, MD, MMSc
Instructor in Medicine
Department of Medicine
Harvard Medical School;
Assistant in Pediatrics
Department of Endocrinology
Children's Hospital Boston
Boston, Massachusetts

Joseph T. Flynn, MD, MS
Professor of Pediatrics
Department of Pediatrics
University of Washington School of Medicine;
Director
Pediatric Hypertension Program
Division of Nephrology
Children's Hospital and Medical Center
Seattle, Washington

J. Dennis Fortenberry, MD, MS
Professor
Department of Pediatrics
Indiana University School of Medicine
Indianapolis, Indiana

Praveen S. Goday, MBBS, CNSP
Assistant Professor
Department of Pediatrics
Medical College of Wisconsin;
Director
Department of Clinical Nutrition
Children's Hospital of Wisconsin
Milwaukee, Wisconsin

Melanie A. Gold, DO
Associate Professor of Medicine
Division of Adolescent Medicine
Department of Pediatrics
University of Pittsburgh School of Medicine;
Director of Adolescent Medicine Research
Director of Family Planning Services
Department of Pediatrics
Division of Adolescent Medicine
Children's Hospital of Pittsburgh
Pittsburgh, Pennsylvania

Neville H. Golden, MD
Professor of Pediatrics
Department of Pediatrics
Stanford University School of Medicine;
Chief of Adolescent Medicine
Department of Adolescent Medicine
Lucile Packard Children's Hospital at Stanford
Stanford, California

Catherine M. Gordon, MD, MSc
Associate Professor of Pediatrics
Department of Pediatrics
Divisions of Endocrine and Adolescent Medicine
Harvard Medical School, Children's Hospital Boston;
Associate in Medicine
Department of Medicine
Divisions of Adolescent Medicine and Endocrinology
Children's Hospital Boston
Boston, Massachusetts

Albert C. Hergenroeder, MD
Professor of Pediatrics
Department of Pediatrics
Baylor College of Medicine;
Chief
Adolescent Medicine & Sports Medicine
Adolescent Medicine & Sports Medicine Service
Texas Children's Hospital
Houston, Texas

Paula J. Adams Hillard, MD
Professor
Department of Obstetrics/Gynecology
Stanford University School of Medicine;
Director of Gynecologic Specialties
Department of Obstetrics and Gynecology
Stanford University Medical Center
Stanford, California

Stephen A. Huang, MD
Assistant Professor
Department of Pediatrics
Harvard Medical School; Director
Thyroid Program
Children's Hospital Boston
Boston, Massachusetts

Loris Y. Hwang, MD
Fellow
Department of Pediatrics
University of California, San Francisco
San Francisco, California

Marc S. Jacobson, MD
Professor
Department of Pediatrics, and Epidemiology and Social
    Medicine
Albert Einstein College of Medicine
Bronx, New York;
Director
Center for Atherosclerosis Prevention
Schneider Children's Hospital
New Hyde Park, New York

Mary Anne Jamieson, MD, FRCSC
Associate Professor
Department of Obstetrics & Gynecology
Queen's University;
Attending Staff
Department of Obstetrics & Gynecology
Kingston General Hospital
Kingston, Ontario

M. Susan Jay, MD
Chief
Adolescent Medicine
Department of Pediatrics
Medical College of Wisconsin
Milwaukee, Wisconsin;
Director
Adolescent Health and Medicine
Children's Hospital of Wisconsin
Wauwatosa, Wisconsin

Alain Joffe, MD, MPH
Director
Department of Student Health and Wellness Center
Johns Hopkins University;
Associate Professor of Pediatrics
Department of Pediatrics
Johns Hopkins Medical Institutions
Baltimore, Maryland

Lisa M. Johnson, MD
Consultant
Adolescent Medicine
Department of Public Health
Nassau, Bahamas

Jessica A. Kahn, MD, MPH
Associate Professor of Pediatrics
Department of Pediatrics
University of Cincinnati College of Medicine;
Director of Research Training
Department of Research Training
Division of Adolescent Medicine
Cincinnati Children's Hospital Medical Center
Cincinnati, Ohio

Debra K. Katzman, MD, FRCP(C)
Associate Professor of Pediatrics
Head, Division of Adolescent Medicine
Department of Pediatrics
The Hospital for Sick Children and University of Toronto
Toronto, Ontario

Sari L. Kives, MD, FRCSC
Assistant Professor
Department of Obstetrics/Gynecology
University of Toronto;
Staff Physician
Department of Obstetrics/Gynecology
St. Michaels Hospital for Sick Children
Toronto, Ontario

Jonathan D. Klein, MD, MPH
Associate Professor
Department of Pediatrics
University of Rochester School of Medicine and Dentistry;
Associate Chair for Community and Government Affairs
Golisano Children's Hospital at Stong
University of Rochester Medical Center
Rochester, New York

John R. Knight, MD
Associate Professor of Pediatrics
Department of Pediatrics
Harvard Medical School;
Director
Center for Adolescent Substance Abuse Research
Children's Hospital Boston
Boston, Massachusetts

Michael R. Kohn, FRACP
Senior Clinical Lecturer
Faculty of Medicine
Sydney University
Camperdown, New South Wales;
Senior Staff Specialist
Division of Adolescent Medicine
The Children's Hospital at Westmead
Westmead, New South Wales

John Kulig, MD, MPH
Professor of Pediatrics
Public Health and Family Medicine
Tufts University School of Medicine;
Director
Adolescent Medicine
Department of Pediatrics
Tufts–New England Medical Center
Boston, Massachusetts

Stan Kutcher, MD, MA
Professor of Psychiatry
Sun Life Chair in Adolescent Mental Health
Department of Psychiatry
Dalhousie University;
Consultant Psychiatrist
Department of Psychiatry
IWK Health Sciences Center
Halifax, Nova Scotia

Judith A. Lacy, MD
Clinical Instructor
Department of Obstetrics and Gynecology
Stanford University
Lucile Packard Children's Hospital
Stanford, California

Sharon Levy, MD, MPH
Assistant Professor
Department of Pediatrics
Harvard Medical School;
Director
Adolescent Substance Abuse Program
Department of Medicine
Children's Hospital, Boston
Boston, Massachusetts

Peter R. Loewenson, MD, MPH
Pediatrics and Adolescent Medicine
Health East Care System
Minneapolis, Minnesota

Patricia A. Lohr, MD, MPH
Medical Director
British Pregnancy Advisory Service
Stratford-upon-Avon, United Kingdom

Keith J. Loud, MD, CM, MSc
Assistant Professor
Department of Pediatrics
Northeast Ohio Universities College of Medicine;
Medical Director
Adolescent Health Services
Akron Children's Hospital
Akron, Ohio

Robert E. Morris, MD, BS
Professor of Clinical Pediatrics and Health Care
Director, Division of Juvenile Justice
Department of Corrections and Rehabilitation
Department of Pediatrics
University of California at Los Angeles
Los Angeles, California

Heather R. Macdonald, MD
Assistant Professor of Clinical Obstetrics & Gynecology and
    Breast Surgery
Department of Obstetrics & Gynecology, Surgery
USC Keck School of Medicine;
Assistant Professor of Clinical Obstetrics & Gynecology and
    Breast Surgery
Department of Obstetrics & Gynecology, Surgery
Norris Comprehensive Cancer Center
Los Angeles, California

Joan M. Mansfield, MD
Assistant Professor of Pediatrics
Department of Pediatrics
Divisions Endocrinology and Adolescent Young Adult Medicine
Harvard Medical School;
Associate in Medicine
Endocrinology and Adolescent/Young Adult Medicine,
Children's Hospital Boston
Boston, Massachusetts

Miguel Martinez, MSW, MPH
Program Manager
Division of Adolescent Medicine
Children's Hospital Los Angeles
Los Angeles, California

Eric Meininger, MD, MPH
Community–University Health Care Center
University of Minnesota
Minneapolis, Minnesota

Jordan D. Metzl, MD
Assistant Professor
Department of Pediatrics
Weill Medical College of Cornell University;
Medical Director
The Sports Medicine Institute for Young Athletes
Hospital for Special Surgery
New York, New York

Catherine A. Miller, MD
Clinical Fellow
Department of Pediatrics
Division of Adolescent Medicine
University of California, San Francisco
San Francisco, California

Melissa D. Mirosh, MD, FRCSC
Attending Staff
Department of Obstetrics and Gynecology
High River Hospital
Alberta, Canada

Laurie A. P. Mitan, MD
Associate Professor of Clinical Pediatrics-Affiliated
Department of Pediatrics
The University of Cincinnati College of Medicine;
Associate Professor
Department of Adolescent Medicine
Cincinnati Children's Hospital Medical Center
Cincinnati, Ohio

Wendy G. Mitchell, MD
Professor
Department of Neurology and Pediatrics
USC Keck School of Medicine;
Pediatric Neurologist
Division of Neurology
Childrens Hospital Los Angeles
Los Angeles, California

Anna-Barbara Moscicki, MD
Professor of Pediatrics
Department of Pediatrics;
Associate Director of Adolescent Medicine
Department of Adolescent Medicine
Pediatrics School of Medicine
University of California, San Francisco
San Francisco, California

Lawrence S. Neinstein, MD, FACP
Professor of Pediatrics and Medicine
Executive Director
USC University Park Health Center
Chief, Division of College Health
Department of Pediatrics
USC Keck School of Medicine
Associate Dean of Student Affairs
University of Southern California
Los Angeles, California

Anita L. Nelson, MD
Professor
Obstetrics and Gynecology
David Geffen School of Medicine at UCLA
Los Angeles, California;
Medical Director
Women's Health Care Programs
Harbor–UCLA Medical Center
Torrance, California

Donald P. Orr, MD
Professor
Pediatrics, Adolescent Medicine
Indiana University School of Medicine
Health Information & Translational Sciences;
Director
Pediatric Adolescent Medicine
Indiana University School of Medicine
Indianapolis, Indiana

Ponrat Pakpreo, MD
Physician
Pediatrics
Sacred Heart Children's Hospital
Spokane, Washington

Mei-Lin T. Pang, MD
Research Fellow
Department of Pediatric and Adolescent Dermatology
Rady Children's Hospital San Diego;
Department of Dermatology
Division of Dermatology
University of California San Diego Medical Center
San Diego, California

Arthur Partikian, MD
Child Neurology Fellow
Department of Neurology
Childrens Hospital Los Angeles;
University of Southern California
Keck School of Medicine
Los Angeles, California

Mari Radzik, PhD
Clinical Assistant Professor of Pediatrics
USC Keck School of Medicine;
Clinical Psychologist
Division of Adolescent Medicine
Childrens Hospital Los Angeles
Los Angeles, California

Gary Remafedi, MD, MPH
Professor
Department of Pediatrics;
Executive Director
Youth and AIDS Projects
University of Minnesota
Minneapolis, Minnesota

Vaughn I. Rickert, PsyD
Professor of Clinical Population and Family Health
Heilbrunn Department of Population and Family Health
Mailman School of Public Health at Columbia University
New York, New York

Arthur L. Robin, PhD
Professor of Psychiatry & Behavioral Neurosciences
Department of Psychiatry & Behavioral Neurosciences
Wayne State University School of Medicine;
Director of Psychology Training, Chief of Psychology
Department of Child Psychiatry and Psychology Department
Children's Hospital of Michigan
Detroit, Michigan

David S. Rosen, MD, MPH
Professor
Departments of Pediatrics and Internal Medicine
University of Michigan Medical School;
Chief
Section of Teenage and Young Adult Health
Department of Pediatrics
University of Michigan Health System
Ann Arbor, Michigan

Owen Ryan, MPH, MIA
Graduate Research Assistant
Heilbrunn Department of Population and Family Health
Columbia University
Mailman School of Public Health
New York, New York

Kiarash Sadrieh, MD
Director
Pediatric Neurology
White Memorial Medical Center
Los Angeles, California

Sandra Loeb Salsberg, MD
Fellow in Endocrinology
Division of Endocrinology
Children's Hospital Boston
Boston, Massachusetts

Marcie B. Schneider, MD, FAAP, FSAM
Associate Clinical Professor of Pediatrics
Department of Pediatrics
Albert Einstein College of Medicine
Bronx, New York;
Associate Attending
Department of Pediatrics
Greenwich Hospital
Greenwich, Connecticut

Howard Schubiner, MD
Clinical Professor
Department of Pediatrics
Internal Medicine and Psychiatry
Wayne State University
Detroit, Michigan;
Faculty Internist
Department of Internal Medicine
Providence Hospital
Southfield, Michigan

Robert Sege, MD, PhD
Professor of Pediatrics
Department of Pediatrics
Boston University School of Medicine;
Director
Division of Ambulatory Pediatrics
Boston Medical Center
Boston, Massachusetts

Mary-Ann B. Shafer, MD
Professor of Pediatrics
Associate Director of Training
Division of Adolescent Medicine
University of California, San Francisco
San Francisco, California

Sara Sherer, PhD
Assistant Professor of Clinical Pediatrics
Keck School of Medicine
University of Southern California;
Director, Psychology Postdoctoral Fellowship
USC UCEDD Mental Health
Department of Pediatrics
Division of General Pediatrics
Director, Behavioral Services
Division of Adolescent Medicine
Department of Pediatrics
Childrens Hospital Los Angeles
Los Angeles, California

Lydia A. Shrier, MD, MPH
Assistant Professor
Department of Pediatrics
Harvard Medical School;
Director of Clinic-Based Research
Division of Adolescent/Young Adult Medicine
Children's Hospital Boston
Boston, Massachusetts

David M. Siegel, MD, MPH
Professor
Departments of Pediatrics and Medicine
University of Rochester School of Medicine and Dentistry;
Chief
Division of Pediatric Rheumatology and Immunology
University of Rochester;
Edward H. Townsend Chief of Pediatrics
Rochester General Hospital;
Department of Pediatrics
Golisano Children's Hospital at Strong
Rochester, New York

Gail B. Slap, MD, MS, FSAM
Professor of Pediatrics
Associate Chair for Fellowship Training
Department of Pediatrics
University of Pennsylvania
Philadelphia, Pennsylvania

Norman P. Spack, MD
Assistant Professor of Pediatrics
Harvard Medical School;
Associate in Endocrinology
Children's Hospital Boston;
Senior Associate
Endocrine Division
Children's Hospital Boston
Boston, Massachusetts

Diane E. J. Stafford, MD
Instructor
Department of Pediatrics
Harvard Medical School;
Assistant Clinical Director
Division of Endocrinology
Children's Hospital
Boston, Massachusetts

Paula L. Swinford, MS, MHA, CHES
Director
Health Promotion and Prevention Services
University of Southern California
Los Angeles, California

Diane Tanaka, MD
Assistant Professor of Clinical Pediatrics
Department of Pediatrics
University of Southern California;
Attending Physician
Division of Adolescent Medicine
Children's Hospital of Los Angeles
Los Angeles, California

Brigid L. Vaughan, MD
Assistant Professor
Department of Psychiatry
Harvard Medical School;
Medical Director
Psychopharmacology Program
Department of Psychiatry
Children's Hospital Boston
Boston, Massachusetts

Emmanuel B. Walter, MD, MPH
Associate Professor
Associate Director Duke Vaccine and Infectious Disease and
  Epidemiology Unit
Department of Pediatrics
Duke University Medical Center
Durham, North Carolina

Shelly K. Weiss, MD
Assistant Professor
Department of Paediatrics
University of Toronto;
Neurologist
Department of Paediatrics
Hospital for Sick Children
Toronto, Ontario

Merrill Weitzel, MD
Instructor in Obstetrics
Department of Gynecology and Reproductive Biology
Harvard Medical School;
Assistant in Surgery
Department of Surgery
Division of Gynecology
Children's Hospital Boston;
Associate
Department of Obstetrics and Gynecology
Brigham and Women's Hospital
Boston, Massachusetts

Elizabeth R. Woods, MD, MPH
Associate Professor
Department of Pediatrics
Harvard Medical School;
Associate Chief
Division of Adolescent/Young Adult Medicine
Department of Pediatrics
Children's Hospital Boston
Boston, Massachusetts

Alan D. Woolf, MD, MPH
Associate Professor
Department of Pediatrics
Harvard Medical School;
Director of Pediatric Environmental Health Center
Division of General Pediatrics
Children's Hospital Boston
Boston, Massachusetts

Kimberly A. Workowski, MD, FACP, FIDSA
Associate Professor of Medicine
Department of Medicine
Division of Infectious Diseases
Emory University;
Chief
Guidelines Unit
Epidemiology and Surveillance Branch
Centers for Disease Control and Prevention
Atlanta, Georgia

FOREWORD

It is our great pleasure to write the foreword to the fifth edition of *Adolescent Health Care: A Practical Guide*. Larry Neinstein and his associate editors provide a wonderful resource for practicing health professionals caring for adolescents, who will use this handy reference guide on a daily basis. This latest volume reflects the changing field of adolescent medicine: It incorporates new ideas and data into earlier versions while adding new perspectives in the field. Most importantly, the very practical approaches of previous editions continue to permeate this latest version of one of the most useful guides written for the medical care of teenagers.

Many faculty members tell us of the very practical ways this book influences their teaching and delivery of care. We also know that many other physicians, nurses, and health practitioners, who see the majority of adolescents in private practice and public health settings, will also find this book of great use.

It is for those who are in training, the many subspecialists now in the field, and the larger health professional audience that this fine volume has been revised. Older sections have been brought up to date and new sections added to reflect the latest in management and care of adolescents and their families.

Dr. Neinstein and his associate editors have provided us with a solid base for the practice of adolescent medicine, adding new chapters on psychosomatic illness, complementary medicine, anxiety disorders, substance abuse, human papillomavirus (HPV), and anogenital warts. Sixty-six new authors and coauthors have contributed to this edition, further recognizing the many leading experts who add their skill and expertise to the field of adolescent health care. They have skillfully distilled and synthesized new knowledge and transformed it into useful and accessible information for the practitioner.

It is hard to believe that it has been more than 23 years since *Adolescent Health Care* was first conceived. During this time, dramatic changes have occurred in the field, including the establishment of adolescent medicine as a subspecialty in pediatrics, family medicine, and internal medicine. This recognition has served to codify special areas of interest and knowledge in the field. Expertise in adolescent health is found in academic health centers, college health centers, community agencies, and school services nationally and internationally.

It is certainly hard to predict where the field will go in the next 50 years. Clearly, adolescence as a period of life will continue to undergo dramatic changes as our young people seek new ways to redefine themselves and to explore new ideas and challenges. We will need to understand how they will influence other teenagers and how young people will have an impact on their families, their communities, and the world at large. Their health care may play a much larger role in understanding how health and illness will change in our society, in an increasingly smaller and smaller world.

One can only wonder how the daily care of teenagers will also change. Clearly, the developmental aspects of this challenging period of time will remain. But with enhanced communication between teenagers and their world, an expanded role of the Internet, iPods, and cell phones in our lives, and the drive toward seeking and improving self-help and self-knowledge, it is hard to conceive of the many new ways by which we will be providing care for these young people.

With that in mind, we are sure that a future edition of *Adolescent Health Care: A Practical Guide* will be around to assist us in meeting the challenges of youth and give us the opportunity to provide the highest quality of health care.

Iris F. Litt, MD
Dale C. Garell, MD

PREFACE

It feels incredible to see the fifth edition of *Adolescent Health Care: A Practical Guide* come to life. A once small project to help with my instruction of residents and adolescent medicine fellows has turned into a comprehensive but practical text whose "life" has now spanned almost a quarter of a century through its five editions. It has been a joy to see the continued development of adolescent health care as an exciting multidisciplinary field and see the increasing interest in this age group among so many different groups in health care. I have continued to be extremely gratified that the text remains so highly utilized among individuals at all levels of training and by so many different disciplines. One of the most satisfying aspects of my professional career has been the continued positive feedback I have received from you about the usefulness and practicality of the book for clinical, teaching, and study purposes. I continue to love seeing heavily worn copies of this book in offices and clinics.

Adolescent health care continues to expand as a field and includes pediatricians, internists, family medicine physicians, gynecologists, nurse practitioners, physician assistants, psychologists, social workers, nurses, health educators, nutritionists, and teachers, among many others. The field has grown to include the health issues among college students, young adults with chronic illnesses transitioning into adult health care systems, adolescents in a variety of institutional settings, and adolescents served in school-based clinics. I thank all of you who are the providers of care to this population. I am always amazed and uplifted by the number of wonderful individuals from so many disciplines involved in the care of youth.

It is at times a daunting task to approach a new edition of this text with the increasing volume of information that continues to change at an ever-rapid rate. To facilitate a wider range of expertise and to broaden the approach, I have added associate editors. Dr. Debra Katzman, Dr. Catherine M. Gordon, Dr. David Rosen, and Dr. Elizabeth Woods are among the most respected names in the field of adolescent health care in North America. They provide a wide range of expertise ranging from gynecology, endocrinology, mental health issues, and prevention health issues to substance abuse and sexually transmitted diseases. They have been an invaluable addition in continuing to raise the standards of this textbook. In addition to these four associate editors, new experts have been added to almost every chapter. I sincerely thank the many contributors who have helped make this fifth edition, which I consider the most complete and the most user- and Web-friendly edition yet.

With the many requests, it is always difficult to decide what special new topics to add to a new edition. Several topics came to the forefront that were important to either add, expand upon, or reorganize. These include the addition of a chapter on anxiety disorders, the total reorganization of the substance abuse chapters, the addition of material on complementary medicine, and the reorganization and expansion of material on HPV and cervical cytology. All other material has been extensively revised to include new information, research, and recommendations as well as new references and Web sites. Web sites, both in the text and in the reference section, have also been expanded to access up-to-date information where relevant. Web sites that are appropriate for teenagers, parents, and professionals have also been included.

I hope that all readers will enjoy this latest edition of *Adolescent Health Care*. Particularly for new readers, the intent is to make the material practical and easy to read, while maintaining a thorough approach that is evidence based but in a concise format. I know that the many tables, figures, statistics, references, and resources will help you in providing care to the many adolescents and young adults that you serve. The appendices cover a wide range of books, magazines, articles, organizations, and Web sites available for this age-group. As always, the hope is to make it easier for you, the reader, to perform appropriate evaluations and workups.

I dedicate this book to young people and to their health care providers. I hope this edition will provide a wealth of information for those who care for youth and young adults. Importantly, I welcome and look forward to feedback on this edition so I can continue to improve this book as the most practical guide to adolescent health issues.

Lawrence S. Neinstein, MD

Adolescent Health Care: A Practical Guide is written for those health-care professionals involved in the care of adolescents, including pediatricians, family practitioners, internists, gynecologists, house staff, nurses, nurse practitioners, and others. The list is long because the challenge of adolescent medicine crosses the specialty boundaries of medicine as well as the lines separating the medical, psychological, and social areas of health care.

This volume is designed for day-to-day office use. Topics are reviewed in a format that outlines and highlights subjects for easy reference. Selection of subject areas was discussed with house staff and other experts in adolescent medicine and primary care medicine in order to assure that pertinent areas of interest were not overlooked. In this connection, many subspecialty concerns have been excluded, as they were felt to be better examined in internal medicine or pediatric texts.

Normal growth and psychosocial development of adolescents is discussed first in the book, in order to provide a framework in which to consider abnormalities. Among the chapters featured, for example, are those on problems unique to adolescence (i.e., gynecomastia); problems exacerbated by adolescence (i.e., suicide, school problems); and problems with unique considerations during adolescence (i.e., thyroid disease, chest pain). In addition, because of the high prevalence of teenage sexual activity, sexually transmissible diseases, and drug use, extensive sections of the book have been devoted to these areas. To assist the health-care practitioner in treating adolescents, other chapters concentrate on developing rapport with teens, legal issues associated with teenage care, and psychosocial problems in teens. Useful doctor's office and hospital materials are furthermore included, such as questionnaires for initial interviews, history and physical examination forms, and patient handouts on contraception. The book's numerous tables provide statistics on the adolescent age group in areas such as morbidity, mortality, hypertension, and hyperlipidemia. These have been drawn from many sources and endeavor to provide the practitioner with age-relevant statistics. Last, to assist the practitioner in finding available community resources, an extensive Appendix has been added.

Working with adolescents is exciting, challenging, and sometimes difficult and frustrating. Adolescence is a time of rapid growth and development of mind and body, presenting difficulties in adjustment for the teenager, the family, and the physician. It is also a time of high risk for many problems such as suicide and sexually transmissible diseases, as well as being a critical period for detecting chronic illnesses and risk factors for cardiovascular disease. Moreover, it is an ideal time to educate adolescents about how to best care for their bodies. This book is dedicated to helping the health-care professional meet these challenges.

ACKNOWLEDGMENTS

It takes a tremendous effort to put together a book as complex and comprehensive as *Adolescent Health Care*. I am forever indebted to the late Adie Klotz, MD, a friend, teacher, and source of inspiration, who helped me realize the excitement of working with young people. I also acknowledge both Richard G. MacKenzie, MD, and Dale Garell, MD, who encouraged my interest in the field of adolescent medicine.

With this fifth edition, I have gained four wonderful colleagues and friends who helped in the completion of this project—my four associate editors. They have all been an incredible pleasure to work with, and have added their unique qualities and expertise to this text. In addition, they have been responsive and eager to add their own input to this text. I sincerely thank Catherine M. Gordon, Debra Katzman, David Rosen, and Elizabeth Woods for their assistance as coeditors.

I also express my deepest appreciation to the many experts who served as authors on the many chapters of this book. Their knowledge, expertise, and dedication have helped to make this the most complete edition yet. I personally thank them for their time and effort in response to our many, many requests, e-mails, and demands.

I want to thank both the wonderful and dedicated staff of the Division of Adolescent Medicine at Children's Hospital of Los Angeles and the staff and students at the USC University Park Center who have taught me so much about adolescents and college students. Many other health care professionals have also given me their assessments and helpful comments in the development of this fifth edition.

Special thanks go to several individuals at the University of Southern California. I would like to thank Lucy Vergara, at the USC University Park Health Center, who was always there to assist in communicating with Lippincott Williams & Wilkins and coauthors. I also wish to thank Michael Jackson, Vice-President of Student Affairs, and Dr. Roberta Williams, Chair of Pediatrics, USC Keck School of Medicine, who continued to encourage my academic pursuits.

Individuals at Lippincott Williams & Wilkins also deserve recognition in the development of this edition.

I thank Ryan Shaw, managing editor, for his assistance in being a kind facilitator to my many requests for edits and changes. I also thank Kimberly Schonberger, marketing manager, Rosanne Hallowell, project manager, and Sonya Seigafuse, acquisitions editor. In addition, I would like to thank, Anitha Rajarathnam, project manager at Laserwords, who also assisted in the copy editing and production of this edition.

These past few years have been personally medically challenging ones. I would like to express my deepest thanks to several physicians whose helpful treatment and advice have kept me healthy. My heartfelt thanks goes to Dr. Gary Dosik, Dr. Brian Durie at Cedars-Sinai Medical Center, Dr. Steve Forman at City of Hope Medical Center, and Dr. Burt Liebross. I also want to thank the caring and supportive nursing staff at all of these facilities and my wonderful friends and family who have been there for me. It was certainly a rewarding experience to work on some of this current edition and communicate with my associate editors while on the transplant unit at the City of Hope Medical Center. So, with all my heart, a deep thank you.

There are also individuals very close to me who deserve special recognition. My parents have shown me what appropriate, loving, and involved parenting can mean during one's tumultuous adolescent years and during adult life. Without their guidance, I would not have had the skills and ability to become the person I am. A second set of parents, Roz and Ben, have also provided unflagging support during the past 35 years. Loving thanks to all of you.

Lastly, I thank my loving wife, Debra, and my children, Yael and Yossi, Aaron, and David. Debbie has continued to support me despite even far more hours and late nights spent preparing this edition. Yael and Yossi, Aaron and David serve to inspire me with wonderful examples of healthy young adults. I love all of you and thank you for your understanding, support, and encouragement with this fifth edition.

PART I

General Considerations in Adolescent Care

CHAPTER 1

Normal Physical Growth and Development

Jeremi M. Carswell and Diane E. J. Stafford

Accelerated growth, maturation of sexual characteristics, and the attainment of adult height and body proportions are the physical hallmarks of adolescence. Underlying these changes are the complicated activation and interplay of several hormonal axes that have been previously quiescent. The teenage years also involve significant developmental changes in the psychosocial area (see Chapter 2). This chapter provides an overview of the normal pubertal process and highlights the wide variation in the onset and duration of puberty in healthy adolescents and between male and female adolescents. Understanding these variations will provide the health care provider a framework for differentiating normal variations from abnormal pubertal development. The focus of Chapter 8 is abnormalities in growth and pubertal development.

THE MAJOR ENDOCRINE AXES AFFECTING GROWTH AND DEVELOPMENT

Although there is activity and change in most hormonal systems during adolescence, there are three primary hormonal axes that influence the physical changes observed. These are the hypothalamic-pituitary-gonadal (HPG) axis, the hypothalamic-pituitary-adrenal (HPA) axis, and the growth hormone (GH) axis.

Hypothalamic-Pituitary-Gonadal Axis

The HPG axis is responsible for the release of estradiol (E2) from the ovary and testosterone (T) from the testes and ultimately responsible for secondary sexual characteristics, menarche (onset of menses), and thelarche (onset of breast development). The initial signal originates from the hypothalamus in the form of gonadotropin-releasing hormone (GnRH) (also called *luteinizing hormone–releasing hormone*, or LHRH) from the so-called GnRH pulse generator, which signals the release of the gonadotropins, luteinizing hormone (LH), and follicle-stimulating-hormone (FSH) from the pituitary gland. Although the exact pubertal triggers are incompletely understood, it is release of inhibition by the central nervous system (CNS) through neurotransmitters that allows the initiation of a positive feedback loop that characterizes pubertal maturation within this system.

Figure 1.1 depicts this system diagrammatically, whereas Figure 1.2 illustrates how the CNS and gonadal steroids influence GnRH pulsatility.

Hypothalamic-Pituitary-Adrenal Axis

Androgens secreted from the adrenal glands are under the control of the HPA axis and are independent of the changes occurring in the HPG axis. The two primary hormones are dehydroepiandrosterone (DHEA) and its sulfate ester, dehydroepiandrosterone-sulfate (DHEA-S), both produced in the zona reticularis of the adrenal gland. These hormones exert their effects by acting as precursors for the more potent androgens, testosterone and dihydrotestosterone, as DHEA and DHEA-S do not appear to activate the androgen

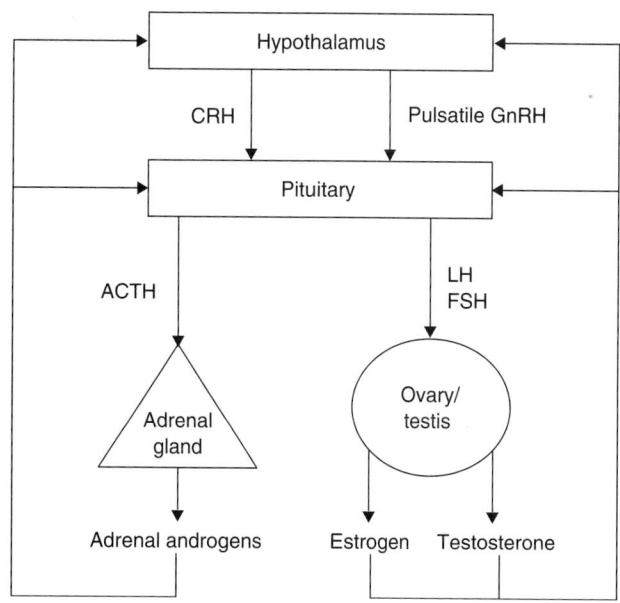

FIGURE 1.1 The hypothalamic-pituitary-gonadal and the hypothalamic-pituitary-adrenal axes. CRH, corticotropin-releasing hormone; GnRH, gonadotropin-releasing hormone; ACTH, adrenocorticotropic hormone; LH, luteinizing hormone; FSH, follicle-stimulating-hormone.

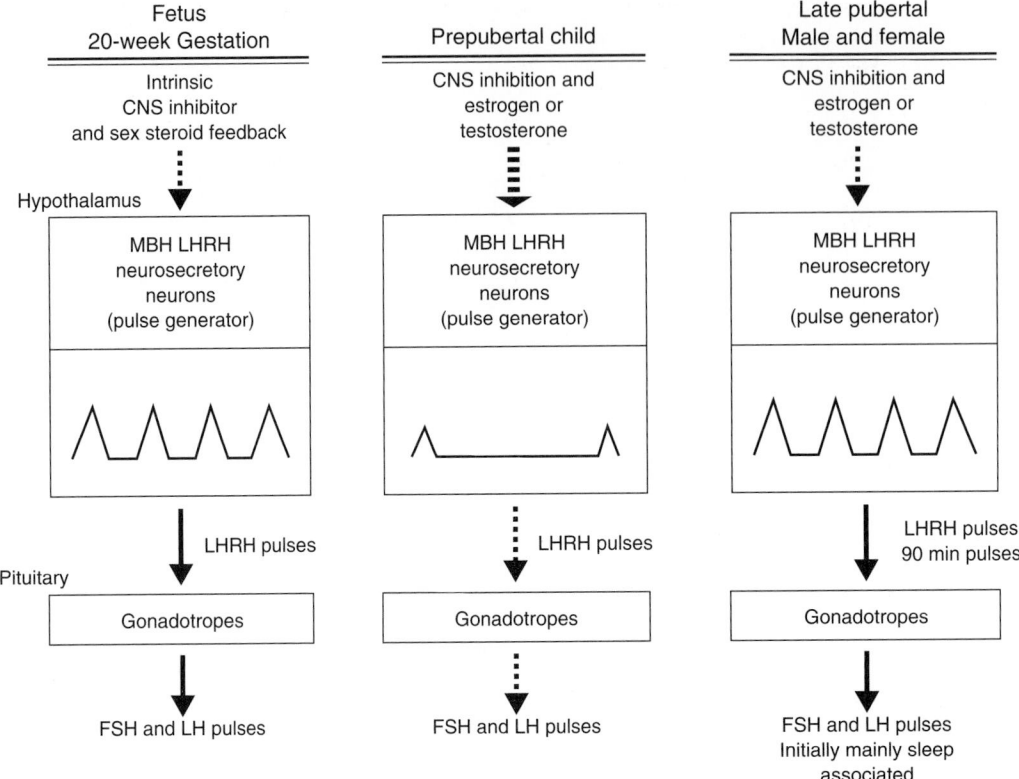

FIGURE 1.2 Postulated influences of the central nervous system and gonadal steroids on gonadotropin-releasing hormone (GnRH) pulsatility and the changes with puberty. Interrupted arrows indicate inhibition. Note the action of both components during the prepubertal phase. CNS, central nervous system; LHRH, luteinizing hormone releasing hormone; MBH, medial basal hypothalamus; FSH, follicle-stimulating-hormone; LH, luteinizing hormone. (Copied with permission from: Grumbach MM, Styne DM. Puberty: ontogeny, neuroendocrinology, physiology, and disorders. In: Larsen RM, Wilson JD, Foster DW, et al. eds. *Williams textbook of endocrinology*, 10th ed. Philadelphia: © 2003 WB Saunders, 2003:1161.)

receptors themselves. The primary physical manifestations of the rise in adrenal hormones (adrenarche) are as follows:

1. Growth of terminal hair in the axillary and pubic areas
2. Development of body odor
3. Increased sebum production and potential development of acne

Growth Hormone Axis

The key hormone influencing growth is GH. Pituitary secretion of this hormone is regulated by growth hormone–releasing hormone (GHRH) and somatostatin, as shown in Figure 1.3. GH secretion is increased by GHRH and decreased by somatostatin. GH is released in a pulsatile manner, with maximum rates at the onset of slow wave sleep. There is negative feedback of GH secretion through GH itself and the insulin-like growth factors (IGFs).

The effects of GH are primarily modulated through the IGFs. The two major types are IGF-I (formerly somatomedin-C) and IGF-II. As the term implies, these hormones have qualitative biological effects that are similar to those of insulin. The major mechanism for growth appears to be through stimulation of IGF-I by GH, which affects bone growth. Serum levels of IGF-I increase with age and pubertal development. However, levels vary widely from individual to individual.

At puberty, both sex steroids and GH participate in the pubertal growth spurt. This is best illustrated by the fact that children with isolated GH deficiency grow throughout puberty, but lack a definitive growth spurt. The cessation of the growth spurt is secondary to epiphyseal closure, due to the action of the sex steroids.

Endocrine Axes through the Life Span

Fetus/Neonate

In fetal life, GnRH, LH, FSH, estrogen, and testosterone (in the male) are detectable by a gestational age of 10 weeks, with hormone levels rising between 10 and 20 weeks. GnRH secretion is intermittent, causing pulsatile LH secretion. After the withdrawal of placental sex steroids, there is an initial fall in sex-steroid levels, but LH and FSH concentrations then rise to midpubertal levels for several months, exhibiting a pattern that is consistent with a mature differentiated hypothalamic-pituitary unit.

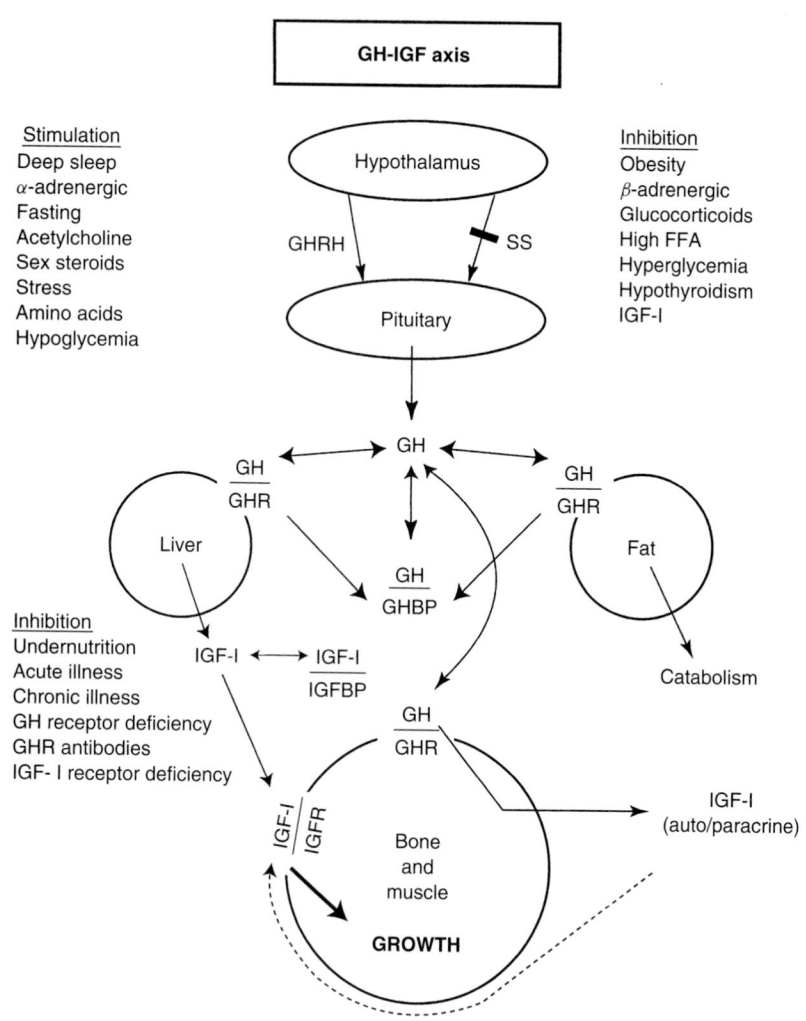

Stimulation
Deep sleep
α-adrenergic
Fasting
Acetylcholine
Sex steroids
Stress
Amino acids
Hypoglycemia

Inhibition
Obesity
β-adrenergic
Glucocorticoids
High FFA
Hyperglycemia
Hypothyroidism
IGF-I

Inhibition
Undernutrition
Acute illness
Chronic illness
GH receptor deficiency
GHR antibodies
IGF- I receptor deficiency

FIGURE 1.3 Simplified diagram of growth hormone–insulin-like growth factor I (GH-IGF-I) axis involving hypophysiotropic hormones controlling pituitary GH release, circulating GH-binding protein and its GH receptor source, IGF-I and its largely GH-dependent binding proteins, and cellular responsiveness to GH and IGF-I interacting with their specific receptors. FFA, free fatty acids; GHRH, growth hormone–releasing hormone. (From Rosenbloom AL, Guevara-Aguirre J, Rosenfield RG, et al. *Trends in endocrinology and metabolism; vol 5. Growth in growth hormone insensitivity*. New York: Elsevier Science, 1994:296, with permission.)

Both testosterone levels and estradiol levels also rise. This period has been referred to as "mini-puberty" and provides a window of opportunity to study the HPG axis to determine whether abnormalities exist that will affect future pubertal/sexual maturation. This period usually ends by age 9 months to 1 year in the male and by 2 years of age in the female, by when the levels of sex hormones have fallen to prepubertal levels in both boys and girls.

Infancy
Growth during infancy is at a higher velocity than at any other time during the life span, with infants growing 25 cm/year on average. It is worth noting that much of the rapid growth seen during infancy is not GH dependent, but nutritionally driven via the effects of insulin. Therefore one cannot make predictions about final height based on an infant's growth curve.

Childhood
During childhood, GnRH pulsatility and the HPG system is restrained, a likely result of tonic inhibition by the CNS from neurotransmitters acetylcholine, γ-aminobutyric acid (GABA), and others. During this quiescent phase, however, both the pituitary gland and the gonads are capable of mature function after appropriate stimulation.

FSH concentrations are relatively higher than LH levels during this time, especially in girls (Apter et al., 1993; Goji, 1993; We et al., 1991), and stimulation of the axis will result in a characteristic FSH-dominant response.

Height velocity during childhood is relatively constant, falling rapidly after the first year of life before increasing during adolescence. On average, children grow 10 cm/year in the second year of life, followed by 8 cm/year and 7 cm/year in the third and fourth years of life, respectively. During the ages of 5 to 10 years, height velocity is at its lowest at 5 to 6 cm/year. It is also important to note that many boys experience a slowing in height velocity before the rapid acceleration seen in puberty. This may be a source of concern to many parents and preteens.

MATURATION OF THE HYPOTHALAMIC-PITUITARY-GONADAL AXIS

Gonadal Steroids

The target tissues of LH and FSH are the ovaries and testes, which produce estradiol (E2) and testosterone (T), respectively. Leydig cells in the testes also produce, but to a much lesser extent, androstenedione, dihydrotestosterone, and estradiol.

Estrogen

Estradiol (E2) from the ovary accounts for most of the circulating estrogens, although there is a small amount of extra-ovarian conversion from androstenedione and testosterone. In addition to stimulating breast growth and maturation of the vaginal mucosa, estrogen has been found to have a major impact on the skeleton, being the primary hormone responsible for epiphyseal closure.

Testosterone

Although the testes represent the primary source of this hormone, a small amount comes from extra-testicular conversion of the adrenal hormone androstenedione in both males and females. Testosterone is the primary hormone responsible for the voice change in males and the attainment of male body habitus, but it is dihydrotestosterone, the product of conversion of testosterone by 5α-reductase, which causes growth of the phallus and prostate.

Gonadotropin-Releasing Hormone Pulse Generator

At the time of puberty, GnRH is secreted from the GnRH pulse generator in the hypothalamus in a pulsatile manner, leading to the secretion of LH and FSH from the pituitary and subsequent secretion of estradiol (E2) from the ovaries or testosterone (T) from the testes. Although the exact triggers are poorly understood, there are three distinct changes that are observed in the hypothalamic-pituitary unit.

1. A nocturnal sleep-related augmentation of pulsatile LH secretion begins as a result of the increase in the pulsatile release of GnRH (Marshall and Kelch, 1986).
2. The sensitivity of the hypothalamus and the pituitary to estradiol (E2) and testosterone (T) decreases so that the gonadotropins, LH and FSH, begin to increase. This is probably the result of sequential maturation of the CNS.
3. In the female, a positive feedback system develops, and critical levels of estrogen trigger a large release of GnRH, stimulating LH to initiate ovulation.

Potential Regulators

In addition, recent research has elucidated new potential regulators and key players in the awakening of this system.

GPR54/KiSS-1

GPR54, a G-protein–coupled receptor, and its ligand, derived from the *KiSS-1* gene, have been recently implicated as regulators of puberty. This was first discovered by examination of a kindred with multiple members with delayed puberty from idiopathic hypogonadotropic hypogonadism, later found to have a mutation in the *GPR54* gene (Seminara et al., 2003). Studies with *GPR54* knockout mice confirmed a role for this receptor and its ligand in pubertal development (Seminara et al., 2003; Funes et al., 2003). *KiSS-1* encodes the ligands for the GPR54 receptor called *kisspeptins*. Kisspeptins appear to stimulate LH through GnRH at the hypothalamic level. This stimulation is both dose- and time-dependent, with effects seen within 10 minutes of administration of minimal doses. Kisspeptins also stimulate FSH, but to a lesser degree (Navarro et al., 2005).

Astroglial-Neuronal Connections

Neuroendocrine glial cells may influence neurons to produce LHRH in an autocrine/paracrine manner using prostaglandin E_2 (PGE2) (Ojeda and Terasawa, 2002). Mice with a specific mutation in the glial receptors erbB-1 and erbB-4 have delayed sexual maturation and diminished reproductive capacity in early adulthood (Prevot et al., 2005).

Leptin

Recent research has focused on the role of leptin, a product of the *ob* gene produced by fat cells, in pubertal development (Zhang et al., 1994). Leptin was discovered to play a key role in the regulation of appetite, food intake, and energy expenditure, providing a signal to the CNS regarding satiety and the amount of energy stored in adipose tissue (Pellymounter et al., 1995; Halaas et al., 1995; Campfield et al., 1995). Animal studies have shown that leptin is also implicated in the control of pubertal development and reproductive function. Mice lacking leptin are obese and infertile, and leptin replacement reverses their obesity and reproductive failure (Chehab et al., 1996).

Although leptin originally was thought to be produced only in white adipose tissue, it has also been shown to be expressed in the hypothalamus and pituitary, among other tissues. Leptin receptors have been found throughout the HPG axis. In vitro, it has been found to accelerate GnRH pulsatility and stimulate GnRH release. (Moschos et al., 2002). Leptin may also have direct stimulatory effects on LH release by gonadotrophs.

The link between adequate nutrition and the timing of puberty has long been recognized. The theory that leptin could be the initiator of puberty was attractive, as researchers had hypothesized that a critical body weight and fat mass were necessary for puberty (Frisch and Revelle, 1970; Frisch, 1984; Johnston et al., 1971). However, there has been an absence of a molecular mechanism to link activation of the HPG axis to adipose cell mass or function. Recent experimental evidence suggests that leptin may play a role in this respect.

There is a significant change in leptin levels during pubertal development and a distinct sexual dimorphism is exhibited. Serum leptin levels peak in boys just before or during early puberty, followed by a decrease to baseline as testosterone levels rise (Mantzoros et al., 1997; Blum et al., 1997; Clayton et al., 1997; Garcia-Mayor et al., 1997; Horlick et al., 2000). In girls, there is a steady rise in leptin levels throughout puberty (Fig. 1.4). The exact interplay between leptin and other hormones, and its effect on the release of the "brake" which results in activation of the HPG axis remains unclear and is an area of active research.

Gonadotropin Secretion in Adults

Pulsatile secretion of GnRH from the hypothalamus continues into adulthood. As is seen during puberty, the frequency and amplitude of the GnRH pulses are critical to the secretion of gonadotropins, as a minor change may inhibit secretion. The control of GnRH secretion is not well understood, but is likely under the influence of a variety of neurotransmitters such as catecholamines (dopamine and norepinephrine), serotonin, and endogenous opioid

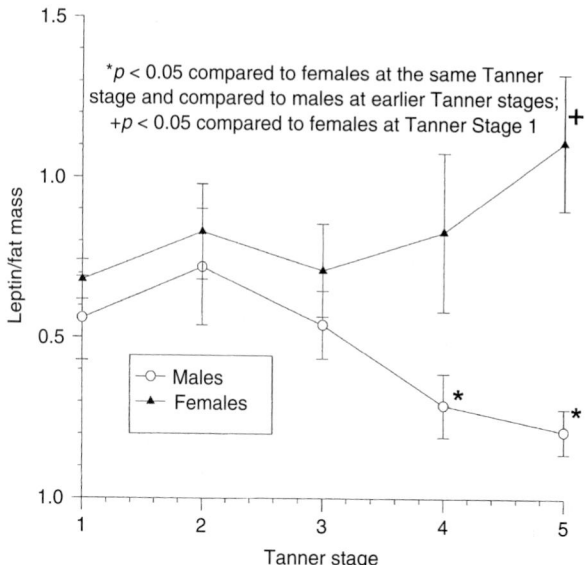

FIGURE 1.4 Standard Error of the Mean (SEM) leptin/Fat Mass (FM) in females and males. *, $p < 0.05$ compared with same-sex subjects at Tanner stage 1; +, $p < 0.05$ compared with girls at the same Tanner stage. (From Horlick MB, Rosenbaum M, Nicolson M, et al. Effect of puberty on the relationship between circulating leptin and body composition. *J Clin Endocrinol Metab* 2000;85:2509, with permission.)

peptides (endorphins and enkephalins). Sex steroids generally have a negative influence on the production of gonadotropins. This negative feedback may occur at the level of the hypothalamus or pituitary, or both. An estradiol level of approximately 200 pg/mL or greater generates positive feedback leading to a surge of gonadotropin secretion and ovulation in the mature female.

SEXUAL DEVELOPMENT IN PUBERTY

What is commonly thought of as pubertal secondary sexual characteristics should be separated into gonadarche and adrenarche, arising from the HPG axis and the HPA axis, respectively. In girls, gonadarche is represented by thelarche (the onset of breast budding), and in boys it is represented by testicular enlargement to 4 mL and above, or 2.5 cm in the longest axis. Pubarche, or the growth of terminal sexual hair in girls, is mainly the result of adrenarche. In boys, both testicular and adrenal androgens contribute. Health care providers should feel comfortable in dealing with the multitude of questions that may arise from adolescents and their parents regarding not only sexual maturation but also the issues of arising sexuality.

Sexual Maturity Rating Scales

Sexual maturity rating (SMR) scales (also called *Tanner staging*) as developed by Marshall and Tanner (Marshall and Tanner, 1969; Marshall and Tanner, 1970) allows for accurate classification of physical pubertal maturation. For both boys and girls there are five stages categorizing secondary sexual characteristics (pubic hair and breast development

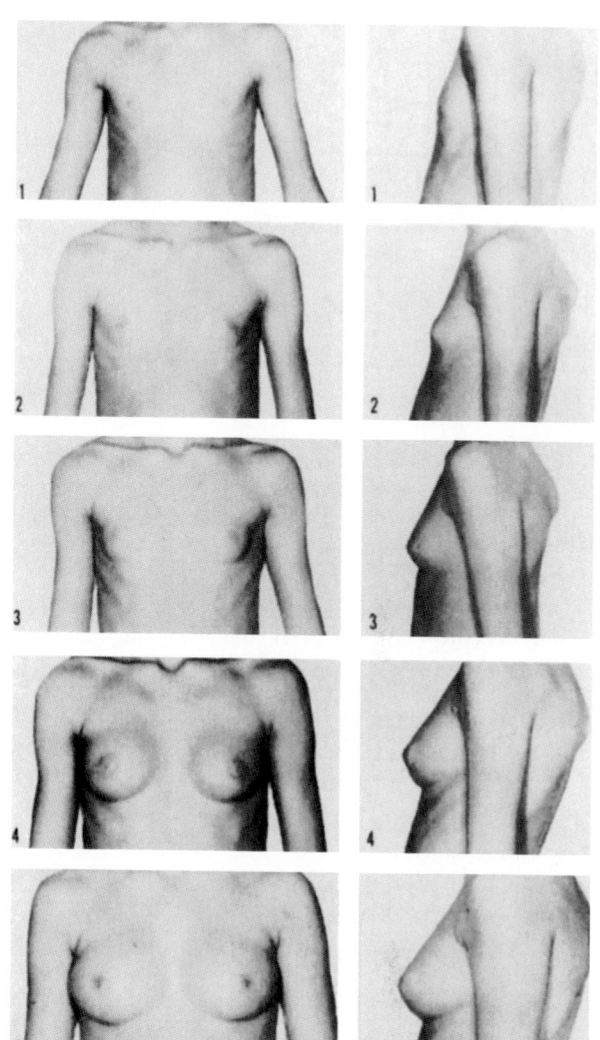

FIGURE 1.5 Stages of breast development. (From Tanner JM. *Growth at adolescence*, 2nd ed. Springfield, IL: Blackwell Scientific Publications, 1962, with permission. Copyright © 1962 by Blackwell Scientific Publications.)

in females and pubic hair and genitalia in males). These stages are described as follows and are shown both in photographs and drawings in Figures 1.5 through 1.11.

Males (testicular volumes as measured by a Prader Orchidometer)
1. Genital stage 1 (G1): Prepubertal
   a. Testes: Volume <4 mL, or long axis <2.5 cm
   b. Phallus: Childlike
2. Genital stage 2 (G2)
   a. Testes: Volume 4 to 8 mL, or long axis 2.6 to 3.3 cm
   b. Scrotum: Reddened, thinner, and larger
   c. Phallus: No change
3. Genital stage 3 (G3)
   a. Testes: Volume 10 to 15 mL, or long axis 3.4 to 4.0 cm
   b. Scrotum: Greater enlargement
   c. Phallus: Increased length

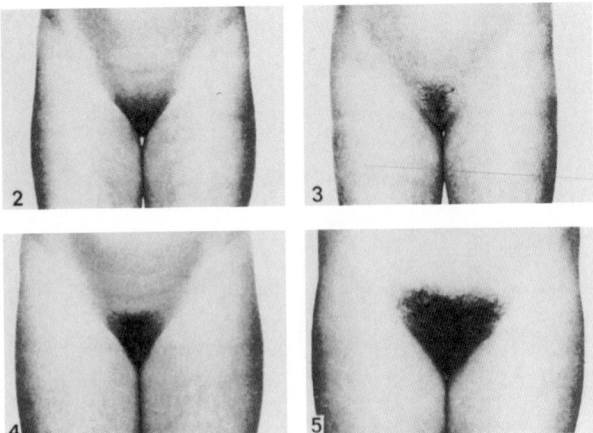

FIGURE 1.6   Stages of female pubic hair development. (Reproduced from Tanner JM. University of London, Institute of Child Health, with permission.)

  4. Genital stage 4 (G4)
     a. Testes: Volume 15 to 20 mL, or long axis 4.1 to 4.5 cm
     b. Scrotum: Further enlargement and darkening
     c. Phallus: Increased length and circumference
  5. Genital stage 5 (G5)
     a. Testes: Volume >25 mL, or long axis >4.5 cm
     b. Scrotum and phallus: Adult
Females
  1. Breast stage 1 (B1)
     a. Breast: Prepubertal; no glandular tissue
     b. Areola and papilla: Areola conforms to general chest line
  2. Breast stage 2 (B2)
     a. Breast: Breast bud; small amount of glandular tissue
     b. Areola: Areola widens
  3. Breast stage 3 (B3)
     a. Breast: Larger and more elevation; extends beyond areolar parameter
     b. Areola and papilla: Areola continues to enlarge but remains in contour with the breast

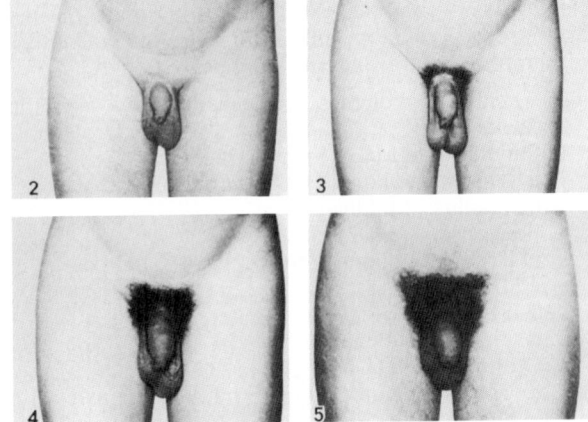

FIGURE 1.7   Stages of male pubic hair development. (Reproduced from Tanner JM. University of London, Institute of Child Health, with permission.)

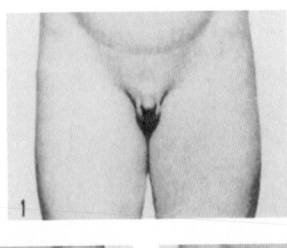
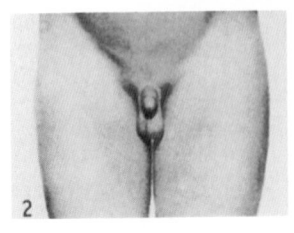
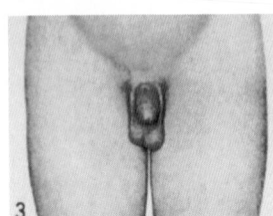
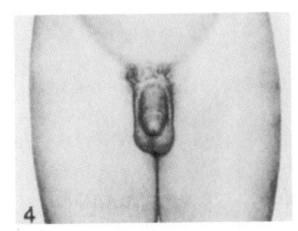
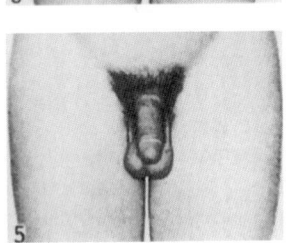

FIGURE 1.8   Stages of male genital development. (Reproduced from Tanner JM. University of London, Institute of Child Health, with permission.)

  4. Breast stage 4 (B4)
     a. Breast: Larger and more elevation
     b. Areola and papilla: Areola and papilla form a mound projecting from the breast contour
  5. Breast stage 5 (B5)
     a. Breast: Adult (size variable)
     b. Areola and papilla: Areola and breast in same plane, with papilla projecting above areola
Male and Female: Pubic hair
  1. Pubic hair stage 1 (PH1)
     a. None
  2. Public hair stage 2 (PH2)
     a. Small amount of long, slightly pigmented, downy hair along the base of the scrotum and phallus in the male or the labia majora in female; vellus hair versus sexual type hair (PH3)
  3. Pubic hair stage 3 (PH3)
     a. Moderate amount of more curly, pigmented, and coarser hair, extending more laterally
  4. Pubic hair stage 4 (PH4)
     a. Hair that resembles adult hair in coarseness and curliness but does not extend to medial surface of thighs
  5. Pubic hair stage 5 (PH5)
     a. Adult type and quantity, extending to medial surface of thighs

Importance of Sexual Maturity Ratings

SMRs should be recorded yearly, as this provides critical information in the identification of an abnormal pubertal progression and also reassurance to the health care provider and the teenager that puberty is progressing normally. The SMR is also critical in evaluating issues such as hematocrit (Fig. 1.12), alkaline phosphatase values (Table 1.1), and menarche (Fig. 1.13).

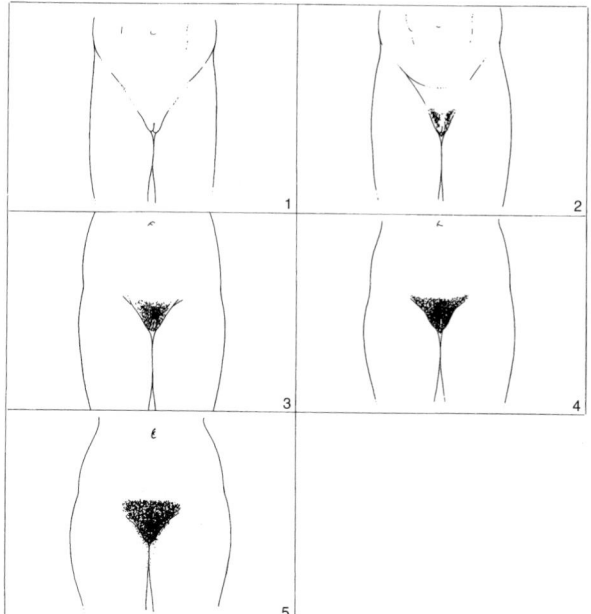

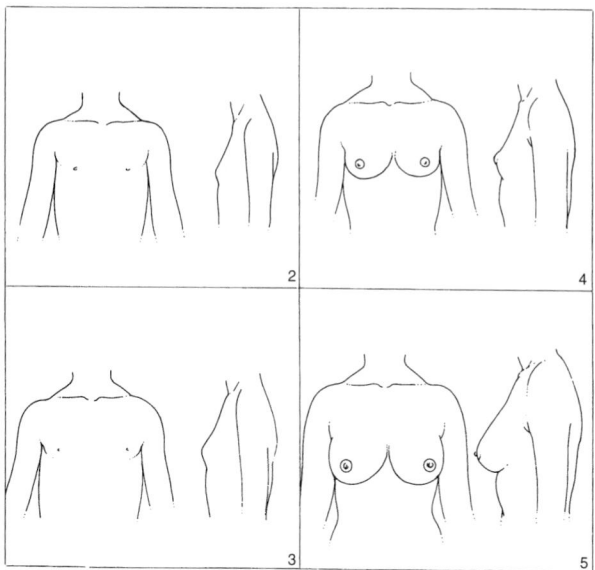

FIGURE 1.9 Female pubic hair development. *Sexual maturity rating 1 (SMR 1):* Prepubertal; no pubic hair. *SMR 2:* Straight hair is extending along the labia and, between ratings 2 and 3, begins on the pubis. *SMR 3:* Pubic hair has increased in quantity, is darker, and is present in the typical female triangle but in smaller quantity. *SMR 4:* Pubic hair has increased in quantity, is darker, and is more dense, curled, and adult in distribution but less abundant. *SMR 5:* Abundant, adult-type pattern; hair may extend onto the medial aspect of the thighs. (From Daniel WA, Palshock BZ. A physician's guide to sexual maturity rating. *Patient Care* 1979;30:122, with permission. Illustration by Paul Singh-Roy.)

FIGURE 1.10 Female breast development. *Sexual maturity rating 1 (SMR 1),* not shown: Prepubertal; elevations of papilla only. *SMR 2:* Breast buds appear; areola is slightly widened and projects as small mound. *SMR 3:* Enlargement of the entire breast with protrusion of the papilla or of the nipple. *SMR 4:* Enlargement of the breast and projection of areola and papilla as a secondary mound. *SMR 5:* Adult configuration of the breast with protrusion of the nipple; areola no longer projects separately from remainder of breast. (From Daniel WA, Paulshock BZ. A physician's guide to sexual maturity rating. *Patient Care* 1979;30:122, with permission. Illustration by Paul Singh-Roy.)

Female Pubertal Changes

Events of Puberty: During puberty, the breasts develop and the ovaries, uterus, vagina, labia, and clitoris increase in size, with the uterus and ovaries increasing in size by approximately fivefold to sevenfold. Winer-Muram et al. (1989) evaluated the ovaries and uterine length in peripubertal females, with uterine length growing to a size of 6.98 ± 1 cm in 15- to 16-year-old girls, and ovarian size reaching 3.5 ± 0.4 cm^3 by the same age. Fifty-nine of the 75 girls had multiple ovarian cysts ranging from 3 to 10 mm^3. Body composition changes as girls accumulate fat mass at an average annual rate of 1.14 kg/year (Roche et al., 2001).

Sequence: Often the earliest physical sign of puberty in girls is thelarche, although few girls have pubic hair development as the first sign (Fig. 1.12). On an average, breast development starts at the age of 10 years for white girls and at 8.9 years for African-American girls, according to a frequently cited large cross-sectional study (Herman-Giddens et al., 1997). These physical findings, however, may be preceded by the growth spurt by approximately 1 year. Therefore, the growth curve is an essential tool in the evaluation of precocious or delayed puberty. The average length of time for completion of puberty is 4 years, but can range from 1.5 to 8 years.

Menarche: Menarche usually occurs during SMR B3 or B4, and approximately 3.3 years after the growth spurt, or roughly 2 years after breast budding. The normal range for menarche varies from 9 to 15 years, and is dependent on such factors as race, socioeconomic status, heredity, nutrition, and culture. It occurs later at higher altitudes, in rural areas, and in larger families. Body composition

TABLE 1.1

Serum Alkaline Phosphatase Levels

Sexual Maturity Rating	Male	Female
1	74 ± 21 IU	79 ± 16
2	89 ± 29	93 ± 21
3	116 ± 41	84 ± 41
4	103 ± 43	39 ± 21
5	70 ± 39	32 ± 12

Adapted from Bennett DL, Ward MS, Daniel WA. The relationship of serum alkaline phosphatase concentrations to sexual maturity ratings in adolescents. *J Pediatr* 1976;88:633–636.

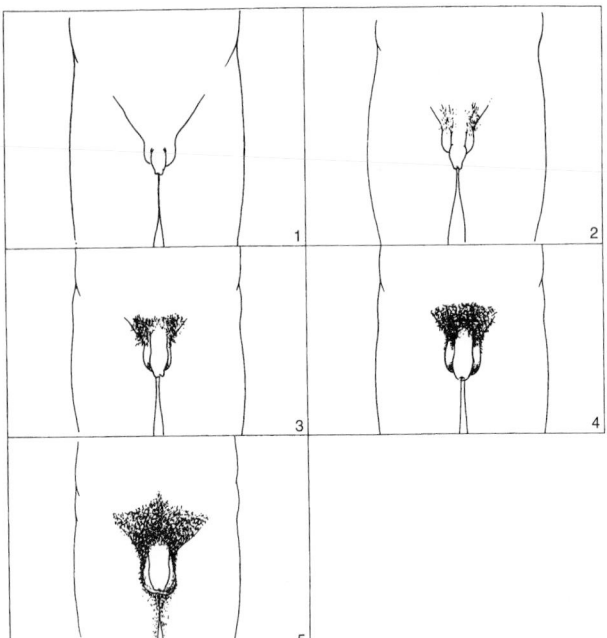

FIGURE 1.11 Male genital and pubic hair development. Ratings for pubic hair and for genital development can differ in a typical boy at any given time, because pubic hair and genitalia do not necessarily develop at the same rate. *Sexual maturity rating 1 (SMR 1):* Prepubertal; no pubic hair. Genitalia unchanged from early childhood. *SMR 2:* Light, downy hair develops laterally and later becomes dark. Penis and testes may be slightly larger; scrotum becomes more textured. *SMR 3:* Pubic hair has extended across the pubis. Testes and scrotum are further enlarged; penis is larger, especially in length. *SMR 4:* More abundant pubic hair with curling. Genitalia resemble those of an adult; glans has become larger and broader, scrotum is darker. *SMR 5:* Adult quantity and pattern of pubic hair, with hair present along the inner borders of the thighs. The testes and the scrotum are adult in size. (From Daniel WA, Paulshock BZ. A physician's guide to sexual maturity rating. *Patient Care* 1979;30:122, with permission. Illustration by Paul Singh-Roy.)

also influences age at menarche, although controversy exists whether there is a necessary amount of adipose mass needed at the time of menarche. For a large population, there appears to be a relationship between height and weight and menarche (Fig. 1.14). This relationship is less meaningful in evaluating a single adolescent.

Earlier menarche is usually correlated with shorter adult height, although this depends upon the degree of estrogen stimulation before menses. Girls with higher or prolonged estrogen levels tend to grow less after menarche. On an average, girls grow 4 to 6 cm after menarche. The sequence of pubertal events in females is found in Figures 1.13 and 1.15B. The age at menarche has gradually decreased during the last century, as illustrated in Figure 1.16. However, this trend has slowed significantly in the past few decades.

Several investigators have examined data from the Third National Health and Nutrition Examination Survey (NHANES III) conducted from 1988 to 1994 (Wu et al., 2002; Sun et al., 2003; Chumlea et al., 2003; Anderson et al., 2003). One study (Anderson et al.) compared data from an earlier U.S. survey 25 years previous to the NHANES III data and found that the average age at menarche had declined only minimally (i.e., by approximately 2.5 months, from 12.8 years to 12.5 years). Another study cited up to a 4-month decrease in age at menarche (Chumlea et al., 2003). All studies that have examined the race have demonstrated that African-American girls reach menarche the earliest, followed by Mexican-American and white girls.

Age at Puberty : There have been several studies in recent years that have examined the age at puberty in U.S. girls (Herman-Giddens et al., 2004 review). Although there are slight differences in the ages of onset, the trend is for earlier pubertal onset, but almost no change in the age at menarche. On an average, girls of African-American descent appear to enter puberty earlier than their Hispanic and white counterparts. The large study from the Pediatric Research in Office Settings group sampled >17,000 white and black girls from around the United States with the Tanner method and found that the earliest signs of puberty are occurring earlier than previously described (Herman-Giddens et al., 1997). In that study, the mean ages at onset of breast development were 8.9 years for African-American girls and 10 for white girls. Pubic hair development started at 8.8 years for African-American girls and at 10.5 years for white girls. Similarly, African-American girls experienced menarche at 12.2 years, and white girls at 12.9 years.

Male Pubertal Changes

Events of puberty: By the end of male puberty, the potential for reproduction will have been achieved. Internal and external genital organs increase in size, and body proportions change so that percentage of body fat actually declines (Roche et al., 2001) versus rising in females. Gynecomastia is a common issue in midpubertal boys that may cause significant concern. True gynecomastia is glandular development of at least 0.5 cm that is palpable. This may not be easily differentiated from pseudogynecomastia, which is an accumulation of fatty tissue. Gynecomastia is covered in detail in Chapter 57.

Sequence: Table 1.2 lists the normal variation of timing of secondary sexual characteristics in adolescent boys. The earliest sign of physical pubertal development in approximately 98% of males is an increase in testicular volume to 4 mL or 2.5 cm in the long axis. However, the most noticeable first event of male puberty is the growth of pubic hair. Midpuberty, or the time of rising testosterone concentrations, is associated with the period of most rapid linear growth, in contrast to the early growth spurt in girls. This is also the time when the voice changes, axillary hair develops, and acne may appear. Ejaculation occurs usually at SMR G3, as does the first evidence of spermarche, but fertility is not usually attained until SMR G4. Facial hair growth typically starts approximately 3 years after pubic hair growth. The hair on the face, chest, back, and abdomen may continue

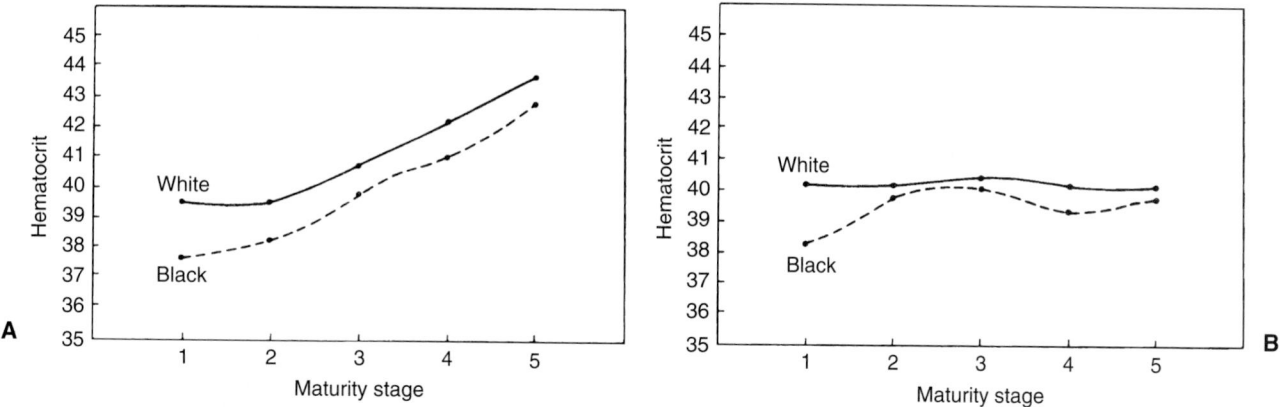

FIGURE 1.12 Hematocrit values for African-American and white boys **(A)** and girls **(B)** during puberty. (From Daniel WA. Hematocrit: maturity relationship in adolescence. *Pediatrics* 1973;52:388, with permission.)

throughout and beyond puberty into adulthood, the amount and distribution being quite variable and dependent on ethnicity and family patterns. The average length of time for completion of puberty is 3 years, but it can range from 2 to 5 years. The sequence of events for an average male is shown in the following text in Figures 1.17 and 1.15B. Table 1.3 lists male genital size by age and Table 1.4 lists testicular volume by SMR.

Age at Puberty: NHANES III data for boys demonstrate a similar trend regarding the initiation of puberty, but no change from earlier studies with regard to the attainment of Tanner stage 5. Also, as with girls, there were noticeable differences noted among racial groups, with African-American boys entering puberty the earliest, followed by white boys, then Mexican-American boys. Overall, *initiation of genital development* was at 10.1 years for white boys, 9.5 years for

African-American boys, and 10.4 years for Mexican-American boys (Herman-Giddents et al., 2001). Marshall and Tanner's classic reference of institutionalized white boys in the United Kingdom in 1969 cited genital development at a mean age of 11.6 years, a full 1.5 years later than current findings (Marshall and Tanner, 1969). However, as with girls, the age at completion of genital development is not significantly different from previous studies (Harlan et al., 1979; Lee, 1980; Villareal et al., 1989; Marshall and Tanner, 1969; Largo and Prader, 1983), with white boys *completing puberty* at 15.9 years, African-American boys at 15.7 years, and Mexican-American boys at 14.9 years. The overall trend, therefore, is earlier entry with prolonged progression. The potential causes of this trend are not entirely known. However, the boys in NHANES III were taller and heavier at the earlier ages of puberty than in the past (Herman-Giddens et al., 2001). It is clear, however, that precocious puberty in boys should always prompt further work-up, as this condition is associated with pathology more often than in girls. Further evaluation should be undertaken if there is evidence of signs and symptoms of pubertal development before the age of 10 years or out of context of family history.

In both sexes, consequences of earlier maturation with regard to teen behavior, sexual activity, and pregnancy need to be addressed with age-appropriate interventions during middle childhood and the preteen years. In addition, the lifetime health consequences of early sexual maturation merit further study.

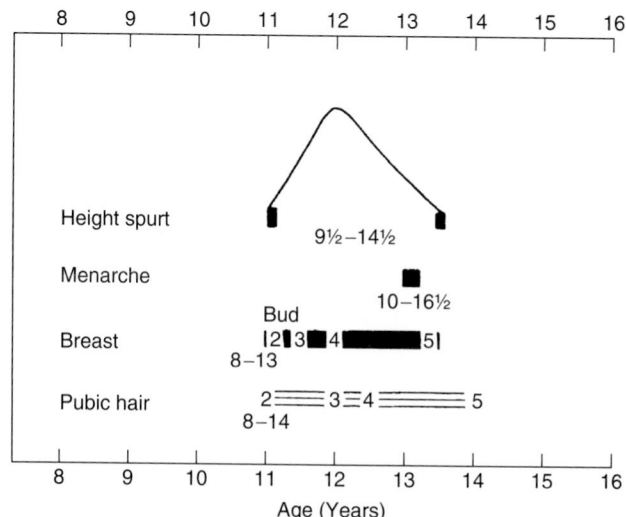

FIGURE 1.13 Biological maturity in girls. (From Tanner JM. *Growth at adolescence*, 2nd ed. Springfield, IL: Blackwell Scientific Publications, 1962, with permission. Copyright © 1962 by Blackwell Scientific Publications.)

ADRENARCHE

The increased secretion of androgens from the adrenal gland, called *adrenarche*, in the prepubertal and pubertal periods is independent of HPG changes. The two events are temporally related, with the increase in adrenal hormones preceding that of the gonadal sex steroids (Ducharme et al., 1976), although the effects are evident later. It is important to note, however, that adrenal androgens are not necessary for pubertal development or the adolescent growth spurt. It is widely believed that adrenarche begins in midchildhood, at around the age of 6 years (de Peretti and Forest, 1976),

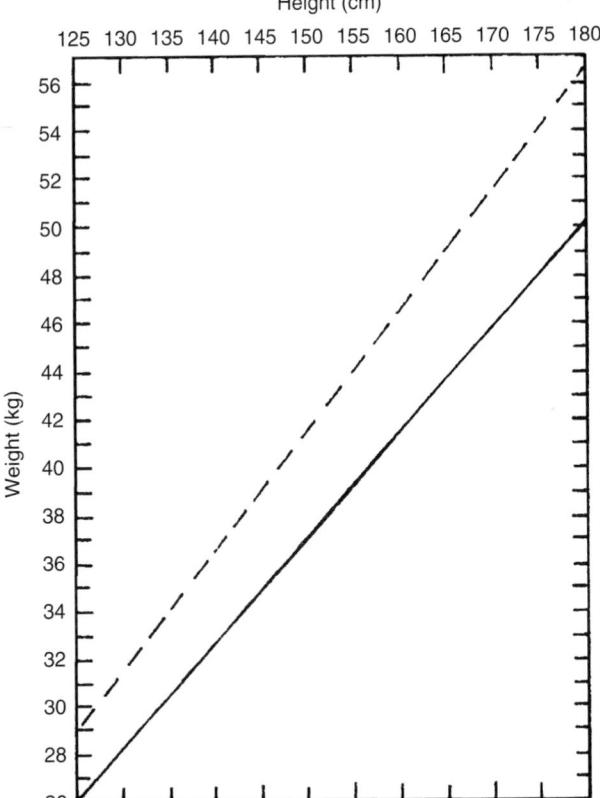

FIGURE 1.14 The weight for height at which menarche is likely to occur (*solid line*) and the weight for height at which regular ovulatory menstrual periods are likely to be maintained (*dashed line*). (From Frisch RE, McArthur JW. Menstrual cycles: fatness as a determinant of minimum weight for height necessary for their maintenance or onset. *Science* 1974;185:949, with permission. Copyright 1974 by American Association for the Advancement of Science.)

and levels continue to rise until the age of 20 to 30 years. Recent evidence, however, has suggested that the rise of DHEA-S is a more gradual process and occurs as early as the preschool years (Palmert et al., 2001; Remer and Manz, 1999; Remer et al., 2005).

Physical Manifestations

Local conversion of DHEA-S to testosterone, then to dihydrotestosterone is responsible for hair growth in the androgen-dependent areas (face, chest, pubic area, axilla). Axillary and pubic areas are most sensitive to the effects of androgens, which is why these areas are the first to develop sexual hair. In addition, local conversion of DHEA-S within the apocrine glands of the axillae causes body odor, and conversion within sebaceous glands is responsible for the development of acne.

PHYSICAL GROWTH DURING PUBERTY

One of the most striking changes in adolescents is their rapid growth velocity. This height spurt is dependent

TABLE 1.2

Means and Normal Variation in the Timing of Adolescent Secondary Sexual Characteristics (Males)

Stage	Mean Age at Onset ±2 SD (yr)	Stage	Time between Stages (yr) Mean	Percentile 5th	Percentile 95th
G2	11.6 ± 2.1	G2–3	1.1	0.4	2.2
G3	12.9 ± 2.1	PH2–3	0.5	0.1	1.0
PH2	13.4 ± 2.2[a]	G3–4	0.8	0.2	1.6
G4	13.8 ± 2.0	PH3–4	0.4	0.3	0.5
PH3	13.9 ± 2.1	G4–5	1.0	0.4	1.9
PH4	14.4 ± 2.2	PH4–5	0.7	0.2	1.5
G5	14.9 ± 2.2	G2–5	3.0	1.9	4.7
PH5	15.2 ± 2.1	PH2–5	1.6	0.8	2.7

[a]Mean is probably too high due to experimental method. From Barnes HV. Physical growth and development during puberty. *Med Clin North Am* 1975;59:1305.

primarily upon GH and the insulin-like growth factors, but many other hormones may influence growth as well, especially the sex steroids. Premature or delayed puberty without prompt recognition and treatment may have marked effects on height.

Growth Hormone during Puberty

Most linear growth is dependent upon GH and its feedback loop, shown graphically in Figure 1.3. As shown, GH secretion is increased by GHRH, and decreased by somatostatin from the hypothalamic arm of the loop. GH concentrations have been shown to double during the pubertal growth spurt. As with many hormones, GH

TABLE 1.3

Male Genital Size by Age

Age (yr)	Testicular Volume (mL) Mean	Range[a]	Phallus Length (cm) Mean	Range[a]
10	1.3	1–3	6.4	4–8
11	1.8	1–3	6.7	4–8
12	4.0	1–6	7.0	5–10
13	7.0	3–11	7.8	5–12
14	10.8	5–16	9.7	6–14
15	12.8	7–18	11.2	8–15
16	14.4	9–18	12.3	10–15
17	17.6	11–19	13.0	10–16
18	18.2	13–23	13.2	11–17

[a]Acceptable normal ranges. From Barnes HV. Recognizing normal and abnormal physical growth and development during puberty. In: Moss AV, ed. *Pediatrics update: reviews for physicians.* New York: Elsevier-North Holland, 1979.

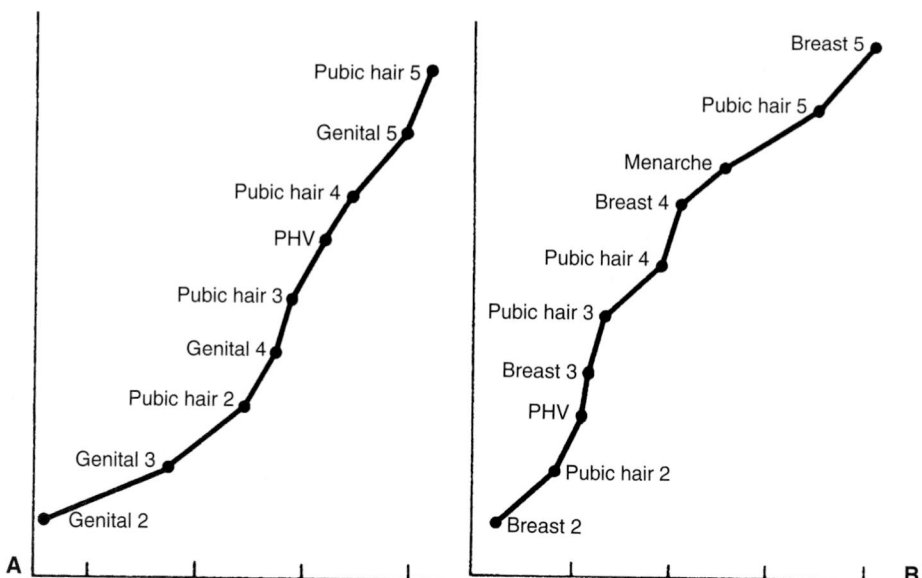

FIGURE 1.15 **A:** Sequence of pubertal events in males. **B:** Sequence of pubertal events in females. PHV, peak height velocity. (From Root AW. Endocrinology of puberty. *J Pediatr* 1973;83:1, with permission.)

is secreted in a pulsatile manner, with maximum rates at the onset of slow-wave sleep. It has been shown that the increased available GH is due to higher pulse amplitude and amount per pulse, as opposed to increased frequency or decreased clearance (Martha et al., 1989; Martha et al., 1992). It is this pulsatile secretion which renders random GH testing unhelpful. GH exerts its effects through insulin-like growth factors, or IGFs, mainly IGF-I (or somatomedin-C) and IGF-II. Serum IGF-I levels increase slowly and steadily during the prepubertal years,

rise more steeply during puberty (Juul et al., 1994), and remain elevated 1 to 2 years past the pubertal growth spurt. IGF levels among males and females must be interpreted with regard to pubertal stage and age.

Height Velocity

Height velocity during the pubertal growth spurt is at its highest levels outside of infancy (Fig. 1.18). It should be noted that when calculating height velocity, it is important to use an interval of 6 to 12 months, as height growth is greatest during the spring and summer months. Although males and females are roughly the same height upon entry into puberty, males emerge taller by 13 cm on average. This is primarily due to the boys' 2-year lag behind girls in

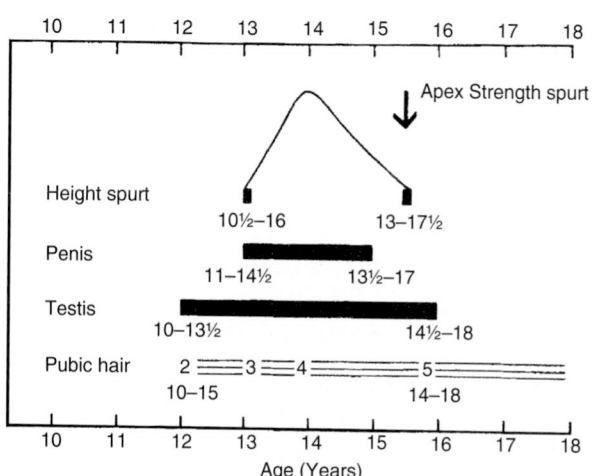

FIGURE 1.16 Secular trend in age at menarche. (From Tanner JM. Fetus into man. Cambridge, MA: Harvard University Press, 1978, with permission. Copyright 1978 by Harvard University Press, Cambridge, MA.)

FIGURE 1.17 Biological maturity in boys. (From Tanner JM. *Growth at adolescence*, 2nd ed. Springfield, IL: Blackwell Scientific Publications, 1962, with permission. Copyright ©1962 by Blackwell Scientific Publications.)

TABLE 1.4

Testicular Volume by Sexual Maturity Rating

Sexual Maturity Rating[a]	Volume (cm³)			
	Left Testis		Right Testis	
	Mean	SD	Mean	SD
1	4.8	2.8	5.2	3.9
2	6.4	3.2	7.1	3.9
3	14.6	6.5	14.8	6.1
4	19.8	6.2	20.4	6.8
5	28.3	8.5	30.2	9.6

[a]Mean of genital and public hair ratings.
Adapted from Daniel WA Jr., Feinstein RA, Howard-Peebles P, et al. Testicular volumes of adolescents. *J Pediatr* 1982;101:1010.

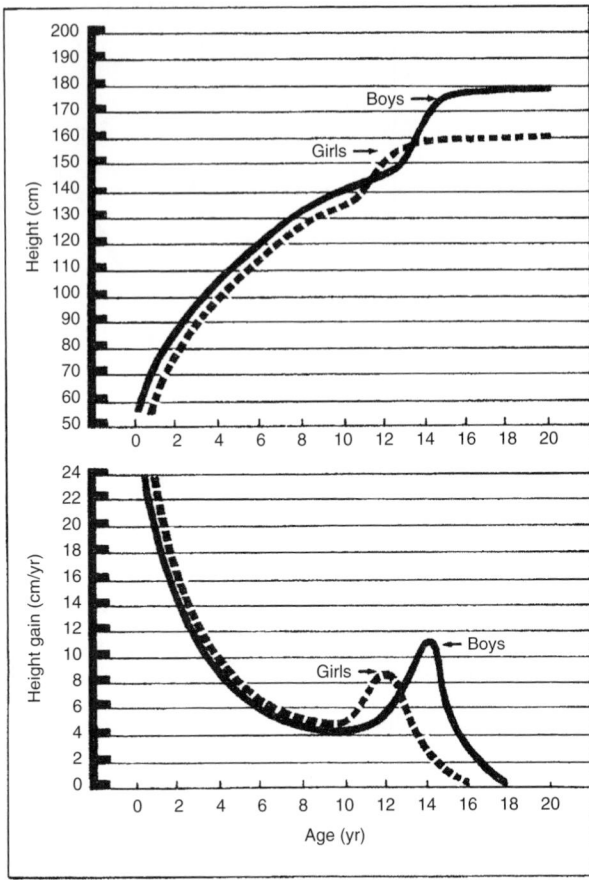

FIGURE 1.18   Typical individual velocity curves for height in boys and girls: height-attained growth curve (*top*) and growth velocity curve for height (*bottom*). (From Hill DE, Fiser RH. Chronic disease and short stature. *Postgrad Med* 1977;62:103, with permission.)

attainment of their peak height velocity, but a small amount of height may be accounted for by the higher peak velocity (Figs. 1.17 and 1.18). Girls gain their peak height velocity of 8.3 cm/year at an average age of 11.5 years and at Tanner stages B2 to B3 whereas boys do not have their peak height velocity of 9.5 cm/year until the age of 13.5 years, at Tanner genital stages 3 to 4. Although there is great inter-individual variation for height, one trend is for the peak height velocity to be higher, but not more sustained, in those who mature early. Therefore, there may not be a difference in final height. There are also curves available for early and late maturers (Figs. 1.19 and 1.20).

Prediction of Final Height

Predicting final height is a difficult task, and it should be emphasized that the methods available provide a general estimate. One method of predicting a general range for adult height is by the average of parental heights, accounting for the height difference of 13 cm (or 5 inches) between men and women. This is referred to as the midparental target height. One standard deviation from midparental height is 2 inches. As a result, 4 inches around the midparental height is within two standard deviations of the mean.
For girls:

$$\frac{(\text{father's height} - 13 \text{ cm or } 5 \text{ inches}) + \text{mother's height}}{2}$$

For boys:

$$\frac{(\text{father's height} + 13 \text{ cm or } 5 \text{ inches}) + \text{mother's height}}{2}$$

The Bayley-Pinneau method uses the bone age to predict final height. This is based on attainment of a bone age, or x-ray of the left hand and wrist that is then matched to standards. Because sex steroids are known to cause bony maturation and epiphyseal fusion, this method is based on the percentage of final height as assessed by bony maturation. In addition, various computer models have used these data to predict adult height. With these programs, basic information (e.g., height, weight, skeletal age) is entered, and the program calculates adult height using several methodologies, including that of Bayley and

Pinneau. See Table 1.5 for calculations of estimated final predicted height with this method.

The Role of Sex Steroids

Gonadal steroids contribute to the growth spurt by inducing an increase in GH secretion and by stimulating local production of IGF-I in cartilage and bone directly (Grumbach, 2000; Attie et al., 1990; Van Wyk and Smith, 1999; Rogol, 1994).

Estrogen

Estrogen is the hormone that is most involved with the growth spurt through its effects on bone and cartilage, in both men and women. Estradiol concentration correlates with the pubertal growth spurt; girls have an estradiol increase, and the corresponding peak height velocity is earlier than boys. Boys' peak estradiol levels also correlate with peak height velocity (Klein et al., 1996). At higher doses, estrogen causes epiphyseal fusion and thereby termination of linear growth. The importance of this hormone in men was underscored by three different case studies: one sexually mature male who had a mutation in the estrogen receptor (Smith et al., 1994), and two cases of men with mutations in *CYP19* gene that encodes aromatase,

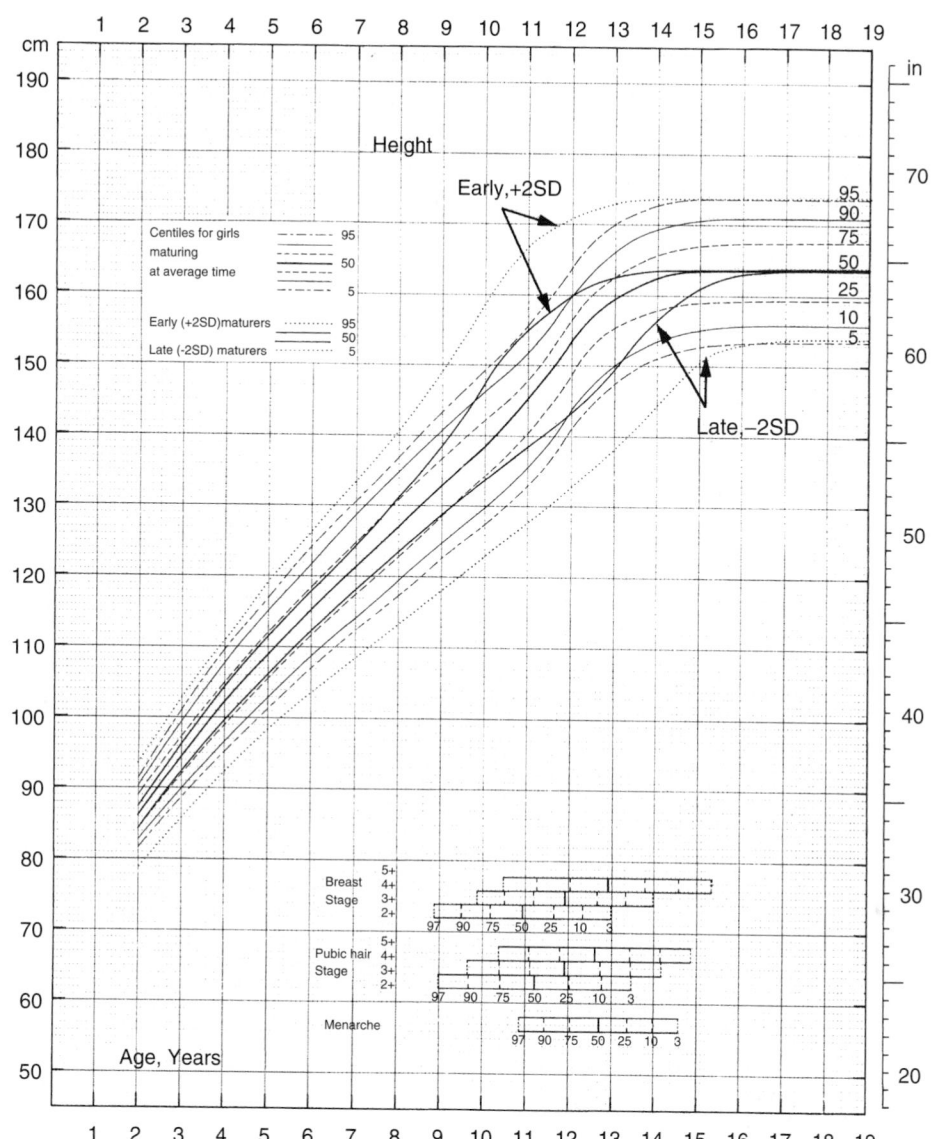

FIGURE 1.19   Height attained for American girls. (From Tanner JM, Davies PW. Clinical longitudinal standards for height and height velocity for North American children. *J Pediatr* 1985;107:317, with permission.)

which converts testosterone to estrogen (Morishima et al., 1995; Morishima et al., 1997; Carani et al., 1997). All had tall stature, eunuchoid proportions, osteopenia, and unfused epiphyses. Treatment with estrogen in the men with aromatase deficiency caused epiphyseal closure and an increase in bone mineralization within 6 to 9 months (Bilezikian et al., 1998). The mechanisms by which this end result is accomplished are manifold, but primarily, estrogen stimulates chondrogenesis in the epiphyseal growth plate, which acts to increase linear growth (Weise et al., 2001).

Androgens

Androgens seem to have little direct effects on pubertal bone growth, as evidenced by the case studies presented in the preceding text, although androgen receptors can be found on developing and mature osteoblasts (Colvard et al., 1989). It is clear that androgens have a role in the sexual

dimorphism of the skeleton (Orwoll, 1996; Bellido et al., 1995; Kasperk et al., 1997; Vanderschueren, 1996; Hofbauer and Khosla, 1999) and are likely responsible for the greater increase in periosteal bone deposition and bone strength in men compared with women (Schoenau et al., 2001). As an example, patients with complete androgen insensitivity syndrome (CAIS) who are karyotype 46XY females have a normal growth spurt and a bone density comparable to normal XX women (Munoz-Torres et al, 1995).

Weight Growth

1. Weight velocity increases and peaks during the adolescent growth spurt.
2. Pubertal weight gain accounts for approximately 50% of an individual's ideal adult body weight.

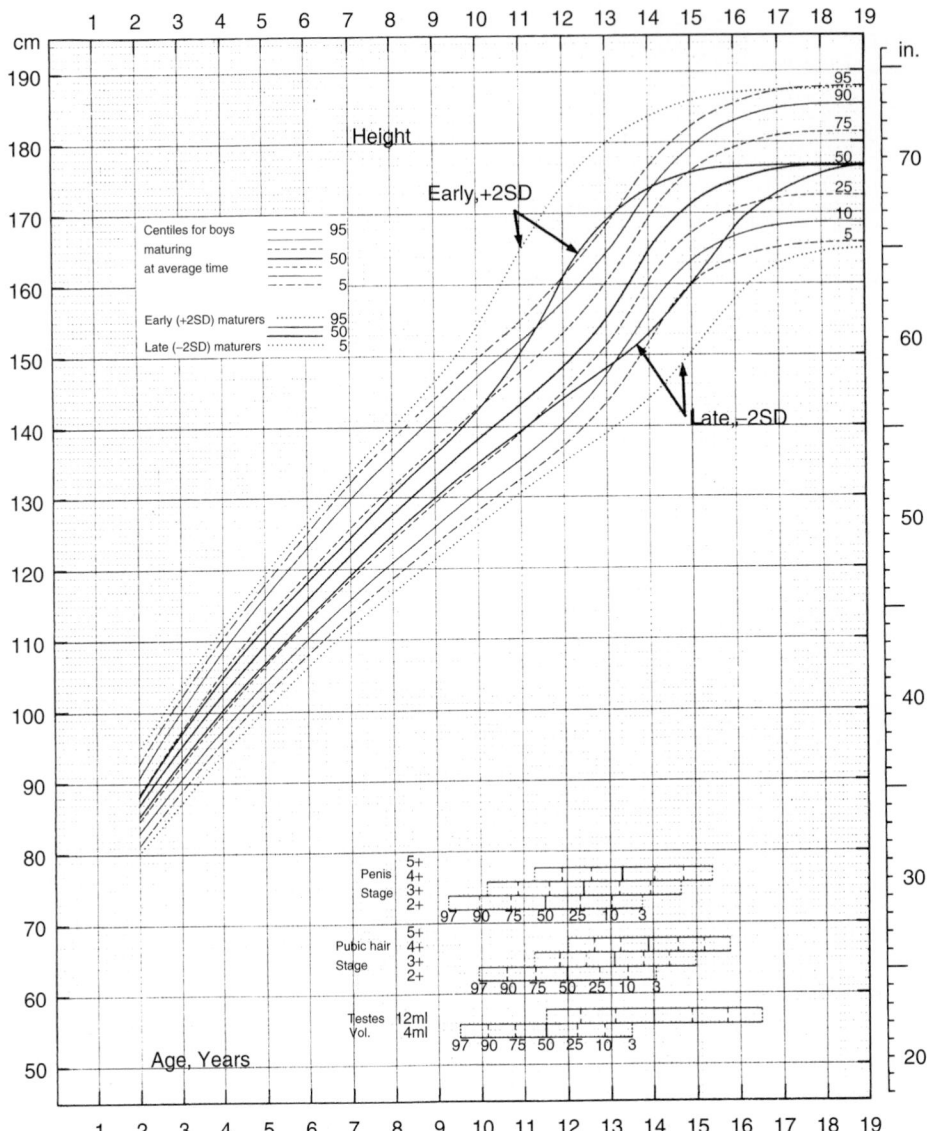

FIGURE 1.20 Height attained for American boys. (From Tanner JM, Davies PW. Clinical longitudinal standards for height and height velocity for North American children. *J Pediatr* 1985;107:317, with permission.)

3. The onset of accelerated weight gain and the peak weight velocity (PWV) attained are highly variable. For example, normal weight gain during the year of PWV can vary from 4.6 to 10.6 kg in girls and from 5.7 to 13.2 kg in boys. (Normal weight-for-age percentile curves are available through the Centers for Disease Control and Prevention [CDC], 6525 Belcrest Road, Hyattsville, MD 20782-2003. They are also available on the CDC Web site: www.cdc.gov/growthcharts/. See also Figs. 1.21– 1.26.)

Pubertal Changes in Body Composition

During childhood, boys and girls have relatively equal proportions of lean body mass, skeletal mass, and body fat. By the end of puberty, however, men have 1.5 times more lean body mass and skeletal mass than women, and women have double the fat mass. Table 1.6 shows the

effects of GH and the sex steroids on different aspects of body composition. The skeleton also undergoes epiphyseal maturation under the influence of estradiol (E2) and testosterone (T), as reviewed in the preceding text.

Lean Body Mass
1. Females

   The lean body mass decreases from approximately 80% of body weight in early puberty to approximately 75% at maturity. The lean body mass increases in total amount, but decreases in percentage because adipose mass increases at a greater rate.
2. Males

   The lean body mass increases from 80% to 85% to approximately 90% at maturity. This primarily reflects increased muscle mass from circulating androgens.

TABLE 1.5

Prediction of Adult Height Using Skeletal Age

Directions:
1. Obtain skeletal age by wrist and hand radiograph using the standards of Greulich and Pyle (1959).
2. Find x for equation in table under skeletal age, using:
   Row A if skeletal age is within 1 year of chronological age;
   Row B if skeletal age is 1–2 years below chronological age; and
   Row C if skeletal age is 1–2 years advanced beyond chronological age.
3. Sole equation:

$$\text{adult height} = \frac{\text{present height}}{x}$$

Skeletal Age

	9–0	9–3	9–6	9–9	10–0	10–3	10–6	10–9	11–0	11–3
Males										
A	0.752	0.761	0.769	0.777	0.784	0.791	0.795	0.800	0.804	0.812
B	0.786	0.794	0.800	0.807	0.812	0.816	0.819	0.821	0.823	0.827
C	0.720	0.728	0.734	0.741	0.747	0.753	0.758	0.763	0.767	0.776
Females										
A	0.827	0.836	0.844	0.853	0.862	0.874	0.884	0.896	0.906	0.910
B	0.841	0.851	0.858	0.866	0.874	0.884	0.896	0.907	0.918	0.922
C	0.790	0.800	0.809	0.819	0.828	0.841	0.856	0.870	0.883	0.887

Skeletal Age

	11–6	11–9	12–0	12–3	12–6	12–9	13–0	13–3	13–6	13–9
Males										
A	0.818	0.827	0.834	0.843	0.853	0.863	0.876	0.890	0.902	0.914
B	0.832	0.839	0.845	0.852	0.860	0.869	0.880	0.890	0.902	0.914
C	0.786	0.800	0.809	0.818	0.828	0.839	0.850	0.863	0.875	0.890
Females										
A	0.914	0.918	0.922	0.932	0.941	0.950	0.958	0.967	0.974	0.978
B	0.926	0.929	0.932	0.942	0.949	0.957	0.964	0.971	0.977	0.981
C	0.891	0.897	0.901	0.913	0.924	0.935	0.945	0.955	0.963	0.968

Skeletal Age

	14–0	14–3	14–6	14–9	15–0	15–3	15–6	15–9	16–0	16–3
Males										
A	0.927	0.938	0.948	0.958	0.968	0.973	0.976	0.980	0.982	0.985
B	0.927	0.938	0.948	0.958	0.968	0.973	0.976	0.980	0.982	0.985
C	0.905	0.918	0.930	0.943	0.958	0.967	0.971	0.976	0.980	0.983
Females										
A	0.980	0.983	0.986	0.988	0.990	0.991	0.993	0.994	0.996	0.996
B	0.983	0.986	0.989	0.992	0.994	0.995	0.996	0.997	0.998	0.999
C	0.972	0.977	0.980	0.983	0.986	0.988	0.990	0.992	0.993	0.994

Skeletal Age

	16–6	16–9	17–0	17–3	17–6	17–9	18–0	18–3	18–6
Males									
A	0.987	0.989	0.991	0.993	0.994	0.995	0.996	0.998	1.0
B	0.987	0.989	0.991	—	—	—	—	—	—
C	0.985	0.988	0.990	—	—	—	—	—	—
Females									
A	0.997	0.998	0.999	0.999	1.0	—	—	—	—
B	0.999	0.999	1.0	—	—	—	—	—	—
C	0.995	0.997	0.998	0.999	0.999	—	—	—	—

From Freidman I, Goldberg E. Reference materials for the practice of adolescent medicine. *Pediatr Clin North Am* 1980;27:193, with permission. Modified from Bayley N. Pinneau Sr. Tables for predicting adult height from skeletal age: revised for use with the Greulich-Pyle hand standards. *J Pediatr* 1952;40:423–441.

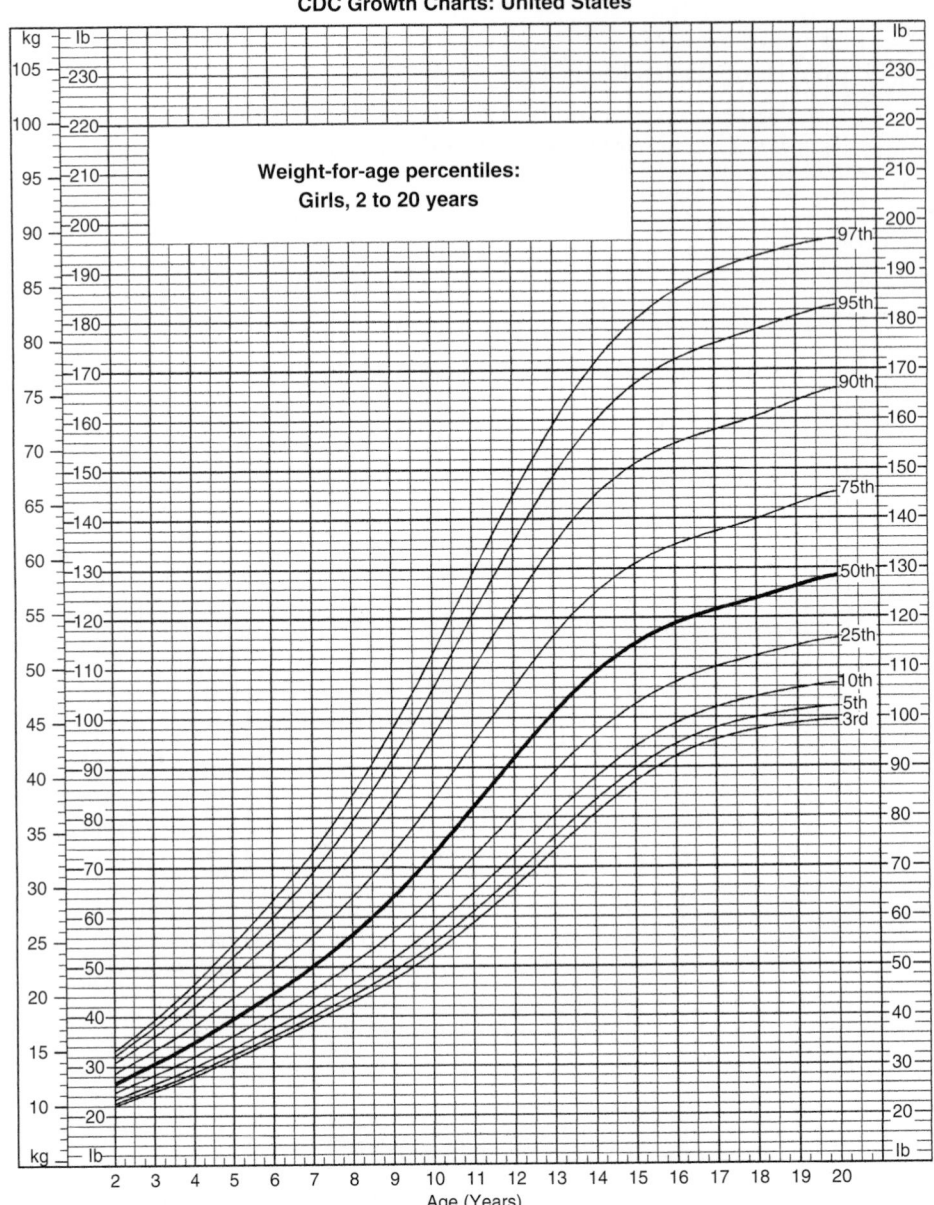

FIGURE 1.21 Weight-for-age percentiles for girls, 2 to 20 years of age. (From CDC. Growth charts: United States—advance data. From vital and health statistics of the Centers for Disease Control and Prevention. *Natl Center Health Stat* 2000;314:1.)

Adipose Mass

The percentage of body fat increases in females during puberty and decreases in adolescent males. Changes in body composition stem from hormonal fluctuations that are part of normal adolescence (Table 1.7).

Pelvic Remodeling in Women

During puberty, the female pelvis widens more rapidly than it increases in the anteroposterior dimension. The forepart of the pelvis also widens and becomes more rounded.

Skeletal Mass

Changes in bone mass, or bone mineral density (BMD), parallel the alterations in lean body mass, body size, and

muscle strength. Major determinants of BMD are physical activity level, heredity, nutrition, endocrine function, and other lifestyle factors. The accretion of skeletal bone mass during puberty is critical. Peak bone mass is acquired by early adulthood, serving as the "bone bank" for the remainder of life (Bachrach, 2000). Skeletal bone mass has been affected by the following:

1. Age at menarche: There is an inverse relation between the age at menarche and the risk of osteoporosis later in life, as demonstrated by epidemiological studies (Ribot et al., 1992; Tuppurainen et al., 1995; Johnell et al., 1995; Melton, 1997).
2. Nutrition: Much has been studied about the effects of calcium and vitamin D, with mixed results, although

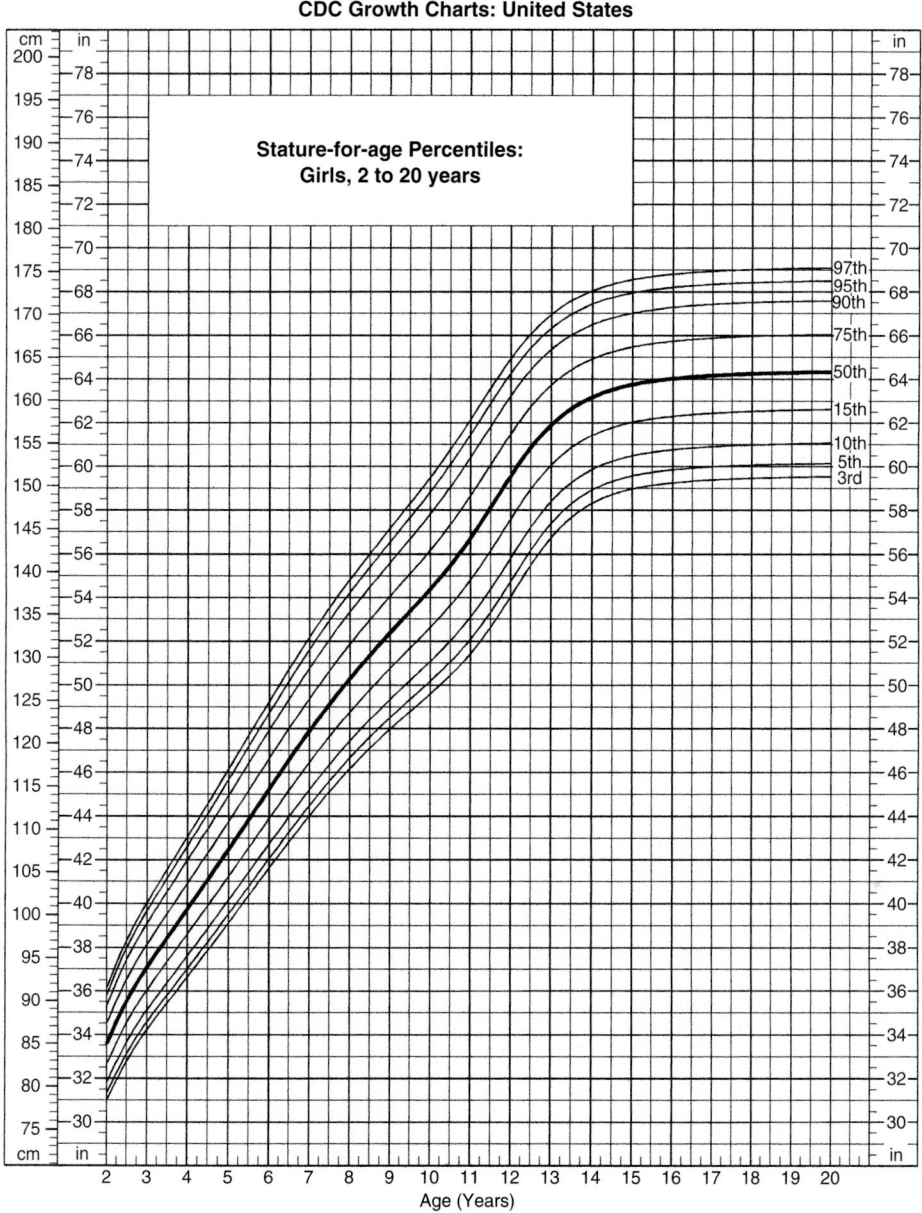

CDC Growth Charts: United States

Stature-for-age Percentiles:
Girls, 2 to 20 years

FIGURE 1.22 Stature-for-age percentiles for girls, 2 to 20 years of age. (From CDC. Growth charts: United States—advance DATA. From vital and health statistics of the Centers for Disease Control and Prevention. *Natl Center Health Stat* 2000;314:1.)

there is a consensus that adequate consumption of both of these nutrients is important for optimal bone mineral accrual. For example, one Swiss study found that supplementing healthy breast-fed infants with vitamin D resulted in higher bone mass later in childhood among girls (Zamora et al., 1999). Several studies have documented that increased calcium intake during childhood and adolescence results in higher peak bone mass (Matkovic et al., 1990; Johnston et al., 1992; Lloyd et al., 1993; Lee et al., 1994; Lee et al., 1995; Lloyd et al., 1996; Bonjour et al., 1997; Nowson et al., 1997; Dibba et al., 2000). A recent study followed a cohort of 144 girls randomized during the prepubertal years to receive either calcium supplementation of 850 g/day or placebo for 1 year (Chevalley et al., 2005). Postmenarchal follow-up showed that even this relatively brief intervention resulted in sustained increases in bone density in those girls who had earlier than average menarche, raising the question of whether higher calcium intake prepubertally may advance menarche. It appears that calcium intakes of between 1,200 and 1,800 mg/day result in maximal calcium absorption for children between age 9 and 18 years (Baker et al., 1999; Abrams and Stuff, 1994; Jackman et al., 1997; Matkovic and Heaney, 1992; Andon et al., 1994; NIH Concensus Conference, 1994; Institute of Medicine, Food and Nutrition Board, 1997).

3. Exercise   Weight-bearing physical activity during pre- and early puberty has been shown to improve bone

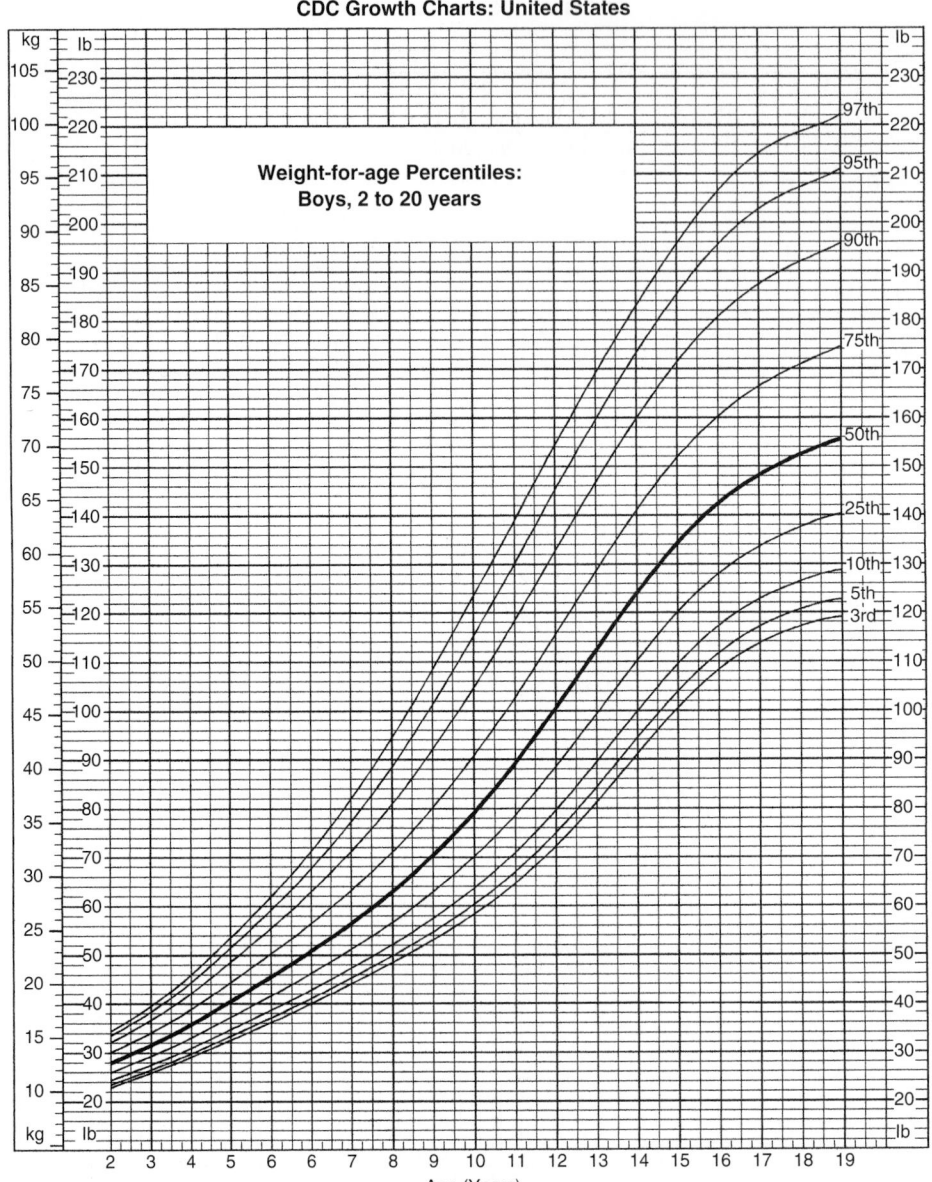

FIGURE 1.23 Weight-for-age percentiles for boys, 2 to 20 years of age. (From CDC. Growth charts: United States—advance data. From vital and health statistics of the Centers for Disease Control and Prevention. *Natl Center Health Stat* 2000;314:1.)

strength, but results have been less promising regarding the effects of exercise on postmenarcheal girls (for review see MacKelvie et al., 2002). In one study, a jumping program integrated into gym class resulted in greater femoral cross-sectional area, reduced endosteal expansion, and greater bending strength in both prepubertal and early pubertal (Tanner stages 2 and 3) girls compared with controls (MacKelvie et al., 2001).

Bone Age
Skeletal maturation, as reflected by bone age measurements, can be determined by comparing a radiograph of an adolescent's hand, wrist, or knee to standards of maturation in a normal population. Bone age is an index of

physiological maturation, providing an idea of the proportion of the total growth that has occurred. For example, if an adolescent is 15 years old and has a bone age of 12 years, there will be more potential growth than if the same adolescent's bone age were 15 years. The use of skeletal age is discussed further in Chapter 8.

Internal Organs
The growth of the brain, heart, liver, and kidneys during puberty is less than that of muscle and bone. Therefore, the percentage of body weight represented by the brain, heart, liver, and kidney decreases from approximately 10% to approximately 5% at maturity.

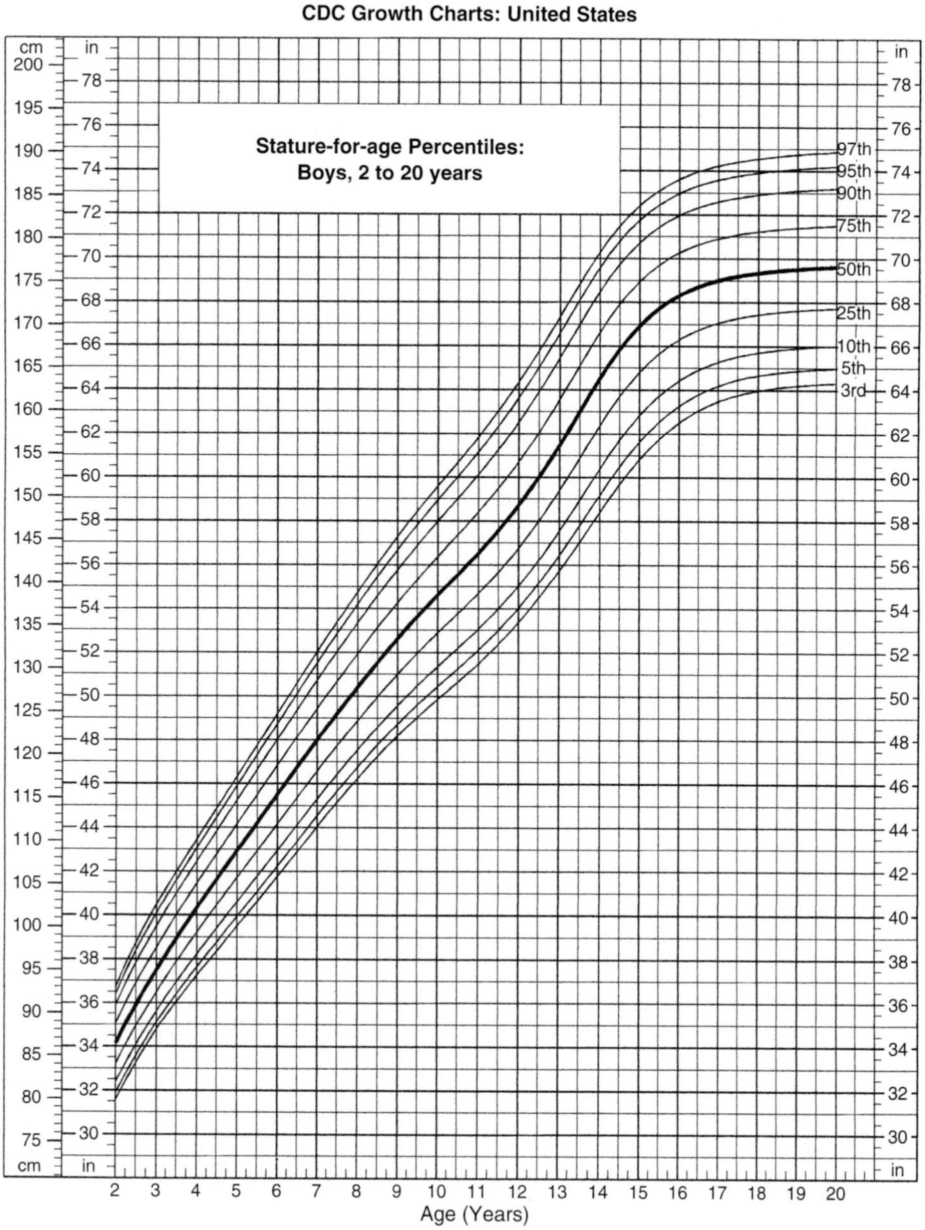

CDC Growth Charts: United States

FIGURE 1.24 Stature-for-age percentiles for boys, 2 to 20 years of age. (From CDC. Growth charts: United States—advance data. From vital and health statistics of the Centers for Disease Control and Prevention. *Natl Center Health Stat* 2000;314:1.)

Body Mass Index

Body mass index (BMI) increases with puberty, although it should be pointed out that BMI does not quantitate body composition. BMI varies with age, gender, and ethnicity. In children and adolescents, BMI must be compared using age-stratified standardized percentiles. Charts and tables for BMI, which should be tracked in all children and teenagers, can be obtained from the National Center for Chronic Disease Prevention and Health Promotion of the CDC (mailing and Web site addresses were listed previously in the section on Weight Growth). See Figures 1.25 and 1.26 to determine the normal BMI for a given age. There is a strong correlation between the timing of puberty and BMI: children with higher mean BMI mature earlier. BMI is determined by the following formula:

$$BMI = \text{Weight in kilograms} \div [\text{height in meters}]^2$$

or

$$BMI = [\text{Weight in kilograms} \div \text{height in centimeters} \div \text{height in centimeters}] \times 10,000$$

The equivalent formula in English units is the following:

$$BMI = [\text{Weight in pounds} \div \text{height in inches} \div \text{height in inches}] \times 703$$

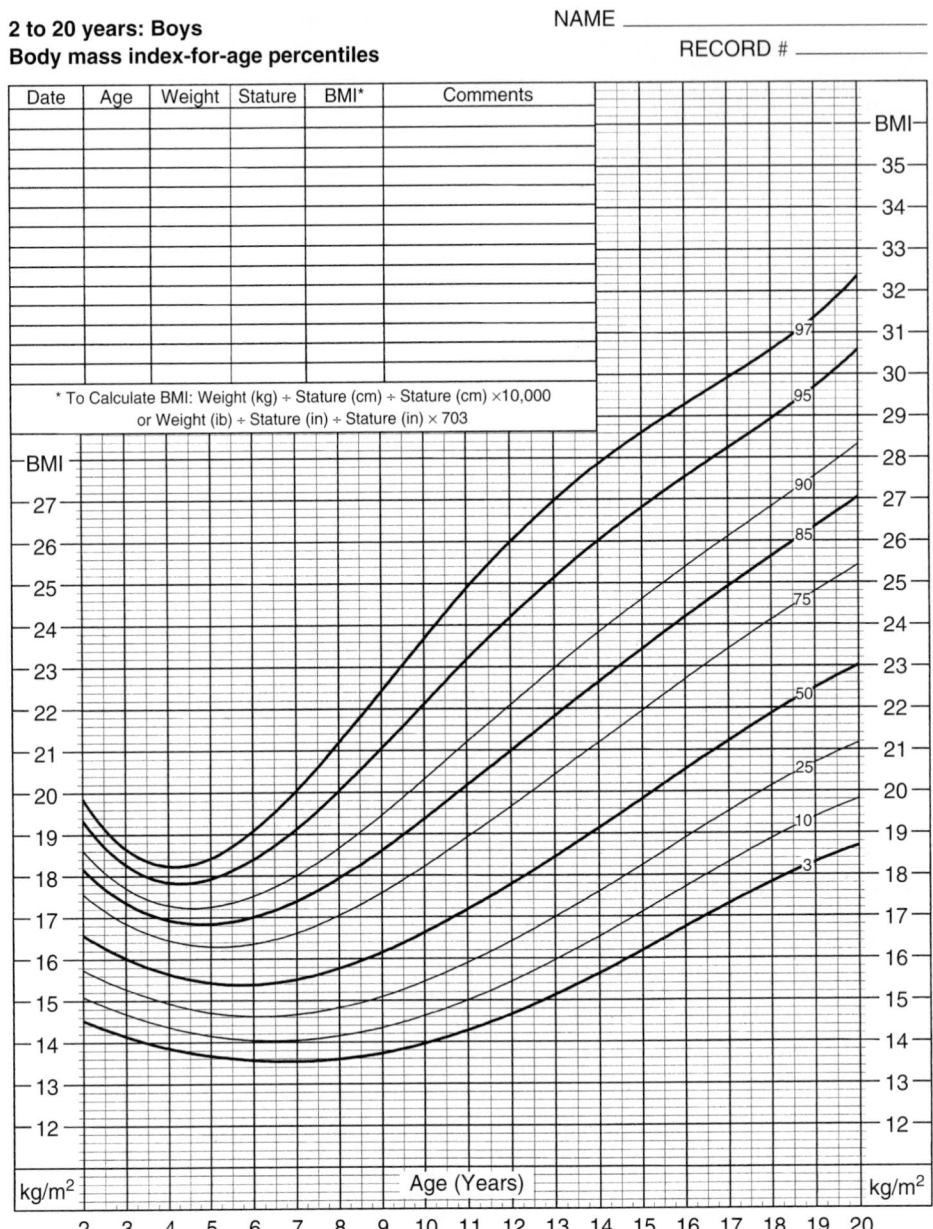

FIGURE 1.25   Body mass index-for-age percentiles for boys, 2 to 20 years of age. (From CDC. Growth charts: United States—advance data. From vital and health statistics of the Centers for Disease Control and Prevention. *Natl Center Health Stat* 2000;314:1.)

The BMI declines from birth and reaches a minimum between 4 and 6 years of age, before gradually increasing through adolescence and adulthood. The upward trend after the lowest point is referred to as the "adiposity rebound." Children with an earlier rebound are more likely to have an increased BMI.

CONCERN ABOUT GROWTH AND DEVELOPMENT

This chapter has discussed most of the features of normal adolescent growth and development. As essential as it is for the health care provider to have a firm grasp of the facts of normal growth and development, a clear understanding and feeling for what these changes mean to the adolescent are also critically important. As their bodies change, adolescents develop tremendous concern about whether their bodies are "normal." The great variation in the timing of puberty, with resultant differences in physical maturity of similar-aged adolescents, serves to heighten teenagers' worries. Practitioners must be adept at detecting the adolescent's concerns about height, weight, pubic hair growth, or phallus size, for example, even if these concerns are not stated overtly in the initial complaint.

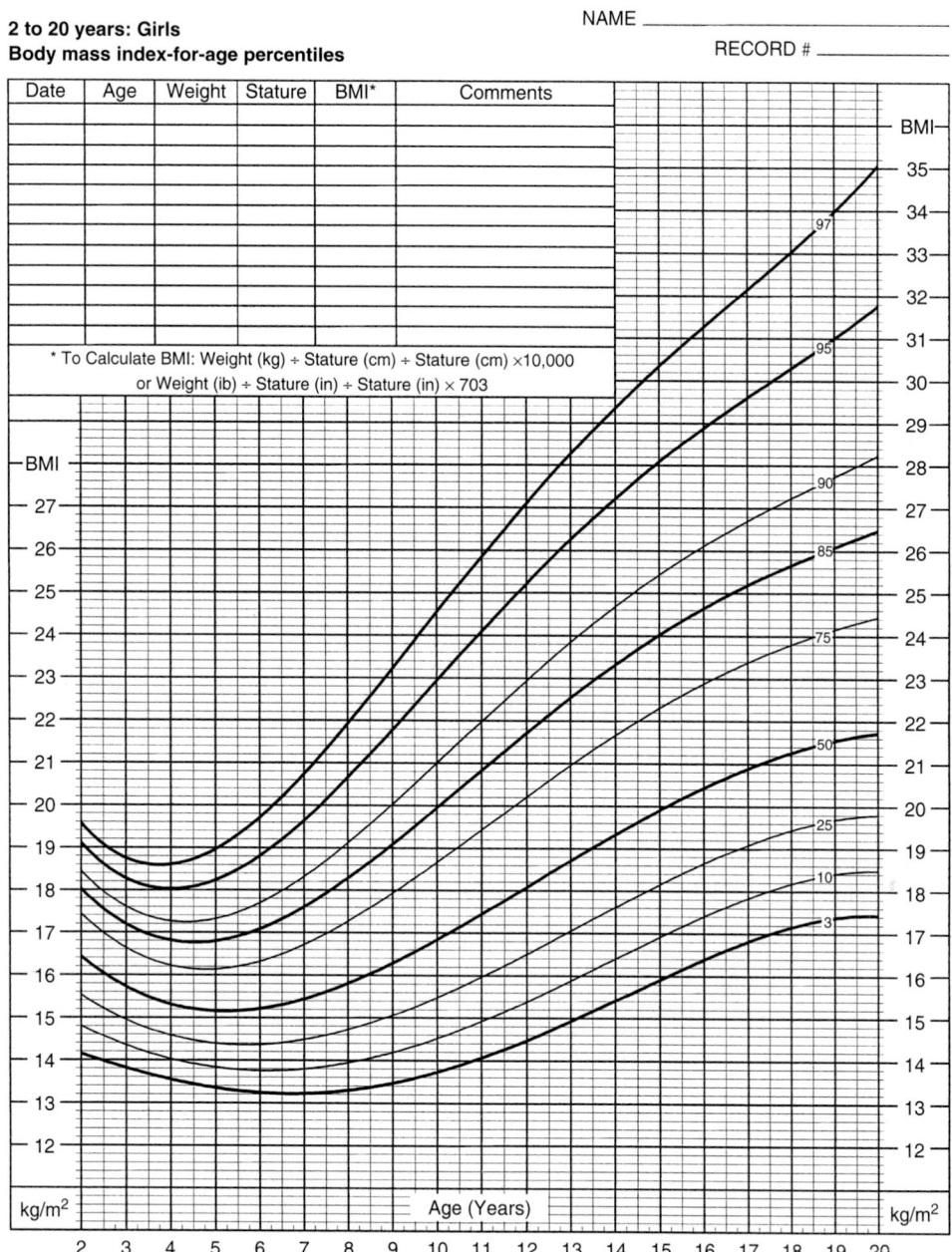

2 to 20 years: Girls
Body mass index-for-age percentiles

NAME _____

RECORD # _____

Date	Age	Weight	Stature	BMI*	Comments

* To Calculate BMI: Weight (kg) ÷ Stature (cm) ÷ Stature (cm) ×10,000
or Weight (ib) ÷ Stature (in) ÷ Stature (in) × 703

Age (Years)

FIGURE 1.26   Body mass index-for-age percentiles for girls, 2 to 20 years of age. (From CDC. Growth charts: United States—advance data. From vital and health statistics of the Centers for Disease Control and Prevention. *Natl Center Health Stat* 2000;314:1.)

SUMMARY

The changes of puberty are a marvel of nature and a testimony to the intricacies and wonders of the human hormonal system. The health care provider must understand these changes and the wide variations of normalcy. He or she must also be able to sense the profound effect these changes have on the adolescent and be prepared to be a source of information, reassurance, and help if abnormalities are detected.

WEB SITES

For Teenagers and Parents

http://www.teenwire.com/. What happens during puberty for guys and girls, from Teen Wire.
http://www.youngwomenshealth.org. From Young Women's Health Center at Boston Children's Hospital.
http://www.puberty101.com/. Information site on puberty and other adolescent questions.
http://www.iwannaknow.org/puberty/. Information on puberty from American Social Health Association.

TABLE 1.6

Primary Actions of GH and Sex Steroids on Body Composition[a]

	GH	Estradiol	Testosterone
Visceral fat[b,c]	↓↓	[d,e]	↓
Subcutaneous fat[b,f]	↓	↑	↓
Bone mineral[b,g]	↑	↑↑	↑↑
Muscle mass[b,f]	↑	[d]	↑↑
Extracellular water	↑ (acutely)	[d]	↑ (acutely)
Linear bone growth[b,f,g]	↑	↑↑	↑↑
Epiphyseal fusion[e,g]	[d]	↑↑	↑↑
Energy expenditure	↑	[d]	↑↑

[a]Refs. 194, 244, 393, 562–571.
[b]Possible synergy between somatotropic and gonadotropic signals.
[c]Nonaromatizable androgens also effectual.
[d]Limited or inconsistent data.
[e]Only in combination with a (synthetic) progestin.
[f]May differ in children and adults.
[g]Maximal effects require aromatization.

http://www.aap.org/healthtopics/stages.cfm#adol. The American Academy of Pediatrics web site with different and rotating issues related to teen health.

http://www.plannedparenthood.org/pp2/portal/medicalinfo/teensexualhealth/pub-period.xlm. Information from Planned Parenthood for girls on puberty and menstruation.

http://www.keepkidshealthy.com/adolescent/puberty.html. Teen health site, puberty section.

TABLE 1.7

Percentage of Body Fat During Puberty

Stage of Puberty	% Body Fat
Female	
1	15.7
2	18.9
3	21.6
4	26.7
Male	
1	14.3
2	11.2

Percentage of body fat remains unchanged in stages 3, 4, and 5 in males.

For Health Professionals

http://www.teachingteens.com/index2.htm. Health education site on teaching teens about puberty.
http://www.cdc.gov/growthcharts. Growth charts on-line.

REFERENCES AND ADDITIONAL READINGS

Abrams SA, Stuff JE. Calcium metabolism in girls: current dietary intakes lead to low rates of calcium absorption and retention during puberty. *Am J Clin Nutr* 1994; 60:739.

Anderson SE, Dallal GE, Must A. Relative weight and race influence average age at menarche: results from two nationally representative surveys of US girls studied 25 years apart. *Pediatrics* 2003;111:815.

Andon MB, Lloyd T, Matkovic V. Supplementation trials with calcium citrate malate: evidence in favor of increasing the calcium RDA during childhood and adolescence. *J Nutr* 1994;124:1412S.

Apter D, Bützow TL, Laughlin GA, et al. Gonadotropin-releasing hormone pulse generator activity during pubertal transition in girls: pulsatile and diurnal patterns of circulating gonadotropins. *J Clin Endocrinol Metab* 1993;76:940.

Attie KM, Ramirez NR, Conte FA, et al. The pubertal growth spurt in eight patients with true precocious puberty and growth hormone deficiency: evidence for a direct role of sex steroids. *J Clin Endocrinol Metab* 1990;71:975.

Bachrach LK. Making an impact on pediatric bone health. *J Pediatr* 2000;136:137.

Baker SS, Cochran WJ, Flores CA, et al. American Academy of Pediatrics. Committee on Nutrition. Calcium requirements of infants, children, and adolescents. *Pediatrics* 1999;104:1152.

Bellido T, Jilka RL, Boyce BF, et al. Regulation of interleukin-6, osteoclastogenesis, and bone mass by androgens. The role of the androgen receptor. *J Clin Invest* 1995;95:2886.

Bilezikian JP, Morishima A, Bell J, et al. Increased bone mass as a result of estrogen therapy in a man with aromatase deficiency. *N Engl J Med* 1998;339:599.

Blum WF, Englaro P, Hanitsch S, et al. Plasma leptin levels in healthy children and adolescents: dependence of body mass index, body fat mass, gender, pubertal stage and testosterone. *J Clin Endocrinol Metab* 1997;82:2904.

Bonjour JP, Carrie AL, Ferrari S, et al. Calcium-enriched foods and bone mass growth in prepubertal girls: a randomized, double-blind, placebo-controlled trial. *J Clin Invest* 1997;99:1287.

Campfield LA, Smith FJ, Guisez Y, et al. Recombinant mouse OB protein: evidence for a peripheral signal linking adiposity and central networks. *Science* 1995;269:546.

Carani C, Qin K, Simoni M, et al. Effect of testosterone and estradiol in a man with aromatase deficiency. *N Engl J Med* 1997;337:91.

Chehab F, Lim M, Lu R. Correction of the sterility defect in homozygous obese female mice by treatment with the human recombinant leptin. *Nat Genet* 1996;12:318.

Chevalley T, Rizzoli R, Hans D, et al. Interaction between calcium intake and menarcheal age on bone mass gain: an eight-year follow-up study from prepuberty to postmenarche. *J Clin Endocrinol Metab* 2005;90:44.

Chumlea WC, Schubert CM, Roche AF, et al. Age at menarche and racial comparisons in US girls. *Pediatrics* 2003;111:110.

Clayton PE, Gill MS, Hall CM, et al. Serum leptin through childhood and adolescence. *Clin Endocrinol* 1997;46:727.

Colvard DS, Eriksen EF, Keeting PE, et al. Identification of androgen receptors in normal human osteoblast-like cells. *Proc Natl Acad Sci U S A* 1989;86:854.

Dibba B, Prentice A, Ceesay M, et al. Effect of calcium supplementation on bone mineral accretion in Gambian children accustomed to a low-calcium diet. *Am J Clin Nutr* 2000;71:544.

Ducharme JR, Forest MG, De Peretti E, et al. Plasma adrenal and gonadal sex steroid in human pubertal development. *J Clin Endocrinol Metab* 1976;42:468.

Frisch RE. Body fat, puberty, and fertility. *Biol Rev Camb Philos Soc* 1984;59:161.

Frisch RE, Revelle R. Height and weight at menarche and a hypothesis of critical body weights and adolescent events. *Science* 1970;169:397.

Funes S, Hedrick JA, Vassileva G, et al. The KiSS-1 receptor GPR54 is essential for the development of the murine reproductive system. *Biochem Biophys Res Commun* 2003;312:1357.

Garcia-Mayor RV, Andrade MA, Rios M, et al. Serum leptin levels in normal children: relationship to age, gender, body mass index, pituitary-gonadal hormones, and pubertal stage. *J Clin Endocrinol Metab* 1997;82:2849.

Gill MS, Hall CM, Tillman V, et al. Constitutional delay in growth and puberty (CDGP) is associated with hypoleptinemia. *Clin Endocrinol* 1999;50:721.

Goji K. Twenty-four-hour concentration profiles of gonadotropin and estradiol (E2) in prepubertal and early pubertal girls: the diurnal rise of E2 is opposite the nocturnal rise of gonadotropin. *J Clin Endocrinol Metab* 1993;77:1629.

Grumbach MM. Estrogen, bone, growth and sex: a sea of change in conventional wisdom. *J Pediatr Endocrinol Metab* 2000;13(Suppl 6):1439.

Halaas JL, Gajiwala KS, Maffei M, et al. Weight-reducing effects of the plasma protein encoded by the obese gene. *Science* 1995;269:543.

Harlan WR, Grillo GP, Cornoni-Huntley J, et al. Secondary sex characteristics of boys 12-17 years of age: the US Health Examination Survey. *J Pediatr* 1979;95:293.

Herman-Gddens ME, Kaplowitz PB, Wasserman RC. Navigating the recent articles on girls' puberty in pediatrics: what do we know and where do we go from here? *Pediatrics* 2004;113:911.

Herman-Giddens ME, Slora EJ, Wasserman RC, et al. Secondary sexual characteristics and menses in young girls seen in office practice: a study from the pediatric research in office settings network. *Pediatrics* 1997;99:505.

Herman-Giddens ME, Wang L, Koch G. Secondary sexual characteristics in boys: estimates from the National Health and Nutrition Examination Survey III, 1988–1994. *Arch Pediatr Adolesc Med* 2001;155:1022.

Hofbauer LC, Khosla S. Androgen effects on bone metabolism: recent progress and controversies. *Eur J Endocrinol* 1999;140:271.

Horlick MB, Rosenbaum M, Nicolson M, et al. Effect of puberty on the relationship between circulating leptin and body composition. *J Clin Endocrinol Metab* 2000;85:2509.

Institute of Medicine, Food and Nutrition Board. *Dietary reference intakes for calcium, phosphorus, magnesium, vitamin D, and fluoride.* Washington, DC: National Academy Press, 1997.

Jackman LA, Millane SS, Martin BR, et al. Calcium retention in relation to calcium intake and postmenarcheal age in adolescent females. *Am J Clin Nutr* 1997;66:327.

Johnell O, Gullberg B, Kanis JA, et al. Risk factors for hip fracture in European women: the MEDOS Study. Mediterranean osteoporosis study. *J Bone Miner Res* 1995;10:1802.

Johnston FE, Malina RM, Galbraith MA, et al. Height, weight, and age at menarche and the "critical weight" hypothesis. *Science* 1971;174:1148.

Johnston CC Jr, Miller JZ, Slemenda CW, et al. Calcium supplementation and increases in bone mineral density in children. *N Engl J Med* 1992;327:82.

Juul A, Bang P, Hertel NT, et al. Serum insulin-like growth factor-I in 1030 healthy children, adolescents, and adults: relation to age, stage of puberty, testicular size, and body mass index. *J Clin Endocrinol Metab* 1994;78:744.

Kaplowitz PB, Oberfield SE. Reexamination of the age limit for defining when puberty is precocious in girls in the United States: implications for evaluation and treatment. Drug and Therapeutics and Executive Committees of the Lawson Wilkins Pediatric Endocrine Society. *Pediatrics* 1999;104:936.

Kasperk C, Helmboldt A, Boercsoek I, et al. Skeletal site-dependent expression of the androgen receptor in human osteoblastic cell populations. *Calcif Tissue Int* 1997;61:464.

Klein KO, Martha PM Jr, Blizzard RM, et al. A longitudinal assessment of hormonal and physical alterations during normal puberty in boys. II. Estrogen levels as determined by an ultrasensitive bioassay. *J Clin Endocrinol Metab* 1996;81:3203.

Largo RH, Prader A. Pubertal development in Swiss boys. *Helv Pediatr Acta* 1983;38:211.

Lee PA. Normal ages of pubertal events among American males and females. *J Adolesc Health Care* 1980;1:26.

Lee WT, Leung SS, Leung DM, et al. A randomized double-blind controlled calcium supplementation trial, and bone and height acquisition in children. *Br J Nutr* 1995;74:125.

Lee WT, Leung SS, Wang SH, et al. Double-blind, controlled calcium supplementation and bone mineral accretion in children accustomed to a low-calcium diet. *Am J Clin Nutr* 1994;60:744.

Lloyd T, Andon MB, Rollings N, et al. Calcium supplementation and bone mineral density in adolescent girls. *JAMA* 1993;270:841.

Lloyd T, Martel JK, Rollings N, et al. The effect of calcium supplementation and Tanner stage on bone density, content and area in teenage women. *Osteoporos Int* 1996;6:276.

MacKelvie KJ, Khan KM, McKay HA. Is there a critical period for bone response to weight-bearing exercise in children and adolescents? A systematic review. *Br J Sports Med* 2002;36:250.

MacKelvie KJ, McKay HA, Khan KM, et al. A school-based loading intervention augments bone mineral accrual in early pubertal girls. *J Pediatr* 2001;139:501.

Mantzoros CS, Flier JS, Rogel AD. A longitudinal assessment of hormonal and physical alterations during normal puberty in boys. Rising leptin levels may signal the onset of puberty. *J Clin Endocrinol Metab* 1997;82:1066.

Marshall JC, Kelch RP. Gonadotropin-releasing hormone: role of pulsatile secretion in the regulation of reproduction. *N Engl J Med* 1986;315:1459.

Marshall WA, Tanner JM. Variations in the pattern of pubertal changes associated with adolescence in girls. *Arch Dis Child* 1969;44:291.

Marshall WA, Tanner JM. Variations in the pattern of pubertal changes in boys. *Arch Dis Child* 1970;45:13.

Martha PMJ, Gorman KM, Blizzard RM, et al. Endogenous growth hormone secretion and clearance rates in normal boys as determined by deconvolution analysis; relationship to age, pubertal status, and body mass. *J Clin Endocrinol Metab* 1992;74:336.

Martha PM Jr, Rogol AD, Veldhuis JD. Alterations in the pulsatile properties of circulating growth hormone concentrations during puberty in boys. *J Clin Endocrinol Metab* 1989;69:563.

Matkovic V, Fontana D, Tominac C, et al. Factors that influence peak bone mass formation: a study of calcium balance and the inheritance of bone mass in adolescent females. *Am J Clin Nutr* 1990;52:878.

Matkovic V, Heaney RP. Calcium balance during human growth: evidence for threshold behavior. *Am J Clin Nutr* 1992;55:992.

Melton LJ III. Epidemiology of spinal osteoporosis. *Spine* 1997;22:2S.

Midyett LK, Moore WV, Jacobson JD. Are pubertal changes in girls before age 8 benign? *Pediatrics* 2003;111:47.

Morishima A, Grumbach MM, Bilezikian JP. Estrogen markedly increases bone mass in an estrogen deficient young man with aromatase deficiency (abstract). *J Bone Miner Res* 1997;12:S126.

Morishima A, Grumbach MM, Simpson ER, et al. Aromatase deficiency in male and female siblings caused by a novel mutation and the physiological role of estrogens. *J Clin Endocrinol Metab* 1995;80:3689.

Moschos S, Chan KL, Mantzoros CS. Leptin and reproduction: a review. *Fertil Steril* 2002;77:433.

Munoz-Torres M, Jodar E, Quesada M, et al. Bone mass in androgen-insensitivity syndrome: response to hormonal replacement therapy. *Calcif Tissue Int* 1995;57:94.

Navarro VM, Castellano JM, Fernàndez-Fernàndez R, et al. Effects of KiSS-1 peptide, the natural ligand of GPR54, on follicle-stimulating hormone secretion in the rat. *Endocrinology* 2005;146:1689.

NIH Consensus Conference. Optimal calcium intake. NIH consensus development panel on optimal calcium intake. *JAMA* 1994;272:1942.

Nowson CA, Green RM, Hopper JL, et al. A co-twin study of the effect of calcium supplementation on bone density during adolescence. *Osteoporos Int* 1997;7:219.

Ojeda SR, Terasawa E. Neuroendocrine regulation of puberty. In: Pfaff D, Arnold A, Etgen A, et al. eds. *Hormones, brain and behavior*, Vol. 4. New York: Elsevier Science, 2002:589.

Orwoll ES. Androgens as anabolic agents for bone. *Trends Endocrinol Metab* 1996;7:77.

Palmert MR, Hayden DL, Mansfield MJ, et al. The longitudinal study of adrenal maturation during gonadal suppression: evidence that adrenarche is a gradual process. *J Clin Endocrinol Metab* 2001;86:4536.

Pellymounter MA, Cullen MJ, Baker MB. Effect of obese gene product on body weight regulation in ob/ob mice. *Science* 1995;269:543.

de Peretti E, Forest M. Unconjugated dehydroepiandrosterone plasma levels in normal subjects from birth to adolescence in humans: the use of a sensitive radioimmunoassay. *J Clin Endocrinol Metab* 1976;43:982.

Prevot V, Lomniczi A, Corfas G, et al. erbB-1 and erbB-4 receptors act in concert to facilitate female sexual development and mature reproductive function. *Endocrinology* 2005;146:1465.

Remer T, Boye KR, Hartmann MF, et al. Urinary markers of adrenarche: reference values in healthy subjects, aged 3-18 years. *J Clin Endocrinol Metab* 2005;90:2015.

Remer T, Manz F. Role of nutritional status in the regulation of adrenarche. *J Clin Endocrinol Metab* 1999;84:3936.

Ribot C, Pouilles JM, Bonneu M, et al. The effect of gynecological risk factors on lumbar and femoral bone mineral density in peri- and post-menopausal osteoporosis using clinical factors. *Clin Endocrinol* 1992;36:225.

Roche AF, Heysfiled SB, Lohman TG, eds. *Human body composition. Total body composition: birth to old age.* Champain, IL: Human Kinetics Publishers, 2001:230.

Rogol AD. Growth at puberty: interaction of androgens and growth hormone. *Med Sci Sports Exerc* 1994;26:767.

Schoenau E, Neu CM, Rauch F, et al. The development of bone strength at the proximal radius during childhood and adolescence. *J Clin Endocriol Metab* 2001;86:613.

Seminara SB, Messager S, Chatzidaki EE, et al. The GPR54 gene as a regulator of puberty. *N Engl J Med* 2003;349:1614.

Smith EP, Boyd J, Graeme RF, et al. Estrogen resistance caused by a mutation in the estrogen-receptor gene in a man. *N Engl J Med* 1994;331:1056.

Strobel A, Issad I, Camion L, et al. A leptin missense mutation associated with hypogonadism and morbid obesity. *Nat Genet* 1998;18:213.

Sun SS, Shumei S, Schubert CM, et al. National estimates of the timing of sexual maturation and racial differences among US children. *Pediatrics* 2003;111:815.

Tuppurainen M, Kroger H, Saarikoski S, et al. The effect of gynecological risk factors on lumbar and femoral bone mineral density in peri- and post-menopausal women. *Maturitas* 1995;21:137.

Vanderschueren D. 1996 Androgens and their role in skeletal homeostasis. *Horm Res* 1996;46:95.

Van Wyk JJ, Smith EP. Insulin-like growth factors and skeletal growth: possibilities for therapeutic interventions. *J Clin Endocrinol Metab* 1999;84:4349.

Veldhuis JD, Roemmich JN, Richmond EJ, et al. Endocrine control of body composition in infancy, childhood and puberty. *Endocr Rev* 2005;26:114.

Villareal SF, Martorell R, Mendoza F. Sexual maturation of Mexican-American adolescents. *Am J Hum Biol* 1989;1:87.

Wu FCW, Butler GE, Kelnar CJH, et al. Patterns of pulsatile luteinizing hormone and follicle-stimulating hormone secretion in prepubertal (midchildhood) boys and girls and patients with idiopathic hypogonadotropic hypogonadism (Kallman's syndrome): a study using an ultrasensitive time-resolved immunofluorometric assay. *J Clin Endocrinol Metab* 1991;72:1229.

Weise M, De-Levi S, Barnes KM, et al. Effects of estrogen on growth plate senescence and epiphyseal fusion. *Proc Natl Acad Sci U S A* 2001;98:6871.

Wu T, Mendola P, Buck G. Ethnic differences in the presence of secondary sex characteristics and menarche among US girls: the Third National Health and Nutrition Examination Survey, 1988–1994. *Pediatrics* 2002;110:752.

Zamora SA, Rizzoli R, Belli DC, et al. Vitamin D supplementation during infancy is associated with higher bone mineral mass in prepubertal girls. *J Clin Endocrinol Metab* 1999;84:4541.

Zhang Y, Proenca R, Maffei M, et al. Positional cloning of the mouse *ob* gene and its human homologue. *Natura* 1994;372:425.

CHAPTER 2

Psychosocial Development in Normal Adolescents

Mari Radzik, Sara Sherer, and Lawrence S. Neinstein

No brief manual can hope to fully illuminate the complicated psychosocial developmental process of adolescence. This chapter offers an elementary framework from which to approach the study of this developmental process and discusses ways to enhance interactions between health care providers and adolescents.

In terms of physical development, adolescence can be described as the period of life beginning with the appearance of secondary sexual characteristics and terminating with the cessation of somatic growth. In modern Western culture, the behavioral aspects of this developmental period have become equally important. Adolescence is, in fact, a biopsychosocial process that may start before the onset of puberty and last well beyond the termination of growth. The events and problems that arise during this period are often perplexing to parents, health care providers, and adolescents. It is a time in which, for example, a previously obedient, calm child may become emotionally labile and act out.

It is vital that health care providers who provide comprehensive care for adolescents understand the adolescent psychosocial developmental process. Such an understanding is not only beneficial in routine adolescent health care but can also help adolescents and their families through problem periods involving, for example, failure in school, depression, suicidal tendencies, and out-of-control behavior. This chapter examines the phases and tasks of normal adolescent psychosocial growth and development, beginning with some general comments about the process of adolescence.

THE PROCESS OF ADOLESCENCE

First, it is important to keep in mind that no outline of psychosocial development can adequately describe every adolescent. Adolescents are not a homogeneous group, but display wide variability in biological, psychological, and emotional growth. Each adolescent responds to life's demands and opportunities in a unique and personal way. Further, adolescents must meet the challenges that arise from their own high-risk behaviors as well as the many social factors that impact their lives (Atav and Spencer, 2002; Galambos and Leadbeater, 2000; Gutgesell and Payne, 2004; Lerner and Galambos, 1998).

Second, the transition from childhood to adulthood does not occur by a continuous, uniform synchronous process. In fact, biological, social, emotional, and intellectual growth may be totally asynchronous (Steinberg, 2005). In addition, growth may be accented by frequent periods of regression. It must be remembered that all of life, from birth to death, is a constant process of change and that adolescence is not the only challenging period.

Third, whereas adolescence has historically been described as a period of extreme instability or "normal psychosis," most adolescents survive with no lasting difficulties, and many are unperturbed by the process (Freud, 1958). This ability to cope is a resiliency that is often overlooked, as the behaviors of adolescents are often the primary focus of attention (Olsson et al., 2003). In actuality, approximately 80% of adolescents cope well with the developmental process. Of these 80%, approximately 30% have an easy continual growth process, 40% have periods of stress intermingled with periods of calm, and 30% have tumultuous development marked by bouts of intense storm and stress. In a national survey, approximately 90% of 16-year-old boys and girls reported that they got along well with their mothers and 75% reported getting along well with their fathers (Rutter, 1980). Only one in five families reported difficult parent–child relationships. Overall, intractable and major conflict between parents and their adolescent children is not a "normal" part of adolescence (Steinberg, 1990; Laursen et al., 1998).

Phases and Tasks of Adolescence

Adolescence can be conceptualized by dividing the process into three psychosocial developmental phases:

1. Early adolescence: approximate ages 10 to 13, or middle school years
2. Middle adolescence: approximate ages 14 to 17, or high school years
3. Late adolescence: approximate ages 17 to 21, or college or 4 years of work after high school

These stages overlap among different adolescents. By the end of adolescence, emerging adults (Arnett, 2000) have become emancipated from parents and other adults and have attained a psychosexual identity and sufficient resources from family, education, and community to begin to support themselves in an emotionally, socially, and financially satisfying way. In addition, they have learned how to appropriately seek support from other individuals when needed.

Several tasks characterize the development of the adolescent and are discussed in the next several sections in conjunction with the various phases of adolescence. These tasks include the following:

1. Achieving independence from parents
2. Adopting peer codes and lifestyles
3. Assigning increased importance to body image and acceptance of one's body image
4. Establishing sexual, ego, vocational, and moral identities

EARLY ADOLESCENCE (APPROXIMATE AGES 10 TO 13)

Early adolescent psychosocial development is heralded by rapid physical changes with the onset of puberty. These physical changes engender self-absorption and initiate the adolescent's struggle for independence. The onset of puberty occurs 1 to 2 years earlier for girls than for boys. Concomitantly, the psychosocial and emotional changes also occur 1 to 2 years earlier in girls. Recent studies have provided evidence for an earlier age at onset of pubertal development in girls.

Independence–Dependence Struggle

Early adolescence is characterized by the beginning of the shift from dependence on parents to independent behavior. Common events at this time include:

1. Less interest in parental activities and more reluctance to accept parental advice or criticism; occasional rudeness; more realization that the parent is not perfect
2. An emotional void created by separation from parents, without the presence of an alternative support group, which can often create behavioral problems (e.g., a decrease in school performance)
3. Emotional lability (wide mood and behavior swings)
4. Increased ability to express oneself through speech
5. Search for new people to love in addition to parents

Body Image Concerns

Rapid physical changes lead the adolescent to be increasingly preoccupied with body image and the question of, "Am I normal?" The early adolescent's concern with body image is characterized by the following four factors:

1. Preoccupation with self
2. Uncertainty about appearance and attractiveness
3. Frequent comparison of own body with those of other adolescents
4. Increased interest in sexual anatomy and physiology, including anxieties and questions regarding menstruation or nocturnal emissions, masturbation, and breast or penis size

Peer Group Involvement

With the beginning of movement away from the family, the adolescent becomes more dependent on friends as a source of comfort (Pugh, 1999; Eccles, 1999). The early adolescent's peer group is characterized by the following:

1. Solitary friendships with a member of the same sex. This idealized friendship may become intense; boys, for example, may become "comrades-in-arms" with sworn pacts and allegiances and young teenage girls may develop deep crushes on men as well as women.
2. Strongly emotional, tender feelings toward peers, which may lead to homosexual exploration, fears, and/or relationships.
3. Peer contact primarily with the same sex, with some contact of the opposite sex made in groups of friends.

Identity Development

At the same time that the rapid physical changes occur, the adolescent's cognitive abilities are improving markedly. According to Piaget's (1969) cognitive theory, this corresponds to the evolution from concrete thinking (concrete operational thoughts) to abstract thinking (formal operational thoughts). During this time, the adolescent is expected to achieve academically and to prepare for the future. This period of identity development is characterized by the following:

1. Increased ability to reason abstractly. This ability is usually turned inward, leading to increased self-interest and fantasy. For example, the young adolescent may feel himself or herself constantly "onstage."
2. Frequent daydreaming, which is not only normal but also an important component in identity development because it allows adolescents an avenue to explore, enact, problem solve, and recreate important aspects of their lives.
3. Setting unrealistic or idealistic (depending on the individual) vocational goals (e.g., musician, airplane pilot, or truck driver).
4. Testing authority is common behavior in adolescents as they attempt to better define themselves and is often one cause of tension between the adolescent and his or her family or teachers.
5. A need for greater privacy, with diary or journal writing often becoming highly important.
6. Emergence of sexual feelings often relieved through masturbation or the telling of dirty jokes. Girls are often ahead at this point in sexual development.
7. Development of the adolescent's own value system, leading to additional challenges to family and others.
8. Lack of impulse control and need for immediate gratification, which may result in dangerous risk-taking behavior.
9. Tendency to magnify one's personal situation (although adolescents often feel that they are continually onstage, conversely, they may also be convinced that they are alone and that their problems are unique).

MIDDLE ADOLESCENCE (APPROXIMATE AGES 14 TO 16)

Middle adolescence is characterized by an increased scope and intensity of feelings and by the rise in importance of peer group values.

Independence–Dependence Struggle

Conflicts become more prevalent as the adolescent exhibits less interest in parents and devotes more of his or her time to peers.

Body Image Concerns

Most middle adolescents, having experienced most of their pubertal changes, are less preoccupied with these changes. Although there is greater acceptance and comfort with the body, much time is spent trying to make it more attractive. Clothes and makeup may become all important. Because of the societal emphasis on youthful body image, eating disorders may become established during this developmental phase.

Peer Group Involvement

The powerful role of peer groups is most apparent during middle adolescence (Pugh, 1999; Eccles, 1999). Characteristics of this involvement include the following:

1. Intense involvement by the adolescent in his or her peer subculture
2. Conformity by the adolescent with peer values, codes, and dress, in an attempt to further separate from family
3. Increased involvement in partnering relations manifested by dating activity, sexual experimentation, and intercourse
4. Involvement with clubs, team sports, gangs, and other groups

Evidence suggests that friends are the primary source of influence on youths' behavior, but estimates of peer pressure are often overstated (Aseltine, 1995). Adolescents' reactions to peer pressure are extremely varied and peer pressures can also involve a desire to excel in school, sports, or other positive activities.

Identity Development

The abilities to abstract and to reason continue to increase in middle adolescence, along with a new sense of individuality. The middle adolescent's ego development is characterized by the following:

1. Increased scope and openness of feelings, with a new ability to examine the feelings of others
2. Increased intellectual ability and creativity
3. Less idealistic vocational aspirations (adolescents with average and below-average intellectual abilities often realize their limitations at this time and may consequently experience lowered self-esteem and depression)
4. A feeling of omnipotence and immortality, leading to risk-taking behavior, which is certainly a factor in the high rate of accidents, suicides, drug use, pregnancies, and sexually transmitted diseases that become prevalent at this stage

LATE ADOLESCENCE (APPROXIMATE AGES 17 TO 21)

Late adolescence is the final phase of the adolescent's struggle for identity and separation. If all has proceeded well in early and middle adolescence, including the presence of a supportive family and peer group, the adolescent will be well on his or her way to handling the tasks and responsibilities of adulthood. If the previously mentioned tasks have not been completed, then problems such as depression, suicidal tendencies, or other emotional disorders may develop with the increasing independence and responsibilities of young adulthood. A new conceptualization of the period from late adolescence through the twenties (specifically the period from 18–25 years of age) is referred to as the "emergent adult" period (Arnett, 2000). These new young adults have begun to accept responsibility for their behaviors, formulate their own decisions, and make an effort to be financially independent.

Independence–Dependence Struggle

For most, late adolescence is a time of reduced restlessness and increased integration. The adolescent has become a separate entity from his or her family and may better appreciate the importance of his or her parents' values. Such an understanding may make it possible for the adolescent to seek and accept parental advice and guidance. However, it is not uncommon for some adolescents to be hesitant to accept the responsibilities of adulthood and to remain dependent on family and peers. Characteristics include the following:

1. Firmer identity
2. Greater ability to delay gratification
3. Better ability to think ideas through and express ideas in words
4. More stable interests
5. Greater ability to make independent decisions and to compromise

Body Image Concerns

The late adolescent has completed pubertal growth and development, and is typically less concerned with this process, unless an abnormality has occurred.

Peer Group Involvement

Peer group values become less important to late adolescents as they become more comfortable with their own values and identity. More time is spent in a relationship with one person. Such relationships involve less exploitation and experimentation and more sharing. The selection of a partner is based more on mutual understanding and enjoyment than on peer acceptance.

Identity Development

Ego development during the late adolescent phase/stage is characterized by the following:

1. The development of a rational and realistic conscience
2. The development of a sense of perspective, with the abilities to delay, compromise, and set limits
3. The development of practical vocational goals and the beginning of financial independence
4. Further refinement of moral, religious, and sexual values

TABLE 2.1

Psychosocial Development of Adolescents

Task	Early Adolescence	Middle Adolescence	Late Adolescence
Independence	Less interest in parental activities Wide mood swings	Peak of parental conflicts	Reacceptance of parental advice and values
Body image	Preoccupation with self and pubertal changes Uncertainty about appearance	General acceptance of body Concern over making body more attractive	Acceptance of pubertal changes
Peers	Intense relationships Same-sex friends	Peek of peer involvement Conformity with peer values Increased sexual activity and experimentation	Peer group less important More time spent in sharing intimate relationships
Identity	Increased cognition Increased fantasy world Idealistic vocational goals Increased need for privacy Lack of impulse control	Increased scope of feelings Increased intellectual ability Feeling of omnipotence Risk-taking behavior	Practical, realistic, and vocational goals Refinement of moral, religious, and sexual values Ability to compromise and to set limits

CONCLUSION

Most adolescents follow the general psychosocial developmental phases as outlined above. An understanding of this general pattern helps health care providers evaluate an adolescent's behavior. Table 2.1 summarizes the developmental tasks for each phase of adolescence.

WEB SITES

http://www.My.webmd.com. Web MD Health, search under "growth and development".

http://www.Connectforkids.org. For adults—parents, grandparents, educators, policy makers and others who want to become more actively involved with youth.

http://www.apahelpcenter.org/. The American Psychological Association's online resource center.

http://www.Generalpediatrics.com. The General Pediatrician's view of the Internet.

http://www.Parent-teen.com. An online magazine for families with teens.

http://www.cpyu.org. Center for Parent Youth Understanding.

http://www.aacap.org/publications/factsfam/develop. htm. American Academy of Child and Adolescent Psychiatry.

REFERENCES AND ADDITIONAL READINGS

Arnett JJ. Emerging adulthood, a theory of development from the late teens through the twenties. *Am Psychol* 2000;5(55): 469.

Aseltine R. A reconsideration of parental and peer influences on adolescence deviance. *J Health Soc Behav* 1995;36(2): 103.

Atav S, Spencer G. Health risk behaviors among adolescents attending rural, suburban, and urban schools: a comparative study. *Fam Community Health* 2002;25(2):53.

Coleman JC. Understanding adolescence today: a review. *Child Soc* 1993;7:137.

Eccles J. The development of children ages 6 to 14. *Future Child* 1999;9(2):30.

Freud A. Adolescence. *Psychoanal Study Child* 1958;13:255.

Galambos NL, Leadbeater BJ. Trends in adolescent research for the new millennium. *Int J Behav Dev* 2000;24(3): 289.

Gutgesell ME, Payne N. Issues of adolescent psychological development in the 21st century. *Pediatr Rev* 2004;25:79.

Hill JP. *Understanding early adolescence: a framework*. Carrboro, North Carolina: Center for Early Adolescence, 1980.

Laursen B, Coy KC, Collins WA. Reconsidering changes in parent-child conflict across adolescence: a meta-analysis. *Child Dev* 1998;69(13):817.

Lerner RM, Galambos NL. Adolescent development: challenges and opportunities for research, programs, and policies. *Annu Rev Psychol* 1998;49:413.

Lipsitz JS. *Sexual development of young adolescents*. Chapel Hill: University of North Carolina, Center for Early Adolescence, 1980.

Litt IF. The interaction of pubertal and psychosocial development during adolescence. *Ped Rev* 1991;12:249.

Mehr M. The psychosocial and psychosexual unfolding of adolescence. *Semin Fam Med* 1981;2:155.

Olsson CA, Bond L, Burns JM, et al. Adolescent resiliency: a concept analysis. *J Adolesc* 2003;26:1.

Piaget J. The intellectual development of the adolescent. In: Caplan G, Lebovici S, eds. *Adolescence: psychological perspectives*. New York: Basic Books, 1969.

Pugh MJV, Hart D. Identity development and peer group participation. *New Dir Child Adolesc Dev* 1999;84: 55–70.

Remschmidt H. Psychosocial milestones in normal puberty and adolescence. *Horm Res* 1994;41(Suppl 2):19.

Rutter M. *Changing youth in a changing society.* Cambridge, Massachusetts: Harvard University Press, 1980.

Sider RC, Kreider SD. Coping with adolescent patients. *Med Clin North Am* 1977;61:839.

Slap GB. Normal physiological and psychosocial growth in the adolescent. *J Adolesc Health Care* 1986;7:139.

Steinberg L. *Understanding families with young adolescents.* Carrboro, North Carolina: Center for Early Adolescence, 1980.

Steinberg L. Autonomy, conflict and harmony in the family relationship. In: S Feldman, G Eliot eds. *At the threshold: the developing adolescent.* Cambridge, MA: Harvard University Press, 1989:255.

Steinberg L. Adolescent development. *Annu Rev Psychol* 2001; 52:83.

Steinberg L. Cognitive and affective development in adolescence. *Trends Cogn Sci* 2005;9(2):69.

CHAPTER 3

Office Visit, Interview Techniques, and Recommendations to Parents

Elizabeth R. Woods and Lawrence S. Neinstein

The style and personality of the provider and his/her philosophy of medical care are particularly important in the medical care of adolescents. The provider should be mature and open-minded, and genuinely interested in teenagers as persons first, then in their problems, and also in their parents. He/she should not only like teenagers but must also feel comfortable with them. He/she should be able to communicate well with his/her patients and their parents. The provider should help enhance family communication while assuring confidentiality when requested around personal issues.

(Adapted from Committee on Care of Adolescents in Private Practice of the Society for Adolescent Medicine.)

Providing care to adolescents in a sensitive, flexible, developmentally and culturally appropriate manner requires interest, time, and experience on the part of health care providers. No book can adequately teach the art of relating to patients or adolescents; it is a skill that is ultimately perfected through practice. A good medical interview with the adolescent is important, because it allows the provider not only to collect information but also to set the tone for future interactions. This chapter contains general guidelines for establishing better rapport with adolescents, as well as suggested interviewing techniques. At the end of the chapter there are some suggestions for parents to improve communication with their teen.

GENERAL GUIDELINES FOR THE OFFICE VISIT

Liking the Adolescent

To provide effective care and establish rapport with the adolescent patient, the health care provider must like adolescents. If the provider dislikes or is extremely uncomfortable with teenagers, it is best to refer them elsewhere. If the particular condition requires more expertise than the provider has or causes personal conflicts about moral or religious issues, the adolescent should be referred elsewhere.

Meeting the Adolescent and Family: The First Session

It is important for the provider to introduce himself or herself to the family and to the adolescent as the adolescent's provider. At about the time of puberty, a transition should be made to allow more of the visit to be focused on the adolescent. Providers should advance along the visit styles described here as the adolescent matures and the family is known and trusts the adolescent-focused visit. One of three basic approaches may be used to start the interview; the choice may depend on the complexity of the visit, nature of the complaints, knowledge of the individual and family, and the age of the adolescent.

Separate Time for Family and Adolescent

For new, complex patients, the provider may need an extensive history from the family and an understanding of their full agenda. The provider should greet the adolescent first, explain the order of the visit, and request a few minutes to meet with the parents alone, "about when you were a child." This gives the parents a few minutes to relate the past history, family history, their agenda, and concerns. Some of these items the parents might not feel comfortable stating in front of the adolescent, such as "I am afraid he has cancer" or "I think she is sexually active and needs birth control." Having this information at the start of the interview will improve the focus of the whole visit, rather than having it spill out at the end of the visit. Next, the adolescent should be seen alone for additional history, discussion of confidentiality, and physical examination. The adolescent should be present from the time he or she meets with the provider, through to the end of the visit so that the adolescent does not feel that the provider is divulging confidential information to the family. This approach allows discussions with the parents about issues they may feel are sensitive. Follow-up visits can start with a very brief meeting with the parents alone, if major issues persist, but should rapidly switch over to one of the other types of visit, described next.

Family Together

Some health care providers prefer to see the family and adolescent together first. This approach can yield a great deal of information in the first few minutes regarding family dynamics. For example, if the adolescent is asked why he or she wants to be seen and the mother quickly answers for the adolescent, a sense of the adolescent–mother relationship is gained. When the family is seen together, it is helpful to have the teen introduce the family members to the provider. This gives the adolescent the message that the provider is primarily interested in him or her. After this part of the interview, the adolescent should be interviewed and examined alone.

Adolescent Alone

Another basic approach is to start by interviewing the adolescent alone. Some health care providers favor this approach in the belief that it quickly helps to establish rapport and a sense of trust. However, it is important to inform the adolescent that some input regarding his or her past history will be required from the parent during the initial interview. At this point, the family may be brought in to continue the interview; however, the adolescent should be present to hear what is stated. This approach is especially important for older adolescents.

Summarizing

At the end of any of the three visit types described, the provider should summarize the issues and plans with the adolescent. Issues that can or must be discussed with the family can be summarized with the family and the adolescent together, so that the adolescent can hear how the information is presented and discussed with the family and all concerns can be addressed. As the adolescent becomes a young adult, the full visit will tend to be with the young person. If family members come with the young adult, they can be included in a brief summary at the end of the visit, if helpful for the support of the young person or to assist the young person with adherence to complex treatment regimens.

Office Setup

Space

Adolescents prefer their own waiting area in a pediatrician's office. They do not like to be treated as young children. It is helpful if the waiting room has materials such as magazines that are appropriate for adolescents and health education brochures. A separate waiting area or corner of the waiting room should be set aside for adolescents and young adults, or separate blocks of time should be used so that age-appropriate materials can be displayed. If the office is used for other age groups, one examination room should be set aside for use with teens. For privacy, the examination table should be facing away from the door or an inner curtain should be added.

The office should have enough room to accommodate the family as well as the adolescent. It is preferable not to interview the adolescent and family in the examination room on the first comprehensive visit. The desk in the office should be oriented so that the health care provider sits beside the desk, not behind it. Placing a large desk between the adolescent and oneself can create an artificial barrier.

Appointments

Usually, initial comprehensive visits for an adolescent should be scheduled to last 1 hour. Obviously, there may be time constraints based on the practice setting if the provider is pressed for time. Most follow-up appointments should be scheduled for after-school hours or early in the morning to minimize missed school time. At the end of the first visit, a decision should be made with the teen and the family as to whether the adolescent can make future visits on his or her own. Transportation needs may limit this option for young adolescents in some practice settings, but the permission to come to visits on his or her own is important.

Billing

The issue of fee payment should be discussed early. This can even be done when the first appointment is made. Confidentiality can be maintained by using nonconfidential or symptom-based billing codes when the parents are paying for services. The adolescent must realize that an insurance payment may result in parents finding out about visits and the diagnosis; however, a neutral diagnosis can be used in most situations. Ideally, a mutual agreement can be reached with the adolescent and parents in this area. Alternatives include:

1. Confidential billing (if the insurance company allows), so that the parents are not aware of the exact nature of the visits
2. Having the adolescent pay for his or her own bills on a flexible installment plan with reduced fees
3. Having the adolescent obtain Medicaid funds for conditions such as pregnancy, family planning, and substance abuse
4. Referral to a clinic that can provide free confidential care

Availability of Educational Materials

It is helpful to place books, pamphlets, hot line numbers, and reliable Web site information in the waiting room or office on topics such as puberty, sexually transmitted diseases, sexuality, and contraception. The presence of such materials helps the adolescent to feel that it is "O.K." to talk about these subjects. Helpful materials and Web sites are listed at the end of this chapter.

Avoiding Interruptions

Constant interruptions or phone calls during the interview tend to decrease rapport. The office staff should hold all nonemergency questions or phone calls until after the interview.

Taking Notes

The provider should take as few notes as possible during the interview. For referred patients, the content of letters to referring primary care providers concerning confidential issues should be discussed with the adolescent.

Establishing Rapport

Establishing rapport with an adolescent, especially with a nonverbal or hostile teenager, can be difficult. Helpful suggestions include the following:

1. Begin the interview by introducing yourself to the teen and parents or guardians. It is helpful to shake the hand of the adolescent.
2. Begin by chatting informally about friends, school, or hobbies. Not only does this decrease tension but it also

enables the provider to gain important insights into the adolescent's personality, mood, and thought content.

3. Let the adolescent talk for a while, even if he or she meanders.
4. Treat the adolescent's comments as seriously as you would an adult's. The teenager should feel you are treating him or her as a person, not as a child or patient.
5. Start with nonthreatening health questions, such as a review of systems, especially if the adolescent is highly tense or suspicious.
6. Explore with the adolescent the issues that concern him or her. These issues may differ radically from concerns expressed by the parents.

Ensuring Confidentiality

It is important to establish a sense of confidentiality with the adolescent. The limits of this confidentiality may vary depending on the type of medical practice and current laws of a particular state (English, 2003; English and Ford, 2004; Ford et al., 2004). The adolescent should be aware of these limits. For example, it should be explained that discussions will be kept confidential unless a problem becomes a threat to the adolescent or to others. When there are concerns about safety, the provider should relay to the adolescent that this is a situation that needs to be shared with the parents. Adolescents are often more willing to discuss topics with their parents in the safer environment of the provider's office, and the provider can help facilitate the discussion of difficult topics.

Many parents are naturally concerned about being separated from their teen during the interview process. One approach is to explain to the parents early the philosophy of your practice, for example: "As we are proceeding in gathering information about John, I would like to tell you both how I work with adolescents. After I finish talking with all of you together, I am going to speak with John alone for a few minutes. Then I will take him to the examination room for a physical examination. When this is done, I will call you back to go over the findings and my recommendations. During this time, I may discuss some matters that John would prefer I keep in confidence. It has been my philosophy to respect that confidence. Certainly, if there were any serious problem that was a threat to John's life or health I would inform you. Now, before we break as a group, are there any other concerns that you have about John that we have not discussed?"

Avoiding a Surrogate Parent Role

Rather than being a surrogate parent, the health care provider should function as an extraparental adult. The emphasis should be on listening, advising, and guiding, using as nonjudgmental an approach as possible.

Avoiding an Adolescent Role

The adolescent is looking for a provider who can be a sensitive and mature resource, not someone who is "one of the gang" and who dresses and talks like an adolescent.

Sidestepping Power Struggles

It is difficult to force adolescents into action. In other words, no one is better at being an adolescent than an adolescent. Teenagers respond better if they can arrive at their own conclusions.

Acting as an Advocate

The adolescent encounters any number of adults who are nonsupportive and who stress the adolescent's negative attributes. Try to emphasize an adolescent's positive characteristics and abilities. Keep in mind, however, that supporting the adolescent in "down" times is not the same as supporting inappropriate behavior.

Importance of Listening

Listening can often be the key to developing rapport with an adolescent. However, listening can be difficult, as thoughts usually wander or focus on the next response. The health care provider should practice his or her listening skills to give full attention to the adolescent's statements and feelings. Good listening skills include:

1. Staying focused on what the teen is telling you
2. Asking questions that help move the conversation along
3. Being cautious about giving advice before being asked
4. Using gender-neutral terms until the adolescent has indicated his or her preferences
5. Trying to understand the teen's perspective

Instilling Responsibility

Adolescents should be made aware that they are responsible for their own care. The more responsibility that adolescents take for their personal progress, the fewer problems that occur with compliance. Adolescents have a great ability to instill guilt in health care providers. The provider can feel overwhelmed with the burden of changing the adolescent's life and habits. This burden should be shifted onto the adolescent.

Displaying Interest and Concern

The adolescent must be able to feel the health care provider's interest and concern. Shrugging off concerns as unimportant is a sure way to alienate the adolescent.

Family and Parents

Although the adolescent may be the primary patient, the parents cannot be overlooked. Parental input and insight are crucial, for in a real sense the family is the patient. Often the full agenda of the visit cannot be understood without initial input from the parents. To ignore the family's involvement in an adolescent's problem can often prolong the problem. Families must be consulted for the following reasons:

1. To elucidate past medical history, family history, and present concerns
2. To understand family dynamics and structure

3. To alleviate the parents' sense of rejection or guilt
4. To help bring about changes in the family unit and in the adolescent
5. To negotiate fair and consistent limits
6. To support the adolescent in complex treatment regimens
7. To ensure consistency of follow-up and referral care

Nonverbal Cues

Much can be learned by observing the adolescent's body language, such as hand movements, manner of sitting, eye movements, or eyes slightly brimming with tears when certain subjects are discussed.

Process Versus Content

Although inappropriate behavior should not be condoned, the health care provider must explore the reasons behind the action. For example, shoplifting may occur secondary to peer pressure or family or school problems. Positive comments supporting the adolescent's health choices can help the adolescent recognize his or her strengths and resist peer pressure.

Hidden Agenda

Adolescents often present with chief complaints that are unrepresentative of their true concerns. A female adolescent presenting with mild sore throat, acne, or pelvic pain may in actuality be afraid she is pregnant or has a sexually transmitted disease. A male adolescent with chest pains may be concerned about gynecomastia. Gentle but persistent exploration of the adolescent's concerns is often necessary before the true chief complaint is evident. If an adolescent girl is extremely reluctant to communicate or has vague symptoms, a pregnancy test should be considered.

Developmentally Oriented Approach

In the course of interviewing and evaluating the adolescent, the health care provider should be conscious of the adolescent's developmental process and tasks. The areas of sex, school performance, family, peer group, identity, and future plans should all be explored. Evaluative expectations should be based on the stage of emotional development the adolescent has attained. Early or middle adolescents, for example, certainly cannot be expected to think and behave as logically as adults. Below are sample questions regarding various adolescent tasks:

1. Body image: Do you have any questions or problems with the physical changes you are experiencing? Do you like yourself as you are? What would you change? Many teens have questions about periods, wet dreams, or changes in breasts or pubic hair; do you?
2. Peer relationships: Who is your best friend? How many close friends do you have? What kinds of activities do you participate in? What do you do for fun?
3. Independence: Do you get along with your parents? Over what issues do family arguments occur? Is your privacy respected at home?

4. Identity: Are you satisfied with the way things are going for you? If you could change certain aspects of your life, what would you do and why? Are you working now? What are your plans for the future?
5. Sexuality: Are you dating? Do you have a particular girlfriend or boyfriend with whom you are serious? Do you have questions or concerns about sexual activities, contraception, sexually transmitted diseases, or pregnancy?

Another approach to obtain psychosocial/developmental information is the HEADSS (*h*ome, *e*ducation/employment, peer group *a*ctivities, *d*rugs, *s*exuality, *s*uicide/depression) (Goldenring and Cohen, 1988; Ehrman and Matson, 1998) or the expanded HEEADSSS (with *e*ating and *s*afety topics added) interview (Goldenring and Rosen, 2004). An advantage of this approach is that the provider moves from less personal questions to more personal and potentially threatening questions.

Home: Where is the teen living? Who lives with the teen? How is the teen getting along with parents, family, and siblings? Have there been any recent moves? Has the teen ever run away or been incarcerated? The provider should not begin with a statement such as, "Tell me about your parents," because this question assumes that the teen has two living parents.

Education: Is the teen in school? What is the teen good and bad at in school? What classes are particularly interesting or boring? What grade average does the teen maintain? Has the teen repeated or failed any classes? Are there subjects that are more difficult or require extra help? Has the teen received any suspensions? How is the teen getting along with teachers? What goals does the teen have when he or she finishes school? If the teen is older or out of school, the provider should ask about employment. The provider should avoid asking, "How is school?" because this will lead to the answer, "O.K."

Eating: What does the teen like or dislike about his/her body? Have there been recent changes in weight? Has the teen dieted to control weight? Has the teen done anything else to control weight? Has the teen every made himself/herself throw up or take diet pills or laxatives to control weight? Does the teen worry about weight? Does the teen eat in front of the television or computer? Does the teen feel that eating is out of control?

Activities: What does the teen do after school? What does the teen do to have fun and with whom? Does the teen participate in any sports activities? Community or church activities? What reading does the teen do? What music does the teen like? Does the teen have or use a car, and does the teen use seat belts? What are the teen's hobbies? Does the teen use a helmet when using a bicycle or roller blades? Does the teen have friends? A best friend? How much time does the teen spend watching television or playing video games?

Drugs: What types of drugs are used by the teen's peers? What types of drugs do family members use? What types of drugs does the teen use and in what amount and frequency? Does the teen use intravenous drugs? What is the source of income to pay for these drugs? The manner in which these questions are asked can significantly alter the responses. Consider the following examples.

MD 1: Do you ever use drugs?
Teen: No!

That probably would end the questioning on drug use.

MD 2: I know that drugs are fairly common on school campuses. What drugs are common on your campus?

Teen: Oh, I don't know, maybe pot and crack.

MD 2: It is not uncommon for some teens to try some of these drugs. Have any of your friends tried them?

Teen: Some of them.

MD 2: How do you handle the situation when your friends are using drugs? Do you ever try?

Teen: Yeah, once in a while. I really have only tried pot, and that was only twice.

MD 2: The two most common drugs that I have seen teens use are often not thought of as drugs. These are alcohol and cigarettes. How much alcohol do you drink in a week?

Teen: Oh, I usually don't drink during the week, but on weekends I really get blasted almost every Friday and Saturday night.

Sexuality:: Is the teen dating? What are the degree and types of sexual experience? Is the teen involved with another individual in a sexual relationship? Is the teen attracted to or prefer sex with the same, opposite, or both sexes? Has the teen had sexual intercourse? How old was the teen during his or her first sexual encounter? How many partners does the teen have? Is there a concern about masturbation? Has the teen had a sexually transmitted disease, and what are the teen's knowledge base and concerns about sexually transmitted diseases? Does the teen use contraception and with what frequency? Does the teen or the partner use condoms and with what frequency? Is there a history of pregnancy or abortion? Does the teen enjoy sexual activity? Sexuality is another area in which the style of questioning can dramatically alter the response. Consider the following examples.

MD 1: Are you sexually active?

Teen: No.

MD 1: Tell me about your boyfriend or girlfriend.

Teen: I don't have one.

In this instance, the teen may not even know what "sexually active" means or may think that the term implies a certain frequency of sexual intercourse. In addition, asking only about heterosexual relations may close the opportunity to find out about homosexual concerns or behavior.

MD 2: Jane, I mentioned that I may be asking you some questions that were personal but very important to your health. Again, this is information that I will be keeping confidential. The area I want to discuss has to do with relationships. Are you going out with anyone right now?

Teen: Yes.

MD 2: What is this person's first name?

Teen: Bill.

MD 2: As you know, there are many teens who are sexually active. By that I mean that they have had sexual intercourse. There are also many teens who have chosen not to have sexual intercourse. How have you handled this part of your relationship with Bill or with other boys you have dated?

Teen: I have not had sex with Bill yet, although we are thinking about it. I did have sex once approximately 6 months ago at a party.

Suicide and depression: Does the teen feel sad or down more than usual? Does the teen cry more than usual? Does the teen feel "bored" all of the time? Has the teen had any prior suicide attempts? Does the teen have any current suicidal ideation? It is very appropriate to ask direct questions about suicidal ideation, such as, "Have you ever thought about killing yourself?" or "Have you ever tried?" or "Would you kill yourself?" or "Do you have a plan?" Direct questions do not precipitate suicidal action and are the best way to obtain such information.

Safety: Does the teen use seatbelts? How much of the time? Has the teen ever been seriously injured? Has the teen ever ridden in the car with someone driving who was high or drunk? Does the teen use safety equipment for sports or other physical activities (such as helmets for biking or skateboarding)? Is there violence in the teen's home, school or neighborhood? Has the teen ever been physically or sexually abused? Have you ever been picked on or bullied? Has the teen ever felt that he/she had to carry a gun or weapon to protect himself/herself? Has the teen ever had to run away to be safe? Questions about physical and sexual abuse can be particularly sensitive, but essential to ask any teen with problems in any of the previous areas, especially those who have run away, had early onset of sexual activity, or have a history of suicide attempts (see Chapters 39 and 79).

Physical Examination

The physical examination provides an excellent opportunity to educate the adolescent about his or her changing body. For example, the young adolescent may be reassured about growth and pubertal development. The adolescent may, in addition, raise concerns not mentioned during the initial interview. The true chief complaint may, in fact, be revealed during the physical examination.

Another issue of concern has been the question of who should be present during the physical examination. In general, the adolescent is examined without the presence of the guardian or parent. However, some younger or developmentally delayed adolescents prefer to have the parent present. The teen could be asked first whether he or she preferred that the parent be in the room during the examination. Male providers should use a chaperon during the breast and genital examination of female patients. Theoretically, the same concept would hold for a female examiner during genital examination of a male patient, although this usually has not occurred in clinical practice.

Closure

At the close of the initial or follow-up visit, the health care provider should address the following issues:

1. Provide a brief summary of the proposed diagnosis and treatment, addressed primarily to the adolescent. Parents who accompany the adolescent to the visit should

be included in a final discussion of the nonconfidential issues, so that they can help support the plans.

2. Discuss any other resources available to the adolescent.
3. Allow the adolescent time to discuss any final questions or concerns.
4. Schedule any follow-up appointments.
5. Inform the adolescent that the health care provider is available at other times. The adolescent should feel free to make follow-up appointments or telephone calls for either medical or emotional reasons.

INTERVIEWING

The following is a list of suggestions to assist the provider during the interview:

1. Shake hands with the adolescent first.
2. Ask questions in context.
3. Avoid lecturing and admonishing.
4. Bring the adolescent into the present. If the adolescent is focusing on his or her homework or on yesterday's date with a girlfriend or boyfriend, the interviewer is unlikely to gather much useful information.
5. Focus initial history taking on the presenting complaints or problems.
6. Identify who has the problem (i.e., is this problem the teen's concern or the parents').
7. Take a neutral stance.
8. Usually, the less the interviewer says the better.
9. Be attentive.
10. Avoid writing during the interview, especially during sensitive questioning.
11. When asking direct questions (a) use less personal questions before more personal questions, (b) use open-ended questions, and (c) use gender-neutral terms.
12. Talk in terms that the adolescent will understand.
13. Do not misinterpret the adolescent's response.
14. Criticize the activity, not the adolescent.
15. Highlight the positive.
16. Assess your own ability to listen. A provider's difficulty in listening may be related to his or her own resentments or opinions of the adolescent's behavior.

Listed next are recommended interviewing techniques. Some aspects of interviewing, such as the initial introduction and establishing of rapport, were mentioned earlier in the general guidelines.

Open-ended Questions

The use of open-ended questions, such as, "Tell me more about it" or "What does your pain prevent you from doing?" or "What was that like for you?" often facilitate communication better than the use of direct questions, such as, "Did that make you feel bad?"

Reflection Responses

The reflection response mirrors the adolescent's feelings. Consider the following example.

MD: How do you like school?
Teen: I hate it.

MD: You hate it?
Teen: Yeah, my teachers always. . . .

Restatement and Summation

Stopping to restate the adolescent's feelings or to summarize the interview may often help clarify the problem or encourage the adolescent to make additional comments. An example might be, "Let me see if I understand. You really like Jim, but you do not want to have sexual intercourse with him. However, you feel if you say no, he will stop liking you and drop you for someone else."

Clarification

Asking the adolescent to clarify a statement or feeling may help crystallize the problem. Asking, "What did you mean by that?" can also be useful in clarifying colloquial jargon. For example:

Teen: My friend and I like to go scamming. We do it most every weekend.
MD: Scamming? Help me out with that one? What does that mean?

Not only does such a question open up communication but it also makes the teen feel like an authority on a subject and that the provider is human too and does not know everything.

Insight Questions

Some questions may give the health care provider better insight into the adolescent: What do you do well? If you had one wish, what would it be? When are you the happiest? What do you do when you're angry? What do you see yourself doing in 1 or in 5 years? What do your mother and father do when *you* are not there? What do you do when you are not in school?

Reassuring Statements

The use of reassuring statements when dealing with embarrassing subjects may often facilitate discussion. For example: "Almost all boys your age masturbate or play with themselves, and this is normal. I wonder if you do this sometimes."

Support and Empathy

A noncriticizing response that recognizes and acknowledges the adolescent's feelings is often helpful during the interview. Examples of this type of response are: "I can really understand how bad that must have felt." "That really must have made you feel sad." "I'm impressed that you have taken care of yourself so well, despite all the problems that you've had." "You are making some really healthy choices."

Special Interview Problems

1. Garrulous adolescent: The overtalkative adolescent can sometimes be directed with a statement such as, "I can see you like talking about this. Why?"

2. Quiet adolescent: With the quiet adolescent, getting him or her to talk about any subject, such as school, sports, or television, can often help break the silence.
3. Anxious adolescent: The use of reassuring statements is frequently effective. An example is, "It is often difficult to talk about———."
4. Angry adolescent: Clarify how you as the provider might be able to help the adolescent, for example, "It sounds as though some help discussing some of these issues with your parents might be useful."

Interview Structure

The interview may meander, but it should have structure, including a beginning, middle, and end:

1. The beginning of the interview should include introductions, attempts to put the adolescent at ease, and an explanation of what will be happening and why.
2. The middle part of the interview should move into defining the adolescent's problems and feelings.
3. The end of the interview should include informing the adolescent about the results of the examination and about what will happen next. Time should be provided for the adolescent to ask questions before summarizing with the adolescent and the parents.

As stated at the beginning of the chapter, developing interviewing skills requires practice and interest on the part of the examiner. Reviewing one's interviews through the use of video equipment is an excellent technique for improving skills. Such techniques are of special value for providers, who rarely undergo observation in their training. Appropriate consent from both the teen and the parent or guardian should be obtained. Alternative techniques such as written questionnaires and computer surveys can also be used in conjunction with the verbal interview to obtain information about the adolescent. Personal questions and answers that could be seen by the parents or others in the waiting area should be avoided.

Written Questionnaires

Several questionnaires are found in Chapter 4. Cavanaugh (1986); Frazar (1998); Suris et al. (2005) have described office questionnaires. If confidential questions are included the forms should be completed privately in a confidential space. Providers may also benefit from written screening tools to increase delivery of preventive services (Ozer et al., 2005).

Computer Surveys

The computer can be a nonthreatening format to some adolescents, and can sometimes increase the disclosure of personal information. Paperny developed interactional questionnaires for teens on areas such as psychosocial risk profile, adolescent pregnancy, and family planning. These are available from David Paperny, Teen Health Computer Programs, 2516 Pacific Heights Road, Honolulu, HI 96813-1027 (Paperny and Hedberg, 1999). A private carrel in the clinical area may be required when sensitive issues are included.

Family Considerations

As noted earlier, the patient is the product of the family. To fully understand the adolescent or to effect change requires interviewing and working with the family. The definition of family has changed over time, and part of understanding a patient includes understanding the patient's definition of family. There are many possible family constellations, including single-parent families, stepfamilies, blended families, foster families, adoptive families, extended families, and families of choice. The dynamics of the family and the relationships among the different subsystems (spouse, parent/child, or sibling) should be understood. Family cultural and ethnic backgrounds are important for providers to understand. Not all health care providers want to or should provide family therapy. But any provider who wishes to provide comprehensive care to adolescents must feel comfortable working with families. The "Other Resources" section at the end of the chapter lists articles that may be especially helpful.

Internal Considerations

Although the health care provider should be careful not to project feelings about his or her own adolescence onto a teenager being treated, remembering one's own adolescence can help the professional empathize with teenagers. Providers need to move beyond their personal experiences, but still remember complexities of their own adolescent experiences, such as: What did I feel at 13 years old? 15 years old? 18 years old? What things embarrassed me the most? What physical problems worried me the most? What was my first date and first sexual experience like? What things did I enjoy most during those years? Who was my best friend? What did we do together? What things started arguments between my parents and me? How did I feel about my parents and my siblings? How much did I confide in my parents? What did I like most about school? What did I like the least? What dreams did I have for the future? How did I develop as an individual separate from my family?

Optimize the Adolescent–Provider Communication

Adolescents' perceptions of their provider's behavior contribute to their willingness to return for follow-up visits and adhere to the treatment regimen. Ginsburg et al. (1995) showed that cleanliness, honesty, respect, carefulness, experience, confidentiality, and equal treatment of all patients rank highest in affecting adolescents' decisions to seek health care. Provider's honesty, listening, answering questions, statements of confidentiality, showing respect, exchanging information enhance satisfaction and return for follow-up (Kahn et al., 2003; Ong et al., 1995; Ford et al., 2004; Woods et al., 2005).

RECOMMENDATIONS TO PARENTS OF ADOLESCENTS

Parents often ask health care providers for suggestions of reference books or of methods for coping better with adolescents. Helpful methods for parents might begin with the same recommendations previously stated for health care providers.

General Guidelines

1. Listen to the teenager.
2. Treat his or her comments seriously.
3. Avoid power struggles.
4. Be flexible.
5. Show interest and concern in the adolescent's activities.
6. Spend time together and time alone together.
7. Show trust in the teenager.
8. Make resources available to the adolescent.
9. Strive for a good communication in the family between working together, playing together, and loving. Playing and having fun together is an important part of establishing good parent-teen relationships.

Challenges of Teen Years

Parents should be aware that although most adolescents do well and go through adolescence without too much distress, it can be a challenging time period. The challenges faced by parents of teenagers include the following:

1. Parents must adapt to change in the relationship with their teen, as the *teen's peers become an increasingly important influence* and the teen seeks increasing independence.
2. Parents must limit testing and *experimentation by teens.* Teens may experiment with many different types of behaviors, including sex, drinking, and using other drugs. However, parents should remember that, despite how teens may act, the vast majority accept their parents' basic values. In one study, more than 75% of adolescents reported accepting their parents' discipline practices (Rutter, 1980). Teen experimentation does not mean that teens reject their parents' basic values.
3. Parents must *not overreact to rejection* of one or both parents by the teen for a time period.
4. Parents must recognize that *separation is difficult for teens and their parents*, and there may be harder and easier times.
5. Adolescents are at *maximal growth velocity and change* and may be more vulnerable to social risks such as drugs, sexuality, domestic violence, and poverty.
6. *Modern family issues*, such as less family support, more divorce, less extended families, and more working families, add additional challenges.
7. Excessive exploitive and violent *messages through the media* add to the challenges of the teen years for parents.
8. Adolescents' *feelings of invulnerability* also add to their willingness to expose themselves to risks.

Daydreaming

Parents worry about teenagers' wasting time and daydreaming. However, parents should be reassured that this is a normal part of the adolescent developmental process. If school and learning issues coincide, concerns about distractibility, impulsivity and poor organizational skills may suggest attention deficit disorder/attention deficit hyperactivity disorder (ADD/ADHD) (see Chapter 80). Depressed mood or anxiety may suggest psychiatric diagnoses (see Chapter 78)

Communication

The provider should encourage parents to avoid barriers to communication, including:

1. Comparison with other teenagers
2. Lecturing or moralizing
3. Minimizing a problem
4. Excessive talking
5. Taking over an adolescent's problem
6. Taking everything too seriously
7. Overreacting, especially reaching conclusions based only on appearance, dress, or language
8. Phrases such as
   a. The trouble with you is....
   b. How could you do this to me?
   c. Is that all? I thought it was something important.
   d. In my day....
   e. You're wrong.
   f. How could you feel like that?
   g. That's a dumb thing to say.
   h. Don't bother me now.
   i. You're stupid...crazy...incompetent.
9. The "shoulds": My child should be what I want him to be, he should satisfy my needs, or she should always feel loving.

The provider should encourage the parents to stress positive aspects of communication:

1. Empathize with the adolescent.
2. Stress the positive attributes of the adolescent. Adolescents get enough negative feedback. A dose of positive feedback and reinforcement when they do good work, such as follow-through on their chores, can go a long way in positive communication.
3. Deliver clear messages.
4. Respect each other's privacy.
5. Keep a sense of humor.
6. Resolve conflicts together. Decisions that occur in the home about the adolescent should involve the adolescent's input. This can take place in the form of weekly family meetings or brainstorming sessions. In this way, the adolescent is much more likely to carry through with the decisions. During brainstorming sessions to resolve conflicts, parents should:
   a. Involve all family members in the process.
   b. Come up with at least five possible solutions.
   c. Write down all possible suggestions even if they seem outrageous.
   d. Avoid criticisms.
   e. Employ some humor when possible.
   f. Take a break if the session becomes too argumentative.
   g. Discuss the pros and cons of the most viable alternative ideas.
   h. After writing down several possible suggestions, try to agree on one solution or a solution that combines two different suggestions. Parents may also wish to ask other families how they solved similar problems and situations. (A good resource on family problem solving is Forgatch and Patterson (1989)
7. Involve teens in topics they like. When several hundred youths were asked what they wished to discuss with their parents, the top eight topics were
   a. Family matters: Discussions about decisions that affected the whole family or themselves, such as allowance, curfew, and rules
   b. Controversial issues locally or nationally
   c. Emotional issues
   d. The "whys" of life
   e. The future

f. Current affairs
g. Personal interests of the teen
h. Parents' life histories

Parents should also remember that, overall, parents may in fact be more bothered and remember conflicts with their teens longer than the teens do and recover more slowly.

Setting Limits

Adolescents need firm, fair, and explicit limits. Again, involvement of the adolescent in the limit-setting process is beneficial.

House Rules

Some families work better together if there is a set of "house rules." These prescribe the expectations for behaviors and guidelines for the family to live together as a group. Well-defined house rules can become quite important during the adolescent years. Having these rules discussed and written down can avoid conflicts over what behaviors are acceptable. If there is a particular problem in following a rule, then the parents may want to implement associated consequences if the rule is broken. However, the rules should be fair and consistent and should involve input from the teen. Adolescents may be eager to participate in the establishment of such rules when they find out that they might include a rule such as, "No one will enter someone else's room without knocking first." Rules are mainly needed for teen or family member behaviors that are a problem. There should probably be a maximum of 5 to 10 rules. Here is a sample set of house rules adapted from Patterson and Forgatch (2005):

1. Dinner will be at approximately 6 p.m. and everyone is expected to be home and ready to eat at that time.
2. Family members are expected to speak courteously to each other.
3. Before opening someone's door, knock and wait for an answer.
4. If you make a mess, you clean it up.
5. Going out on school nights must be discussed in advance. Schoolwork must be caught up beforehand.
6. Parties must be prearranged, and an adult must be present at the party.
7. Without an adult present, only teens of the same sex are allowed in the home.
8. Curfew on weekdays is 10:30 p.m. and midnight on weekends.
9. The car must be returned when borrowed, with the same amount of gas that it had previously.

These are just samples and should be changed to meet each family's needs, expectations, and values.

Requests that Work

A key to making requests that work is limiting their number. Trained observers have found that normal mothers make 17 requests/hour, and mothers from problem families average >27 requests/hour. Lobitz and Johnson (1975) found that when parents were asked to increase the number of requests they made to their children, the rate of problem behaviors and noncompliance doubled. Key components in making useful requests from teens include the following:

1. Decrease or limit the number of requests.
2. Make well-timed requests. Timing of requests or other feedback to adolescents is critical. Poorly timed requests (e.g., while teen is doing homework, on the phone, or in a bad mood) will surely be met with anger, refusal, or rebellion.
3. Make requests in a polite and pleasant manner.
4. Make requests, one at a time. Dumping three or four requests on a teen at once is another behavior sure to trigger noncompliance and anger from the teen.
5. Use statements rather than questions in making a request.
   a. Question approach:

   | *Parent:* | John, how would you like to take out the garbage tonight? |
   | *John:* | No Dad, I'm busy with homework tonight. |

   b. Statement approach:

Parent:	John, please take out the garbage now, it is your turn.
John:	I'm busy Dad.
Parent:	John, take out the garbage.

6. Make requests specific. For example, if giving the teen a time to be home from a movie, it should be a specific time, not "early."

In a study of compliance to parental requests, Patterson and Forgatch (2005) found that the average rate of compliance from normal children to requests from mothers was 57% and from fathers 47%. So parents should expect a 50% to 60% rate of compliance. Providers can refer parents to numerous books, articles, Web sites, and other resources, a sampling of which are listed here.

Supported in part by the Leadership Education in Adolescent Health Training grant #T71MC00009 from Maternal and Children Health Bureau, Health Resources and Services Administration.

WEB SITES

For Teens and Parents

http://www.iwannaknow.org/. American Social Health Association Web site for teens.

http://www.youngwomenshealth.org. Center for Young Women's Health at Children's Hospital Boston with educational information on a broad range of topics.

http://www.adolescenthealth.com. Links to young women's and men's health by Children's Hospital Boston.

http://www.teengrowth.com. TeenGrowth is a Web site specifically tailored toward the health interests and general well-being of the teenage population; it includes information on alcohol, drugs, emotions, health, family, friends, school, sex, and sports.

http://www.awarefoundation.org. AWARE is devoted to educating adolescents about making responsible decisions regarding their wellness, sexuality, and reproductive health.

http://www.kidshealth.org. Health information for teens and parents.

http://www.teenwire.com. Information for teens from Planned Parenthood Federation of America.

http://www.thebody.com. AIDS and HIV information resource.

http://www.glbthealth.org. The Gay Lesbian Bisexual and Transgender Health Access Project is a collaborative project between the Massachusetts Department of Public Health and its founding partners, the Justice Resource Institute, The Medical Foundation, and JSI Research and Training.

http://www.goaskalice.columbia.edu/. Go Ask Alice! is the health question and answer Internet site produced by *Alice!, Columbia University's Health Education Program,* a division of the Columbia University Health Service.

http://TeenHealthFx.com. Site to provide teens with a fun way to get factual health and medical information, funded through the Atlantic Health System's Morristown Memorial Hospital, Overlook Hospital, Mountainside Hospital, and The General Hospital Center at Passaic.

http://TeensHealth.org. Nemours foundation site to answer questions for teens and parents.

http://familydoctor.org/x5575.xml. Family Doctor has components for teens and parents concerning health issues.

For Parents

http://www.tnpc.com. Site dedicated to providing parents with comprehensive and responsible guidance.

http://www.healthfinder.gov. Federal government site to find health information.

http://www.4women.gov. National Women's Health Information Center from Office of Women's Health.

http://ncadi.samhsa.gov. National Clearinghouse on Drug and Alcohol Information.

http://dmoz.org/Kids_and_Teens/Health/Teens/. Cincinnati Children's Hospital site with references on a broad range of topics relating to teens.

http://parentingteens.about.com/parenting/parentingteens/mbody.htm. Parenting site.

http://www.parentingadolescents.com/. Parenting site.

http://www.pflag.org/. Site for Parents, families, and friends of lesbians and gays (PFLAG) provides support and resources for parents.

http://www.childdevelopmentinfo.com/. Site of the Child Development Institute contains information about developmental issues of adolescents.

For Health Professionals

http://aap.org/. Resources and position papers of the American Academy of Pediatrics.

http://www.adolescenthealth.org/. Position papers and information from the Society for Adolescent Medicine; go to links and then categories.

http://www.healthfinder.gov. Finder of health sites from federal government.

http://www.4women.gov. National Women's Health Information Center from Office of Women's Health.

http://www.medlineplus.gov. Medline for health information.

http://ncadi.samhsa.gov. Clearinghouse on drug and alcohol information.

www.usc.edu/adolhealth. Adolescent health online curriculum.

OTHER RESOURCES

Books and Articles for Health Professionals

Malone CA. Child and adolescent psychiatry and family therapy. *Child Adolesc Psychiatr Clin N Am* 2001;10(3):395.

Sargent J. Family therapy in child and adolescent psychiatry. *Child Adolesc Psychiatr Clin N Am* 1997;6(1):151.

Walsh F. The concept of family resilience: crisis and challenge. *Fam Process* 1996;35:261.

Zayas LH. Family functioning and child rearing in an urban environment. *Dev Behav Pediatr* 1995;16:S21.

The following books also provide some excellent references for dealing with families:

Allmond BW, Tanner LJ, Gofman HF. *The family is the patient: using family interviews in children's medical care,* 2nd ed. Baltimore, MD: Lippincott Williams & Wilkins, 1999.

Eron JB, Lund TW. *Narrative solutions in brief therapy.* New York: Guilford Press, 1996.

Fishman HC. *Treating troubled adolescents: a family therapy approach.* New York: Basic Books, 1988.

Patterson GR, Forgatch MS. *Parents and adolescents living together: Part 2: family problem solving,* 2nd Edition. Champaign IL: Research Press, 2005.

Haley J. *Problem solving therapy,* 2nd ed. San Francisco: Jossey-Bass, 1987.

Haley J. *Leaving home: the therapy for disturbed young people.* Philadelphia, PA: Brunner/Mazel, 1997.

Hartman A, Laird J. *Family-centered social work practice.* New York: The Free Press, 1983.

Lobitz WC, Johnson SM. Parental manipulation of the behavior of normal and deviant children. *Child Dev* 1975;46:719.

McGoldrick M, ed. *Re-visioning family therapy: race, culture and gender in clinical practice.* New York: Guilford Press, 1998.

McGoldrick M, Carter B. Understanding the life cycle: the individual, the family, the culture. In Walsh F. *Normal family processes,* 3rd ed. New York: Guilford Press, 2002.

Minuchin P, Colapinto J, Minuchin S. *Working with families of the poor.* New York: Guilford Press, 1998.

Minuchin S. *Family healing: strategies for hope and understanding.* New York: The Free Press, 1998.

Pittman FS. *Turning points: treating families in transitions and crisis.* New York: WW Norton, 1987.

Visher EB, Visher JS. *Old loyalties, new ties: therapeutic strategies with stepfamilies.* New York: Brunner/Mazel, 1988.

White M, Epson D. *Narrative means to therapeutic ends.* New York: WW Norton, 1990.

Woods ME, Hollis F. *Case work: a psychosocial therapy,* Chapters 14 and 15. 5th ed. New York: McGraw-Hill, 2000.

Books for Parents and Families

Fairchild B, Hayward N. *Now that you know: a parent's guide to understanding their gay and lesbian children.* New York: Harcourt Brace, 1998.

Kaufman M, ed. *Mothering teens: understanding the adolescent years.* Charlottetown, PEI: Genergy Books, 1997.

Patterson GR, Forgatch MS. *Parents and adolescents living together: Part 1: The Basics*, 2nd Edition. Champaign IL: Research Press, 2005.

Patterson GR, Forgatch MS. *Parents and adolescents living together: Part 2: family problem solving*, 2nd Edition. Champaign IL: Research Press, 2005.

Pipher MB. *Reviving ophelia: saving the selves of adolescent girls*. New York: Putnam, 1994.

Ponton L. *The sex lives of teenagers*. New York: Dutton, 2000.

Romer D. *Reducing adolescent risk: toward an integrated approach*. Thousand Oaks: Sage Publications Inc, 2003.

Slap GB, Jablow MM. *Teenage health care: the first comprehensive family guide for the preteen to young adult years*. New York: Pocket Books, 1994.

Steinberg L, Levine A. *You and your adolescent: a parent's guide for ages 10 to 20*. New York: Harper Perennial, HarperCollins, 1997.

Books for Teens

Canfield J, Hansen MV, Kirberger K. *Chicken soup for the teenage soul: 101 stories of life, love and learning*. Deerfield Beach, FL: Health Communications, Inc, 1997.

Columbia University Health Education Program. *The "Go Ask Alice" book of answers: a guide to good physical, sexual and emotional health*. New York: Henry Holt & Co., 1998.

Kimball G. *The teen trip: the complete resource guide*. Chicago: Equality Press, 1997.

Madaras L. *What's happening to my body? Book for boys: the new growing up guide for parents and sons*, 3rd ed. New York: Pocket Books, 2000.

Madaras L. *What's happening to my body? Book for girls: the new growing up guide for parents and daughters*, 3rd ed. New York: Pocket Books, 2000.

McCoy K, Wibbelsman C. *Life happens: a teenager's guide to friends, failure, sexuality, love, rejection, addiction, peer pressure, families, loss, depression, change and other challenges of living*. New York: Perigee, 1996.

McCoy K, Wibbelsman C. *Teenage body book*. New York: Perigee, 1999.

Weston C. *Girl talk: all the stuff your sister never told you*. New York: Harper Perennial, HarperCollins, 1997.

REFERENCES AND ADDITIONAL READINGS

Boggio N, Cohall AT. Evaluating the adolescent: the search for the hidden agenda. *Emerg Med* 1990;30:18.

Braverman PK, Strasburger VC. Office-based adolescent health care: issues and solutions. *Adoles Med: State-of-the-Art Rev* 1997;8:1.

Cavanaugh RM Jr. Obtaining a personal and confidential history from adolescents: an opportunity for prevention. *J Adolesc Health Care* 1986;7:118.

Council on Scientific Affairs, American Medical Association. Confidential health services for adolescents. *JAMA* 1993;269:1420.

Elster A, Kuznets N. *AMA guidelines for adolescent preventive services (GAPS): recommendations and rationale*. Baltimore: Williams & Wilkins, 1994.

English A. Changing health care environments and adolescent health care: legal and policy challenges. *Adolesc Med: State-of-the-Art Rev* 1997;8:375.

English A, Ford C. The HIPAA privacy rule and adolescents: legal questions and clinical challenges. *Perspect Sex Reprod Health* 2004;36(2):80.

English A, Kenney KE. *State minor consent laws: a summary*, 2nd ed. Chapel Hill, NC: Center for Adolescent Health & The Law, 2003.

Ehrman WG, Matson SC. Approaches to assessing adolescents on serious or sensitive matters. *Pediatr Clin North Am* 1998;45:189.

Ford C, English A, Sigman G. Confidential health care for adolescents: position paper of the society for adolescent medicine. *J Adolesc Health* 2004;35:160.

Ford CA, Millstein SG, Halpern-Felsher BL, et al. Influence of physician confidentiality assurances on adolescents' willingness to disclose information and seek future health care: a randomized controlled trial. *JAMA* 1997;278:1029.

Frazar GE. A private provider's approach to adolescent problems. *Adolesc Med : State-of-the-Art Rev* 1998;9:229.

Ginsburg KR, Slap GB, Cnaan A, et al. Adolescents' perceptions of factors affecting their decisions to seek health care. *JAMA* 1995;273:1913.

Goldenring JM, Cohen E. Getting into adolescent heads. *Contemp Pediatr* 1988;5:75.

Goldenring JM, Rosen DS. Getting into adolescents heads: an essential update. *Comtemp Pediatr* 2004;21(1):64.

Green M, ed. *Bright futures: guidelines for health, supervision of infants, children and adolescents*. Arlington, VA: National Center for Education in Maternal and Child Health, 1994.

Greydanus DE. *American Academy of Pediatrics: caring for your adolescent—ages 12 to 21*. New York: Bantam, 1991.

Johnson RL, Tanner NM. Approaching the adolescent patient. In: Hofmann AD, Greydanus DE, eds. *Adolescent medicine*, 2nd ed. Norwalk, CT: Appleton & Lange, 1989.

Kahn JA, Goodman E, Huang B, et al. Predictors of papanicolaou smear return in a hospital-based adolescent and young adult clinic. *Obstet Gynecol* 2003;101:490.

Klein JD, Slap GB, Elster AB, et al. Access to health care for adolescents: a position paper of the Society for Adolescent Medicine. *J Adolesc Health Care* 1992;13:162.

Latta RJ, Lee PD. Counseling adolescents in office practice. *J Curr Adolesc Med* 1981;3:15.

MacKenzie RG. Approach to the adolescent in the clinical setting. *Med Clin North Am* 1990;74:1085.

Ong LML, De Haes CJM, Hoos AM, et al. Doctor-patient communication: a review of the literature. *Soc Sci Med* 1995;40(7):903.

Ozer EM, Adams SH, Lustig JL, et al. Increasing the screening and counseling of adolescents for risky health behaviors: a primary care intervention. *Pediatrics* 2005;115(4):960.

Paperny DM, Hedberg VA. Computer-assisted health counselor visits: a low-cost model for comprehensive adolescent preventive services. *Arch Pediatr Adolesc Med* 1999;153(1):63.

Patterson G, Forgatch M. *Parents and adolescents: living together. Part 1: the basics*. Eugene, OR: Castalia Publishing, 1987.

Patterson GR, Forgatch MS. *Parents and adolescents living together: Part 2: family problem solving*, 2nd Edition. Champaign IL: Research Press, 2005.

Perrin EC. *Sexual orientation in child and adolescent health care*. New York: Kluwer Academic/Plenum Publishers, 2002.

Rainey DY, Brandon DP, Krowchuk DP. Confidential billing accounts for adolescents in private practice. *J Adolesc Health* 2000;26:389.

Rutter M. *Changing youth in a changing society*. Cambridge: Harvard University Press, 1980.

Ryan C, Futterman D. Lesbian and gay youth: care and counseling. *Adolesc Med: State-of-the-Art Rev* 1997;8:259.

Suris JC, Nebot M, Parera N. Behavior evaluation for risk-taking adolescents (BERTA): an easy to use and assess instrument to detect adolescent risky behaviors in a clinical setting. *Eur J Pediatr* 2005;164:371.

Society for Adolescent Medicine. Meeting the health care needs of adolescents in managed care: position paper. *J Adolesc Health* 1998;22:271.

Society for Adolescent Medicine. Confidential health care for adolescents: position paper of the Society for Adolescent Medicine. *J Adolesc Health* 2004;35:160.

Thrall JS, McCloskey L, Ettner SL, et al. Confidentiality and adolescents' use of providers for health information and for pelvic examinations. *Arch Pediatr Adolesc Med* 2000; 154:885.

Wender EH, Coupey SM. Interviewing adolescents. In: Hoekelman RA, ed. *Primary pediatric care*, 4th ed. St. Louis, MO: Mosby, 2001:915.

Woods ER, Klein JD, Wingood GM, et al. Development of a new adolescent patient-provider interaction scale (APPIS) for youth at-risk for STDs/HIV. *J Adolesc Health* 2005, 2006;35(6):753.e.1.

CHAPTER 4

Preventive Health Care for Adolescents

David S. Rosen and Lawrence S. Neinstein

The goals of preventive health care for adolescents are to promote optimal physical and mental health and to support healthy physical, psychological, and social growth and development. Because the most common morbidities and mortalities of adolescence today are preventable health conditions associated with behavioral, environmental, and social causes, preventive services for adolescents should reflect these shifts in etiology. Therefore, visits to a health care provider should reinforce positive health behaviors, such as exercise and nutritious eating, while discouraging health-risk behaviors such as those associated with unsafe sexual behaviors, unsafe driving, and use of tobacco or other drugs. Although the incidence of serious medical problems during adolescence is low, adolescence is a time during which lifelong health habits are established. Furthermore, numerous issues and concerns may emerge during adolescence that affect overall health and well-being. Therefore, adolescence becomes an ideal period for health professionals to invest time in health promotion and preventive services.

In the current health care environment, characterized by increasingly limited resources, managed care, and evidence-based medicine, it is essential to determine what constitutes appropriate, cost-effective, and relevant preventive services for any age-group. Unfortunately, little empirical research demonstrates the effectiveness of preventive services for adolescents. Furthermore, methodological issues makes it unlikely that future research will provide robust evidence for the value of preventive services (Downs and Klein, 1995). Therefore, expert opinion drives most of our preventive services recommendations; and a variety of preventive services guidelines have been proposed.

Elster (1998) comprehensively reviewed recommendations for adolescent clinical preventive services developed by national organizations (Table 4.1). In 1989, the U.S. Preventive Services Task Force (USPSTF) (1996), convened by the Office of Disease Prevention and Health Promotion, U.S. Department of Health and Human Services, developed recommendations on periodic health examination based on the health risks of specific age-groups (available at http://www.ahrq.gov/clinic/uspstfix.htm#About). To the extent possible, these recommendations have been evidence-based, but they also rely on expert opinion. Since 1998, the USPSTF has been sponsored by the Agency for Healthcare Research and Quality (AHRQ), and its recommendations are considered the "gold standard" for

clinical preventive services. The recommendations have been periodically updated. A recent analysis of preventive services recommended by the USPSTF considered the cost-effectiveness and the clinically preventable disease burden to produce rankings of relative health impact. Among services relevant for adolescents and young adults, the highest ranking preventive services were the childhood immunization series, screening for tobacco use and brief interventions for tobacco users, screening for "problem drinking" and brief intervention for those at risk, cervical cancer screening with cervical cytology (Pap smears), and Chlamydia screening in sexually active women younger than 25 years. Of these, tobacco use screening, screening for problem drinking, and Chlamydia screening were all estimated to occur <50% of the time (Maciosek et al., 2006). Rankings and article are also available online at: http://www.prevent.org/content/view/49/99/.

In 1992, the American Medical Association (AMA, 1992) released *Guidelines for Adolescent Preventive Services (GAPS)*. GAPS is a comprehensive package of recommendations aimed at the delivery of preventive services in primary care settings (Table 4.2). The GAPS recommendations were developed by the AMA's Division of Adolescent Health, with the assistance of a national scientific advisory board, to address highly prevalent health issues and those most likely to cause serious morbidity. GAPS recommendations cover both the content and delivery of health care to adolescents (Fig. 4.1). Information on these recommendations can be found at the AMA Web site (http://www.ama-assn.org/ama/pub/category/1980.html).

The Bright Futures guidelines for the health care supervision of infants, children, and adolescents were published in 1994 and represent the work of expert panels convened through a collaboration of the Maternal and Child Health Bureau of the Health Resources and Services Administration, and the Medicaid Bureau of the Health Care Financing Administration (http://brightfutures.aap.org/web/). The guidelines are both evidence-based and based on expert opinion. Issues related to normal and abnormal development, nutrition, and mental health are highlighted in the Bright Futures guidelines. A comprehensive revision of Bright Futures is currently underway.

The American Academy of Family Physicians (AAFP) offers age-specific recommendations for periodic health examinations for healthy patients (available at http://www.aafp.org). The AAFP recommendations are derived from

TABLE 4.1

Comparisons among Recommendations for Adolescent Preventive Services

Subject	AAFP	AAP	AMA	BF	USPSTF
Immunizations:					
ACIP recommendations	Yes	Yes	Yes	Yes	Yes
Health guidance for teens:					
Normal development[a,b]	Yes	Yes	Yes	Yes	No
Injury prevention[a,c]	Yes	Yes	Yes	Yes	Yes
Nutrition[a]	Yes	Yes	Yes	Yes	Yes
Physical activity[a]	Yes	Yes	Yes	Yes	Yes
Dental health[a]	Yes	Yes	No	Yes	Yes
Breast or testicular self-examination[a]	Yes	Yes	No	Yes	Yes
Skin protection[a]	Yes	Yes	Yes	Yes	No
Health guidance for parents[a]	No	Yes	Yes	Yes	No
Screening/counseling[d]:					
Obesity[a]	Yes	Yes	Yes	Yes	Yes
Contraception[e]	Yes	Yes	Yes	Yes	Yes
Tobacco use[a]	Yes	Yes	Yes	Yes	Yes
Alcohol use[a]	Yes	Yes	Yes	Yes	Yes
Substance use[a]	Yes	Yes	Yes	Yes	Yes
Hypertension[a]	Yes	Yes	Yes	Yes	Yes
Depression/suicide[a]	No	Yes	Yes	Yes	No
Eating disorders[a]	No	Yes	Yes	Yes	No
School problems[a]	No	Yes	Yes	Yes	No
Abuse[a]	No	Yes	Yes	Yes	No[f]
Hearing[a]	Yes	Yes	No	Yes	No
Vision[a]	No	Yes	No	Yes	No
Tests:					
Tuberculosis[e]	Yes	Yes	Yes	Yes	Yes
Papanicolaou test[e]	Yes	Yes	Yes	Yes	Yes
Human immunodeficiency virus infection[e]	Yes	Yes	Yes	Yes	Yes
Sexually transmitted diseases[e]	Yes	Yes	Yes	Yes	Yes
Cholesterol[e]	Yes	Yes	Yes	Yes	No
Urinalysis[a]	No	Yes	No	No	No
Hematocrit[a]	No	Yes	No	No	No
Periodicity of visits	Tailored	Annual	Annual	Annual	Tailored
Target age range (yr)[g]	13–18	11–21	11–21	11–21	11–24

AAFP, American Academy of Family Physicians; AAP, American Academy of Pediatrics; AMA, American Medical Association; BF, Bright Futures; USPSTF, U.S. Preventive Services Task Force; ACIP, Advisory Committee on Immunization Practices.

[a]Procedure is recommended for all adolescents/parents.

[b]This includes providing adolescents with information on normal physical, psychosocial, and sexual development.

[c]This includes activities such as promoting the use of safety belts and safety helmets, placement of home fire alarms, and reducing the risk of injury from firearms and violence. Organizations differ in the activities they include for injury prevention.

[d]The AAP recommends "developmental/behavioral assessment."

[e]Procedure is recommended for selected adolescents who are at high risk for the medical problem.

[f]Child abuse is not addressed as a separate screening topic, but is included in the general screening for family violence.

[g]The AAP, AMA, and BF make a distinction among developmental stages of adolescence.

From Elster AB. Comparison of recommendations for adolescent clinical preventive services developed by national organizations. *Arch Pediatr Adolesc Med* 1998;152:193, with permission.

the USPSTF report by the Commission on Public Health and Scientific Affairs of the AAFP.

Finally, the American Academy of Pediatrics (AAP) also reviewed preventive care for children and adolescents and published revised recommendations in 1995. These recommendations represent "a consensus by the Committee on Practice and Ambulatory Medicine in consultation with national committees and sections of the American Academy of Pediatrics." Guidelines for Health Supervision III, published by the AAP in 1996 and revised and updated

TABLE 4.2

Guidelines for Adolescent Preventive Services (GAPS) Recommendations

1. From ages 11–21, all adolescents should have an annual preventive services visit.
   a. These visits should address both biomedical and psychosocial aspects.
   b. Complete physical examinations should be done during three of these preventive visits, one each during early (11–14 years), middle (15–17 years), and late (18–21 years) adolescence.
2. Preventive services should be age and developmentally appropriate and should be sensitive to individual and sociocultural differences.
3. Physicians should establish office policies regarding confidential care for adolescents and how parents will be involved in that care. These policies should be made clear to adolescents and their parents.
4. Parents or other adult caregivers should receive health guidance at least once during their child's early adolescence, once during middle adolescence, and preferably once during late adolescence. Health guidance should include the following information:
   a. Normative adolescent development, including physical, sexual, and emotional development
   b. Signs and symptoms of disease and emotional distress
   c. Parenting behaviors that promote healthy adolescent adjustment
   d. Why parents should discuss health-related behaviors with their adolescents, plan family activities, and act as role models
   e. Methods for helping their adolescent avoid potentially harmful behaviors:
      • Monitoring and managing adolescents' use of motor vehicles
      • Avoiding having weapons in the home
      • Removing weapons and potentially lethal medications from the homes of adolescents with suicidal intent
      • Monitoring their adolescent's social and recreational activities for the use of tobacco, alcohol, and other drugs and sexual behavior
5. All adolescents should receive health guidance annually to promote a better understanding of their physical growth, psychosocial and psychosexual development, and the importance of becoming actively involved in decisions regarding their health care.
6. All adolescents should receive health guidance annually to promote the reduction of injuries. Counseling includes the following:
   a. How to avoid use of alcohol or other drugs while using motor or recreational vehicles
   b. How to use safety devices, including seat belts and bicycle helmets
   c. How to resolve interpersonal conflicts without violence
   d. How to avoid the use of weapons
   e. How to promote appropriate physical conditioning before exercise
7. All adolescents should receive health guidance annually about dietary habits, including the benefits of a healthy diet, and ways to achieve a healthy diet and safe weight management.
8. All adolescents should receive health guidance annually about the benefits of exercise and should be encouraged to engage in safe exercise on a regular basis.
9. All adolescents should receive health guidance annually regarding responsible sexual behaviors, including abstinence. Latex condoms to prevent STDs, including HIV infection, and appropriate methods of birth control should be made available, as should instructions on how to use them effectively.
10. All adolescents should receive health guidance annually to promote avoidance of tobacco, alcohol, other abusable substances, and anabolic steroids.
    Screening recommendations:
11. All adolescents should be screened annually for hypertension according to the protocol developed by the National Heart, Lung, and Blood Institute Second Task Force on Blood Pressure Control in Children.
12. Selected adolescents should be screened to determine their risk of developing hyperlipidemia and adult coronary heart disease, following the protocol developed by the Expert Panel on Blood Cholesterol Levels in Children and Adolescents.
13. All adolescents should be screened annually for eating disorders and obesity by determining weight and stature, and by asking about body image and dieting patterns.
14. All adolescents should be asked annually about their use of tobacco products, including cigarettes and smokeless tobacco.

TABLE 4.2

(Continued)

15. All adolescents should be asked annually about their use of alcohol and other abusable substances and about their use of over-the-counter or prescription drugs for nonmedical purposes, including anabolic steroids.
    a. Adolescents whose substance use endangers their health should receive counseling and mental health treatment, as appropriate.
    b. Adolescents who use anabolic steroids should be counseled to stop.
    c. The use of urine toxicology for the routine screening of adolescents is not recommended.
16. All adolescents should be asked annually about involvement in sexual behaviors that may result in unintended pregnancy and STDs, including HIV infections.
    a. Sexually active adolescents should be asked about their use and motivation to use condoms and contraceptive methods, their sexual orientation, the number of sexual partners they have had in the last 6 months, if they have exchanged sex for money or drugs, and their history of prior pregnancy or STDs.
    b. Adolescents at risk for pregnancy, STDs, or sexual exploitation should be counseled on how to reduce this risk.
17. Sexually active adolescents should be screened for STDs. The frequency of screening for STDs depends on the sexual practices of the individual and the history of previous STDs. STD screening includes the following:
    a. Cervical culture (females) or urine leukocyte esterase analysis (males) to screen for gonorrhea
    b. An immunologic test of cervical fluid (female) or urine leukocyte esterase analysis (male) to screen for genital *Chlamydia*
    c. A serological test for syphilis if the individual has lived in an area endemic for syphilis, has had other STDs, has had more than one sexual partner within the last 6 months, has exchanged sex for drugs or money, or is a male who has engaged in sex with other male(s)
    d. Evaluation for human papilloma virus by visual inspection (males and females) and by Pap test.
18. Adolescents at risk for HIV infection should be offered confidential HIV screening with the ELISA and confirmatory test. Testing should be performed only after informed consent is obtained from the adolescent and should be performed in conjunction with both pretest and posttest counseling.
19. Female adolescents who are sexually active or any female 18 years of age or older should be screened annually for cervical cancer by use of a Pap test.
20. All adolescents should be asked annually about behaviors or emotions that indicate recurrent or severe depression or risk of suicide.
21. All adolescents should be asked annually about a history of emotional, physical, or sexual abuse.
22. All adolescents should be asked annually about learning or school problems.
23. Adolescents should receive a tuberculin skin test if they have been exposed to active tuberculosis, have lived in a homeless shelter, have been incarcerated, have lived in or come from an area with a high prevalence of tuberculosis, or currently work in a health care setting.
    Recommendations for immunizations:
24. All adolescents should receive prophylactic immunizations according to the guidelines established by the federally convened Advisory Committee on Immunization Practices.
    a. Adolescents should receive a bivalent Td vaccine 10 years after their previous DTP vaccination.
    b. All adolescents should receive a second trivalent MMR vaccination, unless there is documentation of two vaccinations earlier during childhood. An MMR should not be given to adolescents who are pregnant.
    c. Susceptible adolescents who engage in high-risk behaviors should be vaccinated against hepatitis B virus. Widespread use of the hepatitis B vaccine is encouraged because risk factors are often not easily identifiable among adolescents. Universal hepatitis B vaccination should be implemented in communities where intravenous drug use, adolescent pregnancy, or STD infections are common.

STD, sexually transmitted diseases; HIV, human immunodeficiency virus; ELISA, enzyme-linked immunosorbent assay; DTP, diphtheria and tetanus toxoids and pertussis; MMR, measles-mumps-rubella.
Adapted from GAPS Executive Committee, Department of Adolescent Health. *American Medical Association guidelines for adolescent preventive services*. Chicago: American Medical Association, 1992.

in 2002, more comprehensively describes the elements of health supervision visits for children and adolescents (American Academy Pediatrics, 1996). Updated guidelines for health supervision will be part of the revised Bright Futures guidelines on which the AAP is collaborating. Information is available on their Web site (http://www.aap.org).

The various recommendations for adolescent preventive services are compared in Table 4.1. There appear to be more similarities than differences. All of the recommendations support the immunization schedule of the Advisory Committee on Immunization Practices (ACIP), and all advocate health guidance for teens. The GAPS, Bright Futures,

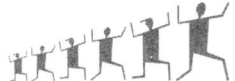

Guidelines for Adolescent Preventive Services

Preventive Health Services by Age and Procedure

Adolescents and young adults have a unique set of health care needs. The recommendations for Guidelines for Adolescents Services (GAPS) emphasize annual clinical preventive services visits that address both the developmental and psychosocial aspects of health, in addition to traditional biomedical conditions. These recommendations were developed by the American Medical Association with contributions from a Scientific Advisory Panel, comprised of national experts, as well as representatives of primary care medical organizations and the health insurance industry. The body of scientific evidence indicates that the periodicity and content of preventive services can be important in promoting the health and well-being of adolescents.

Procedure	Age of Adolescent										
	Early				Middle			Late			
	11	12	13	14	15	16	17	18	19	20	21
Health Guidance											
Parenting*		——— • ———				——— • ———					
Development	•	•	•	•	•	•	•	•	•	•	•
Diet and Physical Activity	•	•	•	•	•	•	•	•	•	•	•
Healthy Lifestyle**	•	•	•	•	•	•	•	•	•	•	•
Injury Prevention	•	•	•	•	•	•	•	•	•	•	•
Screening											
History											
Eating Disorders	•	•	•	•	•	•	•	•	•	•	•
Sexual Activity***	•	•	•	•	•	•	•	•	•	•	•
Alcohol and Other Drug Use	•	•	•	•	•	•	•	•	•	•	•
Tobacco Use	•	•	•	•	•	•	•	•	•	•	•
Abuse	•	•	•	•	•	•	•	•	•	•	•
School Performance	•	•	•	•	•	•	•	•	•	•	•
Depression	•	•	•	•	•	•	•	•	•	•	•
Risk for Suicide	•	•	•	•	•	•	•	•	•	•	•
Physical Assessment											
Blood Pressure	•	•	•	•	•	•	•	•	•	•	•
BMI	•	•	•	•	•	•	•	•	•	•	•
Comprehensive Exam		——— • ———				——— • ———			——— • ———		
Tests											
Cholesterol		——— 1 ———				——— 1 ———			——— 1 ———		
TB		——— 2 ———				——— 2 ———			——— 2 ———		
GC, Chlamydia, Syphilis, & HPV		——— 3 ———				——— 3 ———			——— 3 ———		
HIV		——— 4 ———				——— 4 ———			——— 4 ———		
Pop Smear		——— 5 ———				——— 5 ———			——— 5 ———		
Immunizations											
MMR		—• —									
Td		—• —				—○ —					
Hep B		—• —				— 6 —			— 6 —		
Hep A		——— 7 ———				— 7 —			— 7 —		
Varicella		——— 8 ———				— 8 —			— 8 —		

1. Screening test performed once if family history is positive for early cardiovascular disease or hyperlipidemia.
2. Screen if positive for exposure to active TB or lives/works in high–risk situation, eg homeless shelter, jail, health care facility.
3. Screen at least annually if sexually active.
4. Screen if high risk for infection.
5. Screen annually if sexually active or if 18 years or older.
6. Vaccinate if high risk for hepatitis B infection.
7. Vaccinate if at risk for hepatitis A infection.
8. Offer vaccine if no reliable history of chicken pox or previous immunization.
* A parent health guidance visit is recommended during early and middle adolescence.
** Includes counseling regarding sexual behavior and avoidance of tobacco, alcohol, and other drug use.
*** Includes history of unintended pregnancy and STD.
○ Do not give if administered in last five years.

FIGURE 4.1 Recommended frequency of GAPS preventive services. (From American Medical Association. *Guidelines for adolescent preventive services* [Recommendations monograph]. Chicago: American Medical Association, 1995.)

and AAP recommend health guidance for parents also, as a strategy to assist them in supporting the growth, development, and changing needs of their adolescent. Screening and counseling for various health risks are also a common feature of the recommendations from each of the five organizations, although there is some variability in the specific recommendations for screening. Periodicity may be the most important distinction among the five sets of recommendations. GAPS, Bright Futures, and the AAP specifically recommend *annual* visits for preventive services, whereas the USPSTF and AAFP recommend visits every 1 to 3 years based on the specific needs of the individual.

Although guidelines help standardize and provide structure to the range of preventive services offered to adolescents, service delivery remains an even more challenging issue. Research in the last 2 decades has clearly demonstrated both the limitations of the current delivery system and the value of offering services in a wide range of settings and formats. Still, preventive services remain inconsistently delivered, and in some settings they are delivered at dangerously low rates. These findings are easy to understand but difficult to resolve. It is well known, for example, that adolescents are generally considered "healthy," that they are reluctant health care consumers, and that their access to health care is limited by issues related to reimbursement, confidentiality, transportation, and the training of the providers who care for them.

Solving these problems remains even more vexing. Establishing a broader context for adolescent "health" is a matter for public and professional education. Adolescents report issues that they want and need to discuss with their health care providers but that they often do not. To better serve adolescents, preventive services must be available in a *wide range of health care settings*. These include private physicians' offices within managed care organizations; community-based adolescent health, family planning, and public health clinics; and as part of school-based and school-linked health services. Simple, skills-based *training for clinicians in adolescent preventive services* has been convincingly shown to increase the likelihood of appropriate screening and counseling as well as provider self-efficacy in a variety of clinical settings. *Reimbursement* for these services will continue to be problematic. *National standards of care* such as those discussed in this chapter may increase the likelihood that payers will begin to provide reimbursement for adolescent preventive services. However, for adolescent preventive services to become routinely available to all adolescents a dramatic shift in both health care provider and health care consumer expectations—from a reactive, acute care orientation to a proactive view that values health promotion and disease prevention—will be required.

PREVENTIVE CARE FOR ADOLESCENTS

Many of the most effective health promotion and disease prevention strategies aimed at adolescents are straightforward and consistent among the various recommendations and guidelines discussed earlier (GAPS, Bright Futures, USPSTF, AAP, and AAFP). Furthermore, because health-risk behaviors and health habits have their genesis in adolescence, healthy behaviors and lifestyle choices established during adolescence have the potential to persist into adult life and to have a strongly positive impact on adult health as well. In this context, the Society for Adolescent Medicine has endorsed the use of guidelines as a strategy to improve the delivery of adolescent preventive services (information available at http://www. adolescenthealth.org). The Society for Adolescent Medicine's major recommendations include the following:

1. Educational efforts should be developed to enhance public and professional recognition of the merit and value of adolescent preventive care.
2. Practice guidelines are endorsed as a means to standardize the content of adolescent preventive services, improve quality and promote consistent delivery. They are designed as tools for health care professionals and are not meant to replace individual decision-making or practice styles.
3. Preventive services visits are recommended *annually* for adolescents to promote frequent, repetitive guidance, screening and counseling about risk behaviors and healthy lifestyles.
4. Primary care clinicians and other health care providers should receive appropriate training and preparation to provide comprehensive adolescent preventive services confidently and effectively.
5. Adequate system financing and provider reimbursement are essential for the broad delivery of comprehensive adolescent preventive services.
6. The health outcomes and cost-effectiveness of adolescent preventive services and their individual components should be studied.
7. Adolescent preventive services should be widely available and easily accessible.
8. Comprehensive preventive services for adolescents should be delivered in a manner that meets the needs of adolescents and their families.
9. Innovative approaches should be designed and tested to expand the capacity to deliver comprehensive, cost-effective preventive services.

In addition, in the Society's position paper on adolescent immunizations, it recommended that three distinct adolescent vaccination visit/platforms be developed including 11–12, 14–15, and 17–18 year visits. These would be used to integrate and emphasize the role of vaccinations in the recommended comprehensive health care screening and provision visits. The first visit would be used for ACIP-recommended vaccines, the second visit for catch-up on missed vaccines, and the third as catch-up before college graduation or for newly recommended vaccines while the teen is still covered by third-party payers.

Healthy People 2010 provides national objectives aimed at improving health and well-being. Of the 467 Healthy People 2010 objectives, 107 are relevant for adolescents and young adults and 21 have been identified as critical health objectives. These include the following:

- Decrease deaths among adolescents and young adults
  - Reducing deaths caused by motor vehicle crashes
  - Decreased deaths and injuries caused by alcohol and drug-related automobile crashes
  - Increased and consistent use of seat belts
  - Decreased driving while intoxicated or riding with an intoxicated driver
  - Reduce the suicide rate
  - Reduce the rate of suicide attempts
  - Reduce the homicide rate

- Reduce the rate of fighting and physical violence
- Reduce the rate of weapon carrying by adolescents
- Reduce binge drinking
- Reduce the use of illicit substances
- Decrease use of tobacco
- Reduce rates of depression
- Increase proportion of adolescents with mental illness who receive mental health services
- Increase the proportion of adolescents who abstain from sexual intercourse or who use condoms if sexually active
  - Reduce pregnancies among adolescent females
  - Reduce rates of Chlamydia infection
  - Reduce rates of new human immunodeficiency virus (HIV) diagnoses among adolescents and young adults
- Decrease the proportion of adolescents who are overweight or obese
- Increase physical activity among adolescents

Clinical Settings for Adolescent Preventive Services

Improving the delivery of adolescent preventive services depends on the integration of standards and service delivery across multiple systems and points of access, including public clinics, managed care organizations, private physician offices, school-based and school-linked clinics, and community-based agencies. In fact, there is evidence to suggest that traditional office-based care for teens may fall short of the care they receive in other settings. Blum et al. (1996) studied adolescent preventive services in a variety of practice settings and showed that the highest level of preventive care was delivered in teen clinics whereas the lowest level of preventive care occurred in private pediatric or family practices. Potential explanations for these disparities include the specific teen focus of teen clinics and limitations within the private practices related to provider comfort and/or training addressing teen issues, time pressures, limited reimbursement, and so on. Similarly, a study of a California managed care organization demonstrated better performance with adolescent preventive services than that provided by physicians in private practice settings. Success in this managed care setting may have been related to confidentiality policies, frequently reported recommendations for annual visits, or other factors.

School-based and school-linked health resources have become more important in the overall landscape of health services available to adolescents (see http://www.gwu.edu/~mtg and http://www.nasbhc.org). Adolescents who use school-based health services are highly satisfied with the care they receive. Moreover, school-based and school-linked services seem to play a unique and complementary role in meeting the health needs of some teens. For example, there is evidence to suggest that teens may be more willing to access school-health services rather than traditional health resources to address mental health, substance use, and reproductive health concerns.

Preventive Services Visit

General Suggestions for Providing Adolescent Preventive Services

Caring for adolescents requires a different approach, format, and style than does caring for either children or adults, so it is not surprising that many health care providers report discomfort caring for adolescents. This discomfort is exacerbated when sensitive health concerns must be discussed or treated, or when providers feel ill-trained or ill-equipped to manage the specific issues before them. Although there is no substitute for proper training or a teen-friendly office environment, the following general suggestions provide a framework for the delivery of adolescent health services:

1. Create a comfortable and conducive atmosphere for discussion, disclosure, and counseling by ensuring privacy, minimizing interruptions, and giving the adolescent your full respect and attention.
2. Confidentiality is of paramount importance to teens; therefore, a foundation of confidentiality should be established so that the teen feels comfortable with the provider and trusts him or her enough to discuss sensitive subjects. Especially when discussing sensitive issues, the examiner should be direct, empathetic, and nonjudgmental.
3. Most of the history should be obtained privately and directly from the teenager. Still, it is valuable to obtain additional history from parents, both to corroborate the teen's history and to gather additional information. Ideally, one should have the opportunity to speak with parents both alone and together with the adolescent. Collateral information from others (e.g., school personnel) may be very helpful in some circumstances.
4. Screening for health-risk behaviors (e.g., use of drugs or alcohol, drinking and driving) and providing developmentally appropriate guidance should be an integral and essential component of a preventive services visit.
5. There should be adequate time left at the end of the visit to summarize the session and to answer questions from the adolescent.
6. The physical examination provides an excellent venue to discuss concerns that the adolescent might have about a particular body region. It is especially important to discuss growth and development with younger adolescents. Teaching and encouraging breast or testicular self-examination can be done as part of the physical examination for older adolescents.

Questionnaires and Other Health Screening Tools

Questionnaires and screening forms can be efficient tools for collecting information, thereby reducing the amount of time spent with patients. Some patients also find it easier to disclose sensitive information through questionnaire than face-to-face. Screening questionnaires and personal interviews may therefore be considered complementary, and neither will be adequate in all situations. Many clinics, programs, and practices elect to create their own questionnaires based on their unique knowledge of their individual practice. The AMA's GAPS program has published a series of carefully constructed and updated questionnaires for both adolescents and their parents (Figs. 4.2 to 4.5). There are longer versions best suited to new patients and shorter versions suitable for returning patients. The questionnaires are also available in Spanish and are easily modified for providers who wish to individualize them. They may be obtained from the AMA (http://http://www.ama-assn.org/ama/pub/category/1981.html).

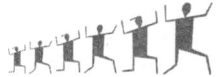

Guidelines for Adolescent Preventive Services
Initial Adolescent Preventive Services Visit Form

Confidential

Name _____   Date _____
          Last   First   Middle Initial

Date of birth _____   Sex M   F   Age _____

Grade in school _____   Year in college _____

Language(s) spoken in your home _____

1. Why did you come to the clinic today? _____
    _____
    _____

Part A

Medical History

2. Are you allergic to any medicines?
    ☐ Yes ☐ No Name of medicine _____

3. Are you taking any medicine now?
    ☐ Yes ☐ No Name of medicine _____

4. Do you have any health problems?
    ☐ Yes ☐ No Problem _____

5. Have you ever been hospitalized overnight?
    ☐ Yes ☐ No If yes, give age hospitalized and describe the problem   Age _____ Problem _____

                                                                            Age _____ Problem _____

6. Have you had any serious injuries or sports-related injuries?
    ☐ Yes ☐ No If yes, give age it occurred and describe the injury   Age _____ Injury _____

                                                                          Age _____ Injury _____

7. Have you ever had any of the following illnesses or problems?

    If yes, write down how old you were when the problem or illness started:

	Yes	No	Age		Yes	No	Age
Allergies	☐	☐	_____	Pneumonia	☐	☐	_____
Anemia or blood disorders	☐	☐	_____	Rheumatic fever or heart disease	☐	☐	_____
Asthma	☐	☐	_____	Scoliosis	☐	☐	_____
Bladder or kidney infections	☐	☐	_____	Seizures	☐	☐	_____
Cancer	☐	☐	_____	Severe acne	☐	☐	_____
Chicken pox	☐	☐	_____	Sports injuries or fractures	☐	☐	_____
Diabetes	☐	☐	_____	Thyroid disease	☐	☐	_____
Endocrine/gland disease	☐	☐	_____	Tuberculosis	☐	☐	_____
Hepatitis	☐	☐	_____	Ulcer or digestive problems	☐	☐	_____
Headaches/migraines	☐	☐	_____	Mental illness or depression	☐	☐	_____
Mononucleosis	☐	☐	_____	Other	☐	☐	_____

FIGURE 4.2 Comprehensive initial preventive services questionnaire for adolescents. (From American Medical Association. *Guidelines for adolescent preventive services* [Recommendations monograph]. Chicago: American Medical Association, 1995.)

Confidential   Name _____

Part B

Family Information

8. With whom do you live? (Check all that apply.)

☐ Mother   ☐ Stepmother   ☐ Brother(s)/ages: _____

☐ Father   ☐ Stepfather   ☐ Sister(s)/ages: _____

                  ☐ Guardian   ☐ Other: (explain) _____

9. Do you have older brothers and sisters who live away from home?........................... ☐ Yes   ☐ No

10. Were you adopted? .... ☐ Yes   ☐ No

11. During the past year, have there been any major changes in your family such as: (Check all that apply.)

☐ Marriage   ☐ Serious illness   ☐ Births

☐ Separation   ☐ Loss of job   ☐ Deaths

☐ Divorce   ☐ Move to a new house ☐ Other: (explain) _____

12. Have you ever lived away from home? .... ☐ Yes   ☐ No

    If yes, please explain: _____

13. Father's/stepfather's occupation or job: _____   Mother's/stepmother's occupation or job: _____

14. Do you have any family problems?... ☐ Yes   ☐ No

15. Have your parents or any of your blood relatives had a stroke or heart attack before age 55? ..... ☐ Yes   ☐ No   ☐ Not sure

16. Do your parents or any of your blood relatives have "high cholesterol"? .... ☐ Yes   ☐ No   ☐ Not sure

Job/Career Information

17. Are you working? .... ☐ Yes   ☐ No

    If yes, what is your job?: _____

18. How many hours do you work each week?_____

19. What are your future plans or career goals? _____

Part C

Specific Health Concerns

20. Please check whether you have questions or concerns about any of the following:

☐ Height/weight   ☐ Mouth/teeth   ☐ Muscle or joint pain   ☐ Diet/food/appetite
                                                     in arms/legs
☐ Blood pressure   ☐ Neck/back   ☐ Future plans/job
                                                  ☐ Frequent or
☐ Skin (rash, acne)   ☐ Chest pain   painful urination   ☐ Physical or sexual abuse

☐ Headaches/migraines   ☐ Coughing/wheezing   ☐ Wetting the bed   ☐ Masturbation

☐ Dizziness/passing out ☐ Breasts   ☐ Sexual organs/genitals   ☐ Cancer

☐ Eyes/vision   ☐ Heart   ☐ Menstruation/periods   ☐ Dying

☐ Ears/hearing/earaches ☐ Stomach pain   ☐ Trouble sleeping   ☐ Other (explain)

☐ Nose   ☐ Nausea/vomiting   ☐ Tiredness   _____

☐ Frequent colds   ☐ Diarrhea/constipation   _____

FIGURE 4.2   *(Continued)*

Confidential   Name _____

Part D

Health Profile

These questions will help us get to know you better. Choose the answer that best describes what you feel or do. Your answers will be seen only by your health care provider and his/her assistant.

Eating/Weight

21. Are you satisfied with your eating patterns? .... ☐ No   ☐ Yes

22. Do you ever eat in secret?... ☐ Yes   ☐ No

23. In the past year, have you tried to lose weight or control your weight by vomiting taking diet pills or laxatives, or starving yourself? .... ☐ Yes   ☐ No

School

24. Are your grades this year worse than your grades the year before? .... ☐ Yes   ☐ No

25. Are you in special education classes?.. ☐ Yes   ☐ No

26. Have you been suspended from school this year?.. ☐ Yes   ☐ No

Friends & Family

27. Do you have at least one friend who you really like and feel you can talk to? .... ☐ No   ☐ Yes

28. Do you think that your parent(s) or guardian(s) *usually* listen to you and take your feelings seriously?.. ☐ No   ☐ Yes

29. In your opinion, is there a lot of tension or conflict in your home? .... ☐ Yes   ☐ No   ☐ Not sure

Weapons/Violence

30. Do you or anyone you live with have a gun, rifle, or other firearm in your home? .... ☐ Yes   ☐ No   ☐ Not sure

31. In the past year, have you carried a gun, knife, club, or other weapon for your protection? .... ☐ Yes   ☐ No

32. Have you been in a physical fight during the *past 3 months*? .... ☐ Yes   ☐ No

33. Have you ever been in trouble with the law? .... ☐ Yes   ☐ No

34. Do you have any questions or concerns about violence or your safety? .... ☐ Yes   ☐ No   ☐ Not sure

Tobacco

35. Do you ever smoke cigarettes or use snuff or chewing tobacco? .... ☐ Yes   ☐ No

36. Do any of your close friends ever smoke cigarettes or use snuff or chewing tobacco?............. ☐ Yes   ☐ No

37. Does anyone you live with smoke cigarettes or use snuff or chewing tobacco? .... ☐ Yes   ☐ No

Alcohol

38. In the past month, did you get drunk or very high on beer, wine, wine coolers, or other alcohol? .. ☐ Yes   ☐ No

39. In the past month, did any of your close friends get drunk or very high on beer, wine, wine coolers, or other alcohol?... ☐ Yes   ☐ No

40. Have you ever used alcohol *and* then done any of the following: • driven a car/truck/van/ motorcycle • gone swimming or boating • gotten into a fight • used tools or equipment • done something that you later regretted? .... ☐ Yes   ☐ No

41. Have you ever been criticized or gotten into trouble because of drinking? .... ☐ Yes   ☐ No   ☐ Not sure

42. In the past year, have you been in a car or other motor vehicle when the driver has been drinking alcohol or using drugs? .... ☐ Yes   ☐ No

43. Does anyone in your family have a problem with drugs or alcohol? .... ☐ Yes   ☐ No

FIGURE 4.2 *(Continued)*

> **Confidential**

Drugs

44. Do you ever use marijuana, other drugs or inhalants? .... ☐ Yes ☐ No ☐ Not sure

45. Do any of your close friends ever use marijuana, other drugs or inhalants? .... ☐ Yes ☐ No ☐ Not sure

46. Some drugs can be bought at a store without a doctor's prescription. Do you ever use
non-prescription drugs to get to sleep, stay awake, calm down, or get high? .... ☐ Yes ☐ No

47. Have you ever used steroids (eg, "roids or juice") without a doctor telling you to? .... ☐ Yes ☐ No ☐ Not sure

Development

48. Do you have any concerns or questions about the size or shape of your body, or
your physical appearance? .... ☐ Yes ☐ No ☐ Not sure

49. Are you physically and emotionally attracted to people of your own sex? .... ☐ Yes ☐ No ☐ Not sure

50. Have you ever had sexual intercourse? .... ☐ Yes ☐ No ☐ Not sure

51. Are you using birth control? .... ☐ Yes ☐ No ☐ Not sure

52. Do you and your partner *always* use condoms when you have sex? .... ☐ No ☐ Yes ☐ Not sure

53. Have any of your close friends ever had sexual intercourse? .... ☐ Yes ☐ No ☐ Not sure

54. Have you ever been told by a doctor or nurse that you had a sexually transmitted disease (STD)
such as herpes, gonorrhea, chlamydia, trichomoniasis ("trick"), hepatitis,
genital warts, HIV infection, or others? .... ☐ Yes ☐ No ☐ Not sure

55. Do you have any questions or concerns about sex, relationships or STDs? .... ☐ Yes ☐ No ☐ Not sure

56. Would you like to receive information or supplies *today* to prevent pregnancy or sexually
transmitted diseases? .... ☐ Yes ☐ No ☐ Not sure

57. Would you like to know how to avoid getting the HIV/AIDS virus? .... ☐ Yes ☐ No ☐ Not sure

Emotions

58. Have you had fun during the past two weeks? .... ☐ No ☐ Yes

59. In general, are you happy with the way things are going for you these days? .... ☐ Yes ☐ No ☐ Not sure

60. During the past few weeks, have you *often* felt sad or down or as though you have
nothing to look forward to? .... ☐ Yes ☐ No

61. Have you ever *seriously* thought about killing yourself, made a plan to kill yourself,
or actually tried to kill yourself? .... ☐ Yes ☐ No

62. Do you have any questions or concerns about being physically, sexually, or emotionally abused? .. ☐ Yes ☐ No ☐ Not sure

Special Circumstances

63. In the past year, have you been exposed to tuberculosis? .... ☐ Yes ☐ No ☐ Not sure

64. In the past year, have you stayed overnight in a homeless shelter, jail, or detention center? ...... ☐ Yes ☐ No

65. Have you ever run away from home overnight? .... ☐ Yes ☐ No

66. Have you ever lived in foster care or an institution? .... ☐ Yes ☐ No

Self

67. What do you like about yourself? _____

68. What do you do best? _____

69. If you could, what would you change about your life or yourself? _____
_____

Thank you for completing this form.

FIGURE 4.2 *(Continued)*

| Guidelines for Adolescent Preventive Services |
| **Initial Parent/Guardian Questionnaire** |

Confidential

Date _____

Adolescent's name _____ Birthdate _____ Age _____

Name of person completing this form _____ Relationship to adolescent _____

Your phone number: Home_____ Work _____

Part A

Adolescent Health History

1. Is your adolescent allergic to any medicine?

    ☐ Yes ☐ No   If yes, what?_____

2. List any medications your adolescent is taking now and the problem for which the medication was given:

    Medication   Reason   How Long

    _____   _____   _____

    _____   _____   _____

    _____   _____   _____

3. Has your adolescent ever been hospitalized overnight?

    ☐ Yes ☐ No   If yes, give the age at time of hospitalization and describe the problem.

    Age   Problem

    _____   _____

    _____   _____

4. Has your adolescent ever had any serious or sports-related injuries?

    ☐ Yes ☐ No   If yes, explain _____

5. Has there been any change in your adolescent's health during the past year?

    ☐ Yes ☐ No   If yes, give the age it occurred and describe the injury. _____

    _____

6. Please check (✔) whether your son/daughter ever had any of the following health problems:
    If yes, at what age did the problem start:

	Yes	No	Age		Yes	No	Age
Allergies	☐	☐	_____	Pneumonia	☐	☐	_____
Anemia or blood disorders	☐	☐	_____	Rheumatic fever or heart disease	☐	☐	_____
Asthma	☐	☐	_____	Scoliosis.........................	☐	☐	_____
Bladder or kidney infections	☐	☐	_____	Seizures.........................	☐	☐	_____
Cancer	☐	☐	_____	Severe acne......................	☐	☐	_____
Chicken pox	☐	☐	_____	Sports injuries or fractures	☐	☐	_____
Diabetes	☐	☐	_____	Thyroid disease	☐	☐	_____
Endocrine/gland disease	☐	☐	_____	Tuberculosis	☐	☐	_____
Hepatitis	☐	☐	_____	Ulcer or digestive problems	☐	☐	_____
Headaches/Migraines	☐	☐	_____	Mental illness or depression	☐	☐	_____
Mononucleosis	☐	☐	_____	Other:...........................	☐	☐	_____

7. If your adolescent received an immunization that has not been recorded with this office/clinic, please indicate the immunization and date it was given. (This includes tetanus, measles (MMR), Hepatitis B or Varicella vaccine.)

    _____   _____
    Immunization   Month/Year

FIGURE 4.3   Comprehensive initial preventive services questionnaire for parents/guardians. (From American Medical Association. *Guidelines for adolescent preventive services* [Recommendations monograph]. Chicago: American Medical Association, 1995.)

Confidential

Adolescent's name _____

Part B

Family History

8. Have you or any of your adolescent's *blood* relatives (parents, grandparents, aunts, uncles, brothers or sisters), living or deceased, had any of the following problems? If the answer is **Yes,** please state the age of the person when the problem occurred and their relationship to your teen.

Condition	Yes	No	Unsure	Age at Onset	Relationship
Alcoholism/Drugs	☐	☐	☐	_____	_____
Allergies/Asthma	☐	☐	☐	_____	_____
Arthritis	☐	☐	☐	_____	_____
Birth defects	☐	☐	☐	_____	_____
Blood disorders/Sickle cell anemia	☐	☐	☐	_____	_____
Cancer (type_____)	☐	☐	☐	_____	_____
Diabetes	☐	☐	☐	_____	_____
Endocrine/gland disease	☐	☐	☐	_____	_____
Heart attack or stoke before are 55	☐	☐	☐	_____	_____
Heart attack or stoke after are 55	☐	☐	☐	_____	_____
High blood pressure	☐	☐	☐	_____	_____
High cholesterol	☐	☐	☐	_____	_____
Kidney disease	☐	☐	☐	_____	_____
Lung disease/Tuberculosis	☐	☐	☐	_____	_____
Mental health/Depression	☐	☐	☐	_____	_____
Mental retardation	☐	☐	☐	_____	_____
Obesity	☐	☐	☐	_____	_____
Seizures/Epilepsy	☐	☐	☐	_____	_____
Smoking	☐	☐	☐	_____	_____

9. With whom does the adolescent live most of the time? (Check all that apply).

☐ Both parents in same household   ☐ Stepmother   ☐ Alone
☐ Mother   ☐ Stepfather   ☐ Brother(s)/ages _____
☐ Father   ☐ Guardian   ☐ Sister(s)/ages _____
                                                          ☐ Other _____

10 **In the past year**, have there been any changes in your family such as:

☐ Marriage   ☐ Serious illness   ☐ Change in school
☐ Separation   ☐ Loss of job   ☐ Births
☐ Divorce   ☐ Move to a new house   ☐ Deaths
                                           ☐ Other _____

FIGURE 4.3   *(Continued)*

Screening tools that have been more formally and rigorously validated can be useful in practice, particularly to screen for behavioral and mental health problems. For example, the Beck Depression Inventory is a well validated and easily administered tool to screen for depression. The 21-question inventory is designed for adolescents and is simple to use and score in a busy clinical setting. A wide variety of other tools are available to screen for family function, behavioral difficulties, and other mental health problems.

Computer-aided Screening and Assessment

In this information age, there is increasing interest in using technology to assist in providing preventive services to adolescents. Computer-aided screening, information kiosks, and Internet-based health information are all being investigated as tools to increase access to information and resources, as well as to deliver preventive services in the most cost-effective manner possible. For example, Paperny and Hedberg (1999) tested a low-cost strategy to provide preventive services to adolescents with the use of computerized health assessments, individualized educational videos, trained health counselors, and nurses. They found that most adolescents preferred the computer-assisted visits to standard office visits, and that preventive services could be delivered at a very modest cost. Further work will be required to assess the utility of this strategy in affecting health outcomes.

History

A comprehensive history is the most important aspect of the preventive services evaluation. As with any history, essential domains include past medical history, family

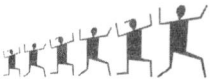

Guidelines for Adolescent Preventive Services

Periodic Adolescent Preventive Services Visit Form

Confidential

Name _____ Date _____
          Last   First   Middle Initial

Date of birth _____ Sex M   F   Age _____ Grade in school _____

Your reason for today's visit _____

Specific Health Concerns

Please check whether you have questions or concerns about any of the following:

☐ Height/weight	☐ Mouth/teeth	☐ Diarrhea/constipation	☐ Tiredness
☐ Blood pressure	☐ Neck/back	☐ Skin (rash, acne)	☐ Diet/food/appetite
☐ Headaches/migraines	☐ Chest pain	☐ Muscle or joint pain in arms/legs	☐ Future plans/job
☐ Dizziness/passing out	☐ Coughing/wheezing	☐ Frequent or painful urination	☐ Physical or sexual abuse
☐ Eyes/vision	☐ Breasts	☐ Wetting the bed	☐ Masturbation
☐ Ears/hearing/earaches	☐ Heart	☐ Sexual organs/genitals	☐ Cancer
☐ Nose	☐ Stomach pain	☐ Menstruation/periods	☐ Dying
☐ Frequent colds	☐ Nausea/vomiting	☐ Trouble sleeping	☐ Other (explain)

Health Profile

These questions will help us get to know you better. Choose the answer that best describes what you feel or do. Your answers will be seen only by your health care provider and his/her assistant.

Eating/Weight

1. Are you satisfied with your eating patterns? .... ☐ No   ☐ Yes
2. Do you ever eat in secret? .... ☐ Yes   ☐ No
3. In the past year, have you tried to lose weight or control your weight by vomiting, taking diet pills or laxatives, or starving yourself? .... ☐ Yes   ☐ No

School

4. Are your grades this year worse than your grades the year before? .... ☐ Yes   ☐ No   ☐ Not in school
5. Are you in special education classes? .... ☐ Yes   ☐ No
6. Have you been suspended from school this year? .... ☐ Yes   ☐ No

Friends & Family

7. Do you have at least one friend who you really like and feel you can talk to? .... ☐ No   ☐ Yes
8. Do you think that your parent(s) or guardian(s) *usually* listen to you and take your feelings seriously? .... ☐ No   ☐ Yes
9. In your opinion, is there a lot of tension or conflict in your home? .... ☐ Yes   ☐ No   ☐ Not sure

Weapons/Violence

10. Do you or anyone you live with have a gun, rifle, or other firearm in your home? .... ☐ Yes   ☐ No   ☐ Not sure
11. In the past year, have you carried a gun, knife, club, or other weapon for your protection? .... ☐ Yes   ☐ No
12. Have you been in a physical fight during the *past 3 months*? .... ☐ Yes   ☐ No
13. Have you ever been in trouble with the law? .... ☐ Yes   ☐ No

Tobacco

14. Do you ever smoke cigarettes or use smokeless tobacco (Snuff or chewing tobacco)? .... ☐ Yes   ☐ No
15. Do any of your close friends ever smoke cigarettes or use smokeless tobacco (snuff or chewing tobacco)? .... ☐ Yes   ☐ No
16. Does anyone you live with smoke cigarettes or use smokeless tobacco? .... ☐ Yes   ☐ No

FIGURE 4.4 Brief periodic preventive services questionnaire for adolescents. (From American Medical Association. *Guidelines for adolescent preventive services* [Recommendations monograph]. Chicago: American Medical Association, 1995.)

Alcohol

17. In the past month, did you get drunk or very high on beer, wine, wine coolers, or other alcohol?   ... ☐ Yes   ☐ No

18. In the past month, did any of your friends get drunk or very high on beer, wine, wine coolers, or other alcohol? .... ☐ Yes   ☐ No

19. Have you ever used alcohol *and* then done any of the following: • driven a car/truck/van/ motorcycle • gone swimming or boating • gotten into a fight • used tools or equipment • done something that you later regretted? .... ☐ Yes   ☐ No

20. Have you ever been criticized or gotten into trouble because of drinking? .... ☐ Yes   ☐ No   ☐ Not sure

21. In the past year, have you been in a car or other motor vehicle when the driver has been drinking alcohol or using drugs? .... ☐ Yes   ☐ No

22. Does anyone in your family have a problem with drugs or alcohol? .... ☐ Yes   ☐ No

Drugs

23. Do you ever use marijuana, other drugs or inhalants? .... ☐ Yes   ☐ No   ☐ Not sure

24. Do any of your close friends ever use marijuana, other drugs or inhalants? .... ☐ Yes   ☐ No   ☐ Not sure

25. Some drugs can be bought at a store without a doctor's prescription. Do you ever use non-prescription drugs to get to sleep, stay awake, calm down, or get high? .... ☐ Yes   ☐ No

26. Have you ever used steroids (eg. "roids or juice")? .... ☐ Yes   ☐ No   ☐ Not sure

Development

27. Do you have any concerns or questions about the size or shape of your body, or your physical appearance? .... ☐ Yes   ☐ No   ☐ Not sure

28. Are you physically and emotionally attracted to people of your own sex? .... ☐ Yes   ☐ No   ☐ Not sure

29. Have you ever had sexual intercourse? .... ☐ Yes   ☐ No   ☐ Not sure

30. Are you using birth control? .... ☐ No   ☐ Yes   ☐ Not sure

31. Do you and your partner *always* use condoms when you have sex? .... ☐ No   ☐ Yes   ☐ Not sure

32. Have any of your friends ever had sexual intercourse? .... ☐ Yes   ☐ No   ☐ Not sure

33. Have you ever been told by a doctor or nurse that you had a sexually transmitted disease (STD) such as genital herpes, gonorrhea (drip), chlamydia, trichomoniasis ("trick"), hepatitis, genital warts, HIV infection, or others? .... ☐ Yes   ☐ No   ☐ Not sure

34. Do you have any questions or concerns about sex, relationships or STDs? .... ☐ Yes   ☐ No   ☐ Not sure

35. Would you like to receive information or supplies *today* to prevent pregnancy or sexually transmitted diseases? .... ☐ Yes   ☐ No   ☐ Not sure

36. Would you like to know how to avoid getting the HIV/AIDS virus? .... ☐ Yes   ☐ No   ☐ Not sure

Emotions

37. Have you had fun during the past two weeks? .... ☐ No   ☐ Yes

38. In general, are you happy with the way things are going for you these days? .... ☐ No   ☐ Yes   ☐ Not sure

39. During the past few weeks, have you *often* felt sad or down or as though you have nothing to look forward to? .... ☐ Yes   ☐ No

40. Have you ever *seriously* thought about killing yourself, made a plan to kill yourself, or actually tried to kill yourself? .... ☐ Yes   ☐ No

41. Have you ever been physically, sexually, or emotionally abused? .... ☐ Yes   ☐ No   ☐ Not sure

Special Circumstances

42. In the past year, have you been exposed to tuberculosis? .... ☐ Yes   ☐ No   ☐ Not sure

43. In the past year, have you stayed over night in a homeless shelter, jail, or detention center? ...... ☐ Yes   ☐ No

44. Have you ever run away from home overnight? .... ☐ Yes   ☐ No

45. Have you ever lived in foster care or an institution? .... ☐ Yes   ☐ No

Self

46. What do you like about yourself? _____

47. What do you do best? _____

48. If you could, what would you change about your life or yourself? _____

Thank you for completing this form.

     <u>**FIGURE 4.4**</u>   *(Continued)*

Guidelines for Adolescent Preventive Services
Periodic Parent/Guardian Questionnaire

Confidential

Today's date ————————————————

Adolescent's name ———————————————————————————— Birthdate ———————— Age —————

Name of person completing this form ———————————————— Relationship to adolescent —————————

Your phone number: Home ———————————————————— Work ————————————————

Family History

1. Please indicate whether you or any of your adolescent's *blood* relatives (parents, grandparents, uncles, aunts, brothers, sisters), living or deceased, have ever had any of the following problems? If the answer is yes please state that person's relationship to the adolescent.

	Yes	No	Relationship
Problems with circulation	☐	☐	_____
High blood pressure	☐	☐	_____
High cholesterol	☐	☐	_____
Heart attack (before age 55)	☐	☐	_____
Heart attack (age 55 or older)	☐	☐	_____
Stroke (before age 55)	☐	☐	_____
Stroke (age 55 or older)	☐	☐	_____
Lung disease/Tuberculosis	☐	☐	_____
Diabetes	☐	☐	_____
Obesity	☐	☐	_____
Eating disorders	☐	☐	_____
Depression/Suicide	☐	☐	_____
Alcohol or drug problems	☐	☐	_____
Smoker or tobacco user in household	☐	☐	_____
Other _____	☐	☐	_____

2. With whom does the adolescent live most of the time? (check all that apply).

☐ Both parents in same household   ☐ Stepmother   ☐ Alone

☐ Mother   ☐ Stepfather   ☐ Brother(s)/ages ————————

☐ Father   ☐ Guardian   ☐ Sister(s)/ages ————————

☐ Other ————————————

3, In the past year, have there been any changes in your family such as:

☐ Marriage   ☐ Serious illness   ☐ Change in school

☐ Separation   ☐ Loss of job   ☐ Births

☐ Divorce   ☐ Move to a new house   ☐ Deaths

☐ Other ————————————

FIGURE 4.5   Brief periodic preventive services questionnaire for parents/guardians. (From American Medical Association. *Guidelines for adolescent preventive services* [Recommendations monograph]. Chicago: American Medical Association, 1995.)

Parental/Guardian Concerns

4. Some parents or guardians have questions or concerns about their adolescent's developemtn. Please review the topics listed below and check (✓) if this is a concern you have about *your* son or daughter, or if you would like to discuss this topic.

	Concern About Your Adolescent	Want to Discuss		Concern About Your Adolescent	Want to Discuss
Recurrent complaints	☐	☐	Lying, stealing, or vandalism	☐	☐
Physical development/ complaints	☐	☐	Violence	☐	☐
			School performance/truancy/dropout	☐	☐
Weight	☐	☐	Smoking cigarettes/chewing tobacco	☐	☐
Change of appetite	☐	☐	Drug use	☐	☐
Sleep patterns	☐	☐	Alcohol use	☐	☐
Diet/nutrition	☐	☐	Dating/parties	☐	☐
Amount of physical activity	☐	☐	Sexual behaviors	☐	☐
Emotional development	☐	☐	HIV/AIDS	☐	☐
Relationships with family members	☐	☐	Birth control	☐	☐
His/her choice of friends	☐	☐	Sexual identity (heterosexual/homosexual)	☐	☐
Self image/self worth	☐	☐			
Excessive moodiness or rebellion	☐	☐	Work or job	☐	☐
Depression	☐	☐	Other:	☐	☐

Questions for Parents/Guardian

5. Do you regularly supervise or keep track of your adolescent's social and recreational activities for the use of alcohol, tobacco, or other drugs? ☐ No ☐ Yes

6. Have you discussed with your adolescent his/her use of alcohol, tobacco, or other drugs? ☐ No ☐ Yes

7. Have you discussed with your adolescent his/her sexual orientation and sexual behavior? ☐ No ☐ Yes

8. Have you discussed with your adolescent safe driving as a passenger and as a driver? ☐ No ☐ Yes

9. Have you discussed bike safety and rules of the road with your adolescent? ☐ No ☐ Yes

10. Have you discussed injury prevention with your adolescent in regard to swimming, on the job safety, sports, and operating machinery? ☐ No ☐ Yes

11. Is there a gun in your household? ☐ Yes ☐ No

12. If yes, have you discussed firearm safety with your adolescent? ☐ No ☐ Yes

13. Do you believe your parenting style and discipline techniques are effective for your adolescent? ☐ No ☐ Yes

14. Do you involve your adolescent in decisions about his/her health? ☐ No ☐ Yes

15. Would you like to receive information today on parenting adolescents? ☐ Yes ☐ No

16. Would you like to receive information today about normal physical and emotional development of adolescents? ☐ Yes ☐ No

17. What do you find most rewarding about being the parent of your adolescent?

_____

18. What is it about your adolescent that makes you proud of him or her?

_____

19. What do you and your adolescent do together on a regular basis (for example, have meals together)?

_____

Parent and Guardian Challenges

Healthy life-styles and preventive measures should be a part of everyone's daily routine. *Your* decisions about alcohol and other drugs, smoking, food choices, safety, and physical activity can strongly influence your adolescent's behavior and decisions. Parents/guardians demonstrate by their actions what they believe or value.

FIGURE 4.5 *(Continued)*

history, psychosocial history, and an age-appropriate review of systems. Any current health concerns should also be sought. When preventive services are delivered in the setting of a visit made with another specific agenda (e.g., sports physical, acute medical problem), the patient's agenda should be fully addressed before preventive services are offered.

Past Medical History

Past medical history is best obtained from both the adolescent and the parents and should include the following:

1. Childhood infections and illnesses
2. Prior hospitalizations and surgery
3. Significant injuries
4. Disabilities
5. Medications, including prescription medications, over-the-counter medications, complementary or alternative medications, vitamins, and nutritional supplements
6. Allergies
7. Immunization history
8. Developmental history, including prenatal, perinatal, and infancy history; history of problems with walking, talking, eating, or learning; peer relations; and school functioning
9. Mental health history, including a history of hospitalization, outpatient counseling, medications, school interventions, or other treatment

Family History

Most information about family history is most accurately obtained from the parents. It should include the following:

1. Age and health status of family members
2. History of significant medical illnesses in the family, such as diabetes, cancer, heart disease, tuberculosis (TB), hypertension, or stroke
3. History of mental illness in the family, such as mood disorders, anxiety disorders, schizophrenia, or alcoholism
4. Vocational status of parents

Psychosocial History

The psychosocial history is obtained primarily from the adolescent while he or she is interviewed alone. Some material will also be gathered from the parents or from interviews with the family together. Obtaining much of this information is dependent on successfully establishing trust and rapport between the practitioner and the adolescent. Many clinicians rely on the *HEADSS* acronym to guide their psychosocial history. The original acronym included *h*ome, *e*ducation, *a*ctivities (including information about peers), *d*rugs, *s*exuality, and *s*uicide (mental health). A more up-to-date incarnation of the acronym—*HEEADSSS*—includes additional questions covering *e*ating and *s*afety (see Chapter 3). A complete psychosocial history includes the following areas:

1. Home: Family configuration and family members; living arrangements; relationships between the adolescent and family members; and relationships among other family members
2. Education/employment: Academic or vocational success; future plans; and safety at school or in the workplace

3. Eating: Brief nutrition history; risk factor for obesity; concerns about weight or body image; or disordered eating behaviors
4. Activities: Friendships with peers of the same and opposite sex; recreational activities; dating activity and relationships; and sexual activity
5. Drugs: Personal use of tobacco, alcohol, illicit drugs, anabolic steroids; peer substance use; family substance use; and driving while intoxicated
6. Sexuality: Sexual orientation; sexual activity; and sexual abuse
7. Suicide (mental health): Feelings of sadness, loneliness, depression; pervasive boredom; inappropriately high levels of anxiety; or suicidal thoughts
8. Safety: Risk of unintentional injury; risk from violence; fighting or weapon carrying

Review of Systems

The review of systems covers the following areas:

1. Vision: Trouble reading or watching television; vision correction
2. Hearing: Infections, trouble hearing, earaches
3. Dental: Prior care, pain, concerns (e.g., braces)
4. Head: Headaches, dizziness
5. Nose and throat: Frequent colds or sore throats; respiratory allergies
6. Skin: Acne, moles, rashes, warts
7. Cardiovascular: Exercise intolerance, shortness of breath, chest pain, palpitations, syncope, physical activity
8. Respiratory: Asthma, cough, smoking, exposure to TB
9. Gastrointestinal: Abdominal pain, reflux, diarrhea, vomiting, bleeding
10. Genitourinary: Dysuria, bed-wetting, frequency, bleeding
11. Musculoskeletal: Limb pain, joint pain, or swelling
12. Central nervous system (CNS): Seizures, syncope
13. Menstrual: Menarche, frequency of menses, duration, menorrhagia or metrorrhagia, pain
14. Sexual: Sexual activity, contraception, pregnancy, abortions, sexually transmitted diseases (STDs) or STD symptoms

Physical Examination

The physical examination is another important component of the screening evaluation of the adolescent. The examination allows the clinician to assess growth and pubertal development and to instruct the adolescent in methods of self-examination and other means of health promotion. The physical examination also affords the adolescent an opportunity to ask about any specific health concerns, and it provides the clinician with the opportunity to detect unnoticed diseases. The examination should be performed in such a way as to preserve the adolescent's modesty. Main elements of the physical examination (Fig. 4.6) include the following topics.

Height, Weight, and Vital Signs Height, weight, blood pressure, and pulse should be measured. The serial measurement of height and weight allows for monitoring of the adolescent's growth and for the earlier detection of risk factors for obesity. Body mass index (BMI) should be calculated and tracked. Gender-specific age-based BMI norms

Guidelines for Adolescent Preventive Services

Adolescent Physical Examination

Name_____   Identification No. _____

Birthdate _____   Age_____   Date_____

Subjective

Date of last: DPT/Td _____   MMR _____   Hepatitis B _____   Varicella _____   LMP_____

CC/HPI_____

_____

Objective

Hearing   (R) _____   (L) _____

Vision   OD_____   OS_____

PE: Ht _____ in/cm   _____%   Wt _____ lbs/kg   _____%

Body Mass Index (BMI) _____   Overwt _____   At Risk _____   Normal _____

T._____   P._____   R. _____   BP._____ / _____

☑ = Normal   ☐ = Not Examined   ☒ = See Notes

☐ General	☐ Ears	☐ Nodes	☐ Lungs	☐ Elbow	☐ Foot	☐ Hip
☐ Skin	☐ Nose	☐ Thyroid	☐ Breasts	☐ Wrist	☐ Neck	☐ Neurological
☐ Head	☐ Throat	☐ Heart	☐ Abd	☐ Hand	☐ Shoulder	
☐ Eyes	☐ Mouth	☐ Pulse	☐ MSK	☐ Knee	☐ Back	
☐ Fundi	☐ Teeth		☐ Extremities	☐ Ankle	☐ Lower Back	

☐ Penis   ☐ Testes   ☐ Female Ext   ☐ Vagina

☐ Uterus   ☐ Rectum

☐ Cervix   ☐ Adnexa

Lab Tests

Assessment

Plan

FIGURE 4.6   Adolescent physical examination form. (From American Medical Association. *Guidelines for adolescent preventive services* [Recommendations monograph]. Chicago: American Medical Association, 1995.)

are available and are used in assessing risk for obesity (Figs. 4.7 to 4.9). Blood pressure should be recorded with an appropriately sized cuff. If blood pressure is elevated, it should be rechecked at least three separate visits before a diagnosis of hypertension is considered (Figs. 4.10 to 4.12).

Vision Screening Among 12- to 17-year-old adolescents, approximately 25% have visual acuity of 20/40 or less. This condition often develops during early adolescence. Adolescents should have a vision screening at the time of their initial evaluation and every 2 to 3 years thereafter. This can be done with a standard Snellen chart or a similar test. To pass a line the adolescent should view the chart with one eye covered and be able to read one half or more of the line correctly. Referral should be made for vision <20/30 in either or both eyes.

Hearing Screening There is increasing concern about threats to hearing and every adolescent should have at least one test for hearing screening performed during the adolescent years. It is important that this test be performed in a quiet room to allow for detection of subtle defects that may be contributing to a learning problem. Screening examinations are usually conducted at frequencies of 1,000, 2,000, and 4,000 Hz at 20 dB. Referral for more comprehensive hearing testing is indicated if there is a failure to hear 1,000 or 2,000 Hz at 20 dB or 4,000 Hz at 25 dB. The more comprehensive threshold test evaluates for the lowest intensity of sound heard at frequencies of 250, 1,000, 2,000, and 4,000 Hz. Evaluation is indicated with a threshold of 25 dB at two or more frequencies or at 35 dB for any frequency.

Sexual Maturity Rating The sexual maturity rating (SMR), discussed in Chapter 1, is the method by which pubertal development is evaluated and described. Because many "normal values" in adolescents depend more on SMR than on age, evaluation of SMR is important not only in describing pubertal milestones but also in adequately assessing many physical parameters (e.g., BMI), and laboratory values (e.g., hemoglobin).

Skin Check for evidence of acne, warts, fungal infections, and other lesions. Carefully inspect moles, especially in patients who are at particular risk for melanoma.

Teeth and Gums Teeth and gums frequently present problems in the adolescent age-group. Check for evidence of dental caries or gum infection. Look for signs of smokeless tobacco use. Enamel erosions are sometimes the first clue to the self-induced vomiting associated with some eating disorders. Regular checkups with a dentist should be encouraged.

Neck Check for thyromegaly or adenopathy.

Cardiopulmonary Check for heart murmurs or clicks.

Abdomen Check for evidence of hepatosplenomegaly, tenderness, or masses.

Musculoskeletal The musculoskeletal examination is especially important in adolescent athletes, in whom instabilities or other evidence of previous injury is the best predictor of future injury. Check for signs of overuse syndromes or osteochondroses. Check for scoliosis, particularly in premenarchal females.

Breasts Examine for symmetry and developmental variations; in girls, assess SMR. Examine for masses or discharge; in boys, identify gynecomastia (present in approximately one third of pubertal males). The value of breast self-examination is unclear, especially in adolescent females in whom the risk of breast cancer is extremely low. If breast self-examination is to be taught and encouraged, it should be done only when developmentally appropriate.

Neurological Test strength, reflexes, and coordination.

Genitalia (Male) Examine the penis and testicles. Assess SMR. Look for signs of STDs. Retract the foreskin in uncircumcised patients. Check for hernia.

Pelvic Examination (Female) A pelvic examination is indicated for female adolescents who have ever been sexually active and for any female adolescent who requests an examination. In addition, pelvic examination is indicated for female adolescents with pelvic pain, an atypical or changing vaginal discharge, or an undiagnosed menstrual disorder. "Annual" pelvic examination and Pap screening, which had previously been recommended for all women beginning at approximately 18 years of age, are now recommended beginning 3 years after coitarche or age 21, whichever comes earlier. Annual screening for STDs (which may or may not require a pelvic examination) is clearly recommended for sexually active female patients (see Chapter 48).

Rectal Examination Rectal examination is not routinely indicated as a *screening* procedure in the male adolescent. It is sometimes, but not always, part of the female pelvic examination.

Laboratory Tests

Laboratory tests should be kept to a minimum in the asymptomatic adolescent. Suggested screening tests are discussed in the following sections.

Hemoglobin or Hematocrit During adolescence there is a significant prevalence of iron deficiency anemia due to rapid growth, poor nutritional habits, exercise, and menstrual losses. A screening hemoglobin or hematocrit is recommended at the first encounter with the adolescent or at the end of puberty, or both. Although the normal levels remain stable for females throughout adolescence, the normal levels in males are dependent on age and, more importantly, on SMR. Lower levels of the normal hematocrit in white male adolescents range from 35.6% at SMR 1 to 40.6% at SMR 5; in African-American male adolescents this range is slightly lower, from 34.9% (SMR 1) to 39.3% (SMR 5).

Urinalysis A routine urinalysis, including a dipstick test for glucose and protein and a microscopical evaluation, is recommended at the first encounter with the adolescent or at the end of puberty, or both. However, up to one third of healthy adolescents have small amounts of proteinuria that is nonpathological and requires no treatment (see Chapter 27). Abnormal pyuria requires further investigation for urinary tract infection and, in males, for *Chlamydia* infection.

Sickle Cell Screening Screening for sickle cell anemia is recommended at the first visit with an African-American adolescent if it has not been documented already.

Guidelines for Adolescent Preventive Services

Body Mass Index for Selected Weight and Stature

Stature m (in)

Weight kg (lb)	1.24 (49)	1.27 (50)	1.30 (51)	1.32 (52)	1.35 (53)	1.37 (54)	1.40 (55)	1.42 (56)	1.45 (57)	1.47 (58)	1.50 (59)	1.52 (60)	1.55 (61)	1.57 (62)	1.60 (63)	1.63 (64)	1.65 (65)	1.68 (66)	1.70 (67)	1.73 (68)	1.75 (69)	1.78 (70)	1.80 (71)	1.83 (72)	1.85 (73)	1.88 (74)	1.90 (75)	1.93 (76)
20 (45)	13	13	12	12	11	11	10	10	10	9	9	9	8															
23 (50)	15	14	13	13	12	12	11	11	10	10	10	9	9	9	9	8												
25 (55)	16	15	15	14	14	13	13	12	12	12	11	11	10	10	10	9	9	9										
27 (60)	18	17	16	16	15	15	14	13	13	13	12	12	11	11	11	10	10	10	9	9								
29 (65)	19	18	17	17	16	16	15	15	14	14	13	13	12	12	12	11	11	10	10	10	10							
32 (70)	21	20	19	18	17	17	16	16	15	15	14	14	13	13	12	12	12	11	11	11	10	10						
34 (75)	22	21	20	20	19	18	17	17	16	16	15	15	14	14	13	13	12	12	12	11	11	11	10					
36 (80)	24	22	21	21	20	19	19	18	17	17	16	16	15	15	14	14	13	13	13	12	12	11	11	11				
39 (85)	25	24	23	22	21	21	20	19	18	18	17	17	16	16	15	15	14	14	13	13	13	12	12	12	11			
41 (90)	27	25	24	23	22	22	21	20	19	19	18	18	17	17	16	15	15	14	14	14	13	13	13	12	12	12		
43 (95)	28	27	25	25	24	23	22	21	20	20	19	19	18	17	17	16	16	15	15	14	14	13	13	13	12	12		
45 (100)	29	28	27	26	25	24	23	22	22	21	20	20	19	18	18	17	17	16	16	15	15	14	14	14	13	13	13	12
48 (105)	31	30	28	27	26	25	24	24	23	22	21	21	20	19	19	18	17	17	16	16	16	15	15	14	14	13	13	13
50 (110)	32	31	30	29	27	27	25	25	24	23	22	22	21	20	19	19	18	17	17	16	16	15	15	15	14	14	13	13
52 (115)	34	32	31	30	29	28	27	26	25	24	23	23	22	21	20	20	19	18	18	17	17	16	16	16	15	15	14	14
54 (120)	35	34	32	31	30	29	28	27	26	25	24	24	23	22	21	20	20	19	19	18	18	17	17	16	16	15	15	15
57 (125)	37	35	34	33	31	30	30	28	27	26	25	25	24	23	22	22	21	21	20	20	19	19	18	17	17	16	16	15
59 (130)	38	37	35	34	32	31	30	29	28	27	26	26	25	24	23	22	22	21	20	20	19	19	18	18	17	17	16	16
61 (135)	40	38	36	35	34	33	31	30	29	28	27	27	25	25	24	23	22	22	21	20	20	19	19	18	18	17	17	16
64 (140)	41	39	38	36	35	34	32	31	30	29	28	27	26	26	25	24	23	22	22	21	21	20	20	19	19	18	18	17
66 (145)	43	41	39	38	36	35	34	33	31	30	29	28	27	27	26	25	24	23	23	22	21	21	20	20	19	19	18	18
68 (150)	44	42	40	39	37	36	35	34	32	31	30	29	28	28	27	26	25	24	24	23	22	21	21	20	20	19	19	18
70 (155)	46	44	42	40	39	37	36	35	33	33	31	30	29	29	27	26	26	25	24	23	23	22	22	21	21	20	19	19
73 (160)	47	45	43	42	40	39	37	36	35	34	32	31	30	29	28	27	27	26	25	24	24	23	22	22	21	21	20	19
77 (170)	50	48	46	44	42	41	39	38	37	36	34	33	32	31	30	29	28	27	27	26	25	24	24	23	23	22	21	21
79 (175)		49	47	46	44	42	40	39	38	37	35	34	33	32	31	30	29	28	27	27	26	25	24	24	23	22	22	21
82 (180)	51	48	47	45	44	42	40	39	38	36	35	34	33	32	31	30	29	28	27	27	26	25	24	24	23	23	22	
84 (185)		50	48	46	45	43	42	40	39	37	36	35	34	33	32	31	30	29	28	27	26	26	25	25	24	23	23	
86 (190)			49	47	46	44	43	41	40	39	37	36	35	34	32	32	31	30	29	28	27	27	26	25	24	24	23	
88 (195)			51	49	47	45	44	42	41	39	38	37	36	35	33	32	31	31	30	29	28	27	26	26	25	25	24	
91 (200)				50	48	46	45	43	42	40	39	38	37	35	34	33	32	31	30	30	29	28	27	27	26	25	24	
93 (205)					50	47	46	44	43	41	40	39	38	36	35	34	33	32	31	30	29	29	28	27	26	26	25	
95 (210)						49	47	45	44	42	41	40	39	37	36	35	34	33	32	31	30	29	28	28	27	26	26	
98 (215)						50	48	46	45	43	42	41	40	38	37	36	35	34	33	32	31	30	29	28	28	27	26	
100 (220)							49	47	46	44	43	42	40	39	38	37	35	35	33	33	31	31	30	29	28	28	27	
102 (225)							51	49	47	45	44	42	41	40	38	37	36	35	34	33	32	31	30	30	29	28	27	
104 (230)								50	48	46	45	43	42	41	39	38	37	36	35	34	33	32	31	30	30	29	28	
107 (235)									49	47	46	44	43	42	40	39	38	37	36	35	34	33	32	31	30	30	29	
109 (240)									50	48	47	45	44	43	41	40	39	38	36	36	34	34	33	32	31	30	29	
111 (245)										49	48	46	45	43	42	41	39	38	37	36	35	34	33	32	31	31	30	
113 (250)										50	49	47	46	44	43	42	40	39	38	37	36	35	34	33	32	31	30	
116 (255)											50	48	47	45	44	42	41	40	39	38	37	36	35	34	33	32	31	
118 (260)												49	48	46	44	43	42	41	39	39	37	36	35	34	33	33	32	
120 (265)												50	49	47	45	44	43	42	40	39	38	37	36	35	34	33	32	
122 (270)													50	48	46	45	43	42	41	40	39	38	37	36	35	34	33	
125 (275)														49	47	46	44	43	42	41	39	38	37	36	35	35	33	
127 (280)															50	48	47	45	44	42	41	40	39	38	37	36	35	34
129 (285)															50	49	47	46	45	43	42	41	40	39	38	37	36	35
132 (290)																50	48	47	46	44	43	42	41	39	38	37	36	35
134 (295)																50	49	47	46	45	44	42	41	40	39	38	37	36
136 (300)																	50	48	47	45	44	43	42	41	40	39	38	37

FIGURE 4.7 Body mass index calculation for selected weight and stature. (From American Medical Association. *Guidelines for adolescent preventive services* [Recommendations monograph]. Chicago: American Medical Association, 1995.)

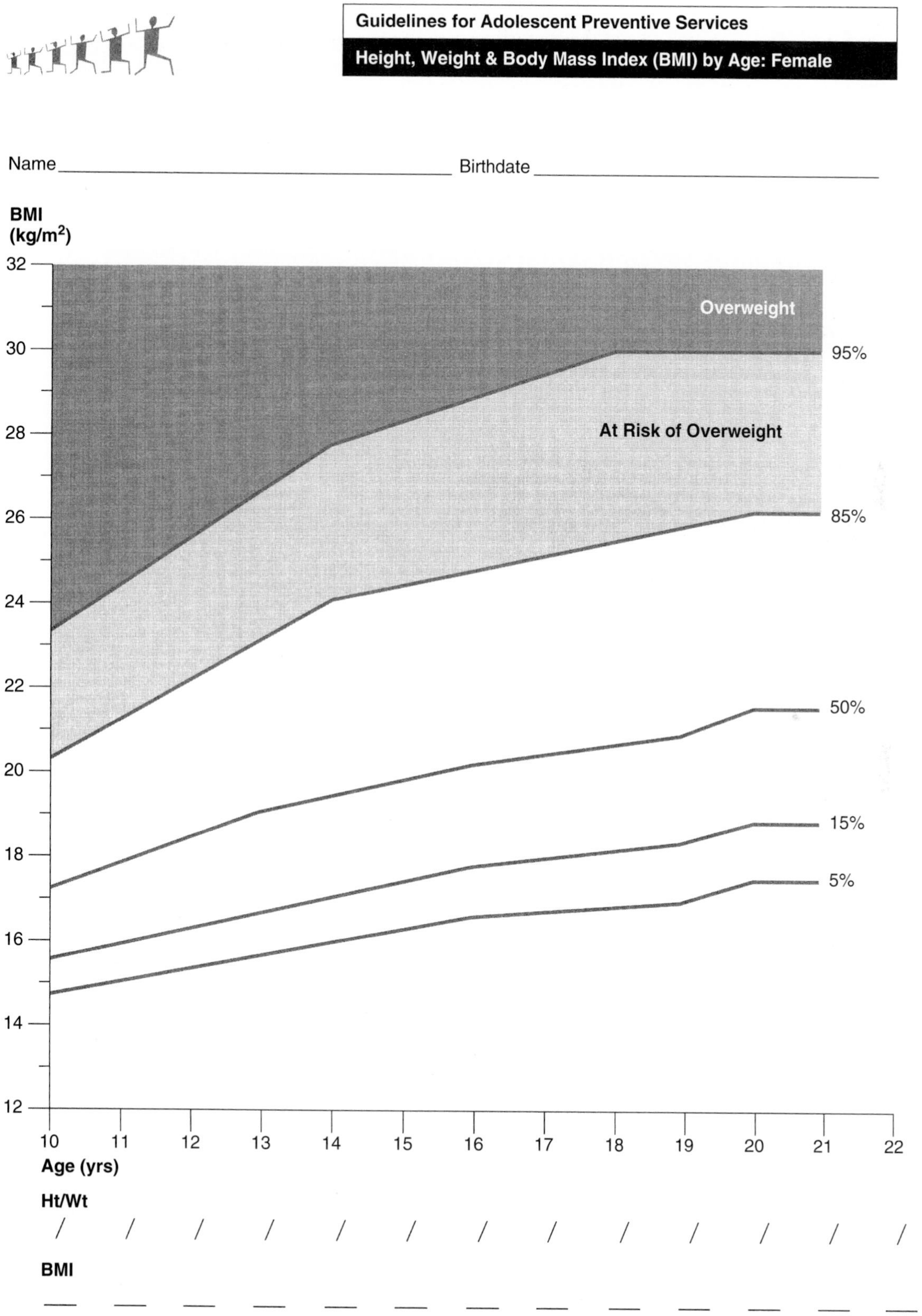

Guidelines for Adolescent Preventive Services

Height, Weight & Body Mass Index (BMI) by Age: Female

Name_____ Birthdate _____

BMI (kg/m²)

Overweight

95%

At Risk of Overweight

85%

50%

15%

5%

Age (yrs)

Ht/Wt

/   /   /   /   /   /   /   /   /   /   /   /   /

BMI

FIGURE 4.8 Tracking of height, weight, and body mass index by age: girls. (From American Medical Association. *Guidelines for adolescent preventive services* [Recommendations monograph]. Chicago: American Medical Association, 1995.)

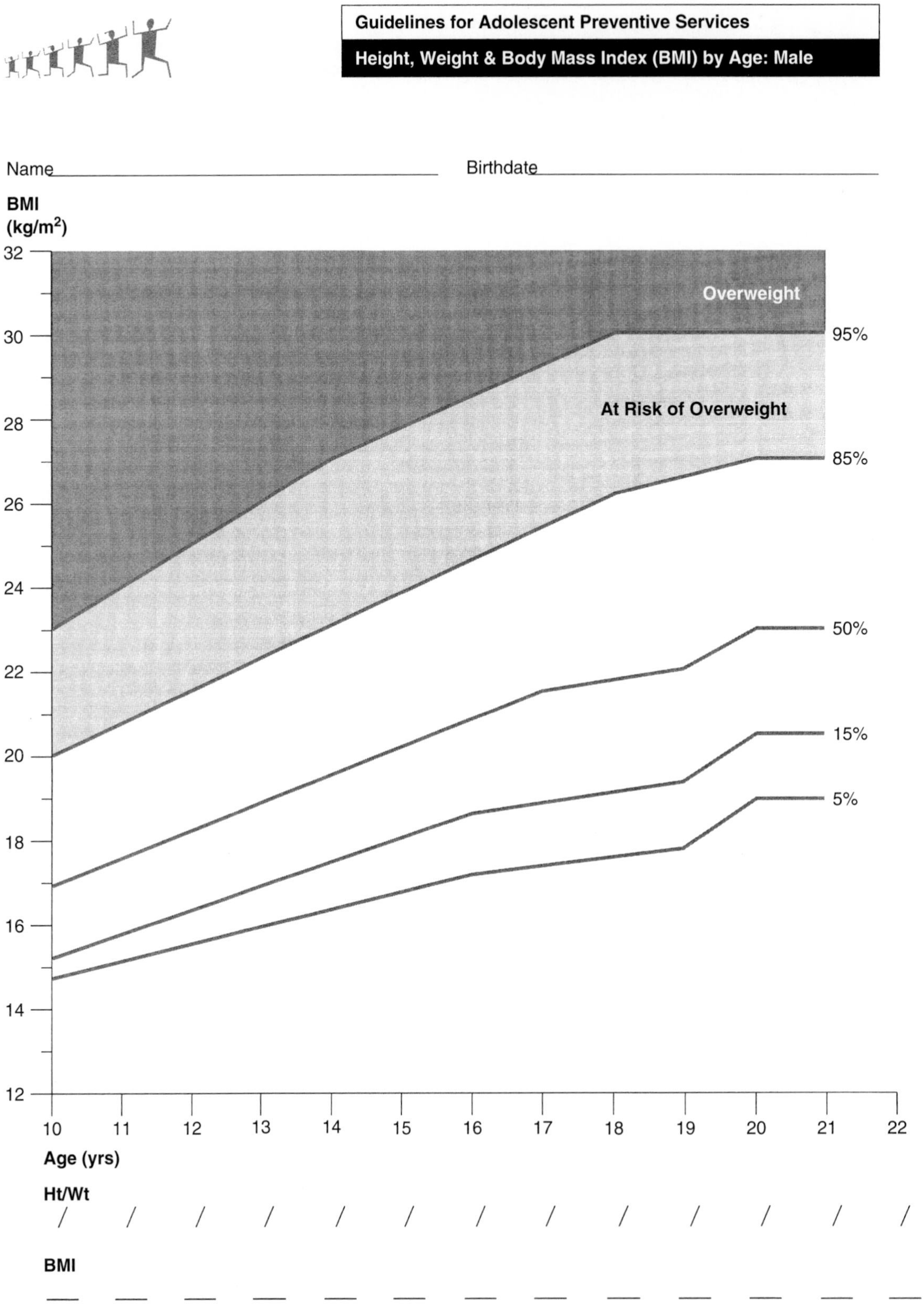

Guidelines for Adolescent Preventive Services

Height, Weight & Body Mass Index (BMI) by Age: Male

Name_____   Birthdate_____

FIGURE 4.9 Tracking of height, weight, and body mass index by age: boys. (From American Medical Association. *Guidelines for adolescent preventive services* [Recommendations monograph]. Chicago: American Medical Association, 1995.)

Guidelines for Adolescent Preventive Services								
Blood Pressure Value (mm Hg) by Age and Gender								
	Males (sitting)				**Females (sitting)**			
	Systolic		**Diastolic**		**Systolic**		**Diastolic**	
Age	**90%**	**95%**	**90%**	**95%**	**90%**	**95%**	**90%**	**95%**
11	119	123	76	80	119	123	77	81
12	122	126	77	81	122	126	78	82
13	124	128	77	81	124	128	78	83
14	126	130	78	82	125	129	81	85
15	129	133	79	83	126	130	82	86
16	132	136	81	85	127	131	81	85
17	133	138	83	87	127	132	81	84
18	136	140	84	88	127	132	80	84

Source: Second Task Force on Blood Pressure Control in Children. National Heart, Lung, Blood Institute, 1987.

FIGURE 4.10   The 90th and 95th percentiles for blood pressure by age and gender. (From American Medical Association. *Guidelines for adolescent preventive services* [Recommendations monograph]. Chicago: American Medical Association, 1995.)

Sexually Active Adolescents Suggested tests for sexually active adolescents are discussed in the following sections.

Females
Cervical gonorrhea and chlamydia culture or nonculture test, and vaginal wet mount are recommended. Syphilis serology should be considered in high-risk populations or where syphilis is prevalent. Screening for the HIV should be offered to all sexually active adolescents and should be encouraged for adolescents with any history of STD. Begin annual Pap smears 3 years after coitarche or at age 21.

Males
A leukocyte esterase test on the first 15 mL of a random urine sample is recommended to screen for *Chlamydia* infection. However, there is concern about the sensitivity and specificity of this test. In high-risk populations, annual urethral screening for gonorrhea and chlamydia by culture or nonculture test can be encouraged. Syphilis serology should be considered in high-risk populations or where syphilis is prevalent. Screening for the HIV virus should be offered to all sexually active adolescents and should be encouraged for adolescents with any history of STD.

Men who have sex with men
Annual syphilis serology, gonorrhea cultures (urethral, rectal, and pharyngeal), *Chlamydia* screening, and HIV screening are recommended. Homosexual males who are not already immunized should be screened for hepatitis B as well. Those with negative surface antigen and antibody tests should receive hepatitis B vaccine.

Liver Function Tests Liver function tests are not a routine screening test but should be obtained as indicated by the drug or alcohol history.

Cholesterol and Fasting Triglyceride Testing Targeted cholesterol and fasting triglyceride testing is indicated in adolescents with heart disease, hypertension, diabetes mellitus, or a family history of heart disease or hyperlipidemia. Intervention is indicated for individuals with a total cholesterol level >180 to 200 mg/dL on repeated testing (see Chapter 12). Some authorities advocate at least one screening cholesterol test during adolescence. Targeted screening in adolescents misses one third to one half of those teens with elevated cholesterol concentrations. However, the recommended intervention for most adolescents with mild to moderate hyperlipidemia is a prudent low-fat diet, which can be taught to all adolescents.

Human Immunodeficiency Virus Antibody Testing Routine screening for antibody to HIV is a controversial matter. Individuals at risk should be encouraged to receive HIV testing after a discussion regarding the benefits and possible negative consequences of the results (see Chapter 31). Individuals with any STD should be screened for others, including HIV infection.

Tuberculin Testing A purified protein derivative (PPD) tuberculin skin test should be considered at the first encounter with the adolescent based on an assessment of individual risk factors and recommendations of the local health department (in high-risk areas, screening is usually recommended yearly).

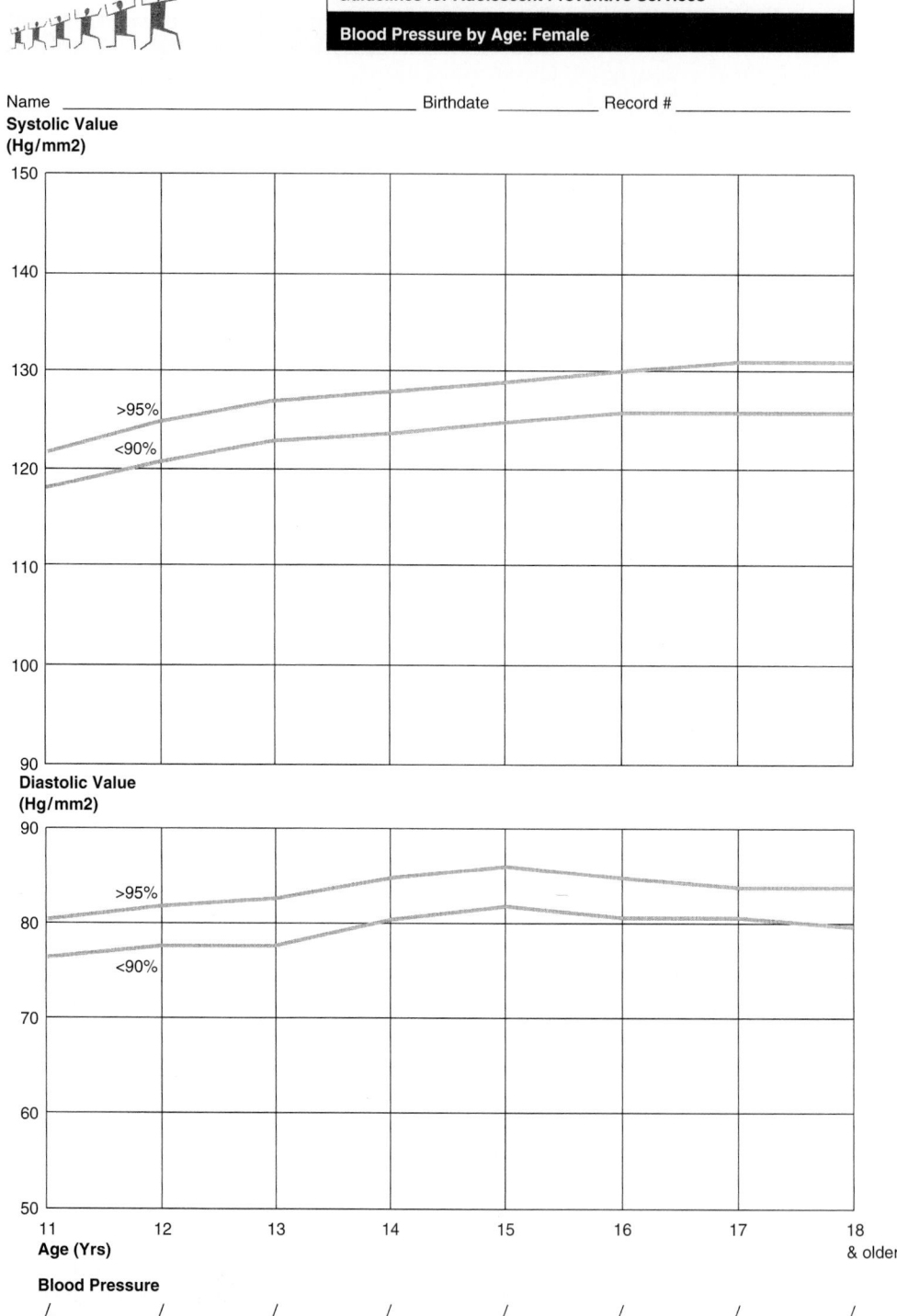

FIGURE 4.11 Tracking of blood pressure by age: girls. (From American Medical Association. *Guidelines for adolescent preventive services* [Recommendations monograph]. Chicago: American Medical Association, 1995.)

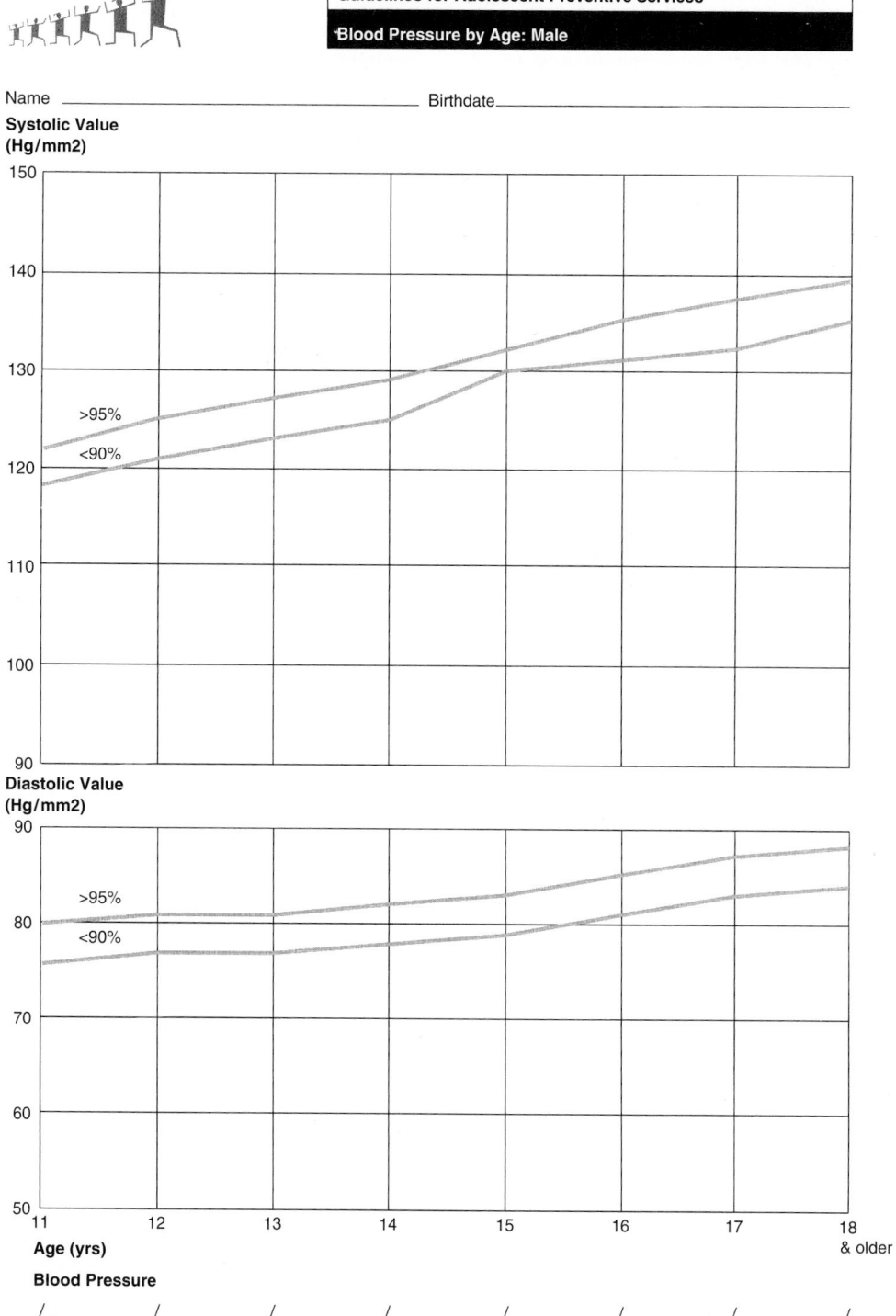

Tracking of blood pressure by age: boys. (From American Medical Association. *Guidelines for adolescent preventive services* [Recommendations monograph]. Chicago: American Medical Association, 1995.)

1. A tuberculin skin test is indicated for adolescents with known or suspected contact with persons with TB; for adolescents with clinical or radiographic findings suspicious for TB; for adolescents emigrating from countries where TB is endemic; and for adolescents traveling to endemic countries or who have contact with persons from those countries.
2. Annual tuberculin skin test is recommended for HIV-infected adolescents, adolescents living in homes with HIV-infected persons, and incarcerated adolescents.
3. Adolescents exposed to HIV-infected individuals, homeless persons, or nursing home residents; institutionalized adolescents; adolescents who use illicit drugs; migrant farm workers; and adolescents exposed to adults with any of these characteristics should have a tuberculin skin test every 2 to 3 years.
4. Tuberculin skin test screening is recommended once during adolescence for teens whose parents migrated from regions of the world with high TB prevalence and for those without specific risk factors who live in high-prevalence areas as determined by local public health agencies.

Recommendations from the Centers for Disease Control and Prevention (CDC) on interpretation of the PPD results include the following points:

1. An induration 5 mm or larger is classified as positive in the following persons:
   a. Those who have HIV infection or risk factors for HIV infection but unknown HIV status
   b. Those who have had recent close contact with persons with active TB
   c. Those with suspected TB based on clinical or radiographic evidence
2. An induration 10 mm or larger is classified as positive in all persons who do not meet any of the previous criteria but who have other risk factors for TB, including the following:
   a. Those in high-risk groups
      • Injection drug users known to be HIV seronegative
      • Persons who have other medical conditions that reportedly increase the risk of progression from latent TB infection to active TB, including:
        Silicosis
        Gastrectomy or jejunoileal bypass
        Being 10% or more below ideal body weight
        Chronic renal failure with renal dialysis
        Diabetes mellitus
        High-dose corticosteroid or other immunosuppressive therapy
        Some hematologic disorders, including malignancies such as leukemias and lymphomas
        Other malignancies
      • Children younger than 4 years
   b. Those in high-prevalence groups
      • Persons born in countries in Asia, Africa, the Caribbean, and Latin America that have high prevalence of TB
      • Persons from medically underserved, low-income populations
      • Residents of long-term care facilities (e.g., correctional institutions, nursing homes)
      • Persons from high-risk populations in their communities, as determined by local public health authorities

3. An induration 15 mm or larger is classified as positive in persons who do not meet any of the earlier criteria. Recent converters are defined on the basis of both size of induration and age of the person being tested:
   a. An increase of 10 mm or more within a 2-year period is classified as a recent conversion for persons younger than 35 years
   b. An increase of 15 mm or more within a 2-year period is classified as a recent conversion for persons 35 years of age or older

IMMUNIZATIONS

Obtaining the immunization history and completing the immunizations properly is increasingly important in the care of adolescents, because a variety of common childhood diseases appear during adolescence and the young adult years. This is a group that still has significant rates for nonimmunization. During 2001 to 2004, persons aged 20 years or older accounted for 50% of reported measles cases, and adolescents (age 10 to 19 years) accounted for 18.6% of cases. The rate of rubella susceptibility and risk for rubella infection are highest among young adults. The number of cases of varicella is falling in all ages with increasing immunization rates in infants and children; however, many adolescents and young adults remain susceptible. With increasing immunization rates, especially among the young, there is a corresponding decrease in the incidence of vaccine-preventable disease, with fewer opportunities for the nonimmunized population to be exposed to these diseases at a young age. As a result, there is an expansion of the nonimmunized, susceptible *adolescent* population.

With the advent of ever-newer vaccines, adolescents previously considered to be fully vaccinated suddenly find themselves "behind." The challenge of ensuring that adolescents' immunizations are up-to-date is compounded by the substantial number of adolescents who have received their immunizations in more than one place; inadequate documentation of prior vaccination remains a significant issue in the adolescent population. The issue of documentation may be resolved over time with the increasing use of vaccine registries. Because vaccination schedules remain a moving target, clinicians are well advised to keep abreast of the latest vaccine recommendations of the ACIP of the CDC. The current immunization schedule is available at http://www.cdc.gov. In addition, international travel information is available at http://www.cdc.gov/travel.

General Vaccination Information

Vaccination of adolescents is safe and should be seen as a high priority for adolescents whose previous immunization is lacking or incomplete. Adolescents who have been partially vaccinated can have their vaccination completed without restarting the series. Likewise, adolescents who begin vaccination can complete it at any time after the vaccination process is interrupted, even if there has been a substantial delay between doses. Vaccines should not be given more frequently than the recommended intervals. Although not every possible combination of vaccines has been explicitly tested, there are no contraindications to giving any or all of these vaccines simultaneously, so long as they are given at separate and appropriate anatomical

TABLE 4.3

Immunization Catch-up Schedule for Adolescents

Vaccine	Dose 1 to Dose 2	Dose 2 to Dose 3	Dose 3 to Booster
Tetanus/diptheria Td (Tdap)[a]	4 wk	6 mo	5 yr
Inactivated poliovirus vaccine (IPV)[b]	4 wk	4 wk	c
Hepatitis B (HBV)	4 wk	8 wk (and 16 wk after first dose)	
Measles, mumps, rubella (MMR)	4 wk		
Varicella	4 wk		

[a]Tdap may be substituted for any dose in the catch-up series or as a booster if age-appropriate for Tdap. A 5-year interval is recommended from the last Td dose when Tdap is used as a booster dose.

[b]IPV is not generally recommended for persons 18 years of age or older.

[c]A fourth dose is recommended only if the patient is younger than 18 years and has received both IPV and oral polio vaccine (OPV) as part of their series.

sites. Nevertheless, many clinicians faced with having to give four or five vaccines choose to offer the patient a return visit to limit the number of simultaneous injections.

Informed Consent

Since 1994, all health care providers who administer measles-mumps-rubella (MMR), polio, diphtheria and tetanus toxoids and pertussis (DTP), and Td vaccines have been required to distribute vaccine information sheets each time a patient is vaccinated. The clinic or office should obtain a signature of either the patient, parent, or guardian to acknowledge having been provided with vaccine information. This should also be noted in the medical record. Appropriate documentation of vaccination includes consent for vaccination, immunization type, date of administration, injection site manufacturer and lot number of vaccine, and name and address of the health care provider administering the vaccine. Helping patients and their families to maintain their own immunization records facilitates proper vaccination of adolescents who may go on to receive immunizations in more than one location. Vaccination registries, which are available online in many states, will also improve this process.

Erroneous Contraindications against Vaccination

In an effort to improve vaccination rates, the ACIP has specifically addressed a variety of situations in which many practitioners have deferred or delayed vaccination. Situations that specifically *do not* represent contraindications to vaccination include the following:

1. Reaction to a previous dose of DTP vaccine with only soreness, redness, or swelling
2. Mild acute illness with low-grade fever
3. Current antimicrobial therapy
4. Pregnancy in the adolescent's mother or in another household contact
5. Recent exposure to an infectious disease
6. Breast-feeding
7. History of nonspecific allergies
8. Allergy to penicillin or other antimicrobials except anaphylactic reactions to neomycin or streptomycin
9. Allergies to duck meat or duck feathers
10. Family history of seizures in children who require vaccination

Furthermore, "minor illnesses" such as mild upper respiratory tract infections, with or without low-grade fever, are not contraindications for vaccination. Inappropriate avoidance of vaccination because of a mild acute illness has contributed to many missed opportunities for vaccinating children and adolescents.

Vaccination during Pregnancy

Because of theoretical risks to the developing fetus, live attenuated virus vaccines are not routinely given to pregnant women or to those who are likely to become pregnant within 3 months of receiving the vaccine. There is no convincing evidence of risk to the fetus after immunization of pregnant women with inactivated virus vaccines, bacterial vaccines, or toxoids. This includes tetanus and diphtheria toxoid. There is also no risk to the fetus from passive immunization of pregnant women with immune globulin. Because MMR vaccine viruses are not transmitted from individuals receiving them, children of pregnant women may receive these vaccines.

Sample Schedule for Nonimmunized Adolescents

Most adolescents seeking preventive health services are either fully or partially immunized. For adolescents who have received no immunizations, a sample immunization schedule is provided in Table 4.3. Immunization recommendations are updated annually by the CDC and can be found at http://www.immunize.org/cdc/child-schedule.pdf.

Adolescents with Human Immunodeficiency Virus Infection

Vaccine recommendations for HIV-infected adolescents are described in the text for individual vaccines and are summarized in Table 4.4.

Diphtheria, Tetanus, Pertussis

It is now well known that adolescents and adults have a higher incidence and prevalence of pertussis than children. In recent years, the highest increase in cases has been in the 10 to 19 years age-group. In adolescents, pertussis infection typically presents clinically as a mild respiratory infection that goes on to produce a protracted (3 or more

TABLE 4.4

Recommendations for Immunization of Human Immunodeficiency Virus–Infected Patients

Vaccine	Asymptomatic	Symptomatic
Tdap/Td	Yes	Yes
IPV	Yes	Yes
MMR	Yes	Yes, consider
Hepatitis B	Yes	Yes
Varicella	No	No
Pneumococcal	Yes	Yes
Meningococcal	optional	optional
Influenza	Optional	Yes

IPV, inactivated poliovirus vaccine; MMR, measles-mumps-rubella.

weeks) cough. Adolescents with pertussis make frequent health care visits and miss considerable school days. In one study, 83% of adolescents with pertussis missed an average of 5.5 days of school. Moreover, in nearly half of households with an ill adolescent, a parent missed many days of work.

Two new tetanus toxoid, diphtheria toxoid, and acellular pertussis (Tdap) vaccines created for use in adolescents and adults have recently been approved for use in the United States. Boostrix is a product of GlaxoSmithKline and is licensed for use in adolescents aged 10 to 18 years. Adacel is a product of Sanofi Pasteur and is licensed for use in adolescents and adults aged 11 to 64 years. Both of these vaccines have been demonstrated to be safe and effective when administered as a single booster dose to adolescents. The ACIP now recommends that adolescents aged 11 to 18 who have completed their primary vaccination series against diphtheria, pertussis, and tetanus now receive a single dose of Tdap instead of the Td. The preferred age for Tdap vaccination is 11 to 12 years; ideally, Tdap should be given concurrently with the new tetravalent meningococcal conjugate vaccine (Menactra; see subsequent text). Tdap can be administered concurrently with other vaccines as well using a separate syringe at a different anatomic site. Adolescents who have already received a single dose of Td should still receive a single dose of Tdap between the ages of 11 and 18 years. An interval of at least 5 years is recommended (but not required) between Td and Tdap to reduce the risk of reactions. After Tdap vaccination, Td boosters continue to be recommended every 10 years throughout life. The dose of Tdap is 0.5 mL administered intramuscularly in the deltoid muscle.

Contraindications

Tdap is contraindicated in those who have had serious allergic reactions to any of its components and in those who have developed encephalopathy associated with previous pertussis vaccination. Tdap should be deferred in patients who developed Guillain-Barré syndrome (GBS) associated with previous tetanus toxoid vaccination and in those with progressive encephalopathies or uncontrolled epilepsy. Vaccination should be postponed in patients who are acutely ill with moderate–serious illnesses until the illness has resolved. Reactions to previous DTP/Tdap vaccination (except those noted earlier) are generally not contraindications to vaccination. Neither are breast-feeding, immunosuppression, or intercurrent minor illnesses. Because pregnant women have been excluded from prelicensure trials, neither Tdap vaccines are approved for use in pregnancy (Pregnancy Category C). However, Td vaccine, also Pregnancy Category C, has been used extensively during pregnancy without any evidence of teratogenicity and pregnancy is not considered a contraindication to Tdap vaccination.

Adverse Effects

The most common side effect of either Tdap vaccine was pain at the injection site. No serious adverse effects related to vaccination have been observed in the first 6 months of postvaccination monitoring with either Boostrix or ADACEL.

Pertussis infection in adolescents is discussed in detail in Chapter 29.

Hepatitis A

The hepatitis A vaccination now offers effective, long-lasting protection against this virus. Two vaccines are available: Havrix (SmithKline Beecham Biologicals) and Vaqta (Merck & Co.). The vaccines are inactivated and come in adult and pediatric formulations, with different dosages and administration schedules. Almost 100% of children, adolescents, and adults develop protective levels of antibody to hepatitis A virus after completing the vaccine series. The vaccine can be administered simultaneously with other vaccines and toxoids, including hepatitis B, diphtheria, and tetanus, without altering immunogenicity or adverse effects. However, other vaccines should be given at separate injection sites. The recommended dosing is described in Table 4.5.

1. Children who should be routinely vaccinated include those who live in states, counties, or communities where the average annual rate of hepatitis A between 1987 and 1997 was $\geq$20 cases per 100,000 (i.e., about twice the national average).
2. Vaccination should be considered for children who live in states, counties, or communities where the average annual rate of hepatitis A between 1987 and 1997 was <20 but $\geq$10 cases per 100,000 (i.e., above the national average but < twice the national average).

TABLE 4.5

Dosing Recommendations for Hepatitis A Vaccine

Age (yr)	ELISA Units	Volume (mL)	No. of Doses	Months
Havrix				
2–18	720	0.5	2	0, 6–12
>18	1,440	1.0	2	0, 6–12
Vaqta				
2–17	25	0.5	2	0, 6–18
>17	50	1.0	2	0, 6

ELISA, enzyme-linked immunosorbent assay.
The Advisory Committee on Immunization Practices (ACIP) (CDC, 1999) recommends these dosages.

Twinrix (GlaxoSmithKline) is also available containing both vaccines for hepatitis A and hepatitis B. Hepatitis A, including others for whom the vaccine is recommended, is discussed in detail in Chapter 30.

Hepatitis B

Two recombinant hepatitis B vaccines (Recombivax HB and Engerix-B) are used currently in the United States. Universal vaccination is now recommended in the United States, and the ACIP recommends the three-dose hepatitis B vaccine series for adolescents at age 11 to 12 years who have not previously been immunized. Vaccination should be a special priority for the following persons:

1. Those with lifestyle risk
   a. Sexually active adolescents with more than one partner in preceding 6 months
   b. Persons with any history of STD
   c. Homosexual and bisexual men
   d. Users of injectable drugs
2. Those with occupational risk
3. Those with environmental risk factors
   a. Household and sexual contacts of carriers
   b. Adoptees from countries with high hepatitis B endemicity
   c. Populations with high endemicity of hepatitis B infection, such as Alaskan Natives, Pacific Islanders, and refugees from endemic areas
   d. Clients and staff of institutions for mentally retarded individuals
   e. Inmates of long-term correctional facilities
   f. Certain international travelers
   g. Other contacts of hepatitis B carriers
4. Special patient groups, such as recipients of hemodialysis treatment or clotting factor concentrates

Persons in casual contact with carriers in settings such as schools and offices are at minimal risk of hepatitis B infection, and vaccine is not routinely recommended.

Hepatitis B is discussed in detail in Chapter 30.

Hepatitis B vaccine is given in a three-dose series. The second dose is given 1 to 2 months after the first, and the third dose is given 4 to 6 months after the first. The series does *not* need to be restarted if it is interrupted. The three-dose hepatitis B vaccine induces protective antibodies (anti-HBs) in >90% of healthy adults and >95% of infants, children, and adolescents through 19 years of age. Protective effects appear to be quite durable and long lasting. Hepatitis B vaccine can be given simultaneously with other vaccines.

Adverse reactions to hepatitis B immunization are unusual. Pain at the injection site and fever are the most commonly reported adverse effects. Anaphylaxis is rare. Anecdotal cases of autoimmune disease, chronic fatigue syndrome, GBS, and CNS diseases associated with hepatitis B vaccination have not been causally linked to immunization.

Haemophilus Influenzae Type B

Haemophilus influenzae type B vaccine is indicated for those adolescents not previously immunized who are at risk because of splenic dysfunction or other conditions. A single dose of 0.5 mL is recommended.

Human Papillomavirus

Two vaccines for prophylaxis against human papillomavirus (HPV) have been developed, a quadrivalent vaccine (Gardasil, Merck & Co.) and a bivalent vaccine (see Chapter 66). The quadrivalent vaccine was licensed in June 2006 by the FDA and the ACIP has recommended that it be routinely given to girls aged 11 to 12 years. The quadrivalent vaccine targets HPV types 16 and 18 (the most common HPV types implicated in cervical cancer) as well as HPV types 6 and 11 (the most common HPV types associated with genital warts). So far, both vaccines have been shown to be safe, highly immunogenic, and to prevent infections with HPV types 16 and/or 18 in randomized, double-blind, placebo-controlled trials. Approximately 70% of cervical cancer is related to HPV types 16 and 18 and 90% of genital warts are related to types 6 and 11. Therefore, the potential is very high to prevent a significant number of both genital warts and cervical cancer. Vaccine-related adverse effects were rare and no serious adverse effects have been reported.

The current recommendation is that the quadrivalent vaccine (Gardasil) be given to girls aged 11 to 12, but the vaccination series of three vaccines can be started as early as age 9 at the discretion of the health care provider. Ideally, vaccination should occur before the onset of sexual activity as the vaccine will not be effective against any HPV subtypes that may have been already acquired. However, women aged 13 to 26, even if they are already sexually active, are thought to benefit from the vaccine as well, acquiring protection from any HPV subtypes to which they have not already been exposed. "Catch-up" vaccination has also been recommended by the ACIP. The vaccine is not currently recommended for males. Time and experience will establish how vigorously the vaccine will be endorsed by health care providers, or how the vaccine will be accepted by patients and families. The longer-term effects of vaccination on cervical cancer are unclear and less is known even about the effect of vaccination on other cancers (e.g., vulvar, penile, anal). Although some individuals have raised concerns that increased or riskier sexual behavior will be an unintended consequence of the vaccine, there is no evidence to support these claims. Finally, widespread deployment of HPV vaccines will likely have an eventual effect of the recommendations for cervical cancer screening. However, the current vaccine offers no protection against 30% of the HPV subtypes currently causing cervical cancer, so some strategy for cancer screening will continue to be required. Despite these unanswered questions, it seems likely that these new vaccines have the potential to dramatically reduce rates of genital warts and cervical and other cancers.

Influenza

Vaccine

Influenza continues to cause major outbreaks of illness, usually beginning in December or January each year. If vaccine is administered, it ought to be given in the fall. Two types of vaccine are available, an inactivated vaccine and a live attenuated vaccine. Both vaccine types contain three virus strains (two type A and one type B), representing the strains most commonly found worldwide and predicted to be most likely to cause infections in the coming year. Vaccines are updated annually. Influenza in adolescents is discussed in detail in Chapter 29.

Indications

Vaccination with inactivated influenza vaccine is recommended for the following adolescents because of their increased risk for complications from influenza:

- Adolescents (and young adults) who are residents of nursing homes and other chronic-care facilities that house persons with chronic medical conditions
- Adolescents (and young adults) who have chronic disorders of the pulmonary or cardiovascular systems, including asthma (hypertension is not considered a high-risk condition)
- Adolescents (and young adults) who have required regular medical follow-up or hospitalization during the preceding year because of chronic metabolic diseases (including diabetes mellitus), renal dysfunction, hemoglobinopathies, or immunosuppression (including immunosuppression caused by medications or by HIV)
- Adolescents (and young adults) who have any condition (e.g., cognitive dysfunction, spinal cord injuries, seizure disorders, or other neuromuscular disorders) that can compromise respiratory function or the handling of respiratory secretions or that can increase the risk for aspiration
- Adolescents (up to age 18 years) who are receiving long-term aspirin therapy and, therefore, might be at risk for experiencing Reye syndrome after influenza infection
- Adolescent and young adult women who are pregnant during the influenza season

Adolescents who might transmit influenza to those at high risk should also be vaccinated. These include the following:

- Adolescents (and young adults) who are household contacts of persons in groups at high risk
- Adolescents (and young adults) who provide home care to persons in groups at high risk

In addition, the vaccine should be administered to any person who wishes to reduce the likelihood of becoming ill with influenza or transmitting influenza to others. Students or other persons in institutional settings (e.g., those who reside in dormitories) should be encouraged to receive the vaccine to minimize disruption to their routine activities during epidemics.

Inactivated influenza vaccine is administered intramuscularly in the deltoid muscle. Only a single dose is required for those older than 9 years. It is contraindicated in persons with anaphylactic reactions to eggs and it should be delayed in those with significant febrile illnesses (but not in those with minor upper respiratory infections).

Live, attenuated influenza vaccine (LAIV) is marketed in the United States as Flumist. It is administered intranasally and is indicated for healthy persons aged 5 to 49 years, including those who may have contact with high-risk groups. It is contraindicated in adolescents with asthma, reactive airways disease, or other chronic condition; in adolescents receiving aspirin or other salicylates (because of the association of Reye syndrome with wild-type influenza infection); in adolescents with a history of GBS; in pregnant women; or in adolescents with a history of hypersensitivity, including anaphylaxis, to eggs. LAIV should not be used in those who will have close contact with severely immunocompromised persons within 7 days of vaccination. LAIV is administered only through the intranasal route, 0.25 mL in each nostril. Only a single dose

is required for those older than 9 years. A refrigerator stable version with broader age indications for both healthy and at-risk individuals may be available by the 2008 influenza season.

Adverse Effects

The most common adverse effects of LAIV include runny nose, nasal congestion, and sore throat. Serious adverse effects are rare (rates <1%).

Chemoprophylaxis

Chemoprophylaxis drugs are also available to help prevent influenza. Chemoprophylaxis is appropriate for individuals who are at high risk and who either have not been immunized or are exposed to influenza before a vaccine response has occurred (2 weeks). It is also useful for immunosuppressed adolescents who may not respond to the vaccine and for adolescents for whom vaccination is contraindicated. Chemoprophylaxis for influenza is discussed in Chapter 29.

Measles

Measles has been decreasing dramatically in the United States, with 441,703 cases in 1960; 47,351 in 1970; 13,506 in 1980; 2,933 in 1988; and 312 in 1993. There was an increase to 963 in 1994, but the number dropped to 288 in 1995, and case numbers in 1997, 1998, and 1999 reached all-time lows. In 2004, only 37 confirmed measles cases were reported to the CDC. Measles is not considered endemic in the United States at this time; the incidence is <0.02 cases per 100,000 population.

Although the potential still exists for measles epidemics on college campuses, reported case numbers are low at present because of cyclical changes in measles incidence, improvement in measles vaccination coverage among preschool-aged children, and increased use of a second dose of vaccine among school- and college-aged youth. Because of the low incidence of measles, suspected cases should be confirmed by serology. Because of the problem of waning immunity, it is now universally recommended that children and adolescents receive a second vaccination either at primary school level or on entry to junior high school. If these opportunities are missed, the vaccine should be caught up whenever the teen presents for health care. Likewise, all young adults who enter college or other institutions of postsecondary education should have documentation of receiving two doses of measles vaccine, and those who do not have such documentation should receive a second dose of vaccine. In practice, measles vaccine is usually administered as MMR vaccine.

Adolescents should be vaccinated if there is no evidence of prior live measles virus immunization received after 1 year of age, unless the adolescent has had physician-diagnosed measles or has laboratory-confirmed immunity. Routine serological testing for immunity to measles is not indicated before immunization.

Exposed Susceptible Adolescents

Unvaccinated adolescents exposed to measles should receive measles vaccine. If more than 5 days has elapsed since exposure, immune serum globulin (IVIG), 0.25 mL/kg, is also given.

Immunosuppressed Adolescents

Vaccination with live measles virus, or any other live virus, is contraindicated in immunosuppressed patients and in those receiving immunosuppressive therapy. At present, information available on MMR vaccination among asymptomatic and symptomatic HIV-infected individuals has not demonstrated serious or unusually adverse events. Therefore, HIV-infected patients can be immunized so long as they are not actively immunocompromised. Adolescents with leukemia in remission can also be vaccinated, as can those who have had short-term (<2 weeks), low- to moderate-dose systemic corticosteroid therapy, topical steroid therapy, or intraarticular steroid injections.

Adverse Effects

Adverse effects of measles vaccine include fever, rash, and, rarely, transient thrombocytopenia. There is no causal link between measles vaccination and seizures, encephalitis, or encephalopathy.

Meningococcal Vaccine

Routine vaccination against meningococcal disease became the recommendation of the ACIP beginning in 2005, coinciding with the availability of a new tetravalent meningococcal polysaccharide-protein conjugate vaccine (MCV4) marketed as Menactra by Sanofi Pasteur. Subsequently, the AAP has also recommended routine vaccination with the new MCV4 vaccine. Like the meningococcal vaccine that preceded it, MCV4 provides immunity against serotypes A, C, Y, and W135. However, unlike the previous meningococcal vaccine, the new vaccine is likely to provide protection that is substantially longer lasting. The current recommendation is for adolescents to be immunized as part of a preadolescent health supervision visit at age 11 to 12 years. For those not receiving the vaccine at age 11 to 12 years, immunization before high school entry is recommended. Routine vaccination for college students living in dormitories, military recruits, and others at high risk continues to be recommended. Because their risk is low, routine vaccination of adults who are not members of high-risk groups is not recommended. However, the vaccine is licensed for use for those aged 11 to 55 years; therefore, adults who wish to reduce their risk of meningococcal disease may elect to be vaccinated. The vaccine is given as a single 0.5 mL dose, administered intramuscularly.

Contraindications

Vaccination with MCV4 is contraindicated in those who have severe allergic reactions to any of its components (which include diphtheria toxoid and natural latex). Vaccination should be postponed in cases of moderate to severe illness; minor acute illnesses are not a contraindication to vaccination. Because MCV4 is inactivated, immunosuppression is not a contraindication (although the protection in immunocompromised patients may be reduced). No data is available on vaccination with MCV4 during pregnancy.

Adverse Effects

Local redness, pain, and swelling were the most common adverse effects. Serious adverse effects have not occurred at rates higher than would be expected in the adolescent population. Concern about a possible association between vaccination with MCV4 and GBS have been raised after seven cases of GBS were identified occurring 11 to 31 days after vaccination. However, the number of cases of GBS is not higher than would be expected in the unvaccinated population. At this time, the CDC is investigating further but has made no changes in the recommendations for vaccination.

Mumps

The number of cases of mumps has declined dramatically in the United States, from 59,647 cases in 1975 to 8,576 in 1980; 2,982 in 1985; 1,537 in 1994; 338 cases in 2000; and 258 cases in 2003. However, a recent mumps outbreak in 2006 highlights the importance of continued vigilance. Many of the involved individuals in this outbreak were college students, indicating the importance of this age-group as susceptible individuals. Approximately 65% of mumps cases now occur in patients between 10 and 19 years of age, with approximately 20% or more of such adolescents developing orchitis. A live mumps virus vaccine was developed in 1967. The vaccine has few side effects, and >90% of susceptible patients develop protective, long-lasting antibodies. Mumps vaccine is usually administered as MMR. Susceptible adolescents should receive a single dose of mumps vaccine alone or as MMR. Susceptible adolescents are those without documented live mumps vaccination beyond the age of 1 year, unless they have had physician-diagnosed mumps or have laboratory evidence of mumps immunity. Tests for immunity are unnecessary, because revaccination is safe.

Exposed Susceptible Adolescents

Nonvaccinated adolescents who are exposed to mumps should be immunized with the vaccine; vaccination has not been shown to prevent disease in such cases, but it will help prevent future infection. There is no evidence of efficacy of immune globulin.

Contraindications

Vaccination should be avoided in adolescents who are pregnant, have a serious febrile illness, have an immunodeficiency, are receiving immunosuppressive therapy, or have leukemia or lymphoma. HIV infection, unless the adolescent is severely immunocompromised, is not a contraindication to mumps vaccination.

Adverse Effects

Adverse reactions to mumps vaccine, including allergic reactions, are extremely rare. Purported reactions to mumps vaccine, including seizures and other CNS events, have not been causally linked to immunization.

Pneumococcal Vaccine

Pneumococcal vaccine is indicated for individuals with a chronic illness, particularly of the cardiovascular or pulmonary system. It is also indicated for those who are at increased risk of pneumococcal disease, including patients with nephrotic syndrome, sickle cell disease, asplenia or functional asplenia, HIV infection, or B-cell immune deficiency, as well as patients at risk for meningitis. The duration of immunity is unclear and revaccination is not currently recommended by the CDC; however, some centers recommend reimmunization with pneumococcal vaccine (Pneumovax 23) 3 to 5 years after primary immunization in patients who are at especially high risk.

Poliovirus

The last reported case of poliomyelitis caused by locally acquired wild-type virus in the United States occurred more than 20 years ago. Killed-virus inactivated poliovirus vaccine (IPV) is now the vaccine of choice, and oral poliovirus vaccine (OPV) is no longer recommended for use in the United States. Routine vaccination of nonimmunized adults is not required unless they are at particularly high risk because of travel to endemic areas, exposure to wild poliovirus, or occupational exposure. The immunization schedule for nonimmunized adolescents consists of three doses of IPV—two doses with an interval of 4 to 8 weeks, and a third dose 6 to 12 months after the second dose. Persons exposed to wild poliovirus may receive an additional dose of IPV. Immunosuppression is not a contraindication to vaccination. There is a theoretical risk during pregnancy, so vaccination of pregnant women should be avoided. There is also a theoretical risk of anaphylaxis in patients with known allergies to streptomycin, polymyxin B, and neomycin. Adverse effects from the currently available IPV vaccine have not been described.

Rubella

The number of cases of rubella in the United States has continued a marked decline, with 46,975 cases in 1966; 16,652 in 1975; 3,904 in 1980; 630 in 1985; 221 in 1988; 200 in 1995; and only 10 cases in 2004! Colleges have been high-risk settings for rubella transmission; cases of rubella have often occurred among nonimmunized adults in outbreaks in colleges and workplaces. Therefore, proof of rubella and measles immunity should continue to be required for attendance from both male and female students. All students who enter institutions of postsecondary education should have documentation of having received at least one dose of rubella vaccine or other evidence of rubella immunity. The diagnosis of acute rubella should be confirmed serologically with either the presence of immunoglobulin M (IgM) antibody or a significant rise in IgG titers. Rubella vaccination is usually administered as MMR.

Vaccination during Pregnancy

In 1979, a new rubella vaccine, RA 27/3 (Meruvax II), was introduced that leads to higher titers with fewer side effects. A review of rubella vaccination for the period 1971–1989, in which 321 known rubella-susceptible pregnant women vaccinated with live rubella vaccine within 3 months before or after conception were monitored, showed that none of the infants had malformations compatible with congenital rubella infection. The estimated risk with 95% confidence limits is from 0% to 1.2% with an observed risk of zero. The U.S. Public Health Service nevertheless recommends that women of childbearing age be asked whether they are pregnant. If they say no, they should be advised of the theoretical risk to a fetus from vaccination and instructed to avoid pregnancy for 3 months; they may then be vaccinated. Routine pregnancy testing before vaccination is not indicated. Certainly, if there is any question whether the adolescent might be pregnant, vaccination can be deferred until the question is resolved. When time and cost are not prohibitive, female adolescents can be tested serologically before vaccination. However, this should no longer be done routinely and should not interfere with immunization programs. Clinical diagnosis should not be relied on as evidence of rubella infection.

Males

Males without evidence of prior vaccination should also be vaccinated to decrease the community prevalence of susceptible individuals and therefore the risk of exposure to susceptible pregnant females.

Immunocompromised Adolescents

Replication of vaccine viruses can be enhanced in persons with immune deficiency diseases and in persons with immunosuppression, such as individuals with leukemia, lymphoma, or generalized malignancy and those receiving immunosuppressants or large doses of corticosteroids. Such persons should not receive live rubella virus vaccine. Asymptomatic HIV-infected persons in need of an MMR vaccination may receive it so long as severe immunocompromise is absent. Vaccinations should not be given to adolescents with serious febrile illnesses but should not be postponed because of a mild illness, such as an upper respiratory tract infection. Adverse effects from rubella vaccination include fever, rash, lymphadenopathy, and transient arthritis or arthralgias. Purported CNS events associated with immunization have not been causally linked to vaccination.

Varicella

There were more than 151,000 reported cases of varicella in 1994, with an estimated 3.7 million cases in the United States each year. With widespread vaccination, fewer than 33,000 cases were reported in 2004. Still, varicella results in more than 9,000 hospitalizations annually, and in 2004, accounted for nine reported deaths. Whereas younger patients usually have uncomplicated chickenpox, older ones have more serious infections with higher rates of complications. The estimate from the CDC is that about $384 million could be saved annually with vaccine usage. A live attenuated varicella vaccination for chickenpox was approved in 1995 for use in children, adolescents, and adults. The vaccine is marketed under the name Varivax and is approximately 70% to 90% effective in preventing varicella. Varicella vaccination is now recommended for persons of all ages without documented chickenpox or measurable levels of protective antibody.

Children and young adolescents between 1 and 13 years of age without documented varicella infection should receive a single dose of varicella vaccine. Adolescents 13 years or older should receive two doses of varicella vaccine, 4 to 8 weeks apart. Immunization is also recommended for susceptible adults, particularly those at residential or occupational risk and those living or working with children. The vaccine can be co administered with MMR vaccine. Varivax is a live attenuated vaccine. It is not recommended for children younger than 1 year of age, pregnant women, people who are hypersensitive to gelatin or other vaccine components, those with a history of anaphylactoid reaction to neomycin, or those with active untreated TB. The vaccine should also be avoided in immunosuppressed patients (including those who are immunocompromised from HIV infection) and those who are receiving immunosuppressive therapy. Approximately 5% to 10% of persons vaccinated develop a rash, which can be contagious. Other adverse reactions include redness, hardness, and swelling at the injection site; fatigue; malaise; and nausea.

PREVENTIVE HEALTH INTERVENTIONS

The practice of medicine is often more of an art than a science, and this is especially true in the care of adolescents. Only through experience do practitioners develop a style that "works" for them. Clinicians working with adolescent patients must feel comfortable in screening for psychosocial morbidity and assessing the level of risk in individual adolescent patients. This includes screening patients for risks associated with sensitive health issues such as sexual behavior, substance use, and mental health concerns. However, adequate screening is insufficient if it is not followed up with appropriate and effective intervention strategies when patients screen "positive" for serious health risks. The next steps—that is, how to deliver relevant health education and offer effective, brief office interventions—are not nearly as straightforward. Some precepts from behavioral medicine are important in designing practical office interventions:

1. Health education should be targeted to the specific needs of the patient.
2. The patient and physician should agree on the goals for behavior change and the approach to be used.
3. Barriers to the proposed change should be explored, and specific strategies to overcome these barriers should be discussed.
4. Monitoring, feedback, and positive reinforcement should be an integral part of the overall plan.
5. Once behavioral change has occurred, a plan for maintenance should be addressed.

Imagine a clinical encounter where a sexually active adolescent patient is asked about condom use. The patient responds that she uses condoms "sometimes." At this point, a not infrequent clinician response is to wax eloquent for a few minutes on the importance and health benefits of condom use, with the patient usually listening respectfully and offering little. The clinician feels good about the "counseling" that has been offered, but the patient generally has gotten almost nothing of value from the interaction. In fact, the patient already understands the value of condoms—after all, she is using them sometimes. For this patient, the problem with condom use lies elsewhere—she can't afford them, her partner refuses to use them, someone is allergic to latex, or, most frequently, there never seems to be a condom available when one is required. None of these potential barriers is likely to emerge while the clinician sermonizes from atop a soapbox. Productive advice for this particular patient does not rest in a general treatise on the value of condoms but rather in addressing directly the specific barriers faced by the individual patient. This requires active listening, explicit questioning, specific strategies, and the willingness to go back and make sure that the intervention has been successful. Inherent in this approach is clinicians' willingness to go beyond screening and on to interventions and solutions, to engage with patients on difficult and sometimes sensitive issues, and, most importantly, to take the time to fully understand the context of health-risk behavior.

The G-A-P-S Algorithm

As part of the GAPS project, the AMA has attempted to develop a standardized method of assessment and intervention that embodies current health education principles but remains practical for office practice. The mnemonic G-A-P-S is used: *gather* information, *assess* further, *problem* identification, and specific *solutions* (Fig. 4.13). A publication from the AMA, *GAPS: Clinical Evaluation and Management Handbook,* includes fully developed algorithms for each of the GAPS recommendations (available at http://www.ama-assn.org/adolhlth).

G: Gather Initial Information Screen for problems using simple trigger questions, such as, "Have you been feeling down and blue?" or "Do you usually wear seat belts while riding in a car?" As has already been discussed,

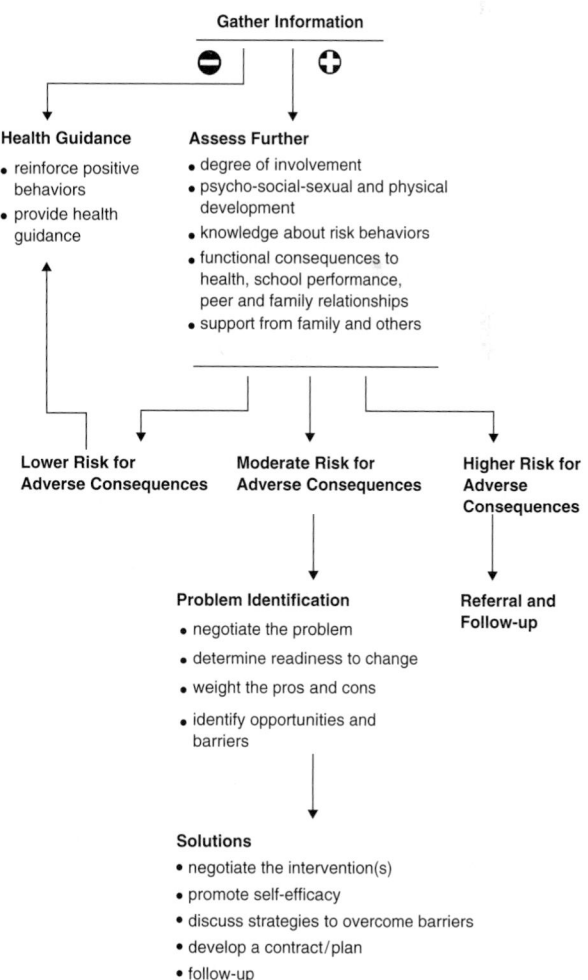

FIGURE 4.13 Algorithm for providing health screening and guidance to adolescents. (From American Medical Association. *Guidelines for adolescent preventive services* [Recommendations monograph]. Chicago: American Medical Association, 1995.)

this initial screening step may be facilitated by use of questionnaires, computers, or nonclinician personnel. If the screening result is negative and no increased risk is identified, basic information and positive reinforcement of the healthy behavior can and should be offered. If the result is positive, proceed to the next level.

A: Assess Further Assess the level and nature of risk in the particular area. Identify the seriousness of the problem by assessing the patient's knowledge and involvement, predisposing and protective factors, the availability of family and other support, and the consequences for the patient's health and function (e.g., school, peer relationships). The intervention offered depends on the assessed risk. Often, low risk can be successfully managed with health information, a few targeted suggestions, and positive reinforcement about the issue. If the patient is at high risk, he or she probably needs an in-depth evaluation that may be beyond the bounds of a preventive services visit. A return visit for more intensive intervention, or referral, is warranted. Patients who are at intermediate risk also require an explicit intervention, such as that suggested in the next step. This can be begun within the context of the preventive services visit if the clinician feels comfortable with the particular issue.

P: Problem Identification This step involves working with the patient toward an agreement on the problem, helping the patient decide to make a change, and working with the patient to develop a specific plan for that change. The goal is to be "patient-centered" in the approach—that is, to help the *patient* decide what is in his or her best interest, rather than forcing the patient to accept the physician's view of the problem or behavior. Problem identification is an attempt to define the problem in terms that the patient accepts. For example, questions such as, "You seem to be down and blue; is that something that is a problem for you right now?" or "Do you think it would be healthier for you if you used condoms?" may help the patient further acknowledge a problem. Once agreement on problem definition is reached, proceed to the next step. If the patient does not agree that there is a problem with a specified behavior, look for areas of agreement and common ground. An adolescent may not accept use of alcohol as being problematical but may acknowledge that binge drinking puts him or her at risk. Clinician perseveration on areas of obvious disagreement is unlikely to be productive and may negatively affect subsequent discussions. On the other hand, adolescent patients are often amenable to "agreeing to disagree," will still accept factual risk information, and are willing to establish criteria that would elevate the issue to "problem" status and justify future discussion and intervention. For example, a question such as, "You clearly don't think that this is a problem area, but when would you consider it might become one?" would assist in setting boundaries that define the problem. Finally, any problem that poses an immediate threat to the adolescent's safety warrants an immediate intervention or referral whether the adolescent is fully prepared for change.

The clinician guides the adolescent to weigh the pros and cons of making a certain change. The adolescent may find several reasons to make (or not make) the change in behavior, and it is helpful to address these reasons explicitly. This technique helps prepare adolescents to deal with the ambivalence that they often feel toward changes in behavior. While beginning to develop a "plan," find out what the adolescent is willing (or not willing) to do. Make sure the plan is concrete and fully detailed. Decisions should be framed as being in the adolescent's hands. If the adolescent is only willing to try using a condom once, that might become an initial plan. However, most adolescents are willing to make more substantive changes (e.g., always wearing seat belts, not drinking alcohol) at least for a specified period, usually a few weeks or months. Try to avoid sweeping changes that are unrealistic, such as avoiding alcohol use for the rest of their lives.

S: Specific Solutions: Self-efficacy, Support, Solving Problems, and "Shaking on a Contract" *Self-efficacy* is assessed by asking whether the adolescent thinks he or she will be able to carry out the proposed plan. If the adolescent is ambivalent, revisit perceived barriers and attempt to redefine specific solutions. Plans should be achievable so that success becomes self-reinforcing. An overly ambitious plan may need to be modified.

Support is important, and adolescents should be encouraged to identify people who can help them carry out their plan. Hopefully, they will be able to call on resources such as trusted adults or close friends. At times, adolescents may want advice on how best to recruit their support system. At times, the clinician can also be helpful in helping adolescents to disclose information to parents or others.

Solving problems reminds us to assess the barriers that the adolescent foresees and to work with the adolescent in developing specific strategies to overcome them. For example, if an adolescent recognizes that he will have difficulty not drinking at an upcoming party, he must have a plan for how to deal with that situation. It is usually most helpful if adolescents come up with their own solutions, but they often can be helped to recognize solutions or options they might not have considered.

"Shaking on a contract" is a crucial step. It serves as a tangible reinforcement of the proposed plan and implies some commitment on the adolescent's part. Written contracts can also be used, especially for younger adolescents, but they are unwieldy as a general rule. It is important to specify the actions agreed to and the time frame in which the actions are to be taken. Make sure that the adolescent feels comfortable with the plan and understands it. If you are able to involve another party in the contract, such as a friend or parent, there is likely to be better compliance. Follow-up is critical and should be arranged in some form—either a visit, telephone contact, or e-mail—in the time frame agreed to in the contract.

WEB SITES

http://odphp.osophs.dhhs.gov. Office of Disease Prevention and Health Promotion.

http://www.ama-assn.org/ama/pub/category/1947.html. Adolescent Health Online (AMA).

http://brightfutures.aap.org/web/. Bright Futures.

http://www.aap.org. American Academy of Pediatrics.

http://www.aafp.org. American Academy of Family Physicians.

http://www.adolescenthealth.org. Society for Adolescent Medicine.

http://www.nasbhc.org. National Association of School-based Health Centers.

http://www.cdc.gov/nccdphp/dash. CDC Department of Adolescent and School Health.

http://www.cdc.gov. Centers for Disease Control and Prevention.

http://www.acha.org. American College Health Association.

http://www.adolescenthealthlaw.org. Center for Adolescent Health and the Law.

http://www.ama-assn.org/ama/pub/category/1980.html. GAPS AMA site.

REFERENCES AND ADDITIONAL READINGS

Advisory Committee on Immunization Practices. prevention of Hepatitis A Through Active or passive immunization: Recommendations of the Advisory Committee on Immunization Practices (ACIP). *MMWR* 1999;48(RR12); 1–37. http://www.cdc.gov/mmwr/preview/mmwrhtml/rr4812a1.htm accessed March 2007.

Advisory Committee on Immunization Practices, Centers for Disease Control and Prevention. Prevention and control of meningococcal disease. *MMWR* 2005;54(RR07); 1. Accessed on 3-25-06 at http://www.cdc.gov/mmwr/preview/mmwrhtml/rr5407a1.htm.

Advisory Committee on Immunization Practices, Centers for Disease Control and Prevention. Preventing tetanus, diphtheria, and pertussis among adolescents: use of tetanus toxoid, reduced diphtheria toxoid and acellular pertussis vaccines. *MMWR* 2006;55(RR03):1. Accessed on 3-25-2006 at http://www.cdc.gov/mmwr/preview/mmwrhtml/rr5503a1.htm.

American Academy of Pediatrics, Committee on Practice and Ambulatory Medicine. Recommendations for pediatric and preventive health care. *Pediatrics* 1995;96:373.

American Academy of Pediatrics, Committee on Psychosocial Aspects of Child and Family Health. *Guidelines for health supervision III. (Updated).* Elk Grove Village, IL: American Academy of Pediatrics, 2002.

American College of Obstetricians and Gynecologists. Primary and preventive health care for female adolescents: ACOG educational bulletin #254. *Int J Gynecol Obstet* 2000;69:181.

American Medical Association. *AMA guidelines for adolescent preventive services (GAPS): recommendations and rationale.* Baltimore: Williams & Wilkins, 1994.

American Medical Association. *AMA guidelines for adolescent preventive services (GAPS): clinical evaluation and management handbook.* Baltimore: Williams & Wilkins, 1995.

Anglin TM, Naylor KE, Kaplan DW. Comprehensive school-based health care: high school students' use of medical, mental health, and substance use services. *Pediatrics* 1996;97:318.

Blum RW, Beuhring T, Wunderlich M, et al. Don't ask, they won't tell: the quality of adolescent health screening in five practice settings. *Am J Pub Health* 1996;86:1767.

Blum RW, Runyan C. The comprehensive health history and physical examination. In: Blum RW, ed. *Adolescent health care.* New York: Academic Press, 1982.

Borenstein PE, Harvilchuck JD, Rosenthal BH, et al. Patterns of ICD-9 diagnoses among adolescents using school-based clinics: diagnostic categories by school level and gender. *J Adolesc Health* 1996;18:203.

Breslow L, Somers AR. The lifetime health monitoring program: a practical approach to preventive medicine. *N Engl J Med* 1977;206:601.

Centers for Disease Control and Prevention. Immunization of adolescents: recommendations of the Advisory Committee on Immunization Practices, the American Academy of Pediatrics, the American Academy of Family Physicians, and the American Medical Association. *MMWR Morb Mortal Wkly Rep* 1996;45:(RR-13) 1.

Committee on Infectious Diseases. *Red book, 2006.* Elk Grove Village, IL: American Academy of Pediatrics, 2006.

Committee on Practice and Ambulatory Medicine, American Academy of Pediatrics. Vision screening and eye examination in children. *Pediatrics* 1986;77:918.

Committee on School Health. School health assessments. *Pediatrics* 1991;88:649.

Downs SM, Klein JD. Clinical preventive services efficacy and adolescents' risky behaviors. *Arch Pediatr Adolesc Med* 1995;149:374.

Elster AB. Comparison of recommendations for adolescent clinical preventive services developed by national organizations. *Arch Pediatr Adolesc Med* 1998;152:193.

Elster AB, Levenberg P. Integrating comprehensive adolescent preventive services into routine medical care: rationale and approaches. *Pediatr Clin North Am* 1997;44:1365.

Frame PS. Health maintenance in clinical practice: strategies and barriers. *Am Fam Physician* 1992;45:1192.

Gadomski A, Bennett S, Young M, et al. Guidelines for adolescent preventive services: GAPS in practice. *Arch Pediatr Adolesc Med* 2003;157:426.

Gans JE, Alexander B, Chu RC, et al. Cost of comprehensive preventive medical services for adolescents. *Arch Pediatr Adolesc Med* 1995;149:1226.

Gilchrist VJ. Preventive health care for the adolescent. *Am Fam Physician* 1991;43:869.

Goldenring J, Rosen DS. Getting into adolescent heads: an essential update. *Contemp Pediatr* 2004;21:64.

Green M. *Bright futures: guidelines for the health supervision of infants, children, and adolescents.* Arlington, VA: National Center for Education in Maternal and Child Health, 1994.

Halpern-Felsher BL, Ozer EM, Millstein SG, et al. Preventive services in a health maintenance organization: how well do pediatricians screen and educate adolescent patients? *Arch Pediatr Adolesc Med* 2000;154:173.

Harris KM, Gordon-Larsen P, Chantala K, et al. Longitudinal trends in race/ethnic disparities in leading health indicators from adolescence to young adulthood. *Arch Pediatr Adolesc Med* 2006;160:74.

Hersch BS, Fine PEM, Kent WK, et al. Mumps outbreak in a highly vaccinated population. *J Pediatr* 1991;119:187.

Kahn JA. Vaccination as a prevention strategy for human papillomavirus-related diseases. *J Adolesc Health* 2005;37:S10.

Kaplan DW, Calonge BN, Guernsey BP, et al. Managed care and school-based health centers: use of health services. *Arch Pediatr Adolesc Med* 1998;152:25.

Klein JD, Allan MJ, Elster AB, et al. Improving adolescent preventive care in community health centers. *Pediatrics* 2001;107:318.

Klein JD, Slap GB, Elster AB, et al. Adolescents and access to health care. *Bull N Y Acad Med* 1993;70:219.

Klein JD, Wilson KM. Delivering quality care: adolescents' discussion of health risks with their providers. *J Adolesc Health* 2002;30:190.

Kollar LM, Rosentahl SL, Biro FM. Hepatitis B vaccine series compliance in adolescents. *Pediatr Infect Dis J* 1994;13:1006.

Lieu TA, Cochi SL, Black SB, et al. Cost-effectiveness of a routine varicella vaccination program for U.S. children. *JAMA* 1994;271:375.

Lustig JL, Ozer EM, Adams SH, et al. Improving the delivery of adolescent clinical preventive services through skills-based training. *Pediatrics* 2001;107:1100.

Maciosek MV, Coffield AB, Edwards NM, et al. Priorities among effective clinical preventive services. *Am J Prev Med* 2006;31:52.

Marks A, Cohen MI. Health screening and assessment of adolescents. *Pediatr Ann* 1978;7:596.

Marks AM, Fisher M. Health assessment and screening during adolescence. *Pediatrics* 1987;80(1 Pt 2):135S.

Millar HEC, ed. U.S. Department of Health, Education and Welfare. *Adolescent health care: a guide for BCHS-supported programs and projects. Publication #NO(HSA)79-5234.* Washington, DC: U.S. Government Printing Office, 1980.

National Vaccine Advisory Committee. The measles epidemic: the problems, barriers, and recommendations. *JAMA* 1991;266:1547.

Ozer EM, Adams SH, Gardner LR, et al. Provider self-efficacy and screening of adolescents for risky health behaviors. *J Adolesc Health* 2004;35:101.

Ozer EM, Adams SH, Lustig LJ, et al. Can it be done? Implementing adolescent clinical preventive service. *Health Serv Res* 2001;36:150.

Ozer EM, Adams SH, Lustig LJ, et al. Increasing the screening and counseling of adolescents for risky health behaviors: a primary care intervention. *Pediatrics* 2005;115:960.

Paperny DMN, Hedberg VA. Computer-assisted health counselor visits: a low-cost model for comprehensive adolescent preventive visits. *Arch Pediatr Adolesc Med* 1999;153:63.

Pastore DR, Juszczak L, Fisher MM, et al. School-based health center utilization: a survey of users and non-users. *Arch Pediatr Adolesc Med* 1998;152:763.

Rosen DS, Elster A, Hedberg V, et al Clinical preventive services for adolescents: position paper of the Society for Adolescent Medicine. *J Adolesc Health* 1997;21:203.

Santelli J, Vernon M, Lowry R, et al. Managed care, school health programs, and adolescent health services: opportunities for health promotion. *J Sch Health* 1998;68:434.

Schubiner HH. Preventive health screening in adolescent patients. *Prim Care* 1989;16:211.

Schubiner H, Eggly S. Strategies for health education for adolescent patients: a preliminary investigation. *J Adolesc Health* 1995;17:37.

Sox HC, Jr. Preventive health services in adults. *N Engl J Med* 1994;330:1589.

Steiner BD, Gest KL. Do adolescents want to hear preventive counseling messages in outpatient settings? *J Fam Pract* 1996;43:375.

Thompson RS, Taplin SH, McAfee TA, et al. Primary and secondary prevention services in clinical practice: twenty years' experience in development, implementation, and evaluation. *JAMA* 1995;273:1130.

U.S. Preventive Services Task Force. *Guide to clinical preventive services: an assessment of the effectiveness of 169 interventions,* 2nd ed. Baltimore: Williams & Wilkins, 1996.

U.S. Preventive Services Task Force. *Guide to clinical preventive services: an assessment of the effectiveness of 169 interventions,* 3rd ed. Accessed online at http://www.ahrq.gov/clinic/gcpspu.htm. 2001–2004.

Zimmerman RK, Clover RD. Adult immunizations—a practical approach for clinicians: part I. *Am Fam Physician* 1995;51:859.

Zimmerman RK, Clover RD. Adult immunizations—a practical approach for clinicians: part II. *Am Fam Physician* 1995;51:1139.

CHAPTER 5

Vital Statistics and Injuries

Ponrat Pakpreo, Jonathan D. Klein, and Lawrence S. Neinstein

Intentional and unintentional injuries are responsible for most morbidity and mortality in adolescents. Injuries are preventable health problems, but the prevention of injuries poses considerable challenges to medical and public health professionals. The public health approach to injury prevention includes educational strategies, environmental modifications, and engineering techniques (Rivara and Aitken, 1998). The success of these interventions also relies on accurate and comprehensive reporting of morbidity and mortality data related to adolescent injury. This chapter presents an overview of mortality and morbidity in adolescents as well as available data on intentional and unintentional injuries. The chapter will be organized in the following manner:

- Demographics of the adolescent population.
- Data sources of vital statistics on adolescents and young adults including demographics, morbidity, and mortality.
- Mortality in adolescents including leading causes, unintentional injuries, intentional injuries, cancer, and trends in mortality.
- Focus on unintentional injuries.
- Recovery from injuries.
- Prevention of injuries.
- Morbidity including hospitalizations and ambulatory visit data.

DEMOGRAPHICS

1. *General:* In 2005, adolescents 10- to 19-years old were more than 42 million or 14.2% of the U.S. population and 20.8 million young adults 20- to 24-years old comprised an additional 7.1%. From 2000 to 2005, the adolescent population aged 10 to 14 years increased 1.4% compared with the 4.7% increase among 15- to 19-year olds. Table 5.1 demonstrates a rise in the actual number of the 10- to 14-year-old adolescent population since 1980 and among those 15- to 19-years old since 1990. However, the percentages of the total U.S. population represented by these age-groups have declined since 1980.
2. *Projections:* It is projected that by 2010, the 10- to 19-year-old population will have decreased to 41.1 million, a decline of just >2% (Table 5.1). It is projected that the 20- to 24-year-old population will increase by 3.4% to

21.7 million. The number of adolescents aged 10- to 19-years is projected to continue to increase through 2050; however, as a percentage of the total U.S. population, the number of adolescents, although decreasing, appears to stabilize by 2010. In the 20- to 24-year-old population, this percentage, although increasing since 1998, is projected to decrease after 2004 and then stabilize by 2020.
3. *Ethnicity:* Hispanic adolescents, 10- to 14-years old, are one of the fastest growing segments of the U.S. population, having increased 19.6% between 2000 and 2004. Hispanic teens aged 10 to 19 years comprise 2.4% of the entire 2004 U.S. population and 17.2% of the U.S. Hispanic population. Hispanic youth are second in overall numbers compared with non-Hispanic whites. African-American youth aged 10 to 19 years are third (U.S. Census Bureau, 2006) comprising 15.7% of that age-group in the United States.

DATA SOURCES

Adolescent demographics, morbidity, mortality, and health behaviors change from year to year. The most current data are typically available on the Internet and can be accessed by readers seeking the most up-to-date information.

Demographic and General Health Data

1. *Health, United States, 2006:* Available at http://www.cdc.gov/nchs/hus.htm. Health, United States is an annual report on trends in health statistics. The report consists of two main sections—a chartbook containing text and figures that illustrate major trends in the health of Americans and a trend tables section that contains 147 detailed data tables. This Web site is updated when new versions of this publication are available. The Web site also includes an executive summary, a highlights section, an extensive appendix, a reference section, and an index.
2. *The 2006 Statistical Abstract, U.S. Census Bureau:* Available at http://www.census.gov/compendia/statab/. Each year the Census Bureau publishes data related to U.S. demographics, health, education, and a wide range of other areas.
3. *The National Health Interview Survey (NHIS):* Available at http://www.cdc.gov/nchs/nhis.htm. The NHIS is a

TABLE 5.1

Actual and Projected Number of Adolescents, United States (in Thousands)

	5–9 yr Number (%)	10–14 yr Number (%)	15–19 yr Number (%)	20–24 yr Number (%)
Actual				
1980	16,700 (7.4)	18,242 (8.1)	21,168 (9.3)	21,319 (9.4)
1990	18,040 (7.3)	17,065 (6.9)	17,893 (7.2)	17,893 (7.2)
1998	20,510 (7.4)	19,825 (7.1)	19,640 (7.2)	18,167 (6.6)
2000	20,550 (7.3)	20,530 (7.3)	20,221 (7.2)	18,961 (6.7)
2004	19,775 (6.8)	21,193 (7.3)	20,477 (7.0)	20,971 (7.1)
2005	19,467 (6.6)	20,838 (7.1)	21,172 (7.2)	20,823 (7.0)
Projected				
2010	20,706 (6.7)	19,767 (6.3)	21,336 (6.9)	21,676 (7.0)
2020	22,564 (6.7)	21,914 (6.5)	21,478 (6.4)	20,751 (6.2)
2030	23,790 (6.5)	23,539 (6.5)	23,503 (6.5)	23,136 (6.4)
2040	25,550 (6.5)	24,953 (6.4)	24,824 (6.3)	24,897 (6.3)
2050	27,521 (6.6)	26,974 (6.4)	26,572 (6.3)	26,297 (6.3)

Adapted from United States Census Bureau. *Statistical abstract of the United States, 2005–2006*, 125th ed. Washington, DC: US Bureau of the Census, 2006.

multistage probability sample survey conducted annually by the National Center for Health Statistics (NCHS) through in-home interviews of the civilian noninstitutionalized U.S. population. The NHIS sample frame is also linked to several other national health survey efforts. The objectives of the NHIS surveys are to monitor the health and health care of the U.S. population through the collection and analysis of data on a broad range of health topics. Current topics include the following (National Center for Health Statistics, 2005):

- Health status and limitations
- Utilization of health care
- Injuries
- Family resources
- Health insurance
- Access to care
- Selected health conditions (including chronic conditions)
- Health behaviors
- Functioning
- Human immunodeficiency virus (HIV)/acquired immunodeficiency syndrome (AIDS) testing
- Immunization

4. *National Vital Statistics System:* Available at http://www.cdc.gov/nchs/nvss.htm. The National Vital Statistics System is the oldest and most successful example of intergovernmental data sharing in public health. These data include births, deaths, marriages, divorces, and fetal deaths that are recorded across the United States.

5. *Healthy People 2010:* Available at http://www.healthypeople.gov/and outlines national health promotion and disease prevention objectives that are monitored and updated over time. Of the 467 *Healthy People 2010* objectives for children and adults, 107 are relevant to adolescents and young adults. Adolescent health experts convened and identified 21 critical health objectives, which reflect some of the leading causes of morbidity and mortality among adolescents and young adults. Table 5.2 lists the 21 critical health objectives as well as baseline data and 2010 target goals.

6. Healthy Campus 2010: Available at http://www.acha.org/info_resources/hc2010.cfm. Healthy Campus 2010 establishes national college health objectives and serves as a basis for developing plans to improve student health. Healthy Campus 2010 is a series of health objectives parallel to Healthy People 2010 but adapted for the college population.

Mortality Data

1. *Health, United States, 2006:* As described in "Demographic and General Health Data" section in the preceding text.

2. *Deaths, Final Data for 2003:* This yearly publication is available at the NCHS Web site. The 2003 final report is at http://www.cdc.gov/nchs/products/pubs/pubd/hestats/finaldeaths03/finaldeaths03.htm.

3. *National Center for Injury Prevention and Control (NCIPC):* Available at http://www.cdc.gov/ncipc/. The NCIPC has a vast array of data and information on injuries and injury prevention in all age-groups. Also at this site are two interactive data tools: WISQARS and injury maps.

- *WISQARS*—Web-based Injury Statistics Query and Reporting System is available at http://www.cdc.gov/ncipc/wisqars/default.htm. This site is the NCIPC's interactive, online database that provides customized injury-related mortality data and nonfatal injury data. One can also stratify results by age, gender, ethnicity, and region of the country.

- *Injury maps,* the NCIPC's interactive mapping system, available at: http://www.cdc.gov/ncipc/maps/default.htm, helps identify and communicate the impact of injury deaths in a particular county, state, region, or the entire United States.

Morbidity Data Including Diseases, Health Risks, and Health Behaviors

1. *The National Health and Nutrition Examination Survey (NHANES):* Available at http://www.cdc.gov/nchs/

TABLE 5.2

National Initiative to Improve Adolescent Health—21 Critical Health Objectives for Adolescents and Young Adults

Objective No.	Objective	Baseline (yr)	2010 Target
16-03 (a, b, c)	Reduce deaths of adolescents and young adults		
	10- to 14-yr-olds	21.5/100,000 (1998)	16.8/100,000
	15- to 19-yr-olds	69.5/100,000 (1998)	39.8/100,000
	20- to 24-yr-olds	92.7/100,000 (1998)	49.0/100,000
Unintentional Injury			
15-15 (a)	Reduce deaths caused by motor vehicle crashes (15- to 24-yr-olds).	25.6/100,000 (1999)	*a*
26-01 (a)	Reduce deaths and injuries caused by alcohol- and drug-related motor vehicle crashes (15- to 24-yr-olds).	13.5/100,000 (1998)	*a*
15-19	Increase use of safety belts (9th–12th grade students).	84% (1999)	92%
26-06	Reduce the proportion of adolescents who report that they rode, during the previous 30 days, with a driver who had been drinking alcohol (9th–12th grade students).	33% (1999)	30%
Violence			
18-01	Reduce the suicide rate		
	10- to 14-yr-olds	1.2/100,000 (1999)	*a*
	15- to 19-yr-olds	8.0/100,000 (1999)	*a*
18-02	Reduce the rate of suicide attempts by adolescents that require medical attention (9th–12th grade students).	2.6% (1999)	1%
15–32	Reduce homicides		
	10- to 14-yr-olds	1.2/100,000 (1999)	*a*
	15- to 19-yr-olds	10.4/100,000 (1999)	*a*
15-38	Reduce physical fighting among adolescents (9th–12th grade students).	36% (1999)	32%
15-39	Reduce weapon carrying by adolescents on school property (9th–12th grade students).	6.9% (1999)	4.9%
Substance Use and Mental Health			
26-11 (d)	Reduce the proportion of persons engaging in binge drinking of alcoholic beverages (12- to 17-yr-olds).	7.7% (1998)	2%
26-10 (b)	Reduce last-month use of illicit substances (marijuana) (12- to 17-yr-olds).	8.3% (1998)	0.70%
06-02	Reduce the proportion of children and adolescents with disabilities who are reported to be sad, unhappy, or depressed (4- to 17-yr-olds).	*b*	*b*
18-07	Increase the proportion of children with mental health problems who receive treatment	59% (2001)	66%
Reproductive Health			
09-07	Reduce pregnancies among adolescent females (15- to 17-yr-olds).	68/1,000 (1996)	43/1,000
13-05	(Developmental) Reduce the number of new HIV diagnoses among adolescents and adults (13- to 24-yr-olds).	16,479 (1998)*d*	*c*
25-01 (a, b, c)	Reduce the proportion of adolescents and young adults with *Chlamydia trachomatis* infections. (15- to 24-yr-olds).		
	• Females attending family planning clinics	5% (1997)	3%
	• Females attending sexually transmitted disease clinics	12.2% (1997)	3%
	• Males attending sexually transmitted disease clinics	15.7% (1997)	3%

(continued)

TABLE 5.2

(Continued)

Objective No.	Objective	Baseline (yr)	2010 Target
25-11	Increase the proportion of adolescents (9th–12th grade students) who: • Have never had sexual intercourse • If sexually experienced, are not currently sexually active • If currently sexually active, used a condom the last time they had sexual intercourse	 50% (1999) 27% (1999) 58% (1999)	56% 30% 65%
Chronic Diseases			
27-02 (a)	Reduce tobacco use by adolescents (9th–12th grade students).	40% (1999)	21%
19-03 (b)	Reduce the proportion of children and adolescents who are overweight or obese (12- to 19-yr-olds)	11% (1988–1994)	5%
22-07	Increase the proportion of adolescents who engage in vigorous physical activity that promotes cardiorespiratory fitness 3 or more d/wk for 20 or more min per occasion (9th–12th grade students).	65% (1999)	85%

HIV, human immunodeficiency virus.Bolded objectives numbers indicate critical health outcomes. Behaviors that substantially contribute to important health outcomes are in normal font.

[a]2010 target not provided for adolescent/young adult age-group.

[b]Baseline and target inclusive of age-groups outside of adolescent/young adult age parameters.

[c]Developmental objective-baseline and 2010 target to be provided by 2005.

[d]Proposed baseline is shown but has not yet been approved by the Healthy People 2010 Steering Committee.

Adapted from the National Adolescent Health Information Center. *21 critical health objectives for adolescents and young adults. Data from the U.S. Department of Health and Human Services. Healthy People 2010,* Vol. 1 and 2. Washington, DC: U.S. Government Printing Office, Available at http://nahic.ucsf.edu/nationalinitiative. November 2000.

nhanes.htm, NHANES is another survey conducted by the NCHS on overall health risks and behaviors. Data collection is unique in that it combines a home interview with objective health measures and a physical examination conducted in a mobile examination center. The goals of this survey include the following:

- To estimate the number and percentage of persons in the U.S. population and designated subgroups with selected diseases and risk factors
- To monitor trends in prevalence, awareness, treatment, and control of selected diseases or conditions including those unrecognized or undetected
- To monitor trends in risk behaviors and environmental exposures
- To analyze risk factors for selected diseases, including heart disease, diabetes, osteoporosis, and infectious diseases
- To study the relationship between diet, nutrition, and health, including a focus on iron deficiency anemia and other nutritional disorders, children's growth and development, and obesity/physical fitness
- To explore emerging public health issues and new technologies
- To establish a national probability sample of genetic material for future genetic testing

2. The National Ambulatory Medical Care Survey and the National Hospital Ambulatory Medical Care Survey: Available at http://www.cdc.gov/nchs/about/major/

ahcd/ahcd1.htm, these surveys focus on characteristics of patients' visits to physicians' offices, hospital outpatient settings, and emergency departments. Additionally, these surveys collect data on diagnoses and treatments, prescribing patterns, and characteristics of clinical facilities.

3. Reproductive health: The *National Survey of Family Growth* is available at http://www.cdc.gov/nchs/nsfg.htm has data about reproductive health behaviors.

4. *National Survey of Children with Special Health Care Needs:* Available at http://www.cdc.gov/nchs/about/major/slaits/cshcn.htm, this survey assesses the prevalence and impact of special health care needs among children in all 50 states and the District of Columbia.

5. Cancer data: *National Cancer Institute, Surveillance Epidemiology and End Results (SEER)* data are available at http://seer.cancer.gov/publicdata/. The SEER Public-Use Data include SEER incidence and population data associated by age, sex, race, year of diagnosis, and geographical areas (including SEER registry and county).

6. Infectious diseases: The *Summary of Notifiable Diseases* is available each year in the MMWR. Available at www.cdc.gov/mmwr.

7. Sports injury data: *The National Center for Catastrophic Sport Injury Research* (http://www.unc.edu/depts/nccsi/) collects and disseminates death and permanent disability sports injury data that involve brain and/or

spinal cord injuries. This research has been conducted at the University of North Carolina at Chapel Hill since 1965. Three annual reports are compiled each spring: (a) Annual Survey of Football Injury Research, (b) Annual Survey of Catastrophic Football Injuries; and (3) Annual Report of National Center for Catastrophic Sports Injury Research.

8. *Youth Risk Behavior Survey (YRBS):* Available at http://www.cdc.gov/HealthyYouth/yrbs/index.htm. The Youth Risk Behavior Surveillance System was developed in 1990 to monitor priority health-risk behaviors that contribute to the leading causes of death, disability, and social problems among youth and adults in the United States. Behaviors studied include tobacco use, unhealthy dietary behaviors, inadequate physical activity, alcohol and other drug use, sexual behaviors that contribute to unintended pregnancy and sexually transmitted diseases (STDs) (including HIV infection), and behaviors that contribute to unintentional injuries and violence. The survey examines the prevalence of health-risk behaviors, trends over time, comparable data among subgroups of adolescents, and progress toward Healthy People 2010 objectives.

The YRBS is conducted by staff members of the state departments of education with assistance from the Centers for Disease Control and Prevention (CDC) every 2 years. The survey includes representative samples of 9th through 12th grade students both in public and private schools. The Youth Risk Behavior Surveillance System also includes three additional national surveys conducted by CDC:

- *YRBS*, conducted in 1992 as a follow-up to the National Health Interview Survey among approximately 11,000 persons aged 12 to 21 years.
- *National College Health-Risk Behavior Survey,* conducted in 1995 among a representative sample of approximately 5,000 undergraduate students.
- *National Alternative High School Youth Risk Behavior Survey,* conducted in 1998 among a representative sample of approximately 9,000 students in alternative high schools.

Some notable statistics reported by the 2003 YRBS are presented in Table 5.3.

9. *National College Health Assessment (NCHA):* Available at http://www.acha-ncha.org/index.html. The American College Health Association (ACHA)-National College Health Assessment (NCHA) is a national research effort organized by ACHA to assist health care providers, health educators, counselors, and administrators in collecting data about college students' habits, behaviors, and perceptions on the most prevalent health topics. Topics include alcohol, tobacco, and other drug use; sexual health; weight, nutrition, and exercise; mental health; and injury prevention, personal safety, and violence. Results of recent studies are reviewed in Chapter 84.

10. *Add Health:* Available at http://www.cpc.unc.edu/addhealth. Add Health is a nationally representative study that explores the causes of health-related behaviors of adolescents in grades 7 through 12 and their outcomes in young adulthood. Add Health examines how social contexts (families, friends, peers, schools, neighborhoods, and communities) influence adolescents' health and risk behaviors. Wave 1 was initiated in 1994, and is the largest, most comprehensive survey of adolescents ever undertaken. Data at the individual, family, school, and community levels were collected in two waves between 1994 and 1996. In 2001 and 2002, Add Health respondents, 18- to 26-years old, were reinterviewed in a third wave to investigate the influence that adolescence has on young adulthood. Numerous public and restricted release datasets are available. Longitudinal data are collected on such attributes as height, weight, pubertal development, mental health status (focusing on depression, the most common mental health problem among adolescents), and chronic and disabling conditions. Data are gathered from adolescents themselves, their parents, and school administrators. Already existing databases provide information about neighborhoods and communities.

11. Substance Abuse: *Monitoring the Future Study* is available at www.monitoringthefuture.org. *Monitoring the Future* (MTF) is an ongoing study of the behaviors, attitudes, and values of American secondary school students, college students, and young adults. Each year, approximately 50,000 8th, 10th, and 12th grade students are surveyed (12th graders since 1975, and 8th and 10th graders since 1991). In addition, annual follow-up questionnaires are mailed to a sample of each graduating class for a number of years after their initial participation. This study provides perhaps the most complete and comprehensive examination of substance use and abuse patterns both cross-sectionally and longitudinally in the United States. Volume I of the annual MTF report focuses on secondary school students and Volume II focuses on college students and young adults. Results are reviewed in Chapters 68 and 84.

Another source of national data is the Fed Stat gateway at http://www.fedstats.gov/. This site has links to more than 70 federal agencies that collect national data on a wide range of areas.

MORTALITY

Quick Facts Regarding Mortality Risks for Adolescents in the United States

- A fatal injury occurs every 5 minutes (National Safety Council [NSC], 2004).
- Gunfire kills a child every 3 hours, 8 children everyday, and 55 children a week (Children's Defense Fund, 2005).
- Every 5 hours a child or adolescent commits suicide (Children's Defense Fund, 2004b).

Leading Causes of Death

The ten leading causes of death for youth aged 10 to 14 years vary slightly from those of older adolescents and young adults. The leading causes of mortality for each age-group (per 100,000) are shown in Table 5.4 (National Center for Injury Prevention and Control, 2006). Unintentional injuries, homicides, and suicides are the top three causes of death in the 15- to 24-year-old population. In the 10 to 14 years age-group both unintentional injuries and suicide are the leading causes. Malignant neoplasms are the second highest cause of mortality. HIV-related deaths are sixth in young adults aged 25 to 34 years and eighth in the leading causes of death among 15- to 24-year olds.

In general, the leading cause of death is the same among different ethnicities in all age-groups except those

TABLE 5.3

Percentage of High School Students Who Engaged in Selected Health-Risk Behaviors, by Grade—United States Youth Risk Behavior Survey, 2005

Behavior	9th Grade	10th Grade	11th Grade	12th Grade	Total
Rarely or never used safety belts[a]	10.9	8.6	10.1	10.8	10.2
Rarely or never wore motorcycle helmets[b]	36.8	31.9	38.2	39.5	36.5
Rarely or never wore bicycle helmets[c]	83.0	84.3	82.2	84.0	83.4
Rode with a drinking driver[d]	27.9	27.8	28.0	30.1	28.5
Participated in a physical fight[e]	43.5	36.6	31.6	29.1	35.9
Carried a weapon[f]	19.9	19.4	17.1	16.9	18.5
Lifetime cigarette use[g]	48.7	52.5	57.5	60.3	54.3
Current cigarette use[h]	19.7	21.4	24.3	27.6	23.0
Current smokeless tobacco use[j]	7.6	7.5	8.4	8.4	8.0
Lifetime alcohol use[k]	66.5	74.4	76.3	81.7	74.3
Current episodic heavy drinking[l]	19.0	24.6	27.6	32.8	25.5
Lifetime marijuana use[m]	29.3	37.4	42.3	47.6	38.4
Lifetime cocaine use[n]	6.0	7.2	8.7	8.9	7.6
Lifetime ecstacy use	5.8	6.0	6.5	6.7	6.3
Lifetime methamphetamine use	5.7	5.9	6.7	6.4	6.2
Ever injected drugs[o]	2.4	2.3	1.7	1.7	2.1
Ever had sexual intercourse	34.3	42.8	51.4	63.6	46.8
Sexual intercourse with four or more partners (lifetime)	9.4	11.5	16.2	21.4	14.3
Used condom during last sexual intercourse[p]	74.5	65.3	61.7	55.4	62.8
Used birth control pills before last sexual intercourse[p]	7.5	14.3	18.5	25.6	17.6
Ate fruits and vegetables[q]	21.3	21.4	18.8	18.3	20.1
Played on a sports team[r]	60.4	58.0	54.9	49.2	56.0
Engaged in moderate physical activity[s]	36.9	38.5	34.4	32.9	35.8
Made a suicide plan in last 12 mo	13.9	14.1	12.9	10.5	13.0

[a]When riding in a car or truck as a passenger.

[b]When riding on a motorcycle.

[c]When riding on a bicycle.

[d]Rode at least once during the 30 days preceding the survey in a car or other vehicle driven by someone who had been drinking alcohol.

[e]Fought at least once during the 12 months preceding the survey.

[f]Carried a gun, knife, or club at least 1 day during the 30 days preceding the survey.

[g]Ever tried smoking, even one or two puffs.

[h]Smoked cigarettes on one or more of the 30 days preceding the survey.

[j]Used chewing tobacco or snuff on one or more of the 30 days preceding the survey.

[k]Ever drank one or more drinks.

[l]Drank five or more drinks of alcohol on at least one occasion during the 30 days preceding the survey.

[m]Ever used marijuana.

[n]Ever tried any form of cocaine (i.e., powder, "crack," or "freebase").

[o]Respondents were classified as injecting-drug users only if they (a) reported injecting-drug use not prescribed by a physician and (b) answered "one or more time" to any of the following questions: "During your life, how many times have you used any form of cocaine including powder, crack, or freebase?" "During your life, how many times have you used heroin (also called *smack, junk,* or *China White*)?" "During your life, how many times have you used methamphetamines (also called *speed, crystal, crank,* or *ice*)?" or "During your life, how many times have you taken steroid pills or shots without a doctor's prescription?"

[p]Among respondents who had sexual intercourse during the 3 months preceding the survey.

[q]Ate five or more servings of fruits and vegetables (fruit, fruit juice, green salad, and cooked vegetables) during the 7 days preceding the survey.

[r]During the 12 months preceding the survey.

[s]Activities that did not cause sweating or hard breathing for at least 30 minutes at a time on five or more of the 7 days preceding the survey.

Adapted from Centers for Disease Control and Prevention. Youth risk behavior surveillance, 2005. *MMWR CDC Surveill Summ* 2006b;55(SS-5):1–108.

TABLE 5.4

Ten Leading Causes of Death, United States, 2004, by Age Group

Rank	All Ages	Age Groups 10 to 14	15 to 24	25 to 34
Total number of deaths	2,397,615	3,946	33,421	40,868
1	Heart disease 652,486 (27.2%)	Unintentional injury 1,540 (39.9%)	Unintentional injury 15,449 (46.2%)	Unintentional injury 13,032 (31.9%)
2	Malignant neoplasms 553,888 (23.1%)	Malignant neoplasms 493 (12.5%)	Homicide 5,085 (15.2%)	Suicide 5,074 (12.4%)
3	Cerebrovascular 150,074 (6.3%)	Suicide 283 (7.2%)	Suicide 4,316 (12.9%)	Homicide 4,495 (11.0%)
4	Chronic low-respiratory disease 121,987 (5.1%)	Homicide 207 (5.2%)	Malignant neoplasms 1,709 (5.1%)	Malignant neoplasms 3,633 (8.9%)
5	Unintentional injuries 112,012 (4.7%)	Congenital anomalies 184 (4.7%)	Heart disease 1,038 (3.1%)	Heart disease 3,163 (7.7%)
6	Diabetes mellitus 73,138 (3.1%)	Heart disease 162 (4.1%)	Congenital anomalies 483 (1.4%)	HIV 1,468 (3.6%)
7	Alzheimer disease 65,965 (2.8%)	Chronic low-respiratory disease 74 (1.9%)	Cerebrosvascular 211 (0.6%)	Diabetes mellitus 599 (1.5%)
8	Influenza and pneumonia 59,664 (2.5%)	Influenza and pneumonia 49 (1.2%)	HIV 191 (0.6%)	Cerebrovascular 567 (1.4%)
9	Nephritis 42,480 (1.8%)	Benign neoplasms 43 (1.1%)	Influenza and pneumonia 185 (0.6%)	Congenital anomalies 420 (1.0%)
10	Septicemia 33,373 (1.7%)	Cerebrovascular events 43 (1.1%)	Chronic low-respiratory disease 179 (0.5%)	Septicemia 328 (0.8%)
All others	533,548 (22.2%)	868 (22.0%)	4,575 (13.7%)	8,089 (19.8%)

HIV, human immunodeficiency virus. Adapted from CDC. Wisqars. at www.cdc.gov/ncipc/wisqars, last accessed 12. 2006.

aged 15 to 44 years. Among individuals aged 15 to 34 years, unintentional injuries are the leading cause of death for all races except African-Americans, in whom homicides are the leading cause of death. Table 5.5 shows the leading causes of death by race among adolescents 10 to 19 years of age. Homicide also ranks higher as a cause of death in this age-group for the Hispanic population compared with the non-Hispanic population.

Unintentional Injuries

Unintentional injuries are the fifth leading cause of death in the United States for the total population, but are the leading cause of death among 1- to 44-year olds. The leading cause of death due to unintentional injury is motor vehicle crashes. In 2004, when adolescents aged 10 to 19 years accounted for 14.3% of the total population in the United States, they also accounted for 15.8% (6,608) of all motor vehicle deaths (U.S. Census Bureau, 2006, National Center for Injury Prevention and Control, 2006a). Of these deaths, two out of every three were male adolescents (Insurance Institute for Highway Safety, 2006a).

The data is particularly striking for adolescent drivers. Although the 12 million adolescent drivers represent only 6% of total drivers, they account for approximately 14% of the fatal crashes (American Academy of Pediatrics, Committee on Injury, Violence, and Poison Prevention and Committee on Adolescence, 2006). Unintentional injuries are discussed later in this chapter.

Intentional Injuries

Homicide

Homicide continues to be a major public health problem in the United States, particularly for young African-American males. Homicide remains the number two cause of death in the 15- to 24-year-old population and the number one cause of death among African-American males aged 15 to 24 years. Between 1990 and 2002, the overall age-adjusted homicide rate for all adolescents decreased by 35% to 6 deaths per 100,000 persons, reversing an upward trend seen in the late 1980s and early 1990s (National Center for Injury Prevention and Control, 2006). Between 1985 and 1993, the homicide victimization rate for 14- to 17-year olds

TABLE 5.5

United States, 2004, Leading Cause of Death among 10- to 19-Year-Olds by Race, Absolute Numbers

Rank	White	Black	Hispanic	All Races
1	Unintentional injury 70,110	Homicide 1,129	Unintentional injury 1,169	Unintentional injury 8,365
2	Suicide 1,642	Unintentional injury 1,013	Homicide 532	Homicide 2,139
3	Malignant neoplasms 959	Malignant neoplasms 217	Suicide 253	Suicide 1,983
4	Homicide 932	Suicide 203	Malignant neoplasms 249	Malignant neoplasms 1,224
5	Heart disease 338	Heart disease 171	Congenital anomalies 63	Heart disease 528
6	Congenital anomalies 325	Congenital anomalies 96	Heart disease 61	Congenital anomalies 441
7	Influenza and pneumonia 91	Chronic low-respiratory disease 79	Influenza and pneumonia 19	Chronic low-respiratory disease 159
8	Cerebrovascular events 82	Anemias 41	Cerebrovascular events 17	Influenza and pneumonia 116
9	Chronic low-respiratory disease 75	HIV 37	Chronic low-respiratory disease 12	Cerebrovascular events 112
10	Benign neoplasms 64	Diabetes mellitus 34	Two-tied benign neoplasias and pregnancy complications 11 each	Septicemia 93

HIV, human immunodeficiency virus. Adapted from the National Center for Injury Prevention and Control, Centers for Disease Control and Prevention, WISQARS, United States, 2006. *Leading causes of death report and from the National Vital Statistics Reports.* Available at http://webappa.cdc.gov/sasweb/ncipc/leadcaus10.html. Last accessed 12. 2006.

increased approximately 170%, and after 1993, adolescent homicide victimization rates declined to levels similar to those seen before 1985.

Trends by race The homicide rate among African-American male adolescents increased by 135% between 1950 and 1990. The rate peaked at 163.21 per 100,000 in 1993 and subsequently decreased by 49% to a rate of 82.8 per 100,000 in 2002. Still, the current rate is eight times that of white males and nearly three times that of Hispanic males in the same age-group. Compared with peak rates in the early 1990s the greatest declines in homicide rates are among Hispanic males and females 15- to 19-years old (57% and 61% reduction, respectively) and black males 15- to 19-years old (61% reduction) (National Center for Injury Prevention and Control, 2006a). Figures 5.1 and 5.2 from the U.S. Department of Justice, demonstrate the trends in homicide victimization by age-group, gender, and race over time. In 2004, the highest homicide rates were among older adolescents and young adults 18- to 24-years old. Males have higher rates of homicide victimization and perpetration compared to females. Adolescent homicide victims most often died due to arson (28.4%), poisoning (26.5%), gang-related killings (25%), and sex-related crimes

(19.8%). Figures 5.3 and 5.4 demonstrate the rates of homicide offenders by age-group, gender, and race over time. Adolescent homicide offenders were more often implicated in gang-related killings (30%) and felony murders (15%). More than 75% of homicides in older adolescents and young adults involved firearms. In 2004, African-American males 18- to 24-years old had the highest homicide victimization rates at 95.5 per 100,000, more than double the rate for black males 25 years and older (38.3 per 100,000) and four times the rate for black males 14- to 17-years old (25.8 per 100,000) (U.S. Department of Justice, 2006). Although rates appeared to be increasing again from 2000 to 2003, there appears to be a drop off in 2004 (U.S. Department of Justice, 2006).

Suicide

Incidence Suicide has changed from a problem of predominantly older persons to one that affects primarily adolescents and young adults. Adolescent suicide rates remained stable between 1900 and 1955 and then began to rise dramatically. Currently, suicide is the third leading cause of death for adolescents and young adults aged 10 to 14 years and 15 to 24 years, respectively (Centers for Disease Control and Prevention, 2006). The rate within that age-group

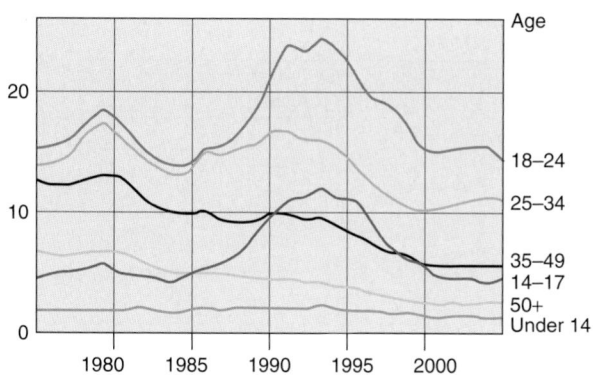

FIGURE 5.1 Homicide victimization rates (per 100,000) by age-group from 1976 to 2004. (Graphs from Fox JA, Zawitz MW. *Homicide trends in the United States*. U.S. Department of Justice, Office of Justice Programs, Bureau of Justice Statistics. Accessed 11/22/06 at http://www.ojp.gov/bjs/homicide/teens.htm. 2006.)

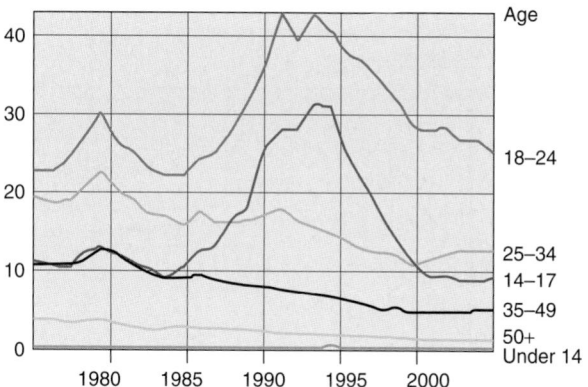

FIGURE 5.3 Homicide offending rates (per 100,000) by age-group from 1976 to 2002. (Graphs from Fox JA, Zawitz MW. *Homicide trends in the United States*. U.S. Department of Justice, Office of Justice Programs, Bureau of Justice Statistics. Accessed 11/22/2006 athttp://www.ojp.gov/bjs/homicide/teens.htm. 2006.)

escalated from 4.5 per 100,000 in 1950 to 13.57 per 100,000 in 1994. Since then, the suicide rate in this age-group has declined. In 2004, the suicide rate was 10.35 per 100,000 accounting for 4,316 deaths within the 15- to 24-year-old population. This represents almost 13% of all suicides as well as almost 13% of all deaths within that age-group. For

both 15 to 19 and 20- to 24-year olds, suicide rates are highest among Native Americans and whites. African-Americans had the lowest rates among 15- to 19-year olds and Asians had the lowest rate among 20- to 24-year olds (National Center for Injury Prevention and Control, 2006). The ratio

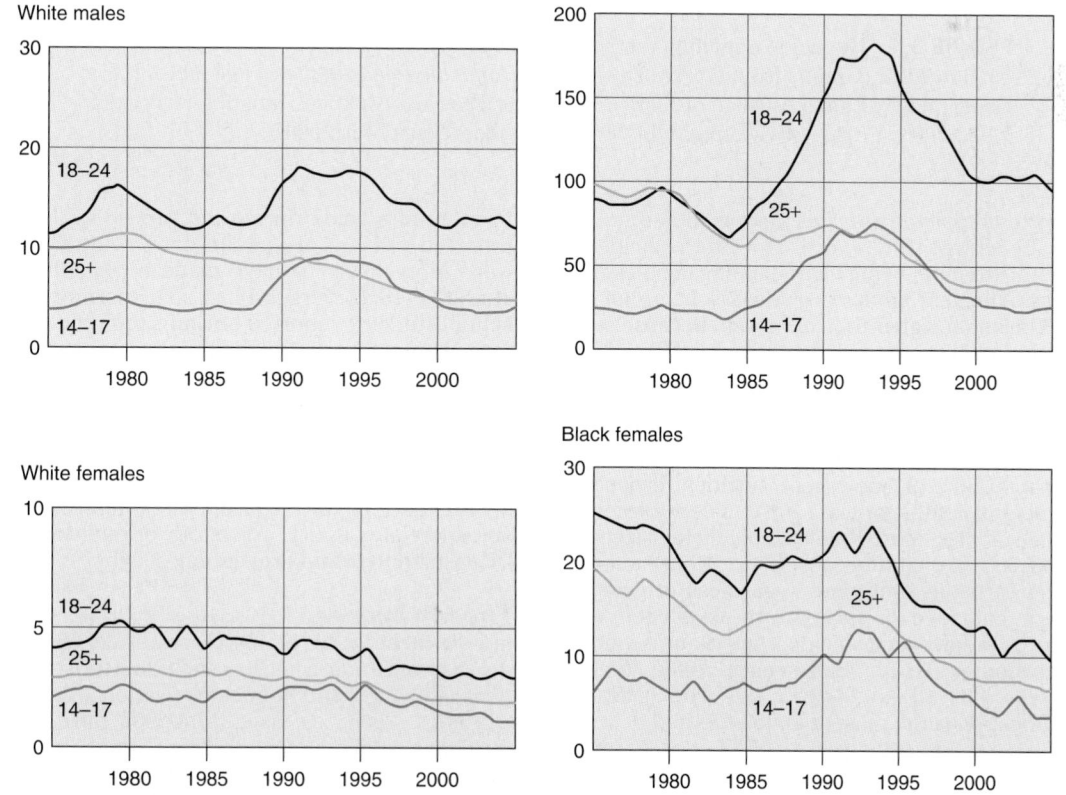

FIGURE 5.2 Homicide victimization rates (per 100,000) by age-group, race, and gender from 1976 to 2004. (Graphs from Fox JA, Zawitz MW. *Homicide trends in the United States*. U.S. Department of Justice, Office of Justice Programs, Bureau of Justice Statistics. Accessed 11/22/2006 at http://www.ojp.gov/bjs/homicide/ageracesex.htm. 2006.)

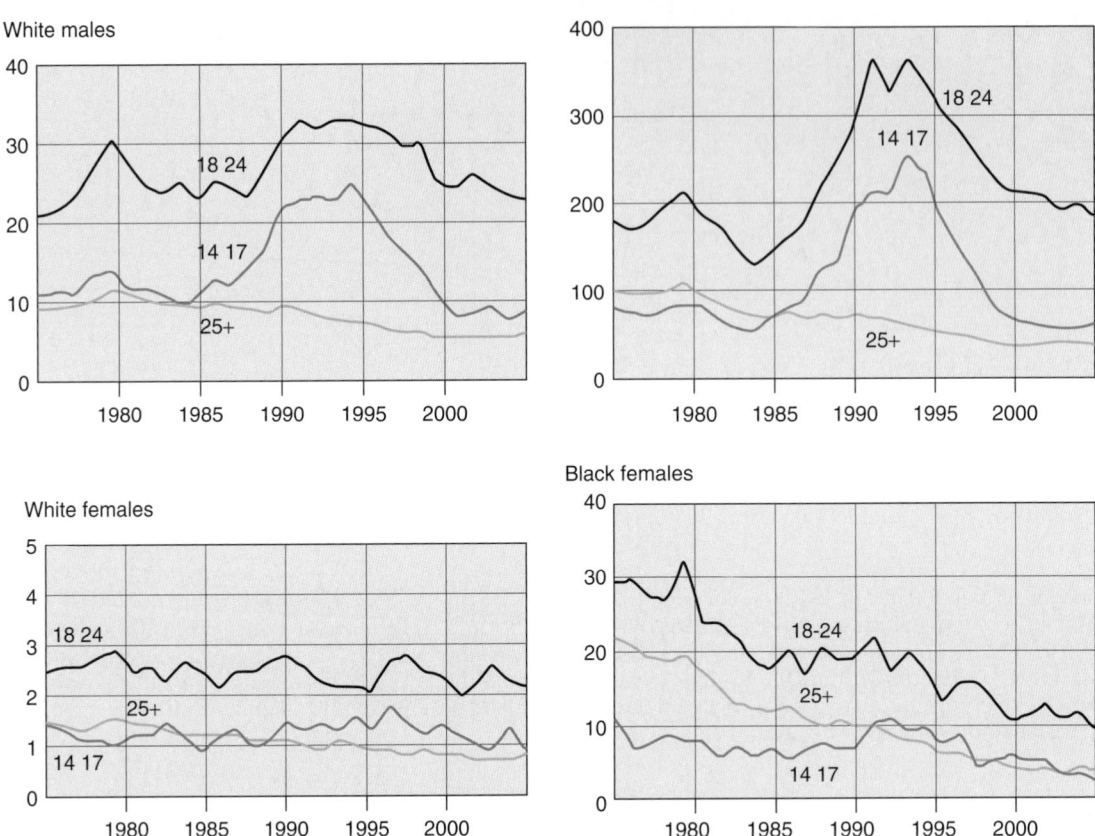

FIGURE 5.4 Homicide offending rates (per 100,000) by age-group, gender, and race from 1976 to 2004. (Graphs from Fox JA, Zawitz MW. *Homicide trends in the United States.*U.S. Department of Justice, Office of Justice Programs, Bureau of Justice Statistics. Accessed 11/22/2006 at http://www.ojp.gov/bjs/homicide/ageracesex.htm. 2006.)

of attempted to completed suicides among adolescents is estimated to be between 50:1 and 100:1, with the incidence of unsuccessful attempts being higher among females than among males. The true number of deaths from suicide may actually be much higher than indicated, because some suicide deaths are recorded as "accidental" (American Academy of Pediatrics Committee on Adolescence, 2000).

Method Ingestion of pills is the most common method among adolescents who *attempt* suicide. Firearms, used in approximately 50% of adolescent suicides, cause the greatest number of deaths for male and female adolescents who *complete* suicides. More than 90% of suicide attempts involving a firearm are fatal because there is little chance for rescue. Firearms in the home, regardless of whether they are kept unloaded or locked, are associated with a higher risk of adolescent suicide (American Academy of Pediatrics Committee on Adolescence, 2000). Among younger adolescents 10- to 14-years old who complete suicides, suffocation is the most common method.

Suicide attempts In a national survey of high school students in 2003, 16.9% reported having seriously considered attempting suicide during the 12 months preceding the survey. Overall, female students (21.3%) were significantly more likely than male students (12.8%) to have considered suicide. More serious ideation, having made a specific plan

to attempt suicide during the preceding 12 months was reported by 16.5% of students nationwide. Female students were more likely to have made a plan than were male students (18.9% versus 14.1%). Furthermore, 8.5% of high school students reported having attempted suicide at least once within the previous 12 months. More female than male students reported having made an attempt (11.5% versus 5.4%). Hispanic and white females most often reported considering suicide, making a suicide plan, and having attempted suicide than other female and male students. Of all students who reported a history of suicide attempts, only 2.9% had been treated by a doctor or nurse for an attempted suicide-related injury, poisoning, or overdose (Centers for Disease Control and Prevention, 2004b).

Firearm Injuries
In 2004, in the United States, there were 29,569 (9.95/100,000) deaths from firearm injuries, including those related to accidents, suicides, and homicides (National Center for Health Statistics, 2006, accessed 12/4/2006, http://webappa.cdc .gov/sasweb/ncipc/mortrate10_sy.html). Table 5.6 reviews firearm mortality rates among those 1 through 34 years of age. Most of the firearm deaths in the adolescent and young adult age-group are related to suicide or homicide. Between 1990 and 2004, the age-adjusted death rate for firearm injuries decreased by 28% and has remained at a rate near 10 per 100,000 since 1999. In 2004, the largest

TABLE 5.6

Firearm Mortality Rates among Children, Youth, and Young Adults, 1- to 34-Year Olds, United States, 2004 (Rates per 100,000)

Cause of Death	<5 yr	5–9 yr	10–14 yr	15–19 yr	20–24 yr	25–29 yr	30–34 yr
Male							
Total							
White	0.14	0.20	1.48	14.41	22.30	19.45	17.01
African-American	1.09[a]	0.99[a]	3.49	55.17	107.64	102.09	64.87
Suicide							
White	0[a]	0[a]	0.49	7.10	11.67	10.25	10.38
African-American	0[a]	0[a]	0.39[a]	3.71	10.69	10.19	7.82
Homicide							
White	0.07[a]	0.14[a]	0.63	6.53	9.68	8.60	6.23
African-American	0.73[a]	0.62[a]	2.88	49.95	94.92	90.24	55.75
Female							
Total							
White	0.13[a]	0.23	0.31	2.35	2.77	2.76	3.53
African-American	0.94[a]	0.58[a]	0.80	5.85	7.9	7.28	6.99
Suicide							
White	0[a]	0[a]	0.10[a]	1.07	1.21	1.45	2.01
African-American	0[a]	0[a]	0.06[a]	0.74[a]	1.08[a]	0.84[a]	0.96[a]
Homicide							
White	0.10[a]	0.20[a]	0.16	1.19	1.48	1.21	1.42
African-American	0.81[a]	0.39[a]	0.74[a]	5.05	6.56	6.37	5.89

Adapted the National Center for Injury Prevention and Control, Centers for Disease Control and Prevention, WISQARS, United States, 2004. *Injury mortality reports.* Available at: www.cdc.gov/ncipc/osp/data.htm., Last accessed 12. 2006.
[a]Figure does not meet standards of reliability or precision.

absolute numbers and rates of firearm-related deaths occurred in the 20- to 24-year (19.29 per 100,000) and the 25- to 29-year age-groups (16.90 per 100,000). Among firearm deaths from individuals aged 10 to 29 in 2004, 47% occurred among white males, 40% among African-American males, 6% among white females, and 3% among African-American females. However, the death rate is highest among African-American males aged 20 to 24 years at 107.64 per 100,000, which is five times that of white males of the same age. American Indian/Alaskan Native males aged 20 to 24 have the next highest death rate at 26.58 per 100,000. Adolescent male (15 to 24 years old) deaths due to firearms were eight times the rate among females (National Center for Injury Prevention and Control, 2006a).

Cancer

Excluding intentional and unintentional injuries, cancer is the leading cause of death in adolescents and is the leading cause of death by disease. It is the second cause of death among younger adolescents 10- to 14-years old and ranks fourth among 15- to 24-year olds (National Center for Injury Prevention and Control, 2006, National Center for Health Statistics, 2006). In 2005, the estimated number of children younger than 15 years old diagnosed with cancer was 9,510 and 1,585 were estimated to have died from cancer (American Cancer Society, 2005). The overall annual incidence of cancer for adolescents has increased from 141.4 per million in 1975–1981 to 162.6 per million in 1996–2002 (Ries et al., 2005). On an average, 1 or 2 of every 10,000 children

in the country develops cancer (National Cancer Institute, 2005, http://www.cancer.gov/cancertopics/factsheet/Sites-Types/childhood.).

The types of tumors that occur in the adolescent population, especially those 15- to 19-years old, differ significantly from those that predominate in younger children and adults. During adolescence, there are increases in incidence and mortality due to Hodgkin disease, germ cell tumors, central nervous system tumors, and non-Hodgkin lymphoma, thyroid cancer, malignant melanoma, and acute lymphoblastic leukemia (Ries et al., 1999). Table 5.7 lists the incidence, mortality, and 5-year survival rates of the top cancer sites among 5- to 19-year olds. Of the 12 major types of childhood cancers, leukemias (blood cell cancers) and brain and other central nervous system tumors account for more than one half of new cases. Leukemias make up approximately one third of childhood cancers and it is the number one cause of death from malignancies among 15- to 24-year olds. Overall 5-year survival rates for adolescents aged 10 to 14 years with cancer have improved from 58.8% (1975–1977) to approximately 80% (1996–2002) and for those aged 15 to 19 the 5-year survivals rates have improved from 67.7% to 79.7% (National Cancer Institute, 2005). This is reflected in a decreasing cancer mortality rate.

Human Immunodeficiency Virus

HIV remains one of the ten leading causes of death in all ages between 15 and 54 years, although each ranking has decreased since 1994 and HIV has fallen out of the top ten

TABLE 5.7

Childhood Cancer, SEER Incidence, Mortality, and 5-Year Survival Rates (per 100,000) for Top Cancer Sites by Age Group 2000–2003

	Incidence	Mortality	5-yr Survival 1975–1977	5-yr Survival 1996–2002
Ages 5–9				
All sites	11.2	2.5	58.2	77.9
Brain and other nervous system	3.2	0.9	58.0	72.4
Leukemia	3.8	0.7	52.0	80.7
Acute lymphocytic	3.2	0.4	55.2	84.0
Ages 10–14				
All sites	12.5	2.5	58.8	79.7
Bone and joint	1.3	0.3	53.8	69.88
Brain and other nervous system	2.6	0.7	59.5	80.1
Hodgkin lymphoma	1.1	0	78.7	95.2
Leukemia	2.8	0.8	35.2	70.5
Acute lymphocytic	1.9	0.4	43.6	80.7
Ages 15–19				
All sites	21.0	3.6	67.7	79.7
Bone and joint	1.5	0.5	51.0	63.3
Melanoma of the skin	1.7	0	75.1	97.5
Testis	3.4	0.1	66.0	91.7
Brain and other nervous system	2.0	0.5	64.7	79.9
Thyroid	1.8	—	100	97.5
Hodgkin lymphoma	3.0	0.1	88.9	94.9
Non-Hodgkin lymphoma	1.7	0.3	45.2	75.5
Leukemia	3.0	1.1	24.4	48.9
Acute lymphocytic	1.7	0.5	29.5	52.7

Adapted from National Cancer Institute. *SEER cancer statistics review, 1975–2003.* Bethesda, MD: National Cancer Institute, Available at http://seer.cancer.gov/cgi-bin/csr/1975_2003/search.pl#results. Accessed 12.3.2006

causes of death in those younger than 15 and older than 54. HIV infection ranks 14th for ages 10 to 14 years, 10th for ages 15 to 24, and 6th for ages 25 to 34 (National Center for Injury Prevention and Control, 2006). HIV mortality in the second and third decades of life often represents infection acquired during the teen years.

Trends in Mortality

Death rates from all causes have actually decreased over the past few decades (Tables 5.8 and 5.9), but the nature of youth deaths has changed drastically. Nevertheless, death rates for adolescents and young adults are still higher in 2004 than they were in 1950 for deaths due to suicides and homicides. Injuries cause more adolescent deaths than all diseases and natural causes combined. At least one U.S. adolescent between 10 and 19 years of age dies as the result of an injury every hour, every day. Unintentional injury accounts for approximately 60% of all adolescent injury-related deaths; the remaining 40% are attributed to violence (National Center for Health Statistics, 2000; Deal et al., 2000). Advanced technology has helped to keep more adolescents alive after experiencing an event that years ago might have been fatal. However, there is ample room for improvement in implementing prevention efforts that will reduce the incidence of adolescent injury altogether. More than 75% of all deaths among

persons 15- to 24-years old are due to four causes—motor vehicle crashes, other unintentional injuries, homicide, and suicide. Additional data regarding adolescent unintentional injuries are discussed in the following section.

UNINTENTIONAL INJURIES

Unintentional injuries account for 44% of all injury deaths to children and adolescents in the United States. Among youth aged 1 to 19 years, unintentional injuries are responsible for more deaths than homicide, suicide, congenital anomalies, cancer, heart disease, respiratory illness, and HIV combined (Deal et al., 2000). Table 5.10 is a summary of unintentional/accidental deaths by age and type in 2004. Tables 5.11 through 5.13 give the death rates and number of deaths due to all intent injuries among adolescents by event, race, ethnicity, and sex in 2003 for 10- to 14-year-old, 15- to 19-year-old, and 20- to 24-year-old adolescents.

National injury surveillance provides more information about treatment of injuries (NSC, 2006). In 2002, in personal household interviews (National Health Interview Survey), 23.7 million people reported seeking medical care for an injury; a survey of hospitals (National Hospital Discharge Survey) found that 2.7 million people were hospitalized for an injury. Additionally, 39.2 million patients in private

TABLE 5.8

Mortality Rates (per 100,000) for Common Causes of Death among Children and Adolescents, United States, Trends over Selected Years 1950–2004

Cause and Age Group (yr)	1950	1960	1970	1980	1985	1987	1992	1998	2002	2004
Accidents, all										
5–14	20.1	26.0	20.1	15.0	12.5	12.3	9.3	8.3	6.6	6.62
15–24	48.2	58.4	68.7	61.7	48.4	48.9	37.8	35.9	38.0	37.86
Motor vehicle accidents										
5–14	8.8	7.9	10.2	7.9	6.8	7.0	5.2	4.8	3.9	3.93
15–24	34.4	38.0	47.2	44.8	36.1	37.8	28.5	26.9	28.2	28.15
Homicide										
5–14	0.5	0.5	0.9	1.2	1.2	1.2	1.6	1.2	0.9	0.87
15–24	6.3	5.9	11.7	15.6	12.1	14.0	22.2	14.8	12.9	12.39
Suicide										
5–14	0.2	0.3	0.3	0.4	0.8	0.7	0.9	0.8	0.6	0.64
15–24	4.5	5.2	8.8	12.3	12.9	12.9	13.0	11.1	9.9	10.35
Malignant neoplasms										
5–14	6.7	6.8	6.0	4.3	3.5	3.3	3.0	2.6	2.6	2.5
15–24	8.6	8.3	8.3	6.3	5.4	5.1	5.0	4.6	4.3	4.0
Human immunodeficiency virus										
5–14	—	—	—	—	—	—	0.6	0.1	0.1	0.1
15–24	—	—	—	—	—	—	3.4	0.5	0.4	0.5
Diseases of the heart										
5–14	2.1	1.3	0.8	0.9	0.9	1.2	0.8	0.8	0.6	0.6
15–24	6.8	4.0	3.0	2.9	2.8	3.6	2.7	2.8	2.5	2.3
Congenital anomalies										
5–14	2.4	3.6	2.2	1.6	1.4	1.3	1.2	0.9	1.0	0.9
15–24	1.8	2.7	2.1	1.4	1.2	1.3	1.2	1.2	1.2	1.2
Pneumonia and influenza										
5–14	3.2	2.6	1.6	0.6	0.4	0.3	0.3	0.3	0.2	0.2
15–24	3.2	3.0	2.4	0.8	0.6	0.7	0.6	0.6	0.4	0.5
Cerebrovascular events										
5–14	0.5	0.7	0.7	0.3	0.2	0.2	0.2	0.2	0.2	0.2
15–24	1.6	1.8	1.6	1.0	0.8	0.6	0.5	0.5	0.4	0.5
Total										
5–14	60.1	46.6	41.3	30.6	26.3	25.6	22.5	19.9	17.4	16.6
15–24	128.1	106.3	127.7	115.4	95.9	99.4	95.6	82.3	81.4	78.9

Adapted from National Center for Health Statistics. *National vital statistics reports. Table 5.7. Deaths and death rates for 10 leading causes of death in specified age groups, United States, 2004,* Vol. 54. No. 19. Hyattsville, MD: US DHHS, June 28, 2006; and CDC. WISQARS, accessed 12/2006.

physicians' offices reported that they were treated in an emergency room for an injury (National Ambulatory Medical Care Survey). In 2003, the estimated cost of fatal and nonfatal injuries was >$607 billion, approximately $5,700 per household (National Safety Council, 2006). The number of nonfatal injuries is significantly greater than fatal injuries, at more than 15,000 per 100,000 for ages 15 to 19, and approximately 13,000 per 100,000 (Centers for Disease Control and Prevention, 2004a). Among 10- to 19-year olds, most nonfatal injuries are due to unintentional injury (90.7%), assault (7.9%), and self-harm (1.3%).

Trends in Injury Deaths

Despite significant reductions in incidence rates since 1979, injuries remain a major health problem (and the leading cause of death) for children and adolescents. In the pediatric age-group, unintentional injury mortality has fallen by >45% since 1979, with the largest decreases among those aged 5 to 9 years and the smallest decrease among teenagers. Table 5.14 reflects changes in childhood and adolescent injury rates by age-group over the last two decades and Table 5.15 shows the trend in unintentional injury and motor vehicle-related death rates throughout the last century (National Safety Council, 2004).

Morbidity

Deaths only partially convey the enormous damage caused by childhood injuries. It is estimated that for every childhood death caused by injury there are approximately 34 hospitalizations, 1,000 emergency department visits,

TABLE 5.9

Mortality Rates (per 100,000) of Adolescents Due to All Causes According to Race, Sex, and Age, United States, Trends in Selected Years 1950–2003

Race, Sex, and Age (yr)	1950	1960	1970	1980	1990	2000	2002	2003
White male								
5–14	67.2	52.7	48.0	35.0	26.4	19.8	18.4	18.4
15–24	152.4	143.7	170.8	167.0	131.3	105.8	109.7	108.9
White female								
5–14	45.1	34.7	29.9	22.9	17.9	14.1	13.7	13.1
15–24	71.5	54.9	61.6	55.5	45.9	41.2	42.4	43.2
African-American male								
5–14	95.1	75.1	67.1	47.4	41.2	28.2	28.9	26.8
15–24	289.7	212.0	320.6	209.1	252.2	181.4	172.6	171.3
African-American female								
5–14	72.8	53.8	43.8	30.5	27.5	20.0	19.9	18.9
15–24	213.1	107.5	111.9	70.5	68.7	58.3	54.4	54.0
Total								
5–14	*60.1*	*46.6*	*41.3*	*30.6*	*24.0*	*18.0*	*17.4*	*17.0*
15–24	*128.1*	*106.3*	*127.7*	*115.4*	*99.2*	*79.9*	*81.4*	*81.5*

Adapted from National Center for Health Statistics. *Health, United States, 2006 with chartbook on trends in the health of Americans. Table35*. Hyattsville, MD: US DHHS, 2006.

many more visits to private physicians and school nurses, and an even larger number of injuries treated at home. Approximately 21 million children in the United States are injured each year. This equates to an injury rate of one in four children, or 56,000 nonfatal injury episodes each day that require medical attention or limit children's activity (Danseco et al., 2000).

Leading Causes of Injuries

Four types of injury—being struck by or against an object or person, falls, motor vehicle traffic-related injuries, and being cut by a sharp object—account for approximately 60% of all injury-related visits to emergency departments by adolescents. Of these four causes, only motor vehicle traffic-related injuries are a significant source of mortality. Sports injuries make up >40% of injuries classified as "being struck by or against an object or person." At each age, the rate of such injuries among males is twice that among females (National Center for Health Statistics, 2000).

- Injuries are the leading cause of death for persons between the ages of 1 and 44 years in the United States.

- Unintentional injuries, suicide, and homicide cause >75% of all deaths in the adolescent age-group. Unintentional injuries cause approximately 42% of all deaths among 5- to 14-year olds and approximately 44% among 15- to 24-year olds. Intentional injuries comprise approximately 10% and 31% of deaths in these age-groups, respectively (National Center for Health Statistics, 2006c).
- The 15 to 24 year age-group has the highest cost related to injury of any age-group in the United States. Estimated costs for this group reach almost $90 million annually. The estimated total cost for unintentional childhood injuries just falls short of $350 billion each year (Danseco et al., 2000).

Epidemiology

Age: Years of monitoring have identified certain risk factors as fairly strong indicators of injury events. First and foremost, the risk of injury is clearly related to the physical, mental, and emotional developmental milestones of children or adolescents; for this reason, age is a predictable risk factor for injury. Infants are at greatest

TABLE 5.10

Unintentional (Accidental) Deaths by Age and Type, United States, 2004

Age (yr)	All Types	Motor Vehicle	Drowning	Fires and Burns	Firearms	Falls	Poisoning
10–14	1,540	1,013	138	87	35	26	47
15–19	6,825	5,224	304	66	80	87	643
20–24	8,624	5,763	270	120	92	154	1,616

CDC. WISQARS. 2006, last accessed 12.4.2006.

TABLE 5.11

Crude Death Rates (per 100,000) and Number of Deaths Due to All Intent Injuries among Adolescents 10- to 14-Year-Olds by Event, Race, Ethnicity (Hispanic, Non-Hispanic), and Sex, United States, 2003

Race	Male		Female		Both	
	No.	Rate	No.	Rate	No.	Rate
All injury deaths						
White	1,006	11.93	460	5.75	1,466	8.92
Black	297	16.43	137	7.82	434	12.20
American Indian/Alaskan Native	37	24.14	13[a]	8.67[a]	50	16.49
Asian Pacific Islander	38	8.20	21	4.80	59	6.55
All races, Non-Hispanic	1,158	12.88	546	6.38	1,704	9.71
All races, Hispanic	218	11.66	85	4.76	303	8.29
All injury and adverse effects deaths						
White	1,007	11.94	462	5.77	1,469	8.94
Black	298	16.49	139	7.94	437	12.28
American Indian/Alaskan Native	37	24.14	13[a]	8.67[a]	50	16.49
Asian Pacific Islander	38	8.2	21	4.8	59	6.55
All races, Non-Hispanic	1,160	12.90	549	6.42	1,709	9.74
All races, Hispanic	218	11.66	86	4.81	304	8.31
Cut/pierce deaths						
White	8[a]	0.09[a]	3[a]	0.04[a]	11[a]	0.07[a]
Black	4[a]	0.22[a]	2[a]	0.11[a]	6[a]	0.17[a]
American Indian/Alaskan Native	0[a]	0[a]	0[a]	0[a]	0[a]	0[a]
Asian Pacific Islander	0[a]	0[a]	0[a]	0[a]	0[a]	0[a]
All races, Non-Hispanic	9[a]	0.10[a]	4[a]	0.05[a]	13[a]	0.07[a]
All races, Hispanic	3[a]	0.16[a]	1[a]	0.06[a]	4[a]	0.11[a]
Drowning deaths						
White	56	0.66	21	0.26	77	0.47
Black	44	2.43	13[a]	0.74[a]	57	1.60
American Indian/Alaskan Native	3[a]	1.96[a]	1[a]	0.67[a]	4[a]	1.32[a]
Asian Pacific Islander	6[a]	1.29[a]	1[a]	0.23[a]	7[a]	0.78[a]
All races, Non-Hispanic	93	1.03	30	0.35	123	0.70
All races, Hispanic	16[a]	0.86[a]	6[a]	0.34[a]	22	0.60
Fall deaths						
White	19[a]	0.23[a]	11[a]	0.14[a]	30	0.18
Black	2[a]	0.11[a]	1[a]	0.06[a]	3[a]	0.08[a]
American Indian/Alaskan Native	0[a]	0[a]	0[a]	0[a]	0[a]	0[a]
Asian Pacific Islander	2[a]	0.43[a]	1[a]	0.23[a]	3[a]	0.33[a]
All races, Non-Hispanic	19[a]	0.21[a]	9[a]	0.11[a]	28	0.16
All races, Hispanic	4[a]	0.21[a]	4[a]	0.22[a]	8[a]	0.22[a]
Fire/burn deaths						
White	24	0.28	27	0.34	51	0.31
Black	20[a]	1.11[a]	15[a]	0.86[a]	35	0.98
American Indian/Alaskan Native	1[a]	0.65[a]	1[a]	0.67[a]	2[a]	0.66[a]
Asian Pacific Islander	1[a]	0.22[a]	0[a]	0[a]	1[a]	0.11[a]
All races, Non-Hispanic	43	0.48	37	0.43	80	0.46
All races, Hispanic	3[a]	0.16[a]	6[a]	0.34[a]	9[a]	0.25[a]
Residential fire/flame deaths						
White	18[a]	0.21[a]	22	0.27	40	0.24
Black	18[a]	1[a]	15[a]	0.86[a]	33	0.93
American Indian/Alaskan Native	1[a]	0.65[a]	1[a]	0.67[a]	2[a]	0.66[a]
Asian Pacific Islander	1[a]	0.22[a]	0[a]	0[a]	1[a]	0.11[a]
All races, Non-Hispanic	36	0.40	33	0.39	69	0.39
All races, Hispanic	2[a]	0.11[a]	5[a]	0.28[a]	7[a]	0.19[a]
Firearm deaths						
White	137	1.62	22	0.27	159	0.97
Black	67	3.71	22	1.26	89	2.50
American Indian/Alaskan Native	5[a]	3.26[a]	1[a]	0.67[a]	6[a]	1.98[a]
Asian Pacific Islander	7[a]	1.51[a]	0[a]	0[a]	7[a]	0.78[a]

(continued)

TABLE 5.11
(Continued)

Race	Male		Female		Both	
	No.	Rate	No.	Rate	No.	Rate
All races, Non-Hispanic	182	2.02	37	0.43	219	1.25
All races, Hispanic	34	1.82	8*	0.45*	42	1.15
Motor vehicle, overall						
White	508	6.02	286	3.57	794	4.83
Black	94	5.20	59	3.37	153	4.30
American Indian/Alaskan Native	19*	12.39*	6*	4*	25	8.24
Asian Pacific Islander	15*	3.24*	10*	2.29*	25*	2.77*
All races, Non-Hispanic	528	5.87	314	3.67	842	4.80
All races, Hispanic	107	5.72	47	2.63	154	4.21
Motorcyclist deaths						
White	21	0.25	3*	0.04*	24	0.15
Black	3*	0.17*	1*	0.06*	4*	0.11*
American Indian/Alaskan Native	0*	0*	0*	0*	0*	0*
Asian Pacific Islander	1*	0.22*	0*	0*	1*	0.11*
All races, Non-Hispanic	24	0.27	3*	0.04*	27	0.15
All races, Hispanic	1*	0.05*	1*	0.06*	2*	0.05*
Pedal cyclist deaths						
White	53	0.63	10*	0.12*	63	0.38
Black	14*	0.77*	2*	0.11*	16*	0.45*
American Indian/Alaskan Native	3*	1.96*	0*	0*	3*	0.99*
Asian Pacific Islander	4*	0.86*	1*	0.23*	5*	0.55*
All races, Non-Hispanic	63	0.70	13*	0.15*	76	0.43
All races, Hispanic	11*	0.59*	0*	0*	11*	0.30*
Pedestrian deaths						
White	102	1.21	41	0.51	143	0.87
Black	22	1.22	18*	1.03*	40	1.12
American Indian/Alaskan Native	3*	1.96*	1*	0.67*	4*	1.32*
Asian Pacific Islander	0*	0*	0*	0*	0*	0*
All races, Non-Hispanic	106	1.18	54	0.63	160	0.91
All races, Hispanic	21	1.12	6*	0.34*	27	0.74
Poisoning deaths						
White	24	0.28	12*	0.15*	36	0.22
Black	9*	0.50*	9*	0.51*	18*	0.51*
American Indian/Alaskan Native	2*	1.30*	1*	0.67*	3*	0.99*
Asian Pacific Islander	1*	0.22*	3*	0.69*	4*	0.44*
All races, Non-Hispanic	33	0.37	20*	0.23*	53	0.30
All races, Hispanic	3*	0.16*	5*	0.28*	8*	0.22*
Suicide deaths						
White	147	1.74	41	0.51	188	1.14
Black	34	1.88	9*	0.51*	43	1.21
American Indian/Alaskan Native	6*	3.91*	1*	0.67*	7*	2.31*
Asian Pacific Islander	1*	0.22*	5*	1.14*	6*	0.67*
All races, Non-Hispanic	156	1.74	44	0.51	200	1.14
All races, Hispanic	31	1.66	12*	0.67*	43	1.18
Homicide deaths						
White	72	0.85	26	0.32	98	0.60
Black	66	3.65	29	1.66	95	2.67
American Indian/Alaskan Native	1*	0.65*	1*	0.67*	2*	0.66*
Asian Pacific Islander	6*	1.29*	1*	0.23*	7*	0.78*
All races, Non-Hispanic	116	1.29	49	0.57	165	0.94
All races, Hispanic	29	1.55	8*	0.45*	37	1.01

[a]Rates based on 20 or fewer deaths may be unstable. Use with caution.

Adapted the National Center for Injury Prevention and Control, Centers for Disease Control and Prevention, WISQARS, United States, *Injury mortality reports*. Available at: www.cdc.gov/ncipc/osp/data.htm. 2003.

TABLE 5.12

Crude Death Rates (per 100,000) and Number of Deaths Due to All Intent Injuries among Adolescents 15- to 19-Year-Olds by Event, Race, Ethnicity (Hispanic, Non-Hispanic), and Sex, United States, 2003

	Male		Female		Both	
Race	No.	Rate	No.	Rate	No.	Rate
All injury deaths						
White	5,830	70.41	2,173	27.86	8,003	49.77
Black	1,580	96.78	300	18.94	1,880	58.44
American Indian/Alaskan Native	163	109.14	73	50.71	236	80.46
Asian Pacific Islander	175	38.01	75	17.20	250	27.89
All races, Non-Hispanic	6,367	72.02	2,276	27.09	8,643	50.12
All races, Hispanic	1,350	80.23	339	21.71	1,689	52.06
All injury and adverse effects deaths						
White	5,845	70.59	2,176	27.90	8,021	49.88
Black	1,582	96.90	300	18.94	1,882	58.51
American Indian/Alaskan Native	164	109.81	73	50.71	237	80.80
Asian Pacific Islander	175	38.01	75	17.20	250	27.89
All races, Non-Hispanic	6,382	72.19	2,278	27.11	8,660	50.22
All races, Hispanic Cut/pierce deaths	1,352	80.35	340	21.77	1,692	52.16
White	71	0.86	15*	0.19*	86	0.53
Black	62	3.80	18*	1.14*	80	2.49
American Indian/Alaskan Native	6*	4.02*	1*	0.69*	7*	2.39*
Asian Pacific Islander	4*	0.87*	1*	0.23*	5*	0.56*
All races, Non-Hispanic	104	1.18	28	0.33	132	0.77
All races, Hispanic	36	2.14	7*	0.45*	43	1.33
Drowning deaths						
White	194	2.34	18*	0.23*	212	1.32
Black	58	3.55	4*	0.25*	62	1.93
American Indian/Alaskan Native	3*	2.01*	1*	0.69*	4*	1.36*
Asian Pacific Islander	18*	3.91*	1*	0.23*	19*	2.12*
All races, Non-Hispanic	224	2.53	23	0.27	247	1.43
All races, Hispanic	46	2.73	1*	0.06*	47	1.45
Fall deaths						
White	82	0.99	23	0.29	105	0.65
Black	8*	0.49*	2*	0.13*	10*	0.31*
American Indian/Alaskan Native	2*	1.34*	2*	1.39*	4*	1.36*
Asian Pacific Islander	6*	1.30*	1*	0.23*	7*	0.78*
All races, Non-Hispanic	86	0.97	27	0.32	113	0.66
All races, Hispanic	12*	0.71*	1*	0.06*	13*	0.40*
Fire/burn deaths						
White	44	0.53	27*	0.35*	71	0.44
Black	13*	0.08*	11*	0.69*	24	0.75
American Indian/Alaskan Native	0*	0*	1*	0.69*	1*	0.34*
Asian Pacific Islander	2*	0.43*	0*	0*	2*	0.22*
All races, Non-Hispanic	49	0.55	35	0.42	84	0.49
All races, Hispanic	10*	0.59*	4*	0.26*	14*	0.43*
Residential fire/flame deaths						
White	27	0.33	16*	0.21*	43	0.27
Black	9*	0.55*	10*	0.63*	19*	0.59*
American Indian/Alaskan Native	0*	0*	1*	0.69*	1*	0.34*
Asian Pacific Islander	1*	0.22*	0*	0*	1*	0.11*
All races, Non-Hispanic	32	0.36	24	0.29	56	0.32
All races, Hispanic	5*	0.30*	3*	0.19*	8*	0.25*
Firearm deaths						
White	1,194	14.42	154	1.97	1,348	8.38
Black	969	59.35	67	4.23	1,036	32.21
American Indian/Alaskan Native	34	22.77	9*	6.25*	43	14.66
Asian Pacific Islander	34	7.39	8*	1.83*	42	4.69

(continued)

TABLE 5.12

(Continued)

	Male		Female		Both	
Race	No.	Rate	No.	Rate	No.	Rate
All races, Non-Hispanic	1,766	19.98	193	2.30	1,959	11.36
All races, Hispanic	454	26.98	44	2.82	498	15.35
Motor vehicle, overall						
White	2,996	36.18	1,532	19.64	4,528	28.16
Black	352	21.56	145	9.15	497	15.45
American Indian/Alaskan Native	78	52.53	43	29.87	121	41.25
Asian Pacific Islander	86	18.68	50	11.47	136	15.17
All races, Non-Hispanic	2,925	33.09	1,546	18.40	4,471	25.93
All races, Hispanic	580	34.47	221	14.15	801	24.69
Motorcyclist deaths						
White	157	1.90	17*	0.22*	174	1.08
Black	12*	0.74*	2*	0.13*	14*	0.44*
American Indian/Alaskan Native	1*	0.67*	0*	0*	1*	0.34*
Asian Pacific Islander	4*	0.87*	1*	0.23*	5*	0.56*
All races, Non-Hispanic	147	1.66	19*	0.23*	166	0.96
All races, Hispanic	27	1.60	1*	0.06*	28	0.86
Pedal cyclist deaths						
White	40	0.48	12*	0.15*	52	0.32
Black	7*	0.43*	0*	0*	7*	0.22*
American Indian/Alaskan Native	4*	2.68*	0*	0*	4*	1.38*
Asian Pacific Islander	2*	0.43*	0*	0*	2*	0.22*
All races, Non-Hispanic	45	0.51	10*	0.12*	55	0.32
All races, Hispanic	8*	0.48*	2*	0.13*	10*	0.31*
Pedestrian deaths						
White	178	2.15	82	1.05	260	1.62
Black	37	2.27	19*	1.20*	56	1.74
American Indian/Alaskan Native	14*	9.37*	4*	2.78*	18*	6.14*
Asian Pacific Islander	6*	1.30*	3*	0.69*	9*	1*
All races, Non-Hispanic	182	2.06	91	1.08	273	1.58
All races, Hispanic	53	3.15	17*	1.09*	70	2.16
Poisoning deaths						
White	499	6.03	180	2.31	679	4.22
Black	14*	0.86*	13*	0.82*	27	0.84
American Indian/Alaskan Native	8*	5.36*	4*	2.78*	12*	4.09*
Asian Pacific Islander	5*	1.09*	2*	0.46*	7*	0.78*
All races, Non-Hispanic	463	5.24	179	2.13	642	3.72
All races, Hispanic	62	3.68	19*	1.22*	81	2.50
Suicide deaths						
White	1,047	12.64	227	2.91	1,274	7.92
Black	107	6.55	14*	0.88*	121	3.76
American Indian/Alaskan Native	37	24.77	13*	9.03*	50	17.05
Asian Pacific Islander	31	6.73	11*	2.52*	42	4.69
All races, Non-Hispanic	1,065	12.05	227	2.70	1,292	7.49
All races, Hispanic	155	9.21	37	2.37	192	5.92
Homicide deaths						
White	660	7.97	138	1.77	798	4.96
Black	962	58.92	106	6.69	1,068	33.20
American Indian/Alaskan Native	23	15.40	8*	5.56*	31	10.57
Asian Pacific Islander	32	6.95	9*	2.06*	41	4.57
All races, Non-Hispanic	1,239	14.02	212	2.52	1,451	8.41
All races, Hispanic	423	25.14	48	3.07	471	14.52

[a]Rates based on 20 or fewer deaths may be unstable. Use with caution.

Adapted the National Center for Injury Prevention and Control, Centers for Disease Control and Prevention, WISQARS, United States, *Injury mortality reports.* Available at: www.cdc.gov/ncipc/osp/data.htm. 2003.

TABLE 5.13

Crude Death Rates (per 100,000) and Number of Deaths Due to All-Intent Injuries among Adolescents 20- to 24-Year-Old by Event, Race, Ethnicity (Hispanic, Non-Hispanic), and Sex, United States, 2003

Race	Male		Female		Both	
	No.	Rate	No.	Rate	No.	Rate
All injury deaths						
White	8,779	103.69	2,240	28.43	11,019	67.41
Black	2,797	180.37	480	30.74	3,277	105.30
American Indian/Alaskan Native	213	148.83	58	43.77	271	98.32
Asian Pacific Islander	261	49.93	88	17.19	349	33.73
All races, Non-Hispanic	9,830	114.15	2,498	29.69	12,328	72.42
All races, Hispanic	2,179	105.19	354	21.16	2,533	67.65
All injury and adverse effects deaths						
White	8,786	103.77	2,252	28.58	11,038	67.53
Black	2,798	180.43	483	30.93	3,281	105.42
American Indian/Alaskan Native	213	148.83	58	43.77	271	98.32
Asian Pacific Islander	261	49.93	88	17.19	349	33.73
All races, Non-Hispanic	9,837	114.23	2,512	29.86	12,349	72.54
All races, Hispanic Cut/pierce deaths	2,180	105.23	355	21.22	2,535	67.70
White	133	1.57	43	0.55	176	1.08
Black	100	6.45	31	1.99	131	4.21
American Indian/Alaskan Native	8*	5.59*	2*	1.51*	10*	3.63*
Asian Pacific Islander	13*	2.49*	2*	0.39*	15*	1.45*
All races, Non-Hispanic	179	2.08	59	0.70	238	1.40
All races, Hispanic	75	3.62	18*	1.08*	93	2.48
Drowning deaths						
White	222	2.62	22	0.28	244	1.49
Black	50	3.22	5*	0.32*	55	1.77
American Indian/Alaskan Native	8*	5.59*	0*	0*	8*	2.90*
Asian Pacific Islander	19*	3.63*	4*	0.78*	23	2.22
All races, Non-Hispanic	229	2.66	28	0.33	257	1.51
All races, Hispanic	70	3.38	3*	0.18*	73	1.95
Fall deaths						
White	158	1.87	28	0.36	186	1.14
Black	14*	0.90*	6*	0.38*	20*	0.64*
American Indian/Alaskan Native	3*	2.10*	1*	0.75*	4*	1.45*
Asian Pacific Islander	6*	1.15*	3*	0.59*	9*	0.87*
All races, Non-Hispanic	144	1.67	33	0.39	177	1.04
All races, Hispanic	37	1.79	5*	0.30*	42	1.12
Fire/burn deaths						
White	78	0.92	50	0.63	128	0.78
Black	16*	1.03*	10*	0.64*	26	0.84
American Indian/Alaskan Native	3*	2.10*	0*	0*	3*	1.09*
Asian Pacific Islander	0*	0*	2*	0.39*	2*	0.19*
All races, Non-Hispanic	88	1.02	54	0.64	142	0.83
All races, Hispanic	8*	0.39*	8*	0.48*	16*	0.43*
Residential fire/flame deaths						
White	45	0.53	31	0.39	76	0.46
Black	8*	0.52*	7*	0.45*	15*	0.48*
American Indian/Alaskan Native	1*	0.70*	0*	0*	1*	0.10*
Asian Pacific Islander	0*	0*	1*	0.20*	1*	0.10*
All races, Non-Hispanic	52	0.60	36	0.43	88	0.52
All races, Hispanic	2*	0.10*	3*	0.18*	5*	0.13*
Firearm deaths						
White	2,022	23.88	240	3.05	2,262	13.84
Black	1,817	117.17	164	10.50	1,981	63.65
American Indian/Alaskan Native	47	32.84	6*	4.53*	53	19.23
Asian Pacific Islander	69	13.20	12*	2.34*	81	7.83

(continued)

TABLE 5.13

(Continued)

Race	Male		Female		Both	
	No.	Rate	No.	Rate	No.	Rate
All races, Non-Hispanic	3,159	36.68	350	4.16	3,509	20.61
All races, Hispanic	780	37.65	68	4.07	848	22.65
Motor vehicle, overall						
White	3,586	42.35	1,167	14.81	4,753	29.08
Black	538	34.69	157	10.05	695	22.33
American Indian/Alaskan Native	99	69.18	35	26.41	134	48.62
Asian Pacific Islander	96	18.36	42	8.21	138	13.34
All races, Non-Hispanic	3,488	40.5	1,232	14.65	4,720	27.73
All races, Hispanic	820	39.58	165	9.86	985	26.31
Motorcyclist deaths						
White	396	4.68	37	0.47	433	2.65
Black	50	3.22	3*	0.19*	53	1.70
American Indian/Alaskan Native	3*	2.10*	0*	0*	3*	1.09*
Asian Pacific Islander	17*	3.25*	0*	0*	17*	1.64*
All races, Non-Hispanic	415	4.82	37	0.44*	452	2.66
All races, Hispanic	50	2.41	3*	0.18*	53	1.42
Pedal cyclist deaths						
White	31	0.37	0*	0*	31	0.19
Black	2*	0.13*	2*	0.13*	4*	0.13*
American Indian/Alaskan Native	0*	0*	0*	0*	0*	0*
Asian Pacific Islander	1*	0.19*	0*	0*	1*	0.10*
All races, Non-Hispanic	22	0.26	2*	0.02*	24	0.14
All races, Hispanic	12*	0.58*	0*	0*	12*	0.32*
Pedestrian deaths						
White	246	2.91	72	0.91	318	1.95
Black	46	2.97	16*	1.02*	62	1.99
American Indian/Alaskan Native	12*	8.38*	1*	0.75*	13*	4.72*
Asian Pacific Islander	8*	1.53*	5*	0.98*	13*	1.26*
All races, Non-Hispanic	232	2.69	84	1	316	1.86
All races, Hispanic	77	3.72	10*	0.60*	87	2.32
Poisoning deaths						
White	1,408	16.63	441	5.60	1,849	11.31
Black	70	4.51	25	1.60	95	3.05
American Indian/Alaskan Native	13*	9.08*	4*	3.02*	17*	6.17*
Asian Pacific Islander	13*	2.49*	11*	2.15*	24	2.32
All races, Non-Hispanic	1,354	15.72	442	5.25	1,796	10.55
All races, Hispanic	148	7.14	38	2.27	186	4.97
Suicide deaths						
White	1,781	21.04	263	3.34	2,044	12.50
Black	278	17.93	48	3.07	326	10.47
American Indian/Alaskan Native	43	30.05	10*	7.55*	53	19.23
Asian Pacific Islander	57	10.90	21	4.10	78	7.54
All races, Non-Hispanic	1,885	21.89	306	3.64	2,191	12.87
All races, Hispanic	266	12.84	33	1.97	299	7.99
Homicide deaths						
White	1,121	13.24	252	3.2	1,373	8.40
Black	1,727	111.37	211	13.51	1,938	62.27
American Indian/Alaskan Native	35	24.46	12*	9.06*	47	17.05
Asian Pacific Islander	64	12.24	8*	1.56*	72	6.96
All races, Non-Hispanic	2,216	25.73	378	4.49	2,594	15.24
All races, Hispanic	716	34.56	99	5.92	815	21.77

[a]Rates based on 20 or fewer deaths may be unstable. Use with caution.

Adapted from the National Center for Injury Prevention and Control, Centers for Disease Control and Prevention, WISQARS (Web-based Injury Statistics Query and Reporting System), United States, *Injury mortality reports*. Available at: www.cdc.gov/ncipc/osp/data.htm. 2003.

TABLE 5.14

Unintentional Injury Mortality Rates (per 100,000 and Number of Deaths by Age Group), United States, 1979, 1996, and 2003

Age Group	1979		1996		2004	
	Rate	Number	Rate	Number	Rate	Number
0–4	27.24	4,377	15.01	2,895	13.42	2,693
5–9	15.97	2,690	8.04	1,564	5.74	1,126
10–14	16.07	2,966	9.61	1,824	7.29	1,540
15–19	59.30	12,664	36.09	6,735	32.93	6,825
All children and adolescents	31.16	22,697	17.04	13,018	14.94	12,184

Adapted from The National Center for Injury Prevention and Control, Centers for Disease Control and Prevention, WISQARS. United States, 2004. *Injury mortality reports.* Available at: www.cdc.gov/ncipc/osp/data.htm. Last accessed 12.4.2006.

risk of burns, drowning, and falls. As children increasingly acquire mobility, poisonings join the list. Young school-aged children are at greatest risk of pedestrian injuries, bicycle-related injuries, motor vehicle occupant injuries, burns, and drowning. Adolescents are most likely to suffer from motor vehicle injuries and injuries resulting from firearms and other forms of violence (Rivara and Aitken, 1998). At 10 years of age slightly fewer than half of all deaths are caused by injury but, by 18 years, >80% are injury related (National Center for Health Statistics, 2006). For every type of injury, except bicycle deaths, there are substantial rate increases between early and late adolescence.

Gender: A second important risk factor for injury is gender. Beginning at approximately 1 or 2 years of age and continuing until the seventh decade of life, males have higher rates of injury than females. This gender difference during childhood does not appear to be caused by differences in developmental or motor skills. In part, it may be related to greater exposure of males to hazards or to gender-based differences in behavior (Rivara and Aitken, 1998). For nearly all injuries in 2003, the male death rate from injuries exceeds the rate in females: 2.1 times among adolescents aged 10 to 14 years, 2.8 times for ages 15 to 19 years, and 3.97 times for young adults aged 20 to 24 years (National Center for Injury Prevention and Control, 2006b).

Race and ethnicity: Injury death rates also vary substantially by race and ethnicity. The highest injury fatality rates are among African-American and Native American adolescents and the lowest rates are among Asian youth, as seen in Tables 5.11, 5.12, and 5.13. In 2003, adolescent African-American males had the highest death rates due to drowning, firearms, and homicide. Although the overall numbers are lower, American Indian and Alaskan Natives have the highest overall death rates among 10- to 19-year olds and the second highest among 20- to 24-year olds. African-American males had the highest death rate among 20- to 24-year olds. Hispanic youth have rates between those of whites and African-Americans, although age and gender also influence those rates. A further explanation for these racial differences appears to be related to poverty, which is another important risk factor in predicting adolescent injuries.

Factors Contributing to Adolescent Injuries

Socioeconomic factors: Poor children are at greatest risk for injury and studies have indicated that their risk level is two to five times that of children who are not poor. This is true for pedestrian injuries, fires and burns, drownings, and intentional injuries. The number of U.S. children living in poverty in 2003 was 12.7 million (Annie E. Casey Foundation, 2005). The injury death rate is consistently higher in nonmetropolitan areas than in cities (Rivara and Aitken, 1998).

Environmental factors: The risk associated with each type of adolescent injury is also influenced by environmental factors. These include hazards such as all-terrain vehicles, backyard swimming pools, firearms, kerosene

TABLE 5.15

Unintentional Injury Death Rates (per 100,000) among Youth by Age Group, United States, 1903–2003

	Total by Age (yr)		Motor Vehicle by Age (yr)	
Year	5–14	15–24	5–14	15–24
1903	46.8	65.0	—	—
1910	39.1	65.3	—	—
1920	44.9	55.5	14.6	8.7
1930	36.9	62.3	14.7	27.4
1940	28.8	53.5	11.5	28.7
1950	22.6	55.0	8.8	34.5
1960	19.1	55.6	7.9	37.7
1970	20.1	68.0	10.2	46.7
1980	15.0	61.7	7.9	44.8
1990	10.3	43.9	5.8	34.2
2000	7.5	36.7	4.5	27.5
2004	6.54	37.05	4.06	26.35

Adapted from National Safety Council. *Injury facts: 2004 edition.* Itasca, IL: National Safety Council, 2004 and CDC. WISQARS, 2006, last accessed 12.4.2006.

heaters, traffic patterns, and gang activity. Policies such as regulations concerning requirements for fences around private pools, smoke detectors in homes, bicycle helmets, and graduated drivers license programs with night restrictions also influence injury rates.

Location—school environment: Because children and adolescents spend much of their day at school, it follows that many of the injuries they sustain occur there. In fact, between 33% and 50% of all child and adolescent injuries happen on school grounds. Playground accidents are the most common source of childhood injury at schools, particularly in the lower grades. However, most such injuries are minor and do not require medical attention (Hudson et al., 1999). Males are injured at school much more often than females. Falls are the most common cause of injury in secondary schools, and they usually result in contusions, abrasions, or local swelling. Also frequent are burns, strains, sprains, and dislocations, especially of the upper extremities. The number of injuries that occur in vocational classrooms and on athletic fields increases with age and grade level. A large number of those injuries involve the improper use or malfunctioning of equipment (Knight et al., 2000).

Developmental factors: Factors contributing to high injury rates in adolescents often relate to the discrepancies between an adolescent's physical development and his or her cognitive and emotional development. Adolescent health is influenced by the strengths and vulnerabilities of individuals and also by the character of the settings in which they live. These settings—the schools they attend, the neighborhoods they call home, their families, and the friends who make up their social network—play an important role in shaping adolescent health, affecting how individuals feel about themselves as well as influencing the choices they make about behaviors that can affect their health and well-being.

As a group, adolescents are physically healthy. They have survived early childhood and are decades away from the diseases associated with aging. Threats to their health stem primarily from their behavior. Several developmental characteristics of the adolescent contribute to risk-taking behaviors and may lead to injuries and death. Some of these characteristics are as follows:

- Experimentation with adult roles
- Experimentation with risky behaviors or situations when opportunities for healthy risk taking are not available or provided
- Challenge of authority or rules
- Desire for peer approval and a tendency to join peer activities and to follow peer norms

Placing these characteristics in an environment where there is alcohol, tobacco, violence, unprotected sex, fast cars, and drugs heightens adolescents' risk of injury and death (Blum and Rinehart, 1999).

Automobile Injuries

Automobile injuries are the leading cause of mortality and morbidity among all Americans aged 1 to 64 years. The transportation environment is the most dangerous setting for the adolescent, whether as a driver, passenger, motorcyclist, bicyclist, or pedestrian. Crashes involving adolescent drivers typically are single-vehicle crashes, primarily run-off-the-road crashes, and involve driver error and/or speeding (Insurance Institute for Highway Safety, 2005). Among youth 10- to 19-years old, motor vehicle traffic–related injuries account for almost 36% of all deaths and 74% of deaths due to unintentional injuries (National Center for Injury Prevention and Control, 2006a). An excellent overall review of the teen driver is in the American Academy of Pediatrics policy statement from December 2006. This policy paper reviews risk factors, proposed interventions, and recommendations for health care providers.

Risk Factors for Automobile Injuries

Teenagers are at particularly high risk for motor vehicle crashes primarily because of their inexperience and risk-taking behaviors. Teenagers are more likely to underestimate the dangers in hazardous situations, and have less experience coping with such situations (Chen et al., 2000; Insurance Institute for Highway Safety, 2005). Research shows that teenagers are more likely than older drivers to speed, run red lights, make illegal turns, tailgate, ride with an intoxicated driver, and drive after using alcohol or other drugs. Males are more likely than females to engage in risky driving behaviors, drive after drinking alcohol, and are less likely to wear seat belts (Centers for Disease Control and Prevention, 2006). Younger age, driving at night, having other teen passengers in the vehicle, and driving after drinking alcohol increases the risk of motor vehicle crashes.

- More than 75% of children aged 5 to 14 years who die in traffic crashes were not wearing a seat belt or other restraint (Federal Interagency Forum on Child and Family Statistics, 2000).
- In 2003, two out of every three adolescents killed in motor vehicle crashes were male.
- The risk of crash involvement per mile driven among drivers aged 16 to 19 years is four times the risk among older drivers.
- Approximately 60% of adolescent passenger deaths in 2003 were in motor vehicles driven by another adolescent.
- In 2003, 42% of motor vehicle–related deaths among adolescents occurred between 9 p.m. and 6 a.m. and 54% of teen motor vehicle crashes occurred on Friday, Saturday, or Sunday (Insurance Institute for Highway Safety, 2005)
- In 2001 to 2002, night time passenger vehicle crashes were three times higher among females and six times higher among male drivers 16- to 19-years old than for those 30- to 59-years old.
- The incidence of motor vehicle crashes fatal to 16- and 17-year-old drivers, in particular, increases with the number of passengers for both male and female drivers, during daytime and at night. Crashes are more likely to be fatal to drivers aged 16 and 17 years when in the presence of male passengers, teenage passengers, and passengers aged 20 to 29 years (Chen et al., 2000).

Alcohol

Alcohol involvement in crashes is highest among men aged 21 to 30 years. Alcohol-related crashes peak at night and are higher on weekends than on weekdays. Among passenger vehicle drivers fatally injured between 9 p.m. and 6 a.m. in 1998, 55% had a blood alcohol concentration (BAC) of 0.10% or greater, compared with 15% of such drivers during other hours. On weekends in 1998 (6 p.m. Friday to 6 a.m.

Monday) 41% of fatally injured drivers had a BAC of 0.10% or higher; during the week, the corresponding measure was 21% (Insurance Institute for Highway Safety, 2005a).

Data analysis shows that at all levels of BAC, the risk of being involved in a motor vehicle crash is greater for teenagers and young people than for older people. In 2003, 16% of fatally injured drivers aged 16 and 17 had BACs at or >0.08%, a 60% decrease from 1982 (Insurance Institute for Highway Safety, 2005a). Teenage male drivers with a BAC in the 0.5% to 0.10% range are 18 times more likely and female drivers 54 times more likely than sober teenagers to be killed in single-vehicle crashes (Insurance Institute for Highway Safety, 2005). Although many states have reduced the BAC for "driving while intoxicated" (DWI) convictions to 0.08%, zero-tolerance policies for adolescents younger than 21 years may further reduce alcohol-related motor vehicle injuries.

In a 2005 national survey of high school students, 28.5% of respondents said that within the last 30 days they had ridden in a motor vehicle driven by someone who had been drinking alcohol (Centers for Disease Control and Prevention, 2006) and 9.9% had driven a motor vehicle after drinking alcohol. This is a decrease from 39.9% and 16.7%, respectively, in 1991.

Air Bags and Seat Belts

For all ages, air bags reduce the risk of death in frontal crashes by 18% and in all crashes by 11%. However, for children younger than 13 years air bags actually may increase the risk of death. A safety device that protects against death in all but a very few specific situations is the safety belt, with which all vehicles are equipped (Rivara, 1999). In the 2005 YRBS, approximately 10% of high school students reported that they rarely or never wear safety belts when riding with someone else (Centers for Disease Control and Prevention, 2006). Male high school students are more likely (12.5%) than female students (7.8%) to rarely or never wear safety belts. Black (13.4%) and Hispanic (10.6%) students are more likely than white students (9.4%) to rarely or never wear safety belts (Centers for Disease Control and Prevention, 2006).

Graduated Licensing Programs

Motor vehicle crashes are highest in the first 2 years that drivers have their license. The crash rate per mile driven is twice as high among 16-year olds as it is among 18- to 19-year olds. Graduated licensing programs are ideally designed to have three phases of supervision including a supervised learning period, an intermediate restricted license, and then an unrestricted license. In the intermediate phase, new drivers have limits on higher risk conditions such as late-night driving and transporting other adolescent passengers while unsupervised. After this phase, the restrictions are removed and the driver is fully licensed. Early data from states that have implemented graduated driving demonstrate a decrease in adolescent motor vehicle–related crashes and fatalities (Marin and Brown, 2005; Hedlund and Compton, 2005). Almost all states have enacted some form of a graduated driver licensing law.

Nonautomobile Injuries

Motorcycle

- Males accounted for nine of every ten motorcycle deaths in 2005.

- A total of 4,439 motorcyclists died in crashes in 2005. Motorcyclist deaths had been declining since the early 1980s but began to increase in 1998 and have continued to increase. Since 1997 motorcyclist deaths have more than doubled.
- In 2005, 32% of all motorcycle deaths occurred among 16- to 29-year olds.
- For each mile traveled, the number of deaths on motorcycles is 27 times greater than in cars (Insurance Institute for Highway Safety, 2005b).

Drowning

Drowning was the second leading cause of unintentional death in children younger than 15 and the third cause of unintentional death in those 15- to 24-years old in 2004. Approximately 1,500 children and adolescents die each year in the United States (Rivara, 1999). Drowning is unique as an injury problem because of its high case-fatality rate and because of the relative lack of impact that medical care has on outcome. Approximately 50% of children and adolescents requiring care for a submersion incident will die (Rivara, 1999). Swimming pools play a role in drowning among young, school-aged children and among adolescents; immersion in natural bodies of water, either while swimming or boating, also plays an increasingly important role (Rivara and Aitken, 1998).

Gender: In 2004, males accounted for almost 80% of fatal drownings in the United States. Males are three times more likely to die from drowning than are females in almost every age-group (National Center for Injury Prevention and Control, 2006c). Males between the ages of 15 and 19 years are more than 10 times likely to drown than females of the same age.

Race: In 2004, the overall age-adjusted drowning rate for African-Americans was 1.25 times higher than that for whites. Black children aged 5 to 19 years drowned at 2.3 times the rate of similar-aged whites.

Alcohol use: Alcohol use is involved in approximately 25% to 50% of adolescent and adult deaths associated with water recreation. It is also a major contributing factor in up to 50% of drownings among adolescent boys in particular (National Center for Injury Prevention and Control, 2006c).

Firearms

Firearms are the sixth leading cause of death due to unintentional injuries in the adolescent age-group. In 2004, 3,635 children and adolescents 20 years and younger died from firearms. This represents an 11% reduction from 1997 and a 47% decrease since 1994. Tables 5.11, 5.12, and 5.13 include the number of death and mortality rates by firearms according to age-group, sex, and race in 2003.

- It is estimated that there are three nonfatal firearm injuries for every death associated with a firearm.
- Adolescents and young adults have the highest rate of unintentional firearm-related fatalities; males between the ages of 20 and 24 years having the highest risk (National Center for Health Statistics, 2006a).
- More than 75% of homicides of older adolescents and young adults are committed with a firearm.
- Among adolescents 15- to 19-years old, one in every four deaths is caused by a firearm (National Center for Injury Prevention and Control, 2006a).

- More than 85% of all firearm-related deaths occur in males (Rivara, 1999).
- Firearm assaults on family members and other intimate acquaintances are 12 times more likely to result in death than assaults with other weapons.
- In 2005, 5.4% of high school students in a national survey reported having carried a gun to school within the last 30 days (Centers for Disease Control and Prevention, 2006).

Bicycle Accidents

- In 2005, 782 bicyclists were killed in crashes with motor vehicles. This is a 38% reduction since 1975 but a 25% increase since 2003.
- In 2005, 21% of bicycle deaths were among riders 14 years and younger (National Highway Traffic Safety Administration, 2005).
- In 2005, 87% of bicycle deaths occurred among males (IIHS 2005c).
- In 2005, 23% of riders who died in a bicycle-related accident had elevated blood alcohol levels.
- Bicycle deaths are most likely to occur in the summer and fall and between the hours of 3 p.m. and 9 p.m. (IIHS, 2005c).
- In 2002, almost 300,000 children 14 years and younger were treated in emergency departments for bicycle-related injuries.
- Approximately 70% of fatal bicycle crashes involve head injuries.
- In 2005, 86% of bicycle-related deaths occurred in riders without helmets (Insurance Institute for Highway Safety 2005c). Bicycle helmets decrease the risk of head injury by 85% and brain injury by 88%.
- Collisions with motor vehicles are responsible for approximately 33% of all bicycle-related brain injuries and 90% of bicycle fatalities.
- In 2005, of all high school students who reported riding a bicycle within the preceding 12 months, 83.4% reported never or rarely wearing a bicycle helmet (Centers for Disease Control and Prevention, 2006).

Skateboards

Skateboarding has experienced intermittent periods of popularity since the 1960s. Along with this popularity, there have been concomitant increases in numerous types of injuries. Most documented cases occur in boys between the ages of 10 and 14 years, with injuries ranging from minor cuts and abrasions to multiple fractures and, in some cases, even death. Head injuries account for approximately 3.5% to 9% and fractures of both upper and lower extremities account for 50% of all skateboarding injuries. Not surprisingly, 33% of those injured on skateboards experience some form of trauma within the first week of participating in the sport. Despite traffic legislation, 65% of injured adolescents sustain injuries on public roads, footpaths, and parking lots (Fountain and Meyers, 1996).

All-Terrain Vehicles

Almost 3,000 deaths have been associated with use of all-terrain vehicles (ATVs) since 1985. The risk of death is approximately 0.8 to 1.0/10,000 ATVs, and has remained fairly steady for the last 10 years. Children younger than 16 years account for 47% of the injuries and 36% of deaths, whereas those younger than 12 years represent 15% of all deaths related to ATVs. Risk factors for injury include rider inexperience, intoxication with alcohol, excessive speed, and lack of helmet use. Head injuries account for most ATV-related deaths. Other nonfatal injuries include head and spinal trauma, abdominal injuries, abrasions, lacerations, and fractures (American Academy of Pediatrics, Committee on Injury and Poison Prevention, 2000a).

Boating Accidents

In 2004, the U.S. Coast Guard received reports for 4,904 boating incidents; 3,363 participants were reported injured and 676 died in boating incidents (National Center for Injury Prevention and Control, 2006c). Among those who drowned, 90% were not wearing life jackets. Most boating fatalities in 2004 (70%) were caused by drowning; the remainder were due to trauma, hypothermia, carbon monoxide poisoning, or other causes. Alcohol was involved in about one third of all reported boating fatalities. Personal watercrafts (PWCs) were involved in 25% of incidents.

The use of PWC has increased dramatically during the last decade, as have the speed and mobility of the watercraft. A similar dramatic increase in PWC-related injury and death has occurred simultaneously. In many states, persons younger than 16 years are not legal operators of PWCs. Nonetheless, 7% of these injuries occur in children aged 14 years and younger and 27% occur in those younger than 17 years. The most common types of PWC-related injuries are head trauma, lacerations, and fractures (American Academy of Pediatrics, Committee on Injury and Poison Prevention, 2000b).

Poisoning

In 2004 alone, more than 2.4 million human exposures to poison were reported to poison control centers in the United States (Watson et al., 2005). U.S. poison centers handled one poison exposure every 13 seconds. Each year, almost 900,000 visits to emergency departments occur because of poisonings (National Center for Injury Prevention and Control, 2006c). Although young children are at particularly high risk for unintentional ingestion, the percentage of unintentional deaths due to poisoning actually increases with age in the adolescent population (National Center for Injury Prevention and Control, 2006b). Adolescent females are more likely to die by poisoning compared to males (55.1% vs. 44.5%). In 2004, there were 90 reported adolescent fatalities, comprising 7.6% of all poison-related fatalities. Of these, >50% were presumed suicides and 27% were caused by intentional abuse (Watson et al., 2005).

Common household items are often the cause of poisonings. For young adolescents between the ages of 10 and 14 years, approximately 80% of all poisoning deaths are from substances other than medications. In contrast, medications cause 58% of all poisoning deaths among adolescents aged 15 to 19 years. The most lethal substances for children of all ages are stimulants, street drugs, cardiovascular drugs, and antidepressants (Grossman, 2000b).

Sports Injuries

In the 2004–2005 school year, the number of high school athletes increased to more than 7 million participants. This is the 16th consecutive year of increased participation (National Federation of State High School Associations, 2005). Such participation also results in approximately 750,000 sports-related injuries each year that require hospital-based emergency treatment. In total, injury rates are reported to be as high as 81% of all participants, with >3 million injuries annually resulting in time lost from sports (Marsh and Daigneault, 1999). Football is associated with the highest number of catastrophic (fatal, permanent severe functional disability, or severe injury without permanent functional disability) injuries. Male athletes account for 84% of all adolescent sports-related injuries, despite the fact that rates are often higher among females, because fewer girls participate overall (Cheng et al., 2000). However, the number of catastrophic injuries among female athletes has increased. According to the National Center for Catastrophic Sports Injury Research, the incorporation of gymnastic type stunts in cheerleading has lead to these sports accounting for 50% of high school and 64% of college female athlete catastrophic injuries (National Center for Catastrophic Sport Injury Research, 2005). Within any given season, it is estimated that 48% of all adolescent athletes sustain at least one injury (Patel and Nelson, 2000). Of all adolescent sports injuries, 17% occur while participating in one of six sports—football, basketball, baseball or softball, soccer, biking, or skating. The event-based injury rate is 25.0 per 1,000 adolescents and the most common mechanisms are falls and being struck by or against objects. Table 5.16 shows the percentages of injury types and body locations in those six high school sports. Hospitalization is required in 2% of all sports-related injury visits; of those cases, 51% involve other persons, 12% are equipment related, and 8% involve poor field or surface conditions (Cheng et al., 2000).

Football

Football accounts for the highest number of injuries in boys (Patel and Nelson, 2000). Of all football injuries, 7% involve being struck by an opponent's helmet and 9% involve inappropriate field conditions. Football has the highest number and rate of mild traumatic brain injury. The chance of sustaining a mild brain injury is 11 times higher during football games than during practices (Powell and Barber-Foss, 1999). In 2004, there were 19 high school and ONE college catastrophic injuries (National Center for Catastrophic Sport Injury Research, 2005). In addition, there were ten indirect fatalities related to

heat stroke and lightning strikes. There were also 13 permanent disabilities—10 cervical spine and 3 head injuries.

Basketball

Basketball causes more facial and dental injuries among adolescents than any other sport (American Academy of Pediatrics, Committee on Sports Medicine and Fitness CSMF, 2000a). The injury rates for boys' and girls' basketball are 28.3 and 28.7 per 100 players, respectively. For both boys and girls, the ankle or foot is the most common site of injury, accounting for 39.3% of injuries in boys and 36.6% in girls. Knee injuries make up 11.1% of all injuries in boys and 15.7% in girls. Boys sustain 42% of their injuries in game situations, whereas 46.8% of girls' injuries happen during games. The types of activities that mostly cause injury during games are dribbling for girls (13.1%) and shooting or related activities for boys (13.3%) (Powell and Barber-Foss, 2000).

Baseball

The adolescent injury rate for baseball is 13.2 per 100 players. Of all baseball injuries, 55% involve ball or bat impact, often to the head (Cheng et al., 2000). Baseball injuries are divided fairly evenly between practices and games. During baseball games, base running accounts for the largest proportion of injuries (25.7%), followed by fielding (23.4%). Approximately 24.6% of baseball injuries occur to the forearm, wrist, or hand, and 19.7% occur to the arms or shoulders. Approximately one in five baseball injuries occur among pitchers (Powell and Barber-Foss, 2000).

Softball

The adolescent injury rate for softball is 16.7 per 100 players. This makes the softball injury rate 27% higher than that of baseball. Practices account for 55.9% of all softball injuries. The types of softball injuries that occur most often are similar to those that occur in baseball. During softball games, base running accounts for the largest proportion of injuries (32.7%), followed by fielding (26.9%). Slightly >10% of softball injuries occur among pitchers. Approximately 22.9% of softball injuries occur to the forearm, wrist, or hand, and 16.3% occur to the arms or shoulders (Powell and Barber-Foss, 2000).

TABLE 5.16

Injuries in Six Sports: Injury Type and Body Location, 1996–1998 (percentage with each sport)

Sport	Injury Type					Body Location			
	Head Injury	Fracture Dislocation	Open Wound	Contusion Abrasion	Sprain Strain	Head	Upper Extremity	Lower Extremity	Torso
Baseball/softball	7	24	17	20	32	37	32	26	3
Basketball	2	23	13	17	44	17	34	45	4
Bicycling	9	20	27	34	8	29	34	29	7
Football	5	29	11	23	31	16	47	28	8
Skating	4	39	9	17	25	10	50	30	9
Soccer	10	26	7	30	25	22	30	41	8

Adapted from Cheng TL, Fields CB, Brenner RA, et al. Sports injuries: an important cause of morbidity in urban youth. *Pediatrics* 2000;105:e32.

Soccer

Soccer is one of the most popular team sports. Of all soccer-related injuries, 45% occur in players younger than 15 years. Injury rates per 1,000 player-hours range from 0.6 to 19.1 per 1,000, depending on the level of play and the definition of injury. Soccer is the second leading cause of facial and dental injuries in sports, preceded only by basketball (American Academy of Pediatrics, Committee on Sports Medicine and Fitness, 2000a). For all sports, soccer accounts for the highest number of injuries in girls (Patel and Nelson, 2000). The injury rates for boys' and girls' soccer are 23.4 and 26.7 per 100 players, respectively. Most soccer injuries happen during game situations, accounting for 59.3% of boys' injuries and 57.8% of girls' injuries. The most common site of soccer injury for both boys and girls is the ankle or foot, accounting for 33.3% of boys' injuries and 33.5% of girls' injuries. Other injuries occur most commonly to the hip, thigh, or leg and then the knee, for both boys and girls. Concussive injuries during soccer often occur because of head–head or head–ground impact (National Center for Catastrophic Sport Injury Research, 2004). The knee injury rate for girls' soccer is 5.2 per 100 players (Powell and Barber-Foss, 2000). In 1999, the Consumer Product Safety Commission announced new safety standards to reduce the risk of soccer goal tip-over. Tip-overs have been associated with a number of soccer participant fatalities (National Center for Catastrophic Sport Injury Research, 2005).

Ice Hockey

Ice hockey is played by approximately 200,000 youth in the United States. Because collisions in this sport occur at high speeds, participants are at risk for serious injury. Among players between the ages of 9 and 15 years, head and neck trauma account for 23% of all injuries. Body checking accounts for 86% of all injuries that occur during games. Of particular concern is that size differences among players often increase with age, with 14- and 15-year-old players showing the most variation. Players in this age-group also sustain the most injuries (54%) (American Academy of Pediatrics, Committee on Sports Medicine and Fitness, 2000b).

RECOVERY FROM INJURIES: CONSIDERATIONS IN THE ADOLESCENT

Children and youth grow and mature both physically and psychologically during the adolescent years. Maturation results in physiological changes that affect performance, health status, and healing. Feeling themselves to be invulnerable, it is not uncommon for adolescents to push themselves psychologically and physically beyond their limits. Increasing peer pressure may encourage adolescents to aspire to be and do what it is they think others expect of them.

Adolescent development may also confound the recovery period in various ways.

1. It is often difficult to distinguish between developmental issues of adolescents and problems secondary to an injury, such as irritability or poor judgment.
2. Peer, family, or team expectations may fail to adjust to changes resulting from an injury.
3. Young people often lack the experience and maturity to make healthy choices and at times this may impede

their rehabilitation and successful recovery after serious injury.

4. Mental changes including impaired judgment, decreased attention span, irritability, short-term memory loss, and memory deficits make it difficult for adolescents to adhere to a treatment regimen.
5. Adolescents who experience athletic injuries and must discontinue sports participation may suffer depression or other psychological symptoms (Marsh and Daigneault, 1999).

PREVENTION OF INJURIES

Most unintentional injury deaths of children can be prevented. The three key approaches to injury prevention are education, environment and product changes, and legislation or regulation. Education can serve to promote changes in individual behaviors that increase the risk of injury and/or death. Environment and product modifications can make the adolescent's physical surroundings, toys, equipment, and clothes less likely to facilitate an injury. Legislation and regulation are among the most powerful tools to reduce adolescent injury, but they also require the most energy and concentrated efforts on the part of individuals and groups.

Successful reductions in future rates of childhood and adolescent injury will require the dedication of individuals to implement evidence for what works, the determination of communities to create environments where children can grow safely, and public and private funds to support injury prevention research and disseminate effective interventions. The following lists are examples of some of the measures that may be taken to reduce injuries to adolescents.

Motor Vehicle Injuries

1. Adopt graduated licensing laws and policies that keep teenage drivers off the streets during late night and early morning hours.
2. Have parents impose restrictions and limitations of driving privileges on their teenage children.
3. Adopt laws restricting the number and age of passengers carried by teenage drivers (Chen et al., 2000; Grossman, 2000a).
4. Promote administrative license revocation that authorizes police to confiscate the licenses of drivers who either fail or refuse to take a chemical test for alcohol.
5. Promote primary safety belt laws that allow police to stop vehicles if the occupants are not using safety belts.
6. Strictly enforce zero-tolerance laws for blood alcohol in drivers younger than 21 years.
7. Evaluate strategies to limit access to alcohol and promote safety belt use among teenagers.
8. Continue to evaluate the separate components of graduated licensing systems to determine which ones are most effective.

Bicycle Injuries

1. Make bicycle helmets mandatory for all riders.
2. Impose bicycle curfews to keep riders off the streets after dark.

3. Disseminate injury control recommendations on bicycle helmets.
4. Distribute written materials addressing all traffic laws and rules of the road in communities and schools.
5. Advise against riding double and freestyle stunt riding.

Drownings

1. Encourage swimming lessons at an early age.
2. Educate parents about the dangers of leaving children unattended in the bathtub or around swimming pools.
3. Establish a buddy system and never swim alone.
4. Educate people about the dangers of mixing alcohol with swimming or boating.
5. Mandate and enforce legal limits for BAC during water recreation activities.
6. Eliminate advertisements that encourage alcohol use during water recreation.
7. Require fencing around all public and private pools.
8. Restrict the sale of alcohol at water recreation facilities.
9. Always wear a personal flotation device while boating in open water (Grossman, 2000a).

Personal Watercraft Injuries

1. Require a PWC operator's license for 16- to 20-year olds.
2. Restrict adolescents younger than 16 years from operating a PWC unless accompanied by an adult.

3. Require PWC driver education for all operators.
4. Require helmets and life jackets for all riders.

Sports Injuries

1. Make the preparticipation athletic examination a requirement for all participants.
2. Encourage weight training and aerobic conditioning before the start of the season.
3. Provide medical coverage for all athletes at sporting events.
4. Appoint only coaches who have been properly trained and certified in youth sports.
5. Ensure that all athletes are properly hydrated throughout sporting events.
6. Appoint only officials who have been properly trained and certified in youth sports.
7. Ensure that all playing equipment, fields, and surfaces are safe and approved for youth sport participation.
8. Document the proper use of sport-specific protective equipment and distribute such items to all participants and their parents before play begins.
9. Check for proper safety equipment before approving players for participation in practice sessions or games.
10. Mandate the attendance of a certified emergency medical professional at all sporting events.
11. Arrange team composition based on body size and skills, not just chronologic age (Cheng et al., 2000).

Suicide

1. Document the risk factors for suicide attempts and disseminate this information to parents and teachers.

TABLE 5.17

Morbidity of Selected Notifiable Diseases in Children, Adolescents, and Young Adults, United States, 2005

Disease	5–14 yr	15–24 yr	25–39 yr	Total (All Ages)
Acquired immunodeficiency syndrome (AIDS)	110	2119	18,932	44,108
Chlamydia	NA	663,484	218,957	929,462
Gonorrhea	NA	189,629	104,451	330,132
Hepatitis A	883	887	1,20	5,683
Hepatitis B	32	664	24,435	6,212
Hepatitis C	2	119	223	720
Lyme disease	3,866	1,804	2,712	19,804
Measles	3	8	3	37
Meningococcal disease	163	275	148	1,361
Mumps	60	37	39	258
Pertussis	8,334	4,806	2,573	25,827
Syphilis (primary and secondary)	NA	1,368	3,878	7,980
Toxic shock syndrome	20	38	9	95
Tuberculosis	405	1,600	3,622	14,517

NA, data not available.

Adapted from Centers for Disease Control and Prevention. Summary of notifiable diseases—United States, 2004. *MMWR* 2006a;53(53):1–79. Published June 16, 2006 http://www.cdc.gov/mmwr/preview/mmwrhtml/mm5353a1.htm.

2. Ask questions about depression, suicidal thoughts, and other risk factors associated with suicide during routine history taking in adolescents.
3. Advocate for health insurance coverage that ensures adolescent access to adequate and appropriate preventive and therapeutic mental health (American Academy of Pediatrics, Committee on Adolescence, 2000).
4. Recommend that guns be removed from the home or, if present, that they be kept unloaded and locked separately from bullets or shells (Grossman, 2000a). Placing cable or trigger locks on locked guns is an added safety feature.

Homicide

1. Encourage use of a skills-building violence prevention and conflict resolution curriculum in the schools, from kindergarten through grade 12.
2. Provide education regarding conflict resolution, negotiation, and anger management skills among adolescents.
3. Advise parents to limit their adolescents' viewing of violence in the media and witnessing or experiencing violence in the home and neighborhood.
4. Encourage parents to remove guns from the home or, if guns are present, to keep them unloaded and locked separately from bullets or shells (Grossman, 2000a). Placing cable or trigger locks on locked guns is an added safety feature.

MORBIDITY

Notifiable Communicable Diseases

Mortality rates for adolescents are low compared with those for adults; nonetheless, there is significant morbidity among teenagers. Table 5.17 lists the morbidity rates for selected diseases among adolescents during 2004. As with adolescent deaths, many of the diseases that are contracted by adolescents are a result of health-related behaviors and lifestyle choices. For example, STDs are more prevalent among adolescents than any other population group.

Several other datasets available for understanding adolescent morbidity are reviewed in the following sections.

Hospitalizations and Outpatient Visits

Hospitalizations

According to the Healthcare Cost and Utilization Project, hospitalizations for youth between the ages of 1 and 17 years represented 4.5% of the total number of hospitalizations in the United States in 2002. Adolescent pregnancy accounts for 3% of all pediatric hospitalizations and for almost 9% of nonneonatal hospitalizations. The ten most common principal discharge diagnoses among all children aged 1 to 17, excluding those for pregnancy and pregnancy

related conditions, are listed here (Merrill and Elixhauser, 2005). For ages 13 to 17, injuries (including leg fractures), medication poisonings, and head injuries, are among the most common discharge diagnoses. Affective disorders are the most common cause of hospitalization for children for nonneonatal or nonpregnancy–related conditions (Owens et al., 2003).

Top Ten Diagnoses	Number of Discharges (in Thousands) for Ages 1–17	Number of Discharges (in Thousands) Ages 13–17
Asthma	128	15
Pneumonia	120	9
Fluid and electrolyte disorders (primarily dehydration and fluid overload)	75	—
Appendicitis	74	31
Affective or mood disorders (depression and bipolar disorder)	60	58
Epilepsy, convulsions	49	—
Acute bronchitis	36	—
Chemotherapy and radiation therapy	34	10
Skin and subcutaneous tissue infections	32	—
Other infections of upper respiratory tract (nose, throat, trachea)	30	—
Other mental disorders	—	26
Fracture of lower limb	—	15
Poisoning by medications and drugs	—	13
Diabetes mellitus with complications	—	12
Head (intracranial) injuries	—	10

Ambulatory Visits

Tables 5.18, 5.19, and 5.20 provide additional data regarding childhood and ambulatory adolescent medical visits. Adolescents and young adults aged 15 to 24 made 70,593,000 office visits in 2004 accounting for approximately 8% of all ambulatory visits in the United States. This group made an additional 17,931,000 emergency room visits. Preventive health care visits comprised 28% of visits in this age-group and 18.5% in the 5- to 14-year age-group. The most common visits in the 13- to 21-year age-group were for normal pregnancy, routine child care, upper respiratory infections, and acne. The most common emergency room visits were for contusions, open wounds, abdominal pain, fractures, and sprains and strains.

TABLE 5.18

Number, Percentage Distribution, and Annual Rate of Office Visits for Children, Adolescents, and Young Adults Aged 5 to 24 Years, United States, 2004

	5–14 yr	15–24 yr	All Ages
Number of outpatient office (in thousands)	76,144	70,593	910,857
% Distribution of all visits	8.4%	7.8%	100%
Acute problem	40,917 (53.7%)	28,587 (40.5%)	316,137 (34.7%)
Chronic problem, routine	13,643 (17.9%)	13,031 (18.5%)	296,569 (13.8%)
Chronic problem, flare-up	4,459 (5.9%)	4,546 (6.4%)	72,741 (8%)
Pre or post surgery	1,542 (2.0%)	2,667 (3.8%)	50,655 (5.6%)
Preventive care	14,078 (18.5%)	19,511 (27.6%)	147,002 (16.1%)
Unknown	1,505 (2.0%)	2,252 (3.2%)	27,754 (3.0%)
Number of ER visits (in thousands)	10,722	17,931	110,216
% Distribution	9.7%	16.3%	100%
Number of visits per 100 persons/yr	26.3	44.1	38.2

ER, emergency room. Adapted from National Ambulatory Medical Care Survey: 2004 Summary. *Advance data; health and vital statistics; number 374: June 23, 2006 and the National Ambulatory Medical Care Survey: 2004 Emergency Department Summary.* Advance Data; Health and Vital Statistics, Number 372: June 23, at http://www.cdc.gov/nchs/products/pubs/pubd/ad/ad.htm. 2006.

TABLE 5.19

Number and Percentage Distribution of Office and Emergency Room Visits for 13- to 21-Year-Olds, According to the Five Leading Primary Diagnosis Groups, United States, 2004

Primary Diagnosis Groups	Number of Visits (in Thousands)	Percentage Distribution (%)	Number of Visits per 100/persons/yr
All visits (office visits)	910,857	100	11.6
All visits, 13–21 yr	65,131	100	10.1
Normal pregnancy	4,033	6.2	4.3
Routine infant or child health check	3,368	5.2	1.7
Acute upper respiratory infection	2,966	4.6	1.5
Acne	2,624	4	1.1
Asthma	a	a	—
All other diagnoses	50,266	77.2	8.4
All visits (emergency room visits)	110,216	100	38.2
All visits, 13–21 yr	14,162	100	38.3
Contusion with intact skin surface	920	6.5	2.5
Open wound, excluding head	728	5.1	2.0
Abdominal pain	557	3.9	1.5
Fractures, excluding lower limb	522	3.7	1.4
Sprains and strains, excluding ankle and back	517	3.6	1.4
All other diagnoses	10,918	77.1	29.5

[a]Figure does not meet standard of reliability or precision.

Adapted from National Ambulatory Medical Care Survey: 2004 Summary. *Advance data; health and vital statistics; number 374: June 23, 2006 and the National Ambulatory Medical Care Survey: 2004 Emergency Department Summary.* Advance Data; Health and Vital Statistics; Number 372: June 23, at http://www.cdc.gov/nchs/products/pubs/pubd/ad/ad.htm. 2006.

TABLE 5.20

Number and Percentage Distribution of Office Visits by Selected Diagnostic and Therapeutic Services According to Age and Sex, United States, 1995–1996

Sexlected Visit Characteristics	Below 15 yr		15–24 yr	
	Number of Visits (1,000s)	Percentage Distribution of all Visits	Number of Visits (1,000s)	Percentage Distribution of All Visits
Diagnostic and screening services:				
All visits	136,200	100	57,682	100
No services Examinations:	76,369	56.1	16,066	27.9
Breast	1,018	0.7	5,066	8.8
Pelvic	729	0.5	8,369	14.5
Rectal	742	0.5	1,449	2.5
Visual	7,701	5.7	2,649	4.6
Tests:				
Blood pressure	17,281	12.7	26,457	45.9
Urinalysis	9,306	6.8	12,008	20.8
Cholesterol	432	0.3	672	1.2
Other blood test	9,077	6.7	6,415	11.1
Other test	9,648	7.1	6,023	10.4
X-ray	5,857	4.3	3,892	6.7
Therapeutic and preventive services:				
All visits	136,200	100	57,682	100
No services	95,314	70	39,140	67.9
Counseling/education:				
Weight reduction	722	0.5	1,342	2.3
Growth/development	22,051	16.2	2,099	3.6
Tobacco use/exposure	3,463	2.5	1,760	3.1
HIV transmission	[a]	[a]	895	1.6
Other counseling	8,593	6.3	5,476	9.5
Other therapy:				
Physiotherapy	1,346	1	1,881	3.3
Psychotherapy	788	0.6	1,247	2.2
Corrective lenses	743	0.5	252	0.4
Other therapy	1,852	1.4	929	1.6
Number of medications:				
Zero	47,717	35	24,220	42
One	48,260	35.4	18,535	32.1
Two	25,658	18.8	9,748	16.9
Three	10,736	7.9	3,329	5.8
Four	2,878	2.1	1,331	2.3
Five	605	0.4	347	0.6
Disposition:				
No follow-up	17,931	13.2	6,165	10.7
Return if needed	56,059	41.2	18,482	32
Return at specified time	61,846	45.4	32,114	55.7
Admit to hospital	654	0.5	377	0.7
Other disposition	4,221	3.1	1,775	3.1

HIV, human immunodeficiency virus. Adapted from Schappert SM, Nelson C. National Ambulatory Medical Care Survey, 1995–1996. Summary. *Vital health statistics,* Vol. 13. No. 142. 1999:59,66,81. Hyattsville, MD: National Center for Health Statistics.
[a]Figure does not meet standard of reliability or precision.

WEB SITES

http://www.childstats.gov. This Web site offers easy access to federal and state statistics and reports on children and their families, including population and family characteristics, economic security, health, behavior and social environment, and education. Reports of the Federal Interagency Forum on Child and Family Statistics include *America's Children: Key National Indicators of Well-Being,* the annual federal monitoring report on the status of the nation's children, and *Nurturing Fatherhood.*

http://hcupnet.ahrq.gov/. From the Agency for Healthcare Research and Quality, a tool for identifying, tracking, analyzing, and comparing statistics on hospitals at the national, regional, and state level.

http://www.iihs.org. Statistics from the Insurance Institute for Highway Safety.

http://www.cancer.gov/. Information from the National Cancer Institute.

http://www.cdc.gov/nccdphp/. Statistics and information on chronic diseases from National Center for Chronic Disease Prevention and Health Promotion.

http://www.cdc.gov/HealthyYouth/. Information on the Youth Risk Behavior Survey from the Centers for Disease Control and Prevention.

http://www.cdc.gov/nchs. Portal for national health statistics from the National Center for Health Statistics.

http://www.cdc.gov/ncipc/ncipchm.htm. Statistics and searching tool from the National Center for Injury Prevention and Control; click either data or facts for information.

http://www.cdc.gov/nchs/about/major/ahcd/ahcd1.htm. Data from the National Center for Health Statistics on ambulatory care.

http://www.health.gov/healthypeople/. Information on Healthy People 2010.

http://www.aecf.org. Annie E. Casey Foundation Web site, which provides national and state-by-state data and analysis on critical issues affecting families and at-risk kids.

http://www.ahrq.gov. Overall Web site for Agency for Healthcare Research and Quality.

http://www.cdc.gov. Overall Centers for Disease Control and Prevention portal for information and statistics including *Mortality and Morbidity Weekly Report.*

http://www.futureofchildren.org. *The Future of Children* is published by the Woodrow Wilson School of Public and International Affairs at Princeton University and The Brookings Institution. Its primary purpose is to disseminate timely information on major issues related to children's well-being.

http://www.guttmacher.org/. Publications and statistics on reproduction from the Allan Guttmacher Institute.

http://www.childtrends.org/. Child Trends is a nonprofit, nonpartisan research organization that studies children, youth, and families through research, data collection, and data analysis.

http://www.nih.gov/health/. Health information from the National Institutes for Health.

http://childhealthdata.org/Content/Default.aspx The Maternal and Child Health Bureau supported Child and Adolescent Health Measurement Initiative Data Resource Center (DRC) on Child and Adolescent Health Web site

puts national, state, and regional survey findings available in a searchable and easily compared and displayed format.

REFERENCES AND ADDITIONAL READINGS

Agency for Healthcare Research and Quality. *Healthcare cost and utilization project (HCUPnet).* Rockville, MD: Agency for Healthcare Research and Quality, Available at www.ahrq.gov/data/hcup/hcupnet.htm. 2000.

American Academy of Pediatrics, Committee on Adolescence. Suicide and suicide attempts in adolescents. *Pediatrics* 2000;105:871.

American Academy of Pediatrics, Committee on Injury and Poison Prevention. All-terrain vehicle injury prevention: two-, three-, and four-wheeled unlicensed motor vehicles. *Pediatrics* 2000a;105:1352.

American Academy of Pediatrics, Committee on Injury and Poison Prevention. Personal watercraft use by children and adolescents. *Pediatrics* 2000b;105:452.

American Academy of Pediatrics, Committee on Injury, Violence, and Poison Prevention and Committee on Adolescence. The teen driver. *Pediatrics* 2006;118:2570.

American Academy of Pediatrics, Committee on Sports Medicine and Fitness. Injuries in youth soccer: a subject review. *Pediatrics* 2000a;105:659.

American Academy of Pediatrics, Committee on Sports Medicine and Fitness. Safety in youth ice hockey: the effects of body checking. *Pediatrics* 2000b;105:657.

American Cancer Society. *Cancer facts and figures 2005.* Atlanta: American Cancer Society, 2005.

Annie E. Casey foundation. *Kids count data book, 2005.* Baltimore, MD: Annie E. Casey Foundation, 2005.

Blum RW, Rinehart PM. *Reducing the risk: connections that make a difference in the lives of youth.* Minneapolis, MN: Division of General Pediatrics and Adolescent Health, University of Minnesota, 1999.

Centers for Disease Control and Prevention. *Healthy youth, youth risk behavior survey.* Available at: http://www.cdc.gov/ HealthyYouth/yrbs/about_yrbss.htm. Accessed 2006.

Centers for Disease Control and Prevention. *Surveillance for fatal and nonfatal injuries, United States, 2001. MMWR Morb Mortal Wkly Rep* 2004a;53(SS07):1.

Centers for Disease Control and Prevention. Youth risk behavior surveillance, 2003. *Morb Mortal Wkly Rep CDC Surveill Summ* 2004b;53(SS-2):1–95.

Centers for Disease Control and Prevention. Summary of notifiable diseases, United States. *MMWR Morb Mortal Wkly Rep* 2006;53(53):1–79.

Centers for Disease Control and Prevention. Youth risk behavior surveillance, 2005. *Morb Mortal Wkly Rep CDC Surveill Summ* 2006b;55(SS-5):1–108.

Centers for Disease Control and Prevention. Summary of notifiable diseases–United States, 2004. *Morb Mortal Wkly Rep* 2006;53(53):1–79.

Chen LH, Baker SP, Braver ER, et al. Carrying passengers as a risk factor for crashes fatal to 16- and 17-year-old drivers. *JAMA* 2000;283:1578.

Cheng TL, Fields CB, Brenner RA, et al. Sports injuries: an important cause of morbidity in urban youth. *Pediatrics* 2000;105:e32.

Children's Defense Fund. *Each day in America*. Washington, DC: Children's Defense Fund, Available at: http://www.childrensdefense.org/data/eachday.aspx. 2004a.

Children's Defense Fund. *Moments in America for children*. Washington, DC: Children's Defense Fund, Available at: http://www.childrensdefense.org/data/moments.aspx. 2004b.

Children's Defense Fund. *Protect children not guns*. Washington, DC: Children's Defense Fund, 2005.

Danseco ER, Miller TR, Spicer RS. Incidence and costs of 1987–1994 childhood injuries: demographic breakdowns. *Pediatrics* 2000;105:e27.

Deal LW, Gomby DS, Zippiroli L, et al. Unintentional injuries in childhood: analysis and recommendations. *The future of children: unintentional injuries in childhood*, Vol. 10. Los Altos, CA: David and Lucile Packard Foundation, 2000:4.

Federal Interagency Forum on Child and Family Statistics. *American's children 2000*. Washington, DC, Available at http://www.childstats.gov. 2000.

Fountain JL, Meyers MC. Skateboarding injuries. *Sports Med* 1996;22:360.

Grossman D. Adolescent injury prevention and clinicians: time for instant messaging. *West J Med* 2000a;172:151.

Grossman DC. The history of injury control and the epidemiology of child and adolescent injuries. *The future of children: unintentional injuries in childhood*, Vol. 10. Los Altos, CA: David and Lucile Packard Foundation, 2000b:23.

Hedlund J, Compton R. Graduated driving research in 2004 and 2005. *J Safety Res* 2005;36:4.

Hudson S, Thompson D, Mack MG. The prevention of playground injuries. *J Sch Nurs* 1999;15:30.

Insurance Institute for Highway Safety. *2005 Fatality facts: teenagers*. Arlington, VA: IIHS, Available at www.iihs.org. 2005.

Insurance Institute for Highway Safety. *2005 Fatality facts: alcohol*. Arlington, VA: IIHS, Available at www.iihs.org. 2005a.

Insurance Institute for Highway Safety. *2005 Fatality facts: motorcycles*. Arlington, VA: IIHS, Available at www.iihs.org. 2005b.

Insurance Institute for Highway Safety. *2005 Fatality facts: bicycles*. Arlington, VA: IIHS, Available at www.iihs.org. 2005c.

Knight S, Junkins Ep Jr, Lightfoot AC, et al. Injuries sustained by students in shop class. *Pediatrics* 2000;106:10.

Marin PS, Brown BV. Are teens driving safer? *Child Trends* 2005:(4)1–10. Available at www.childtrendsdatabank.org.

Marsh JS, Daigneault JP. The young athlete. *Curr Opin Pediatr* 1999;11:84.

Merrill CT, Elixhauser A. *Hospitalization in the United States, 2002: HCUP fact book No. 6*. AHRQ Publication No. 05–0056, June 2005. Rockville, MD: Agency for Healthcare Research and Quality, 2005. http://www.ahrq.gov/data/hcup/factbk6/.

National Campaign to Prevent Teen Pregnancy. *Fact sheet: how is the 34% statistic calculated?* Washington, DC: National Campaign to Prevent Teen Pregnancy, 2004.

National Cancer Institute. *Cancer facts*. Bethesda, MD: NCI, Available at http://www.cancer.gov/cancertopics/factsheet/ accessed 3.15.07. 2005.

National Center for Catastrophic Sports Injury Research. *Twenty-second annual report on catastrophic sports injury research: fall 1982-spring 2004*. Last updated June 2005. Available at: http://www.unc.edu/depts/nccsi/AllSport.htm. 2005.

National Center for Health Statistics. *Health, United States, 2000 with adolescent health chartbook*. Hyattsville, MD. 2000.

National Center for Health Statistics. *Summary of surveys and data systems*. U.S. Department of Health and Human Services, Centers for Disease Control and Prevention, Available at http://www.cdc.gov/nchs/data/NCHS_Survey_Matrix.pdf. June 2004.

National Center for Health Statistics. Available at http://www.cdc.gov/nchs/about/major/nhis/hisdesc.htm. 2005.

National Center for Health Statistics. *Health, United States, 2006 with adolescent health chartbook*. Hyattsville, MD. Available at: http://www.cdc.gov/nchs/hus.htm. 2006.

National Center for Health Statistics. *National vital statistics report. Deaths: preliminary data for 2004*, Vol. 54. No. 19. Hyattsville, MD: U.S. Department of Health and Human Services, 2006a.

National Center for Health Statistics. *National vital statistics report. Deaths: final data for 2003*, Vol. 54. No. 13. Hyattsville, MD: U.S. Department of Health and Human Services, 2006b.

National Center for Health Statistics. *National vital statistics report. Injuries, 2002*, Vol. 54. No. 10. Hyattsville, MD: U.S. Department of Health and Human Services, 2006c.

National Center for Injury Prevention and Control. *Leading cause of death reports*. Atlanta, GA: CDC Web-based Injury Statistics Query and Reporting System (WISQARS), Available at http://webappa.cdc.gov/sasweb/ncipc/leadcaus.html. 2006.

National Center for Injury Prevention and Control. *Injury mortality reports*. Atlanta, GA: CDC Web-based Injury Statistics Query and Reporting System (WISQARS), Available at http://webappa.cdc.gov/sasweb/ncipc/mortrate.html. 2006a.

National Center for Injury Prevention and Control. *Injury mortality reports*. Atlanta, GA: CDC Web-based Injury Statistics Query and Reporting System (WISQARS), Available at www.cdc.gov/ncipc/osp/data.htm. 2006b.

National Center for Injury Prevention and Control. *Water-related injuries: fact sheet*. Atlanta, GA: Centers for Disease Control and Prevention, http://www.cdc.gov/ncipc/factsheets/drown.htm. 2006c.

National Center for Injury Prevention and Control. *Facts about poisoning*. Atlanta, GA: Centers for Disease Control and Prevention, Available at http://www.cdc.gov/ncipc/factsheets/poisoning.htm. 2006d.

National Center for Injury Prevention and Control. *Facts on adolescent injury*. Atlanta, GA: Centers for Disease Control and Prevention, Available at http://www.cdc.gov/ncipc/factsheets/children.htm. 2006e.

National Federation of State High School Associations. 2004–05 *NFHS high school athletics participation survey*. Indianapolis: National Federation of State High School Associations, Available at: www.nfhs.org. 2005.

National Highway Traffic Safety Administration. *Traffic safety facts: bicycle helmet use laws*. Washington, DC: National Center for Statistics and Analysis, Available at www.nhtsa.dot.gov. 2005.

National Safety Council. *Injury facts: 2004 edition*. Itasca, IL: National Safety Council, 2004.

National Safety Council. *Injury facts: 2005–2006 edition*. Itasca, IL: National Safety Council, 2006.

Owens PL, Thompson J, Elixhauser A, et al. *Care of children and adolescents in U.S. hospitals*. HCUP Fact Book No. 4 AHRQ Publication. Rockville, MD: Agency for Healthcare Research and Quality, 2003.

Patel DR, Nelson TL. Sports injuries in adolescents. *Med Clin North Am* 2000;84:983.

Powell JW, Barber-Foss KD. Traumatic brain injury in high school athletes. *JAMA* 1999;282:958.

Powell JW, Barber-Foss KD. Sex-related injury patterns among selected high school sports. *Am J Sports Med* 2000;28:385.

Ries LAG, Eisner MP, Kosary CL, et al. eds. *SEER cancer statistics review, 1975–2002*. Bethesda, MD: National Cancer Institute, Available at http://seer.cancer.gov/csr/1975_2002/. 2005.

Ries LAG, Smith MA, Gurney JG, et al. eds. *Cancer incidence and survival among children and adolescents: United States SEER program 1975–1995*. Bethesda, MD: National Cancer Institute, 1999.

Rivara FP. Pediatric injury control in 1999: Where do we go from here? *Pediatrics* 1999;103:883.

Rivara FP, Aitken M. Prevention of injuries to children and adolescents. *Adv Pediatr* 1998;45:37.

Schappert SM, Nelson C. National Ambulatory Medical Care Survey, 1995–1996: summary. In: *Vital and health statistics*, Vol. 13. No. 142. Hyattsville, MD: National Center for Health Statistics, 1999:17.

U.S. Census Bureau. *Statistical abstract of the United States: 2006*, 125th ed. Washington, DC: U.S. Bureau of the Census, Available at http://www.census.gov/compendia/statab/. 2006.

U.S. Department of Health and Human Services. *Healthy people 2010: understanding and improving health*, 2nd ed. Washington, DC: U.S. Government Printing Office, November 2000.

U.S. Department of Justice. *Homicide trends in the United States*. Last updated: June 29, 2006. Available at http://www.ojp.usdoj.gov/bjs/. 2006.

Watson WA, Litovitz TL, Rodgers GC, et al. 2004 annual report of the American association of poison control centers toxic exposure surveillance system. *Am J Emerg Med* 2005;23(5):589–666.

CHAPTER 6

Nutrition

Michael R. Kohn

This chapter focuses on energy and nutrient requirements as well as deficiency states that develop during adolescence. Adolescent obesity is discussed in Chapter 32.

Nutrition is an essential component of total adolescent health care. Two important transformations occur during adolescence that may cause significant changes in a teenager's nutritional needs. Growth in height and weight and changes in body composition are greater and more rapid than at any other time in life, except during infancy. In general, there is also a significant change in the adolescent's eating habits and food consumption. Adolescents have been found to have the highest prevalence of any age-group for unsatisfactory nutrition. Adolescents are known to reduce regular breakfast consumption, increase consumption of prepared foods, snacks, fried foods, nutrient-poor foods, and sweetened beverages and have a significant increase in portion size at each meal. This is associated with a decrease in the consumption of dairy products, fruits, and vegetables. Furthermore, sodium intake is far in excess of recommended levels, whereas calcium and potassium intakes are below recommended levels (Gidding et al., 2005).

Health care providers should assess nutritional status and provide appropriate nutritional counseling as part of health supervision visits. The MyPyramid Food Guide (www.MyPyramid.gov) is a helpful educational tool that can be used to assist teenagers in improving their diets (Figs. 6.1 and 6.2). MyPyramid incorporates recommendations from the *2005 Dietary Guidelines for Americans* that was released by the United States Department of Agriculture (USDA) and United States (U.S.) Department of Health and Human Services (HHS). The *Dietary Guidelines for Americans* provides authoritative advice for individuals 2 years of age and older on how proper dietary habits can promote health and reduce risk of major chronic diseases. MyPyramid was developed to promote dietary guidance and increase the awareness of the health benefits from simple and modest improvements in nutrition, physical activity, and lifestyle.

POTENTIAL NUTRITIONAL PROBLEMS

Risk Factors

1. Increased nutritional needs during adolescence are related to several factors.

   a. Adolescents gain 20% of their adult height.
   b. Adolescents gain 50% of their adult skeletal mass.
   c. Caloric and protein requirements are maximal.
   d. Gender-specific nutrient needs.
2. Increased physical activity of adolescents makes proper nutrition essential.
3. Poor eating habits contribute to nutritional problems.
   a. Missed meals are common.
   b. High-sugar snacks of low nutritional value are popular. A study of 460 teenage girls (Wyshak, 2000) found that almost 80% consumed soft drinks, most of which were sugar-containing cola drinks. The same study found an association between carbonated beverage consumption and history of bone fracture.
   c. Peer pressure leads to changes in a range of eating behaviors including restrictive and overeating patterns and purging behaviors (Van den Berg et al., 2002).
   d. The adolescent's family may exhibit poor eating habits and meal preparation may be inadequate.
   e. Many meals and snacks are obtained from vending machines or fast-food restaurants. Table 6.1 lists the fat and sodium contents of popular fast foods and ice cream snacks, many of which approach or exceed 50% of their calories from fat. Open access to nutritional information on fast foods is available on the Internet at www.nutritiondata.com.
   f. Inadequate financial resources to purchase food or to prepare nutritious meals.
4. Factors that influence nutritional needs during adolescence are as follows:
   a. Level of activity
   b. Special diets (i.e., vegetarian)
   c. Chronic illness
   d. Substance abuse
   e. Menstruation
   f. Pregnancy
   g. Lactation

All of these factors contributed to the findings of the Food and Drug Administration's (FDA) Ten State Nutritional Survey in the 1960s (U.S. Department of Health, Education and Welfare, 1972), the National Health and Nutrition Examination Survey (NHANES) during 1971–1974 (National Center for Health Statistics [NCHS], 1979), the NHANES III study in 1988–1994 (National Center for Health Statistics,

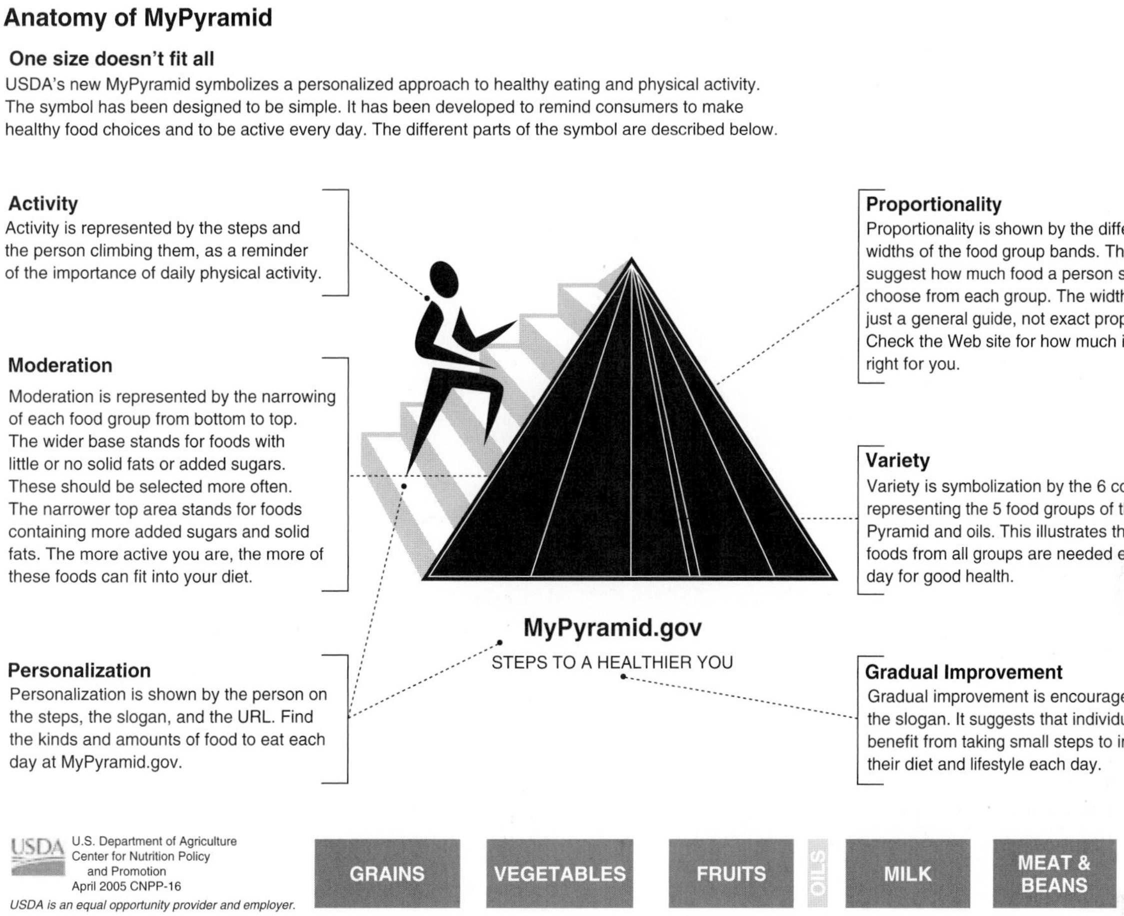

Anatomy of MyPyramid

One size doesn't fit all

USDA's new MyPyramid symbolizes a personalized approach to healthy eating and physical activity. The symbol has been designed to be simple. It has been developed to remind consumers to make healthy food choices and to be active every day. The different parts of the symbol are described below.

Activity
Activity is represented by the steps and the person climbing them, as a reminder of the importance of daily physical activity.

Moderation
Moderation is represented by the narrowing of each food group from bottom to top. The wider base stands for foods with little or no solid fats or added sugars. These should be selected more often. The narrower top area stands for foods containing more added sugars and solid fats. The more active you are, the more of these foods can fit into your diet.

Personalization
Personalization is shown by the person on the steps, the slogan, and the URL. Find the kinds and amounts of food to eat each day at MyPyramid.gov.

Proportionality
Proportionality is shown by the different widths of the food group bands. The widths suggest how much food a person should choose from each group. The widths are just a general guide, not exact proportions. Check the Web site for how much is right for you.

Variety
Variety is symbolization by the 6 color bands representing the 5 food groups of the Pyramid and oils. This illustrates that foods from all groups are needed each day for good health.

Gradual Improvement
Gradual improvement is encouraged by the slogan. It suggests that individuals can benefit from taking small steps to improve their diet and lifestyle each day.

MyPyramid.gov
STEPS TO A HEALTHIER YOU

USDA
U.S. Department of Agriculture
Center for Nutrition Policy and Promotion
April 2005 CNPP-16
USDA is an equal opportunity provider and employer.

GRAINS   VEGETABLES   FRUITS   OILS   MILK   MEAT & BEANS

FIGURE 6.1 USDA new food pyramid. (From U.S. Department of Agriculture Center for Nutrition Policy and Promotion. www.mypyramid.gov. April 2005.)

1994), and the National Health and Nutrition Examination Survey, 1999–2002. These surveys concluded that the highest prevalence of unsatisfactory nutritional status occurs in the adolescent age-group. Of particular note were deficiencies in the intake of calcium, iron, riboflavin, thiamine, and vitamins A and C.

Key Areas

1. Overweight: On the basis of data from National Health and Nutrition Examination Survey, 1999–2002, the prevalence of adolescent overweight ranges from 12.7% to 24% depending on the race (Hedley, 2004).
2. Iron deficiency ranges from 0.6% to 7% in adolescents between 11 and 19 years of age. Rates of iron deficiency depend on gender and socioeconomic status (iron deficiency is higher in low-income families (Donovan, 1995)). Iron deficiency is best indicated by serum ferritin ($<16\,\mu g/L$).
3. Deficiencies in protein, minerals, and vitamins during pregnancy.

NUTRITIONAL ASSESSMENT

Assessing the nutritional status of an adolescent should be part of a comprehensive health evaluation. This becomes even more important in adolescents who are identified as nutritionally at risk. Such adolescents include those with nutritionally related medical conditions, dietary deficiencies, or those with conditions that predispose them to inadequate nutrition. Nutritional assessment requires repeated measurements of nutritional status over time. Methods used in the nutritional assessment of adolescents include dietary and clinical evaluation, measurements of body composition and laboratory data.

Dietary Data

Dietary information can be obtained from a food record kept by the teenager, a dietary history obtained from a nutritionist, a 24-hour recall, or a diet questionnaire. Figure 6.3 is an example of a diet questionnaire for adolescents. Simple screening questions that are quick and easy to ask include the following:

1. How many meals do you usually space eat in a day? Any snacks?
2. Tell me everything you have eaten in the past 24 hours.
3. Are there any foods that you have eliminated from your diet?
4. Are you on a diet?
5. Are you comfortable with your eating habits?
6. Do you ever eat in secret? Do you ever feel you can't stop eating?

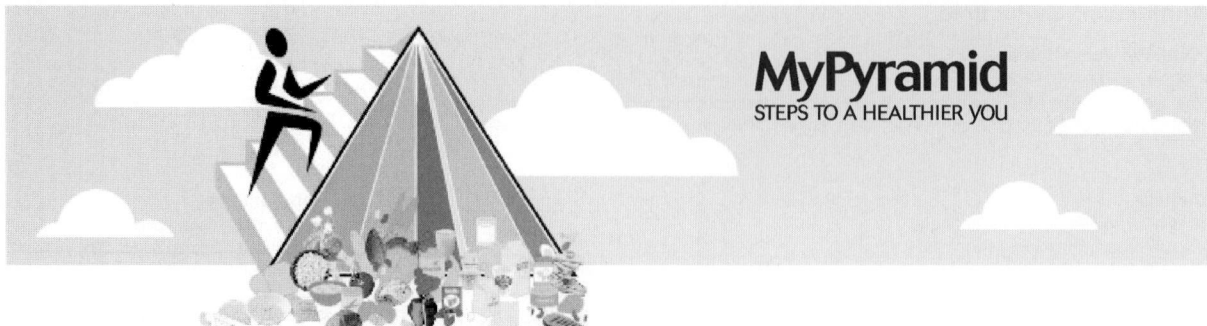

Based on the information you provided, this is your daily recommended amount from each food group.

GRAINS 10 ounces	VEGETABLES 3 1/2 cups	FRUITS 2 1/2 cups	MILK 3 cups	MEAT & BEANS 7 ounces
Make half your grains whole Aim for at least **5 ounces** of whole grains a day	**Vary your veggies** Aim for these amounts each week: **Dark green veggies** = 3 cups **Orange veggies** = 2 1/2 cups **Dry beans & peas** = 3 1/2 cups **Starchy veggies** = 7 cups **Other veggies** = 8 1/2 cups	**Focus on fruits** Eat a variety of fruit Go easy on fruit juices	**Get your calcium-rich foods** Go low-fat or fat-free when you choose milk, yogurt, or cheese	**Go lean with protein** Choose low-fat or lean meats and poultry Vary your protein routine— choose more fish, beans, peas, nuts, and seeds

Find your balance between food and physical activity

Be physically active for at least **60 minutes** every day, or most days.

Know your limits on fats, sugars, and sodium

Your allowance for oils is **8 teaspoons a day.**

Limit extras–solid fats and sugars–to **425 calories a day.**

Your results are based on a 2800 calorie pattern.   Name: _____

This calorie level is only an estimate of your needs. Monitor your body weight to see if you need to adjust your calorie intake.

FIGURE 6.2 USDA new food pyramid, example for 16-year-old male. (From U.S. Department of Agriculture Center for Nutrition Policy and Promotion. www.mypyramid.gov. April 2005.)

7. Have you recently lost or gained weight, or has your weight stayed the same?
8. Do you feel that your weight is too much, too little, or about right?
9. What is the most you have ever weighed, and what would you like to weigh?

Helpful screening questions used in older adolescents and young adults (followed by the associated sensitivity and specificity for disordered eating) include the following (Anstine and Grinenko, 2000):

1. How many diets have you been on in the past year? (Two or three diets, 88% sensitivity and 63% specificity; four or five diets, 69% sensitivity and 86% specificity).
2. Do you feel you should be dieting? (Often, 94% sensitivity and 67% specificity; usually, 87% sensitivity and 82% specificity).
3. Do you feel dissatisfied with your body size? (Often, 96% sensitivity and 61% specificity; usually, 88% sensitivity and 74% specificity).
4. Does your weight affect the way you feel about yourself? (Often, 97% sensitivity and 61% specificity; usually, 91% sensitivity and 74% specificity).

Each of these questions appears to have a very high correlation with the score on the Eating Attitudes Test (EAT-26). This screening test examines attitudes and behaviors regarding food, weight, and body image and has been validated for use in adolescents.

Anthropometric Measurements

1. Weight: Weight is a short-term measurement of nutrition. To accurately measure an adolescent's weight, the young person should remove his or her shoes and heavy clothing. Weight-for-age charts can be obtained from the Centers for Disease Control (CDC) on their website at www.cdc.gov/growthcharts (Figs. 1.21 and 1.23).
2. Height: Height is a long-term indicator of nutrition. A wall-mounted stadiometer is the most accurate method for measuring height. Have the teen remove his or her shoes and stand with heels touching the wall. Height-for-age charts are also available at http://www.cdc.gov/growthcharts/(Figs. 1.22 and 1.24).
3. Body mass index: The body mass index (BMI) is equal to the weight in kilograms divided by the square of

TABLE 6.1

Fat and Sodium Contents of Popular Fast Foods

Food	Serving Size (g)	Calories	Cholesterol (mg)	Sodium (mg)	Calories from Fat (%)
Hamburgers:					
Jumbo Jack (Jack in the Box)	271	550	75	880	49
Big Mac (McDonald's)	219	560	80	1,010	50
Original Whopper (Burger King)	291	710	85	980	50
Famous Star (Carl's Jr.)	254	590	70	910	49
Sandwiches:					
Arby's Roast Beef	154	320	45	950	34
Filet-O-Fish (McDonald's)	156	470	50	730	51
Chicken Sandwich (Jack in the Box)	164	400	40	770	45
Other:					
Large fries (McDonald's)	170	520	0	290	44
Kentucky Fried Chicken Original Recipe breast	161	370	145	1145	49
Taco (Taco Bell)	99	220	25	560	41
Domino's Classic cheese pizza (two slices of 12-in. pizza)	159	375	23	784	27
Small chocolate shake (McDonald's)	333 mL	440	40	250	22
Ice cream:					
Häagen-Dazs ice cream bar (vanilla/milk chocolate)					64
Vanilla ice cream					50
Frozen yogurt					20
Sherbet					29
Gelato					29

A Comparison of Two Fast-Food Meal Choices

Meal Option	Calories	Total Fat (g)	Calories from Fat (%)	Saturated Fat (%)	Cholesterol (mg)
Typical meal:					
McDonald's Quarter Pounder with cheese	510	26	40	46	90
Chocolate shake, small	440	10	20	60	40
Large fries	570	30	47	20	0
Total	1520	66	39	36	130
Lower-fat, lower-calorie alternative:					
McDonald's Grilled Chicken Deluxe without mayonnaise	300	5	15	20	50
Small fries	250	11	40	23	0
Medium Coca-Cola	210	0	0	0	0
Total	760	16	19	22	50

the height in meters or BMI = kg/m². The BMI is easily determined, is highly reliable, and has a correlation of 0.7 to 0.8 with body fat content in adults. The correlation coefficient of BMI with body fat content in children and adolescents is 0.39 to 0.90. Adolescents who are overweight or deemed at risk for overweight have a BMI between the 85th and 95th percentiles for age and gender, and those who are obese have a BMI exceeding the 95th percentile for age and gender. BMI values in adolescents are listed in Chapter 1 (Figs. 1.25 and 1.26). BMI-for-age charts are available at www.cdc.gov/growthcharts/.

4. Skin fold measurements: Triceps skin fold measurement is helpful in evaluating the adipose tissue component and degree of obesity. Barlow and Dietz (1998) published

a chart of triceps skinfold thickness for age and sex (Table 32.1). This measurement does not take into account the regional distribution of body fat, which in adults has been correlated with future obesity-related health risk. However, skin fold thickness is a more direct measure of adiposity than BMI and correlates well with body fat content in both children and adults. This technique requires training and has lower intraobserver and interobserver reliability than height and weight measurements used in the calculation of the BMI.

5. Waist-hip ratio: The waist-hip ratio (WHR) is useful in young adults. The WHR is equal to the circumference of the waist divided by the circumference of the hips. Its reliability is similar to that of the BMI and it

FIGURE 6.3 Diet questionnaire for adolescents. (Adapted from Fomon S. *Nutritional disorders of children: prevention, screening, and follow-up* [DHEW Publication (HSE) 78–5104]. Rockville, MD: U.S. Department of Health, Education, and Welfare, Health Services Administration, 1976.)

DIET QUESTIONNAIRE

1. Do you drink milk? Yes _____ No ____
   If yes, whole milk _____
           2% milk _____
           1% milk _____
           nonfat milk _____

2. Please indicate which of the following foods you eat and how often:

	Never or hardly ever (less than once a week)	Sometimes (not daily but at least once a week)	Every day or nearly every day
Cheese, yogurt, ice cream	_____	_____	_____
Eggs	_____	_____	_____
Dried beans, peas, Peanut butter	_____	_____	_____
Bread, rice, pasta, grits, Cereal, tortillas, potatoes	_____	_____	_____
Fruits or fruit juices	_____	_____	_____
Vegetables	_____	_____	_____

3 If you eat fruits or drink fruit juices every day or nearly every day, which ones do you eat or drink most often? _____
_____

4. If you eat vegetables every day or nearly every day, which ones do you eat most often?
_____

5. Do you usually eat anything between meals? If yes, name the two or three snacks that you have most often: _____
_____

6. Do you take vitamins or iron? yes ____ No ____
   If yes, how often? _____
   What kind? _____

7. Are you on a special diet? Yes ____ No ____
   If yes, what is the reason?
      Allergy—spcify type of diet: _____

      Weight reduction—specify: _____

      Other (such as vegetarian)—specify reason for diet and type of diet: _____

may be a better predictor of the sequelae associated with adult obesity. A WHR >1.0 in adult men or >0.8 in adult women has been shown to predict complications from obesity, independent of BMI. It should be noted that the WHR has not been evaluated in all ethnic groups.

Clinical Evaluation

The clinical evaluation includes examination of skin, eyes, lips, tongue, gums, teeth, hair, and nails. The following is an illustrative list of clinical findings and possible nutritional causes.

1. Skin
   a. Pallor: Iron deficiency
   b. Follicular hyperkeratosis: Vitamin A deficiency or excess
   c. Xanthoma: Hyperlipidemia
   d. Petechiae: Vitamin C deficiency
2. Eyes
   a. Night blindness: Vitamin A deficiency
   b. Angular palpebritis: Riboflavin, niacin deficiencies
3. Lips
   a. Angular stomatitis, cheilosis: Riboflavin, niacin deficiencies
4. Tongue
   a. Glossitis: Niacin, folic acid, vitamin B_{12}, or vitamin B_6 deficiencies
   b. Papillary atrophy: Riboflavin, niacin, folic acid, vitamin B_{12}, or iron deficiencies
   c. Loss of taste: Zinc deficiency
5. Gums
   a. Soft, spongy, or bleeding: Vitamin C deficiency
6. Teeth
   a. Excessive dental cavities: Diet high in refined sugar
7. Hair
   a. Dry, dull, and brittle: Protein–calorie malnutrition
8. Nails
   a. Brittle with frayed borders: Malnutrition, iron or calcium deficiency
   b. Concave or eggshell (free edge curved sharply outward): Vitamin A deficiency
9. Other nutritional signs of general malnutrition
   a. Muscle wasting
   b. Delayed sexual maturation and growth

TABLE 6.2

Recommended Dietary Allowances for Adolescents

	Male (yr)			Female (yr)				Lactating	Lactating
Category	11–14	15–18	19–24	11–14	15–18	19–24	Pregnancy	(first 6 mo)	(second 6 mo)
Weight (kg)	45	66	72	46	55	58			
Height (cm)	157	176	177	157	163	164			
Energy (cal)	2,500	3,000	2,900	2,200	2,200	2,200	+300	+500	+500
Protein (g)	45	59	58	46	44	46	60	65	62
Minerals									
Iron (mg/d)	12	12	10	15	15	15	30	15	15
Zinc (mg/d)	15	15	15	12	12	12	15	19	16
Iodine (µg/d)	150	150	150	150	150	150	175	200	200
Vitamins									
Vitamin A (IU)	10	10	10	10	10	10	10	10	10

Adapted from Food and Nutrition Board, National Research Council. *Recommended dietary allowances*, 10th ed. Washington, DC: National Academy Press, 1989.

c. Amenorrhea
d. Hepatomegaly

Laboratory Tests

Laboratory tests helpful in assessing nutritional status include hemoglobin, hematocrit, ferritin, serum protein, and albumin.

Nutritional Requirements

Dietary reference intakes (DRIs) represent the new approach to providing quantitative estimates of nutrients used to plan and evaluate diets for healthy people. The DRIs are a set of four nutrient reference values that have replaced the 1989 recommended dietary allowances (RDAs).

1. Recommended dietary allowance (RDA): This is the dietary intake level that is sufficient to meet the nutrient requirements of almost all healthy individuals (97%–98%) in the United States.
2. Adequate intake (AI): This is the value based on observed or experimentally determined approximations of nutrient intake by a group—used when RDA cannot be determined.
3. Estimated average requirement (EAR): This is the intake value that is estimated to meet the requirement defined by a specified indicator of adequacy in 50% of an age- and gender-specific group. At this level of intake, the remaining 50% of the specified group would not have its needs met.
4. Tolerable upper intake level (UL): This is the maximum level of daily nutrient intake that is unlikely to pose risks of adverse health effects to almost all of the individuals in the group for whom it is designed.

The DRIs cover the following groups of nutrients:

1. Calcium, vitamin D, phosphorus, magnesium, and fluoride
2. Folate and other B vitamins
3. Antioxidants (e.g., vitamin C, vitamin E, selenium)
4. Macronutrients (e.g., proteins, fats, carbohydrates)
5. Trace elements (e.g., iron, zinc)
6. Electrolytes and water
7. Other food components (e.g., fiber, phytoestrogens)

Energy Requirements Energy requirements are determined by basal metabolic rate, growth status, physical activity, and body composition. Energy requirements of adolescents vary depending on the timing of growth and pubertal development. As such, energy needs are based on height because it provides a better estimate of total daily caloric recommendations. Suggested caloric intakes are listed in Table 6.2, but these will vary widely according to body size and activity level.

Protein Protein provides 4 kcal of energy in each gram. Protein requirements are based on the amount of protein needed to maintain existing lean body mass and the increase in additional lean body mass with growth and development. Protein requirements are highest during the peak height velocity. Most teenagers' diets exceed the RDA for protein.

Carbohydrates Carbohydrates provide 4 kcal of energy in each gram. Carbohydrates are the primary source of dietary energy. Carbohydrates should make up approximately 50% of the daily caloric intake. However, no more than 10% to 25% of calories should come from sweeteners (sucrose and high fructose corn syrup). Beverages with caloric sweeteners, sugars and sweets, and other sweetened foods that provide little or no nutrients are negatively associated with diet quality and can contribute to excessive energy intakes. In fact, 12% of all carbohydrates consumed by adolescents come from the added sweeteners in soft drinks.

Carbohydrate-containing foods include grain products, fruits, and vegetables. Approximately 25 to 35 g of fiber should be consumed daily. Fiber is found in whole grain foods, fruits, vegetables, legumes, nuts, and seeds.

Glycemic index (GI) classifies carbohydrate foods on the basis of the response they bring about in the body, specifically the effect on blood glucose. The GI of foods is

TABLE 6.3

Recommended Dietary Allowances (Light Face Type) and Adequate Intake (Bold Face Type) Values, by Age

Daily Amount	Male (yr)			Female (yr)			Pregnant (yr)		Lactating (yr)	
	9–13	14–18	19–30	9–13	14–18	19–30	<19	19–30	<19	19–30
Calcium (mg)	1,300	1,300	1,000	1,300	1,300	1,000	1,300	1,000	1,300	1,000
Phosphorus (mg)	**1,250**	**1,250**	**700**	**1,250**	**1,250**	**700**	**1,250**	**700**	**1,250**	**700**
Magnesium (mg)	**240**	**410**	**400**	**1,250**	**1,250**	**700**	**1,250**	**700**	**1,250**	**700**
Fluoride (mg)	2	3	4	2	3	3	3	3	3	3
Selenium (pg)	40	55	55	40	55	55	60	60	70	70
Vitamin C (mg)	45	75	90	45	65	75	80	85	115	120
Vitamin D (µg)	5	5	5	5	5	5	5	5	5	5
Vitamin E (mg)	**11**	**15**	**15**	**11**	**15**	**15**	**15**	**15**	**19**	**19**
Thiamine (mg)	**1.2**	**1.2**	**1.2**	**0.9**	**1.0**	**1.1**	**1.4**	**1.4**	**1.5**	**1.5**
Riboflavin (mg)	**0.9**	**1.3**	**1.3**	**0.9**	**1.0**	**1.1**	**1.4**	**1.4**	**1.6**	**1.6**
Niacin (mg)	12	16	16	12	14	14	18	18	17	17
Vitamin B$_6$ (mg)	**1.0**	**1.3**	**1.3**	**1.0**	**1.2**	**1.3**	**1.9**	**1.9**	**2.0**	**2.0**
Folacin (µµg)	**300**	**400**	**400**	**300**	**400**	**400**	**600**	**600**	**500**	**500**
Vitamin B$_{12}$ (µg)	**1.8**	**2.4**	**2.4**	**1.8**	**2.4**	**2.4**	**2.6**	**2.6**	**2.8**	**2.8**
Pantothenic acid (B$_5$) (mg)	4	5	5	4	5	5	6	6	7	7
Biotin (µg)	20	25	30	20	25	30	30	30	35	35
Choline (mg)	375	550	550	375	550	550	450	450	550	550

Adapted from Food and Nutrition Board, National Academy of Sciences. U.S. Department of Agriculture. www.nalusda.gov/fnic/etext/000105.html. 1998.

ranked according to this "glycemic response". The index ranges from 0 to 100; with glucose or other reference standard being 100. Hence, the lower the GI, the lower the expected rise in blood sugar for a given food. In general, foods are classified into low GI (<40), moderate GI (40–70), and high GI (>70).

Alcohol provides 7 calories of energy in each gram and can also be a significant source of calories.

Fat Fat provides 9 kcal of energy in each gram. Adolescents require dietary fat and essential fatty acids for many vital functions in the body. A teenager's diet should contain no more than 30% of calories from fat. Most adolescents' total and saturated fat intake is greater than that recommended.

Minerals

Iron There is an increased need for iron in both males and females during adolescence because of the rapid growth, and increase in muscle mass and blood volume. In addition, females require increase in iron because of menstrual losses. High-iron foods include lean red meats, spinach, green vegetables, and fortified cereals. Nonheme iron, present in plant sources is less bioavailable, but its absorption can be enhanced by concurrent intake of vitamin C.

Calcium Calcium, which is important for attaining skeletal health, is particularly important during adolescent growth and development. Requirements for dietary calcium increase substantially during periods of peak velocity of growth and accrual of bone-mineral content. Adolescents tend to eat a diet deficient in calcium. The DRI for calcium for 9- to 18-year olds is 1,300 mg/day (Table 6.3). Many adolescents have inadequate calcium intakes, in part due to the substitution of carbonated beverages for milk. It is highly likely that current high levels of soft drink consumption are replacing the drinking of milk. Data from the U.S. Department of Agriculture Continuing Surveys of Food Intakes by Individuals indicate a drop in milk intake among adolescent girls from 72% on a given day in 1977 to 1979 to 57% in 1994.

Those adolescents not taking in adequate calcium from food sources may need to take supplemental calcium such as calcium carbonate, citrate, lactate, or phosphate (absorption varies from 25%–35%). Optimal absorption of the calcium supplements occurs when no more than 500 mg/dose is taken with food. In addition to dairy products, calcium is found in tofu, salmon and sardines, dark-green leafy vegetables, and calcium-fortified foods (such as orange juice).

Zinc Zinc is needed for adequate growth, sexual maturation, and wound healing. The RDA for zinc was set at 8 mg/day for adolescents 9 to 13 years old and 9 mg/day and 11 mg/day for females and males 11 to 14 years old, respectively. Good food sources of zinc include lean meats, seafood, eggs, and milk.

Vitamins Vitamin requirements increase during adolescence, especially for vitamin B$_{12}$; folate; vitamins A, C, D, and E; thiamine; niacin; and riboflavin (Table 6.3). It has been shown that supplements of antioxidant vitamins (A, C, E, and β-carotene) probably reduce the risk of cardiovascular disease and certain cancers, but there is no current recommendation to prescribe them routinely.

GUIDELINES FOR NUTRITIONAL THERAPY

General Recommendations

1. Be aware of and sensitive to the family context, lifestyle, and cultural milieu.
2. Motivate lifestyle change by stressing the positive effects of dietary changes, for example, feeling good about oneself, feeling energetic.
3. Use the MyPyramid Food Guide (Fig. 6.1) to recommend the appropriate number of daily servings from each food group.
4. Recommend that teenagers participate in a regular exercise program for at least 30 minutes, at least 4 days of the week. Balance dietary energy intake with physical activity to maintain normal growth and development.
5. Simplify good nutrition concepts by recommending the following to adolescents and their families:
   - Maintain a healthy weight.
   - Eat a wide variety of nutritious foods. Include lean meat, fish, and poultry.
   - Limit solid fats (butter, margarine, shortening, lard) and choose foods low in saturated fat and trans fatty acids. Use more polyunsaturated fats.
   - Broil or bake instead of frying foods.
   - Use nonfat (skim) or low-fat milk and dairy products daily.
   - Eat plenty of vegetables, legumes, and fruits.
   - Eat plenty of cereals (including breads, rice, pasta, and noodles), preferably wholegrain.
   - Drink water instead of soft drinks or fruit drinks. Limit juice intake.
   - Eat meals and snacks regularly. In a recent study, eating family dinner was correlated with improved nutritional intake in early adolescence (Gillman et al., 2000).

Special Conditions

Vegetarian Diets

Adolescents may be vegetarian because of ecological, economic, religious, or philosophical beliefs. Teens who are vegetarians (but not choosing to be vegan) are likely to have an adequate nutritional intake. Nutritional counseling may be of benefit to ensure adequate intake of energy, protein, and micronutrients as well as to assess the need for supplements.

Types of Vegetarians

Semivegetarians eat milk products and limited seafood and poultry but no red meat.

Lactovegetarians consume milk products but no eggs, meat, fish, or poultry.

Ovolactovegetarians consume milk products and eggs but no meat, fish, or poultry.

Vegans consume vegetable foods only and no foods of animal origin (i.e., no eggs, milk products, meat, fish, or poultry).

Fruitarians consume raw fruit and seeds only. Examples of such fruits include pineapple, mango, banana, avocado, apple, melon, orange, all kinds of berries, and the vegetable fruits such as tomato, cucumber, olives; and nuts.

Further information is available from the Vegetarian Resource Group on their Web site: http://www.vrg.org/.

Supplemental Needs of Vegetarians

Potential nutritional issues with vegetarian diets include macronutrient and micronutrient deficiencies such as those of protein, fat, vitamin B_{12}, iron, zinc, calcium, and vitamin D.

Vitamins: Semivegetarians, lactovegetarians, and ovolactovegetarians have no need for supplements if attention is paid to dietary composition. Vegans may need supplemental riboflavin and vitamins B_{12} and D.

Protein: Adequate protein intake has been a traditional concern for vegetarians; however, vegetarians usually meet or exceed protein requirements (except for vegans). There is also mounting evidence that the practice of eating complementary proteins in the same meal is unnecessary.

Minerals: There is no uniform need for supplements, but vegetarians are at increased risk for iron and zinc deficiencies. Vegetarians may need up to 50% more zinc in their diet since phytate (found in plants) and calcium hinder zinc absorption.

Lactose Intolerance

Teens with lactose intolerance are at risk of inadequate calcium intake. Some adolescents with lactose intolerance can tolerate small amounts of milk products including aged cheese or yogurt with active cultures. There are many nondairy foods high in calcium including green vegetables, such as broccoli and kale; fish with edible bones, such as salmon and sardines; calcium-fortified orange juice; and soymilk. Currently, there are a variety of lactose-reduced dairy products in the supermarket including milk, cottage cheese, and processed cheese slices. Teens often find lactase enzyme replacement pills or liquid helpful.

Pregnancy

There is limited information available regarding the nutrition needs in pregnant adolescents. Energy requirements are greater for pregnant adolescents than for nonpregnant adolescents. Younger adolescents may require higher energy intake than older women. Pregnant adolescents should not consume less than 2000 kcal/day and in many cases their needs may be higher. The best gauge of adequate energy intake during pregnancy is satisfactory weight gain. Goals for weight gain are based on prepregnancy weight, height, age, stage of development, and usual eating patterns. Young pregnant women who are below an optimal weight are advised to gain more weight than overweight women.

Folate is essential for nucleic acid synthesis and is required in greater amounts during pregnancy. Recent research suggests that taking folic acid before and during early pregnancy can reduce the risk of spina bifida and other neural tube defects in infants. Because these defects occur early in gestation, it is advised that women of childbearing age and those who are capable of becoming pregnant consume 400 µg/day of folic acid. The DRI for folate during pregnancy is 600 µg/day. Good sources of folate include leafy dark-green vegetables, legumes, citrus fruits and juices, peanuts, whole grains, and some fortified breakfast cereals.

The calcium recommendation during pregnancy is 1,300 mg/day for adolescents. Since most nonpregnant adolescent females consume significantly less than the recommended amount of calcium, pregnant teens should either add calcium-rich foods to their diet or take calcium supplementation.

Dietary counseling can be one of the most important interventions for a pregnant adolescent to ensure a healthy pregnancy and a healthy baby. Teens should be encouraged to obtain their nutrients from food. A low-dose vitamin–mineral supplement is recommended for pregnant adolescents who do not regularly consume a healthy diet. Teens should be counseled against dieting during pregnancy.

Athletes

Risk for Iron and Zinc Deficiency
Both male and female adolescent athletes are at risk for iron deficiency. Athletes (especially menstruating females and those involved in endurance sports such as distance running) should be screened for low hemoglobin or hematocrit levels. Serum ferritin can be helpful in determining loss of iron stores and need for supplementation. A ferritin level of < 16 µg/L corresponds with depleted iron stores. For the athlete who is not anemic but has low iron stores, 50 to 100 mg of elemental iron daily (ferrous gluconate 240 or 325 mg twice daily or ferrous sulfate 325 mg daily or twice daily) should be recommended. For the anemic athlete, 100 to 200 mg of elemental iron daily (ferrous gluconate 325 mg three times daily or ferrous sulfate 325 mg twice daily), should be given. Laboratory measurements should be repeated after 2 to 3 months to document response to therapy. Athletes with iron deficiency anemia may also be zinc deficient. Education regarding good dietary sources of zinc and iron should be provided.

Sodium and Potassium
Athletes need increased intake of sodium and potassium. This requirement will generally be met as they increase their calorie intake.

Calories
The active athlete who engages in 2 hours/day of heavy exercise needs 800 to 1,700 extra calories/day beyond the recommended minimum for age, sex, height, and weight. According to the American Dietetic Association, the approximate distribution of calories should be carbohydrates, 55% to 60%; proteins, 12% to 15%; and fats, 25% to 30%.

Hydration
Attention must be given to hydration before and during activity.

- The athlete should drink 10 to 16 oz of cold water 1 to 2 hours before exercise.
- Repeat 20 to 30 minutes before exercise.
- Drink 4 to 6 oz of cold water every 10 to 15 minutes during exercise.
- Cold fluids are preferable because gastric emptying is more rapid.
- Plain water can be used for exercise periods of <2 hours.
- Sports drinks may be used to provide carbohydrates for longer events. Fructose-containing solutions should be avoided since they are not as well absorbed as solutions with sucrose or glucose and can cause gastrointestinal upset.

Weight Restrictions
Avoid any major weight restriction during the adolescent growth spurt. Alterations in diet to cause rapid weight gain or loss should be discouraged. Eating disorders are prevalent among athletes (especially female athletes), especially in those involved in running, swimming, diving, gymnastics, or dance (Chapter 33). Therefore, carefully question all athletes regarding body image, desired weight, and amenorrhea. The female athlete triad (amenorrhea, disordered eating, and osteoporosis) should be suspected in an athlete with secondary amenorrhea.

Carbohydrate Loading
Diets that are chronically high in carbohydrate are not recommended. For optimal performance, the athlete should train lightly or rest 24 to 36 hours before competition. On the day of competition, the athlete may consider a high-carbohydrate, low-fat meal 3 to 6 hours before an event and an optional snack 1 to 2 hours before the event. Foods high in carbohydrates (60% to 70%) have also been recommended after competition to replace glycogen stores. However, Hawley et al. (1995) pointed out that a diet of 5,000 kcal/day that is only 45% carbohydrate is sufficient to restore muscle glycogen within 24 hours. An initial "depletion phase" consisting of vigorous workouts and low-carbohydrate eating before competition is also no longer recommended.

Ergogenic Nutritional Supplements
The word "ergogenic" is derived from the Greek word *ergon*, which means "to increase work or potential for work." Anecdotal reports suggest that compounds such as bee pollen, caffeine, glycine, carnitine, lecithin, brewer's yeast, and gelatin improve strength or endurance. However, scientific research has failed to substantiate these claims.

Teen athletes who are considering the use of nutritional supplements should be aware that the effects of long-term supplement use have not been studied. In addition, supplement use can be quite costly. Most athletes can maximize their performance through consistent, appropriate training and attention to adequate nutrition rather than relying on supplement use (http://www.drugfreesport.com/choices/supplements/). See Chapter 83 for further discussion on herbal therapies.

WEB SITES

For Teenagers and Parents

http://www.mypyramid.gov/index.html. USDA web site that customizes food pyramids based on age, sex and exercise levels.

http://www.mayohealth.org. Nutrition section from Mayo Clinic.

http://www.fda.gov/fdac/features/795_teenfood.html. How to read a food label.

http://www.vrg.org. Vegetarian Resource Center.

http://www.eatright.org. American Dietetic Association Web site.

http://www.kidshealth.org/teen/food_fitness. Exercise and nutrition site for teens.

http://www.foodsafety.gov. U.S. Food and Drug Administration site on nutrition and food safety.

http://www.nal.usda.gov/fnic/etext/fnic.html. U.S. Department of Agriculture (USDA) food and information center.

For Health Professionals

http://www.mypyramid.gov. MyPyramid from USDA.

http://www.vrg.org. Vegetarian Resource Center.

http://www.americanheart.org. American Heart Association diets.

http://www.nutrition.org. American Society for Nutritional Sciences.

http://www.iom.edu/topic.asp?id=3708. Food and Nutrition Board home page with sections on RDIs.

http://www.drugfreesport.com/choices/supplements. Nutritional supplements, NCAA sponsored site.

REFERENCES AND ADDITIONAL READINGS

Anstine D, Grinenko D. Rapid screening for disordered eating in college-aged females in the primary care setting. *J Adolesc Health* 2000;26:338.

Barlow S, Dietz W. Obesity evaluation and treatment: expert committee recommendations. *Pediatrics* 1998;102(3):e29.

Baynes RD. Iron deficiency. In: Brock JH, Halliday JW, Pippard MJ, et al., eds. *Iron metabolism in health and disease.* London: WB Saunders, 1994:189.

Borrud L, Wilkinson Enns C, Mickle S. What we eat: USDA surveys food consumption changes. *Commun Nutr Inst* 1997;1997:4.

Brown LJ, Wall TP, Lazar V. Trends in total caries experience: permanent and primary teeth. *J Am Dent Assoc* 2000;131:223.

Burke L. Searching for the competitive edge: commonly asked nutrition questions. *Aust Fam Physician* 1999;28:694.

Canadian Paediatric Society Nutrition Committee. Adolescent nutrition: 1. Introduction and summary [Part 1 of 6]. *Can Med Assoc J* 1983;129:419.

Donovan UM, Gibson RS. Iron and zinc status of young women aged 14 to 19 years consuming vegetarian and omnivorous diets. *J Am Coll Nutr* 1995;14(5):463.

Dunger DB, Preece MA. Growth and nutrient requirements at adolescence. In: Grand RJ, Sutphen JL, Dietz WH Jr, eds. *Pediatric nutrition: theory and practice.* Boston: Butterworths, 1987.

Food and Nutrition Board, Commission on Life Sciences, National Research Council. *Recommended dietary allowances,* 10th ed. Washington, DC: National Academy Press, 1989.

Forbes GB. Nutrition and growth. In: McAnarney ER, Kreipe RE, Orr DP, et al., eds. *Textbook of adolescent medicine.* Philadelphia: WB Saunders, 1992.

Garcia-Webb P. Iron in todays laboratory. *Clin Biochemist Rev* 1997;18:113.

Gidding SS, Dennison BA, Birch LL, et al. Dietary recommendations for children and adolescents a guide for practitioners: consensus statement from the American Heart Association. *Circulation* 2005;112:2061.

Gillman MW, Rifas-Shiman SL, Frazier AL, et al. Family dinner and diet quality among older children and adolescents. *Arch Fam Med* 2000;9:235.

Hawley JA, Dennis SC, Lindsay FH, et al. Nutritional practices of athletes: are they sub-optimal? *J Sports Sci* 1995;13:75S.

Hedley A, Ogden CI, Johnson CI, et al. Prevalence of overweight and obesity among U.S. children, adolescents, and adults, 1999—2002. *JAMA* 2004;291:2847.

Himes JH, Dietz WH. Guidelines for overweight in adolescent preventive services recommendations from an expert committee. The Expert Committee on Clinical Guidelines for Overweight in Adolescent Preventive Services. *Am J Clin Nutr* 1994;59:307.

Lifshitz F, Tarim O, Smith MM. Nutrition in adolescence. *Endocrinol Metab Clin North Am* 1993;22:673.

Loosli AR. Reversing sports-related iron and zinc deficiencies. *Phys Sportsmed* 1993;21:70.

Marion DD, King JC. Nutritional concerns during adolescence. *Pediatr Clin North Am* 1980;27:125.

National Center for Health Statistics. *Caloric and selected nutrient values for persons 1–74 years of age: first health and nutrition examination survey 1971–1974 [Vital and Health Statistics Series 11, 209, DREW publication (PHS) 79–1657].* Hyattsville, MD: National Center for Health Statistics, 1979.

Nielsen P, Nachtigall D. Iron supplementation in athletes. *Sports Med* 1998;26:207.

Probart CK, Bird PJ, Parker KA. Diet and athletic performance. *Med Clin North Am* 1993;77:757.

Rees JM, Worthington-Roberts B. Position of the American Dietetic Association: nutrition care for pregnant adolescents. *J Am Diet Assoc* 1994;94:449.

Reynolds RD. Vitamin supplements: current controversies. *J Am Coll Nutr* 1994;13:118.

Squire DL. Heat illness: fluid and electrolyte issues for pediatric and adolescent athletes. *Pediatr Clin North Am* 1990;37:1085.

Steen SN. Nutrition for young athletes: special considerations. *Sports Med* 1994;17:152.

Steen SN. Timely statement of the American Dietetic Association: nutrition guidance for adolescent athletes in organized sports. *J Am Diet Assoc* 1996;96:611.

Story M, Stang J. Nutrition needs of adolescents. In: Stang J, Story M, eds. *Guidelines for adolescent nutrition services.* School of Public Health, University of Minnesota: Center for Leadership, Education, and Training in Maternal and Child Nutrition, Division of Epidemiology and Community Health, 2005:21.

U.S. Department of Agriculture, U.S. Department of Health and Human Services. *Nutrition and your health: dietary guidelines for Americans. Home and garden bulletin 232.* Washington, DC: U.S. Government Printing Office, 1985; revised 1990.

U.S. Department of Health, Education, and Welfare. *Ten state nutrition survey, 1968–1970: highlights.* Washington DC: U.S. Department of Health, Education, and Welfare, Health Services and Mental Health Administration, Centers for Disease Control, U.S. Government Printing Office, 1972.

U.S. Department of Health, Education, and Welfare. Millar HEC, ed. *Adolescent health care: a guide for BCHS-supported programs and projects. DHEW publication (HSA) 79–5234.* Washington, DC: U.S. Government Printing Office, 1979.

U.S. Food and Drug Administration. *FDA consumer special issue on food labeling [S/N 017-017-01200360-5].* Washington, DC: U.S. Government Printing Office, 1993.

Van den Berg P, Wertheim EH, Thompson JK, Development of body image, eating disturbances, and general psychological functioning in adolescent females: a replication using covariance structure modeling in an Australian sample. *Int J Eat Disord* 2002;32:46.

White R, Frank E. Health effects and prevalence of vegetarianism. *West J Med* 1994;160:465.

Wyshak G. Teenaged girls, carbonated beverage consumption, and bone fractures. *Arch Pediatr Adolesc Med* 2000;154:610.

CHAPTER 7

Understanding Legal Aspects of Care

Abigail English

Whenever a health care practitioner treats an adolescent, it is essential for the practitioner to have a clear understanding of the legal framework within which care is to be provided. Because many adolescents are minors—younger than 18 years in almost all states—their legal status differs from that of adults. Therefore, the laws related to their health care have distinct aspects based on their age and legal status.

For adolescents who are 18 years or older, the governing laws are essentially the same as those for other adults. For adolescents who are minors, the laws may be different. The legal issues that arise most frequently in providing health care to adolescents who are minors fall into three specific areas:

1. Consent: Who is authorized to give consent for the adolescent's care and whose consent is required?
2. Confidentiality: Who has the right to control the release of confidential information about the care, including medical records, and who has the right to receive such information?
3. Payment: Who is financially liable for payment and is there a source of insurance coverage or is public funding available that the adolescent can access?

LEGAL FRAMEWORK

Over the past few decades, the legal framework that applies to the delivery of adolescent health care has evolved in several significant ways. First, the courts have recognized that minors, like adults, have constitutional rights, although there has been considerable debate concerning the scope of those rights. Second, all states have enacted statutes to authorize minors to give their own consent for health care in specific circumstances. Third, laws governing the confidentiality of health care information have changed in ways that affect adolescents. Finally, the financing of health care services for all age-groups and income levels is undergoing major change, at an increasingly rapid pace, which has had and will continue to have a significant impact on adolescents' access to health care.

Constitutional Issues

Beginning with *In re Gault,* (1967), in which the U.S. Supreme Court stated that "neither the Fourteenth Amendment nor the Due Process Clause is for adults alone," the Court has held repeatedly that minors have constitutional rights. The *Gault* decision, which accorded minors certain procedural rights when they are charged by the state with juvenile delinquency offenses, was followed by others recognizing that minors had rights of free speech under the First Amendment (*Tinker v. Des Moines Independent School District,* 1969) and that they also had privacy rights (*Planned Parenthood of Central Missouri v. Danforth,* 1976; *Carey v. Population Services International,* 1977). Although the Supreme Court subsequently rendered decisions that were more equivocal about the scope of minors' constitutional rights, the basic principles articulated in the early cases still stand.

The area of most frequent constitutional litigation has been the rights of minors with respect to reproductive health care, particularly abortion. The early cases, *Carey* and *Danforth,* clearly established that the right of privacy protects minors as well as adults and encompasses minors' access to contraceptives and the abortion decision. The subsequent history of constitutional litigation with respect to abortion has been complex. After the decision in the *Danforth* case, which held that parents cannot exercise an arbitrary veto with respect to the abortion decisions of their minor daughters, the U.S. Supreme Court decided a series of cases—beginning with *Bellotti v. Baird* (1979) and continuing more recently with *Planned Parenthood of Southeastern Pennsylvania v. Casey,* (1992)—addressing parental notification and consent issues related to abortion. The collective import of these cases has been that although a state may enact a mandatory parental involvement requirement for minors who are seeking abortions, it must also, at minimum, establish an alternative procedure whereby a minor may obtain authorization for an abortion without first notifying her parents. This alternative most often takes the form of a court proceeding known as a "*judicial bypass.*" In the bypass proceeding, a minor must be permitted, without parental involvement, to seek a court order authorizing an abortion: If she is mature enough to give an informed consent, the court must allow her to make her own decision; and if she is not mature, the court must determine whether an abortion would be in her best interest. Many, but not all, states have enacted such parental involvement or judicial bypass statutes, some of which have been implemented, although others have been enjoined by the courts. As of January 2007, at least 34 states have laws in effect that require either the consent or notification of at least one parent; all but one of these states provides for a judicial bypass and several provide for consent or notification of an adult family member other than a parent.

State and Federal Laws

Although the constitutional litigation concerning minors' rights in the reproductive health care arena has attracted significant attention, most of the specific legal provisions that affect adolescents' access to health care are contained in state and federal statutes and regulations or in "common law" decisions of the courts. These provisions cover a broad range of issues related to consent, confidentiality, and payment and are critical in defining the parameters of what practitioners in the adolescent health field are legally permitted and required to do. Therefore, practitioners providing services to adolescents must develop a familiarity not only with the general constitutional principles that have evolved in recent decades but also with federal laws and state laws, including court decisions, that apply in their own states.

CONSENT

The law generally requires the consent of a parent before medical care can be provided to a minor. There are, however, numerous exceptions to this requirement. In many situations, someone other than a biological parent—such as a caretaker relative, foster parent, juvenile court, social worker, or probation officer—may be able to give consent in the place of the parent. Moreover, in emergency situations, care may be provided without prior consent to safeguard the life and health of the minor, although parents must be notified as soon as possible thereafter.

Highly significant for the adolescent health care practitioner, however, are the legal provisions that authorize minors themselves to give consent for their care. These provisions are typically based on either the status of the minor or the services sought. (See the Appendix at the end of this chapter, which includes a general overview of these provisions in each state.)

All states have enacted one or more provisions that authorize minors to consent to certain services. These services most frequently include contraceptive services; pregnancy-related care; diagnosis and treatment of sexually transmitted disease (STD) or venereal disease (VD); human immunodeficiency virus (HIV), or acquired immunodeficiency syndrome (AIDS), and reportable or contagious diseases; examination and treatment related to sexual assault; counseling and treatment for drug or alcohol problems; and mental health treatment, particularly outpatient care. Not all states have statutes covering all of these services. Among those that do, some of the statutes contain

age limits, which most frequently fall between the ages of 12 and 15 years.

Similarly, all states have enacted one or more provisions that authorize minors who have attained a specific status to give consent for their own health care. Pursuant to these provisions, the following groups of minors may be authorized to do so—emancipated minors, those who are living apart from their parents, minors serving in the armed forces, married minors, minors who are the parents of a child, high school graduates, and minors who have attained a certain age. Moreover, in a few states, explicit statutes authorize minors who are "mature minors" to consent for care. Few states have enacted all of these provisions and laws are frequently amended; therefore, practitioners are advised to consult their state laws and to ensure they have current information.

THE MATURE MINOR DOCTRINE AND INFORMED CONSENT

Even in the absence of a specific statute, "mature minors" may have the legal capacity to give consent for their own care. The mature minor doctrine emerged from court decisions addressing the circumstances in which a physician could be held liable in damages for providing care to a minor without parental consent. Unless a state has explicitly rejected the mature minor doctrine, in most states it means that there is little likelihood a practitioner will incur liability for failure to obtain parental consent provided that the minor is an older adolescent (typically at least 15 years old) who is capable of giving an informed consent and the care is not high risk, is for the minor's benefit, and is within the mainstream of established medical opinion. During the past few decades, diligent searches have found no reported decisions holding a physician liable in such circumstances solely on the basis of failure to obtain parental consent when nonnegligent care was provided to a mature minor who had given informed consent. A few states have rejected application of the doctrine in particular circumstances. The basic criteria for determining whether a patient is capable of giving an informed consent are that the patient must be able to understand the risks and benefits of any proposed treatment or procedure and its alternatives, and must be able to make a voluntary choice among the alternatives. These criteria apply to minors, as well as adults. Again, however, laws do vary from state to state and practitioners must become familiar with local requirements.

PRIVACY AND CONFIDENTIALITY

There are numerous reasons why it is important to maintain confidentiality in the delivery of health care services to adolescents. The most compelling is to encourage adolescents both to seek necessary care on a timely basis and to provide a candid and complete health history when they do so. Additional reasons include supporting adolescents' growing sense of privacy and autonomy and protecting them from the humiliation and discrimination that could result from disclosure of confidential information.

The confidentiality obligation has numerous sources in law and policy. They include the federal and state constitutions; federal statutes and regulations such as those that pertain to medical privacy in general, Medicaid, family planning programs, and federal drug and alcohol programs; state statutes and regulations such as medical confidentiality and medical records laws, privilege statutes, professional licensing laws, and funding programs; court decisions; and professional ethical standards. The federal government has issued extensive medical privacy regulations that affect the care of adolescents and adults, which are known as the *HIPAA Privacy Rule* and are of critical importance. Proposals are also frequently introduced in Congress that would affect confidential health care for adolescents, so practitioners should monitor ongoing developments carefully.

Because these varied provisions sometimes conflict or are less than clear in their application to minors, practitioners must have some general guidelines to follow—or questions to ask—when developing their understanding of how to handle confidential information. Confidentiality protections are rarely, if ever, absolute, so practitioners must understand what may be disclosed (based on their discretion and professional judgment), what must be disclosed, and what may not be disclosed. In reaching this understanding, practitioners may need to consider several questions; a few of the most relevant questions include the following:

- What information *is* confidential (because it is considered private and is protected against disclosure)?
- What information *is not* confidential (because such information is not protected)?
- What *exceptions* are there in the confidentiality requirements?
- What information can be released *with consent*?
- What other mechanisms allow for *discretionary* disclosure without consent?
- What *mandates* exist for reporting or disclosing confidential information?

In general, even confidential information may be disclosed as long as authorization is obtained from the patient or another appropriate person. Often, when minors have the legal right to consent to their own care, they also have the right to control disclosure of confidential information about that care. This is not always the case, however, because there are a number of circumstances in which disclosure over the objection of the minor might be required—if a specific legal provision requires disclosure to parents; if a mandatory reporting obligation applies, as in the case of suspected physical or sexual abuse; or if the minor poses a severe danger to him or herself or to others.

When the minor does not have the legal right to consent to care or to control disclosure, the release of confidential information must generally be authorized by the minor's parent or the person (or entity) with legal custody or guardianship. Even when this is necessary, however, it is still advisable—from an ethical perspective—for the practitioner to seek the agreement of the minor to disclose confidential information and certainly, at minimum, to advise the minor at the outset of treatment of any limits to confidentiality. Fortunately, in many circumstances, issues of confidentiality and disclosure can be resolved by discussion and informal agreement between a physician, the adolescent patient, and the parents without reference to legal requirements.

The HIPAA Privacy Rule

In 2002, the final provisions of the HIPAA Privacy Rule were issued, which affect the health care information of adolescents who are minors, built on the framework of consent and confidentiality laws that had been developed over the past several decades. Specifically, when minors are authorized to consent for their own health care and do so, the Rule treats them as "individuals" who are able to exercise rights over their own protected health information. Also, when parents have acceded to a confidentiality agreement between a minor and a health professional, the minor is considered an "individual" under the Rule.

Generally, the HIPAA Privacy Rule gives parents access to the health information of their unemancipated minor children, including adolescents. However, on the issue of when parents may have access to protected health information for minors who are considered "individuals" under the Rule and who have consented to their own care, it defers to "state and other applicable law."

Therefore, the laws that allow minors to consent for their own health care have acquired increased significance with the advent of the HIPAA Privacy Rule. The Rule must also be understood in the broader context of other laws that affect disclosure of adolescents' confidential health information to their parents. Specifically, if state or other law explicitly requires information to be disclosed to a parent, the regulations allow a health care provider to comply with that law and disclose the information. If state or other law explicitly permits, but does not require, information to be disclosed to a parent, the regulations allow a health care provider to exercise discretion to disclose or not. If state or other law prohibits the disclosure of information to a parent without the consent of the minor, the regulations do not allow a health care provider to disclose it without the minor's consent. If state or other law is silent or unclear on the question, an entity covered by the Rule has discretion to determine whether to grant access to a parent to the protected health information, as long as the determination is made by a health care professional exercising professional judgment.

HIPAA and FERPA

Health care providers should be aware of the confusing and perhaps conflicting rules that may apply to student health centers on college and university campuses. The confusion relates to whether the records at student health centers are covered by HIPAA or FERPA (Family Educational Rights and Privacy Act). FERPA is a complicated statute that deals with privacy issues of educational records of children, adolescents, and college students. However, there has been a split between rulings at different universities on whether a student's health records and information fall under HIPAA or FERPA. They can only fall under one or the other, *not both*.

The HIPAA Privacy rule explicitly excludes from its purview records that are considered education records under FERPA. However, it should also be noted that FERPA specifically states that: the term "education records" does not include "records on a student who is eighteen years of age or older, or is attending an institution of postsecondary education, which are made or maintained by a physician, psychiatrist, psychologist, or other recognized professional or paraprofessional acting in his professional or paraprofessional capacity, or assisting in that capacity, and which are made, maintained, or used only in connection with the provision of treatment to the student, and are not available to anyone other than persons providing such treatment, except that such records can be personally reviewed by a physician or other appropriate professional of the student's choice."

In light of ongoing differences of opinion that exist regarding whether student health records at college or university health centers are governed by HIPAA, FERPA, or state privacy laws, health care providers who provide care to older adolescents and young adults on college campuses should consult with their general counsel on this issue.

PAYMENT

There is an integral relationship among the legal provisions that pertain to consent, confidentiality, and payment in the delivery of health care services to adolescents. A source of payment is essential whether an adolescent needs care on a confidential basis or not. The issue is particularly critical for adolescents from low-income families or those who have no family to support them, and even more critical when a young person needs confidential care.

If an adolescent does not have available a source of free care or access to insurance coverage, legal provisions that allow adolescents to give consent for care and to expect confidentiality protections to apply to that care do not actually guarantee access. Financing for the care is therefore an essential element of confidentiality. Some of the state minor consent laws specify that if a minor is authorized to consent to care, it is the minor rather than the parent who is responsible for payment. In reality, however, few, if any, adolescents are able to pay for health care "out of pocket," unless there is a sliding fee scale with very minimal payments required.

There are some federal and state health care funding programs that enable minors to obtain confidential care with little or no cost to them. Most notable is the federal family planning program funded under Title X of the Public Health Services Act. As significant a role as these programs play, they do not ensure access to comprehensive health services for teens. The financing available through insurance is therefore all the more important.

Adolescents are uninsured and underinsured at higher rates than other groups in the population, although young adults are uninsured at the very highest rates. Those adolescents and young adults living below the poverty level are at the greatest risk for lacking health insurance. Private employer-based coverage for adolescents has declined, but coverage through public insurance programs such as Medicaid and the State Children's Health Insurance Program (SCHIP) has increased. Enrollment of all adolescents who are eligible for these programs would significantly decrease the number of uninsured adolescents and have great potential for improving their access to care. Again, specific requirements—for eligibility and benefits—vary by state, so practitioners need to be familiar with their own state's programs.

However, even when adolescents are covered by public or private insurance, they may be unable to access that coverage without the involvement of their parents. Therefore, more than other age-groups, they may be dependent for specific services on care that is provided at no cost or based on a sliding fee scale through federal-funded and state-funded programs. Although the legal framework for financing of health care services is undergoing dramatic changes in general and not only for adolescents, it is nevertheless essential that practitioners familiarize themselves with all potential options whereby adolescent health services can be paid for, including the available sources of public and private funding.

It is only through a comprehensive understanding by practitioners of the legal framework for adolescent health services, including the relationships among consent, confidentiality, and payment issues, that adolescents' access to the health care they need can be ensured. Extensive resources are available on Web sites and in peer-reviewed journals to assist practitioners in becoming familiar with this legal framework.

ACKNOWLEDGMENTS

The author gratefully acknowledges the support of the Annie E. Casey Foundation, Brush Foundation, Compton Foundation, George Gund Foundation, and Moriah Fund. The views expressed are those of the author alone. The author also gratefully acknowledges the research assistance provided by Elisha Dunn-Georgiou, JD, MS.

DISCLAIMER

Please note that neither this chapter nor the Appendix represents legal advice. Health care practitioners are reminded that laws change and that statutes, regulations, and court decisions may be subject to differing interpretations. It is the responsibility of each health care professional to be familiar with the current relevant laws that affect the health care of adolescents. In difficult cases involving legal issues, advice should be sought from someone with state-specific expertise.

WEB SITES

http://www.cahl.org. The Center for Adolescent Health & the Law (CAHL) is a national nonprofit legal and policy organization that promotes the health of adolescents and their access to comprehensive health care.

http://www.healthlaw.org. The National Health Law Program (NHeLP) is a national public interest law firm that seeks to improve health care for America's working and unemployed poor, minorities, the elderly, and people with disabilities, including children and adolescents.

http://www.youthlaw.org/. The National Center for Youth Law (NCYL) is a national nonprofit law office serving the legal needs of children and their families.

http://www.abanet.org/child/home.html. The American Bar Association (ABA) Center for Children and the Law is a national project of the American Bar Association that works to improve children's lives through advances in law, justice, knowledge, practice, and public policy.

http://www.healthprivacy.org. The Health Privacy Project is dedicated to raising public awareness of the importance of ensuring health privacy in order to improve health care access and quality, both on an individual and a community level.

http://www.hhs.gov/ocr/hippa/. The Office for Civil Rights (OCR) in the U.S. Department of Health & Human Services is the agency charged with implementing the HIPAA Privacy Rule.

http://www.guttmacher.org. The Guttmacher Institute is a nonprofit organization focused on sexual and reproductive health research, policy analysis, and public education.

http://www.familiesusa.org. Families USA is a national nonprofit, nonpartisan organization dedicated to the achievement of high-quality, affordable health care for all Americans.

http://www.cbpp.org. The Center on Budget and Policy Priorities (CBPP) conducts research and analysis to inform public debates over proposed budget and tax policies and to help ensure that the needs of low-income families and individuals are considered in these debates. CBPP also develops policy options to alleviate poverty, particularly among working families.

http://www.aap.org. The American Academy of Pediatrics includes on its Web site a broad array of position papers and policies that are relevant to legal issues in the health care of adolescents.

http://www.adolescenthealth.org. The Society for Adolescent Medicine includes on its Web site numerous position papers and statements that are relevant to legal issues in the health care of adolescents.

REFERENCES AND ADDITIONAL READINGS

American Academy of Pediatrics, Committee on Adolescence. The adolescent's right to confidential care when considering abortion. *Pediatrics* 1996;97:746.

Bellotti v. Baird, 443 US 622 (1979).

Boonstra H, Nash E. Minors and the right to consent to health care. *Guttmacher Report* 2000;3:4.

Brindis C, Morreale MC, English A. The unique health care needs of adolescents. *Future Child* 2003;13:117.

Carey v. Population Services International, 431 US 678 (1977).

Cheng T, Savageau J, Sattler A, et al. Confidentiality in health care: a survey of knowledge, perceptions, and attitudes among high school students. *JAMA* 1993;269:1404.

Council on Scientific Affairs, American Medical Association. Confidential health services for adolescents. *JAMA* 1993;269:1420.

Crosby MC, English A. Mandatory parental involvement/judicial bypass laws: do they promote adolescents' health? *J Adolesc Health* 1991;12:143.

English A. Treating adolescents: legal and ethical considerations. *Med Clin North Am* 1990;74:1097.

English A. Reproductive health services for adolescents. Critical legal issues. *Obstet Gynecol Clin North Am* 2000;27:195.

English A. Financing adolescent health care: legal and policy issues for the coming decade. *J Adolesc Health* 2002; 31(suppl):334.

English A, Ford CA. The HIPAA privacy rule and adolescents: legal questions and clinical challenges. *Perspect Sex Reprod Health* 2004;36:80.

English A, Kenney KE. *State minor consent laws: a summary,* 2nd ed. Chapel Hill, NC: Center for Adolescent Health & the Law, 2003.

English A, Morreale MC, Larsen J. Access to health care for youth leaving foster care: Medicaid and SCHIP. *J Adolesc Health* 2003;32(suppl):53.

English A, Morreale M, Stinnett A. *Adolescents in public health insurance programs: Medicaid and CHIP.* Chapel Hill, NC: Center for Adolescent Health & the Law, 1999.

English A, Simmons PS. Legal issues in reproductive health care for adolescents. *Adolesc Med* 1999;10:181.

Ford CA, Bearman PS, Moody J. Foregone health care among adolescents. *JAMA* 1999;282:2227.

Ford CA, English A. Limiting confidentiality of adolescent health services: what are the risks? *JAMA* 2002;288:752.

Ford CA, English A, Sigman G. Society for Adolescent Medicine. Confidential health care for adolescents: position paper. *J Adolesc Health* 2004;35:160.

Ford C, Millstein S, Halpern-Felsher B, et al. Influence of physician confidentiality assurances on adolescents' willingness to disclose information and seek future health care. *JAMA* 1997;278:1029.

Ford CA, Mitchell RD. Discussing confidentiality with adolescent patients: strategies used by clinician members of the Society for Adolescent Medicine. *J Adolesc Health* 2000; 26(2):129.

Holder A. *Legal issues in pediatrics and adolescent medicine,* 2nd ed. New Haven, CT: Yale University Press, 1985.

In re Gault, 387 US 1 (1967).

Klein J, Wilson KMcNulty M, et al. Access to medical care for adolescents: results from the 1997 Commonwealth Fund survey of the health of adolescent girls. *J Adolesc Health* 1999;25(2):120.

Morreale MC, Dowling EC, Stinnett AJ, eds. *Policy compendium on confidential health services for adolescents,* 2d ed. Chapel Hill, NC: Center for Adolescent Health & the Law, 2005.

Morreale MC, English A. Eligibility and enrollment of adolescents in Medicaid and SCHIP: recent progress, current challenges. *J Adolesc Health* 2003;32(suppl):25.

Morreale MC, Kapphahn CJ, Elster AB, et al. Society for Adolescent Medicine. Access to health care for adolescents and young adults: position paper. *J Adolesc Health* 2004;35: 342.

Morrissey JM, Hoffman AD, Thrope JC. *Consent and confidentiality in the health care of children and adolescents: a legal guide.* New York: The Free Press, 1986.

Planned Parenthood of Central Missouri v. Danforth, 428 US 52 (1976).

Planned Parenthood Federation of America, Inc. *Major U.S. Supreme Court rulings on reproductive health and rights.* Available at http://www.ppfa.org/pp2/portal/files/portal/medicalinfo/abortion/fact-abortion-rulings.pdf. 1965–2003.

Planned Parenthood of Southeastern Pennsylvania v. Casey, 505 US 833 (1992).

Rainey D, Brandon D, Krowchuk D. Confidential billing accounts for adolescents in private practice. *J Adolesc Health* 2000;26:389.

Sigman GS, O'Conner C. Exploration for physicians of the mature minor doctrine. *J Pediatrics* 1991;119:520.

Teare C, English A. Nursing practice and statutory rape: effects of reporting and enforcement on access to care for adolescents. *Nurs Clin North Am* 2002;37:393.

Tinker v. Des Moines Independent School District, 393 US 503 (1969).

APPENDIX

Minor Consent for Health Care in the States*

State	Emancipated Minor[1]	Minor Living Apart[2]	Married Minor[3]	Pregnant Minor[4]	Minor Parent (for Self)[5]	Minor Parent (for Child)[6]	Age, Maturity and Other Factors[7]
States That Allow Minors with a Specific Status to Consent for Health Care[a]							
Alabama	■		■	■	■	■	■[15]
Alaska	■	■	■	■	■	■	■[16]
Arizona	■	■[17]	■				
Arkansas	■		■	■		■	■[18]
California	■	■	■	■			
Colorado		■	■			■	
Connecticut	■		■			■	
Delaware			■	■		■	
Dist. of Columbia	■[19]	■[19]	■[19]	■		■	
Florida	■		■	■		■	
Georgia			■	■		■	
Hawaii			■	■			
Idaho						■	■[20]
Illinois	■		■	■	■		■[21]
Indiana	■	■	■				
Iowa			■				
Kansas				■		■	■[22]
Kentucky	■		■	■	■	■	
Louisiana	■		■	■		■	■[23]
Maine	■	■	■				
Maryland	■		■	■	■	■	■[24]
Massachusetts	■	■	■	■	■	■	■[25]
Michigan	■		■	■		■	
Minnesota		■	■			■	
Mississippi				■		■	
Missouri			■	■	■	■	
Montana	■	■	■	■	■	■	■[26]
Nebraska			■				
Nevada	■	■	■	■[29]	■	■	■[29]
New Hampshire							
New Jersey			■	■	■	■	
New Mexico	■		■	■			
New York	■[31]		■	■	■	■	
North Carolina	■		■	■			
North Dakota							
Ohio							
Oklahoma	■	■	■	■	■	■	
Oregon							■[32]
Pennsylvania			■	■		■	■[33]
Rhode Island			■			■	
South Carolina			■			■	■[34]
South Dakota	■		■				
Tennessee			■[35]	■		■	
Texas	■	■	■	■		■	
Utah	■		■	■		■	
Vermont	■		■				
Virginia	■		■	■		■	
Washington	■			■[36]			

(continued)

APPENDIX

(Continued)

State	Emancipated Minor[1]	Minor Living Apart[2]	Married Minor[3]	Pregnant Minor[4]	Minor Parent (for Self)[5]	Minor Parent (for Child)[6]	Age, Maturity and Other Factors[7]
West Virginia	■		■				
Wisconsin							
Wyoming	■	■	■				
TOTALS	**29**	**14**	**42**	**32**	**12**	**33**	**14**

States That Allow Minors to Consent for Specific Health Care Services[a]

State	Family Planning/ Contraception[8]	Pregnancy Care[9]	STD/ VD[10]	Reportable Disease[11]	HIV/ AIDS[12]	Drug/ Alcohol[13]	Outpatient Mental Health[14]
Alabama	■[15]	■	■	■	■	■	■
Alaska	■	■	■	■[16]	■[16]	■[16]	■[16]
Arizona	■		■		■	■	
Arkansas	■	■	■	■[18]	■[18]	■[18]	■[18]
California	■	■	■	■	■	■	■
Colorado	■		■		■	■	■
Connecticut			■		■	■	■
Delaware	■	■	■	■	■	■	
Dist. of Columbia	■	■	■			■	■
Florida	■	■	■		■	■	■
Georgia	■	■	■			■	
Hawaii	■	■			■	■	
Idaho	■	■[20]	■	■	■	■	■[20]
Illinois	■	■	■		■	■	■
Indiana			■		■	■	
Iowa	■		■		■	■	
Kansas	■	■	■	■[22]	■[22]	■	
Kentucky	■	■	■		■	■	■
Louisiana		■	■	■[23]	■	■	
Maine	■		■		■	■	■
Maryland	■	■	■	■[24]	■	■	■
Massachusetts	■	■	■	■	■	■	■
Michigan		■	■		■	■	■
Minnesota	■	■	■		■	■	■
Mississippi	■	■	■		■	■	
Missouri		■	■			■	
Montana	■[27]	■	■	■	■	■	■
Nebraska			■		■[28]	■	
Nevada	■[29]	■[29]	■	■[29]	■	■	■[29]
New Hampshire			■		■	■	■[30]
New Jersey		■	■			■	
New Mexico	■	■			■	■	■
New York	■	■			■	■	■
North Carolina	■	■		■	■	■	■
North Dakota			■		■	■	
Ohio			■		■	■	■
Oklahoma	■		■	■	■	■	
Oregon	■	■[32]	■	■[32]	■	■	■
Pennsylvania	■[33]	■	■	■	■	■	■

APPENDIX

(Continued)

State	Family Planning/ Contraception[8]	Pregnancy Care[9]	STD/ VD[10]	Reportable Disease[11]	HIV/ AIDS[12]	Drug/ Alcohol[13]	Outpatient Mental Health[14]
Rhode Island			■	■	■	■	
South Carolina	■[34]	■[34]	■[34]	■[34]	■[34]	■[34]	■[34]
South Dakota			■			■	
Tennessee	■	■	■			■	■
Texas		■	■	■	■	■	■
Utah		■	■		■		
Vermont			■			■	
Virginia	■	■	■	■	■	■	■
Washington	■	■[36]	■		■	■	■
West Virginia			■		■	■	
Wisconsin			■		■	■	■[37]
Wyoming	■		■		■		
TOTALS	**34**	**35**	**51**	**20**	**43**	**48**	**31**

*This table indicates for each state the general circumstances in which minors may consent for their own care, either based on their status or based on the services they are seeking. In all columns, "■" indicates states with laws that allow minors to consent to their own care or to receive care without prior parental consent. Specific limitations based on age, provider, type of service, number of visits, or disclosure of information are not included in this table but are contained in many states' laws. This table does not include information about abortion, for which the requirements change frequently. This table should not be relied on in lieu of the laws themselves or more detailed summaries of the laws. This table is adapted from English A, Kenney KE. State minor consent laws: a summary, 2nd ed. Chapel Hill, NC: Center for Adolescent Health & the Law, 2003, a monograph that contains summaries of each state's laws, an explanatory introduction, and appendices. Information in this table is current as of June 2005.

[1]Includes states that expressly allow emancipated minors to consent for health care or specify that emancipated minors have adult status. In these and other states that do not have explicit emancipation statutes, minors who meet common law criteria for emancipation (marriage, military service, or living apart from parents with parental consent or acquiescence and managing their own financial affairs) may be considered emancipated and allowed to consent for their own health care.

[2]Includes states that expressly allow minors who are living apart from their parents to consent for health care. Some states include a requirement that these minors be managing their own financial affairs.

[3]Includes states that expressly allow married minors to consent for health care or specify that married minors are emancipated or have adult status. Some states include minors who are or have been married.

[4]Includes states that expressly allow pregnant minors to consent for all care or for pregnancy-related care; does not include information about minor consent or parental notification or consent for abortion.

[5]Includes states that expressly allow minors who are parents to consent for health care for themselves. In other states, minors who are parents may be able to consent on another basis.

[6]Includes states that expressly allow minors who are parents to consent for health care for their child. Even without an explicit statute, minor parents would likely be able to consent for care for their child based on common law and constitutional principles.

[7]Includes states that expressly allow minors to consent for health care based on their age, high school graduation, or specific criteria of maturity, parental availability, or health-related need; does not include states that allow minors to consent for their own care because they are emancipated minors, minors living apart, married minors, pregnant minors, or minor parents; information about these minors is listed in other columns.

[8]Includes states that expressly allow minors to consent for contraceptive services, family planning services, or services to prevent pregnancy. Also includes states that provide for adolescents to receive these services by allowing them to consent for health care generally, based on age, maturity, or other factors. In other states, minors may be able to consent for these services based on having attained another specific status.

[9]Includes states that expressly allow pregnant minors to consent for all care or expressly allow minors to consent for pregnancy-related care. Does not include information about minor consent or parental notification or consent for abortion. Also includes states that provide for minors to receive these services by allowing them to consent for health care generally, based on age, maturity, or other factors. In other states, minors may be able to consent for these services based on having attained another specific status.

[10]Includes states that expressly allow minors to consent for diagnosis and treatment for sexually transmitted disease (STD) or venereal disease (VD). Also includes states that expressly allow minors to consent for prevention of STD or VD. Minors may be able to consent for these services based on having attained another specific status.

[11]Includes states that expressly allow minors to consent for diagnosis and treatment for reportable, infectious, contagious, or communicable disease. Also includes states that expressly allow minors to consent for prevention of such disease. Includes states that provide for minors to receive these services by allowing them to consent for health care generally based on age, maturity, or other factors. In other states, minors may be able to consent for these services based on having attained another specific status.

APPENDIX

(Continued)

[12]Includes states that expressly allow minors to consent for testing and/or treatment for human immunodeficiency virus (HIV) and/or acquired immunodeficiency syndrome (AIDS); also includes states that expressly allow minors to do so based on the classification of HIV or AIDS as a sexually transmitted or reportable disease; and includes states that provide for minors to receive these services by allowing them to consent for health care generally, based on age, maturity, or other factors. In other states, minors may be able to consent for these services based on having attained another specific status.

[13]Includes states that expressly allow minors to consent for care related to the use of drugs and/or alcohol, substance abuse, or chemical dependence, and states that allow minors to receive this care without parental consent. Includes states that provide for minors to receive these services by allowing them to consent for health care generally based on age, maturity, or other factors. In other states, minors may be able to consent for these services based on having attained another specific status.

[14]Includes states that expressly allow minors to consent for outpatient mental health services. Also includes states that provide for adolescents to receive these services by allowing them to consent for health care generally, based on age, maturity, or other factors. In other states, minors may be able to consent for these services based on having attained another specific status.

[15]Alabama allows minors aged 14 or older and high school graduates to consent for their own care.

[16]Alaska allows minors to consent for their own care if a parent or legal guardian cannot be contacted or is unwilling to grant or withholds consent.

[17]Arizona defines a minor living apart as a homeless minor younger than 18 living apart from his parents who lacks a fixed nighttime residence.

[18]Arkansas allows minors to consent for their own care if they have sufficient intelligence to understand and appreciate the consequences of the proposed surgical or medical treatment or procedures.

[19]District of Columbia does not specify in a statute that an emancipated minor may consent for health care. An emancipated minor includes a minor who has been married or residing apart from his or her parents. *Bonner v. Moran*, 126 F.2d 121 (D.C. App. 1941) suggests that parent/guardian may or may not be required to give consent for an emancipated minor.

[20]Idaho allows minors with sufficient intelligence and awareness to comprehend the need for and risks of care to give their own consent.

[21]Illinois has recognized the mature minor doctrine by court decision. In Re E.G., 549 N.E.2d 322 (Ill., 1989).

[22]Kansas allows minors aged 16 or older to give consent for care when no parent or guardian is immediately available.

[23]Louisiana allows minors to consent for their own care for an illness or disease.

[24]Maryland allows minors to consent for care if delaying to obtain another's consent would adversely affect the life or health of the minor.

[25]Massachusetts has recognized the mature minor doctrine by court decision. Baird v. Attorney General, 360 N.E.2d 288, 296 (1977).

[26]Montana allows non-emergency services to be provided for conditions that will endanger the life or health of the minor if services would be delayed by obtaining parental consent.

[27]Montana state law limits the provision of family planning services to a "minor who is or professes to be pregnant."

[28]Nebraska provides that a person may not be tested for HIV unless he or she has given informed consent. A parent or judicially appointed guardian of a minor may give such consent.

[29]Nevada allows minors who are in danger of suffering a serious health hazard if services are not provided to consent for their own care.

[30]New Hampshire allows minors to apply to an approved community mental health program to receive services from the state mental health services system.

[31]New York allows emancipated minors to consent for outpatient mental health services and treatment for chemical dependency.

[32]Oregon allow minors aged 15 and older to consent for their own care.

[33]Pennsylvania allows high school graduates (as well as married minors and pregnant minors) to consent for their own care.

[34]South Carolina allows minors who are aged 16 or older to consent for their own care, other than operations.

[35]Tennessee allows married minors to consent for contraception and family planning services.

[36]Authority in Washington allowing minor consent for pregnancy-related care comes from *State v. Koome*, 530 P.2d 260 (1975), in which the court held that a minor's privacy right to pregnancy care cannot be subjected to absolute parental veto.

[37]Wisconsin allows minors aged 14 and older to consent for mental health services only if they obtain a waiver of informed parental consent from a mental health review officer.

With permission from Center for Adolescent Health and the Law, 2006.

PART II

Endocrine Problems

CHAPTER 8

Abnormal Growth and Development

Joan M. Mansfield and Lawrence S. Neinstein

Chapter 1 described the varied presentation of the normal physical changes of adolescence. The current chapter focuses on the adolescent whose growth and/or development falls outside the range of normal. These issues are usually of enormous concern to adolescents and their family, and the health care provider must have a clear understanding of how to evaluate and manage these problems.

REVIEW OF NORMAL GROWTH

Chapter 1 covers normal growth and development in detail. Briefly, there are three general phases of growth during childhood and adolescence. In infancy, there is a period of rapid growth. This phase is followed by a relatively steady period of growth during midchildhood, averaging 5 to 6 cm/year with a gradual decrease seen over time. A growth rate of <5 cm/year during this middle childhood phase is considered abnormal. Growth hormone (GH) and thyroid hormone are the primary hormonal determinants of growth during midchildhood. This phase is followed by the adolescent growth spurt, which is caused primarily by the hormones of puberty (estrogen and androgens). GH secretion increases significantly during the pubertal growth spurt under the influence of sex steroids. Thyroid hormone continues to be required for growth. During peak pubertal growth, growth rates increase to the range of 9 cm/year in girls and 10 cm/year in boys. As puberty progresses, estrogen results in the gradual fusion of the epiphyses with eventual termination of growth in height. In evaluating growth during adolescence, it is necessary to assess whether a teen has reached puberty, whether puberty is proceeding normally, and whether the bony epiphyses are still open to permit further growth.

SHORT STATURE WITHOUT DELAYED PUBERTY

Adolescents who are progressing normally through puberty may present with concerns about short stature. Most of these teens have genetic or familial short stature with other major categories including chronic disease, constitutional delay of growth and development, and endocrine diseases. Girls who are short may seek medical attention for this complaint when they have just reached menarche and worry that future growth in height will be limited. Boys may present as their pubertal growth spurt slows and they are still shorter than they had hoped. Most hormonal deficiencies, chronic diseases, and malabsorptive states which slow growth will also cause at least some delay in puberty or failure to progress normally through puberty, so that these are less likely causes for the short stature in teens who have normal puberty.

Definition of Short Stature

Adult height is strongly dictated by genetic factors; therefore, evaluation of short stature must be assessed considering the heights of family members. Generally, the 3rd percentile on a cross-sectional growth chart is used as the lower limit of normal.

Criteria for Evaluation An adolescent should be considered for an evaluation of short stature if:

1. Linear growth rate is <4 to 5 cm/year during the years prior to the normal age for peak linear growth velocity
2. No evidence of a peak linear growth velocity by age 16 years in boys and 14 years in girls.
3. Deceleration below an individual's established growth velocity occurs.
4. The adolescent's height is more than 2 standard deviations (SDs) below the calculated midparental height (see Chapter 1)
5. The adolescent's height is more than 3 SDs below the mean. Consideration should be given to carrying out a full evaluation if an adolescent's height is between 2 to 3 SDs below the mean; at a minimum, a careful history and physical examination, screening laboratory tests and observation of growth for 6 months is warranted.

Differential Diagnosis

1. Familial short stature
2. Chronic illness—can include diseases such as cystic fibrosis, human immunodeficiency virus (HIV) infection, severe asthma, congestive heart failure, renal failure, inflammatory bowel disease, sprue among others
3. Constitutional delay of puberty

4. Endocrine—can include hypothyroidism, isolated GH deficiency, hypercortisolism states and poorly controlled diabetes
5. Congenital syndromes including Down syndrome (trisomy 21), Ullrich-Turner syndrome (45X), Noonan, Hurler, Silver-Russell syndrome, Laron syndrome (GH receptor gene mutations); deletions of the portion of the X chromosome containing genes for stature can present with short stature but normal puberty
6. Intrauterine growth retardation
7. Skeletal disorders—chondrodysplasias (often have abnormally short extremities)

Evaluation

History

1. Maternal pregnancy history—medical illnesses and medication use
2. Birth weight and length, and estimate of gestational age—important because premature infants with appropriate small weight tend to have a normal growth potential, whereas infants with intrauterine growth retardation who are inappropriately small for gestational age may not have catch-up growth
3. Complete review of systems:
   a. Renal—polyuria and polydipsia for hypothalamic and/or pituitary disorders
   b. Cardiac—peripheral edema, murmurs, and cyanosis
   c. Gastrointestinal—diarrhea, flatulence (malabsorption), vomiting, and/or abdominal pain
   d. Pulmonary—sleep apnea, asthma, or symptoms suggestive of cystic fibrosis
   e. Neurological—visual field defects suggesting pituitary neoplasms
4. Growth history—close review of symptoms (Figs. 8.1–8.7, growth charts for various disease states)
5. Family history—adult height and growth and pubertal patterns of all first- and second-degree relatives
6. Dietary history
7. Review of the growth chart

Physical Examination

A complete physical examination is the next step in the evaluation and should include:

1. Height and weight
2. Arm span and upper-to-lower (U/L) body-segment ratio
3. Sexual maturity ratings (SMRs)
4. A general physical examination, with special attention to the thyroid gland, ophthalmological examination, neurological examination, and stigmata of congenital syndromes

Laboratory Evaluation

The laboratory evaluation of short stature should include the following:

1. Routine Laboratory Screening: Includes complete blood cell (CBC) count, sedimentation rate, urinalysis, chemistry profile including serum creatinine and liver enzymes, and also thyroid-stimulating hormone (TSH) and adjusted T_4. If celiac disease is suspected, then antiendomysial antibodies, immunoglobulin A, and anti-transglutaminase immunoglobulin G (IgG),

transglutaminase antibodies, and anti-gliadin IgG titers may be useful.
2. Bone Age: X-ray of the left hand and wrist for bone age (since the bone age can determine if there is more potential for growth and be used to estimate predicted final height).
3. Midparental Height Calculation: It is also useful to obtain the parents' heights and calculate a midparental height (formula provided in Chapter 1). Although there are many genes involved in stature, and an offspring's height frequently varies considerably from midparental height, the midparental or target height can still give a good clue that the short stature is genetic.
4. Karyotype: A karyotype is sometimes useful in evaluating the extremely short child who presents with normal puberty.
5. Other Tests: Other tests may be indicated depending on the history and physical examination and may include:
   a. Central imaging studies
   b. Gastrointestinal studies
   c. Endocrine studies:
      (1) Serum levels of insulin-like growth factor I (IGF-I) formerly named somatomedin C, and also insulin-like growth factor-binding protein 3 (IGFBP-3).
      (2) GH stimulation testing is usually done by a pediatric endocrinologist using one of several protocols (insulin, glucagon, arginine, L-dopa, or clonidine). Two tests are usually carried out together and the patient is considered GH deficient if the GH response is <7 to 10 ng/mL on both tests.

Suggestions for Diagnosis

1. Constitutional Delay of Puberty: Most short stature in adolescents is the result of either constitutional delay of puberty or familial short stature. Guidelines for diagnosis are outlined later in this chapter.
2. Genetic or Familial Short Stature: Genetic or familial short stature is suggested by the following:
   a. Normal history and physical examination findings
   b. Birth weight and length that are often below the 3rd percentile for gestational age
   c. Family history of short stature
   d. Growth curve that generally parallels the 3rd percentile
   e. Bone age that is appropriate for chronological age
3. Chronic Illness: Chronic renal disease and Crohn disease are frequent causes of short stature at tertiary care hospitals. These diseases are usually diagnosed by an abnormal history, physical examination findings, or results of tests including screening CBC, sedimentation rate, urinalysis, and chemistry studies. Renal tubular acidosis can easily be overlooked as a cause of short stature. This process may be suggested by family history, urine pH level, or serum bicarbonate values.
4. Endocrine Causes: Endocrine causes of short stature, such as hypothyroidism, GH deficiency, and adrenocortical excess, are uncommon. Hypothyroidism and adrenocortical excess can usually be detected by the patient's history, physical examination, or screening laboratory tests. Adolescents with classic GH deficiency can be difficult to differentiate from those with constitutional delay of puberty. This is particularly difficult during the

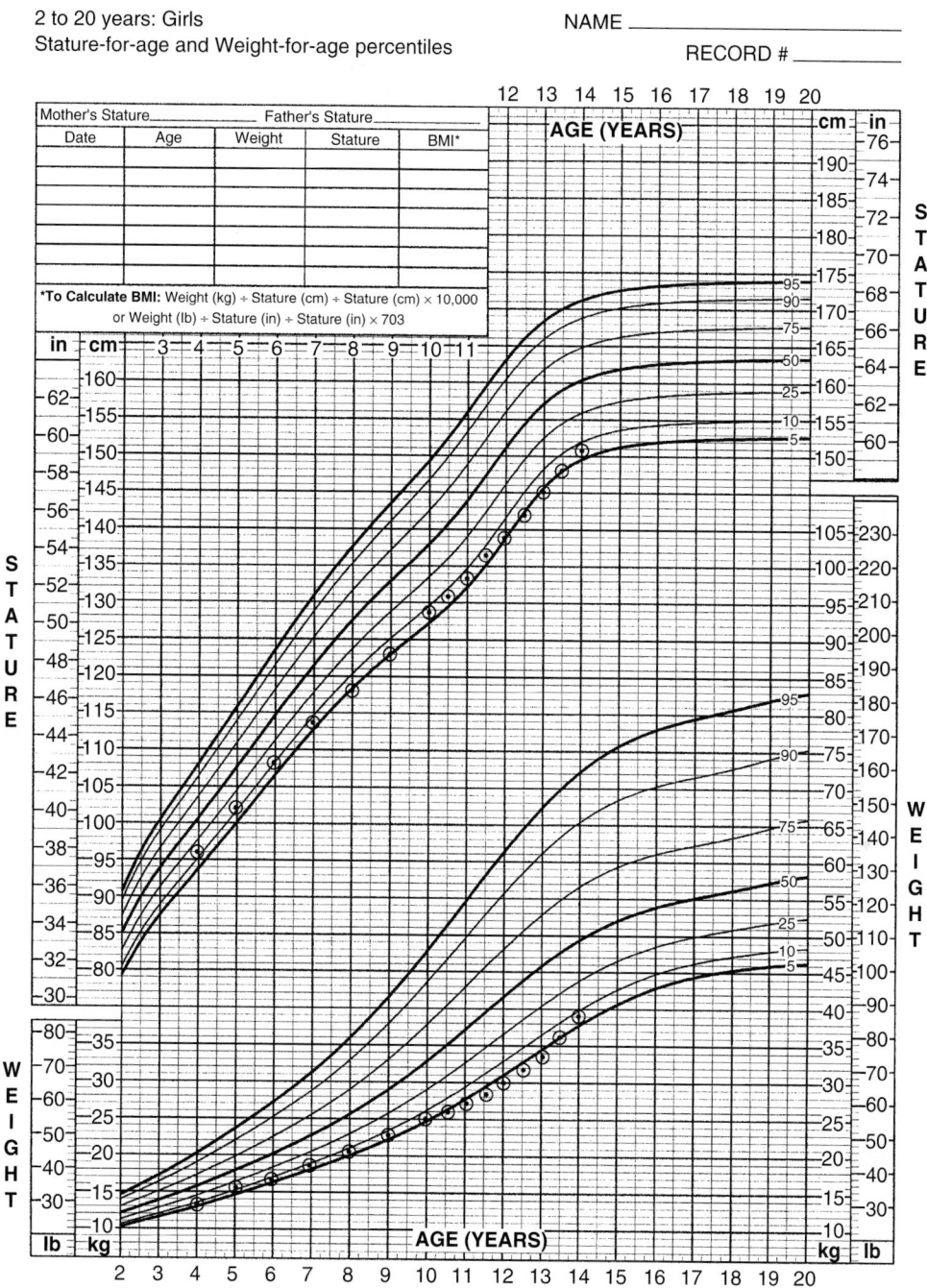

2 to 20 years: Girls
Stature-for-age and Weight-for-age percentiles

NAME _____

RECORD # _____

FIGURE 8.1 Constitutional delay of puberty in girls 2 to 20 years of age (National Center for Health Statistics percentiles). (Adapted from National Center for Health Statistics. *NCHS growth charts.* www.cdc.gov/growthcharts. 2000.)

time of expected peak linear growth velocity, when the growth of an adolescent with constitutional delay of puberty may seem to differ from the normal growth curve as other adolescents accelerate their growth velocities. Individuals with classic GH deficiency have normal body proportions and often a high-pitched voice, a tendency toward hypoglycemia, a microphallus in boys, a childlike face, soft and finely wrinkled skin, and a large prominent forehead.

Treatment of Short Stature with Growth Hormone

Growth Hormone Deficiency

Patients with classic GH deficiency have marked benefit in statural outcome as the result of GH treatment. In addition, those with complete GH deficiency benefit from treatment (from the metabolic effects of GH) with regard to improving bone density, decreasing fat mass, and improving muscle

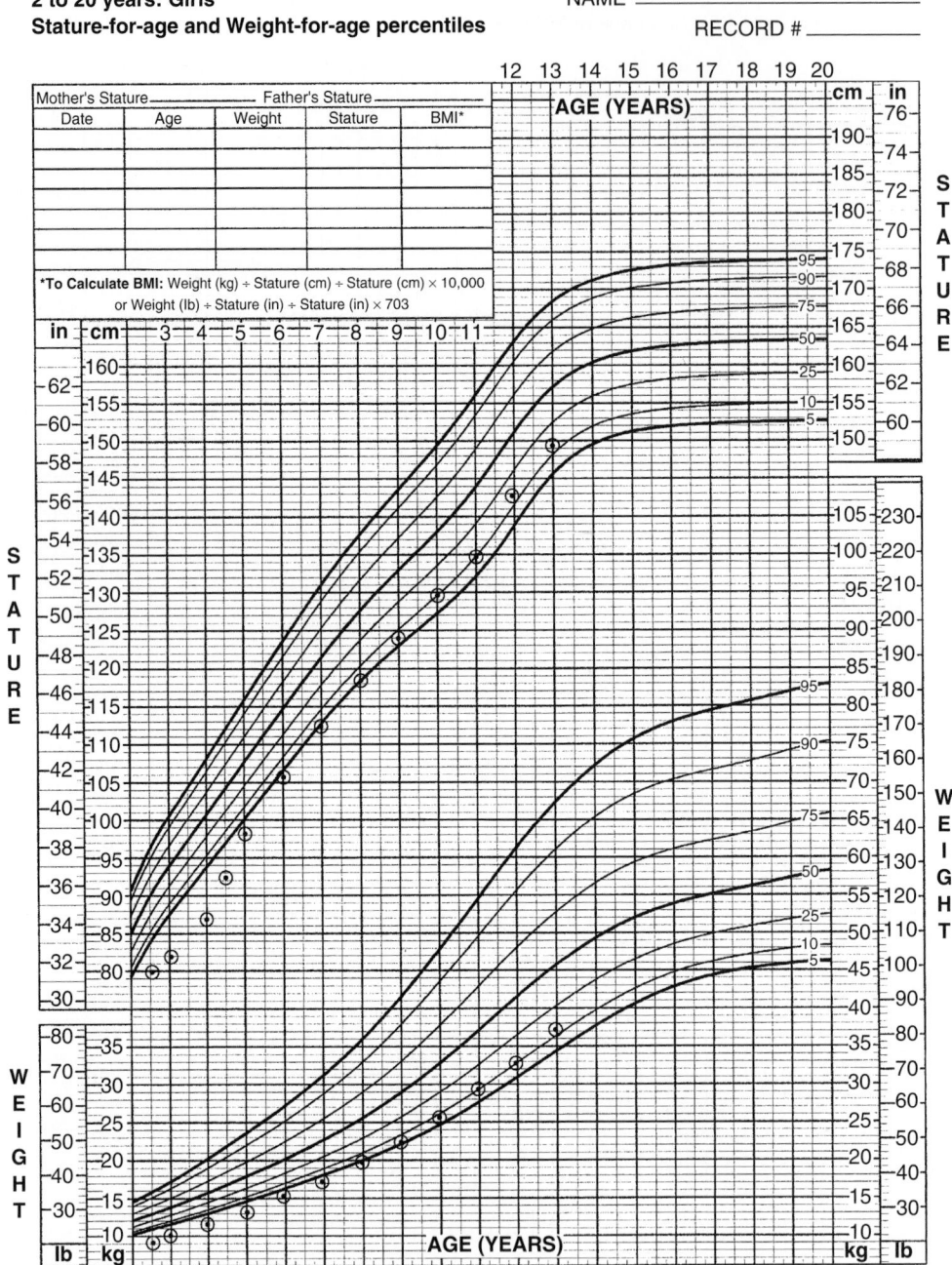

2 to 20 years: Girls
Stature-for-age and Weight-for-age percentiles

NAME _____

RECORD # _____

FIGURE 8.2 Catch-up growth in girls 2 to 20 years of age, with prematurity or deprivation states (National Center for Health Statistics percentiles). (Adapted from National Center for Health Statistics. *NCHS growth charts.* www.cdc.gov/growthcharts. 2000.)

strength, even if epiphyseal fusion has been achieved. It appears these subjects should continue GH treatment at a markedly reduced dose, compared with that used for growth augmentation, throughout life.

Bioengineered human GH has been available since the 1980s and indications for treatment continue to expand. Patients with classical GH deficiency usually present with extreme short stature and slow growth (<4 cm/year) well before adolescence, although acquired GH deficiency,

sometimes due to head trauma, may present in adolescence with slow growth and relatively delayed puberty.

Other Conditions

Turner Syndrome

GH has been used to increase height velocity and increase final adult height in patients who do not have GH deficiency by GH stimulation tests. GH is approved for use in patients with short stature due to Turner syndrome using

2 to 20 years: Girls
Stature-for-age and Weight-for-age percentiles

NAME _____

RECORD # _____

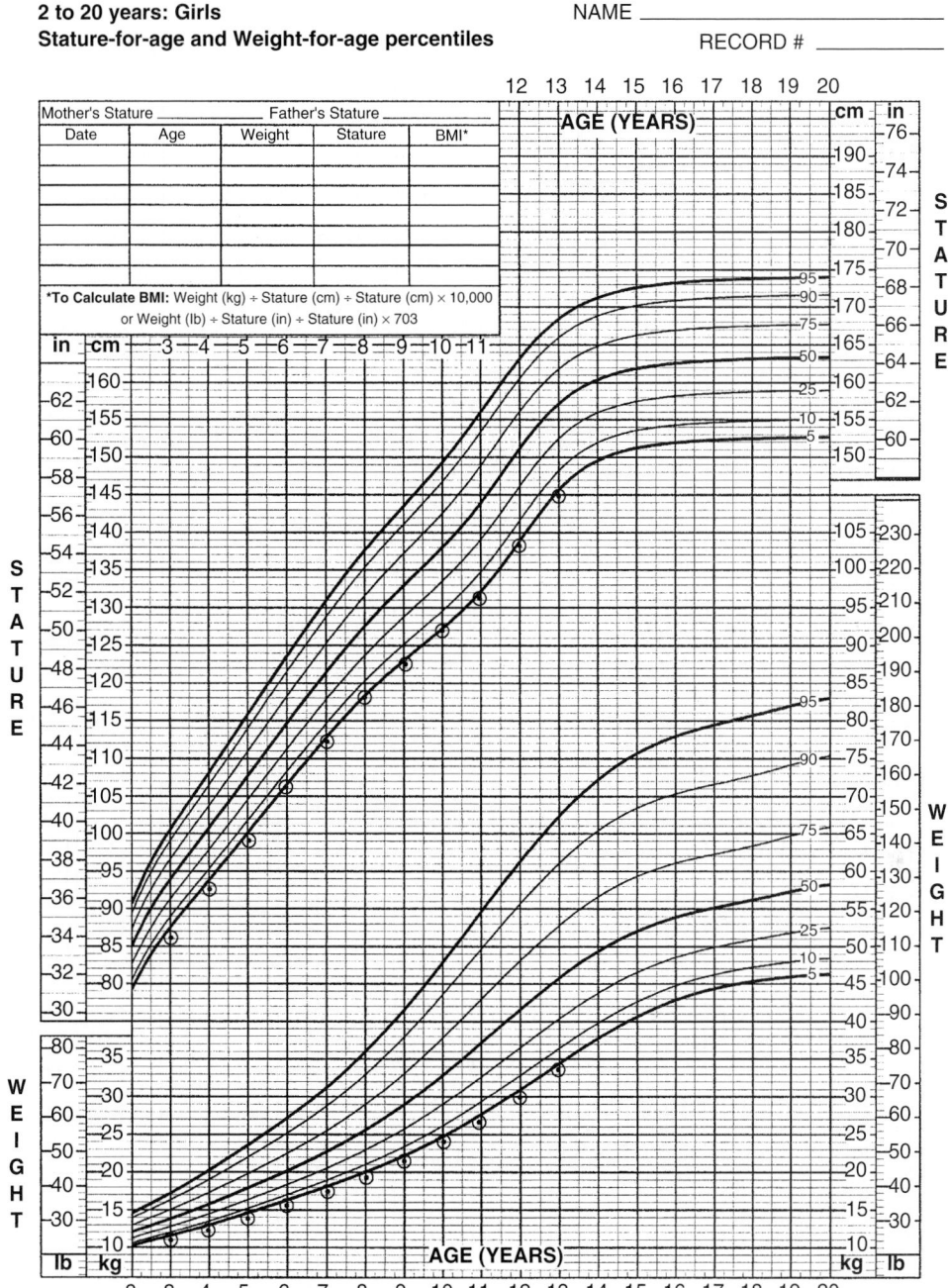

FIGURE 8.3 Low height and low weight in girls 2 to 20 years of age with familial short stature, primordial short stature, with familial short stature or primordial short stature (National Center for Health Statistics percentiles). (Adapted from National Center for Health Statistics. *NCHS growth charts.* www.cdc.gov/growthcharts. 2000.)

a higher dose than is recommended for GH deficiency (0.05 mg/kg/day subcutaneously or 0.35 mg/kg/week for Turner syndrome). IGF-I, thyroid screens, and bone ages by x-ray are monitored during therapy. Patients with Turner syndrome should have baseline renal ultrasonography and periodic echocardiograms to screen for aortic root enlargement. Aortic dissection is a rare but potentially fatal cause of severe chest pain in patients with Turner syndrome. GH treatment should ideally be initiated early in childhood when growth rate begins to fall off. Estrogen replacement is usually delayed to age 12 to 14 or sometimes later to maximize height gain in patients with Turner syndrome. GH has also been used in Noonan syndrome.

Intrauterine Growth Retardation
GH is also approved by the U.S. Food and Drug Administration for use in patients with short stature due to intrauterine growth retardation, Prader-Willi syndrome, and chronic

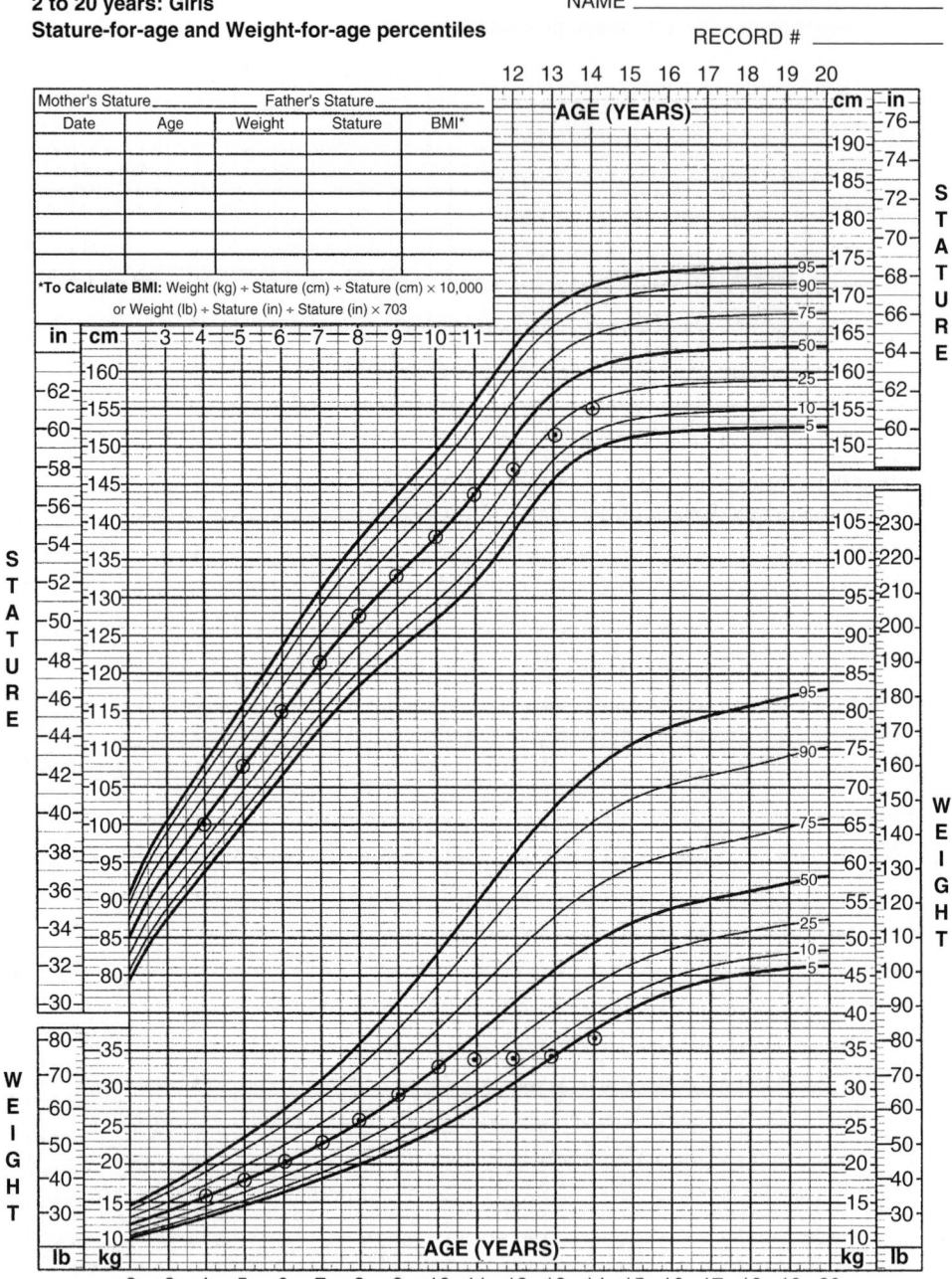

2 to 20 years: Girls
Stature-for-age and Weight-for-age percentiles

NAME _____

RECORD # _____

FIGURE 8.4 Decreased height and markedly decreased weight in girls 2 to 20 years of age with chronic illness states (National Center for Health Statistics percentiles). (Adapted from National Center for Health Statistics. *NCHS growth charts.* www.cdc.gov/growthcharts. 2000.)

renal failure before transplantation. GH has also been approved for treatment of children and adolescents with idiopathic short stature who are more than 2.25 SD below the mean in height and who are unlikely to catch up in height. Patients who qualify for a trial of treatment with human GH for idiopathic short stature must have open epiphyses permitting further height gain. Patients with severe short stature who desire treatment with GH should be referred to a pediatric endocrinologist.

DELAYED PUBERTY

Review of Normal Development

The appearance of secondary sex characteristics is a response to rising levels of sex steroid hormones. As outlined in Chapter 1, in the normal sequence of events, the rise of adrenal androgens known as adrenarche occurs by age 8 years and is followed several years later

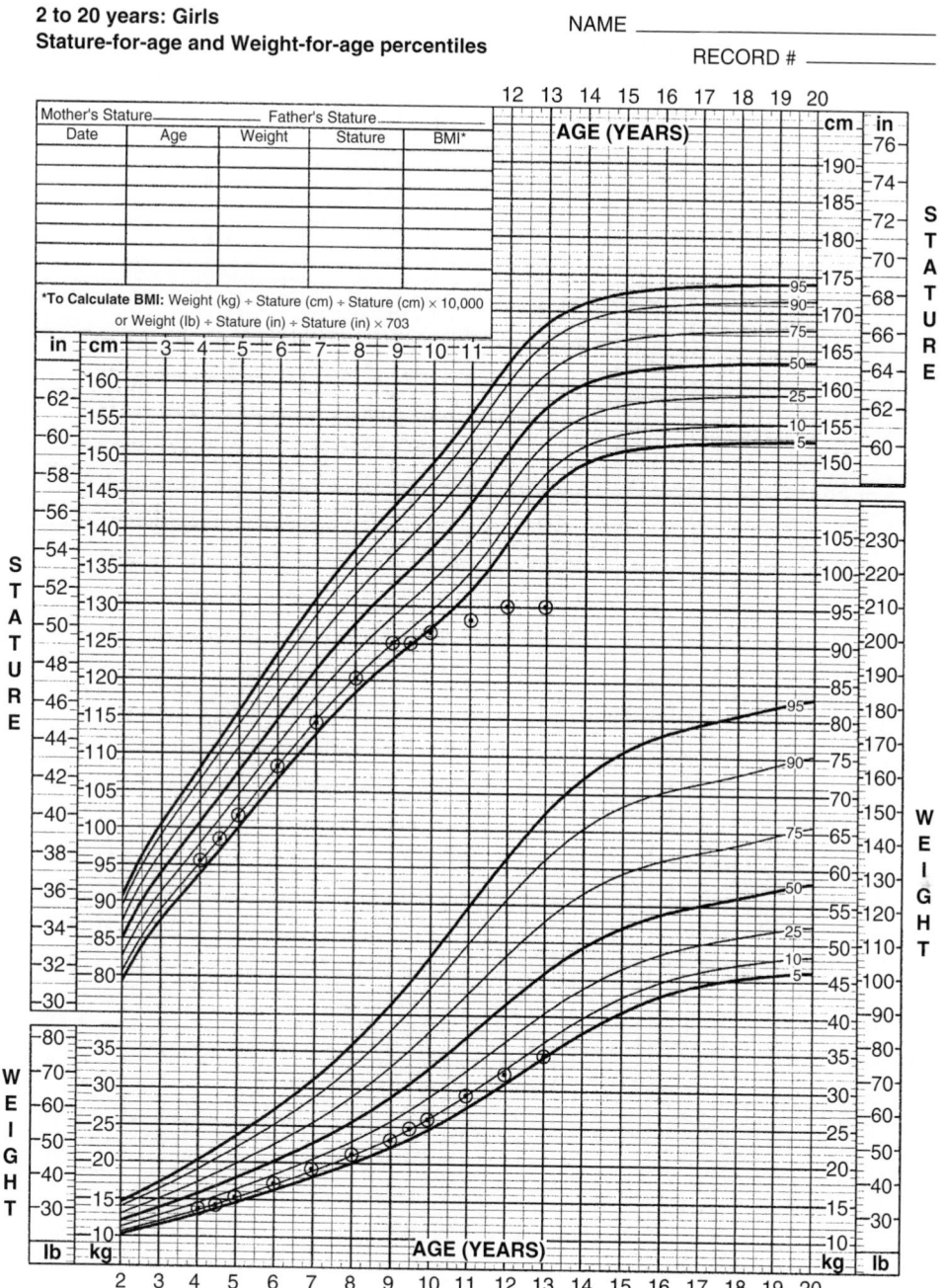

2 to 20 years: Girls
Stature-for-age and Weight-for-age percentiles

NAME _____

RECORD # _____

FIGURE 8.5 Markedly decreased height and decreased weight in girls 2 to 20 years of age with hypopituitary states, metabolic disorders such as rickets, or hypothyroidism (National Center for Health Statistics percentiles). (Adapted from National Center for Health Statistics. *NCHS growth charts*. www.cdc.gov/growthcharts. 2000.)

by an increase of hypothalamic gonadotropin-releasing hormone (GnRH) pulsations that trigger the synthesis and release of luteinizing hormone (LH) and follicle-stimulating hormone (FSH) from the pituitary. LH and FSH stimulate gonadal production of sex steroid hormones and development of the germ cells. The absence of puberty may be the result of failure at any point along the hypothalamic-pituitary-gonadal axis. The challenge of evaluating an adolescent with delayed puberty is to differentiate between constitutional delay of puberty, a normal variation in the tempo of development, and organic diseases such as chronic illness, nutritional insufficiency, tumor, or primary endocrinopathy associated with delayed development.

The pattern of normal puberty is discussed in detail in Chapter 1. Readers are reminded that secondary sexual characteristics usually begin to develop between ages 8 and 13 in girls, and 9 and 14 years in boys.

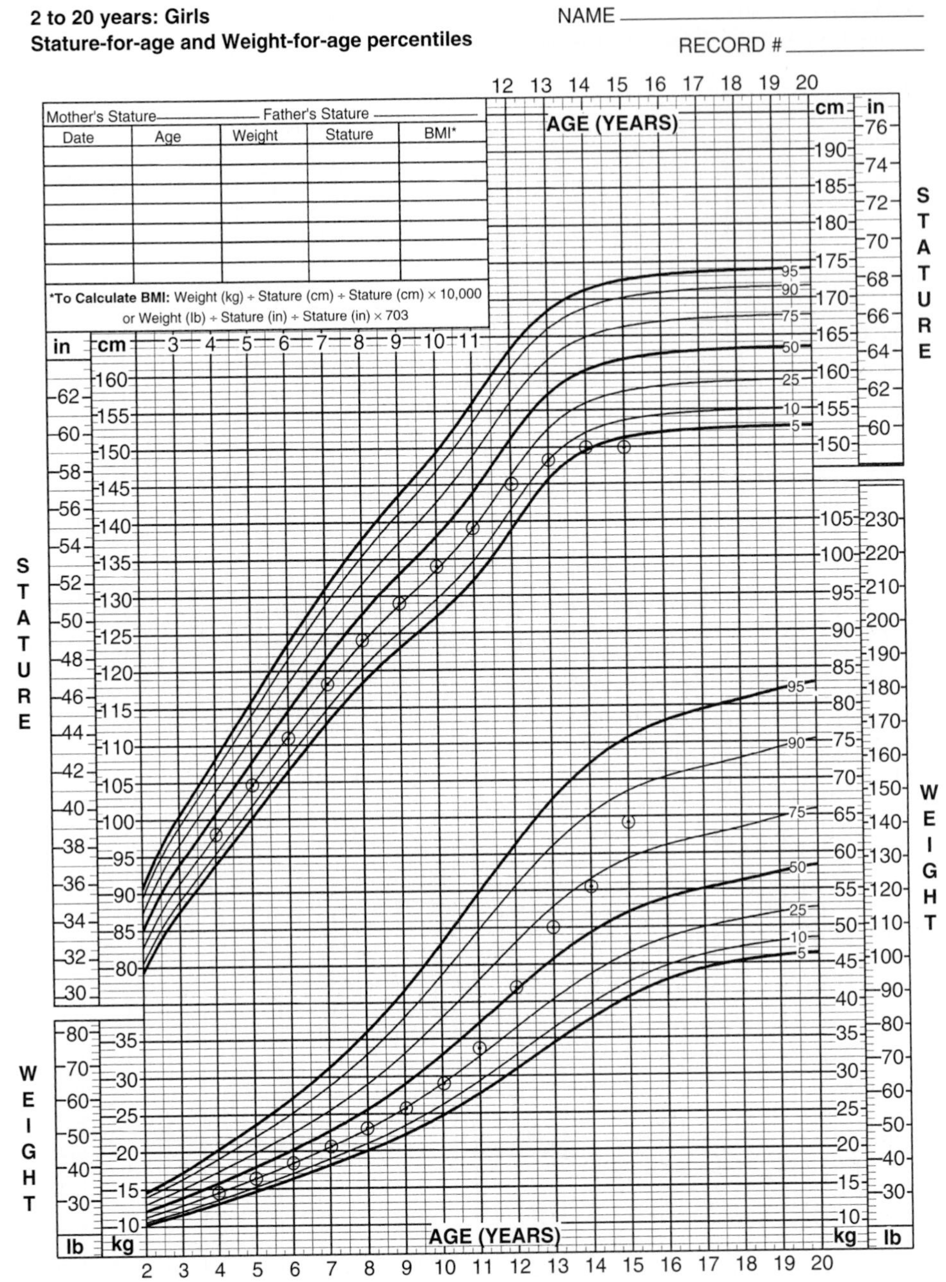

FIGURE 8.6 Decreased height and increased weight in girls 2 to 20 years of age with Cushing syndrome and hypothyroidism (National Center for Health Statistics percentiles). (Adapted from National Center for Health Statistics. *NCHS growth charts.* www.cdc.gov/growthcharts. 2000.)

Females
- Breast budding is the first sign of development in 85% of girls, followed by the appearance of sexual hair. Some normal girls show sexual hair as the first sign of pubertal development.
- Growth acceleration begins early during female puberty, followed by menarche occurring at an average age of 12.5 years, after peak height velocity has passed.
- Girls reach menarche an average of 2.3 ± 1(SD) years after the onset of breast budding.

Males
- The first sign of development in boys is usually enlargement of the testes to >2.4 cm in length (4 mL volume) at an average age of 11.5 years.
- Enlargement of the testes is followed by phallic enlargement, and the appearance of pubic and axillary hair as androgens are secreted, and ultimately an increase in growth rate with peak height velocity being reached approximately 2.5 years after the onset of testicular development.
- Boys usually complete testicular development in 3 ± 2 (SD) years.

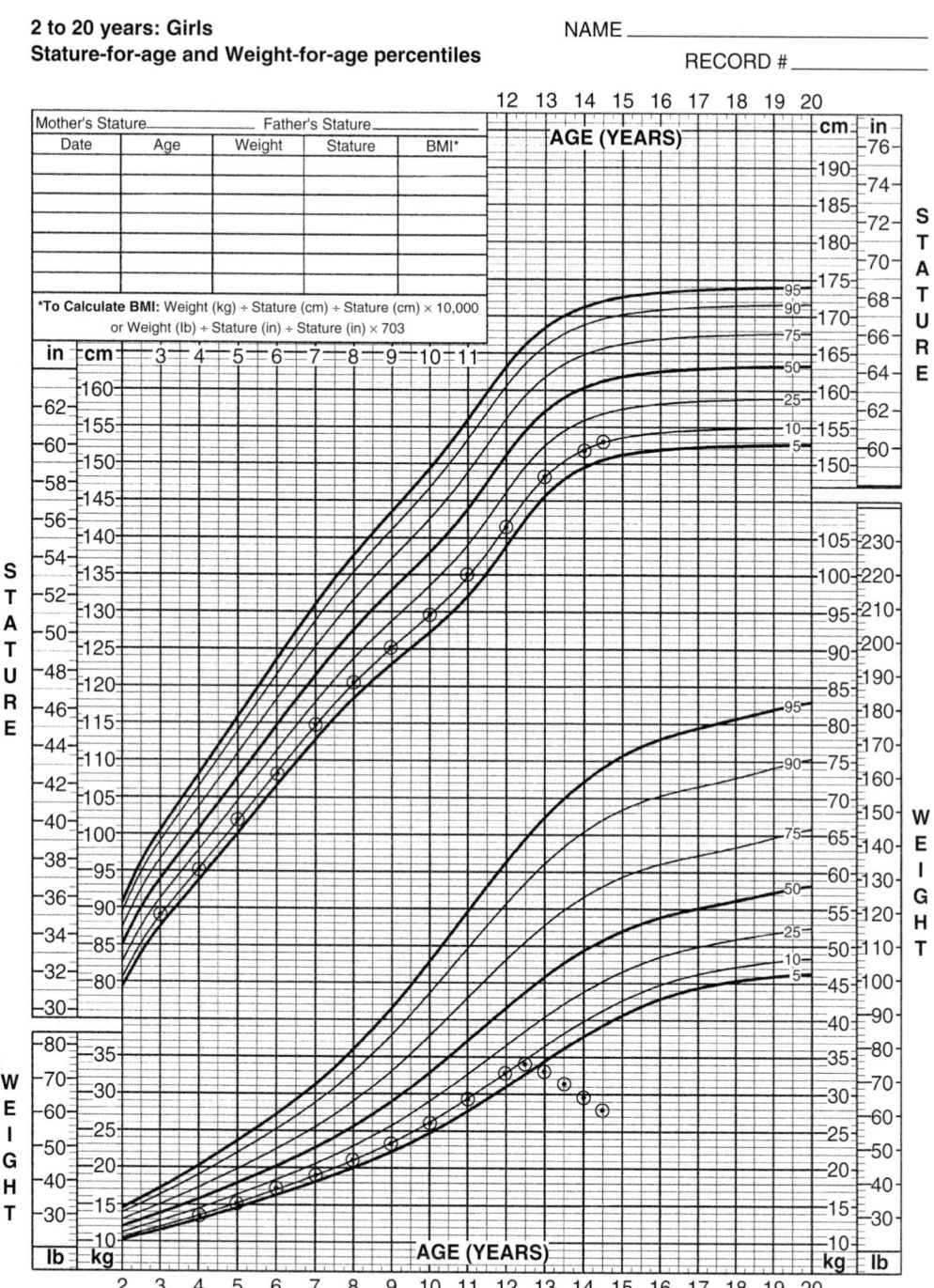

2 to 20 years: Girls
Stature-for-age and Weight-for-age percentiles

NAME _____

RECORD # _____

FIGURE 8.7   Markedly decreased weight in girls 2 to 20 years of age with anorexia nervosa (National Center for Health Statistics percentiles). (Adapted from National Center for Health Statistics. *NCHS growth charts*. www.cdc.gov/growthcharts. 2000.)

Definition

In general, two SDs above and below the mean are used to define the range of normal variability. Chapter 1 is helpful in determining guidelines for evaluation, and further guidelines are discussed subsequently.

Delayed development is defined by the absence of breast budding by age 13 in girls or the lack of testicular enlargement by age 14 in boys, both 2.5 SD beyond the average age at onset of these changes. Alterations in the chronological relationship of pubertal events are also common causes for evaluation. These include phallic enlargement in the absence of testicular enlargement in boys or the absence of menarche by age 16, or 4 years after the onset of breast development, in girls. If puberty is interrupted, there is a regression or failure to progress in the development of secondary sexual characteristics, accompanied by a slowing in growth rate.

General Guidelines for Evaluating Puberty

In Males:
A male adolescent may be considered to have delayed puberty if:

1. Genital stage 1 (G1) persists beyond the age of 13.7 years, or pubic hair stage 1 (PH1) persists beyond the age of 15.1 years.
2. More than 5 years have elapsed from initiation to completion of genital growth.
3. The following SMRs persist past the listed guidelines:

G2 >2.2 years	PH2 >1.0 year
G3 >1.6 years	PH3 >0.5 year
G4 >1.9 years	PH4 >1.5 years

In Females:
A female adolescent may be considered to have delayed maturation if:

1. Breast stage 1 (B1) persists beyond the age of 13.4 years, PH1 persists beyond the age of 14.1 years, or there is failure to menstruate beyond the age of 16 years.
2. More than 5 years have elapsed between initiation of breast growth and menarche.
3. The following SMRs persist past the listed guidelines:

B2 >1.0 year	PH2 >1.3 years
B3 >2.2 years	PH3 >0.9 year
B4 >6.8 years	PH4 >2.4 years

These general guidelines must be considered in the context of the teen's family history as to growth and pubertal development, his or her previous growth pattern, and with regard to the review of systems and physical examination.

Differential Diagnosis

Delayed development occurs more commonly in boys than girls. Most patients who present for an evaluation of slow growth and delayed development are high school–aged boys who are concerned about their short stature, as well as their lack of muscular and secondary sexual development which puts them at a disadvantage among their peers. Most of these boys have constitutionally delayed development; however, the clinical presentation of the patient with constitutional delay may be indistinguishable from that of the patient whose pubertal delay is the result of an organic lesion.

Constitutional Delay of Puberty
Adolescents with constitutional delay of puberty have often been slow growers throughout childhood. In the absence of sex steroids of puberty, growth may slow even further to <5 cm/year as these children reach an age when puberty would normally occur. Growth velocity increases into the normal range when these teens finally enter puberty. Adolescents with constitutional delay of puberty often have a family history of delayed growth and development in relatives. Teens with constitutional delay of puberty eventually enter puberty on their own. Although they have a longer time to grow before their epiphyses close, they tend to have a less exuberant growth spurt than earlier developers so that their final height is often shorter than average.

Functional Causes of Delayed Puberty
GnRH secretion, can be inhibited centrally by

1. Inadequate nutrition, including eating disorders
2. Chronic disease including chronic heart disease, severe asthma, inflammatory bowel disease, celiac disease, juvenile rheumatoid arthritis, chronic renal failure, renal tubular acidosis, sickle cell anemia, diabetes mellitus, systemic lupus erythematosus, cystic fibrosis, and infection with HIV
3. Severe environmental stress
4. Intensive athletic training
5. Hypothyroidism and excess cortisol states
6. Drugs such as opiates and stimulants

Eating disorders associated with self-imposed restriction of caloric intake can delay or interrupt the progression of puberty. Anorexia nervosa most often develops in girls in early to middle adolescence, who have already entered puberty. Young adolescent boys or girls who are dieting because of fear of obesity may present with the complaint of delayed development. Crohn disease or celiac disease may also present with delayed development and poor growth as the major symptoms. Since adolescence is normally a period of rapid growth and weight gain, failure to gain or small amounts of weight loss may be manifestations of significant nutritional insufficiency. Poor growth and delayed puberty are common in cystic fibrosis, thalassemia major, renal tubular acidosis, renal failure, cyanotic congenital heart disease, sickle cell anemia, systemic lupus erythematosus, acquired immune deficiency syndrome, or very poorly controlled asthma or type 1 diabetes. Patients who are on stimulants such as methylphenidate (Ritalin) for treatment of attention deficit disorder may have decreased appetite because of the medication and slower growth rates as a result of nutritional insufficiency.

Hypothyroidism may present in an adolescent with slowing of height velocity (height dropping percentiles on the growth chart) whose weight is well preserved for height or who is mildly overweight, sometimes with delayed or interrupted pubertal development. The classic signs include dull dry skin, perhaps with scalp hair loss, decrease in pulse rate and blood pressure, constipation, and cold intolerance. A goiter is not always present. Autoimmune thyroiditis is the most common cause of hypothyroidism in teens. There may be a family history of hypothyroidism or autoimmune issues.

Cushing syndrome (endogenous glucocorticoid overproduction) or chronic exposure to high doses of glucocorticoids for medical treatment causes excessive weight gain, slowing of height velocity, and may interrupt or delay puberty or, if endogenous sex steroid production is also increased, may present with precocious puberty without a growth spurt.

Hypothalamic Causes of Delayed Puberty
The ability of the hypothalamus to secrete GnRH may be damaged by:

1. Local tumors (germinomas, craniopharyngiomas, astrocytomas, or gliomas)

2. Infiltrative lesions such as central nervous system (CNS) leukemia or histiocytosis X
3. CNS irradiation
4. Traumatic gliosis
5. Mass lesions such as brain abscesses or granulomas due to sarcoidosis or tuberculosis
6. Congenital defects in the ability to secrete GnRH (idiopathic hypogonadotropic hypogonadism may be associated with midline craniofacial defects or olfactory defects [Kallmann syndrome] and may be familial). Other congenital brain malformations associated with inability to secrete GnRH include septooptic dysplasia.

Pituitary Causes of Delayed Puberty

Puberty may not begin or may fail to proceed if the pituitary cannot respond to GnRH stimulation with LH and FSH production. This may be due to:

1. Pituitary tumor
2. Selective impairment of gonadotrope function by hemochromatosis
3. Congenital hypopituitarism, which is usually diagnosed either in the neonatal period or with poor growth during childhood; causes include genetic defects that interfere with pituitary formation and empty sella syndrome
4. Acquired hypopituitarism
5. Prolactinoma—excessive prolactin production by a pituitary adenoma (prolactinoma) or other tumor may interrupt or prevent puberty by interfering with gonadotropin production. Patients with prolactinomas most often present with secondary amenorrhea often with galactorrhea, but may present with stalled puberty. Headaches are sometimes present. Prolactinomas are more common in girls than boys, but can occur in both. Psychotropic drugs such as antipsychotics are a frequent cause of hyperprolactinemia.

Gonadal Failure

If the gonads are unable to respond to LH and FSH, puberty will not proceed.
   The causes of gonadal failure with abnormal karyotype include:

1. Gonadal Dysgenesis: The most common cause of gonadal failure is gonadal dysgenesis, which occurs in association with abnormalities of sex chromosomes. The gonads fail to develop and become rudimentary streaks. These patients are phenotypic females with normal immature female genitalia. The most common phenotype is Turner syndrome which is caused by absence of part or all of a second sex chromosome. These patients are typically short with a final untreated height averaging 143 cm. Other identifying features of Turner syndrome are low set ears, a webbed neck, widely spaced nipples, a trident hairline, an increased carrying angle of the lower arms, and short forth and fifth fingers and toes. Renal abnormalities such as duplications and horseshoe kidney, and left-sided cardiovascular abnormalities such as bicuspid aortic valve, dilatation of the aortic root and coarctation of the aorta are also associated with Turner syndrome. Half of these patients have 45,X karyotypes whereas the rest are mosaics or have various X chromosome abnormalities or deletions.
2. Klinefelter Syndrome: Males with Klinefelter syndrome (47,XXY) may present with poorly progressing puberty caused by partial gonadal failure. Although they lack sperm production, their testes can make some testosterone when driven by high levels of gonadotropins (LH and FSH). In the 47,XXY patient with pubertal development, the testes become small and firm because they become fibrotic. Gynecomastia and eunuchoid body habitus are often seen.

   The causes of gonadal failure with normal karyotype include:

1. Acquired Gonadal Disorders
   a. Infection—viral or tubercular orchitis or oopheritis
   b. Trauma—bilateral testicular torsion resulting in anorchia is another cause of gonadal failure in males
   c. Postsurgical removal
   d. Radiation, chemotherapy with agents such as cyclophosphamide
   e. Autoimmune oophoritis or orchitis (sometimes with multiple autoimmune endocrine abnormalities)
   f. The resistant ovary syndrome
   g. Sarcoidosis
   h. Fragile X may present as secondary amenorrhea in females with ovarian failure
   i. Cryptorchidism—in males who are cryptorchid, the testes may fail to function, particularly if they remain intraabdominal beyond infancy
2. Congenital Gonadal Disorders
   a. Anorchism: In the "vanishing testis syndrome", the testes are absent in a phenotypic male, presumably as a result of destruction in utero.
   b. Pure gonadal dysgenesis: This presents as absent puberty in patients with a normal karyotype (46,XX or 46,XY), normal stature, and a female phenotype.
   c. Enzyme defects in androgen and estrogen production: Enzymatic defects, such as 17α-hydroxylase or 20,22-desmolase deficiency, which render the gonad unable to produce estrogens or androgens, are other rare causes of primary gonadal failure. No specific cause for gonadal failure can be found in many cases.
   d. Gonadal failure is associated with other diseases such as congenital galactosemia in girls and ataxia telangiectasia.
3. Androgen-Receptor Defects
   a. Complete androgen insensitivity (previously referred to as "testicular feminization") presents as a patient who is a phenotypic female with tall stature, absence of sexual hair, normal breast development and timing of puberty, but absence of menarche. The vagina is a short pouch and there is no uterus. The karyotype is 46,XY, and testosterone levels are elevated.
   b. Incomplete (previously referred to as a variety of syndromes, including Reifenstein syndrome)

Syndromes Associated with Pubertal Delay

There are several syndromes that are characterized by extreme obesity, short stature, and delayed puberty. These include the following:

1. Prader-Willi (extreme obesity, developmental delay, small hands and feet, and chromosome 15 deletion)
2. Lawrence-Moon-Bardet-Biedel (obesity, polydactaly, retinitis pigmentosa, genital hypoplasia, developmental delay)
3. Borjeson-Forseeman-Lehman (obesity, severe mental deficiency, microcephaly, epilepsy and skeletal anomalies)

Another congenital syndrome is congenital absence of the uterus and upper vagina (Mayer-Rokintansky-Kuster-Hauser syndrome). This is associated with normal puberty, but absent menses.

WORK-UP OF DELAYED PUBERTY

Most adolescents with delayed maturation have constitutional delay of puberty. However, this diagnosis is made by excluding other causes. Following is a discussion of the evaluation of the adolescent with delayed puberty, including criteria for a provisional diagnosis of constitutional delay of puberty. A detailed history and physical examination will help focus and minimize the laboratory testing needed to evaluate an adolescent with delayed development.

History

1. Neonatal History: The neonatal history should include birth weight, history of previous maternal miscarriages and congenital lymphedema (Turner syndrome). The past medical history should focus on any history of chronic disease, congenital anomalies, previous surgery, radiation exposure, chemotherapy, or drug use.
2. Growth Records: Past growth measurements that are plotted on appropriate developmental charts for height, weight, and body mass index are important in evaluating the adolescent with delayed puberty. The overall pattern of growth and changes in that pattern often lead to a diagnosis. Examples of growth charts in various disease states are provided in Figures 8.1 through 8.7. The child whose delayed puberty is associated with a nutritional deficiency due to an eating disorder, inflammatory bowel disease, celiac disease, or other chronic disease will show a greater decline in weight gain than in height and be underweight for height (Fig. 8.4). In contrast, the child who has delayed puberty on the basis of an endocrinopathy such as acquired hypothyroidism or gonadal dysgenesis will have a greater slowing in height gain than in weight gain, and have weight well preserved for height, often being mildly overweight (Fig. 8.6).
3. Review of Systems: Special attention should be paid to weight changes, dieting, environmental stress, exercise and athletics, gastrointestinal symptoms, headache, neurological symptoms (including abnormal peripheral vision and anosmia), and symptoms suggestive of thyroid disease.
4. Nutritional History and Eating Habits: This helps to discount a problem of chronic malnutrition.
5. Family History: The family history should include the heights, and timing of secondary sexual development and fertility of family members, a history of anosmia, and a history of endocrine disorders.

Physical Examination

A complete physical examination is indicated for the adolescent with delayed puberty, but the following areas are of particular importance:

1. Overall nutritional status and measurements of height, weight and vital signs

2. Body measurements including:
   a. Arm span
   b. Upper to lower segment ratio: This can be measure by measuring symphysis pubis to floor for lower, subtracting lower from total height for upper. This measurement can be useful for patients who have either short extremities (short bone syndromes, congenital short stature syndromes) or long extremities (eunuchoid appearance). The normal U/L ratio is 1.7 at birth, 1.0 at age 10 years, and 0.9 to 1.0 in adulthood in Caucasians, and 0.85 to 0.9 in African-Americans. Hypothyroidism will cause a U/L ratio to remain greater than 1.0, which would be the case in most patients with chondrodysplasia. Hypogonadism will usually have a U/L ratio close to 0.9 or less. A normal ratio is often found in those with GH deficiency, constitutional delay of puberty, and chronic disease states.
3. Congenital anomalies, including midline facial defects
4. Staging of sexual maturity: The patient should be examined for a delay in pubertal development as assessed by staging of breast and pubic hair in girls, and genitalia and pubic hair in boys. Pubic hair may be present, although the genitalia are prepubertal in a boy who had normal adrenarche, but lacks gonadal activation. Any evidence of heterosexual development, such as clitoromegaly or hirsutism in girls or gynecomastia in boys should be noted.
5. Thyroid: Check for evidence of goiter. Absence of goiter can be seen with hypothyroidism.
6. Chest: Check for evidence of chronic pulmonary disease.
7. Cardiac: Check for evidence of congenital heart disease.
8. Abdomen: Check for abdominal distension as a sign of a malabsorptive disease and check for evidence of liver or spleen enlargement as a sign of a chronic systemic disorder.
9. Genital examination: The examination of the external genitalia in girls should focus on obvious congenital anomalies and an assessment of estrogen effect. A pale pink vaginal mucosa with white secretion indicates the current presence of estrogen. A pelvic examination is not necessary as a part of the initial evaluation of a girl with delayed secondary sexual development, but should be done if possible to rule out gynecological congenital anomalies in a girl who has normal pubertal development but delayed menarche. The pelvic examination should be carried out by a practitioner who is familiar with the techniques used for examining nonsexually active teen girls such as assessing the depth of the vagina with a saline-moistened cotton-tipped applicator, and using a one finger bimanual vaginal–abdominal examination if the vaginal introitus comfortably permits. If amenorrhea is a problem, then either a complete pelvic examination is indicated or pelvic ultrasonography can be performed if needed to determine the presence of müllerian structures (uterus and tubes) and to visualize ovaries.
10. Neurological examination: This will help eliminate from consideration any intracranial pathology. Ophthalmoscopic and visual-fields examination is done to rule out abnormalities of the optic nerves and to look for evidence of intracranial hypertension.

Laboratory Tests

Laboratory evaluation should be focused according to the clinical impression (see clue to diagnosis). In the patient who is underweight for height, studies would include screening tests for chronic disease or malabsorptive states such as celiac disease.

Bone Age The most useful initial examination in delayed puberty and slow growth is often an x-ray of the left hand and wrist for a bone age assessment. This information can be used to assess how much height growth potential remains in the patient with short stature and delayed development. A predicted adult height can be obtained using the Bayley-Pinneau tables in the Atlas of Skeletal Maturation by Gruelich and Pyle (or see Table 1.5).

1. Constitutional Delay of Puberty: The patient with constitutional delay of puberty will usually have an equal delay of height age and bone age. Caution should be used in height predictions in patients with constitutional delay of puberty since boys with constitutional delay and short stature frequently reach a final height short of the final adult height predicted by the tables.
2. Delayed Bone Age: Patients with GH deficiency, hypothyroidism, and chronic disease usually have bone ages that are delayed several years behind their chronological age.
3. Normal or Delayed Bone Age: Often seen with Turner syndrome.

    Bone age may also be used in conjunction with height age and chronological age to give clues about a diagnosis as indicated below. *Height age* is determined by locating the corresponding age at which the patient's height would be equal to the 50th percentile. See Table 8.1.

Routine Laboratory Tests Initial laboratory studies to be considered in the adolescent with delayed puberty include a CBC count, erythrocyte sedimentation rate (useful as a screening test for chronic illness such as inflammatory bowel disease) electrolytes, blood urea nitrogen, creatinine, glucose, calcium, phosphorus, albumin, liver enzymes and urinalysis.

Evaluation for Celiac Disease Evaluation for celiac disease (antitissue transglutaminase and total IgA, or celiac panel) should be considered. More extensive testing for inflammatory bowel disease includes an upper gastrointestinal tract series with small bowel follow through and barium enema.

Central Imaging Studies If there is a suspicion of a CNS tumor, cranial magnetic imaging with contrast is the best way to evaluate the hypothalamus and pituitary. A computed tomography (CT) scan is a less sensitive alternative.

Hormonal Tests Hormonal tests to be considered include thyroid function tests (adjusted T_4, TSH), prolactin, LH and FSH, dehydroepiandrosterone sulfate, testosterone or estradiol, and IGF-I and IGFBP-3.

In the early stages (Tanner stage 2) of puberty, breast budding and vaginal maturation in girls and penile and testicular enlargement in boys are more sensitive indicators of pubertal neuroendocrine-gonadal function than a single daytime measurement of gonadotropin (LH and FSH) levels, estradiol or testosterone. LH, FSH, and testosterone or estradiol may be in the prepubertal range on a daytime sample even though these hormones are actively being secreted at night. Testosterone or estradiol levels may be valuable in following the patient whose puberty is not progressing normally by clinical assessment of growth and secondary sexual development.

GH is secreted primarily during sleep, so daytime levels are expected to be low. IGF-I and IGFBP-3 are used to assess GH sufficiency. IGF-I levels should be compared with normals for bone age rather than chronological age since the levels increase during puberty. IGF-I levels are low in patients with nutritional insufficiency. Patients with delayed puberty and slow growth often have temporarily decreased GH secretion simply due to pubertal delay which increases to normal as puberty begins. If GH deficiency is suspected, the patient should be referred to a pediatric endocrinologist for GH stimulation testing. Patients with constitutional delay of puberty who are prepubertal may appear GH deficient on GH stimulation testing unless primed with estrogen before the test.

LH and FSH determinations are only useful if they are elevated since these hormones are secreted primarily during sleep in the early phases of puberty. Early to midpubertal levels (Tanner breast stage 2) are indistinguishable from prepubertal levels, usually with a very low LH and FSH higher than LH. Elevated LH and FSH levels are suggestive

TABLE 8.1

Typical Relationships between Bone Age, Height Age, and Chronological Age for Causes of Delayed Puberty or Short Stature

Cause of Delayed Puberty or Short Stature	Relationship between Bone Age (BA), Chronological Age (CA), and Height Age (HA)
Genetic	HA < BA = CA
Skeletal dysplasia	HA ≤ BA < CA or BA < HA < CA
Constitutional	HA = BA < CA
Hypopituitarism	HA ≤ BA < CA
Hypothyroidism	BA < HA < CA
Hypogonadism	BA ≤ HA < CA
Systemic illness	BA = HA < CA

TABLE 8.2

Criteria for Provisional Diagnosis of Constitutional Delay of Puberty

Required features
  Detailed negative review of systems
  Evidence of appropriate nutrition
  Linear growth of at least 3.7 cm/yr
  Normal findings on physical examination, including genital anatomy, sense of
    smell, and U/L body-segment ratio
  Normal CBC, sedimentation rate, urinalysis results, adjusted T_4 concentration, and
    noncastrate levels of serum LH and FSH
  Bone age delayed 1.5–4.0 yr compared with chronological age
Supportive features
  Family history of constitutional delay of puberty
  Height between 3rd and 25th percentiles for chronological age

---

U/L, upper-to-lower; CBC, complete blood cell; LH, luteinizing hormone; FSH, follicle-stimulating hormone.

From Barnes HV. Recognizing normal and abnormal growth and development during puberty. In: Moss AV, ed. *Pediatrics update: reviews for physicians*. New York: Elsevier–North Holland Publishing, 1979:103, with permission.

---

of primary gonadal failure. If LH and FSH levels are elevated, further laboratory evaluation would include blood karyotyping in search of a chromosomal abnormality such as 45,X. Patients with gonadal dysgenesis who have Y chromosomal material present should have their gonads removed surgically because of an increased risk for gonadoblastoma. If the chromosomes are normal in the patient with gonadal failure, antiovarian antibodies may be obtained to look for autoimmune gonadal damage. Pelvic ultrasonography may be used to visualize the uterus and ovaries, but should be interpreted with caution since the prepubertal uterus is small and may be missed on ultrasonography. A vaginal ultrasonography is usually postponed until adulthood.

If the initial prolactin level is elevated, it should be repeated without a breast examination on the day of the testing, and ideally in a fasting state. Patients with significantly elevated prolactin levels should have a cranial magnetic resonance imaging (MRI) with contrast.

Neuroendocrine Pharmacological Testing If there is a question of multiple pituitary hormone defects, the patient may be referred to an endocrinologist for pharmacological and physiological tests of neuroendocrine function. A GnRH stimulation test with gonadorelin (Factrel), 2.5 µg/kg intravenously, maximum 100 µg, has been used in the past to assess pituitary LH and FSH response in the evaluation of delayed puberty. If the patient has central puberty, there will be a large increase in LH during the 2 hours after GnRH is given (sample can be drawn at 45 minutes). Since GnRH is currently not commercially available, GnRH analog stimulation tests are substituted (leuprolide acetate 500 µg).

Constitutional Delay of Puberty
The chief diagnostic challenge in the patient with pubertal delay is to distinguish between constitutional delay and true GnRH deficiency. About 90% to 95% of delayed puberty is constitutional delay of puberty. No single test reliably separates patients with constitutional delay from those with idiopathic hypogonadotropic hypogonadism.

This diagnosis is made by excluding the other causes, as discussed. However, using the guidelines in Table 8.2, one can confidently make a provisional diagnosis.

Clues to Other Diagnoses

1. Gonadotropin deficiency
   a. Low serum FSH and LH levels, particularly if bone age is more than 13 years
   b. Low response to GnRH
   c. Abnormal central imaging study results
   d. History of neurological symptoms, CNS infections, radiation, or disease
   e. Possible absence of sense of smell (Kallmann syndrome)
      The presence of midline facial defects, anosmia, cryptorchidism, or microphallus strongly suggests idiopathic hypogonadotropic hypogonadism; however the diagnosis cannot be firmly established until the patient reaches the age of 18 years and is still prepubertal. Genes for hypothalamic hypogonadism have been identified, as have some genes for familial pubertal delay.
2. Gonadal disorder
   a. History of genital radiation, surgery, infection, or trauma
   b. Castrate levels of FSH and LH
   c. Abnormal karyotype, such as 46,XY in a phenotypic girl
   d. Low U/L body-segment ratio
   e. Arm span may exceed height by >2 inches
   f. Gynecomastia in a boy
   g. Small testes in boys with genetic hypogonadal disorders: Testes rarely exceed 6 cm^3 in volume
3. Turner syndrome: Excluding constitutional delay of puberty, one of the more common causes of maturation delay is Turner syndrome. The patient may have a 45,X karyotype or a mosaic karyotype such as 45,X/46,XX or ring or isochromosomes. Patients with

Turner syndrome usually have some of the following characteristics:

- Short stature
- Streak gonads
- Absent pubertal growth spurt
- Poor development of secondary sexual characteristics, with less breast development than pubic hair development
- Lymphedema
- Nail dysplasia
- High arched palate
- Strabismus
- Hearing deficit due to chronic otitis

- Cubitus valgus
- Webbing of the neck
- Low hairline
- Shield-shaped chest
- Coarctation of the aorta
- Horseshoe kidneys
- Short fourth metacarpal
- Multiple pigmented nevi
- Normal vagina, cervix, and uterus
- Poor space-form perception with normal overall intelligence

Savendahl and Davenport (2000) recommend a karyotype in all girls with unexplained short stature, delayed puberty, webbed neck, lymphedema, or coarctation of the aorta. Karyotype should also be considered for girls with a height below the 5th percentile and two or more features of Turner syndrome, such as high palate, nail dysplasia, short fourth metacarpal, and strabismus.

4. Chronic illness
   a. Abnormal findings on review of systems or physical examination
   b. Falling off height and weight curves at onset of disease
   c. Abnormal CBC count, sedimentation rate, urinalysis results, or chemistry panel results

MANAGEMENT OF DELAYED PUBERTY

Before age 14 years in girls and age 16 years in boys, if there is no evidence of an underlying disease or neurological abnormality and the initial evaluation reveals normal prepubertal hormone levels, the adolescent can be seen at 6-month intervals for measurements of growth, assessment of pubertal status by physical examination, and reassurance if progression of secondary sexual development is evident. After the first signs of testicular or beast enlargement are observed, follow-up at regular intervals is desirable to reassure the patient and parents that puberty is progressing. Since the testes begin to enlarge in males before increased testosterone production and increased growth velocity occur, support and guidance in dealing with the frustrations of delayed puberty are important, even after there is evidence that secondary sexual development has begun.

If the evaluation reveals primary gonadal failure, cyclic estrogen and progestin therapy in girls or testosterone therapy in boys will be necessary. Adolescents with hypogonadotropic hypogonadism or hypopituitarism will also need estrogen or testosterone replacement, often with replacement of other hormones as well. Short courses of estrogen or testosterone can also to be used to initiate development in constitutional delay of puberty if there is no sign of development by age 14 in girls or 15 in boys.

Treatment for Girls

In girls, there are several regimens for replacing estrogen and progesterone. If growth is desired, estrogen is begun at a low dose, since height velocity is greater at low estrogen doses, and higher doses cause more rapid epiphyseal closure. The three phases of estrogen replacement are:

1. Induction of breast development and increase in height velocity in the patient with no secondary sexual development
2. Establishment of normal menses and increase in bone mineralization
3. Long-term maintenance of a normal estrogen state

Induction of Breast Development

In the first phase, a number of low dose estrogen preparations have been used: estrogen regimens include conjugated estrogens (Premarin) 0.3 mg tablet or less (1/2 tablet) daily by mouth, 0.3 mg estrone sulfate (Estratab), or 0.5 mg micronized estradiol (Estrace) for the first 6 to 12 months of treatment or until linear growth slows. Although lower doses of ethinyl estradiol (10 μg) and transdermal estradiol (5–10 μg) have been used in research studies to induce puberty, the lowest dose estradiol transdermal patch available is 25 μg and the lowest dose of ethinyl estradiol available is 20 μg.

Induction of Menses

In the second phase, the daily dose of estrogen is increased to 0.625 mg conjugated estrogens, 1.0 mg micronized estradiol, 20 μg ethinyl estradiol, or a 50 μg transdermal estradiol patch. After 2 to 3 months, a progestin such as (medroxyprogesterone [Provera] 5–10 mg or norethindrone 0.7–1 mg) or micronized progesterone 200 mg is added initially 5 days each month.

Long-term Estrogen Replacement

In the third phase, 10 mg of medroxyprogesterone or other progestin is given 12 to 14 days a month to decrease the risk of endometrial hyperplasia. Estrogen regimens for long-term replacement include conjugated estrogens 0.625 mg, ethinyl estradiol 20 μg, esterified estrogens 0.625 mg, micronized estradiol 1.0 mg, or transdermal estradiol 50 to 100 μg. Once growth is essentially complete, estrogen can also be replaced as a 20 to 35 μg oral contraceptive pill, or combined estrogen–progestin transdermal patch.

Oral estrogens pass first through the liver which could theoretically increase side effects. Transdermal alternatives include estradiol patches (Vivelle dot, Climera, Alora, and Estraderm) which are changed once or twice a week depending on the preparation. An oral progestin (medroxyprogesterone 10 mg or micronized progesterone 200 mg) is added for 12 to 14 days each month. One transdermal regimen is Vivelle dot (0.05 mg) for 2 weeks each month followed by Combipatch 0.05 mg estradiol/0.14 mg norethindrone acetate for 2 weeks.

Many patients with delayed puberty have decreased bone density for age. The optimal dose of estrogen replacement for increasing bone density in adolescents remains to be established, but it is probably higher than in menopausal women. A bone density by dual-energy x-ray absorptiometry (DXA) of the hip and spine at baseline and every 2 years is commonly carried out in adolescents on estrogen or testosterone replacement. Bone density is compared with age-matched norms. The importance of appropriate calcium (1,300 mg/day) intake by diet or supplements and at least 400 IU vitamin D to support bone calcification should be stressed on each visit. The timing of initiation of sex steroid therapy to achieve maximum height depends on the patient's chronological and skeletal age, and current height velocity.

Treatment for Boys

In boys with constitutional delay of puberty, 3 to 6 month courses of testosterone 1% gel 2.5 to 5 gm daily or intramuscular testosterone enanthate 25 to 50 mg every 2 to 4 weeks can be used to initiate secondary sexual development. Intramuscular hCG is used less commonly. Exposure to testosterone or hCG may speed the onset of the patient's own puberty. Since sex steroids cause fusion of epiphyses, care must be taken in the timing and monitoring of these therapies so that final height is not compromised. These patients should therefore be referred to an endocrinologist for treatment. The timing of such an intervention must take into account such complex issues as psychosocial stress, self-image, and school performance which appear to be more affected by pubertal delay than by short stature alone. Males with gonadal failure, hypopituitarism, or hypothalamic hypogonadism are maintained on long-term testosterone replacement using testosterone gel. They should receive dietary adequate calcium and vitamin D and should have DXA scans for spinal and hip bone density measurements since they are at risk for a low bone mass. In both males and females whose delayed puberty is due to abnormalities in hypothalamic GnRH secretion that do not correct with time, fertility can be achieved using a small pump to deliver pulses of GnRH intravenously or subcutaneously for weeks or months. Some GnRH-deficient males will achieve spermatogenesis with hCG alone or in combination with FSH. Ovulation can be induced by FSH and hCG in GnRH-deficient females.

Treatment of Specific Conditions

Hypothyroidism Treatment is begun with levothyroxine (see Chapter 9 for hypothyroidism). Thyroid function tests are repeated in 6 weeks and the dose is adjusted to maintain the TSH concentration in the midnormal range. The final dose is usually 75 to 100 μg in females and 100 to 125 μg in males. Noncompliance with medication is often the underlying issue in teens whose TSH is elevated despite receiving unusually high doses of thyroid replacement. A 7-day pill package and adult supervision of doses may be helpful. Once the dose is established, thyroid tests are repeated at 6-month intervals. Catch-up growth is expected when thyroid hormone replacement is initiated, but patients who have been untreated for several years will lose some adult height.

Turner Syndrome and Gonadal Dysgenesis Short stature associated with Turner syndrome can be treated with human growth hormone (hGH). The U.S. Food and Drug Administration and other worldwide regulatory agencies have approved the use of hGH for statural improvement in Turner syndrome. The hGH therapy should be started before the adolescent years and before beginning estrogen therapy for feminization. The dose used is approximately double that used for subjects with classic GH deficiency. Data from the National Cooperative Growth Study from Genentech has shown GH to be effective in improving the final height of girls with Turner syndrome and that GH is safe for these patients (Blethen et al., 1996). Oxandrolone (0.075 to 0.25 mg/kg/day) or fluoxymesterone (2.0 mg/day) can be added to GH therapy to improve the growth response. If this is done, it is usually begun after 2 to 3 years of GH therapy alone, before feminization, for a limited time, and with great caution because androgens have the following disadvantages:

a. Potential for hepatic toxic effects
b. Advancement of the bone age
c. Potential for mild androgenic characteristics, such as clitoral enlargement
d. Delay of treatment with estrogen and therefore delay of inducement of female secondary sexual characteristics

Anabolic steroids as the sole therapy for this syndrome are no longer recommended. Secondary sexual characteristics in females are achieved through the use of increasing doses of conjugated estrogens as discussed above. Chernausek et al. (2000) evaluated the timing of estrogen replacement in girls with Turner syndrome with regards to final height outcome. Patients in whom estrogen treatment was delayed until the age of 15 years gained an average of 8.4 cm over their projected height. Those who started estrogen at 12 years of age gained only 5.1 cm. They found that growth was stimulated for 2 years after beginning estrogen replacement therapy and that the timing of estrogen therapy is important for final height. This indicates that for some girls, particularly those who are shortest and in whom GH has not been given for more than 2 years, delaying estrogen therapy may be indicated to improve height outcome.

If there is a Y chromosome present on the initial study done to diagnose Turner syndrome, no further chromosomal analysis is required to anticipate that the patient will require gonadectomy. However, Y chromosomal material, rather than a full Y chromosome, may be present in girls who are virilized, either at birth or with puberty not as the result of androgen therapy. They should have fluorescent in situ hybridization (FISH) for the Y chromosome to ensure that no Y chromosomal material has been translocated. The presence of any Y material is an indication for gonadectomy, to prevent potential malignant neoplasias. Surgery should be followed by hormonal replacement therapy during and after puberty.

Chronic Illness Treatment of pubertal delay caused by chronic illness necessitates treating the underlying disorder. For example, enzyme replacement in cystic fibrosis, gluten-free diet in celiac disease, corrective surgery for congenital heart disease, and hyperalimentation in inflammatory bowel disease usually result in catch-up growth and maturity. Medications such as steroids or antimetabolites can inhibit growth. Catch-up growth can be observed after discontinuation of treatment with these drugs. In some cases, the disease process is irreversible, such as in sickle cell anemia. The pubertal delay in sickle cell anemia is thought to be hypogonadism, possibly caused by a zinc deficiency. Zinc has been used with some early experimental success in alleviating this problem. In patients with chronic renal failure, there may be some growth after improved nutrition and hemodialysis or transplantation. However, many patients with chronic renal failure remain short. Recent studies suggest that GH can be administered to subjects with chronic renal failure before transplantation to improve height, without causing deterioration of underlying renal function (Fine et al., 1994). HIV infected children who have poor growth and body wasting may benefit from the anabolic effects of short-term GH administration; however, long-term use of such agents remains under investigation (Mulligan et al., 1993).

PATIENT EDUCATION

Young adolescents are preoccupied with their physical appearance. Any variation from the normal timing of sexual development is a major source of embarrassment to them and evokes feelings of personal inadequacy. A review of a patient's progress on the growth pubertal growth and growth chart can help reassure him or her that growth is proceeding in a pattern that is appropriate. For patients who have a permanent defect in reproductive function, counseling and support from both the primary health provider and medical specialist can be helpful in enabling the patient to establish a positive self-image of himself or herself as a capable adult. Further counseling by a mental health professional may be necessary. Questions about fertility should be answered as they arise, with emphasis on the patient's ability to function normally as a marriage partner and parent of adopted children. With current technology, pregnancies are possible using *in vitro* fertilization with donor eggs in patients with ovarian failure.

EXCESSIVE GROWTH: TALL STATURE

Tall stature is seldom a complaint in males, but is occasionally a source of concern in adolescent females. This is less common than in the past since the role models of athletes and fashion models have made tall stature more socially acceptable in women now than in the past. Most commonly, tall stature is genetic and one or both parents are also tall.

Differential Diagnosis

1. Constitutional tall stature
2. Excess GH (e.g., GH-secreting tumors)
3. Anabolic steroid excess (exogenous, adrenal tumor, gonadal tumor, congenital adrenal hyperplasia—classic or nonclassical, precocious puberty, premature adrenarche)
4. Hyperthyroidism
5. Miscellaneous
   a. Marfan syndrome
   b. Neurofibromatosis
   c. Hypogonadism in boys
   d. Androgen-receptor deficiency in boys
   e. Estrogen deficiency in boys
   f. Homocystinuria
   g. Hereditary abnormalities of the skeleton
   h. Soto syndrome

Evaluation

Obese girls tend to be taller than average, perhaps due to higher levels of insulin. Many genetically tall girls who are above the 95th percentile for height in the early adolescent period are experiencing an early pubertal growth spurt, but will have a final adult height in the normal range. Review of the growth chart and a bone age are useful. If growth rate is excessive, evaluation might include thyroid function tests looking for hyperthyroidism, and an IGF-I, IGFBP-3, and random GH to exclude GH excess. If GH is low, acromegaly is unlikely. Elevated GH may be a random pulse and should be repeated. IGF-I is elevated in acromegaly. Marfan syndrome is usually diagnosed clinically. The phenotype is characterized by tall stature, lean body habitus and elongated extremities. A slit lamp examination by an opthamologist may detect lens dislocation in 50% of patients. Echocardiogram may reveal a dilated aortic root. The syndrome is caused by a gene abnormality causing deficient fibrillin production.

Treatment

In the past, high doses of estrogen were used to limit height gain in girls whose predicted height would be more than 6 ft (183) cm. Estrogen affects growth by suppressing IGF-I and accelerating epiphyseal fusion. This is seldom done currently since female tall stature has become more socially acceptable. High-dose estrogen treatment in girls is associated with side effects which include nausea, breast soreness, hypertension, and, rarely, blood clots.

The treatment of boys has been studied less extensively. Theoretically, administration of high-dose testosterone could accelerate epiphyseal fusion, but concerns of this therapy would include edema, acne, weight gain and a decrease in testicular volume. Therefore, tall stature in boys is typically not treated.

PRECOCIOUS PUBERTY

Definition

In boys, development before age 9 years or 2.5 SD earlier than average is considered precocious. Early development in boys is rare. There are 10 times as many girls with precocious puberty as boys. There is currently a controversy over the definition of precocious puberty in North American girls. In girls, the cut off has traditionally been 8 years or 2.5 SD below the average of breast development. However, a 1997 study by Herman-Giddens (Herman-Giddens et al., 1997) of 17,000 American girls found a mean age of breast development of just below 10 years in Caucasian girls and 9 years in African-American girls; 15% of African-American girls having the appearance of breast development by 7 to 8 years and 5% of Caucasian girls having breast development by 7 to 8 years. Pubic hair was present in 3% of Caucasian girls and 18% of African-American girls by age 7 to 8 years. This has led to a revision of the definition of precocious puberty by the Lawson Wilkins Pediatric Endocrine Society as the presence of breast or pubic hair before age 7 in Caucasian and before age 6 years in African-American girls. Since then, numerous reports have pointed out that cases of true pathology such as CNS tumors may be missed by excluding 7- to 8-year-old girls from evaluation. Girls who have both pubic hair and breast development at ages 7 to 8, should have at least a bone age for height prediction, a review of growth and history, and consideration of further testing. Girls with rapid progression or unusual progression of puberty, a predicted height below 150 cm or –2 SD below target midparental height, those with neurological symptoms, or girls who are having psychological difficulty due to early puberty should be referred for further evaluation and consideration of possible suppression of puberty with GnRH analog therapy. Puberty is normally held back in humans during childhood by inhibitory connections to the hypothalamus which suppress GnRH pulsations. If these inhibitory connections are damaged, GnRH pulse amplitude increases, and central puberty ensues. There is often a family history of early puberty in girls with precocious puberty; some studies suggest an autosomal dominant pattern with variable penetrance.

The vast majority of girls with central precocious puberty have idiopathic precocious puberty. Boys are much more likely to have a specific lesion causing their precocity.

Causes

Central causes of precocious puberty include the following:

1. CNS tumors (optic gliomas, craniopharyngiomas, dysgerminomas, ependymoma)
2. CNS malformations (hamartomas, arachnoid and suprasellar cysts, hydrocephalus, septooptic dysplasia)
3. Infiltrative lesions (histiocytosis, granulomas, abscess)
4. CNS damage (irradiation, trauma, meningitis, encephalitis)

Gonadotropin-independent causes of precocity in girls include the following:

1. Ovarian cysts, sometimes with McCune-Albright syndrome
2. Ovarian or adrenal estrogen secreting tumors
3. Severe hypothyroidism
4. Exposure to exogenous estrogen

In boys, in addition to the central causes listed above, precocious puberty can be caused by androgen exposure, congenital adrenal hyperplasia, gonadal and adrenal tumors secreting androgens, and familial activating mutations of the LH receptor.

Incomplete Forms of Precocious Puberty

Premature Thelarche
Premature thelarche occurs often in female infants and toddlers. Self-limited breast budding which is also transient occurs in girls aged 6 and above. There is no sustained growth spurt or bone age advancement in these girls. Breast budding may appear and recede several times before sustained puberty ensues.

Premature Adrenarche
Benign premature adrenarche presents with underarm odor, and pubic and/or axillary hair development usually at ages 6 to 8 years. Bone age is often slightly advanced (1 year) and adrenal androgens are in the pubertal range. Twenty percent of the girls with benign premature

adrenarche will go on to have polycystic ovary syndrome as teens. Patients with a history of intrauterine growth retardation followed by excessive weight gain and insulin resistance in childhood may present with premature adrenarche. They are at increased risk for polycystic ovary syndrome and sometimes glucose intolerance as teens. Virilization in girls is rare and can be due to an androgen secreting adrenal or ovarian tumor, topical androgen exposure, or congenital adrenal hyperplasia. Symptoms of virilization include rapid growth and bone age advancement, deepening of the voice, clitoromegaly or muscular development. A thorough evaluation is required.

Evaluation of Precocious Puberty

History
History includes a review of family history of endocrine or pubertal disorders, timing of puberty in family members, use of estrogen or androgen containing gels by family members, and heights of family members. The patient's past history should be reviewed for evidence of predisposing medical conditions. The growth chart should be obtained.

Physical Examination
The physical examination includes careful measurement of height and weight, vital signs, examination of the skin for large irregular café au lait spots suggestive of McCune-Albright syndrome, examination of the fundi, assessment for thyroid enlargement, abdominal examination, Tanner staging (measurement of breast or testicular and phallic dimensions, and pubic hair staging). The vaginal introitus can be examined for signs of estrogen effect on the labia minora and presence of leukorrhea in the frog-leg position. Internal examination is not necessary unless unexplained vaginal bleeding is present in which case an experienced observer can often visualize the vagina and cervix in the knee chest position without instrumentation. In boys, the testicular examination should focus on any testicular asymmetry or masses, or phallic enlargement without testicular enlargement suggesting a source of androgens outside of the testes, such as congenital adrenal hyperplasia.

Laboratory Evaluation
A bone age x-ray of the left hand and wrist is useful. If the bone age is 2 years advanced, more evaluation is usually indicated (Fig. 8.8). A baseline prediction of adult height can be made using the average charts from the Bayley-Pinneau table at the back of the Gruelich and Pyle Atlas of Skeletal maturation (see Chapter 1 for details).

Laboratory evaluation might include an LH, FSH, estradiol, DHEAS, and TSH in girls, and in boys, a testosterone and 8 a.m. 17 OH progesterone and DHEAS, hCG, LH, and FSH. The LH and FSH will be in the prepubertal range (LH less than FSH) in the early stages of central puberty. By the time breast or gonadal development is in Tanner SMR stage 3, LH and FSH are often in the pubertal range. To confirm central puberty, it is sometimes necessary to do a GnRH or GnRH analog stimulation test (GnRH itself has recently been unavailable) using 500 µg leuprolide acetate and obtaining an LH, FSH, and estradiol or testosterone 45 minutes to 2 hours after the injection. If estradiol is markedly elevated (more than 100 pg/mL) and LH and FSH are suppressed, an ovarian cyst or more

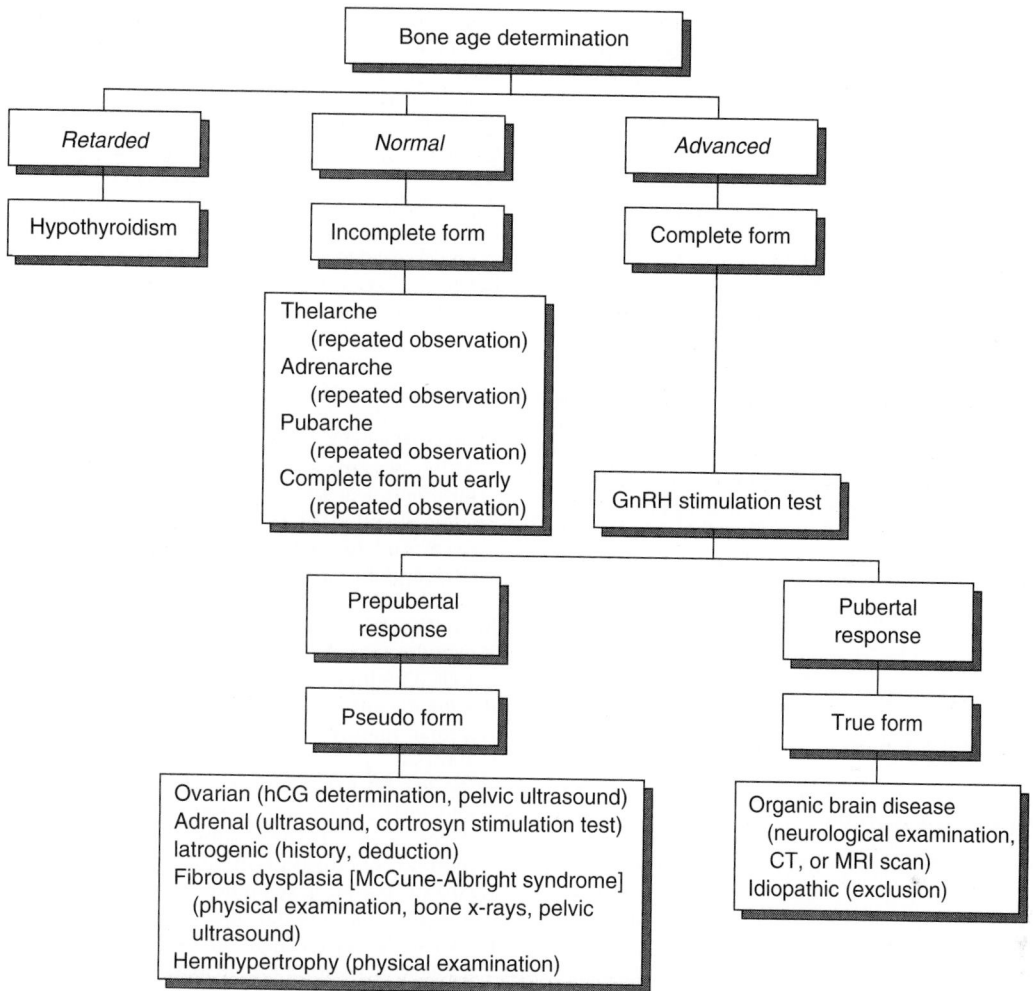

FIGURE 8.8   Flow sheet for evaluation of isosexual precocious puberty. hCG, human chorionic gonadotropin; CT, computed tomography; MRI, magnetic resonance imaging. (Adapted from Brenner PE. Precocious puberty in the female. In: Mishell DR, Davajan VC, eds. *Reproductive endocrinology, infertility, and contraception.* Philadelphia: FA Davis Co, 1979.)

rarely tumor is suspected. A pelvic ultrasonography can be done in girls if an ovarian cyst or tumor is thought to be the cause of the precocity. In boys, a hCG test should be done to rule out a hCG-producing tumor that could be causing testosterone production. A cranial MRI with contrast should be done to rule out CNS lesion in all boys with central precocious puberty, in all girls younger than 6 years, and should be considered in girls between 6 and 8 years of age depending on the clinical history. An adrenocorticotropic hormone (ACTH) stimulation test may be needed if congenital adrenal hyperplasia is suspected as a cause of androgen excess.

Treatment of Precocious Puberty

If the evaluation has not revealed a specific treatable cause of precocious puberty and the child has central precocious puberty, GnRH analog treatment should be considered. Most girls in the 7 to 9 year range do not require treatment for suppression of puberty.

Many girls in this age range have a slow intermittent progression of their puberty and reach a final height which is not short. Early developers take longer on average to reach menarche than later developers. Often parents are most worried about how they will handle menses in a grade school child, and can be reassured that menarche is not imminent in most cases and that menses can be suppressed if necessary using GnRH analog therapy. Untreated girls should be followed up at 6 month to 1 year intervals. If the child has an initial predicted adult height below 62 in. (157 cm), bone age may need to be repeated in 6 months to 1 year because the predicted height can decline with rapid bone age advancement, and therapy may be required to preserve height potential. Depot leuprolide at an initial dose of 0.3 mg/kg can be given q28 days intramuscularly. LH, FSH, and estradiol in girls or testosterone in boys can be obtained 45 minutes to 2 hours after the depot leuprolide to document adequate suppression of puberty on therapy after 2 to 3 months of treatment. Partial suppression of puberty has been achieved in girls with gonadotropin independent puberty (McCune-Albright syndrome) with the aromatase inhibitor testolactone. Similar regimens with antiandrogens and testolactone have been used in boys with familial LH-activating mutations.

WEB SITES

For Teenagers and Parents

http://www.magicfoundation.org. Magic Foundation with information about growth disorders and brochures about many disorders.

http://www.hgfound.org. Human Growth Foundation Web site with information and support for children and adults with growth disorders.

http://www.keepkidshealthy.com/welcome/conditions/delayed_puberty.html. Information from keepkidshealthy on delayed puberty.

http://www.turner-syndrome-us.org/. Information about Turner syndrome.

http://www.humatrope.com. Information from Eli Lilly about synthetic GH.

http://www.novonordisk.com/. Facts from novo on GH deficiency and treatment.

http://www.toosoon.com. Information from Lupron Association on precocious puberty.

For Health Professionals

http://humatrope.com. Information from Lilly on GH.

http://www.aafp.org/afp/990700ap/209.html. Review article from the American Academy of Family Physicians on Evaluation of Growth Disorders.

REFERENCES AND ADDITIONAL READINGS

Adan L, Souberbielle JC, Brauner R. Management of the short stature due to pubertal delay in boys. *J Clin Endocrinol Metab* 1994;78:478.

Albanese A, Stanhope R. Investigation of delayed puberty. *Clin Endocrinol* 1995;43:105.

Albanese A, Stanhope R. Predictive factors in the determination of final height in boys with constitutional delay of growth and puberty. *J Pediatr* 1995;126:545.

Allen DB, Fost N. hGH for short stature: ethical issues raised by expanded access. *J Pediatr* 2004;144:648.

Allen DB, Fost NC. Growth hormone therapy for short stature: panacea or Pandora's box? *J Pediatr* 1990;117:16.

Ankarberg-Lindgren J, Elfving M, Wiklan KA, et al. Nocturnal application of transdermal estradiol patches produces levels of estradiol that mimic those seen at the onset of spontaneous puberty in girls. *J Clin Endocrinol Metab.* 2001;86:3039.

Attie KM, Frane JW. The Genentech Collaborative Study Group. Accuracy of adult height prediction methods for Turner's syndrome using U.S. untreated control data. *Horm Res* 1997;60:60.

August GP, Julius JR, Blethen SL. Adult height in children with growth hormone deficiency who are treated with biosynthetic growth hormone: The National Cooperative Growth Study Experience. *Pediatrics* 1998;102:512.

Bailey JD, Park E, Cowell C. Estrogen treatment of girls with constitutional tall stature. *Pediatr Clin North Am* 1981;28:501.

Baily N, Pinneau SR. Tables for predicting adult height from skeletal age: revised for use with the Gruelich and Pyle hand standard. *J Pediatr* 1952;40:423.

Barbieri RL. Clinical applications of GnRH and its analogues. *Trends Endocrinol Metab* 1992;3:30.

Barnard ND, Scialli AR, Bobela S. The current use of estrogens for growth suppressant therapy in adolescent girls. *J Pediatr Adolesc Gynecol* 2002;15:26.

Barnes N. Excessive growth. *Arch Dis Child* 1983;58:845.

Barnes PD. Imaging of the nervous system in pediatrics and adolescence. *Peditr Clin N Am* 1992;39:743.

Bercu BB, Shulman D, Root AW, et al. Growth hormone provocative testing frequently does not reflect endogenous GH secretion. *J Clin Endocrinol Metab* 1986;63:709.

Bhatia S, Neely EK, Wilson DM. Serum luteinizing hormone rises within minutes after deot leuprolide injection: implications for monitoring therapy. *Pediatrics* 2002;109:30.

Blethen SL, Allen DR, Graves D, et al. Safety of recombinant deoxyribonucleic acid-derived growth hormone: The National Cooperative Growth Study experience. *J Clin Endocrinol Metab* 1996;81:1704.

Blum WE, Rainke MB. Use of insulin-like growth factor-binding protein 3 for the evaluation of growth disorders. *Horm Res* 1990;33(Suppl 4):31.

Borgna-Pignatti C, DeStefano P, Zonta L, et al. Growth and sexual maturation in thalassemia major. *J Pediat* 1985;106:150.

Bramswig JH, Fasse M, Holthoff ML, et al. Adult height in boys and girls with untreated short stature and constitutional delay of growth and puberty: accuracy of five different methods of height prediction. *J Pediatr* 1990;117:886.

Byard PJ. The adolescent growth spurt in children with cystic fibrosis. *Ann Hum Biol* 1994;21:229.

Cameron N. Assessment of growth and maturation during adolescence. *Horm Res* 1993;39:9.

Cara JF. Growth hormone in adolescence: normal and abnormal. *Endocrinol Metab Clin North Am* 1993;22:533.

Chernausek SD, Attie KM, Cara JF, et al. Growth hormone therapy of Turner syndrome: the impact of age of estrogen replacement on final height. *J Clin Endocrinol Metab* 2000;85:2439.

Crawford JD. Treatment of tall girls with estrogen. *Pediatrics* 1978;62:1189.

Cutler L. Editorial: safety and efficacy of growth hormone treatment for idiopathic short stature. *J Clin Endocrinol Metab* 2005;90:5502.

De Waal WJ, Greyn-Fokker MH, Stijnen T, et al. Accuracy of final height prediction and effect of growth-reductive therapy in 362 constitutionally tall children. *J Clin Endocrinol Metab* 1996;81:1206.

Donaghue K, Rodda C, Cameron F, et al. Proceedings of the Australian Pediatric Endocrine Group. In: Laron Z, ed. *Journal of pediatric endocrinological metabolism*. London: Freund Publishing House, 2000.

Dunkel L, Perheentupa J, Virtanen M, et al. Gonadotropin-releasing hormone test and human chorionic gonadotropin test in the diagnosis of gonadotropin deficiency in prepubertal boys. *J Pediatr* 1985a;107:388.

Dunkel L, Perheentupa J, Virtanen M, Maenpaa J. GnRH and HCG tests are both necessary in differential diagnosis of male delayed puberty. *Am J Dis Child.* 1985; 139:494.

Emans SJ, Laufer MR, Goldstein DP, eds. *Pediatric and adolescent gynecology*, 5th ed. Philadelphia: Lippincott Williams and Wilkins, 2005.

Eugster E, Pescovitz OH. Perspective: new revelations about short stature. *N Engl J Med* 2003;349:1110.

Fenton C, Tang M, Pth M. Review of precocious puberty part 1: gonadotropin-dependent precocious puberty. *Endocrinologist* 2000;10:107.

Feuillan PP, Foster CM, Pescovitz OH. Treatment of precocious puberty in the McCune-Albright syndrome with the aromatase inhibitor testolactone. *N Engl J Med* 1986;315:1115.

Fine RN, Kohaut EC, Brown D, et al. Growth after recombinant human growth hormone treatment in children with chronic renal failure: report of a multicenter randomized double-blind placebo-controlled study. *J Pediatr* 1994;124:374.

Finkelstein JS, Neer RM, Biller BMK. Osteopenia in men with a history of delayed puberty. *N Engl J Med* 1992;326:600.

Frasier SD, Lippe BM. The rational use of growth hormone during childhood [Clinical review 11]. *J Clin Endocrinol Metab* 1990;71:269.

Furlanetto RW. Insulin-like growth factor-1 measurements in the evaluation of growth hormone secretion. *Horm Res* 1990; 33(Suppl 4):25.

Gruelich WW, Pyle SI. *Atlas of skeletal development of the hand and wrist*, 2nd ed. Stanford, CA: Stanford University Press, 1959.

Guttman H, weiner Z, Nikolski E, et al. Choosing an oestrogen replacement therapy in young adult women with Turner syndrome. *Clin Endocrinol* 2001;54(2):159.

Heinze HJ. Ovarian function in adolescents with Turner syndrome. *Adolesc Pediatr Gynecol* 1994;7:3.

Herman-Giddens ME, Slora EJ, Wasserman RD, et al. Secondary sexual characteristics and menses in young girls seen in office practice: a study from the pediatric research in office settings network. *Pediatrics* 1997;99:505.

Hill DE, Fisher RH. Chronic disease and short stature. *Postgrad Med* 1977;62:103.

Hoeck HC, Vestergaard P, Jakobsen PE, et al. Diagnosis of growth hormone (GH) deficiency in adults with hypothalamic-pituitary disorders: comparison of test results using pyridostigmine plus GH-releasing hormone (GHRH), clonidine plus GHRH and insulin-induced hypoglycemia as GH secretogogues. *J Clin Endocrinol Metab* 2000;85:1467.

Hoffman AR, Crowley WF Jr. Induction of puberty in men by long-term pulsatile administration of low-dose gonadotropin-releasing hormone. *N Engl J Med* 1982;307:1237.

Ibanez L, Dimartino-Nardi J, Potau N, et al. Premature adrenarche- normal variant or forerunner of adult disease? *Endocr Rev* 2000;21:671.

Kaplan SL, Grumbach MM. Pathophysiology and treatment of sexual precocity. *J Clin Endocrinol Metab* 1990;71:785.

Kaplowitz P, Oberfield S. Reexamination of the age limit for defining when puberty is precocious in girls in the United States: implications for evaluation and treatment. *Pediatrics* 1999;104:936.

Kaplowitz PB, Slora EJ, Wasserman RC, et al. Earlier onset of puberty in girls: relation to increased body mass index and race. *Pediatrics* 2001;108(2):347.

Kemp SF, Kuntze J, Attie KM, et al. Efficacy and safety results of long-term growth hormone treatment of idiopathic short stature. *J Clin Endocrinol Metab* 2005;90:5247.

Klein KO. Editorial: precocious puberty: who has it? Who should be treated?. *J Clin Endocrinol Metab* 1999;84:411.

Kletter GB, Kelch RP. Disorders of puberty in boys. *Endocrinol Metab Clin North Am* 1993;22:45.

LaFranchi S, Hanna CE, Mandel SH. Constitutional delay of growth: expected versus final adult height. *Pediatrics* 1991; 87:82.

Lee PA. Central precocious puberty: an overview of diagnosis, treatment, and outcome. *Endocrinol Metab Clin North Am* 1999;28(4):901.

Lee MM. Clinical practice. Idiopathic short stature. *N Engl J Med* 2006;354:2576.

Legler JD, Rose LC. Assessment of abnormal growth curves. *Am Fam Physician* 1998;58:153.

Lisska MC, Rivkees SA. Daily methylphenidate use slows the growth of children: a community based study. *J Pediatr Endocrinol Metab* 2003;16(5):711.

MacFarlane CE, Brown DC, Johnston LB, et al. Growth hormone therapy and growth in children with Noonan's syndrome: results of 3 years' follow-up. *J Clin Endocrinol Metab* 2001; 86(5):1953.

Mahajan T, Lightman SL. A simple test for growth hormone deficiency in adults. *J Clin Endocrinol Metab* 2000;85:1473.

Mahoney CP. Evaluating the child with short stature. *Pediatr Clin North Am* 1987;34:825.

Marin G, Domene HM, Barnes KM. The effects of estrogen priming and puberty on the growth hormone response to standardized treadmill exercise and arginine-insulin in normal girls and boys. *J Clin Endocrinol Metab* 1994;79:537.

Marti-Henneberg C, Vizmanos B. The duration of puberty in girls is related to the timing of its onset. *J Pediatr* 1997; 131:618.

Martinez A, Heinrich JJ, Domene H, et al. Growth in Turner's syndrome: long-term treatment with low-dose ethinyl estradiol. *J Clin Endocrinol Metab* 1987;65:253.

Midyett LK, Moore WV, Jacobson JD. Are pubertal changes in girls before age 8 benign? *Pediatrics* 2003;111:47.

Mulligan K, Grunfeld C, Hellerstein MK, et al. Anabolic effects of recombinant human growth hormone in patients with wasting associated with human immunodeficiency virus infection. *J Clin Endocrinol Metab* 1993;77:956.

Oberfield SE, Levine IS. The child with short stature. *N Y State J Med* 1986;86:15.

Oerter KE, Uriarte M, Rose SR, et al. Gonadotropin secretory dynamics during puberty in normal girls and boys. *J Clin Endocrinol Metab* 1990;71:1251.

Palmert MR, Malin HV, Boepple PA. Unsustained or slowly progressive puberty in young girls: initial presentation and long-term follow-up of 20 untreated patients. *J Clin Endocrinol Metab* 1999;84:415.

Pearce EN, Farwell AP, Braverman LE. Current concepts: thyroiditis. *N Engl J Med* 2003;348:2646.

Platt OS, Rosenstock W, Espeland MS. Influence of sickle hemoglobinopathies on growth and development. *N Engl J Med* 1984;311:7.

Prader A. Pubertal growth. *Acta Paediatr Jpn* 1992;34:222.

Pugliese MT, Lifshitz F, Grad G, et al. Fear of obesity: a cause of short stature and delayed puberty. *N Engl J Med* 1983;309:513.

Quigley CA, Crowe BJ, Anglin DG, et al. Growth hormone and low dose estrogen in Turner syndrome: results of a United States multi-center trial to near-final height. *J Clin Endocrinol Metab* 2002;87(5):2033.

Quigley CA, Pescovitz OH. Premature thelarche and precocious puberty. *Curr Ther Endocrinol Metab* 1997;6:7.

Reiter EO, Blethen SL, Baptista J, Early initiation of growth hormone treatment allows age-appropriate estrogen use in Turner's syndrome. *J Clin Endocrinol Metab* 2001;86:1936.

Reiter EO, Rosenfield RG. Normal and aberrant growth. In: Larsen R, Kronenberg HM, Melmed S, et al. eds. *Williams textbook of endocrinology*, 10th ed. Philadelphia: WB Saunders, 2003:1003.

Reynolds JM, Wood AL, Eminson DM, et al. Short stature and chronic renal failure: what concerns children and parents? *Arch Dis Child* 1995;73:36.

Richman RA, Kirsch LR. Testosterone treatment in adolescent boys with constitutional delay in growth and development. *N Engl J Med* 1988;319:1563.

Rivkees SA, Bode HH, Crawford JD. Long-term growth in juvenile acquired hypothyroidism: the failure to achieve normal adult stature. *N Engl J Med* 1988;318:599.

Rogers DG. Puberty and insulin-dependent diabetes mellitus. *Clin Pediatr* 1992;31:168.

Rosenbach Y, Dinari G, Zahavi I, et al. Short stature as the major manifestation of celiac disease in older children. *Clin Pediatr* 1986;25:13.

Rosenfeld RG, Frane J, Attie KM, et al. Six-year results of a randomized, perspective trial of human growth hormone and oxandrolone in Turner syndrome. *J Pediatr* 1992; 121:49.

Rosenfield RL. Low-dose testosterone effect on somatic growth. *Pediatrics* 1986;77:853.

Rugarli EI, Ballabio A. Kallmann syndrome: from genetics to neurobiology. *JAMA* 1993;270:2713.

Sas T, De Waal W, Mulder P, et al. Growth hormone treatment in children with short stature born small for gestational age: 5 year results of a randomized, double-blind dose-response trial. *J Clin Endocrinol Metab* 1999;84:3064.

Savendahl L, Davenport ML. Delayed diagnosis of Turner's syndrome: proposed guidelines for change. *J Pediatr* 2000;137: 455.

Schaefer F, Seidel C, Binding A, et al. Pubertal growth in chronic renal failure. *Pediatr Res* 1990;28:5.

Soliman AT, Khadir MM, Asfour M. Testosterone treatment in adolescent boys with constitutional delay of growth and development. *Metabolism* 1995;44:1013.

Spagnoli A, Spadoni GL, Cianfarani S, et al. Prediction of the outcome of growth hormone therapy in children with idiopathic short stature: a multivariate discriminant analysis. *J Pediatr* 1995;126:905.

Street ME, Bandello MA, Terzi C, et al. Luteinizing hormone responses to leuprolide acetate discriminate between hypogonadotropic hypogonadism and constitutional delay of puberty. *Fertil Steril* 2002;77:555.

Sun SS, Schubert CM, Chumlea WC, et al. National estimates of timing of sexual maturation and racial differences among US children. *Pediatrics* 2002;110(5):911.

Sybert VP, McCauley E. Turner's syndrome. *N Engl J Med* 2004; 351:1227.

Takano K, Shizume K, Hibi I. Long-term effects of growth hormone treatment on height in Turner syndrome: results of a 6-year multicentre study in Japan. Committee for the Treatment of Turner Syndrome. *Horm Res* 1995;43:141.

Tillmann V, Buckler JMH, Kibirige MS, et al. Biochemical tests in the diagnosis of childhood growth hormone deficiency. *J Clin Endocrinol Metab* 1997;82:531.

Underwood LE. Growth hormone therapy for short stature: yes or no? *Hosp Pract* 1992;27:192.

Van der Werff ten Bosch JJ, Bot A. Growth of tall girls without and during oestrogen treatment. *Neth J Med* 1981;24:52.

Vance ML, Mauras N. Drug therapy: growth hormone therapy in adults and children. *N Engl J Med* 1999;341:1206.

Visser-van Balen H, Sinnema G, Geenen R. Growing up with idiopathic short stature: psychosocial development and hormone treatment; a critical review. *Arch Dis Child* 2006; 91:43.

Voss LD. Growth hormone therapy for the short normal child: who needs it and who wants it? The case against growth hormone therapy. *J Pediatr* 2000;136:103.

Weaver DS, Own GM. Nutrition and short stature. *Postgrad Med* 1977;62:93.

Wilson DM, Kei J, Hintz RL, et al. Effects of testosterone therapy for pubertal delay. *Am J Dis Child* 1988;142:96.

Wilson TA, Rose SR, Cohen P, et al. Update of guidelines for the use of growth hormone in children: the Lawson Wilkins Pediatric Endocrinology Society Drug and Therapeutics Committee. *J Pediatr* 2003;143:415.

Wilson DM, Rosenfeld RG. Treatment of short stature and delayed adolescence. *Pediatr Clin North Am* 1987;34:865.

Wu T, Mendola P, Buck GM. Differences in the presence of secondary sex characteristics and menarche among US girls: the third National Health and Nutrition examination survey, 1988–1994. *Pediatrics* 2002;110(4):752.

Yanovski JA, Rose SR, Municchi G, et al. Treatment with a luteinizing hormone-releasing hormone agonist in adolescents with short stature. *N Engl J Med* 2003;348(10):908.

CHAPTER 9

Thyroid Disease in Adolescents

Stephen A. Huang and Lawrence S. Neinstein

The prevalence of thyroid abnormalities in adolescents 11 to 18 years of age is cited to be 3.7% (Rallison et al., 1991) with more females than males affected. This chapter presents a summary of thyroid disease that occurs during adolescence, discussing thyromegaly, thyroid dysfunction (hypo- and hyperthyroidism), and nodular thyroid disease, with an emphasis on their clinical management. By maintaining an appropriate index of suspicion, the clinician can often recognize thyroid disease in its early stages. This can be very important during adolescence as thyroid abnormalities can lead to altered growth and development, menstrual irregularities, deterioration in school performance, or changes in behavior. Aspects of thyroid management related to pregnancy and the transition to adult care are also discussed.

CHANGES IN THYROID GLAND SIZE AND FUNCTION DURING ADOLESCENCE

Marked changes in thyroid volume occur during puberty as an adaptation to body and sexual development (Chanoine et al., 1991; Fleury et al., 2001).

Volume and Weight

1. Thyroid volume significantly increases until the age of 8 without being influenced by sex and thereafter varies widely (Chanoine et al., 1991).
2. The volume increases from 2.7 mL (SD = 0.8) in prepubertal subjects aged 8 to 11 years to 11.6 mL (SD = 4.4) in late pubertal subjects older than 17 years. This increase significantly correlates not only with chronological age but also with body weight, height, body mass index (BMI), and with pubertal stage (Fleury et al., 2001; Chanoine et al., 1991).
3. The increase in volume occurs early between the ages of 11 and 15, usually with the onset of the first clinical signs of puberty (Fleury et al., 2001).
4. Weight—several pediatric norms have been published and the equation of $T = 1.48 + 0.054A$, where T is the weight of the thyroid in grams and A is the age in months describes the average thyroid weight from birth to 20 years (Kay, et al., 1966). In North America, the normal adult thyroid weighs approximately 14 to 20 g (average weight 14.4 g for females 20 to 69 years of age and 16.4 g for males 20 to 29 years of age) (Mochizuki et al., 1963; Pankow et al., 1985).

Hormonal Changes

1. From the age of 1 year onwards, the concentration of total thyroxine (T_4), free T_4, and thyroid-stimulating hormone (TSH) tend to decrease until adult age, with the exception of thyroxine binding globulin (TBG) which increases by >60% and reaches a maximum at approximately 5 years of age (Elmlinger et al., 2001).
2. Thyroid hormone levels do not appear to be associated with sexual development, except for TBG, which decreases slightly ($p < 0.04$) between sexual maturity ratings of 1 and 5 (Elmlinger et al., 2001).

CLINICAL EVALUATION FOR THYROID DISEASE

It is critical to take a careful history and perform a thorough physical examination to evaluate adolescents for thyroid dysfunction.

History

Duration and severity of symptoms, fever, swelling, and pain must be recorded.

1. Family history of goiter, thyroiditis, other thyroid problems, or other autoimmune disease
2. Drug history—use of goitrogens, including lithium, iodine excess or anticonvulsants, exposure to radiation
3. Pubertal and menstrual history
4. Change in weight
5. Growth problems
6. Change in behavior, sleep pattern, activity level, or function in school
7. Change in bowel habits

Physical Examination

Important signs to consider in thyroid dysfunction include abnormal changes in:

1. Height, weight, and BMI
2. Pulse, blood pressure
3. Skin texture or lesions
4. Presence of tremor
5. Eye examination—presence of exophthalmos or lid lag
6. Deep tendon reflexes—normal or delayed relaxation phase
7. Thyroid examination

- Normal gland: The normal thyroid gland is bilobed and connected by an isthmus that overlies the second through fourth tracheal cartilages. The main lobes of the thyroid are usually equal in size, but the right lobe tends to enlarge to a greater degree than the left in patients with diffuse thyromegaly.
- Physical examination: Physical examination of the thyroid is best performed with the patient seated and the neck in moderate extension. The health care provider should first inspect the neck visually, and then palpate the thyroid gland and the cervical and supraclavicular lymph nodes. Because the thyroid is ensheathed in the pretracheal fascia, it moves on swallowing and this feature is critical to the differentiation of thyroid tissue from other neck structures. Accordingly, the patient must be provided a cup of water and instructed to swallow sips of water at appropriate intervals during palpation. Some health care providers prefer to stand behind the seated patient and palpate the thyroid with their fingertips. Alternatively, the clinician can face the seated patient and use gentle pressure with the thumb to locate the thyroid isthmus and then move laterally, without release of pressure, to compress the lobe of the thyroid against the trachea as the patient sips water (Larsen and Davies, 2003). With practice, one should be able to palpate the normal thyroid in nearly all adolescents. The assessment of a goiter should take into account the normal thyroid size for age as described earlier. The health care provider should note size/shape/nodularity of the gland, location of any thyroid mass, mobility of any masses, and any tenderness.

Thyroid Tests

Many thyroid tests are available, but only few are typically necessary for appropriate diagnosis. In euthyroid individuals, 99.98% of serum thyroxine (T_4) and 99.7% of serum triiodothyronine (T_3) is bound to serum protein (mostly TBG) and is biologically inactive (Larsen and Hay, 1998). Total thyroid hormone concentrations can therefore be abnormal not only in individuals with thyroid dysfunction but also in those with abnormal binding. This issue can be addressed by measuring serum free T_4 (or free T_3). Such tests are widely available for routine use. Alternatively, one can simultaneously measure total T_4 and the T_3-resin uptake (an estimate of protein binding), and then use the results to calculate a free T_4 index (FT$_4$I) (Baloch et al., 2002). These approaches are detailed in guidelines provided by the National Academy of Clinical Biochemistry at http://www.aacc.org/AACC/members/nacb/LMPG/. For nearly all patients, the simultaneous measurement of serum TSH and free T_4 (or FT$_4$I) is sufficient to diagnosis thyroid dysfunction (or to rule it out).

Common thyroid tests include the following:

1. Serum total T_4: Total T_4 is usually measured by competitive immunoassay.
2. Adjusted T_4: This is a calculation using total T_4 and T_3 resin uptake with adjustment for changes in thyroid-binding capability, including TBG levels. This is also referred to as the *free T_4 index* (FT$_4$I). Adjusted T_4 is generally high in patients with hyperthyroidism and low in patients with hypothyroidism. In individuals with normal hypothalamic-pituitary-thyroid function, conditions that alter thyroid hormone binding and thereby total T_4 concentrations but yield a normal adjusted T_4 (or free T_4) level include the following:
   a. Factors increasing TBG: Oral contraceptives, pregnancy, heredity, heroin, methadone, acute hepatitis.
   b. Factors decreasing TBG: Androgens, cirrhosis, nephrosis, acromegaly, genetic, high-dose steroids (Sarlis, 2006).
   c. Drugs decreasing binding of T_4 and T_3: Salicylates, furosemide, mefenamic acid, heparin, phenytoin, barbital, (Surks and Sievert, 1995).
3. Serum free T_4: Free T_4 can be assayed by methods that employ the physical separation of free hormone from bound hormone (equilibrium dialysis, ultrafiltration, gel filtration). Most routine clinical laboratories estimate free hormone concentrations by a two-test strategy or a ligand assay approach.
4. Serum total T_3: Total T_3 is usually measured by competitive immunoassay. Measurement of T_3 can be useful in the rare thyrotoxic patient with a low serum TSH but a normal serum free T_4. T_3 measurements are generally not useful in evaluating hypothyroidism.
5. Serum free T_3: Measured in a manner similar to that of free T_4.
6. Serum TSH: Serum TSH is usually measured by nonisotopic immunometric assay (IMA) principles. Modern TSH assays are sufficiently sensitive to detect the suppressed TSH concentrations associated with hyperthyroidism. TSH is the most sensitive test for diagnosing primary hypothyroidism (high TSH) or thyrotoxicosis (low TSH, usually <0.1 µU/mL).
7. Thyroid radioiodine uptake (RAIU): A measurement of thyroidal uptake of iodine-131 (^{131}I) or iodine-123 (^{123}I). ^{123}I is preferred because of the lower radiation dose. The chief value of this test is in the differential diagnosis of thyrotoxicosis. The RAIU value is typically high in Graves hyperthyroidism or hyperthyroidism from hyperfunctioning thyroid nodule(s). The RAIU value is low in factitious hyperthyroidism and the thyrotoxic phase of transient thyroiditis. In the United States, dietary iodine intake renders the RAIU values in hypothyroidism indistinguishable from the lower end of the normal range, so RAIU measurements are usually not helpful in the evaluation of hypothyroidism. Addition of a perchlorate discharge test to the RAIU can be used to diagnose defects in iodine organification.
8. Thyroid scan: A thyroid scan evaluates thyroid anatomy and function. It can be useful in the differential diagnosis of thyroid nodules and in the identification of ectopic thyroid tissue. ^{123}I is the preferred radionuclide.
9. Thyroid antibodies: Titers of antithyroglobulin and antimicrosomal (anti-thyroid peroxidase [TPO])

antibodies are elevated in most patients with Hashimoto thyroiditis. Antimicrosomal antibodies are more sensitive (99% sensitivity) than antithyroglobulin antibodies (36% sensitivity) (Nordyke et al., 1993). Titers of thyroid-stimulating immunoglobulin (TSI) and other TSH-receptor antibodies are typically elevated in Graves disease. These antibodies can be assayed at the time of diagnosis of Graves disease and monitored as an indicator of the resolution of the autoimmune process. The sensitivity of serum thyrotropin-receptor antibody (TRAb) assays is cited to be 75% to 96% for TSH-binding inhibitor immunoglobulin (TBII, a competitive binding assay with TSH) and 85% to 100% for thyroid-stimulating antibody (TSAb) measurements (a bioassay of TSH receptor activation) in untreated Graves disease (Saravanan and Dayan, 2001; Weetman, 2000). In practice, the measurement of TRAb is rarely needed to diagnose Graves disease.

10. Reverse T_3 (rT3): Reverse T_3 is an inactive isomer of T_3, produced from the inner-ring deiodination of T_4. In nonthyroidal illnesses, such as starvation and anorexia nervosa, T_3 concentrations can be low and reverse T_3 concentrations can be normal or elevated. In hypothyroidism, levels of both T_3 and reverse T_3 are usually low.
11. Thyroxine binding globulin: TBG can be measured directly by immunoassay.
12. Thyroglobulin level: Serum thyroglobulin is high in hyperthyroidism, thyroiditis (thyroid inflammation), certain types of dyshormonogenesis, and in some patients with differentiated thyroid cancers of follicular cell origin and high tumor burden. Its utility in the monitoring of patients with thyroid cancer is realized only after the normal thyroid gland has been removed.

Thyroid deficiency and thyroid hyperfunction are associated with abnormalities of the hypothalamic-pituitary axis. In hypothyroidism, growth hormone, gonadotropin, and prolactin secretory dynamics are altered. This can cause impaired growth, menstrual irregularities, pseudo-precocity, and galactorrhea. Hyponatremia can occur in hypothyroidism due to impaired free water clearance. In prolonged hyperthyroidism, menstrual irregularities can also occur, and linear growth and bone maturation are accelerated.

THYROMEGALY

Thyromegaly and goiter are synonyms that refer to enlargement of the thyroid gland. These disorders may be categorized by cause.

Causes of Thyromegaly

1. Diffuse thyromegaly
   a. Thyroiditis
      • Autoimmune thyroid disease (Table 9.1): Classic Hashimoto thyroiditis Graves disease
      • Painless sporadic thyroiditis (see "Hyperthyroidism and Thyrotoxicosis" section).

TABLE 9.1

Classification of Autoimmune Thyroiditis

Type 1 autoimmune thyroiditis (Hashimoto disease type 1)
1A Goitrous
1B Nongoitrous
Status: euthyroid with normal TSH

Type 2 autoimmune thyroiditis (Hashimoto disease type 2)
2A Goitrous (classic Hashimoto disease)
2B Nongoitrous (primary myxedema, atrophic thyroiditis)
Status: persistent hypothyroidism with increased TSH
2C Transient aggravation of thyroiditis (e.g., postpartum thyroiditis)
Status: may start as transient, low RAIU thyrotoxicosis, followed by transient hypothyroidism

Type 3 autoimmune thyroiditis (Graves disease)
3A Hyperthyroid Graves disease
3B Euthyroid Graves disease
Status: hyperthyroid or euthyroid with suppressed TSH; stimulatory autoantibodies to the TSH receptor are present (autoantibodies to thyroglobulin and TPO are also usually present)
3C Hypothyroid Graves disease
Status: orbitopathy with hypothyroidism; diagnostic levels of autoantibodies to the TSH receptor (blocking or stimulating) may be detected (autoantibodies to Tg and TPO are also usually present)

Adapted from Larsen PR. Hypothyroidisim and thyroiditis. In: Larsen PR, Melmed S, Polonsky KS, eds. *Williams textbook of endocrinology,* 10th ed. Philadelphia: WB Saunders, 2003.

Because of multiple classification schemes, the terms silent sporadic thyroiditis and subacute lymphocytic thyroiditis are used as synonyms for painless sporadic thyroiditis. (Huang, 2006)
- Postpartum thyroiditis (see "Hyperthyroidism and Thyrotoxicosis" section).
- Painful subacute thyroiditis (see "Hyperthyroidism and Thyrotoxicosis" section).

Because of multiple classification schemes, the terms deQuervain disease, deQuervain thyroiditis, subacute thyroiditis, subacute nonsuppurative thyroiditis, giant-cell thyroiditis, migratory "creeping" thyroiditis, subacute granulomatous thyroiditis, pseudogranulomatous thyroiditis, and struma granulomatosa are all used variably as synonyms for painful subacute thyroiditis. (Huang, 2006)

   b. Environmental goitrogens: Iodine deficiency, medications (thionamides, lithium).
   c. Familial goiter.
   d. Idiopathic: An asymptomatic, euthyroid goiter may be discovered on routine physical examination, noted by a parent, or discovered by the teenager. The incidence is 9 of 1,000 per year, with most affected teens being female.
2. Nodular thyromegaly:
   a. Hypofunctioning thyroid nodules (see "Thyroid Nodules" section).
   b. Hyperfunctioning thyroid nodules (see "Hyperthyroidism and Thyrotoxicosis" section).

Clinical Presentation

Thyromegaly often occurs in combination with thyroid dysfunction, and such patients typically present with hypothyroid or thyrotoxic symptoms. In euthyroid individuals, thyroid enlargement may be noted as a cosmetic issue. Symptoms related to the compression/displacement of the trachea (stridor), esophagus (dysphagia), or recurrent laryngeal nerve (hoarseness) are unusual and generally limited to rare individuals with very large and rapidly growing goiters. Painful subacute thyroiditis can present with thyroid pain or tenderness, sometimes preceded by symptoms of fever or upper respiratory infection.

Evaluation

Although some goiters are idiopathic, the finding of thyromegaly obligates an investigation for underlying pathology and a focused evaluation will identify the cause in most cases. Assessment of goiter should take into account the normal thyroid size for age as described earlier. Thyroid ultrasonography can be used to estimate thyroid size more accurately and to address the possibility of any nodule appreciated by palpation. Because the most common causes of goiter are associated with thyroid dysfunction, thyroid function tests should be obtained in all patients with thyromegaly and monitored every 4 to 6 months through adolescence.

Therapy

The management of nodular thyromegaly focuses on the evaluation for possible malignancy (hypofunctioning

nodules) or hyperthyroidism (hyperfunctioning thyroid nodules). If thyroid dysfunction is present, it should be treated (see "Hypothyroidism" and "Hyperthyroidism and Thyrotoxicosis" sections). There is controversy over the approach to idiopathic goiter as many teenagers remain euthyroid for years and spontaneous resolution is possible. Specialists are divided between the use of exogenous thyroid hormone versus close observation without treatment. Rapid thyroid growth, compressive symptoms, or cosmetic concerns are indications to consider treatment. Thyroid hormone, if indicated, can be given as levothyroxine and titrated to a low normal serum TSH concentration (0.2–0.3 μU/mL).

HYPOTHYROIDISM

Causes

Mostly, congenital hypothyroidism is permanent and requires lifelong hormone replacement. Outside of the newborn period, acquired hypothyroidism is usually due to autoimmune thyroiditis and so chronic autoimmune thyroiditis is the focus of this section. The childhood prevalence of chronic autoimmune thyroiditis peaks in early to mid-puberty and a female preponderance of 2:1 has been reported (Lafranchi, 1992). Improvements in the measurement of circulating autoantibodies have obviated the need for biopsy in the diagnosis of autoimmune thyroid disease and the nomenclature itself has been redefined only during recent years (Table 9.1) (Davies and Amino, 1993; Larsen, 2003). The term thyroiditis is defined as evidence of "intrathyroidal lymphocytic infiltration," with or without follicular damage. Two types of chronic autoimmune thyroiditis (also known as *chronic lymphocytic thyroiditis*) are causes of persistent hypothyroidism, Hashimoto disease (goitrous form, type 2A), and atrophic thyroiditis (nongoitrous form, type 2B).

Clinical Presentation

The presentation of chronic autoimmune thyroiditis includes either hypothyroidism or goiter, or both. Thyromegaly is typically diffuse with a "pebbly" or "seedy" surface that evolves into a firm and nodular consistency. As the disease progresses, subclinical and then clinical hypothyroidism appears. Symptoms of hypothyroidism may be subtle, even with marked biochemical derangement (Table 9.2). Growth and pubertal development may be delayed. Gain in height is usually compromised to a greater degree than weight gain, and the bone age is delayed (Boersma et al., 1996; Chiesa et al., 1998). Hypothyroidism typically causes pubertal delay in teenagers, but in children may also induce a syndrome of pseudoprecocity manifested as testicular enlargement in boys and breast enlargement and vaginal bleeding in girls (Anasti et al., 1995; Castro-Magana et al., 1988; Jannini et al., 1995).

Evaluation

1. Laboratory evaluation
   a. TSH and free T_4: The serum TSH concentration is elevated in primary hypothyroidism. If the differential diagnosis includes central hypothyroidism or if the overall suspicion for hypothyroidism is high, a

TABLE 9.2

Symptoms and Signs of Hypothyroidism

Symptoms
- Constipation
- Cold intolerance
- Fatigue
- Hoarseness
- Slowed mentation (lethargy and impaired school performance)
- Menstrual dysfunction, sometimes as dysfunctional uterine bleeding

Signs
- Abdominal distension
- Bradycardia (decreased cardiac output)
- Coarse facial features
- Coarse, brittle, strawlike hair
- Decreased systolic blood pressure and increased diastolic blood pressure
- Dry, sallow skin
- Delayed deep tendon reflexes
- Dull facial expression
- Fluid retention and weight gain (impaired renal free water clearance)
- Goiter
- Growth retardation
- Hypothermia
- Hyporeflexia with delayed relaxation, ataxia, or both
- Jaundice
- Loss of scalp hair, axillary hair, pubic hair, or a combination
- Macroglossia
- Nonpitting edema (myxedema)
- Pubertal disorders (delay or pseudoprecocity)
- Pallor
- Periorbital puffiness
- Pericardial effusion
- Pitting edema of lower extremities
- Slowed speech and movements
- Skeletal maturational delay

free T_4 measurement should be included. In mild hypothyroidism, serum T_3 can remain in the normal range because of the increased peripheral conversion of T_4 to T_3 and the preferential secretion of T_3 by the gland during hyperthyrotropinemia (elevated TSH). For these reasons, measurement of the serum T_3 concentration is not useful in the diagnosis or monitoring of patients with primary hypothyroidism.

  b. Anti-TPO antibodies and antithyroglobulin antibodies: The presence of goiter or elevated TSH values should prompt the measurement of anti-TPO antibodies. Anti-TPO antibodies are the most sensitive screen for chronic autoimmune thyroiditis (Nordyke et al., 1993). Antithyroglobulin antibodies may be added if anti-TPO titers are negative. The typical patient with hypothyroidism secondary to chronic autoimmune thyroiditis has an elevated TSH level (more than 10 µU/mL), a low free T_4, and positive anti-TPO antibodies (Saravanan and Dayan, 2001). However, in early stages of the disease, TSH may be normal (type 1A) or only modestly elevated. If antithyroid antibodies are absent, less common etiologies of primary hypothyroidism such as transient hypothyroidism (post subacute thyroiditis), external irradiation, and consumptive hypothyroidism should be considered (Hancock et al., 1995; Huang et al., 2002; Huang, 2005).

2. Evaluation after biochemical hypothyroidism is confirmed: The initial history should include inquiry into energy level, sleep pattern, menses, cold intolerance, and school performance. In addition to palpation of the thyroid, the health care provider should assess the extraocular movements, fluid status, and deep tendon reflexes. Chronic autoimmune thyroiditis may be the initial presentation of an autoimmune polyglandular syndrome and the possibility of coexisting autoimmune diseases such as type 1 diabetes, Addison disease, and pernicious anemia must be addressed by the history.

Therapy

Levothyroxine (L-T_4) is the replacement of choice. There are virtually no adverse reactions and its long half-life of 5 to 7 days allows the convenience of daily administration.

1. Initiation of levothyroxine: Some authors advocate a graded approach to the initiation of levothyroxine (Slyper and Swenerton, 1998). Alternatively, a starting dose can be estimated on the basis of the patient's age and ideal body weight with a full dose of thyroxine. The medication's long half-life ensures a gradual equilibration over the course of 5 to 6 weeks. Average daily requirements approximate 2 to 4 µg/kg in 10- to 15-year olds and 1.6 µg/kg during adulthood (average maintenance is between 50 and 200 µg), but dosing needs to be individualized ultimately on the basis of biochemical monitoring (LaFranchi, 1992). Current average replacement doses equal approximately 127 ± 39 µg in adults. Overtreatment with thyroxine should be avoided because it could lead to osteoporosis. Health care providers should counsel adolescents on thyroid hormone supplementation to have adequate calcium intake. However, calcium carbonate has been shown to interfere with thyroid hormone absorption. Patients taking this preparation need to be monitored to ensure that thyroid hormone replacement doses are adequate.

2. Response to levothyroxine and monitoring: TSH normalization is the goal of replacement and we aim for a target range of 0.5 to 3 µU/mL. This will usually be associated with a free T_4 in the upper half of the normal range. Thyroid function tests should be obtained 6 weeks after the initiation or adjustment of the levothyroxine dosage. Once biochemical euthyroidism has been achieved, TSH can be monitored every 4 to 6 months in the growing teenager and yearly once linear growth is complete. If noncompliance is suspected as the cause of treatment failure, a free T_4 may be measured because a serum TSH greater than twice the normal in the context of a normal free T_4 suggests intermittent omission of the medication. A variety of conditions or drugs may

TABLE 9.3

Conditions that Increase Levothyroxine Requirements

Pregnancy	
Gastrointestinal disease	Mucosal diseases of the small bowel (e.g., sprue)
	Jejunoileal bypass and small bowel resection
	Diabetic diarrhea
Drugs which impair L-T$_4$ absorption	Cholestyramine
	Sucralfate
	Aluminum hydroxide
	Calcium carbonate
	Ferrous sulfate
Drugs which may enhance CYP3A4 and thereby accelerate levothyroxine clearance	Rifampin
	Carbamazepine
	Estrogen
	Phenytoin
	Sertraline
	Statins
Drug which impairs T$_4$ to T$_3$ conversion	Amiodarone
Conditions which may block type 1 deiodinase	Selenium deficiency
	Cirrhosis

Adapted from Larsen PR. Hypothyroidisim and thyroiditis. In: Larsen PR, Melmed S, Polonsky KS, eds. *Williams textbook of endocrinology,* 10th ed. Philadelphia: WB Saunders, 2003.

alter levothyroxine requirements (Table 9.3). In theory, levothyroxine should be administered at least 30 minutes before eating or any medication known to impair its absorption. However, from a practical viewpoint, the most important goal is to establish a regular time for levothyroxine administration. Growth and sexual development should be followed systematically as in any pediatric patient.

3. Side effects: Although very rare, case reports have described the development of pseudotumor cerebri around the initiation of levothyroxine in a small number of school-aged children (Van Dop et al., 1983). A temporary reduction in the levothyroxine dose is appropriate to consider in this situation. Reactions to specific dyes or binders can be addressed by switching the levothyroxine preparation/manufacturer.

4. Subclinical hypothyroidism: Subclinical hypothyroidism is defined as TSH elevation with normal serum free T$_4$. The log-linear relation between serum TSH and free T$_4$ explains how small reductions in serum free T$_4$ lead to large deviations in TSH. Most patients with subclinical hypothyroidism are asymptomatic and there is debate as to the need for treatment. Because studies in adults suggest that individuals with the combined risk factors of hyperthyrotropinemia and positive thyroid antibodies are at high risk for progression to overt hypothyroidism, it is our practice to recommend thyroid hormone replacement in patients with TSH values >10 μU/mL or with TSH values >5 μU/mL in combination with goiter or thyroid autoantibodies (Mandel et al., 1993).

5. Counseling issues: Although rare exceptions have been reported, parents of teens with chronic autoimmune thyroiditis should be advised that the hypothyroidism will likely be permanent (Sklar et al., 1986). The

monitoring of thyroid function is lifelong, but after the completion of linear growth, serum TSH measurements can be obtained annually, once euthyroidism has been restored. The initiation of medications which can alter levothyroxine requirements, such as those shown in Table 9.3, warrants additional monitoring.

6. Pregnancy: Levothyroxine requirements increase by an average of 45% to 47% during gestation and untreated maternal hypothyroidism may adversely affect the intellectual development of the fetus (Alexander et al., 2004; Haddow et al., 1999; Mandel et al., 1993). Accordingly, a TSH should be checked if pregnancy is diagnosed and the frequency of monitoring increased. Young women who are treated for hypothyroidism and are euthyroid on replacement can be advised to increase empirically their prepregnancy levothyroxine dose by taking two extra daily doses each week (a 29% increase) beginning with the week pregnancy is confirmed. They should then undergo thyroid function testing and obtain appropriate professional guidance as soon as possible (Alexander et al., 2004).

HYPERTHYROIDISM AND THYROTOXICOSIS

The term *thyrotoxicosis* refers to the manifestations of excessive quantities of circulating thyroid hormone from any source. In contrast, *hyperthyroidism* refers only to the subset of diseases associated with thyrotoxicosis, which are due to hormone overproduction (increased biosynthesis) and secretion by the thyroid gland itself (Table 9.4). Most adolescent and young adult patients have thyrotoxicosis caused by hyperthyroidism, especially

TABLE 9.4

Differential Diagnosis of Thyrotoxicosis

Causes of Thyrotoxicosis

**Thyrotoxicosis associated with sustained hormone
    overproduction (hyperthyroidism):**
    High RAIU
    Graves disease
    Toxic multinodular goiter
    Toxic adenoma
    Increased TSH secretion
Thyrotoxicosis without associated hyperthyroidism:
    Low RAIU
    Thyrotoxicosis factitia
    Subacute thyroiditis
    Chronic thyroiditis with transient thyroiditis
        (painless thyroiditis, silent thyroiditis,
        postpartum thyroiditis)
    Ectopic thyroid tissue (struma ovarii, functioning
        metastatic thyroid cancer)

Adapted from Davies TF. Thyrotoxicosis. In: *Williams
textbook of endocrinology,* 10th ed. Philadelphia: WB
Saunders, 2003.

Graves disease. However, some may have thyrotoxicosis
caused by thyroid gland inflammation causing a release of
stored thyroid hormone (but not accelerated synthesis) or
from ingestion of exogenous thyroid hormone. The ability
to diagnose accurately hyperthyroidism and differentiate
it from thyrotoxicosis is critical as disease management
differs and antithyroid drugs have no role in the treatment
of thyrotoxicosis without hyperthyroidism.

Prevalence

1. Graves disease is the most common cause of hyperthyroidism in the United States and is the focus of most
   of this section. Only 5% of patients with Graves disease
   are younger than 15 years. However, hyperthyroidism
   becomes more common with age, particularly in women,
   affecting approximately 2% of women. The prevalence in
   females increases dramatically during late adolescence
   and young adult ages, with a peak at approximately
   25 years.
2. Graves disease is the most common autoimmune
   disorder in the United States and is associated with
   a five to ten times greater prevalence in women.

Causes of Thyrotoxicosis and
Hyperthyroidism

1. Common
   a. Graves disease: For practical purposes, almost all
      hyperthyroidism in adolescents is caused by Graves
      disease. Graves hyperthyroidism is caused by TSAbs
      that bind and activate the thyrotropin receptor,
      leading to thyromegaly and the hypersecretion of

thyroid hormone. Lymphocytic infiltration of the thyroid is present, hence its classification as a form of
thyroiditis (Table 9.1). Lymphocytic infiltration and
the accumulation of glycosaminoglycans in the orbital
connective tissue and skin cause the extrathyroidal
manifestations of Graves ophthalmopathy and dermopathy (Weetman, 2000). Girls are affected four to
five times more frequently than boys, although no gender difference is noted below 4 years of age (Lavard
et al., 1994; Zimmerman and Lteif, 1998).
2. Uncommon
   a. Transient thyrotoxicosis due to the release of pre-
      formed thyroid hormones from a damaged gland:
      • Painless sporadic thyroiditis
      • Painless postpartum thyroiditis
      • Painful subacute thyroiditis
      These forms of thyrotoxicosis are self-limited be-
      cause the thyroid gland contains a limited quan-
      tity of preformed hormone. It is hypothesized that
      painless postpartum thyroiditis and painless spo-
      radic thyroiditis may result from thyroid autoimmu-
      nity (Pearce et al., 2003). Because painful subacute
      thyroiditis is often preceded by a prodome of infec-
      tious symptoms, a viral etiology has been proposed,
      although definitive evidence is lacking. In practice,
      the precipitating insult of transient thyroiditis in any
      individual patient is usually unknown, but care is unaf-
      fected as thyrotoxicosis is self-limited and supportive
      therapies are nonspecific. These forms of transient
      thyroiditis should be distinguished from acute or sup-
      purative thyroiditis, which refer to infections (usually
      bacterial) of the thyroid gland that often require an-
      tibiotic therapy, but are usually not associated with
      the derangement of thyroid function (Huang, 2006).
   b. Toxic nodular goiter: Single adenoma or multiple
      nodules
3. Rare
   a. Ectopic thyroid tissue (e.g., struma ovarii [ovarian
      teratoma-containing thyroid tissue])
   b. Inappropriate TSH secretion—pituitary tumor
   c. Exogenous iodide intake
   d. Thyroid cancer

Clinical Presentation

The presentation of Graves disease in adolescence may be
insidious and a careful history will often reveal a several-
month history of progressive symptoms (Table 9.5). A goiter is palpable in most cases, with diffuse enlargement that
is smooth, rubbery, and nontender. Extrathyroidal manifestations such as ophthalmopathy and dermopathy are rarer
than in adults and tend to be less severe (Zimmerman and
Lteif, 1998). In adolescents, prolonged hyperthyroidism
from Graves disease may accelerate linear growth and
bone maturation (Buckler et al., 1986; Wong et al., 1999).
Commonly, patients have a family history involving a wide
spectrum of autoimmune thyroid diseases, such as Graves
disease, Hashimoto thyroiditis, or postpartum thyroiditis,
among others.

Evaluation

1. TSH and free T_4: Thyrotoxicosis is recognized by
   an elevation of serum free T_4 with a decreased or
   suppressed serum TSH (typically $<0.1 \mu U/mL$). Free T_4

TABLE 9.5

Symptoms and Signs of Hyperthyroidism in
Children and Adolescents

Goiter
Exophthalmos
Acceleration of linear growth
Nervousness
Increased irritability
Decreased concentration and impaired school
  performance
Headache
Hyperactivity
Fatigue
Muscle weakness
Palpitations
Sinus tachycardia
Increased pulse pressure
Hypertension
Heart murmur
Polyphagia
Increased frequency of bowel movements
Weight loss with increased appetite
Heat intolerance
Increased perspiration
Tremor, hyperreflexia
Warm, moist skin
Sleep disturbance
Pruritus
Menstrual changes—amenorrhea, oligomenorrhea,
  dysfunctional uterine bleeding

Adapted from LaFranchi SHC. Graves' disease in the neonatal period and childhood.

may be normal in early disease or in iodine-deficient patients, so a determination of free T_3 should be added if TSH is suppressed and the serum free T_4 is normal.
2. Duration of disease: Once biochemical derangement has been documented, it is helpful to address the duration of thyrotoxicosis to facilitate the differentiation of Graves disease from painless thyroiditis. Onset may be documented by prior laboratory studies or inferred from the history.
   a. More than 8 weeks: For thyrotoxicosis that has been present for >8 weeks, Graves is by far the most likely etiology. In such patients, the constellation of thyrotoxicosis, goiter, and orbitopathy is pathognomonic for Graves and no additional laboratory or imaging tests are necessary to confirm the diagnosis.
   b. Less than 8 weeks: If thyrotoxicosis has been present for <8 weeks, and if thyromegaly is subtle and eye changes are absent, an ^{123}I uptake should be performed to address the possibility of transient thyrotoxicosis secondary to painless sporadic thyroiditis or painful subacute thyroiditis. The RAIU in these conditions will be low, distinguishing them from the more common Graves disease (Table 9.4). Hyperfunctioning nodules must be large to cause hyperthyroidism

(typically 2–3 cm or more in diameter), so radioiodine thyroid scanning should be reserved for patients in whom a discrete nodule(s) is palpable. [123]I uptake will localize to the hyperfunctioning nodule(s) and radionuclide signal in the surrounding tissue will be low secondary to TSH suppression. Thyrotoxicosis factitia can be recognized by a low RAIU and serum thyroglobulin in the presence of thyrotoxicosis and a suppressed TSH.

Therapy

Therapy for hyperthyroidism (Graves disease) includes medical therapy with antithyroid drugs and definitive therapy with ^{131}I or surgery.

Medical Therapy (Antithyroid Drugs)
Medical therapy is usually the primary modality for adolescent patients.

1. *Symptomatic end-organ therapy with a β-blocker (e.g., propranolol):* The cardiovascular manifestations of hyperthyroidism are generally well-tolerated in the young, so this measure is needed only if symptoms are significant.
2. *Antithyroid medications:* The thionamide derivatives, Tapazole (MMI) and propylthiouracil (PTU), are the most commonly used antithyroid drugs (Cooper, 2005; Franklyn, 1994). Both block thyroid hormone biosynthesis and PTU, when used at doses more than 450 to 600 mg/day, also inhibits the extrathyroidal activation of T_4 to T_3 (Klein et al., 1994). The recommended pediatric starting dose is 0.5 to 1.0 mg/kg/day for MMI and 5 to 10 mg/kg/day for PTU. For adolescent patients, the following rule of thumb is helpful in the determination of a starting dose:

Starting Dose of Tapazole for Adolescent Patients	
Free T_4 (or FT_4I)	Tapazole dose
<1.5 times the upper limit of normal range	10 mg qd
1.5 to 2 times the upper limit of normal range	10 mg b.i.d
>2 times the upper limit of normal range	20 mg b.i.d

Because of its longer half-life, MMI can be administered qd or b.i.d, compared with the t.i.d dosing of PTU, so it is our first choice for initial therapy except for those patients who are pregnant (MMI administration during pregnancy has been associated with aplasia cutis) and those who present with severe hyperthyroidism. For severely hyperthyroid patients, PTU is the preferred thionamide because of its ability to inhibit T_4 to T_3 conversion and a combination of high-dose PTU (up to 1,200 mg/day divided q6 hours) and inorganic iodine (SSKI three drops PO b.i.d for 5–10 days) will speed up biochemical correction (Davies, 2003).
3. *Response to antithyroid drugs and monitoring:* After the free T_4 has fallen to the upper half of normal range, the dose of antithyroid drug should be decreased by one half or one third. Patients should be counseled that clinical response often lags behind biochemical correction,

usually starting 2 to 4 weeks into therapy. Further dose adjustments are guided by serial thyroid function tests, initially relying upon the free T_4. After pituitary TSH secretion recovers from suppression, TSH normalization is the goal of maintenance therapy. For any patient on antithyroid drug, we monitor thyroid function tests every 3 months and also 3 weeks after dose adjustment. Physical examination should focus upon heart rate, puberty, linear growth, and vision.

4. *Side effects:* Antithyroid drugs are usually well-tolerated, but side effects are more common in children than in adults (Lazar et al., 2000; Rivkees et al., 1998).
   a. Common side effects include pruritus, fever, rash, and urticaria. Less common side effects include gastrointestinal distress and change in taste sensation, and production of insulin autoantibodies, causing hypoglycemia.
   b. Agranulocytosis (defined as a granulocyte count $<500/\mu l$) is a serious idiosyncratic reaction that can occur with either MMI or PTU (Cooper et al., 1983). For this reason, a baseline white blood cell count should be obtained before the initiation of antithyroid drugs, and teens and their parents should be counseled that fever, sore throat, or other serious infections warrant the immediate cessation of antithyroid drugs, the notification of the physician, and a determination of white blood cell count with differential.
   c. Hepatitis is another serious but rare adverse reaction associated with the thionamides, so symptoms suspicious of hepatitis (jaundice, right upper abdominal pain, etc.) similarly warrant the immediate discontinuation of drug and medical evaluation including liver function tests.
5. *Remission:* Reports of long-term remission rates in children and adolescents are variable, ranging anywhere from 30% to 60% (LaFranchi, 2005; Raza, et al., 1999; Rivkees et al., 1998; Shulman et al., 1997). If a patient has a normal serum TSH concentration for 6 months to 1 year on a minimal dose of antithyroid medication (5 mg/day of Tapazole or 50 mg/day of PTU), a trial off medication may be offered. Antithyroid drugs can be discontinued and TSH concentrations monitored at monthly intervals. If hyperthyroidism recurs, antithyroid medications should be resumed or definitive therapy provided.
6. *"Block and replace" strategy:* Some authors have advocated a "block and replace" strategy of high-dose antithyroid medication (to suppress all endogenous thyroid secretion) combined with levothyroxine replacement. One report described a lower recurrence rate with this approach, but all subsequent studies have failed to duplicate this finding (Hashizume et al., 1991; Lucas, et al., 1997; McIver et al., 1996). For the purpose of simplifying the patient's regimen and minimizing the risk of adverse drug reactions, we prefer monotherapy with a single antithyroid medication.
7. *Subclinical hyperthyroidism:* The term "*subclinical hyperthyroidism*" refers to patients who have a subnormal serum TSH (usually between 0.1 and 0.3 μU/mL) but normal concentrations of both free T_4 and free T_3. These patients are generally asymptomatic. The differential diagnosis is the same as for overt thyrotoxicosis. In adults older than 60 years, subclinical hyperthyroidism is associated with an increased risk of atrial fibrillation, but the adverse sequelae of untreated subclinical disease in adolescents are not defined (Marqusee et al., 1998). No consensus exists as to the indications for therapy but, assuming there are no specific risk factors such as a history of cardiac disease, asymptomatic adolescents with subclinical hyperthyroidism can be followed without treatment. Thyroid function tests should be obtained every few months with the expectation that TSH suppression that is due to transient thyroiditis will resolve spontaneously and that which is due to Graves disease or autonomous secretion will declare itself over time.

Definitive Therapy

The two options for the definitive treatment of Graves disease are radioiodine (^{131}I) and thyroidectomy. Both are likely to result in lifelong hypothyroidism and there is disagreement in the literature as to their indications. Some centers use them as first-line treatment for pediatric hyperthyroidism (Clark et al., 1995; Moll and Patel, 1997; Ward et al., 1999). However, as a remission of Graves disease occurs in a significant percentage of adolescents, we recommend the long-term use of antithyroid medications until young adulthood. If patient noncompliance prevents the successful treatment of thyrotoxicosis or if both antithyroid medications must be discontinued secondary to serious drug reactions, definitive therapy is appropriate.

1. Radioiodine (^{131}I) ablative therapy: Therapeutic administration of ^{131}I is the definitive treatment of choice in adults. Several studies support that the incidence of secondary malignancy in children or adolescents treated with ^{131}I is not increased, but these study populations are relatively small and the carcinogenic effects of radiation to the thyroid are higher in young children than in adults (Read et al., 2004; Lafranchi, 2005; Baverstock et al., 1992; Nikiforov et al., 1996). This argues for continued study and, for children and teenagers who fail antithyroid medication, the provision of an ^{131}I dose adequate to destroy all thyroid follicular cells. Efficacy is dependent on both thyroid uptake and mass, so we perform an ^{123}I RAIU before treatment and prescribe an ^{131}I dose which will provide approximately 200 μCi/g estimated weight into the gland at 24 hours (limited to a maximum of 11 mCi total into the gland at 24 hours).

   At some point in young adulthood, it is appropriate to revisit the option of definitive therapy for those individuals on medical therapy. For young adults with persistent hyperthyroidism, ^{131}I is our definitive treatment of choice. We perform an RAIU before treatment with the goal of delivering approximately 8 mCi of ^{131}I into the gland at 24 hours. For glands larger than three times normal size, approximately 11 mCi is required (Alexander and Larsen, 2002). Definitive therapy typically results in permanent hypothyroidism, but allows for a simpler regimen of medication and laboratory monitoring (daily levothyroxine and a yearly TSH measurement). Additionally, prior definitive therapy simplifies the management of female patients during pregnancy.

2. Surgery: Thyroidectomy is rarely used electively for the definitive therapy of Graves disease in the United States, except for patients with massive thyromegaly (more than eight times normal size) or for patients who have coexisting cytologically abnormal thyroid nodules. A recent meta-analysis of the pediatric literature reported that thyroidectomy relieved hyperthyroidism in 80% (subtotal thyroidectomy) to approximately 97% (total thyroidectomy) of children with Graves disease, but the

overall complication rates included a 2% incidence of permanent hypoparathyroidism, a 2% incidence of vocal cord paralysis, and a 0.08% mortality (Rivkees et al., 1998). On the basis of these data, the authors suggest that thyroidectomy be considered only for patients who have persistently failed medical management, or those whose parents or physicians do not wish to proceed with radioiodine therapy. The experience of the individual surgeon is the primary determinant of thyroidectomy morbidity and so referral to a surgeon with a low personal complication rate and extensive experience with subtotal thyroidectomy is required, if this is the desired procedure (Sosa et al., 1998). [131]I therapy is an acceptable alternative if the surgical options are undesirable in a given community. [131]I is recommended for all patients who have recurrence following surgery because of the high complication rate of secondary thyroidectomy (Waldhausen, 1997).

Pregnancy-Related Issues

Approximately 0.6% of infants born to mothers with a history of Graves disease will develop neonatal hyperthyroidism due to the transplacental passage of TSI. This can occur even after successful definitive treatment with ^{131}I or thyroidectomy, secondary to the persistence of maternal autoantibodies. The care of such women must be coordinated between a high-risk obstetrician and an endocrinologist. Fetal heart rate and growth should be monitored by regular prenatal ultrasonography, and the measurement of antithyrotropin receptor antibodies during at-risk pregnancies is recommended as a predictor for the development of fetal/neonatal Graves disease (Laurberg et al., 1998). Health care providers should be aware that maternal antithyroid medication use near delivery or the co-transfer of maternal thyrotropin receptor–blocking immunoglobulins may delay the appearance of neonatal hyperthyroidism (McKenzie and Zakarija, 1992; McKenzie and Zakarija, 1983). For high-risk infants, such as those born to mothers with high levels of TSAbs or those with a history of an affected sibling, the authors recommend thyroid function tests at birth, and at 1 and 2 months of age. An additional set of laboratory work at 1 week of age is indicated for infants who have been exposed to maternal antithyroid drugs in the third trimester.

THYROID NODULES

1. Prevalence: The frequency of nodular thyroid disease increases with age. Thyroid nodules are therefore common in adults (lifetime risk of 5% to 10%), but are rare in children (estimated frequency of .05% to 1.8%) (Mazzaferri 1993; Rallison et al., 1975; Trowbridge et al., 1975). The condition affects more women than men. Although nodular disease of the thyroid is common, malignancy of the thyroid occurs in only 0.004% of the American population annually (12,000 new cases per year). In comparison to the 5% to 10% cancer prevalence cited for adults, early pediatric series reported a 40% to 60% prevalence of thyroid cancer in children with thyroid nodules (Rallison et al., 1975; Schlumberger et al., 2002; Trowbridge et al., 1975). More recent studies estimate the cancer prevalence of pediatric thyroid

nodules to be 5% to 33% (Al-Shaikh et al., 2001; Arda et al., 2001; Khurana et al., 1999; Lafferty and Batch, 1997).

2. Causes: High doses of neck irradiation increase the risk of developing thyroid nodules (Cooper et al., 2006). Thyroid nodules are also associated with several genetic disorders including multiple endocrine neoplasia type 2, familial nonmedullary thyroid cancer, the PTEN hamartoma tumor syndromes (Cowden syndrome, Bannayan-Riley-Ruvalcaba syndrome), and familial adenomatous polyposis. Other risk factors are described in subsequent text. In the authors' experience, most children and adolescents with thyroid nodules present without these risk factors.

3. Clinical Presentation: Thyroid nodules may be detected on routine physical examination, as an incidental finding on radiographic studies, or brought to medical attention by the patients or their family. Regardless of how a thyroid nodule is discovered, all nodules of significant size should be evaluated for the possibility of malignancy.

4. Evaluation: Because thyroid cancer prognosis depends in part upon tumor size, the early identification of differentiated thyroid cancer is the primary goal in the evaluation of nodular thyroid disease. Once a nodule has been detected, the medical history should include inquiry into prior neck irradiation, determination of whether there is a family history of thyroid cancer, and if there are extrathyroidal manifestations suspicious of other syndromes associated with thyroid cancer (see preceding text). A complete review of systems should include symptoms of thyroid dysfunction and neck compression (dysphagia, hoarseness, pain, etc.). Physical examination should include palpation of both the thyroid gland and the cervical lymph nodes. Nodules that are hard, large, adherent to adjacent structures, or associated with lymphadenopathy should heighten the suspicion of cancer.
   a. Factors suggesting a malignant diagnosis are as follows (Hegedus, 2004):
      High suspicion
      - Family history of medullary thyroid carcinoma or multiple endocrine neoplasia
      - Rapid tumor growth
      - Hard or firm nodule
      - Fixation of the nodule to adjacent structure
      - Paralysis of vocal cords
      - Regional lymphadenopathy
      - Distant metastasis
      Moderate suspicion
      - Males
      - Age younger than 20 years or older than 70 years
      - Nodule more than 4 cm or partially cystic
      - Symptoms of compression such as dysphagia, dysphonia, hoarseness, dyspnea, and cough
      - History of neck irradiation
   b. Factors suggesting a benign diagnosis are as follows:
      - Family history of autoimmune disease (e.g., Hashimoto thyroiditis)
      - Family history of benign thyroid nodule or goiter
      - Thyroid hormonal dysfunction—either hypo- or hyperthyroidism
      - Pain or tenderness associated with nodule
      - Soft, smooth, and mobile nodule
   c. Laboratory evaluation: The initial laboratory evaluation should include thyroid function testing (serum

TSH) to screen for autonomous/hyperfunctioning nodule(s). Diffuse thyromegaly and/or hyperthyrotropinemia warrant the measurement of antithyroid antibodies to diagnose possible chronic autoimmune thyroiditis. However, it is important to realize that the diagnosis of autoimmune thyroid disease does not exclude the possibility of coexistent thyroid cancer, illustrated by the report of autoimmune thyroiditis in 18% (7 of 39) of pediatric patients with papillary thyroid cancer cited by one study (Gupta et al., 2001).

d. Imaging studies and ultrasonography: Because >90% of thyroid nodules are cold by thyroid scanning and therefore require biopsy, the author recommends that ^{123}I thyroid scanning/scintigraphy to detect benign hyperfunctioning nodules should be reserved for patients with suppressed serum TSH concentrations (Schlumberger et al., 2002). For all others, ultrasonography is the most cost-effective imaging modality to confirm the presence of a thyroid nodule. Because of limitations of physical examination alone, thyroid ultrasonography should be performed in all adolescents with suspected thyroid nodules before any attempt at biopsy. Cytology should be obtained in all patients before considering surgery and ultrasound-guided fine-needle aspiration is the procedure of choice because it improves the diagnostic accuracy of fine-needle aspiration guided by palpation alone and reduces the likelihood of accidental penetration into the trachea or the great vessels (Marqusee et al., 2000).

5. Suggested Approach for the Evaluation and Management of Thyroid Nodules: The serum TSH concentration should be measured before endocrine consultation for nodular thyroid disease. If the patient's serum TSH concentration is suppressed, an ^{123}I scan should be obtained to address the possibility of a hyperfunctioning nodule. The hyperfunctioning nodule might be treated with radioiodine, but alternatives include no treatment, surgery, and ethanol injection. If the serum TSH is normal or high, the patient should be triaged directly to a center with experience in the management of thyroid nodules and cancer, and any thyroid nodule ≥1 cm in diameter requires biopsy by ultrasound-guided fine-needle aspiration. Categorization of biopsy interpretations into cytologic risk categories facilitates the discussion on surgical approach, based on the likelihood of malignancy associated with the patient's specific category and an individual assessment of the child's operative risks. If surgery is indicated, referral to a surgeon with extensive experience in pediatric thyroidectomy and a low personal complication rate is paramount, regardless of the degree of resection (Sosa et al., 1998). Adolescents with thyroid nodules <1 cm or with benign cytology should be followed up chronically by serial ultrasonography every 6 to 12 months, and ultrasound-guided fine-needle aspiration should be repeated if significant interval growth or other concerning sonographic features develop. Clinical practice guidelines were published in Cooper et al, 2006 by the American Thyroid Association (www.thyroid.org/professionals/publications/documents/Guidelinesthy2006.pdf and the American Association of Clinical Endocrinologists (www.aace.com/pub/pdf/guidelines/thyroid_nodules.pdf).

WEB SITES

For Teenagers and Parents

http://www.magicfoundation.org/www/docs/114/thyroid_disorders.html. Information from the Magic foundation on thyroid disorders.

http://www.tsh.org. Thyroid Foundation of America information on thyroid disease; also has links to many more sites.

http://www.thyroid.org. Home page of the American Thyroid Association.

http://www.endocrineweb.com/thyroid.html. From Endocrine Web page, information on many thyroid problems with information on thyroid hormone, tests, disease states, and more.

http://www.nlm.nih.gov/medlineplus/thyroiddiseases.html. The National Institutes of Health search area on thyroid diseases.

http://www.thyroid.about.com/health/thyroid/library/weekly/aa0421001.html. Thyroid 101 with basic information about all thyroid diseases.

For Health Professionals

http://familydoctor.org/flowcharts/514.html. Flowchart on neck swelling evaluation from the American Academy of Family Physicians.

http://www.thyroid.org. The American Thyroid Association website with helpful updates on a variety of topics, including patient information sheets, thyroid hormone assays, and ongoing diagnostic and management controversies.

http://www.aacc.org/AACC/members/nacb/LMPG/. The National Association of Clinical Biochemists provides Guidelines for Laboratory Support for the Diagnosis and Monitoring of Thyroid Disease.

REFERENCES AND ADDITIONAL READINGS

Alexander EK, Larsen PR. High dose of (131)I therapy for the treatment of hyperthyroidism caused by Graves' disease. *J Clin Endocrinol Metab* 2002;87:1073.

Alexander EK, Marqusee E, Lawrence J, et al. Timing and magnitude of increases in levothyroxine requirements during pregnancy in women with hypothyroidism. *N Engl J Med* 2004; 351:241.

Al-Shaikh A, Ngan B, Daneman A, et al. Fine-needle aspiration biopsy in the management of thyroid nodules in children and adolescents. *J Pediatr* 2001;138:140.

Anasti JN, Flack MR, Froehlich J, et al. A potential novel mechanism for precocious puberty in juvenile hypothyroidism. *J Clin Endocrinol Metab* 1995;80:276.

Arda IS, Yildirim S, Demirhan B, et al. Fine needle aspiration biopsy of thyroid nodules. *Arch Dis Child* 2001;85:313.

Baloch Z, Carayon P, Conte-Devolx B, et al. Laboratory Support for the Diagnosis and Monitoring of Thyroid Disease. In NACB Laboratory Medicine Practice Guidelines: National Academy of Clinical Biochemistry. 2002.

Baverstock K, Egloff B, Pinchera A, Ruchti C, Williams D. Thyroid cancer after Chernobyl. *Nature* 1992;359:21.

Belfiore A, Giuffrida D, La Rosa GL, et al. High frequency of cancer in cold thyroid nodules occurring at young age. *Acta Endocrinol (Copenh)* 1989;121:197.

Bindra A. Thyroiditis. *Am Fam Physician* 2006;73:1769.

Boersma B, Otten BJ, Stoelinga GB, et al. Catch-up growth after prolonged hypothyroidism. *Eur J Pediatr* 1996;155:362.

Buckler JM, Willgerodt H, Keller E. Growth in thyrotoxicosis. *Arch Dis Child* 1986;61:464.

Burch HB. Evaluation and management of the solid thyroid nodule. *Endocrinol Metab Clin North Am* 1995;24:663.

Castro MR, Gharib H. Continuing controversies in the management of thyroid nodules. *Ann Int Med* 2005;142:926.

Castro-Magana M, Angulo M, Canas A, et al. Hypothalamic-pituitary gonadal axis in boys with primary hypothyroidism and macroorchidism. *J Pediatr* 1998;112:397.

Chanoine JP, Toppet V, Lagasse R, et al. Determination of thyroid volume by ultrasound from the neonatal period to late adolescence. *Eur J Pediatr* 1991;150:395.

Chiesa A, Gruneiro de Papendieck L, Keselman A, et al. Final height in long-term primary hypothyroid children. *J Pediatr Endocrinol Metab* 1998;11:51.

Clark JD, Gelfand MJ, Elgazzar AH. Iodine-131 therapy of hyperthyroidism in pediatric patients. *J Nucl Med* 1995;36:442.

Cooper DS. Antithyroid drugs. *N Engl J Med* 2005;352:905.

Cooper DS, Doherty GM, Haugen BR, et al. Management guidelines for patients with thyroid nodules and differentiated thyroid cancer. *Thyroid* 2006;16:109.

Cooper DS, Goldminz D, Levin AA, et al. Agranulocytosis associated with antithyroid drugs. Effects of patient age and drug dose. *Ann Intern Med* 1983;98:26.

Davies TF. Thyrotoxicosis. In *Williams Textbook of Endocrinology*. Philadelphia, PA: Saunders. P.R. Larsen, H.M. Kronenberg, S. Melmed, and K.S. Polonsky, editors. Philadelphia, Pennsylvania: Saunders. 2003;372–421.

Davies TF, Amino N. A new classification for human autoimmune thyroid disease. *Thyroid* 1993;3:331.

Degnan BM, McClellan DR, Francis GL. An analysis of fine-needle aspiration biopsy of the thyroid in children and adolescents. *J Pediatr Surg* 1996;31:903.

Elmlinger MW, Kuhnel W, Lambrecht HG, et al. Reference intervals from birth to adulthood for serum thyroxine (T4), triiodothyronine (T3), free T3, free T4, thyroxine binding globulin (TBG) and thyrotropin (TSH). *Chem Lab Med* 2001;39:973.

Fleury Y, Van Melle G, Woringer V, et al. Sex-dependent variations and timing of thyroid growth during puberty. *J Clin Endocrinol Metab* 2001;86:750.

Force TCT. AACE/AAES medical/surgical guidelines for clinical practice: management of thyroid carcinoma. American Association of Clinical Endocrinologists. American College of Endocrinology. *Endocr Pract* 2001;7:202.

Franklyn JA. The management of hyperthyroidism. *N Engl J Med* 1994;330:1731.

Garber JR, Hennessey JV, Liebermann JA III, et al. Clinical upate. Managing the challenges of hypothyroidism. *J Fam Pract* 2006;55:S1.

Guirguis-Blake J, Hales CM. Screening for thyroid disease. *Am Fam Physician* 2005;71:1369.

Gupta S, Patel A, Folstad A, et al. Infiltration of differentiated thyroid carcinoma by proliferating lymphocytes is associated with improved disease-free survival for children and young adults. *J Clin Endocrinol Metab* 2001;86:1346.

Haddow JE, Palomaki GE, Allan WC, et al. Maternal thyroid deficiency during pregnancy and subsequent neuropsychological development of the child. *N Engl J Med* 1999;341:549.

Hancock SL, McDougall IR, Constine LS. Thyroid abnormalities after therapeutic external radiation. *Int J Radiat Oncol Biol Phys* 1995;31:1165.

Hashizume K, Ichikawa K, Sakurai A, et al. Administration of thyroxine in treated Graves' disease. Effects on the level of antibodies to thyroid-stimulating hormone receptors and on the risk of recurrence of hyperthyroidism. *N Engl J Med* 1991;324:947.

Hay ID. Thyroiditis: a clinical update. *Mayo Clin Proc* 1985;60:836.

Hegedus L. The thyroid nodule. *N Engl J Med* 2004;351:1764.

Huang SA. Physiology and pathophysiology of type 3 deiodinase in humans. *Thyroid* 2005;15(8):875.

Huang SA. Thyromegaly. In: Lifshitz F, ed. *Pediatric endocrinology*, 5th ed. New York, NY: Marcel Dekker Inc, 2006.

Huang SA, Fish SA, Dorfman DM, et al. A 21-year-old woman with consumptive hypothyroidism due to a vascular tumor expressing type 3 iodothyronine deiodinase. *J Clin Endocrinol Metab* 2002;87:4457.

Hung W, Anderson KD, Chandra RS, et al. Solitary thyroid nodules in 71 children and adolescents. *J Pediatr Surg* 1992;27:1407.

Hung W, August GP, Randolph JG, et al. Solitary thyroid nodules in children and adolescents. *J Pediatr Surg* 1982;17:225.

Hung W, Sarlis NJ. Autoimmune and non-autoimmune hyperthyroidism in pediatric patients: a review and personal commentary on management. *Ped Endo Rev* 2004;2:21.

Jannini EA, Ulisse S, D'Armiento M. Macroorchidism in juvenile hypothyroidism. *J Clin Endocrinol Metab* 1995;80:2543.

Kay C, Abrahams S, McClain P. The weight of normal thyroid glands in children. *Arch Pathol* 1966;82:349.

Khurana KK, Labrador E, Izquierdo R, et al. The role of fine-needle aspiration biopsy in the management of thyroid nodules in children, adolescents, and young adults: a multi-institutional study. *Thyroid* 1999;9:383.

Klein I, Becker DV, Levey GS. Treatment of hyperthyroid disease. *Ann Intern Med* 1994;121:281.

Lafferty AR, Batch JA. Thyroid nodules in childhood and adolescence–thirty years of experience. *J Pediatr Endocrinol Metab* 1997;10:479.

Lafranchi S. Thyroiditis and acquired hypothyroidism. *Pediatr Ann* 1992;21:29.

Lafranchi SHC. Graves' disease in the neonatal period and childhood. In: Braverman LE, ed. *Werner and Ingbar's the thyroid. A fundamental and clinical text*. Philadelphia: Lippincott Williams & Wilkins, 2005.

Larsen PR. Hypothyroidisim and thyroiditis. In: Larsen PR, Melmed S, Polonsky KS, eds. *Williams textbook of endocrinology*. Philadelphia: WB Saunders, 2003.

Larsen PR, Davies TF. Hypothyroidism and thyroiditis. In: Larsen PR, Kronenberg HM, Melmed S, et al. eds. *Williams textbook of endocrinology*. Philadelphia: WB Saunders, 2003.

Larsen PR, Hay ID. The thyroid gland. In: Foster DW, Wilson JD, Kronenberg HM, et al. eds. *Williams textbook of endocrinology*. Philadelphia: WB Saunders, 1998.

Laurberg P, Nygaard B, Glinoer D, et al. Guidelines for TSH-receptor antibody measurements in pregnancy: results of an evidence-based symposium organized by the European Thyroid Association. *Eur J Endocrinol* 1998;139:584.

Lavard L, Ranlov I, Perrild H, et al. Incidence of juvenile thyrotoxicosis in Denmark, 1982–1988. A nationwide study. *Eur J Endocrinol* 1994;130:565.

Lazar L, Kalter-Leibovici O, Pertzelan A, et al. Thyrotoxicosis in prepubertal children compared with pubertal and postpubertal patients. *J Clin Endocrinol Metab* 2000;85:3678.

Lucas A, Salinas I, Rius F, et al. Medical therapy of Graves' disease: does thyroxine prevent recurrence of hyperthyroidism? *J Clin Endocrinol Metab* 1997;82:2410.

Mandel SJ, Brent GA, Larsen PR. Levothyroxine therapy in patients with thyroid disease. *Ann Intern Med* 1993;119:492.

Marqusee E, Benson CB, Frates MC, et al. Usefulness of ultrasonography in the management of nodular thyroid disease. *Ann Intern Med* 2000;133:696.

Marqusee E, Haden ST, Utiger RD. Subclinical thyrotoxicosis. *Endocrinol Metab Clin North Am* 1998;27:37.

Mazzaferri EL. Management of a solitary thyroid nodule. *N Engl J Med* 1993;328:553.

McIver B, Rae P, Beckett G, et al. Lack of effect of thyroxine in patients with Graves' hyperthyroidism who are treated with an antithyroid drug. *N Engl J Med* 1996;334:220.

McKenzie JM, Zakarija M. Fetal and neonatal hyperthyroidism and hypothyroidism due to maternal TSH receptor antibodies. *Thyroid* 1992;2:155.

Mochizuki Y, Mowafy R, Pasternack B. Weights of human thyroids in New York City. *Health Phys* 1963;65:1299.

Moll GW Jr, Patel BR. Pediatric Graves' disease: therapeutic options and experience with radioiodine at the University of Mississippi Medical Center. *South Med J* 1997;90:1017.

Nikiforov Y, Gnepp DR, Fagin JA. Thyroid lesions in children and adolescents after the Chernobyl disaster: implications for the study of radiation tumorigenesis. *J Clin Endocrinol Metab* 1996;81:9.

Nordyke RA, Gilbert FI Jr, Miyamoto LA, et al. The superiority of antimicrosomal over antithyroglobulin antibodies for detecting Hashimoto's thyroiditis. *Arch Intern Med* 1993;153:862.

Pankow BG, Michalak J, McGee MK. Adult human thyroid weight. *Health Phys* 1985;49:1097.

Pearce EN. Diagnosis and management of thyrotoxicosis. *Br Med J* 2006;332:1369.

Pearce EN, Farwell AP, Braverman LE. Thyroiditis. *N Engl J Med* 2003;348:2646.

Rallison ML, Dobyns BM, Keating FR Jr, et al. Thyroid nodularity in children. *JAMA* 1975;233:1069.

Rallison ML, Dobyns BM, Meikle AW, et al. Natural history of thyroid abnormalities: prevalence, incidence, and regression of thyroid diseases in adolescents and young adults. *Am J Med* 1991;91:363.

Raza J, Hindmarsh PC, Brook CG. Thyrotoxicosis in children: thirty years' experience. *Acta Paediatr* 1999;88:937.

Read CH Jr., Tansey MJ, Menda Y. A 36-year retrospective analysis of the efficacy and safety of radioactive iodine in treating young Graves' patients. *J Clin Endocrinol Metab* 2004;89:4229.

Reid JR, Wheeler SF. Hyperthyroidism: diagnosis and treatment. *Am Fam Physician* 2005;72:623.

Rivkees SA, Sklar C, Freemark M. Clinical review 99: the management of Graves' disease in children, with special emphasis

on radioiodine treatment. *J Clin Endocrinol Metab* 1998;83:3767.

Sarlis NJ. *Thyroid binding globulin deficiency.* emedicine, September 2006.

Saravanan P, Dayan CM. Thyroid autoantibodies. *Endocrinol Metab Clin North Am* 2001;30:315.

Schlumberger M, Filetti S, Hay ID. Nontoxic goiter and thyroid neoplasia. In: Larsen PR, Kronenberg HM, Melmed S, et al. eds. *Williams textbook of endocrinology.* Philadelphia: WB Saunders, 2002.

Segni M, Leonardi E, Mazzoncini B, et al. Special features of Graves' disease in early childhood. *Thyroid* 1999;9:871.

Shulman DI, Muhar I, Jorgensen EV, et al. Autoimmune hyperthyroidism in prepubertal children and adolescents: comparison of clinical and biochemical features at diagnosis and responses to medical therapy. *Thyroid* 1997;7:755.

Silverman SH, Nussbaum M, Rausen AR. Thyroid nodules in children: a ten year experience at one institution. *Mt Sinai J Med* 1979;46:460.

Sklar CA, Qazi R, David R. Juvenile autoimmune thyroiditis. Hormonal status at presentation and after long-term followup. *Am J Dis Child* 1986;140:877.

Slyper AH, Swenerton P. Experience with low-dose replacement therapy in the initial management of severe pediatric acquired primary hypothyroidism. *J Pediatr Endocrinol Metab* 1998;11:543.

Sosa JA, Bowman HM, Tielsch JM, et al. The importance of surgeon experience for clinical and economic outcomes from thyroidectomy. *Ann Surg* 1998;228:320.

Surks MI, Sievert R. Drugs and thyroid function. *N Engl J Med* 1995;333:1688.

Trowbridge FL, Matovinovic J, McLaren GD, et al. Iodine and goiter in children. *Pediatrics* 1975;56:82.

Van Dop C, Conte FA, Koch TK, et al. Pseudotumor cerebri associated with initiation of levothyroxine therapy for juvenile hypothyroidism. *N Engl J Med* 1983;308:1076.

Waldhausen JH. Controversies related to the medical and surgical management of hyperthyroidism in children. *Semin Pediatr Surg* 1997;6:121–127.

Ward L, Huot C, Lambert R, et al. Outcome of pediatric Graves' disease after treatment with antithyroid medication and radioiodine. *Clin Invest Med* 1999;22:132.

Weetman AP. Graves' disease. *N Engl J Med* 2000;343:1236.

Wilson GR, Curry RW Jr. Subclinical thyroid disease. *Am Fam Physician* 2005;72:1517.

Wong GW, Lai J, Cheng PS. Growth in childhood thyrotoxicosis. *Eur J Pediatr* 1999;158:776.

Zakarija M, McKenzie JM. Pregnancy-associated changes in the thyroid-stimulating antibody of Graves' disease and the relationship to neonatal hyperthyroidism. *J Clin Endocrinol Metab* 1983;57:1036.

Zimmerman D, Lteif AN. Thyrotoxicosis in children. *Endocrinol Metab Clin North Am* 1998;27:109.

CHAPTER 10

Diabetes Mellitus

Donald P. Orr

Diabetes mellitus (DM) is a group of metabolic diseases characterized by hyperglycemia resulting from defects in insulin secretion, insulin action, or both. Chronic hyperglycemia is associated with long-term microvascular (retinopathy, nephropathy, and neuropathy) and accelerated macrovascular (coronary artery disease and stroke) complications. The direct and indirect costs of diabetes care in the United States were estimated at $132 billion in 2002; the medical conditions associated with diabetes among older adults account for a significant share of these costs.

If all adults with type 1 DM received intensive treatment with the goal of achieving normal glycemia, it is estimated they would gain approximately 7.7 additional years of sight, 5.8 additional years free from end-stage renal disease, and 5.6 additional years free from lower extremity amputation. Compared with conventionally treated patients (typically those receiving only two insulin injections), the average individual would gain 15.3 years of life free from any significant microvascular or neurological complications. Another computer simulation estimated that for 13- to 24-year olds diagnosed with type 1 DM, intensive therapy would increase life expectancy from 56.51 to 60.87 years. Intensive therapy would be cost-effective at $13,599 per discounted life-year and from $22,576 to $9,626 per discounted quality-adjusted life-year (Meltzer et al., 2000). Comparable clinical trials of intensified treatment for individuals with type 2 DM have demonstrated a significant reduction in risk for microvascular complications; the effect of strict glycemic control on macrovascular complications is less clear. Risk for these is reduced with intensive treatment of hypertension and dyslipidemia.

CLASSIFICATION AND ETIOLOGY

Classification of diabetes is based on the presumed etiology, rather than the mode of treatment (i.e., insulin vs. no insulin) (American Diabetes Association, 2005). The more common types of diabetes include the following (see Table 10.1 for characteristics of type 1, type 2, maturity-onset diabetes of youth [MODY], and atypical forms):

1. Type 1 DM is the result of beta-cell destruction, usually leading to absolute insulin deficiency. Adolescents are usually symptomatic at presentation and at risk for ketoacidosis.

   a. Immune mediation: Type 1 DM is linked to the major histocompatibility genes associated with diabetes, human leukocyte antigen DQ (Devendra et al., 2004). It is believed to be mediated by T cells that recognize beta-cell-specific antigens. The immune changes may be detected many months to years before the onset of diabetes. Multiple antibodies have been observed that are directed against islet cells (islet cell antibody [ICA]), insulin, glutamate decarboxylase (anti-GAD_{65}), receptor-linked tyrosine phosphatases (IA-2, IA-2_β); antibodies are present in 85% to 90% of children and adolescents at the time of diagnosis and persist for years. It appears that African-Americans may have a lower prevalence of these antibodies than whites. A later onset is associated with a longer duration of symptoms, higher serum C-peptide concentrations (more beta-cell reserve), and a lower frequency of ICA.

   b. Idiopathic: Nonimmune mediated diabetes is uncommon and appears to occur more frequently in adults of African or Asian descent. Atypical diabetes mellitus (ADM), once considered a subtype of MODY, has been identified in approximately 10% of African-Americans with youth-onset diabetes; it is also recognized among Asians. ADM presents clinically as acute-onset diabetes often associated with weight loss, ketosis, and even diabetic ketoacidosis (DKA) and requires insulin during the initial treatment. Approximately 50% of patients with ADM are obese. The specific defect(s) remains unknown (Sobngwi et al., 2002).

2. Type 2 DM may range from predominantly insulin resistance with relative insulin deficiency to a predominantly secretory defect that results in insulin resistance. It is characterized by decreased muscle glucose uptake, increased hepatic glucose production, impaired insulin secretion, and probable overproduction of free fatty acids by fat cells, which further stimulates gluconeogenesis, decreases postprandial hepatic glucose uptake, and may increase muscle insulin resistance, further impairing insulin secretion. Dyslipidemia, metabolic syndrome, and a family history of type 2 DM are common.

3. Other specific types are as follows:

   a. Specific genetic defects of beta-cell function have been identified.
   - MODY: MODY is associated with monogenetic defects in beta-cell function, impaired insulin

TABLE 10.1

Characteristics of the Common Types of Diabetes

	Type 1	Type 2	Atypical	Maturity-Onset Diabetes of Youth
Age	Childhood	Pubertal	Pubertal	Child, adolescent (usually age <25)
Onset	Acute; severe	Mild to severe; often insidious	Acute; severe	Mild; insidious
Insulin secretion	Very low	Variable	Moderately low	Variable
Insulin sensitivity	Normal	Decreased	Normal	Normal
Insulin dependence	Permanent	No, until late	Variable	Usually no, until late
Racial/ethnic groups at increased risk	All (low in Asians)	African-Americans, Hispanic-Americans, Native Americans	African-Americans	All
Genetics	Polygenic	Polygenic	Presumed autosomal dominant	Autosomal dominant
Proportion of those with diabetes	10%–20%	~80%	5%–10%	Rare
Association with: Obesity	No	Strong	Variable	No
Acanthosis nigricans	No	Yes	No	No
Autoimmune etiology	Yes (small subset non autoimmune type)	No	No	No

From Rosenbloom AL, Joe JR, Young RS, et al. Emerging epidemic of type 2 diabetes in youth. *Diabetes Care* 1999;22:345, with permission.

secretion with minimal or no defects in insulin action, autosomal dominant inheritance, and onset usually before the age of 25 years (Fajans et al., 2001).

Classic MODY is seen predominantly in nonobese whites, is nonketotic, and is generally not insulin-requiring at diagnosis. It represents <5% of cases of childhood diabetes in whites. It is seen in all racial/ethnic groups. Six specific types have been identified with varying levels of insulin deficiency.

- Mitochondrial DNA: This very rare form of diabetes is a characterized by specific genetic defect and is almost always associated with other symptoms—deafness, neurological disorders, cardiac failure, renal failure, and myopathy. The mutations may be sporadic or maternally inherited.

b. Various genetic defects of insulin action are known. These include type A insulin resistance, leprechaunism, Rabson-Mendenhall syndrome, lipoatrophic diabetes, and others.

4. Diseases of the exocrine pancreas leading to destruction of endocrine function are:

a. Cystic fibrosis: Cystic fibrosis-related diabetes (CFRD) is common among adolescents and young adults with cystic fibrosis with increasing prevalence with age. In one large U.S. study, more than 40% of patients older than 30 years were identified with CFRD (Moran et al., 1998). It is more common among women and those with ΔF508 genotype. CFRD is associated with decreased pulmonary function, protein

catabolism and loss of weight. It results primarily from insulinopenia, although insulin resistance may be observed during periods of infection. Insulin resistance may be severe during steroid treatments for pulmonary inflammation. Insulin treatment is associated with increased body weight and improvement in pulmonary function.

b. Others: Pancreatitis, trauma/pancreatectomy, neoplasia, hemochromatosis, fibrocalculous pancreatopathy.

5. Endocrinopathies including acromegaly, Cushing syndrome, hyperthyroidism, and pheochromocytoma.

6. Drugs including glucocorticoids, pentamidine, protease inhibitors, thyroid hormone, diazoxide and thiazides.

7. Genetic syndromes sometimes associated with diabetes are Down syndrome, Klinefelter syndrome, Turner syndrome, Wolfram syndrome, Friedreich ataxia, Huntington chorea, Laurence-Moon syndrome, myotonic dystrophy, and Prader-Willi syndrome.

8. Gestational diabetes mellitus (GDM). The risk for subsequent development of diabetes is elevated; approximately 17% develop type 1 DM and 17% to 70% develop type 2 DM.

EPIDEMIOLOGY

1. Prevalence

a. Type 1 DM: The prevalence of type 1 DM varies by race/ethnicity and country, with the highest rates in areas most distant from the equator. It is estimated that there are more than 500,000 individuals in the United States with type 1 DM. The prevalence is approximately 1.7 per 1,000 persons younger than 19 years. The incidence is increasing by 3% to 4% annually worldwide. The increase is greatest among younger patients; the ages of peak incidence in the United States remain late childhood and early-to-mid adolescence (Gale, 2002).

   b. Type 2 DM: There has been a steady worldwide increase in the prevalence of type 2 DM. By 2030, the total number of people with diabetes is projected to increase worldwide by 30.3% to 366 million. Type 2 DM accounts for up to 20% of the diabetes cases diagnosed in children and adolescents in some large diabetes centers (Bloomgarden, 2004).
   - Racial distribution: Within the United States, African-Americans have a twofold increased risk; Hispanics, a 2.5-fold increase; and Native Americans, a fivefold increase compared with whites.
   - Gender: The risk is slightly higher for females and those living in poverty, probably secondary to the added risk of obesity.
   - Family history: More than 40% of the children of parents with type 2 DM have a lifetime risk of developing type 2 DM.

2. Emergence of diabetes during adolescence, and glycemic control
   - Insulin sensitivity decreases significantly at sexual maturity rating (SMR) 2, remains constant from SMR 2 through 4, and returns almost to prepubertal levels by SMR 5.
   - Girls and African-Americans are more insulin resistant; this is only partially explained by higher body mass index (BMI). The decreased sensitivity to insulin is not explained by sex steroids and is presumed to be associated with peripheral effects of growth hormone (Amiel et al., 1986; Moran et al., 1999).

- Obesity has increased, with an estimated 16.7% of boys and 15.4% of girls aged 12 to 19 years as overweight (BMI above the 95th percentile). The prevalence of obesity is higher among minority youths and poor populations. Children and adolescents are more sedentary.
- A recent large study demonstrated that more than 14% of moderately obese (average BMI 33.4) and 20% of severely obese (average BMI 40.6) children and adolescents had impaired glucose tolerance (IGT) and 39% and 50% respectively had metabolic syndrome. Metabolic syndrome increased with increasing insulin resistance; it was somewhat less common among African-Americans (Weiss et al., 2004). IGT is a significant risk factor for type 2 DM.

DIAGNOSIS

The level of fasting plasma glucose (FPG) has been recommended for screening and diagnosing DM in most circumstances (Table 10.2). This has replaced the traditional oral glucose tolerance test (OGTT) because it is cumbersome and costly, underutilized, and the repeated test reproducibility of the 2-hour postprandial glucose (PG) level is worse than that of the FPG. Hemoglobin A_{Ic} (HbA$_{Ic}$) (a specific glycated protein) is not recommended for the diagnosis of diabetes. Impaired fasting glucose (IFG) level and IGT results are now considered to indicate prediabetes, but are not, of themselves, diagnostic of diabetes. These groups are at increased risk for developing diabetes and the test should be repeated in 3 months.

- FPG $\leq$100 mg/dL (5.6 mmol/L): normal fasting glucose
- FPG 100 to 125 mg/dL (5.6–6.9 mmol/L): IFG, prediabetes
- 2-hour postload glucose 140 to 199 mg/dL (7.8–11.1 mmol/L): IGT, prediabetes
- FPG $\geq$126 mg/dL (7.0 mmol/L): provisional diagnosis of diabetes (the diagnosis must be confirmed, as described in subsequent text).

TABLE 10.2

American Diabetes Association, 2005, Criteria for the Diagnosis of Diabetes Mellitus

1. Symptoms of diabetes plus casual plasma glucose concentration $\geq$200 mg/dL (11.1 mmol/L); casual is defined as any time or day without regard to time since last meal
   Or
2. FPG $\geq$126 mg/dL (7.0 mmol/L); fasting is defined as no caloric intake for at least 8 hr
   Or
3. 2-hr PG $\geq$200 mg/dL (11.1 mmol/L) during an OGTT; the test should be performed as described by the World Health Organization using a glucose load containing the equivalent of 75 g anhydrous glucose dissolved in water

In the absence of acute metabolic decompensation, these criteria should be confirmed by repeated testing on a different day
The third measure (OGTT) is not recommended for routine clinical use

FPG, fasting plasma glucose; PG, postprandial glucose; OGTT, oral glucose tolerance test.
From The Expert Committee on the Diagnosis and Classification of Diabetes Mellitus. Report of the expert committee on the diagnosis and classification of diabetes mellitus. *Diabetes Care* 2005; 28(Suppl 1):S37, with permission.

SCREENING

1. Type 1 DM: No screening is recommended.
2. Type 2 DM
   a. Screen with FPG testing every other year, starting at 10 years or at onset of puberty, if puberty occurs at a younger age.
   b. Screen
      - Overweight patients (those with a BMI above the 85th percentile for age and sex, those with weight for height above the 85th percentile, or weight of >120% of ideal for height weight) plus
      - Those who have any two of the following risk factors:
         Family history of type 2 DM in first- or second-degree relative
         Race/ethnicity: Native American, African-American, Hispanic, Asian/Pacific Islander
         Signs of insulin resistance or conditions associated with insulin resistance, such as acanthosis nigricans, hypertension, dyslipidemia, and polycystic ovary syndrome

PREVENTION

1. Type 1 DM: There is no effective prevention at this time.
2. Type 2 DM: Several studies of adults with IGT have shown that lifestyle changes (intensive physical activity, reduced intake of carbohydrates and weight loss if indicated) reduce the risk for progression to diabetes by approximately 60%; metformin in combination with standard recommendations for diet and exercise decreased the risk by 31% (Knowler et al., 2002; Tuomilehto et al., 2001).

EVALUATION AND TREATMENT

The initial use of insulin in an adolescent newly diagnosed with diabetes does not commit to extended use if the clinical course suggests type 2 (obese, strong family history of type 2 DM, absence of ketonemia with insulin omission) or MODY. At initial presentation, the state of hydration and acid–base balance determine the need for fluids and insulin. (See any standard textbook of medicine, pediatrics, and endocrinology for treatment of DKA.) It is important to determine the type of diabetes to the extent possible because the underlying diagnosis will guide the management. Measurement of autoantibodies may be useful if the etiology is unclear; for example, obese African-Americans with ketonemia in whom ATM is suspected. If type 1 DM is diagnosed, measurement of thyroid hormone levels is indicated because of associated thyroiditis in 10% to 15% of patients. Type 2 DM usually has an insidious presentation and is suggested by obesity, acanthosis, hypertension, dyslipidemia, or strong family history of type 2 DM. Normal weight and mild symptoms suggest very early type 1 DM or MODY.

1. Education: In addition to the recommended information about diabetes, blood glucose (BG) testing, hypoglycemia, hyperglycemia, and insulin administration, education and periodic education by a certified diabetes educator should include information about alcohol use, use of contraception, and the importance of preconception counseling to decrease risk for pregnancy complications. (See the "Web Sites" section at the end of this chapter for help in identifying an educator.)
2. Meals, food, and nutrition: There is no standard American Diabetes Association (ADA) meal plan; rather, diet is adjusted for the individual to provide sufficient calories and nutrients to grow/maintain weight; limiting fat to 30% or less of total calories is encouraged. Weight reduction and exercise are important for those who are overweight, particularly if they have type 2 DM. "Carbohydrate counting" is replacing the "exchange system" because it permits greater flexibility and offers the potential for adjusting the dose of short-acting and rapid-acting insulin before each meal on the basis of the amount of carbohydrate consumed at each meal. In this system, 15 g of carbohydrate is equivalent to one carbohydrate. This is estimated from package labels that list the carbohydrate content per serving and standard servings of milk (1 cup), fruit, juice (1/2 cup), and starch/bread; vegetables or meat (approximately one third carbohydrate per serving) may or may not be counted depending on the degree of glycemic control targeted. Fast-food carbohydrate counting guides are available from major fast-food companies, often through their corporate Web sites.
3. Accessing glycemic control: The goal is to lower BG level, and resultant HbA_{Ic} to achieve maximum prevention of complications, taking into account patient safety and the ability to carry out the treatment regimen. Although normal levels of BG are the goal (70–120 mg/dL before meals and fasting), most patients (adult and adolescent) are not able to achieve consistently *normal* levels of glycated hemoglobin. Any lowering of glycated hemoglobin will reduce the risks of long-term complications.
   a. Capillary BG testing—testing is recommended before meals and bedtime snack—more frequent if "normal" BG levels are the objective. Testing at 2 to 3 a.m. is useful for evaluating nighttime hypoglycemia and fasting hyperglycemia (the dawn phenomenon). The recommended frequency of testing for type 2 DM is not well defined, but daily fasting blood glucose (FBG) and a random premeal BG test should be sufficient once effective control has been achieved. Devices to measure capillary BG must demonstrate that 95% of the tests are within 10% to 15% of the true BG value. They are usually calibrated to plasma glucose, which is higher than whole BG (see the "Web Sites" section).
   b. Glycated hemoglobin should be measured at each visit (generally quarterly) and the results discussed with the adolescent and parent in relation to BG test results. Glycated hemoglobin values reflect the average BG over the previous 8 to 12 weeks, so BG records must also be examined to identify swings in BG that would not be evident in the percentage of glycated hemoglobin. Several different assays are available, each with its own reference (nondiabetic) range. It has been suggested that all glycated hemoglobin assays be standardized and reported in values equivalent to HbA_{Ic} (which was used in the Diabetes Control and Complications Trial [DCCT]). Point-of-care testing for HbA_{Ic} is available. Having the results of the glycated hemoglobin level available at the time of the visit has been shown to result

in significantly improved control among adults. Discussing the results at the next visit or by telephone is less satisfactory. On the basis of the DCCT HbA$_{Ic}$ values, the target HbA$_{Ic}$ level is $\leq$7%. The need for an individualized approach to insulin therapy in patients with diabetes is important. In addition, certain subgroups of patients with the diagnosis can be differentiated from each other according to the pattern of BGs over the course of a day, as has been recently reviewed (Mooradian et al., 2006). Examples of these patterns include: "round-the-clock" hyperglycemia, fasting hyperglycemia and daytime euglycemia; and daytime hyperglycemia with fasting euglycemia.

4. Insulin: Human insulins (DNA origins) have almost entirely replaced older animal preparations. Insulin analogs in which one or more amino acids have been substituted on the α chain or β chain afford more specific patterns of release. Rapid-acting preparations include lispro (Humalog), aspart (NovoLog) and glulisine (Apidra). They have a more rapid onset and shorter duration of action; they may be given before or immediately after meals, affording less immediate postprandial hyperglycemia and subsequent hypoglycemia. Two extended acting analogs are available; glargine (Lantus) and detemir (Levemir) have an onset of 2 to 4 hours. Glargine provides a peakless duration of >24 hours while detemir has a somewhat shorter duration of 12 to 20 hours and may require twice daily administration. Neither *should be mixed* with other insulin preparations (Table 10.3).
   a. Insulin delivery devices: Many different devices are available, allowing adolescents to manage their diabetes more easily (see the "Web Sites" section).
   b. Insulin syringes: These are available in 0.3-, 0.5-, and 1.0-mL sizes with needles of 28, 29, or 30 gauge and 8.0- or 12.7-mm length. Adolescents usually prefer one type over another.
   c. Insulin pens: These are disposable devices that are prefilled or hold cartridges of 300 units of short-acting, rapid-acting, Neutral Protamine Hagedorn (NPH), 70/30 (70% NPH/30% regular), 75/25 (75% NPH/25% lispro or aspart), and glargine insulins. These devices are approximately the size of a large fountain pen and can be carried easily in a purse or shirt pocket. Disposable needles (29, 30, and 31 gauge, and 12.7, 8, 6, and 5 mm) must be prescribed separately. Pens and insulin cartridges from different manufacturers are not always interchangeable.
   d. Continuous subcutaneous insulin infusion (CSII) (external insulin pumps): These permit ultimate flexibility in designing an insulin regimen, compensating for exercise, variations in carbohydrate intake including delayed meals and the dawn phenomenon. They are particularly useful for individuals who experience severe, recurrent nocturnal hypoglycemia and erratic day-to-day schedules with respect to meal times and exercise. Multiple basal insulin rates can be preprogrammed. The patient must determine the amount of insulin to be delivered for each mealtime or corrective bolus, and instruct the pump to deliver this amount at the correct time. Some systems contain an integrated BG meter and can be programmed to calculate bolus insulin doses based on carbohydrate consumed and level of BG. Candidates for pumps are very motivated, test at least four times daily (and often include 2 to 3 a.m. testing when required), actively monitor carbohydrate intake, adjust insulin doses with each meal and snack, and have frequent contact with the diabetes team. Individuals with serious psychological problems are generally poor candidates for pump therapy. Several studies have demonstrated improved glycemic control among adolescents and adults who desire more intensive diabetes, who are randomly assigned to insulin pumps compared to MDI regimens. Adolescents who wish to use CSII should be referred to a diabetes team experienced with CSII and adolescents (see the "Web Sites" section).
   e. Inhaled insulin: In combination with injected long-acting insulin, inhaled insulin has been demonstrated in phase 3 clinical efficacy trials to be safe and as effective in controlling BG as rapid-acting injectable insulin (Hollander et al., 2004; Quattrin et al., 2004; Rave et al., 2005). This agent is Food and Drug Administration (FDA) approved. It may be useful for individuals with type 2 DM who have difficulty administering rapid-acting insulin by injection.

5. Treatment of patients who require insulin: Insulin therapy is always necessary for type 1 DM, and for those with insulin deficiency. Although insulin remains the recommended pharmacologic treatment for GDM, several studies have demonstrated that among those not controlled by diet, glyburide is safe and as effective as insulin (Saade, 2005).

TABLE 10.3

Characteristics of Human Insulin Preparations

Informal Description	Proprietary or Other Name	Onset (hr)	Peak (hr)	Effective Duration (hr)	Maximum Duration (hr)	Technical Description
Rapid acting	Lispro, aspart, glulisine	0.25	1–2	2–3	4	Insulin analog
Short acting	Regular	0.5–1.0	2–3	3–6	4–6	Insulin
Intermediate acting	Neutral protamine hagedorn (NPH)	2–4	4–10	10–16	14–18	Insulin isophane (suspension)
Long acting	Detemir	1–2	8–11	12–20	14–22	
	Glargine	2–4	None	>24	24–36	Analog

Adapted from Orr DP. Contemporary management of adolescents with diabetes mellitus. Part 2: type 2 diabetes. *Adolesc Health Update* 2000;12(3):3, with permission.

a. Insulin regimens—MDIs of insulin are preferred. The greater number of injections (three or more) offers more flexibility to accommodate varied intake, exercise, and meal times, and has the potential for improved glycemic control. Simply adding prelunch short- or rapid-acting insulin to a standard twice-daily insulin regimen will decrease presupper hyperglycemia, with less risk of hypoglycemia associated with a very large prebreakfast dose of intermediate-acting insulin. With the exception of a bedtime snack to prevent nocturnal hypoglycemia, snacks usually are no longer required with MDI—an advantage for busy adolescents and those who wish to maintain a target weight.

b. Contemporary MDI insulin regimens are based on the use of a longer acting insulin (e.g., glargine or detemir) to provide *basal* insulin requirements (suppression of hepatic glucose production in the fasting state) and premeal *boluses* of rapid-acting insulin to cover the amount of carbohydrate consumed (food dose) and to correct for fluctuations in premeal BG (corrective dose). Descriptions of traditional twice-daily split-mixed insulin regimens using rapid- and intermediate-acting insulins can be found in standard textbooks dealing with diabetes.

BOLUS INSULIN DOSE = FOOD DOSE + CORRECTIVE DOSE

- Food dose to cover carbohydrates at meal or snack
  - One unit of short- or rapid-acting insulin will usually "cover" approximately 8 to 15 g of carbohydrate (carbohydrate to insulin ratio of 8 to 15), meaning that one unit of rapid-acting insulin will be required for each 8 to 15 gm of carbohydrate consumed.
  - To estimate the grams of carbohydrate covered by one unit of short- or rapid-acting insulin use the rule of 450/500 = (450 for short-acting or 500 for rapid-acting insulin)/total daily dose (TDD) of all insulins in 24 hours. Note that if the patient is poorly controlled and TDD is >1.4 U/kg, reduce by 20%.
  - Food dose = grams of carbohydrate consumed/carbohydrate to insulin ratio
- Corrective dose—adjusting the dose of short- or rapid-acting insulin administered before meals takes into account the fact that BG varies from day to day depending on carbohydrate intake at previous meals, the time that previous dose was administered, the amount of interval exercise, and the rate of insulin absorption from subcutaneous tissues. The corrective dose of insulin is added to the food dose and administered before or after that meal. The corrective dose may also be used to correct for hyperglycemia at other times of the day, independent of meals.
  - One unit of rapid- or short-acting insulin will usually lower BG 25 to 100 mg/dL depending on the individual's sensitivity to insulin (insulin sensitivity factor)
  - The rule of 1,500/1,800 may be used to estimate more closely the initial "insulin sensitivity factor" (the estimated point drop in BG per unit of short- or rapid-acting insulin) used for the corrective dose:

The sensitivity factor = (1,500/TDD for short-acting insulin) and (1,800/TDD for rapid-acting insulin) (ADA, 2005)
- Corrective dose = (measured BG—target BG)/insulin sensitivity factor

BASAL INSULIN DOSE

- Basal insulin dose = Approximately 40% to 50% of TDD on previous insulin regimen.
- Administer 40% to 45% of TDD as glargine insulin as single injection once daily or detemir as twice daily injections before breakfast and at bedtime.
- The following is an example to change from twice-daily insulin dosing to multiple dosing for a 15-year-old girl weighing 50 kg and using rapid-acting insulin (current TDD = 50 units of insulin):
  (1) Basal insulin: 20 units of glargine with breakfast, dinner, or bedtime (40% of previous TDD)
  (2) "Insulin sensitivity factor": 1,800/50 = 36-mg drop per unit of rapid-acting insulin.
  (3) Target BG = 120 mg/dL
  (4) Carbohydrate covered by one unit of insulin from the rule of 450/5,000: 450 for rapid-acting insulin/TDD = 450/50 = 9 g of carbohydrate per unit of rapid-acting insulin.
  (5) Bolus insulin doses = (grams of carbohydrate eaten/carbohydrate to insulin ratio) + (BG–target BG)/insulin sensitivity factor.
  (6) For example, to calculate a premeal bolus insulin dose from previous description: if premeal BG = 250 mg/dL and 60 g carbohydrate consumed bolus rapid-acting dose = 60 g of carbohydrate/9 + (250–120)/36 = approximately 10 units of rapid-acting insulin.

Insulin doses are adjusted after 5 to 7 days on the basis of the pattern of BG levels.

6. Treatment of type 2 DM and MODY: Treatment should be based on the known pathophysiology—insulin resistance, hepatic overproduction of glucose, and relative insulin deficiency.

a. Acute management of newly diagnosed symptomatic patients: Individuals who are ketotic and those with significant hyperglycemia at diagnosis (BG >250 mg/dL) will initially require insulin therapy to reduce BG levels. Several studies of adults and adolescents have demonstrated that several months of intensive treatment with insulin results in improved glycemic control 1 year later. Metformin therapy, an insulin-sensitizing agent, is generally begun when the patient is no longer ketotic. Insulin can be slowly withdrawn over the subsequent 3 to 4 months as glycemic control is achieved. Although type 2 DM is a progressive disease that will eventually require exogenous insulin, modifications in diet and exercise are the mainstay of treatment.

b. Patients with insidious onset and mild hyperglycemia can be initially managed with diet and exercise as described in following text.
  - Diet: Carbohydrates should be distributed throughout the day to include snacks. Limiting the amount of carbohydrate takes into account the inherently abnormal insulin secretory pattern. Weight loss will increase insulin sensitivity because it reduces visceral adipose tissue. The effect of carbohydrate restriction (as part of

total caloric reduction) may be seen within 4 days, with a reduction in postprandial BG. The effects of weight loss may take months and will be reflected in lower FBG levels and resultant decreased HbA$_{Ic}$. Studies of obese adults with type 2 DM suggest that an FBG of <180 mg/dL after individuals have lost 2.3 kg has a 62% positive predictive value that diet therapy will be effective in achieving control; the positive predictive value is 79% after 4.5 kg has been lost (Watts et al., 1991).

- Exercise: Exercise will increase insulin sensitivity independent of weight loss. At least 20 to 30 minutes of anaerobic activity at least three times per week is recommended. Vigorous walking is an acceptable introductory activity for the sedentary patient.
- Oral hypoglycemic therapy: Failure to see improvement in FBG (HbA$_{Ic}$≤8%) in the face of substantial weight loss or after 3 months suggests that diet and exercise alone will be insufficient to achieve satisfactory control. Initiate oral hypoglycemic agent or insulin therapy. Approximately 25% of adults will achieve an HbA$_{Ic}$≤8% on monotherapy, 50% will see a partial response, and 25% will fail to respond to a single oral agent. Insulin remains the recommended option for treatment of diabetes during pregnancy in the United States. However, several large studies have demonstrated that glyburide is safe and effective for the treatment of GDM. Referral to a high-risk obstetrical program is indicated.

Oral hypoglycemic agents will generally be required at some point in the treatment of type 2 DM. Many agents are available. Each group targets different metabolic components—insulin secretory defect, elevated hepatic glucose output, and insulin resistance. Key points include the following: The response to oral agents follows a sigmoid curve, with a rapid rise in therapeutic activity, leveling off, and then gradual tapering to maximal therapeutic effect; half the maximal dose yields more than half the maximal effect (60%–80%); and side effects increase slowly at low doses and then more rapidly at higher doses.

- Biguanide (metformin) is the first-line oral hypoglycemic agent for obese adolescents (and those who are unable to achieve acceptable glycemic control with diet and exercise) because it is not associated with weight gain. It lowers FBG, by reducing hepatic glucose output and improves lipid profiles, with a reduction in total cholesterol, low density lipoprotein cholesterol (LDL-C), and triglycerides, as well as an increase in high density lipoprotein cholesterol (HDL-C). The major side effects are mild gastrointestinal (GI) symptoms that generally resolve; side effects may be minimized by increasing the dose slowly. Hypoglycemia is uncommon, and lactic acidosis, a potentially serious condition associated with the predecessor biguanide (phenformin), is extremely rare with the only available agent in this class, *metformin*. Discontinue and ensure adequate hydration before contrast studies that may impair renal function and with dehydration.
- Sulfonylurea (SU) drugs and the related meglitinides (*repaglinide* and *netaglinide*) enhance insulin release from the beta cell and may decrease insulin resistance. Use is often associated with weight gain, which tends to further increase insulin resistance. Potential interactions

with sulfonamides, fluconazole, and ciprofloxacin may result in hypoglycemia. SU drugs generally may be given as a single morning dose. The meglitinides also enhance insulin secretion but operates through a mechanism different from that of SU drugs; they must be administered before each meal.

- Glucosidase inhibitors delay the absorption of carbohydrate from the intestine, reducing the rise in BG levels after a meal. They are most useful when employed in conjunction with other hypoglycemic agents to assist in managing postprandial hyperglycemia. They are not associated with weight gain or hypoglycemia. They must be given before each meal, not exceeding three times per day. Slowly increasing the dose tends to decrease the common GI symptoms (e.g., crampy abdominal pain, loose stools, and flatus).
- Thiazolidinediones ("insulin sensitizers") increase insulin action in muscle, adipose tissue, and probably in the liver. The newer thiazolidinediones (pioglitazone and rosiglitazone) do not appear to be associated with serious hepatotoxicity noted with the predecessor troglitazone. Neither is approved for use in patients younger than 16 years. Thiazolidinediones alone or combined with metformin have demonstrated to increase levels of HDL-C and to decrease levels of free fatty acids with variable effects on levels of triglycerides. Rosiglitazone has been shown to increase levels of LDL-C. Liver enzymes must be periodically monitored. These agents do not represent the initial pharmacotherapeutic agent for adolescents with type 2 DM.

Consider combining oral agents or adding insulin when a single medication has not achieved the desired degree of control. Combining agents takes advantage of their additive effects because each operates through different physiological mechanisms, is generally associated with fewer side effects, and has a lower cost (if doses are lower). When combining oral agents, increase the dose of the first drug until maximum dose has been reached or side effects limit further increases. Add the second medication at the lowest dose and increase slowly, watching out for hypoglycemia. If target levels of BG have not been achieved in 4 to 6 months, the addition of insulin is indicated. Some clinicians would choose to add insulin instead of a second oral agent.

Insulin may be used as a single nighttime dose of an intermediate-acting NPH or single dose of long-acting glargine at any time of day (to lower FBG) or in divided doses as with type 1 DM. Adding a single dose to an oral regimen is advantageous because lower doses of insulin and the oral agent may be used. Begin with a single dose of intermediate-acting insulin with the bedtime snack or long-acting insulin at dinner. An initial dose of 5 to 10 units is safe. Increase the dose until the desired level of FBG is achieved. Adolescents who have a large carbohydrate intake at dinner may benefit from the addition of regular or rapid-acting insulin with this meal; this dose of short-acting insulin is adjusted based on bedtime BG levels.

COMPLICATIONS, ASSOCIATED CONDITIONS, AND FOLLOW-UP CARE

1. Autoimmune disorders (type 1 DM only): Approximately 10% to 15% of patients with type 1 DM develop autoimmune thyroiditis. Initial antithyroid antibody levels

do not predict subsequent involvement. Because presentation is usually asymptomatic, annual thyroid studies to detect hypothyroidism are recommended; thyroid-stimulating hormone is generally sufficient. Other autoimmune diseases affecting the adrenal, pituitary, ovary, or parathyroid are uncommon.

2. Microvascular complications: Microvascular complications are directly correlated with the level of glycemic control and duration of diabetes and are exacerbated by hypertension.
   a. Retinopathy: A yearly dilated funduscopic examination is recommended.
   b. Nephropathy: Annual screening for urinary albumin is recommended. The level of random urinary microalbumin: creatinine ratio is highly correlated with timed specimens. Meticulous attention to blood pressure (BP) is important (both systolic and diastolic); attempt to maintain BP ≤130/80 mm Hg. Angiotensin-converting enzyme (ACE) inhibitors or angiotensin receptor antagonists and improved control represent the treatments for persistent microalbuminuria because they have been shown to delay the progression of nephropathy.
   c. Neuropathy: Neuropathy is rarely symptomatic during adolescence. Examination of the feet for pulses, sensation, deep tendon reflexes, hygiene, calluses, and evidence of infection is indicated. The Semmes-Weinstein monofilament test for sensation is a rapid, sensitive screening test for distal sensory neuropathy. Painful distal neuropathy occurs uncommonly in this age-group. Desipramine and amitriptyline are equally effective treatments (Max et al., 1992). Gabapentin is effective, but more expensive and may be considered as an alternative treatment (Backonja, 1999; Morello et al., 1999).
   Symptomatic autonomic neuropathy (heart rate invariability and/or postural hypotension) and gastroparesis (postprandial nausea or vomiting, postprandial hypoglycemia, and diarrhea or constipation) are very rare in this age-group.

3. Macrovascular complications: Macrovascular complications are rarely symptomatic during adolescence and young adulthood. Diabetes-associated accelerated cardiovascular disease may not be preventable with improved glycemic control, although the risk is decreased with tight control of hypertension and hyperlipidemia (Turner et al., 1998; UK Prospective Diabetes Study Group, 1998).

4. Dyslipidemia: Dyslipidemia is common in type 2 DM and in poorly controlled type 1 DM. It increases the risk for cardiovascular disease twofold to fourfold and reflects various degrees of insulin resistance, obesity, diet, and poor glycemic control. The typical pattern is elevated triglycerides and decreased HDL-C. Although all hypoglycemic agents used in adolescents tend to lower triglycerides and LDL-C, if LDL-C levels of <100 mg/dL have not been attained with better glycemic control, weight loss (if indicated), and reduced intake of saturated fat, treatment with lipid-lowering medications is indicated. New-generation "statin" drugs are generally preferred. Yearly measurement of fasting lipid profiles is recommended among those with previously abnormal profiles or ongoing poor glycemic control. Measurement every 5 years is sufficient if initial LDL-C is <100 mg/dL (American Diabetes Association, 2005).

5. Hypertension: Hypertension, even with mild elevations, (>130/80 mm Hg) is associated with an increased risk of microvascular complications. The appearance often coincides with the onset of persistent microalbuminuria. ACE inhibitors/receptor antagonists are the drugs of choice.

6. Gluten sensitivity: Gluten sensitivity is estimated to be present in 5% of individuals with type 1 DM. The benefit of universal screening of all individuals with type 1 DM is not established. Evaluate with Ig-A antiendomysial or Ig-A antitissue transglutamase antibodies if symptoms are suggestive of malabsorption or unexplained postprandial hypoglycemia.

7. Eating disorders: Eating disorders may complicate treatment of diabetes. Disordered eating (including underdosing or omission of insulin) may be present in up to 30% of women with type 1 DM, but the prevalence of eating disorders mentioned in *Diagnostic and Statistical Manual of Mental Disorders, fourth edition* is probably not higher than expected. The coexistence of eating disorders and diabetes is associated with noncompliance with treatment for diabetes and an increased risk of retinopathy (Rydall et al., 1997). Suspect eating disorders when the HbA$_{1c}$ is high and weight loss or excess concerns about weight are present.

8. Hypoglycemia: Severe hypoglycemia is common with intensified regimens targeting euglycemia. An episode of severe hypoglycemia increases the risk for additional hypoglycemia because it is associated with a reduced magnitude of autonomic and neuroglycopenic symptoms, counterregulatory hormone responses, and cognitive dysfunction during subsequent hypoglycemia. These return to normal with strict avoidance of hypoglycemia.

9. Alcohol use: As with healthy adult populations, moderate alcohol use among individuals with older-onset diabetes (older than 30 years) has been shown to reduce the risk of coronary heart disease-related death (Valmadrid et al., 2000). Alcohol use is not recommended for minor adolescents including those with diabetes. For those who do drink, provide education about its potential to cause hypoglycemia. Alcohol tends to inhibit gluconeogenesis and interfere with the counterregulatory responses to insulin-induced hypoglycemia. It also impairs judgment. Severe hypoglycemia may result many hours after consumption of as little as 2 oz of alcohol, particularly on an empty stomach. Anticipatory guidance should include moderation, eating additional carbohydrates at the time of alcohol consumption, and informing others that they have diabetes.

SPECIAL CONSIDERATIONS FOR COMPLIANCE WITH ADOLESCENTS

Managing teens with DM can be difficult, particularly for those with poorly controlled DM. Some suggestions include the following:

1. Identify the reason for poor control and develop a strategy for remediation. Serious psychopathology (including eating disorders) and recurrent DKA are indications for referral.
2. Identify one reasonable and measurable target behavior for action (number of BG tests, recording carbohydrates at a specific meal, self-insulin adjustment based on BG or carbohydrate intake).

3. Identify short-term reinforcers relevant to the adolescent—fewer symptoms (hypoglycemia or nocturia), improved physical performance, more flexibility in timing and content of meals, rewards from parents, and greater independence.
4. Establish realistic time frame for accomplishment based on behavior and goal (e.g., average FBG will be 20% lower over the next 2 weeks). Remember glycated hemoglobin levels reflect average blood sugar level over 8 to 12 weeks. Even a 1% reduction (12%–11%) over this period is significant.
5. Provide frequent feedback; see the adolescent more frequently.
6. Examine the extent of parental support and monitoring; more support and monitoring by parents of midadolescents is associated with increased BG testing and lower HbA$_{Ic}$ (Anderson et al., 1997).
7. Group coping-skill training improves long-term glycemic control and quality of life (Grey et al., 2000).
8. Consider referral to a diabetes specialist if control has not improved within 6 months.
9. For life-threatening, recurrent DKA or long-standing very poor control (HbA$_{Ic}$ ≥12%) refractory to other measures, consider the use of a single daily dose of insulin, monitored by an adult to prevent recurrent DKA.
   a. Regular 30% TDD, NPH 60% TDD, lantus 10% TDD given as two injections in the morning.
   b. Expect subsequent HbA$_{Ic}$ to be 10% or less.

Portions of this chapter have been previously published (Orr, 2000a, b).

WEB SITES

For Professionals

http://www.diabetes.org. Web site of the ADA.
http://www.jdf.org. Juvenile Diabetes Foundation.
http://diabetes.niddk.nih.gov./ National Institute of Digestive Disease and Kidney.
http://www.aadenet.org. Association of Certified Diabetes Educators.
http://www.aace.com/clin/guidelines/diabetes_2002.pdf. Diabetes Clinical Guidelines of the American Association of Clinical Endocrinologists and the American College of Endocrinology.
Manufacturers of insulin and diabetes supplies have Web sites that provide useful information about products.

For Consumers

http://www.diabetesmonitor.com. Diabetes Monitor.
http://www.childrenwithdiabetes.com. Children with Diabetes.
http://www.childrenwithdiabetes.com/d_06_150.htm. Software to download GB meter results to computer.
http://www.childrenwithdiabetes.com/d_0i_000.htm. Information about BG meters.
http://www.fatcalories.com/. Nutrition in the fast Lane.

For Professionals or Patients

http://www.cdc.gov/diabetes/. Website developed by the Centers for Disease Control and Prevention
http://www.joslin.org/main.shtml. Joslin Diabetes Program

REFERENCES AND ADDITIONAL READINGS

Alberti G, Zimmet P, Shaw J, et al. Consensus Workshop Group. Type 2 diabetes in the young: the evolving epidemic: the international diabetes federation consensus workshop. *Diabetes Care* 2004;27(7):1798.

American Diabetes Association. Type 2 diabetes in children and adolescents. *Diabetes Care* 2000;23:381.

American Diabetes Association. Economic costs of diabetes in the U.S. in 2002. *Diabetes Care* 2003;26:917.

American Diabetes Association. Diagnosis and classification of diabetes mellitus. *Diabetes Care* 2005;28(Suppl 1):S37.

American Diabetes Association. Standards of medical care in diabetes. *Diabetes Care* 2005;28(Suppl 1), S4.

Amiel SA, Sherwin RS, Sinonson DC, et al. Impaired insulin action in puberty. *N Engl J Med* 1986;315:215.

Anderson B, Ho J, Brackett J, et al. Parental involvement in diabetes management tasks: relationships to blood glucose monitoring adherence and metabolic control in young adolescents with insulin-dependent diabetes mellitus. *J Pediatr* 1997;130:257.

Backonja MM. Gabapentin monotherapy for the symptomatic treatment of painful neuropathy: a multicenter, double-blind, placebo-controlled trial in patients with diabetes mellitus. *Epilepsia* 1999;40(Suppl 6):S57.

Bloomgarden Z. Type 2 diabetes in the young: the evolving epidemic. *Diabetes Care* 2004;27:998.

Danne T, Becker RH, Heise T, Bittner C, Frick AD, Rave K. Pharmacokinetics, prandial glucose control, and safety of insulin glulisine in children and adolescents with type 1 diabetes. *Diabetes Care* 2005;28(9):2100.

DeFronzo RA. Pharmacologic therapy for type 2 diabetes mellitus. *Ann Intern Med* 1999;131:281.

Devendra D, Liu E, Eisenbarth GS. Type 1 diabetes: recent developments. *BMJ* 2004;328:570.

The Diabetes Control and Complications Trial Research Group. Lifetime benefits and costs of intensive therapy as practiced in the Diabetes Control and Complications Trial. *JAMA* 1996;276:1409.

Fajans S, Bell GI, Polansky KS. Molecular mechanisms and clinical pathophysiology of maturity-onset diabetes of the young. *N Engl J Med* 2001;375:971.

Fagot-Campagna A, Pettitt DJ, Engelgau MM, et al. Type 2 diabetes among North American children and adolescents: an epidemiologic review and a public health perspective. *J Pediatr* 2000;136:664.

Fanelli CG, Epifano L, Rambotti AM, et al. Meticulous prevention of hypoglycemia normalizes the glycemic thresholds and magnitude of most neuroendocrine responses to, symptoms of, and cognitive function during hypoglycemia in intensively treated patients with short-term IDDM. *Diabetes* 1993;42:1683.

Gale EAM. The rise of childhood type 1 diabetes in the 20th century. *Diabetes* 2002;51:3353.

Grey M, Boland EA, Davidson M, et al. Coping skills training for youth with diabetes mellitus has long-lasting effects on metabolic control and quality of life. *J Pediatr* 2000;137:107.

Hedley AA, Ogden CL, Johnson CL, et al. Prevalence of overweight and obesity among US children, adolescents, and adults, 1999–2002. *JAMA* 2004;291:2847.

Hollander PA, Blonde L, Rowe R, et al. Efficacy and safety of inhaled insulin (Exubera) compared with subcutaneous insulin therapy in patients with type 2 diabetes: results of a 6-month, randomized, comparative trial. *Diabetes Care* 2004;27:2356.

Knowler WC, Barrett-Connor E, Fowler SE, et al. Reduction in the incidence of type 2 diabetes with lifestyle intervention or metformin. *N Engl J Med* 2002;346:3932.

Libman IM, Pietropaolo M, Trucco M, et al. Islet cell autoimmunity in white and black children and adolescents with IDDM. *Diabetes Care* 1998;21:1824.

Max MB, Lynch SA, Muir J, et al. Effects of desipramine, amitriptyline, and fluoxetine on pain in diabetes neuropathy. *N Engl J Med* 1992;326:1250.

Meltzer D, Egleston B, Stoffel D, et al. Effect of future costs on cost-effectiveness of medical interventions among young adults: the example of intensive therapy for type 1 diabetes mellitus. *Med Care* 2000;38:679.

Mooradian AD, Bernbaum M, Albert SG. Narrative review: a rational approach to starting insulin therapy. *Ann Intern Med* 2006;145:125.

Moran A, Doherty L, Wang X, et al. Abnormal glucose metabolism in cystic fibrosis. *J Pediatr* 1998;133:10.

Moran A, Jacobs DR, Steinberger J, et al. Insulin resistance during puberty. Results from clamp studies in 357 children. *Diabetes* 1999;48:2039.

Morello CM, Leckband SG, Stoner CP, et al. Randomized double-blind study comparing the efficacy of gabapentin with amitriptyline on diabetic peripheral neuropathy pain. *Arch Intern Med* 1999;59:1931.

Nepom GT, Kwok WW. Molecular basis for HLA-DQ associations with IDDM. *Diabetes* 1998;47:1177.

Orr DP. Contemporary management of adolescents with diabetes mellitus. Part 2: type 2 diabetes. *Adolesc Health Update* 2000;12(3):3.

Orr DP. Contemporary management of adolescents with diabetes mellitus. 1: type 1 diabetes. *Adolesc Health Update* 2000a;12(2):2.

Orr DP. Contemporary management of adolescents with diabetes mellitus. 1: type 2 diabetes. *Adolesc Health Update* 2000b;12(3):2.

Plank J, Bodenlenz M, Sinner F, et al: A double-blind, randomized, dose-response study investigating the pharmacodynamic and pharmacokinetic properties of the long-acting insulin analog detemir. *Diabetes Care* 2005;28:1107.

Quattrin T, Belanger A, Bohanno NJ, et al. Efficacy and safety of inhaled insulin (Exubera) compared with subcutaneous insulin therapy in patients with type 1 diabetes: results of a 6-month, randomized, comparative trial. *Diabetes Care* 2004;27:2622.

Rave K, Bott S, Heinemann L, et al. Time-action profile of inhaled insulin in comparison with subcutaneously injected insulin lispro and regular human insulin. *Diabetes Care* 2005;28:1077.

Rydall AC, Rodin GM, Olmsted MP, et al. Disordered eating behavior and microvascular complications in young women with insulin-dependent diabetes mellitus. *N Engl J Med* 1997;336:2849.

Saade G. Gestational diabetes: a shot or a pill. *Am J Obstet Gynecol* 2005;105:456.

Sobngwi E, Mauvais-Jarvis F, Vexiau P, et al. Diabetes in Africans. Part 2: Ketosis-prone atypical diabetes mellitus. *Diabetes Metab* 2002;28:5.

Tuomilehto J, Lindstrom J, Eriksson JG, et al. Prevention of type 2 diabetes mellitus by changes in lifestyle among subjects with impaired glucose tolerance. *N Engl J Med* 2001;344:1343.

Turner RC, Cull CA, Frighi V, et al. Glycemic control with diet, sulfonylurea, metformin, or insulin in patients with type 2 diabetes mellitus: progressive requirement for multiple therapies. *JAMA* 1998;281:2005.

UK Prospective Diabetes Study Group. Intensive blood-glucose control with sulfonylureas or insulin compared with conventional treatment and risk of complications in patients with type 2 diabetes. *Lancet* 1998;352:837.

Valmadrid CT, Klein R, Moss SE, et al. Alcohol intake and the risk of coronary heart disease mortality in persons with older-onset diabetes mellitus. *JAMA* 2000;282:239.

Veneman T, Mitrakou A, Cryer P, et al. Induction of hypoglycemia unawareness by asymptomatic nocturnal hypoglycemia. *Diabetes* 1993;42:1233.

Watts NB, Spanheimer RG, DiGirolamo M, et al. Prediction of glucose response to weight loss in patients with non-insulin-dependent diabetes mellitus. *Arch Intern Med* 1991;150:803.

Weiss R, Dziura J, Burgert TS, et al. Obesity and the metabolic syndrome in children and adolescents. *N Engl J Med* 2004;350:2362.

Wysocki T, Tylor A, Hough BS, et al. Deviation from developmentally appropriate self-care autonomy. Association with diabetes outcomes. *Diabetes Care* 1996;19:119.

CHAPTER 11

Gynecomastia

Alain Joffe

DEFINITION

Gynecomastia refers to an increase in the glandular and stromal tissue of the male breast. When identified during puberty, it is usually a benign and transient condition. Even at this stage of development, however, gynecomastia can be due to a serious underlying disorder or can persist long enough that the adolescent seeks treatment. With the increase in obesity that has occurred over the last few decades, true gynecomastia must be distinguished from fatty tissue overlying the pectoral muscles.

EPIDEMIOLOGY

1. Gynecomastia occurs in 19.6% of 10.5-year-old males, reaches a peak prevalence of 64.6% at age 14 years, and becomes less common thereafter. In one study, 17% of males 19 years and younger and 33% of 20- to 24-year-olds had palpable breast tissue at least 2 cm in diameter. Approximately 4% of adolescents will have severe gynecomastia (sometimes know as "type III" gynecomastia; >4.0 cm in diameter or approximately equal to the midpubertal female breast) that persists into adulthood. Mean age at onset is 13 years 2 months (SD 0.8 years).
2. Onset of gynecomastia correlates best with pubertal development; typically, its onset occurs 1.2 years (SD 0.6) after a boy reaches stage 2 genital development and 0.4 (SD 0.7) years after reaching stage 2 pubic hair. Genital stage at onset of gynecomastia is as follows:
   Genital stage 1: 20%
   Genital stage 2: 50%
   Genital stage 3: 20%
   Genital stage 4: 10%

ETIOLOGY

Breast tissue of males and females is similar at birth and responds similar to estrogens during childhood. At puberty, the breast tissue of boys demonstrates both ductal and periductal mesenchymal tissue proliferation. This tissue involutes and atrophies as testicular androgens increase to adult levels. In pubertal females, under the influence of increasing levels of both estrogen and progesterone, breast tissue continues to undergo ductal enlargement, branching, and acini development. The balance between estrogen and testosterone levels determines the extent of breast tissue development in males. As estrogens stimulate and androgens antagonize breast tissue development, an increase in estrogen relative to testosterone can lead to gynecomastia. Because estradiol levels increase by three- to fivefold during puberty whereas testosterone levels increase 30- to 40-fold, peak estradiol levels may be reached before adult testosterone levels. Aromatase (estrogen synthetase) plays a key role in estrogen production among men. The adult male's testes produce only 15% of the estradiol and <5% of the estrone circulating in the blood. The remainder is produced in extraglandular sites through aromatization. Hence, significant increases in extraglandular tissue (such as in obesity) result in significant elevations of circulating estrogens.

Alterations in the ratio of estrogens to androgens have been demonstrated in individuals with gynecomastia related to Klinefelter syndrome, thyrotoxicosis, cirrhosis, adrenal and testicular neoplasms, primary hypogonadism, and malnutrition. Use of various medications or drugs can also alter the hormonal milieu. In many patients with gynecomastia, serum hormone levels are within the reference range; however, there is experimental evidence to suggest that in some of these patients, altered sensitivity of the breast tissue to hormones may be responsible for the breast enlargement.

Mechanisms to account for an increase in estrogen or a decrease in androgen activity include the following:

1. Increase in serum estrogen concentrations
   a. Increase in estradiol secretion from testes (e.g., Leydig cell tumors) or from adrenal tumors
   b. Excessive extraglandular conversion of androgens to estrogens by aromatase
      • Overproduction of adrenal precursors (mainly androstenedione) that are then converted by aromatase into estrone
      • Overproduction of testicular precursors (mainly testosterone) that are then converted to estradiol
      • Enhancement of extraglandular aromatase activity
        – Disease states (hyperthyroidism, liver disease)
        – Increased body fat (obesity)
        – Medication (e.g., spironolactone) or drug use

– Idiopathic (caused by persistence of a fetal form of aromatase)

c. Increase in bioavailability of estrogens: a decrease in the amount of estrogen bound to sex hormone-binding globulin (SHBG) (e.g., use of spironolactone or ketoconazole)

d. Exogenous intake of estrogens, either through oral intake or from use of topical estrogens

2. Decrease in serum androgen concentrations
   a. Impairment of testicular production in Leydig cells
   - Primary hypogonadism (e.g., anorchia, Klinefelter syndrome)
   - Secondary hypogonadism through disorders of hypothalamus or pituitary
   - Congenital enzyme defects
   - Drug-induced inhibition of enzymes needed in testosterone synthesis (e.g., spironolactone or ketoconazole)
   - Chronic stimulation of Leydig cells by high levels of human chorionic gonadotropin (hCG) (e.g., hCG-secreting tumors) can lead to a reduction in testosterone biosynthesis
   - Hyperestrogenic states leading to suppression of luteinizing hormone (LH) and testosterone secretion
   b. Increased hepatic clearance of androgens
   c. Increase in SHBG, leading to a decrease in free testosterone (e.g., liver disease and hyperestrogenic states)

3. Alterations of estrogen and androgen receptors
   a. Androgen-receptor deficiency states (e.g., androgen insensitivity syndromes)
   b. Drug interference with androgen receptors (e.g., spironolactone, flutamide, or cimetidine)
   c. Drugs that mimic estrogens and stimulate estrogen-receptor sites (e.g., digoxin and phytoestrogens in some marijuana preparations)

Sher et al. (1998) reviewed the etiology of gynecomastia in 60 male subjects aged 9 and older referred to a pediatric endocrine clinic for evaluation of significant gynecomastia (more than 4 cm in diameter). Seven patients were determined to have an endocrine disorder (including Klinefelter syndrome, 46,XX maleness, primary testicular failure, partial androgen insensitivity, fibrolamellar hepatocarcinoma, and increased aromatase activity). An additional eight patients had other medical problems, including five with neurological disorders, but it is not clear that these conditions were causally related to the gynecomastia. The 45 remaining subjects were considered to have significant idiopathic gynecomastia (normal follicle-stimulating hormone (FSH), LH, testosterone, and estradiol levels); interestingly, they were noted to be both taller and heavier than average.

CLINICAL MANIFESTATIONS

1. Forms
   a. Type I: One or more subareolar nodules, freely movable
   b. Type II: Breast nodules beneath areola but also extending beyond the areolar perimeter
   c. Type III: Resembles breast development of sexual maturity rating 3 (SMR 3) in girls
2. Occurs bilaterally in 77% to 95% of cases, with concurrent or sequential involvement of both breasts

3. Physical examination
   a. Types I and II are associated with a firm, rubbery consistency of the breasts whereas type III has a consistency similar to that of the female breast
   b. Types I and II gynecomastia are usually associated with tenderness on palpation or when clothing touches the breast

DIFFERENTIAL DIAGNOSIS

Differential diagnosis includes (Braunstein, 1993):

1. Physiological—pubertal gynecomastia
2. Medication or drug use. There is some controversy as to which medications truly cause gynecomastia. More than 300 drugs have been reported as causing gynecomastia to the Committee on Safety of Medicines in the United Kingdom since 1963. Thompson and Carter (1993) believe that sufficient evidence exists to implicate calcium-channel blockers, cancer chemotherapeutic agents, histamine$_2$-receptor blockers, ketoconazole, and spironolactone. Braunstein (1993) considers that a strong relationship exists for those marked with an asterisk (*) in the list that follows:
   a. Hormones: Estrogens*, testosterone*, anabolic steroids*, chorionic gonadotropin*
   b. Psychoactive agents: Phenothiazines, atypical antipsychotic agents, diazepam, haloperidol, tricyclic antidepressants
   c. Cardiovascular drugs: Digoxin*, verapamil, captopril, methyldopa, nifedipine, enalapril, reserpine, minoxidil
   d. Antiandrogens or inhibitors of androgen synthesis: Cyproterone*, spironolactone*, flutamide*
   e. Antibiotics: Isoniazid, metronidazole, ketoconazole*
   f. Antiulcer medications: Cimetidine*, ranitidine, omeprazole
   g. Cancer chemotherapeutics, particularly alkylating agents*
   h. Drugs of abuse: Marijuana, alcohol, amphetamines, heroin, methadone
   i. Other: Phenytoin, penicillamine, theophylline, metoclopramide, saquinavir, indinavir (and other antiretroviral drugs)
3. Underlying medical disorders
   a. Renal failure and dialysis
   b. Recovery from malnutrition
   c. Primary gonadal failure: Including Klinefelter syndrome and Reifenstein syndrome
   d. Secondary hypogonadism
   e. Hyperthyroidism
   f. Liver disease, including cirrhosis and hepatoma
   g. Neoplasms
   - Testicular: Germ cell, Leydig cell, or Sertoli cell
   - Adrenal adenomas and carcinoma
   - Ectopic hCG production (particularly lung, liver, and kidney cancer)
   h. Enzyme defects in testosterone biosynthesis
   i. Androgen insensitivity syndromes
   j. Excessive extraglandular aromatase activity
4. Pseudogynecomastia: Caused by adipose tissue in some obese males or prominent musculature in some physically fit adolescent boys
5. Breast mass because of cancer, dermoid cyst, lipoma, hematoma, or neurofibroma

DIAGNOSIS

1. History: Screen for medication and drug use and clues suggesting systemic illness
2. Physical examination
   a. Differentiation of gynecomastia from pseudogynecomastia caused by prominent musculature or excessive adipose tissue
      - The teen is placed in the supine position, with his hands behind his head; the examiner then places the thumb and forefinger at opposing margins of the breast
      - In gynecomastia, as the fingers are brought together, rubbery or firm breast tissue can be felt as a freely movable, and occasionally tender, disk of tissue concentric to the areola; in pseudogynecomastia, no discrete mass is felt
      - In other conditions, such as a lipoma or dermoid cyst, the mass is usually eccentric to the areola
   b. Findings suggestive of hypogonadism, hyperthyroidism, or hypothyroidism
   c. Testicular mass or atrophy
   d. Findings suggestive of liver disease

Pubertal gynecomastia can be presumed as the etiology of the breast enlargement in adolescents who (a) present with a unilateral or bilateral, subareolar, rubbery or firm mass; (b) are not using any medications or drugs possibly associated with gynecomastia; (c) have a normal testicular examination; and (d) lack any evidence of renal, hepatic, thyroid, or other endocrine disease. No further tests are necessary but the patient should be reevaluated in 6 months. If medication or drug use is suspected, it should be discontinued and the adolescent reexamined in 1 month. At that time, breast tenderness, if present, should decrease and breast size may decrease.

If an endocrine disorder is suspected, the practitioner should order measurements of hCG, LH, serum testosterone, and estradiol (or, as some authors recommend, estrone sulphate). These tests will help in differentiating the cause of nonpubertal gynecomastia.

FINDINGS AND IMPLICATIONS OF SERUM HCG, LH, TESTOSTERONE, AND ESTRADIOL

Evaluate laboratory studies as follows (Braunstein, 1993):

1. Elevated hCG concentration: Perform testicular ultrasonography
   a. Mass found: Testicular germ cell tumor
   b. Normal sonogram: Extragonadal germ cell tumor or hCG-secreting neoplasm likely; chest film and abdominal computed tomography (CT) indicated
2. Decreased testosterone concentration with:
   a. Elevated LH concentration: Primary hypogonadism, including Klinefelter syndrome, and testicular atrophy caused by mumps orchitis
   b. Normal or low LH concentration: Measure serum prolactin
      - Elevated prolactin level: Probably prolactin-secreting pituitary tumor; obtain magnetic resonance imaging (MRI) of hypothalamic pituitary area
      - Normal prolactin level: Secondary hypogonadism

3. Elevated testosterone and LH concentrations: Measure thyroxine (T_4) and thyroid-stimulating hormone (TSH) concentrations
   a. Elevated T_4 and low TSH concentrations: Hyperthyroidism (elevated testosterone is secondary to the increase in SHBG, leading to an increase in total testosterone; the etiology of increased LH levels in association with hyperthyroidism is uncertain)
   b. Normal T_4 and TSH concentrations: Androgen resistance
4. Elevated estradiol with low or normal LH concentrations: Perform testicular ultrasonography
   a. Mass on sonogram: Leydig or Sertoli cell tumor
   b. Normal: Perform adrenal CT or MRI
      - Mass found: Adrenal neoplasm
      - No mass: Increased extraglandular aromatase activity
5. Normal concentrations of hCG, LH, testosterone, and estradiol: Idiopathic gynecomastia

THERAPY

1. Underlying causes should be treated as appropriate. If a medication or drug is suspected, it should be discontinued, if possible.
2. Pubertal gynecomastia: In most individuals with pubertal gynecomastia, particularly with mild to moderate degrees, only reassurance is needed. In most cases, the condition will improve or resolve within 6 to 12 months.
3. Medical intervention
   a. Several drugs have been tried to reduce gynecomastia, including androgens (testosterone, dihydrotestosterone and the androgenic progesterone, danazol), antiestrogens (clomiphene, tamoxifen, and raloxifene), and aromatase inhibitors (testolactone, anastrozole, letrozole, and formestane). None of these is approved by the U.S. Food and Drug Administration for the treatment of adolescent gynecomastia, and studies using these medications in adolescents are limited. Dihydrotestosterone can lead to a reduction in breast volume in 75% of individuals, with 25% having a complete response (Kuhn et al., 1983). However, this medication is not readily available. Danazol has some limited effectiveness but is associated with significant side effects and would not be recommended in the treatment of adolescents. Tamoxifen has been evaluated in a number of studies. At a dose of 10 mg twice a day, tamoxifen resulted in a statistically significant reduction in breast size and pain without side effects. Ting et al. (2000) compared the efficacy of tamoxifen (23 patients) with that of danazol (20 patients) in the treatment of 23 males of a wide age range with idiopathic gynecomastia (mean age, 39.5; range 13 to 82). In this study, either tamoxifen (20 mg/day) or danazol (400 mg/day) was offered and continued until a constant response was obtained. Complete resolution of the gynecomastia occurred in 18 patients (78.2%) treated with tamoxifen but only in 8 patients (40%) in the danazol group. Five patients, all from the tamoxifen group, developed recurrence of breast mass. The wide age range of the patients treated precludes a clear determination as to whether tamoxifen

is completely safe or effective in teens. Lawrence et al. (2004) reviewed their experience in managing 38 patients with persistent pubertal gynecomastia using either tamoxifen (10–20 mg twice daily) or raloxifene (60 mg daily) for 3 to 9 months. Mean reduction in breast diameter was 2.1 cm with tamoxifen versus 2.5 cm with raloxifene. Overall improvement was comparable (tamoxifen, 86%; raloxifene, 91%) but more raloxifene-treated patients (86%) than tamoxifen-treated patients (41%) had at least a 50% reduction in breast size. However, the study was neither randomized nor blinded and there was no true control group. Testolactone, an aromatase inhibitor, has also been found in an uncontrolled study to decrease pubertal gynecomastia without side effects.

b. Medical therapy should be reserved for those individuals who have more than mild to moderate gynecomastia and who are significantly concerned about the condition. Tamoxifen could be used at an oral dosage of 10 to 20 mg twice daily for 3 months. This should lead to a decrease in tenderness and pain, followed by a reduction in the size of breast tissue.

4. Surgical intervention: In older adolescents with moderate to severe gynecomastia associated with psychological sequelae, or in older patients in whom gynecomastia is unlikely to resolve spontaneously, surgical treatment is preferable. Recent surgical advances include the use of ultrasonic liposuction.

PROGNOSIS

Pubertal gynecomastia usually resolves in 12 to 18 months. In 27% of affected adolescents, the condition lasts for >1 year, and in 7.7% >2 years. A small percentage of cases may persist into adulthood. There has been no proven relationship between gynecomastia and the development of breast cancer in male subjects.

WEB SITES

For Teenagers and Parents

http://www.mayoclinic.com/health/gynecomastia/DS00850 .htm. Mayo clinic article on gynecomastia.

http://www.keepkidshealthy.com/adolescent/ adolescentproblems/gynecomastia.html. Teen-oriented site with information about gynecomastia and other health issues.

http://kidshealth.org/teen/question/just_guys/boybrst .html. Teen site with information about gynecomastia and other health issues.

http://www.choc.org/pediatricadvisor/pa/pa_gynecoma _hhg.htm Pediatric Advisor information on gynecomastia.

For Health Professionals

http://155.37.5.42/eAtlas/Breast/1694.htm. Site with pathology slide on gynecomastia.

http://www.emedicine.com/med/topic934.htm. E-medicine site on gynecomastia.

REFERENCES AND ADDITIONAL READINGS

Ardick KR. Holiday gynecomastia related to marijuana? *Ann Intern Med* 1993;119:253.

Bembo SA, Carlson HE. Gynecomastia: its features and when and how to treat it. *Cleve Clin J Med* 2004;71:511.

Biro FM, Lucky AW, Fluster GA, et al. Hormonal studies and physical maturation in adolescent gynecomastia. *J Pediatr* 1990;116:450.

Bowers SP, Pearlman NW, McIntyre RC Jr, et al. Cost-effective management of gynecomastia. *Am J Surg* 1998;176:638.

Braunstein GD. Gynecomastia. *N Engl J Med* 1993;328:490.

Braunstein GD. Aromatase and gynecomastia. *Endocr Relat Cancer* 1999;6:315.

Braunstein GD, Glassman HA. Gynecomastia. *Curr Ther Endocrinol Metab* 1997;6:401.

Brenner P, Berger A, Schneider W, et al. Male reduction mammoplasty in serious gynecomastias. *Aesthetic Plast Surg* 1992;16:325.

Buchanan CR. Abnormalities of growth and development in puberty. *J R Coll Physicians Lond* 2000;34:141.

Derman O, Kannbur NO, Kutluk T. Tamoxifen treatment for pubertal gynecomastia. *Int J Adolesc Med Health* 2003;15:359.

Derman O, Kanbur NO, Tokur TE. The effect of tamoxifen on sex hormone binding globulin in adolescents with pubertal gynecomastia. *J Pediatr Endocrinol Metab* 2004;18: 1115.

Eberle AL, Sparrow JT, Keenan BS. Treatment of persistent pubertal gynecomastia with dihydrotestosterone heptanoate. *J Pediatr* 1986;109:144.

Hodgson ELB, Fruhstorfer BH, Malata CM. Ultrasonic liposuction in the treatment of gynecomastia. *Plast Reconstr Surg* 2005;116:646.

Ismail AAA, Barth JH. Endocrinology of gynaecomastia. *Ann Clin Biochem* 2001;38:596.

Kuhn JM, Roca R, Laudat MH, et al. Studies on the treatment of idiopathic gynaecomastia with percutaneous dihydrotestosterone. *Clin Endocrinol* 1983;19:513.

Large DM, Anderson DC. Twenty-four-hour profiles of circulating androgens and oestrogens in male puberty with and without gynecomastia. *Clin Endocrinol* 1979;11:505.

Lawrence SE, Faught KA, Vethamuthu J, et al. Beneficial effects of raloxifene and tamoxifen in the treatment of pubertal gynecomastia. *J Pediatr* 2004;145:71

Madani S, Tolia V. Gynecomastia with metoclopramide use in pediatric patients. *J Clin Gastroenterol* 1997;24:79.

Mahoney CP. Adolescent gynecomastia: differential diagnosis and management. *Pediatr Clin North Am* 1990;37:1389.

Marynick SP, Nisula BC, Pita JC Jr, et al. Persistent pubertal macromastia. *J Clin Endocrinol Metab* 1980;50:128.

Moore DC, Schlaepfer LV, Paunier L, et al. Hormonal changes during puberty. V. transient pubertal gynecomastia: abnormal androgen-estrogen ratio. *J Clin Endocrinol Metab* 1984; 58:492.

Neuman JF. Evaluation and treatment of gynecomastia. *Am Fam Physician* 1997;55:1835.

Nuttall FQ. Gynecomastia as a physical finding in normal men. *J Clin Endocrinol Metab* 1979;48:338.

Nydick M, Bustos J, Dale JH, et al. Gynecomastia in adolescent boys. *JAMA* 1961;178:449.

Parker LN, Gray DR, Lai MK, et al. Treatment of gynecomastia with tamoxifen: a double-blind crossover study. *Metabolism* 1986;35:705.

Peters MH, Vastine V, Knox L, et al. Treatment of adolescent gynecomastia using a bipedicle technique. *Ann Plast Surg* 1998; 40:241.

Sher ES, Migeon CJ, Berkovitz GD. Evaluation of boys with marked breast development at puberty. *Clin Pediatr* 1998; 37:367.

Thompson DE, Carter JR. Drug-induced gynecomastia. *Pharmacotherapy* 1993;13:37.

Ting AC, Chow LW, Leung YF. Comparison of tamoxifen with danazol in the management of idiopathic gynecomastia. *Am Surg* 2000;66:38.

PART III

Cardiovascular Problems

CHAPTER 12

Cardiac Risk Factors and Hyperlipidemia

Marc S. Jacobson, Michael R. Kohn, and Lawrence S. Neinstein

One of the goals of adolescent health care is early intervention to prevent diseases that occur during adulthood. Atherosclerosis results from the interaction of environmental factors with the genetic endowment and begins in childhood. Much has been learned about identifying early risks for cardiovascular disease although questions remain. Interventions to reduce risk factors in children and adolescents have been demonstrated. Whether there is also a reduction in subsequent cardiac disease remains to be determined. However, it is now advisable to screen for risk factors and to provide appropriate interventions for those risk factors that are remediable (Jacobson, 1998).

CARDIAC RISK FACTORS

The National Cholesterol Education Program (NCEP) is directed by the National Heart, Lung and Blood Institute and issues guidelines to help health care professionals determine the best cholesterol management for patients to reduce their risk of myocardial infarctions.

Among the following risk factors, an asterisk [*] indicates those that are identified by NCEP.

Nonintervenable

1. Age: 45 years and above for men*, 65 years for women*
2. Sex: Male
3. Family history: History of cardiovascular disease in first-degree relatives* (≤55 years of age for men, <65 years for women) with atherosclerosis or its sequelae
4. Parent with elevated cholesterol concentration (>240 mg/dL)

Intervenable

1. Smoking*
2. Hypertension: Systolic or diastolic blood pressure (BP) above the 95th percentile*
3. Diabetes mellitus*
4. Diet high in saturated fats and cholesterol, with total fat intake accounting for >30% of daily caloric intake
5. Dyslipidemia: the following are criteria for lipid abnormalities: (modified from recommendations of the NCEP Expert Panel on Blood Cholesterol Levels in Children and Adolescents [National Cholesterol Education Program, 1992], and the NCEP Expert Panel on Detection, Evaluation and Treatment of High Blood Cholesterol in Adults, the Adult Treatment Panel III [ATP III]) (Stone et al., 2005; National Cholesterol Education Program Expert Panel, http://www.nhlbi.nih.gov/guidelines/cholesterol/atp3_rpt.htm). The following are criteria for lipid abnormalities:
   a. Total cholesterol >170 mg/dL for those younger than 20 years, or >200 mg/dL for those older than 20 years
   b. Low-density lipoprotein cholesterol (LDL-C) >130 mg/dL (for persons older than 20 years see the "Screening in Young Adults" section for new guidelines by the ATP III)
   c. High-density lipoprotein cholesterol (HDL-C) <40 mg/dL*
   d. Triglycerides >150 mg/dL*
   e. Ratio of serum very–low-density lipoprotein (VLDL) cholesterol to triglycerides of >0.3
6. Obesity, that is, >30% above expected weight, or body mass index (BMI) above the 95th percentile for age*
7. Insulin resistance with hyperinsulinemia
8. Homocysteinemia (>10 nmol/L)
9. Serum lipoprotein a (Lp[a]) concentration
10. High serum C-reactive protein (CRP) concentrations

In general, individuals are considered at low risk for atherosclerotic disease if they have zero or one cardiovascular risk factor, moderate risk with more than one risk factor other than diabetes mellitus, and high risk with a presence of diabetes or any evidence of atherosclerosis.

RISK FACTOR INTERVENTION

Important information about the relationship between cardiovascular risk factors and coronary artery disease (CAD) has been revealed by recently published longitudinal studies (Oren et al., 2003; Li et al., 2003; Knoflach et al., 2003). These involve monitoring of arterial disease using high resolution B mode ultrasound to measure carotid-intima media thickness (CIMT). In summary, these studies demonstrate that screening in adolescence is a better predictor of adult disease than childhood screening, and that effective management of risk factors diminishes atherosclerosis.

It remains prudent to recommend a heart-healthy lifestyle to reduce atherosclerosis and arterial disease. This approach includes the following:

1. Promoting regular physical activity
2. Counseling on the importance of maintaining an ideal body weight
3. Advocating smoking prevention or cessation
4. Monitoring BP and treating when persistently elevated
5. Recommending a heart-healthy diet that has <30% of the total calories as fat and a diet low in saturated fat for all individuals
6. Ensuring daily intake of 400 µg of folic acid either through diet or supplementation

Hypertension

The distribution of BP in children and adolescents was described by the Second Task Force on Blood Pressure Control. Hypertension was classified by age as being "significant" or "severe." For adolescents with "significant" hypertension (i.e., diastolic BP higher than 86 mm Hg at age 13 to 15 years or higher than 92 mm Hg at age 16 to 18 years) and no other risk factors, interventions should include a low-salt diet, weight reduction, and relaxation or other biofeedback techniques. Intervention for hypertension is covered in more detail in Chapter 13.

Cigarette Smoking

Cigarette smoke is an atherogenic risk factor due to alterations in lipids and fibrinogen and smoking is associated with more cardiovascular deaths than cancer deaths. Most cigarette smoking begins early in adolescence, suggesting that this is an important period for prevention. Effective education programs must be developed and implemented at the national level, at the local school level, and in the practitioner's office. Every preteen and teen should be questioned regarding his or her smoking habits, and specific interventions should be targeted to prevent or extinguish smoking behavior.

Dyslipidemia

The primary therapy for hyperlipidemia during adolescence is modification of diet, including recommendation for a diet that is low in fat, saturated and trans fats, and cholesterol. Regular physical activity is also indicated. Medications should be reserved for those teenagers with markedly high concentrations of lipids unresponsive to dietary and lifestyle change, and with an extensive family history (see "Therapy for Hyperlipidemia" section).

Obesity

The best therapy for obesity is to prevent it. This requires curbing obesity early and particularly during the adolescent growth spurt. Without intervention, eight of ten obese 12-year-old children will become obese adults (Srinivasan, 1996 and http://www.surgeongeneral.gov/topics/obesity/calltoaction/fact_adolescents.htm). Exercise and other physical activities, combined with dietary modifications, are the best preventive measures, and some studies show positive results in relation to changes in

BMI, as well as metabolic changes. In particular, insulin resistance is decreased, as is BP, and there are positive changes in the lipid profile, all of which mitigate against the development of atherosclerosis.

LIPID PHYSIOLOGY

Cholesterol and triglycerides are the major blood lipids. Cholesterol is a key constituent of cell membranes and a precursor of bile acids and steroid hormones. Cholesterol circulates in the bloodstream in spherical particles called *lipoproteins* containing both lipids and proteins called *apolipoproteins*. These particles consist of a core of triglycerides, cholesterol, and cholesterol esters, in varying amounts, surrounded by an outer shell of cholesterol and phospholipids. The apolipoproteins are embedded in the outer lipid layers (Fig. 12.1).

1. Classification of lipoproteins: Five major classes of lipoproteins act as transport systems for cholesterol and triglycerides. They differ in physical and chemical characteristics and function, as well as in amounts of cholesterol, triglyceride, phospholipid, and protein. The lipoproteins can be separated by ultracentrifugation or electrophoresis, on the basis of differences in densities and surface properties (the characteristics of these particles and their functions are summarized). Ultracentrifugation yields chylomicrons, VLDL,

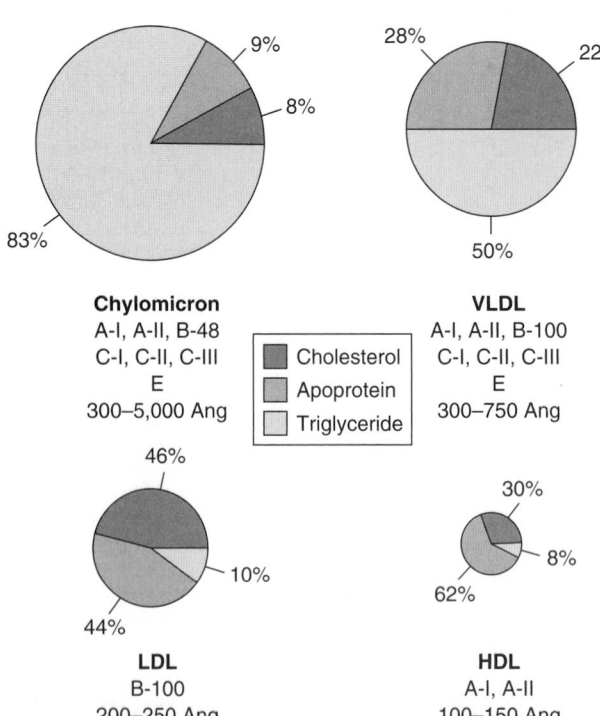

FIGURE 12.1 Characteristics of lipoproteins. Apoproteins and volume are detailed below each lipoprotein. Ang, angstroms; VLDL, very low-density lipoprotein; LDL, low-density lipoprotein; HDL, high-density lipoprotein. (Adapted from Hardoff D, Jacobson MS. Hyperlipidemia. *Adolesc Med State Arts Rev* 1992;3:475.)

low-density lipoproteins (LDLs), and high-density lipoproteins (HDLs).

a. Chylomicrons: Largest and least dense of the lipoproteins; composed mainly of triglycerides with a lipid : protein ratio of 99:1. Chylomicrons carry dietary fat as triglycerides from the intestine to the periphery of the body to be used to meet energy requirements or deposition in fat cells.

b. VLDL: Secreted by the liver and the second major carrier of triglycerides. It is composed largely of triglycerides and contains <10% of the total serum cholesterol concentration.

c. LDL: Major carrier of cholesterol, containing 60% to 70% of the total serum cholesterol concentration, and is an important factor in atherogenesis.

d. HDL: Usually contains 20% to 30% of the total serum cholesterol concentration. It is responsible for the transport of cholesterol back to triglyceride-containing particles for removal in the bile. The calculation of the proportion of LDL is made with the following formula:

$$\text{Total cholesterol} = \text{LDL} + \text{HDL} + \text{VLDL}$$

HDL is measured directly, and VLDL is estimated by dividing the fasting triglyceride concentration by 5 (true so long as the triglyceride concentration is <400 mg/dL). Therefore,

$$\text{LDL} = \text{Total cholesterol} - \text{HDL} - (\text{triglycerides}/5)$$

e. Apolipoproteins: Numerous apolipoproteins are associated with lipoproteins. Each lipoprotein has a characteristic apolipoprotein profile. Lipoproteins may contain several apolipoproteins. These apolipoproteins serve as cofactors for enzymes involved in lipoprotein metabolism, they help in the binding of lipoproteins to cellular receptors, and they facilitate lipid transfer between lipoproteins. Apolipoprotein B-100 (apoB-100) is an important component of VLDL and is the only apolipoprotein in LDL-C. Uptake of LDL by cells is dependent on its binding to the LDL receptor, which is regulated by apoB-100. Abnormalities in both quality and quantity of these proteins, even in the absence of an elevated cholesterol concentration, may contribute to atherosclerosis.

2. Lipoprotein circulation and sources: (Fig. 12.2)

a. Exogenous: Chylomicrons are formed in the gut wall after absorption of dietary fat. They are secreted into the lymph and enter the bloodstream, where the fatty acids are stored in adipose tissue, or are used

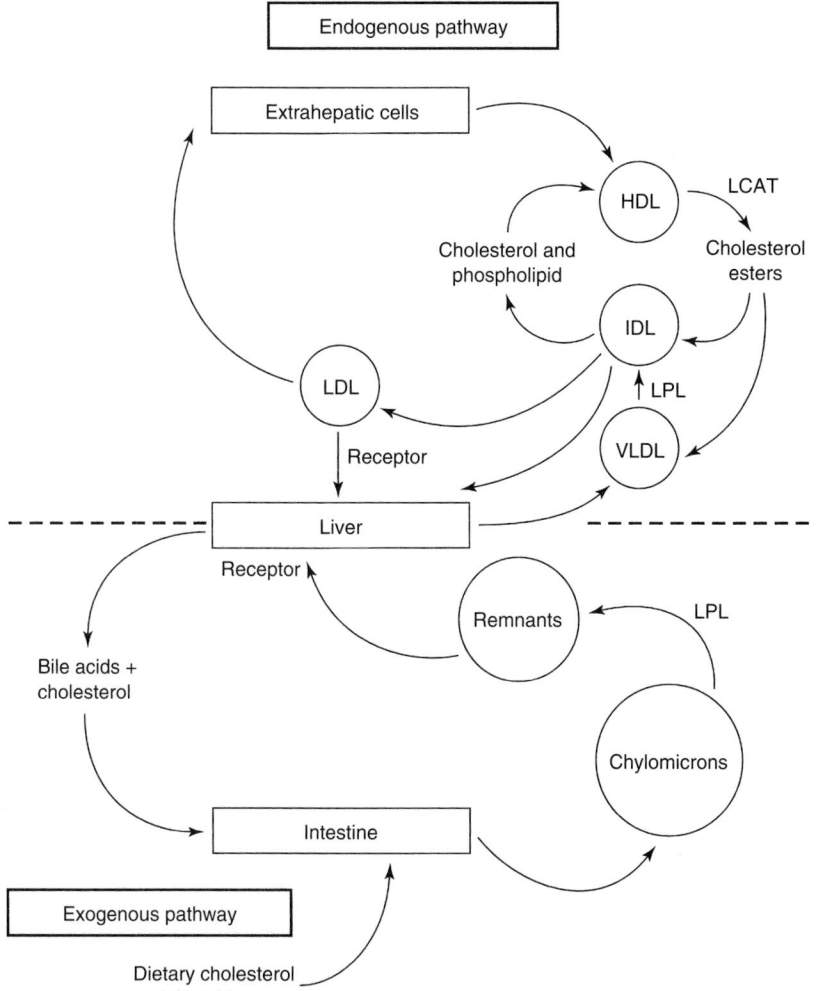

FIGURE 12.2 Pathways of lipoprotein metabolism. LCAT, lecithin-cholesterol acyltransferase; LPL, lipoprotein lipase; HDL, high-density lipoprotein; LDL, low-density lipoprotein; IDL, intermediate density lipoprotein; VLDL, very low-density lipoprotein. (From Weis S, Lacko AG. Role of lipoproteins in hypercholesterolemia. *Pract Cardiol* 1988:12–18.)

in skeletal muscle and myocardium. Eventually, they release almost all of their diet-derived triglycerides. This reaction is catalyzed by lipoprotein lipase. The chylomicron remnants are rapidly absorbed in the liver by specific receptors for these particles. In liver cells, the remnants are degraded to free cholesterol, which is excreted into bile.

b. Endogenous: The endogenous transport system includes VLDL, IDL, LDL, and HDL. Excess calories from carbohydrates and fatty acids are metabolized in the liver into triglycerides. The lipoproteins carrying these triglycerides are primarily VLDL, which moves to adipose tissue, where triglycerides are extracted; the result is the formation of IDL and LDL. The IDL particles are rapidly removed from circulation by LDL receptors in the liver.

- LDL transports cholesterol to peripheral tissues. In addition to the lipid component, LDL particles contain a single apoB-100 molecule, the protein that binds to LDL receptors. After binding to LDL cell surface receptors, the LDL particles deliver cholesterol for synthesis of cell membranes in all cells; for steroid hormones in the adrenal glands, ovary, and testes, and for bile acids in the liver. The LDL-C found in macrophages and smooth muscle cells of atherosclerotic lesions enters by additional mechanisms. This LDL-C is modified by oxidation intravascularly and is taken up in lesions by oxy-LDL receptors and scavenger receptors. This process may provide alternative pathways for therapeutic intervention.

- HDL is secreted from the liver or intestine in a lipid-poor form or is made de novo in the plasma. As it matures, HDL accumulates cholesterol from tissues, including blood vessel walls, and therefore has a major role in removing excess cholesterol and delivering it to the liver by means of the triglyceride-rich lipoproteins and cholesterol ester transfer protein.

LIPID PATHOPHYSIOLOGY AND CAD

1. Epidemiological evidence:
   a. In populations throughout the world, there is a direct correlation between serum cholesterol levels and CAD rates. Individuals moving to a country with higher mean cholesterol levels gradually acquire the dietary habits, cholesterol levels, and CAD rates of their new country. In societies where the total cholesterol concentration is <150 mg/dL, CAD is rare.
   b. Bogalusa Heart Study (Berenson, 1986; Freedman et al., 1999): Observations from this study clearly show that the major risk factors of adult heart disease begin in childhood. Documented atherosclerotic changes (e.g., fatty streak) were seen to occur by age 5 to 8 years. This group noted the significance of environmental factors for hyperlipidemia, hypertension, and obesity. They also showed that the level of risk factors in childhood is different from that in the adult years and that levels change with growth phase. Most importantly, they documented the correlation of risk factor levels with severity of lesions in autopsy material from adolescents who had died of unrelated causes and who had previously been prospectively assessed (Berenson et al., 1998).

   c. Epidemiology: Pathobiological Determinants of Atherosclerosis in Youth (PDAY) study described the relationship between atherosclerosis and serum lipoprotein cholesterol concentrations and smoking in young men. A preliminary report demonstrated an association between commonly accepted risk factors (elevated LDL-C and low HDL-C concentrations and smoking) and the severity of atherosclerotic plaques in adolescents.

2. Genetic evidence:
   a. Familial hypercholesterolemia: Individuals who lack LDL cell surface receptor activity may have very high cholesterol levels. Severe atherosclerosis may develop in the first two decades of life. These individuals are referred to as having familial hypercholesterolemia. Those heterozygous for the LDL-receptor defect account for 15% of premature CAD cases. Clinical manifestations such as xanthomas and other signs of cutaneous lipid deposition are generally seen in the fourth decade of life in heterozygotes and during adolescence in homozygotes.
   b. Familial combined hyperlipidemia (FCHL): Autosomal dominant syndrome that affects approximately 1% to 2% of the population. Most, if not all, patients with this condition have elevated levels of LDL apoB. Abnormal metabolism of VLDL and partial lipoprotein lipase deficiency have also been described in association with this syndrome. Individuals with FCHL account for a significant proportion of early CAD cases.
   c. Apolipoprotein E (apoE): Three common alleles of apoE, at a single-gene locus on chromosome 19, code for three isoforms of apoE: designated as apoE-II, apoE-III, and apoE-IV which are distinguished in the laboratory by isoelectric focusing. Both homozygous and heterozygous genotypes have been found. Increased cardiovascular risk is associated with apoE-II and apoE-IV, in comparison with the more common apoE-III. Type III hyperlipidemia is an uncommon disorder in which >95% of individuals are homozygous for the apoE-II allele. EII-EII occurs in <1% of the population. However, most EII-EII homozygotes are normolipidemic, confounding the relationship between genes and cardiovascular disease.

3. Animal models: Atherosclerosis develops in animals that were fed diets elevating their serum cholesterol concentrations. In other animal experiments, a change of diet and the use of lipid-lowering drugs reduced elevated cholesterol concentrations and caused regression in atherosclerotic plaques.

4. Interventional trials: More than a dozen randomized clinical trials in adults have examined the effects of lowering cholesterol concentrations on CAD. These trials support the conclusion that lowering total and LDL-C concentrations reduces the incidence of CAD events. The degree of benefit is greatest in individuals who have other associated risk factors, such as cigarette smoking, diabetes, and hypertension. Examples of the most significant studies include the following:
   a. Coronary Primary Prevention Trial: A longitudinal double-blind study of asymptomatic men with hypercholesterolemia. This study demonstrated a decreased CAD risk of 2% for every 1% decrease in the serum cholesterol concentrations in adults with levels initially in the 250 to 300 mg/dL range.

b. Helsinki Heart Study: In this study, the use of gemfibrozil lowered LDL-C concentration by 8% and increased HDL-C concentration by 10%. This led to a 34% decrease in the incidence of CAD.

c. Multiple Risk Factor Intervention Trial: This study demonstrated that there is no threshold level of cholesterol for the development of atherosclerotic lesions. The study reported a relative risk of 0.7 with a cholesterol concentration of 150 mg/dL, 1.0 with 200 mg/dL, 2.0 with 250 mg/dL, and 4.0 with 300 mg/dL.

Studies examining the use of 3-hydroxy-3-methylglutaryl coenzyme (HMG-CoA) reductase inhibitors commonly known as "statins" include the following:

• West of Scotland Coronary Prevention Study: In a large cohort of middle-aged men with high cholesterol concentrations, the use of pravastatin significantly reduced the incidence of nonfatal myocardial infarction and cardiac death without increasing the risk of death from other causes (Shepherd et al., 1995).

• Air Force/Texas Coronary Atherosclerosis Prevention Study: This study evaluated the use of cholesterol-lowering therapy in healthy adults with average total cholesterol but below-average HDL-C concentrations. Treatment with lovastatin resulted in a 37% reduction in risk of a first major cardiac event in both men and women (Downs et al., 1998).

• Recent Clinical Trials for the NCEP—ATP III Guidelines, Stone et al., 2005: This updates the ATP III guidelines of the NCEP on the basis of five major clinical trials of statin therapy with clinical end points. These trials confirm the benefit of cholesterol-lowering therapy in high-risk patients and support the ATP III treatment goal of LDL-C <100 mg/dL in high-risk individuals, with an option of <70 mg/dL if the risk is very high.

5. Relationship of particular lipoproteins

a. LDL-C: Studies show a positive relationship between the level of cholesterol, particularly LDL, and the frequency of CAD. There appear to be several outcomes for LDL. Any LDL that is not cleared by LDL receptors is metabolized by nonreceptor mechanisms, which may play a role in atherosclerosis. LDL molecules deposit their excess cholesterol at various tissue sites, including the intima of blood vessels.

b. HDL-C: Population studies suggest an inverse relation between HDL-C and CAD. An HDL-C level of <30 mg/dL carries a significantly increased risk of CAD. A level >50 mg/dL yields a low risk, whereas octogenarians average >75 mg/dL. HDL has two components, HDL2 and HDL3. The former is considered a better indicator of negative CAD risk than is total HDL. Exercise raises the level of cardioprotective HDL2, whereas ethanol raises the level of HDL3. The Framingham Heart Study showed a 10% increase in CAD for each 4-mg/dL decrease in HDL. In addition, low HDL-C levels have been correlated with an increased number of diseased coronary arteries. There also appears to be a higher rate of restenosis after angioplasty in individuals with low HDL-C levels.

c. Apolipoproteins: Preliminary evidence suggests that apolipoproteins A-I (apoA-I), A-II (apoA-II), and apoB may be better than LDL, HDL, and total cholesterol in predicting the risk of CAD. Elevated concentrations of apoA-I and apoA-II are associated with a lower risk, and an elevated apoB concentration is associated with a higher risk of CAD. Isoforms of apoE have also been implicated in cardiovascular risk, as noted previously. In addition, the measurement of the apoB-100 to apoA-I ratio may provide another assessment of cardiovascular risk.

d. Ratios: The correlation between CAD and the LDL:HDL ratio has also been examined in adults. The risk increases sharply with ratios that exceed 3.0. A ratio of >5.0 carries a very high risk of CAD. Individuals with CAD average a ratio of >5:1, whereas newborns have an average ratio of 2:1. Another ratio is that of total cholesterol to HDL-C. A ratio of <4.5 denotes below-average risk, whereas the optimum ratio is 3.5:1. However, the clinical use of ratios is problematic because LDL and HDL represent independent risk factors and respond differently to different interventions. The American Heart Association (AHA) recommends that the absolute numbers for total blood cholesterol and HDL-C be used. The AHA suggests that these are more useful to the physician than the cholesterol ratio, in determining the appropriate treatment for individuals. The ATP III assigns points to various levels of HDL-C as part of the equation that is used to determine LDL-C treatment goals for primary and secondary prevention, rather than focusing on ratios.

6. Other experimental work: Lp(a) is a very large lipoprotein composed of apoB-100 and cholesterol, similar to LDL. In addition, this lipoprotein has a large glycoprotein, homologous to plasminogen, attached through a disulfide bond. It has no known physiological function. Plasma levels appear to be genetically determined and associated with risk of cardiovascular disease and may also increase the risk of thrombotic complications through its interaction with plasminogen. Nicotinic acid has been shown to lower Lp(a) by up to 30% (Knopp, 1999).

CLASSIFICATION OF HYPERLIPIDEMIAS

Historically, patients with hyperlipidemia have been classified into five major groups according to plasma lipoprotein patterns (lipoprotein phenotyping). More recent classifications of hyperlipidemia are either extensions of the earlier models based on more specific data obtained from newer laboratory techniques (Table 12.1) or are based on recently described genetic and metabolic disorders (Table 12.2). The nomenclature remains cumbersome and there is still much overlap, particularly when attempts are made to reconcile these two systems. Previously well-described syndromes, such as familial hypercholesterolemia, have been shown to have a specific genotype and yet may vary in phenotype (i.e., types IIa and IIb). Moreover, type IIa and IIb patterns of hyperlipidemia are associated with another syndrome, FCHL. Finally, the lipoprotein phenotyping system fails to account for children and adolescents at risk of atherosclerosis as a result of hyperapobetalipoproteinemia or hypoalphalipoproteinemia, which have been described in the metabolic classification. Each of the two classification systems has clinical utility at present. It is hoped that as the field of molecular genetics advances, the two systems will be fused into one system on the basis of pathophysiology and the degree of risk (Breslow, 1991).

Although familial forms of hyperlipidemia (Table 12.3), identifiable in the standard clinical laboratory assessment,

TABLE 12.1

Phenotypic Classification

1. Hypercholesterolemia with normal triglycerides	—Secondary: Diabetes mellitus
a. Elevated LDL-C, type IIa	SLE
—Primary: Familial hypercholesterolemia	Alcohol
Familial combined	Nephrotic syndrome

1. Hypercholesterolemia with normal triglycerides
   a. Elevated LDL-C, type IIa
      —Primary: Familial hypercholesterolemia
                   Familial combined
                      hypercholesterolemia
                   Mixed genetic-environmental
                      hypercholesterolemia
      —Secondary: Anorexia nervosa
                   Acute intermittent porphyria
                   Biliary obstruction (lipoprotein X)
   b. Elevated HDL-C
                   Familial hyperalphali-
                      poproteinemia
                   Idiopathic
2. Hypercholesterolemia and hypertriglyceridemia
   a. Elevated LDL-C and VLDL-C, type IIB
      —Primary: Familial hypercholesterolemia
                   Familial combined
                      hypercholesterolemia
                   Familial LCAT deficiency
      —Secondary: Hypothyroidism
                   Nephrotic syndrome
                   Cushing's syndrome/
                      glucocorticoid therapy
   b. Dysbetalipoproteinemia, type III
3. Hypertriglyceridemia with normal cholesterol level
   a. Elevated VLDL only, type IV
      —Primary: Familial hypertriglyceridemia
                   Familial combined hyperlipidemia

—Secondary: Diabetes mellitus
             SLE
             Alcohol
             Nephrotic syndrome
             Pancreatitis
             Pregnancy
             Hypothyroidism
             Idiopathic hypercalcemia
             Medications: Estrogens
   b. Elevated chylomicrons, type I
      —Primary: Lipoprotein lipase deficiency
                   Familial deficiency of
                      apolipoprotein C-II
      —Secondary: Autoimmune
                      hyperchylomicronemia: SLE
                   Diabetes mellitus
                   Alcohol
   c. Elevated VLDL and chylomicrons, type V
      —Primary: Familial hypertriglyceridemia
                   Familial combined hyperlipidemia
                   Apolipoprotein E (apoE-4
                      and apoE-2)
      —Secondary: Diabetes mellitus
                   Alcohol
                   Estrogen
4. Increased risk with normal or elevated cholesterol level
   a. Hyperbetalipoproteinemia
   b. Lp(a) hyperlipoproteinemia

LDL-C, low-density lipoprotein cholesterol; HDL-C, high-density lipoprotein cholesterol; VLDL-C, very low-density lipoprotein cholesterol; LCAT, lecithin-cholesterol acyltransferase; SLE, systemic lupus erythematosus.

From Arden MR. Primary hyperlipidemias. In: Jacobson MS, ed. *Atherosclerosis prevention: identification and treatment of the child with high cholesterol.* London: Harwood Academic Publishers, 1991:30, with permission.

account for only 2% of cases they are responsible for >20% of premature CAD. Most cases of hyperlipidemia occur as a result of diet and lifestyle factors, in association with genetic polymorphism in apoE, lecithin-cholesterol acyltransferase, lipoprotein lipase, and other lipid enzymes and cofactors. Hyperlipidemia also occurs as a result of medical conditions or the use of medications such as estrogens, isotretinoin, and β_3-adrenergic blockers.

1. Familial hypercholesterolemia:
   a. Monogenic: This is an autosomal codominant disorder resulting from insufficient activity of the cell surface receptors for LDL. A number of different mutations in the LDL receptor gene occur in families, all of which result in the same phenotypical disease. Homozygous familial hypercholesterolemia is a rare disease, occurring in approximately one in a million individuals. Typically, individuals homozygous for this condition have coronary atherosclerosis in the second or third decade of life. Clinically, this condition may manifest in childhood and adolescence by the deposition of cholesterol esters in tendons (xanthomas), as well as in soft tissues of the eyelids (xanthelasma) and in the cornea (arcus cornea). The

mean cholesterol concentration in the heterozygous condition ranges from 250 to 500 mg/dL and in the homozygote from 500 to 1,000 mg/dL. Homozygous individuals may respond poorly to drugs and require referral to specialists for consideration of more radical therapies. The heterozygous form has been estimated to occur in 1 of 200 to 500 individuals. A similar clinical presentation is observed in individuals with a heterozygous abnormality; however, the signs and symptoms tend to be milder and develop later, about the fourth or fifth decade of life.
   b. Polygenic: This is a common cause of type IIa hyperlipidemia, probably associated with a combination of multiple genetic abnormalities and environmental factors. Individuals with this condition lack typical features of familial hypercholesterolemia such as xanthelasma, arcus cornea, and tendinous xanthomas.
2. Familial defective apoB-100: This is a mutation in the apoB gene, which results in decreased affinity of LDL to the LDL receptor. The phenotypical expression of this condition in children has not been described. Homozygous and heterozygous genotypes are known. This condition may occur in as many as 1 of 500 people,

TABLE 12.2

Metabolic Classification of Dyslipoproteinemia in Children and Adolescents

1. Disorders of LDL metabolism/disorders with increased LDL
   a. Decreased LDL removal
      —Familial hypercholesterolemia
      —Defective apoB-100
   b. Increased LDL production
      —Familial combined hypercholesterolemia
      —Hyperapobetalipoproteinemia
   c. Other
      —Polygenic hypercholesterolemia
2. Disorders of triglyceride-rich lipoproteins
   a. Decreased removal (type I dyslipoproteinemia)
      —Lipoprotein lipase deficiency
      —ApoC-II deficiency (cofactor for lipoprotein lipase)
   b. Production of abnormal VLDL
      —Familial hypertriglyceridemia (AD)
   c. Decreased removal/increased production
      —Type V dyslipoproteinemia (AD)
      —Dysbetalipoproteinemia
3. Deficiency in HDL
   a. Increased HDL removal
   b. Decreased HDL production

LDL, low-density lipoprotein; VLDL, very low-density lipoprotein; AD, autosomal dominant; HDL, high-density lipoprotein.

From Kwiterovich PO Jr. Diagnosis and management of familial dyslipoproteinemia in children and adolescents. *Pediatr Clin North Am* 1990;37:1489, with permission.

but the defect appears to account for only a small percentage (<2%) of premature CAD.
3. Lipoprotein lipase deficiency: This is a rare condition associated with very high levels of triglycerides and normal cholesterol levels. Eruptive xanthomas may be present. Although the risk of atherosclerosis is not elevated, the individual is at risk of having pancreatitis, particularly when the triglyceride level exceeds 500 mg/dL.
4. Familial dysbetalipoproteinemia: A very uncommon condition, occurring in approximately 1 of 1,000–2,000 persons in the United States; it is seen only rarely in adolescence. In this condition, the catabolism of VLDL remnants and chylomicrons is delayed because an abnormal apoE alters the normal binding of VLDL remnants to LDL receptors. This problem should be suspected when triglyceride levels are some what higher than cholesterol levels in the presence of a significant cholesterol elevation. These individuals have an increased risk of premature CAD and peripheral vascular disease. They are often obese and have glucose intolerance, hyperuricemia, and tuberoeruptive and palmar xanthomas. Caloric restriction is usually effective.
5. Familial hypertriglyceridemia: This is a autosomal dominant trait. Dietary factors, obesity, and a sedentary lifestyle are additional elements involved in the degree of expression.

6. FCHL: Affected individuals have high levels of LDL-C, triglycerides, or both. This condition is usually not associated with tendinous xanthomas but is associated with premature CAD. Multiple lipoprotein phenotypes can occur in a single affected family. Affected individuals may have increases in VLDL alone, LDL alone, or VLDL plus LDL or chylomicrons. The diagnosis is made by a finding of multiple lipoprotein phenotypes in a single family when first-degree relatives are tested or when a typical pattern of modest elevation in concentrations of cholesterol and triglycerides is seen, together with a low HDL-C level. FCHL occurs in approximately 15% of patients with CAD younger than 60 years. The metabolic defect appears to be an overproduction of lipoproteins by the liver, as well as decreased catabolism in the periphery. Dietary therapy, along with physical exercise, plays an important role in treatment.

LIPID SCREENING AND MANAGEMENT

According to NCEP, the process of screening and management differs for adolescents (age 20 years or younger) and young adults (age 20–35 years). In addition to classification of lipid parameters, screening involves the identification of other cardiovascular risk factors by history and physical examination. Once an adolescent with a positive family history is found to have a high total cholesterol, then the algorithm in Figure 12.3 can be used to classify and manage his or her risk.

History

1. Family history of premature cardiovascular diseases (younger than 55 years for male and 60 for female relatives) such as myocardial infarcts or other sequelae of atherosclerosis
2. Family history of dyslipidemia or hypertension
3. History of smoking
4. Dietary history: May use 24 hour recall for dietary history.

Physical Examination

1. Signs of peripheral lipid deposition (xanthoma, xanthelasma, corneal arcus)
2. Weight, height, BP, and sexual maturity rating
3. Body composition indexes: Adjunctively, it may be useful to evaluate body composition by measurement of mid upper arm circumference and standard skin folds. The waist–hip ratio is also an important predictor of lipoprotein levels (Mansfield et al., 1999). A waist circumference of >40 in. (102 cm) in men or 35 in. (80 cm) in women is considered abdominal obesity, a part of the metabolic syndrome highlighted by the ATP III.

Screening in Adolescents

Selective screening of children and adolescents is recommended by the NCEP Expert Panel on Blood Cholesterol Levels in Children and Adolescents, the American Academy of Pediatrics, the Bright Futures guidelines from the National Center for Education in Maternal and Child Health, the Guidelines for Adolescent and Preventive Services

TABLE 12.3

Characteristics of Inherited Hyperlipoproteinemias

Hyperlipoproteinemia	Phenotype	Cholesterol	Triglyceride	Xanthomas	Frequency (%)	Risk of CAD
Familial lipoprotein lipase deficiency	I	Normal	↑	Eruptive	Very rare	0
Familial hypercholesterolemia	IIa IIb	↑	↑	Tendon Tuberous xanthelasma	0.1–0.5	4+
Polygenic hypercholesterolemia	II	↑	Normal	Tuberous	5	2+
Familial dysbetalipoproteinemia	III	↑	↑	Palmar Planar tuberous tendon	Rare	4+
Familial combined hyperlipoproteinemia	IIa IIb IV Rarely V	↑	↑	Any type	1–2	3+
Familial hypertriglyceridemia	IV Rarely V	Normal	↑	Eruptive	1	1+

CAD, coronary artery disease; NL, normal.
From Arky RA, Perlman AJ. Hyperlipoproteinemia. In: Rubenstein E, Federman DD, eds. *Scientific American medicine*. New York: Scientific American, 1988, with permission.

(GAPS) from the American Medical Association, and the American Academy of Family Physicians.

Reference-range values for adolescents and young adults are given in Table 12.4. The NCEP Expert Panel on Blood Cholesterol Levels in Children and Adolescents and the American Academy of Pediatrics Committee on Nutrition (1998) classify risk on the basis of *total cholesterol* levels as follows:

Low risk	<170 mg/dL
Borderline risk	170–199 mg/dL
High risk	200 mg/dL (95th percentile)

Providing dietary treatment for adolescents and young adults with the top 25% of cholesterol values is probably desirable, but this has not been proven to reduce CVD. However, establishing such proof would be extremely difficult, requiring lengthy (30–40 years) longitudinal studies. Recommending drug treatment to the top 10% is even more controversial until more is known about the risk–benefit ratio for drug treatment in a younger population. Several recent studies have proven the short term (1-2yr) safety and efficacy of statins in adolescents with FH so that the FDA has now approved Atrovastatin, Lovastatin, Pravastatin, and Simvistatin for use in 12-18 yr olds with FH (see Drug Theraphy below) (Gotto 2004)

At present, it seems reasonable to recommend that individuals in the borderline-risk group receive hygienic measures, including exercise instruction, nutritional advice such as the NCEP Step 1 prudent diet, and nonsmoking advice. Those in the high-risk group should receive all these measures plus dietary counseling by a dietitian and more frequent follow-up. Although the LDL-C level is more closely correlated with CAD risk, total cholesterol, which can be drawn nonfasting, can be used for follow-up to save on laboratory costs and inconvenience to patients.

1. Who: If possible, all adolescents should be screened once during this age period. If not possible, then the following adolescents should be screened:
   a. Teens whose parents or relatives have had premature CAD or stroke, or clinical evidence of atherosclerosis before the age of 55 years in male members and before the age of 65 years in female members
   b. Teens whose parents have elevated concentrations of lipoproteins
   c. Teens with hypertension, obesity, diabetes, or other significant cardiac risk factors
   d. Smokers
   The optimal screening frequency for high blood cholesterol in this risk group has not been determined and is left to clinical discretion.
2. How: Serum lipids are best measured after a 12- to 14-hour fast; however, the total cholesterol level can be determined in a nonfasting sample because chylomicrons from dietary fat contribute essentially no cholesterol. If a nonfasting cholesterol level is borderline or above, a fasting sample should be obtained and analyzed for triglyceride, total cholesterol, and HDL-C with a calculation of LDL-C. Risk based on LDL-C is as follows:

Acceptable	<110 mg/dL
Borderline	110–129 mg/dL
High risk	>130 mg/dL

The AHA does not recommend mass screenings of plasma cholesterol concentration for all children and adolescents. The reasoning behind this was that such

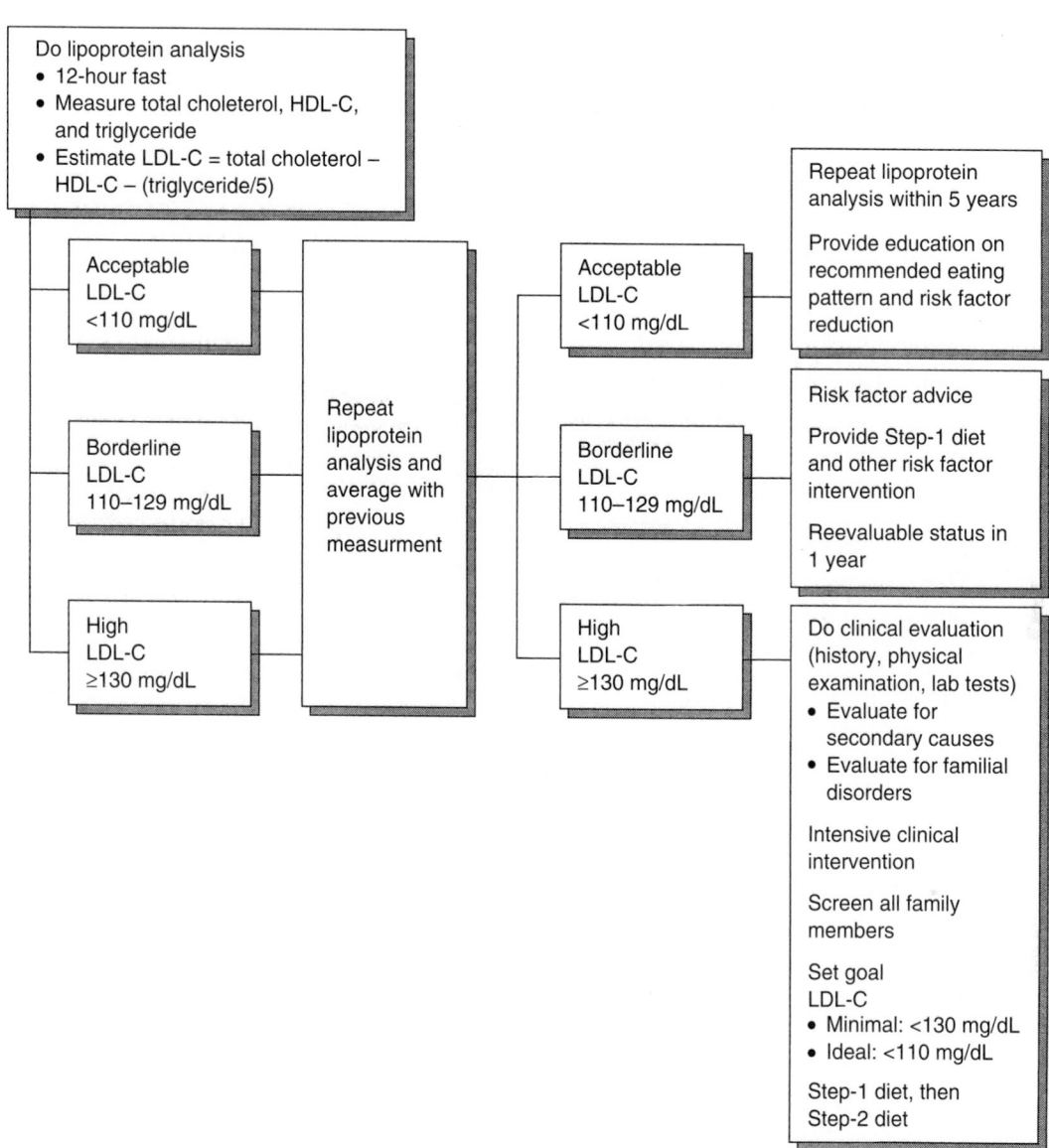

FIGURE 12.3 Classification, education, and follow-up based on LDL-C (low-density lipoprotein cholesterol) in adolescents (<20 years) with elevated total cholesterol. HDL-C, high-density lipoprotein cholesterol. (From the National Cholesterol Education Programs. Report of the expert panel on blood cholesterol levels in children and adolescents. *Pediatrics* 1992;89(suppl):498.)

screenings may reach many individuals who are either at low risk or already know their cholesterol level.

Screening in Young Adults

The ATP III of the NCEP issued an evidence-based set of guidelines on cholesterol management in 2001. Since the publication of ATP III, several major clinical trials of statin therapy with clinical end points have been published (Grundy et al., 2004).

1. ATP III recommendations for young adults between the ages of 20 and 35 years are as follows:
   a. Fasting lipid profile is the preferred method of assessing lipid risk and should be determined in every

young adult regardless of family history at least once every 5 years. Next, the number of risk factors is counted (Table 12.5) for those with two or more risk factors; Framingham scoring is then used to assign 10-year risk of a coronary event. Last, the lipid profile is interpreted by the following guidelines:

- LDL-C

Optimal	<100 mg/dL
Near optimal	100–129 mg/dL
Borderline high	130–159 mg/dL
High	160–189 mg/dL
Very high	190 mg/dL

TABLE 12.4

Lipid Values by Age and Sex

Age (yr)	Cholesterol		Triglycerides		LDL-C		HDL-C	
	75th	90th	75th	90th	75th	90th	10th	25th
Males								
5–9	168	183	58	70	103	117	42	49
10–14	173	188	74	94	109	122	40	46
15–19	168	183	88	125	109	123	34	39
20–24	179	197	107	146	118	138	32	38
25–29	199	223	120	171	138	157	32	37
Females								
5–9	177	190	74	103	115	125	38	47
10–14	171	191	85	104	110	126	40	45
15–19	173	195	84	108	110	127	38	43
20–24	176	202	81	100	113	136	37	43
25–29	192	213	86	108	122	141	40	47

LDL-C, low-density lipoprotein cholesterol; HDL-C, high-density lipoprotein cholesterol.
From The Lipid Research Clinics Population Studies data book. I. *The prevalence study.* Publication No. 80–1527. Bethesda, MD: National Institutes of Health, 1980, with permission.

- Total cholesterol

Desirable	<200 mg/dL
Borderline	200–239 mg/dL
High risk	>240 mg/dL

- HDL-C

Low	<40 mg/dL
High	>60 mg/dL

b. In those without CAD, which will be the vast majority of 20- to 35-year-old adults, the following LDL-C goals and treatments apply: LDL-C goal is <160 mg/dL, at which point therapeutic lifestyle changes (TLC) are indicated. At LDL-C >190 mg/dL, lipid-lowering medications should be considered. At 160 to 189 mg/dL, LDL-C lipid-lowering drugs are optional and based on clinical judgment, which takes into account the presence or absence of two broad classes of additional factors: *life habits* (e.g., obesity, sedentary lifestyle, and atherogenic diet) and *emerging risk factors* (e.g., Lp[a], homocysteine, prothrombotic and proinflammatory plasma factors, as well as impaired glucose tolerance).

2. Results from recent trials have resulted in updated ATP III recommendations as follows (Stone, 2005):
   a. TLC remain an essential modality in clinical management.
   b. The trials confirm the benefit of cholesterol-lowering therapy in high-risk patients and support the ATP III treatment goal of LDL-C <100 mg/dL.
   c. They support the inclusion of patients with diabetes in the high-risk category and confirm the benefits of LDL-lowering therapy in these patients.
   d. The major recommendations for modifications to footnote the ATP III treatment algorithm are the following:

- In high-risk persons, the recommended LDL-C goal is <100 mg/dL, but when risk is very high, an LDL-C goal of <70 mg/dL is a therapeutic option, that is, a reasonable clinical strategy, on the basis of available clinical trial evidence. This therapeutic option extends also to patients at very high risk who have a baseline LDL-C <100 mg/dL.
- Moreover, when a high-risk patient has high triglycerides or low HDL-C, consideration can be

TABLE 12.5

Major Risk Factors (Exclusive of Low-Density Lipoprotein Cholesterol) that Modify Low-Density Lipoprotein Goals[a]

- Cigarette smoking
- Hypertension (blood pressure ≥140/90 mm Hg or on antihypertensive medication)
- Low HDL cholesterol (<40 mg/dL)[b]
- Family history of premature CHD (CHD in first-degree male relative <55 yr; CHD in first-degree female relative <65 yr)
- Age (men ≥45 yr; women ≥55 yr)

[a]Diabetes is regarded as a coronary heart disease (CHD) risk equivalent.

[b] High-density lipoprotein (HDL) cholesterol ≥60mg/dL counts as a "negative" risk factor; its presence removes one risk factor from the total count.

From *JAMA.* Executive summary of the third report of the National Cholesterol Education Program Expert Panel on detection, evaluation, and treatment of high blood cholesterol in adults (ATP III). *JAMA* 2001;285(19):2486–2497, with permission.

given to combining a fibrate or nicotinic acid with an LDL-lowering drug.

- For moderately high-risk persons (2+ risk factors and 10-year risk 10%–20%), the recommended LDL-C goal is <130 mg/dL, but an LDL-C goal <100 mg/dL is a therapeutic option on the basis of recent trial evidence.
- The latter option also extends to moderately high-risk persons with a baseline LDL-C of 100 to 129 mg/dL.
- When LDL-lowering drug therapy is employed in high-risk or moderately high-risk persons, it is advised that intensity of therapy be sufficient to achieve at least a 30% to 40% reduction in LDL-C levels.
- Moreover, any person at high risk or moderately high risk who has lifestyle-related risk factors (e.g., obesity, physical inactivity, elevated triglycerides, low HDL-C, or metabolic syndrome) should make TLC to modify these risk factors regardless of LDL-C level.
- Finally, for people in lower-risk categories, recent clinical trials do not modify the goals and cutpoints of therapy.

A complete report is available online (http://www.nhlbi.nih.gov/guidelines/cholesterol/index.htm), which includes an executive summary, a full report, a quick desk reference, a slide show, an interactive tool for handheld devices, and a 10-year risk calculator from the ATP III on Detection, Evaluation, and Treatment of High Blood Cholesterol in Adults.

Hypertriglyceridemia

Moderate hypertriglyceridemia alone is not independently correlated with CAD. Severe hypertriglyceridemia ($\geq$1,000 mg/dL) is associated with an increased incidence of acute life-threatening pancreatitis and must be aggressively treated with diet, weight loss, and pharmacotherapy. The Framingham study has found that a triglyceride concentration of >150 mg/dL, in combination with a HDL level of <35 mg/dL, is as good a predictor of CAD as LDL elevation. Therefore, in the presence of an elevated triglyceride and a low HDL concentration, treatment with the TLC diet and exercise intervention is recommended. The ATP III now defines hypertriglyceridemia more strictly than previously:

Normal triglycerides	<150 mg/dL
Borderline-high triglycerides	150–199 mg/dL
High triglycerides	200–499 mg/dL
Very high triglycerides	>500 mg/dL

For adolescents, the 90th percentile (Table 12.4) should be used as the upper limit of normal for age and sex.

Nonlipid (Novel) Risk Factor Assessment

Insulin/Glucose Ratio Insulin resistance is indicated by an elevated ratio. It is associated with accelerated atherosclerosis through various mechanisms including lipid oxidation, endothelial dysfunction, and thrombogenic abnormalities (Hayden and Reaven, 2000). It is associated with the metabolic syndrome (syndrome X) (Reaven,

2002), which consists of at least three of the following five: central adiposity, hypertension, elevated triglyceride levels, decreased HDL-C levels, impaired glucose tolerance. In adolescents, the metabolic syndrome is best managed with lifestyle changes aimed at overweight and obesity. ATP III recognizes metabolic syndrome as a secondary target of cardiovascular risk reduction after LDL lowering. Routine screening of fasting insulin is not indicated, rather it should be reserved for individuals with risk factors for type 2 diabetes (such as family history, obesity, or acanthosis nigricans).

Homocysteine Elevated plasma total homocysteine is an independent risk factor for atherosclerotic vascular disease and has been linked to an increased risk of thrombosis. Risk increases continuously across the spectrum of homocysteine concentrations and may become appreciable at levels higher than 10 μmol/L. A compelling case can be made for screening all individuals with atherosclerotic disease or at high risk. Folic acid is the mainstay of treatment, because homocysteine levels can be reduced with folic acid supplementation, but vitamins B_{12} and B_6 may have added benefit in selected patients. The results of ongoing randomized, placebo-controlled trials will help in determining whether lowering the homocysteine concentration reduces the risk of cardiovascular disease (Gerhard and Duell, 1999).

Other potential emerging risk factors explored have included CRP and other inflammatory markers, coagulation factors (such as fibrinogen and factors VIII and VII), deficiency of antioxidant vitamins, and chlamydia infections.

THERAPY FOR HYPERLIPIDEMIA

General Principles

1. Diagnose and treat secondary causes.
2. Reduce risk factors. Intervene with those risk factors that can be altered, including smoking, hypertension, and diabetes.
3. Start a heart-healthy diet. The principal treatment of hyperlipidemia in adolescents and adults is a diet with modified amounts of fat, saturated fat, and cholesterol without increased simple carbohydrates. The goals of dietary therapy are to lower total cholesterol and LDL-C concentration to below the 90th percentile—preferably below the 75th percentile. Nutritional management is described in two steps as recommended by the NCEP Expert Panel on Blood Cholesterol Levels in Children and Adolescents, as shown in Table 12.6. If adherence to the NCEP Step 1 diet fails to achieve the minimal goals of therapy, the Step 2 diet should be prescribed.

The pediatric recommendations differ from those for adults in that careful consideration and monitoring of energy and micronutrient consumption are needed for support of normal growth and development. This is particularly important during the adolescent growth years, when energy, protein, mineral, and vitamin requirements are increased. Nutritional counseling focusing on meeting fat and cholesterol recommendations while ensuring adequate macronutrient and micronutrient intake is needed. The Committee on Nutrition of the American Academy of Pediatrics recently set lower limits on the recommended fat intake of children and adolescents at no more than 30% of the average daily caloric intake and no less than 20% of the average daily caloric intake.

TABLE 12.6

Recommended Diet Modifications to Lower Blood Cholesterol

	Step 1 Diet	
	Choose	*Decrease*
Fish, chicken, turkey, and lean meats	Fish, poultry without skin, lean cuts of beef, lamb, pork or veal, shellfish	Fatty cuts of beef, lamb, pork; spare ribs, organ meats, regular cold cuts, sausage, hot dogs, bacon, sardines, roe
Skim and low-fat milk, cheese, yogurt, and dairy substitutes	Skim or 1% fat milk (liquid, powdered, evaporated), buttermilk	Whole milk (4% fat): regular, evaporated, condensed; cream, half and half, 2% milk, imitation milk products, most nondairy creamers, whipped toppings
	Nonfat (0% fat) or low-fat yogurt	Whole-milk yogurt
	Low-fat cottage cheese (1% or 2% fat)	Whole-milk cottage cheese (4% fat)
	Low-fat cheese, farmer or pot cheese (all of these should be labeled no more than 2–6 g of fat/oz)	All natural cheeses (e.g., blue, roquefort, camembert, cheddar, Swiss), low-fat or "light" cream cheese, low-fat or "light" sour cream, cream cheese, sour cream
	Sherbet, sorbet	Ice cream
Eggs	Egg whites (two whites equal one whole egg in recipes), cholesterolfree egg substitutes	Egg yolks
Fruits and vegetables	Fresh, frozen, canned, or dried fruits and vegetables	Vegetables prepared in butter, cream, or other sauces
Breads and cereals	Homemade baked goods using unsaturated oils sparingly, angel food cake, low-fat crackers, low-fat cookies	Commercial baked goods: pies, cakes, doughnuts, croissants, pastries, muffins, biscuits, high-fat crackers, high-fat cookies
	Rice, pasta	Egg noodles
	Whole-grain breads and cereals (oatmeal, whole wheat, rye, bran, multi-grain, etc.)	Breads in which eggs are a major ingredient
Fats and oils	Baking cocoa	Chocolate
	Unsaturated vegetable oils: corn, olive, rapeseed (canola oil), safflower, sesame, soybean, sunflower	Butter, coconut oil, palm oil, palm kernel oil, lard, bacon fat
	Margarine or shortenings made from one of the unsaturated oils listed above, diet margarine	
	Mayonnaise, salad dressings made with unsaturated oils listed above, low-fat dressings	Dressings made with egg yolk
	Seeds and nuts	Coconut

From The Expert Panel. Report of The National Cholesterol Education Program. *Arch Intern Med* 1988;148:49, with permission.

4. Set dietary goals.
   a. Reduced dietary fats
   b. Reduced saturated fat and improved fatty acid balance
   c. Reduced dietary cholesterol
   d. Increased complex carbohydrates
      Achieving these dietary goals can be difficult for teens, so help from a physician, a dietitian, and the family is crucial. Helpful suggestions include the following:
      • Snacks: Most candies should be limited. Replace with Graham crackers, Rye Krisp, melba toast, soda crackers, bagels, English muffins, and fruits and vegetables. Popcorn should be air popped.

• Desserts: Try fruits, low-fat yogurt, fruit ices, and jello.
• Cooking methods: Choose methods that use little or no fat, such as steaming, baking, or broiling.
• Eating away from home: Order entrées, potatoes, and vegetables without sauces or butter.
• Ask for salad dressings to be served on the side. Limit high-fat toppings such as bacon, crumbled eggs, cheese, and sunflower seeds.
• A regular exercise program is an important adjunct to a change in eating habits.
• Initiate diets that closely correspond to the adolescent's usual eating habits.

- Implement specific goals in a graduated manner, rather than all at once.
- Encourage family participation in the dietary management and the exercise program.
- Stress the maintenance of ideal body weight, an exercise program, and the prevention of nicotine and alcohol use.

Dietary Therapy

Step 1 and Step 2 diets are outlined at the AHA Web site (http://www.americanheart.org). (Table 12.7).

1. Reduce dietary fats: The typical fat intake of children in the United States is 36% of total energy consumption. To meet the goal of 30%, the teen must make several modifications in the intake of "visible" and "invisible" fats. Visible fats include butter, margarine, oils, salad dressing, mayonnaise, cream, and gravies. They are often added to foods or used in preparation (e.g., fried chicken or French fries). Invisible sources of fat include oils and other fats incorporated into baked goods, processed foods (e.g., cold cuts, frozen meats, and franks), whole milk, other dairy products, and snack foods (e.g., chips, doughnuts). Sources of fats should be identified in the adolescent's diet. The amount and frequency of consumption of high-fat food should be reduced and lower-fat alternatives given.

2. Reduce saturated fats and improve fatty acid balance: Saturated fatty acids with chain lengths of 12 carbons (lauric), 14 carbons (myristic), and 16 carbons (palmitic) have the most hypercholesterolemic effect in humans. Stearic acid, an 18-carbon saturated fatty acid, has been found to be less atherogenic than 12- to 16-carbon fatty acids. These 12- to 16-carbon fatty acids are found in certain vegetable oils (e.g., palm or coconut), animal fats, and whole-milk dairy products. The 18-carbon stearic acid is found in chocolate and beef.

    Data from the 1988 Continuing Survey of Food Intakes by Individuals show that 14% of total calories is contributed to the diet from saturated fatty acids, a percentage that is higher than the recommended 10% limit. Therefore, when saturated fats are reduced to <10% of total calories, the balance of monounsaturated and polyunsaturated fatty acids must be considered. Major sources of monounsaturated fatty acids include olive oil, canola oil, peanuts, hazelnuts, avocado, lean beef, and poultry. Substituting these for saturated fatty acids in the context of a low-fat diet can lead to a reduction in LDL-C, no elevation in triglycerides, and preservation of HDL-C.

    The major categories of polyunsaturated fatty acids are ω-6 or ω-3 fatty acids, terms referring to the positions of their double bonds. Linoleic acid, the major ω-6 fatty acid in the diet, is found in vegetable oils such as safflower, sunflower seed, soybean, and corn oils. ω-6 Fatty acids, when used in the context of the other dietary recommendations, lower total cholesterol and LDL-C concentrations without decreasing HDL-C concentration. Taken in amounts higher than 10% of total calories, these fatty acids may cause subsequent lowering of HDL-C levels. The long-term safety of a diet high in polyunsaturated fats, in relation to the incidence of cancers, has not been established.

    ω-3 Fatty acids are primarily found in cold-water fish as eicosapentaenoic acid and docosahexaenoic acid and in soybean and walnut oils as linolenic acid. ω-3 Fatty acids, given as fish-oil supplements, have been shown to lower elevated triglyceride levels in adult patients with hypertriglyceridemia and to improve the dyslipidemia in pediatric patients with systemic lupus erythematosus. Fish-oil supplementation should be monitored medically for side effects such as decreased clotting time. In general, increasing the number of meals with cold-water fish (e.g., salmon, mackerel, bluefish, trout, and sable fish) to a minimum of twice weekly while decreasing fatty beef and poultry dishes would be beneficial.

3. Reduce dietary cholesterol: Dietary cholesterol will elevate both plasma concentrations of total cholesterol and LDL-C. The current consumption of cholesterol by children is <300 mg/day, which is almost within reach of the current recommendations. The following suggestions are given to guide the patient with hyperlipidemia and his or her family:

TABLE 12.7

Dietary Therapy for High Blood Cholesterol Levels: Characteristics of Step 1 and Step 2 Diets for Lowering Blood Cholesterol Levels

Nutrient	Recommended Intake	
	Step 1 Diet	*Step 2 Diet*
Total fat	20% of–30% of total calories	Same
Saturated fatty acids	<10% of total calories	<7% of total calories
Polyunsaturated fatty acids	≤10% of total calories	Same
Monounsaturated fatty acids	Remaining total fat calories	Same
Cholesterol	<300 mg/d	<200 mg/d
Carbohydrates	≈55% of total calories	Same
Protein	≈15%–20% of total calories	Same
Calories	To promote normal growth and development and to reach or maintain desirable body weight	Same

a. Reduce visible egg yolks such as fried eggs and egg yolks used in home recipes and replace with egg whites or egg substitutes.

b. Limit portions of cooked meat, chicken, and fish to 7 to 8 oz daily; if lean cuts of beef and pork and controlled amounts of shellfish (six medium-sized shrimp) are used, they can be incorporated into the diet and can provide a significant source of minerals and vitamins.

c. Use skim milk or the lowest-fat dairy products available. Cholesterol-restricted diets have been shown to be safe in relation to growth and cognitive development in several European studies (Rask-Nissila et al., 2000) and in the United States (Jacobson et al., 1998).

4. Increase complex carbohydrates: When fat is removed from an adolescent's diet, an energy deficit may occur. In the overweight or obese teenager, this may aid in cessation of weight gain, but in the normal-weight to underweight individual, it may result in undesirable weight loss. Therefore, it is important to replace the fat energy with complex carbohydrate sources. Complex carbohydrates are found in fruits, vegetables, and whole-grain products, such as unsweetened cereals, pasta, breads, corn, rice, and crackers.

Fatfree baked products offer a wide variety of snacks for adolescents and encourage adherence to the diet regimen. These products are isocaloric with their full-fat counterparts and thereby contain a significant amount of simple sugar; therefore, their intake must be limited for the patient with elevated triglyceride concentrations, impaired glucose tolerance, or obesity.

What are the Differences between the American Heart Association Diet, and the Step 1 and Step 2 Diets? The Step 1 diet from the AHA is very similar to the diet recommended by the AHA for the general public, with the exception that the Step 1 diet is followed in a medical setting. The Step 2 diet has further reductions in cholesterol and saturated fat for those already on a Step 1 diet or for those with a higher level of cholesterol or more risk factors. Step 1 and Step 2 diets should be combined with regular physical activity in all patients and with weight reduction in the overweight.

What is New in the ATP III Therapeutic Lifestyle Changes Diet? The Step 2 diet's limit on saturated fat of 7% of energy intake has been adopted for all adults and combined with a more liberal total fat intake of 25% to 35%, with the majority coming from monounsaturated fats. These changes recognize the contribution of excess intake of fatfree commercial baked goods with extra sugar, which have contributed to the epidemic of obesity, metabolic syndrome, and type 2 diabetes.

Vitamin Therapy

The ATP III acknowledges the importance of meeting the daily recommended intake (DRI) of vitamins and minerals but does not recommend megavitamin therapy beyond the DRI because of the negative data from clinical trials of β-carotene and antioxidant vitamins. We recommend all adolescents take an over-the-counter multivitamin with 100% of the DRI for folic acid (400 µg), as well as all the other water-soluble and fat-soluble vitamins and minerals for which there are DRIs.

Stanols and Plant Sterols

As adjunctive LDL-C–lowering therapy, the ATP III recommends the addition of plant-derived cholesterol absorption-inhibiting compounds such as esters of cholestanol or other nonabsorbed sterols available as margarine or salad dressing (at two to three servings/day). Studies, mainly from Europe, have shown an additional 10% to 15% LDL-C reduction with daily use of these compounds in persons consuming a low-saturated fat, low-cholesterol diet.

Drug Therapy

The risk-benefit ratio for any drug therapy is unknown in adolescents. However, pharmacotherapy is considered when

1. Xanthomas are present on physical examination or *all of the criteria 2 to 4 are met*
2. Supervised diet modification fails to lower LDL-C to acceptable levels or by at least 15% below baseline, plus
3. A parent has died or had severe atherosclerotic sequelae in his or her forties or younger, plus
4. The adolescent's LDL-C concentration is >190 mg/dL in the absence of other risk factors or >160 mg/dL in the presence of any of the following: smoking, hypertension, diabetes, and clinical signs of atherosclerosis.

In individuals older than 20 years, base the treatment on the ATP III LDL goals outlined previously in the section "Screening in Young Adults."

Table 12.8 summarizes mechanisms of action and major effects and lists recommended doses and side effects of the drugs used for hyperlipidemic conditions. These drugs are further detailed here.

Available Drugs
1. Bile acid sequestrants
   a. Cholestyramine (Questran), a hydrophilic, insoluble anion-exchange resin powder
      - Action: Interrupts the enterohepatic circulation of bile acids and binds bile acids in the intestine to form an insoluble complex, which is excreted in feces and thereby increases hepatic synthesis of bile acids from cholesterol. Depletion of the hepatic pool of cholesterol results in an increase in LDL-receptor activity in the liver. This, in turn, stimulates removal of LDL from plasma and lowers LDL-C concentration. There may be an increase in hepatic VLDL production and thereby an increase in triglyceride concentration. The advantage of this drug in the treatment of adolescents is that there is no systemic absorption or toxic effects. However, the gastrointestinal (GI) side effects are frequent, leading to problems in compliance.
      - Effects: Lowering of both total cholesterol and LDL-C levels by 15% to 30% at 16 to 24 g/day.
      - Side effects
        - GI effects include nausea, bloating, and constipation.
        - Drug is difficult to take because it must be suspended in a liquid vehicle. If water is unsatisfactory, an unsweetened juice may improve palatability. Rapid ingestion may cause air swallowing.

TABLE 12.8

Drug Therapy for Hyperlipidemia

Type of Drug	Mechanism of Action	Major Effects	Example	Starting Dose	Adverse Reactions
Statin	Inhibits cholesterol synthesis in hepatic cells, resulting in increased LDL-receptor activity	Lowers LDL cholesterol and triglyceride, raises HDL-C	Atorvastatin, lovastatin, pravastatin, simvastatin, rosuvastatin	5–20 mg depending on which drug is used	Raised hepatic enzymes, muscle soreness possibly progressing to myolysis
Bile acid sequestrants	Binds intestinal bile acids interrupting enterohepatic recirculation, which in turn results in LDL-receptor up regulation	Lowers LDL-C Raises triglycerides	Cholestyramine, colesevelam	One to two packs of powder or four tablets (1 g) daily, with 8 oz water	Limited to GI tract; gas, bloating constipation, cramps, fat-soluble vitamin deficiency
Fibric acid	Probably inhibits hepatic synthesis of VLDL	Mainly lowers triglycerides and raises HDL-C, with less effect on LDL-C	Gemfibrozil, fenofibrate	Varies with preparation	Dyspepsia, constipation, raised liver enzymes, myositis, rhabdomyolisis, anemia
Nicotinic acid	Upregulates hepatic LDL receptors, decreases hepatic LDL and VLDL production	Lowers triglycerides LDL-C and Lp(a), raises HDL-C	Niaspan	500 mg begin slowly to minimize side effects	Flushing, hepatic toxicity, hyperglycemia
Cholesterol absorption inhibitor	Inhibits cholesterol absorption in small intestine, interferes with enterohepatic recirculation	Lowers LDL-C	Ezetimibe	10 mg	Hepatitis, pancreatitis, cholecystitis, diarrhea, abdominal pain, arthralgia

LDL, low-density lipoprotein; HDL-C, high-density lipoprotein cholesterol; LDL-C, low-density lipoprotein cholesterol; VLDL, very low-density lipoprotein; GI, gastrointestinal.

- Bleeding tendencies, osteoporosis, or iron deficiency may result from poor absorption of vitamin K, calcium, or iron, but these complications are rare.
  - Dose: Available in powder form (16–24 g). Should be started at one pack (4 g of cholestyramine; 5 g of orange-flavored filler) twice a day and gradually increased over a month to the full dose. The average dose is two or three packs (8–12 g) taken orally, twice daily with meals.
  b. Colesevelam (WelChol)
  - Action, effects, and side effects: Are similar to those of cholestyramine but GI side effects are considerably reduced.
  - Dose: Available in pill form, making it more convenient for many teens, although the large size of the tablet can be a deterrent to compliance in some. The average dose is two tablets taken orally twice daily with 8 oz of fluid. The maximum adult dose is seven tablets a day.
2. Nicotinic acid (niacin)
  a. Action: Reduces VLDL production by inhibiting lipoprotein synthesis in the liver. Also has effects on lipoprotein lipase in the adipocyte. Niacin is an effective drug but requires considerable patient education because of flushing. A newer proprietary form, Niaspan has shown increased efficacy and reduced flushing in adults. It is also the least costly of the drugs.
  b. Effects: Primarily reduces triglyceride levels but also lowers LDL-C levels and causes a rise in HDL-C. A dose of 1 to 2 g/day can result in a 40% decrease in triglyceride and VLDL levels, a 20% decrease in LDL levels, and a 30% increase in HDL levels. Nicotinic acid is particularly valuable in combination therapy with a bile acid sequestrant because of the complementary modes of action—niacin inhibiting LDL and VLDL production and the bile acid sequestrant increasing LDL excretion. Statin plus niacin is also effective in mixed dyslipidemias.
  c. Side effects: The vitamin preparation is poorly tolerated in the dose needed for lipid lowering.
  - Gastritis, peptic ulcer disease, vomiting, and diarrhea can occur.
  - Liver function abnormalities can occur.
  - Vasodilatation with flushing is also a troublesome side effect.
  d. Dose: The side effects can be reduced by using the sustained release product and starting with a dose of 500 mg with meals or at bed time and gradually increasing for 1 month to 6 weeks. The average daily dose is 1 to 2 g. The possibility of flushing as a side effect should be discussed in advance with the adolescent and parent. Because the flushing is due to prostaglandin effects, it can be ameliorated by taking one aspirin (81 mg) 30 minutes before each dose. Individuals taking niacin should have regular monitoring of aminotransferase, glucose, alkaline phosphatase, and uric acid values.
3. Inhibitors of HMG-CoA reductase (Table 12.9)
  a. Lovastatin (Mevacor)
  - Action: Competitively inhibits the rate-limiting enzyme in cholesterol biosynthesis. LDL-receptor activity is also increased, leading to an increase in the rate of removal of LDL.

- Effects: Causes an average reduction in the LDL-C concentration of 25% to 45%.
- Side effects: Usually well tolerated. The most common side effects include GI upset, muscle aches, and hepatitis. There is an increase in aminotransferase levels in 1.9% of patients. Careful monitoring of liver function is essential. Myalgias occur in approximately 2.4% of individuals. Others include headaches, nausea, fatigue, insomnia, skin rashes, and myositis. Transient mild elevations in creatinine kinase (CK) are commonly seen; in the few patients in whom markedly elevated CK levels and myositis develop, the drug should be discontinued. Results from the lovastatin adolescent trial on 132 male adolescents with familial hypercholesterolemia show efficacy similar to that seen in adults, with normal growth and development (Stein et al., 1998).
- Dose: Usually, the starting dose is 20 mg once daily with the evening meal, with increases to 40 mg and then 80 mg as a single evening dose or in divided doses. Liver function should be checked at the start of therapy at 4 to 6 weeks, 6 months, and then yearly.
  b. Pravastatin (Pravachol)
  - Action, effects, and side effects: Similar to those of lovastatin.
  - Dose: 10 to 40 mg
  c. Simvastatin (Zocor)
  - Action, effects, and side effects: Similar to those of lovastatin.
  - Dose: 5 to 80 mg
  d. Atorvastatin (Lipitor)
  - Action, effects, and side effects: Similar to those of lovastatin, with the additional effect of lowering triglycerides.
  - Dose: 5 to 80 mg
  e. Simvastatin and atrovastatin have now had several randomized clinical trials in adolescents with familial hypercholesterolemia. They are becoming first-line therapy when TLC fail to lower LDL-C to target ranges in this age-group (Kohn and Jacobson, 2004).
  f. Drugs that interfere with statin metabolism: As indicated in Table 12.9, the cytochrome P-450 CYP3A4 and CYP2C9 pathways are involved in metabolism of some of the statins. This can cause problems, for example, with the following medications:
  - Inhibits CYP3A4 (raises serum drug concentrations): erythromycin, clarithromycin, cyclosporine, ritonavir, fluconazole, verapamil, grapefruit juice
  - Induces CYP3A4 (lowers serum drug concentrations): barbiturates, carbamazepine, nafcillin, phenytoin, primidone, rifampin
  - Inhibits CYP2C9 (may raise serum fluvastatin concentrations): amiodarone, cimetidine, trimethoprim-sulfamethoxazole, fluoxetine, isoniazid, ketoconazole, metronidazole
  - Induces CYP2C9 (may lower serum fluvastatin concentrations): barbiturates, carbamazepine, phenytoin, primidone, rifampin
4. Fibric acid derivatives
  a. Gemfibrozil (Lopid)
  - Action: Increases lipoprotein lipase activity and decreases hepatic triglyceride production and inhibits peroxisome proliferator-activated receptor **gamma** (PPARγ).

TABLE 12.9

Characteristics of Statin Drugs

Characteristic	Lovastatin	Pravastatin	Simvastatin	Atorvastatin	Fluvastatin
Maximum dose (mg/d)	80	40	80	80	80
Maximal LDL cholesterol reduction (%)	40	34	47	60	24
Serum triglyceride reduction produced (%)	16	24	18	29	10
Serum HDL cholesterol reduction produced (%)	8.6	12	12	6	8
Plasma half-life (hr)	2	1–2	1–2	14	1.2
Optimal time of administration	With meals (morning and evening)	Bedtime	Evening	Evening	Bedtime
CNS penetration	Yes	No	Yes	No	No
Hepatic metabolic mechanism	Cytochrome P-450 3A4	Sulfation	Cytochrome P-450 3A4	Cytochrome P-450 3A4	Cytochrome P-450 2C9

LDL, low-density lipoprotein; HDL, high-density lipoprotein; CNS, central nervous system.
Adapted from Knopp RH. Drug treatment of lipid disorders. *N Engl J Med* 1999;341:498, with permission.

- Effects: Reduces both VLDL and triglyceride levels. In some individuals, cholesterol levels may decrease and HDL levels may rise. The drug is primarily used for lowering high levels of triglycerides.
- Side effects: Biliary tract disease, and contraindicated in liver or kidney disease. Abdominal discomfort, diarrhea, muscle ache, and increased appetite can occur.
- Dose: 600 to 1,200 mg/day in two doses.
  b. Fenofibrate (Tricor)
    - Action, effects, and side effects: Similar to those of gemfibrozil.
    - Dose: 48 or 145 mg/day
5. Ezetimibe (Zetia)
  - Action: Blocks cholesterol absorption at the intestinal brush border. Interferes with the enterohepatic reabsorption of cholesterol.
  - Effects: Lowers LDL-C and is synergistic with statins allowing for a lower statin dose with increased efficacy and fewer side effects.
  - Side effects: Hepatitis, pancreatitis, cholecystitis, diarrhea, abdominal pain, and athralgia are reported but rarely seen in clinical practice. Randomized placebo-controlled clinical trials are currently under way in adolescents, which will give further information about efficacy and safety. As of April 2007, ezetimibe is not approved for use in those younger than 18 years.
  - Dose: 10 mg/day
  Generally, in the past the bile acid sequestrants used together with nicotinic acid have been considered first-line agents. Fibrates have been used as a second step. However, they are less effective in lowering LDL-C. Now, inhibitors of HMG-CoA reductase, statins, have become first-line agents. Statins are even more effective when used in conjunction with a bile acid sequestrant, niacin, or ezetimibe.
6. Antioxidants

Research by Steinberg and Witzum (1990) on the effects of oxidized LDL has suggested a therapeutic role for antioxidants in the treatment of elevated levels of LDL-C. These drugs have not been widely accepted in the treatment of adolescents and should be considered investigational.
7. Pancreatic lipase inhibitors: orlistat (Xenical)
  These medications cause fat malabsorption and have been primarily used as an adjunct for weight management. Use of these medications, independent of weight loss, has also been noted to significantly improve cardiovascular risk factors and glycemic control. The usual dose is 120 mg thrice daily approximately 20 minutes before meals. Research into these drugs as lipid-lowering agents for adolescents may provide another method of therapy.

Adherence to Drug Therapy
1. Drug therapy should be considered an adjunct and not a replacement for TLC. Many teens, once they are able to make healthier food choices and get regular vigorous physical activity, can get their LDL-C into the target range without medications.
2. The teen must be well informed about the goals of drug treatment and the side effects.
3. It is important to start with small doses of drugs, particularly with sequestrants or nicotinic acid.
4. The frequency of use of the medication and the impact on lifestyle must be discussed.
5. It is important to maintain regularly scheduled follow-ups with the teen.

SUPPORT MATERIALS

The full report and executive summary of the ATP III, Web-based and Palm software for assessing Framingham risk score, and print materials for professionals and patients are available at http://www.nhlbi.nih.gov/guidelines/cholesterol/index.htm.

The following publications to assist in hypercholesterolemia therapy are available from the AHA (7320 Greenville Ave, Dallas, TX 75231) (many of the handouts are available at the AHA Web site at: http://www.americanheart.org/).

The AHA Diet (publication no. 51-018-B). Moderate, fat-controlled low-cholesterol meal plan.

Cholesterol and Your Heart (publication no. 50-069-A). Explanation of what cholesterol is and why it is a risk factor.

Recipes for Fat-Controlled, Low-Cholesterol Meals (publication no. 50-020-B). Recipes for healthy meals.

AHA Cookbook (publication No. 53-001-A). A fat and cholesterol calorie chart and 250 recipes.

In addition, the following is available from the NCEP, National Heart, Lung, and Blood Institute (Box C-200, Bethesda, MD 20892): *Physician's Kit on High Blood Cholesterol.*

Further dietary information for a heart healthy diet is available in Chapter 6.

WEB SITES

For Teenagers and Parents

http://www.americanheart.org. Topics include cholesterol, cholesterol in children, fiber and oat bran, home testing devices, cholesterol levels, cholesterol ratio, screening, dietary guidelines, drugs, risk factors, and triglycerides.

http://www.cdc.gov/cvh/library/fact_sheets.htm. A list of fact sheets for parents describing types of heart disease and stroke and how to prevent them.

http://www.nhlbi.nih.gov/about/ncep/index.htm. This site is the home page for the National Cholesterol education program and has useful links and information for the public and for professionals

http://www.brightfutures.org. The Bright Futures Organization site presents guidelines for healthy nutrition and physical activity for children and adolescents.

http://www.adolescenthealth.org/Health_Guide_for_Americas_Teens.pdf. This document from the Society for Adolescent Medicine has tips to help teens live a healthy lifestyle.

For Health Professionals

http://www.americanheart.org. Cholesterol screening position paper from the AHA.

http://www.cdc.gov/growthcharts/. The source for the most up-to-date growth charts including the new BMI percentile charts.

http://eurodiet.med.uoc.gr/. This site is useful for a European perspective on healthy lifestyles. It contains consensus statements by a European working group on food-based nutrient guidelines

http://www.usda.gov/. This site is a good place to find the latest dietary guidelines for Americans. Also useful is www.mypyramid.gov for the new food guide pyramid.

http://www.aap.org/policy/re9805.html. American Academy of Pediatrics policy on cholesterol in children.

REFERENCES AND ADDITIONAL READINGS

American Academy of Pediatrics, Committee on Nutrition. Cholesterol in childhood. *Pediatrics* 1998;101:141.

American Academy of Pediatrics, Committee on Nutrition. *Pediatric nutrition handbook*, 5th ed. Elk Grove, IL: American Academy of Pediatrics, 2004.

American Diabetes Association. Management of dyslipidemia in children and adolescents with diabetes. *Diabetes Care* 2003;26:2194.

Anderson KM, Castelli WP, Levy D. Cholesterol and morality: 30 years of follow-up from the Framingham study. *JAMA* 1987; 257:2176.

Ansell BJ, Watson KE, Fogelman AM. An evidence-based assessment of the NCEP adult treatment panel II guidelines. National Cholesterol Education Program. *JAMA* 1999;282:2051.

Arky RA, Perlman AL. Cholesterol and mortality: 30 years of follow-up from the Framingham study. *JAMA* 1987;257:2176.

Baker AL, Roberts C, Gothing C. Dyslipidemias in childhood: an overview. *Nurs Clin North Am* 1995;30:243.

Becque MD, Katch VL, Rocchini AP, et al. Coronary risk incidence of obese adolescents: reduction by exercise plus diet intervention. *Pediatrics* 1988;81:605.

Berenson GS, ed. *Causation of cardiovascular risk factors in children*. New York: Raven Press, 1986.

Berenson GS, Srinivasan SR, Bao W, et al. Association between multiple cardiovascular risk factors and atherosclerosis in children and young adults. The Bogalusa heart study. *N Engl J Med* 1998;338:1650.

Berger S, Utech L, Hazinski MF. Sudden death in children and adolescents. *Pediatr Clin North Am* 2004;51:1653.

Blackett PR, Kittredge D. Hyperlipidemia in children. *South Med J* 1993;86:1083.

Breslow JL. Lipoprotein transport gene abnormalities underlying coronary heart disease susceptibility. *Annu Rev Med* 1991;42:357.

Castelli WP, Garrison RJ, Wilson PWF, et al. Incidence of coronary heart disease and lipoprotein cholesterol levels: the Framingham study. *JAMA* 1986;256:2835.

Castelli WP, Griffin GC. How to help patients cut down on saturated fat. *Postgrad Med* 1988;84:44.

Christensen B, Glueck C, Kwiterovich PO Jr, et al. Plasma cholesterol and triglyceride distributions in 13,665 children and adolescents: the prevalence study of the Lipid Research Clinics Program. *Pediatr Res* 1980;14:194.

Clarke WR, Schrott HG, Leaverton PE, et al. Tracking of blood lipids and blood pressures in school-age children: the Muscatine study. *Circulation* 1978;58:626.

Consensus Conference. Lowering blood cholesterol to prevent heart disease. *JAMA* 1985;253:2080.

Cortner JA, Coates PM, Liacouras CA, et al. Familial combined hyperlipidemia in children: clinical expression, metabolic defects, and management. *J Pediatr* 1993;123:177.

Coughlan BJ, Sorrentino MJ. Does hypertriglyceridemia increase risk for CAD. *Postgrad Med* 2000;108:77.

Deedwania PC. Clinical perspectives on primary and secondary prevention of coronary atherosclerosis. *Med Clin North Am* 1995;79:973.

Department of Health and Human Services. *The surgeon general's call to action to prevent and decrease overweight and obesity*. 2001 Mail Stop SSOP, Washington, DC: U.S. Government Printing Office, 20401-0001; #017-001-00551-7. http://www.surgeongeneral.gov/topics/obesity/calltoaction/fact_adolescents.htm.

Donahue RP, Orchard TJ, Kuller LH, et al. Lipids and lipoproteins in a young adult population: the Beaver County lipid study. *Am J Epidemiol* 1985;122:458.

Downs JR, Clearfield M, Weis S, et al. Primary prevention of acute coronary events with lovastatin in men and women with average cholesterol levels: results of AFCAPS/TexCAPS. Air Force/Texas Coronary Atherosclerosis Prevention Study. *JAMA* 1998;279:1615.

Freedman DS, Dietz WH, Srinivasan SR, et al. The relation of overweight to cardiovascular risk factors among children and adolescents: the Bogalusa heart study. *Pediatrics* 1999; 103(Suppl 6, Pt 1):1175.

Gagliano NJ, Emans SJ, Woods ER. Cholesterol screening in the adolescent. *J Adolesc Health* 1993;14:104.

Gerhard GT, Duell PB. Homocysteine and atherosclerosis. *Curr Opin Lipidol* 1999;10:417.

Gillman MW, Couples LA, Moore LL, et al. Impact of within person variability on identifying children with hypercholesterolemia: Framingham children's study. *J Pediatr* 1992; 121:342.

Ginsberg HN. Insulin resistance and cardiovascular disease. *J Clin Invest* 2000;106:453.

Gosland IF, Crook D, Simpson R, et al. The effects of different formulations of oral contraceptive agents on lipid and carbohydrate metabolism. *N Engl J Med* 1990;323:1375.

Gotto AM Jr. Overview of current issues in management of dyslipidemia. *Am J Cardiol* 1993;71:3B.

Gotto AM Targeting High-risk young patients for statin therapy. *JAMA* 2004;292:377.

Grundy SM. Early detection of high cholesterol levels in young adults. *JAMA* 2000;284:365.

Grundy SM, Cleeman JI, Merz CN, et al. Coordinating Committee of the National Cholesterol Education Program. Implications of recent clinical trials for the national cholesterol education program adult treatment panel III guidelines. *J Am Coll Cardiol* 2004;44:720.

Hardoff D, Jacobson MS. Hyperlipidemia. *Adolesc Med (State Art Rev)* 1992;3:473.

Havel RJ, Hunninghake DB, Illingworth R, et al. Lovastatin (Mevinolin) in the treatment of heterozygous familial hypercholesterolemia: a multicenter study. *Ann Intern Med* 1987; 107:609.

Havel RJ, Rapaport E. Management of primary hyperlipidemia. *N Engl J Med* 1995;332:1491.

Hayden JM, Reaven PD. Cardiovascular disease in diabetes mellitus type 2: a potential role for novel cardiovascular risk factors. *Curr Opin Lipidol* 2000;11:515.

Hunninghake DB, Stein EA, Mellies ML. Effects of one year treatment with pravastatin, an HMG-CoA reductase inhibitor, on lipoprotein a. *J Clin Pharmacol* 1993;33:574.

Jacobson MS, ed. *Atherosclerosis prevention: identification and treatment of the child with high cholesterol*. London: Harwood Academic Publishers, 1991.

Jacobson MS. Heart healthy diets for all children: no longer controversial. *J Pediatrics* 1998;133:1.

Jacobson MS, Copperman N, Haas T, et al. Adolescent obesity and cardiovascular risk: a rational approach to management. *Ann N Y Acad Sci* 1993;699:220.

Jacobson MS, Rees J, Golden NH, et al. Adolescent nutritional disorders. *Ann N Y Acad Sci* 1997;817:179.

Jacobson MS, Tomopoulos S, Williams CL, et al. Normal growth in high risk hyperlipidemic children and adolescents with dietary intervention. *Prev Med* 1998;27:775.

Jones PH. A clinical overview of dyslipidemias: treatment strategies. *Am J Med* 1992;93:187.

Kahn JK. Reversing coronary atherosclerosis: how to put findings of recent trials to practical use. *Postgrad Med* 1993; 94:50.

Kannel WB, Wilson PW. Efficacy of lipid profiles in prediction of coronary disease. *Am Heart J* 1992;124:768.

Kannel WB, Wilson PW. An update on coronary risk factors. *Med Clin North Am* 1995;79:951.

Knoflach M, Kiechl S, Kind M, et al. Cardiovascular risk factors and atheroscl;erosis in young males: ARMY study (Atherosclerosis risk-factors in male youngsters). *Circulation* 2003;108:1064.

Knopp RH. Drug treatment of lipid disorders. *N Engl J Med* 1999; 341:498.

Kohn MR, Jacobson MS. Cholesterol (and cardiovascular risk) in adolescence. *Curr Opin Pediatr* 2004;16:357.

Kottke BA, Zinsmeister AR, Holmes DR Jr, et al. Apolipoproteins and coronary artery disease. *Mayo Clin Proc* 1986;61:313.

Kuritzky L. Dyslipidemia: drugs, diet, and common sense. *Hosp Pract* 1994;29:40.

Kwiterovich PO Jr. Diagnosis and management of familial dyslipoproteinemia in children and adolescents. *Pediatr Clin North Am* 1990;37:1489.

Larsen ML, Illingworth DR. Drug treatment of dyslipoproteinemia. *Med Clin North Am* 1994;78:225.

Laskarzewski P, Morrison JA, deGroot I, et al. Lipid and lipoprotein tracking in 108 children over a four-year period. *Pediatrics* 1979;64:584.

Lauer RM, Clarke WR. Use of cholesterol measurements in childhood for the prediction of adult hypercholesterolemia: the Muscatine Study. *JAMA* 1990;264:3034.

Li SC, Chen W, Srinivasan S, et al. Childhood cardiovascular risk factors and carotid vascular changes: the Bogalusa heart study. *JAMA* 2003;290:2271.

Lipid Research Clinics Program. The lipid research clinics coronary primary prevention trial results I and II. *JAMA* 1984;251:351.

Lovastatin Study Group II. Therapeutic response to lovastatin (Mevinolin) in nonfamilial hypercholesterolemia: a multicenter study. *JAMA* 1986;256:2829.

Lovastatin Study Group III. A multicenter comparison of lovastatin and cholestyramine therapy for severe primary hypercholesterolemia. *JAMA* 1988;260:359.

Malloy MJ, Kane JP, Kunitake ST, et al. Complementarity of colestipol, niacin, and lovastatin in treatment of severe familial hypercholesterolemia. *Ann Intern Med* 1987;107:616.

Manninen V, Elo O, Frick H. Lipid alterations and decline in the incidence of coronary heart disease in the Helsinki heart study. *JAMA* 1988;260:641.

Mansfield E, McPherson R, Koski KG. Diet and waist-hip ratio–important predictors of lipoprotein levels in sedentary and active young men with no history of cardiovascular disease. *J Am Diet Assoc* 1999;99:1373.

National Cholesterol Education Program. Report of the Expert Panel on Blood Cholesterol Levels in children and adolescents. *Pediatrics* 1992;89(suppl):495.

National Cholesterol Education Program, Adult Treatment Panel II. Summary of the second report of the National Cholesterol Education Program (NCEP) Expert Panel on Detection Evaluation and Treatment of High Cholesterol in adults (adult treatment panel II). *JAMA* 1993;269: 3015.

National Cholesterol Education Program Expert Panel. Executive summary of the third report of the National Cholesterol Education Program Expert Panel on detection, evaluation, and treatment of high blood cholesterol in adults (ATP III). *JAMA* 2001;285:2486.

Newman WP, Freedman DS, Voors AW, et al. Relation of serum lipoprotein levels and systolic blood pressure to early atherosclerosis: the Bogalusa heart study. *N Engl J Med* 1986; 314:138.

Orchard TJ, Rodgers M, Hedley A, et al. Changes in blood lipids and blood pressure during adolescence. *Br Med J* 1980; 280:1563.

Oren A, Vos LE, Uiterwaal CS, et al. Change in body mass index from adolescence to young adulthood and increased carotid-intima media thickness at 28 years of age: the ARYA (Arteriosclerosis risk and young adults) study. *Int J Obes Relat Metab Disord* 2003;27:1383.

Osganian SK, Stampfer MJ, Spiegelman D, et al. Distribution of and factors associated with serum homocysteine levels in children: child and adolescent trial for cardiovascular health. *JAMA* 1999;281:1189.

Partinen M, Phil S, Strandberg T, et al. Comparison of effects on sleep of lovastatin and pravastatin in hypercholesterolemia. *Am J Cardiol* 1994;73:876.

Pathobiological Determinants of Atherosclerosis in Youth Research Group. Relationship of atherosclerosis in young men to serum lipoprotein cholesterol concentrations and smoking: a preliminary report from the Pathobiological Determinants of Atherosclerosis Research Group. *JAMA* 1990;264:3018.

Pravastatin, simvastatin and lovastatin for lowering serum cholesterol concentrations. *Med Lett Drugs Ther* 1992;34:57.

Rader DJ. Pathophysiology and management of low high-density lipoprotein cholesterol. *Am J Cardiol* 1999;83:22F.

Rask-Nissila L, Jokinen E, Terho P, et al. Neurological development of 5 year old children receiving a low saturated, low cholesterol diet since infancy: a randomized controlled trial. *JAMA* 2000;284:993.

Reaven G. Metabolic syndrome: pathophysiology and implications for management of cardiovascular disease. *Circulation* 2002;106:286.

Safeer RS, Cornell MO. The emerging role of HDL cholesterol. *Postgrad Med* 2000;108:87.

Safeer RS, Lacivita CL. Choosing drug therapy for patients with hyperlipidemia. *Am Fam Physician* 2000;61:3371.

Schwartz CJ, Valente AL, Sprague EA. A modern view of atherogenesis. *Am J Cardiol* 1993;71:9B.

Shepherd J, Cobbe SM, Ford I, et al. Prevention of coronary heart disease with pravastatin in men with hypercholesterolemia. West of Scotland Coronary Prevention Study Group. *N Engl J Med* 1995;333:1301.

Sorrentino MJ. Cholesterol reduction to prevent CAD: what do the data show?. *Postgrad Med* 2000;108:40.

Srinivasan SR, Bao W, Watigney WA, et al. Adolescent Overweight is associated with Adult overweight. *Metabolism* 1996;45:235.

Stein EA, Illingworth DR, Kwiterovitch PO, et al. Efficacy and safety of lovastatin in adolescent males with familial hypercholesterolemia. *JAMA* 1998;282:137.

Steinberg D, Witzum JL. Lipoproteins and atherogenesis. *JAMA* 1990;264:3047.

Steiner NJ, Neinstein LS, Pennbridge J. Hypercholesterolemia in adolescents: effectiveness of screening strategies based on selected risk factors. *Pediatrics* 1991;88:269.

Stone NJ. Secondary causes of hyperlipidemia. *Med Clin North Am* 1994;78:117.

Stone NJ, Bilek S, Rosenbaum S. Recent National Cholesterol Education Program adult treatment panel III update: adjustments and options. *Am J Cardiol* 2005;22(96):53.

Truswell AS. Food carbohydrates and plasma lipids: an update. *Am J Clin Nutr* 1994;59:7105.

Walden CC, Hegele RA. Apolipoprotein E in hyperlipidemia. *Ann Intern Med* 1994;120:1026.

Yeshurun D, Gotto AM Jr. Hyperlipidemia: perspectives in diagnosis and treatment. *South Med J* 1995;88:379.

CHAPTER 13

Systemic Hypertension

Joseph T. Flynn

Although more than 58 million American adults, or approximately 29% of the population, have systemic hypertension, screening studies in children and adolescents have demonstrated a prevalence of persistent hypertension of between 1% and 2%. Given the impact of the obesity epidemic on the prevalence of hypertension in adolescents, more recent studies, however, have demonstrated a higher prevalence of approximately 5% in obese minority adolescents (Sorof et al., 2004). Most adolescents and adults with hypertension have primary hypertension—that is, no identifiable underlying cause can be found for their blood pressure (BP) elevation. Most hypertensive adolescents, particularly those with primary hypertension, are asymptomatic. Therefore, it is imperative that BP is measured whenever an adolescent is seen for health care. Detection and treatment of hypertension in the adolescent years may prevent later cardiovascular diseases, with their catastrophic consequences (Kavey et al., 2003).

DEFINITION OF HYPERTENSION IN ADOLESCENCE

Definition

The cardiovascular endpoints used to define hypertension in adults (myocardial infarction, stroke, etc.) do not occur in children and adolescents. Therefore, the definition of hypertension in the young is a statistical one derived from analysis of a large database of BPs obtained from healthy children (National High Blood Pressure Education Program Working Group, 2004). The most recent classification of BP in the young is summarized in Table 13.1.

Normative BP values for adolescents ≤17 years of age are listed in Tables 13.2 and 13.3. For these children, height should first be obtained and plotted on a standard growth curve to determine the child's height percentile. Then the gender-appropriate chart should be used to determine the BP percentile. For adolescents ≥18 years of age, the adult BP classification scheme issued by the Joint National Commission (Chobanian et al., 2003) should be followed (Table 13.4).

Prehypertension

Common to both the pediatric and adult BP classification schemes is the recent concept of "prehypertension". This refers to BPs that would have been classified as "high-normal" in prior consensus recommendations. Although the term prehypertension has proved to be controversial, it is meant to serve as a means of alerting patients and physicians alike of the potential for later development of hypertension, and of the need to make lifestyle changes that might prevent this from occurring. The same BP value of >120/80 mm Hg is used in both adolescents and adults to designate prehypertension.

Staging

Also common to both the pediatric and adult BP classification schemes is the concept of "staging" the degree of hypertension. For children and adolescents, this replaces the older terms of denoting higher levels of hypertension, such as "significant" and "severe". As will be discussed later, the staging system also plays a role in determining how rapidly a hypertensive adolescent should be

TABLE 13.1

Classification of Blood Pressure in Adolescents 17 years and Younger

Blood Pressure Classification	Systolic or Diastolic Blood Pressure Percentile[a]
Normal	<90th
Prehypertension	90th–95th; or if BP is >120/80 mm Hg even if <90th
Stage 1 hypertension	95th to 99th plus 5 mm Hg
Stage 2 hypertension	>99th plus 5 mm Hg

[a]See Tables 13.2 and 13.3. taken from National High Blood Pressure Education Program Working Group on High Blood Pressure in Children and Adolescents. The fourth report on the diagnosis, evaluation, and treatment of high blood pressure in children and adolescents. National Heart, Lung, and Blood Institute, Bethesda, Maryland. NIH Publication 05-5267, 2005.

TABLE 13.2

Blood Pressure Values for Adolescent Boys 17 Years or Younger

Age (yr)	BP Percentile	Systolic BP (mm Hg) ← Percentile of Height →							Diastolic BP (mm Hg) ← Percentile of Height →						
		5th	10th	25th	50th	75th	90th	95th	5th	10th	25th	50th	75th	90th	95th
10	50th	97	98	100	102	103	105	106	58	59	60	61	61	62	63
	90th	111	112	114	115	117	119	119	73	73	74	75	76	77	78
	95th	115	116	117	119	121	122	123	77	78	79	80	81	81	82
	99th	122	123	125	127	128	130	130	85	86	86	88	88	89	90
11	50th	99	100	102	104	105	107	107	59	59	60	61	62	63	63
	90th	113	114	115	117	119	120	121	74	74	75	76	77	78	78
	95th	117	118	119	121	123	124	125	78	78	79	80	81	82	82
	99th	124	125	127	129	130	132	132	86	86	87	88	89	90	90
12	50th	101	102	104	106	108	109	110	59	60	61	62	63	63	64
	90th	115	116	118	120	121	123	123	74	75	75	76	77	78	79
	95th	119	120	122	123	125	127	127	78	79	80	81	82	82	83
	99th	126	127	129	131	133	134	135	86	87	88	89	90	90	91
13	50th	104	105	106	108	110	111	112	60	60	61	62	63	64	64
	90th	117	118	120	122	124	125	126	75	75	76	77	78	79	79
	95th	121	122	124	126	128	129	130	79	79	80	81	82	83	83
	99th	128	130	131	133	135	136	137	87	87	88	89	90	91	91
14	50th	106	107	109	111	113	114	115	60	61	62	63	64	65	65
	90th	120	121	123	125	126	128	128	75	76	77	78	79	79	80
	95th	124	125	127	128	130	132	132	80	80	81	82	83	84	84
	99th	131	132	134	136	138	139	140	87	88	89	90	91	92	92
15	50th	109	110	112	113	115	117	117	61	62	63	64	65	66	66
	90th	122	124	125	127	129	130	131	76	77	78	79	80	80	81
	95th	126	127	129	131	133	134	135	81	81	82	83	84	85	85
	99th	134	135	136	138	140	142	142	88	89	90	91	92	93	93
16	50th	111	112	114	116	118	119	120	63	63	64	65	66	67	67
	90th	125	126	128	130	131	133	134	78	78	79	80	81	82	82
	95th	129	130	132	134	135	137	137	82	83	83	84	85	86	87
	99th	136	137	139	141	143	144	145	90	90	91	92	93	94	94
17	50th	114	115	116	118	120	121	122	65	66	66	67	68	69	70
	90th	127	128	130	132	134	135	136	80	80	81	82	83	84	84
	95th	131	132	134	136	138	139	140	84	85	86	87	87	88	89
	99th	139	140	141	143	145	146	147	92	93	93	94	95	96	97

BP, blood pressure.

To use the table, first plot the child's height on a standard growth curve (www.cdc.gov/growthcharts). The child's measured systolic blood pressure and diastolic blood pressure are compared with the numbers provided in the table according to the child's age and height percentile.

National High Blood Pressure Education Program Working Group on High Blood Pressure in Children and Adolescents. The fourth report on the diagnosis, evaluation, and treatment of high blood pressure in children and adolescents. National Heart, Lung, and Blood Institute, Bethesda, Maryland. NIH Publication 05-5267, 2005.

evaluated, and when antihypertensive drug therapy should be instituted.

There are several important considerations in evaluating BP in children and adolescents of any age. They are as follows:

1. Although various methods are available to measure BP, auscultation is the most accurate and is the method of choice. Because of the removal of mercury sphygmomanometers from most health care settings, aneroid devices should be made available and utilized. The stethoscope bell should be used for auscultation, as it is better suited to detect soft, low-pitched Korotkoff sounds than the diaphragm.

2. BP in the young is labile; therefore, hypertension should not be diagnosed on the basis of a single measurement.

At least three elevated readings on separate occasions are necessary to diagnose hypertension. Using one isolated measurement may lead to mislabeling of an individual, with adverse consequences.

3. Proper cuff bladder size is critical. The length of the cuff bladder should be at least 80% of the mid-arm circumference. For practical purposes, use the largest cuff that fits the arm while leaving the antecubital fossa free for auscultation. It is better to choose a cuff slightly too big than one too small, as a cuff that is too small will give a falsely elevated BP, but one that is slightly large will not give a falsely low reading.

4. BP measurements should be taken with the adolescent in the sitting position, with the sphygmomanometer at heart level. The arm (preferably the right) used for the measurement should be recorded in the chart. Ideally,

TABLE 13.3

Blood Pressure Values for Adolescent Girls 17 Years or Younger

Age (yr)	BP Percentile	Systolic BP (mm Hg) ← Percentile of Height →							Diastolic BP (mm Hg) ← Percentile of Height →						
		5th	10th	25th	50th	75th	90th	95th	5th	10th	25th	50th	75th	90th	95th
10	50th	98	99	100	102	103	104	105	59	59	59	60	61	62	62
	90th	112	112	114	115	116	118	118	73	73	73	74	75	76	76
	95th	116	116	117	119	120	121	122	77	77	77	78	79	80	80
	99th	123	123	125	126	127	129	129	84	84	85	86	86	87	88
11	50th	100	101	102	103	105	106	107	60	60	60	61	62	63	63
	90th	114	114	116	117	118	119	120	74	74	74	75	76	77	77
	95th	118	118	119	121	122	123	124	78	78	78	79	80	81	81
	99th	125	125	126	128	129	130	131	85	85	86	87	87	88	89
12	50th	102	103	104	105	107	108	109	61	61	61	62	63	64	64
	90th	116	116	117	119	120	121	122	75	75	75	76	77	78	78
	95th	119	120	121	123	124	125	126	79	79	79	80	81	82	82
	99th	127	127	128	130	131	132	133	86	86	87	88	88	89	90
13	50th	104	105	106	107	109	110	110	62	62	62	63	64	65	65
	90th	117	118	119	121	122	123	124	76	76	76	77	78	79	79
	95th	121	122	123	124	126	127	128	80	80	80	81	82	83	83
	99th	128	129	130	132	133	134	135	87	87	88	89	89	90	91
14	50th	106	106	107	109	110	111	112	63	63	63	64	65	66	66
	90th	119	120	121	122	124	125	125	77	77	77	78	79	80	80
	95th	123	123	125	126	127	129	129	81	81	81	82	83	84	84
	99th	130	131	132	133	135	136	136	88	88	89	90	90	91	92
15	50th	107	108	109	110	111	113	113	64	64	64	65	66	67	67
	90th	120	121	122	123	125	126	127	78	78	78	79	80	81	81
	95th	124	125	126	127	129	130	131	82	82	82	83	84	85	85
	99th	131	132	133	134	136	137	138	89	89	90	91	91	92	93
16	50th	108	108	110	111	112	114	114	64	64	65	66	66	67	68
	90th	121	122	123	124	126	127	128	78	78	79	80	81	81	82
	95th	125	126	127	128	130	131	132	82	82	83	84	85	85	86
	99th	132	133	134	135	137	138	139	90	90	90	91	92	93	93
17	50th	108	109	110	111	113	114	115	64	65	65	66	67	67	68
	90th	122	122	123	125	126	127	128	78	79	79	80	81	81	82
	95th	125	126	127	129	130	131	132	82	83	83	84	85	85	86
	99th	133	133	134	136	137	138	139	90	90	91	91	92	93	93

BP, blood pressure.

To use the table, first plot the child's height on a standard growth curve (www.cdc.gov/growthcharts). The child's measured systolic blood pressure and diastolic blood pressure are compared with the numbers provided in the table according to the child's age and height percentile.

From National High Blood Pressure Education Program Working Group on High Blood Pressure in Children and Adolescents. The fourth report on the diagnosis, evaluation, and treatment of high blood pressure in children and adolescents. National Heart, Lung, and Blood Institute, Bethesda, Maryland. NIH Publication 05-5267, 2005.

the adolescent should have rested for several minutes and should not have smoked or ingested caffeine within 30 minutes before measurement.

5. For apprehensive patients, BP measurements obtained outside of the office setting, such as by a school nurse or at home using a calibrated over-the-counter device may provide insight as to the existence of "white coat" hypertension. However, ambulatory monitoring, in which BP measurements are obtained over a 24-hour period with an automated device, is the preferred technique for diagnosing white coat hypertension. Given the high prevalence of white coat hypertension in

recent studies (Sorof and Portman, 2000), ambulatory BP monitoring should be considered as part of the initial evaluation of an adolescent or young adult with elevated BPs in the office setting.

EPIDEMIOLOGY

As noted in the introduction, the prevalence of hypertension in children and adolescents in screening studies is generally between 0.5% and 2%. The importance of repeated measurements is demonstrated in a study of

TABLE 13.4

Classification of Blood Pressure in Adolescents 18 Years or Older

Blood Pressure Classification	Systolic Blood Pressure (mm Hg)		Diastolic Blood Pressure (mm Hg)
Normal	<120	and	<80
Prehypertension	120–139	or	80–89
Hypertension:			
Stage 1	140–159	or	90–99
Stage 2	≥160	or	≥100

From Chobanian AV, Bakris GL, Black HR, et al. The seventh report of the joint national committee on prevention, detection, evaluation, and treatment of high blood pressure: the JNC 7 report. *JAMA* 2003;289:2560.

3,537 adolescents in New York (Kilcoyne et al., 1974). In this study, 5.4% of adolescents had systolic hypertension and 7.8% had diastolic BPs of >140/90 mm Hg on the first screening. The prevalence dropped to 1.2% and 2.4%, respectively, after a second screening. More recently, screenings conducted in Houston, Texas, public schools have also demonstrated a decreased prevalence of hypertension after repeated measurements (Sorof et al., 2004). Table 13.5 lists various prevalence studies of hypertension in children and adolescents.

FACTORS THAT INFLUENCE BLOOD PRESSURE

Height and Weight

Height has already been mentioned as part of the definition of normative BP in childhood and adolescence (Rosner et al., 1993; National High Blood Pressure Education Program Working Groups, 1996, 2004); this conclusion was based on statistical analysis of the childhood BP database. Others hold that weight is the most important factor in determining BP. Weight has long been held to have a positive relationship with BP, as demonstrated in a study of Minneapolis school children (Leupker et al., 1999). More than half of hypertensive young people are obese. Higgins et al. (1984) suggested that if weight could be reduced in young people to below-obesity levels the prevalence of hypertension would decrease by one third.

Age

BP increases with age in a nonlinear manner through adolescence; this is likely related to growth. Beyond adolescence, BP continues to increase in a significant percentage of individuals as the result of genetic and environmental factors.

Sodium and Other Dietary Constituents

Controversy prevails over the numerous studies concerning the relationship of sodium intake to BP. For most individuals, little correlation exists. However, in certain

TABLE 13.5

Prevalence of Hypertension in Children and Adolescents

Study Location	Number Screened	Age (yr)	Number of Screenings	Threshold BP Value	Prevalence	Reference
Muscatine, IA, United States	1,301	14–18	1	140/90	8.9% sHTN 12.2% dHTN	Lauer et al., 1975
Edmonton, Canada	15,594	15–20	1	150/95	2.2%	Silverberg et al., 1975
Dallas, TX, United States	10,641	14	3	95th percentile	1.2% sHTN 0.4% dHTN	Fixler et al., 1979
Minneapolis, MN, United States	14,686	10–15	1	1987 TF	4.2%	Sinaiko et al., 1989
Tulsa, OK, United States	5,537	14–19	1	1987 TF	6.0%	O'Quin et al., 1992
Buraidah, Saudi Arabia	3,299	3–18	1	1996 WG	10.6%	Soyannwo et al., 1997
Minneapolis, MN, United States	14,686	10–15	2	1996 WG	0.8% sHTN 0.4% dHTN	Androgue and Sinaiko, 2001
Houston, TX, United States	5,102	12–16	3	1996 WG	4.5%	Sorof et al., 2004

BP, blood pressure; dHTN, diastolic hypertension; sHTN, systolic hypertension; TF, Second Task Force Report (1987); WG, Working Group Report (1996).

salt-sensitive individuals, sodium restriction appears beneficial. For example, it has been suggested (Hohn et al., 1983) that African-American children from hypertensive families may be salt sensitive. Obese adolescents also have heightened responsiveness to sodium intake (Rocchini et al., 1989).

Other studies have found a link between potassium intake and both elevated and low BP. However, efforts to correlate calcium and other divalent cations with BP have been equivocal. Similarly, correlations between BP and vitamins A, C, and E, although suggestive, remain to be proved. Falkner et al. (2000) noted that dietary modification of certain nutrients when instituted at an early age could contribute to the prevention of hypertension in urban minority adolescents at risk for hypertension.

Stress

Both physical stress and mental stress evoke changes in BP. Indeed, the degree of change has been thought by some to be useful in predicting later-life hypertension. Early studies by Falkner demonstrated that hypertensive adolescents had significantly greater increases in heart rate, systolic BP, and diastolic BP during mental stress (performance of difficult arithmetic problems) than normotensive adolescents (Falkner et al., 1981). Increased cardiovascular reactivity to the cold pressor test has also been shown to predict the subsequent development of hypertension (Menkes et al., 1989).

Race

Although a significant determinant in adult BP, race is not a factor in teens. Hohn et al. (1983) suggested that certain subgroups of African-American youths have higher BPs than their white counterparts, and Rabinowitz et al. (1993) found a higher prevalence of hypertension among African-American females than among non-Hispanic females. However, Baron et al. (1986) found no significant differences in BP among white, black, and Mexican-American youths. Ethnicity and socioeconomic status have also been related to BP and cardiovascular reactivity (Barnes et al., 2000).

Genetics

Both familial aggregation BP studies, such as those of Lascaux-Lefebvre et al. (1999), and twin studies, such as those of Schieken (1993), indicate a strong positive correlation between hereditary influences and BP measurements. Colhoun (1999) estimated that approximately one third of variations in BP among individuals are due to genetic factors most likely from several genes. Additionally, several single-gene defects have also been recently described (Lifton et al., 2001), which account for hypertension in a small number of children and adolescents, especially those with a family history of severe hypertension of early onset.

Birth Weight and Other Perinatal Factors

The so-called "fetal origins" hypothesis maintains that low birth weight is a risk factor for the subsequent development of primary hypertension in adulthood. This hypothesis is based on the findings of large population studies that demonstrate an inverse correlation between birth weight and adult BP (Barker et al., 1993; Zureik et al., 1996). Proposed explanations for this effect include deficient maternal nutrition, possibly leading to acquisition of a reduced number of nephrons in utero. Other investigators have demonstrated that maternal smoking during pregnancy and bottle-feeding of newborns also may lead to hypertension later in life (Beratis et al., 1996; Singhal et al., 2001), thereby widening the spectrum of possible influences on later BP to include postnatal factors as well. On the other hand, other epidemiological studies have found that adult BP is more closely related to early childhood growth (Falkner et al., 1998) than to birth weight. While more research is clearly needed, it is apparent that at least in some individuals, perinatal and early childhood factors may play an important role in the later development of hypertension.

ETIOLOGY

The causes of hypertension vary among different age-groups. In adolescents, the prevalence of primary hypertension is increased in comparison with younger children. This is particularly true for mild hypertension. Table 13.6 shows an estimation of the causes of hypertension in adolescents from data gathered from a number of population studies. This information shows that primary hypertension is by far the most common cause of hypertension in the adolescent. As in younger children, renal parenchymal diseases are the most common secondary cause in the adolescent age-group.

At least 80% of hypertensive adolescents have no known cause for their disorder and are labeled as having primary or essential hypertension. Primary hypertension in adolescents is frequently characterized by isolated systolic BP elevation (Flynn and Alderman, 2005), whereas diastolic

TABLE 13.6

Estimated Causes of Hypertension in Children and Adolescents

	School-aged Children	Adolescents
Primary/essential	15%–30%	80%–90%
Secondary	70%–85%	10%–20%[a]
Renal parenchymal disease	60%–70%	
Renovascular	5%–10%	
Endocrine	3%–5%	
Aortic coarctation	10%–20%	
Reflux nephropathy	5%–10%	
Neoplastic	1%–5%	
Miscellaneous	1%–5%	

[a]Breakdown of causes is generally similar to that for school-aged children.

BP elevation is more likely to be present in secondary hypertension. Obesity and a positive family history of hypertension are also common in adolescents with primary hypertension.

DIAGNOSIS

Confirmation of Hypertension

Adolescents make fewer visits per year to health care practitioners than other age-groups. However, each visit presents an opportunity to assess the BP. Approximately 10% of these young people will have a high initial BP (at or above the 95th percentile). They should be labeled as having an elevated BP, and not given a diagnosis of hypertension. Before a diagnosis of hypertension can be made, two subsequent BP determinations on different days must also show a high systolic or diastolic pressure or both (National High Blood Pressure Education Program Working Group, 2004). Only 1% to 2% of adolescents will fulfill these criteria and, by definition, have hypertension.

Additionally, determination of "out-of-office BP" to assess possible "white coat hypertension" is increasingly advocated. Recently, however, Vaindirlis et al. (2000) presented data supporting the hypothesis that such "white coat" hypertension may actually be a prelude to permanent hypertension.

Once the diagnosis of hypertension has been confirmed, a diagnostic evaluation and management plan can be initiated. The algorithm in Figure 13.1, although originally designed for children ≤17 years of age, is appropriate for all adolescents and should be followed.

Diagnostic Evaluation

The diagnostic evaluation must be tailored to the individual patient, taking into account the age, sex, race, family history, and level of hypertension. For example, a 12-year-old white female with a past medical history of recurrent urinary tract infections, no family history of hypertension, and a BP of 150/115 mm Hg would be a candidate for an aggressive evaluation for secondary causes, particularly renal parenchymal disease, specifically reflux nephropathy.

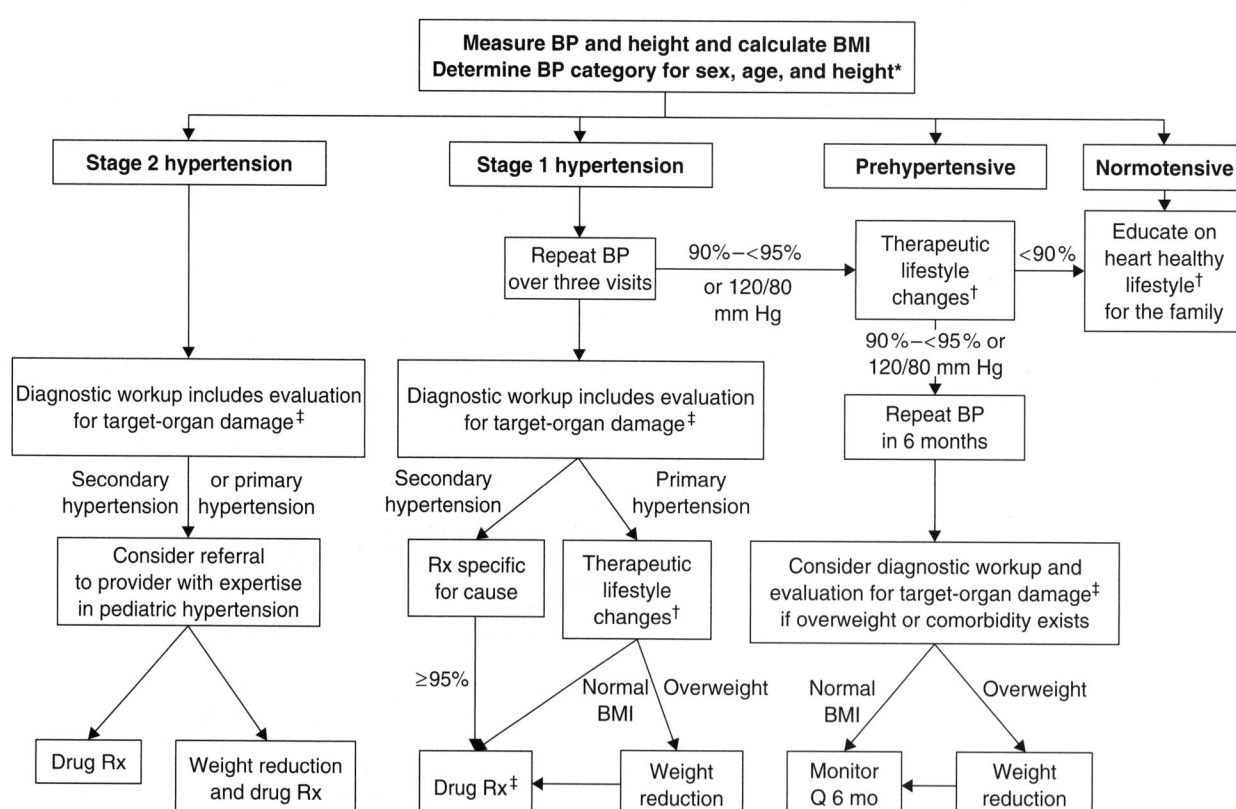

FIGURE 13.1 Algorithm for the identification, diagnosis, and management of hypertension in adolescents. BMI, body mass index; BP, blood pressure; Rx, Treatment.
*See tables 13.2, 13.3 and 13.4.
†Diet modification and physical activity.
‡Especially if younger, very high BP, little or no family history, diabetic, or other risk factors.
Reprinted from National High Blood Pressure Education Program Working Group on High Blood Pressure in Children and Adolescents. The fourth report on the diagnosis, evaluation, and treatment of high blood pressure in children and adolescents. National Heart, Lung, and Blood Institute, Bethesda, Maryland. NIH Publication 05-5267, 2005.

In contrast, invasive studies to look for a secondary cause are unlikely to be helpful in a 17-year-old obese African-American boy with a family history of hypertension and a BP of 150/78 mm Hg. Consultation with someone knowledgeable about hypertension in young people can often be helpful to pursue the most cost-effective and safest diagnostic evaluation.

1. History: Investigating a young person for hypertension requires that a detailed history be elicited. The history should aim at eliciting clues of possible secondary causes, target-organ damage, and other cardiovascular risk factors. Look for symptoms of urinary tract infections or renal disease and for a family history of hypertension or other cardiovascular disease. Activity, dietary, and other habits should be sought. The adolescent with an elevated BP should also be questioned about alcohol, tobacco, and substance use, as many substances may elevate BP (Table 13.7). Also ask about ergogenic aids such as anabolic steroids as well as any complementary or alternative medicine products that they might be using. Clues from the history suggestive of secondary hypertension are listed in Table 13.8.

2. Physical examination: A thorough examination is also an essential part of the diagnostic study. The adolescent in question will often be obese. The examination should include an exploration for evidence of a secondary cause or end-organ damage and an evaluation of the following:
   a. Height, weight, and body mass index (BMI) (calculated)
   b. BP in both arms and a lower extremity
   c. Femoral pulses
   d. Neck: Carotid bruits or an enlarged thyroid gland
   e. Fundi: Arteriolar narrowing, arteriovenous nicking, hemorrhages, exudates
   f. Abdomen: Bruits, hepatosplenomegaly, flank masses
   g. Heart: Rate, precordial heave, clicks, murmurs, arrhythmias
   h. Extremities: Pulses, edema
   i. Nervous system
   j. Skin: Striae, acanthosis nigricans, café au lait spots, neurofibromas

Physical examination findings suggestive of secondary causes of hypertension are listed in Table 13.8. In addition, the clinician should remember that severe hypertension in an adolescent suggests a secondary cause, particularly renal disease. Acute onset may also suggest acute renal disease.

3. Laboratory testing: Some basic/screening studies should be performed in all adolescents with confirmed BP elevation, whereas others should be reserved for those in whom secondary hypertension is suspected or in those with stage 2 hypertension.
   a. *Screening tests*—should be done in all patients and these include:
      • Electrolytes
      • Blood urea nitrogen (BUN) and creatinine
      • Urinalysis
      • Fasting lipid profile
      • Complete blood cell (CBC) count
      • Urine cultures should be done as appropriate based on the history and urinalysis findings. Add a fasting glucose with or without a fasting insulin in obese adolescents to screen for impaired glucose tolerance/hyperinsulinemia.
   b. *Specific laboratory tests* should be done as appropriate to follow up on clues from the history and physical examination, or from the screening test results. These might include an antinuclear antibody (ANA) test and sedimentation rate in a hypertensive female adolescent with a malar rash, thyroid studies if there is a history of thyroid dysfunction for example, heat/cold intolerance, menstrual dysfunction, and so on.
   c. *Echocardiograms* are now recommended to be obtained in all adolescents with confirmed hypertension (National High Blood Pressure Education Program Working Group, 2004). This is to detect left ventricular hypertrophy (LVH), which is a risk factor for sudden cardiac death and an indication to initiate or intensify antihypertensive drug therapy. Recent studies have shown that LVH occurs commonly in hypertensive adolescents (Hanevold et al., 2004; Flynn, 2005).
   d. *Advanced testing* should only be done to confirm suspected secondary causes of hypertension, for

TABLE 13.7

Substances That May Elevate Blood Pressure in Adolescents

Prescription Medications	Nonprescription Medications	Others
Calcineurin inhibitors (cyclosporine, tacrolimus)	Caffeine	Cocaine
Dexedrine[a]	Ephedrine	Ethanol
Erythropoietin	Nonsteroidal antiinflammatory drugs[a]	Heavy metals (lead, mercury)
Glucocorticoids	Pseudoephedrine	MDMA ("Ecstasy")
Methylphenidate[a]		Tobacco
Oral contraceptives		Herbal preparations (*Ephedra, Glycyrrhiza*)
Phenylpropanolamine		
Pseudoephedrine		
Tricyclic antidepressants[a]		

[a]These cause elevated blood pressure relatively infrequently compared with the other agents in the table.

TABLE 13.8

History and Physical Examination Findings Suggestive of Secondary Causes of Hypertension

Present in History	Suggests
Known UTI/UTI symptoms	Reflux nephropathy
Joint pains, rash, fever	Vasculitis, SLE
Acute onset of gross hematuria	Glomerulonephritis, renal thrombosis
Renal trauma	Renal infarct, RAS
Abdominal radiation	Radiation nephritis, RAS
Renal transplant	Transplant RAS
Precocious puberty	Adrenal disorder
Muscle cramping, constipation	Hyperaldosteronism
Excessive sweating, headache, pallor and/or flushing	Pheochromocytoma
Known illicit drug use	Drug-induced hypertension
Present on Examination	Suggests
BP >140/100 mm Hg at any age	Secondary hypertension
Leg BP < arm BP	Aortic coarctation
Poor growth, pallor	Chronic renal disease
Turner syndrome	Aortic coarctation
Café au lait spots	Renal artery stenosis
Delayed leg pulses	Aortic coarctation
Precocious puberty	Adrenal disorder
Bruits over upper abdomen	Renal artery stenosis
Edema	Renal disease
Excessive sweating	Pheochromocytoma
Excessive pigmentation	Adrenal disorder
Striae in a male	Drug-induced HTN

UTI, urinary tract infection; BP, blood pressure; SLE, systemic lupus erythematosus; RAS, renal artery stenosis; HTN, hypertension.

example, plasma normetanephrine to norepinephrine ratio if pheochromocytoma is suspected, or a 24-hour urine collection for proteinuria if there is persistent proteinuria on the urinalysis.

e. *Imaging studies* should only be obtained in specific circumstances. Renal ultrasonography should be obtained in all adolescents with stage 2 hypertension, or in those with stage 1 hypertension and an abnormal urinalysis. Chest x-rays should only be obtained if the cardiac examination is abnormal. More advanced studies such as renal scans or angiography are useful in a very small percentage of hypertensive adolescents and should only be obtained under the direction of the appropriate subspecialist.

THERAPY

Prevention

Optimally, measures to prevent or minimize the effects of hypertension should be applied to those adolescents at risk of developing hypertension later in life. The difficulty lies in finding those at risk and deciding what measures to apply. Data from young people for this purpose are lacking, and long-term follow-up information is unavailable. Nevertheless, a starting point for such a strategy is to consider those with the findings listed in the subsequent text as being at risk. They should be counseled about nonpharmacologic approaches to maintain lower BP and should be periodically monitored:

1. Those with prehypertension (>120/80 mm Hg)
2. Those with BMI >85th percentile, particularly if parents are obese
3. Those with hyperlipidemia or a family history of the disorder, particularly if there is a known family history of coronary artery disease or stroke
4. Those with type 1 or type 2 diabetes mellitus
5. Those with two or more family members with treated hypertension, particularly African-Americans and Hispanics

Nonpharmacologic Interventions

Although the magnitude of change in BP may be modest, weight loss, aerobic exercise, and dietary modifications have all been shown to successfully reduce BP in children and adolescents, at least in research settings. Such "therapeutic lifestyle changes" should therefore be incorporated into the treatment plan for any hypertensive adolescent, whether a secondary cause has been identified, and whether there is an indication to initiate antihypertensive drug therapy (Fig. 13.1).

1. Weight reduction: Excess body weight is correlated closely with increased BP. Weight reduction reduces BP in a large proportion of hypertensive individuals who are >10% above ideal weight.

2. Dietary changes: Moderate sodium restriction in hypertensive individuals has been shown, on average, to reduce systolic BP by 4.9 mm Hg and diastolic BP by 2.6 mm Hg. The benefits of sodium restriction are probably greatest in those with renal disease, those with long-standing hypertension, and possibly also African-Americans. Although there has been some evidence to suggest that potassium, calcium, or magnesium supplementation might theoretically be of benefit, studies have not always confirmed a beneficial effect of supplementing the diet with these minerals. On the other hand, the so-called "DASH diet," which is lower in sodium content and enhanced in potassium and calcium intake, has been demonstrated to be of benefit in hypertensive adults (Appel et al., 1997) and should probably be recommended for hypertensive adolescents.

3. Regular physical exercise: Regular aerobic physical activity, adequate to achieve at least a moderate level of physical fitness, may be beneficial for both prevention and treatment of hypertension. Regular aerobic physical activity ($\geq$30 minutes/session, 4–5 days/week) can reduce systolic BP in hypertensive patients by approximately 10 mm Hg.

4. Other Lifestyle changes: Discontinuance of smoking and avoidance of alcohol excess, medications (except as directed by health care providers), and drugs (e.g., cocaine, amphetamines). In addition to elevating BP, cigarette smoking is a major risk factor for cardiovascular disease and therefore should be avoided by hypertensive individuals. Excessive alcohol intake can raise BP and cause resistance to antihypertensive therapy.

Pharmacologic Treatment

1. Antihypertensive medications are definitely indicated for those who have the following:
   a. Symptoms of hypertension
   b. Stage 2 hypertension
   c. Evidence of hypertensive end-organ damage
   d. Type 1 or type 2 diabetes
   e. Secondary hypertension
   f. Persistent hypertension despite lifestyle changes
2. If none of the above indications are present, drug treatment can be withheld. Lifestyle modifications as discussed in the preceding text should be recommended. If these measures fail to lower BP after a reasonable period of time, then medication should be prescribed.
3. Drug therapy should be simple so that compliance will be increased in what may be a lifelong but asymptomatic problem.
4. Explicit education should be given regarding hypertension and the reasons for therapy.
5. The adolescent should generally be responsible for taking his or her own medication.
6. Antihypertensive agents should be chosen to obtain the maximum benefit with the fewest and least-severe side effects. The ideal hypertensive agent would
   a. Lower BP in almost all hypertensive individuals
   b. Address specific pathogenic mechanisms
   c. Improve hemodynamics
   d. Be associated with few biochemical changes
   e. Be associated with few or no adverse reactions
   f. Be dosed once or, at most, twice daily
   g. Be inexpensive
7. Unfortunately, the ideal antihypertensive agent does not exist. Initial therapeutic regimens have been debated. In adults, diuretics have been advocated as first-line therapy based on the results of the ALLHAT trial (ALLHAT Collaborative Research Group, 2002). However, the findings of this study are not directly applicable to otherwise healthy adolescents with hypertension. Instead, individualized stepped-care approach, as suggested by the National High Blood Pressure Education Program Working Group (2004) and as illustrated in Figure 13.1, should be followed. In this approach, a monotherapy drug regimen is superimposed on nonpharmacologic therapy as initial treatment. Advocates of this approach recommend the following:
   a. Begin with a low dose of the chosen initial drug. Because all classes of antihypertensive agents have now been studied in adolescents, either a diuretic, β-blocker, angiotensin-converting enzyme (ACE) inhibitor, or calcium channel blocker may be chosen as the initial agent. Preparations with once- or twice-daily dosing are available for members of all drug classes and can improve compliance. Increases in the dose of the initial medication may be used to achieve BP control if necessary. If BP control is still not achieved, proceed to combination treatment.
   b. Add a low dose of another drug with a complementary mechanism of action. In many cases, the second agent will be a diuretic. Combination antihypertensive drug treatment with one of the medications being a diuretic is being advocated increasingly in adolescents (Wells and Stowe, 2001). Proceed to a full dose if necessary.
   c. If BP control is still not achieved, one may choose to add a third antihypertensive drug, usually a vasodilator or renin-angiotensin inhibitor, or preferably obtain consultation from an expert on hypertension in adolescents.
   d. Suggested initial and maximum doses of various antihypertensive agents are given in Table 13.9. Many of these now have pediatric-specific Food and Drug Administration (FDA)-approved labeling as a result of recent trials in children and adolescents. More comprehensive references, specifically published clinical trial results, should be consulted for detailed discussion of the specific adverse effects of these medications.
   e. For adolescents younger than 18 years with uncomplicated primary hypertension, target BP should be the 95th percentile for age, gender, and height; for those with secondary hypertension, diabetes, or chronic kidney disease, target BP should be the 90th percentile. In those 18 years or older, BP targets should be <140/90 mm Hg for those with uncomplicated primary hypertension, and <130/80 mm Hg for those with secondary hypertension, diabetes, or chronic kidney disease.
8. Step-down therapy, or drug withdrawal, should not be forgotten. After an extended course of drug therapy and sustained BP control, a gradual reduction in or withdrawal of medication can be attempted. This requires close observation and continuation of nonpharmacologic therapy, and will probably be successful only in the adolescent who has been successful with lifestyle modification.

TABLE 13.9

Antihypertensive Agents for Use in Chronic Treatment of Hypertension in Adolescents

Class	Drug	Starting Dose	Interval	Maximum Dose[a]
Angiotensin-converting enzyme (ACE) inhibitors	Benazepril	0.2 mg/kg/d up to 10 mg/d	q.d.	0.6 mg/kg/d up to 40 mg q.d.
	Captopril	0.3–0.5 mg/kg/dose	b.i.d.–t.i.d.	6 mg/kg/d up to 450 mg/d
	Enalapril	0.08 mg/kg/d	q.d.	0.6 mg/kg/d up to 40 mg/d
	Fosinopril	0.1 mg/kg/d up to 10 mg/d	q.d.	0.6 mg/kg/d up to 40 mg/d
	Lisinopril	0.07 mg/kg/d up to 5 mg/d	q.d.	0.61 mg/kg/d up to 40 mg/d
	Quinapril	5–10 mg/d	q.d.	80 mg/d
	Ramipril	2.5 mg/d	q.d.	20 mg/d
Angiotensin-receptor blockers	Candesartan	4 mg/d	q.d.	32 mg q.d.
	Irbesartan	75–150 mg/d	q.d.	300 mg/d
	Losartan	0.75 mg/kg/d up to 50 mg/d	q.d.–b.i.d.	1.44 mg/kg/d up to 100 mg/d
α- and β-Antagonists	Labetalol	2–3 mg/kg/d	b.i.d.	10–12 mg/kg/d up to 2.4 g/d
	Carvedilol	0.1 mg/kg/dose up to 12.5 mg b.i.d.	b.i.d.	0.5 mg/kg/dose up to 25 mg b.i.d.
β-Antagonists	Atenolol	0.5–1 mg/kg/d	q.d.–b.i.d.	2 mg/kg/d up to 100 mg/d
	Bisoprolol/HCTZ	0.04 mg/kg/d up to 2.5/6.25 mg/d	q.d.	10/6.25 mg q.d.
	Metoprolol	1–2 mg/kg/d	b.i.d.	6 mg/kg/d up to 200 mg/d
	Propranolol	1 mg/kg/d	b.i.d.–t.i.d.	16 mg/kg/d
Calcium channel blockers	Amlodipine	0.06 mg/kg/d	q.d.	0.6 mg/kg/d up to 10 mg/d
	Felodipine	2.5 mg/d	q.d.	10 mg/d
	Isradipine	0.05–0.15 mg/kg/dose	t.i.d.–q.i.d.	0.8 mg/kg/d up to 20 mg/d
	Extended-release nifedipine	0.25–0.5 mg/kg/d	q.d.–b.i.d.	3 mg/kg/d up to 120 mg/d
Central α-agonists	Clonidine	5–10 µg/kg/d	b.i.d.–t.i.d.	25 µg/kg/d up to 0.9 mg/d
	Methyldopa	5 mg/kg/d	b.i.d.–q.i.d.	40 mg/kg/d up to 3 g/d
Diuretics	Amiloride	5–10 mg/d	q.d.	20 mg/d
	Chlorthalidone	0.3 mg/kg/d	q.d.	2 mg/kg/d up to 50 mg/d
	Furosemide	0.5–2.0 mg/kg/dose	q.d.–b.i.d.	6 mg/kg/d
	HCTZ	1 mg/kg/d	b.i.d.	3 mg/kg/d up to 50 mg/d
	Spironolactone	1 mg/kg/d	q.d.–b.i.d.	3.3 mg/kg/d up to 100 mg/d
	Triamterene	1–2 mg/kg/d	b.i.d.	3–4 mg/kg/d up to 300 mg/d
Peripheral α-antagonists	Doxazosin	1 mg/d	q.d.	4 mg/d
	Prazosin	0.05–0.1 mg/kg/d	t.i.d.	0.5 mg/kg/d
	Terazosin	1 mg/d	q.d.	20 mg/d
Vasodilators	Hydralazine	0.25 mg/kg/dose	t.i.d.–q.i.d.	7.5 mg/kg/d up to 200 mg/d
	Minoxidil	0.1–0.2 mg/kg/d	b.i.d.–t.i.d.	1 mg/kg/d up to 50 mg/d

q.d., once-daily; b.i.d., twice-daily; t.i.d., three times daily; q.i.d., four times daily; HCTZ, hydrochlorothiazide.
[a]The maximum recommended adult dose should never be exceeded.

SPECIAL POPULATIONS

1. African-Americans: The frequency of hypertension in African-Americans is among the highest in the world. Hypertension develops at an earlier age and is more severe in African-Americans than in whites. In African-Americans, diuretics have been proved to reduce hypertensive morbidity and mortality rates, so diuretics should be seriously considered for use in the absence of other conditions that prohibit their use. ACE inhibitors used to be considered less effective in African-Americans than in whites, although recent research indicates otherwise (Bakris et al., 2005). Calcium channel blockers and α-receptor blockers are as effective in African-Americans as in whites.

2. Females who take oral contraceptives: Most females who take oral contraceptives have a small increase in systolic and diastolic BPs but usually within the reference range. Hormonal contraceptives, mainly those that contain estrogen, can increase angiotensinogen, leading to an increase in angiotensin II and an increase in BP in some individuals. The risk of overt hypertension appears to increase with age, duration of use, and body mass. Many of the studies of BP and oral contraceptive agents involved higher doses of both estrogen and progesterone than are used currently. If concurrent treatment with an oral contraceptive and antihypertensive medication is needed, consideration should be given to using a low-estrogen or progestin-only contraceptive.

3. Adolescents with asthma: In teens with asthma and hypertension, β-blocking drugs can worsen bronchoconstriction and are therefore relatively contraindicated. Some of the newer, β_1 receptor selective agents such as metoprolol or bisoprolol may be tried, especially in adolescents with mild asthma.

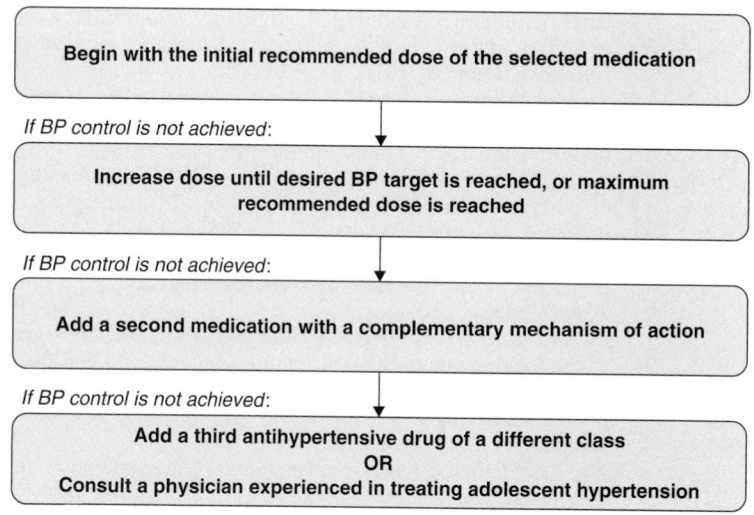

FIGURE 13.2 Stepped-care approach to antihypertensive therapy. BP, blood pressure.

4. Diabetes: As noted in the preceding text, the diagnosis of hypertension or even prehypertension in an adolescent with either type 1 or type 2 diabetes is an indication to initiate antihypertensive drug therapy. ACE inhibitors or angiotensin-receptor blockers should be used as the initial agent in hypertensive diabetic patients because of their potential benefit in slowing the progression of or even preventing diabetic nephropathy.

HYPERTENSIVE EMERGENCIES

Rarely an adolescent will have signs of encephalopathy or heart failure at presentation and be found to have extraordinarily high BP, at levels well above stage 2 hypertension. This constitutes a true emergency and may have disastrous consequences unless efforts to lower the BP are begun at once. Assistance from an expert in hypertension should be sought. Meanwhile, the patient should be hospitalized and an intravenous line placed. Usually, a continuous infusion of either nicardipine or labetalol should be started at a low dose and then titrated up as needed to slowly reduce the BP. The initial reduction should be no more than 25% over the first 8 hours in order to prevent cerebral, cardiac, or renal ischemia from overly rapid BP reduction (Adelman et al., 2000). BP can be further lowered to the 95th percentile over the next 24 hours. When adequate pressure control has been achieved, oral antihypertensive agents can be gradually introduced and the intravenous agents discontinued. A vigorous search for the cause of the hypertension, if not known, must be made once the patient's condition has been stabilized.

SUMMARY

As adolescents mature toward full adulthood, an increasing number will be found to have hypertension. Perhaps this progression can be delayed or avoided through the applications of the principles outlined in this chapter. At the very least, BP should be taken when adolescents are seen for health care, regardless of the complaint.

When pressures are found to be repeatedly elevated, nonpharmacologic antihypertensive measures should be started. They are good general health rules. Initially, in the absence of severe hypertension, a set of basic diagnostic studies should be obtained. Depending on the history, physical examination, and results of the initial studies, other tests may or may not be necessary.

For selected adolescents, drug therapy is indicated. The individualized stepped-care approach displayed in Figure 13.2 is recommended. When hypertension is resistant to initial drug therapies, consultation with an expert on hypertension in adolescents should be sought.

WEB SITES

For Teenagers and Parents

http://www.americanheart.org/presenter.jhtml?identifier=4609. American Heart Association site on childhood hypertension. Free.

http://pediatrichypertension.org. Home of the International Pediatric Hypertension Association. Includes links to additional patient education Web sites about hypertension. Free.

http://www.nhlbi.nih.gov/hbp/index.html. NIH patient education site on hypertension. Free.

http://www.medscape.com/pages/editorial/patiented/index/index-hypertension. WebMD/Medscape patient education site on hypertension. Requires free registration.

http://www.nlm.nih.gov/medlineplus/highbloodpressure.html. "Medline Plus" site on hypertension. Free.

http://www.mayoclinic.com/health/high-blood-pressure/DS00100. Mayo Clinic patient education site on hypertension. Free.

http://monitorbloodpressure.com/. Commercial site to buy home BP monitors.

For Health Care Professionals

http://www.nhlbi.nih.gov/health/prof/heart/hbp/hbp_ped.htm. Home of The Fourth Report on the Diagnosis, Evaluation, and Treatment of High Blood Pressure in Children and Adolescents. Includes link to downloadable PDA application. Free.

http://pediatrichypertension.org. Home of the International Pediatric Hypertension Association. Includes links to additional Web sites about hypertension for health care professionals. Free; membership available for health care professionals.

http://www.who.int/topics/cardiovascular_diseases/en/. World Health Organization site containing links to various cardiovascular disease-related WHO initiatives and resources. Free.

http://www.hdcn.com/fhh.htm. Nephrology-oriented site on hypertension. Contains links to educational lectures and other materials. Requires paid annual subscription to access all content.

REFERENCES AND ADDITIONAL READINGS

Adelman RD, Coppo R, Dillon MJ. The emergency management of severe hypertension. *Pediatr Nephrol* 2000;14:422.

Adrogue HE, Sinaiko AR. Prevalence of hypertension in junior high school-aged children: effect of new recommendations in the 1996 Updated Task Force Report. *Am J Hypertens* 2001;14(5 Pt 1):412.

ALLHAT Officers and Coordinators for the ALLHAT Collaborative Research Group. Major outcomes in high-risk hypertensive patients randomized to angiotensin-converting enzyme inhibitor or calcium channel blocker vs. diuretic: the antihypertensive and lipid-lowering treatment to prevent heart attack trial (ALLHAT). *J Am Med Assoc* 2002;288:2981.

Appel LJ, Moore TJ, Obarzanek E, et al. A clinical trial of the effects of dietary patterns on blood pressure. *N Engl J Med* 1997;336:1117.

Bakris GL, Smith DH, Giles TD, et al. Comparative antihypertensive efficacy of angiotensin receptor blocker-based treatment in African-American and white patients. *J Clin Hypertens* 2005;7:587.

Barker DJP, Gluckman PD, Godfrey KM, et al. Fetal nutrition and cardiovascular disease in adult life. *Lancet* 1993;341:941.

Barnes VA, Treiber FA, Musante L, et al. Ethnicity and socioeconomic status: impact on cardiovascular activity at rest and during stress in youth with a family history of hypertension. *Ethn Dis* 2000;10:4.

Baron AE, Freyer B, Fixler DE. Longitudinal blood pressures in blacks, whites, and Mexican Americans during adolescence and early adulthood. *Am J Epidemiol* 1986;123:809.

Bartosh SM, Aronson AJ. Childhood hypertension: an update on etiology, diagnosis, and treatment. *Pediatr Clin North Am* 1999;46:235.

Beratis NG, Panagoulias D, Varvarigou A. Increased blood pressure in neonates and infants whose mothers smoked during pregnancy. *J Pediatr* 1996;128:806.

Chobanian AV, Bakris GL, Black HR, et al. The seventh report of the joint national committee on prevention, detection, evaluation, and treatment of high blood pressure: the JNC 7 report. *JAMA* 2003;289:2560.

Colhoun H. Commentary: confirmation needed for genes for hypertension. *Lancet* 1999;353:1200.

Couch SC, Daniels SR. Diet and blood pressure in children. *Curr Opin Pediatr* 2005;17:642.

Dickinson HO, Mason JM, Nicolson DJ, et al. Lifestyle interventions to reduce raised blood pressure: a systematic review of randomized controlled trials. *J Hypertens* 2006;24:215.

Falkner B, Kushner H, Onesti G, et al. Cardiovascular characteristics in adolescents who develop essential hypertension. *Hypertension* 1981;3:521.

Falkner B, Hulman S, Kushner H. Birth weight versus childhood growth as determinants of adult blood pressure. *Hypertension* 1998;31(part 1):145.

Falkner B, Sherif K, Michel S, et al. Dietary nutrients and blood pressure in urban minority adolescents at risk for hypertension. *Arch Pediatr Adolesc Med* 2000;154:918.

Falkner B, Gidding SS, Ramirez-Garnica G, et al. The relationship of body mass index and blood pressure in primary care pediatric patients. *J Pediatr* 2006;148:195.

Fernandes E, McCrindle BW. Diagnosis and treatment of hypertension in children and adolescents. *Can J Cardiol* 2000;16:801.

Fixler DE, Laird WP, Fitzgerald V, et al. Hypertension screening in schools: results of the Dallas study. *Pediatrics* 1979;63:32.

Flynn JT. Impact of ambulatory blood pressure monitoring on the management of hypertension in children. *Blood Press Monit* 2000;5:211.

Flynn JT. Evaluation and management of hypertension in childhood. *Prog Pediatr Cardiol* 2001;12:177.

Flynn JT. Drug therapy of childhood hypertension: current status, future challenges. *Am J Hypertens* 2002;15(2 Part2):30S.

Flynn JT. Hypertension in adolescents. *Adolesc Med Clin* 2005;16:11.

Flynn JT, Alderman MH. Characteristics of children with primary hypertension seen at a referral center. *Pediatr Nephrol* 2005;20:961.

Hanevold C, Waller J, Daniels S, et al. The effects of obesity, gender, and ethnic group on left ventricular hypertrophy and geometry in hypertensive children: a collaborative study of the International Pediatric Hypertension Association. *Pediatrics* 2004;113:328.

Higgins MW, Hinton PC, Keller JB. Weight and obesity as a predictor of blood pressure and hypertension. In: Loggie JMH, Horan MJ, Gruskin AB, et al, eds. National Heart, Lung, and Blood Institute workshop on juvenile hypertension. *Proceedings of a symposium.* New York: Biomedical Information, 1984:125.

Hohn AR, Riopel DA, Keil JE, et al. Childhood familial and racial differences in physiologic and biochemical factors related to hypertension. *Hypertension* 1983;5:56.

Kaplan NM. Maximally reducing cardiovascular risk in the treatment of hypertension. *Ann Intern Med* 1988;109:36.

Kavey REW, Daniels SR, Lauer RM, et al. American Heart Association guidelines for primary prevention of atherosclerotic cardiovascular disease beginning in childhood. *Circulation* 2003;107:1562.

Kilcoyne MM, Richter RW, Alsup PA. Adolescent hypertension. I. Detection and prevalence. *Circulation.* 1974;50:758.

Lascaux-Lefebvre V, Ruidavets J, Arveiler D, et al. Influence of parental history of hypertension on blood pressure. *J Hum Hypertens* 1999;13:631.

Lauer RM, Clarke WR. Childhood risk factors for high adult blood pressure: the Muscatine study. *Pediatrics* 1989;84:633.

Lauer RM, Conner WE, Leaverton PE, et al. Coronary heart disease risk factors in school children: the Muscatine study. *J Pediatr* 1975;86:697.

Luepker RV, Jacobs DR, Prineas RJ, et al. Secular trends of blood pressure and body size in a multi-ethnic adolescent population: 1986 to 1996. *J Pediatr* 1999;134:668.

Lieberman E. Pediatric hypertension, clinical perspective. *Mayo Clin Proc* 1994;69:1098.

Lifton RP, Gharavi AG, Geller DS. Molecular mechanisms of human hypertension. *Cell* 2001;104:545.

Menkes MS, Mathhews KA, Krantz DS, et al. Cardiovascular reactivity to the cold pressor test as a predictor of hypertension. *Hypertension* 1989;14:524.

National High Blood Pressure Education Program Working Group. Update on the 1987 task force report on high blood pressure in children and adolescents: a working group report from the National High Blood Pressure Education Program. *Pediatrics* 1996;98:649.

National High Blood Pressure Education Program Working Group on High Blood Pressure in Children and Adolescents. The fourth report on the diagnosis, evaluation, and treatment of high blood pressure in children and adolescents. National Heart, Lung, and Blood Institute, Bethesda, Maryland. *Pediatrics* 2004;114:555.

Neaton JD, Grimm RH Jr, Prineas RJ, et al. Treatment of mild hypertension study: final results. *JAMA* 1993;270:713.

O'Quin M, Sharma BB, Miller KA, et al. Adolescent blood pressure survey: Tulsa, Oklahoma, 1987 to 1989. *South Med J* 1992;85:487.

Pickering TG, Hall JE, Appel LJ, et al. Recommendations for blood pressure measurement in humans and experimental animals: part 1: blood pressure measurement in humans: a statement for professionals from the Subcommittee of Professional and Public Education of the American Heart Association Council on High Blood Pressure Research. *Hypertension* 2005;45:142.

Portman RJ, McNiece KL, Swinford RD, et al. Pediatric hypertension: diagnosis, evaluation, management, and treatment for the primary care physician. *Curr Probl Pediatr Adolesc Health Care* 2005;35:262.

Rabinowitz A, Kushner H, Falkner B. Racial differences in blood pressure among urban adolescents. *J Adolesc Health* 1993;14:314.

Reed WL. Racial differences in blood pressure levels of adolescents. *Am J Public Health* 1981;71:1165.

Rocchini AP, Key J, Bondie D, et al. The effect of weight loss on the sensitivity of blood pressure to sodium in obese adolescents. *N Engl J Med* 1989;321:580.

Rocchini AP. Obesity hypertension. *Am J Hypertens* 2002;15 (2 Pt 2):50S.

Rosner B, Prineas RJ, Loggie JMH, et al. Blood pressure nomograms for children and adolescents, by height, sex and age, in the United States. *J Pediatr* 1993;123:871.

Schieken RM. Genetic factors that predispose the child to develop hypertension. *Pediatr Clin North Am* 1993; 40:1.

Silverberg DS, Nostrand CV, Juchli B, et al. Screening for hypertension in a high school population. *Can Med Assoc J* 1975;113:103.

Sinaiko AR, Gomez-Marion O, Prineas RJ. Prevalence of "significant" hypertension in junior high school-aged children: the Children and Adolescent Blood Pressure Program. *J Pediat* 1989;114(4 Pt 1):664.

Sinaiko AR, Gomez-Marin O, Prineas RJ. Effect of low sodium diet or potassium supplementation on adolescent blood pressure. *Hypertension* 1993;21:989.

Singhal A, Cole TJ, Lucas A. Early nutrition in preterm infants and later blood pressure: two cohorts after randomized trials. *Lancet* 2001;357:413.

Sorof JM, Portman RJ. White coat hypertension in children with elevated casual blood pressure. *J Pediatr* 2000;137:493.

Sorof JM, Lai D, Turner J, et al. Overweight, ethnicity, and the prevalence of hypertension in school-aged children. *Pediatrics* 2004;113:475.

Soyannwo MAO, Gadallah M, Kurashi NY, et al. Studies on preventative nephrology: Systemic hypertension in the pediatric and adolescent population of Gassim, Saudi Arabia. *Ann Saudi Med* 1997;17:47.

Task Force on Blood Pressure Control in Children. Report of the second task force on blood pressure control in children—1987. National Heart, Lung, and Blood Institute, Bethesda, Maryland. *Pediatrics* 1987;79:1.

Vaindirlis I, Peppa Patrikiou M, Dracopoulou M, et al. "White coat hypertension" in adolescents: increased values of urinary cortisol and endothelin. *J Pediatr* 2000;136:359.

Wells T, Stowe C. An approach to the use of antihypertensive drugs in children and adolescents. *Curr Ther Res Clin Exp* 2001;62:329.

Zureik M, Bonithon-Kopp C, Lecomte E, et al. Weights at birth and in early infancy, systolic pressure and left ventricular structure in subjects aged 8 to 24 years. *Hypertension* 1996;27(part 1):339.

CHAPTER **14**

Heart Murmurs and Mitral Valve Prolapse

Amy D. DiVasta and Mark E. Alexander

Cardiac murmurs occur in at least 50% of all normal children and often persist into adolescence. Murmurs are the most frequent reason for referral to a cardiology specialist (Geggel, 2004). The vast majority of these murmurs occur in the absence of an anatomical or physiological abnormality of the heart, and are considered to be "innocent," "normal," or "physiological" in origin. It is the task of the primary care physician to differentiate normal murmurs from those that are pathological. In most patients with a cardiac murmur, a careful history and physical examination serve to establish a diagnosis and/or to guide further referral and evaluation. When a pathological murmur is suspected, pediatric cardiology referral is generally a more effective approach than first obtaining an echocardiogram, particularly if working with adult-focused echocardiogram resources.

HISTORY

Diagnosis begins with a thorough history and physical examination. If a diagnosis of congenital heart disease is already known, the specific diagnoses will drive further cardiology evaluation. Murmurs first heard in childhood or adolescence are more likely to be innocent murmurs than murmurs caused by organic heart disease. Complaints of fatigue, decreased exercise tolerance, exertional chest pain, or palpitations are suggestive of pathological heart disease. Any patient with syncope or near-syncope during exercise merits cardiac evaluation. A thorough family history should also be obtained, including a history of sudden death.

PHYSICAL EXAMINATION

1. Appearance
   a. Growth and maturation should be carefully assessed.
   b. Presence of dysmorphic features is frequently associated with congenital heart disease, as in Trisomy 21, Turner, Noonan, or Marfan syndromes.
   c. Cyanosis and clubbing are strongly suggestive strongly suggestive of uncorrected cyanotic congenital heart disease.
   d. Pectus excavatum deformity (narrow anteroposterior diameter of the chest) is often associated with a normal murmur, but is also associated with systemic connective tissue abnormalities such as Marfan syndrome.

2. Pulses in upper and lower extremities
   a. Observe for any discrepancies in intensity or timing.
   b. Delayed or absent pulses in the lower extremities may indicate coarctation of the aorta.
   c. Bounding pulses due to a wide pulse pressure may indicate structural disease related to "run-off" from a region of higher pressure to one of relatively lower pressure, for example, aortic regurgitation or patent ductus arteriosus.

3. Blood pressures in arm and leg
   a. Sizing of the blood pressure cuff is essential. A good general rule is to size the length of the bladder (the inflatable portion) of the cuff so that it completely encircles the upper arm of the patient. Using a cuff size that is too small leads to falsely high readings. When in doubt, err on the side of a cuff that is *slightly* too large. While a manual blood pressure may be the most accurate office method, automated oscillometric methods have the significant advantages of lacking observer bias, and the ability to delegate the procedure to ancillary office staff.
   b. The leg systolic pressure is normally slightly higher (10 mm Hg) than that of the arm. A lower leg pressure can often indicate coarctation of the aorta.

4. Palpation
   a. Presence of thrill, heave, or lift over the precordium or suprasternal notch is usually an indication of pathology.
   b. The point of maximal impulse (PMI) should be dime-sized, limited to one intercostal space, and located in the midclavicular line. Increased intensity and lateral displacement of the PMI suggests left ventricular (LV) enlargement.

5. Auscultation
   All components of the cardiac cycle should be assessed systematically at the base, at the apex, and along both sides of the sternal border, using both the bell and diaphragm. A dynamic cardiac examination is completed by moving the patient through some combination of positions and maneuvers: supine, sitting, standing, squatting, or isometric hand contraction which allows different cardiac loading conditions to amplify murmurs.

a. First heart sound (S_1): S_1 is produced by closure of the mitral and then the tricuspid valve. It is best heard at the cardiac apex. Splitting of S_1 can be a normal finding. However, auscultation of another sound close to S_1 is usually either a presystolic fourth heart sound (S_4) or an ejection click (see following text).

b. Second heart sound (S_2): The quality of S_2 is of great diagnostic importance. The first component (aortic valve closure, A_2) and the second component (pulmonary valve closure, P_2) of S_2 should be of equal intensity. An accentuated P_2 suggests pulmonary hypertension. Normally, there is respiratory variation or physiological splitting of the S_2, with widening of the separation with inspiration and narrowing or disappearance of the split with exhalation. This is easiest to hear at the upper left sternal border (LSB). Wide, fixed splitting suggests an abnormality of right ventricular (RV) volume overload such as an atrial septal defect. A single S_2 is also abnormal, and may indicate severe stenosis of one of the semilunar valves.

c. Third heart sound (S_3): S_3 corresponds to ventricular filling during early diastole, and is normally heard as a soft sound following S_2 at the cardiac apex. S_3 may be a normal finding in adolescents, and is more prominent in hyperdynamic states.

d. Fourth heart sound (S_4): S_4 is due to atrial contraction. It is heard late in diastole, particularly at the apex, and is almost always pathological in adolescents, although it may be normal in older adults.

e. Clicks: A click is a sharp, high-frequency sound that provides an important clue to the diagnosis of organic disease.
- Early systolic ejection clicks are of either pulmonary or aortic origin, and occur shortly after S_1.
- A pulmonary ejection click is best heard at the upper LSB and is associated with valvular pulmonary stenosis. The intensity of the pulmonary valve ejection click varies with respiration (louder with expiration) and the severity of pulmonary stenosis.
- An aortic ejection click is best heard at the apex and does not vary with respiration. It is associated with a bicuspid aortic valve, which in turn may include aortic stenosis, or coarctation.
- Nonejection clicks are usually midsystolic and are present at the apex. These clicks move within systole as ventricular loading conditions change (with squatting or isometric hand contraction). They are associated with mitral valve prolapse (MVP).

f. Murmurs: The presence of a systolic or diastolic murmur requires careful analysis of its characteristics, including timing, loudness, length, tonal quality, and location. For practical purposes, all diastolic murmurs, except venous hums, should be considered pathological.

DIAGNOSTIC CLUES FOR INNOCENT MURMURS

1. History: Asymptomatic, no family history of cardiac disease
2. Physical examination: Normal, other than the presence of the murmur
3. Timing of murmur: Early systolic; almost never diastolic

4. Duration: Not holosystolic
5. Intensity: Usually grade 1–3/6
6. Radiation: Not extensive
7. Quality: Vibratory; no clicks
8. Location: May vary, but frequently at lower or upper LSB
9. Change with position: Increase in supine position, decrease with sitting or standing
10. S_2: Physiological splitting
11. Laboratory findings: Generally, no laboratory studies are indicated. In the primary care setting, electrocardiograms (ECGs) are obtained only selectively. When obtained, they should be normal.

DIAGNOSTIC CLUES FOR PATHOLOGICAL MURMURS

1. Significant history: Growth failure, decreased exercise tolerance, exertional syncope or near-syncope, exertional chest pain.
2. Physical examination: Clubbing, cyanosis, decreased or delayed femoral pulses, apical heave, palpable thrill, tachypnea, inappropriate tachycardia.
3. Murmur: Diastolic, holosystolic, loud or harsh, extensive radiation, increases with standing, associated with a thrill, abnormal S_2. See Table 14.1.

INNOCENT MURMURS

A number of normal murmurs have been described. They have identifiable characteristics that allow them to be recognized by physical examination alone. Characterizing a murmur as "normal" is not a diagnosis of exclusion; each has definite criteria that should be fulfilled.

Still's Murmur

1. Cause: Turbulence of flow from blood ejected through the LV outflow tract or the presence of ventricular false tendons.
2. Quality
   a. Low- to medium-pitched murmur with vibratory or musical quality.
   b. Grade 1-3/6 early to midsystolic murmur; never holosystolic; S_1 can be clearly distinguished from the murmur.
3. Location: Maximal at lower LSB, extending to the apex.
4. Maneuvers: Murmur decreased on sitting or standing, loudest in supine position.
5. Differential diagnosis: Differentiated from valvular aortic stenosis by the absence of a click or radiation to the upper right sternal border (RSB). Differentiated from hypertrophic cardiomyopathy (HCM) because the murmur decreases with standing. Less harsh than a murmur associated with a ventricular septal defect (VSD).

Pulmonary Flow Murmur

1. Cause: Turbulence of flow in the RV outflow tract across a normal pulmonary valve (the right-sided equivalent

TABLE 14.1

Types of Pathological Murmurs

Murmur Type	Characteristics	Common Defects
Systolic ejection	Crescendo–decrescendo Begins after S_1; ends before S_2 Best heard with diaphragm	Aortic stenosis Pulmonary stenosis Coarctation of the aorta ASD
Holosystolic	Begins with and obscures S_1 Ends at S_2 Heard at LSB or apex	VSD Mitral regurgitation
Early diastolic	Decrescendo Begins immediately after S_2 High–medium pitch	Aortic insufficiency Pulmonary insufficiency
Middiastolic	Low pitch Rumble Best heard with bell	ASD VSD Mitral stenosis
Continuous	Extend up to and through S_2 Continue through all/part of diastole Best heard with diaphragm	PDA

ASD, atrial septal defect; LSB, left sternal border; VSD, ventricular septal defect; PDA, patent ductus arteriosus.

of Still's murmur). Often heard with tachycardia due to fever, anxiety, or exertion. Associated with pectus excavatum or kyphoscoliosis.

2. Quality: Short crescendo–decrescendo midsystolic murmur. Grade 1-3/6. No ejection click. Normal splitting of S_2.
3. Location: Upper LSB, second to third left intercostal space.
4. Maneuvers: Murmur decreased by inspiration and sitting, increased in supine position.
5. Differential diagnosis: Differentiated from valvular pulmonary stenosis by absence of a click; differentiated from an atrial septal defect because S_2 splits normally.

Cervical Venous Hum

1. Cause: Turbulence of venous flow at the sharp angle made between the internal jugular and subclavian veins and the superior vena cava.
2. Quality: Medium-pitched, soft, blowing continuous murmur with diastolic accentuation.
3. Location: Heard best above the sternal end of clavicle, at the base of the neck. May be bilateral or unilateral (right side usually louder; most people have only a right-sided superior vena cava).
4. Maneuvers
   a. Murmur is increased by rotating the head away from the side of the murmur.
   b. Murmur is decreased or obliterated by jugular venous compression.
   c. Murmur *decreased* with supine position—unique for a normal murmur.
5. Differential diagnosis: If murmur is louder over the chest than over the supraclavicular area, and does not

change with the maneuvers described, patent ductus arteriosus or coronary artery fistula must be excluded.

Supraclavicular (Carotid) Bruit

1. Cause: Turbulence at the site of branching of the brachiocephalic arteries from the aortic arch.
2. Quality: Short, high-pitched early systolic murmur, usually grade 2/6.
3. Location: Maximal above the clavicles and lower portion of the sternocleidomastoid muscle, with radiation to the neck.
4. Maneuvers
   a. Murmur is eliminated by compression of the subclavian artery against the first rib.
   b. Murmur is decreased by hyperextending the shoulders (bringing the elbows behind the back).
   c. Murmur is heard in the sitting position with the bell of the stethoscope.
5. Differential diagnosis: Differentiated from aortic or pulmonary stenosis because murmur is louder over the neck than the chest, there is no click, and it changes with the above maneuvers.

MURMURS ASSOCIATED WITH STRUCTURAL HEART DISEASE

Although less common, mildly symptomatic congenital heart disease may not be recognized until adolescence, particularly in underserved populations. Therefore, a careful differential diagnosis must be considered when the examiner first notes a cardiac murmur. A review of these lesions is presented in Table 14.2.

TABLE 14.2

Clues to Specific Organic Cardiac Lesions

Diagnosis	Auscultation	Other Findings	Chest X-ray	ECG
Patent ductus arteriosus	Continuous murmur LUSB and subclavicular area	Wide pulse pressure Bounding pulses	Prominent pulmonary artery	Normal LAE/LVH
Atrial septal defect	Fixed, widely split S_2 Systolic ejection murmur at LUSB Middiastolic rumble at LLSB	RV lift	Prominent RV outflow	Incomplete RBBB (rSR' pattern)
Pulmonary stenosis	Systolic ejection click (mild PS) P_2 delayed and soft SEM at LUSB	RV lift Thrill at LUSB	Prominent RV outflow Poststenotic dilation	RVH RAE
Aortic stenosis	Early systolic murmur RUSB, transmitted to neck Systolic ejection click (mild AS) Soft A_2	LV lift Decreased pulses	LVE	LVH
Mitral regurgitation	Holosystolic murmur with radiation to axilla; soft S_1	LV lift	Large LA and LV	Bifid P waves Left axis deviation
Mitral valve prolapse	Midsystolic click; mid- or late-systolic murmur			Abnormal T waves Arrhythmias
Hypertrophic cardiomyopathy	Midsystolic murmur at LLSB, increased with standing and decreased with Valsalva maneuver	Rapid carotid upstroke	± LVE ± LAE	LVH ± Q waves
Ventricular septal defect	High-pitched, harsh holosystolic murmur at LLSB	Thrill at LLSB	Normal	Normal (if small VSD)
Pulmonary hypertension	Loud P_2 No murmur or regurgitant murmur at LLSB	? Clubbing	Variable	RAE RVH
Coarctation of aorta	Continuous/systolic precordial murmur Systolic ejection click from bicuspid aortic valve	SBP lower in legs than arms Decreased/delayed femoral pulses	Rib notching Increased pulmonary markings	LVH

ECG, echocardiogram; LUSB, left upper sternal border; LAE, left atrial enlargement; LVH, left ventricular hypertrophy; LLSB, left lower sternal border; RV, right ventricular; RBBB, right bundle-branch block; PS, pulmonic stenosis; RVH, right ventricular hypertrophy; RAE, right atrial enlargement; SEM, systolic ejection murmur; RUSB, right upper sternal border; AS, aortic stenosis; LV, left ventricular; LA, left atrium; LVE, left ventricular enlargement; VSD, ventricular septal defect.

Atrial Septal Defect

Other than MVP and bicuspid aortic valve, atrial septal defect is the most common congenital cardiac lesion diagnosed de novo in adolescence or adulthood.

1. Physical examination: Signs and symptoms depend on shunt size.
   a. Hyperdynamic precordium with RV lift with sizable shunt; no thrill.
   b. Widely split and fixed S_2.
   c. Pulmonary flow murmur: Grade 2-3/6 systolic ejection murmur at upper LSB.
   d. Middiastolic rumble at lower LSB (increased flow across tricuspid valve).
2. Further evaluation
   a. ECG: Right axis deviation, RV conduction delay (rSR' pattern), right atrial enlargement, or RV hypertrophy.
   b. Chest radiograph: Mild to moderate cardiomegaly with increased pulmonary vascularity.
   c. Echocardiogram: Diagnostic with visualization of location and size of defect.
   d. Other imaging studies: Both nuclear flow scans and cardiac magnetic resonance imaging (MRI) offer

noninvasive tools that permit quantification of the right to left shunt. Cardiac MRI allows excellent imaging of the atrial septum and RV volume. This information can help in deciding whether defects are good candidates for device closure, or have sufficient right to left shunt to deserve therapy.

3. Management: Both surgical closure and transcatheter device closure are safe, effective, and popular management choices. Transcatheter device closure has the advantages of avoiding cardiopulmonary bypass and preventing a thoracic scar; however, a permanent foreign body is left in place. Conversely, surgical management has now evolved, leading to low postoperative morbidity and rapid recovery. Surgical repair carries with it the inherent risk of bypass, and the postoperative potential for postpericardiotomy syndrome or atrial arrhythmia. Decisions continue to be made on a case-by-case basis.

Ventricular Septal Defect

1. Physical examination: Shunt volume determines findings.
   a. With increasing shunt size, the precordium becomes increasingly hyperdynamic. A thrill may be present with either a large or small shunt.
   b. S_2 is normal with small shunts, accentuated with larger shunts. An S_3 may be present. A loud P_2 (suggesting pulmonary hypertension), particularly with a soft or absent murmur, is a worrisome finding.
   c. Grade 2–3/6 holosystolic murmur at lower LSB (very small defects may be quite localized with a high-frequency, blowing quality).
   d. Middiastolic rumble at the apex with large shunts (increased flow across the mitral valve).
2. Further evaluation
   a. ECG: Normal in small defects; LV hypertrophy with large defects.
   b. Chest radiograph: Normal in small defects; cardiomegaly with increased pulmonary vascularity in large defects.
   c. Echocardiogram: Provides anatomical detail of location and size of defect; color Doppler permits visualization of very small defects.
3. Management: Some patients with small lesions will be lost to follow-up, and have no recollection of this previous diagnosis when being evaluated as a teen. Even large VSDs may not be identified until adolescence. If the echocardiogram confirms low RV pressure, little additional data is required to make appropriate decisions regarding expectant or surgical management. However, when large VSDs are identified in adolescence, pulmonary artery and RV pressures are typically elevated. For these patients, catheterization is critical in assessing pulmonary vascular resistance and reactivity. Some adolescents with late presentation of VSD will need palliative care focused on their pulmonary vascular disease. It is important to note that infectious endocarditis prophylaxis is no longer recommended for VSD.

Patent Ductus Arteriosus

1. Physical examination: Shunt volume determines findings.
   a. Normal precordium with small shunt; hyperdynamic with a thrill with large shunt.
   b. Grade 2–4/6 continuous murmur at upper LSB.
   c. Wide pulse pressure and bounding pulses with large shunt.
2. Further evaluation
   a. ECG: Often normal. LV hypertrophy seen if left to right shunting is significant.
   b. Chest radiograph: Cardiomegaly with increased pulmonary vascularity with large shunt.
   c. Echocardiogram: Visualization with two-dimensional and color Doppler imaging.
3. Management: Cardiac catheterization is rarely required for diagnosis but is commonly done for coil or device occlusion. In the adolescent with a large patent ductus, catheterization is critical in evaluating the level of pulmonary vascular obstructive disease.

Valvular Pulmonary Stenosis

1. Physical examination: Severity of obstruction determines findings.
   a. RV lift with systolic thrill at upper LSB in more severe forms.
   b. Systolic ejection click at upper LSB, which is louder with expiration. In severe pulmonary stenosis, the click becomes more difficult to hear as it moves closer to the S_1.
   c. Normal to soft S_2 or widely split S_2, depending on severity of stenosis.
   d. Grade 2–4/6 harsh systolic ejection murmur at upper LSB; may radiate to the lung fields and back. Intensity and duration of the murmur increase as stenosis severity increases.
2. Further evaluation
   a. ECG: Normal, with progression to RV hypertrophy (upright T wave in lead V1) as stenosis increases
   b. Chest radiogram: Prominent pulmonary artery segment with normal vascularity.
   c. Echocardiogram: Permits evaluation of valve morphology. Doppler evaluation of maximum gradient across the valve has proved to have excellent correlation with cardiac catheterization measurement of gradient.
3. Management: Cardiac catheterization is rarely required for diagnosis. Treatment of choice is balloon pulmonary valvuloplasty.

Valvular Aortic Stenosis

1. Physical examination: Severity of obstruction determines findings.
   a. Prominent apical impulse and systolic thrill (at upper RSB or suprasternal notch) in more severe forms.
   b. Intensity of S_1 may be diminished due to poor ventricular compliance.
   c. Systolic ejection click at lower LSB/apex; does not vary with respiration. Radiates to aortic area at upper RSB. Click is not present in supravalvular or subvalvular types.
   d. Grade 2–4/6 long, harsh systolic crescendo–decrescendo ejection murmur at upper RSB; subvalvular murmur may be heard best at mid-LSB.
   e. High-frequency early diastolic decrescendo murmur of aortic regurgitation.

f. Careful general physical examination looking for features of associated Turner or Williams syndrome.
2. Further evaluation
   a. ECG: Normal to LV hypertrophy, depending on severity of stenosis. Strain pattern (ST segment depression and T wave inversion in left precordium) indicates severe stenosis.
   b. Chest radiograph: Normal heart size with prominent ascending aorta.
   c. Echocardiogram: Permits evaluation of valve morphology and determination of level of stenosis. Seventy percent to 85% of stenotic valves are bicuspid. Mean pressure gradient obtained by Doppler evaluation has good correlation with valve gradient measured by cardiac catheterization.
3. Management: Cardiac catheterization is rarely required for diagnosis. In selective cases, aortic balloon valvuloplasty may be an initial palliative procedure.

Hypertrophic Cardiomyopathy

HCM is the most common unrecognized cause of sudden cardiac death in young people. Although patients with HCM can present with cardiac symptoms (chest pain, dyspnea, palpitations, or syncope), they are frequently asymptomatic. The physical examination is quite dynamic and may either be normal or only transiently abnormal.

1. Physical examination
   a. Careful general physical examination to assess for features of skeletal myopathy.
   b. Normal to hyperdynamic precordium with increased LV impulse, dynamic thrill.
   c. Auscultation may be normal. Adequate examination includes supine, standing, squatting, and repeat examination upon resumption of standing position.
   d. Dynamic aortic stenosis murmur: Systolic ejection murmur at the lower LSB with *increasing* intensity in standing position and with decreasing intensity in squatting or Valsalva maneuver.
   e. Dynamic murmur of mitral insufficiency.
2. Further evaluation
   a. ECG: Normal in some cases. LV and/or septal hypertrophy, T wave discordance, atrial enlargement may be seen.
   b. Chest radiograph: Usually normal. Cardiomegaly may be seen.
   c. Echocardiogram: Diagnostic, with excessive LV wall thickness, impaired ventricular filling, variable degrees of LV outflow tract obstruction, and variable systolic anterior motion of the mitral valve
3. Management: Management of HCM remains controversial. For the symptomatic patient with aborted sudden death (and some with syncope), implantable defibrillators are the primary therapy. Those with severe and symptomatic LV outflow tract obstruction may benefit from either surgical or catheter treatment. Drug therapy is primarily reserved for relief of milder symptoms. Most patients are restricted from competitive sports. Prophylaxis for subacute bacterial endocarditis (SBE) is no longer recommended.

MITRAL VALVE PROLAPSE

MVP is a heterogeneous disorder, with a wide spectrum of pathological, clinical, and echocardiographic manifestations. Although the diagnosis of MVP is common, clinically important MVP is infrequent. The modern understanding of MVP identifies the mitral valve involvement as either part of global connective tissues abnormalities—the most common being Marfan syndrome—or as an isolated finding. Most patients with classic MVP have an excellent prognosis. Other patients, most of whom have other connective tissue disease, are at increased risk for the development of mitral regurgitation, infectious endocarditis, cerebral embolism, life-threatening arrhythmia, and sudden death. Refinement in our approach over the last two decades has led to improved differentiation between the two groups, and recognition of the associated differences in prognosis. This is an important distinction to make to avoid unnecessary anxiety, activity limitations, or antibiotic prophylaxis in otherwise healthy young people. In addition, modern understanding of the potential for over-diagnosis of MVP has led to increased skepticism of symptomatic patients with "MVP syndrome" and minimal cardiac findings.

Normal mechanical function of the mitral valve depends on the relation between the size of the mitral leaflets and the LV cavity. An excess of leaflet tissue or a disproportionately small LV cavity (which can occur with dehydration, cardiomyopathy, or anorexia nervosa) may lead to signs of MVP. MVP also has a well-established association with connective tissue disorders such as Marfan syndrome, Ehlers-Danlos syndrome (EDS), and osteogenesis imperfecta.

Epiemiology

The reported historical prevalence of MVP has ranged from 1% to 35%, depending on the population studied and criteria utilized for diagnosis. Current diagnostic criteria have led to a prevalence estimate of 2% to 3%, with equal distribution among men and women (Freed et al., 1999). MVP may be diagnosed at any age; symptomatic patients tend to be older adolescents or young adults.

Classification

MVP can be divided into three types:

1. Primary (classic) prolapse, an idiopathic but often autosomal dominant disorder (with variable penetrance) affecting the structure of the mitral valve. Valve leaflets are thickened and elongated in association with myxomatous infiltration.
2. Secondary prolapse from myxomatous degeneration of mitral leaflets in individuals with connective tissue diseases such as Marfan syndrome.
3. Prolapse of a normal mitral valve leaflet in individuals with papillary muscle dysfunction related to ischemia, infarction, or cardiomyopathy.

Clinical Manifestations

The true prevalence of the symptoms described in patients with MVP compared with the general population is unknown because prevalence rates are usually based on data from referral centers and/or hospital-based patients.

Historically, many cardiac symptoms were attributed to the presence of MVP. However, the vast majority of adolescents with complaints of chest pain, palpitations, dizziness, syncope, dyspnea on exertion, or fatigue do not have MVP. When true disease is suspected, a dynamic physical examination and two-dimensional echocardiography are the diagnostic standards for MVP. Frequently described symptoms include the following:

1. Palpitations, which may be unrelated to the occurrence of arrhythmias, representing symptomatic sinus tachycardia, orthostatic intolerance and presyncope, or other "noncardiac" causes. Isolated ventricular ectopy, sometimes frequent, does seem to be more common in MVP patients as compared to controls (Kavey et al., 1984; Bobkowski et al., 2002).
2. Chest pain tends to be precordial, nonexertional, and is of longer duration than anginal pain. The cause of the chest pain is unknown, and is likely unrelated to the MVP.
3. Less common symptoms include exertional dyspnea, fatigue, lightheadedness, syncope (common also in adolescents without MVP), and neuropsychiatric symptoms such as anxiety. Historically, comorbidity between MVP and anxiety disorders was suggested. However, recent studies have demonstrated no association between MVP and childhood anxiety disorders (Toren et al., 1999; Arfken et al., 1990).

Physical Findings

1. Click: The mid-to-late systolic click of MVP is best heard with the diaphragm of the stethoscope. This sound is caused by the sudden ballooning of a mitral leaflet into the left atrium during systole. The click often precedes a late systolic murmur of mitral regurgitation. The interval between S_1 and the click varies with LV end-diastolic volume. Maneuvers on physical examination can demonstrate this dynamic variation. As end-diastolic volume increases (supine position, squatting) or as afterload increases (hand-gripping), the click moves later into systole. Conversely, with reduction of end-diastolic volume of the ventricle (standing, Valsalva), the earlier in systole the click occurs. Therefore, the intensity and position of the click may vary in the same individual depending on a variety of factors.
2. Murmur: The murmur of MVP tends to be a high-pitched, late systolic murmur, heard best at the apex of the heart. As with the click, maneuvers that decrease LV volume move the murmur closer to S_1. Maneuvers that increase LV diastolic volume may diminish the murmur. Some patients have no click and only a late systolic murmur.
3. Associated physical abnormalities: An association has been described between MVP and slender body habitus in both adults and children (Arfken et al., 1993). Patients should also be closely examined for stigmata of the commonly associated connective tissue disorders, and evaluated by a clinician who specializes in such disorders if the examination is worrisome. MVP with or without mitral regurgitation is a minor, not major, criterion for determining cardiovascular involvement for the diagnosis of Marfan syndrome (De Paepe et al., 1996). Isolated thoracic bony abnormalities such as scoliosis, pectus excavatum, and decreased anteroposterior diameter have also been associated with MVP.

Further Evaluation

1. Chest x-ray: Generally normal; possible scoliosis.
2. ECG: Usually normal but indicated if a patient complains of palpitations.
3. Holter or event monitoring: Indicated to evaluate for arrhythmia if the patient has palpitations that disrupt activities of daily living or cause serious symptoms (syncope, dizziness).
4. Echocardiogram: If a systolic click or late systolic murmur is heard, an echocardiogram is essential to visualize the mitral valve and to confirm the diagnosis of MVP. The degree of prolapse, amount of mitral regurgitation, severity of the deformity, thickness of the valve leaflets, and LV function can also be evaluated. Certain echocardiographic features have been associated with a poor prognosis, including thickened and redundant mitral valve leaflets. Echocardiogram also allows measurement of the ascending aorta, aortic root diameter, and LVr dimensions for patients with significant mitral insufficiency.

Mild bowing of a mitral leaflet, a normal variant, should not be misdiagnosed as frank prolapse. It is essential that echocardiographic findings that "suggest prolapse" have firm clinical correlation before a healthy person is labeled as having MVP. Patients with less than overt prolapse on echocardiography and absence of a click, murmur, or symptoms should not be misclassified as having MVP. They do not need to follow bacterial endocarditis prophylaxis precautions.

Management

1. Reassurance: The vast majority of adolescents and young adults with MVP are asymptomatic. They should not be restricted in their activities, and serious sequelae need not be discussed. Routine follow-up echocardiography is not recommended, unless new symptoms or new physical examination findings develop.
2. Health maintenance: Studies in adults have demonstrated that increased blood pressure and obesity, two potentially reversible risk factors, place patients with MVP at greater risk for severe mitral regurgitation and the need for valve surgery (Singh et al., 2000).
3. Antibiotic prophylaxis: New recommendations from the American Heart Association significantly reduce the indications for antibiotic prophylaxis of infective endocarditis (Table 14.3–14.6). Routine prophylaxis is no longer recommended for MVP. The complete guidelines are available at: http://www.americanheart.org/presenter .jhtml?identifier=3004539 and a wallet card is available at: http://www.americanheart.org/presenter.jhtml? identifier=11086
4. β-Blocking agents may be indicated for patients with MVP who have significant symptoms from arrhythmias, to provide symptomatic relief or to target a specific arrhythmia. There is no evidence that β-blockade decreases the already low risk of sudden death (Priori et al., 2001).
5. Pregnancy: Mild mitral regurgitation is generally well-tolerated during pregnancy and delivery, with no additional risk to mother or child.
6. Genetic counseling: The first-degree relatives of patients with myxomatous MVP should be screened for MVP using echocardiography because of the high prevalence of the diagnosis within families.

TABLE 14.3

Cardiac Conditions Associated with Endocarditis

Endocarditis Prophylaxis Recommended	*Endocarditis Prophylaxis not Recommended*
Prosthetic cardiac valve	Innocent murmurs
Previous IE	Mitral valve prolapse
Congenital heart disease (CHD)[a]	Hypertrophic cardiomyopathy
Unrepaired cyanotic CHD, including palliative shunts and conduits	
Completely repaired congenital heart defect with prosthetic material or device, whether placed by surgery or by catheter intervention, during the first 6 months after the procedure[b]	
Repaired CHD with residual defects at the site or adjacent to the site of a prosthetic patch or prosthetic device (which inhibit endothelialization)	
Cardiac transplantation recipients who develop cardiac valvulopathy	

[a]Except for the conditions listed above, antibiotic prophylaxis is no longer recommended for any other form of CHD.
[b]Prophylaxis is recommended because endothelialization of prosthetic material occurs within 6 months after the procedure.
Adapted from Wilson W, Taubert KA, Gewitz M, et al. Prevention of Infective Endocarditis: Guidelines from the American Heart Association. *Circulation* 2007;115:1.

7. Exercise: Patients with mild MVP with neither significant mitral insufficiency, ventricular arrhythmias, history of cardiac syncope, nor a family history of premature sudden death need no restrictions to physical activity. Those who have more cardiac manifestations and more significant valvular disease may require some restrictions and careful consideration of athletic choices (Maron and Zipes, 2005).

Complications

Complications of MVP are rare. When complications do develop, they usually occur in patients with a mitral regurgitation murmur, thickened redundant mitral valve leaflets, or an enlarged left atrium or LV. Patients without murmur or echocardiographic evidence of more serious disease have a benign prognosis, and should be considered as a separate group. Complications that can occur include the following:

1. Arrhythmias: The most frequent complication, including premature ventricular contractions, supraventricular tachyarrhythmia, ventricular tachycardia, and bradyarrhythmia.
2. Infectious endocarditis: In the absence of mitral regurgitation, the incidence of infective endocarditis in patients with MVP is similar to that of the general population. However, in patients with MVP *and* a systolic murmur, the risk increases to approximately 0.05% per year (Steckelberg and Wilson, 1993). In the study of risk factors by Nishimura et al. (1985), all patients with endocarditis and MVP had redundant mitral valve leaflets. Although MVP is the most common cause of infective endocarditis, the absolute risk is extremely low and the morbidity is not as severe as in other conditions.

Therefore, SBE prophylaxis is no longer recommended in this population (Wilson et al., 2007).
3. Progressive mitral regurgitation: This complication results from either progressive myxomatous degeneration or chordal rupture, and is rare in otherwise healthy adolescents. Risk factors for regurgitation include advancing age, male gender, hypertension, overweight, thickened leaflets on echocardiogram, and increased LV dimensions (Singh et al., 2000). Patients with connective tissue disorders are at higher risk of mitral valve dysfunction. This may develop and progress without symptoms, but can lead to significant morbidity and mortality by the end of the second decade of life, especially in female patients (van Karnebeek et al., 2001). The severity of mitral regurgitation is an important prognostic indicator for the development of cardiac events in patients with MVP (Kim et al., 1996).
4. Sudden death: Although the risk of sudden cardiac death in patients with MVP is very low (estimated yearly rate of 40 per 10,000), the incidence is still greater than that in the general population (Kligfield et al., 1987). Significant mitral regurgitation, redundant chordae, and depressed LV function increase the risk of sudden death (Kligfield et al., 1987; Nishimura et al., 1985; Grigioni et al., 1999). However, the expected survival is similar to that of the general population (Freed et al., 2002). The cases of sudden cardiac death are likely due to ventricular arrhythmia.
5. Stroke: Early studies demonstrated an association between MVP and cerebrovascular accidents (CVA) in young patients. However, more recent findings have been mixed. Two investigators reported no excess risk of CVA in young patients with MVP (Barnett et al., 1980), whereas another demonstrated a CVA event rate of 0.7% per year, twice the expected rate (Avierinos et al., 2003). These data suggest that MVP may confer a small risk of

TABLE 14.4

Summary of Major Changes in New 2007 AHA Guidelines on Prevention of Infective Endocarditis

Bacteremia resulting from daily activities is much more likely to cause IE than bacteremia associated with a dental procedure.

Only an extremely small number of cases of IE might be prevented by antibiotic prophylaxis even if prophylaxis is 100% effective.

Antibiotic prophylaxis is not recommended based solely on an increased lifetime risk of acquisition of IE.

Recommendations for IE prophylaxis is recommended only to those with conditions listed in Table 14.3.

Antibiotic prophylaxis is no longer recommended for any other form of CHD, except for the conditions listed in Table 14.3.

Antibiotic prophylaxis is recommended for all dental procedures that involve manipulation of gingival tissues or periapical region of teeth or perforation of oral mucosa only for patients with underlying cardiac conditions associated with the highest risk of adverse outcome from IE (Table 14.3).

Antibiotic prophylaxis is recommended for procedures on respiratory tract or infected skin, skin structures, or musculoskeletal tissue only for patients with underlying cardiac conditions associated with the highest risk of adverse outcome from IE (Table 14.3).

Antibiotic prophylaxis solely to prevent IE is not recommended for GU or GI tract procedures.

The writing group reaffirms the procedures noted in the 1997 prophylaxis guidelines for which endocarditis prophylaxis is not recommended and extends this to other common procedures, including ear and body piercing, tattooing, and vaginal delivery and hysterectomy.

Adapted from Wilson W, Taubert KA, Gewitz M, et al. Prevention of Infective Endocarditis: Guidelines from the American Heart Association. *Circulation* 2007;115:1

TABLE 14.5

Dental Procedures for Which Endocarditis Prophylaxis Is Recommended for Patients in Table 14.3

All dental procedures that involve manipulation of gingival tissue or the periapical region of teeth or perforation of the oral mucosa[a]

[a]The following procedures and events do not need prophylaxis: routine anesthetic injections through noninfected tissue, taking dental radiographs, placement of removable prosthodontic or orthodontic appliances, adjustment of orthodontic appliances, placement of orthodontic brackets, shedding of deciduous teeth, and bleeding from trauma to the lips or oral mucosa.

a. Normal to hyperdynamic precordium.
b. Grade 2–4/6 high-frequency holosystolic apical murmur; may radiate toward the base (upper LSB).
c. Low-frequency apical middiastolic rumble with severe regurgitation.

2. Further evaluation
a. ECG: May be normal with mild regurgitation; bifid P wave of left atrial enlargement and even LV enlargement are noted if regurgitation is chronic and severe.
b. Chest radiograph: Normal to cardiomegaly with large left atrium and LV.
c. Echocardiogram: Evaluates cause of valve abnormality and severity of regurgitation.

3. Management: The increased LV volume load induced by the regurgitation gradually increases the ventricular volumes and in turn increases the severity of the mitral regurgitation (mitral regurgitation begets mitral regurgitation). For this reason, patients are serially assessed as to their need for afterload decreasing agents (including angiotensin-converting enzyme (ACE) inhibitors) or for surgery.

SYSTEMIC CONNECTIVE TISSUE DISEASE AND THE HEART

Marfan Syndrome

Marfan syndrome is a global connective tissue disorder with specific ocular, musculoskeletal, and cardiac involvement. In approximately 75% of patients there is parental involvement, confirming the autosomal dominant inheritance. The prevalence of MVP in patients with Marfan syndrome is above 90%; it is due to both histological changes and ventricular-valvar disproportion. Patients with Marfan syndrome have mutations in the *FBN1* gene, and produce abnormal fibrillin protein. Fibrillin is an extracellular matrix protein that contributes to large structures called *microfibrils*. The distorted microfibrils lead to the problems with elastic matrix faced by Marfan syndrome patients. The clinical diagnosis is made using a series of major and minor criteria (De Paepe et al., 1996). MVP with or without mitral insufficiency is a minor cardiac criterion. Aortic root dilation at the level of the sinuses of Valsalva and/or dissection of the ascending aorta are major cardiac criteria.

CVA, but only in older patients with advanced mitral regurgitation. Currently, the American College of Cardiology does not recommend routine prophylactic aspirin treatment.

Mitral Valve Regurgitation

Mitral valve regurgitation is rare in adolescence unless it is associated with MVP, HCM, inflammatory heart disease (such as myocarditis or rheumatic heart disease), or congenital heart disease. A new-onset regurgitant murmur should provoke a thorough investigation.

1. Physical examination: Findings depend on severity of regurgitation.

TABLE 14.6

Regimens for Dental Procedures

| Situation | Agent | Regimen: Single Dose 30 to 60 min Before Procedure | |
		Adults	Children
Oral	Amoxicillin	2 g	50 mg/kg
Unable to take oral medication	Ampicillin **OR**	2 g IM or IV	50 mg/kg IM or IV
	Cefazolin or ceftriaxone	1 g IM or IV	50 mg/kg IM or IV
Allergic to penicillins or ampicillin—oral	Cephalexin[a,b] **OR**	2 g	50 mg/kg
	Clindamycin **OR**	600 mg	20 mg/kg
	Azithromycin or clarithromycin	500 mg	15 mg/kg
Allergic to penicillins or ampicillin and unable to take oral medication	Cefazolin or ceftriaxone[b] **OR**	1 g IM or IV	50 mg/kg IM or IV
	Clindamycin	600 mg IM or IV	20 mg/kg IM or IV

IM indicates intramuscular; IV, intravenous.

[a]Or other first- or second-generation oral cephalosporin in equivalent adult or pediatric dosage.

[b]Cephalosporins should not be used in an individual with a history of anaphylaxis, angioedema, or urticaria with penicillins or ampicillin.

The diagnosis of Marfan syndrome is based on clinical evaluation, with careful anthropometric measurements, detailed physical examination, ophthalmology examination, and echocardiogram. In the absence of family history of documented Marfan syndrome, "major" involvement in two organ systems and minor involvement in a third organ system must be met. For families with clear genetic/familial involvement, the finding of major involvement in any one organ system and at least one minor criterion in a second is sufficient. The specific management of MVP in patients with Marfan syndrome is done in context of the aortic root dilation. β-Blockers are used as prophylaxis to try slow dilation. There may be rapid progression of aortic root dilation in pregnancy. Unlike patients with isolated MVP, patients with Marfan syndrome are generally restricted from high intensity and collision sports (Maron et al., 2004). When the aortic root reaches 5.5 cm, aortic root reconstruction is generally indicated.

Other Connective Tissues Disorders that Include Mitral Valve Prolapse

Ehlers-Danlos Syndromes
EDSs are a range of connective tissue disorders dominated by their musculoskeletal involvement. Approximately 50% of patients with the classic subtype have been demonstrated to have abnormalities in type V collagen resulting from COL5A1 and COL5A2 deletions. MVP is relatively common in the classic subtype of EDS. The hypermobility subtype (EDS type III) is generally considered the least severe type, and less frequently involves MVP.

In all EDS subtypes, aortic root dilation is less severe and less frequent than in Marfan syndrome. As with Marfan syndrome, the genetic diagnosis is not required for the clinical diagnosis. Patients with EDS may demonstrate symptoms of palpitations, presyncope, and syncope associated with the autonomic dysregulation and neurally mediated hypotension of postural orthostatic tachycardia (Rowe et al., 1999). Although screening for cardiac involvement is appropriate, most patients with EDS will not have specific cardiac diagnoses, even if their orthostasis produces sufficient cardiac symptoms to require further evaluation and management.

Fragile X Syndrome
This alteration in the *FMR1* gene is associated with mental retardation, joint laxity, and some incidence of aortic root dilation and MVP. The cardiac involvement may not be apparent until adolescence (Crabbe et al., 1993). Periodic cardiac screening may be warranted.

GENERAL CONSIDERATIONS IN THE MANAGEMENT OF HEART LESIONS

After obtaining a careful history and conducting a thorough physical examination, it should be possible to differentiate normal from pathological murmurs. ECGs and chest radiographs do not add to the accuracy of diagnosis of normal murmurs. The ECG and radiograph are unlikely to be grossly abnormal unless the child has a significant hemodynamic lesion; a patient with such a lesion is unlikely to be asymptomatic. In addition, because pathological disease is not always associated with abnormal test results, normal findings may lead to a false sense of security.

Although often expected to be high yield, echocardiography adds little to the diagnosis of a "normal" murmur. The cost-effective choice between referring to a pediatric cardiologist (which often includes an echocardiogram) and directly obtaining an echocardiogram depends on the relative cost of the test, the accessibility of consultation, and the skill of the individual practitioner in identifying pathological murmurs (Danford et al., 1995). Most adult-oriented laboratories are highly skilled at evaluating LV size and function, but less experienced at diagnosing specific anatomic abnormalities or visualizing coronary artery origins. Pediatric-focused laboratories seem to do better on these imaging tasks (Stanger et al., 1999; Hurwitz et al., 1999). Each clinician will develop a practical approach which reflects his or her personal skills and the availability and cost of specialty referrals.

If diagnosed with structural heart disease, the patient and parents should be informed about the risks of bacterial endocarditis. The recommendations of the American Heart Association for prophylaxis should be provided. New recommendations have recently been published which significantly narrow the indications for antibiotic prophylaxis of IE. Changes in the new 2007 AHA recommendations are summarized in Table 14.4. Prophylactic regimens for dental procedures are outlined in Table 14.5.

Therefore, optimal management of a heart murmur requires a careful and systematic cardiovascular examination; judicious use of laboratory studies; referral, in selected cases, to a pediatric cardiologist; and, in the case of normal murmurs, confident reassurance. If the murmur is deemed innocent, the practitioner should emphasize that the heart is normal. This prohibits the labeling of healthy children with cardiac diagnoses, and prevents needless patient, parental, and provider anxiety.

WEB SITES

For Teens and Parents

http://www.americanheart.org/presenter.jhtml?identifier=4571. American Heart Association Web site describing heart murmurs.
http://www.drkoop.com/ency/93/000180.htm.
http://www.marfan.org. Good resource for both families and professionals on Marfan syndrome.
http://medlineplus.gov. National Library of Medicine on heart murmurs.

Especially for Parents

http://www.kidshealth.org/kid/health_problems/heart/heart_murmurs.html.

Sites to Hear Heart Sounds

http://www.wilkes.med.ucla.edu.

REFERENCES AND ADDITIONAL READINGS

Allen HD, Beekman RH, Garson A, et al. Pediatric therapeutic cardiac catheterization. *Circulation* 1998;97:609.

Arfken CL, Lachman AS, McLaren MJ, et al. Mitral valve prolapse: associations with symptoms and anxiety. *Pediatrics* 1990;85:311.

Arfken CL, Schulman P, McLaren MJ, et al. Mitral valve prolapse and body habitus in children. *Pediatr Cardiol* 1993;14:33.

Avierinos JF, Brown RD, Foley DA, et al. Cerebral ischemic events after diagnosis of mitral valve prolapse: a community-based study of incidence and predictive factors. *Stroke* 2003;34:1339.

Barnett HJ, Boughner DR, Taylor W, et al. Further evidence relating mitral valve prolapse to cerebral ischemic events. *N Engl J Med* 1980;302:139.

Basso C, Corrado D, Thiene G. Cardiovascular causes of sudden death in young individuals including athletes. *Cardiol Rev* 1999;7:127.

Biancaniello T. Innocent murmurs: a parent's guide. *Circulation* 2004;109:e162.

Biancaniello T. Innocent murmurs. *Circulation* 2005;111:e20.

Birkeback NH, Hansen LK, Elle B, et al. Chest roengenogram in the evaluation of heart defects in asymptomatic infants and children with a cardiac murmur: reproducibility and accuracy. *Pediatrics* 1999;103:e15.

Bobkowski W, Wininska A, Zachwieja J, et al. A prospective study to determine the significance of ventricular late potentials in children with mitral valvar prolapse. *Cardiol Young* 2002;12:333.

Bouknight DP, O'Rourke RA. Current management of mitral valve prolapse. *Am Fam Physician* 2000;61:3343.

Cetta F, Graham LC, Lichtenberg RC, et al. Piercing and tattooing in patients with congenital heart disease: patient and physician perspectives. *J Adolesc Health* 1999;24:160.

Cowles T, Gotnik B. Mitral valve prolapse in pregnancy. *Semin Perinatol* 1990;14:34.

Crabbe LS, Bensky AS, Hornstein L, et al. Cardiovascular abnormalities in children with fragile X syndrome. *Pediatrics* 1993;91:714.

Dajani AS, Taubert KA, Wilson W, et al. American Heart Association Committee on rheumatic fever, endocarditis, and kawasaki disease. *JAMA* 1997;277:1794.

Danford DA, Martin AB, Fletcher SE, et al. Echocardiographic yield in children when innocent murmur seems likely by doubts linger. *Pediatr Cardiol* 2002;23:410.

Danford DA, Nasir A, Gumbiner C. Cost assessment of the evaluation of heart murmurs in children. *Pediatrics* 1993;91:365.

De Paepe A, Devereux RB, Dietz HC, et al. Revised diagnostic criteria for the Marfan syndrome. *Am J Med Genet* 1996;62:417.

Driscoll DJ. How to evaluate heart murmurs in children. *Your Patient Fit* 1991;3(2):13.

Driscoll DJ, Allen HD, Atkins DL, et al. Guidelines for evaluation and management of common congenital cardiac problems in infants, children, and adolescents. *Circulation* 1994;90:2180.

Freed LA, Benjamin EJ, Levy D, et al. Mitral valve prolapse in the general population: the benign nature of echocardiographic features in the Framingham Heart Study. *J Am Coll Cardiol* 2002;40:1298.

Freed LA, Levy D, Levine RA, et al. Prevalence and clinical outcome of mitral-valve prolapse. *N Engl J Med* 1999;341:1.

Fukuda N, Oki T, Iuchi A, et al. Predisposing factors for severe mitral regurgitation in idiopathic mitral valve prolapse. *Am J Cardiol* 1995;76:503.

Geggel RL. Conditions leading to pediatric cardiology consultation in a tertiary academic hospital. *Pediatrics* 2004;114:e409.

Grigioni F, Enriquez-Sarano M, Ling LH, Bailey KR, Seward JB, Tajik AJ, et al. Sudden death in mitral regurgitation due to flail leaflet. *J Am Coll Cardiol* 1999;34:2078.

Hayek E, Gring CN, Griffin BP. Mitral valve prolapse. *Lancet* 2005;365:507.

Hurwitz RA, Caldwell RL. Should pediatric echocardiograms be performed in adult laboratories? *Pediatrics* 1998;102:15.

Kavey REW, Blackman MS, Sondheimer HM, et al. Ventricular arrhythmias and mitral valve prolapse in childhood. *J Pediatr* 1984;105:885.

Kim S, Kuroda T, Nishinaga M, et al. Relationship between severity of mitral regurgitation and prognosis of mitral valve prolapse: echocardiographic follow-up study. *Am Heart J* 1996;132:348.

Kligfield P, Levy D, Devereux RB. Arrhythmias and sudden death in mitral valve prolapse. *Am Heart J* 1987;113:1298.

Landzberg MJ, Lock JE. Interventional catheter procedures used in congenital heart disease. *Cardiol Clin* 1993;11:569.

Luisada AA, Haring OM, Aravani C, et al. Murmurs in children: a clinical and echocardiographic study of 500 children of school age. *Ann Intern Med* 1958;48:597.

Mack G, Silberbach M. Aortic and pulmonary stenosis. *Pediatr Rev* 2000;21:79.

MacMahon SW, Roberts JK, Kramer-Fox R. Mitral valve prolapse and infective endocarditis. *Am Heart J* 1987;13:1291.

Maron BJ. Preparticipation screening of competitive athletes. In: Williams RA, ed. *The athlete and heart disease: diagnosis, evaluation, and management.* Philadelphia: Lippincott Williams & Wilkins, 1999.

Maron BJ, Chaitman BR, Ackerman MJ, et al. Recommendations for physical activity and recreational sports participation for young patients with genetic cardiovascular diseases. *Circulation* 2004;109:2807.

Maron BJ, Zipes DP. 31st Bethesda conference: eligibility recommendations for competitive athletes with cardiovascular abnormalities. *J Am Coll Cardiol* 2005;45:1313.

McCrindle BW, Shaffer KM, Kan JS, et al. Cardinal clinical signs in the differentiation of heart murmurs in children. *Arch Pediatr Adolesc Med* 1996;150:169.

McDaniel NL. Ventricular and atrial septal defects. *Pediatr Rev* 2001;22:265.

Meyers DG, Starke H, Pearson PH, et al. Mitral valve prolapse in anorexia nervosa. *Ann Intern Med* 1986;105:384.

Millar BC, Moore JE. Antibiotic prophylaxis, body piercing, and infectious endocarditis. *J Antimicrob Chemother* 2004;54:278.

Moss AI. Clues in diagnosing congenital heart disease. *West J Med* 1992;156:392.

Nishimura RA, Kidd KR. Mitral valve prolapse: implications for the primary care physician. *Am Fam Physician* 2000;61:3238.

Nishimura RA, McGoon MD, Shub C, et al. Echocardiographically documented mitral valve prolapse: long-term follow-up of 237 patients. *N Engl J Med* 1985;313:1305.

Noonan J. Innocent murmur and the pediatrician. *Clin Pediatr* 1999;38:519.

Pelech AN. Evaluation of the pediatric patient with a cardiac murmur. *Pediatr Clin North Am* 1999;46:167.

Pickering TG, Hall JE, Appel LJ, et al. Council on High Blood Pressure Research Professional and Public Education Subcommittee, American Heart Association. Recommendations for blood pressure measurement in humans: an AHA scientific statement from the Council on High Blood Pressure Research Professional and Public Education Subcommittee. *J Clin Hypertens (Greenwich)* 2005;7:102.

Priori SG, Aliot E, Blomstrom-Lundqvist LH, et al. Task force on sudden cardiac death of the European Society of Cardiology. *Eur Heart J* 2001;22:1374.

Rivenes SD, Colon SM, Easley KA, et al. Usefulness of the pediatric electrocardiogram in detecting left ventricular hypertrophy: results from the prospective pediatric pulmonary and cardiovascular complications of vertically transmitted HIV infection (P2C2 HIV) multicenter study. *Am Heart J* 2003;145:716.

Rowe PC, Barron DF, Calkins H, et al. Orthostatic intolerance and chronic fatigue syndrome associated with Ehlers-Danlos syndrome. *J Pediatr* 1999;135:494.

Singh RG, Cappucci R, Kramer-Fox R, et al. Severe mitral regurgitation due to mitral valve prolapse: risk factors for development, progression, and need for mitral valve surgery. *Am J Cardiol* 2000;85:193.

Smythe JF, Teixeira OHP, Demers PP, et al. Initial evaluation of heart murmurs: are laboratory tests necessary? *Pediatrics* 1990;86:497.

Stanger P, Silverman NH, Foster E. Diagnostic accuracy of pediatric echocardiograms performed in adult laboratories. *Am J Cardiol* 1999;83:908.

Steckelberg JM, Wilson WR. Risk factors for infective endocarditis. *Infect Dis Clin North Am* 1993;7:9.

Swenson JM, Fischer DR, Miller SA, et al. Are chest radiographs and electrocardiograms still valuable in evaluating new pediatric patients with heart murmurs or chest pain? *Pediatrics* 1997;99:1.

Toren P, Eldar S, Cendorf D, et al. The prevalence of mitral valve prolapse in children with anxiety disorders. *J Psych Res* 1999;33:357.

Van Karnebeek CD, Naeff MS, Mulder BJ, et al. Natural history of cardiovascular manifestations in Marfan syndrome. *Arch Dis Child* 2001;84:129.

Wilson W, Taubert KA, Gewitz M, et al. Prevention of Infective Endocarditis: Guidelines from the American Heart Association. *Circulation* 2007;115:1.

Zuppiroli A, Rinaldi M, Kramer-Fox R, et al. Natural history of mitral valve prolapse. *Am J Cardiol* 1995;75:102.

PART IV

Orthopedic Problems

CHAPTER 15

Scoliosis and Kyphosis

Matthew J. Bueche

INTRODUCTION

Spinal deformity is a major concern in the adolescent population. Teens with poor posture are frequently brought to the physician by concerned parents, whereas those with more serious structural scoliosis and kyphosis may escape attention. Marked deformity can exist without symptoms. Although the efficacy of school screening programs is controversial, clinicians should routinely examine adolescents for spinal deformity, as treatment may improve the outcome.

Definition

Scoliosis is a lateral curvature of the spine, usually associated with rotational deformity of the spine and trunk. Scoliosis is defined as a curvature of 10 degrees or greater on a frontal radiograph (measured by the Cobb Method [Fig. 15.1]).

Etiology

Scoliosis is a condition rather than a diagnosis. Most adolescents have adolescent idiopathic scoliosis (AIS), a condition with no apparent cause. Scoliosis may be associated with neuromuscular diseases such as spastic quadriplegic cerebral palsy and Duchenne muscular dystrophy. Congenital scoliosis is deformity secondary to vertebral malformations. Nonstructural or functional scoliosis may result from leg length discrepancy or from splinting due to back pain. Scoliosis may be part of a syndrome or disease such as Marfan syndrome, neurofibromatosis, or myelodysplasia.

IDIOPATHIC SCOLIOSIS

Types

There is no known cause of idiopathic scoliosis. It is usually categorized into three age-groups:

1. *Infantile* scoliosis is diagnosed between birth and 3 years, occurs more frequently in males during the first year of life, and may be related to postnatal supine positioning. Most curves resolve spontaneously, although brace treatment or surgery may be necessary. Infantile idiopathic scoliosis is quite rare.
2. *Juvenile* scoliosis manifests between 3 and 9 years of age. Boys and girls are affected equally. Like AIS, the risk

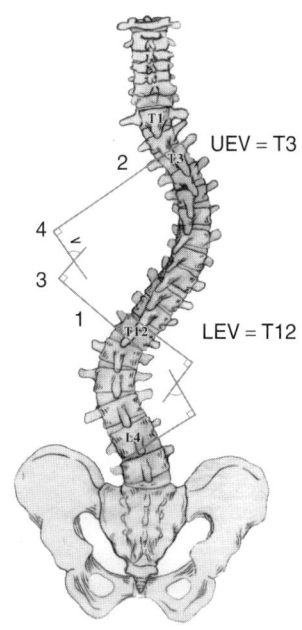

FIGURE 15.1   The Cobb method of radiographic measurement of scoliosis. A line is drawn parallel to the inferior end plate of the lower end vertebra (LEV) (the vertebra that is most tilted) (*1*), another line is drawn at the superior border of the upper end vertebra (UEV) (*3*), perpendicular lines are drawn from each of these previous lines (*2* and *4*), and the intersecting angle is then measured. Drawing the perpendiculars keeps the measurement from running off the edge of the film. A similar method is used on the lateral film to measure sagittal plane curves. (Adapted from O'Brien MF, Kuklo TR, Blanke KM, et al., eds. *Radiographic measurement manual. Spinal Deformity Study Group.* Memphis, Tennessee: Medtronic Sofamor Danek, 2004:110.)

TABLE 15.1

Risk of Progression of Idiopathic Scoliosis

Initial Curve (degrees)	Age at Presentation			
	Girls, 10–12 yr (%)	Girls, 13–15 yr (%)	Girls, >15 yr (%)	Boys (%)
<19	25	1	<1	3
20–29	60	40	10	6
30–59	90	70	30	—
>60	100	90	—	—

From Nachemson A, Lonstein JE, Weinstein SL. Prevalence and natural history committee report. *Read at the Annual Meeting Scoliosis Research Society.* Denver, CO: Scoliosis Research Society, Sept. 25, 1982.

of curve progression increases with curve severity and treatment may be initiated at similar curve magnitudes.

3. *Adolescent* scoliosis is the most frequent form and manifests between 10 years of age and the time of skeletal maturity. It occurs most commonly in girls.

Prevalence

Approximately 2% to 3% of adolescents have a curve >10 degrees and 0.5% have a curve >20 degrees. Although minimal curves occur as often in boys as in girls, curves requiring treatment are found seven times more frequently in girls (Rogala et al., 1978).

Causes

The etiology of AIS is believed to be multifactorial (Miller, 1999):

1. There is an increased incidence of scoliosis in first-degree relatives (Wynne-Davis, 1968). Genomic testing studies to identify markers for AIS are underway (Miller et al., 2005; Bashiardes et al., 2004).
2. Subtle abnormalities in vestibular or other neurological function.
3. Abnormal connective tissue or muscle composition has been noted in subgroups of patients, but these abnormalities may be a result of the disorder rather than a cause.

Natural History

Long-term complications of continued curve progression including cosmetic effects, back pain, neurological compromise, and restrictive pulmonary disease leading to cor pulmonale and death have been described. Fifty-year follow-up of untreated AIS found a tendency toward continued progression of the deformity (Weinstein et al., 2003). Back pain was present more frequently in patients than in the age-matched control group, although most patients reported only mild or moderate pain. Shortness of breath was reported more frequently in the AIS group. In the same study, 3 of the 36 deaths were likely related to the scoliosis.

Adults treated for AIS were found to recall transient body-image dissatisfaction and negative peer interactions during adolescence. Lower body-image scores persisted for several years in surgical patients (Noonan et al., 1997).

Risk Factors for Progression

A combination of the following factors can be helpful in predicting as many as 80% of progressive curves (Peterson and Nachemson, 1995).

1. Age at onset and gender (Table 15.1)
2. Magnitude of the curve: The amount of curvature is measured by the Cobb method (Fig. 15.1). In this method, a line is drawn parallel to the inferior end plate of the lower end vertebra (the vertebra that is most tilted), another line is drawn at the superior border of the upper end vertebra (that most tilted in the other direction), perpendicular lines are drawn from each of these previous lines, and the intersecting angle is then measured. Despite the apparent simplicity of the technique, there is considerable intraobserver and interobserver variability (Carman et al., 1990). Patients with a 20-degree curve have a 20% risk of progression, whereas those with a 50-degree curve have a 90% chance of progression (Lonstein and Carlson, 1984).
3. Skeletal maturity: The Risser stage (0–5) gives a useful estimate of how much skeletal growth remains by grading the progress of ossification of the iliac apophysis. Risser stage is determined by the appearance of the secondary ossification center of the iliac crest. Risser grade zero signifies no ossification whereas Risser grade 5 signifies complete bony fusion of the apophysis (Fig. 15.2). Patients with Risser stage 0 show progression 36% to 68% of the time, whereas those who have a Risser stage 3 or 4 progress only 11% to 18% of the time.

Scoliosis Screening

The American Academy of Orthopedic Surgeons recommends screening girls at ages 10 and 12 (grades 5 and 7) and screening boys once at age 13 or 14 years (grades 8 or 9) (AAOS, 1992). The Scoliosis Research Society concurs with this recommendation. In addition, some state laws mandate school screening for scoliosis. In contrast, the U.S. Preventive Services Task Force's (USPSTF's) *Guidelines for the Guide to Clinical Preventive Services* states that "The

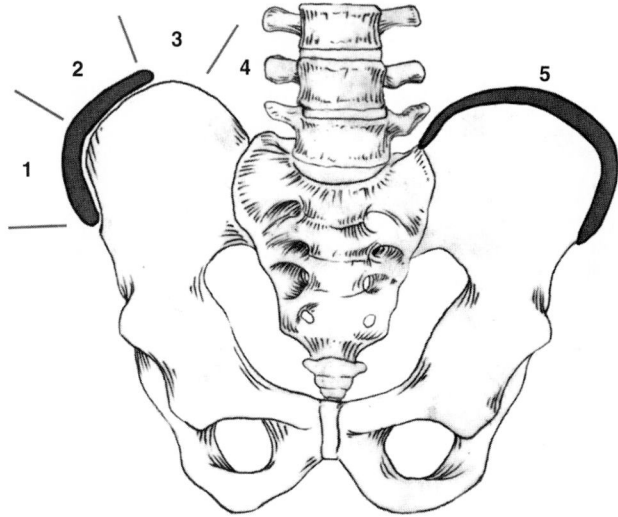

FIGURE 15.2 The Risser sign. The iliac apophysis appears first at the anterior superior iliac spine; ossification then progresses medially toward the posterior superior iliac spine. The crest is divided into four equal quadrants with stages 1 through 4 coinciding with extension of the ossification center into each quadrant and stage 5 being complete fusion of the physis (Risser, 1958). (From O'Brien MF, Kuklo TR, Blanke KM, et al., eds. *Radiographic measurement manual. Spinal Deformity Study Group.* Memphis, Tennessee: Medtronic Sofamor Danek, 2004:110.)

USPSTF found fair evidence that treatment of adolescents with idiopathic scoliosis detected through screening leads to moderate harms, including unnecessary brace wear and unnecessary referral for specialty care. As a result, the USPSTF concluded that the harms of screening adolescents for idiopathic scoliosis exceed the potential benefits" (U.S. Preventive Services Task Force, 2004).

The sensitivity, specificity, and positive and negative predictive value of screening tests depend on the degree of curvature defined as abnormal, the training of the screener, and the prevalence in the population. Properly trained clinicians using an inclinometer (Fig. 15.3) can evaluate the need for scoliosis radiographs. "Schooliosis" or the over-referral of normal adolescents from school screening programs is a known phenomenon. Better communication and proper technique should allow screening to continue at efficient levels (Dvonch et al., 1990).

Clinical Evaluation

History
The patient history should include the following:

1. Age and menarchal status.
2. Presence of pain: Most scoliosis in adolescents is painless and diagnosed secondary to deformity. Significant pain requires a thorough evaluation for an identifiable cause.
3. Neurological symptoms.
4. Family history of scoliosis and spine disorders.

Physical Examination
Evaluation of suspected scoliosis should be directed at the deformity, its cause, and complications. The general examination should include the following:

1. Height: Serial measurements aid in determining risk of progression.
2. Neurological examination: Including reflexes, strength, sensation, and coordination/gait.
3. Skin: Including café-au-lait spots and hairy patches over the spine.
4. Pelvic obliquity: Leg length inequality.
5. Sexual maturity rating: To evaluate risk of progression.

Spinal Examination
Performed with the patient standing, wearing underwear and a gown open in the back

1. Side-to-side symmetry
2. Shoulder height
3. Iliac crest symmetry: They may have to be palpated to ascertain leg length equality.
4. Forward bending: The Adams forward bend test is performed with the adolescent bending forward at the waist until the spine becomes parallel to the horizontal plane, while holding palms together with arms extended and knees straight. The examiner looks along the horizontal plane of the spine from the back and side to detect an asymmetry in the contour of the back for a "rib hump" or paralumbar prominence. This examination may also reveal inflexibility of the spine or muscle spasm. Any rib hump or paralumbar hump should be measured with an inclinometer. The angle of trunk rotation (ATR) is measured by centering the device over the spinous process at the area of greatest asymmetry (Fig. 15.3), with the patient flexed at the waist, such that this area is parallel to the floor. The test may not be specific for spinal deformity, because truncal asymmetry may exist in the absence of measurable scoliosis.
5. Lateral examination: Evaluation for sagittal plane deformity is performed with the examiner at the patient's side. Departures from the normal contours of thoracic kyphosis and lumbar lordosis are noted. The forward bend test is then repeated, noting the smoothness of the thoracic kyphosis (see Scheuermann kyphosis in the subsequent text).

Physical examination signs indicative of nonidiopathic scoliosis are listed in Table 15.2.

Imaging
Recommendations for Radiographs for Suspected Scoliosis
Radiographic studies are recommended for adolescents with an ATR >7 degrees, measured by an inclinometer. This threshold value balances the risks of false-positive and false-negative results (Bunnell, 1993).

Which Radiographs to Order?
The standard films for the evaluation of scoliosis are standing posteroanterior and lateral spinal radiographs using 36-in. films taken at 6-ft distance to allow measurement of the curve using the Cobb method and Risser staging of the iliac apophysis. Directing the beam from posterior to anterior measurably decreases the radiation dose to the breasts and thyroid (Levy et al., 1996).

Skeletally immature patients at risk for curve progression can be followed up with posteroanterior radiographs every 6 to 12 months.

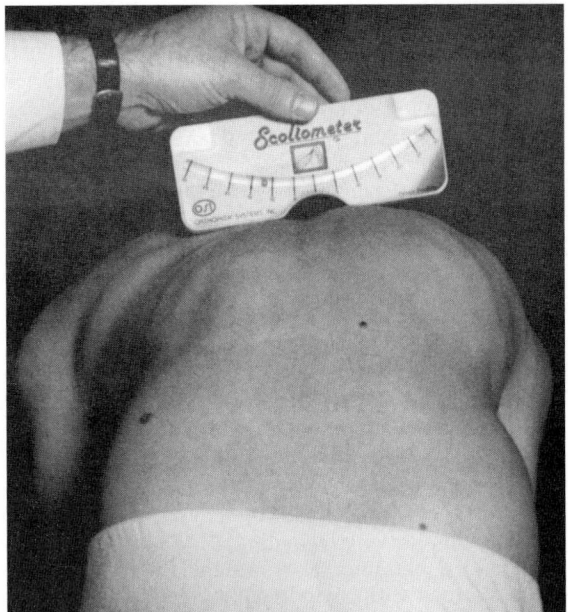 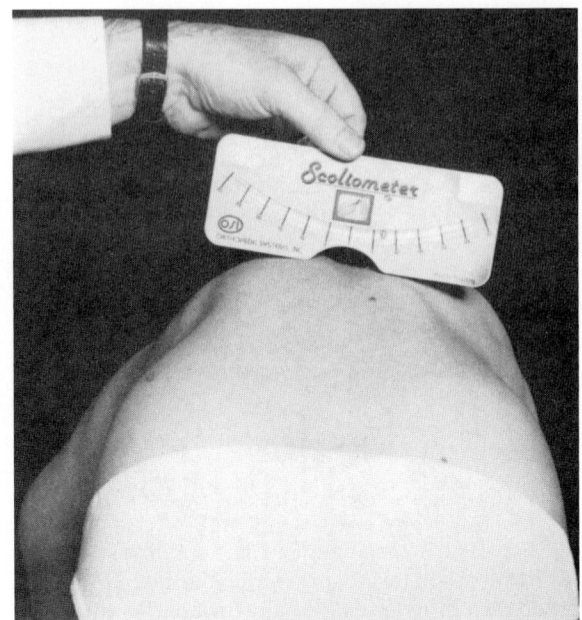

A   B

FIGURE 15.3 The inclinometer (scoliometer). The device is centered over the spinous process at the area of greatest asymmetry. The patient flexes at the waist sufficiently to bring the right thoracic area **(A)** and left lumbar area **(B)** parallel to the floor. (From Weinstein SL, ed. *The pediatric spine. Principles and practice*, 2nd ed. Philadelphia: Lippincott Williams & Wilkins, 2001 Figure 4, page 135.)

Radiographic indications of nonidiopathic scoliosis are listed in Table 15.3.

Magnetic Resonance Imaging
Magnetic resonance imaging (MRI) of the full spine is recommended for adolescents with the following findings:

1. Neurological findings (including café-au-lait spots) on physical examination.
2. Unusual pain.
3. Left major thoracic curve: These are associated (in 10% of cases otherwise thought to be idiopathic) with occult syrinx, Arnold-Chiari malformation, spinal cord tumor, and neuromuscular disorder. Only 2% of adolescent idiopathic thoracic curves are convex to the left (Davids et al., 2004).

Criteria for Referral
Consultation with an orthopedic surgeon (ideally, one who specializes in pediatric orthopedics or orthopedic spinal surgery) should be considered for

a. skeletally immature patients with Cobb angle >20 degrees;
b. skeletally mature patients with Cobb angle >40 degrees.

Treatment

Major treatment options include observation, bracing, and surgery (Table 15.4). Treatment choices in AIS often involve consideration of the teen's physiological (not chronological) maturity, curve magnitude and location, and the potential for progression.

TABLE 15.2

Signs of Nonidiopathic Scoliosis

Region	Finding	Possible Significance
Skin	Hairy patch over spine	Congenital spinal anomaly
	Café-au-lait spots	Neurofibromatosis
Joints	Hyperelasticity	Marfan syndrome/Ehlers-Danlos syndrome
Reflexes (including abdominal)	Abnormal	Neuromuscular disease
Extremities	Excessively long	Marfan syndrome
	Excessively short	Skeletal dysplasias
Pelvis (standing)	Obliquity	Leg length discrepancy

TABLE 15.3

Radiographic Signs of Nonidiopathic Scoliosis

Radiographic Finding	Possible Significance
Sharply angular curve	Neurofibromatosis
Fused ribs	Congenital scoliosis
Widened intrapedicular distance	Syringomyelia
Left thoracic curvature	Neuromuscular etiologies

Brace Therapy

Brace therapy should be considered in the skeletally immature adolescent who has 30 to 40 degrees of curvature or who has a curve >25 degrees with a demonstrated increase of 5 degrees. The primary goal of brace management is to halt curve progression. This treatment modality should not be expected to permanently improve curvature. Although curve magnitude typically decreases during brace treatment, this improvement is often lost in the years following brace weaning.

There are a number of different bracing systems (e.g., Boston, Milwaukee) that have been used to prevent the need for surgery. The Milwaukee brace features a neck ring that may cause cosmetic concerns. Most other scoliosis braces are variants of the thoraco–lumbar–sacral orthosis (TLSO), an underarm brace. It is generally recommended that the braces be worn almost full-time, with removal for bathing and sports participation. Part-time (18 hour/day) programs may be more acceptable to the patient who refuses to wear the brace to school (Green, 1986).

Despite a high incidence of noncompliance, outcomes are better than would be expected from the natural history alone (Nachemson and Peterson, 1995). Less than full-time wear may decrease the psychosocial impact of brace treatment. However, a meta-analysis of brace studies indicated a trend toward decreasing efficacy with decreased time in brace (Rowe et al., 1997). Another study showed that decreasing the prescribed hours of daytime brace wear did not increase compliance (Takemitsu et al., 2004). Nighttime-only braces (e.g., Charleston, Providence) avoid some of the compliance problems associated with daytime braces. Such braces attempt to make up for decreased treatment time by hyper-correcting the curve into the opposite direction (difficult to accomplish in a brace designed for an upright patient, but more feasible when recumbent). These braces have shown promise in

TABLE 15.4

Management of Adolescent Idiopathic Scoliosis

Curve Size (degrees)	Therapy
0–25	Serial observation if immature
25–30 (with progression of 5–10 degrees)	Brace
30–40	Brace
>40	Surgery if immature
>50	Surgery (adult)

patients with specific curve patterns. Among those treated with the Charleston brace, 66% had <5 degrees progression and only 16% required subsequent surgery at long-term follow-up (Price et al., 1997).

Skeletal maturation, defined as no further changes in height and a Risser stage IV, is usually considered the endpoint for brace use.

Surgery

Surgical management is recommended for skeletally immature patients who have a curve >40 to 45 degrees or in skeletally mature patients who have curves >50 degrees, particularly if curve progression has been documented. Surgery fuses the vertebrae in the curve, preventing further progression. Rods are implanted as internal fixation, both stabilizing the spine to allow for reliable fusion and allowing for considerable curve correction. Post-operative bracing is frequently unnecessary. Hospital stays are usually for less than a week and students miss approximately 1 month of school. Although mid- or low-lumbar fusions may cause long-term back stiffness, this does not commonly occur with thoracic fusions.

Other Treatments

Exercise programs have not been shown to alter the natural history of idiopathic scoliosis. Electrical stimulation has proved to be ineffective for scoliosis in multiple studies.

INCREASED KYPHOSIS

Normal sagittal plane posture includes rounded shoulders (thoracic kyphosis) and sway-back (lumbar lordosis). *Increased* kyphosis in adolescents is commonly caused by juvenile postural roundback and less commonly, by Scheuermann kyphosis.

Adolescent Roundback (Juvenile Postural Roundback)

Many adolescents manifest an excessively kyphotic posture. The spine is flexible enough that the adolescent can stand straighter if they desire, although they may complain of muscle pain and fatigue. On forward bending, the spine shows a smooth curvature when viewed from the side. Lateral radiographs may show the increased thoracic kyphosis, but the individual vertebrae and disc spaces will appear normal. It is more common among girls than among boys. It is usually painless.

An exercise program directed by a physical therapist may be helpful if the adolescent is in pain or unhappy with his or her appearance.

Scheuermann Kyphosis

Scheuermann kyphosis is a relatively rigid, abnormally increased kyphosis of the thoracic and thoracolumbar spine that does not correct with hyperextension of the spine. The kyphosis results from anterior vertebral wedging in the affected area of the spine. The matrix of the vertebral end plate has characteristic changes in the ratio of collagen to proteoglycans that leads to an altered ossification process. The exact etiology of Scheuermann disease is unknown but is thought to include excessive stress, genetic predisposition, and congenital malformation of the vertebral end plates. The prevalence is estimated to range from 0.4% to 8.0% in the adolescent population, with a peak age of onset at 12 to 13. There is equal incidence in boys and girls.

Definition and Classification
The radiographic diagnosis of Scheuermann kyphosis is made on a standing lateral 36-in. film. The criteria include the following:

1. More than 5 degrees of anterior wedging of at least three adjacent vertebral bodies
2. Narrowing of the intervertebral disc space
3. Irregularity of the vertebral endplates and Schmorl nodes—abnormal protrusions of intervertebral disc material into the vertebral bodies
4. More than 45 degrees of kyphosis (normal is 20 to 45 degrees), measured by the Cobb method

The classification of Scheuermann kyphosis is made by the location of the kyphosis. Thoracic curves are by far the most common (75%) and thoracolumbar curves are more likely to progress even after skeletal maturity. "Lumbar Scheuermann disease" is distinct from true Scheuermann kyphosis in that it does not have the anterior wedging of the vertebral bodies.

Clinical Manifestations
1. Back deformity: Presenting complaints usually concern the deformity, including the following:
   a. Thoracic kyphosis with secondary lumbar hyperlordosis. On Adams forward bending test the kyphosis has a sharp apex, distinct from the smooth curve seen in adolescent roundback.
   b. Protuberant abdomen.
   c. Forward rounded (protracted) shoulders.
   d. Forward protrusion of the head.
   These deformities are not completely corrected with forward bending or prone hyperextension maneuvers.
2. Pain: *Aching pain* that is usually localized to the apex of the thoracic kyphosis after prolonged sitting or exercise may be present (20%–70%). The incidence of pain increases as the kyphosis progresses. Those with a thoracolumbar kyphosis are more likely to have pain as a presenting complaint.
3. Scoliosis: There is an increased incidence of *scoliosis* (20%–30%), spondylolysis and spondylolisthesis (32%), and thoracic disc herniation.

Differential Diagnosis
In addition to adolescent roundback, there are a number of other processes that must be considered before diagnosing Scheuermann kyphosis.

1. Infectious spondylitis must be considered especially in immunocompromised patients, intravenous drug abusers, and those at risk for tuberculosis. Computed tomography and MRI are helpful in diagnosing and determining the extent of the disease.
2. Compression fractures can be confused with Scheuermann kyphosis from a radiographic perspective, but there is usually a history of trauma or a metabolic bone disease.
3. In congenital kyphosis type II, there are anterior bony bridges between consecutive vertebrae.

4. Juvenile ankylosing spondylitis is seen more frequently in males and is characterized by the loss of lumbar flexibility and painful enthesitis (at points of ligament or tendon insertion) of the feet or knees, or both. In addition, rheumatoid factor (RF) and antinuclear antibody (ANA) are normal. Approximately 90% of those with juvenile ankylosing spondylitis test positive for HLA-B27.
5. Other diagnoses include osteodystrophies (Morquio and Hurler disease), tumors, and postsurgical deformity.

Natural History
Most patients with <75 degrees of kyphosis have a benign progression of their disease with some deformity, back pain, and fatigue. When patients with Scheuermann kyphosis were compared with healthy age- and sex- matched controls, they were found to have more intense back pain, jobs that tended to have lower requirements for activity, less range of motion of extension of the trunk and less strong extension of the trunk, and different localization of the pain. No significant differences were noted between self-esteem, social limitations, and level of recreational activities or preoccupation with physical appearance (Murray et al., 1993).

Treatment
Treatment is controversial and not all patients require intervention. The three main treatment modalities for patients with Scheuermann kyphosis are exercise, bracing, and surgery.

1. Exercise programs to strengthen the low back and improve hamstring and pectoral flexibility may be used for patients with smaller curves (<50 degrees). These programs have not been shown to improve vertebral wedging or the degree of kyphosis. Comfort, and to some extent appearance, may improve with exercise.
2. Bracing treatment has been used for patients with >50 degrees of kyphosis resulting in some short-term improvement. However, most of the improvement is lost during long-term follow-up out of the brace. The Milwaukee brace (which includes the cervical ring) has been recommended for thoracic kyphosis at or above T7. An underarm orthosis (TLSO) can be used for those with lower thoracic or thoracolumbar kyphosis.
3. Operative correction (spinal fusion) is rarely indicated. It is indicated for adolescents with curves >80 degrees that cannot be controlled with brace treatment or for those with chronic pain and curves >70 degrees.

WEB SITES

For Teenagers and Parents

http://www.scoliosis-assoc.org/. Scoliosis Association, Inc., an international information and support organization.
http://www.scoliosis.org/. National Scoliosis Foundation. Patient advocacy and information.
http://orthoinfo.aaos.org/fact/thr_report.cfm?Thread_ID=262&topcategory=Children and http://orthoinfo.aaos.org/brochure/thr_report.cfm?Thread_ID=

14&topcategory=Spine. American Association of Orthopedic Surgeons brochure on Childhood Scoliosis.
http://www.niams.nih.gov/hi/topics/scoliosis/scochild .htm. National Institute of Arthritis and Musculoskeletal and Skin Diseases frequently asked questions about scoliosis.
http://www.mayoclinic.com/health/scoliosis/DS00194. Mayo Clinic information on Scoliosis.

For Health Professionals and Patients

http://www.srs.org. The Scoliosis Research Society.
http://www.nlm.nih.gov/medlineplus/scoliosis.html. Medline plus health information.

REFERENCES AND ADDITIONAL READINGS

AAOS. *AAOS position statement on scoliosis screening.* http://www.aaos.org/about/papers/position/1122.asp. Revised 1992.

Ascani E, Bartolozzi P, Logroscino CA, et al. Natural history of untreated idiopathic scoliosis after skeletal maturity. *Spine* 1986;11:784.

Ashworth M, Hancock J, Ashworth L, et al. Scoliosis screening: an approach to cost/benefit analysis. *Spine* 1988;13:1187.

Bashiardes S, Veile R, Allen M, et al. SNTG1, the gene encoding gamma1-syntrophin: a candidate gene for idiopathic scoliosis. *Hum Genet* 2004;115(1):81.

Bradford DS. Juvenile kyphosis. In: Lonstein JE, ed. *Moe's textbook of scoliosis and other spinal deformities,* 3rd ed. Philadelphia: WB Saunders, 1995:347.

Bradford DS, Moe JH, Montalvo FJ, et al. Scheuermann's kyphosis and roundback deformity: results of Milwaukee brace treatment. *J Bone Joint Surg Am* 1974;56:740.

Bridwell KH. Surgical treatment of idiopathic adolescent scoliosis. *Spine* 1999;24:2607.

Bunnell WP. An objective criterion for scoliosis screening. *J Bone Joint Surg Am* 1984;62:31.

Bunnell WP. Outcome of spinal screening. *Spine* 1993;18(12):1572.

Bunnell WP. Selective screening for scoliosis. *Orthop Relat Res* 2005;434:40.

Carman DL, Browne RH, Birch JG. Measurement of scoliosis and kyphosis radiographs. Intraobserver and interobserver variation. *J Bone Joint Surg Am* 1990;72(3):328.

Chiu KY, Luk KD. Cord compression caused by multiple disc herniations and intraspinal cyst in Scheuermann's disease. *Spine* 1995;20:1075.

Cordover AM, Betz RR, Clements DH, et al. Natural history of adolescent thoracolumbar and lumbar idiopathic scoliosis into adulthood. *J Spinal Disord* 1997;10:193.

Davids JR, Chamberlin E, Blackhurst DW. Indications for magnetic resonance imaging in presumed adolescent idiopathic scoliosis. *J Bone Joint Surg Am* 2004;86-A(10):2187.

Dickson RA. Spinal deformity—adolescent idiopathic scoliosis: nonoperative treatment. *Spine* 1999;24:2601.

Dvonch VM, Siegler AH, Cloppas CC, et al. The epidemiology of "schooliosis". *J Pediatr Orthop* 1990;10(2):206.

Green NE. Part-time bracing of adolescent idiopathic scoliosis. *J Bone Joint Surg Am* 1986;68:738.

Hadley Miller N. Spine update: genetics of familial idiopathic scoliosis. *Spine* 2000;25(18):2416.

Herring JA, ed. Scoliosis and kyphosis. In: *Tachdjian's pediatric orthopaedics,* 3rd ed. Philadelphia: WB Saunders, 2002:213.

Karachalios T, Roidis N, Papagelopoulos PJ, et al. The efficacy of school screening for scoliosis. *Orthopedics* 2000;23:386.

Levy AR, Goldberg MS, Mayo NE, et al. Reducing the lifetime risk of cancer from spinal radiographs among people with adolescent idiopathic scoliosis. *Spine* 1996;21(13):1540.

Lonstein JE, Carlson JM. The prediction of curve progression in untreated idiopathic scoliosis during growth. *J Bone Joint Surg Am* 1984;66:1061.

McMaster MJ. Infantile idiopathic scoliosis: can it be prevented? *J Bone Joint Surg Br* 1983;65:612.

Mack MJ, Regan JJ, McFee PC, et al. Video-assisted surgery for the anterior approach to the thoracic spine. *Ann Thorac Surg* 1995;59:1102.

Mejia EA, Hennrikus WL, Schwend RM, et al. A prospective evaluation of idiopathic left thoracic scoliosis with magnetic resonance imaging. *J Pediatr Orthop* 1996;16:354.

Miller NH. Cause and natural history of adolescent idiopathic scoliosis. *Orthop Clin North Am* 1999;30:343.

Miller NH. Spine update: genetics of familial idiopathic scoliosis. *Spine* 2000;25(18):2416.

Miller NH, Justice CM, Marosy B, et al. Identification of candidate regions for familial idiopathic scoliosis. *Spine* 2005;30(10):1181.

Montgomery SP, Erwin WE. Scheuermann's kyphosis: long term results with Milwaukee brace treatment. *Spine* 1981;6:5.

Murray PM, Weinstein SL, Spratt KF. The natural history and long-term follow-up of Scheuermann kyphosis. *J Bone Joint Surg Am* 1993;75:236.

Nachemson A, Lonstein JE, Weinstein SL. *Prevalence and natural history committee report.* Read at the Annual Meeting Scoliosis Research Society. Denver, CO: Scoliosis Research Society, Sept. 25, 1982.

Nachemson AL, Peterson LE. Effectiveness of treatment with a brace in girls who have adolescent idiopathic scoliosis. A prospective, controlled study based on data from the Brace Study of the Scoliosis Research Society. *J Bone Joint Surg Am* 1995;77:815.

Noonan KJ, Dolan LA, Jacobson WC, et al. Long-term psychosocial characteristics of patients treated for idiopathic scoliosis. *J Pediatr Orthop* 1997;17:712.

O'Brien MF, Kuklo TR, Blanke KM, et al., eds. *Radiographic measurement manual. Spinal Deformity Study Group.* Memphis, Tennessee: Medtronic Sofamor Danek, 2004:110.

Peterson LE, Nachemson AL. Prediction of progression of the curve in girls who have adolescent idiopathic scoliosis of moderate severity: logistic regression analysis based on the data from the Brace Study of the Scoliosis Research Society. *J Bone Joint Surg Am* 1995;77:823.

Price CT, Scott DS, Reed FR, et al. Nighttime bracing for adolescent idiopathic scoliosis with the Charleston bending brace. *J Pediatr Orthop* 1997;17:703.

Renshaw TS. Screening school children for scoliosis. *Clin Orthop* 1988;229:26.

Roach JW. Adolescent idiopathic scoliosis. *Orthop Clin North Am* 1999;30:353.

Rogala EJ, Drummond DS, Gurr J. Scoliosis: incidence and natural history. A prospective epidemiological study. *J Bone Joint Surg* 1978;60-A:173.

Rowe DE, Bernstein SM, Riddick MF, et al. A meta-analysis of the efficacy of non-operative treatments for idiopathic scoliosis. *J Bone Joint Surg Am* 1997;79(5):664.

Takemitsu M, Bowen JR, Rahman T, et al. Compliance monitoring of brace treatment for patients with idiopathic scoliosis. *Spine* 2004;29(18):2070.

U.S. Preventive Services Task Force. *Guidelines for the guide to clinical preventive services*, 2nd ed. Baltimore: Williams & Wilkins, 1996.

U.S. Preventive Services Task Force. *Screening for idiopathic scoliosis in adolescents: a brief evidence update for the U.S. Preventive Services Task Force*. Rockville, MD: Agency for Healthcare Research and Quality, http://www.ahrq.gov/clinic/3rduspstf/scoliosis/scolioup.htm, http://www.ahrq.gov/clinic/3rduspstf/scoliosis/scoliors.htm. June 2004.

Weinstein SL, ed. *The pediatric spine. Principles and practice*, 2nd ed. Philadelphia: Lippincott Williams & Wilkins, 2001.

Weinstein SL, Dolan LA, Spratt KF, et al. Health and function of patients with untreated idiopathic scoliosis: a 50-year natural history study. *JAMA* 2003;289(5):559.

Wever DJ, Tonseth KA, Veldhuizen AG, et al. Curve progression and spinal growth in brace treated idiopathic scoliosis. *Clin Orthop* 2000;377:169.

Wright N. Imaging in scoliosis. *Arch Dis Child* 2000;82:38.

Wynne-Davis R. Familial (idiopathic) scoliosis: a family survey. *J Bone Joint Surg Br* 1968;50B:24.

Yawn BP, Yawn RA, Hodge D, et al. A population-based study of school scoliosis screening. *JAMA* 1999;282(15):142.

CHAPTER 16

Common Orthopedic Problems

Keith J. Loud and Robert J. Bielski

Musculoskeletal problems, including athletic injuries, are among the most common reasons for adolescents to seek medical attention. Appropriate management of these concerns can not only decrease morbidity and prevent sequelae but also earn the valuable and oft elusive confidence of the patient.

GENERAL PRINCIPLES OF MUSCULOSKELTAL CARE

Despite a lack of adequate training, health care providers for adolescents can provide most initial care for orthopedic problems. Recommended resources include:

1. Reference materials
   a. An encyclopedic text such as *Essentials of Musculoskeletal Care*, 3rd Edition, published jointly by the American Academy of Pediatrics (AAP) and American Academy of Orthopedic Surgeons (AAOS)—a comprehensive, practical guide to the diagnosis and treatment of virtually all orthopedic problems encountered in primary care practice.
   b. A diagnostic manual such as *Physical Examination of the Spine and Extremities*, by Stanley Hoppenfield—a classic text that clarifies the musculoskeletal examination.
2. Physical therapy: A strong working relationship with a local physical therapist. Physical therapy is a mainstay in the treatment of many musculoskeletal conditions.
3. Orthopedic care: Easy access to orthopedic specialty care when needed.

General Indications for Referral to an Orthopedic Surgeon for Patients with Acute Trauma of an Extremity

Evaluation, treatment, and criteria for referral for specific injuries are discussed in the following sections. In general, plain radiographs (x-rays) should be considered for any significant unilateral complaint with greater urgency for pain which wakes a patient from sleep, or any unexplained or persistent bilateral complaints.

There are general criteria for immediate consultation regardless of the injury site. They include the following:

1. Obvious deformity
2. Acute locking (joint cannot be moved actively or passively past a certain point)
3. Penetrating wound of major joint, muscle, or tendon
4. Neurological deficit
5. Joint instability perceived by the adolescent or elicited by the health care provider
6. Bony crepitus

If the primary health care provider evaluating the patient has training in the evaluation and functional rehabilitation of musculoskeletal injuries, the threshold for referral will be higher.

Treatment and Rehabilitation of Injuries—General Concepts

The prevention of long-term sequelae of injury depends on complete rehabilitation, characterized by full, pain-free range of motion (ROM) and normal strength, endurance, and proprioception.

There are four phases of rehabilitation:

1. Limit further injury and control pain and swelling.
2. Improve strength and ROM of injured structures.
3. Achieve near-normal strength, ROM, endurance, and proprioception of injured structures.
4. Return to activity (exercise, sport, or work) free of symptoms.

Avoid predicting time frames for return to participation; individuals progress at different rates and disappointment may ensue if goals are not reached as promised.

Phase 1: Limit Further Injury and Control Pain and Swelling

1. The affected part must be rested and protected. Patients should apply whatever devices are necessary (e.g., wrap, splint, crutches, sling) so that they can become pain free and protect the site from further injury.
2. Elevation, compression, and ice should be applied as often as possible during waking hours. *Ice* should be

applied continuously for 20 minutes, directly to the skin and three or four times a day for the first few days.
3. Analgesic medication (e.g., acetaminophen, nonsteroidal antiinflammatory drugs [NSAIDs]), if prescribed, should be dosed regularly to achieve therapeutic steady state levels, not "as needed". Physical therapists can apply electrical stimulation to achieve pain relief in the acute setting.
4. Noninjured structures should be exercised to maintain cardiovascular fitness. For instance, patients with a lower-extremity injury could do seated weight lifting or swim with their arms pulling and without leg action. Those with an upper-extremity injury could ride a stationary bike.
5. Athletes should attend practice sessions so that they are not as likely to withdraw psychologically.

Phase 2: Improve Strength and Range of Motion of Injured Structures
1. Specific exercises should be done within a pain-free ROM. For example, isometric exercises can be started on the first day if there is little pain-free ROM but the subject is able to contract the muscles.
2. Relative rest is the cardinal principle, and that means that the patient should do everything possible, so long as it does not cause pain within 24 hours of the activity.
3. Analgesic medication should be continued, not to mask the pain and allow premature return to play, but to interrupt the cycle of pain, muscle spasm, inflexibility, weakness, and decreased endurance. In addition to reducing swelling, ice pack is a good analgesic modality.
4. General fitness maintenance should continue, as described for phase 1. Other activities, such as water jogging for lower-extremity injuries, may be added.

Phase 3: Achieve Near-Normal Strength, Range of Motion, Endurance, and Proprioception of Injured Structures
1. Exercise is progressed so long as the subject follows the relative rest principle.
2. Healing of ligaments treated nonoperatively manifests as minimal laxity with provocative testing, normal ROM, no tenderness along the ligament or pain with stretching, and progressively less pain with activities of daily living.
3. Healing of muscle tendon units manifests as no tenderness or pain with functional testing, full ROM, and progressively less pain with activities of daily living.

Phase 4: Return to Exercise or Sport Free of Symptoms
1. Premature return is likely to result in further injury or another injury.
2. Successful rehabilitation minimizes the risk of reinjury and returns the injured structures to baseline ROM, strength, endurance, and proprioception.
3. Functional rehabilitation should be sport specific. For example, a baseball pitcher with an upper-extremity injury needs to rehabilitate to normal strength and

ROM, but, before throwing a baseball in a game, he or she should practice throwing gently and work up to full speed over days to weeks, depending on the specific diagnosis and chronicity of the injury.

LARGE MUSCLE CONTUSIONS

The prototype injury in this category is the quadriceps contusion. This injury occurs from a direct blow to the thigh. It occurs in all sports and is very common in football, although the players wear thigh pads.

History

The athlete's presentation can range from feeling a mild discomfort or "Charlie horse" after the game to being unable to bear weight immediately after the trauma. The pathophysiology of the injury is bleeding in and around the quadriceps muscle as a result of the contusion. The quadriceps immediately goes into spasm, resulting in pain and disability. If the bleeding is not arrested immediately, it can be substantial.

Examination

On examination, the health care provider needs to consider a femoral fracture, which would be characterized by severe pain and the inability to bear weight. A quadriceps contusion is characterized by more diffuse tenderness over the quadriceps muscle. The athlete, typically, can bear weight but may not be able to extend the knee actively. With passive flexion of the knee while the athlete is in the prone position, the patient experiences pain as the quadriceps, which is in spasm, is stretched. The injury can be graded according to the degree of passive knee flexion that the patient can permit.

Treatment (Using Quadriceps Contusion as an Example)

- *Stop bleeding and RICE (rest, ice, compression, elevation):* The key is to stop further bleeding by applying ice for 20 minutes. When not applying ice, apply a tight compression wrap around the thigh and have the patient elevate the leg. The player should keep the knee in full flexion as much as possible during the first 24 hours after the injury.
- *Analgesics:* Cyclooxygenase inhibitors should not be given because they might promote decreased clotting. Acetaminophen can be given for pain.
- *Exercise:* The patient should start isometric quadriceps contractions as soon as possible. In moderate to severe injuries, treatment by a sports-trained physical therapist is essential. In experienced hands, the use of ultrasound can promote rapid recovery from this injury. Therapy that is too timid or too aggressive can retard recovery. If the bleeding is extensive and the athlete is reinjured before the hematoma has resolved, he or she is at risk for development of myositis ossificans, which can be career threatening and may require surgical excision if functional ability is compromised.

THE KNEE—GENERAL PRINCIPLES

History of the Injury

On the basis of the description of the mechanism of injury, the events after the injury, and the factors that worsen or improve the pain, the health care provider should be able to prioritize the most likely diagnoses.

1. Knee pain that occurs while running straight, without direct trauma or fall.
   a. Chronic pain: Likely to be patellofemoral syndrome (PFS) or dysfunction.
   b. Acute pain: Consider osteochondritis dissecans (OCD) and pathological fracture. *Any teen with knee pain without a history of trauma and with an equivocal examination that does not pinpoint the diagnosis needs to have a radiographic examination of the knee. In addition, if the hip examination finding is abnormal, radiographs of the hip are needed to rule out slipped capital femoral epiphysis manifested as knee pain.* Osgood-Schlatter disease and patellofemoral dysfunction do not require radiographs to establish a diagnosis.
2. Knee injury that occurs during weight bearing, cutting while running, or an unplanned fall. Consider internal derangement including ligamentous and meniscal tears and fracture. A player who injures the knee while cutting, without being hit or having direct trauma, has an anterior cruciate ligament (ACL) tear until proved otherwise.
3. A valgus injury to the knee (i.e., a force delivered to the outside of the knee, directed toward the midline) is likely to tear the medial collateral ligament, possibly the ACL, and either the medial or lateral meniscus.
4. Chronic anterior knee pain that is worse when going up stairs and/or after sitting for prolonged periods, or after squatting or running, is likely to be patellofemoral dysfunction. *In general*, if the patient does not give a history of the knee giving out or locking, sharp pain, effusion, the sensation of something loose in the knee, or the sensation that something tore with the initial injury, then the injury probably is not significant. If there is hemarthrosis within 24 hours of the injury, then internal derangement is present and a diagnosis must be sought. At the game site, if the patient can be evaluated within 1 hour or so of the injury, the ability to bear weight and walk without pain is the best indicator that he or she has probably not suffered a major injury and does not need to be referred immediately.

Physical Examination

The physical examination should include the following:

1. Observation of gait (weight bearing? antalgic gait?)
2. Inspection for swelling and discoloration
3. Observation of vastus medialis obliquus contraction, looking for reduced bulk and tone
4. Peripatellar palpation (tenderness over the tibial tuberosity is diagnostic of Osgood-Schlatter disease; peripatellar pain is characteristic of patellofemoral dysfunction)
5. Observation of quadriceps and hamstring flexibility

6. Inspection for evidence of meniscal tears (McMurray and modified McMurray tests)
7. Inspection for evidence of ligamentous instability, including valgus and varus testing (for medial collateral and lateral collateral ligaments, respectively)
8. Lachman test and pivot shift test (ACL); sag sign and posterior drawer test (posterior cruciate ligament)

Radiographic Evaluation of Knee Injuries

Any one of the following criteria would be an indication for a radiograph after an acute knee injury:

1. Inability to bear weight
2. Fibular head tenderness
3. Isolated tenderness of the patella
4. Inability to flex the knee beyond 90 degrees

These decision rules, collectively referred to as the *Ottawa Knee Rule*, had a sensitivity of 100% in detecting knee fractures in adults and could potentially reduce the use of plain radiographs by 28% (Steill et al., 1996a).

Anteroposterior and lateral views are standard. The sunrise view details the patellofemoral joint and should be ordered if patellar dislocation is suspected, while the tunnel view should be ordered if suspicious for OCD, ACL injury, or other intraarticular pathology.

Magnetic resonance imaging (MRI) evaluation in the acute or chronically injured knee should not be routine (O'Shea et al., 1996). MRI should be reserved for diagnostic dilemmas and for patients who do not respond to conservative management. The most commonly missed diagnoses are chondral fractures, ACL tears, fibrotic fat pad, and loose bodies (Oberlander et al., 1993). In experienced hands, the MRI added nothing to the diagnosis of knee injuries based on history and physical examination (Oberlander et al., 1993). This emphasizes the clinical (and financial) importance for primary care and emergency room health care providers to have good physical examination skills for diagnosing common musculoskeletal injuries.

Acute Knee Injuries—General Principles of Treatment

1. Establish a working diagnosis.
2. Use the Ottawa Knee Rule.
3. Relative rest: Prescribe use of crutches if the patient cannot bear weight without pain. An elastic wrap is adequate in the initial phase of treatment, or until a definitive diagnosis is made and a treatment regimen planned. Knee immobilizers have a limited role in the management of acute knee injuries because they are bulky and awkward, offer no structural support, and lead to calf strain if the patient tries partial weight bearing with the foot in the plantar-flexed position.
4. Ice: Apply for 20 minutes three or four times a day.
5. Start isometric quadriceps contractions on the first day if possible. If the patient cannot contract the quadriceps and it is anticipated that he or she will be unable to do so for some days, consider an electrical stimulation unit to contract the quadriceps until the patient is able to do so.
6. Maintain elevation of the leg as much as possible.
7. Use a compression wrap.
8. Prescribe analgesic medication.
9. Refer the patient for physical therapy.

THE KNEE—SPECIFIC CONDITIONS

Subluxation and Dislocation of the Patella

Etiology
Instability of the patellofemoral joint may permit the patella to dislocate partially out of the intercondylar groove. The patella then snaps back into place, in contrast to a complete dislocation, in which the patella continues to complete lateral dislocation. These episodes usually occur while the quadriceps is contracting with the knee in flexion and the foot fixed to the ground.

Epidemiology
Subluxation and lateral dislocation of the patella are prevalent in the second and third decades of life, with a slightly higher prevalence in females.

Clinical Manifestations
Symptoms include pain, giving way of the knee, a popping or grinding sensation, and swelling. Physical findings may be similar to those of PFS, which is frequently associated with recurrent subluxation or dislocation. Subluxation of the patella can mimic the clinical picture of a torn meniscus. Complete dislocation is usually a dramatic event and is easy to diagnose, with the patella visible on the lateral side of the joint. Patellar dislocations often reduce spontaneously, so the health care provider may not see the patella in a dislocated position.

Treatment
1. Subluxation of the patella
   a. Prescribe physical therapy for a quadriceps-strengthening program.
   b. Temporarily restrict or modify activity.
   c. Use a patellar sleeve to stabilize the patella. Alternately, the patient may be taught to do McConnell taping to stabilize the patella.
   d. Refer for surgery only if all other therapies fail.
2. Dislocation of the patella
   a. Reduction often occurs spontaneously.
   b. Gentle straightening of the knee by lifting the foot may allow the patella to slide into place. Sedation may be necessary to effect a reduction.
   c. Radiographs should be taken, because the dislocation and reduction generate sufficient force to fracture the bone in up to 10% of cases.
   d. Immobilize the knee in a knee immobilizer for 3 weeks, followed by physical therapy (PT) for range-of-motion and quadriceps-strengthening exercises. Use of a patellar stabilizing brace or McConnell taping is often effective.
3. Recurrent dislocation
   In some nonoperative treatment, therapy and bracing is successful, but when the patient has more than one dislocation, surgical intervention may be needed to realign the extensor mechanism.

Osgood-Schlatter Disease

Definition
Osgood-Schlatter disease is a painful enlargement of the tibial tubercle at the insertion of the patellar tendon. It is a common problem, especially among active adolescent males.

Etiology
During development of the anterior tibial tubercle, a small ossification center develops in the largely cartilaginous tubercle. With developing muscle mass during puberty, this small area comes under great traction stress from the patellar tendon, and small fragments of cartilage or of the ossification center can be avulsed. The problem is often aggravated by activities that involve quadriceps femoris contraction, such as running and jumping, with resultant additional stress on the tubercle.

Epidemiology
1. Males have a greater prevalence than females.
2. Mean age at onset: Onset usually coincides with the period of rapid linear growth.
   a. Females: 10 years, 7 months
   b. Males: 12 years, 7 months
   In a study by Yashar et al. (1995), the average bone age matched chronological age in adolescents with Osgood-Schlatter disease. This is in contrast to slipped capital femoral epiphysis, in which skeletal maturation is often delayed.

Clinical Manifestations
1. Pain and soft tissue swelling over the tibial tubercle.
2. Point tenderness and warmth over the tibial tubercle.
3. Normal knee joint with full ROM.
4. Unilateral involvement more common than bilateral involvement.
5. Duration usually lasts several months but can last longer.

Diagnosis
1. History: Pain at the tibial tubercle, aggravated by activity and relieved by rest.
2. Physical examination: Tenderness and swelling of the tibial tubercle.
3. Radiograph: Not essential for diagnosis but generally done only to eliminate the possibility of other processes. The radiograph may reveal soft tissue swelling anterior to tibial tubercle and/or fragmentation of the tibial tubercle.

Therapy
1. Explanation: Careful explanation of the condition to the adolescent and to his or her parents is essential to alleviate fears and misconceptions.
2. Restriction of activity: If symptoms are mild, the patient may continue in the chosen sport. If symptoms are more severe, curtailing of running and jumping activities for 2 to 4 weeks is usually sufficient.
3. Immobilization: If symptoms are severe or fail to respond to restriction of activity, immobilization with a knee immobilizer for a few weeks is effective. Immobilization should also be strongly considered when the patient has difficulty actively bringing the knee to full extension.
4. NSAIDs and ice: These may provide symptomatic pain relief.
5. Knee pads: Knee pads should be used for activities in which kneeling or direct knee contact might occur.
6. Surgery: Surgery is rarely indicated. If the patient continues to have symptoms after skeletal maturity, he or she may have a persistent ossicle that does not unite with the rest of the tibial tubercle. Simple excision of this fragment may bring relief.

Prognosis

The prognosis is excellent, but adolescents should be informed that the process might recur if excessive activity is performed. Usually, when growth is completed the problem stops, leaving only a prominent tubercle. The patient may still have difficulty kneeling on the prominent tubercle, even into adulthood. Rarely, patients with Osgood-Schlatter disease may fracture through the tibial tubercle.

Patellofemoral Syndrome

Definition

PFS, patellar malalignment syndrome, or patellofemoral dysfunction is a frequent cause of knee pain among adolescents, accounting for as much as 70% to 80% of knee pain problems in females and 30% in males. It is also the leading cause of knee problems in athletes. The term *patellofemoral pain syndrome* may be used currently, because it is a better descriptive term for part of the pathophysiology of the condition. The condition has traditionally been known as *chondromalacia patellae*. However, this term implies actual softening and damage to the patellar articular cartilage, whereas many individuals have no changes in their articular surface, so this term should be abandoned.

Etiology

PFS is often a result of abnormal biomechanical forces that occur across the patella. Even in an individual with normal anatomy, the force that occurs in this area, especially when the body is supported with one leg and the knee is partially flexed, is tremendous. Abnormal forces can result from the following:

1. Quadriceps femoris muscle imbalance or weakness or abnormality in the attachment of the vastus medialis
2. Altered patellar anatomy, such as a small- or high-riding patella
3. Increased femoral neck anteversion, with associated knee valgus and external tibial torsion, which increases lateral stress on the patella
4. Increased Q angle–the angle found between a line drawn from the anterosuperior iliac spine through the center of the patella and a line from the center of the patella to the tibial tubercle (normal, <15 degrees)
5. Variations in the patellar facet anatomy

Epidemiology

PFS is common in both male and female athletes. There is a higher prevalence among females in the general population but a higher prevalence among males in athletic populations.

Clinical Manifestations

1. The pain of PFS is characterized by the following:
   a. Peripatellar or retropatellar location
   b. Relation to activity: The pain usually increases with activities such as running, squatting, or jumping, and decreases with rest. Often the pain is most acute immediately on getting up to start an activity after a period of sitting.
   c. Insidious onset
2. Positive movie or theater sign: Prolonged sitting with flexed knee is uncomfortable.
3. Pain is often severe on ascending or descending stairs.
4. Knees may buckle or give out, especially when going up or down stairs.
5. Crepitus or a grating sensation may be felt, especially when climbing stairs.
6. History of injury to the patella area may be present.
7. Symptoms are bilateral in one third of adolescents.
8. Two thirds of patients have at least a 6-month history of pain.
9. Physical examination
   a. Inspection of the adolescent with PFS may reveal several anatomical abnormalities.
      - Patellar malalignment or squinting patella: With the adolescent's feet together, the two patellae may be displaced anteromedially. This is often found associated with a Q angle of >15 degrees. The Q angle is a measurement of the extensor mechanism alignment and was described previously.
      - External tibial torsion
      - Genu valgum (which increases the Q angle)
   b. Tenderness of the articular surface of the patella is elicited by knee extension and by displacing the patella medially and laterally while palpating the undersurface.
   c. Retropatellar crepitation may be determined by palpating for crepitus with one hand over the knee during flexion and extension. Crepitation is significant only if it is associated with pain.
   d. Dynamic patellar compression test, or "grind sign," may be performed by compressing the superior aspect of the patella between thumb and index finger as the adolescent actively tightens the quadriceps in 10 degrees of flexion. Pain is elicited if chondromalacia patella is present. Direct compression of the patella against the femur with the knee flexed will also elicit pain. This test is somewhat unreliable because it can also elicit pain in the asymptomatic knee.
   e. Knee ROM is usually normal.
   f. Hamstrings are often tight.
   g. Joint effusion usually does not occur but can be present in severe cases.
   h. Decreased bulk of the area around the vastus medialis on the affected side may be present. Thigh circumference should be checked, comparing the normal with the involved side.

Diagnosis

The diagnosis is usually made by compatible history and physical examination. Radiographs usually are of little help but are important in excluding other conditions. They should include anteroposterior, lateral, tunnel (to rule out OCD), and tangential views (also known as *skyline* or *Merchant views*). Other conditions causing knee pain in the adolescent include meniscal lesions, Osgood-Schlatter disease, tendonitis of the patellar tendon, recurrent dislocation of the patella, and OCD. In addition, hip disorders often manifest as vague knee or thigh pain, especially slipped capital femoral epiphysis.

Treatment

1. Control of symptoms
   a. Relative rest—reduction of activities such as running, jumping, climbing, and squatting that produce patellofemoral compression forces. Walking and swimming are good exercises to continue.
   b. NSAIDs, appropriately dosed for a short course.

2. Muscle strengthening: Most patients benefit from a formal physical therapy evaluation and can then be moved to a home program. As soon as tolerated, muscle-strengthening exercises should be performed at least once a day. Initially, these should be isometric quadriceps exercises (straight leg raises). Strengthening of the vastus medialis is particularly important. The exercises should be done with a weighted boot or on an exercise machine with the knee in full extension. The weight should be held for 5 seconds and repeated in three sets of 10 repetitions. Stretching of the hamstrings is an essential component of most therapy programs.

3. Graduated running: After symptoms are controlled and 6-10 lb of weight are held, a graduated running program can be instituted. Ice may be helpful immediately after exercise.

4. Maintenance: When the condition is under control, a maintenance program of quadriceps and hamstring exercises should be done two to three times a week. Most adolescents respond to nonoperative management. An experienced clinician has observed that if a patient can perform straight leg raises of near 15 lb, their symptoms almost invariably disappear.

5. Knee braces: Use of these in patients with PFS is controversial. Theoretically, they help keep the patella from moving too far laterally. However, because the patella moves in various planes, knee braces are best used in patients with lateral subluxation visible on examination. *The knee brace is not a substitute for muscle-strengthening exercises.*

6. Taping the knee: Although this may reduce friction, results are also controversial.

7. Footwear: Athletic shoes have improved in the last decade, but the quality and age of the athletic shoes are more important than a particular brand name.

8. Over-the-counter arch supports or custom orthotics: These can be helpful to some patients. Custom orthotics are expensive and are generally not required, but in some patients these may be more helpful than over-the-counter supports.

9. Surgery: This is considered as a last resort for patellofemoral pain. Occasionally a "lateral release" is appropriate if the problem is clearly related to excessive lateral tracking and other measures are unsatisfactory. This involves cutting the lateral retinaculum to reduce the amount of lateral pull.

Osteochondritis Dissecans (OCD)

Definition

OCD is a condition of focal avascular necrosis in which bone and overlying articular cartilage separate from the medial femoral condyle or, less commonly, from the lateral femoral condyle. The peak incidence is in the preadolescent age-group. The clinical course and treatment vary according to the age at onset, with children and young adolescents having a better prognosis than older adolescents and adults.

Etiology

The exact cause is unknown. Postulated factors include the following:

1. Trauma: Most patients do not report a single traumatic event. There is often a long history of exercise and participation in sports. It is theorized that earlier participation of children in sports has led to the earlier appearance of osteochondritis lesions (Cahill, 1995).

2. Ischemia: Obstruction of blood supply as a cause has been postulated, but evidence is lacking.

3. Epiphyseal development: In younger patients with osteochondritis, an accessory nucleus in the epiphyseal area may make the femoral condyle more vulnerable to trauma. Some adolescents have variants of normal growth that may simulate OCD on radiography, causing the condition to be overdiagnosed in younger adolescents.

4. Heredity: Heredity plays a minor role in some patients.

Clinical Manifestations

1. Onset in childhood and early adolescence
   a. History
      • An intermittent, nonspecific knee pain usually related to activity is a common symptom.
      • Extension movements of the knee may cause swelling and soreness.
      • Symptoms are often present for months to years before consultation.
   b. Examination
      • The adolescent may walk with the tibia in external rotation on the affected side.
      • Localized tenderness over the site of the lesion is best detected with the knee in 90 degrees of flexion and palpation of the femoral condyles. Most lesions are in the posterior femoral condyle, so the knee must be flexed 90 degrees to be able to palpate the OCD lesion.
      • A small, firm, movable mass may be palpable in the joint, indicating the presence of loose bodies.
      • Quadriceps atrophy may be present.
      • Effusion is present on rare occasions.
      • Check for a positive Wilson sign: Flex the knee to 90 degrees; internally rotate the tibia on the femur and extend the knee slowly with the tibia in internal rotation. If the sign is positive, pain will occur as the knee reaches 30 degrees of flexion. This pain is often relieved by external rotation of the tibia.
      • Thirty percent of individuals have bilateral signs.

2. Onset in late adolescence or young adulthood
   a. History
      • Either insidious onset or a history of specific injury with immediate onset of pain and swelling may be present.
      • Locking or acute swelling may occur if a bone fragment becomes loose.
      • Usually, unilateral involvement is seen.
      • Synovial effusion is more common in younger patients than in older ones.
   b. Examination: The findings are similar to those found in younger patients, except that young adults have a higher prevalence of swelling and unilateral involvement.

3. Radiological picture
   Anteroposterior, lateral, and tunnel views should be taken. X-ray examination often reveals a well-circumscribed area of subchondral bone separated from the remaining femoral condyle by a crescent-shaped radiolucent line. The separate bone may appear sclerotic or fragmented. The lesion may not be seen on a standard anteroposterior view; it may be best appreciated on the tunnel view. The medial femoral condyle is involved in 75% to 85% of cases, whereas approximately 15% of

TABLE 16.1

Juvenile Versus Adult Osteochondritis

Characteristic	Juvenile	Adult
Age	5–15 yr	15–30 yr
Epiphyses	Open	Closed
Bilateral	30% of cases	10% of cases
Onset	Insidious	Acute
Injury	Minor factor	Major factor
Prognosis	Excellent	Fair
Complications	Seldom	Occasionally

cases involve the lateral femoral condyle. In addition to the femoral condyle, the patella, femoral head, and talus may be involved.
4. Juvenile versus adult osteochondritis (Table 16.1).

Treatment

1. Children and younger adolescents: Orthopedic or sports medicine referral is recommended for appropriate staging and follow-up, but management is typically nonoperative as listed here:
   a. Restrict symptom-producing activities.
   b. Immobilize with cast or knee immobilizer if symptoms are severe.
   c. Advise regarding use of isometric quadriceps-strengthening exercises.
   d. NSAIDs are not routinely used but are useful if pain or effusion is present.
   e. Healing usually occurs within 6 to 12 months.
   f. If there is a free fragment, surgical intervention is required.
2. Older adolescents and adults: Orthopedic consultation is necessary for possible arthroscopy or surgery for either removal or internal fixation of the fragment. Surgery is particularly important in teenagers with progressive fragment formation, increasing bony sclerosis, or articular changes.

THE LOWER LEG- SHIN SPLINTS AND STRESS FRACTURES

Clinical Manifestations

1. History
   Patients with these conditions experience lower-extremity pain that initially appears toward the end of exercise. If the condition is left untreated and the adolescent continues in the exercise that caused the injury, the pain will occur earlier in the exercise period and persist longer after the exercise is over. It can occur in any adolescent involved in weight-bearing activity but is most common in runners. A common presentation is medial shin pain. The principal two diagnoses to consider are medial tibial stress syndrome (shin splints) and medial tibial stress fracture, which are discussed here. Other diagnostic possibilities include compartment syndromes and vascular abnormalities, which are not discussed and are less common. If these diagnoses

are being considered, referral to a specialist familiar with these conditions is indicated.
2. Examination
   On examination, the pain of shin splints should be more diffuse and tenderness should be closer to the muscle, rather than bone, at the muscle–bone interface along the medial tibia. In stress fractures of the medial tibia, the pain should be more pinpoint and over the bone, not muscle. There is an injury spectrum from shin splints to stress reaction to stress fracture, which can be difficult to distinguish clinically. Further diagnostic studies may be indicated. Stress fractures can occur in any bone and are most common in the tibia and fibula.

Diagnosis

Plain radiographs of patients with shin splints will be normal but, unfortunately, so will most of the plain radiographs of patients with tibial stress fractures, at least during the first few weeks after the injury. The most sensitive test to diagnose stress fractures has been the bone scan. This is being challenged, but has not yet been replaced, by the MRI. If the bone scan is normal, then the health care provider can be more confident that the diagnosis is shin splints due to medial tibial stress syndrome.

Treatment

A single best treatment protocol for shin splints and stress fractures of the medial tibia has not been established. One treatment protocol includes the following:

1. Relative rest and a functional progressive rehabilitation program. This means doing nothing that hurts within 24 hours of the activity. Alternative activities such as swimming, cycling, and pool running (running in the deep end of a pool supported by a buoyant vest or jacket) can be used to maintain the patient's fitness level while the leg injury is recovering. After 7 to 10 days of pain-free activity, the patient can start on a walking program and progress to a jogging program over 10 to 14 days, as long as he or she remains pain free. At any point in this functional rehabilitation progression, if pain reappears, the adolescent should have 2 or 3 pain-free days before resuming the walk–jog program. After jogging for 7 to 10 days, patients can progress to sprinting and then jumping so long as they remain pain free.
2. Apply ice each day for 20 minutes directly to the site.
3. Shoe inserts to control overpronation, if appropriate.
4. Increase the shock absorption of the patient's shoes, if appropriate, for example, if they have a rigid foot.
5. Stretch and strengthen the dorsiflexors (anterior tibialis), plantar flexors (posterior tibialis, gastrocnemius, soleus), and everters (peroneal muscles).
6. Analgesic medication or NSAIDs can be used in shin splints for 7 to 10 days but should not be used chronically as it may mask the pain and the adolescent may return to activity too soon. Analgesic medications should not be used on a regular basis (i.e., daily) for stress fractures because the number of pain-free days is the criterion for return to activity in the functional rehabilitation progression.

It is difficult to predict when an adolescent will recover sufficiently from stress fractures and shin splints to return to exercise or competition. As long as the patient follows a functional rehabilitation program such as the one just outlined, he or she will at least be involved in some rehabilitation toward full activity.

Consideration should be given to bone density evaluation by dual energy x-ray absorptiometry (DXA) in female adolescents with stress fracture, especially in those with a family history or other risk factors for osteoporosis.

THE ANKLE

Ankle injuries are the single most common acute injury in adolescent athletes (Hergenroeder, 1990). The diagnosis and treatment of ankle injuries in adolescents is the same as in adults, with the exception that teens may have open growth plates that may be the primary injury site, whereas in an adult the primary injury is likely to be torn ligaments.

Acute Ankle Injury

Etiology
The mechanism of acute ankle injury in 85% of the cases is inversion (turning the ankle under or in). Injuries resulting from eversion are generally more serious because of the higher risk of syndesmosis injury and fracture.

Clinical Manifestations
1. Physical examination
   Acute injury: The best time to examine any musculoskeletal injury is immediately after the injury, when the examination can be most informative. However, patients commonly present with diffuse swelling, tenderness, and decreased ROM hours to days after the injury. The physical examination will be limited in terms of diagnosing specific lesions at this point. At a minimum the examination should include the following:
   a. Inspect for gross abnormalities, asymmetry, and vascular integrity.
   b. Palpate for bony tenderness specifically at the medial and lateral malleoli, proximal fibula, anterior joint line, navicular, and base of the fifth metatarsal.
   c. Assess ability to bear weight.
   Three to 4 days after injury: The physical examination may be more informative at 3 to 4 days after injury, when the patient has appropriately used rest, ice, compression, and elevation.
   a. Inspect for swelling and ecchymosis.
   b. Assess active ROM in six directions:
      • Plantarflexion; plantarflexion and inversion; plantarflexion and eversion
      • Dorsiflexion; dorsiflexion and inversion; dorsiflexion and eversion
   c. Assess resisted ROM in the same six directions.
   d. Palpate for potential fracture at the sites listed for palpation of bony tenderness.
   e. Attempt passive ROM—plantarflexion and dorsiflexion, talar tilt, anterior drawer test.
   f. Assess for pain-free weight bearing with normal gait and then with heel-and-toe walking.
2. Associated injuries: Complications associated with ankle sprains
   a. Up to 15% of all complete ligament tears have an associated fracture. The most common sites are the talus, fifth metatarsal, fibula, and tibia. If there is bony tenderness in patients with open epiphyses, assume that a fracture is present even if the radiography results are negative. Immobilize without weight bearing for 1 week; if tenderness persists, casting for 2 weeks is required. If a fragment is present, it does not always require casting or surgery. If the fragment is small and does not appear to be in the joint space, then treat conservatively and monitor.
   b. "High ankle sprains"—tibiofibular syndesmosis injury occurs in 6% of ankle sprains. These are more serious injuries than the typical lateral ligament sprain. On examination, there is tenderness proximal to the joint line along the syndesmosis. Pressing the midshaft together and then releasing the pressure may worsen the pain.
   c. Talar fractures occur in 7% of ankle sprains. The patient complains of delayed healing, catching, locking, or persistent pain. Initial x-ray results may be negative; repeat radiographs or computed tomography (CT) scanning may be required.
   d. Peroneal subluxation occurs in 0.5% of ankle sprains. Tenderness is present along the tendon sheath, posterior and superior to the lateral malleolus.

Diagnosis
Radiographical Examination: Ottawa Ankle Rules
An ankle or foot plain radiograph is indicated if there is bone tenderness at the distal/posterior 6 cm of the tibia or fibula (ankle series) or at the navicular or base of the fifth metatarsal (foot series) or if the patient is unable to take four steps both immediately after the injury and during the examination, regardless of limping (Steill et al., 1996b). The Buffalo Modification of the Ottawa Ankle Rules includes the entire distal 6 cm of the tibia and fibula, not just the posterior portions (Leddy et al., 1998). Stress views are typically not indicated in the evaluation of the acute or chronically injured ankle.

Treatment—Acute Phase
1. The goal is to limit disability. Successful treatment is defined not only by the absence of pain but also by return to full ROM, strength, and proprioception.
2. Relative rest: As with rehabilitation of all musculoskeletal injuries, advise the adolescent to do nothing that hurts.
3. Ice: Used in the same manner as for knee injuries, described earlier.
4. Heat during the first 72 hours has a role only if it is applied by an athletic trainer or physical therapist.
5. Compression: If using an elastic wrap, always wrap distal to proximal, from the base of the toes to midcalf. Advise the patient not to sleep with the elastic wrap in place.
6. Compression and stability can be provided by an air stirrup, which should be used for all acute sprains not complicated by fracture.
7. Elevation: For the first 2 to 3 days, elevate the ankle as much as possible.
8. If discussing the injury by telephone, advise the patient not to wait to seek treatment. Athletes should seek treatment immediately.
9. NSAIDs: Use for pain relief and theoretically to control inflammation, but NSAIDs do not affect the outcome per se. Acetaminophen is another alternative.

10. Casting is not indicated for ankle sprains not complicated by fracture (Brostrom, 1966). Casting should not be routine for ankle sprains because it actually worsens the outcome, specifically the time to return to work. The air stirrup provides stability to inversion and eversion but also allows for active dorsiflexion and plantarflexion, which is key in early rehabilitation.

Rehabilitation

Rehabilitation needs to start on the first day of evaluation.

1. Relative rest: Progress off crutches as soon as possible; do pain-free exercise.
2. Stretching: Primarily soleus and gastrocnemius, by doing calf stretches.
3. Strengthening: Band exercises, toe–heel walking, pain free, and progressive (can be done with the air stirrup on).
4. Proprioceptive retraining: Raising on toes with little support (one or two fingers on a chair) and eyes closed for 5 minutes a day.
5. Functional progression of exercise: For instance, toe walking → walking at a fast pace → jogging → jogging and sprinting → sprinting and jogging on curves → figure-of-eight running → back to sports participation.
6. Air stirrup: The air stirrup should be worn in competition sports for 6 months after the injury (Thacker et al., 1999). The air stirrups are most comfortably worn with low-cut or three-fourth height shoes, and they provide excellent stability.

Ankle Instability

The leading causes of chronic ankle stability and pain are as follows:

1. Strength deficits
2. Loss of flexibility
3. Loss of proprioception
4. Intraarticular pathology

All of these need to be considered in the evaluation, and, if deficiencies are found, referral should be made to physical therapy for rehabilitation.

Tarsal Coalition

Definition

Tarsal coalition is a congenital abnormality that results in a partial or complete fusion between two bones of the foot. The fusion may be fibrous, cartilaginous, or bony. It is the most common cause of a painful, stiff, flat foot after the age of 8 years.

Etiology

Tarsal coalition appears to result from a lack of differentiation of mesenchymal tissue in the foot. The condition may be inherited as an autosomal dominant trait.

Epidemiology

1. Prevalence in the United States is approximately 1%.
2. The condition is bilateral in 50% to 60% of patients, but the contralateral side may be asymptomatic.
3. Presentation: Pain manifests between 8 and 12 years of age for calcaneonavicular coalitions, between 12 and 15 years for talocalcaneal coalitions. Although this is a congenital condition, pain does not begin until these later years because the coalition begins to ossify at this age.

Clinical Manifestation

1. Patients often complain of a recurring "ankle sprain."
2. Pain is often felt in the lateral ankle, especially in the sinus tarsi.
3. The heel is generally in valgus.
4. The patient has a rigid, flat foot. The peroneal tendons are often in spasm, leading to the term *peroneal spastic flat foot.*
5. There is lack of hindfoot motion.

Diagnosis

The diagnosis should be suspected in the preteen or teenage patient with insidious or sudden onset of pain in the midfoot to hindfoot associated with a lack of motion in the subtalar joint.

1. Physical examination: The most striking finding is the almost complete lack of inversion and eversion of the subtalar joint. The patient is unable to walk on the lateral border of the foot. Tenderness is often found in the sinus tarsi. The sinus tarsi is the conical-shaped cavity located between the anterosuperior surface of the calcaneus and the inferior aspect of the neck of the talus.
2. Radiographs: If a coalition is suspected, anteroposterior, lateral, 45-degree oblique, and axial (Harris) views of the calcaneus should be obtained.
3. CT and MRI: If the history and physical examination are consistent with a coalition but cannot be demonstrated on plain films, CT or MRI may demonstrate the coalition. MRI is more useful in demonstrating fibrous coalitions. More than one coalition may be present in the same foot.

Treatment

1. Patients who have minimal symptoms or who have only incidental radiographic findings do not require treatment. Longitudinal arch supports may be sufficient to relieve symptoms.
2. When patients have significant symptoms, a short leg walking cast for 3 to 4 weeks, followed by the use of a University of California Berkeley Laboratory (UCBL) orthosis may eliminate the symptoms.
3. If conservative treatment fails, resection of the coalition with interposition of fat or muscle is indicated. Some coalitions of the talocalcaneal joint are so large that they cannot be successfully resected and arthrodesis may be required.

SLIPPED CAPITAL FEMORAL EPIPHYSIS

Definition

Slipped capital femoral epiphysis (SCFE) is a disease in which the anatomical relationship between the femoral head and neck is altered secondary to a disruption of the epiphyseal plate.

Etiology

The femoral head slips posteriorly, inferiorly, and medially on the femoral metaphysis. This occurs through the hypertrophic cell layer of the epiphysis. The condition tends to occur in adolescents because of the following:

1. The increased weight burden at adolescence.
2. A decreased resistance to the added weight burden secondary to a shift in the femoral epiphysis from a horizontal to an oblique position.
3. Increased stress to an area that has not reached bony maturity.

A chronic, gradual slip accounts for 80% or more of cases of slipped capital epiphysis during adolescence and is usually related to the combination of obesity and slow maturation. Acute slips occur secondary to severe trauma, such as a fall or an automobile accident, and are more common in younger children than in adolescents. Most cases of SCFE are unrelated to an endocrine disorder, although the disease has been associated with hypopituitarism, hypogonadism, and hypothyroidism. Endocrine abnormalities are often associated with bilateral slips, and they occur more often in the extremes of the adolescent age-group (before age 9 or after age 16 years).

Epidemiology

1. Sex: The prevalence is two to four times greater in males than in females.
2. Incidence: A representative study (Kelsey, 1971) found the incidence in Connecticut to be 7.79 for African-American males, 6.68 for African-American females, 4.74 for white males, and 1.64 for white females per 100,000 individuals younger than 25 years.
3. Season: Onset of symptoms occurs more frequently in spring and summer.
4. Average age at onset: Usually, symptoms occur shortly before or during the period of accelerated growth (10–13 years of age in girls, 12–15 years in boys).
5. Hip involved: Left hips are affected more commonly in males; no difference is noted in females. Approximately 20% of patients present with a bilateral slip. The contralateral hip should always be examined and visualized radiographically.
6. Weight of affected patients: Approximately 88% of patients are obese, with 50% at or above the 95th percentile of weight for age and the 97th percentile of weight for height.
7. Bone age: Seventy percent of affected patients have skeletal maturation that is delayed by 6 months or more.

Clinical Manifestations

1. Symptoms
   a. Pain: Pain is localized to hip or groin in 80% of patients. However, pain may be strictly in the thigh or knee, referred from the obturator nerve. Some patients present with a painless limp.
   b. Click in the hip occurs.
2. Signs
   a. Internal rotation is diminished and adduction of hip is decreased.
   b. Decreased flexion of the hip is present.
   c. The affected leg is often held in slight external rotation and abduction.
   d. With passive hip flexion, the femur abducts and externally rotates; the leg falls into a "figure of 4" position.
   e. Limp: A limp is present in 50% of patients; the adolescent with acute slippage may not be able to bear weight on the affected extremity.
   f. The family often notices a change in gait. The foot externally rotates during ambulation.

Diagnosis

1. History and physical examination: Consistent signs and symptoms are present. The condition should be considered in any adolescent with hip or knee pain or a limp.
2. Radiographical changes: Anteroposterior and frog-leg lateral roentgenograms of the pelvis should be taken.
   a. In a normal anteroposterior radiograph of the hip, a line drawn on the superior edge of the femoral neck intersects the epiphysis; in a slip, the epiphysis falls below this line (Fig. 16.1).

FIGURE 16.1 In the normal hip on the left, a line drawn on the superior femoral neck intersects the proximal femoral epiphysis. In the hip on the right with a slipped epiphysis, the epiphysis lies completely below a line drawn on the superior femoral neck.

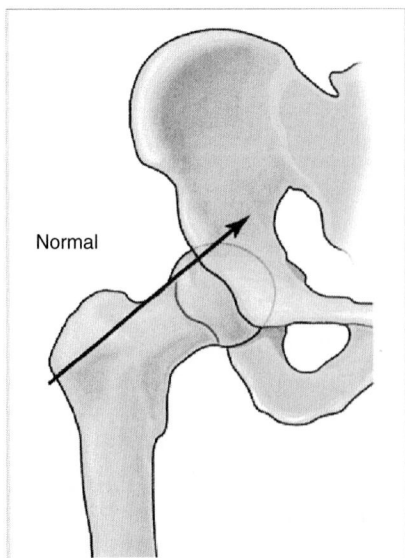
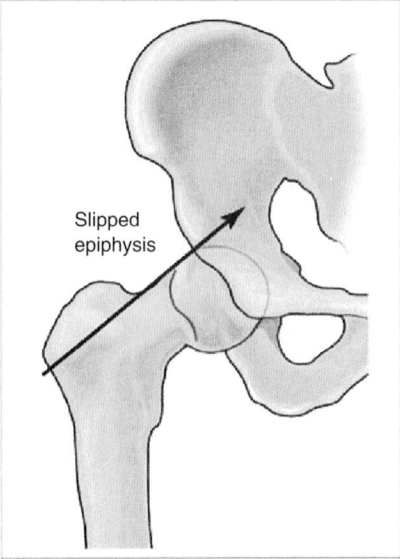

Normal

Slipped epiphysis

b. Earlier and more subtle slips are seen better on the frog-leg lateral views than on the anteroposterior views. More advanced slips show the obvious slippage inferiorly and posteriorly of the femoral head epiphysis on both anteroposterior and frog-leg lateral films. A "true lateral" view can also be helpful.
c. Early changes include epiphyseal widening and rarefaction.
3. Bone scan: A bone scan may show increased uptake at the involved epiphyseal plate.
4. MRI: MRI demonstrates increased blood flow at the epiphysis.
   Most cases of SCFE can be diagnosed with plain radiographs. Bone scan and MRI are rarely needed.

Treatment

Orthopedic referral is required, because surgery is the only reliable treatment. Further slippage can be prevented by the introduction of threaded screws across the epiphyseal plate in situ. (Reduction of the slip is seldom, if ever, indicated.) The condition should be treated promptly, because greater slippage leads to a worse prognosis. Avascular necrosis can occur with acute, large slips. Premature degenerative joint disease is a frequent late development in many patients with severe, chronic slips, even after fixation. For moderate and severe cases, corrective osteotomies can be performed after the growth plate has closed to improve gait and ROM.

LOW BACK PAIN

Low back pain is a common enough presentation in adolescent health care that there is an entire chapter devoted to it in this book (Chapter 17).

"GROWING PAINS"

Definition and Epidemiology

Pain in the lower limbs is common among children and younger adolescents, with a prevalence of "growing pains" reported at between 4% and 50% of children and adolescents, increasing after the age of 5 years, with peaks at ages 13 in boys and 11 in girls.
   Many causes of lower limb pain are possible, including the following:

1. Trauma: Fracture, dislocation, contusion
2. Infection: Osteomyelitis, septic arthritis, abscess, cellulitis
3. Vascular causes: Hemophilia, sickle cell anemia, hemangioma
4. Congenital conditions: Tarsal coalition, dislocation of hip
5. Slipped femoral capital epiphysis
6. Osgood-Schlatter disease
7. Osteochondritis Dessicans
8. Patellofemoral Syndrome
9. Rheumatic disease: Juvenile rheumatoid arthritis, polymyositis
10. Leukemia

Most of these causes are well delineated by history, physical examination, and appropriate laboratory tests. If all of the above diagnoses have been excluded, some practitioners utilize the term "growing pains."

Clinical Manifestations

1. Pain
   a. Intermittent pain or ache is usually localized to the muscles of the legs and thighs. The most common sites are the front of the thighs and calves and behind the knees. Less commonly involved sites include the back, shoulder, arm, and groin.
   b. Bilateral pain is usually present.
   c. Pain usually occurs late in the day, in the evening, or at night.
   d. No loss of mobility
2. No tenderness, erythema, or swelling
3. No fever or symptoms of systemic disease
4. Normal laboratory studies and normal findings on radiography

Diagnosis

There is no simple approach to a definite diagnosis. After a completely normal thorough evaluation, in our clinical practice we may ascribe the discomfort to a relative imbalance between growth in the long bones and inflexibility in the large muscles of the lower extremities, although there is no evidence to support this teleological explanation.

Treatment

Conservative therapy involving reassurance, heat, stretching, massage, and judicious use of NSAIDs is usually sufficient.

WEB SITES

For Teenagers and Parents

http://orthoinfo.aaos.org. Your Orthopaedic Connection from the American Academy of Orthopaedic Surgeons.

Subluxation of Patella

http://orthopedics.about.com/cs/patelladisorders/a/kneecapdisloc.htm. About subluxation of patella.
http://www.med.umich.edu/1libr/sma/sma_subluxin_sma.htm. From University of Michigan.

Osgood-Schlatter Disease

http://orthoinfo.aaos.org/fact/thr_report.cfm?Thread_ID=145&topcategory=Knee.
http://www.mayoclinic.com/health/osgood-schlatter-disease/DS00392. Mayo Clinic article on Osgood-Schlatter.
http://www.nlm.nih.gov/medlineplus/ency/article/001258.htm. Medline Plus article on Osgood-Schlatter.

Osteochondritis Dissecans

http://familydoctor.org/488.xml. American Academy of Family Practice Web site on osteochondritis dissecans.

http://www.mayoclinic.com/health/osteochondritis-dissecans/DS00741. Mayo Clinic article on osteochondritis dissecans.

Shin Splints

http://orthoinfo.aaos.org/. Search on shin splints

http://www.mayoclinic.com/health/shin-splints/DS00271. Mayo Clinic article on shin splints.

Slipped Capital Femoral Epiphysis

http://orthoinfo.aaos.org/fact/thr_report.cfm?Thread_ID=160&topcategory=Hip

http://familydoctor.org/282.xml. From American Academy of Family Practice.

For Health Professionals

www.aaos.org. American Academy/Association of Orthopaedic Surgeons.

http://www.emedicine.com/emerg/topic347.htm. Emedicine article on Osgood-Schlatter disease.

http://www.emedicine.com/radio/topic495.htm. Emedicine article on osteochondritis dissecans.

http://www.emedicine.com/radio/topic673.htm. Emedicine article on tarsal coalition.

http://www.emedicine.com/sports/topic122.htm. Emedicine article on slipped capital epiphysis.

REFERENCES AND ADDITIONAL READINGS

Adams WB. Treatment options in overuse injuries of the knee: patellofemoral syndrome, iliotibial band syndrome, and degenerative meniscal tears. *Curr Sports Med Rep* 2004;3:256.

Aronson DD, Loder RT. Slipped capital femoral epiphysis in black children. *J Pediatr Orthop* 1992;12:74.

Atar D, Lehman WB, Grant AD. Growing pains. *Orthop Rev* 1991;20:133.

Ballas MT, Tytko J, Mannarino F. Commonly missed orthopedic problems. *Am Fam Physician* 1998;57:267.

Binazzi R, Felli L, Vaccari V, et al. Surgical treatment of unresolved Osgood-Schlatter lesion. *Clin Orthop* 1993;289:202.

Brostrum L. Treatment and Prognosis in Recent Ligament Ruptures. *Acta Chir Scand.* 1966;132:537.

Bradley J, Dandy DJ. Osteochondritis dissecans and other lesions of the femoral condyle. *J Bone Joint Surg Br* 1989;71:518.

Busch MT, Morrissy RT. Slipped capital femoral epiphysis. *Orthop Clin North Am* 1987;18:637.

Cahill BR. Osteochondritis dissecans of the knee: treatment of juvenile and adult forms. *J Am Acad Orthop Surg* 1995;4:237.

Calmbach WL, Hutchens M. Evaluation of patients presenting with knee pain: part II. Differential diagnosis. *Am Fam Physician* 2003;68:917.

Canvey BT, Weinstein SL, Noble J. Long-term follow-up of slipped capital femoral epiphysis. *J Bone Joint Surg Br* 1988;70:174.

Causey AL, Smith ER, Donaldson JJ, et al. Missed slipped capital femoral epiphysis: illustrative cases and a review. *J Emerg Med* 1995;13:175.

Davidson K. Patellofemoral pain syndrome. *Am Fam Physician* 1993;48:1254.

Deluca SA, Rhea JT. Slipped femoral epiphysis. *Am Fam Physician* 1984;29:159.

Edmonson AS. Spondylolisthesis. In: Crenshaw AH, ed. *Campbell's operative orthopaedics*, Vol 4. St. Louis: CV Mosby, 1987.

Emery KH, Bisset GS III, Johnson ND, et al. Tarsal coalition: a blinded comparison of MRI and CT. *Pediatr Radiol* 1998;8:612.

Fredericson M, Yoon K. Physical examination and patellofemoral pain syndrome. *Am J Phys Med Rehabil* 2006;85:234.

Fulkerson JP, Kalenak A, Rosenberg TD, et al.. Patellofemoral pain. In: Eilert RE, ed. *Instructional course lectures.* Park Ridge, IL: American Academy of Orthopaedic Surgeons, 1992:57.

Griffin LY, ed. *Essentials of musculoskeletal care*, 3rd ed. Rosemont, IL: American Academy of Orthopaedic Surgeons, 2006.

Henry JH. The patellofemoral joint. In: Nicholas JA, Hershman EB, eds. *The lower extremity and spine in sports medicine.* St. Louis: CV Mosby, 1986.

Hergenroeder AC. Diagnosis and treatment of ankle injuries: a review. *Am J Dis Child* 1990;144:809.

Hinton RY, Sharma KM. Acute and recurrent patellar instability in the young athlete. *Orthop Clin North Am* 2003;34:385.

Hixon AL, Gibbs LM. Osteochondritis dissecans: a diagnosis not to miss. *Am Fam Physician* 2000;61:151.

Hoppenfeld S. *Physical examination of the spine and extremities.* East Norwalk, CT: Appleton-Century-Crofts, 1976.

Horn BD, Moseley CE. Current concepts in the management of pediatric hip disease. *Curr Opin Rheumatol* 1992;4:184.

Katz DA. Slipped capital femoral epiphysis: the importance of early diagnosis. *Pediatr Ann* 2006;35:102.

Kelsey JL. Incidence and distribution of slipped capital femoral epiphysis in Connecticut. *J Chronic Dis* 1971;23:567.

Krause BL, Williams JP, Catterall A. Natural history of Osgood-Schlatter diseases. *J Pediatr Orthop* 1990;1:65.

Kujala UM, Kvist M, Heinonen O. Osgood-Schlatter's disease in adolescent athletes: retrospective study of incidence and duration. *Am J Sports Med* 1985;13:236.

LaBella C. Patellofemoral pain syndrome: evaluation and treatment. *Prim Care* 2004;31:977.

LaBrier K, Oneill DB. Patellofemoral stress syndrome: current concepts. *Sports Med* 1993;16:449.

Leddy JJ, Smolinski RJ, Lawrence J, et al. Prospective evaluation of the Ottawa Ankle rules in a university sports medicine center. *Am J Sports Med* 1998;26:158.

Loder RT, Wittenberg B, Desilva G. Slipped capital femoral epiphysis associated with endocrine disorders. *J Pediatr Orthop* 1995;15:349.

Loud KJ, Gordon CM, Micheli LJ, et al. Correlates of stress fractures among preadolescent and adolescent girls. *Pediatrics* 2005;115:e399.

Manners P. Are growing pains a myth? *Aust Fam Physician* 1999;28:124.

Morita T, Ikata T, Katoh S, et al. Lumbar spondylolysis in children and adolescents. *J Bone Joint Surg Br* 1995;77:620.

Morrissy RT. Slipped capital femoral epiphysis. In: Morrissy RT, ed. *Lovell and winters pediatric orthopaedics*, 3rd ed. Philadelphia: JB Lippincott Co, 1990:885.

Oberlander MA, Shalvoy RM, Hughston JC. The accuracy of the clinical knee examination documented by arthroscopy. *Am J Sports Med* 1993;21:773.

O'Shea KJ, Murphy KP, Heekin RD, et al. The diagnostic accuracy of history, physical examination, and radiographs in the evaluation of traumatic knee disorders. *Am J Sports Med* 1996;24:164.

Oster J. Recurrent abdominal pain, headache, and limb pain in children and adolescents. *Pediatrics* 1972;50:429.

Oster J, Nielsen A. Growing pains. *Acta Paediatr Scand Suppl* 1972;61:329.

Post WR. Patellofemoral pain: results of nonoperative treatment. *Clin Orthop Relat Res* 2005;436:55.

Reynolds RA. Diagnosis and treatment of slipped capital femoral epiphysis. *Curr Opin Pediatr* 1999;11:80.

Roach JW. Knee disorders and injuries in adolescents. *Adolesc Med* 1998;9:589.

Robertson W, Kelly BT, Green DW. Osteochondritis dissecans of the knee in children. *Curr Opin Pediatr* 2003;15:38.

Rosenberg ZS, Kawelblum M, Cheung YY, et al. Osgood-Schlatter lesion: fracture or tendinitis? Scintigraphic, CT, and MR imaging features. *Radiology* 1992;185:853.

Ruffin MT IV, Kiningham RB. Anterior knee pain: the challenge of patellofemoral syndrome. *Am Fam Physician* 1993; 47:185.

Sakellariou A, Claridge RJ. Tarsal coalition. *Orthopedics* 1999; 22:1066.

Sales de Gauzy J, Mansat C, Darodes PH, et al. Natural course of osteochondritis dissecans in children. *J Pediatr Orthop* 1999; 8:26.

Sandow MJ, Goodfellow JW. The natural history of anterior knee pain in adolescents. *J Bone Joint Surg Am* 1985;67:36.

Staheli LT. The lower limb. In: Morrissy RT, ed. *Lovell and winters pediatric orthopaedics*, 3rd ed. Philadelphia: JB Lippincott Co, 1990:741.

Stanitski CL. Anterior knee pain syndromes in the adolescent. *J Bone Joint Surg Am* 1993;75:1407.

Stanitski CL. Knee overuse disorders in the pediatric and adolescent athlete. In: Heckman JD, ed. *Instructional course lectures*. Park Ridge, IL: American Academy of Orthopaedic Surgeons, 1993:483.

Steill IG, Greenberg GH, Wells GA, et al. Prospective validation of a decision rule for the use of radiography in acute knee injuries. *JAMA* 1996a;275:611.

Steill IG, Greenberg GH, McKnight RD, et al. The "real" Ottawa ankle rules. *Ann Emerg Med* 1996b;27:103.

Tachdjian MO. Joints. In: Wickland EH Jr, ed. *Pediatric orthopedics*. Philadelphia: WB Saunders, 1990:1410.

Taylor PM. Osteochondritis dissecans as a cause of posterior heel pain. *Phys Sportsmed* 1982;10:53.

Thacker SB, Stroup DF, Branche CM, et al. The prevention of ankle sprains in sports. *Am J Sports Med* 1999;27:753.

Teitz CC. Sports medicine concerns in dance and gymnastics. *Pediatr Clin North Am* 1982;29:1399.

Tolo V. Foot disorders. In: Pine J, ed. *Pediatric orthopaedics in primary care*. Baltimore: Williams & Wilkins, 1993:103.

Tolo V. Hip and thigh. In: Pine J, ed. *Pediatric orthopaedics in primary care*. Baltimore: Williams & Wilkins, 1993:135.

Tolo V. Knee. In: Pine J, ed. *Pediatric orthopaedics in primary care*. Baltimore: Williams & Wilkins, 1993:169.

Vincent KA. Tarsal coalition and painful flatfoot. *J Am Acad Orthop Surg* 1998;5:274.

Wall E, Von Stein D. Juvenile osteochondritis dissecans. *Orthop Clin North Am* 2003;34:341.

Wechsler RJ, Schweitzer ME, Deely DM, et al. Tarsal coalition: depiction and characterization with CT and MR imaging. *Radiology* 1994;2:447.

Wells D, King JD, Roe IT, et al. Review of slipped capital femoral epiphysis associated with endocrine disease. *J Pediatr Orthop* 1993;13:610.

Williams JS Jr, Bush-Joseph CA, Bach BR Jr. Osteochondritis dissecans of the knee. *Am J Knee Surg* 1998;11:221.

Yashar A, Loder RT, Hemsinger RN. Determination of skeletal age in children with Osgood-Schlatter disease of the knee. *J Pediatr Orthop* 1995;15:298.

CHAPTER 17

Back Pain in the Adolescent

Jordan D. Metzl and Lawrence S. Neinstein

Back pain (in particular, lower back pain) is one of the most common complaints among adult patients and the most common cause of disability in individuals younger than 45 years. Back pain is less common in prepubertal and young adolescent patients; middle, older adolescents and college students more frequently experience back pain. The etiology of adolescent back pain varies although muscular conditions, and bone-related and discogenic problems make up most causes.

PREVALENCE

The prevalence of back pain increases with age, with the lowest prevalence in children and adolescents. However, back pain, particularly lower back pain, can be relatively common in older adolescents. This has been well demonstrated in numerous studies:

1. Balague et al. (1988): Back pain affected 27% of Swiss school students.
2. Fairbanks et al. (1984): Back pain affected 26% of English school students.
3. Burton et al. (1996): Followed up a class of English school children for 4 years. The annual incidence of low back pain rose from 11.8% at age 12 to 21.5% at 15. Lifetime prevalence was 11.6% at age 11, increasing to 50.4% at age 15. By age 15, 59% of the students described their pain as recurrent. Only 15.6% of patients who experienced back pain during the study sought treatment.
4. Olsen et al. (1992): Back pain was experienced by 30.4% of 1,242 American adolescents aged 11 to 17. Of those with back pain, one third had a history of having to restrict their activity, and 7.3% sought medical attention for back pain.
5. College students: In the 2006 National College Health Assessment, 47% listed back pain as a problem in the previous year (American College Health Association, 2006).

It must be noted, however, that back pain may be more common than estimated in these samples, particularly among pediatric and adolescent athletes. This especially includes young gymnasts, ballet dancers, and figure skaters.

ETIOLOGY

The etiology of back pain varies with age. The younger the individual, the more likely that back pain is *not* related to simple musculoskeletal strain. Back pain can be divided into the following categories:

1. Mechanical disorders
   a. Overuse syndromes (including muscle strain)
   b. Herniated nucleus pulposus
   c. Slipped vertebral apophysis
   d. Postural disorders
   e. Vertebral compression fractures
   f. Spondylolysis and spondylolisthesis (acquired)
2. Developmental disorders
   a. Spondylolysis and spondylolisthesis (developmental)
   b. Scheuermann disease
3. Inflammation and infections
   a. Discitis and vertebral osteomyelitis
   b. Disc calcification
   c. Rheumatological conditions including ankylosing spondylitis and reactive spondyloarthropathies such as Reiter syndrome
   d. Sickle cell disease and sickle cell pain crisis
   e. Epidural abscess
4. Neoplastic processes
   a. Vertebral column or spinal canal
   b. Muscular
5. Psychogenic causes

Alternatively, one can also divide back pain in adolescents into those that are muscular in etiology, bone-related, or discogenic.

EVALUATION

In most individuals with acute back pain, the cause is never precisely known but the course is usually benign and self-limited. Nevertheless, a thorough history and physical examination are basic requisites and the history is a key part of the diagnosis. Table 17.1 differentiates muscular, bone-related, and discogenic causes using clues from the history, physical examination, and radiological tests.

TABLE 17.1

Common Causes of Back Pain: Differentiation and Management of Muscular, Bone-Related, and Discogenic Causes Using Clinical Clues

Clues to Pathophysiology	Muscular	Bone-Related	Discogenic
Site of pain	Localized to paraspinous muscles	Localized to center of spine	
Pain during activity	X	X	X
Pain after activity	X	X	X
Pain bending forward		X	X
Pain bending backward		X	
Straight raised leg test elicits pain			X
Pain with twisting	X		
Radiating pain		May occur if there is spondylolisthesis and the degree of slip is sufficient to impinge on the nerve root	X
Strength testing			Strength tests involving the great toe, inverted foot, thigh, and hip flexor may show weakness
Neurosensory examination	Unremarkable	Reflex deficiencies may signal spondylolisthesis that has progressed to compress spinal nerve roots	Reflex deficiencies may signal disk herniation; tingling toes may suggest spinal cord compression
Radiologic tests	Consider x-ray only if pain persists >6 weeks, occult fracture is suspected, or scoliosis is present	X-rays: one AP, one lateral, and two oblique views. Consider MRI if concerned about fracture. If spondylolysis is suspected but not clear on x-ray, MRI will reveal edema	X-rays: one AP and one lateral. MRI considered gold standard; rarely CT if MRI not clear
Activity modification	Patients should be encouraged to return to play as soon as they can, using their judgment and taking nonsteroidal antiinflammatory drugs as needed.	Sports hiatus for younger patients with spondylolysis that may heal with rest. Older patients can play with or without a brace once they are pain free, but must postpone return to play until nerve-related symptoms resolve	Bed rest is not recommended
Indications for referral	Associated scoliosis	Spondylolysis, spondylolisthesis, or pain that persists for more than a month despite physical therapy, regardless of x-ray findings	Always
Treatment plan	Physical therapy, which may include referral to a sports-oriented physical therapist	Referral to a physical therapist and may include referral to a sports-oriented physical therapist and a sports medicine specialist if the individual is an athlete or injury is sports related	Referral to a physical therapist and orthopedist May include sports-oriented specialist if the adolescent is an athlete. Options may include bracing, steroid injection and, if all else fails, microdiscectomy

Modified from Metzel JD. Back pain in the adolescent: a user-friendly guide. *Adolesc Health Update* 2005;17:5

1. History: Key components of the history include the mechanism of injury (if any) and types of movement and activities associated with pain. In addition, ask about prior injuries or periods of back pain, the site of pain, and any pain radiation locations.
   a. General history
      • History of trauma and mechanism of any injury.
      • Characteristics of the pain, including location (lumbar, upper/lower thoracic, midline, paraspinal), severity, type, onset and duration, prior treatment and limitations, and exacerbating and alleviating maneuvers.
      • Severe pain: Severe back pain in an adolescent is more likely associated with a pathological condition than a muscular strain and should be evaluated more carefully. Writhing pain suggests a possible intraabdominal condition. Unrelenting pain suggests tumor or an infectious process.
      • Prior injuries or history of prior back pain.
      • Exercise, athletic, and work history.
      • History of being awoken at night due to the pain.
      • Systemic symptoms: Bowel or bladder problems, abdominal pain, fever, weight loss, malaise, iritis, urethritis, arthritis.
      • Symptoms unrelated to the back, which are suggestive of systemic infection, neoplasm, or a collagen vascular disease.
      • Family history of rheumatological disease including back stiffness or spondylarthropathy.
      • Neurological symptoms, including bladder or bowel changes.
   b. History for specific conditions
      • Tumors: Back pain occurring at rest, especially at night, is a common feature of vertebral involvement with a neoplastic process. Constant back pain, associated neurological deficits, and rigidity of the spine on attempted movement may be associated with tumor or infection. Other suggestive historical information includes prior history of a malignant tumor and unexplained weight loss.
      • Spondylolysis and spondylolisthesis: Back pain may radiate to buttocks or thighs. There may be a history of hyperextension activities of the spine, such as gymnastics or ballet. It is important to note that spondylolysis can be either developmental, or, can also be acquired, as is the case with spondylolysis acquired through repetitive and extension maneuvers.
      • Infection: Discitis and osteomyelitis of a vertebra can lead to significant back pain. Malaise and severe stiffness are common complaints.
      • Spondyloarthropathy: Back pain from spondyloarthropathies is associated with insidious onset, worsening of symptoms in the morning and with rest, decrease in symptoms with activity, onset before 30 years of age, and pain that persists longer than 3 months.
      • Scoliosis: Back pain is not usually a feature of scoliosis and should suggest the possible presence of another disorder.
2. Physical examination: This should include observation of gait and posture followed by testing of motion, strength, and neurosensory testing. The back should also be checked in the standing, sitting, and supine positions.

   a. Gait: Begin examination by asking the patient to walk across the room. See if gait is normal or if there is a tilt to one side.
   b. Standing position
      • Asymmetry: Check for pelvic or leg length discrepancies. Assessment of scapular and hip height while standing is easily done when observing the patient from behind.
      • Curvatures: Check for kyphosis or scoliosis and perform forward-bending examination.
      • Inspect the spine from behind the patient and from the side.
      • Percuss and palpate spine for local tenderness.
      • Palpate the iliac crest, specifically cartilaginous apophysis or growth plates.
      • Range of motion:
         Forward bending: Most adolescents should be able to bend forward to within 15 cm of their toes regardless of the problem. Individuals with paraspinal muscle spasm tend to arch their lumbar area while bending the spine at the hips.
         Backward bending: Also ask the patient to bend backward as pain on backward bending may suggest spondylolysis or a stress fracture.
         Twist back to left and right with hands on hips: Pain with twisting is consistent with muscle spasm or muscle pain.
      • Midline defects: Midline defects including dimpling, hypertrichosis, hemangiomatosis, cutaneous nevi, and soft tissue masses may be related to an underlying spinal abnormality such as spina bifida, lipoma, or diastematomyelia.
   c. Sitting position
      • Test knee and ankle reflexes and Babinski sign.
      • Test muscle strength of lower extremities and reflexes. Specific signs include
         L5 disk herniation: weakness of hallucis longus muscle. Test by asking patient to extend the great tow upward against your resistance.
         L4 weakness: detected by inversion of the foot. Test by asking patient to evert the foot against resistance. L4 nerve root involvement can by assessed by dorsal and plantar flexion of the foot.
         Disk herniation between L3 and L4 would give diminished patellar reflex. Diminished Achilles reflex would indicate a possible disk herniation at L5 level.
      • Perform distraction leg-raising test: Ask the patient to straighten his or her leg while seated. Patients with a disc problem arch backward in tripod position to take pressure off the sciatic nerve. Results of this test should correlate with results of straight leg raising in supine position.
   d. Supine position
      • Measure leg length from anterosuperior iliac spine to medial malleolus. A difference in leg length of >2.5 cm should be evaluated.
      • Check for muscle atrophy by measuring the girth of each leg at fixed measured distances above and below the patella.
      • Perform a sensory examination. Remember to check for "saddle anesthesia," which is indicative of a cauda equina syndrome.
      • Straight leg-raising test: The patient should lie on his or her back. The tested leg is fully extended

while the opposite leg is flexed at the hip and knee with the sole of that foot resting on the table. Pain radiating down the back of the leg when the tested leg is lifted is a positive result. Pain occurring when the angle between the back of the thigh and the table is <60 degrees is an equivocal result. Pain when this angle is >60 degrees may also be caused by muscular irritability. To exclude this, the examiner can also lift the leg to the point of pain and then lower the leg 5 degrees and dorsiflex the foot. This stretches the sciatic nerve; pain indicates nerve impingement and is considered to be a positive result. If pain occurs in the opposite leg while lifting the tested leg, a positive crossed straight leg-raising sign is present. This has been highly correlated with a herniated disc.

- Femoral stretch test: With the teen facing prone and the knees straight, lift one leg backward, extending the hip but keeping the knee straight. This test stretches the femoral nerve, and pain radiating into the anterior thigh indicates L2, L3, and L4 nerve root irritation.
- In patients with chronic back pain, a rectal examination may be indicated to look for decreased sphincter tone, which suggests pressure on nerve roots from a tumor or herniated disc. In addition, the circumferences of the upper and lower legs should be measured to look for muscle atrophy.
- Other red flags on examination include fever, other systemic signs, major motor weakness in lower extremities, focal vertebral tenderness, very limited spinal range of motion, and neurological findings persisting beyond 1 month.

3. Physical examination for specific conditions
   a. Tumors: Neurological deficits may be present, including weakness or bowel and bladder dysfunction.
   b. Spondylolysis and spondylolisthesis: The teen may have hyperlordosis. Stiffness and limited straight leg raising due to hamstring spasm or tautness may be present. Localized tenderness may occur at L5 to S1. Neurological deficits may be present if significant slippage has occurred.
   c. Infections: Tenderness may be well localized over affected vertebrae.
   d. Herniated disc: Pain commonly radiates down the leg. In more advanced cases, a herniated disc is associated with muscle weakness, atrophy, and decrease in sensation and reflexes.
   e. Functional pain: Tests for nonorganic causes are as follows:
      - Press the patient's head with gentle downward pressure. If the patient collapses or complains of severe pain, the problem may be functional.
      - Gently palpate the paraspinous muscles. Complaints of severe pain or falling to the floor may be indicative of a nonorganic problem.
      - Hold the teen's wrists next to his or her hips, and turn the teen's body from side to side. Because this maneuver does not cause stress on the muscles or nerve roots, it should not cause any significant pain.
      - Burns test: Have the teen kneel on a regular chair and touch the floor with his or her fingertips. If teen cannot reach within 15 cm of floor, the test result is considered positive and possibly indicative of a nonorganic cause.

4. Imaging studies: A radiological examination should be performed for an adolescent with chronic back pain (>3 months). Other indications for radiological examination include a history of serious trauma; known history of neoplasia; pain at rest; unexplained weight loss; drug or alcohol abuse; point tenderness; treatment with corticosteroids; temperature >38°C; and clinical manifestations that are consistent with the diagnosis of scoliosis, kyphosis, spondylolisthesis, or ankylosing spondylitis or that demonstrate a neuromotor deficit. In the absence of history or physical findings suggestive of serious disease, spine films have a low diagnostic yield. Lumbar spine radiographs are estimated to be the largest source of gonadal irradiation in the United States. When obtaining radiographs of the lumbar spine, the correct views include anteroposterior (AP), lateral, and oblique views. Consider magnetic resonance imaging (MRI) if there is suspicion of a fracture, if spondylolysis is suspected but not clear on x-ray, or if there are clinical signs suggestive of significant discogenic disease.

DIAGNOSIS AND MANAGEMENT OF SPECIFIC CONDITIONS

Most back pain in adolescents and young adults falls into three general categories: muscular, bone-related, and discogenic (Table 17.1).

Muscular Back Pain

More than 30% of back pain in adolescents, and probably more in older adolescent and young adults, is muscular in origin. The physician must be especially careful to rule out other pathology in the child and young adolescent. In selected cases, the evaluation may require additional imaging studies and/or laboratory tests. Keys to the diagnosis include:

- History of overuse injury, such as heavy backpack
- Paraspinous, not midline pain
- More pain on spinal rotation than with bending forward or backward
- Radicular symptoms are absent

1. Sports-related muscular injury: Muscular back pain is often the result of a sports-related injury. When assessing the adolescent patient with a presumed muscular injury, both the diagnosis and causative factors must be addressed. This means that history and physical examination are important both to help assess cause of pain, and once a diagnosis is established, to create a treatment plan which is specific to the adolescent athlete. This might include the use of a sports-minded physical therapist to address issues such as lack of strength and flexibility, which can predispose athletes to specific injury patterns. In addition, the specific maneuvers that an athlete is performing might also cause back pain. These might include improper form or excessive repetition of a particular movement such as a back bend in gymnastics or a porte-a-bras to the back in ballet.
2. Backpacks: Another possible cause of muscular back pain is the use of backpacks. In a survey of more than 100 orthopedic surgeons conducted by the American

TABLE 17.2

General Recommendations for Acute Back Strain

1. Never bend from the waist only; bend at the hips and knees.
2. When standing for a prolonged period, place one foot on a step to reduce back strain.
3. Never lift a heavy object higher than the waist.
4. Never sleep on the abdomen; it is best to sleep on one side with hips and knees bent. Use a firm mattress or put a 3/4-in. plywood board under a soft mattress.
5. When sitting, place the spine up against the back of the chair, and be sure one or both knees are higher than the hips.
6. Shoes should have low heels.

Academy of Orthopaedic Surgeons, 58% of the respondents reported seeing patients who complained of back and shoulder pain caused by heavy backpacks. Although serious problems due to backpacks are now recognized to be rare, these patients should be encouraged to balance the load over both shoulders, avoid excessive weight, or to use a rolling pack if the backpack continues to cause symptoms.

3. Treatment: Most acute back pain, especially those associated with muscular strain, resolve in a relatively short period: 70% within 1 week, 80% by 2 weeks, and 90% by 2 months. For back pain secondary to muscular strain, the treatment includes back exercise, weight reduction, nonsteroidal antiinflammatory medications, and sometimes a change in activities. Steroids and muscle relaxants are generally not indicated. For acute strain, cryotherapy using ice in a towel or a wet towel that has been kept in the freezer is helpful. It can be applied for 15 to 20 minutes, four times a day, for at least the first 3 days. After that time, cold can be replaced with heat (e.g., heating pad, moist hot towel). Further information can be found in the Tables 17.2 and 17.3 and at the Web sites listed at the end of this chapter. Some adolescents may benefit from referral to a physical therapist for cryotherapy, ultrasound, or electrical stimulation. Usually, the pain will resolve within 4 to 6 weeks.

Bone-Related Back Pain

Bone-related back pain may account for 25% to 50% of back pain in adolescents but is especially common in those who are involved in athletics. This is generally related to overuse syndromes in athletes who perform repetitive extension maneuvers, such as gymnasts, figure skaters, ballerinas, or volleyball players. The common presentation is lumbar pain with extension.

Keys to diagnosis of bone-related pain include:

- Pain on bending backward should be considered bone related until proved otherwise.

TABLE 17.3

Back Exercises

Back exercises should be begun slowly and increased slowly over time.
1. Knee hug
   a. Lie on back with pillow under head; inhale.
   b. Slowly raise knees to chest.
   c. Clasp knees with hands and hold for count of 10.
   d. Repeat three times and build slowly to 20 repetitions per day.
2. Cat backs
   a. Get on all fours on the floor.
   b. Arch back up like a cat and then down as far as possible.
   c. Repeat three times and build slowly to 20 repetitions per day.
3. Leg lifts
   a. Lie on stomach with arms at sides.
   b. Raise each leg in turn, to a height of 1 ft off the floor.
   c. Start with three lifts of each leg and build slowly to 20 per day.
4. Back flattener
   a. Lie on back, knees raised, with feet on floor and hands over head.
   b. Tighten stomach and buttock muscles at the same time to flatten back against floor; hold for a count of 10.
   c. Repeat three times and build slowly to 20 repetitions per day.
5. Shoulder lifts
   a. Lie flat on stomach with arms at side.
   b. Lift both shoulders 6 in. off the floor.
   c. Start with three lifts and build slowly to 20 per day.
6. Posture check
   a. Stand with back to wall; press heels, rump, shoulders, and head against wall.
   b. Move feet forward and bend knees so that the back slides down a few inches.
   c. Tighten abdominal and buttock muscles so the lower back is flat against wall.
   d. Hold this position and walk feet back so that the back slides up the wall.
   e. Standing straight, walk away from wall and around the room.
7. Sit-ups (should be started several weeks after exercises have begun)
   a. Lie flat on back with knees bent.
   b. Sit up to an upright position while grasping knees.
   c. Return to starting position.
   d. Start with three repetitions and build slowly to 20 per day.

- Back pain that awakens the teen from sleep and worsens with sleep and not activity is suspicious for bone neoplasm, most commonly benign osteoid osteoma.

Spondylolysis and Spondylolisthesis

In overuse or repetitive stress injury, bone-related pain is related to edema in the bone and is a sign that could progress to an overt stress fracture—spondylolysis, a crack in the pars interarticularis. In one study of young athletes who presented to a sports medicine clinic with back pain, 50% had spondylolysis (Micheli and Wood, 1995). It should be noted that most individuals though are asymptomatic. In a study of 145 Indiana University football players screened for spondylolysis, 47% with spondylolysis were asymptomatic when they started college and 40% were still pain free at graduation (McCarroll et al., 1986).

1. Etiology: Spondylolysis is a defect of the pars interarticularis, a posterior element of the spine. Spondylolysis can be either acquired or developmental. Spondylolisthesis is the forward slippage of one vertebra on another, almost always L5 on S1. These two conditions often occur together, and they represent the most common cause of chronic low-back pain in the adolescent. Adolescents who participate in athletic endeavors involving large extension forces across the low back are at high risk. These include gymnasts, ballet dancers, wrestlers, and down linemen.
2. Clinical symptoms: Pain localizes in the low back, sometimes radiating into the buttocks. Pain is aggravated with sporting activities or heavy lifting. Hamstring tightness is a hallmark of both of these conditions. A noticeable lordosis may be seen with significant spondylolisthesis.
3. Diagnosis: On physical examination, pain with extension is the hallmark feature of the examination (pain bending backwards). Pain may be present when bending backwards, or patients may have a positive "stork sign" (pain bending backwards while standing supported on one foot). Point tenderness is often present. The radiological diagnosis of spondylolisthesis is simple. Standing lateral films, especially the "spot lateral" film, centered on the L5-S1 junction, demonstrates the slip.

   Diagnosis of spondylolysis is more difficult. Occasionally it can be seen on lateral films, but more commonly it is demonstrated on oblique films that bring out the profile of the pars interarticularis. A bone scan with single-photon emission computed tomography (SPECT) imaging is the most sensitive study for spondylolysis. It demonstrates the early stages of a stress fracture, before the pars interarticularis actually breaks. Increasingly, MRI is being used to evaluate for the presence of spondylolysis.
4. Treatment: Treatment of spondylolysis in the adolescent is largely nonoperative. Modification of activities, especially avoiding hyperextension, along with nonsteroidal antiinflammatory drugs (NSAIDs), physical therapy, and possibly a lumbosacral orthosis have a high rate of success. Patients who fail nonoperative therapy can have an in situ fusion or repair of the pars defect. A 2005 study clearly demonstrated the importance of activity limitation in determining good outcomes in spondylolysis. Patients should be warned that symptom resolution may take 2 to 3 months of activity limitation.

Treatment of spondylolisthesis depends on the percentage of the slip. Meyerding's 5-category classification system is often used to measure the degree of slippage. Meyerding's grade I is a 1% to 25% slip and grade II is a 26% to 50% slip. Slips of 50% or more are considered high grade and include grade III of 51% to 75% slip, grade IV of 76% to 100% slip, and grade V spondyloptosis is a slip >100% (Meyerding, 1947). Those patients with >50% slippage require fusion. If the slip percentage is <50%, treatment can be nonoperative with close monitoring to see whether the slip progresses. Seitsalo et al. (1991) demonstrated that 90% of slip progression had occurred in their patients by the time of the first radiographic study. If pain is refractory to nonoperative measures or progressive slippage is demonstrated, in situ fusion has a high success rate.

Slipped Vertebral Apophysis (Apophyseal Ring Fracture)

This injury is unique to the pediatric population. It is a fracture through the junction of the bony vertebral body and its cartilaginous endplate (apophysis). The apophysis herniates into the canal along with fragments of disc. It is usually seen in adolescent boys who are involved in sports or heavy lifting. Symptoms are acute onset of back pain, often with sciatica. Plain films may show a bony fragment in the canal. In this case, a computed tomographic scan, rather than MRI, shows the pathology better, because it shows cortical bone more clearly. Treatment parallels that for a herniated disc. Nonoperative therapy may bring resolution of symptoms. Neurological compromise or failure of nonoperative therapy is an indication for operative decompression.

Neoplasm

Bone tumors Thankfully, most spinal neoplasms in the adolescent are benign. Osteoid osteoma and osteoblastoma are the most common bone tumors in the pediatric population. Patients may present with back pain that is dramatically improved with NSAIDs. Pain may occur at the same time every day. The neurological examination finding is usually normal. During painful episodes the patient may demonstrate a stiff spine. Because of their small size, osteoid osteomas may be difficult to see on plain films. They show intense uptake on bone scans, and computed tomographic scanning helps delineate the exact location of the tumor. The patient may be treated with long-term NSAID use, because these tumors usually resolve spontaneously after skeletal maturity is reached. However, this may mean years of NSAID use, and the family may be unwilling to follow that course. The tumor can be successfully treated with surgical excision, but that may be difficult depending on its location.

Acute leukemia Back pain may be the presenting symptom of acute leukemia which sometimes may cause vertebral collapse. Approximately 90% of leukemic patients who present with vertebral collapse have an abnormal peripheral smear. Early leukemic infiltration of the vertebral body causes osteopenia before collapse.

Treatment of leukemia is with chemotherapy; a thoracolumbosacral orthosis (TLSO) helps prevent further deformity of the spine.

Spinal cord tumor Spinal cord tumors are most common in the first decade of life. Pain is usually severe and unrelenting. Constant back pain, pain that awakens the teen at night, painful scoliosis, and neurological findings are all warning signs for spinal cord tumors. As many as 90% of patients with spinal cord tumors demonstrate rigidity of the spine. MRI is the imaging modality of choice when a spinal cord tumor is suspected. Astrocytomas and ependymomas are the most common spinal cord tumors.

Discogenic (Nerve-Related) Back Pain

While discogenic back pain is fairly common in adults, it accounts for 10% or less of back pain in adolescents. This pain is related to herniation of an intervertebral disk and subsequent impingement on a central or peripheral nerve. Findings suggestive of discogenic pain include the following:

- Lumbar spine pain that worsens with bending forward
- May be accompanied by pain radiating into the hip or thigh
- Pain that tends to wax and wane
- Positive straight leg-raising test result
- Decrease in patellar or Achilles reflex

Herniated Nucleus Pulposus

Disc herniation in an adolescent is most likely to result from an acute event. Acute onset of back pain, especially with pain radiating into the legs, raises the possibility of a disc herniation. However, discogenic pain may be chronic and have a tendency to wax and wane. An AP and lateral view of the lumbar spine may be helpful in finding an underlying bone cause of discogenic pain; however, MRI is the study of choice for the diagnosis of a herniated disc. Nonoperative treatment is often successful and includes activity restriction (but bed rest is not recommended), NSAIDs, and physical therapy. Epidural steroid injections may also be of value. Disc excision is reserved for those patients with persistent neurological deficit or in whom nonoperative therapy to produce pain relief has failed.

Other Causes

Scheuermann Kyphosis

Scheuermann kyphosis (see Chapter 15) is a rigid kyphosis of the thoracic spine. Patients often present with pain at the apex of their deformity. The cause remains undetermined. It is most often seen in adolescent males who are involved in heavy lifting. Physical examination reveals a sharp, rigid kyphosis that is best seen from the side when the patient is in the forward bend position. Diagnosis is made on standing lateral films of the entire spine. Radiographs reveal irregularities of the endplates, wedging of the vertebrae, and Schmorl nodes (invagination of disc material into the vertebral body).

Treatment depends on the degree of kyphosis, the amount of growth remaining, and the amount of pain. Physical therapy is often helpful in improving symptoms. Brace treatment can produce some correction of the kyphosis, but only in the skeletally immature patients.

For severe kyphosis or intractable pain, spinal fusion with instrumentation may be required.

Atypical or lumbar Scheuermann disease is a painful condition of the lumbar spine. Unlike classic Scheuermann disease, there is no kyphosis, but radiographs show irregularities of the lumbar spine endplates. Treatment is almost always nonoperative. Physical therapy, NSAIDs, and occasional use of an orthosis usually give relief from symptoms.

Discitis and Vertebral Osteomyelitis

Once thought to be separate entities, these two conditions are probably part of the same disease spectrum. Patients present with back pain, malaise, and fever. The physical examination is remarkable for localized tenderness and spine rigidity.

Plain radiographs may reveal disc space narrowing and irregularities of the vertebral body. Laboratory work in a suspected infection should include a complete blood count (CBC) with differential (often normal), erythrocyte sedimentation rate (usually elevated), and blood culture (which reveals an organism in only 41% of cases). In the early stages of infection, plain films may be normal. Technetium bone scanning shows increased uptake in the endplates. However, MRI has the benefit of establishing not only the presence of infection but also the amount of vertebral involvement and the possible presence of an epidural abscess.

Treatment of these conditions is somewhat controversial. Because most of these infections are caused by *Staphylococcus aureus*, the need for vertebral or disc aspiration is unclear. Most patients respond to bed rest and intravenous antibiotics and are then switched to oral antibiotics and mobilization with a TLSO. There is a body of literature that has shown successful treatment of discitis with immobilization without antibiotics. The recurrence rate appears to be higher when antibiotics are not used. Decompression of these infections is usually not needed unless there is neurological compromise or a failure to respond to nonoperative management. The possibility of tuberculosis infection should not be overlooked.

Rheumatologic Disease

Rheumatologic diseases should certainly be considered when the history is unclear, there is no trauma, and systemic symptoms such as fever or fatigue are present. If the history is consistent with a spondyloarthropathy or other arthritic conditions, CBC, sedimentation rate, and human leukocyte antigen (HLA)-B27 tests should be considered.

Psychogenic Pain

This is an important cause of back pain; however, its consideration should not preclude an appropriate investigation for other potential diagnoses. Further evaluation may be required in some teens, including plain films, bone scan, MRI, and laboratory evaluation. However, not all patients need all of these tests, particularly if the history and examination are consistent with psychogenic pain and the mental health history is consistent with the diagnosis. The possibility of back pain referred from other anatomical locations (e.g., pyelonephritis, endometritis) must not be overlooked. When symptoms exceed physical findings, clinical suspicion should be raised. These patients need help, and they will benefit from being referred to appropriate health care providers.

WEB SITES

For Teenagers and Parents

http://www.ninds.nih.gov/health_and_medical/disorders/backpain_doc.htm. National Institutes of Health site on back pain.

http://familydoctor.org/flowcharts/531.html. Patient care flow chart on diagnosis from American Academy of Family Physicians.

http://www.physsportsmed.com/issues/1997/08aug/shiplepa.htm. Exercise photos from Physician and Sportsmedicine.

http://www.physsportsmed.com/issues/1997/01jan/back_pa.htm. Posture recommendations from Physician and Sportsmedicine.

http://orthoinfo.aaos.org/fact/thr_report.cfm?Thread_ID=17&topcategory=Spine&searentry =minimize%20problems. Exercises from American Academy of Orthopaedic Surgeons.

http://orthoinfo.aaos.org/fact/thr_report.cfm?Thread_ID=105&topcategory=Spine. Information on backpacks and back pain in children from the American Academy of Orthopaedic Surgeons.

http://www.spine-health.com. Site for information on spine health.

REFERENCES AND ADDITIONAL READINGS

American College Health Association. *American College Health Association—National College Health Assessment (ACHA-NCHA) Web Summary*. Accessed April 2007 at: http://www.acha-ncha.org/docs/ACHA-NCHA_Reference_Group_Report_Spring2006.pdf.

Balague F, Dutoit G, Waldburger M. Low back pain in schoolchildren. *Scand J Rehabil Med* 1988;20:175.

Bellah RD, Summerville DA, Treves ST, et al. Low back pain in adolescent athletes: detection of stress injury to the pars interarticularis with SPECT. *Radiology* 1991;180:509.

Bodner RJ, Heyman S, Drummond DS, et al. The use of single photon emission computed tomography (SPECT) in the diagnosis of low-back pain in young patients. *Spine* 1988;13:1155.

Bunnell WA. Back pain in children. *Orthop Clin North Am* 1982;13:587.

Burton AK, Clarke RD, McClune TD, et al. The natural history of low back pain in adolescents. *Spine* 1996;21:2323.

Delamarter RB, Sachs BL, Thompson GH, et al. Primary neoplasms of the thoracic and lumbar spine: an analysis of 29 consecutive cases. *Clin Orthop* 1990;256:87.

Deyo RA, Diehl AK. Lumbar spine films in primary care: current use and effects of selective ordering criteria. *J Gen Intern Med* 1986;1:20.

Deyo RA, Rainville J, Kent DL. What can the history and physical examination tell us about low back pain? *JAMA* 1992;268:760.

Dormans JP, Pill SG. Benign and malignant tumors of the spine in children. In: Drummond DS, ed. *Spine: state-of-the-art reviews—strategies in the pediatric spine*, Vol. 14, No. 1. Philadelphia: Hanley & Belfus, 2000:263.

Dyment PG. Low back pain in adolescents. *Pediatr Ann* 1991;20:170.

Ecker ML. Back pain. In: Drummond DS, ed. *Spine: state-of-the-art reviews—strategies in the pediatric spine*, Vol. 14, No. 1. Philadelphia: Hanley & Belfus, 2000:233.

El Rassi G, Takemitsu M, Woratanarat P, et al. Lumbar spondylolysis in pediatric and adolescent soccer players. *Am J Sports Med* 2005;33:1688.

Fairbanks J, Pynsent PB, Poortvliet JA, et al. Influence of anthropometric factors and joint laxity in the incidence of adolescent back pain. *Spine* 1984;9:461.

Frazier LM, Carey TS, Lyles MF, et al. Selective criteria may increase lumbosacral spine roentgenogram use in acute low-back pain. *Arch Intern Med* 1989;149:47.

Ginsburg GM, Bassett GS. Back pain in children and adolescents: evaluation and differential diagnosis. *J Am Acad Orthop Surg* 1997;5:67.

Glazer PA, Hu SS. Pediatric spinal infections. *Orthop Clin North Am* 1996;27:111.

Hall H. A simple approach to back-pain management. *Patient Care* 1992;26:77.

Jones GT, Macfarlane GJ. Epidemiology of low back pain in children and adolescents. *Arch Dis Child* 2005;90:312.

Kayser R, Mahlfeld K, Nebelung W, et al. Vertebral collapse and normal peripheral blood cell count at the onset of acute lymphatic leukemia in childhood. *J Pediatr Orthop B* 2000;9:55.

King HA. Back pain in children. *Orthop Clin North Am* 1999;30:467.

Kneisl JS, Simon MA. Medical management compared with operative treatment for osteoid osteoma. *J Bone Joint Surg Am* 1992;74:179.

Lonstein JE. Spondylolisthesis in children: cause, natural history, and management. *Spine* 1999;24:2640.

McCarroll JR, Miller JM, Ritter MA. Lumbar spondylolysis and spondylo.isthesis in college football players. A prospective stuy. *Am J Sports Med* 1986;14:404.

Metzel JD. Back pain in the adolescent: a user-friendly guide. *Adolesc Health Update* 2005;17:1.

Meyerding H. Low backache and sciatic pain associated with spondylolisthesis and protruded intervertebral disc: incidence, significance and treatment. *J Bone Joint Surg* 1947;23:461.

Micheli LJ, Wood R. Back pain in young athletes: significant differences from adults in causes and patterns. *Arch Pediatr Adolesc Med* 1995;149:15.

Olsen TL, Anderson RL, Dearwater SR, et al. The epidemiology of low back pain in an adolescent population. *Am J Public Health* 1992;82:606.

Pedinoff S, Pinals RS, Schwartz SA, et al. A rational workup for low-back pain. *Patient Care* 1991;25:43.

Ring D, Johnston CE II, Wenger DR. Pyogenic infectious spondylitis in children: the convergence of discitis and vertebral osteomyelitis. *J Pediatr Orthop* 1995;15:652.

Seitsalo S, Osterman K, Hyvarinen H, et al. Progression of spondylolisthesis in children and adolescents: a long-term follow-up of 272 patients. *Spine* 1991;16:417.

Selbst SM, Lavelle JM, Soyupak SK. Back pain in children who present to the emergency department. *Clin Pediatr* 1999;38:401.

Wenger DR, Frick SL. Scheuermann kyphosis. *Spine* 1999;24:2630.

Yeom J, Lee C, Shin HY, et al. Langerhans' cell histiocytosis of the spine: analysis of 23 cases. *Spine* 1999;24:1740.

CHAPTER 18

Guidelines for Physical Activity and Sports Participation

Keith J. Loud and Albert C. Hergenroeder

In 2005, more than half (56%) of students nationwide had played on sports teams sponsored by their school or community groups during the preceding 12 months (Youth Risk Behavior Surveillance [YRBS], Centers for Disease Control and Prevention, 2005). This is a marked increase from 1991 (43.5%) but has remained relatively stable since 1999 at between 55% and 57%.

Beyond organized sports participation, physical inactivity is a priority health risk behavior identified by the Centers for Disease Control and Prevention. The following are two of the objectives from *Healthy People 2010* (Department of Health and Human Services, 2000), which highlight the need for improved physical activity in youth:

1. Increase the proportion of adolescents in grades 9 through 12 who engaged in moderate physical activity for at least 30 minutes on 5 or more of the previous 7 days from 20% in 1997 to 30%.
2. Increase the proportion of adolescents in grades 9 through 12 who engaged in vigorous physical activity that promotes cardiorespiratory fitness for 20 or more minutes per occasion on 3 or more days per week from 64% in 1997 to 85%.

All health care professionals caring for adolescents should therefore be prepared to:

1. Promote physical activity for all adolescents
2. Assess the risks associated with athletic participation for individual adolescents
3. Advise on prevention strategies for athletic injury and illness
4. Diagnose and manage common activity-related morbidities and conditions

IS ATHLETIC PARTICIPATION SAFE FOR ADOLESCENTS IN GENERAL? PROMOTING PHYSICAL ACTIVITY AND FITNESS

Maturational Issues

Although it has been suggested that teens before midpuberty should not play contact sports or that teens playing contact sports should be segregated based on early, middle, or late puberty to reduce the risk of injury, there are no data to support the idea that these interventions decrease injury rates. It has been demonstrated that injury rates increase with pubertal maturation. In contact sports (Table 18.1) this finding is consistent with the understanding that injury is related to the force of impact, which increases with the speed and body mass of the athletes involved. For noncontact sports, this finding may reflect greater force generation related to greater body mass and greater fat-free mass, as well as the increase in training intensity that tends to occur as the level of competition increases with age.

Another issue is whether adult stature could be compromised by excessive sports activities and exercise in the prepubertal and pubertal years. Evidence for reduction in growth potential was reported for a group of adolescent gymnasts with a mean bone age of 12.3 ± 0.2 years who exercised for an average of 22 hour/week, compared with swimmers who exercised for a mean of 8 hour/week (Theintz et al., 1993).

A second study suggested a negative impact of gymnastics training (10–20 hour/week) on statural growth (Lindholm et al., 1994). However, the preponderance of evidence in the literature suggests that short stature in gymnastics is related to selection bias rather than intense training (Daly et al., 2000; Damsgaard et al., 2000).

Intense training by prepubertal and pubertal athletes has raised the concern that repetitive microtrauma to epiphyseal plates could affect ultimate adult height. Runners, figure skaters, and ballet dancers may train as hard as gymnasts. As for gymnasts, the consensus is that participation in sports and exercise does not have adverse effects on adult stature, timing of peak height, or rate of growth (Malina, 1994, 1995).

Physical Fitness and Conditioning

The proportion of high school students attaining the *Healthy People* activity objectives has been described. In addition, 54.2% of students nationwide were enrolled in a physical education class and 33% of students attended such a class daily in the 2005 YRBS (Centers for Diseases Control and Prevention, 2006).

Fitness has four principal components:

1. Body composition
2. Cardiovascular fitness—maximum oxygen consumption (VO_2 max) being the gold standard
3. Strength
4. Flexibility

TABLE 18.1

Classification of Sports by Contact

Contact or Collision	Limited Contact	Noncontact
Basketball	Baseball	Archery
Boxing[a]	Bicycling	Badminton
Diving	Cheerleading	Body building
Field hockey	Canoeing or kayaking (white water)	Bowling
Football	Fencing	Canoeing or kayaking (flat water)
Tackle	Field	Crew or rowing
Ice hockey[b]	High jump	Curling
Lacrosse	Pole vault	Dancing:[d]
Martial arts	Floor hockey	Ballet
Rodeo	Football	Modern
Rugby	Flag	Jazz
Ski jumping	Gymnastics	Field
Soccer	Handball	Discus
Team handball	Horseback riding	Javelin
Water polo	Racquetball	Shot put
Wrestling	Skateboarding	Golf
	Skating:	Orienteering[e]
	Ice	Power lifting
	Inline	Race walking
	Roller	Riflery
	Skiing:	Rope jumping
	Cross-country	Running
	Downhill	Sailing
	Water	Scuba diving
	Snowboarding[c]	Swimming
	Softball	Table tennis
	Squash	Tennis
	Ultimate frisbee	Track
	Volleyball	Weight lifting
	Windsurfing or surfing	

[a]Participation not recommended by the American Academy of Pediatrics.

[b]The American Academy of Pediatrics recommends limiting the amount of body checking allowed for hockey players 15 years and younger to reduce injuries.

[c]Snowboarding has been added since previous statement was published.

[d]Dancing has been further classified into ballet, modern, and jazz since previous statement was published.

[e]A race (contest) in which competitors use a map and compass to find their way through unfamiliar territory.

From Committee on Sports Medicine and Fitness. Medical conditions affecting sports participation. *Pediatrics* 2001;107:1205, with permission.

Body Composition

Although a common notion is that the fitness of today's youth is poor, the only component of fitness that has been documented to have declined in the past three decades is body composition: obesity has increased in both teens and young adults (Gortmaker et al., 1987; National Heart, Lung, and Blood Institute, 1994) (see Chapter 32).

More than one fourth (31.5%) of high school students nationwide thought they were overweight in the 2005 YRBS (Centers for Disease Control and Prevention, 2006). Overall, female students were significantly more likely than male students to consider themselves overweight (38.1% versus 25.1%, respectively). Overall, 45.6% of high school students were trying to lose weight during the 30 days preceding the YRBS survey. Female students were significantly more likely than male students to be trying to lose weight (61.7% versus 29.9%, respectively).

With respect to reducing obesity, adolescents need both reduced caloric intake and increased energy expenditure (Hergenroeder and Phillips, 1994). More adolescents choose to exercise than to diet in an attempt to lose weight in the 2005 YRBS (Centers for Disease Control and Prevention, 2006).

Cardiovascular Fitness

If the goal is to improve cardiovascular fitness, a recommended training program would include *aerobic exercise* (continuous large muscle contractions that involve maintenance of 50% to 85% of the maximum heart rate) for 20 to 25 minutes, three or four times a week. More than two thirds (68.7%) of high school students nationwide had participated in activities that made them sweat and breathe hard (i.e., vigorous physical activity) for at least 20 minutes for 3 or more of the preceding 7 days in the 2005 YRBS (Centers for Disease Control and Prevention, 2006).

Recently, emphasis has been placed on the health benefits of adopting a lifestyle approach to increasing activity, rather than a structured exercise program that may appeal least to sedentary adolescents. The Centers for Disease Control and Prevention and the American College of Sports Medicine guidelines recommend moderate-intensity physical activity on most days—either in a single session or in accumulated multiple bouts, each lasting 8 to 10 minutes (Pate et al., 1995). This involves common activities such as climbing stairs (rather than taking the elevator), brisk walking, doing more house and yard work, and engaging in active recreational pursuits.

The objective is to incorporate moderate physical activity into the lifestyle of those who are sedentary. For those who desire more intensive training, an exercise prescription should be tailored to the adolescent's current level of fitness, desired level of fitness, motivation, and discipline to adhere to a training regime. More detailed goals and practical suggestions for reaching them can be found at the *Bright Futures in Practice: Physical Activity* Online Guide (http://www.brightfutures.org/physicalactivity/).

Strength

Approximately half (51.4%) of students nationwide had done strengthening exercises (e.g., push-ups, sit-ups, weight lifting) on at least 3 of the 7 days preceding the 1997 YRBS survey (Centers for Disease Control and Prevention, 1998). Regarding strength training, it is established that prepubescent and pubescent subjects, like adults, can increase strength safely by resistance training. The training program should include close adult supervision, a preparticipation examination, and the use of well-maintained equipment (including sturdy shoes). Guidelines for resistance training in teens have been reviewed (Blimpke, 1993). Resistance training is associated with strength gains and neuromuscular adaptation in *preadolescents*, but it is not associated with muscle hypertrophy. Short-term resistance training has no effect on somatic growth or body composition and is not associated with increased injury rate or recovery or improved sports performance. Muscle hypertrophy will occur with resistance training in pubertal subjects. The American Academy of Pediatrics (AAP) endorses strength training for children and adolescents, if done properly (see policy statement, American Academy of Pediatrics, Committee on Sports Medicine and Fitness, 2001); a suggested resistance training program could include the following:

1. Establish a 10-repetition maximum (i.e., the maximum weight that can be lifted 10 times), called the *10-rep max*.
2. To start resistance training, perform one set of 10 repetitions at 50% to 75% of the 10-rep max.
3. Then perform a second set of 10 repetitions at 75% of the 10-rep max.
4. Perform a third set at 100% of the 10-rep max, doing as many repetitions as possible.

When 15 repetitions are easily performed during the third set, the weight can be increased by no more than 10% each week. The weight should be lifted through the entire ROM of the joint to avoid loss of flexibility. Warm-up and cool-down periods, which could include stretching exercises, should accompany each session. Three sessions per week on alternate days, allowing for a day of rest in between weight training sessions, is all that is recommended.

One-repetition maximum weight lifting should be avoided because it is a mechanism of injury. Gains in strength are more resistant to detraining than are gains in aerobic fitness, with up to 50% of the strength capacity retained for 1 year or longer in a person who is no longer training.

Flexibility

Nationwide, 51.3% of students had done stretching exercises (e.g., toe touching, knee bending, leg stretching) on 3 or more of the 7 days preceding the 1997 YRBS survey. There is no study demonstrating that stretching in healthy, previously uninjured subjects prevents injuries. However, improving flexibility and strength in previously injured athletes decreases the likelihood of subsequent injuries. A flexibility program for injured joints should include pain-free stretching. If a healthy teen desires a stretching program, the following may be offered: the program should consist of daily stretching. Each stretch should be held statically for 20 seconds, for five to ten repetitions.

IS ATHLETIC PARTICIPATION SAFE FOR *THIS* ADOLESCENT? THE PREPARTICIPATION EVALUATION

While 30 to 40 years ago the preparticipation physical evaluation (PPE) consisted of simply asking the teen, "Are you okay?," listening to the heart, and checking for a hernia, it has evolved in sophistication more recently. In 1992, five major medical organizations (the American Academy of Family Physicians, AAP, American Medical Society for Sports Medicine, American Orthopedic Society for Sports Medicine, and American Osteopathic Academy of Sports Medicine) produced a consensus monograph on the PPE. Updated in 1997 to include the American Heart Association's (AHA) recommendations specifically concerning cardiovascular screening (Maron et al., 1996), it is now in its third edition (Preparticipation Physical Evaluation, American Academy of Family Physicians, American Academy of Pediatrics, American College of Sports Medicine, 2005). The interested reader is directed to the sponsoring organizations' Web sites or the Physician and Sportsmedicine Web site (www.physsportsmed.com) to obtain a copy of what is referred to as *The Monograph*.

The American Medical Association (AMA) *Guidelines for Adolescent Preventive Services* (GAPS) recommends that a comprehensive health evaluation should occur at least every other year during the adolescent period. In addition, the AAP recommends that adolescents involved in strenuous activity should have a sport-specific examination on entry into both junior and senior high school and that this examination should be updated with an annual questionnaire emphasizing recent injuries and any health condition affecting sports participation. Ideally, an adolescent athlete would have an annual to biennial comprehensive health evaluation performed by his or her primary care physician (PCP), with additional sport-specific PPEs performed by a team physician who is responsive to the sponsoring athletic body and knowledgeable about the sport in question. In reality, the PPE monograph acknowledges that the PPE, which is performed primarily to meet legal requirements in 49 of 50 states, is often the only interaction that many adolescents (particularly male adolescents) have with the health care system. Therefore, it is recommended that the PPE be incorporated into a more general health maintenance visit with an established PCP. A multiexaminer, private station-based setup is less preferred, but acceptable alternative; mass screenings in large rooms such as gymnasiums are no longer consered appropriate. Details of how to structure a PPE outside the office setting can be found in *The Monograph*; the remainder of this section highlights the important elements of a history and physical examination to be performed for a PPE within a health maintenance visit. Chapter 4 details the other components of a thorough health maintenance evaluation.

Objectives

The primary objectives of the PPE, as stated in *THE MONOGRAPH*, include the following:

1. Screening for conditions that may be life-threatening or disabling
2. Screening for conditions that may predispose to injury or illness
3. Meeting administrative requirements

Acknowledging that the PPE may "serve as an entry point to the health care system for adolescents," the third edition also lists determining general health and providing opportunity to initiate discussion on health-related topics as objectives, further emphasizing the central role the adolescent primary care provider performs in this evaluation.

Logistical Considerations for the Preparticipation Physical Evaluation

Ideally, the PPE should occur at least 6 weeks before preseason practice begins, to allow time for evaluation, treatment, and rehabilitation of identified problems *before* the first weeks of practice.

History

The medical history form from *The Monograph* is shown in Figure 18.1. An earlier version can be downloaded from the American Academy of Family Physicians at their Web site (http://www.aafp.org/afp/20000815/765.html) to be completed by the athlete and/or parents for review by the physician before the examination. A partnership between the athlete and the parent in completing the form is strongly recommended.

The sport-specific history should be relatively brief to assess for the following factors:

1. Past injuries that caused the athlete to miss a game or practice. The clinician may need to ask, for example: Have you ever had a muscle pull? A pinched nerve? A back injury? The clinician may have to ask the same question in different ways: Have you ever fractured a bone? Have you ever broken a bone? Other athletes may not volunteer information if they think it will result in exclusion from sports participation.

2. Any loss of consciousness or memory occurring after a head injury.
3. Previous exclusion from sports for any reason.
4. Allergies, asthma, or exercise-induced bronchospasm.
5. Medications and supplements, used currently or in the last 6 months.
6. The menstrual history in females.
7. A history of relatively rapid increase or decrease in body weight and the athlete's perception of current body weight.

In addition, the AHA recommends the following questions for cardiovascular screening (Maron et al., 1996):

8. Family history of premature death (sudden or otherwise).
9. Family history of heart disease in surviving relatives; significant disability from cardiovascular disease in close relatives younger than 50 years; or specific knowledge of the occurrence of certain conditions (hypertrophic cardiomyopathy [HCM], long QT syndrome, Marfan syndrome, or clinically important arrhythmias).
10. Personal history of heart murmur.
11. Personal history of systemic hypertension.
12. Personal history of excessive fatigability.
13. Personal history of syncope, excessive or progressive shortness of breath, or chest pain or discomfort, particularly with exertion.

Physical Examination

GAPS does not currently require comprehensive physical examinations at each health maintenance visit. The PPE, however, does necessitate a directed examination to identify medical problems or deficits that could worsen the athlete's performance or conditions that might be worsened by athletic participation.

Many conditions that preclude participation in sports are identified in the preadolescent age-group and are not subtle. For example, congenital heart disease and hemophilia are typically detected before adolescence. However, subtle presentations of congenital defects or acquired diseases may go undetected. The most commonly detected abnormalities on PPEs are previously undetected or unrehabilitated musculoskeletal injuries. The annual PPE, especially for teenagers, should serve as "quality control" for the diagnosis and rehabilitation of injuries. With this in mind, the physical examination should include assessment of the following:

1. Height, weight, and body mass index (BMI): Obesity, by itself, is not a reason for exclusion. However, the increased risk of heat illness and how that risk might be reduced must be mentioned to the athlete, parent, and coach.
2. Blood pressure and pulse: Blood pressure should be taken in the right arm with the athlete sitting. Athletes with hypertension should be evaluated further but not excluded from participation unless the hypertension is severe, as discussed later. Pulse rate can be as low as 25 bpm in highly trained aerobic athletes. A pulse in the 40- to 50-bpm range is routine and does not need evaluation if the athlete is asymptomatic.
3. Visual acuity and pupil equality: Teens with corrected visual acuity worse than 20/40 in one or both eyes should be referred for further evaluation but are not excluded from participation if protective eyewear is worn. It is important that anisocoria be noted before any closed head injury occurs.

Ohio High School Athletic Association
Preparticipation Physical Evaluation

DATE OF EXAM:_____ Page 1 of 4

Name _____ **Sex** _____ **Age** _____ **Date of Birth** _____

Grade_____ **School** _____ **Sport(s)** _____

Address _____ **Phone** _____

Personal Physician_____

In case of emergency, contact: Name _____ *Relationship* _____

Phone (H) _____ *(W)*_____ *(Cell)*_____ *(Cell)*_____

History

This section is to be carefully completed by the student and his/her parent(s) or legal guardian(s) before participation in interscholastic athletics in order to help detect possible risks.

Explain "YES" answers in the space provided. Circle questions you don't know the answer to.

	Question	Yes	No
1.	Has a doctor ever denied or restricted you participation in sports for any reason?	☐	☐
2.	Do you have an ongoing medical condition (like diabetes or asthma)?	☐	☐
3.	Are you currently taking any prescription or nonprescription (over-the-counter) medicines or pills?	☐	☐
4.	Do you have allergies to medicines, pollens, foods, or stinging insects?	☐	☐
5.	Do you think you are in good health?	☐	☐
6.	Have you ever passed out or nearly passed out DURING exercise?	☐	☐
7.	Have you ever passed out or nearly passed out AFTER exercise?	☐	☐
8.	Have you ever had discomfort, pain, or pressure in your chest during exercise?	☐	☐
9.	Does your heart race or skip beats during exercise?	☐	☐
10.	Has a doctor ever told you that you have (check all that apply): ☐ High Blood Pressure ☐ A heart murmur ☐ High Cholesterol ☐ A heart infection		
11.	Has a doctor ever ordered a test for your heart? (for example, ECG, echocardiogram)	☐	☐
12.	Has anyone in your family died for no apparent reason?	☐	☐
13.	Does anyone in your family have a heart problem?	☐	☐
14.	Has any family member or relative died of heart problems or of sudden death before age 50?	☐	☐
15.	Does anyone in your family have Marfan syndrome?	☐	☐
16.	Have you ever spent the night in a hospital?	☐	☐
17.	Have you ever had surgery?	☐	☐
18.	Have you ever had an injury, like a sprain, muscle or ligament tear, or tendinitis, that caused you to miss a practice or game? If yes, circle affected area below:	☐	☐
19.	Have you had any broken or fractured bones or dislocated joints? If yes, circle below:	☐	☐
20.	Have you had a bone or joint injury that required x-rays, MRI, CT, surgery, injections, rehabilitation, physical therapy, a brace, a cast, or crutches? If yes, circle below:	☐	☐

Head	Neck	Shoulder	Upper arm	Elbow	Forearm	Hand / Fingers	Chest
Upper back	Lower back	Hip	Thigh	Knee	Calf/shin	Ankle	Foot / Toes

21.	Have you ever had a stress fracture?	☐	☐
22.	Have you been told that you have or have you had an x-ray for atlantoaxial (neck) instability?	☐	☐
23.	Do you regularly use a brace or assistive device?	☐	☐
24.	Has a doctor ever told you that you have asthma or allergies?	☐	☐

	Question	Yes	No
25.	Do you cough, wheeze, or have difficulty breathing during or after exercise?	☐	☐
26.	Is there anyone in your family who has asthma?	☐	☐
27.	Have you ever used an inhaler or taken asthma medicine?	☐	☐
28.	Were you born without or are you missing a kidney, an eye, a testicle, or any other organ?	☐	☐
29.	Have you had infectious mononucleosis (mono) within the last month?	☐	☐
30.	Do you have any rashes, pressure sores, or other skin problems?	☐	☐
31.	Have you had a herpes skin infection?	☐	☐
32.	Have you ever had a head injury or concussion?	☐	☐
33.	Have you been hit in the head and been confused or lost your memory?	☐	☐
34.	Have you ever had a seizure?	☐	☐
35.	Do you have headaches with exercise?	☐	☐
36.	Have you ever had numbness, tingling, or weakness in your arms or legs after being hit or falling?	☐	☐
37.	Have you ever been unable to move your arms or legs after being hit or falling?	☐	☐
38.	When exercising in the heat, do you have severe muscle cramps or become ill?	☐	☐
39.	Has a doctor told you that you or someone in your family has sickle cell trait or sickle cell disease?	☐	☐
40.	Have you had any problems with your eyes or vision?	☐	☐
41.	Do you wear glasses or contact lenses?	☐	☐
42.	Do you wear protective eyewear, such as goggles or a face shield?	☐	☐
43.	Are you happy with your weight?	☐	☐
44.	Are you trying to gain or lose weight?	☐	☐
45.	Has anyone recommended you change your weight or eating habits?	☐	☐
46.	Do you limit or carefully control what you eat?	☐	☐
47.	Do you have any concerns that you would like to discuss with a doctor?	☐	☐

FEMALES ONLY

48.	Have you ever had a menstrual period?	☐	☐
49.	How old were you when you had your first menstrual period?		_____
50.	How many periods have you had in the last 12 months?		_____

Explain "Yes" Answers Here: (Attach additional sheets as needed)

_____
_____
_____
_____
_____
_____

I (we) hereby state, to the best of my (our) knowledge, my (our) answers to the above questions are complete and correct.

Signature: _____   Signature: _____   Date: _____
         Athlete   Parent or Guardian (If athlete is under 18)

The student has family insurance ☐ Yes ☐ No; If yes, family insurance company name and policy number: _____

NOTE: CONSENT AND HIPAA RELEASE FORMS THAT MUST BE SIGNED BY BOTH THE PARENT AND THE STUDENT ARE ON A SEPARATE SHEET.
NOTE: HISTORY AND ALL CONSENT FORMS MUST BE COMPLETED PRIOR TO PHYSICAL EXAMINATION

Modified from American Academy of Family Physicians, American Academy of Pediatrics, American College of Sports Medicine, American Medical Society for Sports Medicine, American Orthopaedic Society for Sports Medicine, and American Osteopathic Academy of Sports Medicine, 2004. Rev. 03/06

FIGURE 18.1 Preparticipation sports evaluation form. (From the Ohio High School Athletic Association (OHSAA), http://www.ohsaa.org, with permission.)

4. Skin: Infections that are highly contagious (e.g., varicella, impetigo) should be identified. Players with these infections need to be noninfectious before returning to sports in which skin-to-skin contact is possible (Table 18.2).
5. Teeth and mouth: These are examined only if the history suggests an acute problem.
6. Cardiac examination: AHA recommendations for PPE cardiac examination include the following (Maron et al., 1996):
   a. Perform precordial auscultation in supine and standing positions to identify heart murmurs consistent with dynamic left ventricular outflow obstruction.
   b. Assess femoral artery or lower extremity pulses to exclude coarctation of the aorta.
   c. Recognize the physical stigmata of Marfan syndrome; refer the teenager for further evaluation if a male taller than 6 ft or a female taller than 5 ft 10 in. has a family history of two of the following:
      • Kyphosis
      • High-arched palate
      • Pectus excavatum
      • Arachnodactyly
      • Arm span > height
      • Murmur (mitral valve prolapse or aortic)
      • Myopia
      • Lens dislocation
      • Thumb or wrist signs
   d. Assess brachial artery blood pressure in the sitting position.
   e. Document the presence of murmurs, clicks, or rubs (see Chapter 14). Normal or physiological murmurs are characteristically <4/6 systolic murmurs that decrease from supine to standing with no diastolic component, and with a normal physiological split second heart sound (S_2). The murmur of HCM, if one is present, may sound like a normal murmur except that it increases in intensity when the patient moves from the supine to the standing position.
7. Abdomen: Organomegaly is a disqualifying condition for collision/contact or limited-contact sports until definitive evaluation and individual assessment for clearance has been completed.
8. Genitalia: An undescended testicle is not a contraindication to participation in contact sports; however, the player should wear a protective cup to protect the other, descended testis. An evaluation for the unidentified testis is necessary.
9. Sexual maturation stage: Tanner stage assessment for sexual maturity is appropriate for adolescents, but it has no role in deciding whether the teen should play a given sport.
10. Musculoskeletal screening: General musculoskeletal screening should include muscle strength, range-of-motion and joint-stability testing, and evaluation for structural abnormalities of major joints (e.g., ankle, knee, shoulder, elbow, back). An efficient musculoskeletal screening examination is demonstrated in Figures 18.2 to 18.11. A more in-depth examination of the specific body parts should be pursued if there are concerns from the history or general screening examination (listed in parentheses are diagnoses to consider if the examination finding is abnormal):
    a. Body symmetry (Figs. 18.2 to 18.11): Observe the adolescent standing with arms at the sides, dressed in shorts and a shirt that allows inspection of the distal quadriceps muscles and acromioclavicular joints, respectively. Look for the following:
       • Head tilted or turned to side (consider primary cervical spine injury, primary or secondary trapezius, or cervical muscle spasm)
       • Asymmetry of shoulder heights (trapezius spasm, shoulder injury, scoliosis)
       • Enlarged acromioclavicular joint (previous acromioclavicular joint sprain, shoulder separation)
       • Asymmetrical iliac crest heights (scoliosis or leg-length difference, back spasm)
       • Swollen knee; prominent tibial tuberosity (any knee injury, Osgood-Schlatter disease). Ask the athlete to contract ("tighten") the quadriceps muscles, and look for atrophy of the vastus medialis obliquus, a characteristic of any knee or lower extremity injury in which the athlete avoids normal use of that leg.
       • Swollen ankle (unrehabilitated ankle sprain)
    b. Neck examination (Fig. 18.3): This is especially important in players with a previous history of neck injury and brachial plexopathy (referred to as *stingers* or *burners*).
       • Have the athlete do the following maneuvers:
         – Look at the floor (cervical flexion).
         – Look at the ceiling (cervical extension).
         – Look over the left shoulder, then over the right shoulder (left and right rotation, respectively).
         – Put right ear on right shoulder, then left ear on left shoulder (right and left lateral flexion).
       • Look for limited or asymmetrical motion with the maneuvers listed (neck injury, congenital cervical abnormalities). *Any athlete with limitation of range of motion (ROM), weakness or pain on neck examination is excluded from contact or collision sports until further evaluation.*
    c. Shoulder examination (Fig. 18.4)
       • Have the athlete raise the arms from the side and touch the hands above the head, keeping elbows extended (full abduction). Look for the following:
         – Asymmetric elevation of shoulder before arms reach 90 degrees (shoulder weakness due to a brachial plexopathy, shoulder instability, impingement syndrome).
         – Inability to raise arms to full abduction position (shoulder weakness due to brachial plexopathy, impingement syndrome, or apprehension from subluxation or dislocation).
       • Have athlete hold the arms in front of the body (forward flexion) and then to the side (90 degrees abduction); examiner should push the hands down. Look for asymmetrical atrophy or fasciculations of anterior and middle deltoid muscles and pain and/or weakness (may be indicative of a variety of shoulder problems).
       • Have athlete put hands behind head (maximal external rotation/abduction). Look for the following:
         – Inability to get hand behind head (i.e., lack of external rotation of shoulder).
         – Apprehension or inability to pull the elbows, symmetrically, posterior to the shoulder (anterior subluxation or dislocation).
         – An athlete with limitation of motion should be evaluated further before clearance is granted for further participation.

TABLE 18.2

Medical Conditions and Sports Participation[a]

Condition	May Participate?
Atlantoaxial instability (instability of the joint between cervical vertebrae 1 and 2)	Qualified yes
Explanation: Athlete needs evaluation to assess risk of spinal cord injury during sports participation.	
Bleeding disorder	Qualified yes
Explanation: Athlete needs evaluation.	
Cardiovascular diseases	
Carditis (inflammation of the heart)	No
Explanation: Carditis may result in sudden death with exertion.	
Hypertension (high blood pressure)	Qualified yes
Explanation: Those with significant essential (unexplained) hypertension should avoid weight and power lifting, body building, and strength training; those with secondary hypertension (hypertension caused by a previously identified disease) or severe essential hypertension need evaluation. The National High Blood Pressure Education Working group defined significant and severe hypertension.	
Congenital heart disease (structural heart defects present at birth)	Qualified yes
Explanation: Those with mild forms may participate fully; those with moderate or severe forms and those who have undergone surgery need evaluation. The 36th Bethesda Conference defined mild, moderate, and severe disease for common cardiac lesions.	
Dysrhythmia (irregular heart rhythm)	Qualified yes
Explanation: Those with symptoms (chest pain, syncope, dizziness, shortness of breath, or other symptoms of possible dysrhythmia) or evidence of mitral regurgitation (leaking) on physical examination need evaluation. All others may participate fully.	
Heart murmur	Qualified yes
Explanation: If the murmur is innocent (does not indicate heart disease), full participation is permitted; otherwise the athlete needs evaluation (see Congenital heart disease and Mitral valve prolapse discussed earlier).	
Cerebral palsy	Qualified yes
Explanation: Athlete needs evaluation.	
Diabetes mellitus	Yes
Explanation: All sports can be played with proper attention to diet, blood glucose concentration, hydration, and insulin therapy. Blood glucose concentration should be monitored every 30 min during continuous exercise and 15 min after completion of exercise.	
Diarrhea	Qualified no
Explanation: Unless disease in mild, no participation is permitted, because diarrhea may increase the risk of dehydration and heat illness (see "Fever" in this table).	
Eating disorders	Qualified yes
Anorexia nervosa	
Bulimia nervosa	
Explanation: These patients need both medical and psychiatric assessment before participation.	
Eyes	
Functionally one-eyed athlete	Qualified yes
Loss of an eye	
Detached retina	
Previous eye surgery or serious eye injury	
Explanation: A functionally one-eyed athlete has a best corrected visual acuity of <20/40 in the eye with worse activity. These athletes would suffer significant disability if the better eye were seriously injured, as would those with loss of an eye. Some athletes who have previously undergone eye surgery or had a serious eye injury may have an increased risk of injury because of weakened eye tissue. Availability of eye guards approved by the American Society for Testing Materials (ASTM) and other protective equipment may allow participation in most sports, but this must be judged on an individual basis.	

TABLE 18.2

(Continued)

Condition	May Participate?
Fever	No
Explanation: Fever can increase cardiopulmonary effort, reduce maximum exercise capacity, make heat illness more likely, and increase orthostatic hypotension during exercise; fever may rarely accompany myocarditis or other infections that may make exercise dangerous.	
Heat illness, history of	Qualified yes
Explanation: Because of the increased likelihood of recurrence, the athlete needs individual assessment to determine the presence of predisposing conditions and to arrange a prevention strategy.	
Hepatitis	Yes
Explanation: Because of the apparent minimal risk to others, all sports may be played that the athlete's state of health allows. In all athletes, skin lesions should be covered properly and athletic personnel should use universal precautions when handling blood or body fluids with visible blood.	
Human immunodeficiency virus infection	Yes
Explanation: Because of the apparent minimal risk to others, all sports may be played as allowed by the athlete's state of health; in all athletes, skin lesions should be covered properly, and athletic personnel should use universal precautions when handling blood or body fluids with visible blood.	
Kidney, absence of one	Qualified yes
Explanation: Athlete needs individual assessment for contact/collision and limited-contact sports.	
Liver, enlarged	Qualified yes
Explanation: If the liver is acutely enlarged, participation should be avoided because of risk of rupture; if the liver is chronically enlarged, individual assessment is needed before collision/contact or limited-contact sports are played.	
Malignant neoplasm	Qualified yes
Explanation: Athlete needs individual assessment.	
Musculoskeletal disorders	Qualified yes
Explanation: Athlete needs individual assessment.	
Neurological disorders	
History of serious head or spine trauma, severe or repeated concussions, or craniotomy	Qualified yes
Explanation: Athlete needs individual assessment for collision, contact or limited-contacted sports, and also for noncontact sports if deficits in judgment or cognition are present; research supports a conservative approach to management of concussion.	
Seizure disorder, well controlled	Yes
Explanation: Risk of seizure during participation is minimal.	
Seizure disorder, poorly controlled	Qualified yes
Explanation: Athlete needs individual assessment for collision/contact or limited-contact sports. The following noncontact sports should be avoided: archery, riflery, swimming, weight or power lifting, strength training, and sports involving heights. In these sports, occurrence of a seizure may be a risk to self or others.	
Obesity	Qualified yes
Explanation: Because of the risk of heat illness, obese persons need careful acclimatization and hydration.	
Organ transplant recipient	Qualified yes
Explanation: Athlete needs individual assessment.	
Ovary, absence of one	Yes
Explanation: Risk of severe injury to the remaining ovary is minimal.	
Respiratory conditions	
Pulmonary compromise including cystic fibrosis	Qualified yes
Explanation: Athlete needs individual assessment, but generally all sports may be played if oxygenation remains satisfactory during a graded exercise test. Patients with cystic fibrosis need acclimatization and good hydration to reduce the risk of heat illness.	

(continued)

TABLE 18.2

(Continued)

Condition	May Participate?
Asthma	Yes
Explanation: With proper medication and education, only athletes with the most severe asthma will have to modify their participation.	
Acute upper respiratory infection	Qualified yes
Explanation: Upper respiratory obstruction may affect pulmonary function; athlete needs individual assessment for all but mild disease (see "Fever" in this table).	
Sickle cell disease	Qualified yes
Explanation: Athlete needs individual assessment. In general, if status of the illness permits, all but high-exertion, collision, or contact sports may be played. Overheating, dehydration, and chilling must be avoided.	
Sickle cell trait	Yes
Explanation: It is unlikely that individuals with sickle cell trait have an increased risk of sudden death or other medical problems during athletic participation except under the most extreme conditions of heat, humidity, and possibly increased altitude. These individuals, like all athletes, should be carefully conditioned, acclimatized, and hydrated to reduce any possible risk.	
Skin disorders: boils, herpes simplex, impetigo, scabies, molluscum contagiosum	Qualified yes
Explanation: While the patient is contagious, participation in gymnastics with mats, martial arts, wrestling, or other collision, contact, or limited-contact sports is not allowed.	
Spleen, enlarged	Qualified yes
Explanation: Patients with acutely enlarged spleens should avoid all sports because of risk of rupture; those with chronically enlarged spleens need individual assessment before playing collision, contact, or limited-contact sports.	
Testicle, absent or undescended	Yes
Explanation: Certain sports may require a protective cup.	

*a*This table is designed for use by medical and nonmedical personnel.

"Needs evaluation" means a physician with appropriate knowledge and experience should assess the safety of a given sport for an athlete with the listed medical condition. Unless otherwise noted, this is because of the variability of the severity of the disease, the risk of injury for the specific sports listed in the preceding text, or both.

From Committee on Sports Medicine and Fitness. Medical conditions affecting sports participation. *Pediatrics* 2001;107:1205, with permission.

d. Elbow and hand
  - Have athlete extend and flex elbows with arms to the side (90 degrees abduction) (Fig. 18.5). Look for asymmetrical elbow extension or flexion (prior dislocation or fracture, osteochondritis dissecans).
  - With arms at sides and elbows flexed 90 degrees, have the athlete pronate and supinate forearms (Fig. 18.6). Look for asymmetrical loss of motion (residual of forearm fractures, Little League elbow, osteochondritis dissecans of elbow). The cause of a limitation in ROM of the elbow should be established before a young athlete is cleared for participation, especially in throwing sports.
  - In the same position, have the athlete spread fingers, then make a fist (Fig. 18.7). Look for lack of finger flexion, swollen joints, finger deformities (residuals of sprains, fractures). Hand injuries should be evaluated and recommendations for sports participation based on the severity of the injury and the specific sport the athlete desires to play should be made. Typically, the athlete is not excluded from participation unless there is a complication of a previous fracture or tendon rupture that needs further assessment.

e. Back and leg observation
  - Have the patient stand facing away from the examiner (Fig. 18.8). Look for the following:
    - Asymmetry of waist (scoliosis, leg-length difference)
    - Elevated shoulder (scoliosis or trapezius spasm from shoulder or neck injury)
    - Depressed shoulder (scoliosis, muscle weakness)
    - Prominent rib cage (scoliosis)
    - Increased lordosis (spondylolysis, tight hip flexors, weak hamstrings)
    - Idiopathic scoliosis is not a contraindication for sports participation in almost all cases, unless the angle is severe (i.e., a Cobb angle >45 degrees). If pain is present or there is a left major thoracic or lumbar scoliosis, then the diagnosis may not be idiopathic scoliosis and a definitive diagnosis should be established. This should include a neurological examination and magnetic resonance imaging (MRI) of the spine.

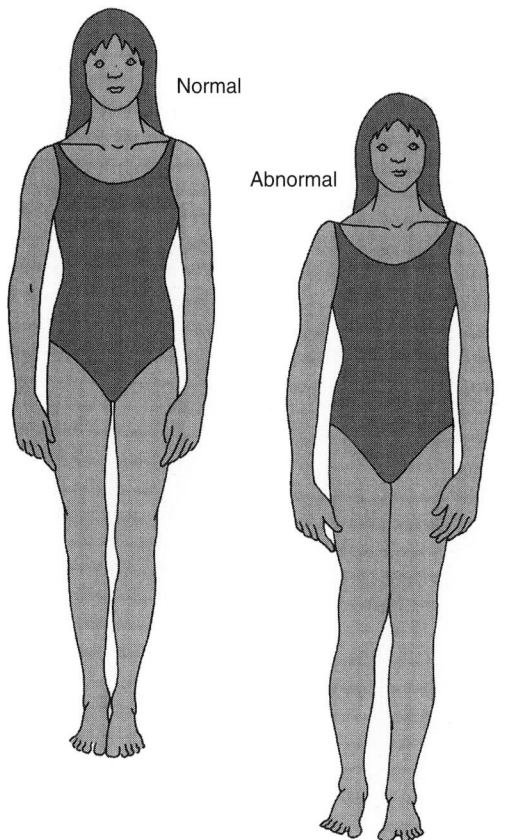

Normal

Abnormal

FIGURE 18.2 Body symmetry. (From Ross Laboratories. *For the practitioner: orthopedic screening examination for participation in sports.* Columbus, OH: Ross Products Division, Abbott Laboratories, 1981, with permission, copyright 1981 Ross Products Division, Abbott Laboratories.)

- Have athlete bend forward at waist/hips (lumbar flexion) to touch toes (Fig. 18.9). Look for the following:
  - Twisting or deviating of side (paraspinous muscle spasm)
  - Asymmetrical prominence of rib cage (scoliosis)
  - Inability to reverse the lumbar lordosis (spondylolysis, paraspinous muscle spasm caused by a chronic inflammatory condition such as ankylosing spondylitis)
- Have athlete stand straight and rise onto toes (Fig. 18.10). Look for the following:
  - Asymmetry of heel elevation (calf weakness, restricted ankle motion from sprain or fracture)
  - Asymmetry of gastrocnemius (atrophy from incompletely rehabilitated ankle or leg injury)
- Have athlete rise onto heels. Look for the following:
  - Asymmetry of elevation of forefoot or toes (weakness of ankle dorsiflexors, limitation of ankle motion from ankle fracture or sprain)
  - If asymmetry on toe or heel raising is detected, further evaluation and treatment is indicated

before the athlete is cleared for full sports participation.

f. Hip, knee, and ankle screening: Have athlete slowly assume a painless squatting position (buttocks on heels) (Fig. 18.11). If the athlete cannot do this, then further evaluation is indicated. Ask athlete to take four steps forward in this squatting position ("duck walk"), then turn 180 degrees in this squatting position and take four more steps. Look for the following:

- Asymmetry of heel height off ground (limited ankle motion or Achilles tendon tightness from tendonitis or injury).
- Asymmetrical knee flexion, that is, difference in heel-to-buttock height from the rear view or inability to get down as far on one side as on the other (knee effusion, residual limitation of motion from sprain, torn meniscus, quadriceps tightness or weakness, patellofemoral pain, Osgood-Schlatter disease).
- Pain at any point in the range of knee flexion. The cause of the pain should be established and the patient rehabilitated before allowing return to participation without restrictions.

g. Ankle screening: Have the athlete hop five times as high as possible on each foot. Inability to do so suggests an undiagnosed or unrehabilitated lower leg, ankle, or foot injury. The ankle should be evaluated and fully rehabilitated before full participation is allowed.

Laboratory Tests

Blood for hemoglobin and a dipstick of the urine for protein, glucose, and blood have been recommended as screening tests for athletic participation. Although the hemoglobin test may be indicated for general health maintenance evaluation, it is not recommended for teens who are asymptomatic. There is a particular problem diagnosing anemia in highly trained aerobic athletes, who have a reduced hematocrit due to intravascular volume expansion but a normal oxygen-carrying capacity. The urine dipstick test is not indicated in the absence of symptoms suggesting genitourinary tract dysfunction (Vehaskari and Rapola, 1982). Screening for iron deficiency in menstruating female athletes, especially those who participate in long-distance events, by measurement of serum ferritin is advocated by some experts. However, empirical iron therapy in the form of a daily multivitamin with iron may be the most cost-effective approach to preventing iron deficiency in healthy female athletes (Elliot et al., 1991).

Some centers use isokinetic or isotonic equipment to screen for muscle weakness, especially quadriceps and hamstring weakness or imbalance. This testing may be reasonable if the equipment is available free of cost to the athletes and to evaluate those with previous injuries where there is question about their recovery. However, its utility in screening all athletes has not been established. Muscle weakness can be determined through the history and physical examination.

Estimating body composition with the use of anthropometric measurements (i.e., skin folds) is indicated in wrestling because prediction equations for minimum wrestling weights have been established. Use of skin-fold measurements as screening tests is not indicated for most

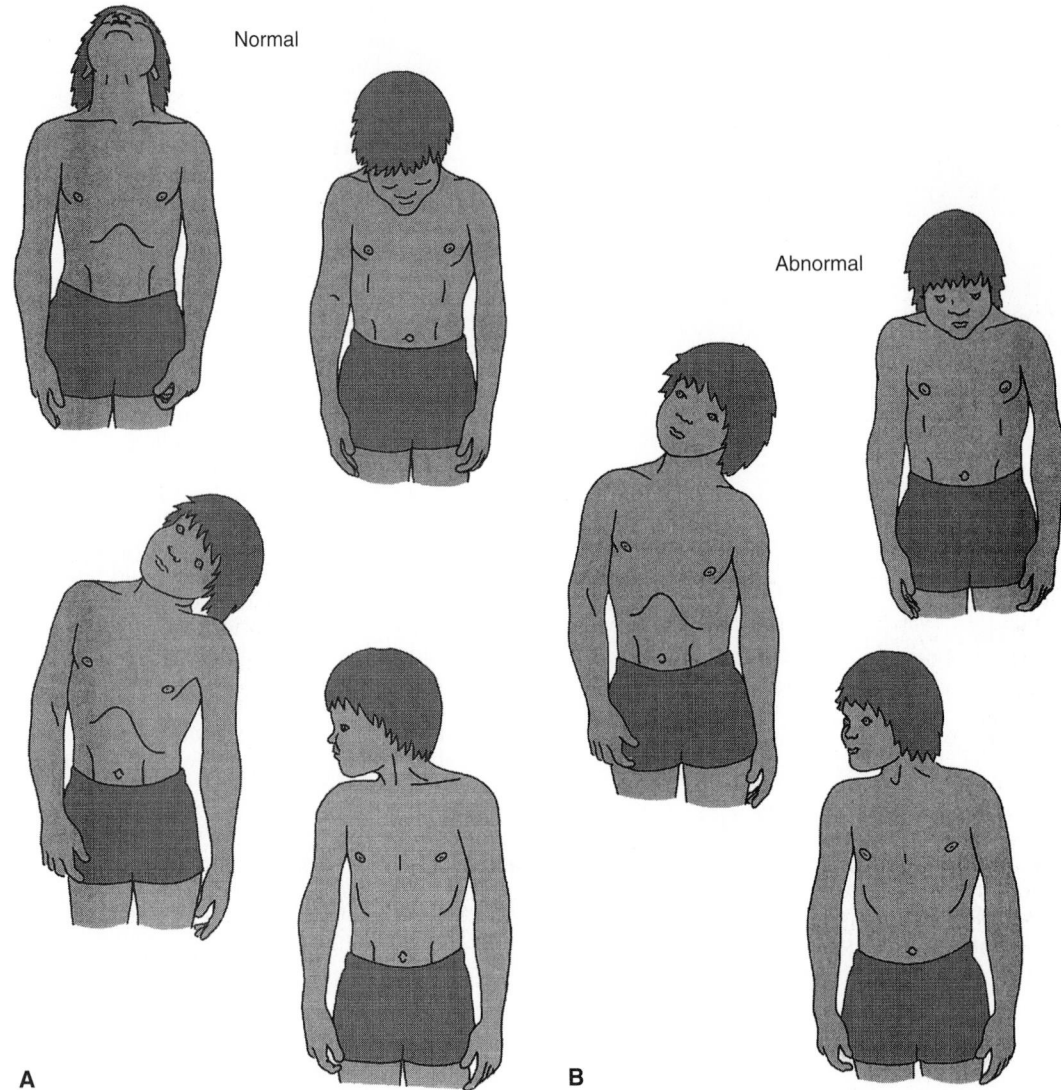

Normal

Abnormal

A B

FIGURE 18.3 Neck symmetry. (From Ross Laboratories. *For the practitioner: orthopedic screening examination for participation in sports.* Columbus, OH: Ross Products Division, Abbott Laboratories, 1981, with permission, copyright 1981 Ross Products Division, Abbott Laboratories.)

athletes. Body weight measurement and BMI calculation is sufficient for tracking patients who choose to gain or lose weight.

CLEARANCE FOR SPORT PARTICIPATION

Table 18.2 lists disqualifying medical conditions for sports participation as recommended by the AAP. These are only guidelines; they may not apply in specific cases. However, it is notable that all except three (carditis, diarrhea, and fever) allow for individualized or modified athletic participation after further evaluation. The goal of the PPE, once again, is promotion of *safe* physical activity for all adolescents.

After the PPE, the patient should be given one of the following recommendations:

1. Cleared without restriction
2. Cleared, with recommendations for further evaluation or treatment
3. Clearance withheld pending further evaluation, treatment, or rehabilitation
4. Not cleared for certain types of sports or for all sports

If there are restrictions on participation, these should be discussed with the athlete and a parent or guardian, with clearly documented recommendations transmitted to a certified athletic trainer or coach. Otherwise, the message to the athlete may be misinterpreted. If a physician is not going to clear an athlete for participation, the physician should be prepared to discuss the risks associated with continued participation. This requires an understanding of the medical problem and the demands placed on the athlete in that sport. For instance, a football lineman with

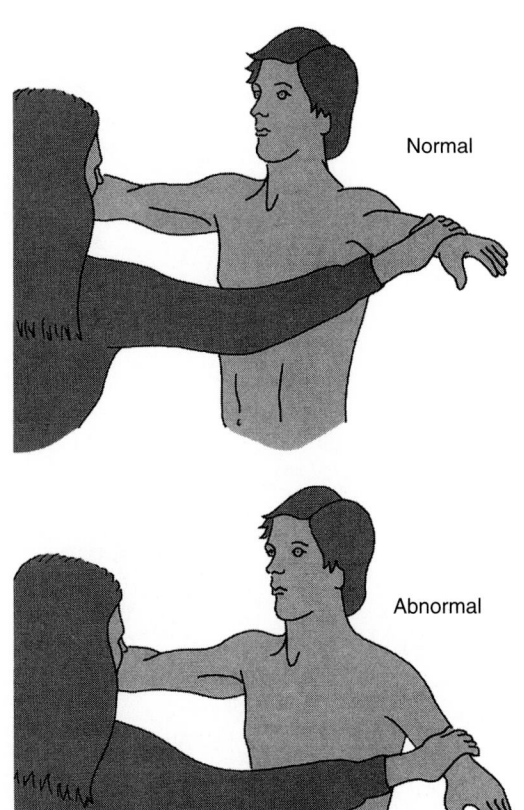

FIGURE 18.4 Shoulder symmetry. (From Ross Laboratories. *For the practitioner: orthopedic screening examination for participation in sports.* Columbus, OH: Ross Products Division, Abbott Laboratories, 1981, with permission, copyright 1981 Ross Products Division, Abbott Laboratories.)

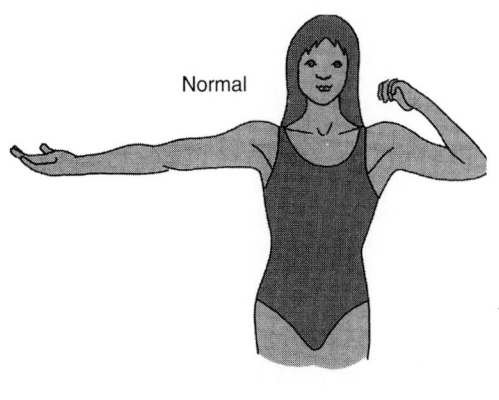

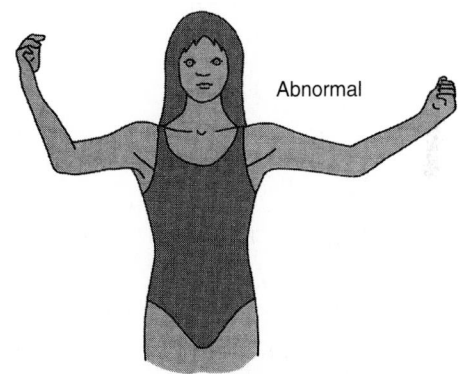

FIGURE 18.5 Elbow and hand symmetry. (From Ross Laboratories. *For the practitioner: orthopedic screening examination for participation in sports.* Columbus, OH: Ross Products Division, Abbott Laboratories, 1981, with permission, copyright 1981 Ross Products Division, Abbott Laboratories.)

an ankle sprain would be able to return to participation earlier than a ballet dancer.

The physician must also consider the importance of this sport compared with another activity; some young athletes may be willing to switch to an activity with a lower risk of reinjury.

Medical–Legal Issues and Exclusion from Sports Participation

Athletes and their parents may seek to participate in a sport against medical advice, citing section 504(a) of the Rehabilitation Act of 1973, which prohibits discrimination against an athlete who is disabled if that person has the capabilities and skills required to play a competitive sport, or the Americans with Disabilities Act of 1990. Athletes with physical disabilities have successfully argued to retain their right to participate in professional athletics using these legal statues. However, an amateur athlete does not have an absolute right to decide whether to participate in competitive sports. Competition in sports is generally

considered a privilege, not a right. The case of *Knapp versus Northwestern University* established that "difficult medical decisions involving complex medical problems can be made by responsible physicians exercising prudent judgment (which will be necessarily conservative when definitive scientific evidence is lacking or conflicting) and relying on the recommendations of specialist consultants or guidelines established by a panel of experts" (Maron et al., 1998). Physicians should clear athletes for participation according to generally agreed-on guidelines for participation with known medical conditions. As Table 18.2 indicates, each decision must be made on an individual basis, and there may not be expert panel guidelines for all conditions. However, such guidelines do exist in many instances, an example being the 36th Bethesda Conference guidelines (see later discussion).

Adolescents with Special Health Care Needs

In addition to identifying in which sports adolescents with special health care needs can participate, the physician should assess current physical fitness activities for these youth. If the fitness activities are inadequate, and the youth and family are interested in more sports or fitness

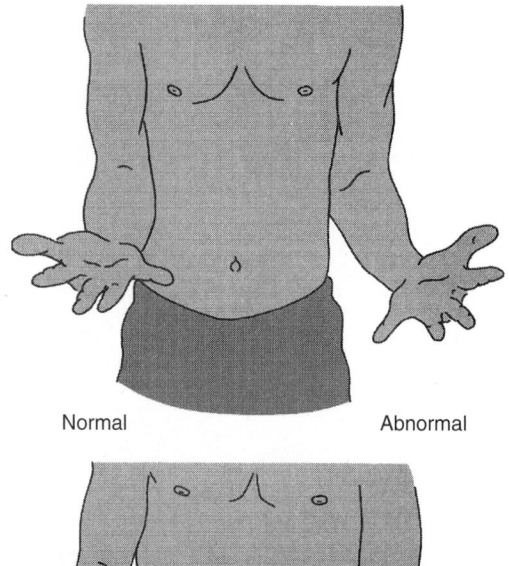

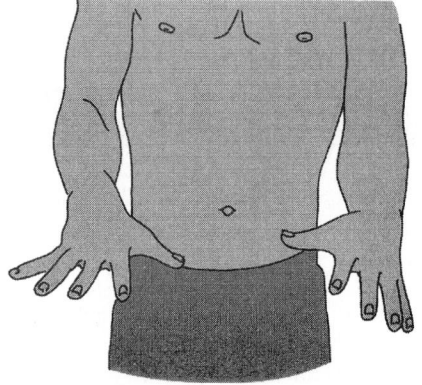

Normal   Abnormal

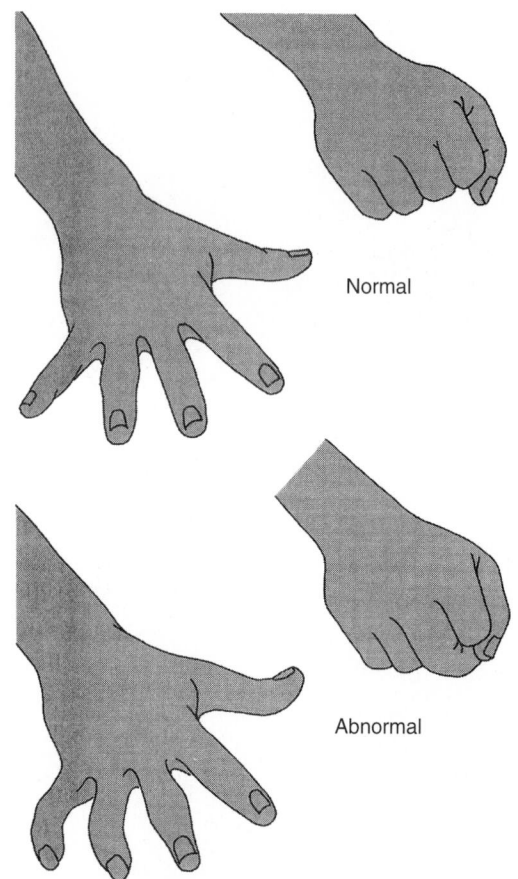

Normal

Abnormal

FIGURE 18.6 Elbow and hand symmetry, continued. (From Ross Laboratories. *For the practitioner: orthopedic screening examination for participation in sports.* Columbus, OH: Ross Products Division, Abbott Laboratories, 1981, with permission, copyright 1981 Ross Products Division, Abbott Laboratories.)

FIGURE 18.7 Elbow and hand symmetry, continued. (From Ross Laboratories. *For the practitioner: orthopedic screening examination for participation in sports.* Columbus, OH: Ross Products Division, Abbott Laboratories, 1981, with permission, copyright 1981 Ross Products Division, Abbott Laboratories.)

opportunities, the physician should either write an exercise prescription for more fitness activities or refer the teen to a physical therapist, physiatrist, exercise physiologist, or sports medicine clinic to design appropriate fitness activities. This should be done in conjunction with the adolescent's subspecialty physicians. Youth with special health care needs have limited access to exercise facilities, and physicians should advocate increasing the availability of facilities for these adolescents.

Clearance for Specific Cardiac Conditions

Mortality during athletic participation is extraordinarily rare (7.8 deaths per million athletes per year—Bundy and Feudtner, 2004), but devastating to the athlete's family, team, and community. Most young athletes who die during sports participation die from sudden cardiac events; most of these athletes are asymptomatic before the event. Therefore, a major focus of the PPE screening is cardiovascular risk conditions.

Any athlete complaining of true angina, syncope, presyncope, or palpitations while exercising, independent of the physical examination, should be excluded from participation until further evaluation. Full evaluation could include, in

consultation with a cardiovascular specialist, a 12-lead electrocardiogram, a continuous ambulatory (Holter) or event capture monitor, a maximal stress test, and a two-dimensional echocardiogram.

The best reference for giving guidance to individual athletes with known cardiac conditions is the 36th Bethesda Conference, 2005 Report: Eligibility Recommendations for Competitive Athletes With Cardiovascular Abnormalities, accessed at http://www.acc.org/clinical/bethesda/beth36/index.pdf. Specific conditions are discussed in the subsequent text.

1. Mitral valve prolapse (see Chapter 14)
   a. Studies of mitral valve prolapse in healthy young adults with no known cardiac disease report a prevalence of 0.6% to 2.7% (Flack et al., 1999; Gilon et al., 1999).
   b. Mitral valve prolapse is generally a benign, asymptomatic condition. Patients can have palpitations, dizziness, supraventricular and ventricular arrhythmias, and chest pain, in which case they should be excluded from sports until they are fully evaluated. Sudden cardiac death in patients with mitral valve

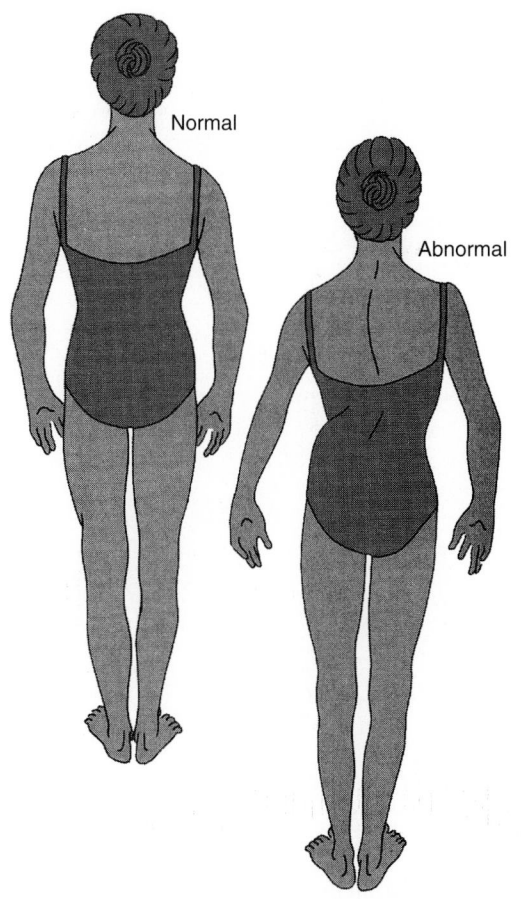

FIGURE 18.8   Back and leg symmetry. (From Ross Laboratories. *For the practitioner: orthopedic screening examination for participation in sports.* Columbus, OH: Ross Products Division, Abbott Laboratories, 1981, with permission, copyright 1981 Ross Products Division, Abbott Laboratories.)

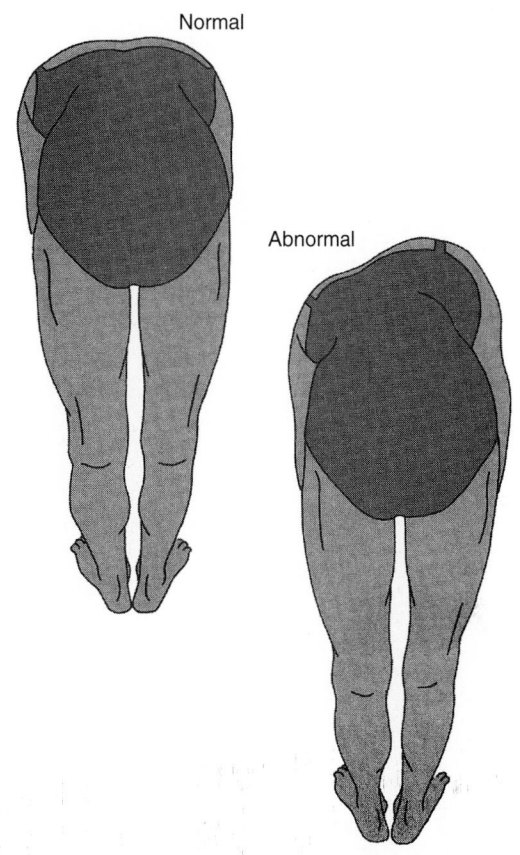

FIGURE 18.9   Back symmetry. (From Ross Laboratories. *For the practitioner: orthopedic screening examination for participation in sports.* Columbus, OH: Ross Products Division, Abbott Laboratories, 1981, with permission, copyright 1981 Ross Products Division, Abbott Laboratories.)

prolapse who die while exercising is rare. A midsystolic click, with or without a late systolic murmur, is the auscultatory hallmark of this condition. However, patient reports of having mitral valve prolapse based on previous physician diagnosis were confirmed definitively on echocardiogram in only 0.45% of cases (Flack et al., 1999). Mitral valve prolapse is a clinical diagnosis generally not requiring echocardiography unless a murmur is present, in which case an echocardiogram is indicated to assess for mitral insufficiency.

   c. Patients with mitral valve prolapse can participate in all competitive sports unless the following exist:
- A history of syncope documented to be arrhythmogenic in origin.
- A family history of sudden death associated with mitral valve prolapse.
- Repetitive forms of supraventricular and ventricular arrhythmias, particularly if exaggerated by exercise.
- Moderate to marked mitral regurgitation.

- Prior embolic event.
- LV systolic ejection fraction <50%.

   d. Athletes with mitral valve prolapse *and* any of the symptoms just listed may participate only in low-intensity sports (i.e., low static, low dynamic—see Figure 18.12, Class IA).

2. Asymmetrical septal hypertrophy or HCM
   a. This is a primary abnormality of the myocardium manifested as an asymmetrically hypertrophied, nondilated left ventricle in the absence of a cardiac or systemic disease that could cause left ventricular hypertrophy (LVH).
   b. The mechanism of sudden death is not established, but a factor may be arrhythmia or myocardial ischemia related to myocardial bridging across coronary arteries. This suggests a role for angiography in patients with HCM (Yetman et al., 1998).
   c. In many cases there are no symptoms before the sudden death. When present, the symptoms include exertional dyspnea, angina pectoris, fatigue, and/or syncope.
   d. There is increased intensity of murmur from supine to standing.

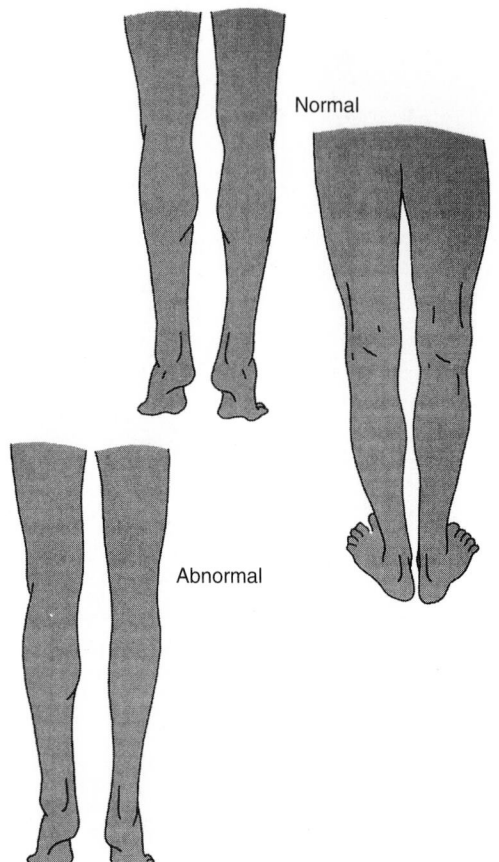

FIGURE 18.10   Leg symmetry. (From Ross Laboratories. *For the practitioner: orthopedic screening examination for participation in sports.* Columbus, OH: Ross Products Division, Abbott Laboratories, 1981, with permission, copyright 1981 Ross Products Division, Abbott Laboratories.)

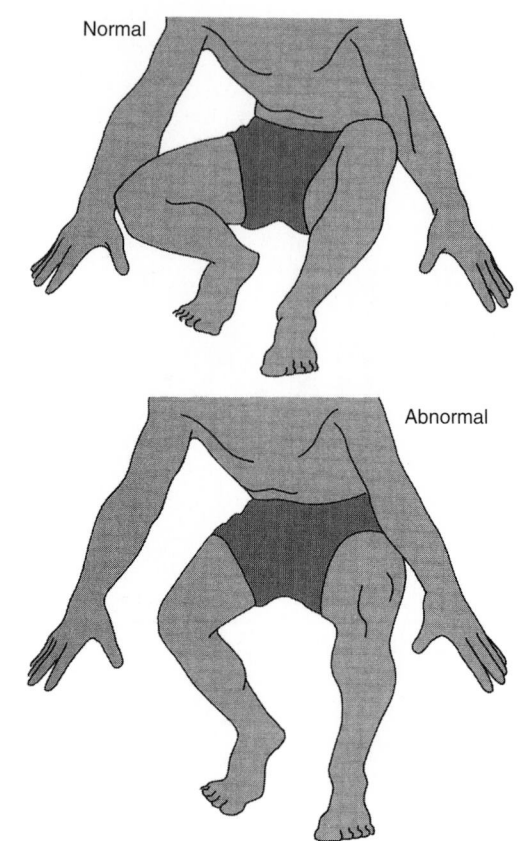

FIGURE 18.11   Leg symmetry, continued. (From Ross Laboratories. *For the practitioner: orthopedic screening examination for participation in sports.* Columbus, OH: Ross Products Division, Abbott Laboratories, 1981, with permission, copyright 1981 Ross Products Division, Abbott Laboratories, with permission.)

e. There may be a family history of early sudden death, particularly related to exercise.

f. The diagnosis is made by demonstrating left ventricular wall thickness >15 mm, although some highly trained athletes can have a left ventricular thickness of up to 16 mm, and some patients with HCM, especially young, growing adolescents, can have a thickness <15 mm.

g. Athletes with HCM must be evaluated by a cardiologist before participation.

h. Recommendations for participation in sports are as follows:
  • Athletes with the unequivocal diagnosis of HCM should not participate in most competitive sports, with the possible exception of low-intensity sports (Fig. 18.12, Class IA). This applies to athletes with and without evidence of left ventricular outflow obstruction.
  • There is currently no compelling evidence to preclude athletes with genotype positive for HCM who do not have phenotypic manifestations (i.e., normal echocardiogram), family history of sudden death, or any cardiac symptoms on history.

3. Coronary artery anomalies
  a. These are rare overall; they should be suspected if the evaluation of syncope or anginal chest pain during exercise is normal.
  b. They may lead to sudden death. Identification before death is difficult because many patients are asymptomatic before the sudden death event.
  c. The cardiac examination is normal.
  d. Cardiac consultation before participation is mandatory if this condition is suspected.
  e. If coronary artery anomalies are identified, there is complete exclusion from sports participation.

4. Myocarditis
  a. The incidence in young athletes is controversial because of the imprecise criteria for diagnosis.
  b. It is a process characterized by an inflammatory infiltrate of the myocardium with necrosis and/or degeneration of myocytes. The disease progresses through active, healing, and healed phases, and arrhythmias may occur at any time.
  c. Recommendations regarding sports participation are as follows:
    • Athletes in whom a presumptive diagnosis has been made should be excluded from all competitive

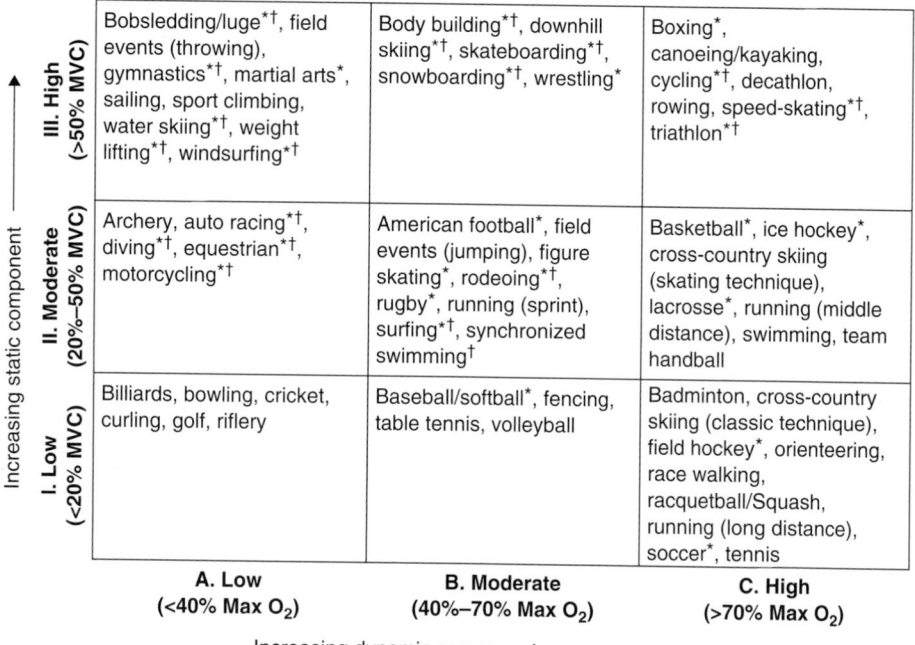

		A. Low (<40% Max O₂)	B. Moderate (40%–70% Max O₂)	C. High (>70% Max O₂)
Increasing static component →	III. High (>50% MVC)	Bobsledding/luge*†, field events (throwing), gymnastics*†, martial arts*, sailing, sport climbing, water skiing*†, weight lifting*†, windsurfing*†	Body building*†, downhill skiing*†, skateboarding*†, snowboarding*†, wrestling*	Boxing*, canoeing/kayaking, cycling*†, decathlon, rowing, speed-skating*†, triathlon*†
	II. Moderate (20%–50% MVC)	Archery, auto racing*†, diving*†, equestrian*†, motorcycling*†	American football*, field events (jumping), figure skating*, rodeoing*†, rugby*, running (sprint), surfing*†, synchronized swimming†	Basketball*, ice hockey*, cross-country skiing (skating technique), lacrosse*, running (middle distance), swimming, team handball
	I. Low (<20% MVC)	Billiards, bowling, cricket, curling, golf, riflery	Baseball/softball*, fencing, table tennis, volleyball	Badminton, cross-country skiing (classic technique), field hockey*, orienteering, race walking, racquetball/Squash, running (long distance), soccer*, tennis

A. Low (<40% Max O₂)   B. Moderate (40%–70% Max O₂)   C. High (>70% Max O₂)

Increasing dynamic component ──────→

FIGURE 18.12   Classification of Sports. This classification is based on peak static and dynamic components achieved during competition. It should be noted, however, that higher values may be reached during training. The increasing dynamic component is defined in terms of the estimated percent of maximal oxygen uptake (MaxO₂) achieved and results in an increasing cardiac output. The increasing static component is related to the estimated percent of maximal voluntary contraction (MVC) reached and results in an increasing blood pressure load. *Danger of bodily collision. †Increased risk if syncope occurs. (From Mitchell JH, Haskel W, Snell P, et al. Task Force 8: Classification of sports. *J Am Coll Cardiol* 2005;45:1364, with permission.)

sports for 6 months and then have their ventricular function evaluated at rest and with exercise before being allowed to return to sports.
- Athletes can return to sports when their ventricular function and dimensions are normal and clinically relevant arrhythmias are absent on ambulatory monitoring.
- There is no strong evidence for endomyocardial biopsy as a precondition for returning to sports participation.

d. Regarding the athlete with an acute febrile illness characterized by fever and myalgia, it seems prudent to withhold that athlete from competition. However, there is no evidence that this precaution protects against sudden death. In athletes diagnosed with sudden death related to myocarditis, there is no clear temporal pattern between the febrile illness and the sudden death.

5. Systemic hypertension (also see Chapter 13)
   a. Although hypertension is associated with an increased risk for sudden death and complex ventricular arrhythmias, to date it has not been incriminated as a cause of sudden cardiac death in young, competitive athletes.
   b. To be consistent with JNC 7 guidelines for adults, classification of hypertension in adolescents has been revised as shown in Table 18.3. Proper measurement of blood pressure and diagnosis of hypertension is discussed in Chapter 13. Athletes with stage 1 or 2 hypertension should be screened for LVH with an echocardiogram.
   c. Athletes with stage 1 hypertension in the absence of end-organ damage, including LVH and heart disease have no restrictions, but should have BP measured every 2 to 4 months to assess the impact of exercise.
   d. Those with stage 2 hypertension should be restricted, especially from high-static sports (Fig. 18.12, Classes IIIA–C), until their blood pressure is controlled.
   e. If athletes have true LVH (in distinction from "athlete's heart") on screening, they should be restricted from participation in high-static sports (Fig. 18.12, Classes IIIA–C) until the hypertension is controlled.

Clearance for Adolescents with Solitary Kidney

Current recommendations of the American Academy of Pediatrics Committee on Sports Medicine and Fitness discuss individual assessments for adolescents with a solitary kidney and their possible disqualification from participating in contact sports. Johnson et al. (2005) evaluated the incidence and outcome of blunt renal injury in

TABLE 18.3

Classification of Hypertension in Adolescents[a]

Classification	Adolescents and Children[b] (mm Hg)	Adults (mm Hg)
Normal		
Systolic	<90th percentile for age, gender, and height[b]	<120
Diastolic		<80
Prehypertension		
Systolic	90th–95th percentile for age, gender, and height[b]	120–139
Diastolic		80–89
Stage 1 hypertension		
Systolic	95th–99th percentile for age, gender, and height plus 5 mm Hg[b]	140–159
Diastolic		90–99
Stage 2 hypertension		
Systolic	>99th percentile for age, gender, and height plus 5 mm Hg[b]	≥160
Diastolic		≥100

[a]Blood pressure values are based on the average of three or more readings taken at each of three or more visits after the initial screening. These definitions apply to individuals who are not taking antihypertensive drugs and are not acutely ill.

[b]Or adult parameters if greater.

Adapted from the National High Blood Pressure Education Program, Working Group on Hypertension Control in Children and Adolescents. Fourth report on the diagnosis, evaluation, and treatment of high blood pressure in children and adolescents. *Pediatrics* 2004;114:555.

children and adolescents by mechanism of injury. Of 49,651 pediatric trauma cases there were 813 involving renal injury. In those individuals with sports-related injuries, there were four nephrectomies and these were associated with sledding (two), skiing (one), and in-line skating (one). There were no kidneys lost in any contact sports, therefore the likelihood of kidney loss related to contact sports is very small.

Effectiveness of the Preparticipation Sports Examination

Pfister et al. (2000) examined 1,110 National Collegiate Athletic Association (NCAA) colleges and universities and found that only 25% had forms that contained at least 9 of the recommended 12 AHA screening guidelines, and 24% contained 4 or fewer of these parameters. Maron (1998) also reviewed this issue and found that 40% of states have no formal screening requirement or approved history and physical examination questionnaires or forms. Authors of the 3rd Edition of the PPE monograph acknowledge that there is a significant need for national standardization of preparticipation screening to better assess its effectiveness and have called for utilization of new technologies such as the Internet for information gathering and sharing. Even with perfect implementation Bundy and Feudtner (2004) cogently argue that the prevalence of sports-related death is too low for the PPE to ever qualify as an effective screening program unless the focus is shifted to and systems created for appropriate rehabilitation of identified musculoskeletal deficits.

CAN WE PREVENT ATHLETIC INJURY AND ILLNESS?

Morbidity and Mortality

Although football has been associated with a high incidence of injuries, the number of injury events resulting in permanent disability or death has been on the decline since the 1970s. However, catastrophic injuries and fatalities still occur in high school and college football and in other sports. A full report is available at the Web site for the National Center for Catastrophic Sports Injury Research, (www.unc.edu/depts/nccsi). At this site, the reader can find a breakdown of injuries and fatalities stratified by high school and college and by type of sport and by year. The sports with the highest incidence of fatalities from direct injuries per 100,000 participants from the 1982–1983 season through 2003–2004 were the following:

High School	Incidence per 100,000 Participants
Males	
Gymnastics	1.12
Ice hockey	0.35
Lacrosse	0.35
Football	0.31
Females	
Softball	0.02
Track	0.01

College	Incidence per 100,000 Participants
Males	
Lacrosse	2.52
Baseball	0.6
Football	0.55
Track	0.39
Baseball	0.32
Females	
Equestrian	89.28
Skiing	7.70

Nonfatal injuries also were similar in regard to the common sports involved. However, for female student-athletes, the leading cause of fatalities and catastrophic injuries between 1982 and 2003 was cheerleading.

There have been dramatic reductions in the number of football fatalities and nonfatal catastrophic injuries since 1976. While football is still associated with the greatest number of catastrophic injuries among all sports, the incidence of injury per 100,000 participants is higher for both gymnastics and ice hockey.

Catastrophic injuries to female athletes have increased over the years from one in 1982 to 1983 to an average of 6.7 in the last 22 years. A major factor in this increase has been the change in cheerleading which increasingly involves gymnastic stunts. Cheerleading now accounts for 50% of all high school catastrophic injuries to female athletes and 64.5% of catastrophic injuries at the college level.

Injury Prediction

Well-defined risk factors for athletic injury are scarce due to the paucity of good epidemiological research in the field. Factors that may predispose the athlete to injury include the following:

1. Weakness and/or inflexibility related to a previous injury.
2. Accelerated growth.
3. Training errors, including too-rapid increases in pace, distance, repetitions, or weight/resistance. *Training errors are the most common factor associated with overuse injuries.*
4. Inappropriate equipment (improper shoes, equipment not sized appropriately).
5. Change in the environment, such as running up hills or on a banked track instead of a flat surface.

Injury Prevention Strategies

There are several ways of preventing injuries.

1. Individual level interventions
   a. Recognize and fully rehabilitate old injuries. As mentioned, the most important function of the PPE may be as a quality control point for injuries and rehabilitation during the past year (Keller et al., 1987).
   b. Stretching is not likely to prevent injuries unless there is an identified deficit. Pope et al. (2000) confirmed this in a group of military recruits. The stretching methods described in that report are typical of a stretching routine for middle school and high school teams, but they are not ideal stretching exercises because they were done only once for 20 seconds.

We recommend stretching of the lower extremities after weight-bearing exercise. This should include gastrocnemius, soleus, hamstring, and quadriceps stretches, held for 20 seconds each, twice per muscle-group.
   c. See "The Female Athlete" section, later in this chapter, regarding prevention of acute knee injuries in female athletes.
2. System or environment-level interventions are far more effective in reducing injury rates.
   a. Breakaway bases (bases in baseball and softball that are not anchored to the ground) have been associated with fewer and less significant ankle and lower-leg injuries from sliding. The incidence of serious neck injuries decreased after the trampoline was removed from gymnastics competition (National Institutes of Health, 1992).
   b. Enforce rules to eliminate behavior that places athletes at high risk for injury. Serious neck injuries in football dropped precipitously after spear tackling was made illegal in football (Mueller and Cantu, 2001). As mechanisms of injury are elucidated, preventive measures can be planned. This underscores the need for continued research into the causes of sports injuries. An excellent review of the approach to the epidemiology of youth sports was published by the Conference on Sports Injuries in Youth (National Institutes of Health, 1992), but its calls have been largely unheeded in the intervening years.
3. Future injury is best prevented by minimizing the consequences of an index injury as it occurs.

Returning to Participation

In general, athletes should not be allowed to return to participation in sports until the following criteria have been satisfied:

1. The injury has been accurately diagnosed.
2. The examiner is reasonably certain that the injury will not significantly worsen with continued play.
3. The examiner is reasonably certain that continued participation (with the injury) will not result in a secondary injury.
4. The athlete has achieved full ROM and strength in the injured joint.
5. The athlete wants to return to play.

The following are examples of injuries or conditions that preclude returning to sports until the criteria just listed have been fulfilled:

1. Unconsciousness, however brief (see "Neurological Concussion" section)
2. Any neurological abnormalities
3. Obvious swelling
4. Limited ROM
5. Pain within the normal ROM
6. Bleeding
7. An injury the examiner does not know how to manage
8. Obvious loss of normal function
9. Athlete's lack of desire to return to play

The physician caring for the athlete should be familiar with common injuries and their therapy. A few are discussed in the following section. For further information on specific injuries, also see Chapter 16 and the References section at the end of this chapter.

DIAGNOSIS AND MANAGEMENT OF SPORTS-RELATED CONDITIONS AND MORBIDITIES

Neurological Concussion

The field of concussion, or sports-related mild traumatic brain injury (MTBI) is evolving rapidly and health care providers should look at recent guidelines to remain up-to-date. A panel of international experts in the field met in Prague in November 2004 to revise and update the consensus recommendations they had made in Vienna in November 2001 (McCrory et al., 2005).

Definition Sports *concussion* is now defined as "a complex pathophysiological process affecting the brain, induced by traumatic biomechanical forces" (McCrory et al., 2005). There are approximately 300,000 sports-related traumatic brain injuries in the United States, annually (Sosin et al., 1996).

Grading The Vienna and Prague groups, which included authors of some of the most widely used concussion grading scales, recommend abandoning such crude systems in favor of individual assessment and guidance based on combined measures of recovery. The grading scales have not reliably correlated with any physiological or psychometric measures so far studied to be useful for predicting risk, sequelae, resolution of symptoms, or return to play.

Classification The consensus panel recommends that clinicians appreciate that concussion in sport may either be simple or complex, but that this classification is made *retrospectively*.

1. Simple concussion: An athlete suffers an injury that progressively resolves without complication over 7 to 10 days.
2. Complex concussion: Cases in which athletes suffer persistent symptoms, any other sequelae (such as seizure), prolonged loss of consciousness (>1 minute), or prolonged cognitive impairment after the injury. Recurrent concussions, especially those triggered by progressively less impact force, fall into this category as well.

Diagnosis and Management Essentially *any* athlete who complains of *any* neurological symptoms or demonstrates *any* neurological signs (Fig. 18.13) or memory loss after *any* bodily contact (not just the head) with another athlete, the ground or other playing surface, or a projectile such as a ball or puck should be managed as an acute concussion.

The Sport Concussion Assessment Tool (SCAT) Card (Fig. 18.13) is a handheld standardized method to evaluate the concussed athlete. It also provides a suggested approach to management, which can be summarized as "When in doubt, sit them out!" In more detail this is as follows:

1. The athlete should not be allowed to return to play in the current game or practice session.
2. The athlete should not be left alone, and regular monitoring for deterioration is essential over the initial few hours after injury.

3. The player should be medically evaluated after the injury.
   a. Any abnormalities on sideline neurological screening necessitate immediate formal neurological evaluation by a physician on-site or at a medical facility.
   b. Neuroimaging may play a part in the assessment of complex sports concussion, but are not essential for simple concussive injury if not indicated by physical examination findings.
4. Return to play must follow a medically supervised stepwise process (i.e., no predetermined time frames for exclusion).

Return to Play Return to play follows a stepwise process, with advance of no more than one step per day:

1. No physical activity. When completely asymptomatic for 24 hours, proceed to step 2.
2. Light aerobic exercise such as walking or stationary cycling, but no resistance (strength) training.
3. Sport-specific exercise may resume—for example skating in ice hockey, running with no pads in football—or beginning of resistance training.
4. Noncontact training drills—for example with helmet and pads in football, shooting and passing in ice hockey—or increased resistance training.
5. After medical clearance (reevaluation by physician), may participate in controlled full-contact training such as practice sessions.
6. Game play.

If *any* postconcussion symptoms occur at a level, the athlete must wait until asymptomatic for at least 24 hours before resuming the progression at the *previous* level.

The minimum time in which such a progression can be completed is a week, but may take much longer depending on the individual case. Lack of progression should prompt referral to a neurologist, neurosurgeon, or sports medicine physician comfortable with the management of sports concussion. Formal neuropsychological testing may be indicated at this time, although its interpretation may be hampered by a lack of baseline assessment. Although they, too, are hindered by issues of validation, particularly in younger age-groups, commercially available computerized neuropsychological batteries performed before participation may be helpful in this regard.

Second Impact Syndrome One of the goals of the above guidelines is to prevent diffuse cerebral swelling with delayed catastrophic deterioration, a known complication of brain trauma. This has been postulated to occur after repeated concussive brain injury in sports and is known as the *second impact syndrome* (SIS). All cases of SIS to date have been diagnosed in adolescent boys. Some authors have suggested a different mechanism of cerebral autoregulation in children and adolescents as compared with adults (Snoek et al., 1984).

However, McCrory (1998) reviewed the 17 cases of SIS reported in the literature as of the year 2000, using strict diagnostic criteria, and established that only 5 were probably SIS. He suggested that, because all of the SIS cases have been reported in North America, because player and teammate recall of traumatic brain injury during sports is poor, and because diffuse cerebral edema after initial traumatic brain injury has been described for <100 years, SIS may in fact be the cerebral response to the

Sport Concussion Assessment Tool

This tool represents a standardized method of evaluating people after concussion in sport. This tool has been produced as part of the Summary and Agreement Statement of the Second International Symposium on Concussion in Sport, Prague 2004

For more information see the "Summary and Agreement Statement of the Second International Symposium on Concussion in Sport" in the: Clinical Journal of Sport Medicine 2005; British Journal of Sports Medicine 2005; Neurosurgery 2005; Physician and Sportsmedicine 2005; this tool may be copied for distribution to teams, groups and organizations.

Sports concussion is defined as a complex pathophysiological process affecting the brain, induced by traumatic biomechanical forces. Several common features that incorporate clinical, pathological and biomechanical injury constructs that may be utilized in defining the nature of a concussive head injury include:

1. Concussion may be caused either by a direct blow to the head, face, neck or elsewhere on the body with an 'impulsive' force transmitted to the head.
2. Concussion typically results in the rapid onset of short-lived impairment or neurological function that resolves spontaneously.
3. Concussion may result in neuropathological changes but the acute clinical symptoms largely reflect a functional disturbance rather than structural injury.
4. Concussion results in a graded set of clinical syndromes that may or may not involve loss of consciousness. Resolution of the clinical and cognitive symptoms typically follows a sequential course.
5. Concussion is typically associated with grossly normal structural neuroimaging studies.

Post Concussion Symptoms

Ask the athlete to score themselves based on how they feel now. It is recognized that a low score may be normal for some athletes, but clinical judgment should be exercised to determine if a change in symptoms has occurred following the suspected concussion event.

It should be recognized that the reporting of symptoms may not be entirely reliable. This may be due to the effects of a concussion or because the athlete's passionate desire to return to competition outweighs their natural inclination to give an honest response.

If possible, ask someone who knows the athlete well about changes in affect, personality, behavior, etc.

Remember, concussion should be suspected in the presence of ANY ONE or more of the following:
- Symptoms (such as headache), or
- Signs (such as loss of consciousness), or
- Memory problems

Any athlete with a suspected concussion should be monitored for deterioration (i.e., should not be left alone) and should not drive a motor vehicle.

The SCAT Card (Sport Concussion Assessment Tool)

What is a concussion? A concussion is a disturbance in the function of the brain caused by a direct or indirect force to the head. It results in a variety of symptoms (like those listed below) and may, or may not, involve memory problems or loss of consciousness.

How do you feel? You should score yourself on the following symptoms, based on how you feel now.

Post Concussion Symptom Scale

	None		Moderate			Severe
Headache	0	1	2	3	4	5	6
"Pressure in head"	0	1	2	3	4	5	6
Neck Pain	0	1	2	3	4	5	6
Balance problems/dizzy	0	1	2	3	4	5	6
Nausea or vomiting	0	1	2	3	4	5	6
Vision problems	0	1	2	3	4	5	6
Hearing problems/ringing	0	1	2	3	4	5	6
"Don't feel right"	0	1	2	3	4	5	6
Feeling "dinged"/"dazed"	0	1	2	3	4	5	6
Confusion	0	1	2	3	4	5	6
Feeling slowed down	0	1	2	3	4	5	6
Feeling like "in a fog"	0	1	2	3	4	5	6
Drowsiness	0	1	2	3	4	5	6
Fatigue or low energy	0	1	2	3	4	5	6
More than emotional	0	1	2	3	4	5	6
Irritability	0	1	2	3	4	5	6
Difficulty concentrating	0	1	2	3	4	5	6
Difficulty remembering	0	1	2	3	4	5	6
(follow up symptoms only)							
Sadness	0	1	2	3	4	5	6
Nervous or anxious	0	1	2	3	4	5	6
Trouble falling asleep	0	1	2	3	4	5	6
Sleeping more than usual	0	1	2	3	4	5	6
Sensitivity to light	0	1	2	3	4	5	6
Sensitivity to noise	0	1	2	3	4	5	6
Other:	0	1	2	3	4	5	6

What should I do?
Any athlete suspected of having a concussion should be removed from play, and told to seek medical evaluation.

Signs to watch for:
Problems could arise over the first 24-48 hours. You should not be left alone and must go to a hospital at once if you:
- Have a headache that gets worse
- Are very drowsy or can't be awakened (woken up)
- Can't recognize people or places
- Have repeated vomiting
- Behave unusually or seem confused; are very irritable
- Have seizures (arms and legs jerk uncontrollably)
- Have weak or numb arms or legs
- Are unsteady on your feet; have slurred speech

Remember, it is better to be safe. **Consult your doctor after a suspected concussion.**

What can I expect?
Concussion typically results in the rapid onset of short-lived impairment that resolves spontaneously over time. You can expect that you will be told to rest until you are fully recovered (that means resting your body and your mind). Then, your doctor will likely advise that you go through a gradual increase in exercise over several days (or longer) before returning to sport.

FIGURE 18.13 Sport Concussion Assessment Tool (SCAT) Card. (From Clinical Journal of Sports Medicine 2005, with permission.)

**The SCAT Card (Sport Concussion Assessment Tool)
Medical Evaluation**

Name: _____ Date: _____

Sport/Team: _____ Mouth guard?   Y N

1) SIGNS
Was there loss of consciousness/unresponsiveness?   Y N
Was there seizure or convulsive activity?   Y N
Was there a balance problem / unsteadiness?   Y N

2) MEMORY
Modified Maddocks questions (check if athlete answers correctly)
- At what venue are we? ____ Which half is it? ____ Who scored last? ____
- What team did we play last? ____: Did we win last game? ____

3) SYMPTOM SCORE
Total number of positive symptoms (from reverse side of the card) = _____

4) COGNITIVE ASSESSMENT (5 word recall)

	(Examples)	Immediate	Delayed
Word 1 ____	cat	_____	_____
Word 2 ____	pen	_____	_____
Word 3 ____	shoe	_____	_____
Word 4 ____	book	_____	_____
Word 5 ____	car	_____	_____

Months in reverse order:
Jun-May-Apr-Mar-Feb-Jan-Dec-Nov-Oct-Sep-Aug-Jul

Digits Backwards (check correct)
5-2-8   3-9-1   _____
6-2-9-4   4-3-7-1   _____
8-3-2-7-9   1-4-9-3-6   _____
7-3-9-1-4-2   5-1-8-4-6-8   _____

Ask delayed 5-word recall now

5) NEUROLOGIC SCREENING

	Pass	Fail
Speech	____	____
Eye Motion and Pupils	____	____
Pronator Drift	____	____
Gait Assessment	____	____

Any neurologic screen abnormality necessitates formal neurologic or hospital assessment

RETURN TO PLAY
Athletes should not be returned to play the same day of injury.
When returning athletes to play they should follow a stepwise symptom-limited program, with stages of progression. For example:
1. rest until asymptomatic (physical and mental rest)
2. light aerobic exercise (e.g stationary cycle)
3. sport-specific training
4. non-contact training drills (start light resistance training)
5. full contact training after medical clearance
6. return to competition (game play)
There should be approximately 24 hours (or longer) for each stage and the athlete should return to stage 1 if symptoms recur. Resistance training should only be added in the later stages. Medical clearance should be given before return to play.

Instructions:
The side of the card is for the use of medical doctors, physical therapists, or athletic therapists. In order to maximize the information gathered from the card, it is strongly suggested that all athletes participating in contact sports complete a baseline evaluation prior to the beginning of their competitive season. This card is a suggested guide only for sports concussion and is not meant to assess more severe forms of brain injury. **Please give a COPY of this card to the athlete for their information and to guide follow up assessment.**

Signs:
Assess for each of these items and circle Y (yes) or N (no).

Memory:
Select any 5 words (an example is given). Avoid choosing related words such as "dark" and "moon" which can be recalled by means of word association. Read each word at a rate of one word per second. The athlete should not be informed of the delayed testing of memory (to be done after the reverse months and/or digits). Choose a different set of words each time you perform a follow-up exam with the same candidate.

Concentration / Attention:
Ask the athlete to recite the months of the year in reverse order, starting with a random month. Do not start with December or January. Circle any months not recited in the correct sequence. For digits backwards, if correct, go to the next string length. If correct, read trial 2. Stop after incorrect on both trials.

Neurologic Screening:
Trained medical personnel must administer this examination. These individuals might include medical doctors, physiotherapists or athletic therapists. Speech should be assessed for fluency and lack slurring. Eye motion should reveal no diplopia in any of the 4 planes of movement (vertical, horizontal and both diagonal planes). The pronator drift is performed by asking the patient to hold both arms in front of them, palms up, with eyes closed. A positive test is pronating the forearm, dropping the arm, or drift away from midline. For gait assessment ask the patient to walk away from you, turn and walk back.

Return to Play:
A structured, graded exertion protocol should be developed, individualized on the basis of sport, age, and the concussion history of the athlete. Exercise or training should be commenced only after the athlete is clearly asymptomatic with physical and cognitive rest. Final decision for clearance to return to competition should ideally be made by a medical doctor.

Notes:
_____
_____
_____
_____
_____
_____

FIGURE 18.13 *(Continued)*

first traumatic brain injury. Nonetheless, it appears most prudent to limit contact sports in adolescent athletes until all postconcussive symptoms have disappeared, regardless of which concussion management protocol is followed.

Sequelae of Chronic Head Trauma There is evidence that traumatic brain injury occurring over an extended period (i.e., months or years) can result in cumulative neurological and cognitive deficits (Gronwall and Wrightson, 1975; Leininger et al., 1990). "Dementia pugilistica" was the description given to the punchy boxer's condition in 1928, and the syndrome also occurs in other sports characterized by repeated head trauma. This syndrome includes the following:

1. Injury in and around the third ventricle, leading to memory deficits, emotion lability, and euphoria.
2. Injury to the inferior cerebellar tonsils, manifested as slurred speech and abnormal balance.
3. Degeneration of the basal ganglia, leading to Parkinson disease.
4. Diffuse neuronal loss, leading to a picture that is similar to Alzheimer disease.

Neuropsychiatric abnormalities can persist for up to 6 months after a concussion (not only in sports). This has led to the definition of the *postconcussional disorder* described in the *Diagnostic and Statistical Manual of Mental Disorders*, 4th ed. (American Psychiatric Association 1994), as follows:.

1. History of head trauma including loss of consciousness and posttraumatic amnesia
2. Evidence of difficulty in attention (concentrating, shifting focus of attention, performing simultaneous cognitive tasks) or memory
3. Three or more of the following occurring shortly after the injury and lasting 3 months or longer:
   a. Easily fatigued
   b. Disordered sleep
   c. Headache
   d. Dizziness
   e. Irritability or aggression with little provocation
   f. Anxiety or depression
   g. Change in personality (social or sexual inappropriateness)
   h. Apathy or lack of spontaneity

Dementia (decreased cognition, memory, or any of the above symptoms) resulting from a single head injury is usually not progressive. If the dementia or behavior grows progressively worse, consider another diagnosis, such as hydrocephalus or major depressive disorder.

Collins et al. (1999) evaluated the relationship between concussion and neuropsychological performance in college football players. They found that both a history of multiple concussions and learning disabilities were associated with reduced cognitive performance, and that the effects were most pronounced in concussed athletes with a history of learning disabilities.

Heading in Soccer The results of cross-sectional, retrospective studies of head injuries in soccer players have been used to suggest that "heading" of the soccer ball by young athletes should be banned. However, it is not the heading of the ball that appears to be the culprit so much as concussions incurred during the course of play. Matser

et al. (1999) found that concussion in soccer players was associated with impaired performance in memory and planned functions. Concussions in soccer players should be managed using guidelines as discussed previously. Other suggestions include the following:

1. Adequate on-site medical care for acute brain injuries
2. Full medical evaluation of concussed players
3. Strict rule enforcement
4. Padding of the goal posts
5. Requiring use of mouth guards
6. Teaching proper heading technique (Green and Jordan, 1998)

Cervical Spinal Injuries

Most catastrophic sports injuries involve the head and neck. The reader is again referred to the Web site for the National Center for Catastrophic Sports Injury Research listed at the end of the chapter.

General Management

1. Initially, when a player's head or neck is injured, a spinal cord injury must be assumed to be present. The patient should not be moved until a diagnosis is established that would allow cervical movement. If a cervical spine injury is suspected, the first priority is to determine that the patient's cardiopulmonary status is normal. If not, basic life support measures must be instituted. The second priority is to do no harm. For a potential unstable cervical spine fracture or dislocation, this means allowing no one to move the athlete, including not taking off the helmet or rolling the patient over, until the appropriate emergency personnel are present. After personnel are present who can prepare the patient for transport, the cervical spine should be stabilized and the patient transported. Physicians who cover football games should be comfortable stabilizing and preparing for the transport of an athlete with a potential cervical spine fracture. This can be learned only through hands-on training. Of special note is the instruction to *not remove any helmets*. In sports where an athlete wears a helmet, they often also wear shoulder pads. Proper alignment of the cervical spine is maintained by the combination of helmet and shoulder padding. Because it is unsafe, typically, to remove the shoulder pads, *it is unsafe to remove the helmet.* Axial traction can be maintained through a properly fit helmet.
2. If the patient is unconscious and has neck pain and/or radiating pain to an extremity, or has paresis or paresthesia, it should be assumed that a cervical spine injury is present. The athlete should be immobilized on a board and transported to an emergency room.
3. If there is no motor or sensory abnormality of the extremities, no neck pain, and the patient is conscious, he/she can be allowed to walk off the field for further evaluation. If at any time the patient complains of radiating pain, paresthesia, or neck pain, the physician should consider that a cervical spine fracture is present and initiate appropriate procedures. If the physician is not comfortable with the above scenarios, then he or she should know what the protocol is for activating emergency medical services.

Cervical Muscle Strain

Cervical muscle strains are common and can be painful. The mechanisms of injury include rapid acceleration of a muscle or muscles as a result of a collision; a quick movement causing the muscle to tear; or repetitive contractions causing muscle fatigue and eventually muscle tearing. There should be no motor or sensory deficits on examination. The athlete will complain of pain typically in the trapezius area. There will be tenderness over the muscle body, limitation of ROM, and pain with resistance. Midline pain and tenderness are consistent with a cervical fracture and should be treated as such in the acute setting. Any player without full ROM and strength is excluded from further contact sports. Ice, analgesic medication, and physical therapy should be initiated immediately. A cervical collar may be used rarely; for example, when the patient is in intractable pain after physical therapy and medication has been started. The physician should reassess the diagnosis if pain is intractable. Once physical therapy has yielded some relief, the player should receive continued physical therapy as needed in the therapist's office, complemented by home exercises. Clearance for return to contact sport requires a normal range of cervical motion and strength.

"Stingers" or "Burners"

A "stinger" is a common injury in American football and is the result of trauma to the brachial plexus that occurs when a player hits another opponent with the head or shoulder. The player describes a burning pain or weakness, or both, in the distribution of a branch of the brachial plexus. The physician who initially evaluates a stinger should first think about the possibility that the paresthesia is secondary to a spinal cord injury, as discussed previously, although unilateral signs and symptoms make this less likely. Once the cervical spine has been cleared (i.e., no midline cervical tenderness and full cervical ROM), then the diagnosis of brachial plexopathy can be made. Typically, these injuries are mild and the player recovers in minutes or less. The athlete may return to full participation if motor and sensory examination of the extremity is normal. However, some patients have dysesthesia and/or weakness that can last days to weeks. We suggest that patients with symptoms persisting longer than 12 hours or weakness documented to be 3/5 or less should be referred to a sports medicine specialist or a neurosurgeon. A nerve conduction or electromyographic study can be considered to assess for the extent of nerve injury after 21 days of symptoms, especially if the patient is not making clinical improvement.

Other Musculoskeletal Injuries and Conditions

The common injuries sustained by athletes and other active (and inactive!) adolescents are detailed in Chapters 16 and 17.

SPECIAL CONSIDERATIONS: THE FEMALE ATHLETE

In general, female athletes have injuries and injury rates similar to those of male athletes in the same sport. The exception to this rule is female athletes in jumping sports, who have a higher rate of anterior cruciate ligament sprains than their male counterparts. The reason for this difference is not established. A reduction in the incidence of acute knee injuries in female athletes after a 6-week neuromuscular training course, compared with a group that did not have this training, has been reported (Hewett et al., 1999). The results of this study and others imply a role for improved neuromuscular control in stabilizing the knee and, potentially, preventing anterior cruciate ligament injuries. It does not establish that neuromuscular control is inadequate in young female athletes as compared with young male athletes, because the latter were not studied with a similar intervention program. The issue of overtraining and adult height in female gymnasts was addressed earlier in this chapter.

Female Athlete Triad

The effects of excessive exercise on the reproductive system in young females deserve special mention. The so-called female athlete triad—disordered eating, amenorrhea, and osteoporosis—highlights the effects of excessive exercise (Yeager et al., 1993). Female athletes with amenorrhea or oligomenorrhea have lower bone mineral density (BMD) and higher rates of stress fracture than eumenorrheic athletes (Barrow and Saha, 1988; Myburgh et al., 1990; Bennell et al., 1999). A long-term consequence of amenorrhea and osteopenia during the second decade may be an increased risk of postmenopausal osteoporosis. Nichols et al., 2006 examined the prevalence rate for the female athlete triad among high schools athletes. They found that among female athletes studied (N = 170), 18.2%, 23.5%, and 21.8% met the criteria for disordered eating, menstrual irregularity, and low bone mass, respectively. Ten girls (5.9%) met the criteria for two components of the triad, and two girls (1.2%) met criteria for all three components.

Evaluation and Treatment

The first step in addressing hypothalamic amenorrhea/oligomenorrhea in female athletes is to make a correct diagnosis. Hypothalamic amenorrhea associated with exercise and/or inadequate caloric intake is a diagnosis of exclusion. The diagnosis is made on the basis of a careful history (menstrual, diet, and exercise history) and appropriate physical examination.

The menstrual history includes the following:

1. Age at menarche
2. Frequency and duration of menstrual cycle
3. Last menstrual period
4. Longest time period without menstruation
5. Physical signs of ovulation, such as dysmenorrhea
6. Prior hormonal therapy

The diet history includes the following:

1. Food history in last 3 days
2. List of any restricted foods

3. Highest and lowest weights since menarche
4. Satisfaction with current weight and perceived ideal weight
5. Bingeing and purging behaviors
6. Use of laxatives, diuretics, appetite suppressants, supplements, or other pathological weight-control behaviors.

The exercise history includes the following:

1. Exercise patterns and training intensity levels
2. Exercise done outside of required training
3. Compulsive exercise
4. History of previous fractures
5. Overuse injuries

The conditions that need to be ruled out in the evaluation of amenorrhea are reviewed in Chapter 52.

If a diagnosis of hypothalamic amenorrhea or oligomenorrhea associated with exercise and/or inadequate caloric intake is made, reductions in training intensity and/or enhanced caloric intake need to be made. Amenorrheic athletes who gain weight through reduced training and improved diet may resume menses spontaneously and increase their BMD (Drinkwater et al., 1986; Lindberg et al., 1987).

If the athlete has a diagnosable eating disorder, then treatment needs to include coordinated medical, nutritional, and psychological therapy. In our experience, this condition is best approached as a chronic condition, with long-term treatment and follow-up (months–years) being typical. Weight gain is the mainstay of treatment in trying to restore BMD in a patient with an eating disorder. However, weight gain is not always associated with improved BMD, and, when BMD is improved, it still tends to be below normal (Hotta et al., 1998; Jonnavithula et al., 1993). Therefore, estrogen replacement should be considered (see "Other Forms of Estrogen and/or Progestin Replacement" section).

The lifestyle changes (i.e., improved caloric intake and reduced exercise training) should be made in consultation with a dietitian. An example of changing the training intensity and dietary intake for a competitive athlete who is at less than 100% of her estimated ideal body weight (IBW) would be to reduce training time by one third and to add a snack containing at least 250 kilocalories (kcal) to the daily diet (Dueck et al., 1996), or at least enough to ensure that available daily energy is >35 kcal/kg fat-free mass (approximately 45–50 kcal/kg of body weight per day). If the athlete weighs 85% to 90% of estimated IBW and is exercising daily, we would recommend more aggressive changes: reduce exercise by one half and add 500 kcal/day (e.g., two dietary supplemental drinks or snacks). We do not recommend exercise if the body weight is <85% of estimated IBW, unless the athlete is >80% of estimated IBW, is eumenorrheic, and her weight is increasing weekly. There appears to be a subgroup of these athletes who have a more robust hypothalamic–pituitary–ovarian axis and maintain their menses better than women with anorexia nervosa, who resume menses only when their weight is >90% of estimated IBW. Exercise may attenuate bone loss in patients with bulimia nervosa compared to those with anorexia nervosa (Sundgot-Borger, 1998). We support exercise in patients with bulimia nervosa if their weight is >90% of the estimated IBW and they are menstruating. Strain on bone (through exercise) and estrogen appear to have additive effects on improving bone strength. The effectiveness of bone modeling through exercise could be limited when estrogen levels are reduced (Damien et al., 1998).

Appropriate Follow-up The athlete should be monitored weekly until weight increases consistently. The visits can then be reduced to once every 2 weeks assuming the teen's weight progresses toward 90% of estimated IBW. This assumes the coach is supportive of the plan. We usually give a written plan to the athlete and encourage her to show it to her coach and ask the coach to call the physician or dietitian with any questions.

Low Bone Density

Measurement of Bone Mineral Density Measurement of the BMD of the lumbar spine and hip by dual-energy x-ray absorptiometry (DXA) should be considered if the patient has been amenorrheic for longer than 6 months or oligomenorrheic, with fewer than 4 menses in the previous year. If the subject has been amenorrheic for longer than 1 year and is malnourished, the DXA scan is more strongly recommended. If DXA scanning is done, it should not be repeated at an interval of <12 months.

World Health Organization Criteria for Osteopenia and Osteoporosis The World Health Organization (1994) has established criteria for the diagnosis of osteopenia and osteoporosis using a T-score. The T-score is the number of standard deviations (SDs) above or below the average peak BMD value for young, healthy women (age 20–29). Osteoporosis is defined as a T-score of −2.5 SD or lower; osteopenia is defined as a T-score between −1 and −2.5 SD. How this designation applies to the risk for subsequent stress fracture, or ultimately to clinical osteoporosis manifested as a fracture, in young athletes with amenorrhea is not known. Therefore, the International Society for Clinical Densitometry (ISCD, www.iscd.org) recommends utilizing only Z-scores (age, gender, and ethnicity matched as best possible) for patients younger than 20 years. Furthermore, because the fracture threshold in children and adolescents has not been established, terminology such as "below the expected range for age" is preferred for Z-scores < − 2.0. Osteoporosis is a clinical, not densitometric, diagnosis in pediatrics. Finally, the physician should exercise caution in interpreting either T-scores or Z-scores in patients with short stature because DXA tends to underestimate BMD in short subjects and overestimate BMD in tall subjects (Leonard et al., 1999).

Hormonal Therapy
Does hormonal therapy reduce stress fractures and/or improve BMD?

It has not been established that estrogen/progestin, in the form of oral contraceptive pills (OCPs), increases BMD more than no treatment. One longitudinal, randomized study (Hergenroeder et al., 1997) demonstrated improvement in total body and lumbar BMD in young amenorrheic females treated for 12 months with OCPs, compared with those treated with medroxyprogesterone or placebo. A second longitudinal, randomized clinical trial (Gibson et al., 1999) reported no improvement in amenorrheic subjects treated over 18 months with an estrogen/progestin preparation (Trisequens) containing 1 to 2 mg estradiol plus

0.5 to 1 mg estriol (equivalent to 35 µg of ethinyl estradiol) every day plus norethisterone (1 mg) for 10 days in a 28-day cycle. Two milligrams of estradiol is estimated to be similar to 25 µg of ethinyl estradiol (Fagan, 1998). The ethinyl estradiol dose that would be equivalent to 1 mg of estriol is not known to us at this time, but the combination of estradiol (2 mg) and estriol (1 mg) appears to be similar.

It has also not been established that OCPs prevent stress fractures (Bennell et al., 1999). Two retrospective cohort studies reported lower rates of stress fractures in women who used OCPs (Barrow and Saha, 1988; Myburgh et al., 1990). One prospective study found no relationship between current or past use of OCPs and the rate of stress fractures of the lower extremity, compared with athletes who had never used OCPs (Bennell et al., 1999).

One study demonstrated that conjugated estrogen (Premarin, 0.625 mg taken daily on days 1 through 25 of each month) and medroxyprogesterone (Provera, 5 mg taken daily on days 16 through 25 of each month) taken for a mean of 1.5 years improved lumbar BMD in females with anorexia nervosa compared with a placebo group if the patient's weight at the initiation of therapy was <70% of the estimated IBW (Klibanski et al., 1995). However, the authors did not state that this study was conclusive that weight <70% of estimated IBW was the criterion for starting this estrogen/progestin therapy. One report demonstrated an improvement of BMD in adult women taking medroxyprogesterone, 10 mg/day, for 10 days a month, but that study has not been replicated and this is not an accepted treatment protocol for adolescents (Prior et al., 1990).

Other Pharmacological Treatments to Prevent Osteoporosis

Selective estrogen receptor modulators (SERMs) have been developed to maximize the effect of estrogen on bone while minimizing the effect of estrogen on the breast and endometrium. Raloxifene is a SERM that has been approved by the U.S. Food and Drug Administration (FDA) for the prevention and treatment of osteoporosis in postmenopausal women. Its effect on the skeletons of adolescent and young adult females is not known.

Bisphosphonates such as alendronate are utilized to improve BMD in postmenopausal women by intercalating into the bone matrix, inhibiting osteoclastic resorption of bone. Because bisphosphonates may remain in the skeleton for a decade or more and may cross the placenta, they are not recommended for women of child-bearing age or younger. Studies are underway to investigate the safety and efficacy of these agents in young women with eating disorders. Recombinant parathyroid hormone and its active polypeptide components have been shown to improve bone density and strength in postmenopausal women and in elderly men as well.

Recombinant insulinlike growth factor has been demonstrated to increase markers of bone turnover in women with anorexia nervosa (Grinspoon et al., 1996). Further research is needed to determine the role of these agents in improving BMD status in young women with amenorrhea.

The effects of all of the above agents on the skeletons of adolescent and young adult females are not known. *Therefore, they must all be considered investigational, to be used only in research settings or by specialized skeletal centers.*

Osteoporosis Prevention with Oral Contraceptive Pills

It has been suggested that use of OCPs in premenopausal women will reduce the risk of postmenopausal osteoporosis (Michaelsson et al., 1999). This effect has not been demonstrated for those who took OCPs at an age younger than 30 years.

With insufficient evidence for clinical benefit, the decision to treat with estrogen/progestin should be individualized. One concern is the psychological effects of taking OCPs. Patients may be falsely reassured by the resumption of menses so as to interfere with recovery. Other patients may be stressed by fears of hormonally mediated weight gain. Some users perceive weight gain even if they do not gain weight (Reubinoff et al., 1995). A prospective, longitudinal, randomized trial is urgently needed to resolve the effect of OCPs on BMD in amenorrheic athletes. However, the dropout rate in studies of amenorrheic subjects treated with hormonal therapy is 25% to 50%, making longitudinal studies difficult to perform (Gulekli et al., 1994; Hergenroeder et al., 1997; Gibson et al., 1999).

The following points should also be considered:

1. Young women with anorexia nervosa and secondary amenorrhea have mean serum estradiol levels that approximate those of postmenopausal women.
2. Osteoporosis is one of the more serious, long-term consequences of prolonged amenorrhea in adolescent athletes.
3. Hypoandrogenemia, reduced serum levels of insulinlike growth factor I (IGF-I), and hypercortisolemia in anorexia nervosa contribute to loss of BMD. These factors improve with weight gain. They are not likely to be affected by estrogen/progestin therapy and unless they are improved, the effect of estrogen/progestin may be limited.

In the absence of compelling evidence and an established standard, the use of combination OCPs should be considered for those female athletes who have been amenorrheic for longer than 6 months, especially if they are malnourished, as manifested by weight <85% of their estimated IBW. In addition, because 60% to 80% of the variance in BMD is likely attributable to heritable factors, a family history of osteoporosis should lower the threshold for hormonal treatment. If the athlete has been amenorrheic for longer than 12 months, stronger consideration should be given to starting OCP treatment, in addition to effecting lifestyle changes discussed earlier (Castro et al., 2000).

Estrogen Therapy in Younger Teens

Some groups have recommended that estrogen replacement must not be prescribed for patients younger than 16 years (American Academy of Pediatrics, 1989). The dilemma is that delaying estrogen therapy may compromise BMD but premature use of estrogen could compromise adult height. Bone age determination may be helpful in the decision to prescribe estrogen/progestin to female adolescents with amenorrhea related to excessive exercise and calorie restriction.

A 15-year old with a bone age of 13 years has achieved 96.4% of her full adult height; with a bone age of 14 years this same teen has achieved 98.3%, and with a bone age of 15 years 99%, of her adult height (Gruelich and Pyle, 1959). The mean height of females in North America is 163 cm at 19 years of age (Tanner and Davies, 1985). If estrogen therapy completely arrested height gain from the onset of therapy, then the adolescent with a bone age of 15 years and a potential adult height of 163 cm could potentially lose only 1.6 cm of height. If statural growth were only partially or minimally arrested, then some additional height growth would occur and any lost height potential would be trivial.

On the other hand, bone loss resulting from an eating disorder occurring before menarche could lead to significant arrest of BMD development, compared with bone loss after menarche. The onset of bone loss in relation to bone development is important in that onset of anorexia nervosa before 15 years of age affects bone size and volumetric BMD more than onset after age 15 does (Seeman et al., 2000). Bone fragility is a function of both bone size and volumetric BMD, and these are partly established during pubertal growth. There is a risk of delaying the start of estrogen/progestin therapy until epiphyseal growth is complete.

It is therefore reasonable to prescribe estrogen/progestin replacement for females with amenorrhea at 15 years of age and a bone age of 15 years, and to consider such therapy for those with a bone age of 14 years, depending on the degree of osteopenia and malnutrition. This is an area that requires further investigation.

Calcium Intake Amenorrheic athletes, like all adolescent females, have a daily elemental calcium recommended daily intake (RDI) of 1,300 to 1,800 mg. It must be noted, however, that in a group of healthy adolescents followed up longitudinally, changes in BMD were independent of calcium intake, which ranged from 500 to 1,500 mg/day (Lloyd et al., 2000).

ERGOGENIC AIDS AND DRUG USE IN ATHLETES

Background

Evidence suggests that substance use among high school and college athletes may be greater in some cases than in nonathletes, with important differences depending on gender and the individual drug being studied (Anderson and McKeag, 1989; Wadler and Hainline, 1989). Specifically, there is recent evidence that marijuana and alcohol use are higher in male students who compete in competitive sports than in those not competing in sports; the reverse is true for female athletes (Ewing, 1998; Aaron et al., 1995). Neither marijuana nor alcohol has ergogenic effects on athletic performance. Cigarettes tend to be used less by athletes (Aaron et al., 1995). Anabolic steroids are used more by athletes. Drugs are often readily available starting in junior high school.

The major categories of drugs used to improve performance by athletes include stimulants, pain relievers, and anabolic steroids (Wadler and Hainline, 1989). In addition, over the last decade there has been increased recognition of the use of dietary supplements as ergogenic aids. These supplements include creatine, androstenedione, and dehydroepiandrosterone (DHEA), γ-hydroxybutyrate, and protein powders.

For more information about drugs of abuse, contact the National Clearinghouse for Alcohol and Drug Information on-line at http://ncadi.samhsa.gov.

Therapeutic Drugs

Over-the-counter analgesics, decongestants, antihistamines, laxatives, antidiarrheal agents, and weight-loss medications are commonly used by athletes. Athletes should be asked specifically about use of these medications during office or training room visits, because they may not perceive them to be as important as prescription drugs and may not report their use. In addition, these medications have important side effects that can affect performance, and some are banned by sports governing bodies (NCAA and United States Olympic Committee). Physicians are encouraged to consult the United States (www.usantidoping.org) and World Anti-Doping Agencies (www.wada-ama.org) when advising athletes, especially college and elite athletes, about medication and prescription drug use.

Performance-Enhancing Drugs

Stimulants
Stimulants have been used extensively to combat psychological and muscular fatigue. These substances are banned by the International Olympic Committee (IOC) and can be detected by urine tests.

Amphetamines Fine motor coordination and performance on tasks requiring prolonged attention have been shown to improve with amphetamine use. Side effects include anxiety, restlessness, tremors, tachycardia, irritability, confusion, and poor judgment, and these effects occur at higher doses.

Cocaine No evidence supports ergogenic effects of cocaine. Effects include increased heart rate, reflexes, and blood pressure, with accompanying euphoria. In the inexperienced user, reflexes are often more rapid but dyssynchronous, leading to a decrement in athletic performance. Lethal toxicity can occur unexpectedly, particularly with intravenous use, because the doses of cocaine available on the street vary widely. Symptoms of acute overdose are difficult to treat and include arrhythmias, seizures, hyperthermia, and death. Metabolites can be found in the urine within 24 to 36 hours of ingestion and up to 4 days after acute ingestion.

Caffeine Caffeine is probably the most commonly used stimulant. Several studies have documented increased muscle work output for endurance activities. Significant side effects mimic those of other stimulants. Caffeine has a direct diuretic effect, potentially complicating fluid and electrolyte status in prolonged exercise activities. Caffeine is banned by the IOC in quantities >12 μg/mL (approximately equivalent to 4–8 cups of coffee or 8–16 cups of cola).

Anabolic Steroids
Anabolic steroid use is associated with increased muscle size and strength, especially in athletes who are weight training when the steroid use is initiated and in those who are consuming a high-calorie diet. Animal models demonstrate that anabolic steroids result in muscle hypertrophy in nonexercising muscle. There is no evidence that steroid use enhances aerobic power. There is evidence that anabolic steroids may aid in the healing of muscle contusion injury, in contrast to corticosteroids, raising potential

ethical issues in the future regarding the use of steroids in muscle healing in response to contusion. FDA-approved uses of anabolic steroids include weight gain in patients with acquired immunodeficiency syndrome (AIDS), severe anemia, hereditary angioedema, metastatic breast cancer, or male adrenal insufficiency.

Anabolic steroids may be injected or taken orally, and they are often freely available from peers and coaches. Buckley et al. (1988) reported that 6.6% of 12th grade male adolescents had used anabolic steroids. Approximately 21% indicated that their primary source was a health professional. The lifetime prevalence of illegal steroid use among high school students in the United States as reported by the YRBS rose from 2.2% in 1993 to 6.1% in 2003 but has since fallen to 4.0%, in the 2005 YRBS (Centers for Disease Control and Prevention, 2006). In the Monitoring the Future study of 12th graders, the lifetime prevalence rates were 2.3% in 1995, 2.9% in 1999, 3.5% in 2003, and 2.6% in 2005(www.monitoringthefuture.org, Johnston et al., 2006). For 8th graders, the lifetime prevalence rates rose from 2.0% in 1995 to 3.5% in 2003, but fell dramatically to 1.7% in 2005.

Side effects of anabolic steroids include the following:

1. Alteration of myocardial textural properties (as detected by ultrasound). These changes are not seen in weight lifters who do not use anabolic steroids, yet nonetheless experience increased left ventricular mass with weight training. The clinical significance and prognostic significance of these changes is unknown.
2. Altered myocardial function: 17α-Methyl testosterone has been associated with reduced myocardial compliance and reduced myocardial function in rats.
3. Risk of hepatic damage (manifested as elevated liver-specific enzymes): The risk of hepatic neoplasms is unknown, because the reports to date are anecdotal.
4. Decreased high-density lipoprotein (HDL) and increased low-density lipoprotein (LDL) cholesterol levels.
5. Oligospermia and azoospermia with decreased testicular size occurs.
6. Premature epiphyseal closure in pubertal athletes.
7. Acne.
8. Masculinization in women: Manifested as deepening of the voice, acne, and hair loss.
9. Feminization in men: Manifested as gynecomastia and a high voice.
10. Adverse psychological effects, including increased aggressiveness and rage in some athletes.
11. Association with the use of other illicit drugs.

Injected steroids are detectable in the urine for 6 months or longer. Orally administered anabolic steroids disappear from the urine after days to weeks. More information on anabolic steroids can be obtained at the NIDA Web site on steroid use: www.steroidabuse.org.

Narcotic Analgesics
Narcotic analgesics may allow an athlete to perform despite pain and/or injury, but they do not enhance athletic performance. In standard doses, there also does not appear to be a detriment. However, they may be abused in an attempt to return to play prematurely. The effects include psychomotor retardation, sedation, dysphoria, and nausea and vomiting.

Dietary Supplements as Ergogenic Aids
The potency, purity, and long-term effects of most dietary supplements (also see Chapter 83) are not known because they are not regulated by the FDA. Unfortunately, the 1994 Dietary Supplement Health and Education Act (DSHEA), which removed the FDA regulation, has lead to an explosion in the availability and use of these products among teens. Reputable information about dietary supplements can be found at *http://dietary-supplements.info.nih.gov*, but our awareness of the "latest" agents likely lags far behind their actual use by our patients. None of these supplements are recommended for use in adolescents.

Androstenedione Androstenedione is an androgen produced by the gonads and adrenal glands. It is a precursor to estradiol and testosterone, yet it is marketed as a prohormone or nutritional supplement and is not regulated by the FDA. Individuals taking androstenedione experience no beneficial effect on strength as compared with controls. It has been associated with increased serum estradiol levels, no change in serum testosterone levels, and an increased LDL:HDL ratio at 12 weeks in healthy adult men (King et al., 1999; Broeder et al., 2000).

There is no medically approved use for androstenedione, and its use is banned by the IOC, the NCAA, the National Football League, and other athletic organizations. However, because of its perceived benefit and because testing for androstenedione is not possible, its use is likely to continue.

Dehydroepiandrosterone DHEA is an adrenal androgen marketed as a food supplement. It is a precursor of androgens and estradiol. Ergogenic effects have not been demonstrated in athletes. DHEA has been reported to increase IGF. The side effects are androgenic, including hair loss and irreversible deepening of the voice in females. Androgens can hasten the growth of prostatic cancer, and estrogens can similarly affect the growth of breast and endometrial cancer. The effects of DHEA on the growth of these tumors are unknown.

Creatine Creatine is synthesized in the liver, kidney, and pancreas. Creatine is supplied in the diet in the form of meat and fish. The usual U.S. diet supplies approximately 1 to 2 g of creatine daily to replenish that which is lost in the urine. Theoretically, creatine works as an ergogenic aid by increasing the cellular concentration of high-energy phosphocreatine, the immediate transport entity in the synthesis of adenosine triphosphate (ATP) from adenosine diphosphate (ADP). It has been suggested that those with lower intracellular creatine concentration may benefit most from creatine supplementation, yet there is no method to assay for low intracellular concentration at this time. There may be some benefit for short-duration (i.e., <30 seconds), high-intensity exercise, but this effect has been demonstrated in laboratory settings and has not translated into improved performance on the athletic field. In addition, there have been case reports of renal injury with the use of creatine and long-term safety has not been established.

γ-Hydroxybutyrate, γ-Hydroxybutyrolactone, and 1,4-Butanediol 1,4-Butanediol (BD) is an industrial solvent that is rapidly converted to γ-hydroxybutyrate (GHB), which is the active metabolite for all three of these compounds. GHB is an endogenous metabolite of γ-aminobutyric acid (GABA), the predominant inhibitory

neurotransmitter in the brain. The clinical use of GHB is limited to trials in patients with narcolepsy. GHB was marketed to bodybuilders in the 1980s as a method to increase muscle and promote fat loss. Although it is a Schedule I drug, it is a common "rave" drug and is readily accessible.

The sale of GHB was banned in 1991 after it was linked to fatal and to serious nonfatal side effects, but DSHEA made it possible to legally sell the precursors of GHB as dietary supplements. Both γ-hydroxybutyrolactone (GBL) and BD were marketed as nontoxic and natural dietary supplements. The FDA subsequently issued warnings about both compounds, the health risks of which included acute intoxication (which can be fatal), addiction, and withdrawal (Zvosec et al., 2001). The FDA has recommended disposing of all supplies of GBL, and there was a voluntary recall of GBL in 1999. Subsequently, BD began being marketed as a "replacement product" despite FDA warnings.

Use of Recreational Drugs by Athletes

Smokeless Tobacco
The incidence of smokeless tobacco use among preprofessional and professional baseball players is estimated to be 30% to 40% (Ernster et al., 1990), compared to 4% to 11% for the same age-group in the general population. Cigarette smoking is less common among baseball players. Complications of smokeless tobacco include oral cancer, periodontal disease, oral leukoplakia, and mouth and gum irritation. Smokeless tobacco may have a performance-enhancing effect on cognitive tasks. There does not appear to be a demonstrable effect on reaction time, and there is no demonstrable ergogenic effect. The perception of benefit and cultural support for smokeless tobacco use in sports such as baseball, football, and rodeo sustain its use.

Alcohol
Alcohol is the leading drug of abuse among high school and college students, regardless of whether they are involved in sports. Alcohol use in college students is better correlated with participation in fraternities and sororities than with participation in athletics. Still, alcohol has become entwined in the fabric of sport in America through sponsorship use of athletic events. Beer producers spend large proportions of their advertising budgets on sports. This financial relationship between alcohol and sports appears unlikely to change, and, to the extent that advertising of alcohol influences drinking behaviors, alcohol abuse will remain a problem for adolescents and young adults.

Alcohol use acutely and chronically impairs athletic performance by impairing cognition and visual-motor coordination. However, athletes who significantly abuse alcohol may not have impaired performance until the problem is chronic. Physicians and trainers should attempt to diagnose and refer patients for treatment at the early and middle stages of alcohol abuse and not wait until performance deteriorates.

Testing for Performance-Enhancing Drugs

Readers are encouraged to contact the NCAA (telephone 1-913-339-1906) or the U.S. Olympic Committee (1-800-233-0393, Drug Control Hotline). The following five components should be included in any drug testing program:

1. Written policy: A written policy regarding the purpose of the drug prevention program, the methods of collection, and consequences. In developing this plan, representatives from coaches, parents, athletes, medical staff, and physicians should be involved.
2. Education: An educational component must be prepared and used.
3. Testing: Actual testing must take place, preferably at random.
4. Discipline for those who test positive: The mechanism of feedback to the player and coaches must be established. The physician should not be in the role of administering any disciplinary action; rather, he or she should work with the athlete to identify a problem if one exists and to facilitate appropriate care.
5. Evaluation of treatment: A process for evaluating the treatment of drug users must be implemented.

The American College Health Association (1994) (http://acha.org/info_resources/guidelines.cfm) has also provided guidelines regarding drug education and testing of student athletes, including the following:

1. The drug education program should reflect the institution's overall commitment to eliminating drug abuse among students, faculty, and staff. The drug education and testing programs should not be restricted to only student athletes.
2. Each institution initiating or evaluating a drug education and testing program should have an advisory committee in place consisting of student athletes and representatives of the athletics department, student health center, counseling center, and student affairs.
3. A single individual should direct and supervise the program.
4. The educational program should target both the athletes and the coaches and staff of the athletic department.
5. Legal counsel should be involved when a drug testing program is instituted.
6. Drug testing should be done only when it is accomplished fairly and accurately.
7. Careful review should be undertaken regarding which athletes will be tested and how often, as well as what sanctions will be imposed.
8. The institution should guarantee that the test results and records will be handled in a strictly confidential manner.
9. It is important that adequate counseling be available for those who test positive.
10. Because alcohol is the most abused drug on campuses, an emphasis on alcohol education should be incorporated into the program.

Given than many jurisdictions that sponsor sports may be limited financially, it may be more cost effective to advocate for balanced educational programs that increase student-athletes' knowledge than to mount an expensive testing program, particularly at the high school and youth sports levels.

WEB SITES

For Teenagers and Parents

http://www.sportsmedicine.com/. Site connecting individuals interested in sports medicine.

http://www.alliedhealthrehab.com/Information/Informational_sheets.htm. Patient information from the Sports Medicine Center, Akron Children's Hospital.

http://orthoinfo.aaos.org. Your Orthopaedic Connection from the American Academy of Orthopaedic Surgeons.

For Health Professionals

http://www.aap.org/sections/sportsmedicine/. American Academy of Pediatrics Council on Sports Medicine and Fitness.

http://www.acsm.org/. American College of Sports Medicine.

http://www.sportsmed.org/. American Orthopaedic Society for Sports Medicine.

http://www.unc.edu/depts/nccsi/. National Center for Catastrophic Sports Injury Research, data on sports injuries and fatalities.

http://www.nata.org/downloads/documents/secondary_school_medcarecommunication.pdf. National Athletic Trainers' Association communication on Appropriate Medical Care for the Secondary School-Age Athlete.

http://www.asmi.org/. American Sport Medicine Institute.

http://www.ipsm.org. Institute for Preventative Sports Medicine.

http://www.newamssm.org. American Medical Society for Sports Medicine.

http://www.cdc.gov/doc.do/id/0900f3ec80017619. U.S. Centers for Disease Control and Prevention Heads Up! Tool Kit on Concussion.

REFERENCES AND ADDITIONAL READINGS

Aaron DJ, Dearwater SR, Anderson R, et al. Physical activity and the initiation on high-risk health behaviors in adolescents. *Med Sci Sports Exerc* 1995;27:1639.

American Academy of Family Physicians, the American Academy of Pediatrics, the American Medical Society for Sports Medicine, the American Orthopedic Society for Sports Medicine and the American Osteopathic Academy of Sports Medicine. Preparticipation physical evaluation. *The Physician and Sports Medicine*, 2nd ed. Minneapolis, MN: A joint publication of the American Academy of Family Physicians, the American Academy of Pediatrics, the American Medical Society for Sports Medicine, the American Orthopedic Society for Sports Medicine and the American Osteopathic Academy of Sports Medicine, 1996.

American Academy of Family Physicians, American Academy of Pediatrics, American College of Sports Medicine. *Preparticipation physical evaluation*, 3rd ed. Minneapolis, MN: McGraw-Hill Healthcare Information, 2005.

American Academy of Pediatrics, Committee on Sports Medicine and Fitness. Mitral valve prolapse and athletic participation in children and adolescents. *Pediatrics* 1995;95;789.

American Academy of Pediatrics, Committee on Sports Medicine and Fitness and American Academy of Ophthalmology. Committee on eye safety and sports ophthalmology. Protective eyewear for young athletes. *Pediatrics* 1996;98;311.

American Academy of Pediatrics, Committee on Sports Medicine and Fitness. Strength training by children and adolescents. *Pediatrics* 2001;107;1470.

American Academy of Pediatrics Committee on Sports Medicine and Fitness. Promotion of healthy weight-control practices in young athletes. *Pediatrics* 2005;116:1557.

American Medical Society for Sports Medicine and American Academy of Sports Medicine. Human immunodeficiency virus and other blood-borne pathogens in sports. *Clin J Sports Med* 1995;5:199.

American Psychiatric Association. *Diagnostic and statistical manual of mental disorders*, 4th ed. Washington, DC: American Psychiatric Association, 1994.

Anderson J. *Stretching*. Bolinas, CA: Shelter Publications, 1980.

Bader RS, Goldberg L, Sahn DJ. Risk of sudden cardiac death in young athletes: which screening strategies are appropriate? *Pediatr Clin North Am* 2004;51:1421.

Batts M. The etiology of spondylolisthesis. *J Bone Joint Surg* 1939;21:879.

Bering JR, Steen SN. *Sports nutrition for the '90s*. Gaithersburg, MD: Aspen Publishers, 1991.

Berger S, Kugler JD, Thomas JA, et al. Sudden cardiac death in children and adolescents: introduction and overview. *Pediatr Clin North Am* 2004;51:1201.

Bergfield JA, Hershman EB, Wilboiurn AJ. Brachial injuries in athletes. *Orthop Trans* 1988;12:743.

236th Bethesda Conference. Eligibility recommendations for competitive athletes with cardiovascular abnormalities. *J Am Coll Cardiol* 2005;45:1313.

Bhasin S, Storer TW, Berman N, et al. The effects of supraphysiologic doses of testosterone on muscle size and strength in normal men. *N Engl J Med* 1996;335:1.

Blimpke CJ. Resistance training during preadolescence. *Sports Med* 1993;15:389.

Bouchard C, Shepard RJ, Stephens T, eds. *Physical activity, fitness, and health: international proceedings and consensus statement*. Champaign, IL: Human Kinetics, 1994.

Broeder CE, Quindry J, Brittingham K, et al. The andro project: physiological and hormonal influences of androstenedione supplementation in men 35 to 65 years old participating in a high-intensity resistance training program. *Arch Intern Med* 2000;160:3093.

Brostrum L. Treatment and prognosis in recent ligament ruptures. *Acta Chir Scand* 1966;132:537.

Buckley WE, Yesalis CE, Friedl KE. Estimated prevalence of anabolic steroid use among male high school seniors. *JAMA* 1988;260:3441.

Bundy DG, Feudtner CF. Preparticipation physical evaluations for high school athletes: time for a new game plan. *Ambul Pediatr* 2004;4:260.

Calfee R, Fadale P. Popular ergogenic drugs and supplements in young athletes. *Pediatrics* 2006;117:e577.

Calin A, Porta J, Fries JF, et al. Clinical history as a screening test for ankylosing spondylitis. *JAMA* 1977;237:2613.

Cantu RC. When to return to contact sports after a cerebral concussion. *Sports Med Dig* 1988;10:1.

Cantu RC, Mueller FO. Fatalities and catastrophic injuries in high school and college sports, 1982–1997. *Phys Sportsmed* 1999;27:35.

Cassas KJ, Cassettari-Wayhs A. Childhood and adolescent sports-related overuse injuries. *Am Fam Physician* 2006;73:1014.

Centers for Disease Control and Prevention. Youth risk behavior surveillance—United States, 1997. *Morb Mortal Wkly Rep* 1998;47(SS-3);1.

Centers for Disease Control and Prevention. Youth risk behavior surveillance—United States, 2005. *Morb Mortal Wkly Rep CDC Surveill Summ* 2006;55(SS05);1. http://www.cdc.gov/HealthyYouth/yrbs/index.htm.

Circulation. Cardiovascular preparticipation screening of competitive athletes. 1996;94:850.

Collins MW, Grindel SH, Lovel MR, et al. Relationship between concussion and neuropsychological performance in college football players. *JAMA* 1999;282:964.

Colorado Medical Society, Sports Medicine Committee. *Guidelines for the management of concussion in sports, revised.* Denver, CO: Colorado Medical Soceity, 1991.

Creatine and androstenedione: two "dietary supplements." *Med Lett Drugs Ther* 1998;40:105.

Dehydroepiandrosterone (DHEA). *Med Lett Drugs Ther* 1996; 38:91.

Department of Health and Human Services, U.S. Public Health Service. *Healthy people 2010: conference edition.* Washington, DC: DHHS, 2000.

DiBello V, Bianchi M, Bertini A, et al. Effects of anabolic-anabolic steroids on weight-lifters' myocardium: an ultrasonic video-densitometric study. *Med Sci Sports Exerc* 1999;31:514.

Drezner JA. Sudden cardiac death in young athletes. *Postgrad Med* 2000;108:37.

Durant RH, Rickert VI, Ashworth CS, et al. Use of multiple drugs among adolescents who use anabolic steroids. *N Engl J Med* 1993;328:922.

Durant RH, Seymore C, Linder CW, et al. The preparticipation examination of athletes: comparison of single and multiple examiners. *Am J Dis Child* 1985;139:657.

Elster A, ed. *American medical association guidelines for adolescent preventive services (GAPS) recommendations and rationale.* Baltimore: Williams & Wilkins, 1994.

Ewing BT. High school athletes and marijuana use. *J Drug Educ* 1998;28:147.

Ernster VL, Grady DG, Greene JC, et al. Smokeless tobacco use and health effects among baseball players. *JAMA* 1990; 264:218.

Faigenbaum AD, Zaichkowsky LD, Gardner DE, et al. Anabolic steroid use by male and female middle school students. *Pediatrics* 1998;101:e6.

Flack JM, Kvasnicka JH, Gardin JM, et al. Anthropometric and physiologic correlates of mitral valve prolapse in a biethnic cohort of young adults: the CARDIA study. *Am Heart J* 1999; 138:486.

Garrick JG, Requa R. Injuries in high school sports. *Pediatrics* 1978;61:465.

Garrick JG, Webb DR. *Sports injuries: diagnosis and management,* 2nd ed. Philadelphia: WB Saunders, 1999.

Gilon D, Buonanno FS, Joffe MM, et al. Lack of evidence of an association between mitral-valve prolapse and stroke in young patients. *N Engl J Med* 1999;341:8.

Glover DW, Maron BJ, Matheson GO. The preparticipation physical examination. *Phys Sportsmed* 1999;27:29.

Goldberg B, Saraniti A, Whitman P, et al. Pre-participation sports assessments: an objective evaluation. *Pediatrics* 1979; 66:736.

Green GA, Jordan SE. Are brain injuries a significant problem in soccer? *Clin Sports Med* 1998;17:795.

Gronwall D, Wrightson P. Cumulative effects of concussion. *Lancet* 1975;2:995.

Hallagan JB, Hallagan LF, Snyder MB. Anabolic-androgenic steroid use by athletes. *N Engl J Med* 1989;321:1042.

Haller CA, Benowitz NL. Adverse cardiovascular and central nervous system events associated with dietary supplements containing ephedra alkaloids. *N Engl J Med* 2000;343:1833.

Hergenroeder AC. Diagnosis and treatment of ankle injuries: a review. *Am J Dis Child* 1990;144:809.

Hergenroeder AC, Garrick JG, eds. Sports medicine. *Pediatr Clin North Am* 1990;37(5).

Hergenroeder AC, Phillips S. Advising teenagers and young adults about weight gain and loss through exercise and diet: practical advice for the physician. In: Shenker IR, ed. *Monographs in clinical pediatrics: adolescent medicine.* London: Harwood Academic, 1994:113.

Jonas AP, Sickles RT, Lombardo JA. Substance abuse. In: Puffer J, ed. *Clinics in sports medicine,* 1992;11:379.

Johnson MD. Anabolic steroid use in adolescent athletes. *Pediatr Clin North Am* 1990;37:1111.

Johnson TS, Rock PB. Current concepts: acute mountain sickness. *N Engl J Med* 1988;319:841.

Johnston LD, O'Malley PM. Bachman JG, et al. *Monitoring the future national survey results on drug use, 1975–2005: volume I, secondary school students* (NIH Publication No. 06–5883). Bethesda, MD: National Institute on Drug Abuse, 2006.

Keller CS, Noyes FR, Buncher R. The medical aspects of soccer injury epidemiology. *Am J Sports Med* 1987;15:230.

Kelly JP, Nichols JS, Filley CM, et al. Concussion in sports: guidelines for the prevention of catastrophic outcome. *JAMA* 1991;266:2867.

King DS, Sharp RL, Vukovich MD, et al. Effect of oral androstenedione on serum testosterone and adaptations to resistance training in young men: a randomized controlled trial. *JAMA* 1999;281:2020.

Kirkwood MW, Yeates KO, Wilson PE. Pediatric sport-related concussion: a review of the clinical management of an oft-neglected population. *Pediatrics* 2006;117:1359.

Landers DM, Crews DJ, Boutcher SH, et al. The effects of smokeless tobacco on performance and psychophysiological response. *Med Sci Sports Exerc* 1992;24:895.

Leddy JJ, Smolinski RJ, Lawrence J, et al. Prospective evaluation of the Ottawa Ankle rules in a university sports medicine center. *Am J Sports Med* 1998;26:158.

Leininger BE, Gramling SE, Fannell HD, et al. Neuropsychological deficits in symptomatic minor head injury patients after concussion and mild concussion. *J Neurol Neurosurg Psychiatry* 1990;53:293.

Leski M. Sudden cardiac death in athletes. *South Med J* 2004; 97:861.

Lyznicki JM, Nielsen NH, Schneider JF. Cardiovascular screening of student athletes. *Am Fam Physician* 2000;62:765.

Maron BJ. Cardiovascular risks to young persons on the athletic field. *Ann Intern Med* 1998;129:379.

Maron BJ, Mitten Matthew J, Quandt EF, et al. Competitive athletes with cardiovascular disease: the case of Nicholas Knapp. *N Engl J Med* 1998;339:1634.

Maron BJ, Roberts WC, McAllister HA, et al. Sudden death in young athletes. *Circulation* 1980;62:218.

Maron BJ, Thompson PD, Puffer JC, et al. Cardiovascular preparticipation screening of competitive athletes. A statement for health professionals from the Sudden Death Committee and Congenital Cardiac Defects Committee, American Heart Association. *Circulation* 1996;94:850; (Addendum appears in *Circulation* 1998;97:2294).

Matser EJT, Kessels AG, Lezak MD, et al. Neuropsychological impairment in amateur soccer players. *JAMA* 1999;282:971.

McClain LG, Reynolds S. Sports injuries in a high school. *Pediatrics* 1989;84:446.

McCrory PR. Second impact syndrome. *Neurology* 1998;50:677.

McGrory PR, Johnston K, Meeuwisse W, et al. Summary and agreement statement of the 2nd International Conference on Concussion in Sport, Prague 2004. *Br J Sports Med* 2005; 39:196.

Metzl JD. Concussion in the young athlete. *Pediatrics* 2006; 117(5):1813.

MMWR Morb Mortal Wkly Rep. Sports-related recurrent brain injuries—U.S. 1997;46:224.

Mueller FD, Cantu RC. *National center for catastrophic injury research: 17th annual report.* Chapel Hill, NC: University of North Carolina, NCCSIR, 2001. Available at www.unc.edu/depts/nccsi.

National Heart, Lung, and Blood Institute. Indexes of obesity and comparisons with the previous national survey data in 9- and 10-year-old black and white girls: the NHLBI Growth and Health Study. *J Pediatr* 1994;124:675.

National High Blood Pressure Education Program, Working Group on Hypertension Control in Children and Adolescents. Fourth report on the diagnosis, evaluation, and treatment of high blood pressure in children and adolescents, *Pediatrics* 2004;114:555.

National Institutes of Health. *Proceedings of the Conference on Sports Injuries in Youth: surveillance strategies.* NIH Publication No. 93–3444. Washington, DC: NIH, Department of Health and Human Services, U.S. Public Health Service, November 1992.

Nickerson HJ, Holubets MC, Weiler BR, et al. Causes of iron deficiency in adolescent athletes. *J Pediatr* 1989;114:657.

Oberlander MA, Shalvoy RM, Hughston JC. The accuracy of the clinical knee examination documented by arthroscopy. *Am J Sports Med* 1993;21:773.

O'Connor FG, Kugler JP, Oriscello RG. Sudden death in young athletes: screening for the needle in a haystack. *Am Fam Physician* 1998;57:2763.

O'Shea KJ, Murphy KP, Heekin RD, et al. The diagnostic accuracy of history, physical examination, and radiographs in the evaluation of traumatic knee disorders. *Am J Sports Med* 1996;24:164.

Pate RR, Long BJ, Heath G. Descriptive epidemiology of physical activity in adolescents. *Pediatr Exerc Sci* 1994;6:434.

Pate RR, Pratt M, Blair SN, et al. Physical activity and public health: a recommendation from the Centers for Disease Control and Prevention and the American College of Sports Medicine. *JAMA* 1995;273:402.

Pfister GC, Puffer JC, Maron BJ. Preparticipation cardiovascular screening for U.S. collegiate student-athletes. *JAMA* 2000;283:1597.

Pope PR, Herbert RD, Kirwan JD, et al. A randomized trial of pre-exercise stretching for prevention of lower-limb injury. *Med Sci Sports Exerc* 2000;32:271.

Powell JW, Barber-Foss KD. Traumatic brain injury in high school athletes. *JAMA* 1999;282:958.

Puffer JC. Drugs and doping in athletes. In: Mellion MB, ed. *Office management of sports injuries and athletic problems.* Philadelphia: Handley & Belfus, 1988.

Purcell JS, Hergenroeder AC. Physical conditioning in adolescents. *Curr Opin Pediatr* 1994;6:373.

Reid DC. *Sports injury assessment and rehabilitation.* New York: Churchill Livingston, 1992.

Reider B, ed. *Sports medicine: the school-age athlete,* 2nd ed. Philadelphia: WB Saunders, 1996.

Ross Laboratories. *For the practitioner: orthopedic screening examination for participation in sports.* Columbus, OH: Ross Laboratories, 1978.

Sallis JF, ed. Physical activity guidelines for adolescents. [Special issue]. *Pediatr Exerc Sci* 1994;6:299.

Semon RL, Spengler D. Significance of lumbar spondylolysis in college football players. *Spine* 1981;6:172.

Shields BJ, Smith GA. Cheerleading-related injuries to children 5 to 18 years of age: United States, 1990–2002. *Pediatrics* 2006; 117:122.

Snoek JW, Minderhoud JM, Wilmink JT. Delayed deterioration following mild head injury in children. *Brain* 1984;107:15.

Soler T, Calderon C. The prevalence of spondylolysis in the Spanish elite athlete. *Am J Sports Med* 2000;28:57.

Sosin DM, Sniezek JE, Thurman DJ. Incidence of mild and moderate brain injury in the United States, 1991. *Brain Inj* 1996;10:47.

Stewart JG, Ahlquist DA, McGill DB, et al. Gastrointestinal blood loss and anemia in runners. *Ann Intern Med* 1984;100:843.

Steill IG, Greenberg GH, Wells GA, et al. Prospective validation of a decision rule for the use of radiography in acute knee injuries. *JAMA* 1996;275:611.

Steill IG, Greenberg GH, McKnight RD, et al. The "real" Ottawa Ankle rules. *Ann Emerg Med* 1996;27:103.

Thacker SB, Stroup DF, Branche CM, et al. The prevention of ankle sprains in sports. *Am J Sports Med* 1999;27:753.

U.S. Department of Health and Human Services, Centers for Disease Control and Prevention, National Center for Chronic Disease Prevention and Health Promotion. *Physical activity and health: a report of the Surgeon General.* Publication No. S/N 017-023-00196-5. Washington, DC: U.S. Department of Health and Human Services, Centers for Disease Control and Prevention, National Center for Chronic Disease Prevention and Health Promotion, 1996.

Valkenburg HA, Haaneen HCM. The epidemiology of low back pain. In: White AA, Gordon SL, eds. *American Academy of Orthopaedic surgeons symposium on idiopathic low back pain.* St. Louis: CV Mosby, 1982:9.

Wadler GI, Hainline B. Ryan AJ, ed. *Drugs and the athlete.* Contemporary Exercise and Sports Medicine Series. Philadelphia: FA Davis Co, 1989.

Zvosec DL, Smith SW, McCurcheon JR, et al. Adverse events, including death, associated with the use of 1, 4-butanediol. *N Engl J Med* 2001;344:87.

The Female Athlete/Maturational Issues

American Academy of Pediatrics, Committee on Sports Medicine. Amenorrhea in adolescent athletes. *Pediatrics* 1989;84:394.

American Academy of Pediatrics, Committee on Sports Medicine and Fitness. Medical concerns of the female athlete. *Pediatrics* 2000;106:610.

Ayers JWT, Gidwani GP, Schmidt IMV, et al. Osteopenia in hypoestrogenic young women with anorexia nervosa. *Fertil Steril* 1984;41:224.

Barrow GW, Saha S. Menstrual irregularity and stress fractures in collegiate female distance runners. *Am J Sports Med* 1988; 16:209.

Bennell KL, Malcolm SA, Thomas SA, et al. Risk factors for stress fractures in track and field athletes. *Am J Sports Med* 1996;24:810.

Bennell K, White S, Crossley K. The oral contraceptive pill: a revolution for sports women? *Br J Sports Med* 1999;33:231.

Bernstein L, Henderson BE, Hanisch R, et al. Physical exercise and reduced risk of breast cancer in young women. *J Natl Cancer Inst* 1994;86:1403.

Birch K. Female athlete triad. *BMJ* 2005;330:244.

Cann CE, Martin MC, Genant HK, et al. Decreased spinal mineral content in amenorrheic women. *JAMA* 1984;251:626.

Castro J, Sazaro L, Pons F, et al. Predictors of bone mineral density reductions in adolescents with anorexia nervosa. *J Am Acad Child Adolesc Psychiatry* 2000;39:1365.

Constantini NW, Warren MP. Physical activity, fitness, and reproductive health in women: clinical observations. In:

Bouchard C, Shepard RJ, Stephens T, eds. *Physical activity, fitness, and health*. Champaign, IL: Human Kinetics, 1994.

Copeland PM, Sacks NR, Herzog DB. Longitudinal follow-up of amenorrhea in eating disorders. *Psychosom Med* 1995; 57:121.

Daly RM, Rich PA, Klein R, et al. Short stature in competitive prepubertal and early pubertal male gymnasts: the result of selection bias or intense training? *J Pediatr* 2000; 137:510.

Damien E, Price JS, Lanyon LE. The estrogen receptor's involvement in osteoblasts' adaptive response to mechanical strain. *J Bone Miner Res* 1998;13:1275.

Damsgaard R, Bencke J, Matthiesen G, et al. Is prepubertal growth adversely affected by sport? *Med Sci Sports Exerc* 2000;32:1698.

Drinkwater BL, Bruemner B, Chesnut CH III. Menstrual history as a determinant of current bone density in young athletes. *JAMA* 1990;263:545.

Drinkwater BL, Nelson K, Chestnut CH, et al. Bone mineral content of amenorrheic and eumenorrheic athletes. *N Engl J Med* 1984;311:277.

Drinkwater BL, Nilson K, Ott S, et al. Bone mineral density after resumption of menses in amenorrheic athletes. *JAMA* 1986;256:380.

Dueck CA, Matt KS, Manore MM, et al. Treatment of athletic amenorrhea with a diet and training intervention program. *Int J Sport Nutr* 1996;6:24.

Elliot DL, Goldberg L, Loprinzi M. Management of suspected iron deficiency: A cost-effectiveness model. *Med Sci Sports Exerc*. 1991;23:1332.

Fagan KM. Pharmacologic management of athletic amenorrhea. *Clin Sports Med* 1998;17:327.

Frisch RE, Wyshak G, Albright NL, et al. Lower prevalence of non-reproductive system cancer among female former college athletes. *Med Sci Sports Exerc* 1989;21:250.

Gibson JH, Mitchell A, Reeve J, et al. Treatment of reduced bone mineral density in athletic amenorrhea: a pilot study. *Osteoporos Int* 1999;10:284.

Goodman LR, Warren MP. The female athlete and menstrual function. *Curr Opin ObstetrGynecol* 2005;17:466.

Gortmaker SL, Dietz WH, Sobol AN, et al. Increasing pediatric obesity in the US. *Am J Dis Child* 1987;14:535.

Grinspoon S, Baum H, Lee K, et al. Effects of short-term recombinant human insulin-like growth factor I administration on bone turnover in osteopenic women with anorexia nervosa. *J Clin Ednocrinol Metab* 1996;81:3864.

Gruelich WW & Pyle SI. Radiographic atlas of the skeltal development of the hand and wrist, 2nd Edition. Stanford, CA: Stanford University Press, 1959.

Gulekli B, Davies MC, Jacos HS. Effect of treatment on established osteoporosis in young women with amenorrhea. *Clin Endocrinol* 1994;41:275.

Haberland CA, Seddick D, Marcus R, et al. A physician survey of therapy for exercise-induced amenorrhea: a brief report. *Clin J Sports Med* 1995;5:246.

Hergenroeder AC, Smith EO, Shypailo R, et al. Bone mineral changes in young women with hypothalamic amenorrhea and oligomenorrhea treated with oral contraceptive pills, medroxyprogesterone, and placebo over 12 months. *Am J Obstet Gynecol* 1997;176:1017.

Hewett TE, Lindenfeld TN, Riccobene JV, et al. The effect of neuromuscular training on the incidence of knee injury in female athletes. *Am J Sports Med* 1999;27:699.

Hobart JA, Smucker DR. The female athlete triad. *Am Fam Physician* 2000;61:3357.

Hotta M, Shibasaki T, Sato K, et al. The importance of body weight history in the occurrence and recovery of osteoporosis in patients with anorexia nervosa: evaluation by dual X-ray absorptiometry and bone metabolic markers. *Eur J Endocrinol* 1998;139:276.

Jonnavithula S, Warren MP, Fox RP, et al. Bone density is compromised in amenorrheic women despite return of menses: a 2-year study. *Obstet Gynecol* 1993;81:669.

Klibanski A, Biller B, Schoenfeld D, et al. The effect of estrogen administration on trabecular bone loss in young women with anorexia nervosa. *J Clin Endocrinol Metab* 1995;80:898.

Kleerekoper M, Briensa RS, Schultz LR, et al. Oral contraceptive use may protect against low bone mass. *Arch Intern Med* 1991;151:1971.

Leonard MB, Properi KJ, Zemel BS, et al. Discrepancies in pediatric bone mineral density reference data: potential for misdiagnosis of osteopenia. *J Pediatr* 1999;135:182.

Loucks AB. Physical activity, fitness, and female reproductive morbidity. In: Bouchard C, Shepard RJ, Stephens T, eds. *Physical activity, fitness, and health*. Champaign, IL: Human Kinetics, 1994.

Lindberg JS, Powell M, Hunt MM, et al. Increased vertebral bone mineral in response to reduced exercise in amenorrheic runners. *West J Med* 1987;146:39.

Lindholm C, Hagenfeldt K, Ringertz B-M. Pubertal development in elite juvenile gymnasts: effects of physical training. *Acta Obstet Gynecol Scand* 1994;73:269.

Lloyd T, Chinchilli VM, Hohnson-Rollings N, et al. Adult female hip bone density reflects teenage sports-exercise patterns but not teenage calcium intake. *Pediatrics* 2000;106:40.

Malina RM. Physical activity and training: effects on stature and the adolescent growth spurt. *Med Sci Sports Exerc* 1994; 26:759.

Malina RM. Issues in normal growth and maturation. *Curr Opin Endocrinol Diabetes* 1995;2:83.

Marcus R, Cann C, Madvig P, et al. Menstrual function and bone mass in elite women distance runners: endocrine and metabolic features. *Ann Intern Med* 1985;102:158.

Michaelsson K, Baron JA, Farahmand BY, et al. Oral-contraceptive use and risk of hip fracture: a case-control study. *Lancet* 1999;353:1481.

Myburgh KH, Hutchins J, Fataar AB, et al. Low bone density is an etiologic factor for stress fractures in athletes. *Ann Intern Med* 1990;113:754.

National Heart Lung and Blood Institute. Indexes of obesity and comparisons with the previous national survey data in 9- and 10-year old black and white girls: The NHLBI Growth and Health Study. *J Pediatr*. 1994;124:675.

Nichols JF, Rauh MJ, Lawson MJ, et al. Prevalence of the female athlete triad syndrome among high school athletes. *Arch Pediatr Adolesc Med* 2006;160:137.

Prior JC, Vigna YM, Schechter MT, et al. Spinal bone loss and ovulatory disturbances. *N Engl J Med* 1990;323:1221.

Recker R, Davies KM, Hinders SM, et al. Bone gain in young adult women. *JAMA* 1992;68:2403.

Rencken ML, Chesnut CH, Drinkwater BL. Bone density a multiple skeletal sites in amenorrheic athletes. *JAMA* 1996; 276:238.

Reubinoff BE, Grubstein A, Meirow D, et al. Effects of low-dose estrogen oral contraceptives on weight, body composition, and fat distribution in young women. *Fertil Steril* 1995;63:516.

Rockwell JC, Sorensen AM, Baker S, et al. Weight training decreases vertebral bone density in premenopausal women: a prospective study. *J Clin Endocrinol Metab* 1990;71:988.

Seeman E, Karlsson MK, Duan Y. On exposure to anorexia nervosa, the temporal variation in axial and appendicular skeletal development predisposes to site-specific deficits in bone size and density: a cross-sectional study. *J Bone Miner Res* 2000;15:2259.

Seeman E, Szmukler GI, Formica C, et al. Osteoporosis in anorexia nervosa: the influence of peak bone density, bone loss, oral contraceptive use, and exercise. *J Bone Miner Res* 1992;7:1467.

Sundgot-Borger J, et al. Normal bone mass in bulimic women. *J Clin Endocrinol Metab* 1998;9:3144.

Theintz GE, Howald H, Weiss U, et al. Evidence for a reduction of growth potential in adolescent female gymnasts. *J Pediatr* 1993;122:306.

Vehaskari V, Rapola J. Isolated proteinuria: Analysis of a school-age population. *J Pediatr.* 1982;101:661.

Warren MP, Brooks-Gunn J, Hamilton LH, et al. Scoliosis and fractures in young ballet dancers: relation to delayed menarche and secondary amenorrhea. *N Engl J Med* 1986; 314:1348.

World Health Organization. *Assessment of fracture risk and its application to screening for postmenopausal osteoporosis.* WHO technical report series. Geneva: WHO, 1994.

Yeager KK, Agostini R, Nattiv A, et al. The female athlete triad: disordered eating, amenorrhea and osteoporosis. *Med Sci Sports Exerc* 1993;25:775.

Yetman AT, McCrindle BW, MacDonald C, et al. Myocardial bridging in children with hypertrophic cardiomyopathy: A risk factor for sudden death. *N Engl J Med.* 1998; 339:1201.

PART V

Dermatologic Disorders

CHAPTER 19

Acne

Mei-Lin T. Pang and Lawrence F. Eichenfield

Acne vulgaris is highly prevalent in adolescents and is the skin disease most often evaluated by adolescent health care providers. Not only is acne common, it also has important psychological consequences, and quality of life is often affected in many individuals.

ETIOLOGY

The sites of acne development, the pilosebaceous units (well-developed sebaceous glands with miniature hairs), are located in highest concentration on the face, upper chest, and upper back. The key pathogenic factors of acne vulgaris are as follows:

1. Androgen-induced increased sebum production
2. Abnormal keratinization of sebaceous and follicular epithelium
3. Proliferation of *Propionibacterium acnes*
4. Inflammation

Androgens and Sebum Production

Acne frequently begins in the prepubertal or early adolescent period as increased adrenal androgens cause increased sebum production. With puberty and gonadal development, androgen production increases even further. Androgenic hormones (gonadal and adrenal) stimulate size and activity of sebaceous glands on the face, neck, and upper trunk, resulting in oily skin and comedones. Sebaceous glands are androgen-sensitive appendages of hair follicles that secrete lipids that lubricate skin and hair. Serum dehydroepiandrosterone sulfate (DHEA-S) appears to be an early marker for the development of acne (Lucky et al., 1991; Stewart et al., 1992). Although increased androgen levels are seen in patients with severe nodulocystic acne, these levels are usually within normal limits in patients with mild-to-moderate acne. One study assessed serum levels of enzyme 5α-reductase type 1, which is responsible for dihydrotestosterone production in patients with and without acne. It found no statistically significant difference in enzyme activity between the two groups; however, the study population was small (Thiboutot et al., 1999). Another study analyzing the effect of androgens and acne severity in adult women failed to show a positive correlation and in fact demonstrated lower values of clinical and laboratory markers of androgenicity in women with a higher grade of acne severity (Cibula et al., 2000).

Abnormal Keratinization

Abnormal keratinization of sebaceous and follicular ducts results in retention hyperkeratosis and microcomedo formation (comedogenesis). The occluded follicle, or microcomedone, is most likely the initial lesion of both inflammatory and noninflammatory acne. Comedones may be closed (whiteheads) or open (blackheads). The whitehead contains inspissated keratin and lipid debris. Blackheads result from the oxidation of tyrosine to melanin through the open pore.

Propionibacterium Acnes

The excessive sebum and the anaerobic environment created by the plugged follicle result in colonization and proliferation of the anaerobic diphtheroid, *Propionibacterium acnes*. This bacteria, although part of normal skin flora, appears to be absent from the skin before puberty. Individuals with acne seem to possess higher concentrations of *P. acnes*.

Immune and Inflammatory Reaction

P. acnes triggers immune and nonimmune inflammatory reactions by a variety of mechanisms, including the following:

1. Lipase production that hydrolyzes sebum triglycerides into irritating and comedogenic free fatty acids that serve as proinflammatory substances
2. Release of chemotactic factors that attract leukocytes. Hydrolytic enzymes released by these neutrophils rupture follicular walls, leaking their contents into the dermis with resultant inflammation, forming papules or pustules, nodules, cysts or abscesses
3. Activation of complement pathways and host response
4. Activation of toll-like receptors (TLRs). TLRs are receptors produced in the innate cell response. Some studies suggest that two well known TLRs, TLR-2 and TLR-4, in keratinocytes are upregulated in acne lesions by *P. acnes* and may play a role in acne-induced inflammation through cytokine release (Jugeau et al., 2005).

EPIDEMIOLOGY

Acne affects 80% to 95% of people between the ages of 11 and 30. Although it is usually a condition of adolescence, acne vulgaris may affect 8% of 25- to 34-year-olds and 3% of the 35- to 44-year-old age-group.

CLINICAL DISEASE

Types of lesions include comedones, inflammatory papules, pustules, nodules, cyst-like lesions, and scars. Each is discussed in this section.

Comedones

Comedones are the earliest sign of acne. They often appear 1 to 2 years before puberty.

1. Microcomedo: Microcomedos are impactions of keratin, lipids, bacteria, and rudimentary hairs within the sebaceous follicle. These subclinical lesions are typically seen with magnification or on biopsy specimens from patients with acne.
2. Open comedo (blackhead): Open comedo consists of an epithelium-lined sac filled with keratin and lipids with a dilated orifice. The black coloration comes from melanin pigment. Usually the keratinous material is sloughed, and no inflammation occurs unless traumatized.
3. Closed comedo (whitehead): Typically 1 to 3 mm in size, with a microscopic opening preventing escape of contents. Active lesions may resolve spontaneously; if the follicular walls rupture superficially, the lesions form inflamed pustules, with deeper inflammation resulting in papules or nodules.

Papules

Papules are inflammatory lesions measuring <5 mm in diameter. Superficial papules usually resolve in 5 to 10 days with little scarring, but may result in postinflammatory hyperpigmentation, especially in adolescents with dark complexions. Deep papules usually have more intense inflammation. They may take weeks to resolve and may result in scarring.

Pustules

Pustules are lesions with a visible central core of purulent material.

Nodules

Nodules are inflammatory lesions measuring 5 mm or larger that last for weeks to months and may heal with scarring.

Cysts

Cysts are deeper lesions filled with pus and serosanguineous fluid.

Scars

Types of scarring include the following:

1. Focal depressed or "ice pick" scars
2. Perifollicular fibrosis
3. Hypertrophic scars and keloids, which tend to form on the chest, back, jaw line, and ears and are more common in dark-complexioned individuals

Location

The face, chest and back are the areas most prominently affected.

Grading

Acne may be classified by the predominant lesion type (e.g., comedonal, papulopustular, nodular, cystic) and severity (mild, moderate, severe). It is also helpful to include the location of the lesions described (e.g., mild comedonal acne on the forehead).

Timing

Acne can appear as early as 5 to 8 years of age and may precede other signs of pubertal maturation. Prevalence and severity of acne increase with advancing pubertal development and peak between the ages of 14 and 17 in females and 16 and 19 years in males. Acne varies from a short, mild course to a severe disease lasting 10 to 15 years or longer. Although less prevalent, acne often persists beyond 20 years of age.

DIFFERENTIAL DIAGNOSIS

Non-Acne Lesions

1. Keratosis pilaris: Hyperkeratotic plugs in hair follicles usually present on the extensor surfaces of upper arms, thighs, and lateral cheeks. Occasional small pustules may be seen. Emollients, lactic acid preparations, and physical debridement may minimize its cosmetic impact.
2. Adenoma sebaceum: This is the most common cutaneous manifestation of tuberous sclerosis, manifesting as pink to red facial papules representing angiofibromas that begin in early childhood and persist through adulthood.
3. Flat warts: These are skin-colored papules or plaques caused by human papillomavirus that may spread (Koebner phenomenon) with trauma.
4. Perioral dermatitis: Small, 1- to 3-mm erythematous papules or papulopustules of the chin, nasolabial folds, or periorbital areas that may be accompanied by scaling. A granulomatous variant exists. Topical corticosteroids can induce or aggravate this condition, which is related to acne rosacea. It is treated with topical and oral antibiotics, such as metronidazole, benzoyl peroxide, combination antibiotics (benzoyl peroxide/erythromycin, benzoyl peroxide/clindamycin), or systemic erythromycin.
5. Hidradenitis suppurativa: A chronic inflammatory disease manifested by multi-headed comedos and deep, tender nodules, tracts and scarring involving primarily the axilla, groin, and buttocks. Treatment is difficult

but may include antibiotics, surgery, and intralesional corticosteroids.

6. Pityrosporum folliculitis: Pruritic follicular papules and pustules on the arms, trunk, and occasionally the face caused by overgrowth of *Pityrosporum orbiculare*. It is most commonly seen in young women.

Subtypes of Acne

1. Neonatal acne: It is caused by stimulation of the sebaceous glands by maternal and neonatal androgens derived from the hyperactive neonatal adrenal gland. The lesions are usually closed comedos on the nose, forehead, and cheeks. Inflammatory acne lesions may also occur. Spontaneous resolution usually occurs in 1 to 3 months. Infantile acne usually manifests between the third and sixth months, and it may be associated with an increased risk of developing acne vulgaris during adolescence (Chew et al., 1990).
2. Gram-negative folliculitis: Usually caused by a secondary colonization with *Escherichia coli, Klebsiella, Pseudomonas, Enterobacter,* or *Proteus spp.* during broad-spectrum antibiotic use, gram-negative folliculitis can produce multiple pustules and nodules with a predilection for the perinasal area. It should be suspected in an adolescent patient with acne who does not improve or continues to have a flare-up while on antibiotics. Culture results should guide diagnosis and therapy. Isotretinoin (Accutane) is also effective.
3. Cosmetic acne: Less common since the advent of noncomedogenic cosmetics (those that do not clog pores), comedonal acne may be created by the use of occlusive moisturizing creams, cocoa butter, vitamin E oil, flavored lip balms, and pomades.
4. Occupational acne: Certain products can cause obstruction to sebaceous follicles, including mineral oil, crude petroleum, coal tar, and pitch. Halogenated aromatic hydrocarbons can also cause an acneform eruption.
5. Drug-induced acne: Drugs that can induce or exacerbate preexisting acne include androgens, adrenocorticotropic hormone (ACTH), steroids (oral and topical), barbiturates, cyclosporine A, phenytoin, carbamazepine, isoniazid, rifampin, lithium, ethionamide, bromides, and iodides. Steroid acne is typically a monomorphous eruption of papules or papulopustules that resolves without scarring. It does not produce comedones, nodules, and scars. It may involve areas, such as the extremities, that are not normally affected in acne vulgaris.
6. Acne conglobata: A severe, suppurative, often chronic form of nodular acne that most often occurs in males. The back is often severely affected, along with the thighs, buttocks, and upper arms.
7. Acne fulminans: This rare form of noduloulcerative acne has an abrupt onset and is often accompanied by fever, leukocytosis, anemia, polyarthritis, and, rarely, osteolytic bone lesions (Karvonen, 1993).
8. Acne mechanica: This form occurs at sites of physical trauma such as the chin from helmet straps and shoulders and upper back from shoulder pads.
9. Acne excoriée des jeunes filles: This is most frequently seen in adolescent girls who excoriate or manipulate the acne lesions; severe scarring and even mutilation may result. It is usually associated with emotional stress.

THERAPY

General

Several considerations are important in treating adolescents with acne:

1. Practitioners must appreciate the significance of this problem to adolescents. The short- and long-term consequences of acne to the adolescent's emotional well-being should not be underestimated. Acne may affect patients' psychosocial and emotional well-being as severely as other more "serious" diseases, such as asthma, epilepsy, or diabetes. Patients with acne have higher rates of unemployment as compared to those without acne and are at higher risk of developing depression and anxiety (Gollnick et al., 2003). However, some adolescents will not explicitly address their concerns about their acne. Therefore, the physician or other health care provider should ask if the acne is bothersome and whether treatment is desired.
2. Perform a thorough history and physical examination. The female patient should be examined for the presence of hirsutism, alopecia, and obesity and should be asked about her menstrual cycle and use of oral contraceptive pills (OCPs).
3. Most adolescents treat themselves and will often heed peer suggestions more readily than those of a physician. Therefore, practitioners must emphasize the role and necessity of compliance.
4. Practitioners must understand the route, timing, and dose of the drugs administered.
5. Make sure the adolescent understands how to use the medications. Written instructions or handouts are very useful.
6. Do not promise instant success. Point out that therapy with topical agents may cause acne to look worse in the first 3 to 4 weeks, and improvement may take months.
7. Explain the side effects of all medications used.
8. Treat according to severity, as follows:
   a. Begin with agents that are easiest to use with the fewest side effects, advancing as needed in a stepwise manner to stronger medications that may be more difficult to use or have more side effects.
   b. Mild acne responds well to topical antibiotic or comedolytic agents. Table 19.1 lists therapeutic options for acne including those that are available as over-the-counter preparations.
   c. Combination therapy may allow medications to work better together, even if the patient feels "they didn't work" when used as monotherapy.
   d. Moderate-severe to severe inflammatory acne may require systemic antibiotics in addition to topical comedolytic agents.
   e. Nodular or nodulocystic acne unresponsive to oral antibiotics or topical retinoids should be treated with systemic isotretinoin (Accutane) by an experienced practitioner.
   f. Combined OCPs may be very useful therapy for all forms of acne in female patients.
9. General measures and misconceptions: It is important to discuss directly with the teen, as well as the parents, common misconceptions about acne:
   a. Diet: No evidence exists that "unhealthy" foods such as carbonated beverages, chocolate, nuts, or French fries increase acne severity. Although stressing that

TABLE 19.1

Topical Therapeutic Options for Acne

Drug	Action	Frequency	Side Effects
Anticomedonal agents			

Tretinoin (Retin-A)
  Cream 0.025%, 0.05%, 0.1%
  Gel 0.01%, 0 .025%,
  Solution 0.05%
Retin-A micro 0.04%, 0.1% gel
Avita 0.025% cream/gel
Generic tretinoin
  0.025%, 0.05%, 0.1% cream,
  0.01%, 0.025% gel
	Normalizes keratinocyte
	  differentiation
	Some anti-inflammatory effect
		q.p.m.	Photosensitivity, drying

Differin (Adapalene) Gel 0.1%,
  cream 0.1%, solution 0.1%,
  pledgets 0.1%
	Normalizes keratinocyte
	  differentiation
	Some anti-inflammatory effect
		q.d.	Less irritating than Retin-A

Tazorac (tazarotene) 0.05%, 0.1% gel; 0.05%, 0.1% cream	Normalizes differentiation Some anti-inflammatory effect	q.d.	
Azelex Cream 20%, Azelaic acid	Normalizes differentiation Antimicrobial	b.i.d.	Less irritating than Retin-A, also appears less effective
Salicylic acid[a]	Mild comedolytic	b.i.d.	Drying
Topical antibiotic			

Benzoyl peroxide (BP)[a]: Many
  forms: 2%–20%, gel, lotion,
  wash
	Comedolytic, antimicrobial,
	  decreases antimicrobial
	  resistance
		q.d.–b.i.d.	Irritation, contact allergy,
			  bleaches clothing

Benzamycin (5% B.P./
  3% Erythromycin)
Benzaclin (5% BP/
  Clindamycin 1%)
	Same as
	  above + anti-inflammatory
		q.d.–b.i.d.	Same as above

Erythromycin (Erycette,
  T-stat, Emgel)
Clindamycin (Cleocin T)
Sodium sulfacetamide
  (Klaron, Novacet, Sulfacet-R)
Topical sulfur[a]: (Fostex,
  Rezamid, SAStid)
	Antimicrobial
	Anti-inflammatory
		q.d.–b.i.d.	Development of resistance,
			  drying, odor

[a]Topical therapeutic options available as over-the-counter preparations.

a "generally healthy" diet is preferable, dietary restrictions are usually unnecessary.

b. Hygiene: Uncleanliness does not cause acne. Overemphasis on compulsive scrubbing is unnecessary and may itself cause dermatitis. Mild soaps or cleansers should be used to wash the face two times a day. Noncomedogenic moisturizers and cosmetics will not interfere with treatment.

c. Stress: Stress can worsen acne and, in turn, increase the adolescent's anxiety levels and impact on self-image. Continued support must be given to the affected adolescent.

d. Neither sexual fantasies nor sexual activity causes acne.

e. Teens should avoid wearing tight headbands or using thick greasy styling products around the forehead; both can exacerbate acne.

f. Premenstrual acne flares can occur.

Topical Agents

The vehicle (cream, gel, lotion, or solution) may be as critical as the active ingredient of the formulation and should be chosen on the basis of the patient's skin type. Overall, solutions and gels are drying, nongreasy, and therefore best for those with oily skin. Creams and lotions are more moisturizing and tend to be preferred by many patients. Creams in particular are appropriate for teens with dry or sensitive skin. Table 19.1 summarizes available topical retinoids and antibiotics.

Benzoyl Peroxide

1. Mechanism of action
   a. Bacteriocidal effect on *P. acnes* with low potential for resistance
   b. Mild comedolytic action; decreases free fatty acids
2. Dosing
   a. Benzoyl peroxide is available in concentrations of 2.5% to 10%.
   b. Benzoyl peroxide comes in gels, lotions, creams, soaps, and washes and is available in both prescription and nonprescription preparations. The aqueous gels are better tolerated than compounds prepared in an alcohol vehicle.
   c. Gradually increase concentration as needed or tolerated. Treatment can be started either every other day, or once to twice daily.
3. Adverse side effects
   a. Peeling, irritation and dryness
   b. Contact dermatitis (1% to 2%)
   c. Bleaching of hair and colored fabrics

Retinoids (Tretinoin, Tazarotene, and Adapalene)

1. Mechanism of action
   a. Retinoids are Vitamin A derivatives that act on retinoic acid receptors, decreasing comedo formation and follicular plugging by reducing hyperkeratosis and decreasing the cohesiveness of follicular epithelial cells, making it very useful in comedonal acne.
   b. Newer preparations of retinoids have included adapalene, tazarotene, and less irritating formulations of tretinoin.
2. Dosing
   a. *Tretinoin (Retin-A, Retin-A Micro, Avita, Altinac):* Tretinoin may be effective as monotherapy in teens with noninflammatory or mild inflammatory acne. Close supervision and instruction are required because of the potential for irritation.
   b. Available concentrations include 0.025%, 0.05%, and 0.1% cream; 0.01% and 0.025% gel, and Retin-A Micro 0.04% and 0.1% gel.
   c. Lower strength creams and microsphere formulations of tretinoin gel contained in a slow-release vehicle are generally less irritating. More potent formulations include, in approximate increasing potency, 0.05% cream, 0.025% gel, 0.1% cream, and the rarely well-tolerated 0.05% solution.
   d. Start with the lower concentrations of cream or Retin-A Micro gel applied every other night to every night approximately 20 minutes after washing the face; gradually increase to a daily regimen. A pea-sized amount of tretinoin should be dotted on the forehead, cheeks, nose and chin then spread in a thin layer across the face to ensure even distribution.
   e. Use of benzoyl peroxide or combination benzoyl peroxide products in the morning and tretinoin in the evening is an effective regimen.
   f. After 3 to 4 weeks, a pustular eruption may occur, indicating the dislodging of microcomedos, which may be perceived as a flare. Patients should be warned about this potential flare and that it indicates that the therapy is working and advised to continue treatment.
   g. Avoid excessive or prolonged sun exposure, because tretinoin may cause photosensitivity. A sunscreen rated SPF-15 or higher may be used.
3. Adverse side effects
   a. Peeling, drying, and irritation, which is increased with higher concentrations
   b. Hyperpigmentation or hypopigmentation, particularly in black and Asian patients
   c. Photosensitivity
   d. Issues concerning potential teratogenicity have been raised, although in at least one study of women exposed to tretinoin in the first trimester of pregnancy there was no increase in the rate of fetal anomalies (Jick et al., 1993).
4. Newer preparations
   a. Tretinoin gel microspheres (Retin-A Micro 0.04% and 0.1%): Tretinoin is incorporated into the macroporous beads or microsponges and gradually released over a sustained period, enhancing delivery to the epidermis and limiting irritation.
   b. Tretinoin polymer cream (Avita): Tretinoin 0.025% cream is combined with a liquid polymer compound called *polyolprepolymer-2* (PP-2) enhancing delivery to the epidermis and within the pilosebaceous unit, limiting irritation. Patch-test studies in humans have demonstrated less irritation with this formulation than with traditional tretinoin formulations.
   c. Adapalene (Differin 0.1% Gel, Cream, Pledgets, and Solution): Adapalene is a derivative of naphthoic acid that behaves like a retinoid but is photostable and causes less irritation. It may be effective for comedonal and inflammatory acne. Adapalene may require up to 8 to 16 weeks of daily use to see optimal results.
   d. Tazarotene (Tazorac 0.1% and 0.05% Gel and Cream): Tazarotene is a synthetic acetylenic retinoid that rapidly penetrates skin and is converted into its active metabolite, tazarotenic acid. This agent binds to nuclear retinoic acid receptors and appears to influence the cohesion of corneocytes and inflammation. Unlike traditional retinoids, tazarotene is a photostable agent applied overnight or as short contact therapy for 5 minutes, and then removed with a mild facial cleanser. Adverse effects are similar to other topical retinoids: erythema, pruritus, burning, dryness, and stinging. It is labeled for use in both psoriasis and mild-to-moderate acne but is not recommended in pregnant women (category X).

Azelaic acid Azelaic acid (Azelex) is used to treat mild-to-moderate inflammatory acne. Azelaic acid is a dicarboxylic acid first developed for benign hyperpigmentation disorders. It is structurally unrelated to other acne therapies and possesses bacteriostatic properties against *P. acnes* and other organisms and appears to normalize keratinization. In some studies, topical azelaic acid was similar in efficacy to topical benzoyl peroxide 5% and 0.05% tretinoin cream, although in clinical use it appears more effective when combined with other topical agents. Azelaic acid is available as a 20% cream (Azelex), which is applied twice daily to clean, dry skin. Side effects are uncommon (<with tretinoin and benzoyl peroxide) but include pruritus, burning and stinging of the skin, rash, and hypopigmentation. It

may be useful in patients with acne and postinflammatory hyperpigmentation.

Topical Antibiotics

Topical antibiotics appear to reduce the counts of *P. acnes* to decrease the percentage of free fatty acids in surface lipids and may have anti-inflammatory effects. The most commonly used topical antibiotics are clindamycin, sulfacetamide, erythromycin, and metronidazole. Topical antibiotics allow direct application and have negligible systemic side effects, but resistance is frequently seen. Although they can be effective for mild-to-moderate inflammatory acne, topical antibiotics cannot replace systemic antibiotics in more severe cases. Preparations include:

1. *Erythromycin 2%* (e.g., *A/T/S solution, T-Stat solution, Erygel, Emgel, Akne-mycin*): Available in solutions, gels, pads, and ointment, applied twice daily.
2. *Clindamycin 1%* (*Cleocin T solution, C/T/S, Clindets, Clindagel, Evoclin*): Available as a solution, lotion, foam, gel, or pledget; applied twice daily. Pseudomembranous colitis has rarely been reported to occur with topical use (Parry and Rha, 1986).
3. *Sodium sulfacetamide (Klaron, Sulfacet-R, Novacet, and Plexion cleanser)*: This antibacterial agent has been used in antiacne preparations for many years. These agents may be more effective for rosacea than for acne. These products should be avoided in sulfa-allergic patients.
4. *Benzoyl peroxide 5% with 3% erythromycin (Benzamycin gel) and clindamycin 1%–benzoyl peroxide 5% gel (Benzaclin and Duac topical gel)*: Preparations that combine a topical antibiotic with benzoyl peroxide are favored because bacterial resistance has not been seen. They may be used as monotherapy for mild to moderate acne, or in combination with topical retinoids and/or oral antibiotics.

Other Agents

1. Keratolytic washes and lotions: Keratolytics such as salicylic acid, sulfur, or resorcinol, are available in non-prescription and prescription preparations. They are not as effective as monotherapy when compared to benzoyl peroxide or retinoids, but may act synergistically when used in combination regimens.
2. Sunlight or ultraviolet light: Potential risks of photoaging and carcinogenesis outweigh benefits.
3. Lasers and light systems: Several lasers and light systems, with or without photodynamic sensitizers have been utilized for acne. This is an evolving therapeutic area, with few studies evaluating the safety and efficacy of the use of lasers and light systems in standard medical therapy.

Systemic Therapy

Table 19.2 summarizes therapeutic options for systemic therapy.

Oral Antibiotics

Oral antibiotics decrease the *P. acnes* population, reduce free fatty acids, and may decrease the inflammatory response. Approximately 3 to 6 months of treatment may be required for a clinical response, at which point, one may attempt transition of the patient to a combination of topical retinoid and antibiotic (benzoyl peroxide, benzoyl peroxide combinations, or other antibiotics.)

1. Tetracycline
   a. Dosing: 250 to 500 mg once or twice daily
   b. Side effects: Gastrointestinal upset
   c. Other considerations: Inexpensive, needs to be taken on an empty stomach
2. Doxycycline
   a. Dosing: 50 to 100 mg once or twice daily
   b. Side effects: Dose-dependent phototoxicity, gastrointestinal upset, lightheadedness
3. Minocycline
   a. Dosing: 50 to 100 mg once or twice daily
   b. Side effects: hyperpigmentation of teeth, oral mucosa, and skin; gastrointestinal upset, lightheadedness, lupus-like reactions, or hepatitis with long-term treatment
4. Trimethoprim–sulfamethoxazole
   a. Dosing: 160 mg trimethoprim/800 mg sulfamethoxazole once daily
   b. Side effects: Toxic epidermal necrolysis and allergic eruptions
5. Erythromycin
   a. Dosing: 250 to 500 mg two to four times daily
   b. Side effects: Gastrointestinal upset

13-cis-Retinoic Acid or Isotretinoin (Accutane)

13-*cis*-Retinoic acid has dramatically reversed the course of acne in many individuals with severe nodulocystic, scarring or recalcitrant disease. Because of significant toxicity, the drug is reserved for treatment of severe nodular or recalcitrant acne by practitioners experienced with its use and involved with government-mandated registry programs. Careful laboratory monitoring is also required.

1. Mechanism of action: Isotretinoin is a synthetic vitamin A derivative that decreases keratinization and sebum production, thereby diminishing *P. acnes* growth and host inflammatory response.
2. Dosing: Isotretinoin is usually given in a daily dose of 0.5 to 1 mg/kg divided into two doses with food. The length of therapy is 16 to 24 weeks, with clinical improvement often continuing after discontinuation of the medication. Relapse is less likely to occur if a total cumulative dose of 120 mg/kg of body weight is reached; however, there appears to be no additional benefit with cumulative doses of >150 mg/kg of body weight. Systemic absorption is increased when isotretinoin is taken with food (40% absorption versus 20% on an empty stomach). The teratogenicity of isotretinoin requires that women of childbearing age not be pregnant or become pregnant while taking the medication. Baseline and monthly pregnancy tests are required during therapy. Female patients should utilize two forms of contraception.
3. Laboratory monitoring
   a. Complete blood count (CBC), liver function tests, cholesterol, triglycerides.
   b. A government-mandated registry program requires baseline and monthly pregnancy tests in females of childbearing age.

TABLE 19.2

Systemic Therapeutic Options for Acne

Systemic Medication	Action	Dosage	Side Effects
Tetracycline	Antimicrobial Anti-inflammatory	250–500 b.i.d. on empty stomach	HA, GI, pseudotumor, yeast infection, OCP interaction, esophagitis, photosensitivity, tooth teratogen
Doxycycline	Same above	50–100 q.d., b.i.d. Can be taken with food	Same as above + increased photosensitivity
Minocycline	Same above	50–100 q.d., b.i.d.	Pigment deposition, dizziness, hypersensitivity, hepatitis, lupus-like reaction
Erythromycin	Antimicrobial, anti-inflammatory	250 q.i.d.	GI distress, drug interactions—Theophylline, Carbamazepine
Oral Contraceptives: norgestimate-ethinyl estradiol (Ortho Tri-Cyclen), norethindrone-ethinyl estradiol (Estrostep), drospirenone-ethinyl estradiol (Yasmin), levonorgestrel-ethinyl estradiol (Alesse)	Antiandrogenic Decreased sebum production		Risk of thromboembolism
Intralesional Steroids	Decrease inflammation	1–5% triamcinolone intralesional	Scarring (usually transient)
Other Antiandrogens (e.g., Spironolactone)		50–100 mg q.d.	Irregular menses, gynecomastia, hypercalcemia, teratogenic
Accutane (Isotretinoin)	Decreases sebum production, normalizes keratinization, decreases inflammation, decreases *Propionibacterium* acnes concentrations	0.5–1.0 mg/kg/d X 16–24 weeks	Many !!! Strong teratogen, drying, cheilitis, hypercholesterolemia, hypertriglyceridemia, paronychia, eczema, alopecia, arthralgia, depression, decreased night vision

HA, headache; GI, gastrointestinal; OCP, oral contraceptive pills.

4. Side effects
   a. Dermatologic: Cheilitis (90%), xerosis (78%), epistaxis (46%), conjunctivitis (40%), desquamation (16%), hair thinning (9%), photosensitivity (5%–10%), occasional pyogenic granuloma-like lesions (hypergranulation tissue), *Staphylococcus aureus* skin colonization and infections
   b. Musculoskeletal: Arthralgias and myalgias (16%), hyperostosis (when used for prolonged periods of time in other dermatological conditions)
   c. Opthalmologic: Decreased night vision
   d. Gastrointestinal: Hypercholesterolemia (7%), hypertriglyceridemia (25%), elevated liver function tests (15%)

TABLE 19.3

Step Therapy for Acne

Acne Severity	Lesion Type	Initial Treatment	If Inadequate Response*
Mild	Comedonal	BP alone q.d.–b.i.d. OR BP/topical antibiotic combo q.d.–b.i.d. OR topical retinoid QHS	Add topical retinoid OR topical antibiotic OR substitute BP/topical antibiotic combination
	Inflammatory/Mixed	BP alone q.d.–b.i.d. OR BP/topical antibiotic combo q.d.–b.i.d. OR topical retinoid QHS	Add topical retinoid or topical antibiotic OR substitute BP/topical antibiotic combination
Moderate	Comedonal	Topical retinoid +/– BP or BP/topical antibiotic combination	Increase strength or change type of topical retinoid OR add BP or BP/topical antibiotic combination to topical retinoid
	Inflammatory/Mixed	BP or BP/combo +/topical retinoid +/– oral antibiotic	Add retinoid or oral antibiotic. Consider oral contraceptive for females. Consider referral to dermatologist
		Oral antibiotic + topical retinoid	Increase strength or change type of topical retinoid. Consider oral contraceptive in females. Add BP or BP/topical antibiotic combination. Consider referral to dermatologist
Severe	Comedonal	Consider referral OR oral antibiotic and topical retinoid OR +/– BP or BP/topical antibiotic combination OR +/– oral contraceptive for female patients	Consider isotretinoin Referral to dermatologist
	Inflammatory/Mixed	Same as above	Same as above

*Determined by physician assessment and patient satisfaction.
BP, Benzoyl peroxide; BP combo, BP–clindamycin (Benzaclin); BP–erythromycin (Benzamycin).
Other topical antibiotic (clindamycin, erythromycin, sodium sulfacetamide) may be substituted if there is irritation, dermatitis, etc. with BP-products.
+Azelaic acid may be substituted.
Low strength retinoid can include Retin-A 0.025% cream, Retin-A Gel Micro 0.04%, Differin 0.1% Cream/Gel or Avita or generic Tretinoin 0.025% cream.

e. Hematologic: Elevated erythrocyte sedimentation rate (40%), leukopenia, elevated platelets (10% to 20%)
f. Genitourinary: Proteinuria, hematuria, vaginal dryness, urethritis
g. Neurologic: Headaches (5%), pseudotumor cerebri (rare)
h. Psychiatric: Depression. Adolescents with a personal or family history of depression may be at increased risk of developing major depression or suicide. A recent literature review did not find any studies to support a causal association between isotretinoin use and increased risk of depression or suicidal behavior, however, a weak association could not be ruled out (Marqueling and Zane, 2005). Physicians should educate patients and their families about this possible side effect and monitor their patients for signs and symptoms of depression or other psychiatric disturbance before, during, and after isotretinoin therapy.

Hormonal Therapy

Women who demonstrate signs of hyperandrogenism (irregular menses, androgenic alopecia, or hirsutism) develop acne resistant to conventional treatment; those who have a relapse soon after finishing a course of isotretinoin, or who have a sudden onset of severe acne require an evaluation for androgen excess, including serum dihydrotestosterone and free testosterone levels. Hormonal therapy with oral contraceptives containing estrogen or androgen antagonists for the treatment of acne may benefit women with hyperandrogenism as well as women with normal serum androgen levels. They may be used in combination with oral antibiotics and topical therapy.

1. Combined oral contraceptives

   Combined OCPs decrease acne lesions by suppressing androgen production and sebaceous gland activity. Norgestimate-ethinyl estradiol (Ortho Tri-Cyclen) and norethindrone acetate-ethinyl estradiol (Estrostep) are approved by the U.S. Food and Drug Administration for the treatment of acne. Studies show that drospirenone-ethinyl estradiol (Yasmin) and levonorgestrel-ethinyl estradiol (Alesse) are also effective. Duration of treatment is usually 6 to 9 months for clinical effect. The effect of injectable and patch systems on acne has not been evaluated. Progesterone-only contraceptives generally worsen acne. Potential side effects include thromboembolism. A more complete list of side effects may be found in the discussion on OCPs in Chapter 43.
2. Antiandrogens

   Spironolactone 50 to 100 mg daily may be added to the patient's regimen if oral contraceptives alone are ineffective. Higher doses are more effective but associated with more adverse effects including menstrual irregularities and breast tenderness. Spironolactone must be used in combination with contraception because of potential teratogenicity.
3. Corticosteroids

   The use of high doses of corticosteroids should be reserved for the treatment of acne conglobata, acne fulminans, and the acute flare of acne precipitated by initiating isotretinoin therapy. Prednisone 5.0 to 7.5 mg or dexamethasone 0.25 to 0.5 mg is effective in reducing adrenal androgen production. Intralesional corticosteroids may be useful for inflammatory cysts and nodules (see the "Acne Surgery" section).

ACNE SURGERY

1. Comedone extraction: Open comedones can be easily removed with a comedo extractor. Closed comedones require puncture with a needle or lancet *first*. Extensive surgical treatment should be avoided, because manipulation can lead to scarring.
2. Incision and drainage: Do not incise acne pustules and nodules, because of possible resultant scarring.
3. Intralesional corticosteroids: Injection of 0.05 to 0.1 mL per lesion of triamcinolone acetate suspension (1.0 to 2.5 mg/mL) into each papulonodular or cystic lesion can lead to rapid improvement in isolated cystic lesions. Individuals should be cautioned that this treatment could lead to atrophy at the injection site, which usually resolves in 4 to 6 months but can be permanent.
4. Rehabilitation: After acne lesions have become quiescent, young adults may explore surgical options for scars. At present, alternatives include punch excision and grafting, chemical peels, dermal fillers, dermabrasion, and laser surgery. Avoid any cosmetic procedures for at least 6 months to 1 year after discontinuing isotretinoin.

SUMMARY

In general, patient education regarding basic skin care should be provided. Treatment regimens using topical and/or systemic therapy should be tailored to the needs of the individual. Mild acne can be treated effectively with topical benzoyl peroxide alone or in combination with a topical retinoid. Moderate or inflammatory acne may require oral antibiotics in addition to a topical retinoid. Isotretinoin should be considered for patients with severe nodulocystic acne or acne refractory to systemic antibiotics. Finally, hormonal therapy may be used in females with signs or symptoms of hyperandrogenism. Table 19.3 provides a stepwise approach to treating acne.

WEB SITES

http://www.skincarephysicians.com/acnenet/. Acne Net: About acne from Roche and American Academy of Dermatology.
http://kidshealth.org.
   Search on acne.
http://www.aad.org/pamphlets/acnepamp.html. American Academy of Dermatology pamphlet on acne.
http://www.niams.nih.gov/hi/topics/acne/acne.htm.
   National Institutes of Health questions and answers about acne.
http://www.healthatoz.com/atoz/HealthUpdate/Alert02182000.asp. Facts about acne from health A to Z.
http://www.ipledgeprogram.com. Registration program for patients on isotretinoin and prescribing physicians.

REFERENCES AND ADDITIONAL READINGS

Aktan S, Ozmen E, Sanli B. Anxiety, depression, and nature of acne vulgaris in adolescents. *Int J Dermatol* 2000;39:354.

Bergfeld WE. The evaluation and management of acne: economic considerations. *J Am Acad Dermatol* 1995;32:552.

Bershad S, Rubinstein A, Patemiti JR Jr, et al. Changes in plasma lipids and lipoproteins during isotretinoin therapy for acne. *N Engl J Med* 1985;313:981.

Berson DS, Shalita AR. The treatment of acne: the role of combination therapies. *J Am Acad Dermatol* 1995;32:531.

Chew EW, Bingham A, Burrows D. Incidence of acne vulgaris in patients with infantile acne. *Clin Exp Dermatol* 1990;15:376.

Cibula D, Hill M, Vohradnikova O, et al. The role of androgens in determining acne severity in adult women. *Br J Dermatol* 2000;143:399.

Corona R. Minocycline in acne is still an issue. *Arch Dermatol* 2000;136:1143.

Cunliffe WJ. Unemployment and acne. *Br J Dermatol* 1986;115:379.

Cunliffe WJ, Holland DB, Clark SM, et al. Comedogenesis: some new aetiological, clinical, and therapeutic strategies. *Br J Dermatol* 2000;142:1084.

Eady EA, Farmery MR, Ross JI, et al. Effects of benzoyl peroxide and erythromycin alone and in combination against antibiotic-sensitive and resistant skin bacteria from acne patients. *Br J Dermatol* 1994;131:331.

Feldman S, Careccia RE, Barham KL. Diagnosis and treatment of acne. *Am Fam Physician* 2004;69:2123.

Goldsmith LA, Bolognia JL, Callen JP, et al. American Academy of Dermatology consensus conference on the safe and optimal use of isotretinoin: summary and recommendations. *J Am Acad Dermatol* 2004;50:900.

Gollnick H, Cunliffe W, Berson D, et al. Management of acne: a report from a global alliance to improve outcomes in acne. *J Am Acad Dermatol* 2003;49:S1.

Gordon PM, Farr PM, Milligan A. Acne fulminans and bone lesions may present to other specialties. *Pediatr Dermatol* 1997;14:446.

Haider A, Shaw JC. Treatment of acne vulgaris—clinical review. *JAMA* 2004;292:726.

Harper JC. An update on the pathogenesis and management of acne vulgaris. *J Am Acad Dermatol* 2004;51:S36.

Healy E, Simpson N. Acne vulgaris. *Br Med J* 1994;308:831.

Hurwitz RM. Steroid acne. *J Am Acad Dermatol* 1989;21:1179.

James WD. Acne. *N Engl J Med* 2005;352:1463.

Jick SS, Terris BZ, Jick H. First trimester topical tretinoin and congenital disorders. *Lancet* 1993;341:1181.

Jordan R, Cummins C, Burls A. Laser resurfacing of the skin for the improvement of facial acne scarring: a systematic review of the evidence. *Br J Dermatol* 2000;142:413.

Jugeau S, Tenaud I, Knol AC, et al. Induction of toll-like receptors by *Propionibacterium acnes*. *Br J Dermatol* 2005; 153:1105.

Karvonen SKL. Acne fulminans: report of clinical findings and treatment of twenty-four patients. *J Am Acad Dermatol* 1993;28:572.

Kaunitz AM. Oral contraceptive health benefits: perception versus reality. *Contraception* 1999;59(Suppl 1):29S.

Koo J. Psychosocial consequences of acne: implications and treatment options for adolescents and adults. *Cosmet Dermatol* 1999;12:35.

Krowchuk DP. Treating acne: a practical guide. *Med Clin North Am* 2000;84:811.

Krowchuk DP, Stancin T, Keskinen R, et al. The psychosocial effects of acne on adolescents. *Pediatr Dermatol* 1991;83:332.

Layton AM. Psychosocial aspects of acne vulgaris. *J Cutan Med Surg* 1998;2(Suppl 3):19.

Layton AM, Henderson CA, Cunliffe WJ. A clinical evaluation of acne scarring and its incidence. *Clin Exp Dermatol* 1994; 19:303.

Layton AM, Knaggs H, Taylor J, et al. Isotretinoin for acne vulgaris: 10 years later—a safe and successful treatment. *Br J Dermatol* 1993;129:292.

Lehucher-Ceyrac D, Weber-Buisset MJ. Isotretinoin and acne in practice: a prospective analysis of 188 cases over nine years. *Dermatology* 1993;186:123.

Leyden JJ, James WE. *Staphylococcal aureus* infections as a complication of isotretinoin therapy. *Arch Dermatol* 1987; 123:606.

Leyden JJ, Shalita A, Thiboutot D, et al. Topical retinoids in inflammatory acne: a retrospective, investigator-blinded, vehicle-controlled, photographic assessment. *Clin Ther* 2004; 27:216.

Lucky AW. Hormonal correlates of acne and hirsutism. *Am J Med* 1995;98:89S.

Lucky AW, Biro FM, Huster GA, et al. Acne vulgaris in early adolescent boys: correlations with pubertal maturation and age. *Arch Dermatol* 1991;127:210.

Lucky AW, Biro FM, Huster GA, et al. Acne vulgaris in premenarchal girls. *Arch Dermatol* 1994;130:308.

Marqueling AL, Zane LT. Depression and suicidal behavior in acne patients treated with isotretinoin: a systematic review. *Semin Cutan Med Surg* 2005;24:92.

Nouri K, Ballard CJ. Laser therapy for acne. *Clin Dermatol* 2006;24(1):26.

Orzolins M, Eady EA, Avery AJ, et al. Comparison of five antimicrobial regimens for treatment of mild to moderate inflammatory facial acne vulgaris in the community: randomized controlled trial. *Lancet* 2004;364:2188.

Parry ME, Rha CK. Pseudomembranous colitis associated with the topical administration of clindamycin phosphate. *Arch Dermatol* 1986;122:583.

Pochi PE, Shalita AR, Strauss JS, et al. Report of the consensus conference on acne classification. *J Am Acad Dermatol* 1991; 24:495.

Poliak SC, DiGiovanna JJ, Gross EG, et al. Minocycline-associated tooth discoloration in young adults. *JAMA* 1985; 254:2930.

Smolinski KN, Yan AC. Acne update: 2004. *Curr Opin Pediatr* 2004;16:385.

Somech R, Arav-Boger R, Assia A, et al. Complications of minocycline therapy for acne vulgaris: case reports and review of the literature. *Pediatr Dermatol* 1999;16:469.

Stainforth JM, Layton AM, Taylor JP, et al. Isoretinoin for the treatment of acne vulgaris: which factors may predict the need for more than one course? *Br J Dermatol* 1993;129:297.

Stem RS. Medication and medical service utilization for acne 1994–1998. *J Am Acad Dermatol* 2000;43:1042.

Stewart ME, Downing DT, Cook JS, et al. Sebaceous gland activity and serum dehydroepiandrosterone sulfate levels in boys and girls. *Arch Dermatol* 1992;128:1345.

Thiboutot D. New treatments and therapeutic strategies for acne. *Arch Fam Med* 2000;9:179.

Thiboutot D, Gilliland K, Light J, et al. Androgen metabolism in sebaceous glands from subjects with and without acne. *Arch Dermatol* 1999;134:1041.

Usatine RP. The science and art of treating acne in adolescence. *West J Med* 2000;172:155.

Webster GF. Inflammation in acne vulgarism. *J Am Acad Dermatol* 1995;33:247.

Weiss JS, Shavin JS. Adapalene for the treatment of acne vulgaris. *J Am Acad Dermatol* 1998;39:S50.

White GM. Acne therapy. *Adv Dermatol* 1999;14:29.

CHAPTER 20

Miscellaneous Dermatological Disorders

Mei-Lin T. Pang and Lawrence F. Eichenfield

Although acne is the most prevalent skin disorder during adolescence, other diseases such as seborrhea, eczematous dermatitis, fungal infections, warts, and several other conditions are also very common. These disorders while variable in severity, may assume the importance of a serious illness in an adolescent concerned about body image and popularity. Effective therapy and understanding of the adolescent's feelings may lead to a strong alliance between the patient and health care provider. Acne is discussed in Chapter 19; this chapter describes other skin problems commonly encountered during adolescence.

ECZEMATOUS DERMATITIS

Eczematous dermatitis is an inflammatory response of the skin to multiple exogenous and endogenous factors and includes a group of problems whose etiology is often either multifactorial or unknown. The two major groups of dermatitis affecting adolescents are contact dermatitis and atopic dermatitis. In a review of the most common dermatological problems seen by internists, dermatitis was the most common diagnosis, making up 15.8% of them (Feldman et al., 1998).

Contact Dermatitis
Clinical Manifestations
1. Distribution: Areas that have been exposed to the inciting agent, often including the hands, eyelids, genitalia, and legs.
2. Lesions: Pruritic, vesicular, erythematous and/or edematous lesions in a well-demarcated area, often corresponding to the distribution of contact. Erythema, edema, and crusting are often present. If chronic, lichenification, scaling, and pigmentary changes are also seen.

Types
Approximately 80% of contact dermatitis is irritant and 20% allergic. Contact and irritant dermatitis may be indistinguishable clinically, but irritant dermatitis usually occurs on the hands. Photoallergic dermatitis usually occurs on sun-exposed areas such as face and neck in response to photosensitization by ingested drugs. Patch testing may be helpful in confirming allergic contact dermatitis if a specific antigen is suspected.

1. Irritant dermatitis: A nonimmunologically mediated dermatitis that can occur in individuals exposed to the agent when exposed to adequate doses. Prior exposure is not required. Common agents include the following:
   a. Alkalis: Soaps, detergents, bleaches, and cleansers
   b. Acids: Hydrochloric acid, nitric acid, oxalic acid, carbolic acid, acetic acid, and salicylic acid
   c. Insecticides
   d. Hydrocarbons: Oils and tars
   e. Fiberglass
   f. Physical irritation or friction
2. Allergic contact dermatitis: A type IV, delayed-type hypersensitivity reaction occurring in patients sensitive to a specific agent (usually an environmental chemical). Prior exposure is required for a reaction. Examples include the following:
   a. Rhus (poison ivy, oak, or sumac)
   b. Nickel and other metals, particularly mercury and chromium
   c. Rubber compounds (latex)
   d. Dichromate: A common cause of shoe dermatitis; also found in metals, paint, cement, and photographic chemicals
   e. Fabric dyes or chemical finishes (e.g., formaldehyde resin)
   f. Adhesives: The rubber component or the glue
   g. Cosmetics: Hair dyes, hair sprays, artificial nails, nail hardeners, lipsticks, eye makeup, preservatives, sunscreens, perfumes, and mouthwashes

Differential Diagnosis
1. Cellulitis
2. Atopic dermatitis
3. Tinea corporis
4. Seborrheic dermatitis
5. Scabies
6. Psoriasis
7. Keratosis pilaris
8. Icthyosis vulgaris

Treatment
1. Identify and avoid the offending agent.
2. Topical corticosteroid creams are applied twice a day to affected areas. Moderate to high potency steroids may be necessary.

3. Antihistamines may help decrease the associated pruritus.
4. Widespread, severe contact dermatitis may require a course of systemic corticosteroids (40–60 mg/day for 7 days, tapered over 2–3 weeks).

Atopic Dermatitis

Atopic dermatitis is a common, chronic, pruritic dermatitis also known as *atopic eczema* and *allergic eczema*. Onset typically occurs in childhood and may improve or continue in adolescence. It appears in approximately 17% of children, with 90% presenting before the first year of life.

Clinical Manifestations

There are many features that may be used for clinical diagnosis.

1. Essential features (must be present)
   a. Pruritus
   b. Eczematous dermatitis (acute, subacute, or chronic)
   - Typical morphology and age-specific patterns. In adolescence, the morphology resembles the adult pattern of flexural lichenification and involvement of the face, neck, and hands. Lesions consist of pruritic, slightly elevated, flat-topped papules that tend to coalesce to form lichenified, scaly plaques. The plaques may become excoriated, exudative, or crusted.
   - Chronic or relapsing history
2. Important features (seen in most cases, adding support to diagnosis)
   a. Early age of onset
   b. Atopy
   - Personal and/or family history. Approximately 50% of individuals concurrently have either asthma or allergic rhinitis. A positive family history of atopy (asthma, allergic rhinitis, and atopic dermatitis) is present in two thirds of individuals.
   - Immunoglobulin E (IgE) reactivity
   c. Xerosis
3. Associated features (suggestive of a diagnosis of atopic dermatitis but are too nonspecific for use in defining or detecting atopic dermatitis for research or epidemiological studies)
   a. Atypical vascular responses (e.g., facial pallor, white dermatographism, delayed blanch response)
   b. Keratosis pilaris/hyperlinear palms/icthyosis
      Keratosis pilaris: Follicular hyperkeratosis on the lateral upper arms and thighs
   c. Ocular/periorbital changes (e.g., Dennie-Morgan lines)
   d. Other regional findings (e.g., perioral changes/periauricular lesions)
      Pityriasis alba: Ill-defined, scaly, hypopigmented patches typically on the face, neck, trunk, and extremities of children and adolescents between the ages of 3 and 16. It is thought to represent a low-grade eczematous dermatitis and is a minor feature of atopic dermatitis. It is typically asymptomatic, however teenagers may complain of pruritus.
   e. Perifollicular accentuation/lichenification/prurigo lesions

Complications

1. Infections: Increased susceptibility to infections with herpes simplex virus, *Staphylococcus aureus*, *Trichophyton rubrum*, warts, and molluscum contagiosum

2. Eye: Increased prevalence of cataracts, keratoconus, recurrent conjunctivitis, periorbital darkening, and retinal detachment
3. Skin: Exfoliative dermatitis

Differential Diagnosis

1. Seborrheic dermatitis: Greasy, scaly scalp; distribution more likely to include scalp, eyebrows, and ears
2. Contact dermatitis: History of contact with an offending agent and patterned distribution of the eruption
3. Tinea corporis or pedis: Sharp margins; confirmed by positive findings from potassium hydroxide examination
4. Scabies: Distribution usually includes web spaces of hands, groin, buttocks, and axilla; skin scraping positive for mites or eggs
5. Psoriasis: Well-demarcated erythematous plaques with silvery scale; predilection for extensor surfaces; nail pitting common, but not specific
6. Keratosis pilaris

Treatment

1. Education: Health care providers should discuss the chronic, recurrent course of atopic dermatitis with patients and their families. They should also review common, exacerbating factors. Written and verbal information as well as treatment plans may be helpful.
2. Hydration: Patients with atopic dermatitis have increased transepidermal water loss secondary to impaired function of the water permeability barrier, and decreased ceramide levels in the skin. Many advocate the "soak and seal" method, consisting of lukewarm to warm baths or showers lasting no more than 10 to 20 minutes using a gentle, nonsoap cleanser. The patient should then moisturize within a few minutes of bathing.
3. Moisturizers: Moisturizers help preserve the stratum corneum barrier and maintain hydration of the skin. Ointments are the most moisturizing but may be too occlusive in hot or humid environments, leading to sterile folliculitis or increased pruritus. Creams and lotions have higher water content than ointments, making them easier to apply. Additives such as fragrances or preservatives can be irritating and should therefore be avoided. Moisturizers can dilute the effect of topical medications and should be applied at least 20 minutes after topical medications.
4. Avoidance of irritants: Patients with atopic dermatitis have increased responsiveness to irritants. Loose fitting, noncoarse clothing is recommended. Patients with severe atopic dermatitis may find using cotton gloves or socks can protect the skin from potential irritants and reduce trauma from scratching. Cleansers with minimal defattening activity and neutral pH are recommended. Products labeled for "sensitive skin" may be better tolerated in patients with atopic dermatitis. Environmental factors such as temperature, humidity, and fabric texture can also contribute to skin irritation. Patients tend to fare better in air-conditioned or temperate environments where sweating is minimized. Sun exposure can also lead to overheating, evaporation, and perspiration.
5. Avoidance of allergens: Some adolescents may be sensitive to dust mites, animal dander, or other airborne triggers. Although food allergies are more common in atopic patients, eczematous flares caused by specific foods occur only in few adolescents.

6. Addressing psychosocial issues: Atopic dermatitis can have a profound effect on the patient and family. Sleep disturbance secondary to pruritus can impact work and school function leading to more missed days at school, increased work absenteeism, household stress, and economic burden of the disease. Sedating antihistamines may be useful in this setting. Behavior modification (e.g., reward system for not scratching) to break the itch-scratch cycle is also recommended.

7. Topical corticosteroids: Topical corticosteroids are a mainstay of therapy in treating acute disease. They range in potency from very mild (1%–2.5% hydrocortisone) to superpotent (clobetasol). They are typically applied twice daily to affected areas.

8. Topical calcineurin inhibitors: Tacrolimus (Protopic) 0.03% ointment is approved for use in patients 2 to 15 years of age, and 0.03% and 0.1% are approved for short-term and intermittent long-term use in adults with moderate-severe atopic dermatitis. Pimecrolimus (Elidel) 1% cream is approved for use in patients at least 2 years of age with mild-moderate atopic dermatitis.

9. Antibacterial therapy: Patients with atopic dermatitis are more prone to secondary skin infections. Systemic antibiotics such as a first- or second-generation cephalosporin (e.g., cephalexin 25–50 mg/kg/day divided b.i.d. to t.i.d., with 2 g maximum total daily dose) for 7 to 10 days are usually recommended. Long-term antibiotic therapy is discouraged as this may select for resistant organisms. Topical antibiotics such as mupirocin (Bactroban, Centany) applied t.i.d. for 7 to 10 days may be used to treat localized infections. Intranasal application of mupirocin twice daily for 5 days can reduce nasal carriage of *S. aureus*. Patients with eczema herpiticum usually require systemic acyclovir in a hospital setting. Bleach baths ($\frac{1}{4}$–$\frac{1}{2}$ cup bleach mixed in a full bath two to three times a week) decrease bacterial colonization and may be useful as adjunctive therapy in patients with recurrent staphylococcal infections.

10. Antihistamine and anxiolytic therapy: Pruritus is one of the most troublesome features of atopic dermatitis. Scratching can lead to excoriation, secondary infection, bleeding, lichenification, or nodular changes. Patients often complain of sleep disturbance, impacting the patient and caregiver's quality of life. Systemic antihistamines such as diphenhydramine and hydroxyzine can be used for their sedating effects when given at bedtime. Doxepin is a tricyclic antidepressant with histamine-blocking properties. It should be used in patients with severe disease.

Other Types of Eczematous Dermatitis

1. Lichen simplex chronicus: One or more lichenified plaques, probably secondary to repeated local trauma such as rubbing or scratching

2. Dyshidrotic eczema (pompholyx): Recurrent crops of vesicles on palms and soles and sides of fingers and toes; exacerbated by stress and frequent exposure to water

3. Seborrheic dermatitis: Greasy scaling patches on scalp, eyebrows, nasolabial area, intertriginous areas, and chest

4. Nummular atopic dermatitis: Minute vesicles and papules that enlarge to form discrete, erythematous, coin-shaped patches.

PYRODERMA

Types

1. Acne: See Chapter 19 for discussion.

2. Folliculitis: Infection of a hair follicle is common and usually involves *S. aureus* or streptococci. Other causes include fungi (*Candida* and *Pityrosporum*), viruses (herpes simplex virus and molluscum), and drugs (corticosteroids, lithium, halogenated compounds). The infection is usually superficial and characterized by tiny pustules near affected hair follicles, surrounded by an area of erythema. Common locations include the scalp, extremities, buttocks, and perioral and perinasal areas. Other areas include the groin or pubic area in patients who shave or wax, especially if the patient does not exfoliate the area on a regular basis. Treatment involves local hygiene with antibacterial soaps or cleansers and a topical antibiotic ointment, solution, or foam (e.g., clindamycin). The differential diagnosis includes culture-negative (normal flora) folliculitis, eosinophilic folliculitis, acne vulgaris, rosacea, keratosis pilaris, and pseudofolliculitis barbae.

Pseudofolliculitis barbae is a noninfectious, inflammatory condition occurring in men with darkly pigmented skin and tightly curled hair, caused by re-entry of curved hairs after shaving. Curative therapy includes avoidance of shaving and letting the beard grow. Although this will eliminate the condition, this is not always practical. Steps to improve the condition include the following:
a. Pretrim hair with clippers, leaving 1 to 2 mm stubble.
b. Wash with a nonabrasive acne soap and rough washcloth, dislodging ingrown hairs with a soft toothbrush. Rinse with warm water and apply warm compresses to the area for at least 2 minutes.
c. Massage a moderate amount of lather and shave in the direction of hair growth with a sharp razor using short, even strokes.
d. Rinse with cool to cold tap water and apply cold compresses for at least 5 minutes.
e. Dislodge any remaining ingrown hairs with a sterile needle or toothpick.
f. Aftershave should be a gentle, moisturizing type. Topical 1% hydrocortisone cream may be used for 1 to 2 weeks if there is any itching or burning. Topical retinoids may also be beneficial.

3. Impetigo: Although most common in children, impetigo does occur in adolescents. Impetigo consists of discrete and coalescent vesicles that quickly become pustular, then rupture, leaving a thick yellowish crust. The lesions are usually related to group A β-hemolytic streptococci or *S. aureus*. Localized infection can be treated with topical mupirocin (Bactroban), but more extensive or recurrent disease requires treatment with systemic antibiotics. Resistance to erythromycin and penicillin is very common. Methicillin-resistant *Staphylococcus aureus* (MRSA) is increasing in frequency. Antibiotics should be prescribed on the basis of community resistance patterns.

4. Pseudomonas folliculitis or hot tub dermatitis: Pruritic papulopustular eruptions appear typically 1 to 2 days after exposure to a whirlpool, hot tub, or swimming pool, with a predilection for areas covered by a swimsuit, the axillae, and the upper arms. Usually self-limited and resolves in 7 to 14 days, is rarely associated with constitutional symptoms or systemic infection.

5. Furuncles: Staphylococcal abscesses develop around hair follicles, typically in areas of friction. Multiple lesions may coalesce and extend into the subcutaneous tissue, forming carbuncles. Treatment includes warm compresses, antistaphylococcal antibiotics, and incision and drainage of fluctuant lesions. Recurrent or chronic furunculosis requires eradication of the staphylococcal carrier state. MRSA should be considered if the patient fails standard antibiotic therapy. Recurrent furuncles in the groin may be secondary to anaerobic bacteria.

PAPULOSQUAMOUS ERUPTIONS

Eruptions consisting of scaly patches and plaques that occur with some frequency during adolescence include psoriasis, pityriasis rosea, seborrheic dermatitis, fungal infections, drug eruptions, and secondary syphilis (for a discussion of syphilis, see Chapter 64).

Psoriasis

Psoriasis affects between 1% and 3% of the population, with the age at onset being between 10 and 20 years in approximately 25% of the cases. Psoriasis is a chronic, genetically influenced, and immunologically-based inflammatory disease of the skin and joints.

Etiology
The cause of psoriasis is unknown; however, heredity seems to play an ever-increasing role. Several human leukocyte antigens (HLA) located on the short arm of chromosome 6 are associated with psoriasis: HLA-B13, HLA-Bw16, HLA-B17, and HLA-B37. White patients who are HLA-Bw16 positive are 13 times more likely to develop psoriasis. Japanese patients are 25 times more likely to develop psoriasis if they are HLA-Bw16 positive (Svejgaard et al., 1975). One study found HLA-Bw16 expressed in 90% of patients with early-onset disease and in 50% of patients with late-onset disease compared to 7.4% in a control group (Schmitt-Egenolf et al., 1996).

Precipitating Factors
Precipitating factors of psoriasis include the following:

1. Certain infections including streptococcal pharyngitis
2. Trauma
3. Stress
4. Cold weather and low humidity
5. Administration of certain medications

Clinical Manifestations
Psoriasis leads to hyperkeratosis and thickening of the epidermis, as well as increased vascularity and infiltration of the dermis with inflammatory cells. The symptoms of psoriasis are highly variable.

1. Appearance: Round, circumscribed erythematous plaques with a silvery "micaceous" scale. The plaques are usually well demarcated and pinpoint bleeding can occur when a scale is removed. Small teardrop-size or guttate lesions are often associated with streptococcal pharyngitis.

2. Distribution: Scalp, trunk, elbows, and knees are common sites. Usually the condition is mild and affects <20% of the skin. In some individuals, local skin trauma (such as tattoo or burn) will precipitate psoriatic lesions in that area (Köbner phenomenon). Inverse psoriasis is limited to the umbilicus and intertriginous areas.
3. Nails may show pitting, onycholysis, and oil spots in approximately 10% of individuals with psoriasis.
4. Psoriatic arthritis: A seronegative oligoarthritis that may present as acute monoarticular disease in childhood, and is fortunately uncommon in adolescence.
5. Depression may be present secondary to the significant skin lesions.

Diagnosis
Diagnosis of psoriasis is based on typical appearance, location of lesions, or rarely skin biopsy results.

Treatment
Psoriasis may remit spontaneously or as a result of therapy, but recurrences are almost certain. There is no cure for psoriasis and treatment is oriented to suppress or ameliorate the disease. Treatment depends on the severity, duration, and site of disease, as well as the emotional state and treatment preference of the adolescent. Many individuals will need some continuing maintenance therapy that includes the following:

1. Evaluation and avoidance of *precipitating factors*.
2. *Topical therapy* should be tried first. Topical therapies are convenient and lack serious side effects of systemic therapy. Their efficacy is debatable.
   a. Topical corticosteroids: A first choice among most dermatologists. A higher strength preparation is usually used for acute flares and areas with thickened plaques, and medium-potency preparations are used for maintenance. Used alone, topical corticosteroids are most appropriate for lesions limited to isolated small areas of the body. Potent steroids should be avoided in thinner areas of the skin such as face, groin, and genital regions. Use of more potent topical steroids should be limited to approximately 2 weeks, at which time a lower potency topical agent should be used. In addition, once the plaques have flattened out, the application can be reduced in frequency (e.g., every 12 hours for three doses, once a week). The health care provider must remember that the topical corticosteroid preparation can vary widely in potency depending on the vehicle. For example, betamethasone dipropionate at a given concentration can vary from midpotent to superpotent depending on the vehicle (Table 20.1). Adverse effects include epidermal atrophy (reversible), dermal atrophy with development of striae especially in intertriginous areas, perioral dermatitis, and rosacea. Allergic contact dermatitis and pituitary-adrenal axis suppression may be seen with prolonged use of potent (class I) corticosteroids.
   b. Calcipotriene (Dovonex) ointment: A synthetic vitamin D_3 analog useful in treating mild to moderate plaque-type psoriasis. The medication can be an effective first- or second-line topical agent for chronic plaque psoriasis. Although not as effective as superpotent topical corticosteroids, it does not have their side effects. In clinical trials, calcipotriene 0.005% ointment was as effective as fluocinonide 0.05% ointment and

TABLE 20.1

Classification of Commonly Used Topical Corticosteroids According to Potency[a]

Group	Generic Name (Vehicle, Concentration)
Group 1 (most potent[b])	Clobetasol propionate (cream, foam, ointment, lotion: 0.05%)
	Betamethasone dipropionate (foam, ointment 0.05%)
	Halobetasol propionate (Ultravate, cream, ointment 0.05%)
	Diflorasone diacetate (Psorcon, ointment 0.05%)
Group 2	Fluocinonide (cream, ointment, gel, solution: 0.05%)
	Mometasone furoate (ointment 0.1%)
	Betamethasone dipropionate (ointment 0.05%)
	Amcinonide (ointment 0.1%)
	Desoximetasone (cream, ointment 0.25%, gel 0.5%)
Group 3	Triamcinolone acetonide (ointment 0.1%)
	Amcinonide (cream, lotion 0.1%)
	Betamethasone dipropionate (cream 0.05%)
	Betamethasone valerate (ointment 0.1%)
	Fluticasone propionate (ointment 0.005%)
	Diflorasone diacetate (cream 0.05%)
Group 4	Mometasone furoate (cream, lotion 0.1%)
	Triamcinolone acetonide (cream 0.1%)
	Fluocinolone acetonide (ointment 0.025%)
	Hydrocortisone valerate (ointment 0.2%)
Group 5	Fluticasone propionate (cream 0.05%)
	Fluocinolone acetonide (cream 0.025%)
	Betamethasone valerate (cream 0.1%)
	Hydrocortisone valerate (cream 0.2%)
	Betamethasone dipropionate (lotion 0.05%)
	Prednicarbate (cream 0.1%)
Group 6	Fluocinolone acetonide (oil 0.01%, solution 0.01%)
	Betamethasone valerate (lotion 0.05%)
	Triamcinolone acetonide (cream 0.1%)
	Desonide (cream, ointment 0.05%)
	Alclometasone dipropionate (cream, ointment 0.05%)
Group 7 (least potent)	Hydrocortisone (cream, ointment, lotion 1.0%, 2.5%)
	Dexamethasone
	Prednisolone
	Methylprednisolone
	Pramoxine hydrochloride (1.0%, 2.5%)

[a]Potency varies according to the corticosteroids, concentration, and vehicle. Ointments are generally more potent than creams.
[b]Use of superpotent steroids should be limited to 2 wk or less.
From Eichenfield LF, Leung DYM. *The eczemas.* New York: Summit Communications, 2004 with permission.

betamethasone valerate 0.1% ointment in decreasing plaque and disease severity (Linden and Weinstein, 1999). The most common adverse side effect was irritant dermatitis (in 10%–15% of individuals).

c. Tazarotene (Tazorac) gel or cream: A synthetic retinoid effective for mild to moderate psoriasis. It may be used as a second-line agent either as monotherapy or in combination with other topical medications. Adverse effects may include local irritation such as pruritus, burning, and erythema in up to 30% of individuals and is increased with higher concentrations of medication. Efficacy may be increased and irritation reduced when used with a mid- to high-potency topical corticosteroid. Tazarotene is used as a once-daily topical gel or cream. It is contraindicated in unstable plaque psoriasis in progress, erythrodermic psoriasis, patients with a history of allergic contact dermatitis to tarazotene, and pregnant or lactating females.

d. Tars: Extremely effective but unpopular agents due to messiness and staining. However, they are inexpensive and mostly free of side effects. Tars are particularly effective for pruritic psoriasis. Some preparations may be more cosmetically pleasing to the adolescent. The most widely used preparation is tar shampoo for scalp psoriasis.

e. Anthralin: Anthralin inhibits enzymes involved in epidermal proliferation. It is useful as a second-line agent as monotherapy or in combination with other agents for moderate to severe psoriasis. It should not be used in plaque, pustular, or erythrodermic psoriasis. Anthralin is often used for short periods such as 15 to 30 minutes/day. Anthralin also can stain skin and clothing. Healthy skin should be avoided.

  f. Keratolytics: Ointments with salicylic acid (2%–10%) can help soften plaques and can be used with topical corticosteroids or coal tar to improve penetration.

  g. Intralesional corticosteroids: Useful for localized psoriatic plaques; potential side effects include atrophy and hypopigmentation.

3. *Systemic therapy* is rarely indicated in adolescents because of the potential long-term side effects. Cases with severe disease should be referred to a specialist and treatment may involve the following:

  a. Phototherapy: Two types of phototherapy are available: ultraviolet B (UVB) and psoralen plus ultraviolet A (UVA). UVA combined with oral or topical psoralens is reserved for severe, recalcitrant psoriasis, because of the increased risk of developing skin cancer.

  b. Systemic therapy can include methotrexate, acitretin (a systemic retinoid), cyclosporine A, and biological agents such as tumor necrosis factor α (TNF-α) inhibitors. All should be used under the care of a specialist.

Pityriasis Rosea

Pityriasis rosea is a self-limited disorder of unknown cause frequently occurring during adolescence.

Clinical Manifestations

1. Lesions: Oval, salmon-colored papular and macular, 1- to 2-cm scaly lesions, whose long axes follow the body's lines of cleavage in a "Christmas tree" distribution. The lesions typically have a fine cigarette paper–like scale peripherally.

2. Herald or mother patch: A large, 2- to 6-cm single lesion that typically precedes the rash by 2 to 21 days.

3. Distribution: Symmetrical, occurring mainly on the trunk, upper arms, and lower neck, with occasional involvement of face, scalp, hands, and feet.

4. Pruritus: Ranges from very mild to severe.

5. Other systemic symptoms: Constitutional symptoms are rare.

Differential Diagnosis

1. Tinea corporis
2. Secondary syphilis
3. Seborrheic dermatitis

Treatment

1. Reassurance: Condition spontaneously resolves within 6 to 8 weeks.

2. Antihistamines or topical corticosteroids: Use if pruritus is significant.

3. Erythromycin for 14 days resulted in complete response in one study (Sharma et al., 2000).

Seborrheic Dermatitis

Seborrheic dermatitis is a chronic inflammatory disease of the skin, limited to areas of excessive sebaceous gland activity.

Clinical Manifestations

1. Distribution: Usually involves the scalp, eyebrows, forehead, lips, ears, nasolabial creases, axilla, chest, inframammary folds, umbilicus, and groin.

2. Appearance: Dry, moist, or greasy scales often crusted with yellow patches of various sizes.

3. Pruritus: May or may not be present.

4. Course: Marked by many remissions and exacerbations.

Differential Diagnosis

1. Psoriasis
2. Tinea corporis
3. Pityriasis rosea
4. Atopic and contact dermatitis

Treatment

1. Scalp should be shampooed two to three times a week with products based on tar, selenium sulfide, sulfur, or zinc, ketoconazole 2% shampoo, or combination scalp treatments.

2. Hydrocortisone 1% to 2.5% or, if necessary, low-potency nonfluorinated topical corticosteroids may be used sparingly for short periods on the face. However, it is best to avoid topical corticosteroids on the face and a trial of ketoconazole 2% cream may be worthwhile. Many topical corticosteroids are available in solutions, shampoos, or foams for the scalp. Topical corticosteroids such as fluocinolone acetonide 0.01%, clobetasol propionate, and betamethasone valerate are some examples.

Fungal Infections

The dermatophytoses are the most common fungal diseases of the skin. The three principal genera responsible are *Trichophyton, Microsporum,* and *Epidermophyton.* These are responsible for tinea capitis, tinea corporis, tinea pedis, tinea barbae, tinea cruris, and tinea unguium (onychomycosis). Other common superficial fungal infections in adolescents include tinea or pityriasis versicolor caused by *Pityrosporum orbiculare* and *Candida albicans,* which is the causative agent in many cases of intertrigo, paronychia, vaginitis, and pruritus ani.

Dermatophytoses

Tinea Capitis

Tinea capitis is a dermatophyte infection of the scalp and hair follicles, most commonly caused in the United States by *Trichophyton tonsurans.* It usually presents as an enlarging scaly patch of alopecia, often consisting of broken hairs (black dots). However, there may be a noninflammatory presentation consisting of dandruff-like scale, minimal pruritus and subtle hair loss which may be mistaken for seborrheic dermatitis. A granulomatous mass, or kerion, can develop in response to the infection. Some of these fungi are spread by contact with objects such as combs, brushes, and hats, and others from cats and dogs.

The diagnosis can be made by either fluorescence of the infected hairs with a Wood's lamp, examination of the hairs with potassium hydroxide, or culture of infected hairs. Some studies show that only one third of individuals will have positive results from examination of a potassium hydroxide specimen, so one cannot necessarily rely on the

TABLE 20.2

Antifungal Agents Available for the Treatment of Common Superficial Fungal Infections

Indications	Antifungal (Trade Name)	Formulation	Frequency
Onychomycosis	Ketoconazole (Nizoral)	Oral	200 mg/d for 2–3 mo
	Terbinafine (Lamisil)	Oral	250 mg/d for 6 wk for fingernails and 12 wk for toenails
Tinea infections	Butenafine (Mentax)	1% Cream	Once or twice daily
	Ciclopirox (Loprox, Penlac)	1% Lacquer, lotion, cream	Twice daily
	Clotrimazole (Lotrimin)	1% Solution, lotion, cream	Twice daily
	Econazole (Spectazole)	1% Cream	Once daily
	Griseofulvin (Fulvicin, Grifulvin, Gris-PEG, Grisactin, Gristatin)	Oral	500 mg/d for 4–6 wk in adults for tinea capitis, corporis, cruris, or pedis; and 10–20 mg/kg/d for 6–8 wk in children for tinea capitis, 2–4 wk for corporis, and 4–8 wk for pedis
	Haloprogin (Halotex)	Solution, cream	Twice daily
	Ketoconazole (Nizoral)	2% Shampoo, 1% cream	Twice weekly, once daily
	Miconazole (Micatin)	2% Solution, lotion, cream, powder	Twice daily
	Naftifine (Naftin)	1% Cream, 1% gel	Once daily
	Oxiconazole (Oxistat)	1% Lotion, cream	Once or twice daily
	Sulconazole (Exelderm)	1% Lotion, cream	Once or twice daily
	Terbinafine (Lamisil)	1% Solution, 1% cream	Once or twice daily
	Tolnaftate (Tinactin)	1% Solution, lotion, cream, or powder	Twice daily
Oral candidiasis	Nystatin (Mycostatin)	Solution	4–6 mL swish and swallow solution four times daily for 2 wk
	Amphotericin B (Fungizone)	Solution	1 mL oral suspension swish and swallow four times daily for 2 wk
	Anidulafungin (LY303366, VER-002)	Intravenous	Unknown
	Fluconazole (Diflucan)	Oral	In non-AIDS patients, 200 mg single dose
	Itraconazole (Sporanox) Micafungin (FK463)	Oral or intravenous	In AIDS patients, 200 mg the first day, then 100 mg for 2 wk 200 mg/d for 2 wk 50 mg/d for 10 d
	Voriconazole (Vfend)	Oral or intravenous	Intravenous: Loading dose 6 mg/kg every 12 hr for 1 d, then maintenance dose at 4 mg/kg every 12 hr Oral: >40 kg body weight: 400 mg orally every 12 hr for 1 d, then 200 mg orally every 12 hr; <40 kg body weight: 200 mg orally every 12 hr for 1 d, then 100 mg orally every 12 hr

AIDS, acquired immunodeficiency syndrome.

potassium hydroxide examination alone. If the diagnosis is in question, a culture can be taken.

Treatment is with systemic griseofulvin, microsize 20 to 25 mg/kg/day or ultramicrosize 10 to 15 mg/kg/day for 6 to 8 weeks or until there is clinical and mycological cure (up to 12–16 weeks.) Terbinafine 250 mg/day for 2 to 4 weeks has been used as an alternative in resistant cases or in patients who cannot tolerate griseofulvin.

Itraconazole capsules may be administered 5 mg/kg/day or oral solution 3 mg/kg/day for 4 weeks as continuous therapy or 5 mg/kg/day for 1 week per month for 2 to 4 months as pulse therapy. In addition, topical selenium sulfide 2.5% or ketoconazole 2% shampoo should be used twice weekly to reduce the shedding of spores. Table 20.2 summarizes antifungal agents used in the treatment of common superficial fungal infections.

Tinea Barbae

This is a dermatophyte infection involving the bearded area. It is more common in adolescents living in rural areas who work with farm animals. There is usually unilateral involvement of the neck or face and results in either deep nodular suppurative lesions or superficial, crusted, partially bald patches. Treatment is with griseofulvin (500 mg daily for 4–6 weeks).

Tinea Corporis

The skin examination is significant for pruritic, annular lesions that spread centrifugally with central clearing involving any area of the body except the hair, nails, palms, and soles. Scales and pruritic vesicles may be present. The condition is commonly seen in wrestlers.

The diagnosis is confirmed by potassium hydroxide examination of a skin scraping or fungal culture. The differential diagnosis includes other papulosquamous eruptions such as dermatoses (nummular eczema, atopic dermatitis, contact dermatitis), pityriasis versicolor, annular psoriasis, and pityriasis rosea.

If the lesions are localized, topical therapy can be chosen from various agents (Table 20.3). If the lesions are widespread or resist local therapy, griseofulvin microsize 500 mg daily for 4 weeks is effective. Systemic fluconazole, itraconazole, and terbinafine are alternative choices but are not approved for the treatment of dermatophytosis. Huang et al. (2004) reviewed oral therapy of common superficial fungal infections of the skin. Treat sources of infection such as pets, infected family members, or other close contacts (including those that occur during sports such as wrestling).

Tinea Cruris

Commonly called *jock itch* or *crotch rot*, this is a common dermatophyte infection of the groin in male adolescents, particularly during summer months. Typical lesions are bilateral or unilateral, crescent shaped, reddish, and scaly, with sharply defined, raised borders on the upper and inner surfaces of the thighs. The scrotum is usually unaffected.

The diagnosis is generally made on the basis of clinical appearance, negative findings from Wood's lamp examination, and the presence of branching hyphae on potassium hydroxide wet mount. Cultures of the scales can be performed, if necessary, for diagnosis.

Differential diagnoses of common groin eruptions include the following:

1. Candidiasis: Eruptions are more inflammatory with less discrete margins and individual satellite papules or pustules outside the confluent area. The scrotum is commonly affected. A potassium hydroxide preparation reveals budding yeast and pseudohyphae. Candidiasis can be treated with topical nystatin, ketoconazole, or miconazole cream two times a day.

TABLE 20.3

Topical Antifungal Drugs and Coverage

Drug	Candida	Dermatophyte	Tinea versicolor
Imidazole compounds			
Clotrimazole (Lotrimin, Mycelex)	+	+	+
Econazole nitrate (Spectazole)	+	+	+
Ketoconazole (Nizoral)	+	+	+
Miconazole nitrate (Monistat Derm, Micatin, Zeasorb-AF powder)	+	+	+
Oxiconazole nitrate (Oxistat)		+	
Sulconazole nitrate (Exelderm)		+	+
Iodinated trichlorophenol			
Haloprogin (Halotex)		+	+
Pyridone-ethanolamine salt			
Ciclopirox olamine (Loprox)	+	+	+
Allylamine compounds			
Butenafine HCL (Mentax)		+	+
Naftifine HCL (Naftin)		+	
Terbinafine HCL (Lamisil)		+	+
Polyenes			
Amphotericin B (Fungizone)	+		
Nystatin (Mycostatin)	+		
Undecylenic acid (Desenex, Pedi-Dri, Pedi-Pro, Cruex)		+	
Tolnaftate (Tinactin, Aftate, Tritin, Ting)		+	?

HCL, hydrochloride.
'+' indicates coverage of drugs.
From Cohn M. Superficial fungal infections. *Postgrad Med* 1992;91:249, with permission.

2. Erythrasma: A superficial bacterial skin infection of intertriginous sites caused by *Corynebacterium minutissimum* (short gram-positive diphtheroid). The rash appears as a well-defined pinkish or brownish patch that may be smooth or covered by a fine scale resembling a cutaneous dermatophytosis. The rash fluoresces a coral red color under a Wood's lamp, caused by porphyrin production. Potassium hydroxide preparation may show negative results, but Gram stain may show gram-positive filamentous rods (*C. minutissimum*). Erythromycin is the treatment of choice and can be used either orally or topically. One gram in divided doses can be given orally for 5 to 7 days or topical erythromycin twice a day can be used. Alternative therapies have included topical 10% to 20% aluminum chloride, 2% clindamycin hydrochloride solution, and miconazole cream. In addition, a single 1-g dose of clarithromycin has been reported to be effective (Wharton et al., 1998).

3. Psoriasis: Often accompanied by psoriatic lesions elsewhere. Potassium hydroxide preparation and Wood's lamp examination are usually negative. Biopsy may be helpful. Topical corticosteroids are the initial treatment of choice.

4. Intertrigo: This skin condition is more common in obese patients, and consists of well-demarcated, red, macerated, foul-smelling skin with a nonraised border in inguinal creases. Findings are negative for potassium hydroxide wet mount and Wood's lamp examination. Patients are advised to keep the affected area dry.

5. Seborrheic dermatitis: Treatment includes low-potency (class VI–VII) topical corticosteroids, ketoconazole 2% cream.

6. Neurodermatitis: Characterized by leathery, lichenified, mottled eruption with ill-defined borders. Potassium hydroxide preparation and Wood's lamp examination are negative. Low-potency topical corticosteroids may be used for treatment.

7. Irritant dermatitis: There is usually a history of use of sprays, soaps, detergents, or medication.

8. Other pruritic groin rashes include scabies, pediculosis pubis, and miliaria.

Treatment of tinea cruris includes loose clothing, drying skin thoroughly after bathing, weight reduction if obese, laundering contaminated clothing and linens, and topical powders. Elimination of coexisting tinea pedis is also important. Topical antifungal creams or oral griseofulvin microsize 500 mg daily for 4 weeks is an effective antifungal regimen.

Tinea Pedis

A dermatophyte infection involving soles of the feet and toe webs. Early signs include scaling, maceration, and fissuring of the toe webs that can extend to scaling, redness, and vesicular eruptions on the soles. Tight-fitting occlusive footwear and warm humid weather are predisposing factors. The infection is often transmitted through shared bath and shower facilities.

Tinea pedis is typically diagnosed clinically. Potassium hydroxide examination will reveal branching hyphae.

Tinea pedis can be confused with pitted keratolysis, juvenile plantar dermatosis, dyshidrosis, psoriasis, and contact dermatitis.

Treatment for tinea pedis consists of the following:

1. Employ a regimen of soaks or wet compresses with Burow or Domeboro solution for 15 to 30 minutes two to four times daily.

2. Secondary bacterial infection should be treated with topical or oral antibiotics depending on severity.

3. A topical antifungal agent can be helpful. If infection is severe or unresponsive, a course of griseofulvin microsize 500 mg/day or ultramicrosize 660 to 750 mg/day for 4 to 8 weeks may be helpful. Oral antifungals should be considered in patients with diabetes, immunocompromised state, or moccasin tinea pedis.

4. If there is a severe inflammatory response or an "id" reaction (see "Dermatophytid" section), a short 1-week course of topical or systemic steroids is helpful.

5. Keep feet dry and well aerated; sandals should be worn if possible or white cotton socks with shoes.

6. Follow a prophylactic program of drying the feet thoroughly after baths, and then use a medicated powder such as Tinactin or Zeasorb-AF, or Lotrimin AF spray once the infection has resolved.

Tinea Unguium

Tinea unguium is a dermatophyte infection of the nail plate. Onychomycosis includes all infections of the nail caused by any fungus, including dermatophytes and yeast. The infection begins with a white or yellow discoloration of the distal part of the nail. The nail subsequently becomes thickened, brittle, elevated, and deformed. Identification of the causative organism is essential for therapy. It is important to sample the subungual debris near the nail bed for culture as various nail dystrophies, including psoriasis, may be confused with onychomycosis.

The following drugs essentially replaced the use of griseofulvin for this condition. Terbinafine (250 mg/day for 3 months) has been approved to treat toenail infections, but only 6 weeks of treatment is necessary for the fingernails. Itraconazole (100 mg twice daily for 3 months) has been approved or it can be given in a pulsed regimen of 200 mg twice daily for 1 week per month repeated for 3 months to treat toenail involvement. The pulsed regimen may be preferable due to shorter treatment duration and rare association of adverse reactions. Treatment for fingernails is shorter, with only 6 weeks of daily therapy or 2 months of the pulsed regimen recommended. When prescribing these newer medications, one must consider potential drug interactions, side effects, and appropriate monitoring. Alternatives to systemic therapy include topical ciclopirox 8% topical solution (Penlac nail lacquer) or avulsion of the nail plate followed by topical therapy.

Dermatophytid

An "id" reaction is a cutaneous or systemic reaction to the fungal antigen borne through the bloodstream from the primary fungal focus to sensitized areas of the skin. The condition is often associated with dermatophytoses of the scalp and feet and rarely causes systemic problems including fever, anorexia, adenopathy, and leukocytosis. The reaction may consist of a widespread follicular scaly eruption or may be limited to a vesiculobullous or scaly eruption of the hands. The former is more commonly associated with tinea capitis and the latter with tinea pedis.

Tinea (Pityriasis) Versicolor

1. Clinical manifestations: Scaly tan, brown, or hypopigmented macules or patches typically located over the

upper trunk and arms, and occasionally on the face and neck, caused by *P. orbiculare*. The lesions are usually asymptomatic.

2. Predisposing factors: Humidity, hyperhidrosis, heredity, diabetes, and systemic corticosteroids.
3. Diagnosis: Made by observation of hyphae and spores (spaghetti and meatballs) on potassium hydroxide wet mount. Wood's lamp examination is helpful in showing yellowish or brownish fluorescence.
4. Differential diagnosis: Pityriasis alba, vitiligo, pityriasis rosea, seborrheic dermatitis, and syphilis.
5. Treatment
   a. Topicals: A study by Lange et al. (1998) found that ketoconazole shampoo used as a single application or applied daily for 3 days was effective in eliminating tinea versicolor. Other agents include selenium sulfide 2.5% shampoo, ketoconazole 2% shampoo, zinc pyrithione shampoo or soap, sulfosalicylic acid, Tinver lotion (25% sodium thiosulfate, 1% salicylic acid, and 10% alcohol), or terbinafine 1% (Lamisil) spray. Usually these agents are used in the shower or overnight as tolerated daily for 2 weeks, then several times a month for maintenance. Topical antifungals of the imidazole class are effective but expensive for large areas of involvement.
   b. Systemic fluconazole and itraconazole: Fluconazole (400 mg as a single dose) and itraconazole (200 mg/day for 5–7 days) have been shown to be effective in the treatment of tinea versicolor. These medications are not U.S. Food and Drug Administration approved for use in the treatment of tinea versicolor.

Drug Eruptions

Drug-associated skin eruptions are very common and mediated by a variety of immunological mechanisms. Hypersensitivity reactions are classified by the Gell and Coombs classification: types I to IV.

- Type I reactions are due to antigen-induced cell activation of mast cells and basophils leading to urticaria or angioedema. A common example is urticaria or anaphylaxis due to penicillin. Anaphylactoid or pseudoallergic reactions mimic type I reactions but are caused by pharmacologic release of histamine from mast cells. Antigen sensitization is not required for these reactions and may therefore occur with first exposure.
- Type II reactions result from interaction of antigen-specific IgG or IgM antibodies with drug antigens on cell membranes. Examples include antibiotic-induced hemolytic anemia or thrombocytopenia.
- Type III reactions occur secondary to circulating soluble drug–antigen–antibody complexes that deposit into tissues. The most common example is serum sickness.
- Type IV delayed-type hypersensitivity reactions are mediated by activated T cells that recognize specific antigens. Reactions include allergic contact dermatitis and fixed drug reactions.

Most drug reactions occur within 1 to 3 weeks of exposure to a new medication and resolve when the offending agent is fully excreted or metabolized.

The following are various common drug eruptions and implicated agents, organized by morphology.

Maculopapular or Morbilliform Rash

These rashes are usually bilateral and symmetrical, starting on the trunk then spreading to the extremities. Exanthematous drug eruptions can mimic viral exanthems with flat and raised "blotchy" areas with maculopapular rashes and "measles-like" pattern for morbilliform eruptions. Common drugs include:

Penicillin	Salicylates
Penicillin derivatives such as ampicillin or amoxicillin with nearly a 90% reaction rate in patients with infectious mononucleosis	Diazepam and related compounds
	Allourinol
	Oral hypoglycemics
Sulfonamides	Captopril
Phenytoin	Thiazides
Barbiturates	Amphoteracin
Carbamazepine	Gentamicin
Nonsteroidal anti-inflammatory drugs (NSAIDs)	

Urticaria

Pruritic, erythematous edematous papules and plaques, also called *wheals*, can occur anywhere on the body. Lesions usually blanch with pressure, although a dusky appearance or areas of central pallor may be seen. Individual lesions typically resolve in <24 hours, although a course of urticaria can last weeks to months.

Examples of drugs associated with non-IgE–mediated urticaria include:

Aspirin	Opiates
Contrast medium	NSAIDs

Examples of drugs associated with IgE-mediated urticaria include:

Penicillin	Sulfonamides
Cyclosporins	Tetracyclines

Erythema Multiforme

Generalized erythematous macules, plaques or bullae, often with targetoid lesions. Mucosae may be involved and fever may accompany more severe reactions. Drugs implicated include the following:

Allopurinol	Hydralazine	Sulfonamides
Barbiturates	Penicillin	Tetanus antitoxin
Bromides	Phenothiazines	Tetracycline
Chloramphenicol	Phenylbutazone	Thiazide diuretics
Gold salts	Phenytoin	Vaccines (measles, polio, diphtheria)
Griseofulvin	Salicylates	

Erythema Nodosum

Deep pink to purple, painful nodules; classically on the anterior tibial surfaces.

Drugs implicated include the following:

Bromides	Oral contraceptives	Salicylates
Codeine	Penicillin	Sulfonamides

Exfoliative Dermatitis

Generalized erythematous eruption with diffuse scaling. Drugs implicated include the following:

Allopurinol	Penicillin	Quinacrine
Barbiturates	Phenyl	Sulfonamides
Codeine	Phenothiazines	Tetracycline
Gold	Phenytoin	Vitamin A
Isoniazid		

Acneform Eruptions

Comedones and inflammatory papules or pustules. Drugs implicated include the following:

Adrenocorticotropic hormone	Corticosteroids
Androgenic hormones	Hydantoins
Bromides	Iodides
Isoniazid	Phenobarbital
Lithium	Vitamin B_{12}
Oral contraceptives	

Photosensitive Eruptions

Rashes of many types with accentuation in photoexposed areas, predominantly on the face and upper extremities. Drugs implicated include the following:

Coal tar	Griseofulvin	Sulfonamides
Disinfectants	Phenothiazines	Tetracyclines
Dyes	Psoralens	Thiazide diuretics
Essential oils	NSAIDs	Methotrexate

Fixed Drug Eruptions

One or a few erythematous, hyperpigmented, or gray-blue ovoid lesions with occasional bullae on the hands, face, lips, feet, and genitalia. They occur in the same location with repeated exposure to the inciting drug. Drugs implicated include the following:

Barbiturates	Penicillin	Opiates
Erythromycin	NSAIDs	Sulfonamides
Dextromethorphan	Pseudoephedrine	Tetracycline
Metronidazole	Trimethoprim	Clindamycin

Secondary Syphilis

For a discussion, see Chapter 64.

SKIN GROWTHS

Warts: Verrucae

1. Etiology: Caused by human papillomavirus (HPV), a DNA virus of Papovaviridae family. Numerous HPV types have been identified (>70). Although there is some association between HPV type and the clinical type of wart, this is not a 100% correlation. HPV types 1, 2, and 4 are associated with common warts and plantar warts. Flat warts appear more related to HPV types 3 and 10.
2. Epidemiology
   a. Age: Ten percent of 2- to 12-year-old children are affected. Peak prevalence is between the ages of 10 and 19; thereafter, the prevalence decreases.
   b. Prevalence: Seven percent to 10% of the general population.
   c. Transmission: Inoculation occurs by direct or indirect contact from one person to another; autoinoculation is common. Local trauma promotes inoculation.
   d. Incubation: 1 to 6 months.
3. Clinical manifestations: The clinical classification and appearance of a wart is dependent on the wart's location on the skin.
   a. *Verruca vulgaris*
      * Single or multiple in occurrence
      * Most frequently occurs on hands, fingers, and periungually but can occur anywhere
      * Usually sharply circumscribed, firm hyperkeratotic papules 1 to 5 mm or larger in diameter
      * Filiform warts with projecting thread-like structures often appear on the neck and face
   b. *Verruca plana (flat warts)*
      * Flat skin-colored or pink lesions, 1 to 3 mm, smooth and slightly raised with a tendency to coalesce
      * Commonly occur on the face, dorsa of hands, wrists, and knees
      * Often numerous and may occur in a linear pattern as a result of trauma (e.g., scratching or shaving) causing viral spread
   c. *Verruca plantaris (plantar warts)*
      * Occur on the plantar surface of the feet, usually at pressure points
      * Typically, do not extend above the skin surface; covered by hyperkeratotic material
      * May occur as an isolated lesion or in groups (mosaic warts)
      * May appear as multiple small black points representing thrombosed blood vessels
   d. *Condylomata acuminata (venereal warts):* Moist, polypoid warts located in the genital area and may be transmitted venereally. These are discussed in Chapter 66.
4. Treatment: Warts vary in natural history. Most regress spontaneously within 1 to 2 years. Some warts remain unchanged or spread. The recurrence rate is high regardless of the choice of therapy. There are no specific antiviral therapies for curing HPV infection, although vaccines for genital herpes viruses are available. Existing treatments for warts aim to destroy visible lesions or induce an immune response to verrucae without causing scarring. Flat warts tend to be resistant to therapy and should be treated minimally to avoid scarring. Light freezing with liquid nitrogen is of value. Topical tretinoin can also be used to treat flat warts.
   a. *Home therapy* with 17% salicylic acid with or without occlusion for up to 12 weeks is effective in treating one half to two thirds of patients. One method of use is as follows:
      * Soak the affected area in hot water for 10 to 20 minutes
      * File away as much skin as possible using a pumice stone or nail file without causing skin irritation
      * Apply salicylic acid to warts, avoiding healthy skin
      * Cover warts with occlusive dressing such as duct tape
      * Remove tape in the morning
      * Repeat nightly
   b. Cryotherapy: Application of liquid nitrogen is an effective method of treating most warts and usually causes less skin scarring than electrodesiccation.

Commercial over-the-counter cryotherapy products are not as strong as liquid nitrogen. Liquid nitrogen may be administered with spray units (cryostats) or with cotton-tipped applicators. Multiple treatments may be necessary.
- Liquid nitrogen should be applied to the wart tissue long enough to create a white rim of 1 to 2 mm, usually approximately 10 to 15 seconds.
- Avoid freezing surrounding tissue, especially near digital vessels and nerves at the sides of fingers.
- Over days to weeks, a blister forms and may be hemorrhagic, and peels off with part or all of the wart.
c. Electrodesiccation and curettage: This treatment requires expert skill due to increased destruction and scarring.
d. Podophyllin: Condylomata acuminatum can effectively be treated with 20% to 25% podophyllin in benzoin, podophyllotoxin (0.5% solution), or trichloroacetic acid solution (various concentrations).
e. *Imiquimod 5% (Aldara) is* a cell-mediated immunological response modifier and has been approved to treat genital warts.
f. Carbon dioxide laser surgery, flash-lamp pulsed dye laser therapy, bleomycin, tretinoin, 5-fluorouracil, and immunotherapy have been used to treat recalcitrant warts.

Molluscum Contagiosum

Molluscum contagiosum is a common condition caused by a poxvirus infection. (For more information, see Chapter 67.)

Parasitic Skin Infections

1. Pediculosis: See Chapter 67 for more information.
2. Scabies: See Chapter 67 for more information.

MISCELLANEOUS SKIN CONDITIONS

Vitiligo

Vitiligo is an acquired, disfiguring disease characterized by well-circumscribed, depigmented plaques. Depigmentation is caused by destruction of melanocytes by an unknown mechanism. It may be associated with autoantibodies, thyroid disease, and leukotrichia (depigmentation of the hair).

Epidemiology
1. Age at onset: Fifty percent of cases experience some pigment loss before age 20.
2. Prevalence: Vitiligo occurs in approximately 1% to 2% of the population.

Etiology
The cause is unknown, but autoimmune mechanisms are speculated.

Clinical Manifestations
1. Depigmented, well-circumscribed macules, several millimeters to several centimeters, appear on the skin. In lighter-skinned individuals, this may be first noticed during the summer as involved skin contrasts with tanned skin.
2. Any area can be affected, but the face and extremities are most common. Areas subjected to repeated trauma, pressure, or friction are often affected.
3. Usually the distribution is bilateral and symmetrical but may be segmental. Segmental vitiligo is usually not associated with other autoimmune diseases.
4. Wood's lamp examination is helpful in identifying early lesions.

Differential Diagnosis
Morphea (localized scleroderma), postinflammatory hypopigmentation, pityriasis alba, and tinea versicolor may be confused with vitiligo.

Treatment
Treatment is only partially satisfactory. Spontaneous repigmentation rarely occurs. Treatment includes the following:

1. Use of sunscreens for photoprotection and avoidance of sun
2. Use of a cover-up cosmetic such as Dermablend or Covermark
3. Mid to high-potency topical corticosteroid or topical calcineurin inhibitor (tacrolimus, pimecrolimus)
4. Ultraviolet B radiation of narrow-band UVB
5. Topical or oral psoralens followed by long wavelength ultraviolet radiation (UVA): Must be used with great caution and administered by a health care provider experienced in their use
6. Autologous skin grafts

Sunburn

Teenagers often spend long days at the beach or are involved in outdoor athletic activities without protecting their skin from the sun. Sunburn can be a frequent summer problem. Recommendations to adolescents include the following:

1. Midday exposure: Avoid unprotected exposure from 10 a.m. to 3 p.m., when the sun's short ultraviolet rays are at their peak. Seek shade when appropriate.
2. Clothing: Wear protective clothing and a hat when possible. Hatch and Osterwalder (2006) reviewed the use of protective clothing as sunscreen material.
3. Sunscreens: Sunscreens may not prevent a tan, but they do lessen burning. Generous application of a sunscreen with a sun protection factor (SPF) of 15 or greater with a broad spectrum of coverage (UVA and UVB) should be used regularly (Table 20.4).
4. Temperature: The cooling effect of water and wind at the beach decreases the ability to detect sunburn; therefore, the adolescent must be educated about the sun's strong effects.
5. Medications: Certain medications can increase photosensitivity. These include tetracycline, NSAIDs, oral contraceptives, sulfonamide, diphenhydramine, phenothiazines, thiazides, griseofulvin, psoralen, and tranquilizers. Photoallergic reactions are uncommon immunologically mediated responses to small amounts of the offending agent. Phototoxic reactions appear as exaggerated sunburns and occur in nearly all individuals with sufficient exposure to the offending drug.

TABLE 20.4

Sunscreens and Protective Spectrum

	Spectrum
Chemical	
PABA	UVB
Cinnamates	UVB
Benzophenones	UVB (some UVA)
Parsol 1789 (butylmethoxy-dibenzoylmethane)	UVA
Physical	
Zinc oxide	UVA/UVB
Titanium dioxide	UVA/UVB

PABA, *p*-aminobenzoic acid; UVA, ultraviolet A; UVB, ultraviolet B.

6. Both tanning and sunburn cause DNA damage and may increase one's risk of developing nonmelanoma and melanoma skin cancer, as well as photoaging. Tanning beds and sunlamps should be avoided. Most tanning beds and sunlamps emit mainly UVA radiation, which may increase one's risk of skin cancer and cause premature skin aging.

Prevention of sunburn is more effective than treatment. Treatment of sunburn includes soothing moisturizers and an oral NSAID as indicated.

Urticaria

Urticaria, or hives, is an extremely common problem, occurring in 15% of all individuals.

Appearance

Characterized by extremely pruritic, transient, discrete, erythematous, edematous wheals, which may coalesce and form large plaques with raised borders. Individual lesions generally last a few hours to <24 hours. Simple urticaria involves only the superficial layers of the skin, whereas angioedema involves edema in the deeper subcutaneous and submucosal tissues, particularly involving the palms of the hands, the soles of the feet, and the head and neck. Angioedema of the throat may cause respiratory obstruction in severe cases. Urticaria is defined as acute if it lasts <6 weeks and chronic if it lasts >6 weeks.

Classifications/Triggers

The triggers involved in urticaria involve many factors; however, in up to 50% of cases of both acute and chronic urticaria and angioedema, no cause is identified.

1. Type I hypersensitivity
   a. Drug induced: Almost any medication can cause urticaria. Antibiotics, pain medications, sedatives, and tranquilizers are the most common drugs involved.
   b. Food: Urticaria after eating most commonly involves ingestion of nuts, fish, eggs, fresh berries, shellfish, or food additives. Some of these reactions are IgE-mediated, whereas others are caused by direct release of histamine.
   c. Insect and arthropod bites and stings
2. Type III hypersensitivity
   a. Infections: Various bacterial, viral, and parasitic infections may cause urticaria.
   b. Autoimmune diseases: Systemic lupus, thyroid diseases, and certain malignancies
   c. Drugs: Penicillin and sulfonamides
3. Direct mast cell degranulation
   a. Food chemicals such as benzoates and tartrazine
   b. Drugs such as aspirin, opiates, and NSAIDs
   c. Hyperosmolar radiocontrast media
4. Physical urticarias
   a. Cholinergic urticaria: This reaction can be triggered by heat, exercise, or stress. Cholinergic urticaria is produced by the reaction of acetylcholine on the mast cell. It is characterized by highly pruritic, punctate wheals 1 to 3 mm in diameter. These wheals are surrounded by large areas of erythema. The palms and soles are spared. Aquagenic urticaria may be a form of cholinergic urticaria that produces a similar reaction on contact with water. The diagnosis can be confirmed by soaking a foot in hot water, exercising the adolescent, or using a methacholine (mecholyl) skin test. All these will reproduce the lesions.
   b. Heat urticaria
   c. Cold urticaria: Localized or generalized hives develop with exposure to cold air or water, rarely accompanied by syncope, hypotension, and drowning. Hereditary and acquired variants exist. The diagnosis may be confirmed in most cases with an ice cube test. Cyproheptadine (Periactin) is helpful, but desensitization may be necessary.
   d. Pressure urticaria: Urticaria in response to slight pressure, such as sitting or clapping
   e. Solar urticaria
   f. Vibratory urticaria
   g. Dermatographism: Characterized by the development of localized wheals and erythema, following stroking of the skin with a blunt instrument
   h. Chronic urticaria: Chronic urticaria can be a serious disabling condition sometimes associated with insomnia and fatigue. The cause of this type of urticaria is usually much more difficult to determine than acute urticaria. Autoimmune diseases such as systemic lupus erythematosus may present with urticaria and should be considered in the differential diagnosis of chronic urticaria.

Evaluation

Acute transient urticarias do not need a further evaluation. Chronic urticarias can be associated with a long list of conditions and further tests should be ordered only after thorough history and physical examination looking for underlying etiologies.

Treatment

1. The best treatment is removal and avoidance of the inciting factor.
2. Antihistamines are effective for suppression of acute urticaria. Hydroxyzine (Atarax) (25 mg three times a day) is the drug of choice in cholinergic urticaria and dermatographism.
3. Topical therapy: Cold baths or showers may be helpful in relieving some of the itching.

4. Epinephrine is useful if the urticaria is associated with angioedema.
5. Systemic steroids are beneficial in severe acute reactions, particularly with associated angioedema.

Hair Loss

Hair loss can be extremely frightening to an adolescent. Evaluating an adolescent with a complaint of hair loss involves a thorough history and physical examination, as well as an understanding of hair physiology.

Hair Physiology

Scalp hair grows at the rate of 0.35 mm/day. The average daily loss is 25 to 100 hairs, from a total of approximately 100,000. Eighty percent to 90% of hair is in the growing, or anagen, phase. Anagen hairs have a heavy external root sheath that looks like a gelatinous capsule around the lower third of the hair. Ten percent to 15% of hair is in the resting, or telogen, phase. These hairs have a smooth shaft, ending in a short bulbous root. Approximately 5% or less of hair is in a transitional or catagen phase.

Hair Conditions

1. Male pattern alopecia: This occurs in genetically susceptible individuals, resulting in a loss of hair secondary to the effects of androgenic hormones. Usually, only scalp hair is involved. Baldness usually does not occur until the late twenties or thirties, but premature alopecia can occur in the teens or early twenties.
2. Telogen effluvium: Acute illness, surgery, or other severe stress can stop hair growth and cause hairs to go into the telogen phase. Several weeks (6–10) later, resting hair is shed. This condition presents as acute general hair loss 2 to 4 months after a stressful event. Illness, surgery, "crash dieting," parturition, discontinuation of oral contraceptives, anticoagulants, and hypervitaminosis A have been known to trigger an episode of telogen effluvium. Thyroid disease may also be a cause.
3. Anagen effluvium: Anagen effluvium is hair loss caused by disruption of hair during the growth phase. Causes include antimitotic drugs used for chemotherapy, immunosuppressive drugs, warfarin (Coumadin), heparin, arsenic, and gentamicin. In anagen effluvium, the hair develops a focal weakness above the bulb, so the anagen bulb is usually not shed with the hair.
4. Alopecia areata: *Alopecia areata* is characterized by complete hair loss in small, round patches, usually involving the scalp, bearded area, eyebrows, or eyelashes. If the hair loss involves the entire scalp, the condition is referred to as *alopecia totalis*, and if the loss includes the whole body, *alopecia universalis*. Alopecia areata may be associated with pitting of the nails. The tendency is for spontaneous recovery, but the prognosis is worse with increasing involvement. In 25% of cases, the condition is permanent.
   a. Etiology: Autoimmunity is probably the cause in most individuals. Activated CD4 and CD8 lymphocytes have been found around the affected anagen hair bulbs. There also appears to be a strong association with certain HLA types including DQB103 and DRB11104. Two other types are associated with alopecia totalis and universalis.
   b. Diagnosis: Clinical presentation of sharply circumscribed patches of alopecia with exclamation point hairs at the periphery of the bald patch
   c. Differential diagnosis: Tinea capitis, early discoid or systemic lupus erythematosus, and trichotillomania
   d. Treatment: Focal alopecia areata often regrows, but the course of the disease is variable and unpredictable. Potent topical, intralesional, or oral corticosteroids have been used to promote hair regrowth, although they are not curative of the condition. Other treatments include anthralin; topical immunotherapy including dinitrochlorobenzene, squaric acid dibutyl ester, diphencyprone; or minoxidil solution. Price (1999) reviewed the therapy for hair loss and the use of these agents. Treatment may take months or years.
5. Hair loss secondary to physical factors
   a. Traction alopecia: Hair loss at the margin of scalp, occurring primarily in African-American females and in women who wear hair tightly braided.
   b. Hot comb alopecia
   c. Trichotillomania: Irregular patches of hair loss secondary to breaking or removal of hairs on the scalp, eyebrows, or eyelashes by plucking, twirling, or rubbing. It is associated with emotional stress, or less commonly a psychiatric disorder.
6. Secondary scalp disease: Hair loss can occur secondary to various scalp diseases, including psoriasis, fungal disease, seborrhea, or eczema.
7. Metabolic disorders: Hair loss can be found with iron deficiency, hypothyroidism, hyperthyroidism, diabetes mellitus, or hypopituitarism.
8. Systemic diseases: Hair loss can be seen with systemic lupus erythematosus.
9. Scarring alopecia: This form of irreversible hair loss is the result of various inflammatory processes or trauma. Some dermatological conditions that may result in scarring include discoid lupus erythematosus, scleroderma, lichen planus, acne keloidalis, folliculitis decalvans, and dissecting cellulitis of the scalp.
10. Hair-shaft structural defects: Various defects in hair structure can result in hair loss. These defects are often associated with abnormalities of the skin, teeth, breast, nails, and bones. Metabolic disorders and mental retardation can also occur. These conditions include pili torti, monilethrix, trichorrhexis, pili annulati, and Menkes kinky-hair syndrome.

Evaluation

1. History: An extensive history is indicated, including the onset and duration of hair loss, drug use, skin or scalp disease, and recent stress, surgery, illness, or dietary changes.
2. Physical examination: Check particularly for evidence of seborrhea, scalp disease, or an endocrine disorder.
3. Pull test: Lightly grasp approximately 20 hairs and pull gently. Normally one or two telogen hairs will come out. In an adolescent with hair-shaft damage, telogen effluvium, alopecia areata, or anagen effluvium, hair pulls out in great quantities. If many hairs pull out,

microscopic examination of the hairs will determine whether anagen or telogen hair loss is present.
4. Examine scalp closely and perform a potassium hydroxide test if indicated. A fungal culture of the hair and scalp may also be productive.
5. A complete blood count, urinalysis, liver function tests, thyroid studies, serum ferritin, and a fasting blood glucose test may be ordered as indicated.
6. Referral to a dermatologist may be necessary for further evaluation and scalp biopsy may be required if diagnosis is in question.

Therapy
Therapy depends on the etiology.

1. Male pattern alopecia: In men, androgenetic alopecia ranges from bitemporal recession of hair to thinning of the frontal area of scalp to complete baldness. Most adolescents have not begun significant hair thinning, but young adults may have significant concerns and early hair thinning. The goal of therapy for young adults with visible hair thinning or balding is to increase coverage of the scalp and retard further hair thinning. The only drugs approved for promoting hair growth in men in the United States are oral finasteride (1 mg/day) and topical solution of 5% and 2% minoxidil. Both can increase scalp coverage by enlarging existing hairs, and both retard further thinning in both the vertex and frontal regions. In general, treatment for 6 to 12 months is needed to improve scalp coverage, and continuous treatment is used to retain a clinical improvement.
2. Telogen effluvium: Generally reassurance is all that is needed, because there is usually no significant hair loss. This condition will usually be self-limited.
3. Alopecia areata: See previous discussion on treatment.
4. Scalp disease: Treat underlying condition.

Tattoos and Body Piercing

Body piercing and tattooing have become more common among adolescents and young adults. Body piercing and tattooing have been practiced in many societies throughout history with influences impacting extent of use and style of "body art" used. Popular piercing sites in addition to ears are the nasal septum, eyebrow, tongue, cheek, nipple, navel, labia, penis, scrotum, and foreskin. Piercing and tattooing may occur in relation to gang activity or peer pressure. Body piercing and tattooing entails infectious risks including hepatitis, tetanus, bacterial infections, as well as rashes, allergies, and scars. In most states, minors cannot consent for body piercing and tattoos without parental consent, although this is not always followed.

Complications include the following:

1. Hypersensitivity to the dye.
2. Unsanitary methods have resulted in bacterial infections, hepatitis, tuberculosis, and syphilis. Concern about transmission of HIV infection exists.
3. Scarring, including keloids can form.
4. Milk ducts may be damaged when piercing a woman's nipple.

Larzo and Poe (2006) reviewed the adverse consequences of tattoos and body piercings in adolescents.

Tattoo Removal
New laser systems can effectively remove many tattoos with minimal scarring or other adverse sequelae. However, not all tattoos can be completely eliminated. Limitations of treatment include the need for multiple treatment sessions, expense, incomplete response of some individuals, and the possibility of pigmentary changes.

It is important to discuss the possibility of HIV and hepatitis transmission. It is also important to promote regulatory control over tattooing and body-piercing establishments to ensure sanitary conditions.

Primary Syphilis and Herpes Simplex

For a discussion of primary syphilis and herpes simplex see Chapters 64 and 65, respectively.

Hyperhidrosis

Hyperhidrosis is excessive sweating in response to heat or emotional stimuli. Treatment with topical aluminum chloride preparations such as Certain Dri, Xerac AC, or Drysol is often beneficial. Systemic anticholinergic agents, glutaraldehyde, and iontophoresis have also been used with varying degrees of success. Referral for botulinum toxin type A (Botox) injection may be warranted in more severe cases. Rarely should surgical intervention be considered.

Bromhidrosis

Bromhidrosis is malodorous sweating that may be apocrine or eccrine in origin and is caused by bacteria. Good hygiene includes the use of antibacterial soaps, topical antibiotics, antiperspirants, Burow solution, or potassium permanganate soaks, and absorbent powders.

Pink Pearly Penile Papules

Pink pearly penile papules are a normal occurrence in approximately 15% of postpubertal males. The lesions appear as elongated papillae, approximately 1 to 3 mm in diameter, located on the coronal margin of the penis, particularly the anterior border. They often appear in one to five rows and are usually of uniform size and shape. The color tends to be pearly white. Microscopically, they have a normal epidermal appearance except for absent pigment in the basal layer. In contrast, condylomata acuminata tend to be of less uniform size and shape, change over time, and are not neatly arranged around the corona of the penis. No treatment is necessary except reassurance.

Acanthosis Nigricans

Acanthosis nigricans appears as a gray-brown thickening of the skin. It is manifested as symmetrical, velvety, papillomatous plaques, with increased skin-fold markings. The lesions are commonly located on the base of the neck, axilla, groin, and antecubital fossa. The lesions may also occur on the dorsum of the hand, elbow, periumbilical skin, and mucous membranes. It may be commonly found during a routine physical examination in an otherwise healthy obese adolescent. Occasionally, a parent is concerned about the "dirty" appearance.

Most acanthosis nigricans lesions in adolescents are associated with insulin resistance secondary to obesity. These individuals may have type 2 diabetes or are at increased risk for type 2 diabetes and hyperlipidemia. Acanthosis nigricans can also be associated with hyperandrogenism, and rarely with malignant conditions.

Weight loss effectively treats obesity-related acanthosis nigricans. Lactic acid or α-hydroxyacid containing emollients, and tretinoin (Retin-A) have been tried but without any controlled studies demonstrating efficacy.

WEB SITES

For Teenagers and Parents

http://www.mckinley.uiuc.edu/health-info/dis-cond/commdis/contderm.html. Contact dermatitis handout from the University of Illinois student health center.

http://my.webmd.com/content/asset/adam_disease_poison_ivy. WebMD on contact dermatitis.

http://www.psoriasis.org/. National Psoriasis Association.

http://www.niams.nih.gov/hi/topics/psoriasis/psoriafs.htm. Questions and answers about psoriasis from the National Institutes of Health (NIH).

http://www.aad.org/pamphlets/tineav.html,

http://www.aad.org/pamphlets/eczema.html,

http://www.aad.org/pamphlets/seborrhe.html,

http://www.aad.org/pamphlets/Vitiligo.html,

http://www.aad.org/pamphlets/warts.html,

http://www.aad.org/pamphlets/Urticaria.html. Handouts on, tinea versicolor, eczema, seborrheic dermatitis, vitiligo, warts, and urticaria from the American Academy of Dermatology.

http://familydoctor.org/handouts/209.html. American Academy of Family Physician handout on warts.

http://www.nlm.nih.gov/medlineplus/warts.html. Information from the NIH on warts.

http://www.alopeciaareata.com. National Alopecia Areata Foundation.

http://www.nvfi.org. National Vitiligo Foundation.

http://www.eczema.org. National Eczema Society.

http://www.dermnet.org.nz/index.html. Information from New Zealand Dermatologic Society on various conditions including atopic dermatitis.

For Health Professionals

http://tray.dermatology.uiowa.edu/DPT/PathBase.html. Dermatology slides from the University of Iowa.

http://www.emedicine.com/EMERG/topic131.htm. E-medicine section on contact dermatitis.

http://www.aafp.org/afp/980700ap/noble.html. American Academy of Family Physicians article on tinea infections.

http://www.emedicine.com/emerg/topic628.htm. E-medicine section on urticaria.

http://www.emedicine.com/derm/topic396.htm. E-medicine section on seborrheic dermatitis.

http://www.emedicine.com/derm/topic300.htm. E-medicine section on onychomycosis.

REFERENCES AND ADDITIONAL READINGS

Adams BB. Tinea corporis gladiatorum: a cross-sectional study. *J Am Acad Dermatol* 2000;43:1039.

Alper BS. SOAP: solutions to often asked problems–choice of antihistamines for urticaria. *Arch Fam Med* 2000;9:748.

Bacelieri R, Johnson SM. Cutaneous warts: an evidence-based approach to therapy. *Am Fam Physician* 2005;72(4):647.

Baxi S, Dinakar C. Urticaria and angioedema. *Immunol Allergy Clin North Am* 2005;25(2):353.

Bertolino AP. Alopecia areata: a clinical overview. *Postgrad Med* 2000;107:81.

Boguniewicz M, Leung DY. Atopic dermatitis. *J Allergy Clin Immunol* 2006;117(2 Suppl Mini-Primer):S475.

Braithwaite RL, Stephens T, Sterk C, et al. Risks associated with tattooing and body piercing. *J Public Health Policy* 1999;20:459.

Bravender T. Index of suspicion. Case: 3. Diagnosis: telogen effluvium. *Pediatr Rev* 2000;21:354.

Brown S, Reynolds NJ. Atopic and non-atopic eczema. *BMJ* 2006;332(7541):584.

Cobb MW. Human papillomavirus infection. *J Am Acad Dermatol* 1990;22:547.

Cohn MS. Superficial fungal infections: topical and oral treatment of common types. *Postgrad Med* 1992;91:239.

Dibbern DA Jr. Urticaria: selected highlights and recent advances. *Med Clin North Am* 2006;90(1):187.

Dunagin WG, Millikan LE. Drug eruptions. *Med Clin North Am* 1980;64:983.

Dunn JF Jr. Vitiligo. *Am Fam Physician* 1986;33:137.

Dunn JF Jr. Pseudofolliculitis. *Am Fam Physician* 1988;38:169.

Eichenfield LF, Leung DYM. *The eczemas.* New York: Summit Communications, 2004:9.

Elder JT, Nair RP, Sun-Wei G, et al. The genetics of psoriasis. *Arch Dermatol* 1994;130:216.

Farber EM, Nall L. Guttate psoriasis. *Cutis* 1993;51:157.

Federman DG, Froelich CW. Topical psoriasis therapy. *Am Fam Physician* 1999;59:957.

Feldman SR, Clark AR. Psoriasis. *Med Clin North Am* 1998;82:1135.

Feldman SR, Fleischer AB, McConnell C. Most common dermatologic problems identified by internists, 1990–1994. *Arch Intern Med* 1998;158:726.

Fenske NA, Johnson SA. Major causes of alopecia, with suggestions for history taking, work up, and therapy. *Postgrad Med* 1976;60:79.

Ferguson H. Body piercing. *BMJ* 1999;319:1627.

Fragola LA Jr, Watson PE. Common groin eruptions: diagnosis and treatment. *Postgrad Med* 1981;69:159.

Friedmann PS. Allergy and the skin. II—contact and atopic eczema. *BMJ* 1998;316:1226.

Friedmann PS. Assessment of urticaria and angio-edema. *Clin Exp Allergy* 1999;29:109.

Galan EB, Janniger CK. Pityriasis alba. *Cutis* 1998;61:11.

Gambichler T, Laperre J, Hoffmann K. The European standard for sun-protective clothing. *J Eur Acad Dermatol Venereol* 2006;20(2):125.

Gonzalez LM, Allen R, Janniger CK, et al. Pityriasis rosea: an important papulosquamous disorder. *Int J Dermatol* 2005;44(9):757.

Greaves MW. Chronic urticaria. *N Engl J Med* 1995;332:1767.

Greaves MW, Weinstein GD. Treatment of psoriasis. *N Engl J Med* 1994;332:581.

Greenberger PA. 8. Drug allergy. *J Allergy Clin Immunol* 2006;117(2 Suppl Mini-Primer):S464.

Grimes PE. Vitiligo: an overview of therapeutic approaches. *Dermatol Clin* 1993;11(20):325.

Guercio-Hauer C, Macfarlane DF, Deleo VA. Photodamage, photoaging and photoprotection of the skin. *Am Fam Physician* 1994;50:327.

Halder RM, Young CM. New and emerging therapies for vitiligo. *Dermatol Clin* 2000;18:79.

Hatch KL, Osterwalder U. Garments as solar ultraviolet radiation screening materials. *Dermatol Clin* 2006;24(1):85.

Headington JT. Telogen effluvium: new concepts and review. *Arch Dermatol* 1993;129:356.

Helm TN. Evaluation of alopecia. *JAMA* 1995;273:897.

Hennino A, Berard F, Guillot I, et al. Pathophysiology of urticaria. *Clin Rev Allergy Immunol* 2006;30(1):3.

Howard R, Frieden IJ. Tinea capitis—new perspectives on an old disease. *Semin Dermatol* 1995;14:2.

Huang DB, Ostrosky-Zeichner L, Wu JJ, et al. Therapy of common superficial fungal infections. *Dermatol Ther* 2004;17:517.

Hurwitz S. *Clinical pediatric dermatology.* Philadelphia: WB Saunders, 1993.

Jackson EA. Hair disorders. *Prim Care (Clin Office Pract)* 2000;27:319.

Jacobs PH. Ketoconazole use in tinea versicolor. *West J Med* 1987;147:547.

Jimbow K. Vitiligo: therapeutic advances. *Dermatol Clin* 1998;16:399.

Kilmer SL. Laser treatment of tattoos. *Dermatol Clin* 1997;15:409.

Kovacs SO. Vitiligo. *J Am Acad Dermatol* 1998;38:647.

Kwong KY, Maalouf N, Jones CA. Urticaria and angioedema: pathophysiology, diagnosis, and treatment. *Pediatr Ann* 1998;27:719.

Lange DS, Richards HM, Guarnieri J, et al. Ketoconazole 2% shampoo in the treatment of tinea verisolor: a multicenter, randomized, double-blind, placebo-controlled trial. *J Am Acad Dermatol* 1998;39:944.

Larzo MR, Poe SG. Adverse consequences of tattoos and body piercings. *Pediatr Ann* 2006;35(3):187.

Laude TA. Approach to dermatologic disorders in black children. *Semin Dermatol* 1995;14:15.

Lebwohl MG. Advances in psoriasis. *Arch Dermatol* 2005;141(12):1589.

Levy ML. Disorders of the hair and scalp in children. *Pediatr Clin North Am* 1991;38(4):905.

Linden KG, Weinstein GD. Psoriasis: current perspectives with an emphasis on treatment. *Am J Med* 1999;107:595.

Madani S, Shapiro J. Alopecia areata update. *J Am Acad Dermatol* 2000;42:549.

Mahmood T. Urticaria. *Am Fam Physician* 1995;51:811.

Malcolm B. Tinea pedis. *Practitioner* 1998;242:225.

Mallory SB, Watts JC. Sunburn, sun reactions, and sun protection. *Pediatr Ann* 1987;16:77.

Mark BJ, Slavin RG. Allergic contact dermatitis. *Med Clin North Am* 2006;90(1):169.

Mathelier-Fusade P. Drug-induced urticarias. *Clin Rev Allergy Immunol* 2006;30(1):19.

McBurnery EL. Vitiligo: clinical picture and pathogenesis. *Arch Intern Med* 1979;139:1295.

Mortz CG, Andersen KE. Allergic contact dermatitis in children and adolescents. *Contact Dermatitis* 1999;41:121.

Muldoon KA. Body piercing in adolescents. *J Pediatr Health Care* 1997;11:298.

Nadalo D, Montoya C, Hunter-Smith D. What is the best way to treat tinea cruris? *J Fam Pract* 2006;55(3):256.

Nielson TA, Reichel M. Alopecia: diagnosis and management. *Am Fam Physician* 1995;51:1513.

Noble SL, Forbes RC, Stamm PL. Diagnosis and management of common tinea infections. *Am Fam Physician* 1998;58:163.

Obrien JM. Common skin problems of infancy, childhood, and adolescence. *Prim Care* 1995;22:99.

Odom R. Diagnosis and treatment of common fungal infections. *Mod Med* 1987;55:34.

Odom R. A practical review of antifungals. *Mod Med* 1987;55:59.

Pardasani AG, Feldman SR, Clark AR. Treatment of psoriasis: an algorithm-based approach for primary care physicians. *Am Fam Physician* 2000;61:725.

Parish LC, Witkowski JA. Cutaneous bacterial infections: how to manage primary, secondary, and tertiary lesions. *Postgrad Med* 1992;91:119.

Plasencia JM. Cutaneous warts: diagnosis and treatment. *Prim Care (Clin Office Pract)* 2000;27:423.

Price VH. Treatment of hair loss. *N Engl J Med* 1999;341:964.

Przybilla B, Eberlein-Konig B, Rueff E. Practical management of atopic eczema. *Lancet* 1994;343:1342.

Rietschel RL, Fowler JF Jr. *Fisher's contact dermatitis,* 4th ed. Baltimore: Williams & Wilkins, 1995.

Roberts BJ, Friedlander SF. Tinea capitis: a treatment update. *Pediatr Ann* 2005;34:201.

Rosen CF. Photoprotection. *Semin Cutan Med Surg* 1999;18:307.

Ross EK, Shapiro J. Management of hair loss. *Dermatol Clin* 2005;23(2):227.

Rupke SJ. Fungal skin disorders. *Prim Care (Clin Office Pract)* 2000;27:407.

Saary J, Qureshi R, Palda V, et al. A systematic review of contact dermatitis treatment and prevention. *J Am Acad Dermatol* 2005;53(5):845.

Satin EE. Alopecia areata in childhood. *Semin Dermatol* 1995;14:9.

Schon MP, Boehncke WH. Psoriasis. *N Engl J Med* 2005;352(18):1899.

Schmitt-Egenolf M, Eierman TH, Boehnke WH. Familial juvenile onset psoriasis is associated with the human leukocyte antigen (HLA) class I side of the extended haplotype Cw6-B57-DRB*0701-DQA1*0201-DQB1*0303: a population and family based study. *J Invest Dermatol* 1996;106:711.

Seville RH. Stress and psoriasis: the importance of insight and empathy in prognosis. *J Am Acad Dermatol* 1989;20:97.

Sex Transm Infect. National guideline for the management of molluscum contagiosum. Clinical effectiveness group (Association of Genitourinary Medicine and the Medical Society for the Study of Venereal Diseases). 1999;75(Suppl 1):S80.

Sharma PK, Yadav TP, Gautam RK, et al. Erythromycin in pityriasis rosea: a double-blind, placebo-controlled clinical trial. *J Am Acad Dermatol* 2000;42:241.

Shapiro J, Madani S. Alopecia areata: diagnosis and management. *Int J Dermatol* 1999;38(Suppl 1):19.

Shenenberger DW. Curbing the psoriasis cascade. Therapies to minimize flares and frustration. *Postgrad Med* 2005;117(5):9.

Simpson EL, Hanifin JM. Atopic dermatitis. *Med Clin North Am* 2006;90(1):149.

Sperling LC, Mezebish DS. Hair diseases. *Med Clin North Am* 1998;82:1155.

Starr NB. Sun smarts: the essentials of sun protection. *J Pediatr Health Care* 1999;13:136.

Sterling GB. Sunscreens: a review. *Cutis* 1992;50:221.

Stuart CA, Driscoll MS, Lundquist KF, et al. Acanthosis nigricans. *J Basic Clin Physiol Pharmacol* 1998;9:407.

Sunenshine PJ, Schwartz RA, Janniger CK. Tinea versicolor. *Int J Dermatol* 1998;37:648.

Svejgaard A, Platz P, Ryder L, et al. HL-A and disease association- a survey. *Transplant Rev* 1975;22:1.

Tariq A, Ross JD. Viral sexually transmitted infections: current management strategies. *J Clin Pharmacol Ther* 1999;24:409.

Thiers BH. Dermatology therapy update. *Med Clin North Am* 1998;82:1405.

Uter W, Johansen JD, Orton DI, et al. Clinical update on contact allergy. *Curr Opin Allergy Clinl Immunol* 2005;5(5):429.

Verbov J. How to manage warts. *Arch Dis Child* 1999;80:97.

Westerhof W. Vitiligo management update. *Skin Ther* 2000;5:1.

Weston WL, Badgett JT. Urticaria. *Pediatr Rev* 1998;19:240.

Wharton JR, Wilson PL, Kincannon JM. Erythrasma treated with single-dose clarithromycin. *Arch Dermatol* 1998;134:671.

PART VI

Neurological Disorders

CHAPTER 21

Epilepsy

Wendy G. Mitchell, Arthur Partikian, and Lawrence S. Neinstein

Epilepsy is the most common chronic neurological condition in adolescents. It is defined as recurrent, usually transient, episodes of disturbed central nervous system (CNS) function (seizures), excluding extracerebral causes such as syncope, hypoglycemia, or episodic psychiatric syndromes. Epilepsy has been reported since biblical times and has been seen differently by various cultures. Views have ranged from veneration of patients with epilepsy as mystics to imprisoning them or placing them in mental hospitals. As recently as 1965, two states prohibited marriage if a person had epilepsy, and until the early 1970s, immigration into the United States was prohibited for people with epilepsy. Most adolescents with epilepsy have the potential for excellent control with medication and a high likelihood of eventual remission of their epilepsy. Recent advances in basic science and neurogenetics have contributed to the understanding of mechanisms of epilepsy and seizures. New medications and surgical techniques have improved the outcome of severe, intractable epilepsy. Despite this, fears, prejudices, and social stigma remain common. Epilepsy is therefore somewhat more challenging to treat in teens than other chronic illnesses.

Epilepsy is a difficult condition for patients of all ages. However, for the adolescent concurrently undergoing the stresses of peer relationships, independence, and body image, epilepsy can be particularly trying. The goals of management of epilepsy include proper diagnosis, evaluation, treatment of underlying etiologies, appropriate use of anticonvulsant drugs, and recognizing and dealing with the many associated psychosocial problems.

ETIOLOGY

Seizures are caused by an excessive discharge of a population of cortical neurons. The location and pattern of spread of activity determine the clinical expression. Seizures may be due to acute physiological or neurological disturbances or due to epilepsy. Recurrent *unprovoked* seizures are the hallmark of epilepsy. The diagnosis of epilepsy does not imply a specific etiological factor in the individual. Epilepsy may be genetic, idiopathic, or secondary, due to remote insult to the nervous system. Infection, trauma, metabolic disturbances, drugs, drug withdrawal, syncope or fever may also provoke seizures

acutely. Seizures that occur *only* in the setting of an acute provocation are not generally classified as epilepsy, although in some epileptics, specific stimuli or situations provoke seizures. Seizures acutely provocable by specific stimuli such as strobe lights (reflex seizures) may be due to genetic epilepsies or may be nonepileptic isolated provoked seizures.

EPIDEMIOLOGY

1. Prevalence: 1 of 200 in the general population, with a higher prevalence in children.
2. Incidence: Annual incidence is 1:1,000.
3. Onset: Peak periods for the onset of idiopathic and age-related primary epilepsies are during the early school years and during adolescence. The onset of secondary (remote symptomatic) seizures is highest during infancy and in the geriatric age-group but may occur at any age.
4. Gender: Epilepsy occurs slightly more often in males than in females (relative risk for males, 1.1–2.4 in various studies).
5. Socioeconomic, racial, and ethnic factors: In the United States and Western Europe, epilepsy is slightly more common among lower socioeconomic groups. Epilepsy is more common in Mexico, South America, and Central America, and in immigrants from these areas in the United States, at least partially due to the high incidence of cerebral cysticercosis. Epilepsy is more prevalent among African-Americans than among Whites in the United States.
6. Mental retardation and cerebral palsy are associated with higher rates of epilepsy, as well as lower rates of remission of childhood-onset epilepsy.
7. Epilepsy is associated with an increased risk of death, including sudden unexplained death, but the risk in adolescents with epilepsy is low.

CLINICAL MANIFESTATIONS

Table 21.1 lists classifications of seizures, based on international classifications.

TABLE 21.1

Classifications of Seizures

Generalized seizures: Bilaterally symmetrical, both in clinical and electroencephalographical manifestations, without focal features.
1. Tonic-clonic, generalized convulsive, grand mal
2. Tonic seizures
3. Clonic seizures
4. Absence seizures
   a. *Simple (impaired consciousness only):* Classic petit mal
   b. *Atypical:* Disturbed consciousness plus myoclonic component, automatisms, autonomic component, or abnormality of postural tone
5. Akinetic (atonic) seizures
6. Myoclonic seizures
Partial seizures: Clinical and electroencephalographical onset is localized to one part of the brain (focal) Simple partial seizures: No impairment of consciousness
1. Motor symptoms
2. Sensory symptoms
3. Autonomic symptoms
4. Special sensory (visual, auditory, olfactory, gustatory)
5. Psychic symptoms (fear, déjà vu, jamais vu, euphoria)
Complex partial seizures: Partial seizure with impairment of consciousness, includes most seizures described as "*psychomotor.*" Seizure may begin with impairment of consciousness or as a simple partial seizure and progress to impaired consciousness.
Partial with secondary generalization: Either partial simple or complex partial seizures may secondarily generalize, producing a tonic-clonic or clonic convulsion similar to a primary generalized convulsion. A partial simple seizure may progress through a complex partial seizure or directly to a secondarily generalized seizure
1. Simple partial seizures progressing to generalized seizures
2. Complex partial seizures progressing to generalized seizures
3. Simple partial seizures progressing to complex partial seizures, progressing to generalized seizures

Seizure Components

The progression of a seizure is characterized by several temporal components, variably present:

1. Prodrome: Altered behavior or mood occurring hours to days before the actual seizure; infrequent.
2. Aura: Altered sensation or psychic symptom occurring just before other ictal manifestations. The aura is actually part of the seizure, representing a simple partial seizure, usually with sensory, special sensory, or psychic symptoms.
3. Ictus: The observed seizure event, usually with motor activity.
4. Postictal state: Altered neurological function ranging from coma to mild lethargy, hemiplegia to minimal focal motor dysfunction, lasting minutes to 24 hours.

Grand Mal Seizures (Generalized Tonic-Clonic Seizures)
1. Aura: May have brief, nondescript aura
2. Ictus
   a. Tonic phase: Forceful, postural contractions in flexion or extension. Usually, the early phase, momentary to several minutes, occasionally longer, may include the following:
      • Deviation of head
      • A cry at the onset
      • Loss of consciousness at the start of the seizure
      • Fall to ground
      • Bites tongue or cheeks
   b. Clonic phase: Bilateral, generally symmetrical, brisk jerking movements. Clonic movements have a discernible fast–slow component, as distinguished from other types of movement (writhing, sustained posturing, random bilateral nonsynchronous movements), which are less likely a part of a convulsion.
   c. After the tonic-clonic phase, the patient usually becomes flaccid, with or without incontinence of urine or stool, as seizure stops.
3. Postictal state
   a. Early: Unconscious state, with decreased tone and reflexes. Patients may have fixed pupils.
   b. Recovery phase: Sleeplike state, but patient is responsive to arousal.
   c. Late phase: Confusion or headache.

Petit Mal and Other Absence Seizures
1. Prodrome: None, but often cluster on rising in the morning.
2. Aura: None; abrupt onset of ictus.
3. Ictus: Brief period (few seconds–30 seconds) of blank staring.
   a. Loss of consciousness, usually without fall.
   b. Typical absence: Minor automatisms; may have blinking of eyes; movement of fingers common. Onset

is abrupt and seizure ends with near-immediate return to normal.

   c. Atypical absence: May be associated with automatisms, myoclonic movements or loss of tone; may be longer than 30 seconds; onset is more likely gradual and end is not as abrupt.

4. Postictal: No postictal confusion, but amnesia of seizure is usual.
5. One third of absence seizures remit during adolescence (most likely in childhood—onset simple absence; less likely in adolescence—onset absence).
6. The electroencephalogram (EEG) is characteristic, showing 3-Hz spike and wave activity in typical petit mal seizure. Other absence syndromes show generalized polyspike wave discharges, slow spike wave (Lennox-Gastaut syndrome), or 4- to 5-Hz spike wave (juvenile myoclonic epilepsy [JME] of Janz).
7. Specific epileptic syndromes with onset in adolescence combine absence with myoclonic seizures and occasional grand mal seizures, most prominent on arising in the morning. Early morning myoclonus may be viewed as "normal" by the patient and not reported without specific questioning (JME of Janz).
8. Patients with absence or absence plus myoclonic seizures are more likely to be photosensitive than those with other seizure types. "Video game"–related seizures are generally limited to these patients.

Myoclonic Seizures

1. Myoclonic jerks are brisk and irregular and may involve the trunk or extremities, symmetrically or asymmetrically. Jerks may be of small amplitude or massive, causing the patient to fall.
2. Patients are generally aware of the jerks if they are isolated. They may be unaware if myoclonic jerks are part of absence seizures.
3. Differential diagnosis includes tics, nonepileptic myoclonus, and other movement disorders.
4. Etiologies
   a. Myoclonus, usually occurring on rising in the morning, with adolescent onset, are a characteristic part of JME. Absence or generalized tonic-clonic seizures often occur in these patients.
   b. Myoclonic seizures may be part of an epileptic encephalopathy, such as Lennox-Gastaut syndrome, beginning in early childhood and continuing in adolescence.
   c. Photomyoclonus may occur with exposure to a strobe or to strobe-like conditions in teens with photosensitive epilepsy. They may have other generalized seizures, or this may be their only symptom.
   d. Various degenerative conditions, including progressive myoclonic epilepsies, sialidosis, and subacute sclerosing panencephalitis, may present in the teen years and may be characterized by myoclonic seizures.
5. There is no prodrome, aura, or postictal period.
6. EEG usually shows bursts of spike wave or polyspike and wave in a generalized distribution. Photosensitivity may be demonstrated on EEG using strobe.

Partial Simple Seizures

1. Benign focal epilepsy of childhood (also known as *benign Rolandic epilepsy*) is the most common cause of focal motor seizures in childhood and early adolescence.

   a. Seizures are partial simple seizures usually involving the face or arm; seizures may secondarily generalize.
   b. Episodes are most likely to occur during drowsiness or sleep onset, or upon awakening.
   c. Seizures usually resolve by the midteen years.
   d. There is no underlying structural lesion.
2. Partial simple seizures with onset in adolescence or adulthood are more commonly associated with structural pathology (e.g., tumor, arteriovenous malformation, head injury, malformation, and stroke).
3. Sensory phenomena (aura) may be the only manifestation of a brief limited seizure.
4. Ictus: Most partial simple seizures are focal motor.
   a. Consciousness is retained. Speech arrest may occur with dominant hemisphere seizure origin (usually with the seizure involving the right face and left brain in the right-handed person). Drooling is common.
   b. Clonic activity may "march" up an extremity or spread from arm to face or arm to leg, and so on (or vice versa).
5. Postictal: Headache, postictal hemiparesis (Todd paralysis).
6. EEG
   a. Benign focal epilepsy of childhood is associated with central temporal spikes, which are more commonly seen in light sleep. EEG abnormality is commonly bilateral, even if all observed seizures were on the same side.
   b. Other partial seizures may be associated with spikes or slowing in a unilateral distribution.

Partial Seizures with Complex Symptomatology

Partial seizures with complex symptomatology are seizures of focal onset with altered consciousness. Older terms include psychomotor seizures and temporal lobe seizures, although not all partial complex seizures originate in the temporal lobe and not all temporal lobe seizures are complex partial (i.e., they may be simple partial).

1. May begin at any age.
2. Structural pathology is more common than in generalized epilepsies or benign focal epilepsy of childhood. Mesial temporal sclerosis may cause seizures of temporal lobe origin with onset in adolescence.
3. Prodrome: Patients may report that "they know a seizure is coming."
   a. May occur hours or days before a seizure.
   b. Includes mood change, headache, and change in appetite.
4. Typical partial complex seizures consist of the following sequence (any of these components may be omitted other than the altered state of consciousness):
   a. Aura: Initial sensory, autonomic, or psychic symptoms lasting seconds to minutes; common phenomena include fear, déjà vu, "rising feeling" in abdomen, tingling, and visual, auditory, olfactory, or gustatory hallucination. Flushing or pallor may be observed. Consciousness is generally retained, and patient remembers this part of the seizure.
   b. Blank stare with impairment of responsiveness and consciousness: The patient is motionless and does not remember events clearly during this phase, if at all.
   c. Automatisms: Hand wringing, picking, lip smacking, walking aimlessly, grunting, gagging, or swallowing. Although destructive or injurious behavior may

TABLE 21.2

Features of Absence and Complex Partial Seizures

Type	Aura	Loss of Consciousness	Duration	Automatisms	Postictal State	Memory of Event	Electro-encephalogram	Associated Abnormalities
Typical absence (Petit Mal)	None	Immediate	5–20 sec	Occasional simple automatisms	None	None	3-Hz spike wave	20% have grand mal seizures as well; mentally normal
Absence atypical	None	Immediate	5–45 sec	Occasional automatisms	None	None	Slow spike wave or polyspike	Myoclonus, drop attacks, grand mal; mental retardation more common
Complex partial	Often	Gradual or partial in some patients	5 sec–5 min	Frequent, more complicated	Frequent	Partial in some patients	Focal spikes	May have secondary generalization; structural lesions may underlie disorder

occur, directed deliberate violence does not. Consciousness is impaired or lost during this phase, and the patient does not remember it. Frontal lobe–origin complex partial seizures may produce thrashing, agitated movements, bicycling leg movements, or pelvic thrusting, which are difficult to distinguish from hysterical behavior.

   d. Postictal state: Confusion, stupor, headache, and lethargy may last seconds to hours.

5. Precipitants: Sleep deprivation, alcohol, or drug ingestion.
6. EEG: Focal spikes in temporal, frontal, or parietal areas, usually unilateral. EEG findings may be normal. Special procedures such as sleep deprivation, special leads, and prolonged monitoring may be useful for diagnosis.

   Features that help differentiate various seizures reported as "little seizures" or "staring spells" (partial complex, petit mal, and atypical absence) are listed in Table 21.2.

DIFFERENTIAL DIAGNOSIS

Seizures

1. Symptomatic seizures (due to acute systemic disturbance or trauma)
   a. Acute metabolic disturbance (e.g., hypoglycemia, hyponatremia, and hypocalcemia)
   b. Acute CNS infection (e.g., encephalitis and meningitis)
   c. Intoxication (e.g., cocaine, alcohol, stimulants, "ecstasy", phencyclidine (PCP), ketamine, and inhalants)
   d. Drug or alcohol withdrawal (e.g., barbiturates, sedatives, and benzodiazepines after prolonged use)
   e. Acute head trauma (impact seizure and seizure in first few days after significant head trauma)
   f. Syncopal seizure: Brief tonic or clonic seizure occurring after primary syncope
   g. Acute stroke
2. Acquired (symptomatic or secondary) epilepsies due to remote history of CNS insult

   a. Cerebral malformations: Macroscopic or microscopic (cortical dysgenesis)
   b. Intrauterine infections (e.g., cytomegalovirus and toxoplasmosis)
   c. Perinatal insults
   d. Postneonatal infections (e.g., meningitis, encephalitis, and brain abscess)
   e. Posttraumatic epilepsy
   f. Tuberous sclerosis
   g. Brain tumors and other mass lesions
   h. Vascular malformations and infarctions
   i. Cysticercosis
   j. Genetic changes due to progressive or degenerative conditions
   k. Unknown but presumed symptomatic: Epileptic encephalopathies such as Lennox-Gastaut syndrome and early myoclonic encephalopathy
3. Idiopathic epilepsy (also called *age-related epilepsies*)
   a. Primary generalized epilepsies
   b. Benign focal epilepsy of childhood

Other Paroxysmal Events That May Suggest Seizure Activity

1. Vasovagal syncope
2. Migraine
3. Cardiac disease
   a. Arrhythmias
   b. Low-output states
   c. Mitral valve prolapse
4. Hyperventilation and anxiety states
5. Orthostatic hypotension
6. Sleep disturbances
   a. Narcolepsy: Catalepsy, sleep attacks, sleep paralysis, and hypnagogic hallucinations
   b. Drowsiness or sleep attacks in patients with obstructive sleep apnea or sleep deprivation
   c. Sleepwalking, rapid eye movement (REM) sleep disturbance, and other parasomnias
   d. Night terrors
   e. Periodic leg movements in sleep

7. Movement disorders
   a. Tics
   b. Paroxysmal kinesiogenic choreoathetosis
   c. Stiff-man syndrome and other syndromes of continuous muscle fiber activity
   d. Dystonias (paroxysmal torticollis, activity-related dystonias, dystonia musculorum deformans, and drug-related)
   e. Pseudohypoparathyroidism: Teens with hypocalcemia secondary to pseudohypoparathyroidism may present with seizure-like episodes that are primarily dystonic.
   f. Restless leg syndrome
8. Pseudoseizures (hysterical symptoms)
9. Episodic "staring" and inattention
   a. Attention deficit disorder
   b. Disorders of arousal

DIAGNOSIS

History

Epilepsy is primarily a clinical diagnosis based on the history. An astute observer of the event is more important than any "test."

1. Review the following with the observers of the event:
   a. What was the teen doing before the episode began—sleeping, quiet, watching television, exercising, reading, or anxious?
   b. Where did the event occur?
   c. At what time of the day?
   d. Relation to sleep state: Did the seizure occur just as the teen was falling asleep, just after awakening, or during deep sleep?
   e. What was the first abnormality noted? Did the teen seem to be aware that something was wrong?
   f. What happened during the seizure?
   g. Could the teen be aroused? Respond to commands? At what point did unresponsiveness start? How long did unconsciousness last?
   h. Was there incontinence of urine or stool?
   i. What happened after the seizure?
2. Review the following with the patient:
   a. What was the last event he or she remembers before the seizure?
   b. Could the patient hear or understand people talking during the seizure? Could he or she respond?
   c. What happened after the seizure? What is the first thing recalled after the event?
   d. Precipitating events: Sensory stimulation, activity, drugs, meals, medications, sleep pattern, stress, and menses.
   e. Earlier seizures or similar events.
3. Family history of epilepsy, neurocutaneous syndromes, and other neurological conditions
4. Perinatal history, particularly birth injury, prematurity, and maternal infections
5. History of CNS infections or trauma
6. Drug history, including prescribed, over-the-counter, and "street" drugs and alcohol
7. Any other recent changes in health or function: Any changes in cognition, motor function, or others to suggest onset of neurological disease other than the seizure

8. Travel history and/or household exposure to recent immigrants from areas with endemic cysticercosis/*Taenia solium*.

Physical Examination

1. Perform general physical examination for evidence of systemic disease.
2. Skin: Look for signs of a neurocutaneous syndrome such as café au lait spots, depigmented macules, adenoma sebaceum, shagreen patch, and subungual fibromas.
3. Eyes: Perform funduscopic examination for optic disc edema (papilledema).
4. Neurological examination: Look for evidence of focal abnormalities. Observe gait and movements at rest and with activity for evidence of movement disorder as alternative explanation of symptoms.
5. Blood pressure: Assess pressure while the teen is lying and standing.
6. Pulse: Check for irregularities, if arrhythmia is suspected.
7. Cardiac examination: Check for evidence of mitral valve prolapse, heart failure, or other abnormalities that might lead to arrhythmias.
8. Hyperventilation: Hyperventilate for 2 to 3 minutes to induce an episode if absence (petit mal) seizures are suspected or if symptoms are thought to be directly due to hyperventilation.

Laboratory Tests

1. Complete blood cell count and routine chemistries including liver function tests are indicated before initiating anticonvulsant therapy (as baseline). Platelet count should be included if valproic acid is to be used.
2. In an apparently well teenager without underlying medical problems, electrolytes, phosphorus, or magnesium have a very low yield for finding a cause of seizures. Rarely, an adolescent presenting with seizure-like episodes is found to have very low blood calcium concentration because of pseudohypoparathyroidism, although the condition is congenital and the calcium concentration is low from infancy. Blood sugar measurements may be helpful if hypoglycemia is suspected only if the blood sample is drawn while the patient is symptomatic. These tests are not indicated on a routine basis in most teens with seizures.
3. EEG: Routine study should consist of waking EEG, hyperventilation, and photic stimulation. Hyperventilation is particularly useful if absence (petit mal) seizures are suspected. Photic stimulation is particularly helpful if the patient reports that seizures occur when exposed to video games, television, rapid flashing lights, or in the car. Sleep deprived EEG increases the yield in patients with complex partial seizures, benign focal epilepsy of childhood, and some generalized epilepsies.
4. Neuroimaging: Computed tomography scan or magnetic resonance imaging is indicated for focal seizures (except clear-cut benign Rolandic epilepsy of childhood), seizures associated with neurological abnormalities, papilledema, neurocutaneous stigmata, or suspected degenerative conditions.
5. Lumbar puncture is indicated if infection or hemorrhage is suspected.

TABLE 21.3

Grand Mal Seizures versus Syncopal Episodes

Component	Grand Mal	Syncope
Preictal	May have prodrome; aura may occur at time of loss of consciousness	Variable—may experience faint or dizzy feeling
Ictal	Violent body spasms; often cries out; sweaty appearance; may have incontinence after tonic-clonic component; coma after seizure	No stereotype; no abrupt onset; slowly falls to floor; cold and clammy May have mild twitching
Postictal	Gradual return to consciousness; confusion	Rarely; confusion

Grand Mal Seizures Versus Syncopal Episode

Table 21.3 compares grand mal seizures with syncopal episodes.

Hysterical Episodes (Pseudoseizures) Versus Epilepsy

Table 21.4 compares pseudoseizures with epilepsy.

THERAPY

After the diagnosis of epilepsy is made, two major components of therapy exist: Drug therapy to control the seizures and counseling regarding psychosocial issues.

Anticonvulsant Therapy

General Guidelines
1. Start with a single anticonvulsant medication. The choice of an anticonvulsant should consider the side effect profile, because this will influence both safety and compliance. For example, sodium valproate, which may be effective in many seizure types, may be associated with some side effects that limit its use by adolescents, particularly female teens. These include an increase in appetite, weight gain, transient hair loss, and menstrual irregularities.
2. Increase the medication slowly by time increments equal to five times the half-life of the drug until seizures are controlled or toxicity occurs, except when control is urgent (frequent seizures or status epilepticus).
3. Use serum levels only as guidelines: Clinical response is more important. Do not evaluate serum levels frequently. At least five half-lives are necessary for medication level to reach steady state after starting or altering the dose.
4. Give medication each day on the basis of half-life. Give a drug more frequently only with refractory seizures, otherwise unmanageable adverse effects or demonstrated rapid metabolism is encountered. Most medications can be given twice a day (b.i.d.), and adherence is better with b.i.d. than thrice-a-day (t.i.d.) schedules.
5. The teen should have close follow-up, including monitoring of seizure frequency, physical examination, and evaluation for drug toxicity. Note that frequent follow-up also allows for early detection of nonmedical effects (social, academic, independence, and vocational).
6. Substitute a second drug only when the first is pushed to tolerance without controlling the seizure, unless allergic or serious idiosyncratic effects are evident. When the second drug is at adequate serum levels, wean the first. Polytherapy is reserved for refractory patients unresponsive to trials of monotherapy with at least two

TABLE 21.4

Hysterical Seizures versus Epilepsy

Hysterical Seizures	Epileptic Seizures
Observers nearby	Observed or unobserved
Bizarre motor activity, back arching, pelvic thrusting	Usually stereotypic for a particular patient; automatisms of complex partial seizures may vary with activity and environment; generalized convulsions, usually tonic-clonic
No incontinence	May be incontinent of urine and stool
During ictus: Active pupillary reflex, normal corneal reflex	May have dilated unreactive pupils and lose corneal reflex during event
May occur in patients with epilepsy; may have abnormal EEG interictally, but no change during episode	Rhythmic spikes, slowing or electrodecremental EEG during episode, but may be normal
	Twofold or threefold increase above baseline serum prolactin after convulsion or partial complex seizure is nearly invariable

to three different anticonvulsants at maximum tolerated levels.

7. Discontinuation criteria: After some time, the clinician must assess the risks and benefits of continued therapy with anticonvulsants. Medications may be tapered and discontinued after the patient is seizure free for 2 to 4 years. The estimated risk for recurrence on tapering is 30% to 40%, greatest during the period of taper or in the first 6 months after discontinuation of the medication. Risk factors for recurrence are somewhat controversial but include the following in at least some studies:
    a. Mental retardation or neurological abnormalities
    b. Long duration of seizures or many seizures before full control with medication
    c. Partial seizures (other than the benign focal epilepsies of childhood such as Rolandic epilepsy)
    d. Abnormal EEG findings despite seizure-free period (highest risk: combination of focal slowing and focal epileptiform spikes)
    e. Adolescent-onset seizures less likely to remit than seizures with onset in earlier childhood

Medication should be tapered one drug at a time (generally sedating drugs first), tapering each drug over 6 weeks to 3 months.

Drugs for Specific Seizure Types

1. Generalized tonic-clonic seizures (grand mal), either primarily or secondarily generalized:
    a. Phenobarbital: Least expensive, can be given once a day. In developing countries, it is often the only drug available. In the United States, it is less often used as first-line therapy due to concerns about cognitive slowing.
    b. Carbamazepine (Tegretol, Carbatrol): Generics are acceptable if same generic is consistently available; avoid switching brands. Two extended-release carbamazepine preparations allow b.i.d. dosing but are more expensive (Tegretol-XR and Carbatrol).
    c. Phenytoin (Dilantin): Brand-name capsules can be used once a day. Using most generic capsules, liquid or chewable tablets, dose must be divided b.i.d. or t.i.d.
    d. Valproic acid (Depakene or Depakote): Depakote is preferred. An extended-release form (Depakote ER) is available that is appropriate for once-a-day use in selected patients.
    e. Primidone (Mysoline): Reserve for refractory patients.
    f. Lamotrigine (Lamictal): Useful for partial and generalized seizures, including adolescents with JME. Generally reserved for teens intolerant of valproic acid and recommended as first-line monotherapy for idiopathic generalized epilepsy among women of reproductive age (including those who are pregnant or breast-feeding).
    g. Topiramate (Topamax): Effective but often significantly sedating and/or cognitively impairing, at least upon initiation. Tendency to cause mild anorexia and weight loss is viewed by some teens as an advantage over other anticonvulsants, which tend to promote weight gain. When used, dosage should be titrated very slowly to avoid cognitive dulling.
    h. Felbamate (Felbatol): is effective for several seizure types including generalized convulsive (tonic-clonic)

seizures, drop attacks, and atypical absence seizures. It is only approved for children with Lennox-Gastaut syndrome (mixed generalized epilepsy). An initial alarming incidence of aplastic anemia associated with felbamate has limited the use of this medication to refractory patients able to give informed consent to its risks and comply with the requirement for frequent laboratory monitoring. Actual risk is probably very low, except in patients with other autoimmune conditions such as systemic lupus erythematosus (SLE).
    i. Other newer anticonvulsants, occasionally useful for generalized convulsions, particularly those thought to be partial with secondary generalization, include levitiracetam (Keppra), and oxcarbazepine (Trileptal).

Many practitioners favor either carbamazepine or valproic acid for first-line use. Phenytoin is an effective medication but may cause unacceptable side effects (e.g., gum hypertrophy and hirsutism), particularly in children and young adolescents. In patients with mixed generalized seizures (i.e., generalized tonic-clonic plus myoclonic or absence seizures), carbamazepine, phenytoin or oxcarbazepine occasionally may induce or exacerbate myoclonic or drop attacks. Valproic acid, preferably in the long-acting capsules (Depakote), or extended-release capsules (Depakote ER) is the drug of choice in mixed generalized epilepsies (grand mal plus myoclonic or absence).

2. Petit mal epilepsy:
    a. Ethosuximide (Zarontin): Standard therapy usually well tolerated for typical childhood petit mal (3-Hz spike wave EEG pattern).
    b. Valproic acid (Depakote): First choice if absence and generalized tonic-clonic seizures coexist, for atypical absence, or for JME.
    c. Clonazepam, clorazepate, or other benzodiazepines: Occasionally effective as monotherapy, but rapid development of tolerance and sedation are significant problems. May increase salivation and respiratory difficulties in adolescents with multiple disabilities.
    d. Felbamate (Felbatol): This is effective for several seizure types but is approved only for children with Lennox-Gastaut syndrome (mixed generalized epilepsy).

3. Simple partial seizures (focal motor, focal sensory) and complex partial seizures with or without automatisms:
    a. Carbamazepine (Tegretol): See previous discussion regarding generic forms and long-acting preparations.
    b. Phenobarbital: See earlier discussion.
    c. Phenytoin (Dilantin): See earlier discussion regarding generic forms.
    d. Primidone (Mysoline): Reserve for refractory patients.
    e. Gabapentin (Neurontin): Approved for monotherapy and adjunctive treatment of partial onset seizures. This anticonvulsant is not metabolized and does not change metabolism of other medications. Consider use in teens with multisystem disease when avoidance of alteration of drug metabolism of other agents is important (i.e., transplant patients, patients on chemotherapy, etc).
    f. Lamotrigine (Lamictal): See earlier discussion. First-line or adjunctive treatment of partial seizures.

g. Topiramate (Topamax): See earlier discussion. First-line or adjunctive treatment of partial seizures.

h. Tiagabine (Gabitril): Adjunctive treatment of partial seizures.

i. Levetiracetam (Keppra): First-line or adjunctive treatment of partial seizures. Often used as first-line therapy in patients with hepatic dysfunction or during chemotherapy because it is excreted by kidneys and is not dependent on the P-450 system for its metabolism. The major concern is the relatively higher risk of behavior disturbance, particularly in teens who already have a history of agitated or aggressive behavior.

j. Zonisamide (Zonegran): First-line or adjunctive therapy for partial seizures. Risks are similar to those of topiramate (sedation, renal stones, acidosis, anorexia, rash, oligohydrosis). Very long half-life makes it appropriate for once-daily dosing.

k. Oxcarbazepine (Trileptal): An alternative to carbamazepine for patients who had an adverse behavioral reaction to carbamazepine at the therapeutic dose. Patients allergic to carbamazepine may also react to oxcarbazepine. Oxcarbazepine does not have an active metabolite. Pharmacokinetic interactions are less problematic than with carbamazepine, making it appropriate for patients on other medications that are affected by or affect the cytochrome P-450 system such as teens with multisystem disease needing many other medications (e.g., during chemotherapy or patients with acquired immunodeficiency syndrome).

l. Felbamate (Felbatol): See earlier discussion. Reserve for refractory patients.

Table 21.5 provides metabolism guidelines for older-generation antiepileptic drugs and Table 21.6 shows metabolism of newer anticonvulsant drugs.

Side Effects of Anticonvulsant Drugs

Adverse effects of anticonvulsants can be divided into two major groups: Dose-related reactions and idiosyncratic reactions unrelated to drug level. Mild sedation is common with initiation of any anticonvulsant. This effect generally wanes after a few weeks. Sedation and ataxia with initiation of treatment is more significant with carbamazepine, so treatment is generally started at low doses and increased over several weeks. Potential reproductive effects are also important to consider in teenage girls of childbearing potential.

Dose-Related Effects

1. Toxic CNS effects are shared among most anticonvulsants.
   a. Excessive levels (or deliberate overdoses) produce ataxia, nystagmus, and sedation progressing to coma, with respiratory and cardiac depression at extremely high doses.
   b. Movement disorders (chorea) and tremor may be seen at toxic drug levels, primarily with phenytoin or carbamazepine.
2. Non-CNS dose-related effects are common.
   a. Alterations in vitamin D metabolism produce "chemical rickets," generally without clinically symptomatic

abnormalities. Clinical rickets is occasionally seen in adolescents with multiple disabilities receiving anticonvulsants but having limited sun exposure and lacking vitamin D supplementation. Osteopenia is frequently found in studies of patients of all ages taking chronic anticonvulsants. Consider supplementing with oral calcium and vitamin D in teens taking anticonvulsants if dietary intake is low.

b. Some anticonvulsants (phenytoin and carbamazepine) may have deleterious effects on bone density by directly interfering with osteoblast proliferation.

c. Folate metabolism is altered, producing megaloblastic changes, usually without anemia. For most adolescents on anticonvulsants physician should consider routinely supplementing with a multivitamin containing at least 400 µg of folic acid. Adolescent girls taking anticonvulsants, particularly those with a potential for future childbearing, should be supplemented with folic acid 1 to 4 mg daily, depending upon which anticonvulsant they are taking. Those taking valproic acid are of particular concern.

d. Thyroid function tests are commonly altered without clinical evidence of hypothyroidism.

e. Gastrointestinal (GI): Gastric distress is common with valproic acid, ethosuximide, and felbamate. These side effects may be minimized if the dose is divided or given with food.

3. Drug interactions are also common.
   a. Virtually all anticonvulsants induce hepatic microsomal enzymes, increasing clearance of themselves (autoinduction), each other, and various other medications including steroids, estrogens, anticoagulants, and so forth. Exceptions are the second-generation anticonvulsants, gabapentin (Neurontin), and levetiracetam (Keppra), which are excreted unchanged in the urine and do not affect other drug metabolisms.
   b. Conversely, several drugs significantly inhibit the metabolism of carbamazepine and to a lesser extent, of phenytoin. The most commonly encountered problematic interaction is with erythromycin (and the newer macrolides), which competitively inhibits carbamazepine metabolism to an extent that previously stable patients may develop significant toxicity <24 hours after the addition of the antibiotic. A similar effect is seen with propoxyphene (Darvon) and with grapefruit juice. Therefore, these drugs and grapefruit juice should be avoided in a patient taking carbamazepine.
   c. Isoniazid (INH) inhibits both carbamazepine and phenytoin metabolism. Because it is generally used on a long-term basis, the anticonvulsant drug can be adjusted to account for the decreased clearance.

Idiosyncratic (Non–Dose-Related Side Effects)
The following side effects may occur with any anticonvulsant:

1. Allergic reactions: Skin rash, Stevens-Johnson syndrome, lupus-like syndromes, and even death can occur with any anticonvulsant, although most reported cases are associated with phenobarbital, phenytoin, or carbamazepine.

TABLE 21.5

Metabolism, Uses, and Dosing Guidelines for Older Antiepileptic Drugs Used as Monotherapy[a]

Generic Name (Brand Name)	Primary Indications	Secondary Indications	Serum Half-Life (hr)	Time to Steady State	Therapeutic Levels	Toxic Levels	Daily Dosage	Preparations
Phenytoin (Dilantin)	Partial onset seizures	Generalized convulsions (avoid in JME)	24 ± 12	5–10 d	10–20 µg	>20 µg/mL	Pediatric: 3–8 mg/kg/d; Adult: 250–400 mg/d	Dilantin capsules: 100 mg, 30 mg (slow release); Dilantin Infatabs: 50 mg; Liquid: 125 mg/5 mL; Generic capsules: 100 mg, rapid release; 300 mg slow release
Phenobarbital (Luminal)		Partial or generalized convulsive epilepsy[b]	72 ± 16	14–21 d	15–40 µg/mL	>40 µg/mL (much higher may be tolerated if used chronically)	Pediatric: 1–5 mg/kg/d; Adult: 90–200 mg/d	Tablets: 15 mg, 30 mg, 60 mg 100 mg (essentially all generic); Liquid: 20 mg/5 mL
Primidone (Mysoline)		Partial or generalized convulsive epilepsy	12 ± 6 for primidone[c]; 72 ± 16 for phenobarbital metabolite	14–21 d for metabolites	8–12 µg/mL primidone 15–40 g/mL phenobarbital metabolite	>15 µg/mL primidone	Pediatric: 10–15 mg/kg/d; Adult: 500–1,000 mg/d	Tablets: 50 mg, 250 mg; Liquid: 250 mg/5 mL
Carbamazepine (Tegretol, Epitol, Carbatrol, Tegretol XR)	Partial onset seizures	Generalized convulsions (avoid in JME)	12 ± 3 chronic; 36 ± 12 naive[d]	3–5 d	5–13 µg/mL	>15 µg/mL	Pediatric: 20 mg/kg/d (start lower); Adult: 400–1,800 mg/d	Tablets: 100 mg, 200 mg carbamazepine (fast release); Liquid: 100 mg/5 mL; Sprinkle capsules, slow release (Carbatrol) 100 mg, 200 mg, 300 mg; Tablets, slow release, Tegretol XR, 100 mg, 200 mg 400 mg

(continued)

TABLE 21.5

(Continued)

Generic Name (Brand Name)	Primary Indications	Secondary Indications	Serum Half-Life (hr)	Time to Steady State	Therapeutic Levels	Toxic Levels	Daily Dosage	Preparations
Ethosuximide (Zarontin)	Typical absence (petit mal)	none	30 ± 6	7–14 d	40–100 μg/mL	>150 μg/mL	Pediatric: 10–40 mg/kg/d; Adult: 500–1,500 mg/d	Capsules: 250 mg; Liquid: 250 mg/5 mL
Valproic acid (Depakene, Depakote, Depakote ER)	Primary generalized seizures, absence (typical or atypical), myoclonic seizures; first line for JME	Partial onset seizures	12 ± 6[e]	2–5 d	50–120 μg/mL	>120 μg/mL	Pediatric: 15–60 mg/kg/d; Adult: 750–3,000 mg/d	Depakote capsules: 125 mg, 250 mg, 500 mg; Depakote ER 250 mg, 500 mg; Depakote sprinkle capsules: 125 mg (may be opened and mixed with food); Depakene or generic capsules 250 mg; Depakene or generic liquid valproic acid, 250 mg/5 mL
Clonazepam (Klonopin)	Absence, myoclonic seizures		24 ± 12	5–10 d	Not helpful[f]	Not helpful	Pediatric: 0.02–0.05 mg/kg/d; Adult: 1–20 mg/d	Tablets: 0.5 mg, 1 mg, 2 mg

JME, juvenile myoclonic epilepsy.

[a]Monotherapy pharmacokinetics differs for chronic-use vs. antiepileptic drug–naïve patient. Patients switched to monotherapy with phenytoin, barbiturates, or carbamazepine from another enzyme-inducing antiepileptic drug generally need higher doses.

[b]Phenobarbital is not considered a first-line medication for most indications despite wide-spectrum coverage, because of the potential for sedation and depression. However, it is first line in most of the developing world due to very low cost and ability to dose once daily.

[c]Primidone has several active metabolites including phenobarbital and PEMA. While primidone has a relatively short half-life, other metabolites have long half-lifes and a steady state may take 14–21 d to achieve.

[d]Carbamazepine metabolism autoinduces in many patients (much more rapid elimination after first few wk of treatment). Repeated dosage adjustments are often necessary in the first few mo of use.

[e]Depakote is of slow release with variable absorption and later peaks but is metabolized to valproic acid with the same elimination kinetics as Depakene and generics.

[f]Serum levels of benzodiazepines are not helpful in predicting therapeutic response. Alterations in receptors produce marked tolerance. Serum levels are occasionally useful in suspected ingestions or overdose, or to check compliance.

TABLE 21.6

Metabolism, Uses and Doses of Newer Anticonvulsant Medications

Generic Name (Brand Name)	Primary Indications	Secondary Indications	Serum Half-Life	Time to Steady State	Daily Dose	Usual Dosing Schedule	Preparations Available in the United States
Gabapentin (Neurontin)	Partial onset seizures, adjunctive	Partial onset seizures, monotherapy	5–7 hr[a]	2–3 d	Pediatric: 15–60 mg/kg/d Adult: 900–4,800 mg/d	t.i.d.–q.i.d.	100 mg, 300 mg, 400 mg, 600 mg, and 800 mg tabs; 250 mg/5 mL solution
Lamotrigine (Lamictal)	Generalized convulsive epilepsy; JME	Partial onset seizures, absence (typical or atypical) monotherapy or adjunctive	30 hr (markedly prolonged by coadministration of VPA; shortened by use of EIAED[b])	5–6 d	Pediatric: 5–15 mg/kg/d (2–5 mg/kg/d in combination with VPA) Adult monotherapy: 100–400 mg/d; up to 700 mg/d with EIAED	b.i.d.	5 mg, 25 mg chewable tabs; 25 mg, 100 mg, 150 mg, and 200 mg tablets
Topiramate (Topamax)	Generalized convulsive epilepsy; partial onset epilepsy (monotherapy or adjunctive)		21 hr	4 d	Pediatric: 5–20 mg/kg/d Adults: 200–400 mg/d	b.i.d.	25 mg, 100 mg, 200 mg tabs; 15 mg and 25 mg sprinkle capsules may be opened onto a spoon of food
Tiagabine (Gabitril)	Partial onset seizures (adjunctive)	Partial onset seizures (adjunctive)	5–8 hr	2 d	Pediatric: 0.5–1 mg/kg/d Adults: 32–56 mg/d	b.i.d.	2 mg, 4 mg, 12 mg, 16 mg, and 20 mg tabs
Zonisamide (Zonegran)	Generalized or partial onset epilepsy (convulsive or nonconvulsive), adjunctive	Generalized or partial onset epilepsy (convulsive or nonconvulsive), monotherapy	60 hr	10–12 d	Pediatric: 5–12mg/kg/d Adults: 100–400 mg/d	q.d. or b.i.d.	25 mg, 50 mg and 100 mg capsules (brand or generic)

(continued)

TABLE 21.6

(Continued)

Generic Name (Brand Name)	Primary Indications	Secondary Indications	Serum Half-Life	Time to Steady State	Daily Dose	Usual Dosing Schedule	Preparations Available in the United States
Levetiracetam (Keppra)	Partial onset seizures (adjunctive)	Partial or generalized onset seizures, (adjunctive or monotherapy)	6–8 hr	1–2 d	Pediatric: 40–60 mg/kg/d Adults: 500–2,500 mg/d	b.i.d.	250 mg, 500 mg, 750 mg tabs; 500 mg/5 mL solution
Felbamate (Felbatol)		Refractory mixed generalized or multifocal seizures; Lennox Gastaut Syndrome (adjunctive or monotherapy)	20–23 hr	5–7 d	Pediatric: 40–60 mg/kg/d Adults: 2,000–4,000 mg/d	b.i.d.	400 mg and 600 mg tabs; 600 mg/5 mL solution
Oxcarbazepine (Trileptal)	Partial onset seizures (adjunctive or monother-apy)		2 hr for parent compound; 9 hr (for active metabolite MHD[c])	2–3 d	Pediatric: 10–40 mg/kg/d Adults: 300–1,800 mg/d	b.i.d.	150 mg, 300 mg, and 600 mg tabs; 300 mg/5 mL solution

JME, juvenile myoclonic epilepsy.
[a]Prolonged with renal dysfunction.
[b]EIAED, enzyme-inducing antiepileptic drugs, typically carbamazepine, phenytoin, phenobarbital or primidone; VPA, valproic acid
[c]MHD, monohydroxy derivative of oxcarbazepine; 10-hydroxycarbazepine is the primary compound.

2. Bone marrow toxicity, usually reversible, has been reported with several anticonvulsants. Fatal aplastic anemia has been reported with carbamazepine and felbamate, primarily in older adults. High serum levels of valproic acid are associated with reversible bone marrow suppression, most commonly thrombocytopenia.
3. Hepatic toxicity and metabolic abnormalities are seen in patients receiving valproic acid, primarily in infants, but can rarely occur with any anticonvulsant, at any age. These may include hyperammonemia, lactic acidosis, and Reye-like syndrome. Carnitine depletion, usually asymptomatic, may occur with valproic acid, particularly with long-term use in patients with poor muscle bulk.
4. Adenopathy, "mononucleosis syndrome," and pseudolymphoma are primarily associated with hydantoin.
5. Hair loss: Moderate hair thinning is relatively common with valproic acid. Frank alopecia does not occur. Other anticonvulsants may produce hair loss as part of allergic reactions.
6. Weight changes: Weight gain is most frequently problematic with valproic acid but has been reported with many anticonvulsants. Weight loss is common with felbamate, particularly at higher doses, and with valproic acid in young children. Topiramate and zonisamide often produce short-term anorexia and weight loss.
7. Pancreatitis: Valproic acid can rarely cause serious pancreatitis. In a patient taking valproic acid with abdominal pain or vomiting, serum lipase should be assessed.

Reproductive There is a moderately increased risk of abnormal pregnancy outcome in women with epilepsy, regardless of specific drug treatment.

1. Facial malformations, particularly cleft palate, microcephaly, congenital heart disease, and minor malformations such as hypoplastic nails have been related to phenytoin, and possibly other anticonvulsants. Some authors feel that these nonspecific malformations are more frequent in offspring of epileptic mothers, regardless of treatment.
2. Open neural tube defects may be more frequent in fetuses exposed to valproic acid and carbamazepine. It is prudent to supplement all female patients taking these anticonvulsants with a multivitamin containing at least 400 μg of folic acid. Some authors advise that female patients on anticonvulsants anticipating pregnancy take 1 to 4 mg/day of folic acid. Unfortunately, a few case reports suggest that even higher doses of periconceptional folic acid may not be protective against the development of malformations.
3. It is difficult to choose an anticonvulsant that is "completely safe." Risk of fetal damage must be balanced against the risk of recurrent convulsions if medications are withdrawn.
4. There is no reason to withhold oral contraceptives from a woman receiving anticonvulsants, but higher estrogen doses may be needed because of more rapid metabolism of the component hormones, because of induction of cytochrome P-450 system.

Other Problems with Anticonvulsant Therapy

1. Because teens in whom epilepsy is well controlled often have no symptoms except for the drug side effects, it is tempting for them to take their medications only intermittently. These and other adherence problems are common (see the suggestions for improving adherence in the "Community Resources" section).
2. Medications may increase preexisting behavioral problems and occasionally cause depression.
3. Some drugs can increase seizure frequency as their dose is increased.

Alternative Treatments of Refractory Epilepsy

Vagal Nerve Stimulation Vagal nerve stimulation (VNS) is a therapeutic option used as an adjunctive treatment for adolescents and adults with medically refractory epilepsy. The VNS device consists of a programmable battery-operated generator and a silastic-coated lead, which are implanted subcutaneously in the chest, with the lead attached to the left vagal nerve. Multicenter trials evaluating the efficacy of the vagal nerve stimulator demonstrated a 50% or more reduction in approximately one third of patients with refractory partial seizures. New uncontrolled data suggests that VNS may be as effective for idiopathic and symptomatic generalized epilepsies. The common side effects include hoarseness of voice, local pain, paresthesias, dyspnea, and dysphagia. Uncommon complications include vocal cord paralysis and lower facial muscle weakness.

The Ketogenic Diet The ketogenic diet is a tightly controlled, high-fat, low-carbohydrate diet used in the treatment of intractable epilepsy. The diet is designed to place the body in a state simulating starvation, which results in the production of high levels of ketone bodies. Undertaking this diet requires a strong commitment from both the patient and care givers and the expertise of a dietician and clinician familiar with the program. Expense may be substantial, including dietitian visits and special foods, which are not generally covered by health insurance.

Epilepsy Surgery Cortical resection or hemispherectomy may result in cessation or dramatic reduction of seizures for selected adolescents with intractable localization-related epilepsy. Key elements of surgical candidacy include intractability, disabling epilepsy; a localized epileptic zone; and a low risk for new postoperative neurological deficits. Surgical options include temporal lobectomy, extratemporal and multilobar resections, functional hemispherectomy, and corpus callosotomy. Teens with uncontrolled or complicated epilepsy warrant referral to specialized centers with extensive pediatric epilepsy surgery experience that can offer comprehensive risk-benefit evaluation for each child. There is some evidence that early temporal lobectomy in teens with intractable complex partial seizures and mesial temporal sclerosis may improve long-term quality of life and overall outcome.

Other Important Treatment Issues

The care of the epileptic teen extends beyond drug therapy. Total care involves dispelling myths and educating, providing for community resources, and providing counseling for the teen's voiced or unvoiced concerns.

Dispelling Myths and Educating

Many myths about epilepsy can be eliminated by reassuring the teenager on the following:

1. Epilepsy is not contagious.
2. The seizures may disappear with age.
3. Most seizures can be prevented with medication.
4. Epilepsy does not lower the teenager's intelligence.
5. He or she can participate in almost all activities.
6. Epilepsy is not a "mental illness."

The parent should also be given these reassurances, in addition to the following:

1. There is no need to feel guilty. It is unlikely that anything the parent did (or did not do) caused the epilepsy.
2. There is no need for special schooling solely because of epilepsy.
3. Neither epilepsy nor anticonvulsants *cause* learning disabilities or cognitive loss, although the prevalence of learning disabilities is higher in children and adolescents with epilepsy as a group.

The teen and family should be educated about the following:

1. Diagnosis.
2. Importance of careful observation and record keeping.
3. Avoidance of precipitating factors, if any.
4. Side effects of medication.
5. Prognosis and follow-up.
6. Precautions and restrictions, particularly regarding driving, swimming, and bicycle and motorcycle riding, until seizure control is ensured: State requirements regarding reports to the Department of Motor Vehicles should be explained. Restrictions may need to be imposed regarding use of hazardous equipment such as power tools.
7. For women and adolescent girls of childbearing age, the need for adequate birth control while receiving most anticonvulsant drugs (see Chapter 42 for recommendations regarding interactions of anticonvulsants and contraceptives). Supplementation with folic acid should be discussed with all women epilepsy patients with childbearing potential.

Family members should be aware of first aid for seizure episodes:

1. Generalized convulsion (tonic, tonic-clonic, and clonic)
   a. Help the person into a lying position if there is adequate warning.
   b. Do not try to restrain the person.
   c. Clear the area of dangerous objects.
   d. Remove glasses and loosen tight clothing.
   e. Turn the head to one side (or roll the person onto his or her side) to allow saliva to drain out.
   f. Do not put anything into the person's mouth.
   g. Report what you observe. Try to time the episode with a watch.
   h. Family members should be given specific criteria to call for paramedic help: If the seizure lasts longer than 5 to 10 minutes, or if seizures cluster without recovery, call for emergency medical help. Specific advice should be individualized, on the basis of the patient's seizure history.
   i. In teens with epilepsy, who have clusters of seizures or prolonged breakthrough seizures that require emergency care, family members can be taught to use a rectal dose of diazepam. In the United States, a rectal gel form of diazepam is available in premeasured syringes as Diastat. The dose for teens is 0.2 mg/kg, rounded up to the next available size, with a maximum of 20 mg/dose. Intranasal or buccal midazolam has also been used to abort prolonged seizures or interrupt seizure clusters, but is "off-label" usage.
2. Partial seizures (simple and complex)
   a. Do not restrain the person.
   b. Remove harmful objects from the area.
3. Petit mal
   a. No first aid is necessary.
   b. Protect from harm if in dangerous situation until the episode passes.

Community Resources Teenagers and parents should be provided with references and should be informed of community resources about epilepsy. Many local epilepsy societies sponsor job search training; some have vocational training and placement programs. Some sponsor teen groups for peer support, camps, and family programs. Local chapters of the Epilepsy Foundation have videotapes, pamphlets, and other educational materials for patients and families.

> Epilepsy Foundation
> 8301 Professional Place
> Landover, MD 20785; http://www.epilepsyfoundation.org
>> Local chapters can be located through the national offices, through an online search, or in telephone directories under "Social Service Organizations."

Miscellaneous Concerns

1. Sports and activity: No need for restriction of activities once seizures are controlled, except for swimming alone, scuba diving, mountain climbing, or bicycling in areas with traffic. Contact sports are generally restricted until seizures are controlled.
2. Medical identification: The teen with epilepsy should wear a medical identification bracelet or necklace. This may avoid unnecessary trips to emergency facilities or unneeded testing if a seizure occurs away from home.
3. Driving: Health care professionals should be aware of their state's driving laws regarding epilepsy. These should be explained to the teen, with the reasons for the laws. The wish to be seizure free to receive a license may enhance compliance. Laws regarding mandatory reporting to the state's Department of Motor Vehicles vary among the states.
4. School: The adolescent's school should be informed if seizures are a recurring problem. If the teenager has been seizure free for an extended time, there is often no need to inform the teachers of diagnosis, because this may cause unnecessary restrictions and lowered expectations.
5. Alcohol: Although abstinence is not always necessary, more than a couple of drinks of alcohol a day may increase the risk of seizures in teens with epilepsy secondary to a lowering of the seizure threshold.
6. Anticipate other concerns: Seizures, because of their unpredictable and abrupt onset, threat of injury, and embarrassment, can have profound effects on the developing adolescent. Try to anticipate and be sensitive to these concerns. Young teens may be concerned

about whether their body is normal. Middle teens will have concerns about their peers, driving, and sports restrictions. Older adolescents will be more concerned regarding vocational planning and perhaps future health insurance. Depression can occur in adolescents with epilepsy and these teens should be assessed for their degree of depression and their suicidality (Baker, 2006).

7. Adherence: As stated earlier, adherence can be a significant problem in dealing with an epileptic teenager. Suggestions for improving adherence include the following:
   a. Provide clear explanations of medications used and their expected side effects.
   b. Give the adolescent the responsibility for taking medications.
   c. Discuss possible consequences of noncompliance with the teen, such as recurrent seizures and inability to get or keep a driver's license.
   d. Referral to a teen group sponsored by a local chapter of the Epilepsy Foundation may be helpful.
   e. "Day-of-the-week" pillboxes, filled and checked weekly, with parental supervision, may enable a young teen to manage his or her own medications.
   f. Attempt to simplify dosing schedules. Use b.i.d. or once-daily dosing if possible.
   g. Use medications with acceptable side effects for the involved teen.

SPECIAL CONSIDERATIONS IN EPILEPSY IN FEMALE PATIENTS

Hormonal Influences on Seizures

Some women with epilepsy experience changes in seizure activity that relate to changes in pubertal status, menstrual cycle, or pregnancy. In general, estrogen increases excitation and reduces inhibition, whereas progesterone has the opposite effect.

Effect of Puberty on Epilepsy

Seizures can have their onset or change in frequency during puberty. Both JME and photosensitive seizures often present during puberty. Childhood absence epilepsy and benign Rolandic epilepsy often remit during puberty.

Effect of Menses on Seizures

As expected, with the rise of estrogen at ovulation and with the fall in progesterone during menses, seizures are more common during these times. Foldvary-Schaefer and Falcone (2003) provide a comprehensive review of catamenial epilepsy.

Reproductive Dysfunctions

Fertility in women with epilepsy is approximately one third that of nonepileptic siblings (Morrell, 1999). This may reflect either a fear of consequences of pregnancy, social pressure not to become a parent, or physiological disruptions to reproductive cycles. Anovulation is more common in women with epilepsy. Women with epilepsy appear to have a higher frequency of reproductive endocrine abnormalities including alterations of daily basal and pulsatile release of luteinizing hormone. Women with epilepsy

may also have hormonal abnormalities, which appear to be reversible with cessation of anticonvulsant medication. Valproic acid in particular is associated with a syndrome similar to polycystic ovary syndrome as well as isolated rise in circulating androgens.

Pregnancy

As discussed earlier, there is an increased risk of abnormal pregnancy outcomes in women with epilepsy regardless of the specific drug treatment.

Contraception

The major issues with the use of contraception in adolescents with epilepsy are the interactions between certain anticonvulsants and their effect on the metabolism of hormonal contraceptives. The most significant problems are with those hormonal contraceptives with low doses of hormones used in combination with anticonvulsants that induce the cytochrome P-450 system (e.g. phenobarbital, primidone, phenytoin, carbamazepine, felbamate, topiramate, and vigabatrin). See Chapter 42 for a full discussion on these interactions and Table 42.4 for World Health Organization guidelines on the appropriateness of each contraceptive device in women on certain anticonvulsants.

WEB SITES

For Teenagers and Parents

http://www.epilepsyfoundation.org. Lots of information from the Epilepsy Foundation including driving laws, e-communities, educational information, and most frequently asked questions. Special sections on living with epilepsy and concerns of adolescents can be accessed via the home page. Detailed information about medications are available.

http://www.epilepsy.org.uk/. Information from the British Epilepsy Association.

http://www.epilepsy.ca/eng/mainSet.html. Much information on epilepsy and links elsewhere from Epilepsy, Canadian site.

http://www.nlm.nih.gov/medlineplus/epilepsy.html. National Institutes of Health search and links on epilepsy, with information forms in Spanish.

http://www.cdc.gov/Epilepsy/index.htm. Information from the Centers for Disease Control and Prevention on epilepsy, including an excellent "Toolkit" entitled "You are not alone" for parents of teens with epilepsy.

For Health Professionals

http://www.aesnet.org/. The American Epilepsy Society's official web site.

REFERENCES AND ADDITIONAL READINGS

Am Fam Physician. Restless legs syndrome: detection and management in primary care. National Heart, Lung, and Blood

Institute Working Group on Restless Legs Syndrome. 2000; 62:108.

Appleton RE, Neville BG. Teenagers with epilepsy. *Arch Dis Child* 1999;81:76.

Baker GA. Depression and suicide in adolescents with epilepsy. *Neurology* 2006;66(6 Suppl 3):S5.

Browne TR. Pharmacokinetics of antiepileptic drugs. *Neurology* 1998;51(Suppl 4):S2.

Buck D, Jacoby A, Baker GA. Factors influencing compliance with antiepileptic drug regimes. *Seizure* 1997;6:87.

Camfield PR, Camfield CS. The prognosis of childhood epilepsy. *Semin Pediatr Neurol* 1994;1:102.

Camfield C, Camfield P. Management guidelines for children with idiopathic generalized epilepsy. *Epilepsia* 2005;46 (Suppl 9):112.

Camfield CS, Camfield PR, Gordon KE, et al. Predicting the outcome of childhood epilepsy: a population-based study yielding a simple scoring system. *J Pediatr* 1993;122: 861.

Carranco E, Kareus J, Co S, et al. Carbamazepine toxicity induced by concurrent erythromycin therapy. *Arch Neurol* 1985;42:187.

Centers for Disease Control and Prevention. Prevalence of self-reported epilepsy—United States, 1986–1990. *JAMA* 1994; 272:1893.

Chadwick D. Do anticonvulsants alter the natural course of epilepsy? *Br Med J* 1995;310:177.

Chigier E. Compliance in adolescents with epilepsy or diabetes. *J Adolesc Health* 1992;13:375.

Cross JH. Update on surgery for epilepsy. *Arch Dis Child* 1999; 81:356.

Dumer M, Greenberg DA, Delgado-Escueta AV. Is there a genetic relationship between epilepsy and birth defects? *Neurology* 1992;42:63.

Engel J Jr. The timing of surgical intervention for mesial temporal lobe epilepsy: a plan for a randomized clinical trial. *Arch Neurol* 1999;56:1338.

Farhat G, Yamout B, Mikati MA, et al. Effect of antiepileptic drugs on bone density in ambulatory patients. *Neurology* 2002;58:1348.

Foldvary-Schaefer N, Falcone T. Catamenial epilepsy: pathophysiology, diagnosis, and management. *Neurology* 2003;61 (Suppl 2):S2.

French J. The long-term therapeutic management of epilepsy. *Ann Intern Med* 1994;120:411.

French JA, Kanner AM, Bautista J, et al. Efficacy and tolerability of the new antiepileptic drugs I: treatment of new onset epilepsy. *Neurology* 2004;62:1252.

French JA, Kanner AM, Bautista J, et al. Efficacy and tolerability of the new antiepileptic drugs II: treatment of refractory epilepsy. *Neurology* 2004;62:1261.

Glauser TA. Behavioral and psychiatric adverse events associated with antiepileptic drugs commonly used in pediatric patients. *J Child Neurol* 2004;19(Suppl 1):S25.

Glauser TA, Pellock JM. Zonisamide in pediatric epilepsy: review of the Japanese experience. *J Child Neurol* 2002; 17:87.

Glauser TA, Pellock JM, Bebin EM, et al. Efficacy and safety of levetiracetam in children with partial seizures: an open-label trial. *Epilepsia* 2002;43:518.

Graf WD, Chatrian GE, Glass ST, et al. Video game-related seizures: a report on 10 patients and a review of the literature. *Pediatrics* 1994;93:551.

Greenwood RS, Tennison MB. When to start and stop anticonvulsant therapy in children. *Arch Neurol* 1999;56: 1073.

Guberman A. Hormonal contraception and epilepsy. *Neurology* 1999;53(Suppl 1):S38.

Hiilesmaa VK. Pregnancy and birth in women with epilepsy. *Neurology* 1992;42:8.

Isojarvi JI. Reproductive dysfunction in women with epilepsy. *Neurology* 2003;61(Suppl 2):S27.

Isojarvi JI, Laatikainen TJ, Knip M, et al. Obesity and endocrine disorders in women taking valproate for epilepsy. *Ann Neurol* 1996;39:579.

Kaplan PW. Reproductive health effects and teratogenicity of antiepileptic drugs. *Neurology* 2004:63(10 Suppl 4):S13.

Loring D, Meador K. Cognitive side effects of antiepileptic drugs in children. *Neurology* 2004;62:872.

MacLeod JS, Austin JK. Stigma in the lives of adolescents with epilepsy: a review of the literature. *Epilepsy Behav* 2003; 4(2):112.

Mattson RH, Cramer JA, Colline JF, et al. Comparison of carbamazepine, phenobarbital, phenytoin, and primidone in partial and secondary generalized tonic-clonic seizures. *N Engl J Med* 1985;313:145.

Mattson RH, Rebar RW. Contraceptive methods for women with neurologic disorders. *Am J Obstet Gynecol* 1993;168: 2027.

Mikkonen K, Vainionpaa LK, Pakarinen AJ, et al. Long-term reproductive endocrine health in young women with epilepsy during puberty. *Neurology* 2004;62:445.

Mitchell WG, Scheier LM, Baker SA. Adherence to treatment in children with epilepsy: who follows "doctor's orders"? *Epilepsia* 2000;41:1616.

Morrell MJ. Guidelines for the care of women with epilepsy [Review]. *Neurology* 1998;51(Suppl 4):S21.

Morrell MJ. Epilepsy in women: the science of why it is special. *Neurology* 1999;53(Suppl 1):S42.

Moshe SL. Mechanisms of action of anticonvulsant agents. *Neurology* 2000;55(Suppl 1):S32.

Nadkarni S, LaJoie J, Devinsky O. Current treatments of epilepsy. *Neurology* 2005;64(Suppl 3):S2.

Nash JL. Pseudoseizures: etiologic and psychotherapeutic considerations. *South Med J* 1993;86:1248.

Neurology. Consensus statements: medical management of epilepsy. 1999;51(Suppl 4):S39.

Nordli DR, DeVivo DC. The ketogenic diet revisited: back to the future. *Epilepsia* 1997;38:743.

Pellock JM, Dodson WE, Blaise FD. *Pediatric epilepsy: diagnosis and therapy.* New York: Demos Publications, 2001.

Sander JW. The use of antiepileptic drugs–principles and practice. *Epilepsia* 2004;45(Suppl 6):28.

Sheth RD, Stafstrom CE. Intractable pediatric epilepsy: vagal nerve stimulation and the ketogenic diet. *Neurol Clin North Am* 2002;20:1183.

Tennison M, Greenwood R, Lewis D, et al. Discontinuing antiepileptic drugs in children with epilepsy. *N Engl J Med* 1994;330:1407.

Vazquez B. Monotherapy in epilepsy: role of the newer antiepileptic drugs. *Arch Neurol* 2004;61:1361.

Wheless JW, Kim HL. Adolescent seizures and epilepsy syndromes. *Epilepsia* 2002;43(Suppl 3):33.

Wyllie E, Comair YG, Kotagal P, et al. Seizure outcome after epilepsy surgery in children and adolescents. *Ann Neurol* 1998;44:740.

Yerby MS. Quality of life, epilepsy advances, and the evolving role of anticonvulsants in women with epilepsy. *Neurology* 2000;55:S21;S54.

Yerby MS. Management issues for women with epilepsy: Neural tube defects and folic acid supplementation. *Neurology* 2003;61(Suppl 2):S23.

Zahn CA, Morrell MJ, Collins SD, et al. Management issues for women with epilepsy: a review of the literature. *Neurology* 1998;51:949.

Zifkin B, Andermann E, Andermann F. Mechanisms, genetics, and pathogenesis of juvenile myoclonic epilepsy. *Curr Opin Neurol* 2005;18:147.

CHAPTER 22

Headaches

Wendy G. Mitchell, Kiarash Sadrieh, and Lawrence S. Neinstein

Recurrent headaches are a frequent problem in adolescents and adults, accounting for numerous physician visits and lost days at work and school. By the age of 15 years, at least 75% of people have experienced at least one headache episode. Most recurrent headaches are not associated with severe organic pathology. In contrast, the single severe acute headache, particularly in a patient without prior headache history, may be due to significant central nervous system (CNS) or systemic disease.

PAIN-SENSITIVE AREAS: WHAT HURTS IN THE HEAD

In general, the brain parenchyma and dura are insensitive to pain. Pain-sensitive areas include the following:

1. Intracranial
   a. Cranial nerves (CN) V, IX, and X (most intracranial structures are innervated by CN V)
   b. Dural arteries
   c. Major venous sinuses
   d. Dura at the base of skull
   e. Intracavernous and proximal intracranial portions of the carotid arteries
2. Extracranial
   a. Skin, fascia, muscles, and blood vessels of the scalp
   b. Upper cervical nerve roots
   c. Muscles of the neck
   d. Sinuses and teeth
   e. Eyes and eye muscles
   f. Ears

MECHANISMS OF PAIN

Vascular Dilation

Distension of pain-sensitive cranial arteries causes headaches. The pain is mediated through the trigeminovascular system, which when depolarized, releases neuropeptides that mediate vasodilation and neurogenic inflammation. This mechanism is involved in migraine headaches and in several headaches associated with fever, systemic infection, metabolic disturbances, and vasodilator drugs. Migraine headaches may be associated with vasoactive agents, including serotonin, bradykinin, norepinephrine, prostaglandins, substance P, neurokinin A, calcitonin gene-related peptide, and histamine. The role of these vasoactive substances may be casual or reactive. There is increasing evidence that migraine is neurally initiated, rather than a direct response of the vascular system, with vascular changes being a secondary phenomena. The "aura" of migraine headaches and the neurological manifestations of complicated migraines may be due to vasoconstriction of intracranial arteries, leading to ischemia in affected areas of the brain.

Muscular Contraction

Increased muscular contraction of the head and neck muscles can lead to a headache. This mechanism of headaches is involved in tension and psychogenic headaches but may be a secondary source of pain in migraines. Patients with a migraine commonly have muscle contraction and tenderness as a result of the headache, rather than as a primary event.

Traction

Traction of pain-sensitive structures intracranially may cause a headache. Examples include mass lesions such as a brain tumor, brain abscess, subdural hematoma, and increased intracranial pressure. Brain tumors rarely cause pain directly unless pain-sensitive CNs are involved, intracranial pressure is increased, or there is traction on the meninges.

Inflammation of Pain-Sensitive Areas

Examples of inflammation of pain-sensitive areas include meningitis (either aseptic or bacterial), sinusitis, dental disease, orbital inflammation, and vasculitic syndromes involving intracranial or extracranial vessels.

EPIDEMIOLOGY

1. Prevalence
   a. Approximately 40% of children have headaches by age 7 years, 66% by age 12, and 75% of adolescents by

age 15 years. Most of these headaches are infrequent and nondisabling.

b. Migraine headaches: Twenty-five percent of migraineurs first develop symptoms during childhood. There is approximately a 4% to 11% prevalence rate among individuals aged 7 years to 11 years and a 8% to 23% prevalence rate among individuals aged 11 years to 15 years and above. However, migraine is commonly underdiagnosed if mild or infrequent, so the prevalence rate may be higher.

2. Sex: Headaches occur in almost equal prevalence among males and females until puberty. At that time, headaches become more common in females.

3. Types: Acute headaches are usually associated with a systemic disease such as a viral illness or sinusitis. Most recurrent headaches in adolescents and adults are either vascular headaches (migraines), muscular contraction headaches, or a combination of both. Other causes, such as a brain tumor, are uncommon. Cluster headaches usually start during late adolescence or later but can start as early as 8 years and are far more common in males. Depressive headaches may present in the preadolescent or adolescent years, at times with denial of other depressive symptoms.

DIFFERENTIAL DIAGNOSIS AND CHARACTERISTICS

See Table 22.1 for characteristics of headaches.

Acute, Nonrecurrent (First or Worst) Headaches

Although this may be the first attack of episodic, recurrent headaches, it is important to rule out the following serious potentially life-threatening etiologies:

1. In the Febrile patient
   a. Meningitis: Bacterial, viral, tuberculosis (TB), and other aseptic causes
   b. Brain abscess, epidural empyema, or other intracranial infection
   c. Encephalitis
   d. Sinusitis
   e. Nonspecific headache due to fever
   f. Associated with other infections: Headache is a common symptom in strep throat, influenza, mononucleosis, and rubeola. Patients with human immunodeficiency virus (HIV) or acquired immunodeficiency syndrome (AIDS) frequently complain of headaches.

2. In the Afebrile patient
   a. Subarachnoid hemorrhage (arteriovenous malformation [AVM], aneurysm with acute bleeding)
   b. Intraparenchymal hemorrhage (AVM, venous angioma, or trauma)
   c. Other (cysticercosis or acute obstructive hydrocephalus)
   d. Headache after a seizure (postictal)
   e. Cerebral ischemia, particularly if other neurological findings or predisposing factors (e.g., sickle cell disease) are present
   f. Severe hypertension
   g. Acute dental disease
   h. Eye or orbit: Acute glaucoma or inflammatory disease of orbit

Recurrent Headaches (Episodic, Complete Recovery between Episodes)

1. Muscle tension headaches: There is currently debate in the neurological literature that primary muscle tension headaches exist, other than in situations of direct neck trauma. Many headache experts consider "tension headaches" to be mostly misdiagnosed vascular headaches. Characteristics are as follows:
   a. Bandlike, bilateral, steady pain, occipital more than temporal
   b. *Lacking the following*: Throbbing, nausea, vomiting, photophobia, and associated neurological symptoms
   c. Often gradual in onset and related to stress or fatigue
   d. May be caused by minor trauma to neck muscles, whiplash, and muscle strain

TABLE 22.1

Headache Presentations

Type of Headache	Onset	Location	Pain Quality
Common migraine	Gradual	Unilateral or bilateral	Throbbing, pulsating
Classic migraine	Gradual	Unilateral	Throbbing, pulsating
Muscle contraction	Variable, usually afternoon	Occipital, bilateral, frontal, bandlike	Steady pressure, dull
Cluster	2 a.m. to 3 a.m., abrupt	Unilateral, orbital, or temporal	Burning, boring, excruciating
Mass lesions	Gradual or sudden, but usually recent	Focal or general	Varied, often dull ache
Pseudotumor (benign increased intracranial pressure)	Variable	Vertex or diffuse	Dull
Depressive	Prolonged, constant	Generalized	Dull, unvarying

e. May be caused by temporomandibular (TMJ) joint dysfunction

2. Migraine: Also known as *vascular headache*
   a. Migraine with aura or "classic migraine": 10% to 15% Characteristics are as follows:
      - "Aura" of sensory disturbances: Visual changes, numbness, tingling, dizziness, vertigo, and syncope are common.
      - Throbbing, unilateral, and usually frontal or temporal pain occurs.
      - Anorexia, nausea, and vomiting are frequent accompanying symptoms.
      - Phonophobia and photophobia are common.
      - Sleep often relieves migraine symptoms.
      - Family history is often positive for migraines. Although a parent may not describe his or her headaches as migraines, more careful history of family members' headache patterns often reveals vascular headaches.
      - A childhood history of motion sickness or cyclic vomiting is common.
      - Pattern of headaches varies over time. Exacerbations or onset may be precipitated by puberty, college, or other life stresses.
      - In some subjects, episodes may be precipitated by certain foods, including chocolate, tyramine-containing cheeses, red wines, and foods containing monosodium glutamate (MSG), nitrates, or nitrites.
      - History of relief with triptans or ergot compounds is supportive of diagnosis.
   b. Migraine without aura or "common migraine": 80% to 90%
      - Characteristics are as previous migraine, but lacking aura
      - May be bilateral and variable in pain distribution
   c. Variant migraine: 5% to 10%
      - Hemiplegic migraine: Often familial and presents with hemiplegia, aphasia, or speech disturbances, followed by headache and associated symptoms as stated earlier. Headache is generally contralateral to hemiplegia. Headache may be less symptomatic than hemiplegia. Some are related to specific channelopathies. For example, genetic abnormalities in the *CACNL1A4* gene (a calcium channelopathy) may present as familial hemiplegic migraine.
      - Confusional migraine: More common in younger children but may continue into the teen years. A period of confusion and disorientation is usually followed by vomiting, deep sleep, and waking up feeling well. Headache may not be reported by the children and is generally not prominent.
      - Abdominal migraine: Episodic abdominal pain with nausea or vomiting, followed by or accompanied by a headache. However, the headache may be minimal or absent, and vomiting is the most prominent symptom. Aura may precede pain. Relief of episodes by sleep or antimigraine therapies supports diagnosis.
      - Basilar migraine: Dizziness, vertigo, syncope, and dysarthria are common, and precede variable headache and vomiting. Headache may be minimal or even absent. Common in adolescent girls.
      - Ophthalmoplegic migraine: Abnormal eye movements, sometimes with near-complete ophthalmoplegia and diplopia, are followed by more typical migraine symptoms.

3. Cluster headaches: Found in <5% of children and adolescents
   a. Male predominance.
   b. Steady burning or pain; usually localized behind one eye; sudden onset; extremely severe but brief.
   c. Rhinorrhea, lacrimation, and conjunctival injection on the same side is common.
   d. Horner syndrome ipsilaterally during attack is common.
   e. During clusters, multiple daily episodes occur, often in early morning hours, awakening patient from sleep.
   f. Differential diagnosis includes occult dental disease, acute glaucoma, and tic douloureux.
      It must be noted that several rare metabolic disorders may mimic a migraine, including mitochondrial diseases such as MELAS (mitochondrial myopathy, encephalopathy lactacidosis, and strokelike episodes syndrome); and several organic acidurias. If metabolic disease is suspected, blood for lactate, pyruvate, and ammonia and urine for organic acids should be collected for tests during the episodes. CADASIL, a familial disorder with slowly progressive vasculopathy and leukoencephalopathy, may present during adolescence with migraine headaches, usually hemiplegic.

Chronic Headaches (Variable but Essentially Continuous or Increasing Since Onset)

1. Intracranial mass lesions
   a. Although many patients with brain tumors have headaches, very few patients with headaches have brain tumors.
   b. Headaches due to brain tumors are usually accompanied by other neurological symptoms such as vomiting, diplopia, gait abnormalities, weakness, neuroendocrine abnormalities, or personality and behavioral changes.
   c. Headaches may be increasing in severity and frequency, and may occur nocturnally.
   d. Findings from neurological examination and funduscopic examination are often abnormal.
2. Hydrocephalus (with or without mass)
   a. May be relatively constant, often worse in the morning.
   b. Aqueductal stenosis may present in adolescents, even if congenital.
   c. Head may be large, but this is not universal.
   d. Pain is usually dull, vertex, and not very severe.
   e. Pain may be increased by straining, bowel movements, coughing, or bending.
3. Postlumbar puncture headaches or spontaneous "low pressure" headaches due to cerebrospinal fluid (CSF) leak
   a. Headache is positional, often abruptly relieved by recumbency.
   b. Headache, nausea, and vomiting may be severe if the patient is upright.
   c. Primary treatment is 1 to 2 days of recumbency.
   d. If severe and not relieved in several days, epidural blood patch provides relief in approximately 90% of cases caused by lumbar puncture, but may cause some lower back discomfort.
   e. Salt and fluid loading and abdominal binders are of limited efficacy.

f. Occasionally, spontaneous or posttraumatic occult CSF leaks may present identically, particularly in patients with Marfan syndrome. Opening pressure on a spinal tap is extremely low.

4. Pseudotumor cerebri (also called benign intracranial hypertension): Increased intracranial pressure without mass effect
   a. Papilledema is common. Visual fields may be abnormal, including enlarged blind spot or constricted peripheral fields.
   b. Visual obscuration (transient dimming or loss of vision with straining or position change) may be present. CN palsies, more frequently of CN VI and VII, may be associated.
   c. Pain is usually dull and vertex.
   d. Pseudotumor cerebri is more common in females and obese patients.
   e. May be caused by excessive vitamin A or vitamin D intake, rapid steroid taper, certain immunosuppressants such as cyclosporin, or tetracycline or minocycline intake (for acne or other indications), or isotretinoin (Accutane).
   f. There is a risk of permanent visual loss if untreated. A patient with headache and papilledema should be treated as an emergency to prevent potential visual loss.
   g. Treatment: Lumbar puncture (postimaging) may be both diagnostic and therapeutic. A careful measurement of opening pressure with the patient in a relaxed position is necessary for diagnosis. Reduction of CSF pressure to 200 mm water or 50% of opening pressure is helpful. Serial lumbar punctations may be needed. Acetazolamide may be useful in some patients provided they tolerate adequate doses of the medication. Corticosteroids are often effective but very difficult to wean without recurrent symptoms. Rarely, a lumboperitoneal shunt needs to be placed. Optic nerve sheath fenestration may be necessary to relieve pressure on the optic nerve.

5. "Transformed migraine": Migraine attacks may go from episodic to chronic, essentially continuous, pain.
   a. Excessive use (usually approximately >14 tablets/week) of symptomatic medication (analgesics, triptans, or ergots) may contribute to transformation to chronic daily headache.
   b. Other migrainous symptoms are usually present but may only be present in retrospect.

6. Depressive headaches
   a. "All day, all the time, every day, no relief."
   b. Other overt depressive symptoms may be absent.
   c. Excessive disability (school absenteeism and social isolation) is common.
   d. Family history is often positive for affective disorders.
   e. Often responsive to antidepressant medications and supportive psychotherapy.

7. Posttraumatic (head trauma)
   a. Headaches usually have mixed migrainous and "tension" quality.
   b. Onset within a few days of head trauma, continuing for weeks to months, but diminishing gradually over time.
   c. Minor head trauma may precipitate episodic migraines.

8. Local extracranial disease.
   a. Chronic sinusitis
   b. Dental disease, including TMJ joint dysfunction
   c. Glaucoma
   d. Other orbital inflammatory lesions
   e. Vasculitis involving extracranial vessels (rare in adolescents)

9. HIV or AIDS
   a. Chronic or recurrent headaches are common.
   b. May be due to HIV, other coexisting infections (intracranial, sinus, or ear), or treatment, including antiretroviral agents.

10. Pregnancy
    a. Early pregnancy may be associated with headache, nausea, and vomiting.
    b. Pregnancy may exacerbate migraines.

11. Chronic meningitis or other inflammatory conditions
    a. CNS sarcoidosis may present with meningeal or parenchymal involvement.
    b. TB, fungal, or recurrent or chronic "aseptic" meningitis may present with sustained or recurrent headaches.

12. Headaches due to substance or drug abuse
    a. Both drug use and drug withdrawal may cause headaches.
    b. Small amounts of alcohol cause intense flushing and headaches in genetically prone individuals, usually of Asian origin.
    c. Alcohol withdrawal causes headaches. Be particularly alert for recurrent morning headaches due to daily alcohol consumption.
    d. Cocaine increases blood pressure and may cause headaches.
    e. Excessive (or even therapeutic) doses of over-the-counter (OTC) stimulants such as ephedrine, pseudoephedrine, caffeine, or "kava" may cause headaches.
    f. Inhalants may cause prominent headache symptoms.
    g. Amphetamines and withdrawal from amphetamines cause headache, as do other stimulants such as "ecstasy".

13. Headaches due to obstructive sleep apnea
    a. Headaches are often worst upon awakening.
    b. History of snoring is common.
    c. History of pauses or gasps during sleep is generally elicited only after asking the parent to observe breathing pattern during sleep.
    d. Large tonsils and adenoids and "mouth breathing" are often apparent on physical examination.

14. Headaches due to other medical conditions: Headaches may be intermittent or continuous. Hypoxia, hypercarbia, significant hypertension, severe anemia, uremia, and dialysis all cause intermittent or continuous headaches in some patients. In addition, multiple medications used for other medical conditions, particularly chemotherapy, antiretroviral therapy, and agents used in organ transplant recipients cause headache. This is particularly important in treating adolescents with other chronic conditions such as cystic fibrosis, chronic pulmonary disease, renal failure, sickle cell anemia, cancer, organ transplantations, or cyanotic congenital heart disease. Treatment is generally aimed at the underlying condition and symptomatic relief of pain. Treatment options may be severely limited by the underlying condition in patients with migraine coexisting with other chronic illnesses.

TABLE 22.2

International Headache Society Criteria for Migraine with Aura

A. At least two attacks that fulfill criteria B
B. Migraine aura fulfilling the following:
  1. Aura consisting of at least one of the following, but no motor weakness:
    a. Fully reversible visual symptoms including positive features (e.g., flickering lights, spots, or lines) and/or negative features (i.e., loss of vision)
    b. Fully reversible sensory symptoms including positive features (i.e., pins and needles) and/or negative features (i.e., numbness)
    c. Fully reversible dysphasic speech disturbance
  2. At least two of the following:
    a. Homonymous visual symptoms and/or unilateral sensory symptoms
    b. At least one aura symptom develops gradually over 5 min and/or different aura symptoms occur in succession over 5 min
    c. Each symptom lasts 5 to 60 min
C. Not attributed to another disorder

From Headache Classification Subcommittee of the International Headache Society. The international classification of headache disorders (2nd edition). *Cephalagia* 2004;8(Suppl 1):9.

DIAGNOSIS

In the evaluation of the patient with headaches, the history is (nearly) everything. The rest is the examination.

(See Tables 22.2 and 22.3 for International Headache Society [IHS] criteria for migraines.)

The history must include the following:

1. Onset: Age at first episode; events or illnesses surrounding onset; temporal pattern of headaches (time of day, day of week, and season); frequency.
2. Pattern and chronology of pain: Have the patient describe a typical headache episode in detail.
  a. Prodrome
  b. Location
  c. Quality (pounding, dull, sharp, or sticking)
  d. Change in quality or location as headache progresses
  e. Associated autonomic symptoms (sweating, pallor, flushing, and palpitations)
  f. Nausea, vomiting, and anorexia
  g. Duration and diurnal variation
  h. Severity and limitation of activities
  i. Response to medications and sleep
3. Preceding and accompanying symptoms, particularly visual or other neurological symptoms.
4. Precipitants of specific episodes or precipitants at onset of headaches.
  a. Stress: Family, school, and peers
  b. Illnesses
  c. Foods/diet/eating pattern: Nitrate- or nitrite-containing foods (cured meats), MSG, chocolate, nuts, cheeses, and other specific suspect foods; skipping meals (true food "allergies" causing migraine are rare)

TABLE 22.3

International Headache Society Criteria for Migraine without Aura

A. At least five attacks that fulfill criteria in B to D
B. Headache attacks that last 4–72 hr (untreated or unsuccessfully treated)
C. Headache has at least two of the following characteristics:
  1. Unilateral site
  2. Pulsating quality
  3. Moderate to severe intensity
  4. Aggravation by or causing avoidance of routine physical activity (e.g., climbing stairs)
D. During headache, at least one of the following symptoms:
  1. Nausea or vomiting (or both)
  2. Photophobia and phonophobia
E. Not attributed to another disorder

From Headache Classification Subcommittee of the International Headache Society. The international classification of headache disorders (2nd edition). *Cephalagia* 2004;8(Suppl 1):9.

d. Medications: Intake of OTC medications (particularly decongestants or diet pills)

e. Exertion and orgasm

f. Caffeine intake or withdrawal

g. Alcohol intake

h. Toxic exposures, particularly lead and hydrocarbons

i. Physical exposures: Bright or flashing lights, temperature changes, and strong odors

5. Other associated illnesses or symptoms, including HIV risks. Changes in menstrual pattern or galactorrhea may suggest pituitary lesion or pregnancy.

6. Medications (prescribed and OTC).
   a. Analgesics
   b. Birth control pills
   c. Other medications used for headaches (acute or prophylactic)
   d. Tetracycline, minocycline, medications for acne

7. Vitamin consumption, particularly fat-soluble vitamins (e.g., vitamins A, D, and E), unusual diets, and supplements.

8. Substance abuse.

9. Depression or mood disorders.

10. School phobia or school avoidance and other secondary gains.

11. Behavior between attacks: Any recent personality change or change in school performance.

12. Family history.
    a. Migraines or other headaches
    b. Epilepsy
    c. Affective disorders
    d. Other neurological conditions

13. Other criteria for migraines: Raskin (1995) identified additional clinical features that suggest the benign nature of a migraine attack. These exceed the IHS criteria (Tables 22.2 and 22.3) of migraine and consist of the following factors: (a) precipitation by menstruation (although the second edition of the IHS classification report does provide criteria for *menstrual migraine* and *menstrual-related migraine*), (b) amelioration with sleep, (c) amelioration during pregnancy, (d) appearance after sustained exertion, and (e) triggers such as alcohol, odors, foods, or changes in the weather.

Physical Examination

The physical examination should include a good general physical examination plus a careful neurological examination. If possible, the patient should be examined both during a typical episode and when free of symptoms. Pertinent physical findings include the following:

1. Vital signs: Elevated blood pressure or temperature.

2. Eyes, ears, nose, and throat: Sinus tenderness, acute or chronic otitis, poor dentition, and refractive error, TMJ pain, or dysfunction.

3. General physical examination: Café au lait spots, depigmented macular lesions suggesting tuberous sclerosis, signs of systemic illness, and galactorrhea.

4. Neck: Nuchal rigidity, spasm or tenderness of cervical neck muscles, or "trigger points."

5. Funduscopic and visual examination: Papilledema, narrowing of vessels, optic atrophy; visual fields, and visual acuity.

6. Neurological examination: Head circumference, mental status, CNs, motor and sensory examination, gait, reflexes, and coordination.

Laboratory Tests

In patients with recurrent headaches separated by periods of complete recovery, laboratory and radiological workups are seldom indicated in the presence of normal physical examination findings. Laboratory and radiological workups should be guided by the history and physical examination results; for example, sinus films may be indicated if facial tenderness or nasal discharge suggest sinusitis. Neuroimaging (computed tomography or magnetic resonance imaging) is indicated if it is an acute severe or increasing headache, if it is an abnormal result on neurological examination, if papilledema is present, or if the head circumference is above the 95th percentile without other explanation. Neuroimaging is *not* generally needed for long-standing recurrent headaches with complete clearing of symptoms between episodes in the face of normal neurological and funduscopic examination results. Other evaluation is guided by physical findings and history. For example, in an adolescent with morning headaches, snoring, and large tonsils, a sleep study to rule out obstructive sleep apnea may be appropriate.

In contrast, an acute severe headache in a patient with no prior headache history must be considered more closely, as underlying systemic or CNS pathology may be life threatening. Neuroimaging and lumbar puncture should be considered to aid in the diagnosis of an acute condition and may be necessary on an emergency basis.

THERAPY

Rule 1A: Not having a headache is better than getting rid of it once it occurs. Rule 1B: Not taking pills every day is better than taking pills. Look for precipitants, particularly avoidable ones.

Rule 2: Take the preferred abortive medication at the onset of the headache, the earlier the better.

Rule 3: Do not underestimate the role of reassurance. Adolescents and parents are often more concerned that the headache is caused by a brain tumor than by the discomfort of the headache itself. Once the adolescent is reassured, treatment beyond simple analgesics may be neither necessary nor desired by the patient.

General strategies for headache management are as follows:

1. Headache diary: The patient should be encouraged to understand the causes and precipitants for headaches. Keeping a headache diary can be therapeutic itself, even if no specific precipitants are ever identified. The diary is kept for a variable period, usually until at least three typical headache episodes have occurred or up to 3 months if no attacks occur while keeping the diary. The adolescent (with the help of a parent) maintains a *detailed* record of headaches, medication intake, and results, as well as activities, foods, stresses, sleep pattern, and physical environment. The following items can be important in uncovering the precipitating factors in recurrent headaches:

a. Foods: Chocolate, nuts, cola, caffeine-containing beverages, and cheeses. (Best to record all food intake in the diary.)

b. Food additives: MSG, nitrates, and nitrites. Nitrates and nitrites are present in nearly all cured meats such as hot dogs, bacon, sausage, ham, and lunch meats. MSG is not always clearly listed on food labels. Foods commonly high in MSG include dried soups and noodles, dried flavoring packets for taco or spaghetti sauces, and some snack foods.

c. Physical stimulants: Exposure to bright lights; rapidly moving or strobe lights (or strobe effect when driving); temperature changes; exercise; and sexual activity.

d. All *medications*, including OTC medications and birth control pills, for headache and any other conditions.

e. Alcohol or other substance intake.

f. Obvious allergic symptoms (rashes, asthma, and allergic rhinitis).

g. Stresses: School, tests, and emotional stressors.

h. Sleep pattern: Deviations from usual pattern, particularly excessive sleep, may precipitate headaches.

2. Treatment of tension headaches

a. A brief period of relaxation or a nap often brings relief.

b. Simple physical measures: Massage or stretching exercises of the neck muscles or warm or cold compresses may help, particularly with relaxation. Biofeedback is occasionally effective but is expensive and requires a very motivated patient and family. Other means of physical relaxation (i.e., yoga, meditation) may be helpful in motivated individuals.

c. Simple analgesics (e.g., acetaminophen, nonsteroidal antiinflammatory drugs [NSAIDs], and aspirin), if not used excessively, are often effective.

d. Combined analgesic-sedative drugs (butalbital [Fiorinal] or other combinations) should be used sparingly, if at all.

e. Mixed tension-vascular headaches, if very frequent and disabling, may be treated on a prophylactic basis with low-dose tricyclic antidepressants, usually amitriptyline.

3. Migraine headaches

Things to do on a *trial* basis for all patients with migraines include the following:

a. Wear sunglasses, brimmed hat, or visor whenever in bright sun. Sunglasses need not be expensive, but should be "100% ultraviolet (UV) protective". In many communities, a "doctor's note" is needed to allow a hat or sunglasses to be worn during outdoor activities at school.

b. Avoid strobe lights or strobelike conditions.

c. Try a diet eliminating MSG and nitrates or nitrites.

d. Stabilize caffeine intake (same amount every day) or wean off completely.

e. Try eliminating all alcohol intake.

f. Try stabilizing sleep pattern to approximately the same amount of sleep daily (i.e., avoid sleep deprivation during the school week followed by "sleeping in" on weekend).

4. Medications for acute episodic migraine treatment (classic, common, or variant) in patients with relatively infrequent headaches

a. Simple analgesics, taken as soon as possible at the onset of the episode (e.g., acetaminophen or NSAIDs such as ibuprofen) often abort the migraine, without the need for stronger medications. American Academy of Neurology (AAN) Practice Parameters recommend ibuprofen as safe and effective. They state that the acetaminophen is probably effective and should be considered. Caffeine (either as a tablet, combined with analgesic, or as a beverage) may potentiate the effect of the analgesic.

b. Antiemetic, either orally, rectally, or parenterally: Promethazine (Phenergan), chlorpromazine (Thorazine), metoclopramide (Reglan), or prochlorperazine (Compazine) combined with or followed by an analgesic is very helpful if nausea or vomiting is prominent. Use of a sedating antiemetic will often allow oral analgesics to be tolerated, promote sleep, and relieve nausea and vomiting.

c. Sedative-analgesic combinations: Small doses of a short-acting sedative such as barbiturate with acetaminophen or aspirin are reasonable if headaches are infrequent and relieved by sleep. Multiple preparations and brands are available.

d. Triptans: Several triptans are available, all selective serotonin receptor agonists. Various preparations (regular tablets, orally dissolvable tablets, nasal sprays, and injections) are marketed. They cannot be mixed (i.e., do not use more than one particular triptan in a given 24-hour period). They should also not be mixed with ergot preparations. They are contraindicated in hemiplegic migraines. Generally, if one triptan does not work, switching to another may not help. If one type works but has unacceptable side effects, or duration of action is too short, another may be better tolerated.

• Sumatriptan (Imitrex), a specific serotonin agonist is administered by subcutaneous injection, nasal spray, or orally.

– Self-injection: The "self-injection" syringes are available only in a 6-mg dose, which may be too high for a smaller adolescent. Fractional doses (2–3 mg) may be used from unit-dose vials using a regular syringe and needle. Because subjective sensory phenomena may be very worrisome to the patient, the first dose should generally be given under direct medical supervision. If successful and well tolerated, the adolescent or the parents may be instructed in administration at home, particularly if episodes are infrequent but very severe.

– Oral: Oral sumatriptan is available as 25- and 50-mg tablets. The adult dose is 25 to 50 mg, given once or twice. Onset of action is in approximately 1 hour, and relief may be long standing if the event is interrupted.

– Nasal spray: Sumatriptan nasal spray is particularly effective for those patients with nausea and vomiting, and can be used at home or school. Nasal sumatriptan is recommended by the AAN for acute migraine treatment. The nasal spray is available in 5- and 20-mg single-dose dispensers. Adolescents generally respond to 10 to 20 mg. The spray generally causes a metallic taste, which lasts for 30 to 60 minutes. Using the spray with the head tilted forward, then compressing the nostrils for a few minutes may partially prevent this effect, which is quite noxious to some patients.

• Zolmitriptan, another serotonin agonist that has been used in adults, is particularly useful for cluster headaches. It comes in 2.5- and 5-mg tablets (maximum dose, 10 mg/24 hours). It also has similar adverse effects such as paresthesias, heaviness, nausea, and tightness.

- Rizatriptan, 5- and 10-mg oral disintegrating tablets. This form is useful for adolescents who cannot or will not swallow a pill during a migraine.
- Naratriptan comes as 1- and 2.5-mg tablets. Has not shown significant efficacy for adolescent migraines. It is longer acting and may be useful in adolescents in whom sumatriptan is effective but has recurrent headaches when a dose wears off.

e. Ergot derivatives are much less commonly used since the introduction of triptans. Ergotamine must be used at the onset of symptoms. Medication should be available to the adolescent at all times, including school. Sublingual, oral, rectal, or inhaled preparations are available, with multiple brand names. Cafergot combines ergotamine and caffeine. Other preparations mostly contain only ergotamine, usually ergotamine tartrate, 1 to 2 mg/dose.

f. Dihydroergotamine (DHE) is available for either intravenous or intramuscular injection or as a nasal spray: DHE-45, given intravenously 10 to 15 minutes after a parenteral dose of antiemetic (commonly metoclopramide [Reglan] or chlorpromazine [Thorazine]), may provide rapid relief of migraine symptoms, even several hours after onset. Several small doses may be given under direct supervision in an emergency department or office. DHE nasal spray (Migranal) may be used at home or school and is sometimes effective in adolescents who do not tolerate or respond to triptans. *Do not use DHE for hemiplegic migraines.*

g. Inhaled high-flow oxygen may relieve cluster headaches rapidly. Patients with cluster headaches often carry a small tank of oxygen with them at all times and become psychologically dependent on the availability of this treatment modality if it is effective at relieving their severe attacks of pain.

h. Chlorpromazine (Thorazine) (10 mg intravenously single dose) has been reported to relieve migraine pain rapidly.

i. Intravenous valproic acid (Depacon) has been used with success as an abortive medication in adolescent migraines. Doses of 1,000 mg to 1,500 mg were efficacious in one series. However, there have been no randomized, controlled studies to date.

Warning: If headaches are frequent (i.e., more than twice a week), beware of analgesic or ergot overuse syndromes. This may convert intermittent migraines to chronic "transformed" migraines.

5. Prophylactic treatment: Adolescents with severe recurrent attacks causing significant school absenteeism or functional limitations should be considered for prophylactic treatment. Prophylactic treatment is generally indicated in migraines accompanied by significant neurological deficits (e.g., hemiplegic migraines), even if the episodes are infrequent. Prophylactic treatment may be preferred even in patients responsive to NSAIDS, triptans, or other agents, due to the inability to carry medications to school. Continue treatment until the headache pattern has markedly improved for approximately 6 months, then consider a trial of tapering-off medication. Current AAN Practice Parameters state that there is insufficient evidence to recommend any drug approved in the United States for migraine prophylaxis.

They do find that flunarizine, a calcium channel blocker not available in the US, is probably effective for migraine prophylaxis in adolescents. There is anecdotal evidence for a number of prophylactic medications, however.

a. β-Blockers: Propranolol is effective in approximately 70% of adolescents with severe migraines, although there have been few well-controlled studies. The initial dose is 40 to 80 mg, divided twice daily (b.i.d.) or three times a day (t.i.d.). A slow-release preparation of propranolol may allow for once daily dosing. Higher doses (up to 240 mg/day) may be used. The effect is not immediate. Usually, a gradual decrease in headache frequency is seen over several weeks to months. Side effects include fatigue, depression, and decreased exercise tolerance, particularly at high doses. Severe asthma, insulin-dependent diabetes, and depression are contraindications. Other β-blockers (e.g., atenolol, nadolol, timolol, and metoprolol) may also be effective.

b. Tricyclic antidepressants (amitriptyline, imipramine, desipramine): Amitriptyline (Elavil) is useful for prophylaxis of migraines or mixed tension-vascular headaches. The initial daily dose is 10 to 25 mg at bedtime, increased gradually as needed to 75 to 100 mg/day. Side effects include sedation, dry mouth, arrhythmias, hypotension, and decreased tolerance of warm environments. At higher doses, electrocardiogram should be monitored.

c. Low-dose aspirin or NSAIDs (e.g., ibuprofen and naproxen) used in chronic low doses may effectively prevent migraine attacks. NSAIDs may be particularly effective in menstrual migraines if started a day or two before expected symptomatic periods.

d. Cyproheptadine (Periactin): The usual dose is 2 to 4 mg t.i.d. A major side effect is sedation. Significant weight gain occasionally occurs.

e. Anticonvulsants: Valproic acid (Depakote), low-dose phenobarbital, topiramate (Topamax), levetiracetam (Keppra), and possibly phenytoin (Dilantin) have been reported to prevent migraines. The dose used often is lower than that necessary for seizure control. Divalproex sodium (Depakote) is currently approved by the Food and Drug Administration for migraine prophylaxis at a dose of 500 mg/day. Topiramate has been shown to be effective in a randomized controlled trial of patients aged 12 to 65 years. The best responses were to doses of 100 mg/day and 200 mg/day. The main adverse effects were paresthesias, fatigue, and nausea. Studies in children show cognitive disturbances as the main side effect.

f. Calcium channel blockers (e.g., verapamil and nimodipine) have been used with limited success for migraine prophylaxis. Flunarizine (not available in the United States) has demonstrated significant headache reduction in a double-blind placebo-controlled trial.

g. Clonidine (Catapres) has occasionally been reported to be useful.

h. Methysergide (Sansert): Significant risks make this a last choice in most circumstances. It should not be used continuously for more than 6 months, because of risk of retroperitoneal and pericardial fibrosis. Close follow-up is essential. However, this is

a very effective modality for patients with refractory, frequent migraines.
  i. Lithium carbonate has been reported to be an effective prophylactic medication for chronic cluster headaches.
  j. Combinations of high-dose riboflavin (vitamin B_2) and magnesium may prevent migraine in some patients. A commercial preparation of magnesium oxide, riboflavin, and the herb feverfew is sold as a food supplement.
6. "Transformed migraines," chronic migraines, rebound headache if severe and disabling.
  a. Intravenous DHE, usually combined with metoclopramide or chlorpromazine, is given over 2 to 4 days on an adjusted q8h schedule. This requires hospitalization, dose supervision, and dose titration over the first few doses.
  b. Short courses of high-dose corticosteroids may end the episode. Usually, high-dose prednisone (2 mg/kg/day) or dexamethasone (Decadron) is used for approximately 5 days, followed by a rapid taper.
  c. Withdrawal of chronic (overused or daily use) nonnarcotic and narcotic analgesics, triptans, and ergots is essential. This may require hospitalization for detoxification.
  d. Psychological supportive therapy, relaxation therapies, and physical exercise programs are often essential to improve the health status of teens with chronic daily headaches.

PROGNOSIS

Guidetti and Galli (1998) studied the evolution of headaches in children and adolescents and found that 34% remitted, 45% improved, 6% worsened, and the condition remained unchanged in 15%. Up to 40% to 50% of childhood-onset migraines may remit during adolescence or young adulthood. Adolescence-onset migraines often continue into adulthood. However, adolescents should be reassured that even people with a strong tendency to have migraines do not have frequent attacks throughout life. Patterns of occurrence are highly variable. The goal is to avoid any offending agents, use effective medication in appropriate doses, and lead a functional lifestyle.

WEB SITES

For Teenagers and Parents

http://www.headaches.org/. Web site of the National Headache Foundation.
http://familydoctor.org/x502.xml. The American Academy of Family Physicians handout on headaches.
http://www.ninds.nih.gov/disorders/headache/headache.htm. National Institutes of Health site on headaches.
http://www.achenet.org/. American Council for Headache Education.
http://www.aan.com/professionals/practice/pdfs/ Headache Peds Patients.pdf. AAN Headache Information.
http://www.emedicinehealth.com/migraine_headache_in_ children/article_em.htm Emedicine patient information.

For Health Professionals

http://www.familydoctor.org/flowcharts/502.html. Flowcharts on headaches from the American Academy of Family Physicians.
http://www.emedicine.com/neuro/topic528.htm.
http://www.emedicine.com/neuro/topic529.htm. Emedicine
http://www.neuropat.dote.hu/pain.htm. Internet Handbook of Neurology.
http://www.ahsnet.org/. American Headache Society— Publisher's of *Headache*.

REFERENCES AND ADDITIONAL READINGS

Ahmed MA, Reid E, Cooke A. Familial hemiplegic migraine in the west of Scotland: a clinical and genetic study of seven families. *J Neurol Neurosurg Psychiatry* 1996;61:616.

Ahonen K, Hamalainen ML, Rantala H, et al. Nasal sumatriptan is effective in the treatment of migraine attacks in children. *Neurology* 2004;62:883.

Annequin D, Tourniaire B, Massiou H. Migraine and headache in childhood and adolescence. *Pediatr Clin North Am* 2000; 47:617.

Brandes JL, Saper JR, Diamond M, et al. Topiramate for migraine prevention: a randomized controlled trial. *JAMA* 2004;291(8):965.

Burton LJ, Quinn B, Pratt-Cheney J, et al. Headache etiology in a pediatric emergency department. *Pediatr Emerg Care* 1997;13:1.

Curran MP, Evans HC, Wagstaff AJ. Intranasal sumatriptan: in adolescents with migraine. *CNS Drugs* 2005;19(4):335.

Deleu D, Hanssens Y. Current and emerging second generation triptans in acute migraine therapy: a comparative review. *J Clin Pharmacol* 2000;40:687.

DuBose CD, Cutlip AC, Cudip WD II Jr. Migraines and other headaches: an approach to diagnosis and classification. *Am Fam Physician* 1995;51:1498.

Edgeworth J, Bullock P, Bailey A, et al. Why are brain tumors still being missed? *Arch Dis Child* 1996;74:148.

Fleisher DR, Matar M. The cyclic vomiting syndrome: a report of 71 cases and literature review. *J Pediatr Gastroenterol Nutr* 1993;17:361.

Gladstein J, Holden EW, Winner P, et al. Chronic daily headache in children and adolescents: current status and recommendations for the future. Pediatric Committee of the American Association for the Study of Headache. *Headache* 1997;37:626.

Golomb MR, Sokol DK, Walsh LE, et al. Recurrent hemiplegia, normal MRI, and NOTCH3 mutation in a 14-year-old: is this early CADASIL? *Neurology* 2004;62:2331.

Guidetti V, Galli F. Evolution of headache in childhood and adolescence: an 8-year follow-up. *Cephalgia* 1998;18(7): 449.

Hamalainen ML, Hoppu K, Santavuori P. Sumatriptan for migraine attacks in children: a double-blind, randomized, placebo-controlled, crossover study. *Neurology* 1997;48: 1100.

Hamalainen ML, Hoppu K, Valkeila E, et al. Ibuprofen or acetaminophen for the acute treatment of migraine in children: a double-blind, randomized, placebo-controlled, crossover study. *Neurology* 1997;48:103.

Headache Classification Subcommittee of the International Headache Society. The international classification of headache disorders (2nd edition). *Cephalagia* 2004;8(Suppl 1):9.

Johannes CB, Linet MS, Stewart WE, et al. Relationship of headache to phase of the menstrual cycle among young women: a daily diary study. *Neurology* 1995;45:1076.

Kaiser RS. Depression in adolescent headache patients. *Headache* 1992;32:340.

Kulig J. Advances in medical management of asthma, headaches, and fatigue. *Med Clin North Am* 2000;84:829.

Lewis DW. Headaches in children and adolescents [Review]. *Am Fam Physician* 2002;65(4):625.

Lewis DW, Ashwal S, Dahl G, et al. Practice Parameter: evaluation of children and adolescents with recurrent headache. *Neurology* 2002;59:490.

Lewis S, Ashwal A, Hershey A, et al. Practice parameter: pharmacological treatment of migraine headache in children and adolescents: report of the American Academy of Neurology Quality Standards Subcommittee and the Practice Committee of the Child Neurology Society. *Neurology* 2004;63:2215.

Lewis DW, Kellstein D, Burke B, et al. Children's ibuprofen suspension for the acute treatment of pediatric migraine headache. *Headache* 2002;42:780.

Lewis DW, Yonker M, Winner P, The treatment of pediatric migraine. *Pediatr Ann* 2005;34(6):448.

Li BU, Murray RD, Heitlinger LA. Is cyclic vomiting syndrome related to migraine? *J Pediatr* 1999;134:567.

Linder SL, Dowson AJ. Zolmitriptan provides effective migraine relief in adolescents. *Int J Clin Pract* 2000;54:466.

Lipton RB, Stewart WE. Migraine in the United States: a review of epidemiology and health care use. *Neurology* 1993;43:S6.

Ojaimi J, Katsabanis S, Bower S, et al. Mitochondrial DNA in stroke and migraine with aura. *Cerebrovasc Dis* 1998;8:102.

Ramadan NM, Schultz LL, Gilkey SJ. Migraine prophylactic drugs: proof of efficacy, utilization, and cost. *Cephalalgia* 1997;17:73.

Rapoport AM. Pharmacological prevention of migraine. *Clin Neurosci* 1998;5:55.

Raskin NH. *Diagnosis and treatment of migraine: update on headache–a comprehensive course in mechanisms and management*. Paper presented at: the Scottsdale Headache Symposium of the American Association for the Study of Headache: January 20-22, 1995; Scottsdale, AZ.

Reiter PD, Nickisch J, Merritt G. Efficacy and tolerability of intravenous valproic acid in acute adolescent migraine. *Headache* 2005;45(7):899.

Rothner AD. Headaches in children and adolescents. *Child Adolesc Psychiatry Clin North Am* 1999;8:727.

Rothner AD. Headaches in children and adolescents: update 2001. *Semin Pediatr Neurol* 2001;8(1):2.

Schulman EA, Silberstein SD. Symptomatic and prophylactic treatment of migraine and tension-type headache. *Neurology* 1992;42:16.

Sorge F, DeSimone R, Marano E, et al. Flunarizine in prophylaxis of childhood migraine. A double-blind, placebo-controlled crossover study. *Cephalalgia* 1988;8:1.

Stewart WF, Linet MS, Celentano DD, et al. Age and sex-specific incidence rates of migraine with and without visual aura. *Am J Epidemiol* 1991;34:1111.

Stewart WF, Lipton RB, Celentano DD, et al. Prevalence of migraine headache in the United States. *JAMA* 1992;267:64.

Ueberall MA, Wenzel D. Intranasal sumatriptan for the acute treatment of migraine in children. *Neurology* 1999;52:1507.

Vanagaite J, Pareja JA, Storen O. Light-induced discomfort and pain in migraine. *Cephalalgia* 1997;17:733.

Wiendels NJ, van der Geest MC, Neven AK, et al. Chronic daily headache in children and adolescents. *Headache* 2005;45:678.

Winner P, Rothner AD, Saper J, et al. A randomized, double-blind, placebo-controlled study of sumatriptan nasal spray in the treatment of acute migraine in adolescents. *Pediatrics* 2000;106:989.

CHAPTER 23

Syncope and Vertigo

Amy D. DiVasta, Wendy G. Mitchell, and Mark E. Alexander

Cardiac symptoms in the adolescent are very common; true cardiac disease is not. Syncope is a frequent complaint, accounting for 1% to 6% of hospitalizations and 3% of emergency room visits annually. These episodes often raise concerns that they could be predecessors to future sudden cardiac death (SCD). The clinician's critical task is to distinguish between presyncopal episodes, vertigo, the benign forms of syncope, and syncope associated with an increased risk of SCD. Each has separate implications for evaluation and therapy. This differentiation is made initially by detailed history, careful physical examination, and, in almost all cases, an electrocardiogram (ECG). Specialized testing may be needed in a minority of patients to confirm these initial conclusions.

SYNCOPE

Etiology

Syncope is a sudden, transient loss of consciousness and postural tone, usually lasting several seconds to a minute, followed by spontaneous recovery. Syncope is common, with a female predominance and a peak incidence between ages 15 to 19 years. Although most episodes are benign, any condition that leads to decreased cerebral perfusion may cause syncope.

Classification

There are three major categories of syncope:

1. Neurocardiogenic
   a. Vasovagal/reflex
   b. Postural orthostatic tachycardia
2. Cardiovascular
   a. Structural
   b. Arrhythmogenic
3. Noncardiovascular
   a. Epileptic
   b. Psychogenic

Both population-based data and pediatric cardiology clinic experience have demonstrated that syncope of unknown origin (often termed *simple syncope*) and neurocardiogenic syncope account for more than 85% to 90% of

events (Driscoll et al., 1997; Ritter et al., 2000; Steinberg et al., 2005). The final common pathway of any true syncopal event is ineffective cerebral blood flow, resulting from inadequate cardiac output. Between 1% and 5% of patients will have significant cardiac disease. Another small minority will have seizures and psychiatric diagnoses including anxiety disorders and pseudoseizures.

History and Physical Examination

The most important step to an accurate diagnosis is a detailed history (including family history) and thorough physical examination.

History

Key elements of the history should include the following:

1. Onset and frequency of episodes.
2. Circumstances: Relation to exercise, posture, and precipitating factors (such as stress, recent infection [labyrinthitis], exercise, position, and environmental factors). Descriptions of the episode help define the nature of the event. If the teen cannot describe the attack, it is helpful to get a description from another witness. Symptoms in others, particularly peers, may be useful in suspected group hysteria.
3. Prodromal symptoms: Dizziness, diaphoresis, nausea, pallor, palpitations, chest pain, and dyspnea. Description of color changes (initial pallor versus cyanosis or flushing) and prodromal sensations is critical and may help distinguish syncope from seizure.
4. Complete or incomplete loss of consciousness, duration, and time to recovery.
5. Abnormal movements, incontinence, or injury. Convulsive activity during the attack, incontinence, or tongue biting suggests epilepsy, although syncope may induce a brief seizure. The order of events is extremely helpful in making this determination. See Table 23.1 for distinguishing features of common fainting versus seizure.
6. Past medical history and medications (including complementary and alternative medications).
7. Family history: Sudden death (particularly if age less than 40 years), similar episodes, early onset heart disease.

The physician should be alert for warning signs that suggest a more serious etiology. These include syncope

TABLE 23.1

Neurocardiogenic Syncope versus Seizure

Characteristics	Neurocardiogenic syncope	Seizure
Warning	Usually prodromal symptoms	Aura common
Duration	Brief	Prolonged
Position at onset	Usually erect	Any position
Color change	Pallor frequent	Flushing or cyanosis
Convulsions	Rare, opisthotonic/myoclonic	Common, may be focal
Urinary incontinence	Rare	Common
Postictal state	Residual symptoms common	Disorientation, headaches

during exercise, syncope while in a supine position, family history of sudden death in a person younger than 30 to 40 years, personal history of cardiac disease, or an event precipitated by a loud noise, intense emotion, or fright.

Physical Examination

The physical examination should include orthostatic vital signs, a careful neurological assessment, and a dynamic cardiac examination performed with the patient in multiple positions to evaluate for a pathological murmur (see Chapter 14).

Neurocardiogenic Syncope

With synonyms including vasovagal syncope, neurocardiac syncope, and reflex syncope, this is the most common form of syncope. The history and physical examination findings should be normal, without any of the warning signs suggestive of a more serious etiology. The physiological basis of the syncopal event represents a temporary derangement of cardiac and vascular regulation.

1. Duration: May last for a few seconds to a few minutes.
2. Onset: Gradual; the patient is generally aware that something is wrong.
3. Etiology: Precipitating factors are usually identifiable. Fear, anxiety, pain, hunger, overcrowding, fatigue, injections, and the sight of blood are common precipitants. Alcohol and exposure to cold or heat can also precipitate an attack. Prolonged upright posture, particularly without movement, may contribute. Group hysteria may precipitate syncopal "epidemics," particularly in schools or other closed populations.
4. Prodromal symptoms: Typical prodromal symptoms include nausea, dizziness, visual spots or dimming, feelings of apprehension, pallor, yawning, diaphoresis, and feelings of warmth.
5. Syncopal event: The loss of consciousness is usually brief, with gradual loss of muscle tone.
6. Syncopal seizures: Rarely, a brief tonic or clonic seizure will be precipitated by syncope. It always follows the preceding syncopal symptoms. A seizure is more likely to happen if the patient faints while sitting or is kept from assuming the recumbent position upon loss of consciousness. Convulsive syncope is also commonly triggered by the sight of blood.
7. Recovery: Consciousness generally returns in <1 minute, often with a brief period of perceived inability to respond despite awareness of the environment. The patient may report residual symptoms of fatigue, malaise, weakness, nausea, and headache for up to an hour after fainting.
8. Pathophysiology: The exact pathophysiology is still not completely understood. With standing position there is significant venous pooling, between 400 to 800 mL. This volume shift leads to decreased ventricular filling and pulse pressure, and activates many homeostatic reflexes (including baroreceptors, carotid body receptors, and C fibers). If the vagal and sympathetic cardiovascular responses are adequate, cerebral perfusion is maintained. However, if responses are exaggerated or ineffective, there can be a paradoxical vagal activation and inappropriate decrease in sympathetic activity. This induces bradycardia and hypotension, further impairs cerebral blood flow, and can lead to syncope.

Diagnostic Evaluation of Neurocardiogenic Syncope

In addition to the history and physical examination, adolescents suffering a true syncopal event should have an ECG performed. The ECG is the ideal screening test for more serious disease in syncopal patients. It allows evaluation of the intervals, rhythm, and ventricular size. Additionally, it is noninvasive, readily available, and inexpensive. A normal diagnostic screen (reassuring history, benign physical examination, and normal ECG) is generally sufficient to exclude the possibility of cardiac disease. Further investigation is warranted only if there are lingering concerns or suspicions of cardiac disease.

1. No laboratory investigations, electroencephalogram (EEG), or intracranial imaging are needed.
2. Echocardiogram: Routine echocardiography has very low yield and is not part of the routine evaluation of a typical syncopal event.
3. Ambulatory ECG monitoring is not generally indicated. If episodes are relatively frequent, temporary memory looping event monitors, which can store 3 to 5 minutes of rhythm during an episode, may be useful.
4. Exercise testing: Required if syncopal episodes occur during exercise.
5. Tilt table testing: Tilt table testing should be reserved for challenging patients with recurrent symptoms, or for patients needing further reassurance. The patient's pulse, blood pressure, and symptoms are monitored first in the supine position, and then in a head-up tilt to 60 to 70 degrees for 12 minutes or more, depending on local protocol. In a positive test, the patient is symptomatic with hypotension ± pulse change. However, tilt testing is not a gold standard; as many as 40% of normal

adolescents will have a positive tilt test. Specificity is poor (35%–100%) and sensitivity is variable (75%–85%).

6. Implantable loop recorder: A subcutaneous device that allows for up to 18 months of monitoring. No patient adherence is required. Can establish a symptom-rhythm correlation in most patients. However, these are invasive and therefore reserved for patients who experience severe, recurrent episodes.

Management of Neurocardiogenic Syncope

The mainstay of treatment is reassurance, and educating patients and parents regarding the benign nature of the condition as well as ways to prevent further episodes. Adolescents should take adequate oral fluids to prevent volume depletion, and avoid caffeine. Postural techniques (including isometric contractions of the extremities, folding the arms, or crossing the legs) help increase systemic blood pressure and venous return to the heart, and can help abort a syncopal episode. If patients begin to experience prodromal symptoms, they should ideally assume a supine position. Upright, weight-bearing exercise may also be helpful in decreasing the frequency of events. Most adolescents outgrow their episodes over time, even if they are highly symptomatic. Drug therapy may be needed for refractory cases that do not respond to supportive therapy. Options are summarized in Table 23.2. Pharmacological therapy is largely driven by tradition, rather than data, in the adolescent population. Pediatric experience suggests that fludrocortisone and β-blockers are comparable in efficacy. Generally, a 12-month symptom-free interval is considered a reasonable duration of treatment; subsequently, a trial off medication is warranted.

Postural Orthostatic Tachycardia Syndrome

Postural orthostatic tachycardia syndrome (POTS) is a heterogeneous disorder of autonomic regulation. POTS is well described in adolescence, and has a female predominance. Patients commonly complain of fatigue, dizziness, and exercise intolerance with upright position.

1. POTS is characterized by a marked pulse change (>30 bpm) or excessive tachycardia (>120 bpm) in response to being upright during a 6-minute stand test.
2. There is little or no blood pressure change.
3. Mechanisms of abnormal autonomic regulation, both acquired and genetic, are as follows:
   a. Enhanced noradrenergic tone at rest, but blunted sympathetic response to standing
   b. Partial sympathetic denervation
   c. Impaired synaptic norepinephrine clearance
   d. Decreased cardiac vagal baroreflex sensitivity
   e. Impaired regulation of cerebrovascular tone
4. There is significant overlap between chronic fatigue syndrome and POTS. In one study by Stewart et al., 25 of 26 chronic fatigue patients had severe orthostatic symptoms on tilt test, compared with only 4 of 13 age-matched controls.
5. Treatment: Fluids and vasoconstrictors relieve symptoms in most patients. β-Blockers are also commonly used for treatment.

Orthostatic Hypotension

Orthostatic hypotension is uncommon in adolescents. It is defined as a drop in systolic blood pressure >20 mm Hg and a drop in diastolic pressure >10 mm Hg with assumption of upright posture. Etiologies of orthostatic hypotension include the following:

1. Inadequate homeostatic mechanisms: Prolonged bed rest, exhaustion after intense exercise, pregnancy, anorexia nervosa, heat exposure, fever, and marijuana use.

TABLE 23.2

Pharmacological Treatment Options for Neurocardiogenic Syncope

Drug	Dose	Proposed Mechanism of Action	Side Effects	Quality of Data
Fludrocortisone	0.1–0.2 mg/d	↑ Renal Na^+ absorption ↑ Circulating blood volume	Bloating or edema Hypokalemia Hypertension	+
Midodrine	5–10 mg q4h Maximum four doses/d	α-Agonist ↑ Peripheral vascular resistance	Piloerection Scalp pruritus Hypertension Urinary retention Difficult adherence to treatment	++

β-Blockers
  Atenolol
  Metoprolol
	25–50 mg daily
	25–50 mg b.i.d.
		Blocks excess sympathetic response (paradoxical effect)	Fatigue
			Depression
				±

SSRIs
  Fluoxetine
  Sertraline
	20 mg daily
	50 mg daily
		↑ Extracellular serotonin leads to down-regulation of receptor density	Headache
			Insomnia
			GI effects
				±

SSRIs, serotonin reuptake inhibitors; GI, gastrointestinal.
+, moderate data to support efficacy; ++: strong data to support efficacy; ± mixed data to support efficacy.

2. Reduced effective blood volume: Hemorrhage, dehydration, burns, diabetes insipidus, hemodialysis, adrenal insufficiency, and varicose veins.
3. Medications and illicit drugs: Antihypertensives, phenothiazines, antidepressants, narcotics, sedatives, calcium channel blockers, and alcohol.
4. Autonomic neuropathies: Pure autonomic neuropathies may be autoimmune or familial (familial dysautonomia). Mixed motor and sensory neuropathies may be genetic or acquired due to autoimmune phenomena (e.g., Guillain-Barré syndrome and chronic immune demyelinating polyneuropathy), diabetes, nutritional deficiencies, uremia, metabolic causes, heavy metal poisoning, porphyria, pernicious anemia, vincristine toxicity, or chronic hydrocarbon toxicity (secondary to inhalant abuse).
5. Central Nervous System: Spinal cord injury, transverse myelitis, spinal cord tumor, or syringomyelia may cause autonomic dysfunction. Orthostatic hypotension (and positional hypertension) is particularly common with acute paraplegia due to spinal injury from any cause. Hydrocephalus and posterior fossa tumors may occasionally cause orthostatic hypotension.
6. Miscellaneous: Syndromes of neurotransmitter excess including carcinoid syndrome, systemic mastocytosis, and pheochromocytoma.

Cardiovascular Syncope

Cardiac syncope is characterized by an acute collapse with few premonitory symptoms, often in association with exercise or exertion. Occurs secondary to either arrhythmia or hemodynamic events, including obstructed left ventricular (LV) filling, obstructed LV outflow, or ineffective myocardial contraction. Cardiac syncope should be suspected when any of the "warning signs" are present (see preceding text). The physical examination or ECG *may* be abnormal. See Table 23.3 for a listing of the more common electrical and structural cardiac conditions that can lead to syncope. A few key conditions are summarized in the subsequent text.

Hypertrophic Cardiomyopathy

1. Definition: An inherited cardiac muscle disorder leading to myocardial hypertrophy. Prevalence estimated at 1 in 500.
2. Natural history and prognosis: Symptoms generally begin during periods of rapid somatic growth, such as adolescence. Genetically and phenotypically heterogeneous, with wide variation in terms of symptom status, LV wall thickness, and arrhythmia risk. Most patients are asymptomatic. If symptoms develop, usual complaints include exertional chest pain, exercise intolerance, shortness of breath, and syncope.
3. Diagnostic findings in hypertrophic cardiomyopathy (HCM):
   a. Physical examination findings include a systolic ejection murmur at the left lower sternal border (with increasing intensity in standing position and decreasing intensity with squatting) and a prominent LV lift.
   b. ECG may reveal signs of LV hypertrophy, ST-T wave changes, or atrial enlargement. However, ECGs are problematic, as there are many false negatives and false positives. The ECG may be abnormal in up to 25% of patients with HCM.
   c. The echocardiogram is close to the "gold standard" for identifying affected individuals. Key findings include thickened interventricular septum and LV free wall, asymmetric septal hypertrophy, systolic anterior motion of the mitral valve, and dynamic LV outflow tract obstruction. A small number of competitive male athletes may have ECG findings suggestive of HCM; they may require 1 to 3 months of deconditioning to prove they have "athletic heart syndrome," which is a benign adaptation to systematic athletic training with no adverse cardiovascular consequences.
4. Sudden death: HCM is the most common cause of SCD for the 15- to 35-year old age group, but is still rare. SCD due to previously undiagnosed cardiomyopathy accounts for <1 death per 1,000,000/year. Patients develop myocardial ischemia from increased myocardial oxygen demand and reduced myocardial perfusion.

TABLE 23.3

Differential Diagnosis of Cardiac Syncope

Electrical	*Structural*
Heart block	Inadequate LV filling
Congenital	Pulmonary hypertension
Acquired	Pulmonic stenosis
Wolff-Parkinson-White syndrome	Inadequate LV output
Dysrhythmias	Aortic stenosis
Long QT syndrome	Hypertrophic cardiomyopathy
Inherited	Dilated cardiomyopathy
Secondary	Coronary artery anomalies
Brugada syndrome	Myocarditis
Postoperative congenital heart disease	Tumors
Arrhythmogenic right ventricular dysplasia	Marfan syndrome

LV, left ventricle.

Mechanism of cardiac arrest is ventricular fibrillation. Risk factors for sudden death are as follows:

a. Previous cardiac arrest
b. Positive family history of sudden death
c. Exertion-related syncope
d. Severe ($\geq$3 cm) hypertrophy
e. Nonsustained ventricular tachycardia during Holter monitoring
f. Abnormal blood pressure response to upright exercise testing

5. Treatment: May be inherited in autosomal dominant manner, so all family members should be screened. Course is variable, but even asymptomatic patients should avoid athletic participation. Symptomatic relief is difficult, and may be treated with medications such as B-blockers, calcium channel antagonists, and disopyramide. Surgical options include catheter ethanol ablation of the hypertrophic septum and surgical septectomy. These may not change the risk of SCD, but can achieve long-term symptom relief in up to 70% of patients. For patients at high risk of SCD, implantable defibrillator therapy is recommended; some patients choose implantable cardioverter-defibrillator (ICD) therapy simply based on combinations of family history and LV wall thickness.

Long QT Syndrome

1. Definition: Disorder of delayed ventricular repolarization. Patients are at risk for development of arrhythmias (such as torsades de pointes or ventricular fibrillation), syncope, seizure, and SCD. Patients may be asymptomatic, or present with recurrent syncopal episodes, palpitations, dizziness, or even sudden death.
2. Hereditary long QT syndrome (LQTS): Both autosomal recessive and autosomal dominant patterns of inheritance have been described. Currently, seven genes and >150 mutations have been described. LQT1, LQT2, and LQT3 account for >95% of identified mutations. Genetic testing is available commercially with approximately 70% sensitivity. The tests cost approximately $5,000; insurance coverage is variable.
3. Acquired LQTS: May be related to underlying disease state, or secondary to drug effect. See Table 23.4 for a list of the more common conditions and medications associated with acquired LQTS. Current recommendations are to monitor ECG before starting select psychotropic agents.
4. Diagnosis: ECG is the diagnostic tool of choice.
   a. Long QT interval $\geq$0.46 second (has a positive and negative predictive value of 95%) is most accurate in identifying gene carriers
   b. Notched/bifid T wave in V_2 to V_4
   c. May present with syncope, seizure, or sudden death
   d. May be asymptomatic
   e. ECG should be obtained on all primary relatives of those patients diagnosed with LQTS
   f. Holter monitors, exercise testing, and drug challenges are of limited utility. Electrophysiologic (EP) testing is not useful.
5. Treatment of LQTS: Although no treatment is perfect, all patients who carry the diagnosis should be referred to a cardiologist and treated, even if asymptomatic. Mortality rate has been estimated to be 1% to 20% annually in patients not receiving treatment; this rate decreases to 1% to 2% per year if therapy is initiated.

TABLE 23.4

Conditions/Medications Associated with QT Interval Prolongation

Conditions	Medications
Coronary artery disease	Cisapride[a]
Myocarditis	Amitriptyline
Alcoholism	Ketoconazole
Eating disorders	Terfenadine[b]
Electrolyte abnormality	Erythromycin
Liquid protein diets	Arsenic
Hypothyroidism	Risperidone
CVA	Haloperidol
Encephalitis	Quinidine
Traumatic brain injury	Procainamide
Subarachnoid hemorrhage	Thioridazine

CVA, cerebrovascular accident.
[a]Limited availability.
[b]Off the market.

Therapy for LQTS includes the following:
a. Restriction from competitive athletics, and prudent changes in recreational activities
b. Avoidance of drugs/medications known to prolong the QT interval (for frequently updated information, see www.torsades.org)
c. Avoidance of loud noises, emotional stressors, or vigorous activity which may precipitate a syncopal episode
d. ECG evaluation of all family members
e. β-Blockers: The initial treatment of choice, B-blockers decrease adrenergic triggers. β-Blocker treatment significantly decreases cardiac events, but does not change the QT interval nor provide absolute protection against sudden death. No absolute reduction in deaths is proven. Medication compliance is essential to prevent rebound receptor catecholamine hypersensitivity, which can precipitate a life-threatening arrhythmia if the medication is suddenly discontinued. There is increasing use of long-acting agents to improve adherence to therapy, for example, using nadolol rather than atenolol.
f. Left cervicothoracic sympathetic ganglionectomy
g. ICDs
h. Gene-specific LQTS therapy: not yet available

Other Ion Channel Defect Disorders

Although LQTS is the most common genetic ion channel disorder, defects in other channels can also lead to syncope. Brugada syndrome is a distinctive mutation of the cardiac sodium channel gene (*SCN5A*) located on chromosome 3. The mutation leads to dynamic right ventricular conduction delays. Patients often present with syncope or cardiac arrest. Other ion channel defects include catecholaminergic ventricular tachycardia, and a newly described short QT syndrome. Although not an ion channel defect, a similar range of genotype–phenotype variation is seen in hereditary cardiomyopathies, such as arrhythmogenic right ventricular dysplasia, in which syncope may be the sentinel symptom.

Management of Suspected Cardiac Syncope

If cardiac disease is suspected as the etiology of a syncopal episode, referral to a pediatric cardiologist is in order. Patients with high-risk presentations should be restricted from competitive athletics until evaluated by the cardiologist. Adolescents should avoid driving a motor vehicle until their evaluation is complete. In many states an episode of cardiac syncope, like a seizure, invalidates the individual's driver's license for a period of several months.

Noncardiovascular Syncopes

1. Hyperventilation: Hyperventilation is a frequent cause of dizziness in the adolescent, although a true syncopal episode occurs only rarely. Attacks often occur during stressful situations, and the adolescent may be unaware of the hyperventilation. Symptoms of hyperventilation include the following:
   a. Respiratory: Subjective shortness of breath secondary to increased thoracic respiratory efforts; chest pain either secondary to pressure on the diaphragm from gastric distension or related to thoracic muscle strain; and increased thoracic breathing, sighing, and yawning.
   b. Cardiovascular: Palpitations, tachycardia, and precordial chest pain.
   c. Neurological: Perioral or peripheral paresthesias, lightheadedness, dizziness, disorientation, impaired thinking, tetany, seizures, syncope, and headaches.
   d. Gastrointestinal: Epigastric pain (usually related to aerophagia), dry mouth, belching, bloating, and flatulence.
   e. Musculoskeletal: Muscle pains and cramps, tremors, stiffness, and muscle spasm.
   f. Psychiatric: Anxiety, depression, phobias, insomnia, sensations of unreality, and nightmares.
   g. General: Fatigue, weakness, and exhaustion, particularly as attack subsides.
   h. Pathophysiology: The alkalosis from hyperventilation leads to cerebral vasoconstriction and decreased cerebral perfusion. It is estimated that cerebral blood flow is decreased by 2% for each 1 mm Hg decrease in $PaCO_2$. The alkalosis also leads to a decrease in peripheral release of oxygen (secondary to the Bohr effect on oxyhemoglobin), decreased ionized calcium level, hypophosphatemia, and possible coronary vasospasm.
   i. Treatment of hyperventilation includes reassurance, education about the physiology of hyperventilation, and teaching of strategies to deal with any identifiable precipitating stressors and to manage the hyperventilation itself. Interventions can include having the patient breathe into a paper bag or teaching diaphragmatic breathing. For example, the teenager should be instructed to place one hand on the abdomen and the other on the chest and to practice breathing so that the lower hand moves while the upper hand is held still.
2. Metabolic disturbances: Hypokalemia and hypomagnesemia can lead to syncope. Hypoglycemia is characterized by a gradual onset of anxiety, weakness, sweating, palpitations, and tremor. Recovery is prompt with carbohydrate intake, but no relief is obtained on recumbency. Symptomatic hypoglycemia other than in the context of insulin-dependent diabetes is very rare

in adolescents and is over-diagnosed by patients and families.
3. Psychogenic syncope: "Hysterical syncope" is typically characterized by a patient who, almost always in the presence of others, gracefully slumps or swoons to the floor, usually without injury. The patient is not anxious. There are generally no blood pressure or pulse alterations or associated physiological changes. Other psychiatric causes include pseudoseizure and panic disorder. Many of these patients may have had an episode of typical syncope that is embellished so that those symptoms dominate the pseudofits, similar to epileptic patients who present with pseudoseizure.
4. Subclavian steal syndrome: An uncommon cause of syncope related to occlusion in the proximal subclavian artery. This can lead to reversal of blood flow in the adjacent vertebral artery if vascular resistance in the arm decreases (during exercise), causing blood to flow away from the brain.
5. Micturition syncope: Reported in older adolescents and young adults, but more common in older populations. Usually not associated with any serious illnesses when it occurs in this age-group. Episodes most frequently occur after the patient rises at night for urination. Rapid emptying of the bladder leads to a reflex vasodilation and a resultant decrease in cerebral blood flow, with a sudden loss of consciousness.
6. Cough syncope: Uncommon in the adolescent, except in patients with chronic lung disease (cystic fibrosis or severe asthma). Episodes are caused by a prolonged bout of severe coughing, leading to increased intrathoracic pressure and a secondary decrease in cardiac output.
7. Cerebrooclusive disease: Extremely rare in the adolescent, unless some predisposing factor such as sickle cell anemia, vasculitis, or vascular anomaly exists.
8. Migraine: Adolescents with migraines can have syncope, vertigo, or dizziness, either preceding or accompanying the headaches. These symptoms may be the presenting complaint, and more prominent than the headache itself (see Chapter 22). Migraines characterized by vertigo, dizziness, or ataxia are generally classified as *basilar artery migraines*.

VERTIGO

Vertigo is a sensation of rotary movement. The world seems to revolve around the patient or the patient senses that he or she is spinning. In contrast, dizziness is generally a sensation of movement or instability without a directional rotary component. Vertigo is much less common in the adolescent than nonspecific dizziness, lightheadedness, or syncope. Causes of true vertigo may be either peripheral or central. Occasionally, vertigo may be the primary or initial symptom of a complex partial seizure (see Chapter 21).

Peripheral Etiologies

Most peripheral vertigo is accompanied by tinnitus and/or hearing loss.

1. Vestibular neuritis (acute labyrinthitis): Usually a result of an acute viral or bacterial infection or local trauma. This usually resolves over several days. Vertigo is

TABLE 23.5

Peripheral versus Central Vertigo

Characteristics	Peripheral Vertigo	Central Vertigo
Onset	Usually paroxysmal	Seldom paroxysmal
Intensity	Severe	Seldom severe
Duration	Usually short	Longer
Influence of head position	Frequent	Seldom
Autonomic nervous system symptoms	Definite	Less intense or absent
Tinnitus	Frequent	Seldom present
Hearing loss	Frequently present	Seldom present
Disturbances of consciousness	Seldom present	More frequently present
Focal neurological deficits	Infrequent	Frequent
Associated symptoms	Nausea, vomiting	Visual, headaches

generally intense, position sensitive, and accompanied by nausea and vomiting.

2. Benign positional vertigo: Characterized by a spinning sensation after quick movements of the head or body. The attacks last seconds to minutes, occur abruptly, and are generally not associated with nausea or vomiting. The cause is unknown in most patients. In older patients, canaliths (small accretions in the semicircular canals) may cause positional vertigo and may respond to maneuvers to alter their position.

3. Ototoxic drugs: Aminoglycosides, diuretics (furosemide), aspirin, caffeine, phenytoin (Dilantin), and alcohol may cause transient or permanent vertigo.

4. Acoustic neuromas: Vertigo with or without tinnitus and hearing loss in the affected ear. Bilateral acoustic neuromas are associated with neurofibromatosis type 2, often with onset in adolescence.

5. Méniére disease: Rare in adolescents. This is characterized by vertigo, tinnitus, and hearing loss secondary to an increase in endolymph. Symptoms are generally intermittent.

6. Perilymphatic fistulas: Are commonly associated with sudden onset of vertigo and hearing loss.

7. Otitis media: Occasionally associated with true vertigo in adolescents.

8. Motion sickness.

9. Ear obstruction (i.e., cerumen compacted against the tympanic membrane).

Central Etiologies

Central lesions of the brain stem or cerebellar tracts involving vestibular input or vestibuloocular pathways may cause vertigo. Central lesions causing true vertigo are often accompanied by ataxia or other motor signs due to involvement of adjacent structures. Cerebellar or brain stem lesions may be caused by the following:

1. Tumors, including lesions of the brain stem and cerebellum.

2. Demyelinating diseases (e.g., multiple sclerosis).

3. Vasculitis (lupus, isolated central nervous system [CNS] angiitis).

4. Cerebral infarctions (stroke).

5. Infections of the nervous system (encephalitis) or postinfectious inflammatory demyelination.

6. Migraine: Basilar migraine may include symptoms of vertigo, although nonspecific dizziness is more common.

7. Brain injury due to head trauma.

History

History is crucial to the evaluation of vertigo, because it allows differentiation of vertigo from syncope and seizures. The history may also be helpful in identifying the specific etiology for the vertigo. In most cases, the diagnosis is established by history and negative physical and neurological examination findings.

1. Descriptions of the episode and any previous attacks help define the nature of the attack.

2. Circumstances preceding the attack.

3. Precipitating factors.

4. Alleviating factors: Recumbency; food, fresh air, and sudden movements.

5. The history may also be helpful in differentiating peripheral from central vertigo (Table 23.5).

Physical Examination

General physical examination with special emphasis on the following:

1. Neurological examination:
   a. Evidence of cranial nerve deficits, particularly III, IV, VI, VII, and VIII; funduscopic examination
   b. Focal motor deficits
   c. Tendon reflexes: Loss, asymmetry, and hyperreflexia
   d. Cerebellar function: Truncal or appendicular ataxia
   e. Nystagmus with straight gaze: Horizontal suggests peripheral etiology, whereas a vertical and diagonal nystagmus is more suggestive of central etiology
   f. Sensory abnormalities: Peripheral sensory loss suggests neuropathy
   g. Skin color, temperature, response to "scratch" to check for evidence of autonomic neuropathy

2. Special examination procedures for vertigo:
   a. Quick head turn
   b. The Valsalva maneuver
   c. Sudden turn while walking

d. Nylen-Bárány test: Have the adolescent sit at the edge of a table. Holding on to the adolescent's head, have the adolescent abruptly lie back as you place his or her head 45 degrees below the table and at a 45-degree angle to one side. Repeat the test with his head at a 45-degree angle to the opposite side. Elicitation of nystagmus indicates a "positive" test result, suggesting benign positional vertigo.

Further Evaluation

For sustained vertigo unassociated with an acute infection or vertigo that seems positional in origin, referral to a neurologist or otolaryngologist is advisable for further evaluation and testing. Patients with abrupt onset of vertigo and hearing loss should be promptly evaluated by an otolaryngologist.

Management

Dizziness and vertigo associated with migraine should be treated as migraine (see Chapter 22). Treatment of vertigo is difficult. For the short-term treatment of vertigo and vomiting associated with acute labyrinthitis, antiemetics or mild sedatives may be useful, but they all cause drowsiness.

Benign positional vertigo may respond to deconditioning maneuvers (e.g., repeatedly provoking the vertigo with position changes to gradually suppress the response). Benign positional vertigo due to canaliths may respond to maneuvers for repositioning the canalith.

Vertigo associated with significant CNS disease is problematic, because long-term treatment with sedating medication is generally unacceptable, and nonsedating medications are usually ineffective. Central vertigo due to acute CNS lesions such as strokes generally decreases or abates entirely, but this process may take months or years. Epileptic vertigo is rare but generally responds to anticonvulsant drugs (see Chapter 21).

SUDDEN DEATH IN ADOLESCENTS AND YOUNG ADULTS

Accidents, suicide, and homicide are the most frequent causes of sudden death in adolescents. After these traumatic events, exacerbations of chronic medical conditions—notably asthma and epilepsy—are significant, with SCD representing only approximately 10% of the overall sudden death rate (Driscoll and Edwards, 1985). The incidence of SCD is approximately 1/100,000 patient-years in the pediatric and young adult population, whereas the overall U.S. mortality rate is 17/100,000 patient-years for 15- to 19-year olds (Wren et al., 2000) (http://www.childtrendsdatabank.org/figures/63-Figure-2.gif). HCM is the most common cause of SCD in the 15- to 35-year old age group, yet it is still rare, with an incidence of <1 death per 1,000,000/year (Wren, 2002). Despite the rarity of SCD, sudden death due to HCM, LQTS, and other potentially occult cardiac conditions occurs in several hundred adolescents in the United States each year.

Etiologies of Sudden Unexpected Cardiac Death in Children and Adolescents

1. Structural or functional abnormalities: Many of these conditions may have a familial component
   a. HCM (described in the preceding text)
   b. Arrhythmogenic right ventricular dysplasia
   c. Coronary artery abnormalities, including aberrant left and right coronary arteries, hypoplastic coronary artery syndrome, Kawasaki syndrome, and Williams syndrome with coronary ostial stenosis
   d. Primary pulmonary hypertension
   e. Myocarditis/dilated cardiomyopathy
   f. Restrictive cardiomyopathy
   g. Marfan syndrome with aortic dissection
   h. Aortic valve stenosis
2. Primary electrical abnormalities
   a. LQTSs, acquired or congenital (described in the preceding text)
   b. Brugada syndrome
   c. Wolff-Parkinson-White syndrome
   d. Primary or idiopathic ventricular tachycardia/fibrillation
   e. Catecholamine-exercise ventricular tachycardia
   f. Heart block, congenital or acquired
3. Acquired conditions
   a. Commotio cordis
   b. Drug abuse: Cocaine, stimulants, inhalants ("sudden sniffing death syndrome")
   c. Secondary pulmonary artery hypertension (Eisenmenger syndrome)
   d. Atherosclerotic coronary artery disease (CAD)
4. Postoperative congenital heart disease
   a. Tetralogy of Fallot
   b. Transposition of the great arteries (after Mustard/Senning repair or after the arterial switch operation)
   c. Fontan surgery
   d. Hypoplastic left heart syndrome
   e. Coarctation of the aorta (after patch angioplasty, aneurysm at repair site)
   f. Cardiac transplantation

Each of these cardiac abnormalities carries differing levels of risk for SCD or other morbidity. Any patient with a suspected cardiac condition should be referred to a cardiologist for a full evaluation, and determination of appropriate athletic and recreational activities.

Evaluation

Important historical details include a history of syncopal episodes, significant exercise intolerance, exertional chest discomfort, and a family history of premature CAD, sudden death in a person younger than 40 years, syncope, or hypertension.

Physical Examination

Clues to cardiac disease include hypertension, abnormal cardiac rhythm, heart murmur, or a body habitus suggestive of Marfan syndrome. However, most patients at risk of sudden death will have a completely normal physical examination.

Laboratory Tests

The ECG is a convenient screening tool, but is often normal. Exercise electrocardiography is useful in an adolescent with symptoms of exertional chest discomfort, syncope, exercise intolerance, or worrisome palpitations. Routine screening with echocardiography or chest x-ray offers little additional value, and is not recommended. For further recommendations on athletic limitations associated with these conditions, see Chapter 18.

Prevention

SCD in children, adolescents, and young adults may be prevented by both primary and secondary prevention programs. The accuracy of presymptomatic diagnostic testing and cost-effectiveness of a widespread preparticipation screening program are controversial issues. Current opinion in the United States is that existing data do not demonstrate that screening with ECGs, echocardiograms, or exercise testing prevents sudden death. In 1996, the American Heart Association concluded that the best screening for cardiovascular disease in athletes is a complete personal history, with thorough evaluation of cardiac or exercise-associated symptoms, a thorough family history, and a careful physical examination (Maron, 2003). Pilot studies continue with the use of screening echocardiography. Secondary prevention programs include chest protectors, maintenance of adequate hydration, the use of automatic electrical defibrillators, emergency response plans for schools, and training of personnel in basic cardiopulmonary resuscitation (CPR).

WEB SITES

For Teenagers and Parents

http://cpmcnet.columbia.edu/dept/syncope/. A comprehensive clinical center for patients who have fainted, who are recurrently lightheaded, or who have related cardiovascular disease. Much information on syncope.

http://www.americanheart.org. American Heart Association site. Search for syncope.

For Health Professionals

http://www.acponline.org. Links to July 1997 *Annals of Internal Medicine* position paper with informed, adult-oriented but relevant clinical guidelines for diagnosing syncope.

http://www.torsades.org. A comprehensive, and frequently updated, list of drugs affecting the QT interval.

REFERENCES AND ADDITIONAL READINGS

Abu-Arafeh I, Russell G. Paroxysmal vertigo as a migraine equivalent in children: a population-based study. *Cephalalgia* 1995;15:22.

Aysun S, Apak A. Syncope as a first sign of seizure disorder. *J Child Neurol* 2000;15:59.

Benditt DL, Fahy GJ, Lurie KG, et al. Pharmacotherapy of neurally mediated syncope. *Circulation* 1999;100:1242.

Boehm KE, Morris EJ, Kip KT, et al. Diagnosis and management of neurally mediated syncope and related conditions in adolescents. *J Adolesc Health* 2001;28:2.

Bower CM, Cotton RT. The spectrum of vertigo in children. *Arch Otolaryngol Head Neck Surg* 1995;121:911.

Cadman CS. Medical therapy of neurocardiogenic syncope. *Cardiol Clin* 2001;19:203.

D'Agostino R, Tarantino V, Melagrana A, et al. Otoneurologic evaluation of child vertigo. *Int J Pediatr Otorhinolaryngol* 1997;40:133.

DiVasta AD, Alexander ME. Fainting freshmen and sinking sophomores: cardiovascular issues of the adolescent. *Curr Opin Pediatr* 2004;16:350.

Driscoll DJ, Edwards WD. Sudden unexpected death in children and adolescents. *J Am Coll Cardiol* 1985;5:118B.

Driscoll DJ, Jacobsen SJ, Porter CJ, et al. Syncope in children and adolescents. *J Am Coll Cardiol* 1997;29:1039.

Goroll AH, May LA, Mulley AG. Evaluation of dizziness. In: Goroll AH, May LA, Mulley AG, eds. *Primary care medicine*. Philadelphia: JB Lippincott Co, 1995.

Grubb BP. Clinical practice. Neurocardiogenic syncope. *N Engl J Med* 2005;352:1004.

Hanna DE, Hodgens JB, Daniel WA Jr. Hyperventilation syndrome. *Pediatr Ann* 1986;15:708.

Heaton JM, Barton J, Ranalli P, et al. Evaluation of the dizzy patient: experience from a multidisciplinary neurology clinic. *J Laryngol Otol* 1999;113:19.

Ishiyama A, Jacobson KM, Baloh RW. Migraine and benign positional vertigo. *Ann Otol Rhinol Laryngol* 2000;109:377.

Kentala E. Characteristics of six otologic diseases involving vertigo. *Am J Otol* 1996;17:883.

Lanzi G, Balottin U, Fazzi E, et al. Benign paroxysmal vertigo of childhood: a long-term follow-up. *Cephalalgia* 1994;14:458.

Lee PW, Leung PW, Fung AS, et al. An episode of syncope attacks in adolescent schoolgirls: investigations, intervention, and outcome. *Br J Med Psychol* 1996;69(Pt 3):247.

Lewis DA, Dhala A. Syncope in the pediatric patient. The cardiologist's perspective. *Pediatr Clin North Am* 1999;46:205.

Linzer M, Varia I, Pontinen M, et al. Medically unexplained syncope: relationship to psychiatric illness. *Am J Med* 1992;92:185.

Mathias CJ, Kimber JR. Postural hypotension: causes, clinical features, investigation, and management [Review]. *Annu Rev Med* 1999;50:317.

McLeod KA. Syncope in childhood. *Arch Dis Child* 2003;88:350.

Moss AJ. Long QT syndrome. *JAMA* 2003;289:2041.

Nishimura RA, Holmes DR Jr. Clinical practice. Hypertrophic obstructive cardiomyopathy. *N Engl J Med* 2004;350:1320.

Ritter S, Tani LY, Etheridge SP, et al. What is the yield of screening echocardiography in pediatric syncope? *Pediatrics* 2000;105:E58.

Russell G, Abu-Arafeh I. Paroxysmal vertigo in children—an epidemiological study. *Int J Pediatr Otorhinolaryngol* 1999;49 (Suppl 1):S105.

Salim MA, Di Sessa TG. Effectiveness of fludrocortisone and salt in preventing syncope recurrence in children: a double-blind, placebo-controlled, randomized trial. *J Am Coll Cardiol* 2005;45:484.

Soteriades ES, Evans JC, Larson MG, et al. Incidence and prognosis of syncope. *N Engl J Med* 2002;347:878.

Steinberg LA, Knilans TK. Syncope in children: diagnostic tests have a high cost and low yield. *J Pediatr* 2005;146: 355.

Stewart JM. Transient orthostatic hypotension is common in adolescents. *J Pediatr* 2002;140:418.

Stewart JM, Gewitz MH, Weldon A, et al. Orthostatic intolerance in adolescent chronic fatigue syndrome. *Pediatrics* 1999;102:116.

Sung RY, Du ZD, Yu CW, et al. Cerebral blood flow during vasovagal syncope induced by active standing or head up tilt. *Arch Dis Child* 2000;82:154.

Willis J. Syncope. *Pediatr Rev* 2000;21:201.

Wren C. Sudden death in children and adolescents. *Heart* 2002;88:426.

Wren C, O'Sullivan JJ, Wright C. Sudden death in children and adolescents. *Heart* 2000;83:410.

CHAPTER 24

Sleep Disorders

Shelly K. Weiss

Sleep is one of our basic needs. It is important for our physical, intellectual, and emotional health. Lack of sleep makes us tired and irritable, decreases short-term memory, and can result in mistakes at work and school, as well as sleep-related accidents. Sleep disturbances are common in adolescents. Many young people acknowledge difficulties with sleep (often not obtaining adequate sleep) when specifically asked, although it may not be their chief complaint.

Sleep disorders are classified into four categories—*dyssomnias* cover a wide range of disorders including difficulty initiating or maintaining sleep, early morning waking (insomnias), and excessive sleepiness; *parasomnias* are disorders associated with undesirable physical (motor or autonomic) phenomena that occur exclusively or predominantly during sleep; *sleep disorders associated with medical/psychiatric disorders,* and *proposed sleep disorders* (Table 24.1) (International Classification of Sleep Disorders [ICSD-R], 2001). Sleep disturbances in adolescents may represent a reaction to anxiety or depression, inadequate sleep due to busy school or work schedules, and drug use (e.g., stimulants, barbiturates, or use of caffeine, nicotine, alcohol, hallucinogens, or other nonprescription substances). In addition, sleep disturbances can be secondary to a specific sleep disorder.

SLEEP PHYSIOLOGY

Sleep is divided into rapid eye movement (REM) sleep and nonrapid eye movement (NREM) sleep. Studies of sleep physiology are carried out using polysomnography, which usually includes electroencephalogram (EEG), electrooculogram, electromyogram, and measures of respiratory function such as airflow, oxygen saturation, and end-tidal P_{CO_2} levels.

Rapid Eye Movement Sleep

REM sleep occupies 20% to 30% of sleep time in adolescents and is characterized by a high autonomic arousal state including increased cardiovascular and respiratory activity, very low voluntary muscle tone, and rapid synchronous nonpatterned eye movements. The EEG pattern shows a low-voltage variable frequency resembling the awake state. Most dreams occur during REM sleep.

Nonrapid Eye Movement Sleep

NREM sleep occupies 70% to 80% of sleep time in adolescents and is divided into four stages:

1. Stage 1: Very light sleep, characterized on EEG by alpha waves similar to the quiet awake state.
2. Stage 2: Medium-deep sleep, characterized on EEG by the presence of sleep spindles, K-complexes, and a change from alpha waves to slower, higher amplitude brain waves compared to stage 1.
3. Stages 3 and 4: Also called *slow-wave sleep*; progressively deeper sleep, characterized on EEG by a general slowing of frequency and an increase in amplitude (delta waves). Muscular and cardiovascular activity are decreased and little dreaming occurs.

SLEEP PATTERN AND CHANGES DURING ADOLESCENCE

Normal sleep usually consists of a brief period of stage 1 and stage 2, followed by a lengthier interval of stages 3 and 4. After approximately 70 to 100 minutes of NREM sleep, a 10- to 25-minute REM period occurs. This cycle is repeated four to six times approximately every 90 minutes throughout the night. The REM periods usually increase by 5 to 30 minutes each cycle.

There are developmental changes in sleep patterns that occur between infancy and adulthood. A meta-analysis of age-related changes in objectively recorded sleep patterns reported a decrease in slow-wave sleep of 7% per 5-year period between the ages of 5 and 15 years. There was a concurrent increase in the lighter stage of NREM (stage 2) sleep (Ohayon et al., 2004).

Another documented change in sleep during adolescence is a delay in the circadian timing system. With progressive adolescent development (documented by increasing sexual maturity ratings), there is a tendency for lengthening the internal day. This coupled with the increasing time devoted to academic, employment, social, and extracurricular activities can cause progressive delay in bedtime (Carskadon et al., 1998).

Adolescents require a minimum of 8.5 to 9.5 hours of sleep per night to awake refreshed and rested. A research study has documented that on school nights, 10- to 11-year

TABLE 24.1

Classification of Sleep Disorders

Dyssomnia: disorders that produce complaints of insomnia (difficulty initiating or maintaining sleep or early morning awakening) and/or excessive daytime sleepiness	Parasomnia: disorders in which unusual behavior occurs during sleep, which may not necessarily produce insomnia or complaints of sleepiness	Sleep disorders associated with medical/psychiatric disorders	Proposed sleep disorders

From International Classification of Sleep Disorders Revised (ICSD-R). *Diagnostic and coding manual.* American Sleep Disorders Association, 2001.

olds sleep an average of 9.5 hours, 12- to 13-year-olds sleep 9 hours, 14- to 15-year-olds sleep 7.75 hours, 16- to 17-year-olds sleep 7.5 hours, and 18-year-old college freshmen sleep 7 hours. The adolescent often tries to make up for the sleep deficit accumulated during the week by sleeping much longer on weekends.

Sleep History

Any adolescent with a sleep disturbance should be asked about the following:

a. Sleep complaint
   - Both the adolescent and the parent should describe the presenting sleep complaint. This is to determine if the perception of the complaint differs between people in the family.
   - A description of the complaint should include age at onset, timing during sleep, duration, frequency, and intermittent or continuous nature of the complaint.
   - Treatment previously tried, length of trial, and result.
b. General sleep history
   - Prior sleep problems
   - Description of bedroom environment, bedtime (weekdays and weekends) and bedtime routines—what is done before sleep, sleep onset location, presence of light, noise, television, or computer in bedroom.
   - Description of sleep—time to fall asleep, amount of sleep, regularity of sleep and wake schedules.
   - Nocturnal arousals—frequency, timing, duration, behavior during arousal, presence of amnesia for event, and response to intervention at time of arousal.
   - Snoring, restlessness (this question must be asked of someone who observes the adolescent while sleeping).
   - Daytime symptoms—time and mood upon waking, daytime naps, daytime sleepiness, timing and regularity of exercise, intake of caffeine, nicotine, ethanol, and nonprescription drugs.
c. Medical history
   - Medical, psychiatric, and surgical history (including history of tonsillectomy and adenoidectomy).
   - Medication history including over-the-counter medications, herbal products, dietary supplements, weight-loss products, performance-enhancing substances, and other stimulants.
d. Psychosocial and academic history
e. Family history, including history of sleep problems

Physical Examination

A targeted physical examination should be done depending on the particular sleep complaint.

Sleep Diary

Have an adolescent keep a 1- to 2-week sleep diary, listing bedtimes, nighttime symptoms, time on awakening, daytime fatigue or sleepiness, and daytime naps, can be a very helpful tool in evaluating a sleep disturbance (Fig. 24.1).

SLEEP DISORDERS IN ADOLESCENTS

In order to appropriately evaluate and manage an adolescent with a sleep disorder, the specific sleep disorder must be determined. Examples of adolescent sleep disorders include the following:

Dyssomnias

Dyssomnia Due to Inadequate Sleep
The most common cause of excessive daytime sleepiness in adolescents (and people of all ages) is inadequate sleep. Inadequate sleep may be due to poor sleeping habits or late bedtimes (often due to busy schedules). Adolescents may have rigorous schedules with academic, employment, and extracurricular activities that result in their having less than the required hours of sleep. In addition, in some school districts, high school starting times are earlier than middle school leaving even less time for sleep. This chronic sleep deprivation may cause complaints of fatigue or difficulty staying awake during school or work, adversely affecting performance. This may result in stimulant use to stay awake, moodiness, and even automobile accidents related to falling asleep at the wheel. Drowsiness or fatigue is associated with >100,000 automobile accidents each year and are especially common in the 16- to 25-year-old driver.

Other causes of inadequate sleep include difficulty falling asleep as a result of stress, anxiety, or depression. Adolescents with depression frequently have sleep onset or sleep maintenance insomnia. Other less common causes of insomnia include any physical illness associated with pain or discomfort and substance abuse or withdrawal (particularly stimulants, alcohol, or sedatives). Medications may

Fill out days 1–7 below	**COMPLETE IN MORNING**						
	I went to bed last night at:	I got out of bed this morning at:	Last night I fell asleep in:	I woke up during the night: (Record number of times)	When I woke up for the day I felt: (Check one)	Last night I slept a total of: (Record number of hours)	My sleep was disturbed by: (List any mental, emotional, physical, or environmental factors that affected your sleep, e.g., stress, snoring, physical discomfort, temperature)
DAY 1 day _____ date _____	PM/AM	PM/AM	Minutes	Times	___Refreshed ___Somewhat Refreshed ___Fatigued	Hours	
DAY 2 day _____ date _____	PM/AM	PM/AM	Minutes	Times	___Refreshed ___Somewhat Refreshed ___Fatigued	Hours	
DAY 3 day _____ date _____	PM/AM	PM/AM	Minutes	Times	___Refreshed ___Somewhat Refreshed ___Fatigued	Hours	
DAY 4 day _____ date _____	PM/AM	PM/AM	Minutes	Times	___Refreshed ___Somewhat Refreshed ___Fatigued	Hours	
DAY 5 day _____ date _____	PM/AM	PM/AM	Minutes	Times	___Refreshed ___Somewhat Refreshed ___Fatigued	Hours	
DAY 6 day _____ date _____	PM/AM	PM/AM	Minutes	Times	___Refreshed ___Somewhat Refreshed ___Fatigued	Hours	
DAY 7 day _____ date _____	PM/AM	PM/AM	Minutes	Times	___Refreshed ___Somewhat Refreshed ___Fatigued	Hours	

FIGURE 24.1 Sleep diary. (From The National Sleep Foundation. *1999 sleep in America poll results*. Washington, DC: The National Sleep Foundation, 1999, with permission.)

also cause insomnia, including selective serotonin reuptake inhibitors (SSRIs), stimulants, sympathomimetics, and corticosteroids.

Dyssomnia Due to Delayed Sleep Phase Syndrome

Daytime sleepiness can result from delayed bedtime resulting in extreme difficulty in waking in the morning. Adolescents are particularly prone to this problem because of their busy evening schedules and an intrinsic biological preference for a later bedtime.

A delayed sleep phase syndrome is a circadian phase disorder in which the timing of sleep is delayed. The adolescent has difficulty falling asleep and waking at an expected time; the person tends to fall asleep 3 to 6 hours later than the desired bedtime. If the adolescent is allowed to sleep for a normal length of time, he/she will wake refreshed but will have a difficult time waking for work, school, or social needs because the timing of waking will also be delayed by 3 to 6 hours. If the adolescent is awakened to attend school, he/she may have difficulty arising and may experience daytime sleepiness due to inadequate sleep. If the adolescent is asked to fall asleep at a normal bedtime, he/she will have sleep-onset insomnia.

Dyssomnia Due to Obstructive Sleep Apnea Syndrome

The main cause of sleep-disordered breathing (SDB) is obstructive sleep apnea syndrome (OSAS). This is the presence of complete or partial obstruction of the upper airway during sleep and is associated with the following history:

• Habitual snoring with labored breathing
• Observed apnea
• Restless sleep
• Daytime neurobehavioral abnormalities or sleepiness

Even if obstructive sleep apnea is present, there may be no abnormalities seen on physical examination. Physical examination may reveal evidence of the following (American Academy of Pediatrics, 2002):

• Growth abnormalities
• Signs of nasal obstruction
• Adenoidal facies
• Enlarged tonsils
• Increased pulmonic component of second heart sound

Risk factors include obesity, African-American heritage, and other respiratory factors such as chronic cough, occasional and persistent wheezing, sinus problems, and asthma.

Fill out days 1–7 below	COMPLETE AT END OF DAY				
	I consumed caffeinated drinks in the: (e.g. coffee, tea, cola)	I exercised at least 20 minutes in the:	Approximately 2-3 hours before going to bed, I consumed:	Medication(s) I took during the day: (List name of medication/drugs):	About 1 hour before going to sleep, I did the following activity: (List activity: e.g. watch TV, work, read)
DAY 1 day _____ date _____	___Morning ___Afternoon ___About 2–3 hrs. before going to bed ___Not applicable	___Morning ___Afternoon ___About 2–3 hrs. before going to bed ___Not applicable	___Alcohol ___A heavy meal ___Not applicable	_____ _____ _____	_____ _____ _____
DAY 2 day _____ date _____	___Morning ___Afternoon ___About 2–3 hrs. before going to bed ___Not applicable	___Morning ___Afternoon ___About 2–3 hrs. before going to bed ___Not applicable	___Alcohol ___A heavy meal ___Not applicable	_____ _____ _____	_____ _____ _____
DAY 3 day _____ date _____	___Morning ___Afternoon ___About 2–3 hrs. before going to bed ___Not applicable	___Morning ___Afternoon ___About 2–3 hrs. before going to bed ___Not applicable	___Alcohol ___A heavy meal ___Not applicable	_____ _____ _____	_____ _____ _____
DAY 4 day _____ date _____	___Morning ___Afternoon ___About 2–3 hrs. before going to bed ___Not applicable	___Morning ___Afternoon ___About 2–3 hrs. before going to bed ___Not applicable	___Alcohol ___A heavy meal ___Not applicable	_____ _____ _____	_____ _____ _____
DAY 5 day _____ date _____	___Morning ___Afternoon ___About 2–3 hrs. before going to bed ___Not applicable	___Morning ___Afternoon ___About 2–3 hrs. before going to bed ___Not applicable	___Alcohol ___A heavy meal ___Not applicable	_____ _____ _____	_____ _____ _____
DAY 6 day _____ date _____	___Morning ___Afternoon ___About 2–3 hrs. before going to bed ___Not applicable	___Morning ___Afternoon ___About 2–3 hrs. before going to bed ___Not applicable	___Alcohol ___A heavy meal ___Not applicable	_____ _____ _____	_____ _____ _____
DAY 7 day _____ date _____	___Morning ___Afternoon ___About 2–3 hrs. before going to bed ___Not applicable	___Morning ___Afternoon ___About 2–3 hrs. before going to bed ___Not applicable	___Alcohol ___A heavy meal ___Not applicable	_____ _____ _____	_____ _____ _____

FIGURE 24.1   *(Continued)*

Sleep studies are used to evaluate for apnea (defined as the absence of any effective airflow into the lungs) or hypopneas (defined as incomplete apnea). A sleep study in a person with obstructive sleep apnea demonstrates a pause in breathing, lasting >10 seconds with an associated decrease in oxygen saturation. An apnea-hypopnea index (AHI) divides the number of respiratory events by the estimated sleep time. Different thresholds are used with little consensus. An AHI of 10 is a reasonable cutoff for adolescents.

Narcolepsy

Narcolepsy is a chronic neurological disorder characterized by two major abnormalities—excessive and overwhelming daytime sleepiness and intrusion of REM sleep phenomenon into wakefulness. The age at onset is usually between 10 and 25 years.

Symptoms

The first and primary manifestation of narcolepsy is excessive daytime sleepiness. The disorder is characterized by the following four classic symptoms:

- Sleep attacks: Intrusive and debilitating periods of sleep during the day that may last anywhere from a few seconds to 30 minutes. These periods are often precipitated by sedentary, monotonous activity, and are more frequent after meals and later in the day. Sleepiness is transiently relieved after short naps, but will gradually increase again within the 2 to 3 hours following the nap.
- Cataplexy: Abrupt, brief (seconds to minutes), bilateral loss or reduction of postural muscle tone while conscious, precipitated by intense emotions (e.g., anger, fright, surprise, excitement, or laughter). This is the most valuable symptom in the diagnosis of narcolepsy.
- Sleep paralysis: Temporary loss of muscle tone occurring with the onset of sleep or upon awakening.
- Hypnagogic and hypnopompic hallucinations: Hallucinations that can be visual, auditory, tactile, or kinetic (with sensation of movement) with the onset of sleep (hypnagogic) or upon awakening (hypnopompic). People without narcolepsy may have occasional sleep paralysis and/or hypnagogic hallucinations. In addition, people with narcolepsy may have automatic activity during periods of altered consciousness.

Frequency of components:
- Sleep attacks: 100%
- Sleep attacks and cataplexy: 70%
- Sleep paralysis: 50%
- Hallucinations: 25%
- All four: 10%

Etiology of Narcolepsy

Narcolepsy is a genetically complex disorder. The close association between narcolepsy–cataplexy and the human leukocyte antigen (HLA) allele DQB1*0602 suggests an autoimmune etiology. Recent studies have identified abnormalities in hypothalamic hypocretin (orexin) neurotransmission (important in regulating the sleep–wake cycle) and in the pathophysiology of narcolepsy (Chabas et al., 2003).

Diagnosis of Narcolepsy

Narcolepsy is diagnosed by history and documentation of objective findings using both overnight polysomnography and daytime multiple sleep latency test (MSLT). The overnight polysomnography will exclude other sleep disorders, such as sleep apnea. The MSLT is the most specific test for narcolepsy. It will show a shortened time to sleep onset (sleep latency) and early onset of REM sleep.

Parasomnias

Sleepwalking and Night Terrors (Disorders of Partial Arousal)

Sleepwalking (somnambulism) and night terrors (sleep terrors, pavor nocturnus) are both disorders of impaired and partial arousal from deep slow-wave sleep.

- Both conditions occur in the first one third of the sleep episode, during the rapid transition from deep NREM sleep to light NREM sleep.
- Both conditions usually begin in childhood or early adolescence and disappear by older adolescence.
- Approximately 40% of 6- to 16-year-old children have at least one episode of sleepwalking and 1% to 3% experience night terrors.
- A positive family history is found in one or both parents in >60% of cases.
- Characteristics
  Sleepwalking (somnambulism):
  – Usually lasts from 1 to 30 minutes.
  – The person usually has a low level of awareness manifested by clumsiness.
  – The individual usually has a blank expression with indifference to the environment.
  – There is usually no recall of the experience.
  Night terrors (sleep terrors, pavor nocturnus):

  – Intense anxiety, fear, and sensation of doom that starts suddenly.
  – Autonomic discharge (tachycardia, tachypnea, and sweating).
  – Vocalizations in the form of screams, moans, or gasps.
  – There is usually no recall of the experience.
- Psychological disturbances are thought to be a more likely cause of night terrors or sleepwalking if the onset is after age 12 years, the condition has persisted for several years, there is a negative family history, and there is maladaptive daytime behavior.
- Hysterical phenomena such as fugue states are suggested by a more alert state, more purposeful movements, and longer duration.

Rapid Eye Movement–Related Parasomnia

1. *Nightmares (dream anxiety attacks)*: This is the most common type of REM–related parasomnia (Table 24.2).
   a. Frequent nightmares affect approximately 5% of the population and are more common in children than adults. There is an increased incidence with insomnia.
   b. Onset is usually before age 10 years. Onset after this age is more suggestive of psychological cause.
   c. Often associated with fear of attack, falling, or death.
   d. Nightmares occur in the last one third to one half of the sleep episode.
   e. Drug withdrawal, particularly from benzodiazepines, barbiturates, or alcohol can lead to nightmares.
2. *Sleep paralysis, hypnagogic and hypnopompic hallucinations.*

   Although frequently seen in narcolepsy, they can occur in nonnarcoleptics.

Nocturnal Enuresis

a. Approximately 2% to 3% of 12-year-old children and 1% to 3% of older adolescents are enuretic (enuresis is discussed in Chapter 26).
b. Enuresis is independent of stage of sleep.
c. Enuresis may be primary or secondary.
d. Etiology of primary enuresis. The cause is likely mutifactorial:
   - There is probably a genetic component as a positive family history is often found in most young people with this condition.
   - Maturational delay in neuromuscular control of the bladder.

TABLE 24.2

Characteristics of Night Terrors (Arousal Disorder) versus Nightmares (Rapid Eye Movement–Related Parasomnia)

Characteristic	Night Terrors	Nightmares
Vocalization	Intense	Limited
Autonomic activity	Marked increase	Slight increase
Arousal	Difficult	Easy
Motility	Marked	Limited
Recall	Minimal	Vivid
Sleep stage	NREM sleep	REM sleep

NREM, nonrapid eye movement; REM, rapid eye movement.

- Blunting of the diurnal antidiuretic hormone secretion, resulting in an increased nocturnal urine production that exceeds the functional bladder capacity.
e. Sleep apnea has also been associated with enuresis.

TREATMENT OF SLEEP DISORDERS

Prevention

Preventive counseling can preclude the development of certain sleep disorders that are secondary to poor sleep habits. The sleep-smart tips for teens from the National Sleep Foundation (www.sleepfoundation.org) are useful for adolescents with and without complaints of sleep difficulties.

Sleep-Smart Tips for Teens

1. Sleep is food for the brain: Get enough of it, and get it when you need it. Even mild sleepiness can hurt your performance—from taking school exams to playing sports or video games. Lack of sleep can make you look tired and feel depressed, irritable, and angry.
2. Keep consistency in mind: Establish a regular bedtime and wake-time schedule, and maintain it during weekends and school (or work) vacations. Don't stray from your schedule frequently, and never do so for two or more consecutive nights. If you must go off schedule, avoid delaying your bedtime by more than 1 hour, awaken the next day within 2 hours of your regular schedule, and, if you are sleepy during the day, take an early afternoon nap.
3. Learn how much sleep you need to function at your best. You should awaken refreshed, not tired. Most adolescents need between 8.5 and 9.25 hours of sleep each night. Know when you need to get up in the morning, then calculate when you need to go to sleep to get at least 8.5 hours of sleep a night.
4. Get into bright light as soon as possible in the morning, but avoid it in the evening. The light helps to signal to the brain when it should wake up and when it should prepare to sleep.
5. Understand your circadian rhythm. Then, you can try to maximize your schedule throughout the day according to your internal clock. For example, to compensate for your "slump (sleepy) times," participate in stimulating activities or classes that are interactive, and avoid lecture classes or potentially unsafe activities, including driving.
6. After lunch (or after noon), stay away from coffee, colas with caffeine, and nicotine, which are all stimulants. Also avoid alcohol, which disrupts sleep.
7. Relax before going to bed. Avoid heavy reading, studying, and computer games within 1 hour of going to bed. Don't fall asleep with the television on—flickering light and stimulating content can inhibit restful sleep. If you work during the week, try to avoid working night hours. If you work until 9:30 p.m., for example, you will still need to plan time to unwind before going to sleep.
8. Say no to all-nighters. Staying up late can cause chaos to your sleep patterns and your ability to be alert the next day ... and beyond. Remember, the best thing you can do to prepare for a test is to get plenty of sleep. All-nighters or late-night study sessions might seem to give you more time to cram for your exam, but they are also likely to drain your brainpower.

Insomnia/Excessive Daytime Sleepiness Due to Inadequate Sleep

The treatment of insomnia/excessive daytime sleepiness will differ depending on the cause. Some general management strategies include:

1. Counseling regarding any existing situational stresses.
2. Regularize bedtime and awakening hours. Try to have the adolescent wake up at a similar hour each day. Avoid excessive sleep on weekends. Avoid trying to force sleep when the adolescent is not tired.
3. Encourage regular mealtimes, especially breakfast in the morning. Avoid heavy late-night meals. A light carbohydrate snack may help induce sleep at bedtime.
4. Teach relaxation techniques.
5. Daily exercise, but not close to bedtime.
6. Curtail nicotine, alcohol, food, or beverages that contain caffeine and other stimulants.
7. Bedroom environment should be for sleep only (i.e., no television or computer in the bedroom).
8. Keep bedroom dark and as quiet as possible. Morning exposure to bright light is also helpful.
9. Avoid daytime naps.
10. Medications. Behavioral techniques should be used to treat adolescents with insomnia unless there are specific medical, psychiatric, or other sleep disorders (e.g., restless leg syndrome) that require medications. There has been a paucity of research on the use of medications for sleep disorders in adolescents. There remains a significant lack of knowledge concerning the efficacy, tolerability, and safety profiles of these medications in adolescents. As such, there are no formal guidelines for the use of these medications alone or as an adjunct in the treatment of adolescent sleep disorders (Owens et al., 2005).

Insomnia Due to Delayed Sleep Phase Syndrome

1. Review all of the above suggestions for the treatment of insomnia.
2. Another treatment for delayed sleep phase syndrome is chronotherapy which involves advancing bedtime by 15-minute intervals or by delaying the bedtime by 2- to 4-hour adjustments every few days, forcing the adolescent to sleep around the clock until reaching an appropriate bedtime with 8.5 to 9.5 hours of sleep. An expert in sleep disorders usually performs this adjustment of sleep-waking schedule. There has been limited research on the efficacy of this treatment either alone or in combination with other treatments.
3. Referral to psychologist or psychiatrist may be required for evaluation of underlying psychological issues contributing to the development and perpetuation of the delayed sleep phase syndrome.
4. Referral to a sleep specialist may be needed for adolescents who do not respond to treatment.

Insomnia Due to Obstructive Sleep Apnea Syndrome

The treatment of OSAS requires a team effort. Weight loss, tonsillectomy and adenoidectomy, constant positive airway pressure, and bi-level pressure ventilation are all modalities used to treat SDB. Consultation with pulmonology, a sleep laboratory or center, and head and neck surgery is suggested. A cardiac echocardiogram, looking for pulmonary artery hypertension or right ventricular hypertrophy, and a lateral x-ray of the soft tissues of the neck are useful studies.

Narcolepsy

1. Arrange life (school, extracurricular activities, time with friends, work, long-term career planning) to accommodate the condition.
2. Ensure regular nocturnal sleep habits, with attention to sleep hygiene.
3. Short scheduled naps during the day may prevent sleep attacks.
4. Avoid dangerous activities (driving or participating in sports when sleepy).
5. Medication for sleepiness—modafinil (a nonamphetamine central nervous system [CNS] stimulant) is effective for treating excessive daytime sleepiness. Amphetamine-like stimulants can also be used but the new treatments (modafinil and sodium oxybate) are decreasing the need for these medications (Mignot, 2004). Any of these medications should be titrated to the lowest effective dose, avoiding late afternoon or evening doses.
6. Medication for cataplexy—tricyclic antidepressants such as protriptyline, imipramine, desipramine, and clomipramine are known to suppress REM sleep. SSRIs are also effective. Sodium oxybate (also known as γ-hydroxybutyrate [GHB]) has efficacy for cataplexy and daytime sleepiness. It is a known drug of abuse associated with CNS adverse events, including death.

Parasomnias

1. Arousal disorders (sleepwalking and night terrors)
   a. Take precautions to prevent injury (e.g., limiting access to staircases, open doors and windows, harmful objects).
   b. Reassure, educate, and explain the phenomena (night terrors in preschool children should resolve with time).
   c. Evaluate precipitating factors (e.g., sleep deprivation, irregular sleep–wake schedule, medications).
   d. There is some evidence to suggest that scheduled awakenings may be helpful (fully waking an adolescent 15 to 30 minutes before expected time of arousal).
   e. Encourage stress reduction/relaxation.
   f. Refer for psychological evaluation and treatment when there is evidence of psychopathology.
   g. Pharmacotherapy is rarely needed. Some medications (e.g., benzodiazepine, tricyclic antidepressant) have been reported to have efficacy when used for a short term to "break the cycle" or to decrease arousals.

2. Nightmares (Sleep Anxiety Attacks)
   a. Evaluate and treat any underlying psychological stresses or fears.
   b. Evaluate and treat any associated alcohol or other drug abuse problems.
3. Nocturnal Enuresis
   The treatment of primary enuresis (with no organic etiology) is reviewed in Chapter 26.

Sleep Disorder Clinics

For severe sleep disorders or diagnostic dilemmas, referral to a sleep disorder clinic can help. Appendix II contains a partial list of institutions specializing in the treatment of sleep disorders.

The National Sleep Foundation keeps an updated state-wise list of accredited sleep disorder centers (www.sleepfoundation.org). In addition, clinics in the United States accredited by the American Academy of Sleep Medicine (listed by state) are available at www.aasmnet.org and clinics in Canada (listed by province) are available at www.css.to/sleep/centers.htm.

RESOURCES

Organizations

American Academy of Sleep Medicine
6301 Bandel Road, Suite 101
Rochester, MN 55901; www.asda.org
Canadian Sleep Society
www.css.to

National Center on Sleep Disorders Research
National Heart, Lung, and Blood Institute
National Institutes of Health (NIH)
9000 Rockville Pike, Bldg 31
Bethesda, MD 20892; www.nhlbi.nih.gov/about/ncsdr/index/htm

National Sleep Foundation
1522 K Street, NW, Suite 500
Washington, DC 20005; www.sleepfoundation.org

WEB SITES

For Teenagers and Parents

http://www.sleephomepages.org. Sleep Home Pages.
http://www.nhlbi.nih.gov/about/ncsdr/. NIH site about sleep disorders.
http://www.sleepnet.com/disorder.htm. Information about various sleep disorders.

For Health Professionals

http://www.aasmnet.org/. American Academy of Sleep Medicine.
http://www.css.to. Canadian Sleep Society.

REFERENCES AND ADDITIONAL READINGS

Acebo C, Wolfson AR, Carskadon MA. Relationship among self-reported sleep patterns, health, and injuries in adolescents. *Sleep Res* 1997;26:149.

Aldrich MS. Narcolepsy. *Neurology* 1992;42(Suppl 6):34.

American Academy of Pediatrics. Section on Pediatric Pulmonology, Subcommittee on Obstructive Sleep Apnea Syndrome. Clinical practice guideline: diagnosis and management of childhood obstructive sleep apnea syndrome. *Pediatrics* 2002;109:704.

American Academy of Sleep Medicine. *International classification of sleep disorders, revised: diagnostic and coding manual.* Chicago, Ill: American Academy of Sleep Medicine, 2001.

Andrade MM, Benedito-Silva AA, Domenice S, et al. Sleep characteristics of adolescents: a longitudinal study. *J Adolesc Health* 1993;14:401.

Attarian HP. Helping patients who say they cannot sleep. *Postgrad Med* 2000;107:127.

Banerjee D, Vitiello MV, Grunstein RR. Pharmacotherapy for excessive daytime sleepiness. *Sleep Med Rev* 2004;8:339.

Carskadon MA. When worlds collide: adolescent need for sleep versus societal demands. *Phi Delta Kappan* 1999;80:348.

Carskadon MA. Sleep difficulties in young people. *Arch Pediatr Adolesc Med* 2004;158:597.

Carskadon MA, Acebo C, Jenni OG. Regulation of adolescent sleep, implications for behavior. *Ann N Y Acad Sci* 2004;1021:276.

Carskadon MA, Acebo C, Richardson GS, et al. An approach to studying circadian rhythms of adolescent humans. *J Biol Rhythms* 1997;12:278.

Carskadon MA, Labyak SE, Acebo C, et al. Intrinsic circadian period of adolescent humans measured in conditions of forced desynchrony. *Neurosci Lett* 1999;260:129.

Carskadon MA, Vieira C, Acebo C. Association between puberty and delayed phase preference. *Sleep* 1993;16:258.

Carskadon MA, Wolfson AR, Acebo C, et al. Adolescent sleep patterns, circadian timing, and sleepiness at a transition to early school days. *Sleep* 1998;21:871.

Chabas D, Taheri S, Renier C, et al. The genetics of narcolepsy. *Annu Rev Genomics Hum Genet* 2003;4:459.

Dahl RE. The development and disorders of sleep. *Adv Pediatr* 1998;45:73.

Dahl RE. The consequences of insufficient sleep for adolescents: links between sleep and emotional regulation. *Phi Delta Kappan* 1999;80:354.

Dahl RE, Carskadon MA. *Sleep and its disorders in adolescence. Principles and practices of sleep medicine in the child.* Philadelphia: WB Saunders, 1995:19.

Evans JHC, Meadow SR. Desmopressin for bed wetting: length of treatment, vasopressin secretion, and response. *Arch Dis Child* 1992;67:184.

Fallone G, Owens JA, Deane J. Sleepiness in children and adolescents: clinical implications. *Sleep Med Rev* 2002;6(4):287.

Ferber R. Sleep schedule-dependent causes of insomnia and sleepiness in middle childhood and adolescence. *Pediatrician* 1990;17:13.

Frank NC, Spirito A, Stark L, et al. The use of scheduled awakening to eliminate childhood sleepwalking. *J Pediatr Psychol* 1997;22:345.

Friman PC, Warzak WJ. Nocturnal enuresis: a prevalent, persistent, yet curable parasomnia. *Pediatrician* 1990;17:38.

Fritz G, Rockney R. Practice parameter for the assessment and treatment of children and adolescents with enuresis. *J Am Acad Child Adolesc Psychiatry* 2004;43(12):1540.

Garcia J, Wills L. Sleep disorders in children and teens: helping patients and their families get some rest. *Postgrad Med* 2000;107:161.

Hjalmas K, Bengtsson B. Efficacy, safety, and dosing of desmopressin for nocturnal enuresis in Europe. *Clin Pediatr* 1993;July, (Special ed):19.

Hogg RJ, Husmann D. The role of family history in predicting response to desmopressin in nocturnal enuresis. *J Urol* 1993;150:444.

Houghton WC, Scammell TE, Thorpy M. Pharmacotherapy for cataplexy. *Sleep Med Rev* 2004;8:355.

Kates A, Soldatos CR, Kates JD. Sleep disorders: insomnia, sleepwalking, night terrors, nightmares, and enuresis. *Ann Intern Med* 1987;106:582.

Kelman BB. The sleep needs of adolescents. *J School Nurs* 1999;15:14.

Knudsen UB, Rittig S, Norgaard JP, et al. Long-term treatment of nocturnal enuresis with desmopressin. *Urol Res* 1991;19:237.

Lackgren G, Lilja B, Neveus T, et al. Desmopressin in the treatment of severe nocturnal enuresis in adolescents: a 7-year follow-up study. *Br J Urol* 1998;81(Suppl 3):17.

Lee KA, McEnany G, Weekes D. Gender differences in sleep patterns for early adolescents. *J Adolesc Health* 1999;24:16.

Liu X, Uchiyama M, Okawa M, et al. Prevalence and correlates of self-reported sleep problems among Chinese adolescents. *Sleep* 2000;21:27.

Mahowald MW, Rosen GM. Parasomnias in children. *Pediatrician* 1990;12:17.

Mercer PW, Merritt SAL, Cowell JM. Differences in reported sleep need among adolescents. *J Adolesc Health* 1998;23:259.

Mignot E. An update on the pharmacotherapy of excessive daytime sleepiness and cataplexy. *Sleep Med Rev* 2004;8:333.

Mignot E. A year in review- basic science, narcolepsy and sleep in neurologic diseases. *Sleep* 2004;27(6):1209.

Milter MM, Hajdukovic R, Erman MK. Treatment of narcolepsy with methamphetamine. *Sleep* 1993;16:306.

Mindell JA, Owens JA, Carskadon MA. Developmental features of sleep. *Child Adolesc Psychiatr Clin North Am* 1999;8:695.

Morrison DN, McGee R, Stanton WR. Sleep problems in adolescence. *J Am Acad Child Adolesc Psychiatry* 1992;31:94.

National Highway Traffic Safety Administration, US Department of Transportation. *Crashes and fatalities related to driver drowsiness/fatigue.* Research Note; 1994.

National Institutes of Health, National Center on Sleep Disorders and Research and Office of Prevention, Education, and Control. *Working group report on problem sleepiness.* August 1997.

National Institutes of Health, National Institute of Neurological Disorders and Stroke. *Understanding sleep.* NIH publication no 98–3440-c, 1998.

The National Sleep Foundation. *1999 sleep in America poll results.* Washington, DC: The National Sleep Foundation, 1999.

The National Sleep Foundation. *Adolescent sleep needs and patterns. Research report and resource guide.* Washington, DC: The National Sleep Foundation, Available at www.sleepfoundation.org. 2000.

Norgaard JP, Djurhuus JC. The pathophysiology of enuresis in children and young adults. *Clin Pediatr* 1993;July, (Special ed):5.

Ohayon MM, Carskadon MA, Guilleminault C, et al. Meta-analysis of quantitative sleep parameters from childhood to old age in healthy individuals: developing normative sleep values across the human lifespan. *Sleep* 2004;27:1238.

Owens J, Babcock D, Blumer J, et al. The use of pharmacotherapy in the treatment of pediatric insomnia in primary care: rational approaches. A consensus meeting summary. *J Clin Sleep Med* 2005;1:49.

Pagel JF. Nightmares and disorders of dreaming. *Am Fam Physician* 2000;61:2037.

Redline S, Tishler PV, Schuluchter M, et al. Risk factors for sleep-disordered breathing in children. *Am J Respir Crit Care Med* 1999;159:1527.

Reid K, Chang AM, Zee P. Circadian rhythm sleep disorders. *Med Clin North Am* 2004;88:631.

Rivinus TM, Ferber R. Practical approaches to sleep disorders in childhood. *Med Times* 1979;107:71.

Roberts RE, Roberts CR, Chen IG. Ethnocultural differences in sleep complaints among adolescents. *J Nerv Ment Dis* 2000; 188:222.

Schenck CH, Mahowald MW. Parasomnias. *Postgrad Med* 2000;107:145.

Silber MH. Chronic insomnia. *N Engl J Med* 2005;353(8):803.

Stepanski E, Zayyad A, Nigro C, et al. Sleep-disordered breathing in a predominantly African-American pediatric population. *J Sleep Res* 1999;8:65.

Taylor DJ, Jenni OG, Acebo C, et al. Sleep tendency during extended wakefulness: insights into adolescent sleep regulation and behavior. *J Sleep Res* 2005;14:239.

Terho P. Desmopressin in nocturnal enuresis. *J Urol* 1991;145: 818.

Tomoda A, Mike T, Yonamine K, et al. Disturbed circadian core body temperature rhythm and sleep disturbance in school refusal children and adolescents. *Biol Psychiatry* 1997;41: 810.

Tynjala J, Kannas L, Levalahti E. Perceived tiredness among adolescents and its association with sleep habits and use of psychoactive substances. *J Sleep Res* 1997;6:189.

US Xyrem [R]Rmulticenter Study Group. Sodium oxybate demonstrates long-term efficacy for the treatment of cataplexy in patients with narcolepsy. *Sleep Med* 2004;5;119.

Vgontzas AN, Kales A. Sleep and its disorders. *Annu Rev Med* 1999;50:387.

Wahlstrom KL, Freeman CM. *School start time study: report summary*. Minneapolis, MN: The Center for Applied Research and Educational Improvement, College of Education and Human Development, University of Minnesota, 1997.

Wolfson AR, Carskadon MA. Sleep schedules and daytime functioning in adolescents. *Child Dev* 1998;69:875.

Wolfson AR, Carskadon MA. Understanding adolescents' sleep patterns and school performance: a critical appraisal. *Sleep Med Rev* 2003;7(6):491.

Wyatt JK. Delayed sleep phase syndrome. *Sleep* 2004;27: 1195.

Zeman A, Britton T, Douglas N, et al. Narcolepsy and excessive daytime sleepiness. *BMJ* 2004;329:724.

Genitourinary Disorders

CHAPTER 25

Genitourinary Tract Disorders

Lawrence J. D'Angelo and Lawrence S. Neinstein

Genitourinary tract infections are common in adolescents. Those types most often diagnosed include cystitis, pyelonephritis, urethritis, and asymptomatic bacteriuria.

CYSTITIS

Epidemiology

1. Over the course of a lifetime, cystitis is likely to occur three to five times more commonly in women than men. For adolescents, this difference may be as great as 50-fold!
2. Ten percent to 20% of girls have at least one episode of acute cystitis during adolescence or young adulthood. Hooton et al. (1996) defined the annual incidence of a lower urinary tract infection (UTI) in female patients as 0.7 infections/person-year in a cohort of sexually active female university students. One infection appears to predispose an individual to more, with Foxman (1990) finding that 27% of young women had at least one recurrence within 6 months of the first infection, and 2.7% had a second recurrence in this same period.
3. Risk factors for infection
   a. Females: Females are at greater risk than males because of a short urethra, which has close proximity to vaginal and rectal microorganisms. Risk factors for a UTI have been reported to include the following, although many of these risks are not well substantiated in the literature:
      - Poor perineal hygiene
        - Infrequent cleansing
        - Incorrect "wiping technique"
        - Tight panty hose
      - Coitus and coital behaviors
        - Diaphragm use (relative risk (RR) = 5.68 in subjects using a diaphragm five times a week)
        - Coital frequency (RR = 4.81 in subjects reporting five coital episodes a week)
        - Use of spermicide-coated condoms (odds ratio = 5.65 for use more than twice weekly) (Fihn et al., 1996)
        - Not voiding soon after intercourse (Strom et al., 1987)
      - Pregnancy

      - Nonsecretor of ABO blood group antigens (bind bacteria to vaginal epithelial cells)
      - Catheterization or instrumentation of the urethra
      - Anatomical abnormalities (e.g., urethral stenosis, neurogenic bladder, and nephrolithiasis)
   b. Males: Because UTIs in general and cystitis in particular are so much less frequent in males, risk factors and pathophysiology are less well understood. In nonsexually active male adolescents, bladder and renal infections are more likely to be a result of structural or functional abnormalities of the urinary tract. Additional factors in any male adolescent may include the following:
      - Blood group B or AB nonsecretor
      - P_1 blood group phenotype (epithelial cell receptors facilitate bacterial attachment)
      - Insertive anal intercourse
      - Sexual partner with vaginal colonization by uropathogens
      - Lack of circumcision (possibly by greater colonization of glans)

Microbiology

Females The most common organism in female adolescents with acute cystitis is *Escherichia coli* (75%–90%). *Staphylococcus saprophyticus* is probably the second most common cause of UTI in young women (5%–15%). Other gram-negative organisms cause most of the remainder of the infections. In chronic or recurrent infections, *Klebsiella* species, enterococci, *Pseudomonas aeruginosa, Enterobacter* and *Proteus* species, *Staphylococcus aureus,* group B streptococcus, *Streptococcus faecalis,* and *Serratia marcescens* may play a more common role than in acute infections.

Males Approximately three fourths of UTIs in male adolescents and young adults are due to gram-negative bacilli, but *E. coli* infections are not nearly as common as in girls. Gram-positive organisms, particularly enterococci and coagulase-negative staphylococci, account for approximately one fifth of infections. *Trichomonas vaginalis* is a rare cause of pyuria in men, usually involving an infection of the urethra or prostate. *Gardnerella vaginalis* can also occasionally cause infections in boys.

Symptoms and Signs

Females
1. Dysuria
2. Frequency, hesitancy, and urgency
3. Suprapubic pain
4. Pyuria
5. Hematuria

Symptoms caused by infections in the genitourinary tract are difficult to localize. For example, dysuria and dyspareunia in the female patient can be related to infections in the bladder, the urethra, or the vulva and vaginal tract. However, the location and timing of the dysuria is occasionally helpful. The dysuria associated with cystitis or urethritis is often described as internal pain and is usually worse when a patient initiates micturition. External pain or "terminal pain" (at the end of micturition) is more often associated with other conditions such as a vulvar inflammation, upper genital tract infection, or a herpes simplex infection.

Males
Apart from the preceding symptoms, male patients may also have symptoms associated with genitourinary infections in the prostate (perineal or rectal pain), epididymis (tender epididymis), or testicles (testicular pain and swelling).

Differential Diagnosis of Acute Dysuria

The most common complaint arousing suspicion of cystitis is dysuria. Dysuria may be a symptom of infection elsewhere in the urinary tract or infection of the genital tract, particularly in adolescents (Demetriou et al., 1982). The following are considerations in the differential diagnosis of cystitis and dysuria:

Females Table 25.1 lists the pathogens, incidence of pyuria and hematuria, urine culture findings, and signs and symptoms of acute dysuria in women.

1. Acute vaginitis and possible associated Skene glands infection secondary to *Chlamydia trachomatis, Neisseria gonorrhoeae,* or herpes simplex virus.
2. Vulvovaginitis due to *Candida* or *Trichomonas.*
3. Local dermatitis: Includes irritation from chemicals and other agents such as soap, contraceptive agents and foams, and feminine hygiene products.
4. Subclinical pyelonephritis: Some females with only dysuria have an upper UTI. These infections may be more difficult to eradicate. There are no reliable and simple methods to distinguish them from lower UTIs.
5. Acute urethral syndrome: The presence of frequency and dysuria in women with urine cultures showing between 10^2 and 10^5 colony-forming units (CFU)/mL has been termed the *acute urethral syndrome* or the *dysuria–pyuria syndrome.* However, studies have shown that many women with symptomatic cystitis have fewer than 10^5 CFU/mL. Therefore, this lower figure of 10^2 CFU/mL may be the appropriate microbiological criteria for determining the presence of a UTI. Kunin et al. (1993) reevaluated acute urinary symptoms and "low-count" bacteriuria ($>10^2$–10^4 CFU/mL) in women. *E. coli* and *S. saprophyticus* were the only microorganisms statistically associated with urinary tract symptoms and pyuria. This revision of bacterial counts has lessened or eliminated the need for a discrete acute urethral syndrome or dysuria–pyuria syndrome. The small group of symptomatic women with no growth on urine culture deserves evaluation for urinary or genital tract infections with *C. trachomatis, Mycobacterium tuberculosis,* herpes simplex virus, *Candida,* or *T. vaginalis.*

Males In males, the major diseases in the differential diagnosis of cystitis and dysuria include the following:

1. Urethritis (secondary to sexually transmitted organisms including *N. gonorrhoeae, C. trachomatis, T. vaginalis,* and others)
2. Prostatitis
3. Irritation from agents such as spermicidal foam
4. Trauma (usually associated with masturbation)

TABLE 25.1

Differential Diagnosis of Acute Dysuria in Women

Condition	Pathogen	Pyuria	Hematuria	Urine Culture	Signs, Symptoms
Cystitis	*Escherichia coli, Staphylococcus saprophyticus, Proteus, Klebsiella* sp	Usually	Sometimes	10^2 to $>10^5$	Acute onset, severe symptoms, dysuria, frequency, urgency, suprapubic or low back pain, suprapubic tenderness
Urethritis	*Chlamydia trachomatis, Neisseria gonorrhoeae,* herpes simplex virus	Usually	Rarely	$<10^2$	Gradual onset, mild symptoms, vaginal discharge or bleeding, lower abdominal pain, new sexual partner, cervical or vaginal lesions on examination
Vaginitis	*Candida* sp, *Trichomonas vaginalis*	Rarely	Rarely	$<10^2$	Vaginal discharge or odor, pruritus, dyspareunia, external dysuria, no frequency or urgency, vulvovaginitis on examination

From Stamm WE, Hooton TM. Management of urinary tract infections in adults. *N Engl J Med* 1993;329:1329, with permission.

Diagnosis

1. History
   a. In females, are there symptoms suggestive of vulvo-vaginitis, such as an abnormal vaginal discharge or vaginal itching? With a vaginal infection, symptoms of frequency and urgency are less common. In males, is there a history of sexual exposure, past urinary tract problems, or trauma?
   b. Does the patient use any medications or irritants such as douches, feminine hygiene products, strong soaps, bubble bath, or contraceptive products that could cause a local dermatitis? Is there a history of mechanical irritation including frequent masturbation?
   c. Is the teen sexually active? If so, sexually transmitted diseases (STDs), including a cervicitis or urethritis caused by *C. trachomatis, N. gonorrhoeae,* or *T. vaginalis,* become a concern.
   d. Are there signs of upper genitourinary tract disease? Fever and flank pain suggest acute pyelonephritis.
   e. Are there factors suggestive of a subclinical pyelonephritis, such as underlying urinary tract disease, diabetes mellitus, urinary infections in childhood, three or more previous UTIs, or acute pyelonephritis in the past?
2. Physical examination
   a. In both sexes, an examination of the abdomen and flank for tenderness should be performed. In addition, the genital area should be examined for a local dermatitis.
   b. In girls, a pelvic examination should be considered if the teen is sexually active or if there is history of a vaginal discharge.
   c. In boys, the physical examination should include inspection and palpation of the genitals to check for urethral discharge, meatal erythema, inflammation of the glans penis, penile lesions, an enlarged or tender epididymis or testis, or inguinal lymphadenopathy. A rectal examination is necessary if a diagnosis of prostatitis is under consideration.
3. Laboratory studies
   a. Microscopic examination of urine
      • The presence of one or more bacteria/oil immersion field of *uncentrifuged* urine has an 80% to 95% correlation with bacteriuria in which the bacteria count is 10^5/mL. This examination may also be performed on a gram-stained specimen of unspun urine.
      • A count of more than ten organisms/oil immersion field on a *centrifuged* unstained sediment also correlates with positive culture results. Pyuria with five or more leukocytes/high-power field of urine sediment on spun urine has a poorer correlation. Sources of error with the latter include variable volumes of urine, variable time and speed of centrifugation, and inconsistent resuspension volume. However, analysis of unspun urine for leukocytes in a counting chamber does give reproducible results and is significant if the count is > ten leukocytes/mm^3. Urine should be examined within 2 hours of collection. Presence of pyuria is a good indicator that antibiotic therapy will be necessary. A positive finding with a leukocyte esterase dipstick has a sensitivity of approximately 75% to 96% and specificity of 94% to 98% in detecting pyuria associated with an infection.
   b. Urine culture
      • A bladder or renal infection is usually characterized by a urine culture with a colony count of >100,000 CFU/mL of a typical urinary pathogen. However, it is now well established that a colony count of >100 CFU/mL of a pure culture of an organism indicates an infection in the presence of symptoms and pyuria. A urine culture is not mandatory for the diagnosis and treatment of a female adolescent with signs and symptoms of a UTI, particularly with a first episode. If therapy fails, if the infection represents a reoccurrence within the 3 months of an initial infection, or if the patient is a male, a culture is recommended. Cultures are also indicated for female patients with pyuria without bacteriuria.
      • In patients who become asymptomatic with therapy, posttreatment cultures are unnecessary. Follow-up cultures are indicated for patients with acute pyelonephritis, a complicated infection, or during pregnancy.
   c. Culture alternatives: Several rapid culture kits available for office use include:
      • Dipslide: Best studied and most reliable kit culture technique. The test is inexpensive and yields high sensitivity and specificity rates (generally <1% false-positive and false-negative results).
      • Filter-paper techniques yield false-negative rates of 3% to 20% and false-positive rates of 2% to 23%.
      • Several other chemical tests use nitrate glucose oxidase or catalase to detect the presence of bacteriuria. These tests are neither highly sensitive nor specific.
4. Other tests
   a. Females: In girls, three infections within 1 to 2 years may be an indication for a more complete evaluation of the patient's urinary tract, which may include a renal ultrasound and a voiding cystourethrogram. However, in postpubertal female young adults with uncomplicated cystitis, evaluation after recurrent episodes is unlikely to reveal significant abnormalities that would change either therapy or prognosis. Figure 25.1 is a flow diagram for the evaluation of women with internal dysuria.
   b. Males: Although some authorities recommend a full investigation after the first infection, this is probably of greater importance in the young child or infant. In male adolescents, an investigation with more invasive tests is probably not indicated after the first infection, unless there is evidence in the history or physical examination of a possible renal abnormality or if there is no response to therapy. This is particularly true for male adolescents who are sexually active. Krieger et al. (1993) evaluated acute UTI in healthy university men. The incidence was 5 per 10,000 men per year. Of this group of men, 92% responded to a single course of antibiotics. None of them had neurological or anatomical abnormalities, and all the radiographic findings were normal. The major risk factor was a history of sexual activity in the previous month.

Recurrent Infections in Female Adolescents

Approximately 20% of young women will have recurrent infections. Most of these adolescents and young

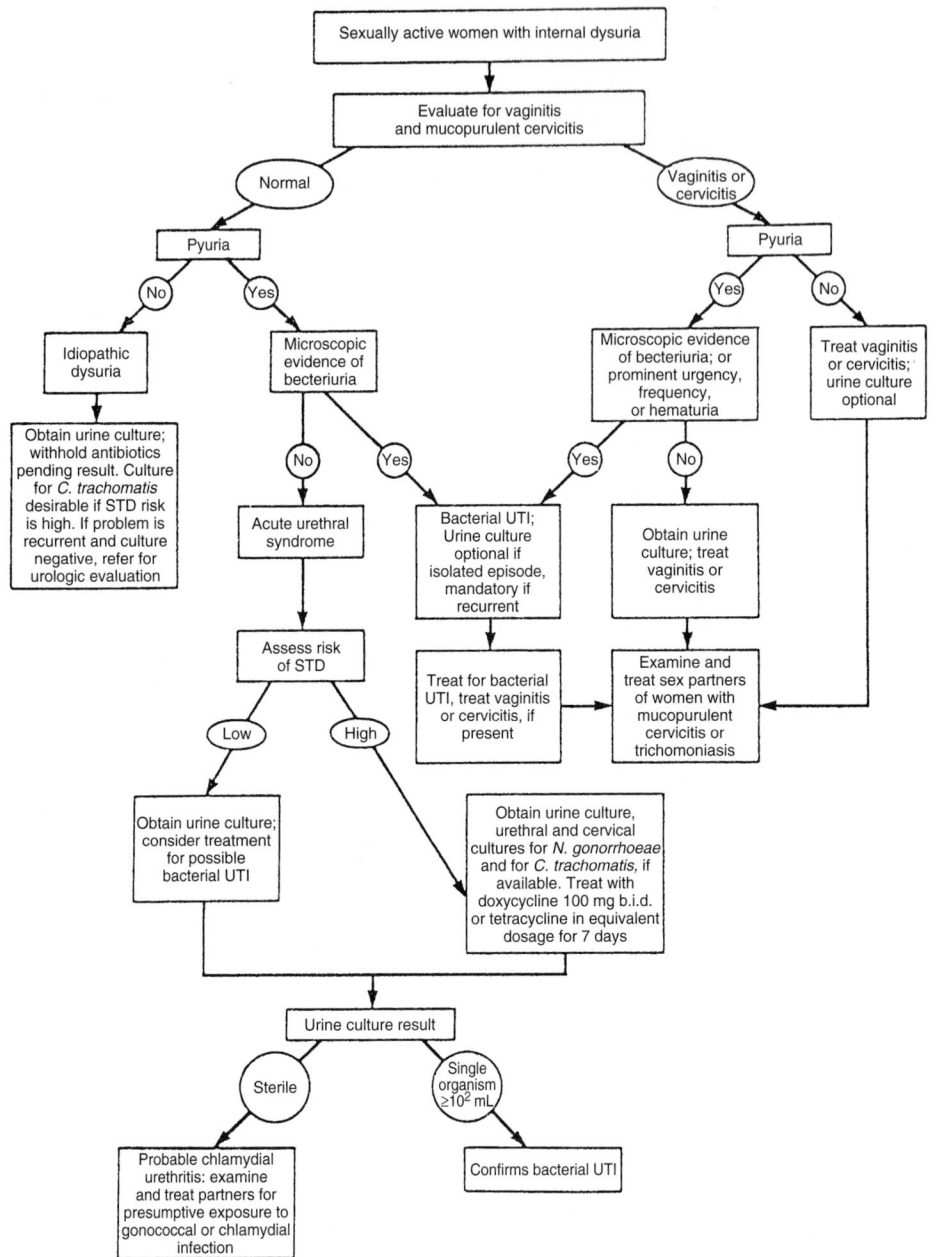

FIGURE 25.1 Flow diagram for the evaluation of women with internal dysuria. STD, sexually transmitted disease; UTI, urinary tract infection. (From Holes KK. Lower genital tract infection in women: cystitis, urethritis, vulvovaginitis, and cervicitis. In: Holmes KK, Mardh PA, Sparling PF et al., eds. *Sexually transmitted diseases.* New York: McGraw-Hill, 1990, with permission.)

women do not have anatomical or functional abnormalities of the urinary tract. However, recurrent cystitis within 3 months of the original infection should call for a urine culture. Those female patients with a relapse (recurrent infection with original pathogen within 2 weeks of completion of therapy) should also have their urine cultured and in either case should have careful follow-up. Continued infections should result in an evaluation for an occult source of infection or urological abnormality.

PYELONEPHRITIS

Pyelonephritis is an infection of the renal pelvis and medulla. Risk factors for pyelonephritis are similar to those for UTI but also include maternal history of UTI and diabetes (Scholes et al., 2005). There are approximately 250,000 cases of acute pyelonephritis each year, resulting in >100,000 hospitalizations. Women are five times more likely than men to be hospitalized. Most infections occur from bacterial ascent through the urethra and bladder.

The clinical and laboratory manifestations usually include the following:

1. Symptoms of acute cystitis
2. Fever
3. Costovertebral tenderness
4. Elevated leukocyte count and erythrocyte sedimentation rate
5. Urinalysis revealing leukocytes and bacterial casts
6. Positive urine culture result

The range of symptoms varies from mild flank pain to those of septicemia. Most cases of acute pyelonephritis in young women are caused by *E. coli* infection (>80%). Pyuria and gram-negative bacteria are usually present on examination of the urine. Urine culture specimens should always be obtained. Blood culture specimens should also be obtained from those whose diagnosis is uncertain, from immunosuppressed patients, from those in whom a hematogenous source is suspected, or from those who are ill enough to be hospitalized. If fever and flank pain persist after 72 hours of treatment, then cultures should be repeated and ultrasonography or computed tomography should be considered to evaluate for an abscess. Additional indications for imaging studies include recurrent pyelonephritis, persistent hematuria, or poor response to treatment. Indications for hospitalization include persistent vomiting, suspected sepsis, uncertain diagnosis, and urinary tract obstruction. Other relative indications include anatomical urinary tract abnormalities, immunocompromised status, and inadequate access to follow-up care.

TREATMENT OF GENITOURINARY INFECTIONS

1. Acute, uncomplicated infections in females (usually caused by organisms such as *E. coli, S. saprophyticus, Proteus mirabilis, Klebsiella pneumoniae,* and others): A growing number of urinary tract pathogens have begun to develop resistance to commonly used antibiotics, particularly trimethoprim-sulfamethoxazole and amoxicillin. Resistance to the latter and its clinical failure rate are now so high that amoxicillin is no longer considered an appropriate "first choice" antibiotic, even if combined with clavulanate (Hooton et al., 2005). Local resistance patterns should be consulted before prescribing any antibiotics as first-line treatment of UTIs. Assuming appropriate sensitivity of organisms:
    a. No complicating factors: Use a 3-day oral regimen of one of the following:
        • Trimethoprim-sulfamethoxazole (160/800 mg every 12 hours) or trimethoprim (100 mg every 12 hours)
        • Cefpodoxime (200 mg every 12 hours)
        • Nitrofurantoin (100 mg every 6 hours)
        • In older adolescents (older than 16 years), a 3-day regimen of a quinolone would also be appropriate. Appropriate regimens include the following:
            – Norfloxacin (400 mg every 12 hours)
            – Ciprofloxacin (250 mg every 12 hours)
            – Ofloxacin (200 mg every 12 hours)
    b. For patients with potentially complicating problems such as diabetes, sickle cell disease, a history of a previous UTI, or symptoms for >1 week, use a 7-day regimen of a previously mentioned medication.
    c. Pregnancy: Use a 7-day regimen of the following:
        • Nitrofurantoin (100 mg four times a day)
        • Cefpodoxime (200 mg every 12 hours)
        • Trimethoprim-sulfamethoxazole (160/800 mg every 12 hours)
    d. 3-day course versus single-dose antibiotics: Although there was great interest in the possibility of treating uncomplicated UTIs in women with a single dose of antibiotics, a 3-day course of antibiotics appears to ensure greater success than the single-dose antibiotic regimens in a number of studies. The exception to this may be the use of fosfomycin in a single 3-g dose for infections in women older than 18 years (minimum age approved).
    e. 3-day course versus longer course of antibiotics: Michael et al. (2006) evaluated ten trials in children up to age 18. There was no significant difference in the frequency of positive urine cultures between the short (2–4 days) and standard duration oral antibiotic therapy (7–14 days) for UTI at 0 to 10 days after treatment and at 1 to 15 months after treatment. There was also no difference in the development of resistant organisms. A 2005 meta-analysis by Katchman et al.(2005) addressed this question in adults with UTIs. Antibiotic therapy for 3 days was similar to prolonged therapy in achieving symptomatic cure for cystitis; however, the prolonged treatment was slightly more effective in obtaining bacteriological cure both short-term (RR = 1.37) and longer term (RR = 1.47). If elimination of bacteriuria is important in an adolescent, a longer treatment time than 3 days, could be considered.
2. Acute, uncomplicated pyelonephritis in female patients (usually caused by organisms such as *E. coli, P. mirabilis, K. pneumoniae, S. saprophyticus*): Avoid amoxicillin and first-generation cephalosporins because 25% to 35% of organisms are resistant to these antibiotics.
    a. Mild to moderate illness with no nausea or vomiting: Initial outpatient oral therapy is acceptable in adolescents with a community-acquired infection not associated with severe systemic symptoms or known complications. Oral therapy can include any of the following, with each regimen administered for 10 to 14 days.
        • Trimethoprim-sulfamethoxazole (160/800 mg every 12 hours)
        • Cefpodoxime (200 mg every 12 hours)
        • Quinolones that can be utilized in older adolescents and young adults:
            – Norfloxacin (400 mg every 12 hours for 10–14 days)
            – Ciprofloxacin (500 mg every 12 hours for 10–14 days)
            – Ofloxacin (200–300 mg every 12 hours for 10–14 days)
            – Levofloxacin (500 mg daily for 10–14 days)
    b. Severe pyelonephritis or other complicated UTI requiring hospitalization (e.g., patients with diabetes, sickle cell disease, or immunodeficiency): Parenterally administered antibiotics, including one of the following:
        • Trimethoprim-sulfamethoxazole (160/800 mg every 12 hours)
        • Ceftriaxone (1–2 g/day)

- Ciprofloxacin (200–400 mg every 12 hours)
- Gentamicin (1 mg/kg every 12 hours [with or without ampicillin])
- Ticarcillin/clavulanate (3.1 g every 8 hours)
- Imipenem (500 mg every 8 hours)

Use these until fever has resolved for 24 to 48 hours and then treat with oral antibiotics for 14 days using one of the following (limit use of quinolones in patients younger than 16 years):
- Trimethoprim-sulfamethoxazole (160/800 mg every 12 hours)
- Cefpodoxime (200 mg every 12 hours)
- Norfloxacin (400 mg every 12 hours)
- Ciprofloxacin (500 mg every 12 hours)
- Ofloxacin (200–300 mg every 12 hours)

  c. Pregnancy: Hospitalization is highly recommended, with parentally administered antibiotics, including one of the following:
- Ceftriaxone (1–2 g/day)
- Aztreonam (1 g every 8–12 hours)
- Gentamicin (1 mg/kg every 12 hours)

Use these until fever has resolved for 24 to 48 hours and then treat with oral antibiotics for 14 days, using one of the following:
- Cefpodoxime proxetil (200 mg every 12 hours)
- Trimethoprim-sulfamethoxazole (160/800 mg every 12 hours)

3. Recurrent infections: Recurrent cystitis in female patients should be managed by either continuous prophylaxis, postcoital prophylaxis, or therapy initiated by the patient.
   a. Continuous prophylaxis: Use one of the following:
- Trimethoprim (100 mg daily)
- Trimethoprim-sulfamethoxazole (40/200 mg daily)
- Nitrofurantoin (50–100 mg daily)
- Norfloxacin (200 mg daily)
- Cephalexin (250 mg daily)
   b. Postcoital prophylaxis: Use one of the following:
- Trimethoprim-sulfamethoxazole (40/200 mg)
- Nitrofurantoin (50–100 mg)
- Cephalexin (250 mg)
   c. Patient-administered therapy: An alternative to prophylaxis in the compliant individual is self-medication initiated at the time the symptoms appear, with a 3-day regimen (Gupta et al., 2001). Patient-initiated therapy is best for individuals with only one or two episodes per year.
   d. Nonantibiotic measures: Nonantibiotic prevention of recurrent UTIs includes the following:
- Voiding after intercourse
- Discontinuing use of a diaphragm
- Emptying the bladder frequently
- Acidifying the urine
4. Treatment of UTIs in male patients: Less information is known about short-term or single-dose therapy in males. Male patients should probably receive a 7- to 10-day course of antibiotics. However, in less compliant male patients, a 3-day regimen of trimethoprim-sulfamethoxazole or a quinolone such as norfloxacin in age-appropriate patients could be used.
5. Cautions and contraindications
   a. Fluoroquinolone antibiotics are not approved for use in adolescents younger than 16 years and *should not be used in pregnancy.*
   b. Trimethoprim-sulfamethoxazole is not approved in pregnancy but has been widely used.
   c. Gentamicin should be used with great caution in pregnancy because of the possibility of toxicity to the eighth nerve of the developing fetus.
   d. Local resistance patterns will influence the ultimate choice of antibiotics.

ASYMPTOMATIC BACTERIURIA

The prevalence of asymptomatic bacteriuria (reproducible growth of $>10^5$ CFU/mL) ranges from approximately 1% to 7%. There is a tendency toward spontaneous cure. However, women with this condition are at increased risk of an overt UTI (8% in the week after documented bacteria in the urine [Hooton et al., 2000]), and in individuals whose infection begins in childhood, there is a suggestion that their infection can lead to renal impairment. Asymptomatic bacteriuria during pregnancy is a risk factor for the development of acute pyelonephritis, for lower fetal birth weight, and for a higher incidence of prematurity. Treatment is mainly indicated for the following individuals:

1. Those who are pregnant
2. Male patients
3. Female patients with either an underlying renal tract abnormality or an immunocompromising disease

Treatment should be with appropriate antibiotics selected on the basis of culture sensitivities.

NONGONOCOCCAL URETHRITIS

Nongonococcal urethritis (NGU) is an infectious inflammation of the urethra characterized by dysuria and by a mucopurulent penile discharge. As its name implies, it is unassociated with infection by *N. gonorrhoeae*. Asymptomatic infections are quite common.

Etiology

1. *C. trachomatis:* There is clear evidence that certain genotypes cause approximately 40% to 50% of the cases of NGU.
2. *Ureaplasma urealyticum:* Reliable data implicate this organism as a cause of approximately 20% to 30% of additional cases of NGU.
3. In the remainder of cases, the cause is uncertain: Other possibilities include *Mycoplasma genitalium, G. vaginalis,* herpes simplex virus, *S. saprophyticus, E. coli,* and *T. vaginalis.*

Epidemiology

1. Incidence: Extremely common among sexually active men. In the United Kingdom, it is the most frequently recorded STD and this would probably be true in the United States if all jurisdictions required reporting of NGU and chlamydial infection. It is estimated that 3 to 4 million cases occur yearly in the United States.
2. Transmission: Sexual contact

Clinical Manifestations

1. Discharge: Usually scanty or moderate, watery discharge; some patients have no discharge, whereas others have copious, purulent discharge, which usually starts 8 to 14 days after contact.
2. Dysuria
3. Rarely, hematuria
4. Complications of untreated infection include epididymitis, prostatitis (rare), and Reiter syndrome (very rare).

Diagnosis

1. Clinical history
2. Gram stain of urethral discharge
   a. More than five polymorphonuclear cells/oil immersion field indicates urethritis.
   b. The lack of intracellular gram-negative diplococci suggests NGU.
3. Urine
   a. A leukocyte count of more than ten cells/high-power dry field of the urine sediment from the first 10 to 15 mL of a urine stream indicates urethritis.
   b. A leukocyte esterase dipstick test result is positive.
   c. The urine sediment test, although often unnecessary if a discharge is present, is helpful in determining the presence or absence of urethritis.
4. Urethral culture if Gram stain result of the discharge is negative; culture or nonculture technique for gonorrheal and chlamydial infection

Therapy

1. Recommended regimen
   a. Doxycycline (100 mg orally twice daily for 7 days) or
   b. Azithromycin (1 g orally in a single dose) or
   c. Ofloxacin (400 mg orally twice daily for 7 days)
2. Alternative regimens
   a. Erythromycin base (500 mg given orally four times daily for 7 days) or
   b. Erythromycin ethylsuccinate (800 mg orally four times daily for 7 days)
   c. For a patient who cannot tolerate high-dose erythromycin schedules: Use one of the following regimens:
      • Erythromycin base (250 mg given orally four times a day for 14 days)
      • Erythromycin ethylsuccinate (400 mg orally four times a day for 14 days)

Note that patients with persistent or recurrent objective signs of urethritis after adequate treatment of themselves and their partners warrant further evaluation for less common causes of urethritis. In addition, in some individuals with persistent infections, a longer (14–21 days) course of antibiotics may be effective. Finally, sexual partners must be treated.

PROSTATITIS

Etiology

Prostatitis is an inflammatory reaction confined to the prostate gland. In adolescents, prostatitis is an unusual condition. Acute prostatitis in adolescents is usually caused by an infection, which probably started as a urethral infection and reached the prostate through the reflux of infected urine into the prostatic ducts or by lymphogenous or hematogenic spread. Although it is often assumed that STDs, and particularly infection with *N. gonorrhoeae* and *C. trachomatis*, cause a large percentage of the cases of acute prostatitis in adolescents and young adults, evidence to support this is inadequate. Coliform bacteria, *S. saprophyticus*, *Mycoplasma hominis*, *U. urealyticum*, and *T. vaginalis*, have also been implicated as causative agents. In one study of 409 patients with prostatitis—boys age 19 years and older—the most frequent organism isolated was *U. urealyticum* (de la Rosette et al., 1993). The cause or causes of noninfectious prostatitis and chronic prostatitis are even more unclear.

Diagnosis

1. In acute bacterial prostatitis, symptoms include the following:
   a. Pain: Penile/scrotal, suprapubic, perineal, groin, or back pain or pain that occurs during ejaculation
   b. Bladder symptoms: Frequency, dysuria, and hesitation
   c. Systemic symptoms: Chills, fever, and malaise
   d. Other symptoms: Hematospermia and hematuria
2. In nonacute prostatitis, the symptoms are less dramatic and may include frequency, urgency, and dysuria.
3. The only method for documenting prostatitis is the segmental culture technique.
   a. Four specimens are collected, including the following:
      • First-voided 10-mL urine
      • Midstream urine
      • Prostatic secretions during prostatic massage
      • First-voided 10 mL after prostatic massage
   b. In individuals with bacterial prostatitis, the third and fourth specimens should grow more colonies than the first two. The presence of more leukocytes in the first specimen suggests urethritis, and growth primarily in the second specimen suggests cystitis. *However, because the meaning and interpretation of this test are not standardized and the test is time consuming, expensive, and uncomfortable, it should not be performed routinely in adolescents.*

Treatment

In the acutely inflamed prostate gland, antibiotics have good penetration; however in adolescents with recurrent prostatic infections, treatment is hampered by the lack of good antibiotic penetration. The best antibiotic choices for empirical treatment of prostatic infections include the following:

Trimethoprim-sulfamethoxazole (160/800 mg every 12 hours for 7 days) or
Ofloxacin (400 mg every 12 hours for 7 days) or
Doxycycline (100 mg every 12 hours for 7 days) or
Erythromycin (500 mg every 6 hours for 7 days)

If symptoms persist, more aggressive attempts to obtain specific diagnostic samples need to be undertaken, including the segmental culture technique described above.

HEMATOSPERMIA

Bloody ejaculate is an unusually reported condition which can occur in male adolescents. The adolescent may notice a reddish discoloration of his semen either after masturbation or on removing a condom after intercourse. This condition may cause extreme anxiety or feelings of guilt. The teen may be concerned about a malignancy or fear that his behavior has caused the condition. In adolescents, the condition is usually either idiopathic and self-limited or related to an infection such as a gonococcal or chlamydial urethritis. Apart from evaluation for a UTI, prostatitis, or sexually transmitted urethritis, an extensive investigation is not required unless the condition is persistent and the initial findings are negative.

WEB SITES

For Teenagers and Parents

http://familydoctor.org. Good general reference for a range of health problems, including UTIs.

http://youngwomenshealth.org/resourcenter.html. Comprehensive site for young women's health issues.

http://womenshealth.gov/faq/Easyread/uti-etr.htm Patient-friendly government handout on UTIs.

http://my.webmd.com/content/article/1680.50565. WebMD article on UTIs.

http://www.drreddy.com/uti.html. Good explanation for teens and parents.

http://www.mayohealth.org. Mayo Clinic site on UTIs. Search for UTIs.

For Health Professional

http://www.urologychannel.com/uti/index.shtml. Discussion of urinary tract health issues, including UTIs.

http://www.niddk.nih.gov/health/urolog/pubs/cpwork/cpwork.htm. National Institutes of Health information on prostatitis.

http://kidney.niddk.nih.gov/kudiseases/pubs/utiadult/. National Institutes of Health information on urinary tract infections.

REFERENCES AND ADDITIONAL READINGS

Abrahamsson A, Hansson S, Jodal U, et al. Staphylococcus saprophyticus urinary tract infections in children. *Eur J Pediatr* 1993;152:69.

Ansbach RK, Dybus KR, Bergeson R. Uncomplicated E. coli urinary tract infection in college women: a retrospective study of E. coli sensitivities to commonly prescribed antibiotics. *J Am Coll Health* 1995;43:183.

Bergeron MG. Treatment of pyelonephritis in adults. *Med Clin North Am* 1995;79:619.

Bonny AE, Brouhard BH. Urinary tract infections among adolescents. *Adolesc Med Clin* 2005;16:149.

Brumfitt W, Hamilton-Miller JM. A comparative trial of low dose cefaclor and macrocrystalline nitrofurantoin in the prevention of recurrent urinary tract infection. *Infection* 1995;23:98.

Davison IM, Sprott MS, Selkon JB. The effect of covert bacteriuria in schoolgirls on renal function at 18 years and during pregnancy. *Lancet* 1984;2:651.

Demetriou E, Emans SJ, Masland RP Jr. Dysuria in adolescent girls: urinary tract infection or vaginitis? *Pediatrics* 1982;70:299.

Fihn SD, Boyko EJ, Normand EH, et al. Association between use of spermicide-coated condoms and Escherichia coli urinary tract infection in young women. *Am J Epidemiol* 1996;144:512.

Fletcher MS, Herzberg Z, Pryor JP. The aetiology and investigation of haemospermia. *Br J Urol* 1981;53:669.

Foxman B. Recurring urinary tract infection: incidence and risk factors. *Am J Public Health* 1990;80:331.

Gupta K, Hooton TM, Roberts PL, et al. Patient-initiated treatment of uncomplicated recurrent urinary tract infections in young women. *Ann Intern Med* 2001;135:9.

Holmes KK, Stamm W. Lower genital tract infection in women. In: Holmes KK, Sparling PE, Mardh PA et al., eds. *Sexually transmitted diseases*, 3rd ed. New York: McGraw-Hill, 1999.

Hooton TM, Scholes D, Gupta K, et al. Amoxicillin-clavulanate vs ciprofloxacin for the treatment of uncomplicated cystitis in women. A randomized trial. *JAMA* 2005;293:949.

Hooton TM, Scholes D, Hughes JP, et al. A prospective study of risk factors for symptomatic urinary tract infection in young women. *N Engl J Med* 1996;335:468.

Hooton TM, Scholes D, Stapleton AE, et al. A prospective study of asymptomatic bacteriuria in sexually active young women. *N Engl J Med* 2000;343:992.

Hooton TM, Winter C, Tiu F, et al. Randomized comparative trial and cost analysis of 3-day antimicrobial regimens for treatment of acute cystitis in women. *JAMA* 1995;273:41.

Joly-Guillou ML, Lasry S. Practical recommendations for the drug treatment of bacterial infections of the male genital tract including urethritis, epididymitis, and prostatitis. *Drugs* 1999;57:743.

Katchman EA, Milo G, Paul M. Three-day vs longer duration of antibiotic treatment for cystitis in women: systematic review and meta-analysis. *Am J Med* 2005;118:1196.

Komaroff AL. Urinalysis and urine culture in women with dysuria. *Ann Intern Med* 1986;104:212.

Krieger JN, Ross SO, Simonsen JM. Urinary tract infections in healthy university men. *J Urol* 1993;149:1046.

Kunin CM, White LV, Hua Hua T. A reassessment of the importance of "low count" bacteriuria in young women with acute urinary symptoms. *Ann Intern Med* 1993;119:454.

Latham RH, Running K, Stamm WE. Urinary tract infections in young adult women caused by Staphylococcus saprophyticus. *JAMA* 1983;250:3063.

Leigh DA. Prostatitis—an increasing clinical problem for diagnosis and management. *J Antimicrob Chemother* 1993;32 (Suppl A):1.

Lipsky BA. Prostatitis and urinary tract infection in men: what's new; what's true? *Am J Med* 1999;106:327.

Merrick MV, Notghi A, Chalmers N, et al. Long-term follow-up to determine the prognostic value of imaging after urinary tract infections. Part 1: reflux. *Arch Dis Child* 1995;72:388.

Merrick MV, Notghi A, Chalmers N, et al. Long-term follow-up to determine the prognostic value of imaging after urinary tract infections. Part 2: scarring. *Arch Dis Child* 1995;72:393.

Michael M, Hodson EM, Craig JC, et al. Short versus standard duration oral antibiotic therapy for acute urinary tract infection in children. *Cochrane Database Syst Rev* 2006;1.

Millar LK, Wing DA, Paul RH, et al. Outpatient treatment of pyelonephritis in pregnancy: a randomized controlled trial. *Obstet Gynecol* 1995;86:560.

Ohkawa M, Yamaguchi K, Tokunaga S, et al. Ureaplasma urealyticum in the urogenital tract of patients with chronic prostatitis or related symptomatology. *Br J Urol* 1993;72:918.

Ramakrishnan K, Scheid DC. Diagnosis and management of acute pyelonephritis in adults. *Am Fam Physician* 2005; 71:933.

de la Rosette JJMCH, Hubregtse MR, Meuleman EJH, et al. Diagnosis and treatment of 409 patients with prostatitis syndromes. *Urology* 1993;41:301.

Rouse DJ, Andrews WW, Goldenberg RL, et al. Screening and treatment of asymptomatic bacteriuria of pregnancy to prevent pyelonephritis: a cost-effectiveness and cost-benefit analysis. *Obstet Gynecol* 1995;86:119.

Scholes D, Hooton TM, Roberts PL, et al. Risk factors associated with acute pyelonephritis in healthy women. *Ann Intern Med* 2005;142:20.

Semeniuk H, Church D. Evaluation of the leukocyte esterase and nitrite urine dipstick screening tests of bacteriuria in women with suspected uncomplicated urinary tract infections. *J Clin Microbiol* 1999;37:3051.

Sheffield JS, Cunningham FG. Urinary tract infection in women. *Obste Gynecol* 2005;106:1085.

Sheinfeld J, Schaeffer AI, Cordon-Cardo C, et al. Association of the Lewis blood-group phenotype with recurrent urinary tract infections in women. *N Engl J Med* 1989;320:773.

Silber TJ, Kastrinakas M. Hematospermia in adolescents and young adults. *Pediatrics* 1986;78:708.

Smellie JM, Rigden SP, Prescod NP. Urinary tract infection: a comparison of four methods of investigation. *Arch Dis Child* 1995;72:247.

Stapleton A, Latham RH, Johnson C, et al. Postcoital antimicrobial prophylaxis for recurrent urinary tract infection: a randomized, double-blind, placebo-controlled trial. *JAMA* 1990;264:703.

Stein GE. Comparison of single-dose fosfomycin and a 7-day course of nitrofurantoin with uncomplicated urinary tract infection. *Clin Ther* 1999;21:1864.

Strom BL, Collins M, West SL, et al. Sexual activity, contraceptive use, and other risk factors for symptomatic and asymptomatic bacteriuria: a case-control study. *Ann Intern Med* 1987;107:816.

Weir M, Brien J. Adolescent urinary tract infections. *Adolesc Med (State Art Rev)* 2000;11:293.

Zhanel GG, Harding GKM, Guay DRP. Asymptomatic bacteriuria: which patients should be treated? *Arch Intern Med* 1990; 150:1389.

CHAPTER 26

Enuresis

Diane Tanaka

Enuresis is defined as the involuntary passage of urine, usually during sleep, occurring more than once a month. Although often considered a childhood problem, enuresis is also found in adolescents, causing major emotional problems and family stress. Current urology literature uses the following terminology regarding enuresis:

Primary nocturnal enuresis: Nighttime wetting without prior periods of dryness.

Secondary nocturnal enuresis: Nighttime wetting that occurs in patients who have a history of 6 months of dryness.

Monosymptomatic nocturnal enuresis (MNE): Isolated nocturnal enuresis. No daytime symptoms and no other symptoms suggestive of problems or abnormalities of the urogenital tract.

Diurnal enuresis: Involuntary or intentional urination into clothing while awake.

Polysymptomatic nocturnal enuresis (PNE): Nighttime wetting associated with other bladder symptoms such as urgency, frequency, instability, or voiding dysfunction.

Dysfunctional voiding: Nocturnal enuresis with daytime symptoms, which can range from urgency and frequency, to daytime incontinence. This is also known as *complex* or *complicated enuresis*. Diurnal enuresis is linked with dysfunctional voiding.

Dysfunctional elimination syndrome: Nocturnal enuresis with urinary and bowel symptoms.

ETIOLOGY OF MONOSYMPTOMATIC NOCTURNAL ENURESIS

Most cases of MNE are related to nonorganic causes. The causes may be multifactorial, with maturational delay as an important etiology.

Organic Causes

Only 2% to 3% of patients have a true organic cause. Five percent to 10% of the enuresis cases are associated with urgency (polysymptomatic enuresis).

1. Neurological lesions
   a. Myelomeningocele, the most common neurological cause of enuresis
   b. Mental retardation
   c. Spinal cord injury
2. Urological abnormalities: Controversy exists over the role and prevalence of urological lesions in enuresis. The prevalence of urological abnormalities in enuretic patients ranges from 2% to 97% in different studies. Described problems include the following:
   a. Recurrent urinary tract infections (UTIs)
   b. Obstructive lesions: Urethral obstruction or posterior urethral valves
   c. Detrusor instability: Khan et al. (1993) found that the mean threshold volume at which detrusor instability was demonstrated was 200 mL in enuretic patients. The mean bladder capacity of age-matched nonenuretic patients was 325 mL.
   d. Incomplete bladder emptying: The common symptom of incomplete bladder emptying is urinary frequency. Common causes of incomplete bladder emptying are lower urinary tract obstruction, neurogenic bladder, and dysfunctional voiding. Adolescents who voluntarily withhold urination during the day and only impartially void at bedtime suffer from dysfunctional voiding. These patients are prone to develop reflux and renal damage.
3. Renal concentrating defects (e.g., sickle cell anemia)
4. Diabetes mellitus and diabetes insipidus: Chronic polyuria is associated with diabetes insipidus and diabetes mellitus. Alcohol, caffeine, and some medications can cause a transient polyuria.

Genetic Causes

The evidence for genetic transmission explains the common occurrence of a positive family history in enuretic patients. The prevalence of enuresis in families is as follows:

Relatives with Enuresis	Prevalence of Enuresis in Offspring
Both parents	77%
One parent	44%
No parents	15%

Twin studies not only provide evidence that there is a genetic etiology to enuresis but they also show that the genetics of enuresis is modulated by environmental factors.

The prevalence in an identical twin of an enuretic twin ranges from 43% to 68%. Prevalence in a fraternal twin of an enuretic twin ranges from 19% to 36%. Genetic studies have shown that the most common mode of inheritance is autosomal dominant with high penetrance. Autosomal dominant inheritance with low penetrance is the next common mode of inheritance, followed by autosomal recessive inheritance. One third of cases appear to be due to sporadic occurrence. Arnell et al. (1997) revealed evidence of sex-linked or sex-influenced factors, which would account for the ratio of affected males to females of 3:1. Possible gene loci that have been identified include 13q, 8q, 12q, and 22q.11.

Sleep Disorder

Enuresis may be associated with incomplete sudden arousal from a deep sleep. In these cases, there is difficulty in arousing the patient. Parents of affected teens often report that their child sleeps too soundly or deeply. Often, the adolescent fails to awaken due to the sensation of a full bladder or even when the bedding becomes wet. However, some studies have demonstrated that enuretic patients are normal sleepers. Sleep studies have shown that sleep patterns are similar between patients with enuresis and those without. Enuretic episodes can occur at random throughout the night and can occur in all stages of sleep, but enuresis primarily occurs during nonrapid eye movement (non-REM) sleep (which occurs in the early part of the sleep cycle).

Maturational Delay

It has been postulated that a developmental delay in adequate neuromuscular maturation of the bladder, as well as an immaturity of the central nervous system inhibition of the micturition reflex, is responsible for enuresis. Further evidence for maturational delay is the fact that enuretic patients become dry with time, whether or not there is a therapeutic intervention.

Small Functional Bladder Capacity

The current thinking among enuresis experts is that affected teens either produce large nighttime volumes of urine with a normal bladder capacity or produce a large nighttime volume with a small bladder capacity. Symptoms of a small bladder capacity include daytime frequency, wetness every night, occasional wetness several times per night, and the presence of the problem since birth.

Psychological Factors

Most enuretic patients are psychologically normal and psychological stressors do not cause enuresis. It is important to remember that the teen is not deliberately wetting the bed. An increased prevalence of emotional difficulties, including poor self-esteem, family stress, and family isolation, has been described in affected adolescents. However, this may often be a result of suffering from enuresis, rather than a causative factor.

Vasopressin Levels

Normally, vasopressin levels rise during the night, resulting in a smaller volume of more concentrated urine at night. Although first postulated in 1985 that MNE is due to nocturnal polyuria with relative nocturnal deficiency of antidiuretic hormone (ADH), more recent studies have questioned this theory with 25% to 100% of adolescents having a lack of nocturnal rise in ADH. This wide variability suggests the presence of other etiological factors.

Another theory postulates that as children approach adolescence, a faulty circadian rhythm of arginine vasopressin (AVP) secretion may be the paramount pathogenetic factor.

Detrusor Instability

When adolescents with MNE were compared to normal children, a 3% to 5% incidence of uninhibited bladder activity was found in both populations. However, if a patient has refractory primary MNE, bladder dysfunction should be considered.

ETIOLOGY OF DIURNAL ENURESIS

Primary Diurnal Enuresis

1. Neurogenic bladder: Myelomeningocele is the most common neurological cause of enuresis. Other causes of a neurogenic bladder include cerebral palsy, sacral agenesis, transverse myelitis, spina bifida, and spinal cord trauma.
2. Congenital urethral obstruction: Characterized by a weak or interrupted urinary stream and the patient may need to push to initiate urination.
3. Ectopic ureter: Patients complain of constant wetness or dampness.
4. Congenital diabetes insipidus

Secondary Diurnal Enuresis

1. Constipation: It has been postulated that the pressure effect of stool in the descending or sigmoid colon triggers uninhibited contraction of the detrusor muscle, resulting in enuresis.
2. UTIs: Enuresis due to UTIs is most commonly seen in preschool children, but can affect girls of any age.
3. Giggle incontinence: Giggling or laughter results in complete involuntary emptying of the bladder. It can develop in up to 8% of girls. It is seen most commonly in school-aged girls and can be familial. Although it tends to improve with age, it can persist into adulthood.
4. Stress incontinence: This occurs in situations associated with increased intraabdominal pressure. If the bladder outlet and proximal urethra fail to compensate for the increased pressure, then wetting occurs. It can occur with jumping, running, and high-impact landing, which is why it is seen more frequently in athletic adolescents. It can be managed by bladder emptying before exercising.
5. Emotional stress: An isolated episode of stress can result in wetting, as can prolonged stress, such as with child abuse.

6. Hinman syndrome: The bladder behaves like a neuropathic bladder, although there are no neurological deficits. Boys are affected more commonly and it is an acquired behavior, usually during toilet training. There is inappropriate voluntary contraction of the striated urinary sphincter during the process of micturition. This results in a functional urinary obstruction that eventually causes UTIs, myogenic bladder failure, hydronephrosis, and renal insufficiency.
7. Traumatic or infectious urethral obstruction: Traumatic strictures of the urethra can occur after traumatic urethral catheterization, presence of a foreign body in the urethra, or pelvic trauma. Infectious strictures can result from purulent urethritis due to bacteria such as *Neisseria gonorrhoeae.*
8. Diabetes mellitus
9. Acquired diabetes insipidus
10. Myogenic detrusor failure: Seen commonly in neurogenic bladders and in patients with posterior urethral valves. It develops over time, so it is usually not recognized until early adolescence. Affected teens suffer from residual urine in the bladder, which makes them prone to UTIs. As there is a hyperreflexic state of the detrusor, hydronephrosis develops before decompensation.

EPIDEMIOLOGY

1. Prevalence: Decreasing prevalence occurs with increasing age.
   a. Age 4: 30%
   b. Age 5: 14% to 20%
   c. Age 6: 10%
   d. Age 10: 5% to 10%
   e. Age 12: 3%
   f. Age 15: 2%
   g. Age 18: 1% to 2%
   h. Army recruits: 0.1% to 2.5% (according to studies of this group)
2. Sex: Male to female ratio is 3:2.
3. Race: More African-American teens are affected than white teens.
4. Timing: Eighty percent to 85% of teens have nocturnal enuresis only, whereas 15% to 20% of teens have nocturnal and daytime enuresis. Eighty percent of adolescents have primary MNE and 20% have secondary MNE.

DIAGNOSIS

A thorough history, a focused physical examination, and simple laboratory tests are all that are usually needed to evaluate enuresis, because significant organic lesions are infrequent. The prevalence of organic lesions is higher in adolescents than children. The prevalence of a psychological or organic cause is higher in secondary and daytime enuresis.

History

The history should include the following:

1. Severity of enuresis: How many dry nights per month, most consecutive dry nights, frequency of urination, urgency of urination, evening fluid intake, and whether the bladder is emptied at bedtime.
2. Type of enuresis: Primary or secondary, polysymptomatic or monosymptomatic.
3. Symptoms of organic disease: Dysuria, intermittent daytime wetness, polydipsia, central nervous system trauma, constipation, or encopresis can indicate an organic disease. Patients with ectopic ureter will complain of constant wetness or dampness. Spinal tumors cause a change in gait, constipation, or encopresis.
4. History of UTIs
5. Toilet-training history
6. Family history of enuresis or small bladders
7. Awakening to use toilet at night: Self-awakens to full bladder, self-awakens to wetness, never awakens spontaneously, awakened by parent, evidence of deep sleep, sleepwalking.
8. Prior therapeutic modalities and results
9. Functional bladder capacity measurement
10. Adolescent's and family's adjustment to the problem
11. Family member responsible for changing sheets and laundry
12. History of any sleep disorders, such as night terrors or unusually deep sleep
13. General psychosocial review of family, peers, and school
14. Timing of wetting: Adolescents who suffer from vaginal reflux of urine, labial fusion, or postvoid dribble syndrome wet after voiding. Other etiologies of enuresis cause wetting before voiding.
15. Voiding history: Teens with urethral obstruction need to push to initiate or sustain voiding. The urinary stream is often weak, interrupted, or of narrow caliber. A history of dribbling or hesitancy suggests posterior urethral valves.
16. Urgency of urination: The common causes of urgency of urination are UTIs, bacteria without dysuria (which can irritate bladder mucosa and cause urinary urgency), or constipation. Rare causes include a bladder calculus, a bladder foreign body, and hypercalciuria.

Physical Examination

1. Check blood pressure.
2. Abdomen: Check for masses.
3. Genitourinary tract: Check the urethral meatus for evidence of stenosis. Observe the urinary stream to see whether it is full and forceful or narrow and dribbling.
4. Look for midline defects in the lumbosacral area, abnormalities of the gluteal fold, or abnormal tufts of hair.
5. Perform a neurological examination including:
   a. Gait
   b. Lower extremity: Motor and sensory
   c. Deep tendon reflexes
   d. Perineal sensation
   e. Rectal sphincter tone
   f. Bulbocavernosus reflex

Laboratory Tests

1. Urinalysis: Every patient should have a urinalysis. This simple, noninvasive test can screen for UTIs, diabetes mellitus, and diabetes insipidus (a specific gravity of

>1.015 g or a specific gravity >1.025 g after a 14-hour fluid restriction rules out diabetes insipidus). Look for the presence of glucose, protein, or white blood cells, and assess the specific gravity. Urethral obstruction can be associated with hematuria.

2. Urine culture: Obtain a urine culture if the urinalysis suggests a UTI.

3. Uroflowmetry: A noninvasive measure of urine flow rate. It can assist in screening for patients with neurogenic bladder and urethral obstruction. Patients void into a special toilet with a pressure-sensitive rotating disk at the base. A normal uroflow study shows a single bell-shaped curve with a normal peak and average flow velocity for age and size. Patients with urethral obstruction or neurogenic bladder have a prolonged curve or an interrupted series of curves and a low peak and average urine flow velocity.

4. Bladder capacity: The teen and his or her family can measure their bladder capacity at home or in the office. The patient drinks 12 oz of water and then the volume of urine is measured when the patient needs to void. Although the formula, age in years plus 2, for calculating the bladder capacity applies to measuring children's bladder capacity, it does not apply to adolescents. Normal adult bladder capacity is 10 to 15 oz.

5. Imaging studies: Radiological studies are not needed routinely. If a urethral obstruction or a neurogenic bladder is suspected, then a voiding cystourethrogram is indicated (the neurogenic bladder will appear as a trabeculated "Christmas tree" or "pine cone" configuration). If a neurogenic bladder is suspected and there is no obvious cause, then obtain a spinal magnetic resonance image to look for spinal cord abnormalities. Ultrasonography is indicated for patients with persistent daytime wetness or for patients with failure to empty the bladder (whether due to urge syndrome, urethral obstruction, or neurogenic bladder). A prevoiding and postvoiding bladder ultrasonography can be obtained to rule out partial emptying (normal residual bladder volume is <10 mL).

THERAPY

If a urological lesion is discovered, then referral to an urologist for appropriate management is recommended. If an occult spinal dysraphism is detected, then neurosurgical referral is warranted. As stated, most affected adolescents are without organic lesions. In most teens, the cause of enuresis is generally multifactorial and includes genetic predisposition, small bladder capacity, a sleep disorder, maturational delay, detrusor instability, nocturnal polyuria, or abnormal secretion of ADH. Because of the multifactorial causes of enuresis, treatment requires several months before improvement or resolution is achieved. The parents must be willing to participate and the family environment should be supportive. Both the parents and the teen need to understand that relapses can be expected and that short-term failure is possible. A goal-oriented therapeutic approach is more successful and the patient needs to be motivated to participate in treatment.

Therapy includes the following:

1. Motivational counseling: Regardless of any other modalities chosen, motivational counseling is helpful. Studies indicate that counseling alone leads to a 25% to 70% remission rate. The relapse rate is 5%. If there is a lack of improvement after 3 to 6 months, other methods should be tried. Through motivational counseling, the teen learns to assume responsibility and become an active participant in the management program. In such a program, the practitioner does the following:

a. Reassures the adolescent and family members that this problem is common to many teens. The parents and the teen should not feel guilty about "causing" the problem.

b. Gives the adolescent an active role by putting him or her in charge of changing the sheets and placing them in the laundry machines. The parents should be encouraged to take a backseat position in dealing with the problem.

c. Reduces secondary friction caused by enuresis.

d. Gives positive reinforcement for dryness.

e. Provides close initial follow-up with the practitioner.

2. Self-awakening or parent-awakening programs: These programs work by training adolescents to recognize when their bladder is full, awakening, and walking to the bathroom. It is useful to inform the teens that they do not need to "hold" their urine all night.

a. Self-awakening programs: This method can be taught in several ways. One technique is to have the teen lie in bed with eyes closed and pretend it is the middle of the night and his or her full bladder is trying to wake him. The teen then goes to the bathroom and empties her bladder. Another technique has the teen go to bed when he or she has the urge to urinate. The teen then pretends to sleep, "awakens," and walks to the bathroom to urinate. A third technique has the teen use self-hypnosis at bedtime with the posthypnotic suggestion that the teen will wake up and use the bathroom during the night.

b. Parent-awakening programs: If self-awakening is not effective, then parent awakening can be used. The parent awakens the patient, but the teen must locate the bathroom alone. It is recommended that the parent use the minimal prompt necessary to awaken the teen. Parents need to awaken their child at the parent's bedtime each night until the teen awakens quickly to sound for seven consecutive nights. At that point, the patient is either cured or ready for an enuresis alarm.

c. Dry bed training: This is a more labor-intensive parent-awakening program. The teen needs to be awakened once an hour until 1 a.m. on the first night. When the teen is awake enough to speak coherently, the parent asks him or her if she needs to use the bathroom. The teen is praised if she is dry. If wet, the teen is encouraged to change the clothes and bedding. At 1 a.m., the teen is instructed to try voiding, even if dry. For the next five nights, the teen is awakened only once. The teen is awakened 3 hours after falling asleep the first night. The second night, the teen is awakened 2.5 hours after falling asleep. By the fifth night, the teen should be awakened 1 hour after falling asleep. On the sixth night, the teen is instructed to self-awaken from then on. If the teen relapses (defined as three consecutive wet nights), then repeat the six nights of awakening. One study found that the cure rate was 92% using this technique and that the relapse rate was 20% (with all patients who relapsed responding to a second trial of training).

3. Alarm systems: Enuresis alarms have the highest cure rate of any available treatment for enuresis. Several

studies have shown comparable cure rates between medications and alarms in the short term. However, these same studies showed persistent effectiveness only with the alarm. The teen has the choice of either wearing an audio alarm or a tactile alarm. The alarms are comfortable, convenient, and inexpensive. The disadvantages to the alarm are that they are time intensive (they need to be used for 2 to 3 months and continued until 3 weeks after dryness has been achieved) and the teen and parent must be motivated to use them properly. By learning to awaken as quickly as possible to the alarm, the teen eventually learns to awaken to the internal stimulus of a full bladder.

  a. Types: Older alarms required elaborate pad-and-bell systems. Newer alarms are lightweight, easy to use, and relatively inexpensive ($40–$90). The alarms consist of two clips attached to the teen's underwear and connected to a wrist alarm or pajama collar alarm. The alarm buzzes if a small amount of wetness occurs on the underwear. Alarms are available from:

Nytone ($69.50)	Wet-Stop ($72)
Medical Products, Inc.	Palco Laboratories
2424 South 900 West	8030 Soquel Drive
Salt Lake City, UT 84119	Santa Cruz, CA 95062
801-973-4090	800-346-4488
www.nytone.com	www.wet-stop.com

  If the teen's family cannot afford to buy an enuresis alarm, then a clock radio, alarm clock, or wristwatch alarm set for 3 hours after going to sleep can be used.

  b. Basis for using alarm: The alarm awakens the teen and usually leads to a contraction of the external bladder sphincter. In order for enuresis alarms to be effective, the teen needs to be able to awaken to touch or sound. Therefore, it is worthwhile to see whether the patient can respond to parent awakening or alarm clock awakening. Further, the teen must want to use the alarm. This technique is ineffective for teens indifferent to using the alarm. The alarm should be continued until 3 weeks after dryness has been achieved.

  c. Results: Long-term cure rates average 70%. Alarm failure rates range from 20% to 30%. Common reasons for alarm failure include the following:
  • The parents discontinue the alarm too soon.
  • The teen fails to hear the alarm because he or she is such a deep sleeper.
  • The teen refuses to use the alarm.
  • The teen refuses to try any technique.
  • The teen suffers from polysymptomatic enuresis (may need oxybutynin in addition to an alarm).
  • The teen wets during deep sleep when it is difficult to awaken the teen (combined treatment with drugs may be necessary; once the teen is dry on drugs, the alarm can be restarted and the drug tapered).

4. Fluid restriction: Have the teen take 40% of their daily fluid intake in the morning hours (7 a.m.–12 noon), 40% in the afternoon (12 p.m.–5 p.m.), and only 20% in the evening (after 5 p.m.). Beverages consumed in the evening should be caffeine free.

5. Other behavioral methods: Biofeedback and pelvic floor muscle retraining have been tried, with varying degrees of success. Bladder exercises have been used to increase bladder tone and size for patients (primarily children) with small bladder capacity. Hypnosis has been shown to be effective in curing enuresis in noncontrolled studies (Olness, 1979; Johnson, 1981). Hypnosis may be successful in treating enuretic patients who are highly motivated. The technique involves suggestions that the adolescent wake up when the urge to urinate occurs and go to the bathroom.

6. Medications: No drug exists that is adequately safe and effective for curing enuresis. However, most pediatricians agree that intermittent use of drugs is appropriate for teens when needed for camping trips, school trips, vacations, or overnights. The major drugs available include the following:

  a. Desmopressin (DDAVP)
  • Action: DDAVP is a synthetic analog of vasopressin. The mechanism of action of the drug is the reduction of urine production by increasing water retention and urine concentration in the distal tubules. Treatment of enuresis using DDAVP is based on the hypothesis that ADH secretion at night is insufficient.
  • Dose: DDAVP is tasteless and odorless and can be administered either intranasally or orally. It is given in the late evening to reduce urine production during sleep. The medication comes as a nasal spray that delivers 10 μg per spray or as a graduated intranasal tube (Rhinal Tube) that delivers doses of 5, 10, 15, and 20 μg per spray. The usual initial dose is 20 μg, or one spray in each nostril, at bedtime. The dose can be increased by 10 μg weekly to a maximum dose of 40 μg. Some individuals may respond to a dose as low as 5 μg/day. The Rhinal Tube must be used if 5-μg doses are required. If the patient remains completely dry on a particular dose, then a dose of 10 μg less should be tried. The duration of action is 10 to 12 hours.
  • Results: DDAVP was approved for the treatment of nocturnal enuresis at the end of 1989. The response to DDAVP improves with increasing age in patients with nocturnal enuresis. Therefore, the best results are seen in patients older than 10 years. A family history of nocturnal enuresis at ages older than 10 years and a normal bladder capacity are also predictors of a positive response to DDAVP. Seventy percent of patients with nocturnal enuresis who receive DDAVP stop their bed-wetting completely or reduce it significantly. A positive effect of the medication is seen within a few days and is maintained as long as the drug is administered. Most patients have a relapse after drug withdrawal, particularly if the drug is stopped abruptly (relapse rates can be as high as 50%–95%). Therefore, the drug should be tapered off slowly. Long-term treatment lasting at least 1 year is becoming more routine. Several long-term studies have found that 50% to 85% of patients on long-term treatment halved the number of wet nights and 40% to 70% became almost completely dry during treatment. The efficacy of DDAVP continued or improved throughout the treatment period, suggesting that patients did not develop tolerance to DDAVP. During long-term therapy, treatment-free windows of approximately 3-month intervals are essential to avoid treating a child who has become dry.

- Side effects: Side effects are infrequent but can include symptomatic hyponatremia (limit fluid intake to 8 oz in the evening hours to avoid this adverse effect), headache, abdominal discomfort, nausea, nasal congestion, rhinitis, nosebleeds, abdominal cramps, and sore throats. These symptoms usually disappear with a reduction in the dose.
- Oral DDAVP: Stenberg and Lackgren (1993) found that oral DDAVP is as effective as intranasal DDAVP and as safe, with similar adverse effects (e.g., headache and abdominal pain). However, at least a tenfold increase in the DDAVP dose is required, compared with the intranasal dose. The initial dose is 0.2 mg (one tablet), given 1 hour before bedtime. If there is no response within a week, increase the dose by 0.2 mg up to a maximum of 0.6 mg nightly.

b. Imipramine (Tofranil)
  - Action: This drug combines an anticholinergic effect that increases bladder capacity with a noradrenergic effect that decreases bladder detrusor excitability. Imipramine is also thought to increase excretion of ADH from the posterior portion of the pituitary gland.
  - Dose: Imipramine is taken 1 hour before bedtime. The duration of action is 8 to 12 hours. Start the patient at 50 mg/day and increase the dose weekly, as needed, to a maximum dose of 75 mg/day. A sustained-release form of imipramine, Tofranil-PM, is also available.
  - Results: Response rate is 25% to 40%; relapse rate can be as high as 75%. The relapse rate is higher when the drug is stopped abruptly or prematurely. The maximal effect of imipramine usually occurs in the first week of therapy. However, one should continue therapy for 1 to 2 weeks before deciding on efficacy and whether to adjust the dose. The current recommendation is to treat for 3 to 9 months and then taper the drug by decreasing the dose by 25 mg decrements over 3 to 4 weeks. If the patient has a relapse, one can repeat a course of therapy. The drug is most beneficial for occasional use when dryness is necessary (e.g., trips, vacations, sleepover parties). Imipramine and DDAVP have been found to be equivalent in effectiveness (Glazener and Evans, 2000). An advantage of imipramine is that it is inexpensive ($5/ month for generic formulations versus $150–250/ month for DDAVP).
  - Side effects: Nervousness, gastrointestinal distress, syncope, and anxiety can occur. Because of imipramine lethality when taken in overdose, both parents and teens need to be aware of its toxicity.

c. Oxybutynin (Ditropan)
  - Action: Oxybutynin provides an anticholinergic, antispasmodic effect that reduces uninhibited detrusor muscle contractions and increases bladder capacity. Therefore, it may be most beneficial for patients with small capacity bladders who also have daytime frequency or enuresis associated with uninhibited bladder contractions.
  - Dosage: A sustained-release formulation of oxybutynin is available (10 mg/day), as well as a conventional formulation (5 mg twice daily). Birns et al. (2000) found that the effectiveness and side effect profile are comparable with either formulation.
  - Results: A success rate of 90% was reported in one study of individuals with daytime enuresis, bladder instability, or both. The drug is rarely helpful in treating patients with MNE. It is to be used in teens with PNE, urge syndrome, or neurogenic bladder.
  - Side effects: Dry mouth, flushing, drowsiness, and constipation.

d. Combined drug therapy with enuresis alarms: Combining drugs with an alarm is very effective in the treatment of enuresis. Glazener and Evans (2000) found that combining drugs with alarms is more effective than using alarms alone. Teens who have frequent enuresis are candidates for this therapy. The drug can both prevent the necessity of awakening to use the bathroom and delay the filling of the bladder until early morning. The enuresis alarm is the backup system. After the adolescent is dry for 3 weeks, the drug is tapered gradually (if using DDAVP, decrease by one spray every 2 weeks; if using imipramine, decrease by 25 mg every 2 weeks).

TREATMENT RELAPSES AND FAILURES

Treatment relapse is defined as the recurrence of enuresis after having been dry for at least 1 month. The remedy is to reinstitute the treatment that was effective previously. Treatment failure occurs when the patient cannot remain dry despite using the alarm or combined therapy. For adolescents, the best approach is to put the teen in charge of solving the problem and emphasize that he or she will become dry once she learns to self-awaken.

PROGNOSIS

Reported spontaneous cure rates (Forsythe and Redmond, 1974) are as follows:

1. Ages 5 to 9: 14%/yr
2. Ages 10 to 14: 16%/yr
3. Ages 15 to 19: 16%/yr
4. After age 20: 3%/yr

WEB SITES

For Teenagers and Parents

http://www.kidney.org/patients/bw/. The National Kidney Foundation's Web site. This link connects to the patient section of the Web site, where information is provided on enuresis in children, teens, and young adults.

http://www.childrensmemorial.org/depts/urology/ enuresis.asp. Children's Memorial Hospital of Chicago's enuresis Web site. It provides good information for parents and teens on enuresis, medications, recommended readings, and related web links.

http://www.eric.org.uk/. A Web site based in the United Kingdom. It provides good information on the etiology, epidemiology, and treatment of enuresis.

http://www.parenthood.com/articles.html?article_id=5351. A Web site aimed at parents. It provides links to pertinent

Web sites about enuresis with a helpful rating system of the Web sites.

http://www.parenthood.com/articles.html?article_id=5351. The Web site of the International Children's Continence Society. It offers a free membership area with relevant research articles pertinent to the field of enuresis, offers a message board, and offers links to support groups and recommended readings.

REFERENCES AND ADDITIONAL READINGS

Arnell H, Hjalmas K, Jagervall M, et al. The genetics of primary nocturnal enuresis: inheritance and suggestion of a second major gene on chromosome 12q. *J Med Genet* 1997;34:360.

Austin PF, Ritchey ML. Dysfunctional voiding. *Pedr Rev* 2000; 21(10):336.

Banerjee S, Srivastav A, Palan BM. Hypnosis and self-hypnosis in the management of nocturnal enuresis: a comparative study with imipramine therapy. *Am J Clin Hypn* 1993;36: 113.

Birns J, Lukkari E, Malone-Lee JG. Oxybutynin CR Clinical Trial Group. A randomized controlled trial comparing the efficacy of controlled-release oxybutynin tablets (10 mg once daily) with conventional oxybutynin tablets (5 mg twice daily) in patients whose symptoms were stabilized on 5 mg twice daily of oxybutynin. *BJU Int* 2000;85:793.

Bloom D. The American experience with desmopressin. *Clin Pediatr* 1993;July (Spec No):28.

Derman O, Kanbur NO, Kinik E. The evaluation of desmopressin in treatment of adolescent nocturnal enuresis. *Int J Adolesc Med Health* 2004;16:377.

Devitt H, Holland P, Butler R, et al. Plasma vasopressin and response to treatment in primary nocturnal enuresis. *Arch Dis Child* 1999;80:448.

Eggert P, Kuhn B. Antidiuretic hormone regulation in patients with primary nocturnal enuresis. *Arch Dis Child* 1995;73: 508.

Forsythe WI, Redmond A. Enuresis and spontaneous cure rate. *Arch Dis Child* 1974;49:259.

Fritz GK, Rockney RM, Yeung AS. Plasma levels and efficacy of imipramine treatment for enuresis. *J Am Acad Child Adolesc Psychiatry* 1994;33:60.

Glazener C, Evans J. Desmopressin for nocturnal enuresis in children. *Cochrane Database Syst Rev* 2000;2:CD002112.

Gonzales ET. *Approach to the child with nocturnal enuresis and management of nocturnal enuresis in children.* Up To Date 2005.

Hogg RJ, Husmann D. The role of family history in predicting response to desmopressin in nocturnal enuresis. *J Urol* 1993; 150:444.

Janknegt R, Zweers H, Delaere K, et al. Oral desmopressin as a new treatment modality for primary nocturnal enuresis in adolescents and adults: a double-blind, randomized, multicenter study. *J Urol* 1997;157:513.

Johnson RL. Use of hypnosis with enuretic adolescents. *J Curr Adolesc Med* 1981;2:39.

Key DW, Bloom DA, Sanvordenker J. Low-dose DDAVP in nocturnal enuresis. *Clin Pediatr* 1992;31:299.

Khan Z, Starer P, Singh VK, et al. Role of detrusor instability in primary enuresis. *Urology* 1993;41:189.

Kodman-Jones C, Hawkins L, Schulman SL. Behavioral characteristics of children with daytime wetting. *J Urol* 2001;166: 2392.

Lawless M, McElderry D. Nocturnal enuresis: current concepts. *Pedr Rev* 2001;22(12):399.

Lee T, Suh HJ, Lee HJ, et al. Comparison of effects of treatment of primary nocturnal enuresis with oxybutynin plus desmopressin, desmopressin alone or imipramine alone: a randomized controlled clinical trial. *J Urology* 2005;174: 1084.

Matthiesen TB, Rittig S, Djurhuus JC, et al. A dose titration and an open 6-week efficacy and safety study of desmopressin tablets in the management of nocturnal enuresis. *J Urol* 1994; 151:460.

McKenna P, Herndon C, Connery S, et al. Pelvic floor muscle retraining for pediatric voiding dysfunction using interactive computer games. *J Urol* 1999;162:1056.

Miller K. Concomitant nonpharmacologic therapy in the treatment of primary nocturnal enuresis. *Clin Pediatr* 1993;July (Spec No):32.

Monda J, Husmann D. Primary nocturnal enuresis: a comparison among observation, imipramine, desmopressin acetate and bed-wetting alarm systems. *J Urol* 1995;154:745.

Nappo S, Del Gado R, Chiozza ML, et al. Nocturnal enuresis in the adolescent: a neglected problem. *Pedr Urol* 2002;90:912.

Neveus T, Lackgren G, Tuvemo T, et al. Desmopressin resistant enuresis: pathogenetic and therapeutic considerations. *J Urol* 1999;162:2136.

Norgaard JP, Djurhuus JC. The pathophysiology of enuresis in children and young adults. *Clin Pediatr (Phila)* 1993;July (Spec No):5.

Olness K. The use of self-hypnosis in the treatment of childhood nocturnal enuresis. *Clin Pediatr* 1979;14:273.

Porena M, Costantini E, Rociola W, et al. Biofeedback successfully cures detrusor-sphincter dyssynergia in pediatric patients. *J Urol* 2000;163:1927.

Pretlow R. Treatment of nocturnal enuresis with an ultrasound bladder volume controlled alarm device. *J Urol* 1999; 162:1224.

Robson WL. Diurnal enuresis. *Pediatr Rev* 1997;18:407.

Robson WL, Leung AKC, Van Howe R. Primary and secondary nocturnal enuresis: similarities in presentation. *Pediatrics* 2005;115(4):956.

Rushton HG. Older pharmacologic therapy for nocturnal enuresis. *Clin Pediatr* 1993;July (Spec No):10.

Rushton HG. Evaluation of the enuretic child. *Clin Pediatr* 1993;July (Spec No):14.

Schmitt BD. Overcoming bed-wetting in the teen years. *Contemp Pediatr* 1992;9:77.

Schmitt BD. Nocturnal enuresis. *Pediatr Rev* 1997;18:183.

Schulman S, Colish Y, von Zuben F, et al. Effectiveness of treatments for nocturnal enuresis in a heterogenous population. *Clin Pediatr* 2000;39:359.

Shu SG, Lili YP, Chi CS. The efficacy of intranasal DDAVP therapy in children with nocturnal enuresis. *Chung-Hua I Hsueh Tsa Chih* 1993;52:368.

Skoog S, Stokes A, Turner K. Oral desmopressin: a randomized double-blind placebo controlled study of effectiveness in children with primary nocturnal enuresis. *J Urol* 1997;158:1035.

Stenberg A, Lackgren G. Treatment with oral desmopressin in adolescents with primary nocturnal enuresis: efficacy and long-term effect. *Clin Pediatr* 1993;July (Spec No):25.

Van Kampen M, Bogaert G, Feys H, et al. High initial efficacy of full-spectrum therapy for nocturnal enuresis in children and adolescents. *BJU Int* 2002;90(1):84.

Van Kerrebroeck PEV. Experience with the long-term use of desmopressin for nocturnal enuresis in children and adolescents. *BJU Int* 2002;89(4):420.

Von Gontard A, Schaumburg H, Hollmann E, et al. The genetics of enuresis: a review. *J Urol* 2001;166:2438.

Von Gontard A, Schmelzer D, Seifen S, et al. Central nervous system involvement in nocturnal enuresis: evidence of general neuromotor delay and specific brainstem dysfunction. *J Urol* 2001;166:2448.

CHAPTER 27

Asymptomatic Proteinuria and Hematuria

Lawrence J. D'Angelo and Lawrence S. Neinstein

ASYMPTOMATIC PROTEINURIA

Asymptomatic proteinuria, defined as proteinuria not associated with hematuria, hypertension, other symptoms or renal insufficiency, is a common finding on a screening urinalysis in adolescent patients. For most of these teens, no significant renal disease is present and the long-term prognosis is excellent. Therefore, except for patients at high risk, screening for proteinuria is not felt to be cost-effective (Boulware et al., 2003). Unfortunately, because testing the urine for protein is so common, many patients with no provable renal disease are identified as having proteinuria. Even in the absence of significant renal disease, proteinuria can cause problems for adolescents by interfering with employment, insurance, or the armed service or by causing anxiety or concerns about long-term prognosis. The objective in evaluating these adolescents is to establish the significance of the proteinuria, search noninvasively for underlying treatable conditions, and select those few patients who need referral for more extensive evaluation, including renal biopsy. Most adolescents can be reassured that they are healthy and that their proteinuria is of no clinical consequence.

Etiology

1. Increased glomerular permeability, as in primary or secondary glomerulopathies (e.g., minimal change disease, systemic lupus erythematosus [SLE], membranous nephropathy)
2. Increased production of abnormal proteins (e.g., monoclonal gammopathies)
3. Decreased tubular reabsorption of proteins, as in tubular disease (e.g., Fanconi syndrome, aminoglycoside nephrotoxicity) or chronic interstitial nephritis
4. Miscellaneous—functional proteinuria (e.g., fever, exercise, congestive heart failure) and orthostatic proteinuria

Epidemiology

Up to 10% to 19% of healthy adolescents have protein in their urine on a dipstick test of a random urine sample. This prevalence falls with repeated testing, and a diagnosis of persistent proteinuria should be based on three separate urine tests. The prevalence peaks at approximately 16 years of age.

Clinical Manifestations

Small amounts of protein in the urine are normal, and most individuals excrete 30 to 130 mg of protein/day. Although the maximum "normal" amount for adolescents and adults is 150 mg/day, completely healthy adolescents may excrete up to 300 mg/day of protein without any evidence of clinical or histopathological renal disease. Nonetheless, "isolated asymptomatic proteinuria" refers to protein excretion of >150 mg/day by a person without clinical signs or symptoms. The leading causes of this condition are "benign persistent proteinuria" and orthostatic proteinuria. Orthostatic (postural) proteinuria, which is proteinuria while upright but not while recumbent, is common in adolescents. The etiology is unclear, although exaggerated hemodynamic response to the upright position and functional compromise of the left renal vein have been postulated as two possible causes (Shintaku et al., 1990). The condition is characterized by the following:

1. An asymptomatic state
2. Age at onset: 10 to 20 years
3. Dipstick urine findings:
   a. In the p.m.: 1 to 3+
   b. In the a.m.: Negative finding
   c. Urine sediment: Negative finding
4. Quantitative protein excretion
   a. Supine: A protein/creatinine ratio of <0.2 on a spot urine sample (<75 mg in 12 hours)
   b. Upright: A spot urine value of 0.3 to 2.0 (150–1,000 mg in 12 hours)
5. Renal function: Normal
   The presence of hypertension, edema, hypoalbuminemia, or hyperlipidemia suggests more significant renal abnormalities.

Differential Diagnosis

1. Mild asymptomatic proteinuria (expected excretion of protein: <500 mg/m^2 in 24 hours)
   a. Benign persistent proteinuria
   b. Orthostatic or postural proteinuria (proved with split 24-hour urine collection)

c. Pyelonephritis (usually with fever and pyuria)
d. Renal tubular disorders
e. Chronic interstitial nephritis
f. Congenital dysplastic lesions
g. Other: Exercise, trauma (with hematuria), fever, congestive heart failure (severe)
2. Moderate proteinuria (expected excretion of protein: 500–2,000 mg/m^2 in 24 hours)
   a. Acute poststreptococcal glomerulonephritis (PSGN)
   b. Primary glomerulonephritis
   c. Hereditary chronic nephritis (Alport syndrome)
   d. Systemic diseases: SLE
3. Severe proteinuria (expected excretion of protein: >2,000 mg/m^2 in 24 hours; usually >3.5 g), typically associated with edema, hypoalbuminemia, and hypercholesterolemia (nephrotic syndrome)
   a. Idiopathic glomerulonephritis: Minimal change disease, focal sclerosis, membranous or membranoproliferative glomerulonephritis
   b. Systemic disease: SLE; amyloidosis (in the setting of chronic inflammatory disease or familial Mediterranean fever)
   c. Less common
      • Infections: Bacterial endocarditis, hepatitis, malaria, human immunodeficiency virus infection
      • Toxins: Mercury, heroin, gold, penicillamine
   d. Uncommon
      • Allergens: Bee stings
      • Mechanical: Pericarditis, renal vein thrombosis
      • Cancer: Hodgkin disease, lymphoma
      • Pregnancy
      • Congenital: Fabry disease and Alport syndrome

Diagnosis

The qualitative dipstick test for protein will detect protein levels as low as 10 to 30 mg/dL. An initial positive test result should be confirmed on two more tests, because many individuals have transient proteinuria and then have negative findings on subsequent evaluation. False-positive test results should be considered (Table 27.1). If proteinuria is confirmed, then a more thorough history, physical examination, and laboratory evaluation are indicated to rule out significant disease. Currently, the most practical method of estimating total urinary protein excretion is a spot urine protein/creatinine ratio. A random urine sample is analyzed for protein and creatinine. When both are expressed in milligram amounts, a ratio of <0.2 is normal and a ratio >1.0 signifies nephrotic-range proteinuria. This test is also useful for monitoring the course of proteinuria without performing the more burdensome timed urine collections.

History Inquire about the following:

1. Recent upper respiratory tract infection or skin infections
2. Edema
3. Skin rashes, arthralgias, or photosensitivity
4. Flank pain, diabetes mellitus (10–14 years of diabetes is usually required before clinical detection of proteinuria; detection of microalbuminuria is possible at earlier stages of disease)
5. Intoxications, drug history, bee stings, and other allergic history
6. Family history of renal disease

Physical Examination Check for the following:

1. Blood pressure; height and weight percentiles
2. Vision and hearing screening, especially if hereditary nephritis is a consideration
3. Edema
4. Rash
5. Abdominal mass
6. Joint examination
7. Cardiac examination
8. Signs of systemic diseases

Laboratory Tests Include the following in the evaluation:

1. Urinalysis
   a. Dipstick tests: Protein, glucose, and blood should be tested. If the dipstick test result is positive for protein, a repeated dipstick test should be performed another one or two times. If protein is still present, a spot urine test for protein/creatinine should be performed.
   b. Microscopical examination for casts and cells: Examination of sediment is crucial because abnormal results suggest an underlying renal problem. Red

TABLE 27.1

Causes of False-Positive Test Results for Proteinuria

Cause	Dipstick Method	Protein Precipitation Methods
Highly concentrated urine[a]	+	+
Gross hematuria	+	+
Contamination with antiseptic (chlorhexidine or benzalkonium)	+	−
Highly alkaline urine	−	−
Radiographic contrast media (affects specific gravity more than proteinuria	−	+
High levels of cephalosporin or penicillin analogs	−	+
Sulfonamide metabolites	−	+

[a]Because the dipstick provides only a qualitative reading, proteinuria (2+) in a highly concentrated urine with a specific gravity of 1.030 may have different (less) significance than proteinuria (2+) in a dilute urine of specific gravity 1.010.
Adapted from Abuelo JF. Proteinuria: diagnostic principles and procedures. *Ann Intern Med* 1983;98:186.

blood cell (RBC) casts suggest glomerulonephritis; white blood cell casts suggest pyelonephritis or interstitial nephritis.

2. Spot urine for protein/creatinine: This simple test has replaced timed urine collections for screening purposes. A ratio of 1.0 closely correlates with the daily excretion of protein of 1.73 g/m^2. This is based on the fact that the average daily excretion of creatinine is approximately 1,000 mg/24 hours/1.73 m^2. To screen for orthostatic proteinuria, a first void specimen obtained immediately on arising is compared with a second specimen obtained at least 4 hours after arising. If the later is at least five times the first specimen, this supports a diagnosis of orthostatic proteinuria.

    Follow-up should be done every 6 to 12 months to monitor for increasing proteinuria, a rising serum creatinine concentration, or the development of hematuria or hypertension. Although it is unusual, significant glomerulopathies can begin with orthostatic proteinuria that later becomes persistent.

3. If the urine protein/creatinine ratio is >0.5 with no definitive postural change, then further evaluation is indicated. This may include a timed urine collection (ideally 24 hours), serum urea nitrogen and creatinine concentrations; complete blood cell count; concentrations of albumin, antinuclear antibody, and cholesterol; hepatitis B screening tests; complement levels (CH$_{50}$, C3, C4); and an antistreptolysin O (ASO) titer. Not all tests need be done at once. The clinical history and physical examination should direct the order and amount of testing. Perform the following if signs or symptoms are suggestive of hepatitis, streptococcal infections, or SLE:
   a. Hepatitis: Measure liver enzymes and hepatitis B surface antigen.
   b. Recent streptococcal infection: Determine serum complement and antistreptococcal enzyme titers.
   c. SLE: Determine antinuclear antigen (ANA) and complement levels.

4. Renal ultrasonography: Order if renal function is abnormal or nonpostural proteinuria is present. This test yields useful information, such as the number of kidneys present (1 in every 1,000 people is born with a single kidney, a finding that could influence subsequent evaluation and treatment), the size of the kidneys (small kidney size reflects chronic disease), and echogenicity. Although the test is nonspecific, increased renal echogenicity reflects "medical renal disease" that may require further evaluation.

5. Renal biopsy: Because of the limited number of treatment options for many renal lesions, the frequent use of therapeutic trials, and the ability to diagnose common lesions on the basis of the history and laboratory findings, the indications for a renal biopsy are now more limited than in the past. A biopsy can help define the nature of the renal disease if the history, physical examination, and laboratory tests are not revealing. A biopsy can also define the severity of the lesion and help in determining its prognosis. This information is very important for teens and their families who are confronted with a diagnosis of renal disease. Refer the patient to a nephrologist for further evaluation and consideration for renal biopsy in the following situations:
   a. A spot urine protein/creatinine ratio of >1.0 (suggesting the 24-hour protein concentration is >1,000 mg).
   b. The diagnosis is unclear and significant disease is suspected because of the presence of proteinuria, hematuria, hypertension, or renal insufficiency.
   c. Nephrotic syndrome is present and has not responded to a therapeutic trial of corticosteroids for minimal change disease.
   d. Renal function is deteriorating.
   e. The patient, family, or both express a need for prognostic information.

With a careful history, physical examination, urinalysis, and 24-hour urinary protein test, one should be able to identify those adolescents with significant proteinuria and thereby determine which teenagers need follow-up only and which need referral for more expert monitoring or renal biopsy.

Prognosis and Follow-up

Isolated Proteinuria In general, the prognosis for asymptomatic orthostatic or persistent proteinuria (excretion of <500 mg protein in 24 hours) is good. A study of the 1937 Yale University class revealed a prevalence of proteinuria of 13.8% (Baskin et al., 1972). On 30-year follow-up, the group with proteinuria had a mortality rate similar to that of the rest of the class. Another study of patients observed

TABLE 27.2

Risk of Chronic Renal Disease and Recommended Follow-up

Pattern of Protein Excretion	Risk of Chronic Renal Failure	Recommended Evaluation	Interval (yr)
Transient	None		
Intermittent		None	
<150 mg/day	None		
150 mg/day	Very slight, if any	Blood pressure, urinalysis	1
Constant	20% after 10 yr (depending on exact lesion)	Blood pressure, urinalysis, blood urea nitrogen, serum creatinine	0.5–1
Orthostatic	Very slight, if any	Blood pressure, urinalysis, monitor change in pattern or amount of proteinuria	1–2

Adapted from Abuelo JF. Proteinuria: diagnostic principles and procedures. *Ann Intern Med* 1983;98:186.

for 20 years showed only 17% with persistent proteinuria, with the decrease being progressive over time (Springberg et al., 1982). Table 27.2 addresses the risk of chronic renal disease based on the pattern of proteinuria and suggests recommendations for follow-up.

Nonisolated Proteinuria The prognosis depends on the underlying cause of the proteinuria and is rarely dictated by the level of the proteinuria. The exception to this is proteinuria seen as a part of diabetic nephropathy—the ultimate prognosis is worse as the level of protein excretion rises.

Microalbuminuria There is some evidence that abnormal urinary microalbumin excretion may be a marker for renal disease in "healthy" children and adolescents. It has been documented to be a risk factor for renal complications in those with hypertension and diabetes mellitus. Assaid (2005) found that in those children and adolescents with hematuria, the presence of microalbuminuria (microalbumin/creatinine [MA/Cr] μg/mg ratio >30) had a 91% prevalence of abnormal renal biopsies. This may be a useful screen in those individuals with microscopic hematuria to evaluate for higher risk categories.

HEMATURIA

Hematuria is defined as the excretion of abnormal quantities of RBCs in the urine. Most authorities accept 2 to 4 erythrocytes per high-power field (HPF) on a resuspended centrifuged urine sediment specimen as normal. The orthotoluidine-impregnated paper strips give a positive result with a urine specimen that contains as few as 2 to 5 RBCs/HPF. Hematuria must be differentiated from pigmenturia caused by myoglobinuria, hemoglobinuria, porphyrinuria, or exogenous pigments.

Epidemiology

Fewer than 3% of healthy individuals excrete >3 RBCs/HPF. Several studies have examined the prevalence of hematuria in school-aged children and young adults and these have ranged from 0.5% to 5.6% (Vehaskari et al., 1979; Dodge et al., 1976; Froom et al., 1984).

Clinical Manifestations

Like proteinuria, hematuria in adolescents is usually asymptomatic. When present, however, the symptoms often suggest a cause. Lower urinary tract infections cause dysuria and frequency, whereas upper tract infections are accompanied by fever and flank pain. Renal stones are often heralded by colicky flank pain, whereas "loin-pain hematuria" is characterized by episodic unilateral or bilateral loin pain. Rash and joint pain often accompany SLE, whereas abdominal pain and "palpable purpura" are seen with Henoch-Schönlein disease. Intrinsic renal disease may be accompanied by edema, hypertension, and symptoms of uremia. Decreased hearing or vision may indicate the presence of familial nephritis.

Differential Diagnosis

Although the differential diagnosis of hematuria is extensive, the common conditions in adolescents are much fewer

and are listed and discussed here separately. In addition, use of a systematic evaluation will narrow the diagnostic possibilities. The causes of hematuria can be divided into renal parenchymal, urinary tract, and systemic coagulation disturbances. False hematuria must also be considered.

Renal Parenchymal Diseases
1. Glomerular diseases
   a. Primary
      - Immunoglobulin A (IgA) nephropathy (Berger disease)
      - Membranous or membranoproliferative glomerulonephritis
      - Focal glomerulonephritis or glomerulosclerosis
   b. Secondary
      - Glomerulonephritis associated with connective tissue diseases, hemolytic uremic syndrome, or Henoch-Schönlein purpura
      - Glomerulonephritis associated with infections such as streptococcal infection, shunt infections, or infective endocarditis
   c. Hereditary: Alport syndrome, polycystic kidney disease, medullary sponge kidney
   d. Benign familial hematuria: Primary renal hematuria with thin basement membrane
2. Nonglomerular diseases
   a. Vascular diseases
      - Malignant hypertension
      - Loin-pain hematuria syndrome
      - Arteriovenous malformation
      - Renal arterial emboli
   b. Papillary necrosis: Sickle cell disease, diabetes mellitus, alcoholism, analgesic abuse
   c. Trauma: Usually significant trauma, as from motor vehicle accidents or contusions from contact sports
   d. Acute pyelonephritis
   e. Neoplasms

Urinary Tract Disease
1. Hypercalciuria or renal calculi
2. Inflammatory: Urethritis, cystitis, or prostatitis
3. Neoplasms or arteriovenous malformation within the bladder
4. Trauma

Coagulopathies Rarely, hematuria is caused by coagulopathy without structural abnormalities in the genitourinary tract and without the use of instruments such as Foley catheters. Such causes include:

1. Thrombocytopenia
2. Congenital or acquired coagulation defect
3. Use of heparin or warfarin sodium (Coumadin)

False Hematuria False hematuria can be caused by vaginal bleeding, factitious hematuria, or pigmenturia, including endogenous (porphyrinuria, hemoglobinuria, myoglobinuria) and exogenous (foods and drugs) forms of pigmenturia.

Etiology

The most common causes of microscopic hematuria in adolescents are acute lower or upper tract urinary infections, trauma, overexercise, hypercalciuria and renal stones, benign recurrent hematuria, and hereditary nephritis. The most common causes of gross hematuria are IgA nephropathy, trauma, hypercalciuria, and cystitis.

Diagnosis

The health care practitioner must first differentiate between true hematuria and false hematuria.

1. True hematuria: Positive dipstick finding, RBCs on spun urine, clear spun urine, and clear spun serum (unnecessary unless myoglobinuria or hemoglobinuria is suspected)
2. False hematuria
   a. Hemoglobinuria: Positive dipstick finding, negative result of microscopical examination, red spun urine, and pink spun serum
   b. Myoglobinuria: Positive dipstick finding, negative result of microscopic examination, orange-red or brown spun urine, clear spun serum
   c. Porphyrins or exogenous pigments: Negative dipstick finding, negative result of microscopical examination, red spun urine, clear spun serum
   d. Menstruation: Must be ruled out because menstrual blood can easily contaminate urine specimens

History
1. Pattern of hematuria: Microscopic versus macroscopic. Macroscopic, or gross, hematuria is more likely with severe trauma, severe cystitis, or IgA nephropathy. The relationship to intercurrent illnesses may indicate possible PSGN or IgA nephropathy.
2. Family history of renal disease or hematuria: Suggestive of hereditary nephritis, benign familial hematuria, or polycystic kidneys. Family history of vision problems or hearing loss with renal disease may indicate hereditary nephritis.
3. Associated symptoms include the following:
   a. Dysuria, frequency: Cystitis, urethritis, or (rarely) hypercalciuria
   b. Colic: Renal stones
   c. Weight gain: Nephrotic syndrome
   d. Fever: Cystitis, pyelonephritis, or a systemic illness
   e. Joint pain and rashes: SLE or Henoch-Schönlein purpura
   f. Hearing loss: Hereditary nephropathy
   g. Bleeding tendency: Coagulopathy
   h. Previous heart murmurs or a history of tooth extractions: Endocarditis
   i. Loin pain: Loin-pain hematuria syndrome
   j. Blood clots: Lower genitourinary tract disease
4. Drug history: Analgesic abuse; use of warfarin (Coumadin), heparin, or oral contraceptives.
5. Relation to exercise: Short-term hematuria after long-distance running or heavy exercise is suggestive of "athletic hematuria."

Physical Examination
1. Blood pressure: Elevated blood pressure associated with hematuria suggests renal abnormality.
2. Skin: Rashes may indicate connective tissue disease. Ecchymosis is suggestive of Henoch-Schönlein purpura. Petechiae are suggestive of thrombocytopenia.
3. Corneal and lens abnormalities and hearing loss suggest hereditary nephritis.
4. Abdomen: Abdominal masses and renal enlargement may suggest polycystic disease.

Laboratory Tests As with proteinuria, the occurrence of true hematuria is determined with repeated examinations. Therefore, significant hematuria should be confirmed on repeated urinalyses before an extensive evaluation is undertaken. Urine should be examined to determine the presence or absence of RBC casts and proteinuria. RBC casts and >10% dysmorphic RBCs suggest a renal parenchymal origin, usually either glomerulonephritis or interstitial nephritis, and the need for further evaluation. Significant associated proteinuria would also suggest a glomerular cause and the need for further evaluation. Although blood in the urine can cause some proteinuria, even heavy bleeding usually results in <1 g/24 hour. If there are no RBC casts or a qualitative proteinuria (>1+), the evaluation will depend on the history and the physical examination findings. Because idiopathic hypercalciuria is now recognized as an important cause of microscopic hematuria, it is useful to obtain a calcium/creatinine ratio on a spot, random urine sample. A ratio of <0.2 is normal. If the ratio is greater, hypercalciuria is overwhelmingly likely to be the cause of the hematuria and no further evaluation is required.

1. With signs or symptoms suggestive of infection, obtain a urine specimen for culture.
2. Basic laboratory tests should be ordered, as discussed earlier for proteinuria, and should include a complete blood cell count, platelet estimation, and determinations of blood urea nitrogen, creatinine, and complement levels.
3. If coagulopathy is suspected, order determinations of the prothrombin time, partial thromboplastin time, platelet count, and bleeding time, as indicated.
4. For African-American patients, order sickle cell screening or hemoglobin electrophoresis to evaluate for sickle cell trait.
5. In adolescents with signs and symptoms suggestive of connective tissue disease or proteinuria and RBC casts, order the following tests: ANA, anti-DNA antibody, third and fourth components of complement (C3 and C4), ASO titer, audiography, serum albumin, cholesterol, quantitative urinary protein, and creatinine clearance.
6. Check urine of first-degree relatives for hematuria. The presence of hematuria in a parent, sibling, or child of an adolescent may indicate either benign familial hematuria (if family members are well) or hereditary nephritis (if family members have renal disease).

Additional Tests If, after evaluation, the diagnosis is unclear and hematuria is persistent or recurrent, then one should obtain a renal sonogram to look for structural causes of hematuria such as cysts or hydronephrosis. If the diagnosis is still unclear and the patient has lower tract symptoms of dysuria or urgency and the RBC morphological features are normal, the next step is cystoscopy. In the presence of RBC casts and significant proteinuria a renal biopsy is indicated, as is done if hypertension accompanies either of these two symptoms. Without such a history, almost all individuals will have either normal biopsy findings or changes not indicative of significant pathological changes. If gross hematuria persists without an obvious cause, renal angiography can be considered while looking for vascular causes of the hematuria.

Specific Conditions

Marathon Runner's (Athlete's) Hematuria
Gross or microscopic hematuria is associated with many forms of exercise, including baseball, track, football, hockey, boxing, cross-country skiing, swimming, crew, lacrosse, rugby, and military training (Hoover and Cromie, 1981). The typical history is one of normal urine before exercise, with hematuria on the first specimen voided after exercise, lasting up to 24 to 48 hours, possibly in association with dysuria and suprapubic discomfort. The cause is unclear, but the condition seems unrelated to the duration of sustained activity. It may be caused by a decrease in renal plasma flow, local trauma to the bladder, or leakage of blood from spiral vessels in the adventitia of minor calyces. It is less of a problem in children than in older adolescents and adults. The prognosis is excellent unless another renal problem is the underlying cause.

Loin-Pain Hematuria Syndrome
This is a cause of hematuria found mainly in young females receiving oral contraceptives (Burke and Hardie, 1996). The condition occurs with recurrent bouts of gross or microscopic hematuria with or without dysuria but almost always with unilateral or bilateral loin pain. The blood pressure and renal function are normal. Protein excretion is usually <1 g/day. The renal biopsy shows C3 deposits in arterioles by fluorescence microscopy. Treatment has not been satisfactory, although nonsteroidal antiinflammatory agents and calcium channel blockers may be of some use. The use of birth control pills should be discontinued.

IgA Nephropathy (Berger Disease)
IgA nephropathy is a relatively common cause of gross hematuria in young adults. It is associated with IgA and IgG deposits in the mesangium. Eighty percent of patients are between 16 and 35 years of age. The male to female ratio is 6:1. Symptoms include recurrent bouts of hematuria (usually gross) after upper respiratory tract infections. The disease may be associated with dysuria and flank pain. The urinary protein excretion is usually >1 g/day. Renal function is usually normal, but a substantial proportion of individuals (40%) may progress to renal insufficiency over the long term. Poor prognostic signs include hypertension, renal insufficiency, and persistent proteinuria (protein excretion >1 g/day). Serum IgA levels are elevated in 50% of patients. The diagnosis is made by characteristic history or renal biopsy. No treatment is available. Henoch-Schönlein purpura can cause similar renal lesions, but it is associated with nonthrombocytopenic vasculitic purpura, arthralgias, and abdominal pain. These two conditions may represent different parts of the spectrum of a similar pathogenic process.

Hereditary Nephritis (Alport Syndrome) and Polycystic Kidney Disease
The adult form of polycystic kidney disease usually manifests in the second or third decade of life with hematuria and hypertension. It is an autosomal dominant disease. Familial nephritis in males often causes an early onset of renal insufficiency. The renal disease is often accompanied by abnormalities of the lens and retina and high-frequency hearing loss.

Benign Familial Hematuria
This is a condition characterized by glomerular hematuria (RBC casts), nonprogressive renal disease, and normal renal function in many affected family members. It is often associated with thinning of the glomerular basement membrane. The inheritance is autosomal dominant. The diagnosis is suggested by (a) the presence of hemoglobin or RBC casts in the urine of the adolescent and in that of a parent or sibling, (b) absence of renal insufficiency in the patient, and (c) no history of renal failure or auditory abnormalities in the affected family members. The disease is more common in females.

WEB SITES

Proteinuria

For Teenagers and Parents
http://kidney.niddk.nih.gov/kudiseases/pubs/proteinuria/index.htm. National Institutes of Health (NIH) site on proteinuria.
http://www.kidney.org/news/newsroom/fsitem.cfm?id=9. National Kidney Foundation site on proteinuria.

For Health Professionals
http://www.aafp.org/afp/981001ap/loghman.html. American Academy of Family Physicians (AAFP) article on proteinuria in children.
http://www.aafp.org/afp/20000915/1333.html. AAFP article on proteinuria in adults.

Hematuria

For Teenagers and Parents
http://kidney.niddk.nih.gov/kudiseases/pubs/hematuria/index.htm. NIH Education site on hematuria.
http://www.urologychannel.com/Hematuria/. Information site on hematuria.
http://www.keepkidshealthy.com/welcome/commonproblems/hematuria.html. Information site for parents on hematuria in children.

For Health Professionals
http://www.duj.com/hematuria.html. Digital Urology Journal on hematuria.
http://www.aafp.org/afp/20010315/1145.html. AAFP article on workup of microscopic hematuria.

REFERENCES AND ADDITIONAL READINGS

Proteinuria

Abitbol C, Zilleruelo G, Freundlich M, et al. Quantitation of proteinuria with urinary protein/creatinine ratios and random testing with dipsticks in nephrotic children. *J Pediatr* 1990;116:243.

Ahmed Z, Lee J. Asymptomatic urinary abnormalities: hematuria and proteinuria. *Med Clin North Am* 1997;81:641.

Assadi FK. Value of urinary excretion of microalbumin in predicting glomerular lesions in children with isolated microscopic hematuria. *Pediatr Nephrol* 2005;20:1131.

Baskin AM, Freedman LR, Davis JS, et al. Proteinuria in Yale students and 30-year mortality experience. *J Urol* 1972;108:617.

Bergstein JM. A practical approach to proteinuria. *Pediatr Nephrol* 1999;13:697.

Boulware LE, Jaar BG, Tarvar-Carr ME, et al. Screening for proteinuria in US adults: a cost-effectiveness analysis. *JAMA* 2003;290:3101.

Carroll MF, Temte JL. Proteinuria in adults: a diagnostic approach. *Am Fam Physician* 2000;62:1333.

Dodge WE, West EE, Smith EH, et al. Proteinuria and hematuria in school children: epidemiology and natural history. *J Pediatr* 1976;88:327.

Ginsberg JM, Chang BS, Matarese RA, et al. Use of single voided urine samples to estimate quantitative proteinuria. *N Engl J Med* 1983;309:1543.

Gulati S, Sural S, Sharma RK, et al. Spectrum of adolescent-onset nephritic syndrome in Indian adolescents. *Pediatr Nephrol* 2001;16:1045.

Keane WF. Proteinuria: its clinical importance and role in progressive renal disease. *Am J Kidney Dis* 2000;35(4 Suppl 1):S97.

Levey AS, Lau J, Pauker SG, et al. Idiopathic nephrotic syndrome: puncturing the biopsy myth. *Ann Intern Med* 1987;107:697.

Mahan JD, Turman MA, Mentser MI. Evaluation of hematuria, proteinuria, and hypertension in adolescents. *Pediatr Clin North Am* 1997;44:1573.

Park YH, Choi JY, Chung HS. Hematuria and proteinuria in a mass school urine screening test. *Pediatr Nephrol* 2005;20:1126.

Potter EV, Lipschultz SA, Abidh S, et al. Twelve- to seventeen-year follow-up of patients with poststreptococcal acute glomerulonephritis in Trinidad. *N Engl J Med* 1982;307:725.

Shintaku N, Takahashi Y, Akaisha K, et al. Entrapment of left renal vein in children with orthostatic proteinuria. *Pediatr Nephrol* 1990;4:324.

Springberg PD, Garrett LE, Thompson AL, et al. Fixed and reproducible orthostatic proteinuria: results of a 20-year follow-up study. *Ann Intern Med* 1982;97:516.

Stapleton FB. Morphology of urinary red blood cells: a simple guide in localizing the site of hematuria. *Pediatr Clin North Am* 1987;34:561.

Stapleton FB, Noe HN, Roy S, et al. Hypercalciuria in children with urolithiasis. *Am J Dis Child* 1982;136:675.

Thompson AL, Durrett RR, Robinson RR. Fixed and reproducible orthostatic proteinuria: results of a 10-year follow-up evaluation. *Ann Intern Med* 1970;73:235.

Wingo CS, Clapp WL. Proteinuria: potential causes and approach to evaluation. *Am J Med Sci* 2000;320:188.

Hematuria

Ahmed Z, Lee J. Asymptomatic urinary abnormalities: hematuria and proteinuria. *Med Clin North Am* 1997;81:641.

Blumenthal SS, Fritsche C, Lemann J Jr. Establishing the diagnosis of benign familial hematuria. *JAMA* 1988;259:2263.

Burke JR, Hardie IR. Loin pain hematuria syndrome. *Pediatr Nephrol* 1996;10:216.

Cilento BG Jr, Stock JA, Kaplan GW. Hematuria in children: a practical approach. *Urol Clin North Am* 1995;22:43.

Dodge WF, West EE, Smith EH. Proteinuria and hematuria in schoolchildren: epidemiology and early natural history. *J Pediatr* 1976;88:327.

Fairly KF, Birch DE. Hematuria: a simple method for identifying glomerular bleeding. *Kidney Int* 1982;21:105.

Froom P, Ribak J, Benbassat J. Significance of microhaematuria in young adults. *Br Med J* 1984;288:20.

Gordon C, Stapleton FB. Hematuria in adolescents. *Adolesc Med Clin* 2005;16:229.

Hogg RJ. Adolescents with proteinuria and/or the nephrotic syndrome. *Adolesc Med* 2005;16:163.

Hoover DL, Cromie WJ. Theory and management of exercise-related hematuria. *Phys Sportsmed* 1981;9:91.

Mohr DN, Offord KP, Owen RA, et al. Asymptomatic microhematuria and urologic disease: a population-based study. *JAMA* 1986;256:224.

Mokulis JA, Arndt WF, Downey JP, et al. Should renal ultrasound be performed in the patient with microscopic hematuria and a normal excretory urogram? *J Urol* 1995;154:1300.

Praga M, Alefre R, Hernandez E, et al. Familial microscopic hematuria caused by hypercalciuria and hyperuricosuria. *Am J Kidney Dis* 2000;35:141.

Topham PS, Jethwa A, Watkins M, et al. The value of urine screening in a young adult population. *Fam Pract* 2004;21:18.

Trachtman H, Weiss RA, Bennett B, et al. Isolated hematuria in children: indications for a renal biopsy. *Kidney Int* 1984;25:94.

Vehaskari VM, Rapola J, Koskimies O, et al. Microscopic hematuria in schoolchildren: epidemiology and clinicopathologic evaluation. *J Pediatr* 1979;95:676.

CHAPTER **28**

Scrotal Disorders

William P. Adelman and Alain Joffe

MALE GENITAL EXAMINATION

Examination of the male genitalia is a crucial part of the examination of the teenager. It is a relatively easy examination to learn because the male genitalia are readily accessible for palpation and the anatomy is straightforward (Fig. 28.1). Once the anatomy is understood, a history and physical examination is often all that is required to make an accurate diagnosis. If the anatomy of the presenting condition is unclear, because of inability to perform a complete examination, or loss of usual landmarks, ultrasonography is a simple, noninvasive method. Female examiners should note that in a study of male adolescents (Neinstein et al., 1989), males felt equally comfortable with either male or female examiners during this part of the examination. Before beginning the examination, the examiner should make sure that his or her gloved hands are warm.

Inspection

1. Inspect pubic hair area and underlying skin: Note sexual maturity rating (Tanner stage) and local pathological conditions such as folliculitis, herpes, scabies, crabs, warts, or molluscum contagiosum. Shaving of the pubic hair is becoming more prevalent, often aiding the practitioner in visual diagnosis, but confounding pubic hair sexual maturity rating.
2. Inspect groin and inner aspect of thighs: Note swelling from lymphadenopathy or hernias or the presence or absence of fungal or bacterial infection.
3. Inspect penile meatus: Check for presence of discharge, erythema, warts, or hypospadias.
4. Inspect prepuce: Check for phimosis.
5. Inspect penile glans: Check for redness (*Candida* infection, balanitis, contact dermatitis) or ulcerations (herpes, syphilis, trauma). Uncircumcised males have higher prevalence rates of pearly penile papules as well as ulcerative sexually transmitted infections. It is best to have the uncircumcised patient retract his own foreskin. Male genital piercing is becoming more prevalent. Observe for signs of infection or contact dermatitis.
6. Inspect corona: Check for pink, pearly penile papules. These are benign, uniform-sized papules that arise most commonly along the corona, during Tanner stage 2 or 3, in as many as 15% of teenagers (Neinstein and Goldenring, 1984).
7. Inspect shaft: Check closely for ulcers or warts.
8. Inspect scrotum: Check for redness, scabies, candidiasis, folliculitis, or epidermal inclusion cysts. Contraction of the dartos muscle of the scrotal wall produces folds or rugae, most prominent in the younger adolescent. An underdeveloped scrotum may indicate an ipsilateral undescended testicle. With a retractile testicle, the scrotum is normally developed.
9. Inspect testes: The left testicle is usually lower than the right. Check for gross enlargement (tumor, infection, hydrocele, hernia) or for gross asymmetry suggesting possible atrophy or cryptorchidism on one side or unilateral enlargement as seen in tumor. Check for a "transverse lie" or "horizontal lie" of the testis suggesting a "bell clapper deformity" and increasing the risk for torsion.

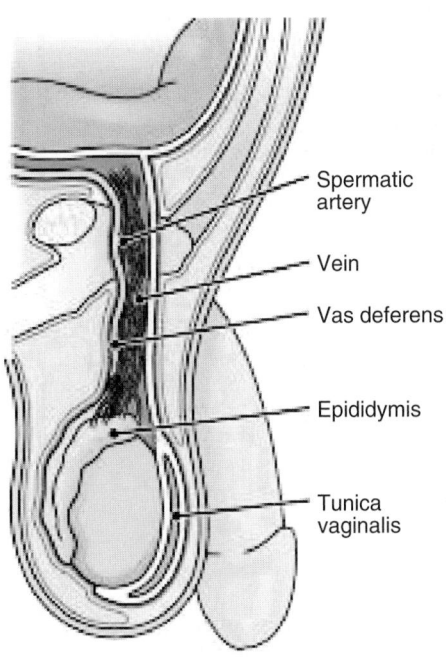

FIGURE 28.1 Male genitalia showing inguinal area, spermatic cord, epididymis, and testis.

Spermatic artery · Vein · Vas deferens · Epididymis · Tunica vaginalis

Palpation

1. Palpate inguinal area: Check for lymphadenopathy or hernia.
2. Palpate the spermatic cord: This fascial-covered structure contains blood vessels, lymphatics, nerves, the vas deferens, and the cremaster muscle. Apply gentle traction on the testis with one hand and palpate the structures of the cord with the index or middle finger and thumb of the opposite hand. The vas deferens feels like a smooth, rubbery tube and is the most posterior structure in the spermatic cord. Absence of the vas deferens bilaterally is associated with cystic fibrosis. Unilateral absence of the vas deferens is associated with ipsilateral renal agenesis. Thickening and irregularity of the vas deferens may be caused by infection. Check for a varicocele (dilated pampiniform plexus of veins) within the spermatic cord.
3. Palpate epididymis: The epididymis lies along the posterolateral wall of the testes. The head of the epididymis attaches at the superior pole of the testicles and runs down the back of the testicles to the tail that lies near the inferior pole. The epididymis becomes the vas deferens and leaves the testicle as part of the spermatic cord. The easiest way to find the epididymis is to follow the vas deferens toward its junction with the tail of the epididymis. Tenderness, induration, and swelling in this area usually indicate epididymitis. A well-localized, nontender, spherical enlargement of the epididymal head is a spermatocele.
4. Palpate testes: Check size, shape, and presence of tenderness or masses. The adult testes are approximately 4 to 5 cm long and 3 cm wide but vary from one person to another. Stabilize the testis with one hand and use the other hand's thumb and first two fingers to palpate the entire surface. The testes should be roughly the same size (within 2 mL in volume of each other). Testicular volume could be quantified with the use of an orchidometer, or by ultrasound. See Chapter 1 for testicular volumes at different pubertal stages. *Any induration within the testis is suspicious of testicular cancer until proved otherwise.* The appendix testis, present in 90% of males, can sometimes be palpated at the superior pole of the testis.
5. Palpate external inguinal ring: Palpate the external inguinal ring by sliding your index finger along the spermatic cord above the inguinal ligament while having the patient cough or strain to check for a hernia.

CRYPTORCHIDISM

Cryptorchidism refers to an undescended testis that cannot be drawn into the scrotum. The normal testicular descent occurs in the eighth month of gestation. If a testis cannot be drawn into the scrotum by the third or fourth month of life, there is little evidence to suggest that it will spontaneously descend later.

Epidemiology

The prevalence of cryptorchidism in newborns is 3.4%, decreasing to 0.7% by 9 months of age. This prevalence remains the same throughout childhood and adolescence. Cryptorchidism is the most common genitourinary disorder of childhood.

Diagnosis

When a testis is not palpable in the scrotum, gentle massage should be performed along the line of descent from the anterosuperior spine, medially, and downward to the pubic tubercle. If the testis is not truly undescended, it should become palpable in the scrotum. If cryptorchidism is present, the teen should be examined for stigmata of associated disorders (i.e., Noonan, Klinefelter, or Kallmann syndrome or trisomy 13, 18, or 21).

Complications

Infertility Data suggest that potential fertility in the cryptorchid testis may be significantly impaired compared with normal testicular fertility, regardless of patient age at the time of discovery of the undescended testis. The fertility index of the descended mates of unilateral undescended testes may also be somewhat impaired in certain age-groups. Fertility is significantly hampered in patients with bilateral cryptorchid testes if the condition is not corrected by 6 years of age. In one study of 100 azoospermic, nonvasectomized men referred to a Danish fertility clinic, 27% had infertility secondary to cryptorchidism (Fedder et al., 2004).

Malignancy Five percent to 12% of all malignant testicular tumors occur in males with a history of an undescended testis. The relative risk of tumors in such individuals is increased approximately 10 to 40 times that of a male without cryptorchidism. Moreover, the risk is increased even if the testis is brought down into the scrotum. In the United Kingdom Testicular Cancer Study (1994), a significant association of testicular cancer with undescended testis (odds ratio, 3.82; 95% confidence interval, 2.24 to 6.52) was found. In this study, the excess risk associated with undescended testis was eliminated in men who had had an orchidopexy before the age of 10 years.

Therapy

Therapy for cryptorchidism in teenagers should be corrective surgery. These teens should be aware of the increased risk of testicular cancer and should be taught testicular self-examination (TSE).

SCROTAL SWELLING AND MASSES

Evaluation

This section discusses the general approach to the adolescent with a scrotal mass or a painful scrotum (Fig. 28.2).

History

The adolescent should be questioned regarding the following:

1. Pain: Abrupt onset is suggestive of torsion; gradual onset suggests epididymitis or orchitis; lack of pain suggests a tumor or cystic mass.
2. Trauma

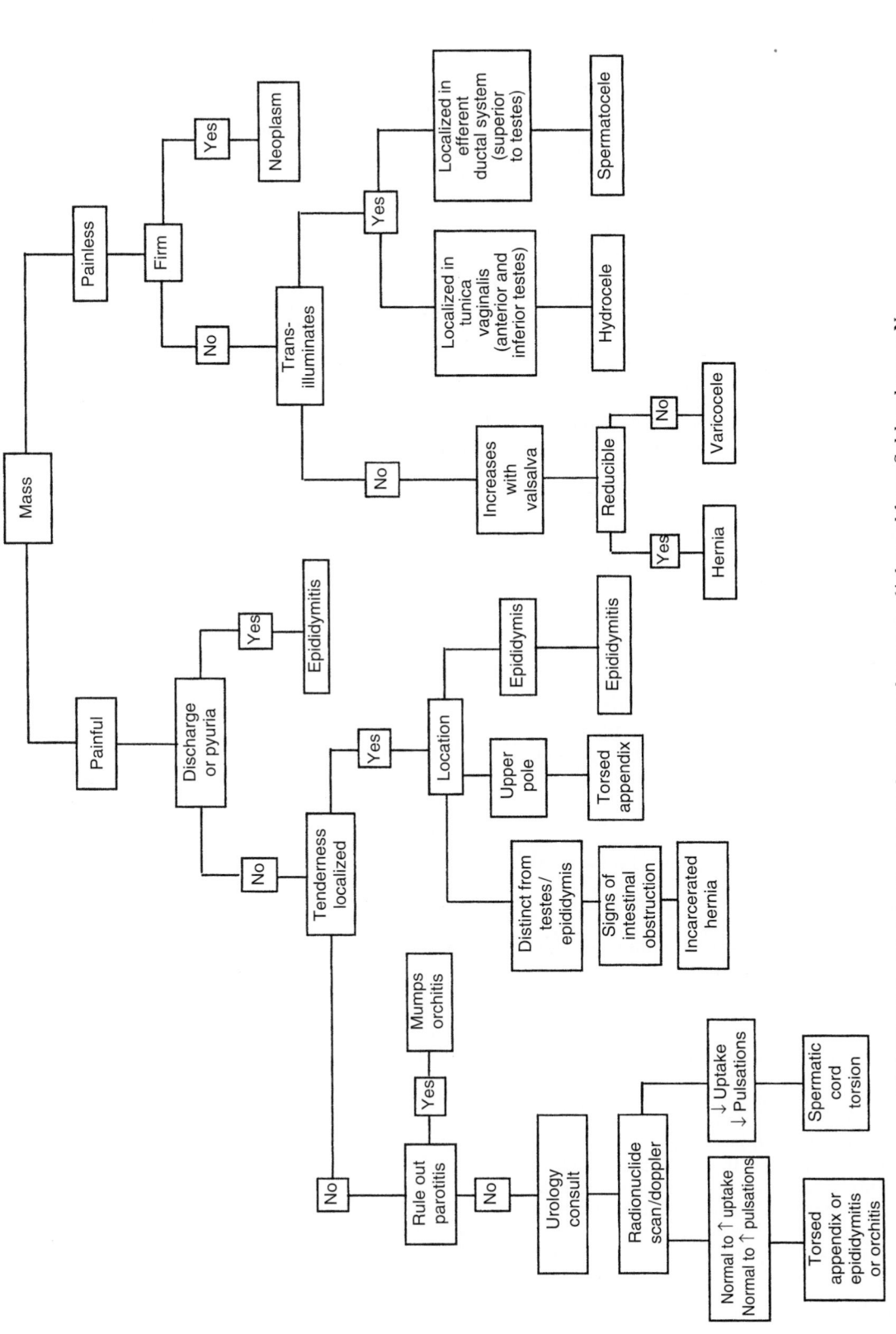

FIGURE 28.2 Diagnostic approach to scrotal masses. (Adapted from Schlossberger N. Male reproductive health: I. Painful scrotal masses. *Adolesc Health Update* 1992;4:1; Klein BL, Ochsenschlager DW. Scrotal masses in children and adolescents: a review for the emergency physician. *Pediatr Emerg Care* 1993;9:351.)

3. Recent change in testicular size or scrotum. Reactive hydroceles are common secondary to trauma, orchitis, testicular cancer, and epididymitis.
4. Sexual activity: Epididymitis in adolescence is usually sexually transmitted.
5. Prior history of pain: Torsion is often preceded by episodes of mild pain.

Physical Examination

1. Inspect testes.
   a. In torsion, the affected testis is often higher than on the contralateral side. With infections, the affected testis is often lower.
   b. In torsion, the affected testis and often the contralateral testis lie horizontally instead of in the usual vertical position, secondary to the congenital defect involved.
   c. In torsion, the epididymis is usually displaced anteriorly, as the testis twists on its vascular pedicle.
2. Carefully palpate the testicular surfaces, the epididymis and cord (posterior structures), and the head of the epididymis (lateral structure).
   a. Isolated swelling and tenderness of the epididymis suggests epididymitis.
   b. A tender, pea-sized swelling at the upper pole of the testis suggests torsion of the appendix testis.
   c. Generalized swelling and tenderness of both the testis and the epididymis can be found in either testicular torsion or epididymitis with orchitis.
   d. Presence of a cremasteric reflex makes torsion unlikely. However, it is often present in torsion of the appendix testis.
   e. Prehn sign: Relief of pain with elevation of the testis suggests epididymitis. Lack of pain relief with elevation of the testis is not a reliable test for torsion.
   f. Nausea or vomiting with testicular pain is usually caused by torsion.
3. If a painless mass is present (Fig. 28.2):
   a. Palpate to assess location.
      • A mass within the testis is a tumor until proved otherwise.
      • A mass palpable separate from the testis is unlikely to be a tumor.
      • A "bag of worms" or "squishy tube" on left spermatic cord is a varicocele.
      • A mass located near the head of the epididymis, above and behind the testis is probably a spermatocele.
      • A mass anterior to the testis or surrounding the testis is probably a hydrocele.
      • A mass that is separate from the testis/epididymis, intensifies with straining (Valsalva), and is reducible is probably a hernia.
   b. Transilluminate the mass with a light source: clear transillumination suggests a hydrocele or a typical spermatocele. Absence of transillumination suggests a testicular tumor or, if the mass is separate from the testis/epididymis, a hernia, or a large spermatocele.

Laboratory Evaluation

1. Urinalysis: In cases of a painful scrotum, or dysuria, a urine dipstick test that is positive for leukocyte esterase or the presence of leukocytes on microscopy (especially if there are >20 white blood cells/high-power field) is suggestive of epididymitis rather than torsion.
2. Gram stain: In cases of a painful scrotum and a history of urethritis or dysuria, a urethral Gram stain is helpful. Gram-negative diplococci suggest a gonococcal epididymitis. A Gram stain with white blood cells without gram-negative bacteria, suggests a chlamydial epididymitis; a gram-negative stain suggests an orchitis, or torsion.
3. Color flow Doppler ultrasound and nuclear scans: In cases of a painful scrotum where torsion is suspected, a Doppler flow study, a nuclear scan, or both can be used in equivocal cases, but should be obtained only after consultation with a urologist. If a reasonable suspicion of torsion exists, the primary therapy should be surgical exploration, without delaying to order diagnostic tests. In cases of torsion, the scan and Doppler study will show a decreased flow to the affected side.

Differential Diagnosis

1. Painless scrotal mass or swelling (Fig. 28.2)
   a. Hydrocele
   b. Spermatocele
   c. Varicocele
   d. Hernia
   e. Testicular tumor
   f. Idiopathic scrotal edema
2. Painful scrotal mass or swelling
   a. Torsion of spermatic cord
   b. Torsion of appendix testis
   c. Epididymitis
   d. Orchitis
   e. Trauma resulting in hematoma
   f. Hernia—incarcerated
   g. Henoch-Schönlein syndrome
   h. Cellulitis or infected piercing
   i. Hymenoptera sting or insect bite
   j. Testicular tumor with bleeding or infarction

TORSION

Etiology

Testicular torsion is a twisting of the testis and spermatic cord that results in venous obstruction, progressive edema, arterial compromise, and, eventually, testicular infarction. Normally, the testes are covered anteriorly with a mesothelial structure, the tunica vaginalis. In some males, the tunica vaginalis is abnormally enlarged and engulfs the testes. This causes the testis to lie like a "bell clapper" in the scrotal cavity. With this deformity, a testis can twist on the spermatic cord, compromising circulation. Aside from torsion at the spermatic cord, appendages of the testes or of the epididymis can occasionally undergo torsion (Fig. 28.3A). Torsion can be difficult to differentiate from epididymitis (Table 28.1).

Epidemiology

Two thirds of cases occur between 12 and 18 years, with incidence peaking at 15 to 16 years. The risk of developing torsion by age 25 is estimated to be approximately 1 in 160.

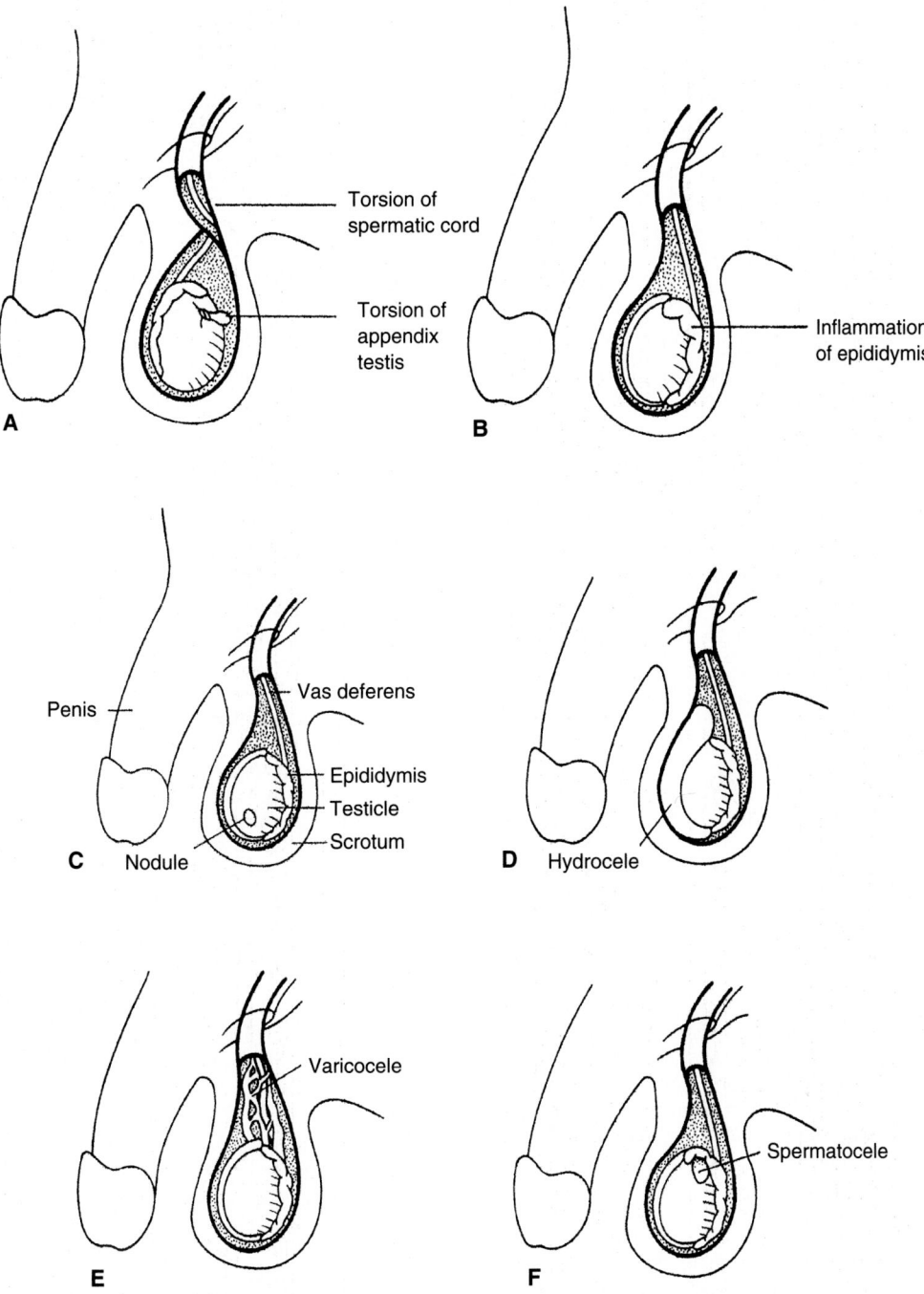

FIGURE 28.3   **A:** Torsion. **B:** Epididymitis. **C:** Testis tumor. **D:** Hydrocele. **E:** Varicocele. **F:** Spermatocele. (From Kapphahn C, Schlossberger N. Male reproductive health: I. Painful scrotal masses. *Adolesc Health Update* 1992;4:1.)

Clinical Manifestations

1. Onset is usually abrupt.
2. Fifty percent of teenagers have had brief prior episodes of scrotal pain.
3. Pain may be isolated to the scrotum or may radiate to the abdomen.
4. Nausea and/or vomiting may occur.
5. Physical examination shows the following:

a. The testis is tender and swollen.
b. The affected side is often higher than the contralateral side because of the elevation from the twisted spermatic cord. The testis that undergoes torsion usually twists so that the anterior portion turns medially. In inflammatory conditions, the affected side is often lower.
c. The epididymis, if palpable, is often out of the usual posterolateral location.

TABLE 28.1

Differentiating Torsion from Epididymitis

Symptoms and Other Findings	Torsion	Epididymitis
Pain	Severe	Severe
Onset	Sudden/abrupt	Hours to days
Prior episodes	50% of cases	Usually not
Nausea or vomiting	Frequent	Less frequent
Time to presentation	Short (<24 hr)	Longer (>24 hr)
Cremasteric reflex	Usually absent	Usually present
Epididymal abnormality	Obscured or anterior	Palpable and tender
Prehn sign	Absent: No relief of or increase in pain with elevation of the scrotum	Present: Pain relief with elevation of the scrotum
Urethral symptoms	Absent	May have dysuria, discharge
Urethral Gram stain	Negative	May be positive for gram-negative intracellular diplococci or white blood cells
Urinalysis	Usually negative	First-catch urine positive for white blood cells and/or leukocyte esterase

d. The affected testis and often the contralateral testis lie in a horizontal plane rather than in the normal vertical plane.
e. The cremasteric reflex is absent.
f. Fever and scrotal redness are usually absent.

Diagnosis

Testicular torsion is a surgical emergency. The diagnosis of torsion should be suspected in any adolescent with a painful swelling of the scrotum. If the history (acute onset of pain, nausea or vomiting, prior episodes of pain, lack of fever, lack of dysuria or urethral discharge) and physical examination (patient in distress, high-riding testis, horizontal position of testis, generalized swelling of the testis) are consistent with torsion, a urology consultation should be immediately obtained and decisions made for further testing or direct surgical exploration (Table 28.1).

Therapy

Therapy involves immediate surgery. Saving testicular function depends on early surgical intervention. If surgery is performed within 6 hours of onset of symptoms, recovery is the rule; if surgery is performed between 6 and 12 hours, 62% of patients have recovery of testicular function. After 12 hours, the success rate falls to 20% to 38% and after 24 hours, only up to 11% of testicles survive.

EPIDIDYMITIS

Etiology

Epididymitis is an inflammation of the epididymis caused by infection or trauma; it is primarily a problem of sexually active adolescents and is usually caused by *Chlamydia trachomatis* or *Neisseria gonorrhoeae*. Epididymitis due to *Escherichia coli* or other bowel flora can be secondary to unprotected insertive anal intercourse. Uncommonly, it can be caused by urinary pathogens in males with or without genitourinary abnormalities.

Non–sexually transmitted epididymitis may be caused by instrumentation, surgery, catheterization, or anatomical abnormalities. Epididymitis can be difficult to differentiate from torsion (Table 28.1).

Epidemiology

1. Uncommon in prepubertal males
2. Uncommon in non–sexually active males without a history of genitourinary tract abnormalities

Diagnosis

The diagnosis is suggested by the presentation of a sexually active teenager with subacute onset of pain in the hemiscrotum, inguinal area, or abdomen with epididymal swelling and tenderness, a reactive hydrocele, urethral discharge, dysuria, possibly fever, and pyuria (Fig. 28.3B). Approximately two thirds of individuals see a physician after 24 hours of pain—later than those who have testicular torsion. Swelling of the epididymis alone is more common with epididymitis than with torsion of the testes (59% versus 15%). The laboratory evaluation should include:

1. Gram staining of an endourethral swab specimen for diagnosis of urethritis and for presumptive diagnosis of gonococcal infection
2. A culture of intraurethral exudates or a nucleic acid amplification test on an intraurethral swab or urine for *N. gonorrhoeae* and *C. trachomatis*
3. Examination of first void urine for leukocytes. If the urethral Gram stain is negative, then send urine for Gram stain and culture.

4. Syphilis serology and human immunodeficiency virus (HIV) counseling and testing

In the absence of a urethral discharge, leukocytes on a gram-stained endourethral swab specimen (on microscopy) or urine dip for leukocyte esterase, or pyuria, an urgent urology consultation is called for as the likelihood of torsion increases. If one of the preceding tests shows abnormal findings but the teen has any risk factors suggesting torsion (i.e., prepubertal teen, non–sexually active teen, elevated or rotated testes, history of prior pain episodes, or acute onset with rapid progression), an immediate urology consultation should be obtained and a nuclear scan or a color flow Doppler ultrasonography should be considered. Orchitis can cause similar symptoms, but it usually occurs without dysuria or urethral discharge. Mumps infection is the most common cause. Mumps orchitis is usually unilateral and occasionally occurs without a history of parotitis. Other viruses (e.g., adenovirus, Coxsackie virus, ECHO virus, Epstein-Barr virus) may also cause orchitis, but with less frequency.

Therapy

Information on sexually transmitted disease (STD) guidelines is available from the Centers for Disease Control and Prevention (CDC) at http://www.cdc.gov/std/treatment.

1. Scrotal support, bed rest, and analgesics are an adjunct to antimicrobial therapy.
2. Ceftriaxone, 250 mg, is given intramuscularly once, and doxycycline, 100 mg, is given orally twice a day for 10 days. If the problem is thought to be caused by enteric organisms or the patient is allergic to ceftriaxone or tetracyclines, alternative drugs are ofloxacin 300 mg twice daily for 10 days, or levofloxacin 500 mg orally once a day for 10 days.
3. Failure to improve within 3 days requires reevaluation.
4. Sexual partners should be treated.
5. In HIV/acquired immunodeficiency syndrome (AIDS) infection or for other immunocompromised states, therapy is the same except that fungal and mycobacterial infections are more common than in immunocompetent patients.

TESTICULAR TUMORS

Etiology

Most testicular neoplasias are malignant and of germ-cell origin (95%). Seminomas are the most common testicular cancer of a single cell type (40% of germ-cell tumors) with a peak incidence in the 25 to 45 year age-group; nonseminoma tumors (embryonal cell, choriocarcinoma, teratoma, yolk sac, and mixed forms) peak in the 15 to 30 year age-group (Fig. 28.3C).

Epidemiology

1. Testicular tumors are the most common solid tumor in males aged 15 to 35 years.
2. The incidence is 2.3 to 10 in 100,000 males.
3. Testicular cancer is 4.5 times more common among White men than African-American men.

4. The risk of a testicular tumor is increased 10 to 40 times in a teenager with a history of cryptorchidism.

Diagnosis

The diagnosis of tumor should be suspected in any male with a firm, circumscribed, painless area of induration within the testis that does not transilluminate. Swelling is noted in up to 73% of cases at presentation, but is usually considered asymptomatic by the patient. Testicular pain is the presenting symptom in 18% to 46% of patients who have germ-cell tumors.

Therapy

Therapy involves a direct biopsy for confirmative diagnosis and cell type. Definitive therapy is beyond the scope of this book and involves a coordinated effort among the urologist, the primary care specialist, and the oncologist.

HYDROCELE

Etiology

This mass is actually a collection of fluid between the parietal and visceral layers of the tunica vaginalis, which lies along the anterior surface of the testicle and is a remnant of the processus vaginalis—the embryonic sleeve through which the testes descend. If the processus vaginalis remains fully open, an inguinal hernia will result. If a small opening remains, a hydrocele will form in the scrotum (Fig. 28.3D). If an opening remains proximally but is closed distally before the scrotum, a hydrocele of the spermatic cord will form.

Diagnosis

A hydrocele is usually a soft, painless, fluctuant, scrotal mass that is anterior to the testis, transilluminates, and appears cystic on ultrasonography. Hydroceles often decrease in size by morning and increase in size by evening. Longstanding hydroceles are usually benign. The presence of a new hydrocele should alert the examiner to check for a possible underlying cause such as a hernia, testicular tumor, trauma, or infection.

Therapy

Usually, no therapy is required for an asymptomatic longstanding hydrocele. Indications for treatment include a painful or tense hydrocele that might reduce circulation to the testis, a bulky mass that is uncomfortable and uncosmetic for the teenager, or a hydrocele associated with a hernia (a communicating hydrocele). Definitive therapy involves resection of the parietal tunica vaginalis.

VARICOCELE

Etiology

A varicocele, or dilated scrotal veins, results from increased pressure and incompetent venous valves in the internal spermatic veins (Fig. 28.3E). Anatomical reasons explain why varicocele is most often noted on the left side. Recent studies suggest that the incidence of bilateral varicocele is underestimated and that percutaneous retrograde venography usually reveals bilateral disease in those with clinically evident unilateral disease.

Epidemiology

1. Varicocele is common in the 10 to 20 year age-group, with a prevalence of 15%.
2. Eighty-five percent of varicoceles are clinically evident on the left side, and 15% are bilateral.

Diagnosis

Varicoceles are detected in adolescents either on routine examination or secondary to a patient's discovery of more "stuff" filling one hemiscrotum than the other. Occasionally, a patient complains of an ache or pain from the varicocele. On examination, a visible varicocele (grade 3 or large) has a "bag of worms" appearance and feel above the testes. A varicocele that is palpable but not visible is classified as grade 2 (moderate). More subtle varicoceles may feel like a thickened or asymmetric spermatic cord. The distension usually decreases when the patient lies down. If there is no decrease in the size of a varicocele in the supine position, an ultrasonogram or intravenous pyelogram is indicated to eliminate the possibility of intraabdominal disease.

Therapy

It is reasonable to obtain a semen analysis, the true test of potential fertility, on willing patients once they reach Tanner stage 5. An adolescent with a normal semen analysis need not be referred for treatment of his varicocele. However, semen analysis is not often a practical test to perform on teenage boys.

Loss of testicular volume or failure of the testis to grow during puberty has been the traditional indication for surgical correction of a varicocele during adolescence. Several recommendations have been suggested as indications for varicocele repair, but definitive answers to who should be referred and when during adolescence, remain elusive.

Kass and Reitelman (1995) recommended varicocele repair in adolescents in the following instances:

1. The results of semen analysis are abnormal.
2. The volume of the left testis is at least 3 mL less than that of the right.
3. The response of either luteinizing hormone (LH) or follicle-stimulating hormone (FSH) to gonadotropin-releasing hormone stimulation is supranormal.
4. Bilaterally palpable varicoceles are detected.
5. A large, symptomatic varicocele is present.

Skoog et al. (1997) recommended surgery for patients with any of the following findings:

1. A difference of >2 mL in testicular volume as noted on serial ultrasonic examinations
2. A testicular size that is smaller by 2 standard deviations when compared with normal testicular growth curves
3. Scrotal pain

A recent study by Guarino et al. (2003) suggests that nonstimulated LH and FSH levels may be helpful in identifying patients with testicular dysfunction in association with varicocele, who may benefit from varicocelectomy. It is also common practice to refer those with varicocele associated with one testis to urology, but little evidence exists to support or refute such a practice.

The earlier in life the varicocele appears, the higher the risk of testicular growth arrest; varicocelectomy during adolescence usually results in "catch-up growth" of the involved testis. Although varicoceles may cause a progressive loss of fertility during the reproductive years in some men, >80% of men with varicoceles are fertile. Although a preponderance of the literature supports a favorable effect of varicocelectomy on fertility, several recent articles, including a systematic review, have questioned whether there is any such effect. A definitive statement about which adolescents need surgery cannot be made.

There are a variety of surgical techniques in addition to nonsurgical embolization and sclerotherapies. A review of the various techniques, as well as a full discussion of the controversies inherent to varicocele management is beyond the scope of this chapter. However, the "References and Additional Readings" section contains several articles addressing these subjects.

SPERMATOCELE

A spermatocele is a retention cyst of the epididymis that contains spermatozoa. Most are small (<1 cm in diameter), painless, cystic, freely movable, and will transilluminate (Fig. 28.3F). If large, the patient may present complaining of a "third testicle," and turbidity from increased spermatozoa may prevent transillumination. It is usually felt as a smooth, cystic sac located above and posterior to the testis, at the head of the epididymis. No therapy is indicated, unless it is large enough to annoy the patient, in which case a urologist may excise it.

TESTICULAR SELF-EXAMINATION

TSE is simple to teach, simple to perform, has negligible cost, and is of unproven effectiveness. There are inconsistent national recommendations regarding implementing TSE as a screening tool for testicular cancer because it is unknown whether screening by either physician examination or patient self-examination actually affects the stage of cancer at detection, or impacts morbidity or mortality from the disease. Although females are commonly taught to examine their own breasts, fewer than 10% of men have been taught how to examine their testicles. However, teaching of TSE by a physician increases the likelihood of performing TSE. Testicular cancer is the most common solid tumor in young adults, and the American Medical Association and the American Urological Association promote and support public awareness and education of TSEs for early detection of testicular cancer. The recommendations for TSE by the American Cancer Society are as follows:

1. Examine the testes during or after a hot bath or shower.
2. Examine each testicle with the fingers of both hands, using the index and middle fingers on the underside of the testicle and the thumbs on the top of the testicle.

3. Gently roll the testicle between the thumbs and fingers.
4. Be on the lookout for lumps, irregularities, change in size, or pain in the testicles.
5. The epididymis should not be mistaken for an abnormality.
6. If any abnormality such as a lump is found, it should be reported immediately.
7. TSE should be performed once a month.

WEB SITES

For Teenagers and Parents

http://www.nlm.nih.gov/medlineplus/testiculardisorders. html. Epididymitis and male reproductive system.

http://tcrc.acor.org/tcexam.html. Testicular Cancer Self Examination.

http://keepkidshealthy.com/adolescent/ adolescentproblems/varicocele.html. Varicocele information from keepkidshealthy.com.

http://kidshealth.org/teen/sexual_health/guys/tse.html. Testicular Cancer Self-Examination.

http://www.emedicine.com/emerg/topic573.htm. Testicular torsion information.

REFERENCES AND ADDITIONAL READINGS

Adelman WP, Joffe A. The adolescent male genital examination: what's normal and what's not. *Contemp Pediatr* 1999;16:76.

Adelman WP, Joffe A. The adolescent with a painful scrotum. *Contemp Pediatr* 2000;17:111.

Adelman WP, Joffe A. Controversies in male adolescent health: varicocele, circumcision, and testicular self-examination. *Curr Opin Pediatr* 2004;16:363.

Adelman WP, Joffe A. Genitourinary issues in the male college student: a case-based approach. *Pediatr Clin North Am* 2005; 52:199.

Baker LA, Sigman D, Mathews RI, et al. An analysis of clinical outcomes using color Doppler testicular ultrasound for testicular torsion. *Pediatrics* 2000;105:604. Available at http://www.pediatrics.org/cgi/content/full/105/3/604.

Berger RE. Epididymitis. In: Holmes K, Sparling PF, Mardh PA et al., eds. *Sexually transmitted diseases*. New York: McGraw-Hill, 1999.

Burgher SW. Acute scrotal pain. *Emerg Med Clin North Am* 1998;16:781.

Cass AS, Cass BP, Veeraraghan K. Immediate exploration of the unilateral acute scrotum in young male subjects. *J Urol* 1980;124:829.

Cayan S, Kadioglu A, Orhan I, et al. The effect of microsurgical varicocelectomy of serum follicle stimulating hormone, testosterone, and free testosterone levels in infertile men with varicocele. *BJU Int* 1999;84:1046. Available at http://www.blackwell-synergy.com/journals.

Centers for Disease Control and Prevention. Sexually transmitted diseases treatment guidelines 2002. *MMWR Morbid Mortal Wkly Rep* 2002;51(RR-6):1.

Chehval MJ, Purcell MH. Deterioration of semen parameters over time in men with untreated varicocele: evidence of progressive testicular damage. *Fertil Steril* 1992;57:174.

Colodny AH. Undescended testes: is surgery necessary? *N Engl J Med* 1986;314:510.

Cornud F, Belin X, Amar E, et al. Varicocele: strategies in diagnosis and treatment. *Eur Radiol* 1999;9:536.

Diamond DA. Adolescent varicocele: emerging understanding. *BJU Int* 2003;92(Suppl 1):48.

Docimo SG. The results of surgical therapy for cryptorchidism: a literature review and analysis. *J Urol* 1995;154:1148.

Dunne PJ, O'Loughlin BS. Testicular torsion: time is the enemy. *Aust N Z J Surg* 2000;70:441. Available at http://www.blackwell-synergy.com/journals.

Evers JLH, Collins JA. Assessment of efficacy of varicocele repair for male subfertility: a systematic review. *Lancet* 2003; 361:1849.

Fedder J, Cruger D, Oestergaard B, et al. Etiology of azoospermia in 100 consecutive nonvasectomized men. *Fertil Steril* 2004;82:1463.

Galejs LS, Kass EJ. Color doppler ultrasound evaluation of the acute scrotum. *Tech Urol* 1998;4:182.

Gat Y, Zukerman Z, Bachar GN, et al. Adolescent varicocele: is it a unilateral disease? *Urology* 2003;62:742.

Gerscovich EO. High-resolution ultrasonography in the diagnosis of scrotal pathology: I. Normal scrotum and benign disease. *J Clin Ultrasound* 1993;21:355.

Gershbein AB, Horowitz M, Glassberg KI. The adolescent varicocele: I. Left testicular hypertrophy following varicocelectomy. *J Urol* 1999;162:1447.

Goldenring JM, Purtell E. Knowledge of testicular cancer risk and need for self-examination in college students: a call for equal time for men in teaching of early cancer detection techniques. *Pediatrics* 1984;74:1093.

Gorelick JI, Goldstein M. Loss of fertility in men with varicocele. *Fertil Steril* 1993;59:613.

Goroll AH, May LA, Mulley AG, eds. Evaluation of scrotal pain, masses, and swelling. In: *Primary care medicine: office evaluation and management of the adult patient*. Philadelphia: JB Lippincott Co, 1995.

Guarino N, Tadini B, Bianchi M. The adolescent varicocele: the crucial role of hormonal tests in selecting patients with testicular dysfunction. *J Pediatr Surg* 2003;38:120.

Gutierrez CS. Cryptorchidism. *West J Med* 1995;163:67.

Hadziselimovic F, Herzog B, Jenny P. The chance for fertility in adolescent boys after corrective surgery for varicocele. *J Urol* 1995;154:731.

Hamm B. Differential diagnosis of scrotal masses by ultrasound. *Eur Radiol* 1997;7:668. Available at http://link.springer-ny .com/link/service/journals/00330/papers/7007005/70070668 .pdf.

Hoover DL. How I manage testicular injury. *Phys Sportsmed* 1986;14:127.

Horstman WG, Haluszka MM, Burkhard TK. Management of testicular masses incidentally discovered by ultrasound. *J Urol* 1994;151:1263.

Jefferson RH, Perez LM, Joseph DB. Critical analysis of the clinical presentation of acute scrotum: a 9-year experience at a single institution. *J Urol* 1997;158:1198.

Joly-Guillou ML, Lasry S. Practical recommendations for the drug treatment of bacterial infections of the male genital tract including urethritis, epididymitis, and prostatitis. *Drugs* 1999;57:743.

Junnila J, Lassen P. Testicular masses. *Am Fam Physician* 1998;57:685.

Kadish HA, Bolte RG. A retrospective review of pediatric patients with epididymitis, testicular torsion, and torsion of testicular appendages. *Pediatrics* 1998;102:73. Available at http://pediatrics.org/cgi/content/full/102/1/73.

Kapphahn C, Schlossberger N. Male reproductive health: I. Painful scrotal masses. *Adolesc Health Update* 1992;4(3):1–8.

Kapphahn C, Schlossberger N. Male reproductive health: II. Painless scrotal masses. *Adolesc Health Update* 1992;5(1): 1–8.

Kass EL, Freitas JE, Salisz JA, et al. Pituitary gonadal dysfunction in adolescents with varicocele. *Urology* 1993;42:179.

Kass EJ, Lundak B. The acute scrotum. *Pediatr Clin North Am* 1997;44:1251.

Kass EL, Reitelman C. Adolescent varicocele. *Urol Clin North Am* 1995;22:151.

Klein BL, Ochsenschlager DW. Scrotal masses in children and adolescents: a review for the emergency physician. *Pediatr Emerg Care* 1993;9:351.

Lau MW, Taylor PM, Payne SR. The indications for scrotal ultrasound. *Br J Radiol* 1999;72:833.

Laven JSE, Haans LCF, Mal WPTM, et al. Effects of varicocele treatment in adolescents: a randomized study. *Fertil Steril* 1992;58:756.

Lewis AG, Bukowski TP, Jarvis PD, et al. Evaluation of acute scrotum in the emergency department. *J Pediatr Surg* 1995;30:277.

Mazzoni G, Fiocca G, Minucci S, et al. Varicocele: a multidisciplinary approach in children and adolescents. *J Urol* 1999;162:1755.

McAleer IM, Packer MG, Kaplan GW, et al. Fertility index analysis in cryptorchidism. *J Urol* 1995;153:1255.

Nagar H, Mabjeesh NJ. Decision-making in pediatric varicocele surgery: use of color Doppler ultrasound. *Pediatr Surg Int* 2000;16:76. Available at http://link.springer-ny.com/link/service/journals/00383/bibs/0016001/00160075.htm.

Neinstein LS, Goldenring JG. Pink pearly papules: an epidemiological study. *J Pediatr* 1984;105:594.

Neinstein LS, Shapiro J, Rabinowitz S, et al. Comfort of male adolescents during general and genital examination. *J Pediatr* 1989;115:494.

Noske HD, Weidner W. Varicocele: a historical perspective. *World J Urol* 1999;17:151. Available at http://link.springer-ny.com/link/service/journals/00345/papers/9017003/90170151.pdf.

Paltiel HJ, Connolly LP, Atala A, et al. Acute scrotal symptoms in boys with an indeterminate clinical presentation: comparison of color Doppler sonography and scintigraphy. *Radiology* 1998;207:223.

Papanikolaou F, Chow V, Jarvi K, et al. The effect of adult microsurgical varicocelectomy on testicular volume. *Urology* 2000;56:136. http://www.sciencedirect.com/science/journal/00904295.

Pinto KJ, Kroovand RL, Jarow JP. Varicocele-related testicular atrophy and its predictive effect upon fertility. *J Urol* 1994; 152:788.

Podesta ML, Gottlieb S, Medel R Jr, et al. Hormonal parameters and testicular volume in children and adolescents with unilateral varicocele: preoperative and postoperative findings. *J Urol* 1994;152:794.

Pyorealea S, Huttunen NP, Uhari M. A review and meta-analysis of hormonal treatment of cryptorchidism. *J Clin Endocrinol Metab* 1995;80:2795.

Rabinowitz R, Hulbert WC Jr. Acute scrotal swelling. *Urol Clin North Am* 1995;22:101.

Rajfer J. Congenital anomalies of the testes and scrotum. In: Walsh PC, Retik AB, Vaughn ED Jr et al., eds. *Campbell's urology*. Philadelphia: WB Saunders, 1998:2172.

Rozanski TA, Bloom DA. The undescended testis: theory and management. *Urol Clin North Am* 1995;22:107.

Schlesinger MD, Wilets IF, Nagler HM. Treatment outcome after varicocelectomy: a critical analysis. *Urol Clin North Am* 1994;21:517.

Siegel MJ. The acute scrotum. *Radiol Clin North Am* 1997;35: 959.

Silber SJ. New concepts in operative andrology: a review. *Int J Androl* 2000;23(Suppl 2):66. Available at http://www.blackwell-synergy.com/journals.

Singer AJ, Tichler T, Orvieto R, et al. Testicular carcinoma: a study of knowledge, awareness, and practice of testicular self-examination in male soldiers and military physicians. *Mil Med* 1993;158:640.

Skoog SJ, Roberts KP, Goldstein M, et al. The adolescent varicocele: what's new with an old problem in young patients? *Pediatrics* 1997;100:112.

United Kingdom Testicular Cancer Study Group. Aetiology of testicular cancer: association with congenital abnormalities, age at puberty, infertility, and exercise. United Kingdom Testicular Cancer Study Group. *Br Med J* 1994;308:1393.

Watkin NA, Reiger NA, Moisey CU. Is the conservative management of the acute scrotum justified on clinical grounds? *Br J Urol* 1996;78:623.

Wilbert DM, Schaerfe CW, Stem WD, et al. Evaluation of the acute scrotum by color-coded Doppler ultrasonography. *J Urol* 1993;149:1475.

Witt MA, Lipshultz LT. Varicocele: a progressive or static lesion? *Urology* 1993;42:541.

PART VIII

Infectious Diseases

CHAPTER 29

Infectious Respiratory Illnesses

Terrill Bravender and Emmanuel B. Walter

INFECTIOUS MONONUCLEOSIS

Infectious mononucleosis (IM) is usually an acute, self-limited, and benign lymphoproliferative disease caused by the Epstein-Barr virus (EBV) and commonly occurs in adolescence or young adulthood. Although EBV is responsible for IM in approximately 90% of cases, the syndrome may also be caused by other infectious agents, such as cytomegalovirus (CMV), toxoplasmosis, human herpes virus 6, and adenovirus. EBV is most often transmitted through direct saliva contact, hence its reputation among adolescents as "the kissing disease." The virus replicates in the lymphoreticular system, where it provokes an intense immunological response frequently involving lymph nodes, spleen, liver, and bone marrow. It is this immune response that is responsible for the clinical symptomatology.

Etiology

EBV is a fragile, enveloped DNA herpes virus. Humans and a few other primates are the only known reservoirs, and the virus cannot survive long outside of the host. Transmission occurs primarily through exposure to oropharyngeal secretions, and the incubation time is 30 to 50 days. The virus initially infects oral epithelial cells, and then spreads to B lymphocytes which disseminate the infection throughout the lymphoreticular system. During this time, there is a polyclonal B-cell proliferation and a vigorous T-cell response. In reaction to infected and transformed B cells, atypical lymphocytes appear in the peripheral blood. These atypical cells are mainly cytotoxic or suppressor (CD8) cells. This immunological response is responsible for many of the clinical manifestations of IM, including lymphadenopathy, hepatomegaly, and splenomegaly.

Acute infection with EBV stimulates production of antibodies directed against EBV antigens as well as non-EBV–specific antibodies that react with antigens found on sheep and horse erythrocytes. These heterophil antibodies form the basis of rapid diagnostic tests for IM. Antibodies to EBV viral capsid antigen (VCA-IgM, and VCA-IgG) are produced slightly earlier than the heterophil antibody, and are more specific for EBV infection. VGA-IgG antibodies persist after acute infection, and represent the development of immunity.

During an acute infection, approximately 0.001% to 0.01% of circulating B cells are infected. Over the next 3 to 4 months, this rate declines to 0.00001%, which persists indefinitely. EBV remains in the body for life, replicating as an extrachromosomal plasmid in a subset of B cells. Virus is shed by 70% to 90% of individuals for 8 to 24 weeks after resolution of the clinical syndrome. After this, 60% to 100% of normal, asymptomatic EBV seropositive individuals shed virus intermittently.

Epidemiology

More than 90% of adults have serological evidence of past EBV infection. The highest rates of acute infection in the United States are in older adolescents and young adults, particularly those living in close proximity to one another, such as in college or the military. EBV is present in the oropharyngeal secretions of up to 20% of asymptomatic adults in the United States.

1. Age: In developing countries, tropical areas, and areas of high population density in industrialized countries, infection usually occurs early in life and is usually subclinical. In these areas, up to 90% of children seroconvert by the age of 6. However, if infection does not occur in childhood, infection with EBV in adolescents and young adults results in the clinical syndrome of IM in 30% to 75% of cases. In one study of first-year university students, 13% of those susceptible had developed EBV antibodies within 9 months of starting classes, and IM developed in 75% of the seroconverters. In the United States, the annual incidence of IM for those between the ages of 15 and 19 is between 345 and 671 cases per 100,000 person-years. In contrast, the incidence for those aged 35 years and older is only two to four cases per 100,000 person-years.
2. Gender: There are no gender differences in prevalence.
3. Race: IM is more prevalent among whites than blacks in the United States. This may be a reflection of earlier subclinical infection in black children living in areas of higher population density.
4. Season: There is no seasonal variation, although there may be an increased incidence in spring and fall among college students, and in summer in military personnel, but these variations are likely population specific.
5. Contagiousness: Because the virus is shed in oropharyngeal secretions, and cannot live outside the host for long, direct contact with saliva is the main vehicle for transmission of EBV. Hence, kissing is an important

modality of transmission in adolescents and young adults. In families, 10% to 40% of susceptible members will develop EBV infection from a household contact. EBV is also detectable in the genital tracts of men and women; therefore the possibility of sexual transmission exists, although salivary contact likely plays a much more prominent role. Because EBV resides in the B lymphocytes, transmission through blood products has also been reported.

Clinical Manifestations

The majority of EBV infections are either asymptomatic or associated with mild, nonspecific symptoms such as malaise, fever and chills, and anorexia. Even in adolescents and young adults in whom classic IM is common, a significant number of EBV infections are subclinical.

The traditional triad of IM includes:

1. Fever, lymphadenopathy, and pharyngitis
2. Lymphocytosis with atypical lymphocytes
3. Antibody response demonstrated by the presence of heterophil antibodies or EBV-specific antibodies

In those who develop clinical symptoms, there is often a prodromal period of 3 to 5 days of malaise, headache, anorexia, myalgia, and fatigue, followed by more severe symptoms and signs as the immune response mounts.

Signs and Symptoms

The common presentation includes fever, which may persist for several weeks. A prominent symptom is sore throat, which can be severe, and may include an exudative pharyngitis in up to 50% of individuals. Palatal petechiae may be seen at the junction of the hard and soft palate. Periorbital or facial edema occurs in approximately 25% of teens with IM. Adenopathy is usually significant and is most commonly symmetrical, with posterior cervical lymph nodes more prominent than anterior ones. Splenomegaly and hepatomegaly may occur by the second week of the illness. Approximately 10% of individuals have a rash that may take on a number of different appearances—erythematous, maculopapular, morbilliform, urticarial, or erythema multiforme. Approximately 90% of patients who receive ampicillin or amoxicillin will develop an erythematous maculopapular rash, which typically does not appear until approximately 1 week after antibiotic therapy has been initiated. Although the exact mechanism for the development of this rash is unknown, it appears that a true drug sensitization does occur in these patients. Whether this sensitization persists following resolution of IM is unknown.

Symptoms	Prevalence (%)
Sore throat	70–80
Malaise	50–90
Anorexia	50–80
Nausea	50–70
Headache	40–70
Myalgia	12–30
Cough	5–15
Abdominal pain	2–14
Arthralgia	5–10
Photophobia	5–10

Signs	Prevalence (%)
Lymphadenopathy	93–100
Fever	80–100
Tonsillopharyngitis	69–91
Palpable splenomegaly	11–60
Hepatomegaly	10–25
Palatal petechiae	25–35
Periorbital edema	25–35
Liver or splenic tenderness	15–30
Jaundice	5–10
Rash (usually maculopapular)	3–15[a]
Pneumonitis	<3

[a]Risk of rash is higher if ampicillin or amoxicillin has been given.

Complications

Occasionally, patients will present with a major complication of IM as their only manifestation of the disease, and the typical clinical symptoms may not appear until later in the course of the illness. Overall, the complication rate is approximately 1% to 2%.

Complication	Prevalence
Neurological:	<1%
Seizures	
Facial or peripheral nerve palsies	
Meningoencephalitis	
Aseptic meningitis	
Optic neuritis	
Reye syndrome	
Coma	
Brachial plexus neuropathy	
Transverse myelitis	
Guillain-Barré syndrome	
Acute psychosis	
Acute cerebellar ataxia	
"Alice in Wonderland" syndrome	
Hematological:	
Autoimmune hemolytic anemia (mild)	0.5%–3%
Thrombocytopenia purpura	Rare
Coagulopathy	Rare
Aplastic anemia	Rare
Hemolytic-uremic syndrome	Rare
Eosinophilia	Rare
Profound thrombocytopenia	Rare (mild thrombocytopenia is common)
Cardiac:	1.7%–6%
Pericarditis	
Myocarditis	
Electrocardiogram changes (nonspecific ST and T wave abnormalities)	
Splenic rupture	0.1%–0.2%
Pulmonary:	
Airway obstruction	Rare (more common in young children)
Pneumonitis	Rare
Pleural effusions	Rare
Pulmonary hemorrhage	Rare

Gastrointestinal:	
Mild elevation of	80%–90%
hepatocellular enzymes	
Pancreatitis	Rare
Hepatitis with liver necrosis	Rare
Malabsorption	Rare
Dermatological:	3%–10%
Dermatitis	
Urticarial rash	
(may be cold-induced)	
Erythema multiforme	
Renal:	
Glomerulonephritis	Rare
Nephrotic syndrome	Rare
Mild hematuria or proteinuria	Up to 13%
Ophthalmological:	Rare
Conjunctivitis,	
Episcleritis	
uveitis	
Superimposed infections:	
β-Hemolytic streptococcus	4%–33%
Staphylococcus aureus	Rare
Mycoplasma pneumoniae	Up to 5%
Other:	Uncommon
Bullous myringitis	
Orchitis	
Genital ulcerations	
Parotitis	
Monoarticular arthritis	

Specific Complications

1. Splenic rupture: Splenic rupture is seen in approximately 0.1% to 0.2% of cases, and at least half of cases are spontaneous without any history of trauma or unusual physical exertion. Typically, there is abrupt abdominal pain in the left upper quadrant that radiates to the top of the left shoulder, known as *Kehr sign*. This is followed by generalized abdominal pain, pleuritic chest pain, and signs and symptoms of hypovolemia. However, the onset may be insidious. Splenic rupture occurs between the 4th and 21st days of the illness, with approximately half of cases occurring during the height of the acute illness, and the other half in the early convalescent phase. Only approximately 50% of cases of splenic rupture have clinically significant splenomegaly noted before the rupture. All patients with IM should be considered at risk for splenic rupture, because clinical severity, laboratory results, and physical examination are not reliable predictors of risk. Because of this, as well as the morbidity and mortality risk associated with splenic rupture, patients should refrain from vigorous physical activity for at least 1 month after the onset of symptoms, or until palpable splenomegaly resolves, whichever is later. Some have advocated using ultrasound to assess for splenomegaly before allowing patients to return to contact sports such as football or hockey, but there is little evidence to support this.
2. Airway obstruction: Airway obstruction is an uncommon but life-threatening complication of IM related to massive lymphoid hyperplasia and mucosal edema. This tends to be more common in younger teens and typically occurs approximately 1 week after the initial symptoms begin. Corticosteroids have been used in an attempt to reduce the edema and hypertrophy of the lymphoid tissue. In more severe cases, acute tonsillectomy may be indicated, and, in emergency situations, intubation or tracheostomy may be necessary.
3. Streptococcal pharyngitis: Although EBV infection may potentiate the ability of β-hemolytic streptococci to adhere to epithelial cells membranes, there are widely varying reported rates of coinfection. Studies from 30 to 40 years ago reported coinfection rates as high as 33%. The most recent studies available are from approximately 20 years ago, and noted a coinfection rate of 4%.

Laboratory Evaluation

Hematological Features There are a number of distinctive hematological abnormalities observed with IM. Generally, the total white blood cell count is elevated, in the range of 10,000 to 20,000/mm^3. Approximately 95% of patients will demonstrate a lymphocytosis, with >50% of the leukocytes being lymphocytes, and 10% or more being atypical lymphocytes. The atypical lymphocytes are usually activated CD8 T lymphocytes, or occasionally EBV-transformed B lymphocytes. Although atypical lymphocytes may be seen in a variety of other viral illnesses, including human immunodeficiency virus (HIV), acute viral hepatitis, rubella, mumps, and rubeola, they typically do not comprise >10% of the total leukocyte count. However, this level of atypical lymphocytosis may also be seen with CMV and toxoplasmosis infections. Other common hematological abnormalities include a mild granulocytopenia and thrombocytopenia (usually in the range of 100,000 to 140,000/mm^3) in approximately half of individuals with IM. Anemia is uncommon, although a mild hemolytic anemia may occur in up to 3% of cases.

Other Laboratory Findings Evidence of mild hepatitis is very common, and is seen in approximately 90% of individuals. Transaminase levels may be as high as 2 to 3 times the normal, and alkaline phosphatase and lactate dehydrogenase levels may also be elevated. Less commonly, bilirubin levels may be mildly elevated, to the range of 1 to 3 mg/dL. These liver function test abnormalities peak at approximately the second or third week of symptoms, and usually resolve by the end of the fourth week. Entirely normal findings from liver chemistries may suggest a diagnosis other than EBV infection.

Serological Features
Heterophil Antibodies The classic test for EBV-associated IM is the presence of heterophil antibodies. These tests detect immunoglobulin M (IgM) antibodies induced by EBV infections that cross-react with phylogenetically unrelated antigens, typically sheep, horse, or bovine erythrocytes. Although the presence of heterophil antibodies is the hallmark of IM, heterophil antibodies can be found in normal human serum in low titers, as well as in higher titers in individuals with malignant disease, serum sickness, or a variety of other viral infections. Additionally, some patients with IM, particularly young children, may be heterophil antibody negative.

Slide and card tests, such as MonoSpot®, exploit the fact that IM heterophil antibodies agglutinate sheep and horse erythrocytes after preabsorption with guinea pig kidney, but not after preabsorption with bovine erythrocytes. These tests are rapid, simple to perform, and inexpensive. The MonoSpot test has a sensitivity of 86% and a specificity of 88% to 99%, but the sensitivity is lower during the first week of illness, and is lower (~80%) in adolescents younger than 16 years. Children younger than 4 years with EBV-associated IM are even less likely to produce heterophil antibodies—only approximately 30% will test positive for heterophil antibody. Individuals who do test positive will have a persistently positive heterophil antibody result for approximately 3 to 6 months following the acute infection and sometimes even longer in low titers.

If EBV-associated IM is suspected, but the heterophil antibody result is negative, one may perform EBV-specific antibody tests.

Specific Epstein-Barr Virus Antibodies Antibody responses to several EBV antigens have been well studied. These antibodies include viral capsid antigen (VCA), early antigen (EA), and Epstein-Barr nuclear antigen (EBNA). Commercially-available enzyme immunoassay (EIA) tests are readily available. Figure 29.1 shows the characteristic EBV antibody responses to various EBV antigens. Table 29.1 shows the pattern of serological results in various EBV stages.

1. VCA antibody: Antibodies against VCA are composed of both IgG and IgM. Antibody levels for both peak at approximately 3 to 4 weeks after the clinical onset of the disease. IgM declines rapidly and is undetectable by 3 months. IgG declines somewhat with time but persists for life. High persistent levels of IgG antibodies against VCA can indicate remote EBV infection as well as systemic lupus, chronic renal failure, lymphoma, nasopharyngeal carcinoma, leukemia, sarcoidosis, rheumatoid arthritis, or any other immunodeficiency state.

2. EA antibody: Antibodies against EA are induced in 70% to 90% of individuals with acute EBV IM. The antibodies are produced very early in the infection and usually persist for 8 to 12 weeks. However, as many as 30% of individuals with past infections have positive titers for EA. These antibodies have been divided into two patterns of staining—diffuse and restricted. Most adolescents and young adults with IM have antibodies against the D (diffuse) component.

3. Nuclear antigen antibody: Antibodies against EBNA develop 2 to 3 months after the onset of infection and tend to persist indefinitely. Positive titers usually indicate an infection at least 1 to 2 months in the past. Absent EBNA titers in patients with an EBV infection are associated with immunodeficiency states and rheumatoid arthritis.

Acute EBV-associated IM is characterized by the presence of both IgM and IgG VCA and EA antibodies. Older and remote infections are characterized by the absence of IgM VCA antibodies and the appearance of IgG EBNA antibodies (Table 29.1). EBV serology is best reserved for measurement in adolescents when (a) clinical IM is present and a heterophil test result is negative; or (b) the clinician is investigating clinical situations such as thrombocytopenia, pneumonia, or a neurological condition to exclude the diagnosis of acute EBV disease.

Epstein-Barr Viral Detection Specific polymerase chain reaction (PCR) assays that quantify EBV DNA in serum have been developed. The assays are specific for EBV DNA, have high sensitivity early in the course of illness including in young children, and the magnitude of the viral load has been correlated with the severity of illness. However, EBV PCR tests are not yet readily available for clinical use.

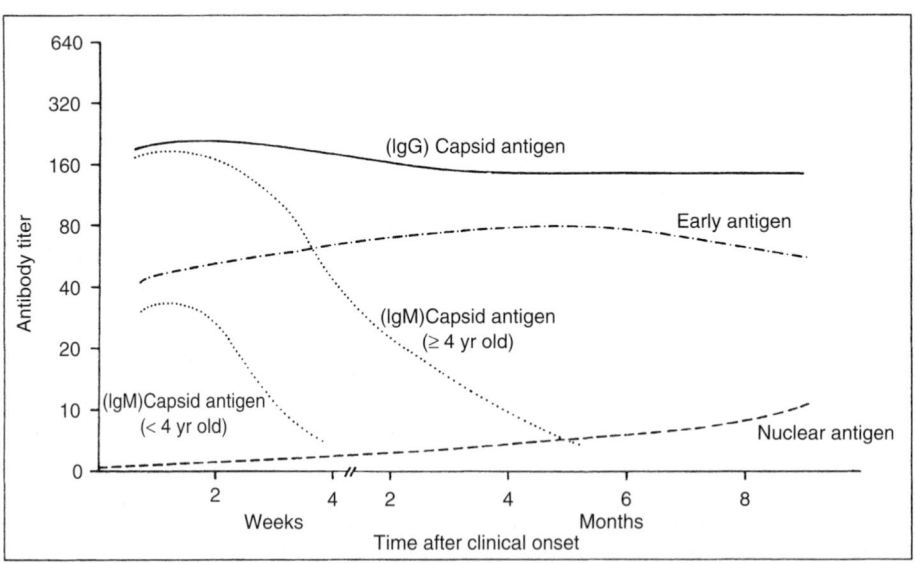

FIGURE 29.1   The evolution of antibodies to various Epstein-Barr virus (EBV) antigens in patients with infectious mononucleosis (IM) is shown in the figure. The titers are geometric mean values expressed as reciprocals of the serum dilution. Immunoglobulin M (IgM) and IgG antibody responses to EBV capsid antigen develop during the acute phase, as does an IgG response to EBV early antigen in most cases. The IgG response lasts for life, but the IgM response is transient and is shortest in very young children. Antibody response to nuclear antigen lasts for life and is typically quite late in onset. (From Sumaya CV. Epstein-Barr serologic testing: diagnostic indications and interpretations. *Pediatr Infect Dis* 1986;5:337.)

TABLE 29.1

Patterns of Serology

Type of Infection	Heterophil Antibody	VCA-IgG	VCA-IgM	Early Antigen D-EA	R-EA	EBNA
Susceptible (nonimmune)	−	−	−	−	−	−
Acute primary infection	+	++	+	+	−	−
Remote past infection	−	+	−	−	−	+
Reactivated infection	+/−	+++	−	+	++	+/−

D-EA, diffuse early antigen; EBNA, Epstein-Barr nuclear antigen; Ig, immunoglobulin; R-EA, restricted early antigen; VCA, viral capsid antigen.

Differential Diagnosis

1. Causes of EBV-negative mononucleosis-like syndrome include:
   a. CMV
   b. Toxoplasma gondii
   c. Rubella
   d. Adenovirus
   e. Herpes simplex virus 6
   f. Drug side effects
   g. Acute HIV infection
2. Other considerations include:
   a. Group A β-hemolytic streptococcal pharyngitis
   b. Viral tonsillitis
   c. Mycoplasma pneumonia
   d. Vincent angina (necrotizing ulcerative gingivitis)
   e. Diphtheria
   f. Viral hepatitis
   g. Lymphoproliferative disorder or leukemia

Diagnosis

The diagnosis is based on the following considerations:

1. Clinical symptoms: IM should be suspected in an adolescent with fatigue, fever, splenomegaly, adenopathy, and pharyngitis.
2. Abnormal white blood cell count: Patients will usually have the following:
   a. Relative lymphocytosis >50%.
   b. Absolute lymphocytosis >4,000/mm^3.
   c. Relative atypical lymphocytosis >10%.
3. Positive serology: Almost all adolescents with IM have positive heterophil antibodies. If a patient continues to be symptomatic and heterophil antibodies are negative, titers for EBV (including VCA and EBNA) should be evaluated.
4. A throat culture is indicated in patients with pharyngitis or tonsillitis, but a positive result does not exclude IM.

Management

Only supportive care is required for most patients with IM.

1. Symptomatic care
   a. Rest as needed should be provided during the acute phase. Adolescents and their parents should be made aware that the acute symptoms usually resolve over 1 to 2 weeks, although the associated fatigue may persist for 2 to 4 weeks, or sometimes longer. Many patients require up to 2 months to achieve a stable level of recovery. Between 9% and 22% of those with IM have reported persistent fatigue 6 months after the onset of symptoms.
   b. Nonsteroidal antiinflammatory agents or acetaminophen may be used as needed for fever and pain. Aspirin should be avoided, because there is a rare association between EBV and Reye syndrome.
2. Antimicrobials: In the absence of coinfection with group A streptococcus or Mycoplasma pneumoniae, antibiotics serve no purpose. Acyclovir is not indicated; although it may reduce viral shedding, it does not impact the clinical syndrome.
3. Corticosteroids: Steroids have not been shown to be effective and are not indicated for routine cases. However, corticosteroids are recommended in patients with significant pharyngeal edema that threatens or causes respiratory compromise. Prednisone, initially 40 to 60 mg daily, then tapered over 1 to 2 weeks may be used in these situations.
4. Return to activity
   a. Light, nonimpact activities may be resumed after 3 weeks of illness, as symptoms permit. Full participation in nonimpact activities may be resumed after 4 weeks of illness.
   b. Contact sports should be delayed for 4 to 6 weeks, even in the absence of splenomegaly. If there is a concern for persistent splenomegaly, ultrasound may be used to assess and monitor splenic size. However, data on the utility of splenic ultrasound to prevent rupture is lacking.

Chronic Epstein-Barr Virus Infection

The vast majority of patients with EBV-associated IM develop lifelong immunity. There are rare individuals who have very high titers of EBV antibodies and have chronic persistent active EBV infection. This is characterized by the following:

1. Severe illness lasting >6 months
2. Histological evidence of end-organ disease, such as hepatitis, uveitis, or pneumonitis
3. Evidence of EBV antigen or DNA in tissue

Despite some clinical similarities, there is little evidence that EBV causes chronic fatigue syndrome, and a positive IgG test for EBV does not imply a causal relationship.

EBV infections can be associated with lymphoproliferative disorders, particularly in individuals with underlying abnormal immune responses. For example, patients with acquired immunodeficiency syndrome (AIDS) have a 10- to 20-fold increase in circulatory EBV-infected B cells as compared with persons without HIV infection. This has implications for such disorders as virus-associated hemophagocytic syndrome, lymphomatoid granulomatosis, and the X-linked lymphoproliferative syndrome in which affected males die from EBV disease, sometimes in a matter of days. When EBV leaves the latent state and becomes chronically active, it can potentially trigger lymphoid malignancies, such as Burkitt lymphoma, Hodgkin lymphoma, and nasopharyngeal carcinoma.

MYCOPLASMA PNEUMONIA

M. pneumoniae is a common cause of upper respiratory infections and pneumonia in adolescents that is often referred to as *walking pneumonia*. It may also cause pharyngitis, tracheobronchitis, and otitis media, but at other times the infection may be asymptomatic.

Etiology

Mycoplasma are approximately 150 to 250 nm, or about the same size as large viruses. More than 100 species have been identified, with at least 13 infecting humans. Mycoplasma are prokaryotes that do have not cell walls, rather, they are bounded by cell membranes containing sterols. Because they lack cell walls, they are resistant to β-lactam antimicrobials. However, they are sensitive to antibiotics that interfere with protein synthesis, such as macrolides and tetracyclines. They appear to cause infection primarily as extracellular parasites, but may also contaminate cell cultures as intracellular parasites.

By means of attachment proteins, *M. pneumoniae* adheres to ciliated and nonciliated respiratory epithelium, causing cellular damage to the trachea, bronchi, and bronchioles. The organism also causes ciliostasis, which may lead to prolonged cough. Transmission to the respiratory tract is through aerosolized inhalation. There is a high rate of transmission to family members and other close contacts, with an incubation period of 3 to 4 weeks.

Epidemiology

Each year there are approximately 2 million cases of *Mycoplasma* pneumonia in the United States, resulting in 100,000 hospitalizations. *M. pneumoniae* infects patients of all ages, but lower respiratory disease is of particular importance in adolescents and young adults. Highest rates of infection are in those between the ages of 5 and 20 years. The illness is responsible for up to 20% of all pneumonias in middle and high school, and up to 50% among college students and military recruits. Epidemic infection occurs at 3 to 7 year intervals in the United States, with low-level endemic disease in the intervals. These epidemics typically occur in the fall, and can persist for months.

Clinical Manifestations

1. Symptoms: The onset of symptoms can be insidious.
   a. General: Malaise, fever, chills, and headache occur early in the course
   b. Respiratory
      - A cough develops 3 to 5 days after the onset of general symptoms. It usually starts as nonproductive, but may lead to the production of frothy white sputum. Sputum production is not as copious as in typical bacterial pneumonias. The cough may become paroxysmal, and occasionally chest pain and hemoptysis occur.
      - Dyspnea is common
      - In those who are predisposed, infection may lead to reactive airway disease
      - Nasal congestion and rhinorrhea are uncommon
      - Bilateral bullous myringitis is highly suggestive, but rare
2. Signs: Patients do not generally appear very ill.
   a. Pharyngitis: 75%
   b. Conjunctivitis: 50%
   c. Lymphadenopathy: 25% to 50%
   d. Chest examination: Findings are often minimal. If pneumonia is present, there may be isolated crackles or areas of wheezing over one or both of the lower lobes. Wheezing may be present in those with reactive airway disease. Signs of pleural effusion are occasionally present.

Complications

Nonrespiratory infections and complications may occur 1 to 21 days after initial symptoms. One must use caution in the diagnosis of an *M. pneumoniae* infection in individuals with extrapulmonary manifestations and no respiratory tract symptoms. In the past, the failure to isolate *M. pneumoniae* from nonrespiratory clinical specimens led to the conclusion that extrapulmonary complications were due to cross-reacting antibodies or by an unidentified toxin. However, through the use of PCR testing, *M. pneumoniae* has been identified in cerebrospinal fluid and serum, both of which are indicative of dissemination. Cross-reacting antibodies may still be the cause for hemolysis and cutaneous manifestations.

1. Musculoskeletal: Arthralgias, myalgias, arthritis, and rhabdomyolysis. The arthritis is usually monoarticular, but may be migratory and polyarticular.
2. Gastrointestinal: Gastroenteritis, hepatitis, and pancreatitis.
3. Dermatological: Most common are erythematous maculopapular lesions or vesicular exanthemas. Other rashes may be vesicular-pustular, petechial, or urticarial. Stevens-Johnson syndrome can occur.
4. Hematological: Hemolytic anemia, splenomegaly, thrombocytopenia, and disseminated intravascular coagulopathy.
5. Cardiovascular: Myocarditis, pericarditis, heart block, congestive heart failure, and acute myocardial infarction.
6. Central nervous system (CNS): Meningitis, Guillain-Barré syndrome (GBS), cranial nerve involvement, sensorineural hearing loss, transverse myelitis, focal encephalitis, cerebellar involvement, and psychosis.

7. Renal: Acute glomerulonephritis and interstitial nephritis.
8. Ophthalmologic: Conjunctivitis, anterior uveitis, optic papillitis, and rarely optic neuropathy.

Laboratory Evaluation

1. Serological testing, although not routine, is the most useful of the laboratory tests.
   a. Cold agglutinins—cold agglutinins are elevated to a titer of >1:32 in 75% of cases. This test is nonspecific, and cold agglutinins may be elevated in patients with other disorders such as infection with EBV, or CMV, lymphoma, or hemolytic anemias. For patients younger than 12 years, cold agglutinins are insensitive and nonspecific.
   b. Complement-fixation serology—this test is more specific than cold agglutinins, but requires paired acute and convalescent titers and so is of little value in the acute setting.
   c. Enzyme-linked immunoassay (EIA) detects IgM and IgG antibodies against *M. pneumoniae*. The IgM test does not become positive until 7 to 10 days after the onset of symptoms, so may not be useful in guiding initial therapy.
2. Direct antigen testing is increasingly available.
   a. Direct antigen testing in sputum may be performed using antigen-capture indirect EIA.
   b. Detection of *M. pneumoniae* ribosomal RNA using radioactive iodine–labeled complementary DNA.
   c. PCR assays are the most promising, being rapid with high sensitivity and specificity.
3. White blood cell count—this is usually normal, although a mild leukocytosis may be present.
4. Chest x-ray examination—variable; appearance is usually a non-lobar, patchy or interstitial pattern; occasionally a pleural effusion is present. Major consolidation is rare. The radiographic findings often appear worse than the clinical findings.
5. Bacterial cultures—these are of little use, because *M. pneumoniae* must be grown in cell culture, has fastidious growth requirements, and growth takes at least 3 weeks.

Differential Diagnosis

1. Streptococcal pneumonia
2. Viral pneumonia, including adenoviral infections, parainfluenza, and influenza
3. *Chlamydia pneumoniae* is a gram-negative intracellular pathogen that is a relatively common cause of pneumonia in adolescents and young adults. Between 35% and 45% of adolescents have been previously infected. Clinical symptoms are quite similar to those of *M. pneumoniae*. Diagnosis is based on serological testing, but specific testing for *C. pneumoniae* is difficult to obtain and requires acute and convalescent sera. Culture is even more difficult for *C. trachomatis* than for *M. pneumoniae*, and direct antigen detection does not appear to work well. Various PCR assays have been investigated, but none are as of yet standard. Treatment is with erythromycin, doxycycline, clarithromycin, or azithromycin.
4. *Legionella* pneumonia—more than 40 *Legionella* species have been identified, but *L. pneumophila* accounts for approximately 2% to 6% of community-acquired pneumonias in adults. Pneumonic illness usually begins abruptly with malaise, headache, myalgia, and weakness. Approximately 24 hours later, a high fever develops in more than half of infected individuals. Nonproductive cough is most common. Other symptoms include pleuritic chest pain, dyspnea, nausea, vomiting, and abdominal pain. Diarrhea is common. Physical findings on chest examination are mild compared with the radiographic findings, but in general, patients appear quite ill. There are numerous pulmonary and extrapulmonary complications including lung abscesses, hypotension, disseminated intravascular coagulation, and renal failure.
5. Less common causes of pneumonia in adolescents include tuberculosis infection, Q fever *(Coxiella)*, rickettsial infections, and fungal infections. Other causes of pneumonia are rare in nonimmunosuppressed teenagers.

Diagnosis

The diagnosis of *Mycoplasma* infections is most often presumptive and based on the patient's clinical presentation. In some instances, a more precise diagnosis may be required, and cold agglutinin tests may be performed quickly, even at the bedside. To perform the rapid test, add approximately 0.3 to 0.4 mL of blood to a standard laboratory collection tube containing 3.8% sodium citrate (a blue-stoppered Protime [PT] tube). Place the tube in ice-cold water for 15 to 30 minutes. Tilt on one side and examine for agglutination. The presence of coarse, floccular agglutination is a positive sign that correlates with a cold agglutinin titer of >1:64. Between 66% and 85% of adolescent patients with a positive cold agglutinin test result have *M. pneumoniae* infection. Other tests are described in the preceding text. PCR assays will likely become the diagnostic test of choice once they become more available.

Management

Although most infections with *M. pneumoniae* are self-limited and resolve without treatment, antibiotic therapy has been shown to decrease the length and severity of illness.

1. Rest, supportive care, and appropriate management of underlying or exacerbated reactive airway disease are important.
2. Antibiotics
   a. Azithromycin: 500 mg on day 1, then 250 mg daily on days 2 through 5.
   b. Clarithromycin: 500 mg twice a day for 7 days.
   c. Erythromycin: 500 mg four times a day for 7 days.
   d. Tetracycline: 500 mg four times a day for 7 days.
   e. Doxycycline: 100 mg twice a day for 7 days

PERTUSSIS

Pertussis, meaning "intense cough," is widely unrecognized and under diagnosed in adolescents and young adults. The term *pertussis* is more appropriate than "whooping cough," because many patients, particularly adolescents and adults, do not "whoop." Pertussis infection continues to cause fatal illness in vulnerable neonates and incompletely immunized infants, and adolescents and young adults are likely a major source of infection for these vulnerable populations.

Etiology

Bordetella organisms are small gram-negative coccobacilli. *Bordetella pertussis* is the sole cause of epidemic pertussis, and the usual cause of sporadic pertussis. Only *B. pertussis* produces pertussis toxin (PT). *B. parapertussis* may occasionally cause pertussis, but accounts for fewer than 5% of *Bordetella* isolates in the United States.

Pertussis is primarily a toxin-mediated disease with PT playing a major virulence role. Besides PT, *B. pertussis* produces other biologically active products and cytotoxins that impact the severity of the illness and induce protective immune responses. Transmission is through close contact with respiratory secretions, and intrafamilial spread is quite common in both immunized and nonimmunized individuals. The incubation period is commonly 5 to 10 days but may be as long as 21 days. Pertussis is primarily a mucosal disease, and although the organism may invade alveolar macrophages, there is no systemic invasion nor bacteremic phase of the illness.

Epidemiology

Each year approximately 60 million cases of pertussis occur worldwide, resulting in >500,000 deaths. The incidence of pertussis demonstrates a cyclic pattern, with peaks occurring every 2 to 5 years—this was true in the prevaccine era, as well as today. Over the past decade, pertussis has increased significantly, even in highly immunized populations. Before widespread vaccine use, pertussis was the leading cause of death due to infectious disease in children younger than 14 years. Routine childhood vaccination resulted in a significant decrease in disease burden, and the rate of pertussis infection reached its lowest level in 1976. Since that time, there have been numerous epidemic outbreaks in the United States, and even the interepidemic rates have not returned to the low levels of 1976. The number of reported cases in the United States went from 4,570 in 1990, to 7,796 in 1996, 9,971 in 2001, 11,647 in 2003, and 25,827 in 2004. Most of the recent increase in pertussis illness has been attributed to disease in adolescents and adults, who now account for approximately half of all cases in the United States. From 1990 to 2004, there has been an 18.8-fold increase in the diagnosis of pertussis in 10- to 19-year olds and 15.5-fold increase in those 20 years and older. Seventy-six percent of illness in infants (who are most at risk for serious illness) is contracted from adolescents and adults (Bisgard et al., 2004). The increase in rate is thought to be a combination of waning immunity (immunity to whole cell pertussis and acellular pertussis is approximately 6 years or perhaps slightly longer) and improved recognition and diagnosis of the illness. In adolescents with prolonged cough illness, between 13% and 20% are due to *B. pertussis* infection.

Clinical Manifestations

The clinical severity of pertussis varies widely, and may be influenced by patient age, immunization history, degree of exposure, past antibiotic administration, and concomitant infections. Classic pertussis is divided into three stages:

1. Catarrhal: This begins after the incubation period with nasal congestion and rhinorrhea that are sometimes accompanied by low-grade fever, sneezing, and watery eyes. Patients are most contagious at this time, but the symptoms are indistinguishable from a routine upper respiratory tract infection. These symptoms begin to wane after 1 to 2 weeks, as the paroxysmal stage begins.
2. Paroxysmal: The onset of cough marks the beginning of the paroxysmal stage. The cough begins as dry and intermittent, which then evolves into the coughing paroxysms that are characteristic of pertussis. An otherwise well-appearing patient will have episodic coughing fits with choking, gasping, and feelings of strangulation and suffocation. A forceful inspiratory gasp sounding like a "whoop" is most frequently seen in young infants. Posttussive emesis is common. At its peak, these episodes may occur hourly.
3. Convalescent: During this stage, the number, severity, and duration of the coughing paroxysms diminish.

The duration of classic pertussis is 6 to 10 weeks. Adolescents, particularly those who have been immunized, are unlikely to show distinct stages of illness. The adolescent may complain only of coughing episodes, with no history of fever or upper respiratory congestion, but the illness often leads to days or weeks of interrupted sleep and time away from school. The physical examination in between coughing episodes may be completely normal.

Pertussis is most contagious from approximately 1 to 2 weeks before the onset of cough and for 2 to 3 weeks after coughing begins. Therefore, in most cases, the person may have transmitted the disease to others before they are diagnosed and treated.

Complications are primarily seen in infants and young children and may include seizures, pneumonia, apnea, encephalopathy, and death. Adolescents rarely develop serious complications, but secondary bacterial pneumonia and adult-respiratory distress syndrome have been reported. Adolescents may develop subconjunctival hemorrhages due to increased intraabdominal and intrathoracic pressures when coughing.

Laboratory Evaluation

1. Profound leukocytosis: Profound leukocytosis with white blood cell counts from 15,000 to as high as 100,000/mm^3 due to an absolute lymphocytosis may be seen, particularly in the catarrhal phase. The platelet count may also be elevated, and significant thrombocytosis as well as extreme leukocytosis have been correlated with a more severe clinical course.
2. Culture: Culture requires nasopharyngeal secretions obtained either by aspiration or with a Dacron (polyethylene terephthalate) or calcium alginate swab that are then plated on special media. The incubation period is 10 to 14 days, and so culture rarely guides treatment decisions. False-negative cultures may occur after the second week of illness, or if antibiotics have been administered.
3. Direct immunofluorescence assay *(DFA)*: DFA of nasopharyngeal secretions may help guide early treatment decisions, but the test is unreliable due to variable sensitivity and low specificity, and culture confirmation of the test should be attempted.

4. Serology: Pertussis infection elicits a heterogeneous antibody response that differs between individuals depending on immune status, age, and history of previous infection. No single test is diagnostic, and to achieve acceptable sensitivity and specificity, acute and convalescent titers must be obtained.
5. DNA amplification: If available, the PCR for the diagnosis of pertussis has shown great promise, being rapid, and having a sensitivity of 97% and specificity of 93%.

Differential Diagnosis

1. Adenoviral infection
2. Mycoplasma pneumonia
3. Chlamydia pneumonia
4. Influenza

Diagnosis

Pertussis should be suspected in any adolescent with a complaint of a cough lasting >1 to 2 weeks, regardless of immunization status. A history of posttussive vomiting and a lymphocytosis on laboratory evaluation support the diagnosis, as do the absence of other symptoms, such as fever, and lack of findings on physical examination. Because laboratory confirmation of pertussis may be delayed or unavailable, the diagnosis is often made based on clinical evaluation. Increasing use of PCR as a diagnostic tool may change the ability of health care providers to make a more timely diagnosis.

Management

All cases of suspected or confirmed pertussis should receive appropriate antibiotic therapy. Treatment may provide some clinical benefit, and clearly decreases the spread of infection.

1. Erythromycin 500 mg 4 times daily for 14 days has been the traditional treatment.
2. Azithromycin has been shown to be as effective as erythromycin and is better tolerated. Dose is given daily for 5 days; 500 mg on day 1 and 250 mg on days 2 to 5.
3. Clarithromycin 500 mg twice daily for 7 days is another alternative.
4. Trimethoprim-sulfamethoxazole is an alternative for those who are unable to tolerate treatment with macrolides. Dose is 1 double-strength tablet twice daily for 14 days.

Control Measures
1. Treatment with a full course of antibiotics is indicated for all household contacts regardless of immunization status. Prompt treatment can limit secondary transmission, because pertussis immunity is not absolute and even those with subclinical disease may be able to transmit the illness to others. Treatment is particularly important for those who have close contact with infants and other young children.
2. Close contacts younger than 7 years who have received fewer than four doses of pertussis vaccine should be immunized appropriately.
3. Others who have been in contact with the infected individual should be monitored for symptoms for 21 days after the most recent contact.

4. Students with pertussis should be excluded from school. Patients are considered no longer infectious after 5 days of antibiotic therapy, and may return to school at that time. If they are unable to take antibiotics, they are considered infectious for 21 days after the onset of cough.

Immunization

Universal pertussis immunization is recommended for children starting at 2 months of age and has been widely used in combination with diphtheria and tetanus toxoids (diphtheria, tetanus, pertussis [DTP]) since the 1940s. Whole cell pertussis vaccines (DTwP) were utilized in the United States until the mid-1990s. These vaccines frequently caused local reactions as well as significant fever and were uncommonly associated with more severe systemic effects such as convulsions and hypotonic and hyporesponsive episodes. Less reactogenic acellular pertussis vaccines (DTaP), containing purified inactivated components of the B. pertussis organism, are highly effective and they have replaced the use of the whole cell vaccine in the United States. The primary series of four doses of DTaP are administered at 2, 4, 6, and 15 to 18 months of age. A fifth dose of DTaP vaccine is recommended before school entry to assure protection of school-aged children.

Natural and vaccine-induced immunity to pertussis wane over time, leaving adolescents and adults susceptible to infection. Two acellular pertussis vaccines have recently been licensed for use in adolescents (Tdap). In order to decrease vaccine reactogenicity, the adolescent pertussis formulations are combined with lower concentrations of tetanus toxoid, diphtheria toxoid, and PT than are present in the infant formulations. Acellular pertussis vaccine in adolescents induces comparable levels of tetanus and diphtheria antibody as the tetanus and diphtheria toxoids (Td) booster as well as antibody responses to pertussis that are higher than those seen in infants who were shown to be protected from pertussis in previous efficacy studies. Tdap has demonstrated effectiveness at reducing pertussis disease in adolescents and adults. Tdap is indicated for:

1. Routine use in adolescents at 11 to 12 years replacing the standard Td booster previously administered at this age.
2. Older adolescents, young adults, and older adults up to 64 years, who have not received a dose of Tdap provided that it has been at least 2 years since a previous dose of Td vaccine.

Tdap should not be administered to those with a severe allergic reaction or an immediate life-threatening reaction after receipt of a prior dose of a vaccine containing the same substances (DTaP, DTP, DT, Td), or to those with encephalopathy not attributable to another identifiable cause within 7 days of a prior dose of a pertussis-containing vaccine.

INFLUENZA

Influenza is an acute respiratory illness that is highly contagious, affects all age-groups, and has caused epidemics for hundreds of years. Although most influenza infections in adolescents are self-limited, those patients with chronic illness such as asthma or cardiac disease may develop a serious life-threatening infection.

Etiology

Influenza viruses are orthomyxoviruses that are enveloped with two important surface glycoproteins: hemagglutinin (HA) and neuraminidase (NA). Influenza viruses are classified as A, B, or C. Influenza A and B viruses are responsible for seasonal epidemics, whereas C virus is responsible for mild, common cold–like illnesses. Influenza A viruses are further categorized into subtypes on the basis of HA and NA. Since 1977 there have been two predominant circulating subtypes, influenza A (H1N1) and influenza A (H3N2). Influenza B is not subtyped. Influenza A and B are indistinguishable clinically, but influenza A (H3N2) viruses are generally associated with the most severe epidemics.

Influenza viruses are negative-sense RNA viruses that contain eight separate gene segments. During virus replication, point mutations in the gene segments can lead to minor antigenic virus variants. Minor antigenic changes occur frequently and lead to yearly epidemics of influenza illness. Novel influenza subtypes are due to genetic reassortment and lead to episodic influenza pandemics. Reassortment between animal and human influenza viruses may occur if a suitable host such as a pig is coinfected by human and animal influenza viruses. Occasionally, an animal virus may begin infecting humans, such as in Hong Kong in 1997 when avian influenza A (H5N1) seen in poultry began infecting humans.

Transmission is person to person through respiratory droplets or by direct contact with articles recently contaminated by nasopharyngeal secretions. The incubation period is only 1 to 4 days, and a single infected person may transmit the virus to a large number of susceptible individuals. Patients are most infectious during the 24 hours before and through the peak of symptoms. Viral shedding continues for approximately 7 days after the onset of symptoms. Seasonal epidemics typically occur during the winter. Local outbreaks can peak within 2 weeks of onset and last 4 to 8 weeks.

Epidemiology

Although influenza may be sporadically identified through the year, epidemics typically occur annually during the winter months. Influenza A generally occurs annually, whereas influenza B recurs every 3 or 4 years. Changes in viral HA and, to a lesser extent, NA account for ability of influenza to cause regular epidemics. Different strains of influenza are associated with varying severities of illness—H3N2 appears to be more virulent than the H1N1-associated illness, and both strains of influenza A appear to be more virulent than influenza B. Despite this, there is no way to clinically differentiate between the various strains.

Local epidemics are maintained by high infection rates in young children. During these outbreaks, infection rates may be as high as 40% for school-aged and preschool children, as opposed to infection rates in young adults of 10% to 20%. Although for most adolescents, influenza may be nothing more than a bad cold, it is a cause of morbidity, particularly for younger children and those with underlying medical conditions. Among those aged 5 to 14 years, influenza accounts for a hospitalization rate of 20 to 40 per 100,000 population, but 200 per 100,000 in those with high-risk conditions such as asthma or heart disease.

Clinical Manifestations

1. Symptoms
   a. Sudden onset of fever and chills
   b. Nonproductive cough
   c. Myalgias
   d. Sore throat
   e. Malaise
   f. Headache
   g. Nausea, vomiting, diarrhea are more common in younger patients
2. Signs
   a. Patient appears unwell
   b. Hyperemic mucous membranes
   c. Injected conjunctiva
   d. Clear rhinorrhea

The fever is often as high as 40°C, peaks within 24 hours of the onset of symptoms, and may last up to 5 days. The dry, hacking cough may persist for up to 1 week after the other symptoms have resolved.

Complications

1. Primary viral pneumonia
2. Encephalitis
3. Encephalopathy
4. Guillian-Barre Syndrome
5. Reye syndrome
6. Myositis

Laboratory Evaluation

1. White blood cell count is usually normal, although there may be a relative neutrophilia and lymphopenia.
2. Viral culture: The time needed for this test renders it impractical for use in clinical care.
3. DFA and indirect fluorescent antibody (IFA) staining.
   a. Viral antigen detection.
   b. Antibodies are either directly or indirectly conjugated to a fluorescein compound. These antibodies bind to influenza antigen, and are then detected under a fluorescent microscope.
   c. Must be performed at a hospital or reference laboratory.
   d. Results are available in 2 to 4 hours.
   e. Tests have low sensitivity (62%–74%), but high specificity (97%–98%). Therefore, it is unusual to have false-positive test results, but false-negative results are more common.
4. Rapid diagnostic test: Immunoassay
   a. Viral nucleoprotein detection.
   b. Antibodies bind to the viral nucleoprotein, and are detected by visualizing a color change.
   c. May be performed in the hospital or reference laboratory, or in a medical office.
   d. Results are available in approximately 15 minutes.
   e. Sensitivity varies widely, from 40% to 100%, as does specificity, ranging from 63% to 100%.
5. Rapid diagnostic test: Viral NA detection
   a. Viral NA catalyzes a chemical reaction that is detected by visualizing a color change.
   b. May be performed in the hospital or reference laboratory, or in a medical office.
   c. Results are available in approximately 30 minutes.

d. Sensitivity varies from 48% to 96%, and specificity ranges from 63% to 93%.

Differential Diagnosis

1. Bacterial infections
   a. Streptococcal pneumonia
   b. Chlamydia pneumonia
   c. Mycoplasma pneumonia
2. Other viral infections
   a. Adenovirus
   b. Parainfluenza
   c. Respiratory syncytial virus
   d. Rhinovirus

Diagnosis

The clinical diagnosis of influenza can be difficult, even during peak influenza activity, because many other circulating respiratory viruses exhibit similar symptoms. During episodes of peak disease activity it is impractical to test every patient with signs and symptoms of influenza. Therefore, the diagnosis is often made based on the clinical presentation of the patients, as well as the prior probability of influenza based on local rates of influenza activity. There is little data examining the validity of the clinical diagnosis of influenza in adolescents, but the reported positive predictive value of the clinical diagnosis in adults varies widely, from 18% to 87% as compared with laboratory-confirmed influenza. During a seasonal outbreak, the diagnosis should be considered in any adolescent who presents with the sudden onset of fever and a dry, nonproductive cough.

Management

Most adolescents who contract influenza will require supportive care only. Ibuprofen or acetaminophen may be used for fever, headache, and myalgia. Patient should be cautioned against the use of aspirin because of the potential for the development of Reye syndrome. Patients who have underlying illness or otherwise healthy patients who present for treatment within 48 hours of the onset of symptoms may benefit from treatment with antiviral medications. These medications have been shown to decrease the time to symptom resolution to 1 to 2 days.

1. Amantadine
   a. Approved for treatment of influenza A in children 1 year and older
   b. Interferes with M2 protein function
   c. May cause CNS disturbance
   d. Adolescent treatment dose: 100 mg by mouth twice a day for 5 days
   e. May be unhelpful in the treatment of resistant strains; it is important to be aware of local patterns of resistance
2. Rimantadine
   a. Approved for treatment of influenza A in adults; approved for chemoprophylaxis of influenza A in children 1 year and older
   b. Interferes with M2 protein function
   c. Causes less CNS disturbance than amantadine
   d. Adolescent treatment dose: 100 mg b.i.d. by mouth twice a day for 5 days
   e. May be unhelpful in the treatment of resistant strains; it is important to be aware of local patterns of resistance
3. Oseltamivir
   a. Approved for treatment of influenza A and B in children 1 year and older; approved for chemoprophylaxis of influenza A and B in adolescents 13 years and older
   b. Inhibits viral NA
   c. Adolescent treatment dose: 75 mg by mouth twice a day for 5 days
4. Zanamivir
   a. Approved for treatment of influenza A and B in children 7 years and older
   b. Inhibits viral NA
   c. Orally inhaled powder
   d. Should not be used in patients with underlying respiratory diseases such as asthma because bronchospasm may occur
   e. Adolescent dose: Two inhalations (5 mg each inhalation) twice a day for 5 days

Immunization

Although antiviral agents may be used for the prevention of influenza, the primary means is through immunization. Vaccines are currently trivalent, containing two A antigens (representing both the H1N1 and H3N2 subtypes) and a B antigen. In years when there is an ample vaccine supply, influenza vaccine should be given to any adolescent and young adult requesting vaccination. Vaccine should be prioritized for adolescents who are at increased risk of developing severe complications due to influenza including:

1. Those with chronic disorders of the pulmonary or cardiovascular systems, including asthma
2. Those who had required regular medical follow-up or hospitalization during the preceding year for the following conditions:
   a. Chronic metabolic diseases (including diabetes mellitus)
   b. Renal dysfunction
   c. Hemoglobinopathies
   d. Immunosuppression
3. Those who have any condition that can compromise respiratory function or the handling of respiratory secretions or that can increase the risk for aspiration
4. Those who are receiving long-term aspirin therapy and, therefore, might be at risk for experiencing Reye syndrome after influenza infection
5. Those who will be pregnant during the influenza season

There are two options for immunization—trivalent inactivated influenza vaccine (TIV) and live attenuated influenza vaccine (LAIV). Both vaccines are trivalent and both vaccine viruses are grown in chicken eggs. TIV is a killed virus product administered by intramuscular injection, whereas LAIV is a live attenuated virus product administered using an intranasal sprayer. Neither vaccine should be given to those with a history of an anaphylactic hypersensitivity to eggs or to other specific vaccine components. TIV can be used for both healthy adolescents as well as those with high-risk medical conditions. Use of LAIV should be restricted to healthy adolescents only and should not be administered to those with the high-risk medical conditions noted in the preceding text. In addition,

LAIV should not be administered to those with a history of Guillian-Barre Syndrome (GBS). The decision to use TIV in patients with a history of GBS should be made on an individual basis. For those at low risk of complications due to influenza and for those who experienced GBS within 6 weeks of receipt of a prior influenza vaccine, TIV should be avoided.

WEB SITES

For Parents and Teens

www.cdc.gov/flu. Mass of information available for both adolescents, parents and health care providers.

www.familydoctor.org. The American Academy of Family Practice has a number of patient-education handouts available including mononucleosis and influenza, and Spanish translations are available.

www.aap.org/parents.html. The American Academy of Pediatrics has patient education information primarily listed by symptom rather than condition.

For Health Care Providers

www.cdc.gov/flu/weekly. Every week from October through mid-May, the Centers for Disease Control and Prevention publishes weekly influenza surveillance reports.

www.cdc.gov/flu. Mass of information available for both adolescents, parents and health care providers.

There are a variety of commercial Web sites available that offer patient handouts, as well as information for clinicians. Two of these include Up to Date, available at http://uptodate.com, and MDConsult, available at http://mdconsult.com. Many academic institutions have subscriptions, but they are subscription services for individuals.

REFERENCES AND ADDITIONAL READINGS

Ambinder RF. Epstein-Barr virus-associated lymphoproliferative disorders. *Rev Clin Exp Hematol* 2003;7(4):362.

Anikster Y, Glustein JZ, Weill M, et al. Extrapulmonary manifestations of *Mycoplasma pneumoniae* infections. *Isr J Med Sci* 1994;30:412.

Auwaerter PG. Infectious mononucleosis in middle age. *JAMA* 1999;281(5):454.

Baum SG. Introduction to mycoplasma diseases. In: Mandell GL, Bennett JE, Dolin R, eds. *Principles and practice of infectious diseases*, 5th ed. New York: Churchill Livingstone, 2000:2015.

Baum SG. Mycoplasma pneumoniaae and atypical pneumonia. In: Mandell GL, Bennett JE, Dolin R, eds. *Principles and practice of infectious diseases*, 5th ed. New York: Churchill Livingstone, 2000:2018.

Biscardi S, Lorrot M, Marc E, et al. *Mycoplasma pneumoniae* and asthma in children. *Clin Infect Dis* 2004;38:1341.

Bisgard KM, Pascual FB, Ehresmann KR, et al. Infant pertussis: Who was the source? *Pediatr Infect Dis J* 2004;23:985.

Boivin G, Hardy I, Tellier G, et al. Predicting influenza infections during epidemics with use of a clinical case definition. *Clin Infect Dis* 2000;31:1166.

Burroughs KE. Athletes resuming activity after infectious mononucleosis. *Arch Fam Med* 2000;9(10):1122.

Candy B, Chalder T, Cleare AJ, et al. Recovery from infectious mononucleosis: a case for more than symptomatic therapy? A systematic review. *Br J Gen Pract* 2002;52:844.

Carrat F, Tachet A, Rouzioux C, et al. Evaluation of clinical case definitions of influenza: detailed investigation of patients during the 1995–1996 epidemic in France. *Clin Infect Dis* 1999;28:283.

Centers for Disease Control and Prevention. Pertussis: United States, 1997–2000. *MMWR Morb Mortal Wkly Rep* 2002;51:73.

Centers for Disease Control and Prevention. Prevention and control of influenza: recommendations of the Advisory Committee on Immunization Practices (ACIP). *MMWR Morb Mortal Wkly Rep* 2005;54(RR-8):1.

Chan SC, Dawes PJ. The management of severe infectious mononucleosis tonsillitis and upper airway obstruction. *J Laryngol Otol* 2001;115(12):973.

Chatterjee A. *Mycoplasma infections. eMedicine.* August 1, 2002. Available at www.emedicine.com/ped/topic1524.htm. accessed November 19, 2005.

Chen CJ, Huang YC, Jaing TH, et al. Hemophagocytic syndrome: a review of 18 pediatric cases. *J Microbiol Immunol Infect* 2004;37(3):157.

Cherry JD. The epidemiology of pertussis: a comparison of the epidemiology of the disease pertussis with the epidemiology of bordetella pertussis infection. *Pediatrics* 2005;115:1422.

Cherry JD, Grimprel E, Guiso N, et al. Defining pertussis epidemiology: clinical, microbiologic, and serologic perspectives. *Pediatr Infect Dis J* 2005;24(5):S25.

Cherry JD, Heininger U. Pertussis. In: Feigin RD, Cherry JD, eds. *Textbook of pediatric infectious diseases*, 5th ed. Philadelphia: WB Saunders, 2003.

Cimolai N. Mycoplasma pneumoniae respiratory infection. *Pediatr Rev* 1998;19(10):327.

Collins M, Fleisher GR, Fager SS. Incidence of beta hemolytic streptococcal pharyngitis in adolescents with infectious mononucleosis. *J Adolesc Health* 1984;5(2):96.

Cooper MJ, Sutton AJ, Abrams KR, et al. Effectiveness of neuraminidase inhibitors in treatment and prevention of influenza A and B: systematic review and meta-analyses of randomized controlled trials. *Brit Med J* 2003;326:1235.

Cox NJ, Subbarao K. Influenza. *Lancet* 1999;354:1277.

Cromer BA, Goydos J, Hackell J, et al. Unrecognized pertussis infection in adolescents. *Am J Dis Child* 1993;147:575.

Cunha BA. Influenza: historical aspects of epidemics and pandemics. *Infect Dis Clin North Am* 2004;18(1):141.

Dragsted DM, Dohn B, Madsen J, et al. Comparison of culture and PCR for detection of Bordetella pertussis and Bordetella parapertussis under routine laboratory conditions. *J Med Microbiol* 2004;53(Pt 8):749.

Ebell MH. Epstein-Barr virus infectious mononucleosis. *Am Fam Physician* 2004;70(7):1279.

Edwards KM. Is pertussis a frequent cause of cough in adolescents and adults? Should routine pertussis immunization be recommended? *Clin Infect Dis* 2001;32:1698.

Epstein MA. Reflections of Epstein-Barr virus: some recently resolved old uncertainties. *J Infect* 2001;43(2):111.

Esposito S, Bosis S, Faelli N, et al. Role of atypical bacteria and azithormycin therapy for children with recurrent respiratory tract infections. *Pediatr Infect Dis J* 2005;24(5):438.

Foreman BH, Mackler L. Can we prevent splenic rupture for patients with infectious mononucleosis? *J Fam Pract* 2005;54(6):547.

Ginevra C, Barranger C, Ros A, et al. Development and evaluation of Chlamylege, an new commercial test allowing simultaneous detection and identification of Legionella, Chlamydophila pneumoniae, and mycolasma pneumoniae in clinical respiratory specimens by multiplex PCR. *J Clin Microbiol* 2005;43(7):3247.

Glezen WP, Greenberg SB, Atmar RL, et al. Impact of respiratory virus infections on persons with chronic underlying conditions. *JAMA* 2000;283:499.

Godshall SE, Kirchner JT. Infectious mononucleosis: complexities of a common syndrome. *Postgrad Med* 2000;107(7):175.

Goetz MB, Rhew DC, Torres A. Pyogenic bacterial pneumonia, lung abscess, and empyema. In: Mason RJ, Murray JF, Broaddus VC et al., eds. *Murray & Nadel's textbook of respiratory medicine*, 4th ed. Philadelphia: Elsevier Science, WB Saunders, 2005:920.

Grayston JT, Campbell La, Kuo CC, et al. A new respiratory tact pathogen: *Chlamydia pneumoniae* strain TWAR. *J Infect Dis* 1990;161:618.

Grotto I, Mimouni D, Huerta M, et al. Clinical and laboratory presentation of EBV positive infectious mononucleosis in young adults. *Epidemiol Infect* 2003;131:683.

Halperin SA, Bortolussi R, Langley JM, et al. A randomized, placebo-controlled trial of erythromycin estolate chemoprophylaxis for household contacts of children with culture-positive *Bordetella perussis* infection. *Pediatrics* 1999;104:e42.

Hammerschlag MR. Pneumonia due to Chlamydia pneumoniae in children: epidemiology, diagnosis, and treatment. *Pediatr Pulmonol* 2003;36:384.

Hardegger D, Nadal D, Bossrt W, et al. Rapid detection of Mycoplasma pneumoniae in clinical samples by real-time PCR. *J Microbiol Methods* 2000;41(1):45.

Hijazi Z, Pacsa A, Eisa S, et al. Laboratory diagnosis of acute lower respiratory tract viral infectious in children. *J Trop Pediatr* 1996;42:276.

van der Horst C, Joncas J, Ahronheim G, et al. Lack of effect of peroral acyclovir for the treatment of acute infectious mononucleosis. *J Infect Dis* 1991;164(4):788.

Jefferson T, Smith S, Demicheli V, et al. Assessment of the efficacy and effectiveness of influenza vaccines in healthy children: systematic review. *Lancet* 2005;365:773.

Kindernecht JJ. Infectious mononucleosis and the spleen. *Curr Sports Med Rep* 2002;1(2):116.

Lahat E, Berkovitch M, Barr J, et al. Abnormal visual evoked potentials in children with "Alice in Wonderland" syndrome due to infectious mononucleosis. *J Child Neurol* 1999;14(11):732.

Langly JM, Halperin SA, Boucher FD, et al. Azithromycin is as effective as and better tolerated than erythromycin estolate for the treatment of pertussis. *Pediatrics* 2004;114:96.

Long SS. Pertussis (*Bordetella pertussis* and *B. Parapertussis*). In: Behrman RE, Kliegman R, Jenson HM, eds. *Nelson's textbook of pediatrics*, 17th ed. Philadelphia: WB Saunders, 2004.

Long SS, Welkin CJ, Clark JL. Widespread silent transmission of pertussis in families: antibody correlates of infection and symptomatology. *J Infect Dis* 1990;161:473.

Lorenzo CV, Robertson WS. Genital ulcerations as presenting symptom of infectious mononucleosis. *J Am Board Fam Pract* 2005;18(1):67.

Merriam SC, Keeling RP. Beta-hemolytic streptococcal pharyngitis: uncommon in infectious mononucleosis. *South Med J* 1983;76(5):575.

Monto AS, Gravenstein S, Elliot M, et al. Clinical signs and symptoms predicting influenza infection. *Arch Intern Med* 2000;160:3243.

Morais-Almeida M, Marinho S, Gaspar A, et al. Cold urticaria and infectious mononucleosis in children. *Allergol Immunopathol (Madr)* 2004;32(6):368.

Morozumi M, Hasegawa K, Chiba N, et al. Application of PCR for Mycoplasma pneumoniae detection in children with community-acquired pneumonia. *J Infect Chemother* 2004; 10(5):274.

Morris MC, Edmunds WJ. The changing epidemiology of infectious mononucleosis. *J Infect* 2002;45:107.

Mullooly JP, Barker WH. Impact of type A influenza on children: a retrospective study. *Am J Public Health* 1982;72:1008.

Murray BJ. Medical complications of infectious mononucleosis. *Am Fam Physician* 1984;30(5):195.

Nicholson AG, Wotherspoon AC, Diss TC, et al. Lymphomatoid granulomatosis: evidence that some cases represent Epstein-Barr virus-associated B-cell lymphoma. *Histopathology* 1996;29(4):317.

Niesters HGM, van Esser J, Fries E, et al. Development of a real-time quantitative assay for detection of Epstein-Barr virus. *J Clin Microbiol* 2000;38:712.

Pichichero ME, Casey JR. Acellular pertussis vaccines for adolescents. *Pediatr Infect Dis J* 2005;24(6):S117.

Pickering LK, ed. American Academy of Pediatrics. *Red Book: 2003 report of the committee on infectious diseases*, 26th ed. Elk Grove Village, IL: American Academy of Pediatrics, 2003.

Pitetti RD, Laus S, Wadowsky RM. Clinical evaluation of a quantitative real time polymerase chain reaction assay for diagnosis of primary Epstein-Barr virus infection in children. *Pediatr Infect Dis J* 2003;22(8):736.

Rea TD, Russo JE, Katon W, et al. Prospective study of the natural history of infectious mononucleosis caused by Epstein-Barr virus. *J Am Board Fam Pract* 2001;14:234.

Renn CN, Straff W, Dorfmuller A, et al. Amoxicillin-induced exanthema in young adults with infectious mononucleosis: demonstration of drug-specific lymphocyte reactivity. *Br J Dermatol* 2002;147:1166.

Rennels MB, Meissner HC. Technical report: reduction of the influenza burden in children. *Pediatrics* 2002;110:e80.

Rodriguez WJ, Schwartz RH, Thorne MM. Evaluation of diagnostic tests for influenza in a pediatric practice. *Pediatr Infect Dis J* 2002;21:193.

Stenfors LE, Bye HM, Raisanen S, et al. Bacterial penetration into tonsillar surface epithelium during infectious mononucleosis. *J Laryngol Otol* 2000;114(11):848.

Strebel P, Nordin J, Edwards K, et al. Population-based incidence of pertussis among adolescents and adults, Minnesota, 1995–1996. *J Infect Dis* 2001;183:1353.

Sumaya CV, Ench Y. Epstein-Barr virus infectious mononucleosis in children: part I. Clinical and general laboratory findings. *Pediatrics* 1985;75(6):1003.

Sumaya CV, Ench Y. Epstein-Barr virus infectious mononucleosis in children: part II. Heterophil antibody and viral-specific responses. *Pediatrics* 1985;75(6):1011.

Teo SSS, Nguyen-Van-Tam JS, Booy R. Influenza burden of illness, diagnosis, treatment, and prevention: what is the evidence in children and where are the gaps? *Arch Dis Child* 2005;90:532.

Terebuh P, Uyeki T, Fukuda K. Impact of influenza on young children and the shaping of United States influenza vaccine policy. *Pediatr Infect Dis J* 2003;22:S231.

Torre D, Tambini R. Acyclovir for treatment of infectious mononucleosis: a meta-analysis. *Scand J Infect Dis* 1999; 31:543.

Tozzi AE, Celentano LP, degli Atti ALC, et al. Diagnosis and management of pertussis. *Can Med Assoc J* 2005;172(4):509.

Tsai HP, Kuo PJ, Liu CC, et al. Respiratory viral infections among pediatric inpatients and outpatients in Taiwan from 1997 to 1999. *J Clin Microbiol* 2001;39:111.

Uyeki TM. Influenza diagnosis and treatment in children: a review of studies on clinically useful tests and antiviral treatment for influenza. *Pediatr Infect Dis J* 2003;22:164.

Vincent MT, Celestin N, Hussain A. Pharyngitis. *Am Fam Physician* 2004;69(6):1465.

Waits KB, Talkington DF. Mycoplasma pneumonia and its role as a human pathogen. *Clin Microbiol Rev* 2004;17(4): 697.

Ward JI, Cherry JD, Chang S, et al. Efficacy of acellular pertussis vaccine among adolescents and adults. *N Engl J Med* 2005;353:1555.

Weiner LB, McMillan JA. Mycoplasma pneumoniae. In: Long SS, Pickering LK, Prober CG, eds. *Principles and practice of pediatric infectious diseases*, 2nd ed.Philadelphia: Churchill Livingstone, 2003.

Yuen KY, Chan PKS, Peiris M, et al. Clinical features and rapid viral diagnosis of human disease associated with avian influenza A H5N1. *Lancet* 1998;351:467.

Zambon M, Hays J, Webster A, et al. Diagnosis of influenza in the community: relationship of clinical diagnosis to confirmed virological, serologic, or molecular detection of influenza. *Arch Intern Med* 2001;161:2116.

Zambon MC, Stockton JD, Clewley JP, et al. Contribution of influenza and respiratory syncytial virus to community cases of influenza-like illness: an observational study. *Lancet* 2001;358:1410.

CHAPTER 30

Hepatitis

Praveen S. Goday

ETIOLOGY

Hepatitis may be caused by viral agents such as hepatitis A virus (HAV), hepatitis B virus (HBV), hepatitis C virus (HCV), delta virus (HDV), hepatitis E virus (HEV), Epstein-Barr virus, cytomegalovirus, or noninfectious causes such as hepatotoxins. This chapter discusses primarily hepatitis A, hepatitis B, and hepatitis C.

1. HAV: Hepatitis A is caused by an RNA virus belonging to the family Picornaviridae.
2. HBV: Hepatitis B is caused by a 42-nm diameter virus, with an outer lipid envelope surrounding the inner core containing the DNA genome (Fig. 30.1). Several components of this virus can be detected by electron microscopy:
   a. Dane particle: This is the whole 42-nm diameter virus.
   b. A 7-nm thick shell contains the hepatitis B surface antigen (HBsAg).
   c. A 28-nm nucleocapsid: This central core contains the hepatitis B core antigen (HBcAg).
   d. Peripheral blood also contains 20- to 22-nm spherical and tubular particles that contain HBsAg and represent excess virus coat material.
3. HCV: This is an RNA virus of the Flaviviridae family. It has great genetic heterogeneity, with at least six major genotypes, more than 80 subtypes, and numerous minor variants called *quasispecies*. There is a genotype-dependent differential response to therapy.
4. HDV: This is an HBsAg-coated 35- to 37-nm diameter particle that is a "defective" pathogen because it is dependent on the presence of hepatitis B to cause an infection.
5. HEV: This is an RNA virus that causes fecal-orally transmitted hepatitis in developing countries.

EPIDEMIOLOGY

Table 30.1 outlines the epidemiology of the hepatitis viruses. A more detailed discussion follows.

Hepatitis A

Hepatitis A is transmitted primarily by the fecal-oral route and through contaminated food or water. Infection through personal contact may occur during sexual intercourse or close contact within households. Percutaneous or transfusion-related transmission is extremely rare. Children generally shed the virus longer than adults and asymptomatically infected young children excreting HAV are an important source. Maximum concentrations of virus are excreted in the 2 weeks before the onset of symptoms. Patients are usually considered noninfectious 1 week after onset of jaundice. In the United States, approximately 10% to 20% of individuals have evidence of prior infection by 20 years of age, and approximately 50% by age 50.

Hepatitis B

HBV has been documented in almost all bodily secretions, including tears, stools, saliva, blood, bile, breast milk, vaginal secretions, urine, sneeze droplets, and semen. Transmission occurs through percutaneous or permucosal routes, by infective blood or body fluids, through sexual contact, by contaminated needles, or perinatally from mother to infant. Infection can also occur in settings of continuous close personal contact (such as institutions for persons with developmental disabilities or in households), presumably through inapparent or unnoticed contact of infective secretions with skin lesions or mucosal surfaces.

In the United States, the prevalence of HBsAg is 0.3% and the number of chronically infected persons is estimated at 1.25 million. From 1990 through 2004, the incidence of reported acute hepatitis B in all ages declined by 68% reflecting the success of the national strategy to eliminate hepatitis B, which included screening of pregnant women and postexposure prophylaxis to appropriate infants, routine vaccination of all infants and children younger than 19, and vaccination of others at increased risk of hepatitis B. Since 1990 through 2004, rates among adolescents aged 14 to 18 years have declined approximately 94%, but the 2004 rate (0.4 per 100,000 population) remains substantially higher than the rate for children younger than 13 years (0.07/100,000). Age-specific rates of hepatitis B in the United States increase through adolescence, peaking among young adults. Similar to adults, the most frequently reported risk factors for hepatitis B among adolescents are sexual contact and injection drug use. Risk factors for infection are not always identified.

FIGURE 30.1 Hepatitis B virion (Dane particle) and spherical and tubular HBsAg particles found in serum of infected persons. HBcAg, and HBsAg: hepatitis B core, and surface antigens, respectively. (Adapted from Kalser MH, Howard RB. Hepatic and pancreatic disorders. *Postgrad Med* 1986;79:199.)

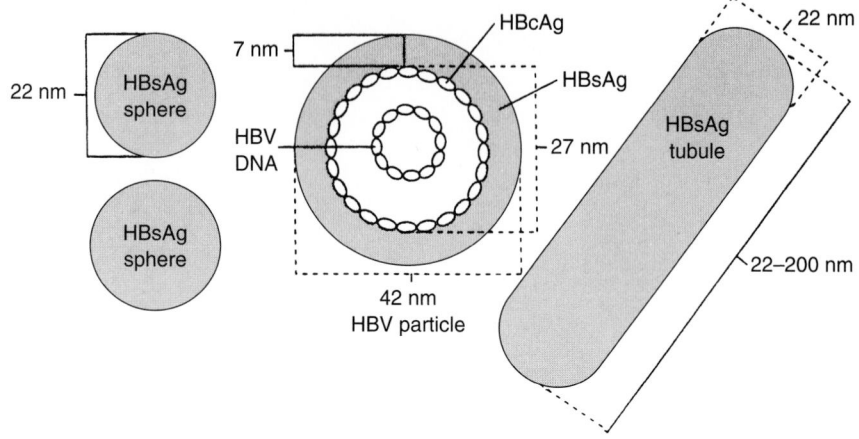

TABLE 30.1

Clinical and Epidemiological Comparison of Hepatitis Viruses

Characteristics	Hepatitis A	Hepatitis B	Hepatitis C	Hepatitis D	Hepatitis E
Transmission					
Usual	Fecal-oral	Parenteral	Parenteral	Parenteral	Fecal-oral
Alternative	Parenteral (rare)	Frequently nonparenteral (venereal, perinatal)	Venereal, perinatal	Venereal	Possibly parenteral
Distribution	Point-source outbreaks, random cases	Prevalent in young adults and urban populations	Injection drug use, venereal, perinatal	Worldwide; not highly endemic in the United States	Primarily Asia, Africa, Mexico; rare in the United States
Incubation period (d)	15–50	45–160	49–63	Coinfection, 45–60 Superinfection, 14–136	15–60
Onset	Acute	Often insidious	Insidious	Acute or insidious	Acute
Severity	Usually mild, often anicteric	More severe than hepatitis A; less often anicteric	Mild to moderate	Often severe or fulminant	Variable; severe in pregnancy
Chronic disease	None	90% of perinatal cases; 10% of adult cases	50%–60% of cases	Yes	None
Carrier state	None	Yes	Yes	Yes	None
Case-fatality rate	0%–0.2%	0.3%–15%	Unknown	Unknown	Unknown
Estimated incidence trend in the United States	Decreasing	Decreasing	Decreasing	Unknown	Not endemic in the United States
Estimated proportion of acute hepatitis cases in the United States	~25%	~50%	~20%	Unknown	None

From Koff RS. Hepatitis B today: clinical and diagnostic overview. *Pediatr Infect Dis J* 1993;12:428. Adapted from Hoofnagle JH. Type B hepatitis: virology, serology, and clinical course. *Semin Liver Dis* 1981;1:1.

Hepatitis C

The prevalence of antibodies to HCV in the United States is approximately 2%. Injection drug use is currently responsible for most HCV transmission in the United States. The prevalence of antibodies to HCV in most studies of injection drug users is 80% to 90%, and incidence rates generally range from 10% to 20%/year. Currently, 68% of HCV transmission in the United States is attributable to injection drug use, 18% is associated with sexual exposure, 4% is associated with occupational exposure, 1% is from other exposures (iatrogenic and perinatal), while 9% of transmissions have no definable source. Approximately 5% of infants born to infected mothers become infected. Screening of organ, tissue, and blood donors for HCV has essentially eliminated the risk of transmission in transplantation and transfusion. Likewise, inactivation procedures introduced in the manufacture of clotting factor concentrates have virtually eliminated the risk of infection in the hemophilic population.

Delta Hepatitis

HDV can cause disease only if HBV is present. The transmission of the virus is usually similar to that of HBV (i.e., blood or body fluids). Risk groups include intravenous drug users, male homosexuals, hemodialysis workers and patients, and recipients of blood products.

Hepatitis E

Hepatitis E is a fecal-orally transmitted form of viral hepatitis seen primarily in developing countries in central Asia, Africa, and Mexico. It has a variable presentation but is somewhat more severe than hepatitis A, with fulminant hepatitis occurring in 1% to 3% of patients overall, but in 20% of pregnant women. Although reported cases of hepatitis E have been identified in the United States, transmission is rare here. HEV will not be discussed further in this chapter.

CLINICAL MANIFESTATIONS

Symptoms

It is not possible to distinguish among the types of hepatitis on the basis of clinical manifestations. If the date of exposure is known, incubation periods may be helpful in diagnosis:

Hepatitis A	15–50 d, average 28 d
Hepatitis B	42–168 d, average 112 d
Hepatitis C	14–182 d, average 49 d
Hepatitis E	15–60 d, average 40 d

The incubation periods of the three major hepatitis viruses can be remembered more readily as hepatitis A: 2 to 6 weeks, hepatitis B: 2 to 6 months, and hepatitis C: 2 weeks to 6 months.

Common early symptoms of viral hepatitis include fatigue, lassitude, anorexia, nausea, dark urine, drowsiness, low-grade fever, right upper abdominal discomfort, myalgia, and arthralgias. In hepatitis A, approximately 20% of individuals have a history of diarrhea. In viral hepatitis B, immune complexes can lead to arthralgias, arthritis, and a rash. The arthritis of hepatitis B may precede the jaundice. It is usually a symmetrical polyarthritis affecting small joints. Larger joints may be affected, but the feet are usually spared. The rash accompanying hepatitis B occurs in up to 50% of patients and is usually urticarial in nature but may be maculopapular or petechial.

Signs

1. Icteric sclera
2. Tender hepatomegaly
3. Splenomegaly (10% of cases)
4. Arthritis
5. Skin rash

Laboratory Findings

1. Relative lymphocytosis
2. Elevated serum transaminases
3. Elevation in total and conjugated bilirubin
4. Mild elevation in serum alkaline phosphatase
5. Severe disease: Decreased serum albumin and prothrombin time. Prothrombin time is the only test that has prognostic significance in hepatitis.
6. Hepatitis B arthritis: Decreased serum and joint complement. White blood cell count in joint fluid ranges between 2,000 and 90,000/ mL.

VIRAL ANTIGENS AND ANTIBODIES

To understand the clinical course and diagnosis of viral hepatitis, one must understand the various antigens and antibodies and their clinical significance.

1. Hepatitis A (Fig. 30.2 and Table 30.2)
   a. Immunoglobulin M (IgM) anti-hepatitis A viral antibody (IgM anti-HAV): This antibody is detected early in the illness and remains detectable for approximately 2 to 3 months.
   b. Immunoglobulin G anti-hepatitis A viral antibody (IgG anti-HAV): This antibody rises more slowly and persists for years. It indicates a past infection and the presence of immunity to HAV.
   c. HAV in stool: This is usually present before the onset of clinical symptoms and is of little clinical utility.
2. Hepatitis B (Fig. 30.3 and Table 30.2)
   a. HBsAg: The surface antigen becomes positive during the incubation period and disappears in most patients during the course of the clinical disease. However, in certain patients, this antigen may remain positive for life. A positive test result for HBsAg indicates either an acute hepatitis B infection or a chronic carrier state and signifies that the patient is capable of transmitting HBV.
   b. Anti-hepatitis B surface antigen (anti-HBs): This antibody usually becomes positive months after the onset of the clinical disease. A positive blood test result indicates past infection or immunity from immunization. If acute hepatitis is present, the patient probably has hepatitis of another etiology.
   c. HBcAg: The core antigen is not routinely assayed for in peripheral blood.

FIGURE 30.2 Course of hepatitis A infection. ANTI-HAV, anti-hepatitis A viral antibody; IgG, immunoglobulin G; IgM, immunoglobulin M; SGPT, alanine transaminase. (Adapted from Centers for Disease Control and Prevention. *Hepatitis Surveillance Report No. 42.* June 1978.)

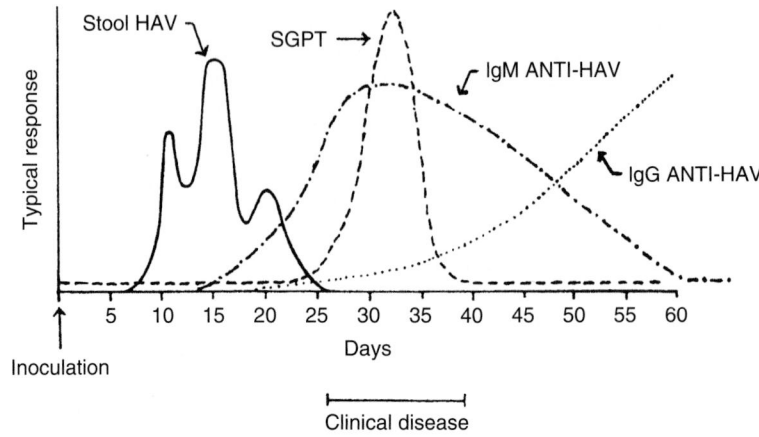

TABLE 30.2

Interpretation of Hepatitis Antibody Test Results

IgM Anti-HAV	IgG Anti-HAV	HBsAg	Anti-HBc (IgM)	Anti-HBc (IgG)	Interpretation
+	−	−	−	−	Acute hepatitis A
−	+	−	−	−	Prior hepatitis A infection • Person is immune to hepatitis A
−	−	+	−	−	Acute hepatitis B; early state or chronic carrier with hepatitis of another origin
−	−	+	+	+	Acute hepatitis B
−	−	+	−	+	Chronic carrier state
−	−	−	+	+	Recent hepatitis B
−	−	−	−	−	Non-A, non-B hepatitis, other viruses, or other causes

Anti-HAV, antibody to hepatitis A virus; anti-HBc, antibody to hepatitis B core antigen; HBsAg, hepatitis B surface antigen; Ig, immunoglobulin.

FIGURE 30.3 Course of hepatitis B infection. Pattern of symptoms and serological tests. ALT, alanine aminotransferase; Anti-HBc, hepatitis B core antibody; Anti-HBe, hepatitis B e antibody; Anti-HBs, hepatitis B surface antibody; HBeAg, hepatitis B e antigen; HBsAg, hepatitis B surface antigen; HBV, hepatitis B virus; Ig, immunoglobulin. (From Hollinger FB. Hepatitis markers: guide to test selection. *Diagnosis* 1986;Aug:58.)

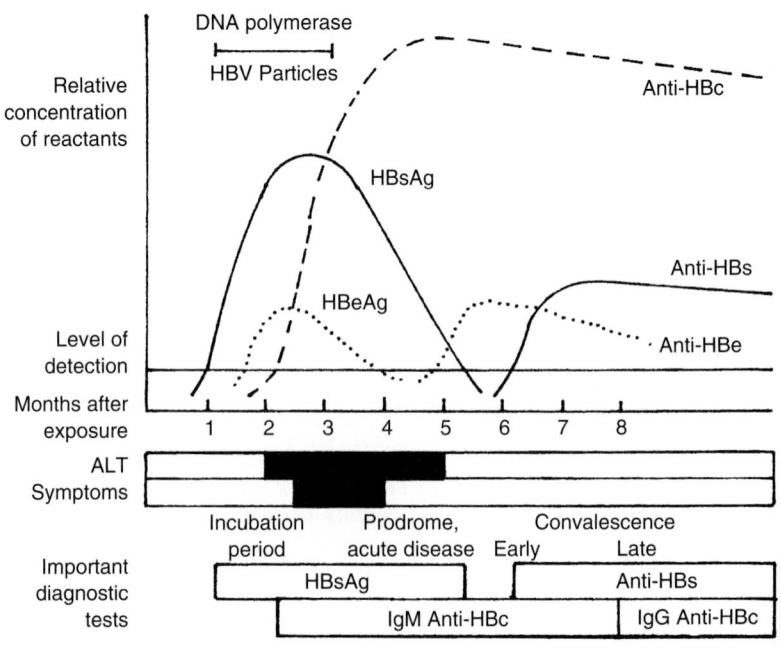

d. Anti-hepatitis B core antigen (anti-HBc): This antibody appears as HBsAg is falling and before anti-HBs appears. Anti-HBc can be fractionated into IgM and IgG components. This is extremely helpful in differentiating between acute and past infections. Anti-HBc (IgM) rises during clinical hepatitis, persists for 2 to 8 months, and then declines, whereas anti-HBc (IgG) rises at the same time to a much higher level and persists for a long time. The detection of anti-HBc (IgM) indicates an acute infection, whereas if only anti-HBc (IgG) is present, the illness must be of at least 6 months' duration. Anti-HBc may be the only test that is positive in some individuals during the window period when HBsAg has become negative and before anti-HBs has become positive.

e. Hepatitis e antigen (HBeAg): HBeAg is closely associated with the nucleocapsid of HBV. It is usually seen during the incubation phase and correlates with increased viral replication. Persistence of HBeAg beyond 10 to 12 weeks is probably indicative of progression to a chronic carrier state. Persistent presence of HBeAg indicates the following:
   • Presence of active viral replication.
   • Development of chronic active hepatitis.
   • Patient is highly infectious. The risk of infectivity in an individual who is positive for HBeAg and HBsAg may be as high as 30,000 times the risk in an individual with only HBsAg positivity. Approximately 10% to 15% of long-term carriers who are HBeAg positive convert each year to negative with the development of anti-HBe titers. These individuals are generally less contagious and have less active liver disease. Conversely, an individual can have reactivation of the disease, especially with immunosuppression, so that anti-HBe titers become negative and HBeAg becomes positive.

f. Anti-hepatitis B e antigen (anti-HBe): This antibody appears with the disappearance of HBeAg and suggests resolving or reduced viral replication. It usually indicates a lower state of infectivity.

3. Hepatitis C
   a. Serological tests for hepatitis C include antibody screening tests and confirmatory tests that measure HCV RNA.
   b. Enzyme immunoassay (EIA) detects antibodies to HCV (anti-HCV). The third-generation EIA test has enhanced sensitivity and a specificity >99% in immunocompetent patients. A negative EIA excludes chronic HCV in patients with normal immune systems. Antibodies against HCV may not be found in the acute illness phase, in patients on hemodialysis, and in those who are profoundly immunodeficient. Conversely, patients with autoimmune diseases may show false-positive results. The EIA test should be followed by a qualitative RNA test to confirm the diagnosis of HCV infection.
   c. Direct measurement of viral RNA in serum remains the "gold standard" in the diagnosis of HCV infection. Qualitative and quantitative tests are available. The qualitative test is used to confirm the diagnosis of hepatitis C infection whereas the quantitative test is used to monitor the effectiveness of therapy.

4. Delta hepatitis
   a. Delta antigen: Detectable in 20% of cases with acute delta infection.
   b. Delta antibody (anti-HDV): Both IgM and IgG antibodies can be measured.
   c. HDV RNA can be measured by polymerase chain reaction (PCR).
   d. Laboratory diagnosis in acute infection is based on serological tests for anti-HDV IgM or HDV RNA or delta virus antigen (HDVAg) in serum. In chronic infection, total (IgM + IgG) antibody is elevated with or without presence of HDVAg in the serum. High titers of IgG antibody suggest active replication. Detection of HDVAg by immunohistochemical analysis of liver tissue is considered the gold standard for diagnosis of persistent HDV infection.

COURSE

1. Viral hepatitis A: The clinical course is summarized in Figure 30.2.
   a. More than 75% of adults and adolescents are symptomatic, while in children <3 years of age it is asymptomatic >80% of the time.
   b. Ninety-five percent of patients have a 4- to 6-week course.
   c. Stool isolates for HAV are the first positive finding.
   d. As IgM antibodies and liver enzymes rise, clinical symptoms appear.
   e. As clinical symptoms disappear and IgM antibodies fall, IgG antibodies rise.
   f. Rarely, individuals can have a relapsing course lasting up to 1 year, which can cause confusion with other causes of chronic liver disease. Also, autoimmune hepatitis can be a rare sequel to hepatitis A.

2. Viral hepatitis B: The clinical course of a typical case is summarized in Figure 30.3.
   a. HBsAg and HBeAg titers rise 4 to 8 weeks after exposure and 4 to 8 weeks before clinical symptoms appear.
   b. Liver transaminases rise, and clinical symptoms appear.
   c. HBsAg may peak and fall in uncomplicated cases or remain positive in long-term carriers.
   d. Anti-HBc titers rise as HBsAg titers fall.
   e. Anti-HBs appears weeks to months after HBsAg disappears.
   f. A "window phase" may exist in which HBsAg is negative before anti-HBs appears. During this phase, anti-HBc IgM will be positive.
   g. Acute phase: After HBV infection the likelihood of developing acute hepatitis is age dependent. Perinatal HBV infection is almost always asymptomatic, whereas 5% to 15% of children 1 to 5 years of age and 33% to 50% of older children, adolescents, and adults develop acute hepatitis after HBV infection.
   h. Chronic HBV infection: Chronic HBV infection is defined as either the presence of HBsAg in serum for at least 6 months or the presence of HBsAg in a person who tests negative for anti-HBc IgM. The likelihood that a newly infected person will develop chronic HBV infection is also dependent on the age at the time of infection.
      • Ninety percent of adolescent and adult patients with hepatitis B recover without sequelae including chronic infections. However, >90% of infected infants, and 25% to 50% of younger children infected

between 1 and 5 years of age develop chronic infection.

- Hepatocellular carcinoma (HCC): Adults who have had chronic HBV infection since childhood develop HCC at a rate of 5% per decade. Up to 25% of infants and older children who acquire HBV infection eventually develop HBV-related HCC or cirrhosis.

3. Hepatitis C
   a. The clinical course varies from asymptomatic infection (up to 70%) to icteric hepatitis (25%) to fulminant liver failure (rare).
   b. Antibody test results remain negative for several weeks after onset of disease.
   c. Chronic disease develops in approximately 55% to 85% of patients, unrelated to mode of transmission or clinical presentation.
   d. Ten percent to 25% of patients with chronic disease develop cirrhosis.
   e. Once cirrhosis develops, HCC develops at a rate of 2% per year.

4. Delta hepatitis
   At least three clinical pictures can occur:
   a. Coinfection: Acute hepatitis caused by a combination of both HDV and HBV—often leading to a more severe form of acute hepatitis than that caused by HBV alone.
   b. Superinfection: Acute hepatitis with HDV acquisition in a long-term carrier of HBV. This may cause a second episode of clinical hepatitis and accelerate the course of the chronic liver disease, or cause overt disease in asymptomatic HBsAg carriers.
   c. Chronic infection: Chronic infection with both HDV and HBV, leading to a more rapid progression in liver disease and a higher mortality rate.

DIFFERENTIAL DIAGNOSIS

1. Drug-induced hepatitis
2. Alcoholic hepatitis
3. Toxic hepatitis
4. Nonalcoholic steatohepatitis (NASH)
5. Viral hepatitis
   a. Hepatitis A
   b. Hepatitis B (with or without delta coinfection or superinfection)
   c. Hepatitis C
   d. Hepatitis E

e. Herpes simplex
f. Cytomegalovirus infection
g. Epstein-Barr virus infection
h. Varicella
i. Enteroviral (Coxsackie B and ECHO virus) infections
j. Rubella
k. Adenoviral infection

DIAGNOSIS

1. What causes acute hepatitis?
   a. Clinical history may suggest toxin, drug, or risk factors for hepatitis A, B, or C.
   b. Order IgM anti-HAV, HBsAg, anti-HBc IgM, anti-HCV EIA, and a mononucleosis spot test. Table 30.2 provides an interpretation of results from the first three of these tests. If hepatitis C is suspected as a cause of acute hepatitis, a qualitative RNA test will be needed as there is high likelihood of a false-negative EIA in this scenario.
2. Acute hepatitis B: What is the infectivity of the patient? Table 30.3 summarizes the infectivity risk of HBV.

THERAPY

General Measures

1. Restriction of physical activity is not needed and teenagers with acute viral hepatitis can be as active as tolerated.
2. Diet: There is no evidence that any special diet affects the course of the disease.
3. Adolescents should avoid alcoholic beverages until transaminases return to normal.
4. Adolescents should avoid oral contraceptives, steroids, and all hepatotoxic drugs.
5. Severe disease is indicated by the following findings:
   a. Elevated prothrombin time
   b. Albumin <2.5 g/dL
   c. Evidence of ascites, edema, or encephalopathy
6. Most cases of hepatitis in adolescents can be managed at home. If hydration cannot be maintained in the outpatient because of nausea and vomiting, hospitalization should be considered. If the home environment is not supportive or the disease activity is particularly severe (see previous discussion), hospitalization may be indicated.

TABLE 30.3

Infectivity for Acute Hepatitis B Virus

HBsAg	Anti-HBc	HBeAg	Anti-HBe	Infectivity
+	+	+	−	Acute infection or chronic carrier; very infectious
+	+	−	−	Acute or recent infection; possible chronic carrier state; moderately infectious
+	+	−	+	Recent infection or chronic carrier state; good prognosis; probably low infectivity

Anti-HBc, antibody to hepatitis B core antigen; anti-HBe, antibody to hepatitis B e antigen; HBeAg, hepatitis B e antigen; HBsAg, hepatitis B surface antigen.

7. When the prothrombin time is elevated, it needs to be followed up closely and the patient may need to be hospitalized. If the prothrombin time is normal or once it returns to normal, the concentrations of serum bilirubin and transaminases should be monitored weekly during the acute illness, then every 2 to 3 weeks as the teen improves and enzymes fall. Monitoring can be stopped when liver enzymes return to normal.

Chronic Hepatitis

Treatment of chronic hepatitis is beyond the scope of this book. Therapy should be conducted by a specialist who is experienced in the treatment of chronic hepatitis.

1. Agents for treatment of chronic hepatitis B
   a. Interferon-α (IFN-α): Interferon treatment is successful in 33% of patients, with success being defined as loss of HBeAg. Interferon therapy has fairly severe side effects.
   b. Lamivudine: Lamivudine therapy can suppress HBV replication. It needs to be used long term and the incidence of viral resistance increases with increasing duration of therapy.
   c. Adefovir dipivoxil is a newer agent that is recommended for lamivudine-resistant HBV infection.
   d. Pegylated IFN α-2a is a recently approved medication for HBV treatment.
2. Agents for treatment of chronic hepatitis C
   Hepatitis C is treated with a combination of pegylated interferon and ribavirin. The dosages and length of treatment depend on the HCV genotype and response to treatment.

COMPLICATIONS

1. Acute hepatitis
   a. Pancreatitis
   b. Myocarditis
   c. Atypical pneumonia
   d. Aplastic anemia
   e. Transverse myelitis
   f. Glomerulonephritis
   g. Arthritis
2. Fulminant hepatitis
3. Chronic carrier state (HBsAg positive for longer than 6 months)
4. Chronic hepatitis
5. Cirrhosis and its complications including:
   a. Chronic liver failure
   b. Hepatocellular carcinoma

PREVENTION

Disinfection

1. Heat sterilization
   a. Boiling in water at 100°C for 10 minutes
   b. Steam autoclaving at 121°C and 15 lb/in³ for 15 minutes
   c. Dry heat of 160°C for 2 hours
2. Other presumed effective modalities
   a. Sodium hypochlorite 2.5% for 30 minutes
   b. Formalin 40% for 12 hours
   c. Glutaraldehyde 2% for 10 hours

Prophylaxis

Hepatitis A Good hand hygiene is central to the prevention of hepatitis A when working in environments with possible exposure (e.g., day-care centers). Effective public water sanitation and food hygiene are also important.

Hepatitis A Prophylaxis
1. Agents: Agents available for preexposure prophylaxis for hepatitis A include human immune serum globulin (HISG) and hepatitis A vaccine. Whenever postexposure prophylaxis is attempted, HISG should be used as there are limited data on the effectiveness of the vaccine alone under such conditions.
   a. HISG: HISG is a concentrated solution of antibodies prepared from pooled plasma. It is at least 85% effective in preventing hepatitis A when given intramuscularly within 2 weeks of exposure and also affords short-term protection against hepatitis A for international travelers. HISG should be given along with hepatitis A vaccine (at a separate anatomical site) for those with risk for further exposures to hepatitis A.
   b. Hepatitis A vaccine: Hepatitis A vaccines offer active immunization and therefore longer and more effective protection than that provided by HISG. Two vaccines are available, Havrix (SmithKline Beecham Biologicals, Research Triangle, NC) and Vaqta (Merck, Inc., White Station, NJ). Havrix is approved for children older than 2 years and Vaqta is approved for children older than 12 months. The vaccines are both inactivated and come in adult and pediatric formulations, with different dosages and administration schedules. Immunogenicity studies indicate that almost 100% of children, adolescents, and adults develop protective levels of antibody to HAV after completing the vaccine series. Estimates suggest that protective levels can last at least 20 years. The vaccine can be administered simultaneously with other vaccines and toxoids. However, if other vaccines are given simultaneously, they should be given at separate injection sites. In addition to the above vaccines Twinrix is also available, which includes both hepatitis A and hepatitis B vaccines in one. Using three doses of Twinrix produces similar seroprotection for hepatitis A and B as using vaccines for A and B separately. Recommended dosing is at 0, 1, and 6 months.
2. Recommended dosing schedules are as follows:
   HAVRIX

Age (yr)	Dose (ELISA units)	Volume (mL)	No. of Doses	Schedule (mo)
2–18	720	0.5	2	0, 6–12
>18	1,440	1.0	2	0, 6–12

VAQTA

Age (yr)	Dose (units)	Volume (mL)	No. of Doses	Schedule (mo)
1–18	25	0.5	2	0, 6–18
>18	50	1.0	2	0, 6–18

TABLE 30.4

Persons Needing Hepatitis A Vaccine or Immune Globulin

Hepatitis A vaccine

Children at least 2 years of age living in a state (Alaska, Arizona, California, Idaho, Nevada, New Mexico, Oklahoma, Oregon, South Dakota, Utah, or Washington) or a county with a high rate of infection ($\geq$20 cases per 100,000 population from 1987 through 1997)

Travelers at least 1 year of age to countries with high or intermediate rates of disease

Men who have sex with men

Users of illicit drugs, both injecting and noninjecting

Persons who have chronic liver disease

Persons who use clotting factor concentrates

Laboratory personnel who work with the hepatitis A virus

Military personnel

Day care attendees older than 1 yr

Immune globulin

Persons who will be traveling to countries with high or intermediate rates of disease within the next 2 wk

Children younger than 1 yr who will be traveling to countries with high rates of disease

People who need the vaccine but are allergic to it or do not wish to take it

For postexposure prophylaxis, within 14 d of exposure:

a. Persons who have been exposed to food that was handled by someone with acute hepatitis A, who had either poor hygiene or diarrhea

b. Persons exposed to a family member with acute hepatitis A

Adapted from Craig AS, Schaffner W. Prevention of hepatitis A with the hepatitis A vaccine. *N Engl J Med* 2004;350:476.

Persons are considered to be protected by 4 weeks after the initial dose of hepatitis A vaccine. For long-term protection, a second dose is needed 6 to 12 months later. For persons who will travel to high-risk areas <4 weeks after the initial vaccine dose, HISG should be administered simultaneously with the first dose of vaccine but at a different injection site. A single dose of HISG (0.02 mL/kg of body weight) provides effective protection against hepatitis A for up to 3 months.

Recommendations for who should be given HISG and hepatitis A vaccine are outlined in Table 30.4. Additional information about hepatitis A vaccine is available from the CDC's Hepatitis Branch, Division of Viral and Rickettsial Diseases, National Center for Infectious Diseases, telephone 1-404-371-5910 or 9+1-404-371-5460 or at the Web site www.cdc.gov/mmwr/preview/mmwrhtml/rr4812a1.htm.

Hepatitis B

Hepatitis B Preexposure Prophylaxis

1. Agents: Two types of products are available for prophylaxis against hepatitis B. Hepatitis B vaccines provide active immunization against hepatitis B infection and are recommended for both preexposure and postexposure prophylaxis. Hepatitis B immune globulin (HBIG) provides temporary, passive protection and is indicated only in certain postexposure settings.
   a. HBIG: HBIG is prepared from plasma preselected to contain a high titer of anti-HBs. The plasma used has been both screened for human immunodeficiency virus (HIV) antibodies and treated to inactivate and eliminate HIV from the final product.
   b. Hepatitis B vaccine: There are two recombinant hepatitis B vaccines licensed in the United States: Recombivax-HB (Merck, Inc.) and Engerix-B (Smith-Kline Beecham).
2. Indications: The strategy of preventing hepatitis B transmission in the United States by identifying and vaccinating persons who were in major risk groups for acquiring the infection did not succeed. So, starting in the late 1980s, a comprehensive strategy to eliminate transmission of HBV during infancy and childhood, as well as during adolescence and adulthood, was devised. This included the following steps:
   a. Prevention of perinatal HBV infection through routine HBsAg screening of all pregnant women and appropriate postexposure immunoprophylaxis of children born to HBsAg-positive women (1988; see "Considerations During Pregnancy" section)
   b. Routine immunization of infants (1992). Recommended schedules for immunoprophylaxis to prevent perinatal transmission of hepatitis B and for vaccination of newborns are listed in Tables 30.5, 30.6, and 30.7.
   c. Routine immunization of adolescents not previously immunized (1995).
   d. Routine immunization of all previously unvaccinated children 0 to 18 years of age (1999). Adolescents are at higher risk of infection because of their risky sexual behavior and drug use during this developmental period. Because adolescents and young adults are not easily identified with regard to high-risk behavior, universal immunization of all preadolescents, adolescents, and young adults—and in

TABLE 30.5

Recommended Doses of Currently Licensed Hepatitis B Vaccines[a]

Group	Recombivax-HB		Engerix-B	
	μg	mL	μg	mL
Infants of HBsAg-negative mothers, children, and adolescents (<20 yr)	5	0.5	10	0.5
Infants of HBsAg-positive mothers; (HBIG [0.5 mL] also recommended)	5	0.5	10	0.5
Adults (>20 yr)	10	1.0	20	1.0
Dialysis patients and other immunocompromised persons	40	1.0[b]	40	2.0[c]

HBsAg, hepatitis B surface antigen; HBIG, hepatitis B immune globulin.

[a]Both vaccines are routinely administered in a three-dose series. Engerix-B has also been licensed for a four-dose series administered at 0, 1, 2, and 12 mo.

[b]Special formulation.

[c]Two 1-mL doses administered at one site, in a four-dose schedule at 0, 1, 2, and 6 mo.

Adapted from American Academy of Pediatrics. Committee on Infectious Diseases. *Red Book 2003*. AAP, 2003:318.

particular those living in areas where high-risk behavior is prevalent—is recommended. The appropriate dose for age should be used (Table 30.5) and the schedule of vaccination at 0, 1, and 6 months is preferred.

e. Table 30.8 lists other groups who should be considered for HBV vaccination.

3. Immunogenicity and efficacy

a. When given in a three-dose series, recombinant vaccines induce protective anti-HBs antibodies in >90% of healthy adults and in >95% of infants, children, and adolescents from birth through 19 years of age. The deltoid muscle is the recommended site for the vaccination in adults and adolescents, because immunogenicity of the vaccine for adults is substantially lower when injections are given in the buttock. Hemodialysis patients and other immunocompromised persons in general develop a poorer response to the vaccines than healthy individuals do, and they require a larger dose. The

TABLE 30.6

Recommended Schedule of Hepatitis B Immunoprophylaxis to Prevent Perinatal Transmission of Hepatitis B Virus Infection[a]

Condition	Age of Infant
Infant born to mother known to be HBsAg positive[a]	
First vaccine dose	Birth (within 12 hr)
HBIG[b]	Birth (within 12 hr)
Second dose	1–2 mo
Third dose	6 mo[c]
Infant born to mother not screened for HBsAg[d]	
First vaccine dose	Birth (within 12 hr)
HBIG[b]	If mother is found to be HBsAg positive, administer dose to infant as soon as possible, not later than 1 wk after birth
Second dose	1–2 mo[e]
Third dose	6 mo[c]

HBsAg, hepatitis B surface antigen.

[a]See Table 30.3 for appropriate vaccine dose.

[b]Hepatitis B immune globulin (HBIG) 0.5 mL administered intramuscularly at a site different from that used for vaccine.

[c]If four-dose schedule (Engerix-B) is used, the third dose is administered at 2 mo of age and the fourth dose at 12–18 mo.

[d]First dose for infant of HBsAg-positive mother (see Table 30.3).

[e]Infants of women who are HBsAg negative can be vaccinated at 2 mo.

From Centers for Disease Control and Prevention. Hepatitis B virus: a comprehensive strategy for eliminating transmission in the United States through universal childhood vaccination. Recommendations of the immunization practices advisory committee (ACIP). *MMWR Morb Mortal Wkly Rep* 1991;40(RR-13):1.

TABLE 30.7

Recommended Schedules of Hepatitis B Vaccination for Infants Born to HBsAg-Negative Mothers[a]

Hepatitis B Vaccine	Age of Infant
Dose 1	Birth (before hospital discharge)
Dose 2	1–4 mo[b]
Dose 3	6–18 mo

HBsAg, Hepatitis B surface antigen.

[a]Hepatitis B vaccine can be administered simultaneously with diphtheria-tetanus-pertussis, *Haemophilus influenza* type conjugate, measles-mumps-rubella, and oral polio vaccines at the same visit.

[b]At least 1 mo should elapse between the two doses.

From Centers for Disease Control and Prevention. Recommended childhood immunization schedule—United States 1995. *MMWR Morb Mortal Wkly Rep* 1995;44(RR-5):1.

vaccine has been shown to be 80% to 95% effective in preventing infection or hepatitis among susceptible persons.

b. Although protection during the first years is excellent, there is evidence that by 7 years 30% to 50% of individuals develop low levels of antibodies, and 10% to 15% have undetectable antibodies. However, protection against viremic infection and clinical disease appears to persist. Persons younger than 20 years seem to have a higher peak response and longer persistence of detectable levels of antibodies.

4. Vaccine dosage and safety
   a. Adults and older children (Table 30.5): Primary vaccination includes three intramuscular doses of vaccine, with the second and third doses given 1 and 6 months after the first. Adults and adolescents should receive a full dose; children younger than 11 years should receive half of the full dose. For patients undergoing hemodialysis and for other immunosuppressed patients, higher doses or an increased number of doses is required. In addition, as noted previously, Twinrix (combined hepatitis A and B vaccine) is also available. Recommended dosing is at 0, 1, and 6 months.
   b. Data are not available on the safety of hepatitis vaccines for the developing fetus. However, because the vaccines contain only noninfectious HBsAg particles, there should be no risk to the fetus. Hence, pregnancy or lactation should not be considered a contraindication to the use of the vaccine.
   c. Side effects—17% of individuals experience soreness at the site. Fifteen percent experience mild systemic symptoms including fever, headache, fatigue, and nausea.

5. Prevaccination serological screening: Screening for past infection is probably only cost-effective in groups with a prior high risk of infection (>20%), and only if the cost of testing is not prohibitive. For groups with a low expected prevalence, such as health professionals in their training years, screening is not cost-effective. For routine screening, either anti-HBc or anti-HBs should be used. Anti-HBs screening identifies those previously infected, except carriers. Anti-HBc screening identifies all previously infected persons, both carriers and noncarriers. Vaccination without prevaccination testing is the most cost-effective approach in preadolescents and adolescents.

6. Postvaccination serology and revaccination
   a. Testing for immunity is not recommended routinely but is advised for individuals who are expected to have a suboptimal response, such as those who received the vaccine in the buttock, those older than 50 years, those with known HIV infection, and individuals whose subsequent management depends on knowing their immune status, such as patients and staff of dialysis units. When necessary, the testing should be done between 1 and 6 months after completion of the vaccine series.

TABLE 30.8

Persons Needing Hepatitis B Vaccine

All newborns, at birth
All children, aged 0–18 yr, who have not been vaccinated
Heterosexuals with >1 partner in the previous 6 mo or with any sexually transmitted infection
Clients and staff of institutions for the developmentally disabled
Homosexual and bisexual men
Injecting drug users
Persons with jobs involving contact with human blood
Hemodialysis patients
Recipients of clotting factor concentrates
Household and sexual contacts of carriers
Adoptees from countries of high hepatitis B endemicity
Inmates of long-term correctional facilities
International travelers who plan to stay in an endemic area for >6 mo

b. Testing of infants born to HBsAg-positive mothers who received immunoprophylaxis should be performed 3 to 9 months after completion of the vaccination series.

c. Revaccination in nonresponders produces adequate antibody in 15% to 25% after one additional dose and in 30% to 50% after three additional doses, when the primary vaccination was given in the deltoid muscle. If the primary vaccine was given in the buttock, revaccination in the arm induces adequate antibodies in >75%. Revaccination should be considered for nonresponders who received the vaccine in the deltoid muscle, and it is recommended for nonresponders who received the primary vaccine in the buttock.

Hepatitis B Postexposure Prophylaxis

Prophylactic treatment to prevent hepatitis B infection after exposure should be considered in the following situations:

1. Perinatal exposure of an infant born to an HBsAg-positive mother: A regimen that combines one dose of HBIG at birth with the hepatitis B vaccine series started soon after birth is 85% to 95% effective. (See "Considerations during Pregnancy" section.)

2. Persons with acute exposure to blood: Decision on prophylaxis depends on whether the source of the blood is available, the hepatitis status of the exposed person, and the status of the source. After such an exposure, a blood sample should be obtained from the person who was the source of the exposure and tested for HBsAg. For greatest effectiveness, passive prophylaxis with HBIG, when indicated, should be given as soon as possible after exposure (the value beyond 7 days after exposure is unclear). A summary of recommendations is given in Table 30.9. Updated U.S. Public Health Service Guidelines for the Management of Occupational Exposures to HBV, HCV, and HIV and Recommendations for Postexposure Prophylaxis can also be obtained at: http://www.cdc.gov/mmwr/PDF/rr/rr5011.pdf.

3. Sexual contacts of HBsAg-positive persons: These individuals are at increased risk of infection, and HBIG is 75% effective in preventing such infections. Screening of sexual partners for hepatitis antibodies (anti-HBc or anti-HBs) before treatment is recommended but should not delay treatment beyond 14 days after last exposure.

TABLE 30.9

Recommendations for Hepatitis B Prophylaxis after Percutaneous Exposure to Blood That Contains (or Might Contain) HBsAg

Exposed Person	Treatment When Source Is		
	HBsAg-Positive	HBsAg-Negative	Unknown or Not Tested
Unimmunized	Administer HBIG[a] 1 dose and initiate hepatitis B vaccine	Initiate hepatitis B vaccine series	Initiate hepatitis B vaccine series
Previously immunized			
Known responder	No treatment	No treatment	No treatment
Known nonresponder	HBIG 2 doses or HBIG 1 dose and initiate immunization[b]	No treatment	If known high-risk source, treat as if source were HBsAg positive
Response unknown	Test exposed person for anti-HBs[c] 1. If adequate, HBIG 1 dose and vaccine booster dose[d] 2. If adequate, no treatment	No treatment	Test exposed person for anti-HBs[c] 1. If inadequate, vaccine booster dose[a] 2. If adequate, no treatment

HBsAg, hepatitis B surface antigen; HBIG, hepatitis B immune globulin; anti-HBs, antibody to HBsAg.

[a]Dose of HBIG, 0.06 mL/kg intramuscularly.

[b]Persons known NOT to have responded to a three-dose vaccine series and to reimmunization with three additional doses should be given two doses of HBIG (0.06 mL/kg), one dose as soon as possible after exposure and the second 1 mo later.

[c]Adequate anti-HBs is ≥10 mIU/mL.

[d]Evaluate for antibody response after the vaccine booster dose. For persons who received HBIG, anti-HBs testing should be done when passively acquired antibody from HBIG is no longer detectable (e.g., 4–6 mo); if they did not receive HBIG, anti-HBs testing should be done 1–2 mo after the vaccine booster dose. If anti-HBs is inadequate after the vaccine booster dose, two additional doses should be administered to complete a three-dose reimmunization series.

Modified from the Centers for Disease Control and Prevention. Immunization of health care workers: recommendations of the Advisory Committee on Immunization Practices (ACIP) and the Hospital Infection Control Committee (HICPAC). *MMWR Morb Mortal Wkly Rep* 1997;46(RR-18):22.

Treatment consists of HBIG (0.06 mL/kg), followed by the hepatitis vaccine series, which may be started at the same time if exposure continues.

4. Household contacts of persons with acute infection: Prophylaxis is not indicated unless there is exposure to blood of the index case (e.g., sharing of toothbrushes or razors). If indicated, treatment is with both HBIG and vaccine. If the index patient becomes a carrier, all household contacts should receive hepatitis B vaccine. Treatment with HBIG and hepatitis B vaccine is also indicated for infants younger than 12 months whose primary caregivers have an acute hepatitis B infection.

Delta Hepatitis Because HDV is dependent on HBV for replication, prevention of HBV infection suffices to prevent delta hepatitis. Exposures of individuals with known positivity for both HDV and HBV should be treated exactly as such exposures to HBV alone.

Hepatitis C Immune globulin is not recommended for postexposure prophylaxis of hepatitis C.

Hygiene

Recommended guidelines include the following:

1. No sharing of razors, toothbrushes, food utensils, or towels.
2. Careful personal hygiene; hand washing after patient contact.
3. Careful handling of secretions of the hepatitis B patient, including saliva, blood, and urine, with needle precautions.
4. Hepatitis A: Isolate the patient until jaundice peaks; use stool precautions.

CONSIDERATIONS DURING PREGNANCY

1. Hepatitis A
   a. There is no maternal–fetal transmission.
   b. Transmission can occur during delivery.
   c. Positive IgM antibodies in the infant indicate acute infection.
2. Hepatitis B
   a. Transmission of HBV from mother to infant during the perinatal period is one of the most efficient modes of hepatitis B infection. This often leads to severe long-term sequelae.
   b. The transmission rate to infants from mothers who are positive for both HBsAg and HBeAg is 70% to 90%, and 85% to 90% of infected infants become chronic hepatitis B carriers.
   c. Infants born to mothers who are HBsAg positive and HBeAg negative have 10% risk of acquiring perinatal infection.
   d. Prenatal screening of all pregnant women identifies those who are HBsAg positive and allows treatment of their newborns with HBIG and hepatitis B vaccine, which prevents development of the chronic carrier state in 90% to 95% of these infants. The Advisory Committee on Immunization Practices (Centers for Disease Control and Prevention, 1991 and CDC, 2005) advises the following:

- All pregnant women should be routinely tested for HBsAg during the first prenatal visit in each pregnancy. If the mother has a particularly high-risk behavior, an additional HBsAg test can be ordered later in the pregnancy. No other serological tests are necessary for maternal screening.
- If the woman was not screened prenatally, HBsAg testing should be done at the time of admission for delivery. If the mother is identified as HBsAg positive 1 month or more after giving birth, the infant should be tested for HBsAg. If the infant is HBsAg negative, he/she should be given HBIG and hepatitis B vaccine.
- When HBsAg testing of pregnant women is not feasible (i.e., in remote areas without access to a laboratory), all infants should receive hepatitis B vaccine <12 hours of birth and should complete the hepatitis B vaccine series according to a recommended schedule for infants born to HBsAg-positive mothers.
- Infants born to HBsAg-positive mothers should receive HBIG (0.5 mL) intramuscularly once they are physiologically stable, preferably within 12 hours of birth. Hepatitis B vaccine should be administered intramuscularly at the appropriate infant dose. The first dose should be given concurrently with HBIG but at a different site. Subsequent doses should be given as recommended for the specific vaccine (Tables 30.5 and 30.6). Testing of infants for HBsAg and anti-HBs is recommended when they are 9 to 15 months of age to monitor the success or failure of therapy. If HBsAg is not detectable and anti-HBs is present, the child can be considered protected. HBIG and hepatitis B vaccination do not interfere with routine childhood vaccinations.
- Obstetric and pediatric staff should be notified directly about HBsAg-positive mothers so that the neonates can receive therapy without delay.
- Breastfeeding can be allowed even before the first dose of HBIG and can continue following immunizations. The mother should ensure that her nipples do not get traumatized.
- Household members and sexual partners of HBV carriers should be tested, and, if susceptible, should receive hepatitis B vaccine.

3. Hepatitis C
   a. An anti-HCV EIA should be performed at the first prenatal visit for pregnant women at high risk for exposure. HCV RNA testing should be performed if anti-HCV is positive. Women at high risk include those with a history of injection drug use, repeated exposure to blood products, prior blood transfusion, or organ transplantations.
   b. The rate of mother-to-infant transmission is 4% to 7% per pregnancy in women with HCV viremia. Coinfection with HIV increases the rate of transmission 4- to 5-fold. The actual time and mode of transmission are not known.
   c. Breastfeeding poses no important risk of HCV transmission if nipples are not traumatized and maternal hepatitis C is quiescent.
   d. Infants of mothers with hepatitis C should be tested for HCV RNA on two occasions, between the ages of 2 and 6 months and again at 18 to 24 months, along with serum anti-HCV.

WEB SITES

For Teenagers and Parents

http://www.cdc.gov/ncidod/diseases/hepatitis/. CDC hepatitis resource page.

http://www.liverfoundation.org. Numerous informational pieces from American Liver Foundation.

http://www.niddk.nih.gov/health/digest/pubs/hep/hepa/hepa.htm. What I Need to Know About Hepatitis A from National Institute of Diabetes and Digestive and Kidney Disease.

http://www.hepnet.com. Canadian hepatitis information network.

For Teens

http://www.nfid.org/factsheets/hbagadol.html. Hepatitis B: What Every Teen Should Know—National Foundation for Infectious Diseases.

http://www.kidshealth.org/teen/infections/stds/hepatitis.html. How Hepatitis Can Hurt You—The Nemours Foundation.

For Health Professionals

http://www.nlm.nih.gov/medlineplus/. Thirty five sites and links to MedLine, National Library of Medicine.

http://www.cdc.gov/ncidod/diseases/hepatitis/. CDC hepatitis resource page.

REFERENCES AND ADDITIONAL READINGS

Atkins M, Nolan M. Sexual transmission of hepatitis B. *Curr Opin Infect Dis* 2005;18:67.

Becherer PR. Viral hepatitis: what have we learned about risk factors and transmission? *Postgrad Med* 1995;98:65.

Belfeler AS, Di Besceglie AM. Hepatitis B. *Infect Dis Clin North Am* 2000;14:617.

Broderick A, Jonas MM. Management of hepatitis B in children. *Clin Liver Dis* 2004;8:387.

Centers for Disease Control and Prevention. Hepatitis B virus: a comprehensive strategy for eliminating transmission in the United States through universal childhood vaccination. Recommendations of the immunization practices advisory committee (ACIP). *MMWR Morb Mortal Wkly Rep* 1991;40(RR-13):1.

Centers for Disease Control and Prevention. Licensure of inactivated hepatitis A vaccine and recommendations for use among international travelers. *MMWR Morb Mortal Wkly Rep* 1995;44:559.

Centers for Disease Control and Prevention. Update: recommendations to prevent hepatitis B virus transmission—United States. *JAMA* 1995;274:603.

Centers for Disease Control and Prevention. Recommendations for prevention and control of hepatitis C virus infection and HCV-related chronic disease. *MMWR Morb Mortal Wkly Rep* 1998;47(RR-19):1.

Centers for Disease Control and Prevention. Prevention of hepatitis A through active or passive immunization. *MMWR Morb Mortal Wkly Rep* 1999;48(RR-12):1.

Centers for Disease Control and Prevention. Notice to readers: alternate two-dose hepatitis B vaccination schedule for adolescents aged 11–15 Years. *MMWR Morb Mortal Wkly Rep* 2000;49:261.

Centers for Disease Control and Prevention. Acute hepatitis B among children and adolescents—United States, 1990–2002. *MMWR Morb Mortal Wkly Rep* 2004;53:1015.

Centers for Disease Control and Prevention: A Comprehensive Immunization Strategy to Eliminate Transmission of Hepatitis B Virus Infection in the United States. *MMWR Morb Mortal Wkly Rep* 2005;54:1.

Clemens R, Safary A, Hepburn A, et al. Clinical experience with an inactivated hepatitis A vaccine. *J Infect Dis* 1995;171(Suppl 1):S44.

Craig AS, Schaffner W. Prevention of hepatitis A with the hepatitis A vaccine. *N Engl J Med* 2004;350:476.

Cuthbert JA. Hepatitis A: old and new. *Clin Microbiol Rev* 2001;14:38.

Dienstag JL, Schiff ER, Wright TL, et al. Lamivudine as initial treatment for chronic hepatitis B in the United States. *N Engl J Med* 1999;341:1256.

Fung SK, Lok AS. Update on viral hepatitis in 2004. *Curr Opin Gastroenterol* 2005;21:300.

Ganiats TG. Hepatitis B immunization for adolescents. *West J Med* 1995;163:70.

Gershon AA. Present and future challenges of immunizations on the health of our patients. *Pediatr Infect Dis J* 1995;14:445.

Gibb DM, Goodall RL, Dunn DT, et al. Mother-to-child transmission of hepatitis C virus: evidence for preventable prepartum transmission. *Lancet* 2000;356:904.

Goldberg D, Anderson E. Hepatitis C: who is at risk and how do we identify them? *J Viral Hepat* 2004;11(Suppl 1):12.

Heathcote J, Main J. Treatment of hepatitis C. *J Viral Hepat* 2005;12:223.

Hess G. Virological and serological aspects of hepatitis B and the delta agent. *Gut* 1993;34:51.

Hill L, Henry B, Schweikert S. Prevention Practice Committee, American College of Preventive Medicine. Screening for chronic hepatitis C: American College of Preventive Medicine practice policy statement. *Am J Prev Med* 2005;28:327.

Karayiannis P, Main J, Thomas HC. Hepatitis vaccines. *Br Med Bull* 2004;70:29.

Kemmer NM, Miskovsky EP. Hepatitis A. *Infect Dis Clin North Am* 2000;14:605.

Kew M, Francois G, Lavanchy D, et al. Prevention of hepatitis C virus infection. *J Viral Hepat* 2004;11:198.

Kwan-Gett TS, Whitaker RC, Kempter KJ. A cost-effectiveness analysis of prevaccination testing for hepatitis B in adolescents and preadolescents. *Arch Pediatr Adolesc Med* 1994;148:915.

Lavanchy D. Hepatitis B virus epidemiology, disease burden, treatment, and current and emerging prevention and control measures. *J Viral Hepat* 2004;11:97.

Leach CT. Hepatitis A in the United States. *Pediatr Infect Dis J* 2004;23:551.

Mondelli MU, Cerino A, Cividini A. Acute hepatitis C: diagnosis and management. *J Hepatol* 2005;42(Suppl 1):S108.

Niro GA, Rosina F, Rizzetto M. Treatment of hepatitis D. *J Viral Hepat* 2005;12:2.

Pearlman BL. Hepatitis C infection: a clinical review. *South Med J* 2004;97:364.

Petermann S, Ernest JM. Intrapartum hepatitis B screening. *Am J Obstet Gynecol* 1995;173:369.

Schwarz KB, Balistreri W. Viral hepatitis. *J Pediatr Gastroenterol Nutr* 2002;35(Suppl 1):S29.

Shepard CW, Finelli L, Fiore AE, et al. Epidemiology of hepatitis B and hepatitis B virus infection in United States children. *Pediatr Infect Dis J* 2005;24:755.

Shukla NB, Poles MA. Hepatitis B virus infection: co-infection with hepatitis C virus, hepatitis D virus, and human immunodeficiency virus. *Clin Liver Dis* 2004;8:445.

Thomson EC, Main J. Advances in hepatitis B and C. *Curr Opin Infect Dis* 2004;17:449.

Tovo PA, Lazier L, Versace A. Hepatitis B virus and hepatitis C virus infections in children. *Curr Opin Infect Dis* 2005;18:261.

Trepo C, Zoulim F, Alonso C, et al. Diagnostic markers of viral hepatitis B and C. *Gut* 1993;34:S20.

Wagner G, Lavanchy D, Darioli R, et al. Simultaneous active and passive immunization against hepatitis A studied in a population of travelers. *Vaccine* 1993;11:1027.

Weinstock HS, Bolan G, Moran JS, et al. Routine hepatitis B vaccination in a clinic for sexually transmitted diseases. *Am J Public Health* 1995;85:846.

CHAPTER 31

Human Immunodeficiency Virus Infections and Acquired Immunodeficiency Syndrome

Marvin E. Belzer, Miguel Martinez, and Lawrence S. Neinstein

Acquired immunodeficiency syndrome (AIDS) is one of the largest pandemics to hit modern society and the focal point of intense national and international debate. The last decade has seen a dramatic reduction in the mortality due to AIDS in developed countries. When taken correctly, combinations of antiretroviral medications called *highly active antiretroviral therapy* (HAART) enable most infected patients to have long healthy lives. The greatest challenges for care providers of adolescents with human immunodeficiency virus (HIV) infection involve identifying infected youth, engaging them in care, and assisting them with long-term adherence to these medications. Unfortunately, in only a fraction of the estimated 20,000 annual new cases of HIV infection in 13- to 25-year olds in the United States does the patient have access to care while still an adolescent or young adult. Internationally, the impact on youth is even higher, with an estimated 50% of new HIV infections occurring in youth. Developing countries have very limited access to the life-saving medications now routinely available in the United States.

Special issues are important to consider in relation to the adolescent population and infection with HIV, including a host of legal and ethical dilemmas regarding testing, disclosure of information, and consent for treatment in research protocols. For HIV-infected adolescents there is also the problem of availability of age-appropriate services.

Adolescents are in danger of contracting HIV because of their risky sexual behaviors, drug use, or both. Because most adolescents are not yet infected but may be involved in high-risk behaviors, they are a high-priority target group for HIV preventive measures.

Information about HIV infection is developing rapidly. Several thousand articles are published yearly with information that often becomes quickly outdated. The treatment of HIV has become so complex that recommendations have been made that all HIV-infected persons should be treated by physicians with expertise in HIV medications, their side effects and interactions, as well the psychosocial interventions required to maintain adherence. This chapter includes an overview of HIV and AIDS, with a focus on considerations that are important in the adolescent. It is essential for the practicing physician to keep up to date through the literature or continuing medical education on the many aspects of HIV infection, including HIV prevention, psychosocial issues, legal issues, diagnosis, evaluation, and treatment.

ETIOLOGY, PATHOGENESIS, AND NATURAL HISTORY

The causative agent of AIDS is HIV, a single-stranded RNA retrovirus. This virus was isolated at the Pasteur Institute in Paris in 1983. HIV-1 is the cause of most cases of AIDS in the world. HIV-2, another retrovirus related to HIV-1, is found primarily in Central Africa. HIV-2 generally has a much slower progression (20 years versus 5–10 years with HIV-1) but a similar spectrum of disease.

HIV-1 infects and leads to the destruction of CD4$^+$ T lymphocytes. A flu-like illness occurs in most patients 2 to 6 weeks after infection. The illness typically lasts 1 to 2 weeks and typically causes fever, fatigue, myalgias, lymphadenopathy, and sore throat (Table 31.1). The phase of illness after the acute infection was once characterized as one of latency, but it is now clear that viral production is steady at an estimated 10 billion virions daily. T-cell production and destruction remain precariously balanced. A slow but steady depletion of CD4$^+$ T cells occurs in all but a small percentage of patients, who are referred to as long-term nonprogressors. Most patients develop AIDS (severe immune deficiency), without treatment, over a period of 8 to 10 years. Approximately 10% of individuals will rapidly progress to an AIDS diagnosis within 4 years. Both host factors like human leukocyte antigen (HLA) type and other genetic factors and host immune response to HIV-1 have been correlated with disease progression. Viral factors like HIV-fitness and ability to be "syncytium-inducing" have also been associated with disease progression. Numerous studies indicate that HAART can suppress the viral load to undetectable levels in most patients. Viral suppression is associated with a steady immune reconstitution in most patients. Even patients with severe depletion of their immune systems can often return to excellent health after months to years of successful treatment. Preliminary studies of adolescents indicate that their "thymic reserve" may allow for even better immune restoration than in adults.

TABLE 31.1

Characteristics of 25 Individuals with Acute Primary Human Immunodeficiency Virus Infection at the Johns Hopkins Hospital, 1993–1995[a]

Characteristic	No. of Individuals (%)
Sex	
Male	15 (60)
Female	10 (40)
Risk exposure	
Injection drug use	11 (44)
Heterosexual	9 (36)
Homosexual/bisexual	3 (12)
Undetermined	2 (8)
Symptoms	
Fever	24 (96)
Fatigue	23 (92)
Myalgia or arthralgia	18 (72)
Adenopathy	16 (64)
Pharyngitis	16 (64)
Diarrhea	12 (48)
Headache	11 (44)
Rash	10 (40)
Weight loss	9 (36)
Nausea or vomiting	8 (32)
Mucocutaneous ulcerations	5 (20)
Thrush	3 (12)

[a]All patients were diagnosed by a p24 antigen level >30 pg/mL. All had a negative or indeterminate Western blot test with later evidence of seroconversion.

From Quinn TC. Acute primary HIV infection. *JAMA* 1997;278:58, with permission.

Unfortunately, even when the best therapy is strictly adhered to for several years, patients have been unable to eliminate HIV from their body (i.e., a cure is not currently possible). Reservoirs of latent virus are effectively hidden from the effects of the potent antiretrovirals. Patients, who go off HAART after several years of treatment, usually develop viremia within a couple weeks. Current research is focused on whether some type of immune modulation with medication or vaccines can nullify the inevitable rebound in HIV viremia.

Although the natural history of HIV has changed from a lethal illness to that of a chronic disease, it is unclear whether lifelong viral suppression is feasible. Many adolescents are unable to adhere to or tolerate complex medication regimens. Some patients develop resistance to medications due to nonadherence, and some patients are being infected with HIV that has extensive resistance to many medications (studies in recent seroconverters indicate that many regions in the United States have 10% to 15% with baseline resistance to at least one antiretroviral medication). Patients with multiple drug resistance can eventually have immune depletion and succumb to the opportunistic infections and neoplasms that were so prevalent before the advent of HAART.

EPIDEMIOLOGY

1. Number of cases
   a. Total cases: As of December 2004, 944,306 cases of AIDS have been reported to the Centers for Disease Control and Prevention (CDC). Also, by the end of 2003, an estimated 1,039,000 to 1,185,000 persons in the United States were living with HIV/AIDS.
   b. Annual cases: The number of AIDS cases reported annually has increased each year for teens aged 13 to 19 between 1998 and 2003 but dropped in 2004 (Fig. 31.1). For those aged 20 to 24 there has been an increase every year from 2000 to 2004 (Fig. 31.2). In 2004, for all age-groups there were 38,730 cases of HIV/AIDS diagnosed in the 33 states and Guam and U.S. Virgin Islands (with long-term, confidential name-based HIV reported). CDC estimates that 40,000 persons become infected with HIV each year. The estimated rate of AIDS cases in the United States in 2004 was 14.1 per 100,000.
2. Age: In all years through 2004, an estimated 40,049 youth aged 13 to 24 or 4% of the total number of cases received an AIDS diagnosis. With a median incubation period of 7 to 10 years from HIV infection to AIDS, most of the cases in young adults aged 25 to 29 (11.4%) were also acquired as adolescents. In 2004, approximately 1% of cases of AIDS were in ages 13 to 19 and 4.2% in those aged 20 to 24. From 2001 through 2004, the estimated number of HIV/AIDS cases decreased in children younger than 13 years, and in 30 to 34, 13 to 14, 30 to 34, 35 to 39, 40 to 44, and 45 to 49 age-groups. Cases increased in the age-groups 15 to 19, 20 to 24, and in those older than 50. Cases remained stable in those young adults aged 25 to 29.
3. Ethnicity: African-Americans are dramatically overrepresented, making up 70% of all cases of HIV/AIDS in youth aged 13 to 19 years (Fig. 31.3) and 50% of adolescents and adults diagnosed during 2004.
4. Gender: Figures 31.4 and 31.5 show that numbers of reported HIV and AIDS cases are higher in males than females but that the difference increases with age. For all adults 25 and older, 74% were males with diagnosed HIV/AIDS in 2004.
5. Transmission: Figure 31.6 shows the common routes of transmission for males and females diagnosed with HIV/AIDS from 2001 to 2004. Although youth with Hemophilia made up 25% of 13- to 19-year olds diagnosed with AIDS in the past, these cases are no longer occurring. Most new cases in males are in men-who-have-sex-with men and/or injection drug users. Figure 31.7 illustrates how heterosexual contact is the main reported mode of transmission in female youth.

Human Immunodeficiency Virus Staging

In 1993, the Centers for Disease Control and Prevention (1992) expanded their AIDS definition criteria and changed their staging system (Table 31.2). The system uses the lowest-ever CD4$^+$ T-cell count (rows 1 through 3) in combination with clinical staging (columns A through C in Table 31.2) based on symptoms. The problem with this current system is that it reflects the most advanced stage a

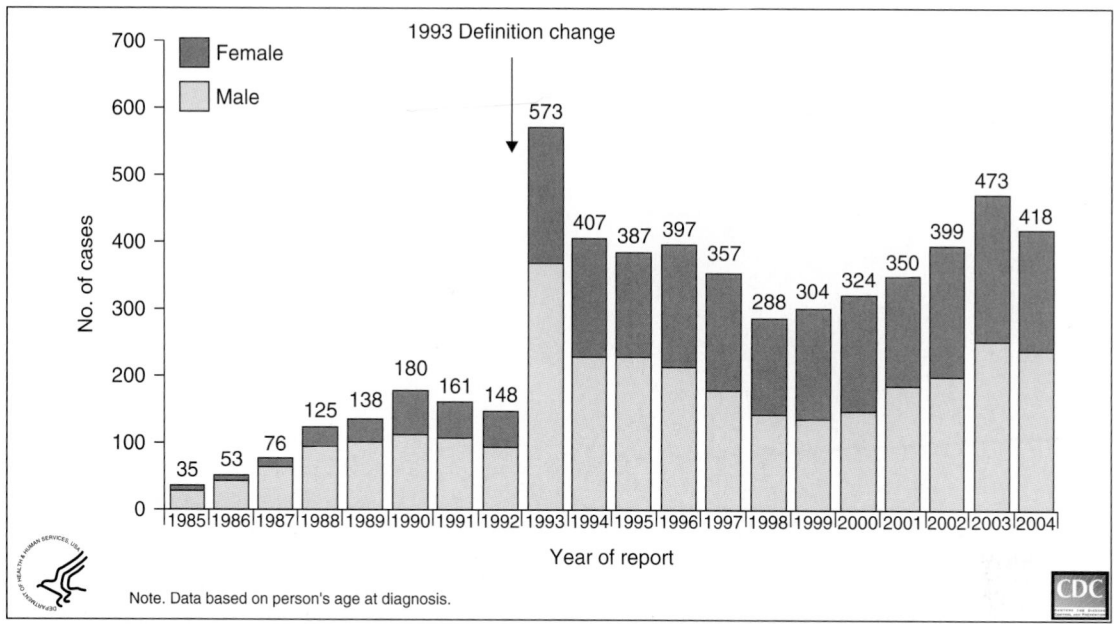

FIGURE 31.1 Reported AIDS cases among adolescents 13 to 19 years of age, by sex, 1985 to 2004—United States (N = 5,593). (From Centers for Disease Control and Prevention. *Adolescents and HIV*. Slide set at http://www.cdc.gov/hiv/topics/surveillance/resources/ slides/adolescents/index.htm. Accessed 2006.)

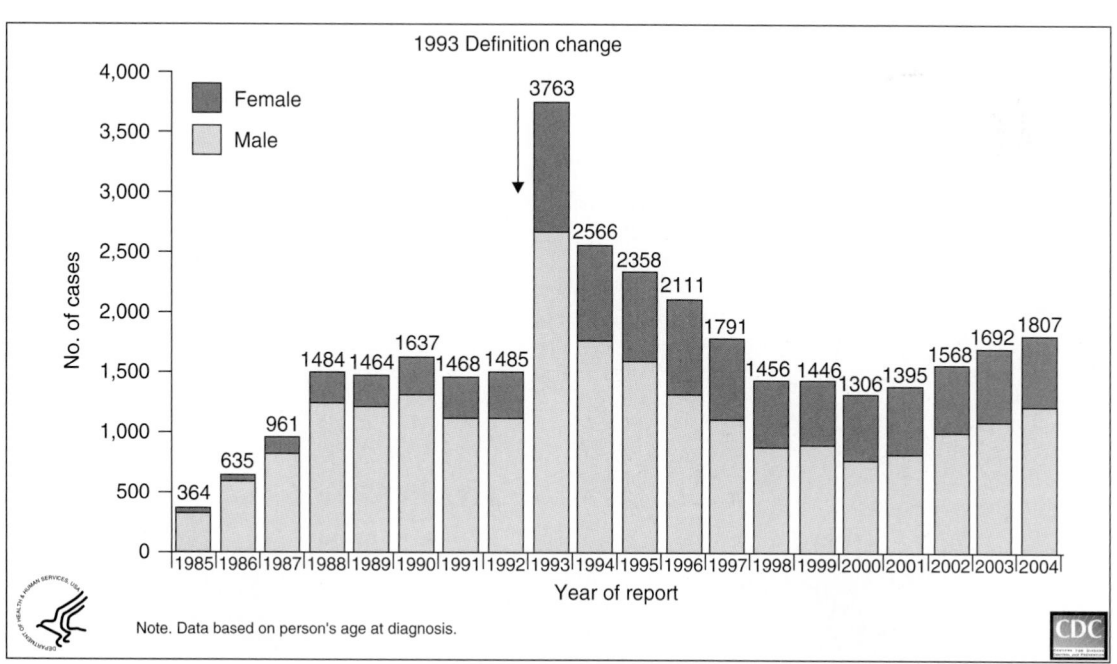

FIGURE 31.2 Reported AIDS cases among young adults 20 to 24 years of age, by sex, 1985 to 2004—United States (N = 32,757). (From Centers for Disease Control and Prevention. *Adolescents and HIV*. Slide set at http://www.cdc.gov/hiv/topics/surveillance/resources/ slides/adolescents/index.htm. Accessed 2006.)

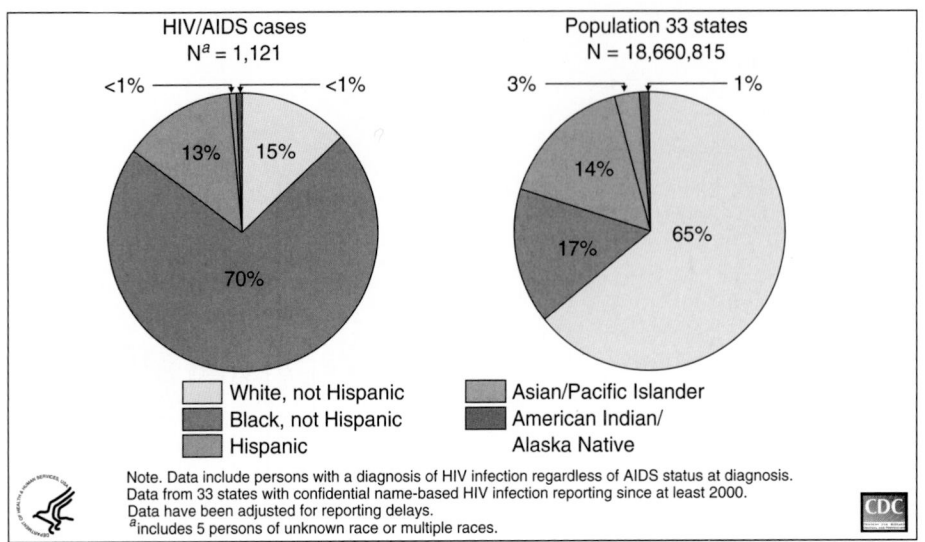

FIGURE 31.3 Proportion of HIV/AIDS cases and population among adolescents 13 to 19 years of age by race/ethnicity, diagnosed in 2004—33 states. (From Centers for Disease Control and Prevention. *Adolescents and HIV*. Slide set at http://www.cdc.gov/hiv/topics/surveillance/resources/slides/adolescents/index.htm. Accessed 2006.)

patient has reached but not the patient's current condition. A patient who once had advanced AIDS with life-threatening infections but who then successfully starts HAART and is asymptomatic with a CD4$^+$ T-cell count higher than 500/mL will still be staged as a 3C (the mostly severely ill stage).

Transmission

HIV can be transmitted only by the exchange of body fluids. Blood, semen, vaginal secretions, and breast milk are the only fluids documented to be associated with HIV infection. Although HIV is found in saliva, tears, urine, and sweat, no case has been documented that implicates these fluids as agents of infection.

HIV is easily transmitted by the sharing of needles. The Centers for Disease Control and Prevention (2005) has provided guidelines for reducing the spread of HIV and hepatitis through the sharing of needles (http://www.cdc.gov/ncidod/dhqp/bp_hiv.html).

- The best way for you to prevent HIV, hepatitis B virus (HBV), and hepatitis C virus (HCV) transmission is to NOT inject drugs.
- Starting substance abuse treatment can help you reduce or stop injecting. This will lower your chances of infection.
- Get vaccinated against hepatitis A and hepatitis B. You can prevent these kinds of viral hepatitis if you get vaccinated.

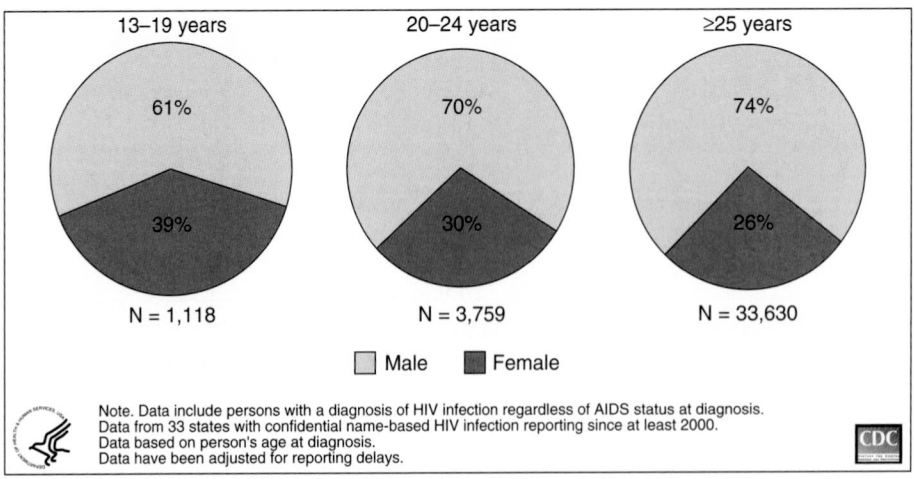

FIGURE 31.4 Proportion of HIV/AIDS cases among adults and adolescents by sex and age-group diagnosed in 2004—33 states. (From Centers for Disease Control and Prevention. *Adolescents and HIV*. Slide set at http://www.cdc.gov/hiv/topics/surveillance/resources/slides/adolescents/index.htm. Accessed 2006.)

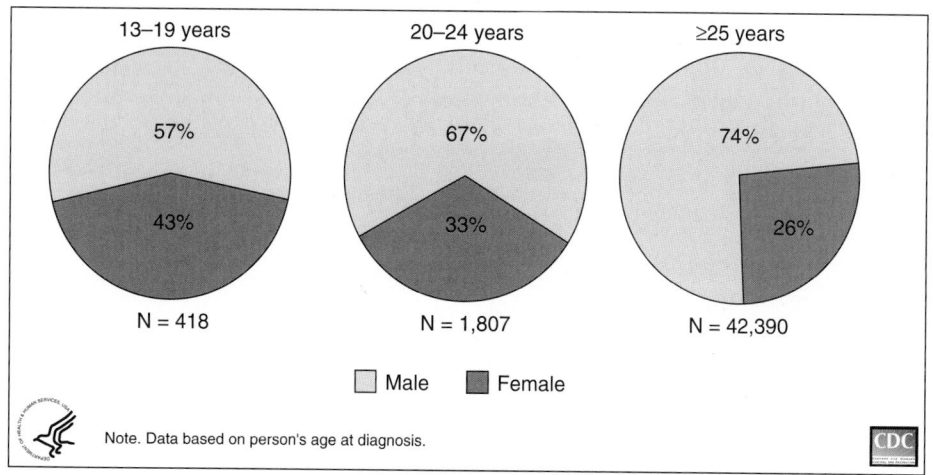

FIGURE 31.5 Proportion of AIDS cases among adults and adolescents by sex and age-group, reported in 2004—United States. (From Centers for Disease Control and Prevention. *Adolescents and HIV*. Slide set at http://www.cdc.gov/hiv/topics/surveillance/resources/slides/adolescents/index.htm. Accessed 2006.)

Transmission category	13–19 years N	13–19 years %	20–24 years N	20–24 years %
Male-to-male sexual contact	1,723	76	6,485	74
Injection drug use (IDU)	185	8	734	8
Male-to-male sexual contact and IDU	85	4	448	5
High risk heterosexual contact[a]	278	12	1,121	13
Other/not identified[b]	11	<1	32	<1
Total	2,282	100	8,820	100

Note. Data include "persons" with a diagnosis of HIV infection regardless of AIDS status of diagnosis. Data from 33 states with confidential name-based HIV infection reporting since at least 2000. Data have been adjusted for reporting delays.
[a] Heterosexual contact with a person known to have or at high risk for HIV infection
[b] Includes hemophilia, blood transfusion, perinatal, and risk factor not reported or not identified.

FIGURE 31.6 HIV/AIDS cases among male adolescents and young adults by transmission category from 2001 to 2004—33 states. (From Centers for Disease Control and Prevention. *Adolescents and HIV*. Slide set at http://www.cdc.gov/hiv/topics/surveillance/resources/slides/adolescents/index.htm. Accessed 2006.)

Transmission category	13–19 years N	13–19 years %	20–24 years N	20–24 years %
Injection drug use	285	14	697	15
High risk heterosexual contact[a]	1,739	85	3,929	84
Other/not identified[b]	22	1	46	1
Total	2,046	100	4,672	100

Note. Data include person's with a diagnosis of HIV infection regardless of AIDS status at diagnosis. Data from 33 states with confidential name-based HIV infection reporting since at least 2000. Data have been adjusted for reporting delays.
[a] Heterosexual contact with a person known to have or at high risk for HIV infection.
[b] Includes hemophilia, blood transfusion, perinatal, and risk factor not reported or not identified.

FIGURE 31.7 HIV/AIDS cases among female adolescents and young adults by transmission category from 2001 to 2004—33 states. (From Centers for Disease Control and Prevention. *Adolescents and HIV*. Slide set at http://www.cdc.gov/hiv/topics/surveillance/resources/slides/adolescents/index.htm. Accessed 2006.)

TABLE 31.2

1993 Revised Classification System for Human Immunodeficiency Virus (HIV) Infection and Expanded Acquired Immunodeficiency Syndrome (AIDS) Surveillance Case Definition for Adolescents and Adults

	Clinical Categories		
CD4+ T-cell Categories	(A) Asymptomatic, Acute (Primary) HIV or PGL	(B) Symptomatic, not (A) or (C) Conditions	(C) AIDS-Indicator Conditions[a]
1. ≥500/μL	A1	B1	C1
2. 200–400/μL	A2	B2	C2
3. <200/μL AIDS-indicator T-cell count	A3	B3	C3

PGL, persistent generalized lymphadenopathy.

[a]Conditions included in the 1993 AIDS Surveillance Case Definition (AIDS indicator conditions) are:

- Candidiasis of bronchi, trachea, or lungs
- Candidiasis, esophageal
- Cervical cancer, invasive
- Coccidioidomycosis, disseminated or extrapulmonary
- Cryptococcosis, extrapulmonary
- Cryptosporidiosis, chronic intestinal (>1 month's duration)
- Cytomegalovirus disease (other than liver, spleen, or nodes)
- Cytomegalovirus retinitis (with loss of vision)
- Encephalopathy, HIV-related or extrapulmonary
- Herpes simplex chronic ulcer(s) (>1 month's duration); or bronchitis, pneumonitis, or esophagitis
- Histoplasmosis, disseminated or extrapulmonary
- Isosporiasis, chronic intestinal (>1 month's duration)
- Kaposi sarcoma
- Lymphoma, Burkitt (or equivalent term)
- Lymphoma, immunoblastic (or equivalent term)
- Lymphoma, primary, of brain
- *Mycobacterium avium* complex or *Mycobacterium kansasii*, disseminated or extrapulmonary)
- *Pneumocystis carinii* pneumonia
- *Mycobacterium tuberculosis*, any site
- *Mycobacterium*, other species or (pulmonary or extrapulmonary) unidentified species, disseminated or extrapulmonary
- Pneumonia, recurrent
- Progressive multifocal leukoencephalopathy
- *Salmonella* septicemia, recurrent
- Toxoplasmosis of brain
- Wasting syndrome due to HIV infection

Adapted from 1993 revised classification system for HIV infection and expanded surveillance case definition for AIDS among adolescents and adults. Center for Disease Control and Prevention. Staging of HIV/AIDS. *MMWR Morb Mortal Wkly Rep* 1992;41:1.

- If you cannot or will not stop injecting, you should:
  - Use a new, sterile syringe obtained from a reliable source to prepare and divide drugs for each injection.
  - Never reuse or share syringes, water, cookers, or cottons.
  - Use sterile water to prepare drugs each time, or at least clean water from a reliable source.
  - *Keep everything as clean as possible* when injecting. If you can't use a new, sterile syringe and clean equipment each time, then disinfecting with bleach may be better than doing nothing at all:
  - Fill the syringe with clean water and shake or tap.
  - Squirt out the water and throw it away. Repeat until you don't see any blood in the syringe.
  - Completely fill the syringe with fresh, full-strength household bleach.
  - Keep it in the syringe for 30 seconds or more.
  - Squirt it out and throw the bleach away.
  - Fill the syringe with clean water and shake or tap.
  - Squirt out the water and throw it away.
- If you don't have any bleach, use clean water to vigorously flush out the syringe:
  - Fill the syringe with water and shake or tap it.
  - Squirt out the water and throw it away.
  - Do this several times.

Because of the unreliability and frequent unacceptance of needle bleaching and unacceptance or inaccessibility of drug treatment, almost all public health organizations support needle exchange. At these sites, injection drug users can turn in dirty needles for clean ones while at the same time gaining access to condoms, bleach, and referral resources. Programs in San Francisco, California, and New Haven, Connecticut, as well as others in the United States and Europe, have shown that injection drug use does not increase in the community or in an individual user when needle exchange is available. Moreover, HIV and other blood-borne disease transmissions (e.g., Hepatitis) are markedly reduced with the availability of needle exchange programs.

Sexual transmission of HIV is thought to have a hierarchy of relative risk. Within this hierarchy, receptive anal intercourse without condoms is riskiest, followed by insertive anal intercourse and vaginal intercourse. Oral sex is categorized as less risky in this model but has been shown to transmit HIV. Studies have shown that the proper and consistent use of latex condoms or dental dams can markedly reduce the risk for HIV transmission during sex.

The risk to health professionals of infection caused by needle sticks from HIV-infected patients is estimated to be 1 in 200 to 1 in 500. Injuries involving injection of blood are much riskier than simple pricks. In a preliminary study from the Centers for Disease Control and Prevention (1995), zidovudine (AZT) was found to be possibly helpful in reducing the risk of HIV infection to health care workers after accidental needle stick with needles contaminated with an infected patient's blood. For the health care workers in this study, the use of AZT decreased the risk 79%. Current CDC recommendations include consideration of rapid treatment within hours, with multiple medications, after the occurrence of a needle stick from a known HIV-infected patient (referred to as *postexposure prophylaxis*) (http://www.ucsf.edu/hivcntr/PEPline/index.html). Other considerations include whether the patient has been receiving effective HIV therapy and whether there is any known drug-resistant virus in the patient involved. The availability of clinicians with expertise in HIV transmission is essential to assist health care personnel exposed to a needle-stick injury to make complicated decisions regarding the risks and benefits of treatment. Information on occupational exposures and postexposure prophylaxis is available from the CDC and other Web sites (included at the end of this chapter) as well as the postexposure prophylaxis hotline (888-448-4911).

Nonoccupational exposure including sexual exposure prophylaxis: Antiretroviral postexposure prophylaxis after injection drug use, sexual, or other nonoccupational exposure to HIV is recommended when persons seeking care within 72 hours of exposure to blood, genital secretions, or other potentially infectious body fluids of a person known to be infected with HIV and the exposure represents a substantial risk for transmission. Treatment with HAART for 28 days is recommended but seeking expert guidance (see phone number in the preceding text or Web sites at the end of this chapter) to help practitioners determine if the exposure represents substantial risk is strongly advised. It is unknown if treatment for exposures after 72 hours provide any reduction in HIV risk and the U.S. Department of Health and Human Services (DHHS) does not take a stance on this. For exposures from persons of unknown HIV status DHHS does not make a recommendation other than recommending consideration of treatment on a case-by-case basis if the exposure is less that 72 hours old.

DEVELOPMENTAL ISSUES RELATED TO HIV INFECTIONS IN ADOLESCENTS

Although most youth do not undergo extreme turmoil and distress in their teenage years, adolescence provides many opportunities for risk for youth with regard to HIV infection. These additional opportunities for risk can be categorized in the following areas as outlined in the subsequent text: (a) cognitive and emotional development; (b) social, behavioral, and physiological development; and (c) family relationships.

Cognitive and Emotional Development

Cognitive and emotional development factors that put teens at increased risk for AIDS include:

1. Greater experimentation and greater degree of influence by peer behaviors
2. Naïveté and lack of good judgment
3. Feelings of immortality and invulnerability
4. Ignorance of modes of AIDS transmission and prevention
5. Denial of personal risk
6. Identification with moral codes (i.e., those of peers) other than those of their parents

Social, Behavioral, and Physiological Development

Adolescent behaviors that increase teens' risk for HIV infection include the following:

1. Sexual activity: A high percentage of adolescents engage in sexual intercourse, often without a barrier contraceptive or any contraceptive. In 2005, 46.8% of high school students reported that they had had sexual intercourse (Centers for Disease Control and Prevention, 2006), http://www.cdc.gov/HealthyYouth/yrbs/index.htm). Teens in urban areas, and particularly inner-city teens and those in group homes and detention centers, seem to have the earliest onset of sexual activity. Many adolescent males (17% to 37%) report having had at least one same-sex experience. A 1994–1998 CDC-sponsored study of urban young men (age 16–22) who have had sex with men reported that 41% had engaged in unprotected anal sex in the preceding 6 months (7% were HIV infected). Although, reported condom use at last sex in high school students has increased from 46.2% in 1991 to 62.8% in 2005, this still leaves many youth at risk for HIV infection through unprotected intercourse (Centers for Disease Control and Prevention, 2006).
2. Sexually transmitted diseases (STDs): The high prevalence of STDs in adolescents is an indicator of both high-risk behavior among teenagers and the lack of condom use. One in four sexually experienced teens contracts STD, annually.
3. Illicit drug use: Although there are no adequate national statistics on injection drug use among teenagers, estimates are that 1 in 50 high school juniors and seniors have injected drugs. Youth who have dropped out of school or are homeless have even higher rates. Millions of youth have used cocaine, stimulants, or opiates, all of which can be used intravenously. Teens may also be sharing needles in other ways, such as piercing ears, tattooing, or using steroids (i.e., athletes). Crack cocaine users appear to have an especially high rate of HIV infection. In addition, any drug use impairs a youth's ability to make good decisions concerning sexuality. In 2005, 23.3% of high school students reported use of alcohol or drugs before their last sexual activity (Centers for Disease Control and Prevention, 2006).
4. Runaway behavior: Approximately 1 million teenagers run away each year, and many of these are involved in high-risk behaviors, including injection drug use and survival sex (sex for money, food, or a place to stay). AIDS-related risks are high but are often ignored in the context of the immediate crises of survival (i.e., housing, food, and clothing).
5. Physiological factors: Adolescent girls may be at increased risk of HIV infection because of several physiological features, including:
   a. Differences in the cervix of adolescents (more columnar epithelium)
   b. Alterations of the vaginal pH as compared with adults
   c. Differences in menstrual patterns (less ovulation, less progesterone, and therefore less thick cervical mucus).

Family Relationships

Unresolved issues can lead to powerful conflicts between parents and adolescents. Sometimes the dysfunctional nature of the teen's family significantly increases the chances of the teen's involvement in high-risk behavior.

HUMAN IMMUNODEFICIENCY VIRUS TESTING

Most laboratories offer enzyme immunosorbent assay (EIA) screening with a confirmatory Western blot analysis for any blood specimen with two consecutive positive EIA test results. A positive EIA test result should never be reported to a patient as a positive test result for HIV. A positive Western blot has almost 100% specificity. Western blot tests can be indeterminate. This is common for patients in the window phase between acute infection and seroconversion. However, many patients with indeterminate tests will later test HIV negative by EIA or Western blot. It is recommended that testing be repeated until a definitive positive or negative result occurs. This can be performed after 1, 3, and 6 months for an indeterminate Western blot. The time delay from HIV infection to positive Western blot averages 21 days with newer test reagents. Rare cases of prolonged seroconversion (6 months or longer) have been reported. False-positive serology results may occur in 1 of 200,000 cases. Factitious reporting of HIV infection has been reported as well. In confusing cases, including indeterminate results, false reporting, and patients who are potentially in the window period, HIV DNA or RNA determination by polymerase chain reaction (PCR) may be helpful in clarifying serostatus.

The technology for HIV testing has expanded greatly. In addition to blood tests, tests of oral secretions and urine are approved by the U.S. Food and Drug Administration (FDA). Oral secretion tests have sensitivity and specificity similar to blood whereas urine tests are slightly less sensitive. In the United States, there are four rapid HIV tests currently licensed that can be used on serum, whole blood, and oral secretions. Positive test results must be confirmed like other screening tests and this must be incorporated into pretest counseling. The Centers for Disease Control and Prevention (2004a) Web site (http://www.cdc.gov/hiv/rapid_testing/) has extensive information on the use of rapid HIV testing, including specific recommendation for providers regarding the Clinical Laboratory Improvement Amendments (CLIA) program, counseling, and quality assurance guidelines. Rapid test technology can change frequently, so health care providers should check the CDC Web site for updates. However, as of 2006, the current tests included:

- OraQuick Advance Rapid HIV-1/2 Antibody test (Oral fluid, whole blood, or plasma)
- Reveal G-2 Rapid HIV-1 Antibody test (serum or plasma)
- Uni-Gold Recombigen HIV test (Whole blood, serum, or plasma)
- Multispot HIV-1/HIV-2 Rapid test (serum or plasma)

All of these tests had sensitivities in the 99% to 100% range and specificities in the 98.6% to 99.9% range. One benefit to rapid testing is that it nearly eliminates the problem of youth not returning for their results. Most rapid tests have CLIA waivers and clinicians can perform these in their offices, although some states may have additional regulations.

Consent and Confidentiality

Health care practitioners must balance the protection of adolescents' rights against the amount of information needed to deliver proper care.

1. Individuals older than 18 years who are competent: These individuals must make an informed consent for HIV testing, which involves a dialogue concerning the risks and benefits of the test, the implications of the test, and alternatives to the test. However, the CDC has recommended that patients in all health care settings get HIV testing after being informed and given a chance to opt-out. They recommend that separate informed consent (from the general medical consent) not be done and that prevention counseling should not be required for HIV diagnostic testing or as part of HIV screening programs.
2. Individuals between 12 and 17 years: The laws vary widely from state to state. In most states, the adolescent can and must give his or her own consent; however, as with any informed consent, the individual must be considered by the practitioner as competent to give an informed consent.
3. Individuals younger than 12 years and incompetent adolescents: For these individuals, a third party (parent or guardian) authorizes the testing. However, this authorization may be restricted by state laws.

An increasing number of states have statutes governing HIV testing. Without such a statute, general laws regarding minors apply. In most states, adolescents can give their own consent for diagnosis and treatment of STDs or contagious diseases. It is not clear whether HIV testing would fall under this category in states that do not declare AIDS to be an STD. In some states, adolescents are authorized and must give their own consent. Generally, those adolescents who are judged to have the right to consent are also considered to have the right to refuse testing and the right of confidentiality.

The physician should be aware of the current local laws regarding the following:

1. Consent for testing: Who can consent? What is the required informed consent? Are pretest and posttest counseling available?
2. Who can get the results of these tests?
3. Where can the test results be recorded?
4. Can results be disclosed to other involved individuals and under what circumstances?
5. What can be written in the chart regarding testing and test results?

To Whom Should Human Immunodeficiency Virus Testing Be Offered?

In 2006, as indicated in the preceding text, the CDC modified its recommendations to advise that HIV testing be routinized for all sexually active adolescents and adults younger than 64 years when they access health care. Youth should be advised that they will be tested and given the option to decline. Once initially tested, persons at high risk should be screened annually. Separate written consent is no longer recommended by the CDC but many states have laws requiring written informed consent. Prevention counseling is not required but does continue to offer benefit for health care systems that have the ability to provide this service. The following groups are at high risk and should have repeat testing at least annually:

1. Men who have sex with other men regardless of sexual orientation (as many youth in this group may not self-identify as gay or bisexual)
2. Youth who share needles (including tattooing, ear piercing, steroid injection, and recreational drugs)
3. Youth with partners from the above two groups
4. Youth who have had intercourse or shared needles with HIV-infected persons
5. Youth with STDs
6. Sexually active youth from inner city or economically disadvantaged areas or areas of known high seroprevalence
7. Youth with multiple sexual partners

Who Should Have Human Immunodeficiency Virus Testing Deferred?

1. Suicidal teens and those who seriously state they would be suicidal if HIV positive
2. Intoxicated and drug-withdrawing youth
3. Severely mentally ill youth who cannot provide consent for testing

When Should Testing Be Repeated for Youth with Positive Confirmatory Human Immunodeficiency Virus Test Results?

Testing should be repeated for the following persons:

1. Any youth who desires a second test
2. Any youth who is claiming to be HIV positive but has unreliable documentation
3. Youth who are at extremely low risk and have a single positive test result
4. Youth with normal CD4$^+$ T cells and undetectable viral load, who are not taking antiretroviral medications and have had only a single positive test result in the past

Methods for Human Immunodeficiency Virus Testing

1. Anonymous testing: Patients are not identified by name but are given a number. Many adolescents prefer this method because of confidentiality issues, but it may lower the rate of return for posttest counseling or the rate of follow-up for medical care if the adolescent is found to be HIV positive.
2. Confidential testing: Pretest and posttest counseling are done, and the results are part of the medical record. Normal laws regarding patient confidentiality still protect clients. Because the counselor or physician probably knows the patient's name and address, he or she can follow-up with HIV-positive clients to ensure they receive adequate care.
3. Youth-specific testing: Many testing sites now have counselors (including peers) who are specifically trained to work with adolescents. These testing sites may therefore be perceived as youth friendly. The counselors may have more time for complete evaluations of risky behaviors and have knowledge of how to help youth change unhealthy behaviors. Often, these sites are located where

other services or activities are available for teens (e.g., homeless shelters, free clinics, schools, recreational centers, mobile testing vans). Youth-specific testing should be recommended whenever possible, because it can be an effective component of prevention education.

HUMAN IMMUNODEFICIENCY VIRUS COUNSELING AND TESTING

The primary goals of HIV testing include identifying patients who are infected with HIV and linkage to appropriate health care and supportive services. The CDC is moving in a direction of increasing the ability and frequency of detecting HIV and avoiding prevention counseling as a possible impediment to HIV testing. Clinicians must weigh the need for HIV testing and HIV prevention counseling for patients. Although HIV prevention counseling is no longer required for HIV testing, Donna Futterman has developed the ACTS (Assess, Consent, Test, Support) system to assist practitioners with brief HIV counseling and testing (Table 31.3) (http://www.adolescentaids.org/healthcare/acts.html). This instrument was specifically designed with adolescents in mind. For some adolescents, the screening test may be a highly "teachable" moment and risk behavior assessment and counseling may be appropriate.

Posttest Counseling for Positive Test Results

Posttest counseling should be given in person and should include the following:

1. Provide the results of the test: This should be done in a direct manner at the beginning of the posttest session.
2. Allow the adolescent time to express feelings and reactions: It is important to give the adolescent hope by reiterating the advances in medical treatment discussed during the pretest session. As discussed in the preceding text, if rapid testing has been employed youth should be reminded that a second test must be conducted for confirmation.
3. Assess the adolescent's understanding of the result: This is best assessed by asking the teen directly what the test result means to him or her. The teen should be supported in identifying behavior change goals to reduce their risk of transmitting the virus to others. The teen should also understand that although the virus is probably present for life, a positive antibody test does not mean one has AIDS. Antibody-positive adolescents should be advised as follows:
   a. Do not donate blood, semen, or body organs.
   b. Employ safer sex practices.
   c. Inform physicians and dentists of HIV status.
   d. Encourage sexual partners, children, and needle contacts to seek evaluation and testing (many counties have anonymous partner notification programs).
   e. No evidence exists that HIV is transmitted to family household members or to close contacts by routes other than sexual intercourse, exposure to infected blood, and perinatal transmission.
   f. Household items may be shared by HIV-infected individuals and household members. Dishes and eating utensils should be routinely washed in hot water and a detergent. Personal hygiene items (i.e., razors and toothbrushes) should not be shared.

TABLE 31.3

ACTS: A Rapid System for HIV Counseling and Testing

Assess need for HIV testing, care, or prevention counseling
- Explain benefits of testing for patient's health and prevention.
- Discuss modes of HIV transmission (e.g., sex, needles, perinatal).
- Review risk assessment form or explain to patient that HIV testing is advisable if the patient has: (a) ever had sex, (b) has had inter-course without a condom, (c) has ever used recreational drugs intra-venously, or (d) shared intravenous syringes and works.
- Recommend testing, discuss HIV prevention, and provide referrals as appropriate.

Counsel and obtain consent
- Clarify the meaning of positive and negative results and explore patient's potential reactions.
- Assess readiness for immediate testing, including patient's social support network.
- Review health department requirements, such as the difference between confidential and anonymous testing and names reporting, partner notification, and domestic violence screening.
- Obtain consent.

Test
- Describe/provide HIV test (e.g., blood, oral, urine, rapid).
- Make appointment to deliver results in person, by phone, or have patient wait for rapid results.

Support during testing and afterward

HIV-negative patients
- Clarify need to retest in 3 months (e.g., window period, based on risk assessment).
- Provide prevention strategies and referrals; HIV testing alone is not prevention.

HIV-positive patients
- Provide support and link to care and prevention.
- Review HIV reporting, partner notification, and domestic/partner violence issues.

Complete ACTS training materials are available at www.adolescentaids.org.

HIV, human immunodeficiency virus.
From Futterman DC. HIV and AIDS in adolescents. *Adolesc Med Clin* 2004;15:369 with permission.

g. The HIV-seropositive individual's blood and other body fluids should be handled with care. Soiled clothes or linen should be washed with a detergent or bleach.
h. Bathroom facilities may be used by all household members.
4. Refer the patient to an HIV specialist who is experienced with adolescents. Ideally, the clinic will have a multidisciplinary team that includes a physician, social worker, nurse, and other caregivers to assist the patient with treatment and in coping with the illness.

MANAGEMENT OF HUMAN IMMUNODEFICIENCY VIRUS INFECTION IN ADOLESCENTS

Initial Assessment

History and Physical Examination
The history and physical examination should stress the following:

1. Prior exposure to diseases that are likely to reactivate in individuals with HIV, including tuberculosis (TB), syphilis, herpes genitalis, herpes zoster, and cytomegalovirus (CMV) infections
2. Number of children, their ages, and their health status
3. Injection drug-use history and history of alcohol and other drug use
4. Travel history to find out about possible exposure to fungal infections that are endemic in certain areas, such as histoplasmosis, coccidioidomycosis, or blastomycosis
5. Sexual history, including sexually transmitted infections
6. Prior immunizations
7. A review of systems, focusing particularly on the following:
   a. Systemic: Anorexia, weight loss, fevers, night sweats
   b. Skin: Pruritis, rashes, pigmented lesions
   c. Lymphatic: Increased size of lymph nodes
   d. Head, eyes, ears, nose, and throat: Headache, change in vision, sinus congestion
   e. Cardiopulmonary: Cough, dyspnea
   f. Gastrointestinal: Dysphagia, abdominal pain, and diarrhea
   g. Musculoskeletal: Myalgias, arthralgias
   h. Neurological: Memory loss, neuralgias, motor weakness, depression, and headache
   i. Genitourinary: Bumps, ulcers, burning, or discharge
8. Careful measurement of weight at each visit

9. Careful examination particularly focusing on the following:
   a. Skin: Seborrhea, folliculitis, Kaposi sarcoma (KS) lesions, psoriasis, tinea, herpetic lesions, and molluscum contagiosum
   b. Eye: Visual acuity and fields, cotton-wool and hemorrhagic exudates on funduscopic examination
   c. Mouth: Periodontal disease (gingivitis), oral hairy leukoplakia (white plaques along lateral aspect of tongue), thrush, oral ulcers, and KS lesions
   d. Lymphatic: Asymmetrical, tender, enlarged nodes, particularly posterior cervical, axillary, and epitrochlear nodes
   e. Cardiopulmonary: Rales, murmurs (in injection drug users)
   f. Gastrointestinal: Hepatosplenomegaly
   g. Genitourinary: Herpetic lesions, warts, and penile discharge in males; cervical or vaginal discharge in females
   h. Rectal: Perianal herpes, condyloma, fissures, and proctitis
   i. Neurological: Focal findings, altered mental status

Laboratory Evaluation
Initial assessment should include the following:

1. Complete blood count, looking for anemia, leukopenia, or pancytopenia
2. Platelet count
3. Chemistry panel, looking for hypergammaglobulinemia, hypoalbuminemia, hypocholesterolemia, increased liver enzymes, or decreased renal function
4. Urinalysis
5. CD4$^+$ T-cell count and percentage
6. Viral load (HIV RNA by PCR)
7. Consider HIV resistance testing (genotyping is less expensive than phenotyping) in patients with acute or recent seroconversion
8. Purified protein derivative (PPD) of tuberculin skin test
9. Serology for syphilis, hepatitis A, B, and C, toxoplasmosis, and varicella if previous infection or immunization status is not known
10. Chest radiograph
11. Tests for gonorrhea and chlamydia infections if sexually experienced
12. Papanicolaou test (Pap smear) in women

Vaccinations

1. Hepatitis A: Recommended for all at-risk individuals.
2. Hepatitis B: Recommended for all patients without evidence of hepatitis B immunity or chronic infection. Retrospective studies demonstrate that many youth with HIV do not develop antibodies to hepatitis B after three immunizations. Physicians can consider a fourth immunization or repeating the series after the patient begins HAART.
3. Human papillomavirus (HPV): HIV infection is not a contraindication (it is not a live vaccine), and in the HIV-infected population, it could be a real positive. However, it is not clear if the efficacy in the immune suppressed population will be as high as that in the nonimmunosuppressed population. Although HPV vaccine is currently FDA approved only for females aged 9 to 26, the significant morbidity and even mortality associated with HPV-related disease in men-who-have-sex-with men argues for its early adoption into clinical practice.
4. Influenza: Should be offered annually in October or November to all HIV-infected individuals. In patients not receiving HAART, the viral load may increase transiently after vaccination, but it returns to baseline in approximately 1 month. Intranasal vaccination is contraindicated.
5. Measles-mumps-rubella (MMR): All patients should have received two MMR vaccinations in their lifetime. MMR is considered safe in patients with HIV but should not be used if severe immunosuppression is present. (Severe immunosuppression is not defined but one might use a CD4$^+$ below 200 in this setting.)
6. Meningococcal vaccination: Persons with HIV are likely at increased risk for meningococcal disease. They may elect to receive the conjugate quadrivalent vaccine although its efficacy in this population is unknown.
7. Pertussis (acellular pertussis): Adolescents and young adults are being recommended to be revaccinated with Tdap. HIV is not a contraindication (it is not a live virus) but the response in those immunosuppressed might be suboptimal.
8. Pneumococcal: Should be given once to previously unimmunized individuals.
9. Polio: Patients requiring primary or booster immunizations should receive the inactive form, inactivated poliovirus (IPV), not the oral poliovirus vaccine (OPV).
10. Tetanus-diphtheria: Same as if uninfected.
11. Varicella (chickenpox): The vaccine for prevention of varicella (varivax—live attenuated varicella virus vaccine) is *NOT* advised for use in those with acquired or primary immunodeficiencies. Research using this vaccine in persons previously infected with varicella is in progress. Currently, the new vaccine Zostavax (live attenuated varicella/zoster vaccine) for prevention of shingles is approved only for individuals older than 60 and is contraindicated in those with immunosuppressive diseases including AIDS.

Follow-up

Patients should have their medical and social needs assessed at least every 3 months. Most patients on HAART should be seen monthly, because adherence issues frequently arise. These appointments should focus on signs and symptoms of disease progression, coping skills, and secondary prevention education. Antiretroviral management is reviewed later in this chapter. Secondary prevention focuses on preventing the spread of HIV to others but also in preventing unplanned pregnancy and STDs that are commonly seen in youth. Follow-up should include the following:

1. Complete blood count with platelet count and CD4$^+$ T-cell count every 3 months
2. HIV RNA by PCR every 3 months
3. PPD yearly
4. Venereal disease research laboratory (VDRL) or a rapid plasma reagin (RPR) test for syphilis, yearly. These tests should be conducted more frequently for young-men-who-have-sex-with men in high prevalence regions.
5. Pap smear annually in sexually experienced women
6. Regular discussion of safer sex and family planning

7. Discussion of disclosure including options for partner notification
8. Discussion of nutrition, exercise, disease progression, medication options, and potential clinical trials
9. Regular evaluation of emotional status
10. Focused interval history and physical examination, concentrating on illnesses common for the patient's stage of HIV disease

Early Manifestations of Human Immunodeficiency Virus Infection

Early manifestations of HIV disease may include the following:

Chronic lymphadenopathy	Pruritic papular eruptions
Unexplained weight loss	Oral hairy leukoplakia
Xerosis	Frequent tinea
Severe molluscum contagiosum	Leukopenia
Seborrheic dermatitis	Exacerbations of psoriasis
Isolated thrombocytopenia	Fatigue and malaise

Opportunistic diseases, including infections and neoplasms, typically occur after immune suppression reaches a certain level. Table 31.4 lists some common diseases and the corresponding CD4$^+$ T-cell count associated with these illnesses.

The management of conditions associated with HIV is beyond the scope of this chapter, changes frequently, and is frequently left to HIV specialists. Updated treatment information is available on several Web sites listed at the end of this chapter.

Management of Sexually Transmitted Infections

1. Uncomplicated chlamydia, gonorrhea, trichomonas, and syphilis are generally treated in the same manner as in adolescents without HIV.
2. Pelvic inflammatory disease can be more difficult to treat in women with HIV, especially if immune dysfunction is pronounced (low CD4$^+$ T-cell count). In general, the CDC treatment guidelines (http://www.cdc.gov/STD/treatment/) are followed, but the threshold for hospitalization for administration of intravenous antibiotics is reduced.
3. Cervical dysplasia has been shown to be very prevalent in women with HIV. High-risk serotypes such as HPV-16 seem to be more common, and spontaneous regression appears to be less common. Still, annual screening after initiating sexual activity (rather than delaying for 3 years as now recommended for HIV-negative patients) and referral for colposcopy for both low-grade and high-grade squamous intraepithelial lesions or recurrent atypical results on Pap smears are recommended. Treatment and follow-up recommendations for abnormal findings on colposcopic biopsies are generally the same as in

---

TABLE 31.4

Opportunistic Diseases

CD4$^+$ T-cell Count (per mm^3)	Condition
200–500	Thrush
	Kaposi sarcoma
	Tuberculosis reactivation
	Herpes zoster
	Bacterial sinusitis/pneumonia
	Herpes simplex
100–200	*Pneumocystis carinii* pneumonia
	All of the above
50–100	Systemic fungal infections
	Primary tuberculosis
	Cryptosporidiosis
	Cerebral toxoplasmosis
	Progressive multifocal leukoencephalopathy
	Peripheral neuropathy
	Cervical carcinoma
0–50	Cytomegalovirus disease
	Disseminated *Mycobacterium avium* complex
	Non-Hodgkin lymphoma
	Central nervous system lymphoma
	AIDS dementia complex

AIDS, acquired immunodeficiency syndrome.
From Phari JP, Murphy RL. *Contemporary diagnosis and management of HIV/AIDS infections.* Newton, PA: Handbooks in Health Care, 1999 with permission.

women not infected with HIV. Whenever possible, refer adolescents with HIV and abnormal Pap smear results to care providers with HIV experience.

Management of Family Planning

Risk of Maternal-Child Transmission With the marked improvements in prevention of maternal-child transmission of HIV, family planning has changed. Many youth now acknowledge their interest in having children despite having HIV. Physicians should be honest about the risks of maternal-child transmission. The risk of maternal-child transmission of HIV is approximately 23% without antiretroviral treatment. The current standard of care is to treat infected women who desire pregnancy, with HAART (minimum of three antiretrovirals). The risk of transmission has been shown to be <4% for women taking HAART, and it is probably <1% when a patient conceives while following an effective HAART regimen (i.e., viral load is undetectable) and maintains the program during pregnancy. The CDC has developed specific guidelines on the prevention of maternal-child transmission; these are available on their Web site (http://www.cdc.gov/mmwr/PDF/rr/rr5118.pdf).

Contraception Although the prevention of maternal-fetal transmission of HIV is no longer the primary reason for birth control, the typical issues of adolescence and being prepared for parenting are still critical. Unplanned pregnancies can disrupt an already complex situation for youth infected with HIV. Providing contraceptive counseling in these youth is complicated by the competing desires to prevent transmission of HIV to sexual partners by using condoms and to prevent unplanned pregnancy (usually with a more effective hormonal method). Studies of adult women with HIV have shown that patients using hormonal methods of contraception were less likely to use condoms. However, those using condoms frequently reported using them irregularly. Data from a cohort of HIV-infected adolescents indicated that most adolescents reported condoms as their main method of contraception (Belzer et al., 2001). Unfortunately, the rate of conception was >20% during the first year in the study, and it was high in those reporting contraception use as well. Contraception needs to be addressed frequently and adherence to the method of choice discussed. Contraceptives utilizing estrogen may be less effective in patients using protease inhibitors (which increase estrogen metabolism), and contraceptive pill use adds to the pill burden in patients taking other medications.

Common Psychosocial Problems

Common psychosocial problems in HIV-infected adolescents include, but are not limited to, the following:

1. Depression and suicidal ideation
2. Substance use
3. Self-blame
4. Social isolation, including family and peers
5. Unsafe sex
6. Distress/negative reactions regarding sexual identity
7. Homelessness
8. Survival sex
9. Denial
10. Unplanned pregnancy
11. HIV disclosure

The cornerstone to good care is the availability of a strong health care team, including physicians, nurses, social workers, psychologists or psychiatrists, nutritionists, substance abuse counselors, and medical subspecialists as needed. Coordinating the team to focus on the *patient's identified needs* improves compliance and facilitates normal adolescent development.

Travel

Visiting regions outside one's normal community can expose an individual to many pathogens. In developing countries, opportunities for exposure to enteric pathogens, including *Cryptosporidium* and *Isospora*, increase. Risk for certain respiratory infections such as coccidioidomycosis, histoplasmosis, and TB also increases in many developing countries and in certain geographic regions of the United States. The CDC offers an international travelers' hotline (telephone 877-FYI-TRIP) and a Web site http://www.cdc.gov/travel/. Patients planning significant travel should discuss preventive strategies with their physician.

1. Avoid contaminated food and drink (i.e., tap water).
2. Receive appropriate immunizations.
3. Extended travel should be accompanied by appropriate medications and telephone numbers for emergency care.
4. Seek medical attention promptly if fever, diarrhea, or other illness occurs during or after travel.

Sports Participation

When Ervin "Magic" Johnson announced that he was infected with HIV, many questions surrounding the advisability of vigorous exercise occurred. To date there have been no studies documenting a positive or negative impact of exercise on HIV. Currently, we recommend using common sense in guiding infected youth on sports participation.

There have been no documented cases of HIV transmission during athletic participation. We would not withhold a youth from competitive sports (even full-contact sports like wrestling or football) solely on the basis of HIV-positive status. The principal risks athletes have for acquiring HIV are related to off-the-field settings (Mast et al., 1995). However, all participants, whether infected with HIV or uninfected, should not compete with open wounds, and universal precautions should always be followed when bleeding occurs.

Evaluation of Specific Syndromes

Pulmonary (Cough or Shortness of Breath)
1. If the CD4+ T-cell count is 200/mL or less or the percentage of CD4+ T cells is 14% or less, the patient requires the following:
   a. Chest radiographic examination: Look for interstitial or other infiltrates
   b. Pulse oximetry or arterial blood gas determination for hypoxemia
   c. Consider induced sputum for *Pneumocystis carinii* pneumonia (PCP)
   d. Consider bronchoscopy for PCP evaluation
2. In patients with a CD4+ T-cell count higher than 200/mL and a percentage higher than 14%, it is unlikely to be PCP. These patients require the following:
   a. Consider evaluation for bronchitis, sinusitis, TB, and bacterial pneumonia

b. Chest radiographic examination or sinus films
c. Subsequent PPD
d. Sputum for culture and sensitivity, acid-fast bacillus

Fever Evaluation in patients who have severe immuno-suppression (CD4$^+$ T-cell count <200/mL) but lack of specific organ system signs or symptoms should include the following:

1. Chest radiographic examination: Interstitial infiltrates are consistent with PCP, infection with *Mycobacterium avium* complex (MAC) or CMV; focal infiltrates are consistent with TB or bacterial pneumonia
2. Complete blood count: Anemia is common in MAC
3. Chemistry panel: Elevated lactate dehydrogenase is common in PCP; elevated alkaline phosphatase is common in MAC
4. Blood cultures for bacteria, virus (CMV), fungus, and acid-fast bacillus
5. Serum cryptococcal antigen

If fever persists and above tests are inconclusive, consider the following:

1. Lumbar puncture: May pick up cryptococcal infection
2. Bone marrow biopsy: May pick up disseminated MAC, CMV, or fungus
3. Ophthalmology consultation: Looking for CMV
4. Body computed tomography (CT): Looking for lymphoma
5. Sinus films

In patients with mild immunosuppression (CD4$^+$ T-cell count 200–500/mL), look for common illnesses (viral or bacterial) and consider looking for TB, sinusitis, and pneumonia.

In patients with minimal immune suppression (CD4$^+$ T-cell count >500/mL), avoid costly workups unless conservative evaluation fails.

Diarrhea Always assess whether this could be medication related. In patients with severe immunodeficiency (CD4$^+$ T-cell count <200/mL):

1. If diarrhea is mild, consider empiric treatment with diphenoxylate (Lomotil) or loperamide (Imodium).
2. If diarrhea is severe, check stool for ova and parasites, culture and sensitivity, *Cryptosporidium, Cyclospora,* or *Isospora* infection.
3. If these tests are inconclusive, consider colonoscopy looking for CMV, MAC, *Microsporidia,* and *Isospora.*

In patients without severe immunodeficiency:

1. Diarrhea is usually self-limited, and costly evaluations should be avoided.
2. Consider stool ova and parasites, stool for *Clostridium difficile* toxin, and bacterial culture and sensitivity if the patient is sexually active, is homeless, or has traveled abroad recently.

Neurological (New Headaches, Seizures, Focal Neurological Signs) In patients with severe immunodeficiency (CD4$^+$ T-cell count <200/mL):

1. Emergency CT or magnetic resonance imaging (MRI) of head: Multiple enhancing ring lesions are usually indicative of toxoplasmosis; primary central nervous system lymphoma is also common.

2. Lumbar puncture for cell count, protein, cryptococcal antigen, Gram stain, routine acid-fast bacillus and fungal cultures, and VDRL.

Dysphagia In patients with severe immunodeficiency (CD4$^+$ T-cell count <200/mL):

1. If oral thrush is present, consider empiric treatment for *Candida* organisms with fluconazole or ketoconazole.
2. If there is no oral thrush or empiric treatment fails, try endoscopy with evaluations for fungus, CMV, and herpes simplex virus.

Prophylaxis

Prophylaxis is one of the most important ways that patients with severe immunosuppression can maintain their health. Patients who have severe immune suppression but are not ready for HAART should still be encouraged to use prophylaxis.

Primary Prophylaxis The CDC frequently publishes updated guidelines for primary prophylaxis and can be found on their Web site (http://aidsinfo.nih.gov/ContentFiles/OIpreventionGL.pdf).

1. *Pneumocystis:* Initiate when the CD4$^+$ T-cell count is 200/mL or less. Patients who start HAART and in whom the CD4$^+$ T-cell count rises above 200/mL for 3 to 6 months may safely discontinue prophylaxis.
   a. Drug of choice: Trimethoprim-sulfamethoxazole double-strength tablet, daily or three times weekly (patients with allergies to sulfa can usually be desensitized).
   b. Alternatives: Dapsone 100 mg/day orally (check for glucose-6-phosphate dehydrogenase [G6PD] deficiency before using); nebulized pentamidine 300 mg every 4 weeks through Respirgard II nebulizer (may be the method of choice in noncompliant youth); Atovaquone 1,500 mg orally a day with meals.
2. *Tuberculosis:* Initiate in teens who are PPD positive (>5 mm), have recent TB exposure, or have a history of inadequately treated TB that healed.
   a. Drug of choice: Isoniazid 300 mg plus pyridoxine 50 mg daily or Isoniazid 900 mg plus pyridoxine 100 mg twice a week for 9 months.
   b. Alternative: Rifampin 600 mg plus pyrazinamide 15 to 20 mg/kg daily for 60 doses (rifampin is contraindicated in patients taking protease inhibitors).
3. *Mycobacterium avium complex:* Initiate when the CD4$^+$ T-cell count is 50/mL or less. Prophylaxis can probably be discontinued if the cell count rises above 100/mL for 3 to 6 months after initiation of HAART.
   a. Drug of choice: Clarithromycin 500 mg twice daily or azithromycin 1,200 mg orally once a week.
   b. Alternative: Rifabutin 300 mg orally once a day.
4. *Toxoplasma gondii* risk: Initiate when the CD4$^+$ T-cell count is <100/mL and serology results are positive for *T. gondii* immunoglobulin G.
   a. Drug of choice: Trimethoprim-sulfamethoxazole, one double-strength tablet/day.
   b. Alternative: Dapsone 50 mg orally once a day plus pyrimethamine 50 mg/week plus leucovorin 25 mg/week.

Antiretroviral Therapy The CDC regularly updates guidelines on the use of antiretrovirals for adolescents and adults (http://aidsinfo.nih.gov/ContentFiles/

AdultandAdolescentGL.pdf) and should be consulted with the assistance of an HIV specialist in determining whether a patient should be treated with HAART. In addition, the Health Resources and Service Administration has published a report titled, *Helping Adolescents with HIV Adhere to HAART* (available through the National AIDS Clearinghouse http://www.cdc.gov/mmwr/preview/mmwrhtml/00001789.htm). Although a full discussion of the use of antiretrovirals is beyond the scope of this chapter, some basic principles pertaining to youth are important.

Initiating Highly Active Antiretroviral Therapy

Although the United States Department of Health Services publishes guidelines for the initiation of HAART in adolescents and adults, which are based primarily on a patient's immune status (CD4$^+$ T-cell count) and risk for disease progression (viral load, HIV RNA), there has been considerable attention to the issue of a patient's ability to adhere strictly to a regimen for many years and perhaps for the rest of the patient's life. Decisions to initiate therapy must be made jointly by a well-informed patient and his or her health care providers. Empowering patients through education on their ability to control HIV through the proper use of medications, while at the same time helping them develop a realistic time frame and plan for initiating therapy, is the key to eventual adherence and the reaching of mutual agreement on treatment.

There are currently 22 FDA-approved antiretroviral drugs that belong to one of four classes based on their mode of preventing HIV replication. New medications in each class are currently in development, and new classes are also being researched. There are also an increasing number of medication formulations that allow 2 to 3 different medications to be placed into one single pill or fewer pills per medication. These have allowed for considerable simplification of antiretroviral regimens.

1. Nucleoside/nucleotide reverse transcriptase inhibitors
   a. Zidovudine (Retrovir or AZT)
   b. Didanosine (Videx or DDI)
   c. Stavudine (Zerit or D4T)
   d. Lamivudine (Epivir or 3TC)
   e. Abacavir (Ziagen)
   f. Zalcitabine (Hivid or DDC)
   g. Emtricitabine (Emtriva or FTC)
   h. Tenofovir (Viread)
   i. Combivir, a combination pill with both zidovudine and lamivudine
   j. Trizivir, a combination of zidovudine, lamivudine, and abacavir
   k. Epzicom, a combination of abacavir and lamivudine
   l. Truvada, a combination of tenofovir and emtricitabine
2. Nonnucleoside reverse transcriptase inhibitors
   a. Nevirapine (Viramune)
   b. Efavirenz (Sustiva)
   c. Delavirdine (Rescriptor)
3. Protease inhibitors
   a. Ritonavir (Norvir)
   b. Saquinavir (Fortovase)
   c. Indinavir (Crixivan)
   d. Nelfinavir (Viracept)
   e. Fosamprenavir (Lexiva)
   f. Lopinavir/ritonavir (Kaletra)
   g. Atazanavir (Reyataz)
   h. Tipranavir (Aptivus)
   i. Darunavir (Prezista)
4. Entry (fusion) inhibitors
   a. Enfuvirtide (Fuzeon)

The general principles of HAART therapy are listed in Table 31.5. The primary aim is to initiate a regimen (frequently described to patients as a cocktail) containing a minimum of three antiretroviral medications with the goal of reducing the patient's viral load to an undetectable level on a highly sensitive assay for HIV RNA. Incomplete suppression, through either inadequate medication or nonadherence, can lead to the development of HIV strains that are resistant to the antiretrovirals. Because of potential cross-resistance, second- and third-line treatment is often more complex, more toxic, and less effective. An increasing number of persons newly infected with HIV are being infected with strains that are already resistant to one or more antiretroviral medications. Physicians should consult their local health departments to determine if assaying for baseline antiretroviral resistance is cost effective for any particular region.

The patient's need for HAART must be balanced with the ability to adhere to the drug regimen. Research has indicated that physicians are notoriously poor at predicting how likely a patient is to take his or her medication. Table 31.6 reviews some factors that may influence patients' decisions to start taking medication. Table 31.7 reviews some basic concepts about adolescents and adherence to HAART. Predictors of poor adherence include psychosocial problems such as poor support, mental health problems (depression was shown to be a predictor of nonadherence in adolescents with HIV in one study), substance abuse, and homelessness. In addition, factors such as patients' trust in their health care providers or concerns that taking medication might inadvertently disclose their HIV status to family, friends, roommates, or coworkers must be considered. Also critical are medication-inherent factors such as the number of pills, the frequency of dosing, the size or taste of pills, potential side effects (many youth fear rashes because they might disclose their HIV status), and food and timing requirements. In general, one would try to keep regimens as simple and tolerable as possible. Regimens as simple as one pill daily or one pill twice daily are available. Because studies have demonstrated that adolescent adherence to antiretroviral therapy is often poor, it is important to choose regimens such that, if resistance develops, options can still be maintained for the future. Close monitoring for nonadherence by multiple providers including psychosocial support staff is critical and monthly follow-up appointments are needed for most patients. The use of pill boxes, alarms, or pagers can help youth stay organized although these methods have yet to be studied in randomized trials. As stated earlier, helping patients to prepare for HAART and to maintain it once begun is a challenging task and one that should be reserved as much as possible for physicians with expertise in HIV and adolescent care. Many adolescent-HIV specialists have adapted the stages of change model developed by Prochaska and DiClemente (1983). Table 31.8 reviews the stages from precontemplation through maintenance and provides the goals for health practitioners and the key objectives for each stage.

In summary, the need for HAART in HIV-infected adolescents must be balanced against the potential for benefit from the medications and the potential for harm

TABLE 31.5

Summary of the Principles of Therapy of Human Immunodeficiency Virus (HIV) Infection

1. HIV replication results in immune system damage and progression to AIDS. HIV infection is always harmful. Regular, periodic measurement of HIV RNA levels (viral load measurements)
   a. Determines the risk for HIV disease progression
   b. Guides decisions to initiate and change antiretroviral treatment regimens (HAART) Measurement of CD4$^+$ T-cell counts monitors the extent of immune dysfunction
2. Treatment decisions are individualized based on both viral load levels and CD4$^+$ T-cell counts
3. The goal of HAART is maximum achievable suppression of HIV replication to below the levels of detection by sensitive viral load assays. The most effective means of maximizing suppression of HIV replication is through treatment with simultaneous initiation of combinations of antiretroviral drugs that
   a. The patient has not received before
   b. Are not cross-resistant with drugs the patient has received
4. Each antiretroviral drug used in combination therapy should always be used according to optimum schedules and dosages
5. Any changes in therapy reduce future treatment options because the number of drugs is limited and cross-resistance occurs
6. Women should receive optimal antiretroviral therapy regardless of pregnancy status
7. These principles apply to HIV-infected children, adolescents, and adults, although the treatment of HIV-infected children involves unique pharmacological, virological, and immunological considerations
8. Persons identified with acute primary HIV infection should also be treated with combination antiretroviral therapy to achieve viral load levels below detectable levels with sensitive plasma HIV RNA assays
9. HIV-infected persons should be considered infectious even with undetectable viral load levels, and should be counseled to avoid sexual or drug-use behaviors that would transmit HIV or other infectious pathogens

AIDS, acquired immunodeficiency syndrome; HAART, highly active antiretroviral therapy.
Adapted from U.S. Department of Health and Human Services. Report of the NIH panel to define principles of therapy of HIV infection. *MMWR Morb Mortal Wkly Rep* 1998;47(R-55):1.

from the development of resistance due to nonadherence. It is not unreasonable to initiate a short trial of practice medication for 1 to 4 weeks. If the patient cannot take the medication regularly or even follow-through with the next appointment, the initiation of medication can be delayed while more preparation can occur. It is very reasonable to hold off on HAART, even for patients with highly advanced AIDS, if the patient and physician conclude that adherence is unlikely. Medication has been demonstrated in many cases to produce immune reconstitution in even the most damaged immune systems as long as the virus is sensitive to the medication and the patient has not developed a terminal or untreatable complication.

HUMAN IMMUNODEFICIENCY VIRUS PREVENTION

Primary

Until a vaccine is found, behavioral interventions, comprehensive school-based health education, blood supply screening, postexposure prophylaxis, and access to sterile needles are the main tools to reduce the risk of infection. Current primary prevention efforts include the use of counseling, HIV testing and referral, increasing the proportion of individuals with known HIV status, and the referral of individuals at high risk of HIV infection into appropriate prevention programs, including evidenced-based interventions.

Appropriate educational interventional goals for HIV-negative adolescents include the following:

1. Reducing misinformation and prejudice against HIV-infected persons
2. Helping to reduce high-risk behavior, including recommendations to decrease sexual activity, numbers of sexual partners, and experimentation with drugs
3. Supporting adolescents who choose abstinence
4. Increasing the use of condoms in adolescents who are having intercourse
5. Encouraging adolescents in sexual relationships to get HIV tested with their partners and to maintain monogamy

HIV/AIDS prevention education needs to be conducted at schools, religious organizations, youth organizations, medical facilities, and meetings with parents. Media (television, radio, magazines) are powerful methods to impart information that may change adolescents' attitudes. Meeting youngsters, where they congregate, by outreach workers can be an especially effective method of reaching high-risk populations such as homeless youth, gang youth, or out-of-school youth. Topics for HIV prevention include the following:

1. Epidemiology of HIV/AIDS and myths about AIDS
2. Sexual transmission and prevention, including abstinence, safer sex, and condom use
3. Transmission through needles, drug use prevention
4. HIV and pregnancy
5. Testing and counseling

TABLE 31.6

Medication Adherence Assessment[a]

Factors that may influence decision to take medication

Client perception of health status	1. What is the meaning of the HIV infection to the patient?
	2. What is his or her perception of his or her level of wellness and illness?
	3. What does taking medicine mean to the patient?
	   a. Does he or she believe medicine will help him or her?
	   b. What are his or her past experiences with medicines, including those taken by family members?

Social support network	1. Who is the most significant person in the patient's life? 2. Is this person aware of the patient's diagnosis? Is this person involved in the patient's care? 3. With whom does the patient live? 4. Who in the patient's home knows the diagnosis? 5. Who doesn't know? 6. What is the patient's relationship with the clinic team?

Living arrangements and financial situation	1. Housing
	   a. Does the patient have stable housing?
	   b. Does the patient have a space he or she calls his or her own?
	   c. Does the patient have access to a refrigerator and a secure place to store his or her medications?
	2. Health insurance
	   a. Does the patient have health insurance that will pay for his or her medications?

Presence of psychopathology and problems with substance use	1. Does the patient have an active psychiatric diagnosis (e.g., manic depressive disorder, poor impulse control, major depression, suicidality)? 2. Is the patient an active substance user (e.g., marijuana, alcohol, crack, cocaine, heroin, Valium, Xanax)?
Developmental level	1. What is the patient's developmental stage? 2. What are the patient's developmental goals?

Factors that may influence ability to perform the work of taking medications

Time orientation and organization	1. Ability to remember recent past
	2. Ability to organize self toward immediate future
	3. Routine organization of activities of daily living both during the week and on the weekend
	   a. What time does the patient awake?
	   b. What does he or she do on awakening?
	   c. Meal schedule, etc.
	4. Future plans and goals

Physical abilities	1. Visual acuity 2. Reading ability 3. Ability to open bottles 4. Ability to take out correct number of pills 5. Ability to take pills at the correct time of day 6. Ability to put pills in mouth 7. Ability to swallow pills 8. Ability to follow directions 9. Ability to prepare medications in advance
Ability to recognize and tolerate side effects	1. Ability to distinguish between major and minor sides 2. Ability to tolerate discomforts of individual medications
Medical regimen complexity	1. Number of pills 2. Number of doses 3. Additional directions for dosing 4. Mechanical actions necessary for preparation (e.g., crushing pills, mixing powder with liquid)

HIV, human immunodeficiency virus.

[a]This assessment was developed in 1998 by Alice Myerson, MSN, PNP of the Adolescent AIDS Program at the Montefiore Medical Center in New York.

TABLE 31.7

Barriers to Adherence

Barriers for the general patient population	1. Complexity of medical regimen 2. Lack of social support 3. Adverse effects of treatment 4. Distrust of health providers 5. Lack of understanding about the medication 6. Difficulty coming to terms with a life-threatening illness

Additional barriers for adolescents	The developmental capacities of adolescence can create barriers to adherence
	1. Early adolescence
	   a. Concrete, not yet abstract, thinking (undeveloped problem-solving skills)
	   b. Preoccupation with self and questions about pubertal changes
	2. Middle adolescence
	   a. Need for acceptance from peers (desire not to appear different)
	   b. Present-orientation (decreased ability to plan for future doses and future implications of disease)
	   c. Busy, unstructured lives (difficulty remembering to take pills)
	3. Late adolescence
	   a. Establishment of independence (the need to challenge authority figures and restructure regimens)
	   b. Feelings of immortality (disbelief that HIV can hurt them)

Additional barriers for adolescents with HIV	1. For most, fear of disclosure of their HIV status to family and friends 2. For many, lack of adult or peer support to reinforce their adherence 3. For youth establishing independence, the conflict between needing to challenge authority figures and needing to depend on adult providers for support in taking HAART 4. For asymptomatic adolescents, difficulty accepting the implications of a serious illness when they still feel well 5. For some who still think concretely, difficulty grasping the concept that there is a connection between strict adherence to HAART and prevention of disease progression 6. For youth who live in the inner city, fear that they will die from violence, not AIDS 7. For homeless and transient youth, lack of refrigeration or a place to store medicines and lack of a daily routine

HIV, human immunodeficiency virus; HAART, highly active antiretroviral therapy; AIDS, acquired immunodeficiency syndrome.

6. Biology of HIV/AIDS
7. Medical aspects of HIV/AIDS
8. Peer pressure and dating skills
9. Community resources

It is important to offer HIV/AIDS education in a language that the adolescent can understand. The information must be simple, accurate, and direct. In recent years, the federal government has put a lot of resources into *abstinence-only* prevention education. Unfortunately, there has never been any research documenting the long-term benefit from abstinence-only prevention education. In fact, in one study abstinence-only education was shown to increase the level of sexual activity in youth. *Abstinence-based* education, which also provides information on how to reduce risk if sexually active, has been shown to delay the onset of sexual activity in some studies. The CDC (http://www.cdc.gov/hiv/pubs/hivcompendium/hivcompendium.htm) posts information on their Web site, including "Programs that Work" and a "Compendium of Effective Interventions to Reduce HIV." They include only strategies that have been documented in the peer-reviewed literature as effective.

Kirby et al. (1994) reviewed the characteristics of school-based sexuality education programs. Effective programs were those that reflected the following key aspects:

- Used social learning theory as a foundation for program development.
- Included a narrow focus on reducing sexual risk-taking behaviors that may lead to HIV, STDs, or pregnancy.
- Provided basic, accurate information about the risks of unprotected intercourse and methods of avoiding unprotected intercourse through experiential activities designed to personalize this information.
- Included activities that address social or media influences on sexual behavior.
- Reinforced clear and appropriate values to strengthen individual values and group norms against unprotected sex.
- Provided modeling and practice in communication and negotiation skills.

TABLE 31.8

Stages of Behavioral Change

Stage	Definition	Goal	Objectives
Precontemplation	Not thinking about starting HAART	To shift the decisional balance regarding taking HAART from negative to positive	To assist youth to • Become aware of the HIV disease process and the potential value of HAART • Understand their personal reluctance to taking HAART • Consider the possibility of taking HAART
Contemplation	Thinking about starting HAART in the next 6 months	To complete the shift of decisional balance regarding taking HAART from negative to positive	To enable adolescents to • Assess their psychosocial and behavioral readiness to begin HAART • Enhance their self-esteem • Overcome their misgivings about their ability to adhere to HAART
Preparation	Planning to begin HAART in next 30 days or has made a recent attempt to begin	To maximize readiness to initiate HAART	To assist adolescents to • Overcome the barriers and strengthen the supports in their lives for adherence to HAART • Enhance their capacity for adherence • Build skills for taking medicines successfully
Action	Has been taking HAART for less than 6 months	To maintain successful adherence to HAART	To assist teens to • Maintain the therapeutic alliance • Continue to solicit the support they need in their lives to remain adherent • Determine and monitor progress toward shared therapeutic goals
Maintenance	Has been taking HAART for 6 months or more	To continue to maintain successful adherence to HAART	To continue to assist teens to • Maintain the therapeutic alliance • Continue to solicit the support they need in their lives to remain adherent • Determine and monitor progress toward shared therapeutic goals

HAART, highly active antiretroviral therapy.

Many youths are not at school and are therefore not reachable through school programs. Street youth service workers who have regular contact with these teens may be effective AIDS educators. Involving peers in the education process can also be helpful. Principles of youth development have shown promise in the prevention of a variety of adolescent high-risk behaviors. These programs:

• Build competencies and self-efficacy (the belief that trying will result in success).
• Help families and communities send consistent messages about standards for positive behavior.
• Expand opportunities and recognition for youth who engage in positive behavior and activities.
• Provide structure and consistency in program activities.
• Last a minimum of 9 months.
• Offer opportunities for engagement of youth in the development and implementation of services.

Secondary

Since the onset of the HIV epidemic, prevention efforts in the United States have largely targeted persons at risk for becoming infected with HIV and have been aimed at reducing sexual and drug-using risk behaviors. Although efforts continue to include primary prevention of HIV transmission, new efforts have also been initiated that target HIV-positive individuals as targets of HIV prevention. Launched in 2003, the CDC's new initiative, *Advancing HIV Prevention: New Strategies for a Changing Epidemic*, aims to reduce barriers to early diagnosis of HIV infection and increase access to quality medical care, treatment, and ongoing prevention services for those diagnosed with HIV. Advancing HIV Prevention includes four main areas:

1. Incorporating HIV testing as a routine part of care in traditional medical settings

2. Implementing new models for diagnosing HIV infections outside medical settings (e.g., rapid testing)
3. Preventing new infections by working with people diagnosed with HIV and their partners
4. Further decreasing mother-to-child HIV transmission

For physicians working with HIV-positive youth, it is important to assess, monitor, and attempt to influence potential risk behaviors while building a trusting provider/patient relationship in order to influence behavior change. The following key steps have been identified:

- Be persistent in efforts to engage and retain youth in services.
- Conduct a comprehensive interview at intake and update every 6 months (or as needed).
- Ask HIV-positive adolescents about their social life at every visit.
- Ask the same question in a variety of ways.
- Talk to youth about your concerns regarding their health.
- Explore the reasons for risky behavior and discuss common issues preventing youth from changing their behavior and disclosing their status (from *Developing Responsive Prevention Programs Targeting Youth living with HIV: A Guide for Medical Providers*).

Recommendations for Primary Care Physicians

Primary care practitioners should:

1. Obtain a sexual history and perform counseling on safer sexual behaviors.
2. Be able to perform pretest and posttest HIV antibody counseling.
3. Be able to co-manage individuals with HIV infections with HIV specialists (especially if the HIV care provider is not familiar with youth issues).
4. Know how to initiate the evaluation of common AIDS-related symptoms such as fever, lymphadenopathy, headache, and diarrhea.
5. Be familiar with community resources for adolescents in need of more intensive HIV prevention interventions.

Controlling Transmission

Blood and body fluid precautions should be consistently used for all patients, because medical history and examination cannot reliably identify all patients who are infected with HIV.

WEB SITES

General Resources

http://AIDSinfo.nih.gov. DHHS HIV treatment guideline for Adolescents and Adults (Oct 2004), Use of antiretrovirals in pregnancy (June 2004).
http://www.ucsf.edu/hivcntr/Clinical_Resources/.
http://www.cdc.gov/hiv/pubs/hivcompendium/hivcompendium.htm. Information on HIV prevention: "Programs that Work."

http://www.cdcnpin.org. National Prevention Information Network–Provides in-depth information about HIV/AIDS and STDs.
http://www.cdc.gov/HealthyYouth/YRBS/. Information on youth risk behaviors in 2005.

Information on Human Immunodeficiency Virus Counseling and Testing

http://www.cdc.gov/hiv. Guidelines for counseling and testing.
http://www.fda.gov/cber/products/testkits.htm. Licensed/approved HIV tests. Information on rapid testing including guidelines, sample consents, quality assurance, and CLIA application information. Consumer-oriented Treatment Information.
http://www.projinf.org/. Project Inform, with numerous articles on many aspects of HIV and AIDS.
http://www.thebody.com. The Body–An HIV and AIDS education site.

Occupational Exposure Issues and Information on Prevention of Human Immunodeficiency Virus and Other Occupational Needle-Stick Exposures

http://www.cdc.gov/mmwr/preview/mmwrhtml/rr5402a1.htm. CDC information on Postexposure prophylaxis.
http://www.cdc.gov/hiv/resources/guidelines/index.htm#occupational. Information on exposure to blood, preventing needlestick injuries, universal precautions.
http://www.cdc.gov/niosh/bbppg.html. Bloodborne Infectious Diseases, HIV/AIDS, Hepatitis B Virus, and Hepatitis C Virus.
http://www.cdc.gov/niosh/2000-108.html. Preventing Needlestick Injuries in Health Care Settings.

Information on Human Immunodeficiency Virus and Other Bloodborne Pathogens in Health Care Workers

http://www.cdc.gov/niosh/. Overview of State Needlestick Legislation (June, 2002).

Postexposure Prophylaxis

http://www.cdc.gov/mmwr/PDF/rr/rr5011.pdf. Updated U.S. Public Health Service Guidelines for the Management of Occupational Exposures to HBV, HCV, and HIV and Recommendations for Postexposure Prophylaxis.
http://www.cdc.gov/hiv/resources/guidelines/index.htm#occupational/. HIV postexposure prophylaxis registry.
National clinicians 24-hour hotline on postexposure prophylaxis (PEP)—telephone 1-888-HIV-4911, 1-888-448-4911 (project of the University of California at San Francisco).

Selected National Human Immunodeficiency Virus Resources

National Pediatric and Family HIV Resource Center, 30 Bergen Street, ADNC #4, Newark, NJ 07103, telephone 973-972 0410, fax 1-973-972-0399.

Magic Johnson Foundation, 6167 Bristol Parkway, Suite 450, Culver City, CA 90230, telephone 1-310-338-8110, fax 1-310-338-8563.

AIDS Alliance for Children, Youth and Families, 1600 K St. NW Suite 200, Washington, DC 20006, telephone 1-202-785-3564, fax 1-202-785-3579.

Advocates for Youth Media Project, telephone 310-234-0454, fax 310-441-6553, website-http://www.themedia-project.com. Advocates for Youth–National Office, 2000 M St. NW Suite 750 Washington, DC 20036, telephone 1-202-419-3420. Website www.advocatesforyouth.org.

AIDS Hotline, United States Public Health Service, telephone 1-800-342-2437 or 1-800-344-7432 in Spanish or 1-800-243-7889 for hearing-impaired persons. National Center for Youth Law–Adolescent Health Care Project, 405 14th Street, Suite 1500, Oakland, CA 94612, telephone 1-510-835-8098, fax 1-510-835-8099. Website www.youthlaw.org.

CDC AIDS Prevention Information Clearinghouse, telephone 1-800-458-5231.

Pacific AIDS Education–Training Center: For help with a clinical HIV problem, telephone 1-800-933-3413.

World Health Organization, Appropriate Health Resources and Technologies Action Group–Essential AIDS Information Resources: For catalog, write to CH 1211 Geneva 27, Switzerland or telephone +41-22-791-4652.

Educational Resources

ETR Associates: Has comprehensive Health Education Resources for grades K-12. Includes HIV or AIDS, STDs, Drugs, Family Life Education, and Reproductive Health. Telephone 1-800-321-4407. Web site www.etr.org.

Project SNAPP–Skills and Knowledge for AIDS and Pregnancy Prevention: An 8-session curriculum and video for middle school students. From Division of Adolescent Medicine, Children's Hospital Los Angeles; published by ETR Associates, telephone 1-800-321-4407.

CDC AIDS Prevention Clearinghouse: Has lists of HIV or AIDS materials. Telephone 1-800-458-5231.

Advocates for Youth: Has fact sheets on youth sexuality including HIV or AIDS and many educational materials. Telephone 1-202-419-3420. Web site www.advocatesforyouth.org.

Alfred Higgins Production, Inc. (video): Teens At Risk: Breaking the Immortality Myth. Telephone 1-310-440-3232.

San Francisco Study Center (video): Between Friends. Telephone 1-415-626-1650.

REFERENCES AND ADDITIONAL READINGS

American Academy of Pediatrics. AAP statement on adolescents and HIV American Academy of Pediatrics [News]. *Am Fam Physician* 1993;48:346.

Barns PE, Le HQ, Davidson PT. Tuberculosis in patients with HIV infection. *Med Clin North Am* 1993;77:1369.

Belzer ME, Fuchs DN, Luftman GS, et al. Antiretroviral adherence issues among HIV-positive adolescents and young adults. *J Adolesc Health* 1999;25:316.

Belzer ME, Rogers AS, Camarca M, et al. Adolescent medicine HIV/AIDS research network. Contraceptive choices in HIV-infected and HIV at-risk adolescent females. *J Adolesc Health* 2001;29(suppl):93.

Bozzette SA, Finkelstein DM, Spector SA, et al. A randomized trial of three antipneumocystis agents in patients with advanced human immunodeficiency virus infection. *N Engl J Med* 1995;332:693.

Braun L. Role of human immunodeficiency virus infection in the pathogenesis of human papillomavirus-associated cervical neoplasia. *Am J Pathol* 1994;144:209.

Brown LK, Lourie KJ, Pao M. *Children and adolescents living with HIV and AIDS: a review.* Great Britain: Cambridge University Press, 2000.

Brown LK, Schultz JR, Gragg RA. HIV-infected adolescents with hemophilia: adaptation and coping. The Hemophilia Behavioral Intervention Evaluation Project. *Pediatrics* 1995;96:459.

Burke DS, Brundage JF, Goldenbaum M, et al. Human immunodeficiency virus infections in teenagers: seroprevalence among applicants for U.S. Military Service. *JAMA* 1990;263:2074.

Cao Y, Qin L, Zhang L, et al. Virologic and immunologic characterization of long-term survivors of human immunodeficiency virus type 1 infection. *N Engl J Med* 1995;332:201.

Centers for Disease Control and Prevention. HIV-related beliefs, knowledge, and behaviors among high school students. *MMWR Morb Mortal Wkly Rep* 1988;37:717.

Center for Disease Control and Prevention. Staging of HIV/AIDS. *MMWR Morb Mortal Wkly Rep* 1992;41(RR-17):1.

Centers for Disease Control and Prevention. Case-control study of HIV seroconversion in health-care workers after percutaneous exposure to HIV infected. *MMWR Morb Mortal Wkly Rep* 1995;44:929.

Centers for Disease Control and Prevention. Guidelines for preventing opportunistic infections among HIV-infected persons-2002 recommendations of the USPHS and the Infectious Disease Society of America. *MMWR Morb Mortal Wkly Rep* 2002;51:RR–R8.

Centers for Disease Control and Prevention. Protocols for confirmation of rapid HIV tests. *MMWR Morb Mortal Wkly Rep* 2004a;53:329.

Centers for Disease Control and Prevention. Youth risk behavior surveillance—United States, 2003. *MMWR Morb Mortal Wkly Rep* 2004b:53(SS-2):1. (Available at: http://www.cdc.gov/HealthyYouth/yrbs/index.htm, accessed November 13, 2005).

Centers for Disease Control and Prevention. Summary of notifiable diseases—United States, 2004 *MMWR Morb Mortal Wkly Rep* 2005;53:1.

Centers for Disease Control and Prevention. *HIV/AIDS surveillance report, 2004,* Vol. 16. Atlanta. US Department of Health and Human Services, Centers for Disease Control and Prevention. 2005. Also available at http://www.cdc.gov/hiv/stats/hasrlink.htm.

Center for Disease Control and Prevention. Trends in HIV/AIDS diagnoses—33 United States, 2001–2004. *MMWR Morb Mortal Wkly Rep* 2005a;54(45):1149.

Centers for Disease Control and Prevention. *Comprehensive HIV prevention messages for young people.* http://www.cdc.gov/nchstp/od/news/compyout.htm. 2005b.

Centers for Disease Control and Prevention. *HIV/AIDS statics and surveillance.* www.cdc.gov/hiv/topics/surveillance/basic.htm. Accessed 2006.

Centers for Disease Control and Prevention. Revised recommendations for HIV testing of adults, adolescents, and pregnant women in health-care settings. *MMWR Morb Mortal Wkly Rep* 2006;55:RR–14.

Centers for Disease Control and Prevention. Youth risk behavior surveillance—United States, 2005. *Morb Mortal Wkly Rep CDC Surveill Summ* 2006;55(SS05);1.

Chaisson RE, Keruly JC, Moore RD. Race, sex, drug use, and progression of human immunodeficiency virus disease. *N Engl J Med* 1995;333:751.

Chesney Margaret. Adherence to HAART regimens. *AIDS Patient Care STDs* 2003;17(4):169.

Chu QD, Medeiros LJ, Fisher AE, et al. Thrombotic thrombocytopenic purpura and HIV infection. *South Med J* 1995;88:82.

Clark LR, Brasseux C, Richmond D, et al. Effect of HIV counseling and testing on sexually transmitted diseases and condom use in an urban adolescent population. *Arch Pediatr Adolesc Med* 1998;152:269.

Concorde Coordinating Committee. Concorde: MRC/ANRS randomised double-blind controlled trial of immediate and deferred zidovudine in symptom-free HIV infection. *Lancet* 1994;343:871.

Connor EM, Sperling RS, Gelber R, et al. Reduction of maternal-infant transmission of human immunodeficiency virus type 1 with zidovudine treatment. *N Engl J Med* 1994;331:1173.

Consortium for Retrovirus Serology Standardization. Serological diagnosis of human immunodeficiency virus infection by Western blot testing. *JAMA* 1988;260:674.

Constantine NT, Zhang X, Li L, et al. Application of a rapid assay for detection of antibodies to human immunodeficiency virus in urine. *Clin Microbiol Infect Dis* 1994;101:157.

Conway GA, Epstein MR, Hayman CR, et al. Trends in HIV prevalence among disadvantaged youth: survey results from a National Job Training Program, 1988 through 1992. *JAMA* 1991;265:1709.

Cote J, Godin G. Efficacy and interventions in improving adherence to antiretroviral therapy. *Int J STD AIDS* 2005;16:335.

D'Angelo LJ. Adolescents and HIV infection: a clinician's perspective. *Acta Paediatr* 1994;400:88S.

Daar ES, Little S, Pitt J, et al. Diagnosis of primary HIV-1 infection. *Ann Intern Med* 2001;134:25.

Daul CB, DeShezo RD, Andes WA. Human immunodeficiency virus infection in hemophiliac patients. *Am J Med* 1988;84:801.

Denning PH, Jones JL, Ward JW. Recent trends in the HIV epidemic in adolescent and young adult gay and bisexual men. *J Acquir Immune Defic Syndr Hum Retrovirol* 1997;16:374.

Douglas SD, Rudy B, Muenz L, et al. Peripheral blood mononuclear cell markers in antiretroviral therapy-naïve HIV-infected and high-risk seronegative adolescents. *AIDS* 1999;13:1629.

English A. AIDS testing and epidemiology for youth: recommendation of the work group. *J Adolesc Health Care* 1989;10:52.

Fahey JL, Taylor JMG, Detels R, et al. The prognostic value of cellular and serologic markers in infection with human immunodeficiency virus type 1. *N Engl J Med* 1990;322:166.

Feldblum PJ, Fortney JA. Condoms, spermicides, and the transmission of human immunodeficiency virus: a review of the literature. *Am J Public Health* 1988;78:52.

Fowler MG, Melnick SL, Mathieson BJ. Women and HIV epidemiology and global overview. *Obstet Gynecol Clin North Am* 1997;24:705.

Freedberg KA, Samet JH. Think HIV: why physicians should lower their threshold for HIV testing. *Arch Intern Med* 1999;159:1994.

French MA, Price P, Stone SF. Immune restoration disease after antiretroviral therapy. *AIDS* 2004;18:1615.

Futterman DC. HIV and AIDS in adolescents. *Adolesc Med Clin* 2004;15:369.

Futterman D, Hein K, Reuben N, et al. Human immunodeficiency virus-infected adolescents: the first 50 patients in a New York City program. *Pediatrics* 1993;91:730.

Gallant JE. HIV counseling, testing, and referral. *Am Fam Physician* 2004;70:295.

Gallant M, Maticka-Tyndale E. School-based HIV prevention programmes for African American youth. *Social Sci Med* 2004;58:1337.

Gayle HD, D'Angelo LJ. Epidemiology of acquired immunodeficiency syndrome and human immunodeficiency virus infection in adolescents. *Pediatr Infect Dis J* 1991;10:322.

Gordon SM, Eaton ME, George R, et al. The response of symptomatic neurosyphilis to high-dose intravenous penicillin G in patients with human immunodeficiency virus infection. *N Engl J Med* 1994;331:1469.

Gross KL, Porco TC, Grant RM. HIV-1 superinfection and viral diversity. *AIDS* 2004;18:1513.

Hammer SM. Management of newly diagnosed HIV infection. *N Engl J Med* 2005;353:1702.

Havens PL. Postexposure prophylaxis in children and adolescents for nonoccupational exposure to human immunodeficiency virus. *Pediatrics* 2003;111:1475.

Hayman C, Peterson L, Miller C. *HIV infection in underprivileged teenagers: update from the Job Corps [Abstract]. Sixth International Conference on AIDS*. San Francisco, 1990.

Health Resources and Services Administration HIV/AIDS Bureau. *Helping adolescents with HIV adhere to HAART*. U.S. Department of Health & Human Services, 1999.

Hein K, Dell R, Futterman D, et al. Pediatrics: comparison of HIV+ and HIV- adolescents. Risk factors and psychosocial determinants. *Pediatrics* 1995;95:96.

Ho DD. Viral counts count in HIV infection. *Science* 1996;272:1124.

Ho DD, Neumann AU, Perelson AS, et al. Rapid turnover of plasma virions and CD4 lymphocytes in HIV-1 infection. *Nature* 1995;373:123.

Holland CA, Ellenberg JH, Wilson CM, et al. Adolescent medicine HIV/AIDS research network. Relationship of CD4+ T cell counts and HIV type 1 viral loads in untreated, infected adolescents. *AIDS Res Hum Retroviruses* 2000;16:959.

Holland CA, Yong MA, Moscicki AB, et al. Adolescent medicine HIV/AIDS research network. Seroprevalence and risk factors of hepatitis B, hepatitis C, and human cytomegalovirus among HIV-infected and high-risk uninfected adolescents. *Sex Trans Dis* 2000;27:296.

Holtgrave DR, Qualls NL, Curran JW, et al. An overview of the effectiveness and efficiency of HIV prevention programs. *Public Health Rep* 1995;110:134.

Hoth DF, Bolognesi DP, Corey L, et al. HIV vaccine development: a progress report. *Ann Intern Med* 1994;121:603.

Johnston LD, O'Malley PM, Bachman JG. *National survey of American high school seniors [Press release]*. Ann Arbor, MI: News and Information Services, University of Michigan, 2000.

Jones JL, Hanson DL, Chu SY, et al. Surveillance of AIDS-defining conditions in the United States. Adult/Adolescent Spectrum of HIV Disease Project Group. *AIDS* 1994;8:1489.

Kamb M, Fishbein M, Douglas J, et al. Project RESPECT Study Group. Efficacy of risk-reduction counseling to prevent human immunodeficiency virus and sexually transmitted diseases. *JAMA* 1998;280:1161.

Keusch GT, Thea DM. Malnutrition in AIDS. *Med Clin North Am* 1993;77:795.

Kipke MD, O'Connor S, Palmer R, et al. Street youth in Los Angeles: profile of a group at high risk for human immunodeficiency virus infection. *Arch Pediatr Adolesc Med* 1995; 149:513.

Kirby D, Short L, Collins J, et al. School-based programs to reduce sexual risk behaviors: a review of effectiveness. *Public Health Rep* 1994;109:339.

Kordi R, Wallace WA. Blood borne infections in sport: risks of transmission, methods of prevention, and recommendations for hepatitis B vaccination. *Br J Sports Med* 2004;38:678.

Laine L, Bonacini M. Esophageal disease in human immunodeficiency virus infection. *Arch Intern Med* 1994;154:1577.

Levy JA. The transmission of HIV and factors influencing progression to AIDS. *Am J Med* 1993;95:86.

Letvin NL. Strategies for an HIV vaccine. *J Clin Invest* 2002; 110:15.

Lifson AR. Do alternate modes for transmission of human immunodeficiency virus exist? A review. *JAMA* 1988;259:1353.

Lindegren ML, Hanson C, Miller K, et al. Epidemiology of human immunodeficiency virus infection in adolescents, United States. *Pediatr Infect Dis* 1994;13:525.

Little SJ, Holte S, Routy JP, et al. Antiretroviral-drug resistance among patients recently infected with HIV. *N Engl J Med* 2002;347:389.

Lyon ME, D'Angelo LJ. *Teenagers, HIV and AIDS.* Ed. Lyon ME and D'Angelo LJ. Westport, Conneticut: Praeger Publishers, 2006.

Lyons C. HIV drug adherence: special situations. *J Assoc Nurses AIDS Care* 1997;8:29.

Main DS, Iverson DC, McGloin J, et al. Preventing HIV infection among adolescents: evaluation of a school-based education program. *Prev Med* 1994;23:409.

Mahoney EM, Donfield SM, Howard C, et al. HIV-associated immune dysfunction and delayed pubertal development in a cohort of young hemophiliacs. *J AIDS* 1999;21:333.

Markovitz DM. Infection with the human immunodeficiency virus type 2. *Ann Intern Med* 1993;118:211.

Martinez J, Bell D, Camacho R, et al. Adherence to antiretroviral drug regimens in HIV-infected adolescent patients engaged in care in a comprehensive adolescent and young adult clinic. *J Natl Med Assoc* 2000;92:55.

Mast EE, Goodman RA, Bond WW, et al. Transmission of blood-borne pathogens during sports: risk and prevention. *Ann Intern Med* 1995;122:283.

Medical News and Perspectives. When sports and HIV share the bill, smart money goes on common sense. *JAMA* 1992;267: 1311.

Mellors JW, Kingsley LA, Rinaldo CR Jr, et al. Quantitation of HIV-1 RNA in plasma predicts outcome after seroconversion. *Ann Intern Med* 1995;122:573.

Mellors JW, Rinaldo CR, Gupta P, et al. Prognosis in HIV-1 infection predicted by the quantity of virus in plasma. *Science* 1996;272:1167.

Millstein SG, Moscicki AB, Broering JM. Female adolescents at high, moderate, and low risk of exposure to HIV: differences in knowledge, beliefs, and behavior. *J Adolesc Health Care* 1994;15:133.

Moodley J, Moodley D. Management of human immunodeficiency virus infection in pregnancy. *Best Pract Res Clin Obstet Gynecol* 2005;19:169.

Moscicki AB, Millstein SG, Broering J, et al. Risks of human immunodeficiency virus infection among adolescents attending three diverse clinics. *J Pediatr* 1993;122:813.

Moss N. Behavioral risks for HIV in adolescents. *Acta Paediatr* 1994;400:81S.

Murphy DA, Belzer ME, Durako SJ, et al. Longitudinal antiretroviral adherence among adolescents infected with human immunodeficiency virus. *Arch Pediatr Adolesc Med* 2005; 159:764.

Murphy DA, Durako SD, Muenz L, et al. Marijuana use among HIV+ and high-risk adolescents: a comparison of self-report through audio computer-assisted self-administered interviewing and urinalysis. *Am J Epidemiol* 2000;152:805.

Murphy DA, Moscicki AB, Vermund SH, et al. Psychological distress among HIV-positive adolescents in the REACH study: effects of life stress, social support, and coping. *J Adolesc Health* 2000;27:391.

Murphy DA, Rotheram MJ, Reid HM. Adolescent gender differences in HIV-related sexual risk acts, social-cognitive factors, and behavioral skills. *J Adolesc* 1998;21:197.

Murphy DA, Sarr M, Durako SJ, et al. Barriers to HAART adherence among human immunodeficiency virus-infected adolescents. *Arch Pediatr Adolesc Med* 2003;157:249.

Murphy DA, Wilson CM, Durako SD, et al. Antiretroviral medication adherence among the REACH HIV-infected adolescent cohort. *AIDS Care* 2001;13:27.

Niu MT, Stein DS, Schnittman SM. Primary human immunodeficiency virus type 1 infection: review of pathogenesis and early treatment intervention in humans and animal retrovirus infections. *J Infect Dis* 1993;168:1490.

O'Connor PG, Selwyn PA, Schottenfeld RS. Medical care for injection-drug users with human immunodeficiency virus infection. *N Engl J Med* 1994;331:450.

Office of National AIDS Policy. *Youth and HIV/AIDS 2000: a new American agenda.* Washington, DC: Office of National AIDS Policy, 2000.

Osmond D, Charlebois E, Lang W, et al. Changes in AIDS survival time in two San Francisco cohorts of homosexual men, 1983 to 1993. *JAMA* 1994;271:1083.

Palefsky J. Anal cancer in HIV infection. *Int AIDS Soc* 2000;8:14.

Pao M, Lyon M, D'Angelo L, et al. Psychiatric diagnoses in adolescents seropositive for the human immunodeficiency virus. *Arch Pediatr Adolesc Med* 2000;154:240.

Peckham C, Gibb D. Mother-to-child transmission of the human immunodeficiency virus. *N Engl J Med* 1995;333:298.

Pedlow CT, Carey MP. HIV sexual risk-reduction interventions for youth: a review and methodological critique of randomized controlled trials. *Behav Modif* 2003;27:135.

Pedlow CT, Carey MP. Developmentally appropriate sexual risk reduction interventions for adolescents: rationale, review of interventions, and recommendations for research and practice. *Ann Behav Med* 2004;27:172.

Pennbridge JN, Belzer ME, Schneir AS, et al. *AIDS: a complete guide to psychosocial intervention.* In: Land H, ed. *Adolescents, HIV, and AIDS.* Milwaukee, WI: Family Service of America, 1992:169.

Perrin EC. *Sexual orientation in child and adolescent health care.* New York: Kluwer Academic/Plenum Publishers, 2002.

Perrin EC, Sack S. Health and development of gay and lesbian youths: implication for HIV/AIDS. *AIDS Patient Care STDs* 1998;12:303.

Prochaska JQ, DiClemente CC. Stages and process of self change of smoking: toward an integrative model of change. *J Consult Clin Psychol* 1983;51:390.

Quinn TC. Acute primary HIV infection. *JAMA* 1997;278:58.

Raj R, Verghese A. Human immunodeficiency virus infections in adolescents. *Adolesc Med* 2000;11:359.

Rawitscher LA, Saitz R, Friedman LS. Adolescents' preferences regarding human immunodeficiency virus (HIV)-related physician counseling and HIV testing. *Pediatrics* 1995; 96:52.

Remafedi G, Lauer T. Survival trends in adolescents with human immunodeficiency virus infection. *Arch Pediatr Adolesc Med* 1995;149:1093.

Robin L, Dittus P, Whitaker D, et al. Behavioral interventions to reduce incidence of HIV, STD, and pregnancy among adolescents: a decade in review. *J Adolesc Health* 2004;34:3.

Robinson EK, Evans BG. Oral sex and HIV transmission. *AIDS* 1999;13:737.

Rogers AS. AIDS and adolescents: exploring the challenge. *J Adolesc Health Care* 1989;10(Suppl 3):15.

Rogers AS, Ellenberg JH, Douglas SD, et al. The prevalence of anergy in human immunodeficiency virus infected adolescents and in the association of delayed-type hypersensitivity with subject characteristics. *J Adolesc Health* 2000;27:384.

Rogers AS, Futterman D, Levin L, et al. A profile of human immunodeficiency virus-infected adolescents receiving health care services at selected sites in the United States. *J Adolesc Health* 1996;19:401.

Rogers AS, Futterman D, Moscicki AB, et al. Adolescent Medicine HIV/AIDS Research Network. The REACH project of the adolescent medicine HIV/AIDS research network: design, methods, and selected characteristics of participants. *J Adolesc Health* 1998;22:300.

Rogers AS, Schwarz DF, Weissman G, et al. A case study in adolescent participation in clinical research: eleven clinical sites, one common protocol, and eleven IRBs. IRB. *A Rev Human Subj Res* 1999;21:6.

Rotheram-Borus MJ, Futterman D. Promoting early detection of human immunodeficiency virus among adolescents. *Arch Pediatr Adolesc Med* 2000;154:435.

Rotheram-Borus ML, Koopman C, Haignere C, et al. Reducing HIV sexual risk behaviors among runaway adolescents. *JAMA* 1991;266:1237.

Samet J, Winter M, Grant L, et al. Factors associated with HIV testing among sexually active adolescents: a Massachusetts survey. *Pediatrics* 1997;100:371.

Schoeberlein DR, Woolston JL, Brett J. School-based HIV prevention. *Child Adolesc Psychiatr Clin N Am* 2000;9:389.

Schneir A, Wilson E. *Developing responsive prevention programs targeting youth living with HIV: a guide for medical providers.* Los Angeles: Los Angeles County Health Department, Office of AIDS Programs and Policy, 2003.

Sellers DE, McGraw SA, McKinlay JB. Does the promotion and distribution of condoms increase teen sexual activity? Evidence from an HIV prevention program for Latino youth. *Am J Public Health* 1994;84:1952.

Sewell DD, Jeste DV, Atkinson JH. HIV associated psychosis: a study of 20 cases. San Diego HIV Neurobehavioral Research Center Group. *Am J Psychiatry* 1994;151:237.

Sikkema KJ, Bissett RT. Concepts, goals, and techniques of counseling: review and implications for HIV counseling and testing. *AIDS Educ Prev* 1997;9(suppl):14.

Society for Adolescent Medicine. HIV infection and AIDS in adolescents: a position paper of the society for adolescent medicine. *J Adolesc Health Care* 1994;15:427.

Stamm WE, Handsfield HH, Rompalo AM, et al. The association between genital ulcer disease and acquisition of HIV infection in homosexual men. *JAMA* 1988;260:1429.

Strathdee SA, O'Shaughnessy MV, Montaner JSG, et al. A decade of research on the natural history of HIV infection: Part 1. Markers. *Clin Invest Med* 1996;19:111.

Stricof RL, Novick LE, Kennedy JT. *HIV-1 seroprevalence in facilities for runaway and homeless adolescents in four states [Abstract].* Sixth International Conference on AIDS, San Francisco, 1990.

Sullivan KE, Cutilli J, Piliero LM, et al. Measurement of cytokine secretion, intracellular protein expression and messenger RNA in resting and stimulated peripheral blood mononuclear cells. *Clin Diagn Lab Immunol* 2000;7:920.

Sullivan PS, Lansky A, Drake A. Failure to return for HIV test results among persons at high risk for HIV infection: results from a multistate interview project. *J AIDS* 2004;35:511.

Sweeney P, Lindegren ML, Buehler JW, et al. Teenagers at risk of human immunodeficiency virus type 1 infection: results from seroprevalence surveys in the United States. *Arch Pediatr Adolesc Med* 1995;149:521.

United Nations Programme on HIV/AIDS (UNAIDS). *AIDS epidemic update 2004.* Available at: http://www.unaids.org. December 2004.

U.S. Department of Health and Human Services. Antiretroviral postexposure prophylaxis after sexual, injection-drug use, or other nonoccupational exposure to HIV in the United States: recommendations from the U.S. Department of Health and Human Services. *MMWR Morb Mortal Wkly Rep* 2005; 54(RR02):1.

Valdiserri RO. HIV counseling and testing: its evolving role in HIV prevention. *AIDS Educ Prev* 1997;9:2.

Valleroy LA, MacKellar DA, Karon JM, et al. Young men's survey group: HIV prevalence and associated risks in young men who have sex with men. *JAMA* 2000;284:198.

Varghese GK, Crane LR. Evaluation and treatment of HIV-related illnesses in the emergency department. *Ann Emerg Med* 1994;24:503.

Walters AS. HIV Prevention in street youth. *Soc Adolesc Med* 1999;25:187.

Wang CY, Snow JL, Su WP. Lymphoma associated with human immunodeficiency virus infection. *Mayo Clin Proc* 1995;70:665.

Weiss RA. How does HIV cause AIDS? *Science* 1993;260:1273.

Wendell DA, Onorato IM, McCray E, et al. Youth at risk: sex, drugs and human immunodeficiency virus. *Am J Dis Child* 1992;146:76.

Wilfert CM, Wilson C, Luzuriaga K, et al. Pathogenesis of pediatric human immunodeficiency virus type 1 infection. *J Infect Dis* 1994;170:286.

Woods ER, Samples CL, Singer B, et al. Young people and HIV/AIDS: the need for a continuum of care: findings and policy recommendations from nine adolescent focused projects supported by the Special Projects of National Significance Program. *AIDS Public Policy J* 2002;17(3):90.

Zhang L, Ramratnam B, Tenner-Racz K, et al. Quantifying residual HIV-1 replication in patients receiving combination antiretroviral therapy. *N Engl J Med* 1999;340:1605.

PART IX

Conditions Affecting Nutrition and Weight

CHAPTER 32

Obesity

Marcie B. Schneider

Obesity is a serious medical problem that is increasing in prevalence in the adolescent and adult population. Almost two thirds (65.7%) of adults are overweight or obese. Obesity is associated with up to 325,000 deaths/year and a shortened lifespan.

Obesity is a now a common problem among adolescents. In children and adolescents, the term obesity has been replaced by overweight. The prevalence of overweight in American adolescents ranges from 12.7% to 24.7%, depending on gender and race. It is a condition in which the psychobiological cues for eating are discordant with energy requirements. Both genetic and environmental factors contribute to overweight problems. Studies on fraternal twins raised apart suggest a strong genetic influence on body mass index (BMI). Genetic mutations have also been identified. Endocrine and metabolic causes such as hypothyroidism, hypercortisolism, and Prader-Willi syndrome occur infrequently in adolescents.

The Expert Committee on Clinical Guidelines for Overweight in Adolescent Preventive Services (Himes and Dietz, 1994) recommends screening adolescents for overweight and at risk for overweight by using the BMI. The BMI is equal to the weight in kilograms divided by the square of the height in meters:

$$BMI = Weight\ in\ kilograms/height\ in\ meters^2$$

Adolescents' body fatness changes over the years with growth and development. Teenage girls and boys differ in their body fatness as they mature. This is why BMI for adolescents, also referred to as *BMI-for-age*, is gender and age specific. It is an easy index to calculate and has a correlation of 0.7 to 0.8 with body fat content in adults. The correlation coefficient of BMI with body fat content is 0.39 to 0.90 in children and adolescents.

For children and adolescents, at risk for overweight is defined as a BMI between the 85th and 95th percentiles for age and gender, while overweight is defined as BMI exceeding the 95th percentile for age and gender. BMI values in adolescents are listed in Chapter 1 (Figs. 1.25 and 1.26). Chapter 4 (Figs. 4.8 and 4.9) also shows height, weight, and BMI by age and gender. BMI-for-age charts can be obtained from the Centers for Disease Control and Prevention (CDC) on their Web site: www.cdc.gov/growthcharts/.

The standards for defining obesity in adults 20 years and older were changed in 1998, following changes to the World Health Organization (WHO) definitions in 1995.

This has increased the number of adults identified in the United States as being overweight or obese. The definition changed the lower limit for BMI for overweight persons from 27.8 kg/m^2 in adult men and 27.3 kg/m^2 in women to 25 kg/m^2.

The criteria published in 1998 by the National Heart, Lung and Blood Institute (NHLBI) of the National Institutes of Health (NIH) (1998) in Clinical Guidelines for Identification, Evaluation, and Treatment of Overweight and Obesity in Adults (Archives of Internal Medicine, 1998) include the following:

NHLBI Classification	BMI Range (kg/m^2)
Underweight	<18.5
Normal	18.5–24.9
Overweight	25–29.9
Obesity class I	30–34.9
Obesity class II	35–39.9
Extreme obesity class III	≥40

Although total body fat can be measured indirectly by a variety of techniques, its use is limited to the research laboratory or clinical studies. However, a clinically useful method is the measurement of triceps skinfold thickness. Barlow and Dietz (1998) published a chart of triceps skinfold thickness for age and gender where greater than the 95th percentile suggests excessive fatness (Table 32.1).

To measure triceps skinfold, calipers are placed 1 centimeter above the midpoint between the acromion and olecranon process on the posterior (triceps area) of a relaxed right arm and measured 3 times, using the average as the thickness. This measurement does not take into account the regional distribution of body fat, which in adults has been correlated with future obesity-related health risk. Potentially useful measurements in adults older than 20 years are the waist circumference and the waist-hip ratio. Many studies have demonstrated distribution of body fat as an independent risk factor for cardiovascular disease. Visceral abdominal fat is more likely to contribute to elevated blood cholesterol and other lipid abnormalities, glucose intolerance, and hypertension. Normal values for waist circumference in children and adolescents are being studied. A recent study using these norms correlated waist circumference with risk for insulin resistance (Hirschler et al., 2005).

TABLE 32.1

Triceps Skinfold Measurements in Children and Adolescents

Age in Years	95% Skinfold Thickness in Males (mm)	95% Skinfold Thickness in Females (mm)
6–6.9	14.6	16
7–7.9	16.7	18
8–8.9	17	20
9–9.9	19.9	22
10–10.9	21	24
11–11.9	22	26
12–12.9	23	28
13–13.9	24	30
14–14.9	23	31
15–15.9	22	32
16–16.9	22	33
17–17.9	22	34
18–18.9	22	34
19–19.9	22	35

Adapted from Barlow SE, Dietz WH. Obesity evaluation and treatment: expert committee recommendations. *Pediatrics* 1998;102:e29.

In summary, methods that use just height and weight are inexpensive and easy to use but do not reflect regional body fat distribution. Skinfold measurements can be inaccurate due to interobserver error. Further research on waist circumference in children and adolescents may prove to be a useful measure. The current developmentally based BMI percentile curves overcome many of the difficulties found in the past height-for-weight charts, but still do not reflect important body fat distribution characteristics.

PUBERTAL CHANGES

Effects of Puberty on Body Composition

During adolescence, lean body mass increases in both sexes. The increase is greater in males because of their greater increase in skeletal muscle. The maximum increase in muscle mass occurs at about the time of peak height velocity (PHV) in both sexes, whereas the maximum fat deposition occurs 2 years before PHV. However, in females, fat deposition continues throughout puberty and females ultimately have more body fat than males.

Effects of Obesity on Puberty

1. Overweight adolescents tend to be taller and larger in skeletal mass and more advanced in skeletal development. Shortness in an overweight preadolescent or early adolescent should raise a "red flag" for possible endocrine disease.

2. Overweight female adolescents tend to have earlier sexual maturation. Black females however, have earlier menarche than whites even after adjustment for weight and height. A recent study (Sun et al., 2005) demonstrated that over that past 30 years menarche has occurred 0.46 and 0.25 years earlier in black and white girls respectively; the current median age of menarche in black girls is 12.06 years and in white girls is 12.55 years.

3. Menstrual irregularities are often seen in overweight adolescents. Aromatization of androgens to estrogen occurs in adipose tissue and is a significant source of extragonadal estrogen. Therefore, excessive body fat, through its effect on peripheral estrogen metabolism, may lead to suppression of follicle-stimulating hormone (FSH) and sensitization of the pituitary gland to release gonadotropin-releasing hormone, with a resultant increase in luteinizing hormone (LH). The resultant changes in FSH and LH can stimulate androstenedione and testosterone production in the ovary and can be associated with the anovulatory cycles characteristic of polycystic ovarian syndrome.

ETIOLOGY

Many theories have been advanced, but the cause of obesity is still unclear. Obesity is a chronic condition with multiple factors contributing to its etiology. Genetic, cultural, socioeconomic, behavioral, and situational factors all play a role in establishing dietary habits and thereby weight control. At some time in future, obesity may be divided into different disease classifications, with therapies tailored to match the underlying cause. At present, only 5% of overweight children and adolescents have an underlying cause identified. This includes approximately 3% with endocrine problems (hypothyroidism, Cushing syndrome, hypogonadism) and 2% with rare syndromes (Prader-Willi, Laurence-Moon-Biedl, Fröhlich, Alström, Kallmann).

INFLUENCING FACTORS

Familial or Genetic

1. There is an increased incidence of obesity among those with obese parents. In one study of Swedish twins, if one parent was obese, there was a 30% risk for the child to be overweight; if both parents were obese, there was a 70% risk for the child to be overweight. Despite the genetic implications, these findings may also be partially environmentally influenced.

2. Stunkard et al. (1990) found a high correlation of BMI between twins, even when reared apart.

3. Stunkard et al. (1986) also demonstrated that there was a strong relationship between the weight class of adoptees and the BMI of their biological parents. There was no relationship between the weight class of the adoptees and the BMI of their adoptive parents.

4. Identified genes linked to obesity include mutations in leptin, leptin receptor, neuropeptide Y, proopiomelanocortin, prohormone convertase 1, and melanocortin receptor MC4R. Obesity loci have been found on chromosomes 2, 5, 10, 11, and 20.

Activity and Energy Expenditure

There are conflicting reports regarding energy expenditure in obese individuals. Obese individuals filmed in time-lapse photography seem to move less than normal-weight individuals. Although some studies show no evidence to implicate a decrease in energy utilization in those who are overweight, Ravussin et al. (1988) found that the rates of energy expenditure were lower in obese individuals and that these rates of expenditure seem to cluster in families. Dietz (1993), drawing from longitudinal data collected in the National Health and Nutrition Examination Surveys (NHANES) study, stated that the most powerful predictor of the development of overweight in adolescence was the time that a child (6–11 years) spends viewing television, even after controlling for other known variables associated with overweight in childhood. For every extra hour of television watched by 12- to 17-year olds, there is a 2% increase in prevalence of overweight. Hernandez et al. (1999) found a 12% increase in prevalence of overweight for each hour of television watched and a 10% decrease in overweight prevalence with every hour of daily exercise in Mexican children. Recently, Epstein et al. (2005) reported that decreasing sedentary behaviors led to a decrease in energy intake, and Gutin et al. (2005) found that adolescents who regularly engaged in exercise were more likely to be fit and lean.

Caloric Intake

Caloric intake is variably elevated in overweight adolescents and is dependent on where they eat. In one study, overweight adolescent boys ingested more calories at school than at home, compared with their lean counterparts. Retrospective diet histories tend to underreport caloric intake in both overweight and nonoverweight adolescents, but more so in the overweight.

Behavior

Overweight adolescents often exhibit the following behaviors:

1. Eating fast
2. Skipping breakfast and lunch and ingesting most of their food at night
3. Eating not when *hungry* but when food is available or when their *appetite* is stimulated by environmental cues
4. Eating when depressed or anxious
5. Eating in association with other activities, such as watching television
6. Underestimating the total number of calories ingested
7. Overindulging in "fast foods"
8. Participation in unhealthy weight control practices
9. Increased sedentary behavior

EPIDEMIOLOGY

1. Data from the NHANES from 1999 to 2002 showed that a substantial proportion of children and adolescents in the United States were overweight (Table 32.2). Of adolescents between 12 and 19 years old, 16.1% were overweight (BMI >95%) and 14.8% were at risk for overweight (BMI 85%–95%). Therefore, a total of 30.9% of adolescents had a BMI > the 85th percentile. More Mexican-Americans were overweight (22.5%) than non-Hispanic blacks (21.1%) or non-Hispanic whites (13.7%). More Mexican-American males were overweight than Mexican-American females; more non-Hispanic white males were overweight than non-Hispanic white females; and more non-Hispanic black females were overweight than non-Hispanic black males.
2. Trends (Table 32.3): Data from the NHANES done in 1976 to 1980, 1988 to 1994, and 1999 to 2002 have shown that the prevalence of overweight in 12- to 19-year olds increased from 5% to 10.5% to 16.1%, respectively; the prevalence of overweight in males increased from 4.8% to 11.3% to 16.7%, respectively and the prevalence of overweight in females increased from 5.6% to 9.7% to 15.4%, respectively.
3. Adults: NHANES data for adults aged 20 through 74 years have also shown an increase in prevalence of obesity. In the period 1988 to 1994, 23.3% of American adults

TABLE 32.2

Prevalence of at Risk for Overweight and Overweight in Children by Sex, Age and Racial/Ethnic Group NHANES 1999–2002

Sex	Age, yr	All BMI >85%	Non-Hispanic White BMI >85%	Non-Hispanic Black BMI >85%	Mexican-American BMI >85%	All BMI >95%	Non-Hispanic White BMI >95%	Non-Hispanic Black BMI >95%	Mexican-American BMI >95%
Boys and girls	6–11	31.2	28.6	33.7	38.9	15.8	13.5	19.8	21.8
Boys and girls	12–19	30.9	27.9	36.8	40.7	16.1	13.7	21.1	22.5
Boys	6–11	32.5	29.3	29.7	43.9	16.9	14.0	17.0	26.5
Boys	12–19	31.2	29.2	32.1	41.9	16.7	14.6	18.7	24.7
Girls	6–11	29.9	27.7	37.9	33.8	14.7	13.1	22.8	17.1
Girls	12–19	30.5	26.5	41.9	39.3	15.4	12.7	23.6	19.9

From Hedley AA, Ogden CL, Johnson CL, et al. Prevalence of overweight and obesity among US children, adolescents and adults, 1999–2002. *JAMA* 2004;291:2847.

TABLE 32.3

Overweight in Children Aged 6 to 11 and Adolescents Aged 12 to 19 Years (United States National Health and Nutrition Examination Surveys)

	NHANES II 1976–1980	NHANES III 1988–1994	NHANES 1999–2002
Females 6–11	6.4	11.0	14.7
Females 12–19	5.3	9.7	15.4
Males 6–11	6.6	11.6	16.9
Males 12–19	4.8	11.3	16.7
Males/females 6–11	6.5	11.3	15.8
Males/females 12–19	5.0	10.5	16.1

Adapted from Ogden CL, Flegal KM, Carroll MD, et al. Prevalence and trends in overweight among US children and adolescents, 1999–2000. *JAMA* 2002;288:1728, and Hedley AA, Ogden CL, Johnson CL, et al. Prevalence of overweight and obesity among US children, adolescents, and adults, 1999–2002. *JAMA* 2004;291:2847.

20 years or older were estimated to be obese while in NHANES 1999 to 2002, 30.4% of adults were obese. There was a dramatic increase from prior studies in all race and sex groups.

4. Fifty percent to eighty-five percent of overweight adolescents will be obese adults. If a child is overweight at 12 years of age, the odds are 4:1 against that child attaining an ideal body weight (IBW); if overweight after adolescence, the odds are 28:1 against attaining an IBW. The persistence and severity of overweight as measured by BMI and triceps skinfold thickness in adolescents predicts the severity of obesity in adulthood.

5. Premature death in women has been associated with higher BMI at age 18 years (van Dam, 2006). From the Nurses Health Study II, a BMI of 30 kg/m^2 or more at age 18 carried with it almost three times the risk of premature death compared with a BMI between 18.5 and 21.9 kg/m^2, and double the risk of those with a BMI of 25 to 29 kg/m^2.

6. Weight-loss practices among American adolescents: In a national study, Serdula et al. (1993) found that 44% of female students and 15% of male students reported that they were trying to lose weight. Students had used the following weight control methods in the 7 days preceding the survey—exercise (51% of female students and 30% of male students), skipping meals (49% and 18%), taking diet pills (4% and 2%), and vomiting (3% and 1%). In a study of 30,000 adolescents in Minnesota (Neumark-Sztainer, 1998), 12% of females and 2% of males reported chronic dieting whereas 30% females and 13% males reported binging, 12% females and 6% males reported self-induced vomiting, and 2% females and 0.5% males reported diuretic or laxative use. In a more recent study of 4,746 Minnesota adolescents, 3.1% of females and 0.9% males stated that they met the criteria for binge eating disorder; 41.2% males and 15% females who identified themselves as meeting criteria for binge eating disorder had BMI >95%. Eighty-five percent to 90% had dieted in the past year and 70% to 80% were currently trying to lose weight (Ackard et al., 2003).

INFLUENCE OF OBESITY ON HEALTH

Complications due to obesity in adolescents include:

1. Cardiovascular: Dyslipidemias, hypertension.
2. Endocrinologic: Hyperinsulinism, insulin resistance, impaired glucose tolerance, type 2 diabetes mellitus, menstrual irregularity, and polycystic ovarian syndrome. Metabolic syndrome is a combination of dyslipidemias (high density lipoprotein [HDL] <40 mg/dL, triglycerides >110 mg/dL), elevated blood pressure, fasting glucose >110 mg/dL, and overweight.
3. Orthopedic: Slipped capital femoral epiphysis, Blount disease.
4. Respiratory: Sleep apnea, snoring, Pickwickian syndrome, asthma, and obesity hypoventilation syndrome.
5. Gastroenterologic: Gall bladder disease, steatohepatitis.
6. Psychological: Depression, eating disorders, social isolation, poor self-esteem.

Future medical problems are usually not a concern of the overweight adolescent, who is more preoccupied with the psychosocial consequences. The overweight adolescent who becomes an obese adult will have more severe obesity than those adults whose obesity began in adulthood. A 50-year follow-up study of overweight adolescents found that the rate of morbidity and mortality from cardiovascular disease was significantly increased compared to their lean counterparts (Must et al., 1992). Moreover, the influence of adolescent overweight on adult morbidity and mortality was independent of the effects of adolescent overweight on adult weight. Excess weight is associated with an increased incidence of cardiovascular disease, type 2 diabetes mellitus, hypertension, stroke, dyslipidemia, sleep apnea, osteoarthritis, and some cancers. However, >80% of the mortality related to complications of obesity occurs in people with a BMI >30 kg/m^2.

MEDICAL EVALUATION

Medical evaluation includes the assessment of factors that contribute to weight gain, inhibit weight loss, and comorbid factors that exist and can benefit from weight loss or maintenance.

1. History
   a. Family history of obesity, cardiovascular disease, hyperlipidemia, hypertension, type 2 diabetes mellitus, thyroid disease, and colorectal or breast cancer
   b. Past weight loss efforts
   c. Onset of obesity
   d. Triggers for weight gain (e.g., illness or injury, depression, medication use)
   e. Diet history including diet recall, family-eating patterns
   f. Unhealthy eating attitudes and weight-related behaviors including dieting, binge eating, purging
   g. Exercise history
   h. Sedentary activity time including evaluation of screen time (computer, video games, handheld electronic games)
   i. Medication use or abuse
   j. History of potential secondary causes (e.g., thyroid disease, Cushing disease)

k. Full review of systems including headaches (i.e., pseudotumor cerebri), orthopedic complaints, snoring, daytime sleeping, abdominal pain, hip pain, urinary frequency, polydipsia, polyuria, and irregular menses or amenorrhea
2. Physical examination
   a. Weight, height, and BMI calculation should be plotted on the appropriate CDC growth curves published in 2000 (Ogden, 2002).
      • Short stature suggests hypothyroidism or Cushing syndrome.
   b. Blood pressure should be checked with the appropriate sized cuff.
   c. Waist circumference may be helpful in those older than 20 years.
   d. Triceps skinfolds can be done if the examiner has expertise with this measurement (Table 32.1).
   e. Sexual maturity rating should be determined.
      • Undescended testicles are seen in males with Prader-Willi syndrome.
      • Delayed puberty in females suggests Turner syndrome.
   f. Skin, hair, and ligaments.
      • Acanthosis nigricans suggests insulin resistance and polycystic ovarian syndrome.
      • Striae that are violet in color and located on the abdomen, buttocks, and thighs are suggestive of Cushing syndrome.
      • Hirsutism is suggestive of polycystic ovarian syndrome.
      • Polydactyly suggests Bardet-Biedl syndrome as does mental retardation.
   g. Papilledema suggests pseudotumor cerebri.
   h. Thyromegaly suggests hypothyroidism.
   i. Developmental delay suggests Prader-Willi syndrome or other genetic syndromes.
3. Laboratory tests
   a. Thyroid-stimulating hormone, thyroxine, fasting blood glucose, fasting lipid profile, and liver function tests.
   b. For evaluation for insulin resistance and type 2 diabetes, particularly if there is acanthosis nigricans or a strong family history of diabetes, a fasting plasma glucose is recommended by the American Diabetes Association. A fasting plasma glucose of 100 to 125 mg/dL represents impaired glucose tolerance, whereas levels of 126 mg/dL or above represents diabetes. Alternative tests include a 2-hour glucose tolerance test and a casual glucose. After the ingestion of a 75-g glucose load, a blood glucose >140 mg/dL at 2 hours reflects impaired glucose tolerance and a blood glucose >200 mg/dL is likely representative of diabetes. A casual glucose of above 200 mg/dL plus polyuria, polydipsia, and weight loss reflect diabetes. Fasting insulin levels and glucose/insulin ratios have also been used to predict insulin resistance.
   c. Patients with polycystic ovarian syndrome may have amenorrhea or irregular menstrual periods, hirsutism, and acne. An elevated free testosterone, DHEAS or androstenedione is helpful in the diagnosis of polycystic ovarian syndrome. An LH : FSH ratio of >3.0 is present in only half of these patients and lacks sensitivity and specificity.
   d. If cushingoid, then 24-hour urine free cortisol and overnight dexamethasone suppression test are in order.
   e. If obstructive sleep apnea is present, overnight oximetry or a sleep study is warranted.

TREATMENT

Therapy for obesity is a challenge for both the health care provider and the patient of any age. Young adolescents are often more difficult to treat than older adolescents because of the lack of abstract thought and motivation. In general, treatment focuses on control rather than cure, as is so often the case with chronic medical conditions. When is it appropriate to strongly recommend weight reduction? Certainly, adolescents with morbid obesity (those with twice normal weight, BMI >40 kg/m^2, or >100 lb [45.5 kg] overweight) are at significant risk for medical problems and need to be encouraged to lose weight. The weight goal should be <85% BMI for age and sex. For many adolescents this can be accomplished by weight maintenance over a period of time, whereas for others a slow 1 lb/month weight loss should be encouraged. It is essential to remember that severe caloric restriction during adolescence, particularly during a growth spurt can halt growth and the progression of puberty. Therefore, understanding where an adolescent is with respect to his or her pubertal development and more specifically to their growth spurt, is critical in developing appropriate weight goals.

Critical areas in assessing treatment readiness in the adolescent include:

1. Motivation: This is critical for success. Is the teen motivated? Is the desire for weight loss or maintenance someone else's idea?
2. Support: Is there a supportive social and family framework for weight reduction or maintenance?
3. Compliance: Is the teen willing to increase physical activity? Is the teen prepared to modify diet?
4. Realistic goals: Are there realistic goals for weight reduction?

Diet, exercise, behavior modification, and support are still the mainstay of treatment for obesity in adolescents and young adults. The role of medication and bariatric surgery for overweight adolescents is still being evaluated.

Diet

An energy deficit is needed for active weight loss and is a critical part of management. However, diet alone is rarely successful in achieving permanent weight loss. Predicting weight loss for an individual teenager based on caloric intake is difficult and can vary widely. For older adolescents and young adults, a deficit of 250 to 500 kcal/day is associated with a loss of approximately 0.5 to 1 lb/week (0.23–0.45 kg). Greater caloric restrictions are very difficult to maintain. The type of caloric restriction should be well planned and should take into account current food types and intake, eating habits, situation-dependent eating, and family and cultural preferences. To support normal growth and development, there must always be good nutritional balance among the food groups.

Approximate daily energy needs in the postpubertal adolescent can be calculated from the weight in kilograms

(*W*) as follows:

$$\text{Males} = [900 + (10 \times W)] \times \text{activity factor}$$
$$\text{Females} = [800 + (7 \times W)] \times \text{activity factor}$$

The activity factor is 1.2 for a low activity level, 1.4 for a moderate activity level, or 1.6 for a high activity level. The energy requirement to maintain each extra kilogram of body weight is approximately 22 kcal. Therefore, an adolescent who weighs 20 kg more than another needs an additional 440 kcal to maintain that weight.

Various nutritional approaches to weight loss exist and some have been studied. The ketogenic diet or low-carbohydrate diet has been studied in adolescents. Sondike et al. (2003) published a 12-week randomized controlled trial comparing a low-fat diet to a low-carbohydrate diet in adolescents. The low-carbohydrate diet was effective for short-term weight loss without affecting the lipid profile. However, the sample size was small with a brief follow-up period. This diet has not been studied in younger adolescents and the long-term benefits require further study.

A balanced weight reduction diet focusing on healthy lifestyle practices is recommended for the adolescent population and should include the following:

1. Foods from all five food groups (milk, meat, bread, fruits, and vegetables).
2. Instructions to eat at least three meals/day.
3. Instructions to eat less food or calories than previously.
4. Instructions on ways of preparing low-calorie foods and of substituting foods with fewer calories for high-calorie foods.

One simplification of this diet is the "Traffic Light" approach (Epstein et al., 1998). Green light foods can be eaten freely (nonfat foods, low-fat foods, fruits, vegetables). Yellow light foods are those eaten with caution (low-to-moderate fat foods such as breads, pastas). Red light foods are those to be eaten rarely (nuts, candy). This concrete view can be helpful to both children and adolescents.

Physical Activity

Every weight reduction program should include an increase in physical activity. This can include the following:

1. Changes in regular activity, such as walking instead of using the bus, using stairs instead of elevators, walking to the television set instead of using a remote control (even minor increases in activity can make a difference overall).
2. An exercise prescription.
3. Participation in regular physical activity. Although no specific recommendations for the amount of physical activity has been established for adolescents, the position statement of the American Academy of Pediatrics Committee (2003) on Nutrition on Prevention of Pediatric Overweight and Obesity (2003) clearly encourages families, schools, and communities to promote physical activity.

Cognitive Behavioral Therapy or Behavior Modification Techniques

Cognitive behavioral therapy (CBT) or behavior modification techniques can be effective when used in combination with diet and medical therapies. Penich et al. (1971)

and Stunkard et al. (1970) have reviewed this approach. These programs usually contain several components:

1. A contract and reward system for weight loss.
2. An initial food diary that contains items such as time spent eating, place, hunger rating, mood, other activity done while eating, food consumed, and amount consumed.
3. A change in current behavior through eating awareness and a food diary.
   a. Eat three regular meals instead of overeating at dinner and evening.
   b. Eat more slowly; allow the body to signal when it is full.
   c. Eat only at places that are meant for eating (e.g., at the dinner table, in restaurants).
   d. Do not watch television while eating.
   e. Do not eat on the go; sit down to eat.
   f. Learn to differentiate between appetite and hunger.
   g. Eat only when hungry and not just when food is available.
   h. Have a breakout activity when feeling out of control or when eating is related to depression, anxiety, or unhappiness.
   i. Be honest about lapses in control.

Groups

Group participation as part of the weight-loss program may be beneficial. Groups provide encouragement, support, and an opportunity for release of feelings, peer contact, and acceptance.

Although there is no evidence for the effectiveness of structured commercially based weight-loss programs in adolescents, such programs have been shown to provide modest weight loss compared with self-help groups in adults (Heshka et al., 2003). All the structured commercial weight-loss programs studied (ranging from moderately to very restrictive diets) led to a similar amount of weight loss at 1 year, with poor dietary adherence with the more restrictive diets (Dansinger et al., 2005).

Medications for the Treatment of Obesity

The two medications studied in the treatment of adolescent obesity are sibutramine and orlistat. A meta-analysis of pharmacological treatments of adult obesity is available from Li et al. (2005).

1. Sibutramine—a serotonin, norepinephrine, and dopamine reuptake inhibitor has been studied in overweight adolescents aged 16 years and older.
   a. Dosage: The starting dose is 10 mg once daily, which may be increased after 4 weeks to 15 mg once daily. Daily dosages of 10 and 15 mg have been associated with a weight loss of 10.6 lb (4.8 kg) and 13.4 lb (6 kg), respectively, compared with 4 lb (1.8 kg) for placebo. Individuals are more likely to lose weight if weight loss is demonstrated in the first 4 weeks. Improvement has also been documented in levels of triglyceride, HDL cholesterol, and insulin, and in insulin sensitivity.
   b. Adverse effects: These include headaches, dry mouth, constipation, insomnia, and increases in heart rate and blood pressure. There is no evidence of an association with cardiac valve abnormalities. The medication does not appear to have a high abuse potential.

Contraindications include anorexia nervosa, hypersensitivity to drug, therapy with monoamine oxidase inhibitors or other serotonergic drugs, coronary heart disease, congestive heart failure, stroke, arrhythmia, uncontrolled hypertension, severe hepatic or renal disease, pregnancy, and lactation. Caution is advised in individuals with a history of seizures. This medication is not indicated for mildly or moderately overweight individuals in the absence of medical complications.

2. Orlistat—acts as a lipase inhibitor, blocking the absorption of dietary fat by inhibiting gastrointestinal lipases. The medication has no effect on the absorption of carbohydrates, proteins, or phospholipids. It increases fecal fat from 5% to 30%. The use of orlistat has been studied in overweight adolescents aged 12 and older and if tolerated, increases short-term weight loss.
   a. Dosage: 120 mg orally three times a day. In one study in adults, 120 mg of orlistat three times a day was associated with loss of 8.8% to 10.2% of body weight after 1 year, compared with 5.8% to 6.1% for placebos.
   b. Adverse effects: The incidence of adverse effects is similar to that of placebo with the exception of more frequent gastrointestinal complaints. There are no reports of vitamin deficiencies. However, individuals should take a daily multivitamin 2 hours before or after orlistat. Contraindications include malabsorption syndromes, cholestasis, known hypersensitivity, pregnancy, and lactation.

Finally, many of the selective serotonin reuptake inhibitors (SSRIs), including fluoxetine, fluvoxamine, sertraline, and citalopram have been used to decrease binging in patients with binge eating disorder. Sibutramine and topiramate have been found to decrease binging in this population as well.

Gastrointestinal Procedures: Bariatric Surgery

A multidisciplinary group of pediatric and surgical specialists published guidelines for bariatric surgery in adolescents (Inge et al., 2004). Potential candidates include:

1. Skeletally mature adolescents who have failed at least 6 months of dietary weight management
2. Adolescents whose BMI is >40 kg/m^2 with serious comorbid conditions that would resolve with sustained weight loss
3. Adolescents who have a supportive family and personal maturity

Those with BMI >50 kg/m^2 with less serious comorbid conditions could be considered. A multidisciplinary team including the bariatric surgeon and specialists in adolescent obesity, psychology, and nutrition are essential to the process. Potential procedures include Roux-en-Y gastric bypass and laparoscopic adjustable gastric banding. The Roux-en-Y gastric bypass is performed laparoscopically, separating the stomach into a small-volume upper pouch (limiting oral intake) and connects the stomach to a limb of jejunum. Approximately 85% of individuals lose at least 50% of their excess weight at 4 years. Micronutrient supplementation is needed. The laparoscopic adjustable band uses a small silastic band around the upper stomach that is inflated with saline through a subcutaneous

port. Although reversible and removable, there have been technical issues as well as patient management problems. A meta-analysis of surgical treatment of obese adults is available from Maggard et al. (2005).

Although similar guidelines are not available for adolescents, the American College of Physicians published evidence-based practice guidelines for the treatment of obesity in adults (Snow et al., 2005). The following are the recommendations:

- Counsel obese adults about lifestyle and behavioral changes in order to achieve the patient's goal for weight loss.
- Offer pharmacological therapy to those obese adults who have not reached their weight loss goal through diet and exercise.
- Discuss the pros and cons of approved medications used for weight loss including side effects, lack of evidence for long-term safety, and temporary nature of weight loss with these medications.
- Consider bariatric surgery for obese adults with BMI >40 kg/m^2 who have failed a weight-loss program or who have obesity-related comorbid medical problems.
- Refer patients who choose to have bariatric surgery to a medical center with experienced surgeons who perform this surgery frequently.

PREVENTION

- Encourage healthy nutritional practices in early puberty when there is programmed propensity to increase fat cells. This includes encouraging adequate intake of calcium, increased fruits and vegetables, and decreased amount of saturated fat. Reduce the intake of soft drinks and caloric dense food.
- Identify unhealthy eating attitudes and harmful eating behaviors including dieting, overeating, and binging, all of which are associated with overweight.
- Encourage a lifestyle of activity and participation rather than one of inactivity and observation. Increase the frequency and intensity of activity during physical education classes in schools. Increase access to recreational facilities within communities.
- Discourage television viewing and other sedentary pastimes. Reducing television, videotape, and video game use may be a promising population-based approach to prevention of childhood obesity.
- Support better food choices in schools including school lunches and vending machines.
- Encourage family time including meals and activities.

WEB SITES

For Teenagers and Parents

http://www.health.gov/dietaryguidelines/. Dietary guidelines.
http://win.niddk.nih.gov/. Weight-control Information Network (WIN), national information service of the NIH, National Institute of Diabetes and Digestive and Kidney Diseases.
http://www.nhlbi.nih.gov/health/public/heart/hbp/dash. DASH, the Dietary Approaches to Stop Hypertension.

http://www.shapeup.org/sua. Shape up America! Founded by former Surgeon General Everett Koop, M.D., promoting healthy weight and increased physical exercise.

http://www.usda.gov/cnpp. Center for Nutrition Policy and Promotion.

http://www.eatright.org. American Dietetic Association Web site for nutrition information, food pyramid and good nutrition reading list

http://www.kidshealth.org/teen/food_fitness/dieting/obesity.html. Information for teens reviewed by physicians, sponsored by Nemours Foundation.

http://www.kidshealth.org/parent/nutrition_fit/nutrition/overweight_obesity.html. Information for parents, reviewed by physicians, sponsored by Nemours Foundation.

http://www.aap.org/obesity/family.htm. Information for parents on childhood obesity.

http://www.bam.gov. CDC Web site for teens on health issues including obesity and nutrition.

For Health Professionals

http://www.nhlbi.nih.gov/guidelines/obesity/ob_home.htm. Clinical Guidelines on the Identification, Evaluation, and Treatment of Overweight and Obesity in Adults, from NIH.

http://www.niddk.nih.gov/health/nutrit/nutrit.htm. National Institute for Diabetes and Digestive and Kidney Diseases, publications on weight control.

http://www.aafp.org/afp/990215ap/861.html. From American Family Physician, evaluation and treatment of childhood obesity.

http://www.obesity.org/subs/childhood/. American Obesity Association.

http://www.aap.org/obesity. Resources for physicians on obesity.

http://www.nasso.org. The obesity society, a scientific society for research, education, advocacy and organizational development whose journal is Obesity Research.

http://www.obesityonline.org. Online collection of evidence based obesity education resources.

REFERENCES AND ADDITIONAL READINGS

Ackard DM, Neumark-Sztainer D, Story M, et al. Overeating among adolescents: prevalence and associations with weight-related characteristics and psychological health. *Pediatrics* 2003;111:67.

Allison DB, Fontaine KR, Manson JE, et al. Annual deaths attributable to obesity in the United States. *JAMA* 1999;282:1530.

Alpert MA, Hashimi MW. Obesity and the heart. *Am J Med Sci* 1993;306:117.

Appolinario JC, Bacaltchuk J, Sichieri R, et al. A randomized, double-blind, placebo-controlled study of sibutramine in the treatment of binge-eating disorder. *Arch Gen Psychiatry* 2003;60(11):1109.

Arnold LM, McElroy SL, Hudson JI, et al. A placebo-controlled, randomized trial of fluoxetine in the treatment of binge-eating disorder. *J Clin Psychiatr* 2002;63(11):1028.

Balsinger BM, Luque-de Leon E, Sarr MG. Surgical treatment of obesity: who is an appropriate candidate? *Mayo Clin Proc* 1997;72:551.

Barlow S, Dietz W. Obesity evaluation and treatment: expert committee recommendations. *Pediatrics* 1998;102:e29.

Berkowitz RI, Fujioka K, Daniels SR, et al. Effects of Sibutramine treatment in adolescents: a randomized trial. *Ann Intern Med* 2006;145(2):81.

Berkowitz RI, Wadden TA, Tershakovec AM, et al. Behavior therapy and sibutramine for the treatment of adolescent obesity. *JAMA* 2003;289:1805.

Braunschweig CL, Gomez S, Liang H, et al. Obesity and risk factors for the metabolic syndrome among low-income urban African American schoolchildren: the rule rather than the exception? *Am J Clin Nutr* 2005;81:970.

Bray GA, Blackburn GL, Ferguson JM, et al. Sibutramine produces dose-related weight loss. *Obes Res* 1999;7:189.

Brownell KD, Rodin J. The dieting maelstrom: is it possible and advisable to lose weight? *Am Psychol* 1994;49:781.

Bullen BA, Reed RB, Mayer J. Physical activity of obese and non-obese adolescent girls appraised by motion picture sampling. *Am J Clin Nutr* 1964;14:211.

Callahan T, Mansfield J. Type II diabetes mellitus in adolescents. *Curr Opin Pediatr* 2000;12:310.

Canadian Task Force on the Periodic Health Examination. Periodic health examination, 1994 update: 1. Obesity in childhood. *Can Med Assoc J* 1994;15:871.

Chanoine JP, Hampl S, Jensen C, et al. Effect of orlistat on weight and body composition in obese adolescents. *JAMA* 2005;293:2873.

Clement K, Boutin P, Froguel P. Genetics of obesity. *Am J Pharmacogenomics* 2002;2:177.

Consensus Development Conference Panel. Gastrointestinal surgery for severe obesity. *Ann Intern Med* 1991;115:956.

van Dam RM, Willett WC, Manson JE, et al. The relationship between overweight in adolescence and premature death in women. *Ann Intern Med* 2006;145(2):91.

Daniels SR, Khoury PR, Morrison JA. The utility of body mass index as a measure of body fatness in children and adolescents: differences by race and gender. *Pediatrics* 1997;99:804.

Dansinger ML, Gleason JA, Griffith JL, et al. Comparison of the Atkins, Ornish, Weight Watchers, and Zone diets for weight loss and heart disease risk reduction; a randomized trial. *JAMA* 2005;293:43.

Davidson MH, Hauptman J, DiGirolamo M, et al. Weight control and risk factor reduction in obese subjects treated for 2 years with orlistat: a randomized controlled trial. *JAMA* 1999;281:235.

Dennison BA, Erb TA, Jenkins PL. Television viewing and television in bedroom associated with overweight risk among low-income preschool children. *Pediatrics* 2002;109:1028.

Dickerson LM, Carek PJ. Drug therapy for obesity. *Am Fam Physician* 2000;61:2131.

Dietz WH. Therapeutic strategies in childhood obesity. *Horm Res* 1993;39:86.

Dietz WH. What constitutes successful weight management in adolescents? *Ann Intern Med* 2006;145(2):145.

Dietz WH, Bellizzi MC. Introduction: the use of body mass index to assess obesity in children. *Am J Clin Nutr* 1999;70:123s.

Dietz WH, Robinson TN. Overweight children and adolescents. *N Engl J Med* 2005;352(20):2100.

DuRant RH, Baranowski T, Johnson M, et al. The relationship among television watching, physical activity, and body composition of young children. *Pediatrics* 1994;94:449.

Epstein LH, Myers MD, Raynor HA, et al. Treatment of pediatric obesity. *Pediatrics* 1998;101(suppl):554.

Epstein LH, Roemmich JN, Paluch RA, et al. Influence of changes in sedentary behavior on energy and macronutrient intake in youth. *Am J Clin Nutr* 2005;81:361.

Farooqi IS, O'Rahilly S. Recent advances in the genetics of severe childhood obesity. *Arch Dis Child* 2000;83:31.

Flegal KM. Defining obesity in children and adolescents: epidemiologic approaches. *Crit Rev Food Sci Nutr* 1993;33:307.

Flegal KM, Graubard BI, Williamson DF, et al. Excess deaths associated with underweight, overweight and obesity. *JAMA* 2005;293:1861.

Fontaine KR, Redden DT, Wang C, et al. Years of life lost due to obesity. *JAMA* 2003;289:187.

Freedman DS, Khan LK, Serdula MK, et al. Relation of age at menarche to race, time period, and anthropometric dimensions: the Bogalusa heart study. *Pediatrics* 2002;110(4):e43.

Freedman DS, Khan LK, Serdula MK, et al. The relation of childhood BMI to adult adiposity: the Bogalusa heart study. *Pediatrics* 2005;115(1):22.

Galuska DA, Will JC, Serdula MK, et al. Are health care professionals advising obese patients to lose weight. *JAMA* 1999;282:1576.

Gortmaker SL, Must A, Perrin JM, et al. Social and economic consequences of overweight in adolescence and young adulthood. *N Engl J Med* 1993;329:1008.

Gutin B, Yin Z, Humphries MC, et al. Relations of moderate and vigorous physical activity to fitness and fatness in adolescents. *Am J Clin Nutr* 2005;81:746.

Hannon TS, Rao G, Arslanian SA. Childhood obesity and type 2 diabetes mellitus. *Pediatrics* 2005;116:473.

Hedley AA, Ogden CL, Johnson CL, et al. Prevalence of overweight and obesity among U.S. children, adolescents, and adults, 1999–2002. *JAMA* 2004;291:2847.

Herbold N, Frates S. Update of nutrition guidelines for the teen trends and concerns. *Curr Opin Pediatr* 2000;12:303.

Hernandez B, Gortmaker SL, Colditz GA, et al. Association of obesity with physical activity, television programs and other forms of video viewing among children in Mexico City. *Int J Obes Relat Metab Disord* 1999;23:845.

Heshka S, Anderson JW, Atkinson RL, et al. Weight loss with self-help compared with a structured commercial program; a randomized trial. *JAMA* 2003;289:1792.

Heyden S, Hames CG, Bartel A, et al. Weight and weight history in relation to cerebrovascular and ischemic heart disease. *Arch Intern Med* 1971;128:956.

Heymsfield SB, Greenberg AS, Fujioka K, et al. Recombinant leptin for weight loss in obese and lean adults: a randomized, controlled, dose-escalation trial. *JAMA* 1999;282:1568.

Hill J, Peters J. Environmental contributions to the obesity epidemic. *Science* 1998;280:1371.

Himes JH, Dietz WH. Guidelines for overweight in adolescent preventive services: recommendations from an expert committee. *Am J Clin Nutr* 1994;59:307.

Hirschler V, Aranda C, de Lujan Calcagno M, et al. Can waist circumference identify children with the metabolic syndrome? *Arch Pediatr Adolesc Med* 2005;159:740.

Hubert HB, Feinleib M, McNamara PM, et al. Obesity as an independent risk factor for cardiovascular disease: a 26-year follow-up of participants in the Framingham Heart Study. *Circulation* 1983;67:968.

Hudson JI, McElroy SL, Raymond NC, et al. Fluvoxamine in the treatment of binge-eating disorder: a multicenter placebo-controlled, double-blind trial. *Am J Psychiatry* 1998; 155(12):1756.

Inge TH, Krebs NF, Garcia VF, et al. Bariatric surgery for severely overweight adolescents: concerns and recommendations. *Pediatrics* 2004;114:217.

Janz KF, Nielsen DH, Cassady SL, et al. Cross-validation of the Slaughter skinfold equations for children and adolescents. *Med Sci Sports Exerc* 1993;25:1070.

Kannel WB, Brand N, Skinner JJ Jr, et al. Relationship of adiposity to blood pressure and development of hypertension: Framingham study. *Ann Intern Med* 1967;67:48.

Kimm SYS, Barton BA, Obarzanek E, et al. Racial divergence in adiposity during adolescence: the NHLBI growth and health study. *Pediatrics* 2000;107(3):e34.

Krebs NF, Jacobson MS. American Academy of Pediatrics Committee on Nutrition. Prevention of pediatric overweight and obesity. *Pediatrics* 2003;112:424.

Lean ME. Sibutramine: a review of clinical efficacy. *Int J Obes Relat Metab Disord* 1997;21(Suppl 1):S30.

Lee IM, Manson JE, Hennekens CH, et al. Body weight and mortality: a 27-year follow-up of middle -aged men. *JAMA* 1993; 270:2823.

Leibel RL, Rosenbaum M, Hirsch J. Changes in energy expenditure resulting from altered body weight. *N Engl J Med* 1995;332:621.

Li Z, Maglione M, Tu W, et al. Meta-analysis: pharmacologic treatment of obesity. *Ann Intern Med* 2005;142:532.

Lowe MR, Miller-Kovach K, Frye N, et al. An initial evaluation of a commercial weight loss program: short-term effects on weight, eating behavior, and mood. *Obes Res* 1999;7:51.

MacMahon SW, Wilcken EEL, MacDonald GJ. The effect of weight reduction on left ventricular mass: a randomized controlled trial in young, overweight hypertensive patients. *N Engl J Med* 1986;314:334.

Maggard MA, Shugarman LR, Suttorp M, et al. Meta-analysis: surgical treatment of obesity. *Ann Intern Med* 2005;142:547.

McCarthy HD, Jarrett KV, Crawley HF. The development of waist circumference percentiles in British children aged 5.0–16.9 y. *Eur J Clin Nutr* 2001;55:902.

McElroy SL, Shapira NA, Arnold LM, et al. Topiramate in the long-term treatment of binge-eating disorder associated with obesity. *J Clin Psychiatry* 2004;65(11):1463.

Must A, Jacques PF, Dallal GE, et al. Long-term morbidity and mortality of overweight adolescents: a follow-up of the Harvard growth study of 1922–1935. *N Engl J Med* 1992;327: 1350.

Must A, Spandano J, Coakley EH, et al. The disease burden associated with overweight and obesity. *JAMA* 1999;282:1523.

National Heart, Lung and Blood Institute, National Institutes of Health. Clinical guidelines on the identification, evaluation, and treatment of overweight and obesity in adults [Executive Summary]. *Arch Intern Med* 1998;158:1855. Available at www.nhlbi.nih.gov/nhlbi/nhlbi.htm.

National Institutes of Health, Consensus Development Panel on the Health Implications of Obesity. Health implications of obesity. *Ann Intern Med* 1985;103:147.

National Institutes of Health Technology Assessment Conference. Methods for voluntary weight loss and control. *Ann Intern Med* 1993;119:641.

National Task Force on the Prevention and Treatment of Obesity. Very low-calorie diets. *JAMA* 1993;270:967.

Neumark-Sztainer D, Story M, Resnick MD, Blum RW. Lessons learned about adolescent nutrition from the Minnesota Adolescent Health Survey. *J Am Diet Assoc.* 1998;98(12):1449–56.

Ogden CL, Flegal KM, Carroll MD, et al. Prevalence and trends in overweight among US children and adolescents, 1999–2000. *JAMA* 2002;288:1728.

Ogden CL, Kuczmarski RJ, Flegal KM, et al. Centers for Disease Control and Prevention 2000 growth charts for the United States: improvements to the 1977 National Center for Health Statistics version. *Pediatrics* 2002;109:45.

Penich S, Filion R, Fox S, et al. Behavior modification in the treatment of obesity. *Psychosom Med* 1971;33:49.

Pietrobelli A, Faith MS, Allison DB, et al. Body mass index as a measure of adiposity among children and adolescents: a validation study. *J Pediatr* 1998;132:204.

Pinhas-Hamiel O, Zeitler P. Type II diabetes in adolescents: no longer rare. *Pediatr Rev* 1998;19:434.

Rand CS, Macgregor AM. Adolescents having obesity surgery: a 6-year follow-up. *South Med J* 1994;87:1208.

Ravussin E, Lillioja S, Knowler WC, et al. Reduced rate of energy expenditure as a risk factor for body weight gain. *N Engl J Med* 1988;318:467.

Revicki DA, Israel RG. Relationship between body mass indices and measures of body adiposity. *Am J Public Health* 1986;76:992.

Robinson TN. Reducing children's television viewing to prevent obesity: a randomized controlled trial. *JAMA* 1999;282:1561.

Robinson TN, Hammer LD, Killen JD, et al. Does television viewing increase obesity and reduce physical activity? Cross-sectional and longitudinal analyses among adolescent girls. *Pediatrics* 1993;91:273.

Rosenblatt E. Weight-loss programs: pluses and minuses of commercial and self-help groups. *Postgrad Med* 1988;83:137.

Rumpel C, Harris TB. The influence of weight on adolescent self-esteem. *J Psychoso Res* 1994;38:547.

Sargent JD, Blanchflower DG. Obesity and stature in adolescence and earnings in young adulthood: analysis of a British birth cohort. *Arch Pediatr Adolesc Med* 1994;148:681.

Schapira DV, Clark RA, Wolff PA, et al. Visceral obesity and breast cancer risk. *Cancer* 1994;74:632.

Serdula MK, Collins ME, Williamson DF, et al. Weight control practices of U.S. adolescents and adults. *Ann Intern Med* 1993;119:667.

Sinha R, Fisch G, Teague B, et al. Prevalence of impaired glucose tolerance among children and adolescents with marked obesity. *N Engl J Med* 2002;346:802.

Slaughter MH, Lohman TG, Boileau RA, et al. Skinfold equations for estimation of body fatness in children and youth. *Hum Biol* 1988;60:709.

Smith JC, Sorey WH, Quebedeau D, et al. The use of body mass index to monitor treatment of obese adolescents. *J Adolesc Health* 1997;20:466.

Snow V, Barry P, Fitterman N, et al. Pharmacologic and surgical management of obesity in primary care; a clinical practice guideline from the American College of Physicians. *Ann Intern Med* 2005;142:525.

Sondike SB, Copperman N, Jacobson MS. Effects of a low-carbohydrate diet on weight loss and cardiovascular risk factors in overweight adolescents. *J Pediatr* 2003;142: 253.

Sterner TG, Burke EL. Body fat assessment: a comparison of visual estimation and skinfold techniques. *Phys Sportsmed* 1986;14:101.

Stunkard A. New theories for eating disorders: behavior modification of obesity and anorexia nervosa. *Arch Gen Psychiatry* 1972;26:391.

Stunkard AJ, Harris JR, Pedersen NL, et al. The bodymass index of twins who have been reared apart. *N Engl J Med* 1990;322: 1483.

Stunkard A, Levine H, Fox S. The management of obesity. *Arch Intern Med* 1970;125:1067.

Stunkard A, Mendelson M. Obesity and the body image: parts 1 and 2. *Am J Psychiatry* 1967;123:1296,1443.

Stunkard AJ, Sorensen TI, Hanis C, et al. An adoption study of human obesity. *N Engl J Med* 1986;314:193.

Styne DM. Obesity in childhood: what's activity got to do with it? *Am J Clin Nutr* 2005;81:337.

Sun SS, Schubert CM, Liang R, et al. Is sexual maturity occurring earlier among U.S. children? *J Adolesc Health* 2005;37: 345.

Swallen KC, Reither EN, Haas SA, et al. Overweight, obesity, and health-related quality of life among adolescents: the national longitudinal study of adolescent health. *Pediatrics* 2005; 115(2):340.

Troiano RP, Flegal KM. Overweight children and adolescents: description, epidemiology and demographics. *Pediatrics* 1998;101:497.

Tsai AG, Wadden TA. Systematic review: an evaluation of major commercial weight loss programs in the United States. *Ann Intern Med* 2005;142:56.

Volkmar FR, Stunkard AJ, Woolston J, et al. High attrition rates in commercial weight reduction programs. *Arch Intern Med* 1981;141:426.

Vuguin P, Saenger P, Dimartino-Nardi J. Fasting glucose insulin ration: a useful measure of insulin resistance in girls with premature adrenarche. *J Clin Endocrinol Metab* 2001;86:4618.

Weiss R, Dziura J, Burgert TS, et al. Obesity and the metabolic syndrome in children and adolescents. *N Engl J Med* 2004;350: 2362.

Willi S, Oexmann M, Wright N, et al. The effects of a high-protein, low-fat, ketogenic diet on adolescents with morbid obesity: body composition, blood chemistries, and sleep abnormalities. *Pediatrics* 1998;101:61.

Yanovski SZ, Yanovski JA. Obesity. *N Engl J Med* 2002;346:591.

Yanovski JA, Yanovski SZ. Treatment of pediatric and adolescent obesity (editorial). *JAMA* 2003;289:1851.

CHAPTER 33

Anorexia Nervosa and Bulimia Nervosa

Debra K. Katzman and Neville H. Golden

This chapter describes the major eating disorders encountered during adolescence including anorexia nervosa, bulimia nervosa, and eating disorders not otherwise specified (EDNOS). The latter group accounts for most adolescents seeking treatment for an eating disorder and refers to those patients not meeting full Diagnostic and Statistical Manual of Mental Disorders, Fourth Edition (DSM-IV) criteria for either anorexia nervosa or bulimia nervosa. In one study, using the DSM-IV criteria, >50% of children were classified as having EDNOS (Nicholls et al., 2000).

ANOREXIA NERVOSA

Anorexia nervosa is an eating disorder that primarily affects adolescent girls and requires a comprehensive and integrated approach to assessment and treatment. This disorder is a classic biopsychosocial syndrome because the psychological and physiological manifestations are intertwined. The core features are self-induced weight loss accompanied by distorted body image, intense fear of weight gain, denial of the seriousness of weight loss, and amenorrhea (absence of at least three consecutive menstrual periods in the postmenarcheal female). Anorexia nervosa is subdivided into a restrictive subtype and a binge eating and purging subtype (Table 33.1). Adolescents diagnosed with anorexia nervosa are reported to have a good prognosis with 76% having a full recovery (Strober et al., 1997).

Etiology

The etiology of anorexia nervosa is multifactorial with a combination of biological, psychological, and sociocultural factors contributing to the development of the disorder. The specific etiology may be different for different individuals. The biopsychosocial model for anorexia nervosa described by Lucas (1981) is shown in Figure 33.1. This figure demonstrates how biological vulnerability, psychological predisposition, and sociocultural influence precipitate dieting and weight loss in a vulnerable individual. This weight loss, in turn, leads to malnutrition, which contributes to the physical, psychological, and emotional changes. Over the last decade, research has focused on the contributions of genetics to biological vulnerability, the personality type associated with anorexia nervosa, and the potential role of neurotransmitters in the etiology of the disorder.

There is a familial predisposition to eating disorders, with female relatives most often affected. There is a higher rate of anorexia nervosa among identical twins compared to fraternal twins. In addition, relatives of individuals with an eating disorder are at higher risk of developing an eating disorder. These findings suggest that genetic factors may predispose some people to eating disorders. To date, no single gene or combination of genes have been identified. Recent research has suggested that certain areas of the human genome may harbor susceptibility genes for anorexia nervosa on chromosome 1 (Grice et al., 2002).

Certain personality traits such as perfectionism, low self-esteem, obsessionality, social isolation, and feelings of ineffectiveness often predate the onset of the illness and persist to a varying degree after recovery. Researchers have discovered disturbances in a number of different neurotransmitters including serotonin, norepinephrine, and dopamine in those with anorexia nervosa. There is evidence that starvation, binging, and excessive exercising can lead to changes in neurotransmitters and conversely, there is evidence that neurotransmitter abnormalities can lead to these behaviors. The role of disturbances in transmission of serotonin, a neurotransmitter that is known to play a role in modulating appetite, obsessional behavior, and impulsivity, has received particular interest in recent years (Kaye et al., 1991, 2003).

Weight concerns and societal emphasis on thinness are pervasive in westernized societies and adolescent girls tend to be more vulnerable to these influences. The slim body ideal is thought to be the key contributor to the gender differences seen in both anorexia nervosa and bulimia nervosa. In the typical situation, in a biologically predisposed individual, feelings of ineffectiveness and loss of control during adolescence, compounded by societal pressures to be thin, lead to dieting to obtain a sense of control. Dieting itself, leads to further preoccupation with shape and weight, perpetuating the cycle. Many of the behaviors, physical signs, and symptoms seen in anorexia nervosa can be attributed to malnutrition.

Epidemiology

1. Prevalence: Most recent data suggest that the estimated prevalence for anorexia nervosa in young women is 0.3% to 0.5% (Hoek and van Hoeken, 2003). The incidence

TABLE 33.1

DSM-IV Diagnostic Criteria for Anorexia Nervosa

1. Refusal to maintain body weight at or above a minimally normal weight for age and height (e.g., weight loss leading to maintenance of body weight <85% of that expected), or failure to make expected weight gain during period of growth, leading to body weight <85% of that expected.
2. Intense fear of gaining weight or becoming fat, although underweight.
3. Disturbance in the way in which one's body weight or shape is experienced, undue influence of body shape and weight on self-evaluation, or denial of the seriousness of current low body weight.
4. In postmenarcheal females, amenorrhea, that is, the absence of at least three consecutive menstrual cycles. (A woman is considered to have amenorrhea if her periods occur only following hormone, e.g., estrogen administration.)

Specify type
Restricting type: During the current episode of anorexia nervosa, the person has not regularly engaged in binge eating or purging (i.e., self-induced vomiting or the misuse of laxatives, diuretics, or enemas).
Binge eating/purging type: During the current episode of anorexia nervosa, the person has regularly engaged in binge eating or purging (i.e., self-induced vomiting or the misuse of laxatives, diuretics, or enemas).

Reprinted with permission from the American Psychiatric Association. *Diagnostic and statistical manual of mental disorders*, 4th ed. Text Revision, Copyright, 2000.

rate is estimated at 8 cases per 100,000 population. Incidence rates for anorexia nervosa are highest in 15- to 19-year-old girls, and have increased dramatically over the last 50 years in this age-group (Lucas et al., 1999). There are anecdotal reports of increasing presentations in prepubertal children. Rates for partial syndrome anorexia nervosa are typically higher.
2. Age: Most eating disorders begin during adolescence and more than 90% of individuals with eating disorders are diagnosed before the age of 25 years. The peak age at onset is midadolescence (13–15 years). However, the age range for the development of anorexia nervosa is

approximately 10 to 25 years old. Increasing numbers of younger children and adolescents are being referred for assessment and treatment.
3. Gender: Females are more likely than males to develop eating disorders. Approximately 85% to 90% of adolescents with eating disorders are female. Recent research has shown that eating disorders are more widespread in males than previously thought. In fact, one in eight adolescents with anorexia nervosa younger than 14 years are boys (Katzman et al., 2005).
4. Comorbidity: Anorexia nervosa may coexist with other psychiatric conditions such as anxiety disorders, depression, obsessive-compulsive disorder (OCD), and

FIGURE 33.1 Biopsychosocial model for anorexia nervosa. (From Lucas AR. Toward the understanding of anorexia nervosa as a disease entity. *Mayo Clin Proc* 1981;56:254, with permission.)

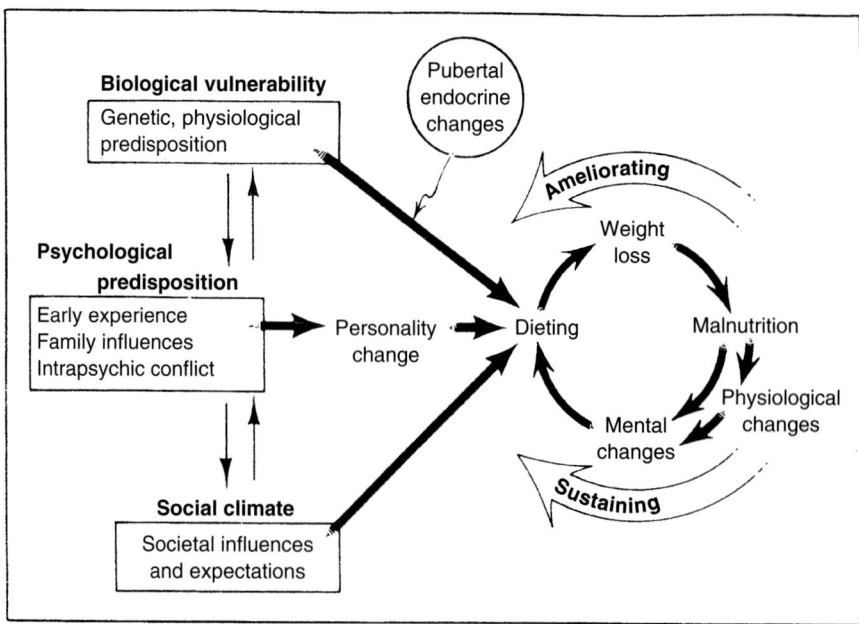

substance abuse disorders. It may also coexist with medical conditions such as diabetes mellitus and cystic fibrosis.

Risk Factors

Risk factors for anorexia nervosa are factors that do not seem to be a direct cause of the disorder but increase the probability of developing the disorder. The absence of any risk factor or the presence of a protective factor does not necessarily protect one against developing anorexia nervosa. According to a recent review (Walsh et al., 2005), potential risk factors predisposing an adolescent to anorexia nervosa include:

1. Age and gender: See preceding text. Anorexia nervosa usually develops during adolescence. Being female, is probably the most reliable risk factor for anorexia nervosa.
2. Early childhood eating problems: Picky eating, anorexic symptoms in childhood, digestive and early eating-related problems, eating conflicts, struggles concerning meals are thought to be risk factors for anorexia nervosa.
3. Weight concerns/negative body image/dieting: Studies have shown that there is a link between dieting and the development of eating disorders in teenagers. Adolescent girls who diet are more likely to develop an eating disorder than girls who do not diet.
4. Perinatal events: Perinatal adverse events (prematurity, small for gestational age, and cephalohematoma) may increase the risk of developing anorexia nervosa. Furthermore, young women with a past history of anorexia nervosa may have an increased risk of experiencing adverse perinatal events.
5. Personality traits: The personalities of adolescents with anorexia nervosa are characterized by perfectionism, anxiety, low self-esteem, and obsessionality.
6. Early puberty: There is a greater risk for developing an eating disorder in girls who experience early puberty. Puberty is a time for biological changes in body weight, shape, and size with increased deposition of body fat.
7. Chronic illness: Teenagers with chronic illness, such as diabetes mellitus, are at greater risk for developing an eating disorder.
8. Physical and sexual abuse: Research suggests that adolescents who have been sexually abused have about the same or only slightly higher incidence of anorexia nervosa as those who have not been abused.
9. Family history/family psychopathology: There are elevated rates of psychiatric disorders (anxiety disorders and affective disorders) in first-degree relatives of patients with anorexia nervosa.
10. Competitive athletics: Participation in certain sports or activities that place a high emphasis on body weight and appearance (e.g., ballet and gymnastics) put young people at risk for anorexia nervosa.

Clinical Manifestations—Typical Presentation

The common behaviors, signs, and symptoms associated with adolescents with anorexia nervosa are outlined in the subsequent text.

Behaviors

1. Dieting: Dieting in young people may be the result of a comment about body weight, shape, or size by a family member, teacher, coach, physician, or peer. Young people can often identify exactly when the dieting began.
2. Relentless pursuit of thinness: Initially, weight loss may be reinforced by positive comments from parents or peers who admire the patient's will power and sense of control. Eventually, preoccupation with food, shape, and weight progress and the patient loses control over eating.
3. Distorted body image: The distortion of body image and denial of feelings of hunger result in continued weight loss, eventually leading to a state of emaciation.
4. Unusual eating attitudes and behaviors: Low-calorie foods (e.g., salad with vinegar and no oil, diet foods, and soft drinks) or foods low in fat are preferred. Foods previously enjoyed by the adolescent with anorexia nervosa are avoided. Adolescents with eating disorders tend to eat the same foods at the same time each day. Adolescents with anorexia nervosa may break food into small portions, eat foods of the same color, hide food, or secretly throw food away. Often large amounts of water or diet sodas with caffeine are consumed to satisfy hunger or to cause diuresis. Many adolescents with anorexia nervosa enjoy reading cookbooks, collecting recipes, watching cooking shows on television, cooking, and preparing food for others, although they themselves will not eat.
5. Increased physical activity: Some adolescents will engage in increased physical activity as a means to control their weight. They may stand constantly, move their arms and legs, run up and down stairs, jog, do floor exercises or calisthenics in an effort to expend energy. As weight loss continues, activity level often increases.
6. Purging behaviors: Some patients with anorexia nervosa purge to augment weight loss. Purging may take the form of vomiting, diuresis, food restriction, excessive exercise, or the use of herbal remedies or complementary and alternative medicines (CAM).
7. Frequent weighing: Adolescents with anorexia nervosa may weigh themselves daily or multiple times a day. The weight on the scale often determines how the adolescent feels about him or herself.
8. Wearing baggy clothes: Often adolescents with anorexia nervosa will wear baggy or layered clothing to conceal their weight loss or because they are cold.
9. Poor self-esteem: Adolescents with anorexia nervosa often have feelings of insecurity and helplessness when dealing with people or certain situations. Many young people will control their weight and eating habits in an attempt to reduce these negative feelings.
10. Isolation: Young people with anorexia nervosa usually withdraw from friends and family. This may reflect an attempt to minimize contact with criticizing or teasing peers. It is also a manifestation of low self-esteem and impaired social skills. The teen with anorexia nervosa tends to avoid social situations, as these circumstances are often associated with food.
11. Inflexibility: There is a strong sense of "right and wrong" to the point of not accepting individual differences.
12. Irritability and mood changes: It is not uncommon for parents to describe their adolescent with anorexia

nervosa as moody or irritable. Starvation can cause some of these changes in mood.

Signs and Symptoms

Signs and symptoms may be minimal but can include the following:

1. Signs
   a. Weight loss: Adolescence is a time of intense growth and development. There is great variability in the rate, timing, and magnitude of weight gain, changes in height, and sexual maturation during normal puberty. The diagnostic criteria for anorexia nervosa outlined in the DSM-IV includes weight loss defined as refusal to maintain body weight at or above a minimally normal weight for age and height (e.g., weight loss leading to maintenance of body weight <85% of that expected or failure to make expected weight gain during period of growth, leading to body weight <85% of that expected). There are concerns about this weight criterion, especially the threshold when considering an adolescent underweight. Although formalized diagnostic criteria can be helpful, it is essential to consider the multiple and varied aspects of normal pubertal growth and adolescent development when diagnosing anorexia nervosa. Therefore, any significant or unexpected weight loss in an adolescent is cause for concern. The signs of malnutrition include loss of subcutaneous tissue, temporal wasting, loss of muscle mass, and prominence of bony protuberances.
   b. Amenorrhea: This is one of the diagnostic criteria outlined in the DSM-IV for postmenarcheal females. In 20% to 25% of patients with anorexia nervosa, the amenorrhea precedes the weight loss; in approximately 50%, the amenorrhea occurs at about the same time as the weight loss; and in approximately 25%, the amenorrhea occurs after substantial weight loss. One study found that amenorrhea did not discriminate between women with anorexia nervosa and those with all the features except amenorrhea across a number of relevant variables. As such, the utility of amenorrhea as a diagnostic criterion has been questioned in the postmenarcheal female (Garfinkel et al., 1996). Finally, an increasing number of patients are being seen with premenarcheal onset of the disorder. Resumption of menses usually occurs within 3 to 6 months of achieving goal weight when normal hypothalamic-pituitary-ovarian function is restored (Golden et al., 1997).
   c. Pubertal delay: Anorexia nervosa can delay the start or progression of puberty in adolescents. An episode of anorexia nervosa before or during pubertal development has the potential for long-term adverse effects on sexual maturation (in particular breast development), menarche, or normal menstrual function. Early treatment is critical to avoid delay or irreversible effects on pubertal growth and development.
   d. Lack of growth or poor growth: An adolescent who develops anorexia nervosa before growth is complete may develop growth retardation (Lantzouni et al., 2002; Modan-Moses et al., 2003). It is important to review the growth chart to determine whether the patient has crossed growth percentiles. Lack of growth or poor growth is more likely to occur in males because of the longer growth period of males.
   e. Changes in body hair: Young people with anorexia nervosa often develop lanugo hair, a fine downy hair commonly seen on the back, stomach, or face. They may also complain of hair loss or thinning.
   f. Skin: The skin is often dry with hyperkeratotic areas. There may be yellow or orange discoloration, most noticeable on the palms of the hand. Nail changes have been described in the form of pitting and ridging.
   g. Recurrent fractures
   h. Hypothermia: Decreased oral body temperature that may be as low as 35°C.
   i. Bradycardia: The most common cardiac finding.
   j. Hypotension: Hypotension often associated with significant postural changes can be observed in adolescents with anorexia nervosa.
   k. Acrocyanosis
   l. Edema, usually dependent
   m. Systolic murmur sometimes associated with mitral valve prolapse
2. Symptoms
   a. Cold intolerance: Young people with anorexia nervosa may report that they feel cold when others around them feel fine.
   b. Postural dizziness and fainting
   c. Early satiety, abdominal bloating, discomfort, and pain.
   d. Constipation (secondary to reduced fluid and dietary intake and lack of response to the usual enteroceptive cues to defecation).
   e. Fatigue, muscle weakness, and cramps
   f. Poor concentration

Laboratory Features

Laboratory findings in patients with anorexia nervosa can include the following:

1. Hematological
   a. Leukopenia: May be a relative lymphocytosis
   b. Anemia: Not common and usually a late finding
   c. Thrombocytopenia
   d. Decreased serum complement C3 levels (but reference range levels of C4) and granulocyte killing defect; no evidence for increased susceptibility to bacterial infection
   e. Decreased erythrocyte sedimentation rate (ESR <4 mm/hour); if the ESR is elevated, consider another diagnosis
2. Chemistry
   a. Increased blood urea nitrogen (BUN) concentration
   b. Mildly increased serum glutamic-oxaloacetic transaminase and serum glutamic-pyruvic transaminase levels
   c. Hypophosphatemia
   d. Depressed serum magnesium and calcium concentrations
   e. Increased cholesterol
   f. Increased serum carotene level in 15% to 40% of patients
   g. Decreased vitamin A level
   h. Decreased serum zinc and copper levels
3. Endocrine: The hormonal changes in anorexia nervosa reflect an adaptive response to malnutrition.
   a. Thyroid
      • Thyrotropin (TSH): Within the reference range

- Thyroxine (T_4): Within the reference range or slightly low
- 3,5,3'-Triiodothyronine (T_3): Often low, probably representing increased conversion of T_4 to reverse T_3
- The thyroid changes represent adaptation to starvation, do not require thyroid hormone replacement, and will reverse with weight gain.

b. Growth hormone (GH):
- Decreased insulin-like growth factor 1 (IGF-1) levels
- GH levels normal or elevated

c. Prolactin: Reference range levels

d. Gonadotropins
- Basal levels of luteinizing hormone (LH) and follicle-stimulating hormone (FSH): Usually low.
- Twenty-four-hour LH secretory pattern: Prepubertal with low LH levels and no spikes or occasional nocturnal spikes
- FSH and LH response to gonadotropin-releasing hormone (GnRH): Often a severely blunted response to GnRH, particularly if weight loss is severe

e. Sex steroids
- Estradiol: Low in females (<30 pg/mL)
- Testosterone: Low in males

f. Cortisol: Normal secretion on stimulation. Basal levels are within the reference range or occasionally slightly high. A decreased response of adrenocorticotropic hormone (ACTH) to corticotropin-releasing hormone has been noted. This resolves by 6 months after weight gain has occurred. This abnormality of ACTH response is not found in individuals with bulimia and normal weight.

4. Cardiac
   a. Electrocardiogram (ECG): Bradycardia, low-voltage changes, prolonged QTc interval, T-wave inversions, and occasional ST-segment depression
   b. Echocardiogram: Decreased cardiac size and left ventricular wall thickness, increased prevalence of mitral valve prolapse (Johnson et al., 1986), and pericardial effusion.

5. Gastrointestinal (GI)
   a. Upper GI tract series: Usually normal findings; with occasional decreased gastric motility. May demonstrate features of the superior mesenteric artery syndrome.
   b. Barium enema: Normal findings

6. Renal and metabolic
   a. Decreased glomerular filtration rate
   b. Elevated BUN concentration
   c. Decreased maximum concentration ability (nephrogenic diabetes insipidus)
   d. Metabolic alkalosis
   e. Alkaline urine

7. Low bone mineral density (BMD) (osteopenia or osteoporosis)

Diagnosis and Differential Diagnosis

The diagnosis of anorexia nervosa should be suspected in any adolescent with unexplained weight loss and food avoidance. The diagnosis is based not only on the absence of a defined organic cause but also on the presence of certain characteristics. The most commonly used diagnostic criteria for anorexia nervosa are outlined in the American Psychiatric Association's *DSM-IV* (Table 33.1).

The differential diagnosis includes both medical and psychiatric conditions:

1. Medical conditions
   a. Inflammatory bowel disease
   b. Malabsorption
   c. Endocrine conditions—hyperthyroidism, Addison's disease, diabetes mellitus
   d. Collagen vascular disease
   e. Central nervous system (CNS) lesions—hypothalamic or pituitary tumors
   f. Malignancies
   g. Chronic infections—tuberculosis, human immunodeficiency virus (HIV)
   h. Immunodeficiency
2. Psychiatric conditions
   a. Mood disorders
   b. Anxiety disorders
   c. Somatization disorder
   d. Substance abuse disorder
   e. Psychosis

Evaluation

The evaluation of the patient with a suspected eating disorder should include a comprehensive history and physical examination and certain preliminary laboratory tests.

History
Helpful questions regarding eating, weight-control behavior, and other issues include:

1. Why has the teen and/or family come for an assessment?
2. How does the teen feel about the way she/he looks?
3. Is the teen trying to change the way she/he looks?
4. Has there been any change in the teen's weight? If yes, what methods has the teen used to control his or her weight?
5. How much does the teen want to weigh?
6. Does the teen binge? Describe a "binge"? How often does the teen binge?
7. Are there any purging behaviors such as vomiting, laxative abuse, diuretic use, ipecac use, diet pills, herbal medications or other CAM?
8. What was the most and least the teen has weighed and when was that?
9. Does the teen's feelings about her/his body affect her/his mood?
10. Is there any particular part of the teen's body that he or she is uncomfortable with and why (e.g., buttocks or thighs)?
11. How much does the disordered eating interfere with the teen's life? How much time does he or she spend preparing food, exercising, and weighing him or herself?
12. How much does the teen worry about eating or her/his weight?
13. Exercise history? Type, amount, and frequency?
14. What has the teen eaten in the last 24 hours?
15. Has the teen ever had a menstrual period? If yes, when was her last normal menstrual period? How often does she get her period? Has there been any change in her periods? Is the teen on oral contraceptive pill (OCP)?
16. Family medical and psychiatric history including teen or other family members with an eating disorder, mental illness, or substance abuse problem/disorder.

17. Any prior or current history of sexual, physical, or emotional abuse?
18. How does the family understand the teen's eating problem? What have the parent(s)/caregiver/family members done to support the teen?
19. Where does the teen get help? With whom does he or she share information?

Instruments

Several instruments have been developed to aid in the diagnosis of eating disorders and the differentiation of anorexia from bulimia nervosa. These include the following:

1. *Eating Attitudes Test (EAT-26)*: This screening test is a 26-item self-report questionnaire that examines attitudes and behaviors regarding food, weight, and body image. A score >21 is suggestive of an eating disorder and warrants further evaluation (Garner and Garfinkel, 1979).The EAT-26 has been validated for use in adolescents.
2. *Eating Disorders Inventory*: A 91-item questionnaire that can be used both for screening and monitoring the emergence of an eating disorder in a high-risk group but not for diagnosis. It assesses drive for thinness, body dissatisfaction, bulimic behaviors as well as other dimensions associated with eating disorders including ineffectiveness, perfectionism, interpersonal distrust, interoceptive awareness, and maturity fears. Scores reflect percentiles for normal populations (Garner et al., 1983).
3. *Eating Disorders Examination Questionnaire (EDE-Q)*: The EDE-Q (Fairburn and Beglin, 1994) is a 38-item self-report version of the Eating Disorders Examination administered to assess eating disorder pathology. The questionnaire assesses restraint and concerns about eating, body weight, and shape.
4. *Kids' Eating Disorders Survey (KEDS)*: The KEDS (Childress et al., 1993) is a 14-item self-report instrument requiring a 2nd grade reading level. It includes a three-point scale and eight figure drawings for assessing body shape concerns. Normal values are available.

Physical Examination

The physical examination should focus on the signs of malnutrition previously described. Height and weight should be carefully measured and plotted on the Centers for Disease Control and Prevention (CDC) growth charts. Previous growth curves are very helpful. Abnormal growth in weight and height may be an indication that there is a medical problem, such as anorexia nervosa. Weight should be measured in a hospital gown or light clothing after the patient has emptied her bladder. Body mass index (BMI) should be calculated (BMI = weight in kilograms divided by height in meters squared) and plotted on the CDC growth charts. The percentage of ideal or standard body weight should be determined from the National Center for Health Statistics Tables (the original data sets from which the growth curves were drawn). For the adolescent, these are readily available at www.Pocket-Doc.com. Finally, sexual maturity rating (SMR) should be determined on each adolescent in order to make sure that puberty is proceeding in a predictable and normal manner.

Laboratory Assessment

Suggested laboratory tests are listed in the subsequent text:

1. Complete blood cell (CBC) count and platelet count
2. ESR
3. BUN and serum creatinine
4. Urinalysis
5. Serum electrolytes and liver function tests: Hypokalemia with an increased serum bicarbonate level may indicate frequent vomiting or use of diuretics, whereas nonanion gap acidosis is common with laxative abuse. Caloric restriction alone, without any purging behavior, does not usually cause hypokalemia. Hyponatremia is common and may be secondary to excess water intake. Mild elevations of serum transaminases occur in 4% to 38% of patients with anorexia nervosa.
6. Serum calcium, phosphate, magnesium, and phosphorus concentrations
7. Serum albumin level (usually normal)
8. Carotene level
9. T_3, T_4, and TSH levels
10. LH, FSH, estradiol, and prolactin level if amenorrheic
11. ECG
12. BMD should be measured in females with anorexia nervosa who have been amenorrheic for >6 months. The most frequently used test is dual energy x-ray absorptiometry (DXA).

Optional laboratory tests include:

1. Upper GI tract series and small bowel series
2. Barium enema
3. Celiac screen
4. Computed tomography or magnetic resonance imaging (MRI) of the head

Nutritional Assessment

The nutritional assessment should include a 24-hour dietary recall, an assessment of both foods and beverages consumed, and anthropometric measurements such as height, weight, BMI, and skinfold measures. A 24-hour recall, including portion sizes and the types of food products used can highlight whether the diet is sufficient, balanced, and structured. Adolescents should be asked to describe which foods they consume from each food group. Adolescents with eating disorders may consume a large quantity of diet products and avoid entire food categories such as fats, carbohydrates, or protein. They may also drink an excessive amount of fluids including caffeinated products such as coffee, tea, iced tea, or soda to reduce hunger and alter body weight. An assessment of dietary calcium intake should be made. Adolescents require 1200 to 1500 mg of calcium/day and may require calcium supplementation should their dietary calcium intake fall below their requirements.

Treatment

1. Team approach: Treatment is best conducted by an interdisciplinary team of individuals who are skilled and knowledgeable in working with adolescents with eating disorders and their families. The treatment team typically consists of a physician, therapist, and nutritionist. It is critical that there is excellent communication among the members of the team and that information is shared as appropriate.
2. Diagnosis: The most critical step in treating anorexia nervosa is to recognize and address the eating disorder as soon as possible. It is important to inform the

adolescent and the family of the diagnosis and treatment plan.

3. Medical and nutritional intervention: The goals of medical intervention are nutritional rehabilitation, weight restoration, and reversal of the acute medical complications. Once there is improvement in the physiological symptoms of starvation, psychological treatment can begin.

4. Psychological intervention: Psychotherapy is an important component of the treatment of adolescents with anorexia nervosa. For the adolescent to be involved in a psychotherapeutic treatment program, he or she needs to be motivated to some extent. The psychological therapies currently used for the treatment of anorexia nervosa include family psychoeducation, interpersonal therapy, and family therapy. Recently, family-based treatment has been found to be effective in the adolescent age-group (Le Grange et al., 2003). It is also important to remember that teens with eating disorders may suffer from a coexisting mental illness such as an anxiety disorder or depression and this needs to be considered in making treatment recommendations.

5. Pharmacological treatment: Some adolescents with eating disorders may benefit from the use of psychotropic medications. Fluoxetine does not appear to be effective in treating the primary symptoms of anorexia nervosa (Attia et al., 1998). Other studies have explored the efficacy of medication after weight restoration, with differing results. One study reported that fluoxetine prevented relapse in older adolescents with anorexia nervosa who have attained 85% of their expected body weight (Kaye et al., 2001), whereas a recent study failed to demonstrate any benefit from fluoxetine in weight restored patients with anorexia nervosa (Walsh et al., 2006). The most common medications used have included the SSRIs such as: fluoxetine, sertraline, paroxetine, fluvoxamine, and citalopram. These medications are also useful in treating comorbid depression or OCD. Health care providers need to be aware that the U.S. Food and Drug Administration has required manufacturers of these medications to include a "black box" warning label that alerts health care providers and consumers to an increased risk of suicidal thinking and behavior in adolescents being treated with the medications (Lock et al., 2005). In addition, there are some recent reports that the atypical neuroleptic medications such as risperidone, olanzapine, and quetiapine may be effective in adolescents with anorexia nervosa. Case reports and small cohort studies have shown that these medications have been helpful in reducing anxiety and obsessional thinking and enhancing weight gain. Further research is required to understand the benefits of these medications in the treatment of anorexia nervosa in adolescents.

6. Treatment setting: The actual treatment setting for the adolescent with anorexia nervosa may involve inpatient treatment, outpatient treatment, partial hospitalization, or residential treatment. Indications for hospitalization are outlined in Table 33.2 (Golden et al., 2003).The goals of hospitalization should be weight gain and reversal of the acute medical complications such as electrolyte disturbances and vital sign instability. Attempts should be made to achieve weight gain through the oral route, if possible. Short-term nasogastric feeding may be necessary in those with severe malnutrition. Behavioral contracts have been helpful and are used in most inpatient programs. Nutritional rehabilitation needs to be performed slowly to prevent the "refeeding syndrome"—a constellation of cardiac, hematological, and neurological symptoms associated with refeeding a

TABLE 33.2

Indications for Hospitalization in an Adolescent with an Eating Disorder

One or more of the following justify hospitalization:
1. Severe malnutrition (weight ≤75% average body weight for age, sex, and height)
2. Dehydration
3. Electrolyte disturbances (hypokalemia, hyponatremia, hypophosphatemia)
4. Cardiac dysrhythmia
5. Physiological instability
   Severe bradycardia (heart rate <50 beats/min daytime; <45 beats/min at night)
   Hypotension (<80/50 mm Hg)
   Hypothermia (body temperature <96°F)
   Orthostatic changes in pulse (>20 beats/min) or blood pressure (>10 mm Hg)
6. Arrested growth and development
7. Failure of outpatient treatment
8. Acute food refusal
9. Uncontrollable binging and purging
10. Acute medical complications of malnutrition (e.g., syncope, seizures, cardiac failure, pancreatitis)
11. Acute psychiatric emergencies (e.g., suicidal ideation, acute psychosis)
12. Comorbid diagnosis that interferes with the treatment of the eating disorder (e.g., severe depression, obsessive-compulsive disorder, severe family dysfunction)

Reprinted with permission from Golden NH, Katzman DK, Kreipe RE, et al. Eating disorders in adolescents. Position paper of the Society for Adolescent Medicine. *J Adolesc Health* 2003;33:496.

FIGURE 33.2 Timeline for resolution of the medical complications of anorexia nervosa. (Reprinted with permission from Golden NH, Meyer W. Nutritional rehabilitation of anorexia nervosa. Goals and dangers. *Int J Adolesc Med Health* 2004;16(2):131. Freund Publishing House Ltd.)

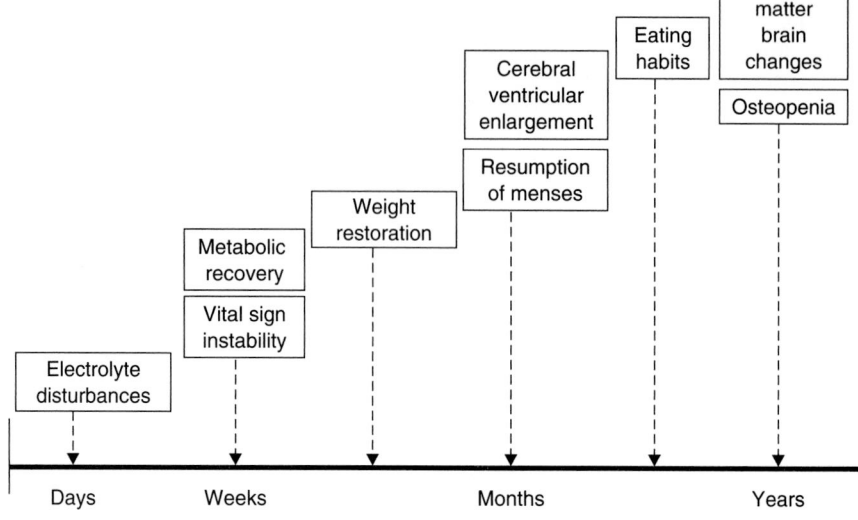

malnourished patient. The most serious feature of this syndrome is sudden unexpected death associated with hypophosphatemia and cardiac arrhythmias. A weight gain of 2 to 3 lb a week is optimal. Most, but not all, of the medical complications are reversible with nutritional rehabilitation (Golden and Meyer, 2004). Those conditions that may not be reversible include growth retardation, osteopenia, and structural brain changes (Katzman, 2005). A timeline for resolution of the medical complications of anorexia nervosa is shown in Figure 33.2.

7. Advice for parents or other caretakers: Several suggestions may be helpful in advising parents who have teenagers with an eating disorder. These include the following:
   a. Be patient: The recovery from anorexia nervosa is a long and hard process. There is no quick or easy cure. The recovery often takes 5 to 6 years.
   b. Avoid blaming: It is helpful for family members to avoid blaming themselves or others for the cause of the eating disorder.
   c. Avoid comments: Avoid comments about your adolescent's weight and appearance. This is often perceived as criticism. Also, avoid comments about your own weight and appearance and the weight and appearance of others. Focus on traits that are not appearance-related.
   d. Promote a positive body image and healthy attitude toward eating and activity.
   e. Encourage family meals as often as reasonably possible.
   f. Avoid making food the struggle. Food often becomes the central topic of discussions and arguments. Parents often become concerned and frustrated when their adolescent refuses to eat. As the adolescent loses weight, it becomes more difficult to change the adolescent's eating attitudes and behaviors.
   g. Work *with* your health care team. The health care team consists of skilled professionals who can treat the adolescent with the eating disorder and support the family through the course of the illness.

Complications

1. Fluid and electrolytes related
   a. Dehydration
   b. Hypokalemia
   c. Hyponatremia
   d. Hypophosphatemia
   e. Hypomagnesemia
   f. Hypoglycemia
2. Cardiovascular
   a. Sinus bradycardia; sinus arrhythmia
   b. Orthostatic hypotension
   c. Ventricular dysrhythmias
   d. Reduced myocardial contractility
   e. Sudden death, secondary to arrhythmias
   f. Cardiomyopathy secondary to ipecac use
   g. Mitral valve prolapse
   h. ECG abnormalities including low voltage, prolonged QTc interval, and prominent U waves
   i. Pericardial effusion
   j. Congestive heart failure
3. Renal
   a. Increased BUN
   b. Decreased glomerular filtration rate
   c. Renal calculi
   d. Edema
   e. Renal concentrating defect
4. GI
   a. Delayed gastric emptying
   b. Constipation
   c. Elevated liver enzymes (acute fatty necrosis)
   d. Superior mesenteric artery syndrome
   e. Rectal prolapse
   f. Gallstones
5. Hematological
   a. Anemia
   b. Leukopenia
   c. Thrombocytopenia
6. Endocrine or metabolic
   a. Primary or secondary amenorrhea
   b. Pubertal delay
   c. Thrombocytopenia

d. Euthyroid sick syndrome (Low T_3 syndrome)
e. Hypercortisolism
f. Decreased serum testosterone level
g. Partial diabetes insipidus
h. Elevated cholesterol level
7. Osteopenia
   a. Fractures: Females with anorexia nervosa have reduced bone mass (osteopenia) and increased fracture risk (Golden et al., 2003). Osteopenia at one or more sites occurs in approximately 90% of patients who meet DSM-IV criteria for anorexia nervosa (Golden et al., 2002; Grinspoon et al., 2000) and the degree of osteopenia is more severe than that seen in hypothalamic amenorrhea (Grinspoon et al., 1999). Body weight is the most important determinant of BMD and weight gain is associated with an increase in BMD (Bachrach et al., 1991), although levels may not revert to normal. Hormone replacement therapy has not been proven to be effective in increasing BMD in adults (Klibanski et al., 1995) or in adolescents (Golden et al., 2002). Recent studies have demonstrated a positive effect of treatment with IGF-1 (Grinspoon et al., 2002), dehydroepiandrosterone (Gordon et al., 2002), and bisphosphonates (Golden et al., 2005) although these modalities are still being studied and are not yet recommended for general use. Current recommendations include weight restoration and resumption of spontaneous menses, calcium, and vitamin D supplementation and moderate weight-bearing exercise.
8. Neuromuscular
   a. Generalized muscle weakness
   b. Seizures secondary to metabolic abnormalities
   c. Peripheral neuropathies
   d. Cardiomyopathy secondary to ipecac abuse
   e. Syncope in absence of orthostatic hypotension
   f. Movement disorders
   g. Structural brain changes—MRI studies have demonstrated enlargement of the lateral ventricles and sulci and significant deficits in both gray- and white-matter volumes in the low-weight stages. Increases in sulcal volume and decreases in gray-matter volume may not be fully reversible with weight recovery.

Clinical and Laboratory Findings Associated with Sudden Death

a. Prolonged QTc interval
b. Decreased serum phosphate concentration
c. Ipecac cardiomyopathy
d. Severe emaciation ($<70\%$ of ideal body weight)
e. Suicide

Outcome

More than 100 studies have been conducted on the outcome of anorexia nervosa over the last 50 years with wide variability in the results. Comparisons among studies are limited by differences in definitions of "cases," length of follow-up, and type of data collected (Fisher, 2003). General consensus is that the prognosis for adolescents with anorexia nervosa is better than that for adults, due in part to the shorter duration of symptoms in adolescents. Approximately 50% of adolescents have a "good" outcome, approximately 30% have a "fair" outcome, and 20% a "poor" outcome.

In a well-designed prospective study, 95 adolescents with anorexia nervosa (ages 12–17) were followed up at 6- to 12-month intervals for 10 to 15 years (Strober et al., 1997). There was full recovery in 75.8%, partial recovery in an additional 10.5%, and chronicity or no recovery in 13.7%. However, the time to full recovery was prolonged and ranged from 57 to 79 months. Readmission to the hospital within the first year of treatment occurred in 30% of patients but did not portend a poor prognosis. Adolescents with anorexia nervosa can fully recover, but the time to recover may take many years and the path may be difficult. The following are some of the findings pertaining to recovery:

1. Weight restoration: At follow-up, 22% to 79% were normal weight, 15% to 43% were 11% to 21% below normal, 2% to 10% were overweight.
2. Menses: Sixty-five percent to 95% of patients with anorexia nervosa were menstruating at follow-up.
3. Eating difficulties: Only a third of subjects were eating normally at follow-up (Hsu, 1980); 23% to 67% had restricted food intake, 11% to 50% were still vomiting or abusing laxatives.
4. Psychological disturbances: Psychiatric comorbidity was common in follow-up studies. Important findings include a lifetime incidence of depression in 50% to 68%; anxiety disorders (especially OCD and social phobia) in 30% to 65%; substance abuse in 12% to 21%; and comorbid personality disorders in 20% to 80%. Estimates of good or satisfactory psychosocial functioning ranged from 22% to 73%. Approximately one third of patients with anorexia nervosa develop bulimia nervosa.
5. Psychosocial: Most patients were engaged in full-time employment, with good work attendance.
6. Mortality: The mortality rate ranges from 2% to 8% with longer-term studies revealing a mortality as high as 15% (Ratnasuria et al., 1991). Patients with anorexia nervosa are 12 times more likely to die than women of a similar age in the general population (Keel et al., 2003). The most common causes of death are suicide and the medical complications of starvation.

Certain factors seem to relate to a good prognosis or poor prognosis:

1. Good prognosis
   a. Short duration of illness
   b. Early identification and intervention
   c. Early onset (<14 years old)
   d. No associated comorbid psychological diagnoses
   e. No binging and purging
   f. Supportive family
2. Poor prognosis
   a. Longer duration of illness
   b. Binging and purging
   c. Comorbid mental illness (affective disorder, substance abuse)
   d. Lower body weight at diagnosis

Anorexia nervosa appears to have lower recovery rates than bulimia nervosa. Weight restoration and resumption of menses seem to respond well to treatment. Psychological improvements also occur but take much longer.

BULIMIA NERVOSA

Bulimia nervosa is an eating disorder characterized by binge eating coupled with compensatory behaviors intended to promote weight loss such as self-induced vomiting, laxative abuse, excessive exercise, or prolonged fasting. The profound emaciation associated with anorexia nervosa is not present in adolescents with bulimia nervosa, and most individuals have a normal weight. Menses are usually normal but may be irregular. The adolescent with bulimia nervosa is usually quite aware of the abnormal eating attitudes and behaviors and is quite distressed by them. The DSM-IV diagnostic criteria for bulimia nervosa are listed in Table 33.3. Adolescents who meet the criteria for anorexia nervosa but also binge or purge are classified as anorexia nervosa, binge eating/purging type. Approximately one third of patients with anorexia nervosa "cross over" to bulimia nervosa at some time in their illness.

Epidemiology

1. Prevalence: Large-scale studies from several countries have found that up to 15% of adolescents report binge eating or purging behaviors (Schneider, 2003). The numbers are even higher for college students. Zuckerman et al. (1986) found that 23% of college women and 14% of college men reported binging at least once each week, and 23% of the females and 9% of the males used vomiting, laxatives, or diuretics for weight control. However, most of these young people do not meet DSM-IV criteria for bulimia nervosa. The lifetime prevalence of bulimia nervosa in young females living in western industrialized countries is estimated to be 1% to 4%.
2. Age: Onset is usually during late adolescence or early adulthood with a modal age at onset of 18 to 19 years old. Bulimia nervosa developing in patients younger than 14 years is rare.
3. Gender: Ninety percent to 95% are female, although recently there has been a reported increased prevalence in males, particularly in those who must weight qualify for interscholastic events (e.g., wrestlers).

4. Comorbidity: Approximately 80% of patients with bulimia nervosa report a lifetime prevalence of another psychiatric condition (Fichter and Quadfling, 1997). The major comorbid conditions are affective disorders (50%–80%), anxiety disorders (13%–65%), personality disorders (20%–80%), and substance abuse (25%) (Walsh et al., 2005). Patients with bulimia nervosa tend to be more impulsive than those with anorexia nervosa and may engage in shoplifting, stealing, self-destructive acts, and sexual acting out.

Risk Factors

As for anorexia nervosa, risk factors for bulimia nervosa are not a direct cause of the disease, but increase the likelihood of developing the condition.

1. Age and gender: Bulimia nervosa is more likely to develop during adolescence. Females are more likely to be affected than males.
2. Early childhood eating and health problems: Some studies have shown that early childhood eating problems (pica, early digestive problems, and weight reduction efforts) are associated with the later development of bulimia nervosa.
3. Weight concerns, negative body image, and dieting: Body dissatisfaction, perceived pressure to be thin, and dieting have all been identified as risk factors for the development of bulimic symptoms.
4. Personality traits: Negative affect, impulsivity, stressful life events, and family conflict have been associated with increased risk of developing bulimia nervosa.
5. Early puberty: Some studies have shown that early menarche increases the risk of developing bulimia.
6. Family history: As for anorexia nervosa, there is an increased risk of developing bulimia nervosa if a family member has an eating disorder. Concordance rates are higher for monozygotic than for dizygotic twins and

TABLE 33.3

DSM-IV Diagnostic Criteria for Bulimia Nervosa

1. Recurrent episodes of binge eating. An episode of binge eating is characterized by both of the following:
   a. Eating, in a discreet period of time (e.g., within any 2 hour period), an amount of food that is definitely larger than most people would eat during a similar period of time and under similar circumstances.
   b. A sense of lack of control over eating during the episode (e.g., a feeling that one cannot stop eating or control what or how much one is eating).
2. Recurrent inappropriate compensatory behavior to prevent weight gain, such as self-induced vomiting; misuse of laxatives, diuretics, enemas, or other medications; fasting; or excessive exercise.
3. The binge eating and inappropriate compensatory behaviors both occur, on average, at least twice a wk for 3 mo.
4. Self-evaluation is unduly influenced by body shape and weight.
5. The disturbance does not occur exclusively during episodes of anorexia nervosa.

Two types have been identified:
1. Purging type: During the current episode of bulimia nervosa, the person has regularly engaged in self-induced vomiting or the misuse of laxatives, diuretics, or enemas.
2. Nonpurging type: During the current episode of bulimia nervosa, the person has used other inappropriate compensatory behaviors, such as fasting or excessive exercise, but has not regularly engaged in self-induced vomiting or the misuse of laxatives, diuretics, or enemas.

Reprinted with permission from the American Psychiatric Association. *Diagnostic and statistical manual of mental disorders*, 4th ed. Text Revision, Copyright, 2000.

range from 27% to 83%. A susceptibility locus for bulimia nervosa has been identified on chromosome 10p (Bulik et al., 2003).

7. Childhood sexual abuse: Childhood sexual abuse is sometimes associated with the later development of bulimia nervosa (Wonderlich et al., 2001).

Clinical Manifestations—Typical Presentation

The common behaviors, signs, and symptoms associated with adolescents with bulimia nervosa are outlined in the subsequent text.

Behaviors

1. Binging and purging: The most important behaviors in adolescents with bulimia nervosa are the binging and purging. The binge episode is the rapid consumption of a large amount of high calorie food in a short period of time and associated with self-perceived loss of control over eating. The most common triggers for binge eating include negative mood, interpersonal stress, hunger due to dietary restriction, and negative feeling related to one's body image. The individual often experiences feelings of being "out of control" during the binge episode. Binging occurs after a short period of starvation, typically in the afternoon after having skipped breakfast or lunch, or late in the evening. Binges can be enormously large in caloric content (as high as 3,000–5,000 kcal). After a binge, feelings of guilt and shame together with fear of weight gain result in purging. Methods of purging include vomiting, excessively exercising, fasting for a day or days after a binge, taking laxatives, diuretics, ipecac, diet pills, herbal remedies, or CAM. The binging and purging is often done secretly. Purging may initially have a calming effect and relieve guilt over a binge episode. This may lead to recurrent cycles of binging and purging in an attempt to manage feelings of depression and anxiety.

    Initially, the binge–purge activity may be infrequent, but with time, it may increase to daily or even several times a day. In addition, as the condition progresses, some individuals with bulimia nervosa will purge even after ingesting normal or small amounts of any food that might be considered high in calories or fat. Therefore, over time, what began as a diet or weight-control measure turns into a means of mood regulation with the binging and purging behaviors becoming a source of coping.

2. Evidence of purging: Some adolescents will make frequent trips to the bathroom, particularly after eating. In addition, there may be signs and/or smells of vomit, presence of empty food containers, or packages of laxatives or diuretics.

3. Evidence of binge eating: Often family members of adolescents with bulimia nervosa report the disappearance of food or the presence of empty wrappers and containers indicating the consumption of large amounts of food. In addition, adolescents with bulimia nervosa may steal, hoard, or hide food, and eat in secret.

4. Frequently weighing self
5. Preoccupation with food
6. Overly concerned with food, body weight, shape, and size.

Signs and Symptoms

Signs and symptoms may be minimal but can include the following:

1. Signs
    a. Body weight is usually normal or above normal.
    b. Skin changes: Calluses on the dorsum of the hand secondary to abrasions from the central incisors when the fingers are used to induce vomiting. This physical sign is known as *Russell sign's*.
    c. Enlargement of the salivary glands, particularly the parotid glands; usually bilateral and painless.
    d. Dental enamel erosion (perimolysis): Usually occurs in the lingual, palatal, and posterior occlusal surfaces of the teeth.
    e. Weight fluctuations.
    f. Edema (fluid retention).
2. Symptoms
    a. Weakness and fatigue
    b. Headaches
    c. Abdominal fullness and bloating
    d. Nausea
    e. Irregular menses
    f. Muscle cramps
    g. Chest pain and heartburn
    h. Easy bruising (from hypokalemia/platelet dysfunction)
    i. Bloody diarrhea (in laxative abusers)

Table 33.4 contrasts anorexia nervosa with bulimia nervosa.

Diagnosis and Differential Diagnosis

The most commonly used diagnostic criteria used for the diagnosis of bulimia nervosa are outlined in the American Psychiatric Association's DSM-IV (Table 33.3). The differential diagnosis includes both medical and psychiatric conditions:

1. Medical conditions
    a. Chronic cholecystitis
    b. Cholelithiasis
    c. Peptic ulcer disease
    d. Gastroesophageal reflux disease
    e. Superior mesenteric artery syndrome
    f. Malignancies (including CNS tumors)
    g. Infections—acute bacterial and viral GI infections, parasitic infections, and hepatitis
    h. Pregnancy
    i. Oral contraceptives: Nausea can be a side effect of oral contraceptives and hormone replacement therapy
    j. Medications—some medications have side effects that may include nausea and vomiting, or food cravings
2. Psychiatric conditions
    a. Anorexia nervosa-binge/purge subtype
    b. Binge eating disorder
    c. Major depressive disorder, with atypical features
    d. Borderline personality disorder
    e. Kleine-Levin syndrome

Evaluation

Evaluation includes a complete history and physical examination.

TABLE 33.4

Anorexia Nervosa versus Bulimia Nervosa: Similar and Contrasting Features

Area	Anorexia Nervosa	Bulimia Nervosa
Epidemiology	90% Female patients	Same
	Increased prevalence of eating disorders and depression in families	Same
	Onset early to midadolescence	Slightly older onset
	Prevalence <1%	Prevalence 1%–4%
Psychopathology	Intense fear of gaining weight or becoming fat	Same
	Introverted, obsessional, perfectionistic, rigid	More outgoing, impulsive, prone to acting-out behaviors (shoplifting, sexual promiscuity, self-destructive acts)
	Poor self-esteem	Same
	Secretive about behaviors	Same
	Binge eating not necessary	Binge eating must be present
	Level of denial high	Aware of problem; wants help
Physical signs		
Weight	Underweight; must be <85% expected weight	Usually of normal weight
		Weight can be normal, high, or low
Menses	Must be amenorrheic	May have normal, irregular, or absent menses

Laboratory screening includes:

1. CBC count
2. BUN and creatinine, electrolytes, glucose, calcium, phosphorus
3. Serum amylase
4. ECG with rhythm strip
5. Urinalysis—specific gravity

Treatment

Like adolescents with anorexia nervosa, the treatment of young people with bulimia nervosa requires an interdisciplinary team approach. The first step is to make a diagnosis and address the eating disorder as soon as possible. The principles of treatment include the following:

1. Medical and nutritional intervention: The goals of medical intervention include careful medical monitoring and the correction of any medical complication, in particular electrolyte abnormalities. A structured meal plan developed with the help of a nutritionist can be very helpful. Eating three normal meals a day will reduce the physiological drive to binge in the late afternoon or evening. The adolescent should be encouraged and supported to avoid foods that trigger a binge (e.g., ice cream or baked goods). Promoting moderate exercise can also be helpful. Adolescents should have routine dental care and consultation should be sought for those teens with dental damage secondary to vomiting.
2. Psychological intervention: In adults, multiple studies have shown that cognitive-behavioral therapy (CBT) reduces binge eating and purging activity in approximately 30% to 50% of patients. Attitudes about body shape and weight are also improved. Treatment with CBT is time limited and problem oriented. It focuses on strategies to cope with the emotional triggers that lead to binge eating and purging and addresses ways to modify abnormal attitudes to eating, body shape, and weight. In individuals with bulimia nervosa, treatment with CBT has been found to be more effective than other psychological treatments such as supportive psychotherapy, interpersonal therapy, or stress management (Walsh et al., 2005).
3. Pharmacologic treatment: Multiple studies have demonstrated a positive effect of a number of different antidepressants for treating bulimia nervosa. The SSRIs are better tolerated and have fewer side effects than earlier generations of antidepressants. Fluoxetine is the only medication approved by the FDA for the treatment of bulimia nervosa and is most effective at a dose of 60 mg daily (Fluoxetine Bulimia Nervosa Collaborative Study Group, 1992; Walsh et al., 1997). Treatment with fluoxetine results in a decrease in binge-eating and purging episodes in 55% to 65% of subjects. A combination of antidepressant medication and CBT appears to be superior to either modality alone (Nakash-Eisikovits et al., 2002).
4. Treatment settings: The treatment settings for adolescents with bulimia nervosa are similar to those outlined for anorexia nervosa. The majority of adolescents with bulimia nervosa can be treated in an outpatient setting (outpatient clinic or partial hospitalization).

Complications

1. Fluid and electrolytes related
   a. Dehydration
   b. Hypokalemia (the most frequently seen electrolyte abnormality—either from vomiting or from laxative or diuretic use)
   c. Hyponatremia
   d. Hypophosphatemia (especially when binging occurs after a prolonged period of dietary restriction)
2. Cardiovascular
   a. Cardiac arrhythmias
   b. Ipecac cardiomyopathy

3. GI
   a. Parotid gland enlargement and increased serum amylase levels
   b. Esophagitis
   c. Mallory-Weiss tears
   d. Rupture of the esophagus or stomach
   e. Acute pancreatitis
   f. Paralytic ileus secondary to laxative abuse
   g. Cathartic colon
   h. Barrett Esophagus
4. Pulmonary
   a. Aspiration pneumonia secondary to vomiting
   b. Pneumomediastinum secondary to vomiting
5. Dental
   a. Erosion of dental enamel
   b. Dental caries

Outcome

Most adolescents with bulimia nervosa recover over time with recovery rates ranging from 35% to 75% at 5 years of follow-up (Fichter and Quadfling, 1997). Bulimia nervosa tends to be a chronic relapsing condition and approximately one third of patients relapse in 1 to 2 years. Comorbidity is frequent but mortality is low.

In one study, after a 90-month follow-up period, the full recovery rate in women with bulimia nervosa (74%) was significantly higher than that of women with anorexia nervosa (33%) (Herzog et al., 1999). No predictors of recovery emerged among bulimic subjects. Eighty-three percent of women with anorexia nervosa and 99% of those with bulimia nervosa achieved partial recovery. Approximately one third of both groups relapsed after full recovery. No predictors of relapse emerged. Bulimia nervosa was characterized by higher rates of both partial and full recovery.

EATING DISORDERS NOT OTHERWISE SPECIFIED

EDNOS refers to the diagnostic category of patients who have problems with eating or body image but who do not meet full DSM-IV criteria for either anorexia nervosa or bulimia nervosa. This category accounts for most adolescents presenting for treatment (Fisher et al., 2001; Nicholls et al., 2000). Importantly, these adolescents suffer from the same medical complications and similar degree of psychological distress as those who meet full criteria. Some of the individuals in the EDNOS category represent those with subthreshold anorexia nervosa or bulimia nervosa, but others represent qualitatively distinct disorders. This heterogeneous diagnostic category is likely to undergo further refinement in the near future.

Examples of individuals with EDNOS include:

1. Teens with all the criteria for anorexia nervosa but who have regular menses
2. Individuals who appear to have anorexia nervosa, but despite significant weight loss, their present weight is in the normal range
3. Individuals who meet all the criteria for bulimia nervosa except that the frequency of binging or purging is less than twice a week or lasts for <3 months

4. Teens who purge daily but never binge
5. Adolescents who repeatedly chew and spit out but do not swallow their food
6. Individuals who binge-eat but do not purge (see Binge Eating Disorder)

An alternative classification for the range of eating disorders of childhood and younger adolescents is outlined in the Great Ormond Street (GOS) criteria (Lask and Bryant-Waugh, 1993; Nicholls et al., 2000). The diagnoses within this classification not only consist of anorexia nervosa and bulimia nervosa but also include the following diagnostic categories:

1. Food avoidance emotional disorder (FAED): FAED refers to a condition seen in children 8 to 13 years old where the child refuses to eat. There is no fear of becoming fat and no distortion in body image. This condition may be accompanied by growth retardation and weight loss.
2. Selective eating disorder (SED): SED refers to those younger patients who will limit their foods to one or two foods for a prolonged period of time. They are unwilling to try new foods, which can be a major source of frustration for their parents. Similar to those with FAED, they do not have the cognitive distortions regarding weight or shape. Their weight and height are usually appropriate for age.
3. Functional dysphagia: Functional dysphagia refers to children and younger adolescents who will avoid certain foods because of a fear of swallowing, choking, or vomiting. Often there is a history of an episode of choking on a specific food.
4. Pervasive food refusal: Pervasive food refusal refers to children and younger adolescents who have a profound refusal to eat, drink, walk, and talk or self-care and are resistant to efforts to help.

The overriding similarities among these diagnostic criteria are the lack of abnormal cognitions and morbid preoccupation with weight and shape.

BINGE EATING DISORDER

Binge eating disorder is a newly recognized disorder and only recently appeared in the DSM-IV (1994) under the category of EDNOS and is also listed as a category for proposed diagnoses and further research. The *DSM-IV* proposed criteria include the following:

1. Recurrent episodes of binge eating. An episode of binge eating is characterized by both of the following:
   a. Eating, in a discrete period of time (e.g., within any 2-hour period), an amount of food that is definitely larger than what most people would eat during a similar period and under similar circumstances
   b. A sense of lack of control over eating during the episode (e.g., a feeling that one cannot stop eating or control what or how much one is eating)
2. The binge eating episodes are associated with three or more of the following:
   a. Eating more rapidly than normal
   b. Eating until feeling uncomfortably full
   c. Eating large amounts of food when not physically hungry
   d. Eating alone because of embarrassment

   e. Feeling disgusted with self and depressed
3. Marked distress regarding binge eating is present.
4. The binge eating occurs, on an average, at least 2 days a week for 6 months.
5. The binge eating is not associated with the regular use of inappropriate compensatory behaviors (e.g., purging, fasting, and excessive exercise) and does not occur exclusively during the course of anorexia nervosa or bulimia nervosa.

This type of eating pattern can lead to significant weight problems and obesity. Some of these individuals start these behaviors after a period of weight-loss diets and restrictive eating, whereas others use the binge as a calming mechanism unrelated to prior dietary restrictions.

Because it is only a recently recognized disorder, there is very little research on binge eating disorder in this age-group. Community-based surveys suggest that binge eating disorder occurs in 1% to 2% of adolescents between the ages of 10 to 19 (Johnson et al., 1999; Zaider et al., 2000; Johnson et al., 2002). Most people with binge eating disorder are obese, but normal-weight people can also be affected (Schneider, 2003). Epidemiological studies in children and adolescents have shown that more boys report having binges than girls (19%–33% of boys versus 6%–7% of girls) (Whitaker et al., 1989; Childress et al., 1993); however, when the symptom of loss of control is included in the definition of binging, more girls than boys report binging (25.6% versus 12.5%) (Croll et al., 2002). Up to 20% of individuals who present with treatment for obesity meet the criteria for binge eating disorder. In contrast to anorexia nervosa and bulimia nervosa, binge eating disorder affects a more diverse population including more male and nonwhite individuals.

The causes of binge eating disorder are still unknown. Up to half of all people with binge eating disorder have a history of depression. The impact of dieting on binge eating disorder is also unclear.

The major complications of binge eating disorder are the complications that are often associated with obesity. Obese adolescents with binge eating disorder are at higher risk for poor self-esteem and depression.

Most young people with binge eating disorder are extremely distressed by their binge eating. Those who try to control the binge eating are not successful over the long term. Treatment approaches currently being studied include CBT, interpersonal psychotherapy, and psychotropic medications such as antidepressants.

MALES AND EATING DISORDERS

Approximately 10% of older adolescents suffering from eating disorders are male. The percentage of males with eating disorders is higher in young adolescent males than in adult males. The reasons for the growing prevalence in younger adolescent males remains unclear. Research indicates that eating disorders in adolescent males are clinically similar to eating disorders in females. Body image concerns appear to be one of the strongest variables in predicting eating disorders in males. Adolescent males at increased risk for developing an eating disorder include those:

1. Involved in athletic activities where there is a focus on body weight and body image—body builders, wrestlers, dancers, swimmers, runners, rowers, gymnasts, and jockeys

2. Struggling with sexual identity conflict
3. Diagnosed with comorbid mental disorders
4. With a family history of an eating disorder

Although males of all types of sexual orientation develop eating disorders, several studies report that there is an increased incidence of homosexuality among males with eating disorders.

FEMALE ATHLETE TRIAD

The female athlete triad is a syndrome consisting of disordered eating, amenorrhea, and osteoporosis in female athletes. The key feature is that in these athletes, caloric intake is insufficient for energy expenditure. The resulting "energy deficit" causes hypothalamic amenorrhea (primary or secondary) and a low estrogen state. The low estrogen state is associated with osteoporosis and increased fracture risk.

Females at greatest risk are those participating in sports that emphasize a lean physique (e.g., figure skating, gymnastics, ballet, long distance running, and swimming). The triad is not restricted to elite athletes but is also seen with increasing frequency in recreational athletes. Frequent weigh-ins, consequences for weight gain, and pressure from parents or athletic coaches may also increase an athlete's risk.

Many female athletes with the triad do not meet the strict DSM-IV criteria for anorexia nervosa or bulimia nervosa, but engage in similar disordered eating behaviors such as dietary restriction, prolonged fasting, self-induced vomiting, or the use of laxatives, diuretics, or diet pills to lose weight or maintain a thin physique. Body weight can be low, but often is in the normal range and usually there is no body image distortion.

This disorder often goes unrecognized because of the subtlety of the symptoms, the secretive nature of the disorder, and the belief that amenorrhea is a common consequence of athletic training. The exact prevalence of the female athlete triad is unknown. The prevalence of disordered eating behavior in female college athletes ranges between 15% and 62%. In addition, the prevalence of amenorrhea is between 3.4% and 66% among female athletes, compared to 2% to 5% in the general population.

Early recognition of the female athlete triad is important and therefore requires careful screening and assessment. Every female athlete with amenorrhea should have a complete history and physical examination to evaluate for an underlying eating disorder and to rule out other treatable causes of amenorrhea. Principles of treatment include increasing caloric intake, calcium and vitamin D supplementation, restricting the intensity of training (if necessary), and monitoring for resumption of menses. Adolescent athletes, their parents, and coaches should be educated about this disorder and the associated health risks.

WEB SITES

For Teenagers and Parents

http://www.cswd.org/. Council on Size and Weight Discrimination Web site attempts to change public opinion and policy regarding weight issues.

http://www.anad.org/. The National Association of Anorexia Nervosa and Associated Disorders operates an international network of support groups for patients and families and offers referrals to health care professionals who treat eating disorders across the United States and in 15 other countries.

http://www.edreferral.com/anorexia_nervosa.htm. Eating disorder referral and information center of the International Eating Disorder Referral Organization.

http://www.aacap.org/about/glossary/anorexia.htm. The American Academy of Child and Adolescent Psychiatry.

http://www.mentalhealth.com/book/p45-eat1.html. Information from the National Institute of Mental Health.

http://www.somethingfishy.org. The Something Fishy Web site on eating disorders has resources of all kinds, including information and online support.

For Health Professionals

http://www.aedweb.org. The Academy for Eating Disorders Web site that promotes effective treatment.

http://www.edap.org/. The National Eating Disorders Association (NEDA) is a nonprofit organization in the United States working to prevent eating disorders and provide treatment referrals to those suffering from anorexia, bulimia, and binge eating disorder and those concerned with body image and weight issues.

http://www.adolescenthealth.org/Eating_Disorders_in _Adolescents.pdf. The Society for Adolescent Medicine (SAM) position paper on adolescent eating disorders.

http://www.nationaleatingdisorders.org. The National Eating Disorders Association (NEDA) Web site offers information about eating disorders and body image; referrals to treatment centers, doctors, therapists, and support groups; opportunities to get involved in prevention efforts; prevention programs for all ages; and educational materials.

http://www.anred.com. Anorexia Nervosa and Related Eating Disorders Inc. (ANRED) is a nonprofit organization that provides information about eating disorders. The material includes self-help tips and information about recovery and prevention.

http://www.iaedp.com. International Association of Eating Disorder Professionals' mission is to promote a high level of professionalism among practitioners who treat those suffering from eating disorders by emphasizing ethical and professional standards.

http://www.psych.org/psych_pract/treatg/pg/eating _revisebook_index.cfm. Practice guidelines for patients with eating disorders from the American Psychiatric Association–second edition, 2000.

http://www.mentalhealth.com/book/p45-eat1.html. Information from National Institute of Mental Health.

http://www.Pocket-Doc.com/IBW.htm. A palm pilot-based program to calculate ideal body weight based on age and height using the NCHS charts. It also calculates BMI and plots BMI on the new CDC charts.

http://www.nedic.ca. The National Eating Disorder Information Centre (NEDIC) is a Canadian organization that provides information and resources on eating disorders and weight preoccupation.

REFERENCES AND ADDITIONAL READINGS

American Academy of Pediatrics. Policy statement. Identifying and treating eating disorders. *Pediatrics* 2003;111:204.

Am J Psychiatry. Practice guideline for the treatment of patients with eating disorders. American Psychiatric Association. *Am J Psychiatry;*third edition, 2006;163(suppl):4–54.

American Psychiatric Association. *Diagnostic and statistical manual of mental disorders*, 4th ed. Washington, DC: American Psychiatric Association, 1994.

Attia E, Haiman C, Walsh BT, et al. Does fluoxetine augment the inpatient treatment of anorexia nervosa? *Am J Psychiatry* 1998;155:548.

Bachrach LK, Katzman DK, Litt IF, et al. Recovery from osteopenia in adolescent girls with anorexia nervosa. *J Clin Endocrinol Metab* 1991;72(3):602.

Becker AE, Grinspoon SK, Klibanski A, et al. Eating disorders. *N Engl J Med* 1999;340:1092.

Brown JM, Mehler PS, Harris RH. Medical complications occurring in adolescents with anorexia nervosa. *West J Med* 2000;172:189.

Bulik CM, Devlin B, Bacanu SA, et al. Significant linkage on chromosome 10p in families with bulimia nervosa. *Am J Hum Genet* 2003;72:200.

Childress AC, Brewerton TD, Hodges EL, et al. The kids' eating disorders survey (KEDS): a study of middle school students. *J Am Acad Child Adolesc Psychiatry* 1993;32:843.

Connors ME, Morse W. Sexual abuse and eating disorders: a review. *Int J Eat Disord* 1993;13:1.

Croll J, Neumark-Sztainer D, Story M, et al. Prevalence and risk and protective factors related to disordered eating behaviors among adolescents: relationship to gender and ethnicity. *J Adolesc Health* 2002;31:166.

Crow SJ, Mitchell JE. Rational therapy of eating disorders. *Drugs* 1994;48:372.

Davis C, Katzman DK, Kirsh C. Compulsive physical activity in adolescents with anorexia nervosa: a psychobehavioral spiral of pathology. *J Nerv Ment Dis* 1999;187:336.

Drewnowski A, Hopkins SA, Kessler RC. The prevalence of bulimia nervosa in the U.S. college student population. *Am J Public Health* 1988;78:1322.

Fairburn CG, Beglin SJ. Assessment of eating disorders: interview or self-report questionnaire? *Int J Eat Disord* 1994; 16:363.

Fairburn CG, Cooper Z, Doll HA, et al. The natural course of bulimia nervosa and binge eating disorder in young women. *Arch Gen Psychiatry* 2000;57:659.

Fairburn CG, Norman PA, Welch SL, et al. A prospective study of outcome in bulimia nervosa and the long-term effects of three psychological treatments. *Arch Gen Psychiatry* 1995;52:304.

Fisher M. The course and outcome of eating disorders in adults and in adolescents: a review. *Adolesc Med* 2003;14:149.

Fisher M, Schneider M, Burns J, et al. Differences between adolescents and young adults at presentation to an eating disorders program. *J Adoles Health* 2001;28:227.

Fichter MM, Quadfling N. Six-year course of bulimia nervosa. *Int J Eat Disord* 1997;22:361.

Fluoxetine Bulimia Nervosa Collaborative Study Group. Fluoxetine in the treatment of bulimia nervosa. *Arch Gen Psychiatry* 1992:49:139.

Garfinkel PE, Lin E, Goering P, et al. Should amenorrhea be necessary for the diagnosis of anorexia nervosa? *Br J Psychiatry Suppl* 1996;168:500.

Garner DM, Garfinkel PE. The eating attitudes test: an index of the symptoms of anorexia nervosa. *Psychol Med* 1979;9:273.

Garner DM, Olmstead MJ, Polivy J. Development and validation of a multidimensional eating disorder inventory for anorexia nervosa and bulimia. *Int J Eat Disord* 1983;2:15.

Gillbert IC, Rastam M, Gillberg C. Anorexia nervosa outcome: six-year controlled longitudinal study of 51 cases including a population cohort. *J Am Acad Child Adolesc Psychiatry* 1994; 33:729.

Golden NH. A review of the female athlete triad (amenorrhea, osteoporosis and disordered eating). *Int J Adolesc Med Health* 2002;14:9.

Golden NH. Osteopenia and osteoporosis in anorexia nervosa. *Adolesc Med* 2003;14:97.

Golden NH, Iglesias EA, Jacobson MS, et al. Alendronate for the treatment of osteopenia in adolescents with anorexia nervosa: a randomized double-blind placebo-controlled trial. *J Clin Endocrinol Metab* 2005;90:31.

Golden NH, Jacobson MS, Schebendach J, et al. Resumption of menses in anorexia nervosa. *Arch Pediatr Adolesc Med* 1997;151:16.

Golden NH, Katzman DK, Kreipe RE, et al. Eating disorders in adolescents: position paper of the Society for Adolescent Medicine. *J Adolesc Health* 2003;33:496.

Golden NH, Lanzkowsky L, Schebendach J, et al. The effect of estrogen-progestin treatment on bone mineral density in anorexia nervosa. *J Pediatr Adolesc Gynecol* 2002;15:135.

Golden NH, Meyer W. Nutritional rehabilitation of anorexia nervosa. Goals and dangers. *Int J Adolesc Med Health* 2004; 16:131.

Golden NH, Shenker IR. Amenorrhea in anorexia nervosa: neuroendocrine control of hypothalamic dysfunction. *Int J Eat Disord* 1994;16:53.

Gordon CM, Grace E, Emans SJ, et al. Effects of oral dehydroepiandrosterone on bone density in young women with anorexia nervosa: a randomized trial. *J Clin Endocrinol Metab* 2002;87:4935.

Gowers SG, Weetman J, Shore A, et al. Impact of hospitalization on the outcome of adolescent anorexia nervosa. *Lancet* 2000; 355:717.

Grice DE, Halmi KA, Fichter MM, et al. Evidence for a susceptibility gene for anorexia nervosa on chromosome 1. *Am J Hum Genet* 2002;70:787.

Grinspoon S, Miller K, Coyle C, et al. Severity of osteopenia in estrogen-deficient women with anorexia nervosa and hypothalamic amenorrhea. *J Clin Endocrinol Metab* 1999;84: 2049.

Grinspoon S, Thomas E, Pitts S, et al. Prevalence and predictive factors for regional osteopenia in women with anorexia nervosa. *Ann Intern Med* 2000;133:790.

Grinspoon S, Thomas L, Miller K, et al. Effects of recombinant human IGF-I and oral contraceptive administration on bone density in anorexia nervosa. *J Clin Endocrinol Metab* 2002; 87:2883.

Heebink DM, Sunday SR, Halmi KA. Anorexia nervosa and bulimia nervosa in adolescence: effects of age and menstrual status on psychological variables. *J Am Acad Child Adolesc Psychiatry* 1995;34:378.

Heinmaa M, Pinhas L, Katzman DK, et al. *Alternative predictors of inpatient readmission in adolescents with eating disorders. 2004 Academy for Eating Disorders International Conference.* Orlando, FL, 2004.

Herzog DB, Dorer DJ, Keel PK, et al. Recovery and relapse in anorexia and bulimia nervosa: a 7.5-year follow-up study. *J Am Acad Child Adolesc Psychiatry* 1999;38:829.

Herzog DB, Sacks NR, Keller MB, et al. Patterns and predictors of recovery in anorexia nervosa and bulimia nervosa. *J Am Acad Child Adolesc Psychiatry* 1993;32:835.

Hoek HW, van Hoeken D. Review of the prevalence and incidence of eating disorders. *Int J Eat Disord* 2003;34:383.

Hsu LK. Outcome of anorexia nervosa: a review of the literature. *Arch Gen Psychiatry* 1980;37:1041.

Isner JM, Roberts WC, Heymsfield SB, et al. Anorexia nervosa and sudden death. *Ann Intern Med* 1985;102:49.

Johnson GL, Humphries LL, Shirley PB, et al. Mitral valve prolapse in patients with anorexia nervosa and bulimia. *Arch of Intern Med* 1986;146:1525–1529.

Johnson WG, Grieve FG, Adams CD, Measuring binge eating in adolescents: adolescent and parent versions of the questionnaire of eating and weight patterns. *Int J Eat Disord* 1999; 6(3):301.

Johnson WG, Rohan KJ, Kirk AA, et al. Prevalence and correlates of binge eating in White and African American adolescents. *Eat Behav* 2002;3:179.

Katzman DK. Medical complications in adolescents with anorexia nervosa: a review of the literature. *Int J Eat Disord* 2005;37(Suppl):S52.

Katzman DK, Morris A, Pinhas L. *Early-onset eating disorders.* http://www.phac-aspc.gc.ca/publicat/cpsp-pcsp03/page6_e .html.

Katzman DK, Zipursky RB, Lambe EK, et al. A longitudinal magnetic resonance imaging study of brain changes in adolescents with anorexia nervosa. *Arch Pediatr Adolesc Med* 1997;151:793.

Kaye WH, Barbarich NC, Putnam K, et al. Anxiolytic effects of acute tryptophan depletion in anorexia nervosa. *Int J Eat Disord* 2003;33:257.

Kaye WH, Gwirtsman HE, George DT, et al. Altered serotonin activity in anorexia nervosa after long-term weight restoration. Does elevated cerebrospinal fluid 5-hydroxyindoleacetic acid level correlate with rigid and obsessive behavior? *Arch Gen Psychiatry* 1991;48:556.

Kaye WH, Nagata T, Weltzin TE, et al. Double-blind placebo-controlled administration of fluoxetine in restricting- and restricting-purging-type anorexia nervosa. *Biol Psychiatry* 2001;49:644.

Keel PK, Dorer DJ, Eddy KT, et al. Predictors of mortality in eating disorders. *Arch Gen Psychiatry* 2003;60:179.

Klibanski A, Biller BM, Schoenfeld DA, et al. The effects of estrogen administration on trabecular bone loss in young women with anorexia nervosa. *J Clin Endocrinol Metab* 1995; 80:898.

Kreipe RE, Birndorf SA. Eating disorders in adolescents and young adults. *Med Clin North Am* 2000;84:1027.

Lantzouni E, Frank GR, Golden NH, Reversibility of growth stunting in early onset anorexia nervosa: a prospective study. *J Adolesc Health* 2002;31:162.

Lask B, Bryant-Waugh R. *Childhood onset anorexia nervosa and related eating disorders.* Melksham, Wiltshire, UK: Redwood Press Limited, 1993.

Le Grange D, Lock J, Dymek M. Family-based therapy for adolescents with bulimia nervosa. *Am J Psychother* 2003;57:237.

Lock J, Agras WS, Bryson S, et al. A comparison of short- and long-term family therapy for adolescent anorexia nervosa. *J Am Acad Child Adolesc Psychiatry* 2005;44(7):632.

Lucas AR. Toward the understanding of anorexia nervosa as a disease entity. *Mayo Clin Proc* 1981;56:254.

Lucas AR, Beard CM, O'Fallon WM, et al. 50-Year trends in the incidence of anorexia nervosa in Rochester, Minnesota: a population-based study. *Am J Psychiatry* 1991;148:917.

Lucas AR, Crowson CS, O'Fallon WM, et al. The ups and downs of anorexia nervosa. *Int J Eat Disord* 1999;26(4):397–405.

Mitchell JE, Seim HC, Colon E, et al. Medical complications and medical management of bulimia. *Ann Intern Med* 1987;107:71.

Modan-Moses D, Yaroslavsky A, Novikov I, et al. Stunting of growth as a major feature of anorexia nervosa in male adolescents. *Pediatrics* 2003;111:270.

Nakash-Eisikovits O, Dierberger A, Westen D. A multidimensional meta-analysis of pharmacotherapy for bulimia nervosa: summarizing the range of outcomes in controlled clinical trials. *Harv Rev Psychiatry* 2002;10:193.

National Center for Health Statistics. Height and weight of youths 12–17 years, United States. *Vital and health statistics. Series 11, No. 124. Health services and mental health administration.* Washington, DC, United States Government Printing Office, 1973.

Nicholls D, Chater R, Lask B. Children into DSM don't go: a comparison of classification systems for eating disorders in childhood and early adolescence. *Int J Eat Disord* 2000;28:317.

Nilsson E, Gillberg C, Gillberg I, et al. Ten-year follow-up of adolescent-onset anorexia nervosa: personality disorders. *J Am Acad Child Adolesc Psychiatry* 1999;38:11.

Palla B, Litt IF. Medical complications of eating disorders in adolescents. *Pediatrics* 1988;81:613.

Palmer EP, Guay AT. Reversible myopathy secondary to abuse of ipecac in patients with major eating disorders. *N Engl J Med* 1985;313:1457.

Panagiotopoulos C, McCrindle BW, Hick K, et al. Electrocardiographic findings in adolescents with eating disorders. *Pediatrics* 2000;105:1100.

Ratnasuriya RH, Eisler I, Szmukler GI, et al. Anorexia nervosa: outcome and prognostic factors after 20 years. *Br J Psychiatry* 1991;158:495.

Robin AL, Gilroy M, Dennis AB, et al. Treatment of eating disorders in children and adolescents. *Clin Psychol Rev* 1998;18:421.

Robin AL, Siegel PT, Koepke T, et al. Family therapy versus individual therapy for adolescent females with anorexia nervosa. *J Dev Behav Pediatr* 1994;15:111.

Rock CL, Curran-Celentano J. Nutritional disorder of anorexia nervosa: a review. *Int J Eat Disord* 1994;15:187.

Schneider M. Bulimia nervosa and binge-eating disorder in adolescents. *Adolesc Med* 2003;14:119.

Sherman P, Leslie K, Goldberg E, et al. Hypercarotenemia and transaminitis in female adolescents with eating disorders: a prospective, controlled study. *J Adolesc Health* 1994;15:205.

Siddiqui A, Ramsay B, Leonard J. The cutaneous signs of eating disorders. *Acta Dermatol Venereol* 1994;74:68.

Siegel JH, Hardoff D, Golden NH, et al. Medical complications in male adolescents with anorexia nervosa. *J Adolesc Health* 1995;16:448.

Soyka LA, Grinspoon S, Levitsky LL, et al. The effects of anorexia nervosa on bone metabolism in female adolescents. *J Clin Endocrinol Metab* 1991;84:4489.

Steiner H, Lock J. Anorexia nervosa and bulimia nervosa in children and adolescents: a review of the past 10 years. *J Am Acad Child Adolesc Psychiatry* 1998;37:4.

Steinhausen HC. Treatment and outcome of adolescent anorexia nervosa. *Horm Res* 1995;43:168.

Steinhausen HC, Seidel R. Outcome in adolescent eating disorders. *Int J Eat Disord* 1993;14:487.

Stice E, Agras WS, Hammer LD. Risk factors for the emergence of childhood eating disturbances: a five-year prospective study. *Int J Eat Disord* 1999;25:375.

Stice E, Killen JD, Hayward C, Age of onset for binge eating and purging during late adolescence: a 4-year survival analysis. *J Abnorm Psychol* 1998;107:671.

Strober M, Freeman R, Morrell W, et al. The long-term course of severe anorexia nervosa in adolescents: survival analysis of recovery, relapse, and outcome predictors over 10–15 years in a prospective study. *Int J Eat Disord* 1997;22:339.

Sullivan PE. Mortality in anorexia nervosa. *Am J Psychiatry* 1995;152:1073.

Touyz SW, Liew VP, Tseng P, et al. Oral and dental complications in dieting disorders. *Int J Eat Disord* 1993;14:341.

Walsh BT, Bulik CM, Fairburn CG, et al. Defining eating disorders. In: Evans DL, Foa EB, Gur RE, eds. *Treating and preventing adolescent mental health disorders; what we know and what we don't know.* New York: Oxford University Press, The Annenberg Foundation Trust at Sunnylands, and the Annenberg Public Policy Center of the University of Pennsylvania, 2005.

Walsh BT, Kaplan AS, Attia E, et al. Fluoxetine after weight restoration in anorexia nervosa: a randomized controlled trial. *JAMA* 2006;295:2605.

Walsh BT, Wilson GT, Loeb KL, et al. Medication and psychotherapy in the treatment of bulimia nervosa. *Am J Psychiatry* 1997;154:523.

Whitaker A, Davies M, Shaffer D, et al. The struggle to be thin: a survey of anorexic and bulimic symptoms in a non-referred adolescent population. *Psychol Med.* 1989 Feb;19(1):143–63.

Wonderlich SA, Crosby RD, Mitchell JE, et al. Eating disturbance and sexual trauma in childhood and adulthood. *Int J Eat Disord* 2001;30:401.

Zaider TI, Johnson JG, Cockell SJ. Psychiatric comorbidity associated with eating disorder symptomatology among adolescents in the community. *Int J Eat Disord* 2000;28:58.

Zuckerman DM, Colby A, Ware NC, et al. The prevalence of bulimia among college students. *Am J Public Health* 1986;76:1135.

For Adolescents, Parents, and Teachers

Bruch H. *The golden cage: the enigma of anorexia nervosa.* Cambridge, MA: Harvard University Press, 1978.

Crisp AH. *Anorexia nervosa: let me be.* New York: Grune & Stratton, 1980.

Hornbacher M. *Wasted. A memoir of anorexia and bulimia.* New York: HarperCollins, 1998.

Katzman DK, Pinhas L. *Help for eating disorders. A parent's guide to symptoms, causes and treatments.* Toronto, Canada: Robert Rose Inc, 2005.

O'Neill CB. *Anorexia nervosa: starving for attention.* New York: Chelsea House, 1998.

Roth G. *Feeding the hungry heart: the experience of compulsive eating.* New York: Dutton, 1993.

Sacker IM, Zimmer MA. *Dying to be thin: understanding and defeating anorexia nervosa and bulimia—a practical lifesaving guide.* New York: Warner Books, 1987.

PART X

Psychosomatic Illnesses and Other Medical Disorders

CHAPTER 34

Psychosomatic Illness in Adolescents

David M. Siegel

The patient who presents with physical and/or physiological symptoms for which an identifiable biomedical etiology cannot be found is a diagnostic and therapeutic challenge known to all experienced clinicians. It is therefore important to have an organized and consistent approach to such situations, with goals of carrying out a judicious, yet complete diagnostic evaluation as well as formulating a management plan that ameliorates symptoms and maintains (or restores) function and quality of life. Pitfalls of excessive, invasive, and inconclusive testing, possible worsening of symptoms, and provider frustration and resentment toward the patient and family are familiar and prudent concerns. However, an effective strategy for handling these cases can and should be developed by those caring for adolescents. In this chapter, a categorization for psychosomatic illness is described, including a framework for understanding how these conditions fit into a person's life. In addition, a plan for management is outlined.

Adolescent adjustment reaction: It is important to remember that adolescence is a time of change and transition. The physical changes of puberty, the cognitive developmental progression from concrete to formal operational thinking, and the changing demands and expectations in the family, and social, academic, and vocational realms, make the journey to young adulthood varied and challenging. Because of these demands, some teens will experience periods of significant struggle as they try to adapt. The resulting emotional upheaval, if sufficiently disruptive, can be characterized as an adjustment disorder and can sometimes be expressed in somatic terms. Milder and more time-limited psychological disequilibrium can also precipitate bodily discomfort. This can lead to physical complaints such as light-headedness, nausea, headache, palpitations, and so on. All of these are commonly associated with emotional distress and may serve in the patient's mind as "legitimate" reasons to see the doctor or nurse practitioner; more acceptable to the patient and family than overtly expressed psychological problems.

CLASSIFICATION

As stipulated in the Diagnostic and Statistical Manual—Text Revision (DSM-IV-TR, 2000) (American Psychiatric Association, 2000) there are three broad categories of psychosomatic disorders:

1. Psychophysiological: Psychological conflict affects the development or recurrence of an existing physical condition.
2. Somatoform: Somatic complaints and/or dysfunctions are not under conscious control and physical findings are absent or insufficient to explain all symptoms and complaints.
3. Factitious: Somatic and/or psychological symptoms are consciously controlled.

Psychophysiological Disorders

In psychophysiological disorders, physical symptoms are observable and often fall into biological processes that are understood by the clinician. In addition, the disease course is clearly influenced by psychological function. For example, the patient with asthma experiences increased bronchospasm when under stress, leading to coughing, wheezing, and shortness of breath. Although, managing and optimally preventing these exacerbations is not necessarily easy or rapidly accomplished, the connection between the psychological and the physical, once shared with and understood by the patient and family, is not typically rejected or denied. The "medical legitimacy" of the primary physiological disorder (i.e., asthma) represents a common ground of acceptance between clinician and patient/family and also provides the clinician with a familiar and well-understood template for medical treatment. Beyond the strictly medical treatment, however, the clinician must attempt to facilitate the adolescent and parent(s) successfully identifying sources of stress and anxiety that contribute to inadequate control of the primary disease and its symptoms. This exploration may very well be enigmatic and may require open-ended questions, thoughtful probing, and multiple visits. Sometimes, referral to a health psychologist or medical family therapist is productive. In any case, the nature of the doctor–patient interaction in psychophysiological disorders is not typically one characterized by conflict or frustration.

Somatoform Disorder

Somatoform and factitious disorders are the more difficult of the psychosomatic illnesses. The discussion in the subsequent text focuses primarily on somatoform disorder

TABLE 34.1

Diagnostic Criteria for 300.82 Undifferentiated Somatoform Disorder

A. One or more physical complaints (e.g., fatigue, loss of appetite, gastrointestinal or urinary complaints)
B. Either (1) or (2):
   (1) After appropriate investigation, the symptoms cannot be fully explained by a known general medical condition or the direct effects of a substance (e.g., a drug of abuse, a medication)
   (2) When there is a related general medical condition, the physical complaints or resulting social or occupational impairment is in excess of what would be expected from the history, physical examination, or laboratory findings
C. The symptoms cause clinically significant distress or impairment in social, occupational, or other important areas of functioning
D. The duration of the disturbance is at least 6 months
E. The disturbance is not better accounted for by another mental disorder (e.g., another somatoform disorder, sexual dysfunction, mood disorder, anxiety disorder, sleep disorder, or psychotic disorder)
F. The symptom is not intentionally produced or feigned (as in factitious disorder or malingering)

From American Psychiatric Association. Somatoform disorders. In: *Diagnostic and statistical manual—text revision* (DSM-IV-TR, 2000), 4th ed. Washington, DC: American Psychiatric Association, 2000.

as it is more likely to be encountered by the adolescent health care provider. However, it is important to remember that factitious disorders especially those that are chronic, such as Munchausen syndrome and particularly Munchausen syndrome by proxy (Von Hahn et al., 2001), are serious and in some instances difficult to distinguish from somatoform conditions. Conscious falsification of symptoms and signs is a different behavior from the unconscious process of somatoform disorders. The intentional creation of the sick role is thought to be motivated by the unconscious need to be cared for. By contrast, symptoms in somatoform disorders are seen as associated with, or reflective of, *unconscious* conflict.

Somatoform disorders include:
1. *Somatization disorder*
2. *Undifferentiated somatoform disorder*
3. *Conversion disorder (hysteria)*
4. *Hypochondriasis*
5. *Body dysmorphic disorder*
6. *Somatoform pain disorder*

In working with adolescents, it is much more common to encounter patients with undifferentiated somatoform disorder (Table 34.1) as opposed to those who meet the restrictive criteria for full-fledged somatization disorder (Table 34.2).

EVALUATION

1. Comprehensive biopsychosocial assessment: The initial encounter with the adolescent complaining of single or multiple somatic symptoms begins with a comprehensive biopsychosocial assessment. Both biomedical and psychosocial factors should be evaluated from the beginning. This will allow the clinician to understand the psychological stressors and conflicts, as well as the biomedical elements that together serve to pare down the differential diagnosis associated with the adolescent's complaints. It also makes the eventual diagnosis of a psychosomatic disorder more acceptable to families in that this conclusion does not arise late in the evaluation process only as a diagnosis of exclusion. Elements of the biopsychosocial assessment include:
  a. Detailed history focused on the presenting symptoms: It is important not to neglect the symptoms that brought the teen and family to the provider. Focusing on the symptoms does not reinforce the illness but can give the teen the message that the provider is taking their symptoms seriously. However, both medical and psychosocial issues should be examined together.
  b. Physical examination focused on symptoms
  c. Laboratory and imaging studies: These should be chosen on the basis of the history and physical examination and should be limited to the least number of minimally-invasive tests required to clarify the diagnosis.
2. Evaluation for psychiatric disease: When this careful biopsychosocial assessment (including the physical examination and laboratory/imaging investigations) leads the clinician away from a discernible biological, pathophysiological abnormality to explain the patient's symptom(s), and somatizing is suspected, an initial consideration should be whether this represents psychiatric disease. Mood disorders (especially major depression), anxiety disorders (e.g., panic disorder), and even schizophrenia can all manifest with somatization, and sometimes physical symptoms may be the only complaints with which the adolescent initially presents. When further questioning and interaction with the patient and family support the presence of significant psychiatric illness, formal mental health consultation is

TABLE 34.2

Diagnostic Criteria for 300.81 Somatization Disorder

A. A history of many physical complaints beginning before 30 years of age that occur over a period of several years and result in treatment being sought or significant impairment in social, occupational, or other important areas of functioning

B. Each of the following criteria must have been met, with individual symptoms occurring at any time during the course of the disturbance:

   (1) Four pain symptoms: A history of pain related to at least four different sites or functions (e.g., head, abdomen, back, joints, extremities, chest, rectum, during menstruation, during sexual intercourse, or during urination)

   (2) Two gastrointestinal symptoms: A history of at least two gastrointestinal symptoms other than pain (e.g., nausea, bloating, vomiting other than during pregnancy, diarrhea, or intolerance of several different foods)

   (3) One sexual symptom: A history of at least one sexual or reproductive symptom other than pain (e.g., sexual indifference, erectile of ejaculatory dysfunction, irregular menses, excessive menstrual bleeding, vomiting throughout pregnancy)

   (4) One pseudoneurological symptom: A history of at least one symptom or deficit suggesting a neurological condition not limited to pain (conversion symptoms such as impaired coordination or balance, paralysis or localized weakness, difficulty swallowing or lump in throat, aphonia, urinary retention, hallucinations, loss of touch or pain sensation, double vision, blindness, deafness, seizures; dissociative symptoms such as amnesia; or loss of consciousness other than fainting)

C. Either (1) or (2):

   (1) After appropriate investigation, each of the symptoms in criterion 2 cannot be fully explained by a known general medical condition or the direct effects of a substance (e.g., a drug of abuse, a medication)

   (2) When there is a related general medical condition, the physical complaints or resulting social or occupational impairment are in excess of what would be expected from the history, physical examination, or laboratory findings

D. The symptoms are not intentionally produced or feigned (as in factitious disorder or malingering)

From American Psychiatric Association. Somatoform disorders. In: *Diagnostic and statistical manual—text revision* (DSM-IV-TR, 2000), 4th ed. Washington, DC: American Psychiatric Association, 2000.

warranted. Less severe mood or anxiety disorder uncovered during the evaluation of somatization may be managed by the adolescent care provider as outlined elsewhere in this chapter.

3. Evaluation for personality disorders: Beyond Axis I psychiatric diagnoses, somatization can also be associated with certain personality (Axis II) disorders. Those patients with enduring attitudes and habitual patterns of response that characterize obsessive-compulsive personality disorder or histrionic personality disorder are at higher risk for developing somatization. In the case of the former, hypochondriasis may be a more likely predisposition. Adolescents with personality traits of dependency or neurotic preoccupation with self also have a greater tendency to experience and describe unexplained physical symptoms.

4. Evaluation of environmental factors: In addition to personality disorders, environmental factors can also underlie the emergence and perpetuation of somatization. Somatizing in parents, family members, or peer contacts should be examined as possible models for, and contributors to, the teen's own symptoms and behaviors. Cultural norms and expectations might also reinforce a form of illness and an expression of distress that emphasizes and serves to support somatization. An awareness on the part of providers as to the adolescent's cultural milieu is critical in placing somatization (and other) behaviors in appropriate context.

Other aspects of a teen's present or past experience might also bear on somatization and provide insights for the provider into the possible meaning for the behavior. For example, a patient whose early life experience did not include consistent parental support and caretaking might develop physical symptoms as a means to meet dependency needs. When these patients become increasingly demanding about diagnostic evaluations, and angry and hostile with the clinician about the lack of a physical diagnosis or the inadequacy of treatment, these emotions may actually be expressions of deeper and unconscious feelings about early caretakers that are now displaced onto the clinician.

In summary, important areas to help the practitioner understand somatization include:

- Symptoms of mental illness or psychiatric diagnosis
- Association with personality traits or disorder
- Modeling or reinforcement of somatizing behavior by the family, peer, or cultural environment
- Placement of somatizing in the context of the patient's present or past experiences and circumstances

APPROACH TO THE PATIENT

Most teens and parent(s) are unaware of the connection between their physical symptoms and underlying distress and conflict, and hence it is the somatic complaint that brings the adolescent to the health care provider. The clinician's initial history taking not only considers a differential diagnosis of physiological causes but also includes sensitivity for psychosomatic etiology. Screening questions about affect and recent life change or stress (both for the individual and family) are included in the history as the clinician considers a possible association between the physical complaints and the psychological inventory. As the physical examination proceeds, a lack of positive physical findings may elevate the likelihood of emotional distress as a major contributor to the symptoms, and also helps guide the clinician's diagnostic testing. At the conclusion of the initial visit, it is important that the clinician describe her/his formulation and plan with regard to the adolescent's physical complaint. Even if questioning directed toward emotional upset has proved positive, the clinician should avoid statements that suggest that this is the exclusive cause of the physical problem. For many patients, such an attribution, especially at the first encounter, will not only be unacceptable but may also threaten the clinician's credibility and thereby compromise effectiveness of future intervention. When an adolescent comes to see the doctor for a specific and disruptive symptom (for example, 3 months of persistent and severe headache), it is important that the problem be addressed in the terms expressed by the patient, and any diagnostic or therapeutic recommendations be presented in that context. When a psychological element is suspected as contributory, this can be constructively introduced to the patient and family without discrediting or trivializing the identified symptoms.

Sample Dialogues

The clinician might say the following:

> It is very clear to me that you have been experiencing some pretty bad headaches for quite some time and I'm glad you came to see me about this. My goal is to identify which illnesses or diagnoses can cause your headaches and then figure out which ones we should pursue and which ones we can cross off the list. You've had severe pain for a good while and we both know that making all of that pain go away in a short period of time, isn't very likely to happen. We need to put together an initial plan that decreases your headaches enough such that they don't interfere so much with your life, like with all the school you've missed due to the pain.
>
> The other thing we both know is that anyone trying to deal with several months of all this discomfort can't help but get at least a little down, depressed, and discouraged about it. When we talked earlier about your mood, you did a good job of giving me a real sense of how depressing these headaches are. Who wouldn't start feeling down with all the pain and missed school you've had to cope with! So, at the same time that we're putting together a strategy for what is and is not the cause of your pain, and how to get these headaches under better control so they stop influencing your life so much, you can count on me not to ignore how this physical problem is also affecting your mood and emotions. We need to take a comprehensive approach to helping you feel and function better.

With this kind of dialogue and framing of the problem, the adolescent and family are assured that the clinician

takes the symptoms seriously, intends to pursue a methodical approach for ruling in or out various diagnoses, and is not discounting their concerns by saying that it is "all in your head." The critical groundwork has been laid, however, for incorporating a psychological health aspect to the problem. In our adolescent practice setting, we have clinical psychologists available on-site for consultation and I will often let patients and families know about this if I think mental health referral is likely at a subsequent visit.

For example I might say the following:

> The emotional stress of all these headaches can get to be pretty tough, so I want you to know we have psychologists right here in our office who know about the psychological part of being sick and can work with us to help you and your family cope with the problem. These psychologists are experts at helping patients, just like you, figure out the best ways to get through those tough times while we continue to work on getting on top of the headaches. After all, for some people stress itself can turn out to be a cause of a headache.

Of course, if depression or anxiety screening have revealed serious risk and dysfunction, then mental health consultation should be made more urgently.

As discussed earlier, some theories of psychosomatic illness hypothesize that physical symptoms can result from psychological conflict and distress. In any complex biopsychosocial problem, such as a psychosomatic or somatizing illness, the initial cause of a symptom can be difficult to discern. The clinician statements quoted in the examples above focus on the emotional distress of patients and parents that is an understandable consequence of trying to cope with the symptom(s). Although this may be only part of the emotional story, it is an acceptable place to start. The aim is to let the patient know that the clinician is well aware of the teen's emotional distress, and to foster acceptance by the adolescent and parent(s) of a psychological dimension that will be integrated into the treatment. As strategies for symptom management and restoration of function develop, and further history gathering and counseling elaborate on significant emotional concerns, the patient/family may or may not come to endorse the psychological process as primary and the physical symptoms as secondary. This insight by the patient may be valuable but is not essential to successful symptom management. Identifying sources of stress, depression, and emotional distress and how to cope with them through an appropriate mix of individual and family counseling, cognitive behavioral therapy, and medication may be seen by the adolescent and parent(s) as a parallel (rather then integrated) process to improvement in the symptom. Both the somatic and psychological realms have, nonetheless, been addressed. In these resistant patients, the emotional/psychological/physical connection is framed in terms that fit the parents' and/or patient's insight, defensive structure, and level of sophistication. It also facilitates overall improvement in a manner that is experienced as supportive or acceptable (rather than provocative or confrontational) for the adolescent and parent(s).

The vast majority of somatizing adolescents can be successfully managed as outpatients, making full use of appropriate consultation. The team includes not only mental health expertise but other inputs as well. For example, if a patient whose somatic complaint is back pain states that she/he is having great difficulty with weight bearing and walking, physical therapy should be instituted early. Therefore, while any psychological issues require explicit delineation and intervention, the physically compromised patient also requires effective treatment such as a physical modality to restore range of motion, strength, and endurance. These physical treatments often have psychological benefit (just as the reverse is true). Even in the case of conversion disorder, wherein the loss of a normal body function (often neurological) occurs in the face of clear evidence of a psychological conflict, the specific medical disability must be addressed through appropriate rehabilitation techniques, along side psychiatric consultation and care. Simultaneous collaborative and integrated medical and psychological attention is key in achieving both patient and family acceptance, as well as a positive treatment outcome.

Inpatient admission should be reserved for the small minority of patients who fail a multidisciplinary outpatient program and/or for those whose deterioration places them at significant risk for chronicity. Factitious disorder, particularly Munchausen syndrome by proxy, may be an indication for hospitalization and/or out-of-home placement depending on severity. The strategy of hospitalizing a somatizing patient with the goal of expediting the diagnostic evaluation and convincing the patient and family that the problem is psychological rather than physical carries the risk of setting up a confrontation with the clinician that is unlikely to facilitate either short-term improvement or a successful long-term outcome. If the clinician feels that all reasonable biomedical causes for a symptom have not been eliminated, and pursuit of necessary testing and referral will be prolonged in the ambulatory setting, then a well planned, highly structured, and organized inpatient admission might be advantageous. However, in many institutions, such well-intentioned strategies often encounter delays and inefficiencies, not to mention the iatrogenic risks posed by an inpatient stay. Furthermore, although the admitting physician may be reassured by the many negative test results and consultations garnered in-hospital, patients and families paradoxically view the decision to admit the adolescent as a statement of physiological severity and therefore have increased resistance to any subsequent psychological explanation and intervention. Therefore, for some patients being hospitalized can be associated with worsening of symptoms.

CONCLUSION

Psychosomatic illness in the adolescent is commonly encountered, and can be fascinating, yet challenging. Its understanding, diagnosis, and treatment represent the clinical enactment of Engels' biopsychosocial approach. Those caring for teens should remain alert for the occurrence of psychosomatic illness, take a methodical and pragmatic approach to its identification, and develop a steadily practiced and multidisciplinary structure for its management. Although patience and persistence on the part of clinicians and patients/families are often called for as treatment progresses, eventual improvement is a realistic expectation in most instances.

REFERENCES AND ADDITIONAL READINGS

American Psychiatric Association. Somatoform disorders. In: *Diagnostic and statistical manual—text revision (DSM-IV-TR, 2000)*, 4th ed. Washington, DC: American Psychiatric Association, 2000.

Brown LK, Bruning K, Fritz GK, et al. Somatoform disorders. In: Wiener JM, Dulcan MK, eds. *Textbook of child and adolescent psychiatry*, 3rd ed. Washington, DC: American Psychiatry Publishing, 2004:751.

Engel GL. The clinical application of the biopsychosocial model. *Am J Psychiatry* 1980;137:5.

Kreipe RE. The biopsychosocial approach to adolescents with somatoform disorders. *Adolesc Med Clin* 2006;17:1.

Mayou R, Kirmayer LJ, Simon G, et al. Somatoform disorders: time for a new approach in DSM-V. *Am J Psychiatry* 2005; 162:847.

McDaniel SH, Campbell TL, Hepworth J. Integrating the mind-body split: a biopsychosocial approach to somatic fixation. In: McDaniel SH, Campbell TL, Hepworth J, et al. eds. *Family oriented primary care*, 2nd ed. New York: Springer-Verlag, 2005:326.

Roca RP. Somatization. In: Barker LR, Burton JR, Zieve PD, eds. *Principles of ambulatory medicine*. Philadelphia: Lippincott Williams & Wilkins, 2003:252.

Servan-Schreiber D, Kolb NR, Tabas G. Somatizing patients: part I. Practical diagnosis. *Am Fam Physician* 2000;61: 1073.

Servan-Schreiber D, Kolb NR, Tabas G. Somatizing patients: part II. Practical management. *Am Fam Physician* 2000;61: 1423.

Silber TJ, Pao M. Somatization disorders in children and adolescents. *Pediatr Rev* 2003;24:255.

Von Hahn L, Harper G, McDaniel SH, et al. A case of factitious disorder by proxy: the role of the health-care system, diagnostic dilemmas and family dynamics. *Harv Rev Psychiatry* 2001;9:124.

CHAPTER 35

Fatigue and the Chronic Fatigue Syndrome

Martin Fisher

The complaint of fatigue is common among adolescents. In studies of teenagers, up to 70% indicate that they are sleepy during the day (Hansen et al., 2005). In most instances, fatigue in adolescence is due to a deficit in hours of sleep. Accordingly, most adolescents sleep more on weekends, when they have time for catch-up, than they do during the week, when they are usually scheduled with multiple activities. In some instances, however, fatigue can be due to medical or psychological causes. The key to the evaluation of the adolescent with fatigue is to distinguish those cases that need merely reassurance and perhaps a change in schedule, from those who require further management for organic or psychiatric disorders or who are exhibiting signs and symptoms of the chronic fatigue syndrome (CFS).

CAUSES OF FATIGUE

Adolescent Sleep Patterns

The most common cause for fatigue in adolescents is insufficient sleep. Recent studies have demonstrated the following:

1. Total sleep duration decreases from a mean of 10.1 hours at 9 years of age to a mean of 8.1 hours at 16 years (Iglowstein et al., 2003).
2. Adolescents sleep as much as 2 hours less per night on weekdays during the school year than during the summer; weekend sleep is an average of 30 minutes more per night during the school year (Hansen et al., 2005).
3. Fifteen percent of adolescents report falling asleep in the car or bus on the way to school; 25% report falling asleep on the way home (Lee et al., 1999).
4. As adolescence progresses, bedtimes get later on both school days and nonschool days; wake-up times on weekends and holidays also get later (Millman, 2005).

Psychological Causes

In adolescents, psychological causes are responsible for most cases of fatigue that is unrelated to too little sleep and/or too much activity. Psychological causes of fatigue include:

1. Depression
2. Anxiety
3. Stressful situations
4. Other psychiatric disorders

Organic Causes

Organic causes of fatigue are infrequent during adolescence, but the differential diagnosis is very broad. Fatigue may result from any of the following:

1. Medications, illicit drugs, and poisonings
   a. Antihistamines, sedatives
   b. Alcohol, drug use
   c. Other medications (including antidepressants and other psychotropic medications)
   d. Heavy metal intoxication
2. Infectious diseases
   a. Mononucleosis (see Chapter 29)
   b. Hepatitis (see Chapter 30)
   c. Influenza, mycoplasma (see Chapter 29)
   d. Cytomegalovirus, parvovirus infections
   e. Chronic infectious diseases, for example, human immunodeficiency virus (HIV), tuberculosis, Lyme disease, brucellosis
   f. Bacterial endocarditis
   g. Parasitic infections
3. Endocrine disorders
   a. Hypothyroidism, hyperthyroidism (see Chapter 9)
   b. Diabetes mellitus, hypoglycemia
   c. Addison disease, Cushing syndrome
   d. Hypopituitarism, hypoparathyroidism
4. Systemic illness
   a. Allergies
   b. Connective tissue diseases
   c. Anemia
   d. Neoplasms
   e. Congenital heart disease
   f. Asthma
   g. Inflammatory bowel disease
   h. Renal failure
   i. Liver failure

Sleep Disorders

Although still relatively uncommon, sleep disorders are increasingly being recognized as a cause of fatigue and/or daytime sleepiness in adolescents. Included in this category are those with:

1. Insomnia—Defined as decreased sleep quality and/or quantity due to trouble falling asleep and/or maintaining sleep. Insomnia can be:
   a. A symptom of an underlying medical or psychological disorder
   b. Due to no readily apparent cause, referred to as *psychophysiological insomnia*
   c. Part of a delayed sleep phase syndrome (DSPS), "a circadian based disorder in which an individual's internal circadian pacemaker is not in synchrony with internal or environmental time." DSPS is thought to occur in up to 7% of adolescents (Millman, 2005).
2. Obstructive sleep apnea (also referred to *as sleep disordered breathing*, SDB) occurs in up to 1% to 3% of adolescents (Millman, 2005).
   a. Most commonly caused by enlarged tonsils and adenoids
   b. Increasingly being reported in obese adolescents
   c. Can also be due to retrognathia or nasal obstruction
3. Other sleep disorders, which are uncommon but which can occasionally be seen in adolescents include the following:
   a. Narcolepsy
   b. Idiopathic hypersomnia
   c. "Periodic leg movements during sleep"
   d. "Restless leg syndrome"

CHRONIC FATIGUE SYNDROME

CFS is a poorly understood and often controversial diagnosis that is seen mostly in adults but has increasingly been reported in adolescents. It involves chronic and debilitating fatigue seen in association with other symptoms. Details of this syndrome, as seen in adolescents, are as follows:

Definition

The Centers for Disease Control and Prevention has developed a working definition of CFS (Fukuda et al., 1994):

1. Fatigue of at least 6 months duration
2. Limits the individual to 50% of premorbid activity levels
3. May be persistent or recurrent
4. No other cause found to account for the fatigue
5. Additional symptoms (four or more are required to meet the criteria for CFS)
   a. Recurrent pharyngitis
   b. Tender lymph nodes
   c. New-onset headaches
   d. Impaired memory or concentration
   e. Joint pains
   f. Muscle pains
   g. Nonrefreshing sleep
   h. Postexertion fatigue

Epidemiology

Studies in adults and adolescents have shown the following:

	Adults (Cho and Stollerma, 1992)	Adolescents (Marshall, 1999)
Female	59%–77%	60%–70%
Mean age	35–41 yr	14–15 yr
Ethnicity	Mostly white	Mostly white
Premorbid	Most employed before illness	Some with school attendance problems
Symptoms	0.5–14 yr before presentation	0.6–2.2 yr before presentation
Sudden onset	85%	60%–70%

Symptoms

Patients often have many symptoms of CFS simultaneously. One study of 59 children and adolescents showed the following symptoms (Krilov et al., 1998):

Fatigue	100%
Headache	74%
Sore throat	59%
Abdominal pain	48%
Fever	36%
Impaired cognition	33%
Myalgia	31%
Diarrhea	29%
Adenopathy	29%
Anorexia	28%
Nausea or vomiting	26%
Dizziness	17%
Arthralgia	17%
Sweats	9%
Chills	7%
Depression	7%

Etiology

No specific etiology has been determined to be the cause of the CFS. Many possibilities have been considered. It is likely that the underlying cause may be a combination of factors, including an acute infectious illness that acts as a precipitant, a background of psychological distress, and an underlying physiological vulnerability (in the cardiovascular, neurological, endocrine, and/or immune systems). It is also likely that no two individuals with CFS have exactly the same relative ratio in the combination of underlying factors. Etiologies that have been considered include the following:

1. Infection
   a. Several infectious diseases, most notably Epstein-Barr virus (EBV) infection and influenza, can serve as the precipitant for the onset of CFS. In other parts of the world, other viral infections have been implicated as triggers for CFS.
   b. Any acute illnesses can cause an exacerbation of symptoms during the course of the syndrome.

c. No specific infectious agent has been found to account for continuation of the symptoms.
2. Cardiovascular system
   a. Orthostatic symptoms are common in patients with CFS (Stewart et al., 1999a).
   b. Tilt-table testing is often positive in patients with CFS.
   c. Underlying cardiovascular instability, in those with a tendency toward hypotension, may be a factor in the cause of CFS.
3. Endocrine system
   a. Decreased hypothalamic-pituitary-adrenal axis function has been suspected as an etiology in CFS but never clearly documented (McKenzie et al., 1998).
   b. No other endocrine disorders have been consistently demonstrated in CFS.
4. Neurological
   a. Headaches and impaired cognition are prominent symptoms in many patients with CFS.
   b. Computed tomography (CT) scans and magnetic resonance imaging (MRI) do not show abnormalities in patients with CFS.
   c. No other reproducible neurological abnormalities have been found to be a cause of CFS.
5. Immune function
   a. Studies have shown *in vitro* abnormalities in lymphocyte function and cytokine production in CFS (Conti et al., 1998).
   b. Reproducible abnormalities and opportunistic infections have not been found.
   c. Treatment with immunoglobulins and other immune modulators have not shown clear benefits in CFS.
6. Depression
   a. A history of depression is found in many adults with CFS; depression may create a psychological vulnerability necessary for the onset of CFS.
   b. Depression may be one physiological consequence of changes in the brain that occur in CFS.
   c. Depression may be a natural reaction to feeling ill and fatigued for a long time.
   d. Some have suggested that CFS is merely an alternate expression of depression.
   e. There is substantial overlap in the symptoms of CFS and depression leading to the possibility that some patients with depression will be misdiagnosed as having CFS and vice versa.
7. Other psychological variables
   a. Separation anxiety and/or school phobia may be a factor in some children and adolescents with CFS.
   b. Some have considered CFS to be in the realm of conversion reaction.
   c. Psychosomatic symptoms may be found premorbidly in some children and adolescents with CFS.

EVALUATION OF FATIGUE

Evaluation of the adolescent with a complaint of fatigue is aimed at distinguishing those who are merely not getting enough sleep from those who may have a specific disorder of sleep or other psychological or medical causes. A complete history and thorough physical examination, selected laboratory tests, and occasionally other studies, are performed.

History

The history is geared toward evaluating the adolescents' sleep patterns and activity levels; looking for evidence of medical, psychological, or sleep disorders; and determining whether a diagnosis of CFS may apply:

1. Sleep patterns and activity levels
   a. Hours of sleep at night, naps during the day
   b. Time going to sleep, time arising
   c. Difficulty falling asleep, waking up during the night
   d. Patterns on weekdays, patterns on weekends
   e. School schedule, out-of-school schedule
   f. Alcohol use, illicit drug use
   g. Dietary patterns, caffeine intake
2. Medical history
   a. Past medical history, review of systems
   b. Medications: over the counter, prescription
   c. History of fever, weight loss, night sweats
   d. Symptoms consistent with endocrinopathy, infection, or neoplastic process
   e. Snoring in patient or family, unexplained leg movements
3. Psychological history
   a. Relationships with family and friends
   b. School performance and attitude
   c. Evidence of depression and/or anxiety
   d. Signs of stress at home or in school
   e. Psychiatric disorders in patient or family
   f. Acting out behaviors, social withdrawal
4. Criteria for diagnosis of CFS
   a. Fatigue persists for >6 months
   b. Activity is limited to <50% of premorbid levels
   c. Accompanying symptoms present
   d. No other cause of fatigue
   e. Fatigue on exertion, nonrefreshing sleep

Physical Examination

Fatigue associated with nonorganic causes is usually accompanied by normal physical examination results. Important areas to examine include the following:

1. General appearance: Evidence of chronic illness
2. Height, weight, and body mass index (BMI)
3. Lymph nodes: Evidence of adenopathy
4. Thyroid gland: Presence of goiter
5. Cardiac: Evidence of abnormal heart murmur
6. Abdomen: Hepatosplenomegaly
7. Extremities: Evidence of arthritis, rash
8. Sexual maturity rating: Puberty advancement normal or not
9. Mental status examination to identify abnormalities in mood, intellectual function, memory, and personality—in particular, signs of depression or anxiety

Laboratory Testing and Other Studies

1. Screening tests: Most adolescents with fatigue will have to undergo baseline screening tests consisting of:
   a. Complete blood count, erythrocyte sedimentation rate
   b. Urinalysis
   c. Comprehensive metabolic panel (electrolytes, liver, kidneys)

TABLE 35.1

Techniques to Reverse Sleep–Wake Cycle in Adolescents with Delayed Sleep Phase Syndrome

1-Day Plan[a]	1-Week Plan[b]
1. Fall asleep at usual time (e.g., 4 a.m.)	1. Stay awake until 3 hr after usual sleep time (e.g., go to sleep at 7 a.m.)
2. Set alarm and wake up 6 hr later (e.g., 10 a.m.)	2. Day 2, stay awake until 3 hr after previous bedtime (e.g., go to sleep at 10 a.m.)
3. Remain awake all day	3. Day 3, go to sleep 3 hr later than previous day (e.g., 1 p.m.)
4. Go to sleep at midnight (will have slept only 6 hr in last 36 hr so should be tired)	4. Day 4, again go to sleep 3 hr later (e.g., 4 p.m.)
5. Set alarm and wake up at 8 a.m. (will again need to be active to stay awake 2 d in a row)	5. Day 5, go to sleep 3 hr later (e.g., 7 p.m.)
	6. Day 6, go to sleep 3 hr later (e.g., 10 p.m.)
	7. Day 7, go to sleep 2 hr later (e.g., at midnight) and wake up 8 hr later (at 8 a.m.)

[a]Fisher R. *personal communication* 2005.
[b]Czeisler CA, Richardson GS, Coleman RM, et al. Chronotherapy: resetting the circadian clocks of patients with delayed sleep phase insomnia. *Sleep* 1981;4:1, Czeisler et al. (1981).

d. T$_4$ and thyrotropin (TSH)
e. Mononucleosis testing (Monospot/heterophile ± EBV titers)
2. Additional tests: As called for, based on the history and physical examination, other tests may include:
   a. Tuberculosis testing (purified protein derivative [PPD])
   b. Electrocardiogram (ECG), chest x-ray
   c. Sinus x-rays
   d. HIV testing
   e. Antinuclear antibody (ANA)/rheumatoid factor (RF)
   f. Cortisol level
   g. Lyme titers (in endemic areas or with a positive travel history)
3. Other studies
   a. Sleep studies (polysomnography) may be performed in a sleep laboratory if a sleep disorder is suspected.
   b. Tilt-table testing may be considered in those with orthostatic symptoms, especially in CFS. However, caution is required in interpreting tilt-table testing because positive results are frequent in adolescence and are nonspecific.
   c. Neurological studies (MRI or CT of the brain) may be necessary in those with headaches or other accompanying symptoms.

TREATMENT

General Causes of Fatigue

Guiding and managing the adolescent with fatigue follows directly from determination of the cause of the fatigue:

1. Adolescent sleep patterns
   a. Reassurance that there are no medical or psychological problems may be provided.
   b. Guidance regarding more appropriate sleep patterns and day time schedules may be offered.
   c. Changing school start times are being considered in some local and national discussions.

2. Medical and psychological causes
   a. Patients with mononucleosis are encouraged to return to school as soon as they are able and they should not participate in contact sports to avoid the potential of splenic rupture (see Chapter 29).
   b. Appropriate treatment is provided to those with other medical causes of fatigue.
   c. Psychological treatment is provided to those with stress, depression, anxiety, or other psychological disorders.
3. Sleep disorders
   a. Guidance on changing sleeping patterns is provided to those with the DSPS (Table 35.1). Both the 1-day and 1-week plans require significant motivation to be successful.
   b. Use of melatonin and/or bright lights have been studied for the treatment of DSPS, but results are inconsistent, these approaches must be used with caution, they are not yet widely accepted, and effects do not appear to be long lasting (Millman, 2005).
   c. Sleep studies may be performed in those with suspected sleep disorders.
   d. Use of continuous positive airway pressure (CPAP) and/or orthodontic appliances at night, may help some adolescents with obstructive sleep apnea syndromes.

Chronic Fatigue Syndrome

No specific treatment has been found to shorten the course of CFS in adolescents; however, certain management approaches can help adolescents and their families cope better with the illness and decrease morbidity associated with CFS. They include the following:

1. Explanation and reassurance
   a. Provide a detailed explanation of CFS (including etiology and management, course and outcome).
   b. Reassure patients and families that symptoms are real and generally improve with time.

c. Guide families on minimizing "doctor shopping," unnecessary testing, and unproven therapies.

d. Do not turn CFS into a chronic illness with secondary problems and secondary gain.

e. Emphasize that the prognosis for adolescent CFS has generally been shown to be substantially better than the prognosis for adult CFS.

2. Symptomatic treatment

a. Antidepressant medication may be used to decrease symptoms of depression in CFS but studies do not show that they change the course or outcome of the illness.

b. Antiinflammatory medications can be used for treatment of symptoms; medications for sleep should be used sparingly.

c. Patients with neurally mediated hypotension and/or a positive tilt-test result may benefit from medication—an α-agonist or β-blocker, fludrocortisone, or an increase in salt and water intake.

d. Multiple vitamins, minerals, herbs, and supplements have been tried in patients with CFS without definitive benefits.

3. Lifestyle changes and coping skills

a. Many adolescents with CFS require home tutoring or partial school programs to function educationally.

b. Studies have shown graded exercise programs to be beneficial in some adolescents with CFS (Viner et al., 2004).

c. Patients and families need to develop realistic expectations while an adolescent is experiencing the symptoms of CFS.

4. Psychological management

a. Studies have shown cognitive-behavioral therapy to provide benefit for some adolescents with CFS (Whiting et al., 2000).

b. Individual and/or family therapy may also be helpful (Krilov and Fisher, 2002).

c. Self-help groups may be more appropriate for adults than for adolescents.

5. Follow-up care

a. Follow-up visits are provided (every 3–6 weeks) to monitor physical symptoms and psychological issues and to provide on-going guidance and reassurance.

b. Although adolescents with CFS generally improve over time, exacerbations may be caused by intercurrent illness, a change in schedule or stressful situations.

c. Studies have shown that more than 80% of adolescents with CFS have significant improvement within 1 to 3 years of onset of illness; this contrasts with adults who generally have a longer course and worse prognosis (Krilov et al., 1998).

WEB SITES

http://www.cdc.gov/ncidod/diseases/cfs/index.htm. The CDC Web site for CFS.

http://www.cfids.org. Chronic Fatigue and Immune Dysfunction Syndrome Association of America has information for patients and families. To receive information, call its resource line at 704-365-2343, or send e-mail at cfids@cfids.org.

http://www.niaid.nih.gov/publications/cfs.htm. NIH state of the art consultation.

REFERENCES AND ADDITIONAL READINGS

Bates DW, Buchwald D, Lee J. Clinical laboratory test findings in patients with chronic fatigue syndrome. *Arch Intern Med* 1995;155:97.

Bates DW, Schmitt W, Buchwald D, et al. Prevalence of fatigue and chronic fatigue syndrome in a primary care practice. *Arch Intern Med* 1993;153:2759.

Blacker CVR, Greenwood DT, Wesnes KA, et al. Effect of galantamine hydrobromide in chronic fatigue syndrome. A randomized controlled trial. *JAMA* 2004;292:1204.

Carter BD, Edwards JF, Kronenberger WG, et al. Case control study of chronic fatigue in pediatric patients. *Pediatrics* 1995; 95:179.

Cho WK, Stollerma GIL. Chronic fatigue syndrome. *Hosp Pract* 1992;27:221.

Conti F, Pittoni V, Sacerdote P, et al. Decreased immunoreactive beta-endorphin in mononuclear leucocytes from patients with chronic fatigue syndrome. *Clin Exp Rheumatol* 1998;16:729.

Czeisler CA, Richardson GS, Coleman RM, et al. Chronotherapy: resetting the circadian clocks of patients with delayed sleep phase insomnia. *Sleep* 1981;4:1.

Dale JK, Strauas SE. The chronic fatigue syndrome: considerations relevant to children and adolescents. *Adv Pediatr Infect Dis* 1992;7:63.

Demitrack MA. Chronic fatigue syndrome and fibromyalgia: dilemmas in diagnosis and clinical management. *Psychiatr Clin North Am* 1998;21:71.

Epstein KR. The chronically fatigued patient. *Med Clin North Am* 1995;79:315.

Evengard B, Schacterie RS, Komaroff AL. Chronic fatigue syndrome: new insights and old ignorance. *J Intern Med* 1999; 246:455.

Feder HM, Dworkin PH, Orkin C. Outcome of 48 pediatric patients with chronic fatigue: a clinical experience. *Arch Fam Med* 1994;3:1049.

Forsyth LM, Preuss HG, MacDowell AL, et al. Therapeutic effects of oral NADH on the symptoms of patients with chronic fatigue syndrome. *Ann Allergy Asthma Immunol* 1999;82:185.

Fukuda K, Straus SE, Hickie I, et al. The chronic fatigue syndrome: a comprehensive approach to its definition and study. *Ann Intern Med* 1994;121:953.

Gill AC, Dosen A, Ziegler JB. Chronic fatigue syndrome in adolescents: a follow-up study. *Arch Pediatr Adolesc Med* 2004;158:225.

Goodnick PJ, Sandoval R. Psychotropic treatment of chronic fatigue syndrome and related disorders. *J Clin Psychiatry* 1993; 54:13.

Guilleminault C, Lee JH, Chan A. Pediatric obstructive sleep apnea syndrome. *Arch Pediatr Adolesc Med* 2005;159:775.

Haines LC, Saidi G, Cooke RW. Prevalence of severe fatigue in primary care. *Arch Dis Child* 2005;90(4):367.

Hansen M, Janssen I, Zee P, et al. The impact of school daily schedule on adolescent sleep. *Pediatrics* 2005;115:1555.

Iglowstein I, Jenni OG, Molinari L, et al. Sleep duration from infancy to adolescence: reference values and generational trends. *Pediatrics* 2003;111:302.

Jain S, DeLisa J. Chronic fatigue syndrome: a literature review from a psychiatric perspective. *Am J Phys Med Rehabil* 1998; 77(2):160.

Jason LA, Jordan KM, Richman JA, et al. A community-based study in prolonged fatigue and chronic fatigue. *J Health Psychol* 1999;4:9.

Jordan K, Landis D, Downey M, et al. Chronic fatigue syndrome in children and adolescents: a review. *J Adolesc Health* 1998; 22:4.

Krilov LR, Fisher M. Chronic fatigue syndrome in youth: maybe not so chronic after all. *Contemp Pediatr* 2002;19:61.

Krilov L, Fisher M, Friedman S, et al. Course and outcome of chronic fatigue in children and adolescents. *Pediatrics* 1998; 102:360.

Lee KA, McEnany G, Weekes D. Gender differences in sleep patterns for early adolescents. *J Adolesc Health* 1999;24:16.

Marshall GS. Report of a workshop on the epidemiology, natural history, and pathogenesis of chronic fatigue syndrome in adolescents. *J Pediatr* 1999;134:395.

McKenzie R, O'Fallen A, Dale J, et al. Low dose hydrocortisone for treatment of chronic fatigue syndrome. *JAMA* 1998;280: 1061.

Melnick A. When an adolescent is tired all the time. *Consultant* 1981;July:150.

Mercer PW, Merritt SL, Cowell JM. Differences in reported sleep need among adolescents. *J Adol Health* 1998;23:259.

Millman RP. Working Group on Sleepiness in Adolescents/Young Adults, American Academy of Pediatrics Committee on Adolescence. Excessive sleepiness in adolescents and young adults: causes, consequences, and treatment strategies. *Pediatrics* 2005;115:1774.

Morehouse RL, Flanigan M, MacDonald DD, et al. Depression and short REM latency in subjects with chronic fatigue syndrome. *Psychosom Med* 1998;60:347.

Natelson BH. Chronic fatigue syndrome. *JAMA* 2001;285:2557.

Nisenbaum R, Reyes M, Mawle AC, et al. Factor analysis of unexplained fatigue and interrelated symptoms: overlap with criteria for chronic fatigue syndrome. *Am J Epidemiol* 1998;148:72.

Peterson PK, Pheley A, Schroeppel J, et al. A preliminary placebo-controlled crossover trial of fludrocortisone for chronic fatigue syndrome. *Arch Intern Med* 1998;158:914.

Powell P, Bentall RP, Nye FJ, et al. Randomized controlled trial of patient education to encourage graded exercise in chronic fatigue syndrome. *Br Med J* 2001;322:387.

Prins JB, van der Meer JW, Bleijenberg G. Chronic fatigue syndrome. *Lancet* 2006;367:346.

van de Putte EM, Uiterwaal CS, Bots ML, et al. Is chronic fatigue syndrome a connective tissue disorder? A cross-sectional study in adolescents. *Pediatrics* 2005;115(4):e415.

Rangel L, Garralda E, Levin M, et al. Personality in adolescents with chronic fatigue syndrome. *Eur Child Adolesc Psychiatry* 2000;9:39.

Reid S, Chalder T, Cleare A, et al. Chronic fatigue syndrome. *Br Med J* 2000;320:292.

Rowe PC. Orthostatic intolerance and chronic fatigue syndrome: new light on an old problem. *J Pediatr* 2002;140:387.

Rowe PC, Bou-Holaigah I, Kan JS, et al. Is neurally mediated hypotension an unrecognized cause of chronic fatigue? *Lancet* 1995;345:623.

Rowe PC, Calkins H, DeBusk K, et al. Fludrocortisone acetate to treat neurally mediated hypotension in chronic fatigue syndrome. *JAMA* 2001;285:52.

Ruffin MT, Cohen M. Evaluation and management of fatigue. *Am Fam Physician* 1994;50:625.

Sharpe M. Chronic fatigue syndrome. *Psychiatr Clin North Am* 1996;19:549.

Smith MS. Adolescent chronic fatigue syndrome. *Arch Pediatr Adolesc Med* 2004;158:207.

Smith MS, Mitchell J, Corey L, et al. Chronic fatigue in adolescents. *Pediatrics* 1991;88:195.

Stewart J, Gewitz M, Weldon A, et al. Orthostatic intolerance in adolescent chronic fatigue syndrome. *Pediatrics* 1999a;103:116.

Stewart J, Gewitz M, Weldon A, et al. Patterns of orthostatic intolerance: the orthostatic tachycardia syndrome and adolescent chronic fatigue. *J Pediatr* 1999;135:218.

Stones G, Fry A, Crawford C. Sleep abnormalities demonstrated by home polysomnography in teenagers with chronic fatigue syndrome. *J Psychosam Res* 1998;45:85.

Strauss SE. Pharmacotherapy of chronic fatigue syndrome: another gallant attempt. *JAMA* 2004;292:1234.

Tanaka H, Matsushima R, Tamai H, et al. Impaired postural cerebral hemodynamics in young patients with chronic fatigue with and without orthostatic intolerance. *J Pediatr* 2002;140:412.

Tillet A, Glass S, Reeve A, et al. Provision of health and education services in school children with chronic fatigue syndrome. *Ambul Child Health* 2000;6:83.

Vercoulen JH, Swanink CM, Zitman FG, et al. Randomized, double-blind, placebo-controlled study of fluoxetine in chronic fatigue syndrome. *Lancet* 1996;347:858.

Vereker MI. Chronic fatigue syndrome: a joint pediatric-psychiatric approach. *Arch Dis Child* 1992;67:550.

Viner R, Gregorowski A, Wine C, et al. Outpatient rehabilitation treatment of chronic fatigue syndrome. *Arch Dis Child* 2004;89:615.

Whiting P, Bagnall A-M, Sowden AJ, et al. Interventions for the treatment and management of chronic fatigue syndrome: a systematic review. *JAMA* 2000;286:1360.

Wilson A, Hickie I, Lloyd A, et al. Longitudinal study of outcome of chronic fatigue syndrome. *Br Med J* 1994;308:756.

Wright JB, Beverley DW. Chronic fatigue syndrome. *Arch Dis Child* 1998;79:368.

CHAPTER 36

Chronic Abdominal Pain

Paula K. Braverman

Chronic abdominal pain is a common complaint among teenagers and young adults. Efforts to treat chronic abdominal pain can lead to intense frustration among patients, families, and health care providers alike. The approach to this problem is particularly challenging in the adolescent population as there is often no specific organic abnormality found in most cases (~90%–95%).

DEFINITION

Patients with chronic abdominal pain have been commonly diagnosed as having "recurrent abdominal pain (RAP)". RAP (Apley and Naish, 1958) was defined as three or more separate episodes of pain for at least 3 months, which interfered with normal function and activities. However, RAP was a descriptive term rather than a specific diagnosis, and clinicians commonly used this terminology to refer to patients with chronic abdominal pain that was functional, psychogenic, or nonorganic in nature.

In 2005, the Subcommittee on Chronic Abdominal Pain of the North American Society for Pediatric Gastroenterology, Hepatology, and Nutrition published a report suggesting that chronic abdominal pain can be long lasting, intermittent, or constant. They further suggested that pain exceeding 1 or 2 months in duration can be considered chronic and recommended that the term *RAP* no longer be used, calling their technical report "Chronic Abdominal Pain" (Di Lorenzo et al., 2005). The differential diagnosis of chronic abdominal pain includes functional gastrointestinal disorders (FGIDs) and organic disorders related to anatomic abnormalities, inflammation, or tissue damage. This chapter will focus on the diagnosis and treatment of chronic abdominal pain highlighting FGID.

DIFFERENTIAL DIAGNOSIS AND CLINICAL MANIFESTATIONS OF CHRONIC ABDOMINAL PAIN

Functional Gastrointestinal Disorders

Epidemiology
The epidemiology of FGID is still in its infancy, as definitions of the various FGIDs in children and adolescents have

recently been categorized and standardized. Older studies commonly used the previously established terminology of RAP to refer to entities which are now being described as FGIDs. Although the exact prevalence of FGID in adolescents is unknown, the following studies summarize what is known to date.

In a study by Oster (1972), the prevalence of RAP in patients between 6 and 19 years of age was as follows:

1. Males: 12.1%
2. Females: 16.7%
3. Peak prevalence occurred at age 9 (21% male, 30% female)
4. Prevalence at age 16 to 17 was approximately 5% of all adolescents

A more recent study by Hymans et al. (1996) found similar results in a community-based study of abdominal pain in 7th and 10th graders attending a suburban middle and high school. This study surveyed students on self-reported gastrointestinal (GI) symptoms but did not provide clinical evaluation to rule out organic disorders or specifically identify the cause of pain in a particular adolescent. In this study, there were no significant differences related to gender.

1. Middle school: Mean age 12.6 years
   a. At least weekly pain: 13%
   b. Pain six or more times in last year: 32%
   c. Pain severe enough to affect activities: 24%
2. High school: Mean age 15.6 years
   a. At least weekly pain: 17%
   b. Pain six or more times in last year: 37%
   c. Pain severe enough to affect activities: 17%

Etiology of Functional Gastrointestinal Disorders
Proposed etiologies of FGID include:

1. Visceral hypersensitivity or hyperalgesia with a decreased threshold for pain
2. Altered GI motility including altered contractile response to a meal
3. Autonomic dysfunction with abnormal processing of signals at the level of central nervous system and disordered brain–gut communication

Altered bowel reactivity may occur secondary to the following:

1. Physiological phenomena such as postprandial gastric/intestinal distension, intestinal gas, or GI reflux

2. Physical stress factors such as constipation, lactose intolerance, gastritis, mucosal inflammation from infection, or aerophagia
3. Psychological stress factors such as parental separation, peer relationship problems, school problems, or anxiety

Diagnostic Criteria

During the last decade, FGIDs have been specifically defined by the Rome criteria for adults and subsequently the Rome II criteria for children and adolescents. The Rome II criteria define FGID as abdominal pain lasting for at least 12 weeks (not necessarily consecutive weeks) during the previous 12 months. Categories of FGID in children and adolescents include:

1. Functional abdominal pain
2. Functional dyspepsia
3. Irritable bowel syndrome (IBS)
4. Abdominal migraine
5. Aerophagia

Many of the disorders causing chronic abdominal pain are the same for the child/adolescent and the adult classifications. However, the Rome II criteria divide the functional disorders by symptoms or complaints whereas the adult Rome classification is divided by the targeted organ (Table 36.1). A description of the disorders listed in Rome II criteria under the category "abdominal pain" (Rasquin-Weber et al., 1999) follows in subsequent sections.

Functional Abdominal Pain

1. Epidemiology: Functional abdominal pain is the most common FGID.
2. Diagnostic criteria
   a. At least 12 weeks of continuous or nearly continuous pain either not related or only occasionally related to physiological events such as eating, menses, and defecation.

   b. The pain is not malingering.
   c. Loss of some daily functioning may occur.
   d. Criteria for other FGIDs not met.
3. Associated symptoms can include
   a. Nausea without vomiting
   b. Headaches
   c. Dizziness
   d. Fatigue
   e. Light-headedness
4. Other factors
   a. The pain is usually periumbilical.
   b. Pain does not usually awaken the patient from sleep but may prevent the patient from falling asleep.
   c. Is associated with individuals who are perfectionistic, have high expectations of achievement, and may have unrecognized learning problems.

Irritable Bowel Syndrome

1. Epidemiology
   IBS occurs in 10% to 20% of adolescents and adults (Lynn and Friedman, 1993; Rasquin-Weber et al., 1999).
   a. In a community-based sample, symptoms consistent with IBS were found in 6% of 7th graders and 14% of 10th graders (Hymans et al., 1996).
   b. Prevalence in females is slightly higher than in males.
   c. Although symptoms increase with stress, an etiological link has not been proved.
   d. Cause of symptoms is probably multifactorial and related to motility and sensory abnormalities.
   e. Symptoms have been found after infective gastroenteritis.
2. Diagnostic criteria
   a. Abdominal pain/discomfort without metabolic or structural abnormalities associated with disordered defecation and meets two of the following three criteria:
   • Pain relief with defecation

TABLE 36.1

Rome Criteria for Functional Gastrointestinal Disorders

Adult Criteria with Selected Subcategories	Child/Adolescent Criteria with Selected Subcategories
Esophageal disorders	Vomiting
Gastroduodenal disorders	Cyclic vomiting syndrome
Functional dyspepsia	Abdominal pain
Aerophagia	Functional dyspepsia
Functional vomiting	Irritable bowel syndrome
Bowel disorders	Functional abdominal pain
Irritable bowel syndrome	Abdominal migraine
Functional constipation	Aerophagia
Functional diarrhea	Functional diarrhea
Functional abdominal pain	Disorders of defecation
Biliary disorders	Functional constipation
Anorectal disorders	Nonretentive fecal soiling
Functional fecal incontinence	

Adapted from: Rasquin-Weber A, Hyman PE, Cucchiara S, et al. Childhood functional gastrointestinal disorders. *Gut* 1999;45(Suppl II):II60.

- Pain onset with associated changes in stool frequency
- Pain onset with associated changes in form or appearance of stool

3. Associated symptoms can include
   a. Abnormal stool passage including straining, urgency, or a feeling of incomplete evacuation
   b. Passage of mucus
   c. Bloating or feeling of abdominal distension
   d. Abnormal stool frequency: Greater than three bowel movements a day or less than three bowel movements a week
   e. Abnormal stool form: Loose/watery or hard/lumpy stools

4. Other factors
   a. Symptoms do not awaken the patient from sleep

Functional Dyspepsia

1. Description: Pain or discomfort centered in upper abdomen
2. Epidemiology: The exact prevalence in adolescents is unknown
3. Diagnostic criteria
   a. Pain in upper abdomen above the umbilicus
   b. No evidence of organic disease (e.g., normal upper endoscopy)
   c. Pain not relieved by defecation and not associated with change in stool frequency or form
4. Types of dyspepsia
   a. Ulcer-like dyspepsia—predominant symptom is upper abdominal pain
   b. Dysmotility-like dyspepsia—nonpainful discomfort in upper abdomen with upper abdomen fullness, early satiety, bloating, or nausea
   c. Nonspecific dyspepsia—symptomatic patients not fitting the criteria for ulcer-like or dysmotility type

Abdominal Migraine

1. Description: Acute incapacitating, noncolicky, midline abdominal pain, lasts for hours to days, associated with pallor and anorexia.
2. Epidemiology: The exact prevalence in adolescents is unknown.
3. Diagnostic criteria
   a. Must have at least three episodes in 12 months. Asymptomatic for weeks to months between episodes.
   b. Must have two of the following:
      - Headache during episode
      - Photophobia during episode
      - Family history of migraine
      - Unilateral headache
      - An aura with either visual, sensory, or motor disturbance
   c. No evidence of metabolic, GI, or central nervous system structural or biochemical diseases.
4. Other factors: Diagnosis in the absence of a history of migraine headaches is presumptive.

Aerophagia

1. Description: Excessive air swallowing resulting in abdominal distension and sometimes in limited oral intake because of discomfort.

2. Epidemiology: The exact prevalence in adolescents is unknown.
3. Diagnostic criteria: At least 12 weeks in the preceding 12 months of at least two of the following:
   a. Air swallowing
   b. Abdominal distension from intraluminal air
   c. Belching and/or flatus
4. Other factors: Abdominal distension resolves during sleep.

Organic Causes of Chronic Abdominal Pain

Causes of Chronic Pain Commonly Associated with Dyspepsia

1. Gastroesophageal reflux: Characterized by heartburn and acid regurgitation.
2. Peptic ulcer disease: Characterized by midepigastric burning pain that can decrease with the ingestion of food or antacids. Peptic ulcers are usually associated with *Helicobacter pylori* gastritis.
3. Biliary tract obstruction: Can result in recurrent episodes of epigastric and right upper quadrant (RUQ) abdominal pain, often with nausea and tenderness in the RUQ of the abdomen. Most adolescents with gallbladder stones have one of the following risk factors—use of oral contraceptives, recent pregnancy, family history of gall bladder disease, obesity, hemolysis, and teens receiving parenteral nutrition (Adye and Ryan, 1983; Reif et al., 1991). Approximately 8% of adolescents with gallstones develop pancreatitis (Reif et al., 1991).
4. Gallbladder dyskinesia: Acalculous biliary colic which is associated with delayed gallbladder emptying.
5. Chronic pancreatitis: Characterized by midepigastric pain radiating to the back and associated with nausea and vomiting.
6. Gastroparesis: Can be associated with epigastric pain, nausea, and vomiting and can occur after a viral infection.
7. Chronic hepatitis

Causes of Chronic Pain Commonly Associated with Altered Bowel Pattern

1. Lactose intolerance: Caused by a maturational decline in functional lactase activity associated with crampy abdominal pain, diarrhea, flatulence, and belching. It is common in individuals of African-American, Asian, Hispanic, Native American, and Jewish descent.
2. Inflammatory bowel disease (IBD): IBD can be manifested by the following:
   a. Poor growth
   b. Anemia and elevated erythrocyte sedimentation rate (ESR)
   c. Bloody stools—although stools may be positive for hemoccult without signs of diarrhea
   d. Systemic symptoms—arthritis, iritis, hepatitis, and erythema nodosum
   e. Abnormal findings on radiological contrast studies
3. Celiac disease: One of the most common genetic diseases occurring in approximately 1 in 250 individuals in the United States and 1 in 18 if a first-degree relative is affected. This disease is often under recognized and under diagnosed by health care providers. Celiac disease can be symptomatic, asymptomatic, or latent. Symptoms include diarrhea, abdominal pain, weight loss, flatulence,

and nutritional deficiencies. However, 70% to 80% of individuals have silent disease and may only manifest the disease through non-GI symptoms such as dermatitis, osteopenia, short stature, delayed puberty, iron deficiency anemia resistant to oral iron, hepatitis, arthritis, aphthous stomatitis, and epilepsy. Associated conditions include diabetes mellitus, thyroiditis, and Down syndrome. Diagnosis is dependent on suspecting the disease, screening with serological testing, and then small bowel biopsy for confirmation in those with positive serology.

4. Colitis
5. Complications of constipation: Encoporesis, megacolon
6. Infection: Parasites (e.g., *Giardia lamblia, Blastocystis hominis*) and bacteria (e.g., *Clostridium difficile, Yersinia, Campylobacter*)
   a. Giardiasis, in particular, may mimic cases of FGID. Individuals with giardiasis may complain of subacute or chronic abdominal pain with bloating, as well as flatulence with or without diarrhea.
   b. Parasitic disease may also present with chronic pain in the absence of an alteration in bowel pattern.
   c. *C. difficile* can be established in the GI tract after the normal flora have been altered by antibiotic use.

Causes of Chronic Pain Commonly Associated with Paroxysmal Abdominal Pain

1. Musculoskeletal pain: Costochondritis, myositis, or abdominal wall muscle strain may be the cause of abdominal pain. Abdominal wall pain and tenderness are not uncommon in teens who are into athletic training.
2. Obstructed viscus: Bowel obstruction caused by adhesions or volvulus.
3. Ureter obstruction: Caused by kidney stones, results in colicky pain, often radiating to the groin.

Gynecological Conditions Associated with Chronic Pain

1. Pelvic adhesions—sometimes secondary to pelvic inflammatory disease
2. Mittelschmerz
3. Dysmenorrhea
4. Endometriosis
5. Obstructive müllerian anomalies
6. Ovarian mass
7. Hydrosalpinx of fallopian tube
8. Fibroids

Other Conditions Associated with Recurrent Abdominal Pain

1. Capsular distension
   a. Hepatomegaly or splenomegaly
2. Referred pain
   a. May be a result of involvement of the lower lobes of the lung (e.g., pneumonia).
   b. An uncommon source of referred pain is from spinal cord tumors (Neinstein, 1989) or discitis (Leahy et al., 1984).
3. Systemic conditions
   a. Diabetic ketoacidosis
   b. Sickle cell crisis
   c. Hereditary angioneurotic edema—may occur without cutaneous or oropharyngeal edema
   d. Polyarteritis nodosa
   e. Lead intoxication
   f. Acute intermittent porphyria

DIAGNOSIS

The Subcommittee on Chronic Abdominal Pain in Children reviewed the existing literature and was unable to produce an evidence-based procedural algorithm for the diagnostic evaluation of chronic abdominal pain. Clinicians attempt to distinguish organic causes of abdominal pain from functional disorders on the basis of the history, physical examination, and results of simple screening laboratory tests. The conclusions drawn by the subcommittee regarding the diagnostic value of these components (Di Lorenzo et al., 2005) are detailed in the following sections.

History

1. Functional abdominal pain disorders have different phenotypic manifestations. There is credible evidence of separate entities that include functional dyspepsia, IBS, and abdominal migraine. Some patients have features of more than one entity.
2. Functional and organic disorders cannot be distinguished by the pain frequency, severity, location, or impact on lifestyle. Timing of the symptoms including postprandial pain and night-time awakening, were not found to be helpful. Although chronic abdominal pain has been associated with headache, joint pain, anorexia, vomiting, nausea, excessive gas, and altered bowel symptoms, there is insufficient evidence to indicate that these associated symptoms are helpful in distinguishing between functional and organic disorders.
3. "Alarm symptoms or signs" suggestive of organic disease requiring further diagnostic testing include but are not limited to the following:
   a. Involuntary weight loss
   b. Family history of IBD
   c. Deceleration in linear growth
   d. Unexplained fever
   e. GI blood loss
   f. Significant vomiting—cyclical vomiting, bilious emesis
   g. Chronic severe diarrhea
   h. Persistent RUQ or right lower quadrant pain
4. Family history
   a. Although parents of patients with FGID have more anxiety, depression, and somatization, such a history is not helpful in distinguishing between functional and organic disorders.
   b. Families of patients with FGID do not differ from families of patients who are healthy or have an acute illness, with respect to overall family functioning (e.g., cohesion, conflict, marital satisfaction).
   c. A family history of metabolic or hematological problems may suggest organic disease, for example, porphyria, diabetes, or sickle cell anemia.
5. Issues regarding the relationship of pain to current stress and emotional and behavioral concerns include:
   a. Patients with FGID have more anxiety, depression, and negative life event stress. However, the presence of recent negative life events, anxiety, and depression

do not distinguish functional from organic abdominal pain.

b. There is a relationship between daily stressors and pain episodes as well as increased negative life events and persistent symptoms.

c. There is no evidence to support the concept of emotional/behavioral symptoms predicting the severity of pain, course of the pain episode, or response to treatment.

d. There is evidence to support that adolescents with FGID are at risk for emotional problems and psychiatric disorders (e.g., anxiety and depression) later in life.

e. Examples of stress areas to investigate in adolescents and young adults include:
  • Home
    Parental arguments, separation, or divorce
    Illness or chronic handicap in a family member/loss of family member
    Move to another location
  • Peers
    Loss of friends
    Teasing by friends
    Pressure by friends
  • School
    Change of school
    School failure
    Pressure in school
    Teacher–pupil problems

Additional history elements not mentioned in subcommittee report:

6. Pain diary: It may be helpful to have the teen keep a diary of the pain, describing the pattern, timing, severity, and precipitating factors for 1 to 3 weeks. It is also useful to include documentation of fast foods, fried foods, milk products, carbonated beverages, dietary starches, and sorbitol-containing products and to ask about any foods that may precipitate pain. In addition to helping the clinician work through the differential diagnosis, this type of diary provides a way for the teen to be directly involved in their care plan.

Physical Examination

FGIDs are usually associated with normal findings on physical examination or mild pressure tenderness without rebound commonly located in the upper abdomen. Signs of organic disorders mentioned by the subcommittee include the following:

1. Lack of growth—evidence of weight loss, decreased growth
2. Hepatosplenomegaly
3. Abdominal masses or localized fullness with mass effect
4. Perianal area—fistulas, fissure, or abscesses
5. Pelvic examination—ovarian masses, adnexal tenderness
6. Spine or costovertebral angle tenderness

Additional signs and symptoms suggestive of organic abdominal pain not specifically referred to in the subcommittee report include:

1. Well-localized pain with location remaining constant
2. Jaundice

3. Skin rash
4. Oral aphthous ulcer lesions
5. Arthritis
6. Delayed puberty, short stature—often early signs of organic disease

Laboratory Tests/Radiological Studies/Diagnostic Tests

The Subcommittee on Chronic Abdominal Pain reached the following conclusions regarding laboratory, radiological, and other diagnostic tests:

1. No studies have been done to specifically evaluate the use of laboratory tests to distinguish between functional and organic abdominal pain even in the face of alarm signals.
2. There is no evidence that ultrasonography of the abdomen or pelvis, endoscopy, and biopsy, or pH monitoring in the absence of alarm signals significantly detects organic disease.
   a. Ultrasonography of the abdomen and pelvis detects abnormalities without "alarm signals" <1% of the time compared with 10% when atypical symptoms exist.
3. FGID can be diagnosed by a primary care clinician when there are no alarm symptoms, the physical examination is normal, and there is a negative stool sample for occult blood. Testing is sometimes necessary to reassure the patient and his or her family when the pain is significantly affecting the patient's quality of life.

Testing for Organic Disorders

The following tests should be considered in the evaluation of a possible organic disorders (Boyle, 2004; Rasquin-Weber et al., 1999):

1. Primary screening tests
   a. Complete blood count with differential
   b. ESR
   c. Urinalysis with or without culture
   d. Chemistry profile with liver function tests
   e. Stool samples obtained for evidence of occult blood, ova, and parasites (including stool for Giardia antigen).
2. If diarrhea is present additional studies to be considered include:
   a. Stool for *C. difficile* toxin
   b. Lactose breath test
   c. Celiac panel
3. If dyspepsia is present additional studies to be considered include:
   a. Serological testing for *H. pylori* antibody (enzyme-linked immunosorbent assay [ELISA])
   b. Serum amylase and lipase
   c. If dyspepsia is associated with recurrent vomiting then an upper GI series with small bowel follow through and abdominal ultrasonography should be considered.
   d. If dyspepsia is associated with RUQ pain then an abdominal ultrasonography may need to be considered. Hepatobiliary scintigraphy with cholecystokinin infusion to evaluate ejection fraction of gallbladder may also be considered.

e. Endoscopy—if symptoms are not consistent with functional dyspepsia or are unresponsive to treatment.
4. If RUQ pain suggesting gall bladder disease or right lower quadrant pain suggesting IBD is present
   a. Abdominal ultrasonography
   b. Upper GI and small bowel follow through
5. If symptoms suggest obstruction
   a. Upper GI and small bowel follow through
6. Indications for colonoscopy include the following:
   a. GI bleeding
   b. Profuse diarrhea
   c. Involuntary weight loss
   d. Growth deceleration
   e. Elevated ESR
   f. Iron deficiency
   g. Other signs of IBD including rash, joint pain, fever, and aphthous ulcers
      Colonoscopy is considered superior to barium enema in further evaluation for diagnoses of IBD and colitis.
7. Other tests depending on history and initial laboratory evaluation are as follows:
   a. Renal ultrasonography if renal or urinary abnormalities are detected.
   b. Pelvic ultrasonography for gynecological complaints or findings.
   c. Sickle cell screening for African-American patients.
   d. Urine porphyrins if unusual, recurrent, severe abdominal pain exists.

Approach to the Evaluation of Functional Gastrointestinal Disorders

If after a careful history and physical examination there is no obvious organic source for the chronic abdominal pain, the practitioner should explain to the teen that the evaluation seems to indicate a FGID. Although a serious underlying disease is not suspected, the teen should appreciate that the symptoms they are experiencing are real. It is also useful to explain the concepts of visceral hypersensitivity, altered motility, and autonomic dysfunction with disordered brain–gut communication in terms that the adolescent and family can understand. A good analogy would be an explanation of the physiological response to "blushing." Blushing is physiological response to the feelings of embarrassment or stress, which cause physical symptoms that are not under the complete control of the patient. Other examples include the increased sensitivity of a healing scar or diarrhea during stressful situations. If further clarification of the history is needed, the teen should be asked to keep a pain diary with a follow-up appointment scheduled in 1 to 3 weeks. If there are alarm signals or further diagnostic tests are necessary for reassurance, selected screening utilizing laboratory tests and/or radiological studies can be performed.

TREATMENT OR THERAPEUTIC APPROACH

FGIDs are best treated in the context of a biopsychosocial model which may include psychological interventions, dietary changes, and some specific pharmacological therapy to reduce the frequency and severity of the symptoms. There are limited studies of pharmacological therapy in children and adolescents. Pharmacological therapy should be used judiciously for specific symptomatology and specific functional GI conditions. Psychological and physical pain triggers should be identified so that they can be modified or reversed. The goal of treatment is to resume normal functioning and return to daily activities rather than focusing on the pain itself.

The Subcommittee on Chronic Abdominal Pain Conclusions on Treatment

The Subcommittee on Chronic Abdominal Pain in Children found a paucity of studies evaluating pharmacological and dietary treatments in children and adolescents (Di Lorenzo, 2005). They concluded the following:

1. Two weeks of treatment with peppermint-oil capsules may be beneficial for children with IBS.
2. Evidence for benefit of H_2 receptor antagonists is inconclusive but may be beneficial in patients with severe dyspepsia.
3. Evidence for benefit of fiber supplementation in decreasing frequency of pain attacks is inconclusive but a small controlled study showed a small statistically significant decrease in pain episodes in children.
4. Lactose intolerance and recurrent pain appear to be two different entities. The evidence that a lactose-free diet decreases symptoms for patients with RAP is inconclusive.

Treatment Options For Functional Gastrointestinal Disorders

Treatment options include the following (Boyle, 2004; Weydert et al., 2003; Di Lorenzo et al., 2005; Rasquin-Weber et al., 1999; Lesbros-Pantoflickova et al., 2004).

Pharmacological Treatments

The following medications have some evidence of effectiveness from pediatric and adult studies:

1. Enteric coated peppermint-oil capsules—thought to have smooth muscle relaxing properties. A 2-week trial in children with IBS revealed a reduction in pain (Kline et al., 2001). A meta-analysis of studies in adults has shown conflicting results (Lesbros-Pantoflickova et al., 2004).
2. H_2 receptor antagonists—Placebo-controlled studies in adults have shown that acid reduction therapy may relieve some symptoms of ulcer-like dyspepsia. As such the subcommittee report stated that there may be some benefit in a 4- to 6-week trial of H_2 receptor antagonists in patients with severe dyspepsia. One pediatric study conducted with famotidine demonstrated efficacy (See et al., 2001).
   a. Failure to respond or relapse with a step-down of therapy should prompt further evaluation with upper endoscopy.
   b. Proton pump inhibitors can be tried in those with confirmed functional dyspepsia who do not respond to H_2 receptor antagonists.
3. Pizotifen—a serotonin antagonist has been effective prophylactically for abdominal migraine. This drug has not yet been approved for use in United States. In

some studies, propanolol and cyproheptadine have been shown to be effective.

4. 5-HT$_4$ antagonist (tegaserod) has been helpful in adult women with constipation-predominant IBS.

5. 5-HT$_3$ antagonist (alosteron) has been helpful in adult women with severe diarrhea-predominant IBS. Because of potential side effects (severe constipation, ischemic colitis, bowel perforation) it is only available under a restricted prescribing program.

6. Tricyclic antidepressants (imipramine, amitriptyline) have been used at low doses with improvement in controlled studies in adults with IBS and appear particularly useful in cases of IBS with refractory diarrhea.

Other symptomatic treatment options:

7. Metoclopramide—there is limited testing in adults with functional dyspepsia but a short course could be tried for dysmotility-like dyspepsia.

8. Nonstimulating laxatives—mineral oil, milk of magnesia, lactulose—may be helpful in constipation-predominant IBS.

9. Antispasmodic or anticholinergic agents may be used for symptomatic relief on short-term basis. Efficacy is controversial for visceral pain and a meta-analysis of studies in patients with IBS has shown conflicting results (Lesbros-Pantoflickova et al., 2004).

10. Treatment for *H. pylori*-positive patients in the absence of peptic ulcer disease is controversial and not proved. However, some pediatric gastroenterologists would treat cases of functional dyspepsia (Boyle, 2004).

Fiber and Dietary Modifications

1. High-fiber diet has been recommended in both constipation-predominant and diarrhea-predominant IBS as well as functional abdominal pain. It is important to note however, that both the Subcommittee on Chronic Abdominal Pain in Children and the meta-analysis of studies on adults with IBS did not provide strong evidence of clinical efficacy of fiber in IBS. Excessive fiber should be avoided because it may cause gas and distension. Foods high in fiber are listed in Table 36.2.

2. Fiber supplements—if foods high in fiber are unsuccessful, one teaspoon of psyllium seed (Metamucil or Citrucel) in orange juice, one to three times a day, can be used. Fiber supplements are also available in tablet form.

3. Patients with IBS having excessive gas or flatulence may benefit from eating slowly, eliminating gum chewing, and avoiding carbonated beverages, legumes, cabbage, and foods with aspartame.

4. Dietary carbohydrates—malabsorption may be a provocative stimulant. Avoid excessive carbonated beverages (fructose), starches, and sorbitol products.

Psychological Interventions

Counseling consists of reassuring the adolescent and his or her family that the abdominal pain which accompanies FGID is real and that no specific organic disease has been found. The practitioner should stress that the pain is not "in the adolescent's head" but is a real manifestation which can be exacerbated by stress. It is important to reassure the adolescent that he/she is physically healthy and can continue with all activities. Often teens with FGID miss a lot of school. If this is the case, the family, teachers, and school nurse should work together with the teen to keep him/her in school. Significant changes in or atypical characteristics of the pain should prompt reevaluation.

TABLE 36.2

Examples of High-Fiber Foods

Food	Amount	Plant Fiber (g)
Bran cereal	$\frac{1}{2}$ cup	33.1
Popcorn	3 cups	15.5
Wheat cereal	$\frac{3}{4}$ cup	13.1
Cornflakes	$\frac{3}{4}$ cup	11.0
Rye bread	1 slice	10.8
Graham crackers	2 crackers	10.1
Pinto beans	$\frac{1}{2}$ cup	10.0
Peas	$\frac{1}{2}$ cup	7.8

If significant depression, anxiety, or family problems are uncovered, the teen and family can be referred for further psychological or family assessment. However, psychological intervention may be helpful even in less severe cases. Cognitive behavioral therapy has been demonstrated to be successful for treating functional disorders in children and adolescents. Other techniques which have been tried include teaching relaxation, self management, coping, and behavior management techniques. Ultimately, the goal is to reduce illness behavior and to help the parents reinforce good coping behavior.

Studies have shown a better response to treatment in adolescents who had signs and symptoms for <6 months compared to those who had complaints for 2 years (Silverberg, 1991; Apley and Hale, 1973). Prompt recognition and intervention is important. Long-term follow-up studies have shown that >25% to 50% of adolescents with functional chronic abdominal pain continue to have symptoms as adults (Hotopf et al., 1998). Children and adolescents with functional abdominal pain are at increased risk for somatic complaints and psychiatric disorders (anxiety and depressive disorders) as adults (Hotopf et al., 1998; Campo et al., 2001; Walker et al., 1995; Magni et al., 1987).

WEB SITES

For Teenagers and Parents

http://www.acg.gi.org. Home page for American College of Gastroenterology.

http://www.iffgd.org/. Home page for the International Foundation for Functional Gastrointestinal Diseases.

http://www.naspgn.org. Home page for North American Society for Pediatric Gastroenterology and Nutrition.

For Health Professionals

http://www.acg.gi.org. Home page for American College of Gastroenterology.

http://www.iffgd.org/. Home page for the International Foundation for Functional Gastrointestinal Diseases.

http://www.merck.com. *Merck Manual* on line. Enter topic of interest.

http://www.naspgn.org/. Home page of North American Society for Pediatric Gastroenterology and Nutrition.

Position papers on various topics online including Functional Abdominal Pain.

REFERENCES AND ADDITIONAL READINGS

Adye B, Ryan JA Jr. Cholecystitis in teenage girls. *West J Med* 1983;139:471.

Al-Homaidhi HS, Sukerek H, Klein M, et al. Biliary dyskinesia in children. *Pediatr Surg Int* 2002;18:357.

Ament ME, Zeltzer L. Chronic abdominal pain in children. *Clin Perspect Gastroenterol* 2000;3:40.

Apley J, Hale B. Children with recurrent abdominal pain: how do they grow up? *Br Med J* 1973;3:7.

Apley J, Naish N. Recurrent abdominal pains: a field survey of 1,000 schoolchildren. *Arch Dis Child* 1958;33:165.

Barr RG, Levine MD, Watkins JB. Recurrent abdominal pain of childhood due to lactose intolerance. *N Engl J Med* 1979;300:1449.

Boyle JT. Abdominal pain. In: Walker WA, Goulet O, Kleinman RE et al., eds. *Pediatric gastrointestinal disease.* Ontario: BC Decker Inc, 2004:225.

Campo JV, Bridge J, Ehmann M, et al. Recurrent abdominal pain, anxiety, and depression in primary care. *Pediatrics* 2004;113:817.

Campo JV, Di Lorenzo C, Chiappetta L, et al. Adult outcomes of pediatric recurrent abdominal pain: do they just grow out of it? *Pediatrics* 2001;108:E1.

Di Lorenzo C, Colleti RB, Lehman HP, et al. Chronic abdominal pain in children, Subcommittee on Chronic Abdominal Pain. *Pediatrics* 2005;115:370, (Technical Report) and 812 (Clinical Report).

Di Lorenzo C, Youseff NN, Sigurdsson L, et al. Visceral hyperalgesia in children with functional abdominal pain. *J Pediatr* 2001;139:838.

Drumm B, Rhoads JM, Stringer DA, et al. Peptic ulcer disease in children: etiology, clinical findings, and clinical course. *Pediatrics* 1988;82:410.

Feldman W, McGrath P, Hodgson C, et al. The use of dietary fiber in the management of simple, childhood, idiopathic, recurrent, abdominal pain. *Am J Dis Child* 1985;139:1216.

Finney JW, Lemanek KL, Cataldo MF, et al. Pediatric psychology in primary health care: brief targeted therapy for recurrent abdominal pain. *Behav Ther* 1989;28:283.

Gold BD, Colletti RB, Myles A, et al. *Helicobacter pylori* infection in children: recommendations for diagnosis and treatment. *J Pediatr Gastroenterol Nutr* 2000;31:490.

Greene JW, Walker LS, Hickson G, et al. Stressful life events and somatic complaints in adolescents. *Pediatrics* 1985;75:19.

Hodges K, Kline JJ, Barbero G, et al. Life events occurring in families of children with recurrent abdominal pain. *J Psychosom Res* 1984;28:185.

Hofopf M, Carr S, Mayou R, et al. Why do children have chronic abdominal pain, and what happens to them when they grow up? Population based cohort study. *Br Med J* 1998;316:1196.

Hyams JS, Burke G, Davis PM, et al. Abdominal pain and irritable bowel syndrome in adolescence: a community-based study. *J Pediatr* 1996;129:220.

Hyams JS, Davis P, Francisco A, et al. Dyspepsia in children and adolescents: a prospective study. *J Pediatr Gastroenterol Nutr* 2000;30:413.

Hyams JS, Hyman PE. Recurrent abdominal pain and the biopsychosocial model of medical practice. *J Pediatr* 1998;133:473.

Kline RM, Kline JJ, DiPalma J, et al. Enteric-coated, pH-dependent peppermint oil capsules for the treatment of irritable bowel syndrome in children. *J Pediatr* 2001;138:125.

Konzen KM, Perrault J, Moir C, et al. Long-term follow-up of young patients with chronic hereditary or idiopathic pancreatitis. *Mayo Clin Proc* 1993;68:449.

Leahy AL, Fogarty EE, Fitzgerald RJ, et al. Discitis as a cause of abdominal pain in children. *Surgery* 1984;95:412.

Lembo T, Wright RA, Bagby B, et al. Alosetron controls bowel urgency and provides global symptom improvement in women with diarrhea-predominant irritable bowel syndrome. *Am J Gastroenterol* 2001;96:2662.

Lesbros-Pantoflickova D, Michetti P, Fried M, et al. Meta-analysis: the treatment of irritable bowel syndrome. *Aliment Pharmacol Ther* 2004;20:1253.

Liebman WM. Recurrent abdominal pain in children. *Clin Pediatr (Phila)* 1978;17:149.

Lugo-Vincente HL. Gallbladder dyskinesia in children. *JSLS* 1997;1:61.

Lynn RB, Friedman LS. Irritable bowel syndrome. *N Engl J Med* 1993;329:1940.

Lynn RB, Friedman IS. Irritable bowel syndrome: managing the patient with abdominal pain and altered bowel habits. *Med Clin North Am* 1995;79:373.

Magni G, Pierri M, Donzelli E. Recurrent abdominal pain in children: a long-term follow-up. *Eur J Pediatr* 1987;146:72.

McGrath PJ, Feldman W. Clinical approach to recurrent abdominal pain in children. *J Dev Behav Pediatr* 1986;7:56.

Muller-Lissner S, Holtmann G, Rueegg P, et al. Tegaserod is effective in the initial and retreatment of irritable bowel syndrome with constipation. *Aliment Pharmacol Ther* 2005;21:11.

Neinstein LS. Abdominal and flank pain as presenting symptoms of schwannoma. *J Adolesc Health Care* 1989;10:143.

Oh JJ, Kim CH. Gastroparesis after a presumbed viral illness: clinical and laboratory features and natural history. *Mayo Clin Proc* 1990;65:636.

Oster J. Recurrent abdominal pain, headache, and limb pains in children and adolescents. *Pediatrics* 1972;50:429.

Pineiro-Carrero VM, Andres JM, Davis RH, et al. Abnormal gastroduodenal motility in children and adolescents with recurrent functional abdominal pain. *J Pediatr* 1988;113:820.

Rappaport L. Recurrent abdominal pain: theories and pragmatics. *Pediatrician* 1989;16:78.

Rasquin-Weber A, Hyman PE, Cucchiara S, et al. Childhood functional gastrointestinal disorders. *Gut* 1999;45(Suppl II):II60.

Reif S, Sloven DG, Lebenthal E. Gallstones in children: characterization by age, etiology, and outcome. *Am J Dis Child* 1991;145:105.

Routh DK, Ernst AR. Somatization disorders in relatives of children and adolescents with functional abdominal pain. *J Pediatr Psychol* 1984;9:427.

Russell G, Abu-Arafeh I, Symon DNK. Abdominal migraine evidence for existence and treatment options. *Pediatr Drugs* 2002;4:1.

Sanders MR, Rebgetz M, Morrison M, et al. Cognitive-behavioral treatment of recurrent nonspecific abdominal pain in children: an analysis of generalization, maintenance, and side effects. *J Consult Clin Psychol* 1989;57:294.

Sanders MR, Shepherd RW, Cleghorn G, et al. The treatment of recurrent abdominal pain in children: a controlled comparison of cognitive-behavioral family intervention and standard pediatric care. *J Couns Clin Psychol* 1994;62:306.

See MC, Birnbaum AH, Schechter CB, et al. Double-blind, placebo-controlled trial of famotidine in children with abdominal pain and dyspepsia. *Dig Dis Sci* 2001;46:985.

Sigurdsson L, Flores A, Putnam PE, et al. Postviral gastroparesis: presentation, treatment, and outcome. *J Pediatr* 1997; 131:751.

Silverberg M. Chronic abdominal pain in adolescents. *Pediatr Ann* 1991;20:179.

Talley NJ, Phillips SE. Non-ulcer dyspepsia: potential causes and pathophysiology. *Ann Intern Med* 1988;108:865.

Wald A, Chandra R, Fisher SE, et al. Lactose malabsorption in recurrent abdominal pain of childhood. *J Pediatr* 1982;100:65.

Walker LS, Garber J, Greene JW. Somatization symptoms in pediatric abdominal pain patients: relation to chronicity of abdominal pain and parent somatization. *J Abnorm Child Psychol* 1991;19:379.

Walker LS, Garber J, Smith CA, et al. The relation of daily stressors to somatic and emotional symptoms in children with and without recurrent abdominal pain. *J Couns Clin Psychol* 2001;69:85.

Walker LS, Garber J, Van Styke DA, et al. Long-term health outcomes in patients with recurrent abdominal pain. *Pediatr Psychol* 1995; 20:233.

Walker LS, Greene JW. Children with recurrent abdominal pain and their parents: more somatic complaints, anxiety, and depression than other patient families? *J Pediatr Psychol* 1989;14:231.

Weydert JA, Ball TM, Davis MF, et al. Systematic review of treatments for recurrent abdominal pain. *Pediatrics* 2003; 111:1.

Zighelboim J, Talley NJ. What are functional bowel disorders? *Gastroenterology* 1993;104:1196.

CHAPTER 37

Chest Pain

John Kulig and Lawrence S. Neinstein

Chest pain is reported by as many as 5% of patients attending adolescent clinics and accounts for approximately 650,000 physician visits annually from patients aged 10 to 21 years.

In contrast to adults, acute chest pain of cardiac origin is uncommon among adolescents. Yet 44% of adolescents with complaints of chest pain fear heart attack, 12% fear heart disease, and 12% fear cancer.

DIFFERENTIAL DIAGNOSIS

The underlying cause of chest pain in adolescents includes several diverse etiologies. The following sections provide a broad classification, in order of frequency, based on several studies.

Musculoskeletal (31%)

In general, musculoskeletal pain is a well-localized, sharp, nagging pain. The onset is often insidious. Movement and breathing may increase the intensity of the pain.

1. Precordial catch/"stitch": A common cause of chest pain, with sudden onset of a sharp needle-like or stabbing pain, lasting 30 seconds to 3 minutes, usually localized at the left sternal border or cardiac apex. The pain most often occurs at rest, is increased with deep breathing, and may be relieved by stretching. The cause is attributed to irritation of the parietal pleura or intercostal nerves.
2. Muscle strain/overuse: Strain of the chest wall, upper back, or shoulder muscles after exercise or lifting can result in chest pain. Localized tenderness is frequently present. Movement of the arms and chest often increases the pain. Prolonged coughing can also lead to muscle strain.
3. Costochondritis (8%): Costochondral pain is well-localized with focal tenderness, usually anywhere from the second through the sixth ribs, on the anterior chest wall. The pain is more often unilateral and in multiple locations. The pain may radiate to the back or abdomen. Deep breathing may increase the pain. The clue to the diagnosis is tenderness over the involved articulations at the costochondral junction. Actual swelling is not characteristic. Costochondritis may be preceded by an upper respiratory tract infection or by exercise.
4. Tietze syndrome: This rare cause of costochondral pain is associated with a tender solitary swelling or nodule, usually located at the second or third costal cartilage. The swelling is typically unilateral, with either a sudden or gradual onset. The pain is often increased with breathing and movement, and may persist for days to months or longer.
5. Slipping rib syndrome: An unusual cause of lower chest pain. This syndrome is caused by slipping of the eighth, ninth, or 10th rib on the immediately superior rib. These three ribs do not attach to the sternum. A tear in the connecting fibrous tissue between these ribs can cause this slippage. The pain is sharp, stabbing, and located in the upper quadrant of the abdomen or at the inferior costal margin. It is usually insidious in onset, unilateral, and worsens with exercise. Occasionally, a click is heard with movement.
6. Fibromyalgia syndrome: Chronic, persistent pain associated with aching, fatigue, and morning stiffness. Symmetric, bilateral, localized tender points present at the top of the shoulders and adjacent to the upper sternum.
7. Thoracic outlet obstruction: Brachial plexus compression may be due to a cervical rib.
8. Malignant disease of bone: Primary or metastatic. A rare cause of chest pain in adolescents.

Idiopathic/Psychogenic (25%)

1. Stress or anxiety: Adolescents under stress may describe a tightness or heaviness in the chest, with or without hyperventilation. Anxiety may also induce intermittent sharp, knife-like pains, or persistent precordial aching unrelated to exertion.
2. Hyperventilation: Hyperventilation syndrome may cause chest pain associated with light-headedness, shortness of breath, paresthesias, and syncope. Is more common in female adolescents.
3. Depression: Chest pain may occur among multiple somatic complaints.
4. Bulimia nervosa: Esophagitis or Mallory-Weiss tear from frequent self-induced emesis.

Pulmonary (21%)

Most pulmonary causes of chest pain in adolescents are associated with other symptoms such as cough, fever, pain on inspiration, and dyspnea. The pain associated with pleural and pulmonary causes is usually more diffuse and difficult for the adolescent to describe.

1. Cough (10%): Persistent cough is a frequent cause of chest pain.
2. Asthma (4%): Asthma is another relatively common cause of chest pain.
3. Pneumonia/bronchitis (7%): Pulmonary infection, particularly when the infection involves the pleura.
4. Pleural effusion: Seen in 10% of *Mycoplasma* infections in the lower respiratory tract; may be a presenting sign of pulmonary tuberculosis.
5. Pleurodynia: Infection with type B coxsackievirus often leads to paroxysmal pain in the intercostal muscles. The onset follows a typical viral prodrome.
6. Spontaneous pneumothorax/pneumomediastinum: Symptoms include an acute onset of pleuritic chest pain and dyspnea. Individuals with cystic fibrosis, asthma, or Marfan syndrome are at increased risk of this complication.
7. Acute chest syndrome in sickle cell disease: May be difficult to distinguish from pulmonary infection, infarction, or embolization.
8. Pulmonary embolism/infarction: A pulmonary embolism can give rise to the acute onset of dyspnea, hemoptysis, and chest pain. This is an uncommon problem in teenagers, unless predisposing factors exist, such as obesity, immobilization, coagulopathy, pregnancy, or use of combined hormonal contraception, particularly with disorders of coagulation.
9. Lemierre syndrome: Pharyngeal abscess complicated by thrombophlebitis of the internal jugular vein and embolic pulmonary abscesses. Presents with throat, neck, and chest pain.

Gastrointestinal (7%)

Numerous gastrointestinal (GI) disorders can cause chest pain. However, these conditions are relatively uncommon among adolescents. Included in this group are the following:

1. Reflux esophagitis
2. Esophageal foreign body, including pill-induced esophagitis/ulceration
3. Esophageal spasm
4. Caustic ingestion
5. Gastritis, including alcoholic gastritis
6. Peptic ulcer disease
7. Nonulcer dyspepsia
8. Cholecystitis
9. Pancreatitis

Trauma (5%)

1. Rib contusion or fracture
2. Sternal contusion or separation
3. Clavicular contusion or fracture
4. Hepatic or splenic trauma

Breast (5%)

1. Pubertal gynecomastia: May be associated with tender and painful breast tissue. Male adolescents may believe that this physiological breast tissue represents cancer or a serious anomaly in their pubertal development.
2. Premenstrual or pregnancy-associated breast tenderness.
3. Fibrocystic breast changes.
4. Breast mass, especially fibroadenoma.
5. Mastitis.

Cardiac (4%)

Pain related to cardiac disease is among the least common causes of chest pain in adolescents. The pain may be associated with exertion. Other symptoms may include syncope, palpitations, and dizziness.

1. Mitral valve prolapse: A controversial cause of either exertional or nonexertional chest pain.
2. Dysrhythmias: Supraventricular tachycardia, prolonged QT interval, atrioventricular block, sick sinus syndrome, and ventricular ectopy can cause palpitations and chest pain.
3. Pericarditis: Pericardial pain is usually sharp and aggravated by respiratory motion, yawning, or swallowing. Sitting up and leaning forward often lessens the pain. Distant heart sounds, a friction rub, tachycardia, and a recent viral infection suggest pericarditis.
4. Myocarditis or cardiomyopathy: May progress to congestive heart failure.
5. Left ventricular outflow obstruction: Severe aortic stenosis or hypertrophic obstructive cardiomyopathy can cause chest pain. Both conditions have been associated with syncope and sudden death in athletes.
6. Ischemic heart disease: Ischemic heart pain is almost nonexistent in the adolescent age-group. Ischemic heart disease in unlikely, unless there are predisposing factors such as a strong family history, severe hyperlipidemia, prolonged hypertension, or local arteritis.
7. Coronary arteritis in Kawasaki disease.
8. Dissecting aortic aneurysm: Dissecting aortic aneurysm is an extremely rare problem during adolescence, except with a predisposing connective tissue disorder such as Marfan syndrome or Ehlers-Danlos syndrome.
9. Anomalous origin of the coronary arteries.

Miscellaneous (2%)

1. Mediastinitis
2. Mediastinal mass
3. Herpes zoster (shingles)
4. Cigarette smoking
5. Carbon monoxide poisoning
6. Illicit drug use: Cocaine, Ecstasy (MDMA), amphetamine, anabolic steroids

Massin et al. (2004) evaluated 168 older Belgian children and young adolescents and also found that chest wall pain was the most common (64%) followed by pulmonary causes (13%), psychological (9%), cardiac (5%), traumatic (5%), and GI problems (4%). Of interest was that the organic causes were all identified by history and physical examination and in no cases were organic diseases diagnosed by ancillary studies.

DIAGNOSIS

History

A careful history is the most effective means of determining the cause of chest pain in adolescents. The history should include questions regarding the following:

1. Characterization of the pain
   a. Quality: A localized sharp or aching pain suggests a chest wall etiology, whereas a deep, gnawing pain suggests a visceral cause.
   b. Onset: Patients with sudden, acute onset of chest pain are more likely to have organic disease.
   c. Severity: Does the pain restrict the patient's usual activities?
   d. Location: Pain in the T1 to T4 dermatome distribution is often referred from the myocardium, pericardium, aorta, or esophagus. Pain in the T5 to T8 distribution may arise from the diaphragm, gallbladder, liver, pancreas, duodenum, or stomach. This pain may also be referred to the back and right scapula. Is the pain positional?
   e. Timing and duration: Brief pain may have a musculoskeletal or chest wall origin. Deep, long-lasting pain suggests a visceral origin. Is the pain related to meals?
   f. Precipitating and alleviating factors: Substernal pain increasing when lying down suggests reflux esophagitis. Pain decreasing with antacids suggests gastritis. Pain increasing with breathing, cough, or movement suggests pleural or chest wall pain. Pain increasing with stress suggests anxiety with or without hyperventilation. Pain that increases at night or awakens the adolescent suggests an organic cause.
2. Recent activity: This includes activity that could cause chest wall strain, such as lifting weights, exercising, athletic competition, or performing household chores.
3. Recent trauma: Has the adolescent sustained an injury?
4. Recent infections or systemic illness: Are there any systemic illnesses such as asthma or sickle cell disease that could contribute to the chest pain? Has there been persistent coughing or vomiting?
5. Medications or drugs. Are there any prescribed medications that could account for the chest pain? Any tobacco or alcohol use? Any illicit drug use?
6. Associated symptoms: Is there light-headedness, paresthesias, or tingling in the extremities, suggesting hyperventilation syndrome?
7. Previous treatment: What treatment has been tried in the past? What has worked?
8. Family history: Known cardiovascular disease? Hypertension? Lipid disorder? Coagulopathy? Sudden deaths?
9. Recent stress: A thorough psychosocial evaluation is important, including questions about functioning at home, at school, and with peers. Recent deaths in the family? Any history of abuse?
10. Fears and concerns: Interview patients alone to determine if they are worried about conditions such as heart disease or cancer.

Physical Examination

A detailed examination, with particular attention to the chest wall, is essential for diagnosis and reassuring for the patient.

1. General state: Evidence of anxiety or hyperventilation? Normal respiratory pattern? Cyanosis? Pallor?
2. Vital signs: Tachypnea, tachycardia, or fever? Hypertension?
3. Chest wall palpation: Examine the adolescent for localized tenderness or swelling along the ribs and intercostal spaces. Check for evidence of trauma, such as swelling or ecchymoses. Individual sternocostal and costochondral junctions should be palpated. Is there asymmetry, kyphosis, or scoliosis? Check for supraclavicular crepitus, a sign of subcutaneous air. Perform the hooking maneuver to check for "slipping" rib. Pain or subluxation can be reproduced by hooking the examiner's fingers under the affected ribs and pulling anteriorly. In males, examine the areolae for palpable breast tissue.
4. Cardiopulmonary examination for the following:
   a. Heaves or thrills/peripheral pulses
   b. Asymmetrical breath sounds: Pneumothorax, pleural effusion, and empyema
   c. Rales: Pneumonia and pulmonary embolism
   d. Pleural friction rub: Pleurisy and pulmonary embolism
   e. Cardiac friction rubs/distant heart sounds: Pericarditis and effusion
   f. Mid-systolic click, late-systolic murmur: Mitral valve prolapse
   g. Other cardiac murmurs: Aortic stenosis, for example
   h. Cardiac dysrhythmia
5. Breast examination: Symmetry, masses, tenderness, discharge.
6. Abdominal examination: Epigastric tenderness may suggest a GI etiology.

Laboratory Testing

Most adolescents require no evaluation other than a detailed history and physical examination. Unless these findings are suggestive of a specific organic cause, testing is usually not helpful in diagnosing chest pain. An electrocardiogram and chest radiograph almost always show no abnormalities in this situation. Indications for further evaluation include acute chest pain that is precipitated by exercise, interferes with sleep, or is associated with dyspnea, palpitations, dizziness, or syncope. Adolescents with a history of cardiac disease, asthma, sickle cell disease, or Marfan syndrome may also require diagnostic studies, as will those patients with specific abnormal physical findings. Studies to consider include the following:

Chest radiograph
Electrocardiogram
Echocardiography
24-hour Holter monitoring
Exercise stress testing
Cardiac enzymes (troponin 1, CPK-MB)

Lipid profile
Urine drug screening
Pulse oximetry
D-dimer
Abdominal ultrasonography
Upper GI tract endoscopy

THERAPY

Chest pain is rarely life threatening in adolescents and rarely necessitates emergent intervention. Because the diagnosis is usually based on the history and physical examination findings, adolescents rarely need referral to a subspecialist. In most instances, the adolescent needs reassurance that he or she does not have a significant cardiac problem and, in addition, that spontaneous resolution of the chest pain is likely. Consider advising the patient to keep a pain diary for further evaluation if the chest pain is chronic or recurrent.

Therapy depends on the specific diagnosis.

1. Musculoskeletal pain
   a. Education and reassurance
   b. Analgesics: Nonsteroidal antiinflammatory drugs (NSAIDs)
   c. Application of heat to affected area
2. Psychogenic
   a. Education and reassurance
   b. Stress-reduction techniques
   c. Referral for counseling
   d. Consider prescribing sertraline if symptoms are chronic
3. Pulmonary
   a. Pleurodynia: Analgesics
   b. Pneumothorax
      • Small pneumothorax in healthy adolescents: May be well tolerated and managed with observation. Consider treatment with 100% oxygen.
      • Large pneumothorax: Immediate insertion of a chest tube to allow reexpansion of the lung; alternatively, a small opening in the chest wall can be created with a large-bore needle as an emergency, temporary measure.
      • Evaluate for Marfan syndrome or other connective tissue disorder.
   c. Community-acquired pneumonia: Macrolide antibiotic or doxycycline
   d. Pulmonary embolism: Hospitalization and anticoagulation
4. GI
   a. Esophagitis and gastritis: Antacids, histamine (H_2) antagonists, gastric acid pump inhibitors
   b. Dietary modification
5. Trauma
   a. Analgesics: NSAIDs
   b. Binder or sling as needed
6. Breast: Education and reassurance
7. Cardiac
   a. Mitral valve prolapse
      • Education and reassurance
      • Endocarditis prophylaxis in the presence of significant mitral insufficiency
      • Severe chest pain or chest pain associated with dysrhythmias: May benefit from a β-blocker
   b. Pericarditis: Analgesics

WEB SITES

For Teenagers and Parents

http://www.cincinnatichildrens.org/health/heart-encyclopedia/signs/chest.htm.Causes of chest pain and advice for parents.
http://familydoctor.org/523.xml.
http://familydoctor.org/x2586.xml.
http://familydoctor.org/x2587.xml. Self-help flowcharts (3) for chest pain.

For Health Professionals

http://www.obgyn.net/femalepatient/?mcfee_tfp Clinical approach to chest pain in female adolescents.
http://www.emedicine.com/ped/topic487.htm. Review of costochondritis as a cause of chest pain.

REFERENCES AND ADDITIONAL READINGS

Anzai AK, Merkin TE. Adolescent chest pain. *Am Fam Physician* 1996;53:1682.
Basso C, Maron BJ, Corrado D, et al. Clinical profile of congenital coronary artery anomalies with origin from the wrong aortic sinus leading to sudden death in competitive athletes. *J Am Coll Cardiol* 2000;35:1493.
Cava JR, Sayger PL. Chest pain in children and adolescents. *Pediatr Clin North Am* 2004;51:1553.
Daley WR, Smith A, Paz-Argandona E, et al. An outbreak of carbon monoxide poisoning after a major ice storm in Maine. *J Emerg Med* 2000;18:87.
Gumbiner CH. Precordial catch syndrome. *South Med J* 2003;96:38.
Hotopf M, Mayou R, Wadsworth M, et al. Psychosocial and developmental antecedents of chest pain in young adults. *Psychosom Med* 1999;61:861.
James LP, Farrar HC, Komoroski EM, et al. Sympathomimetic drug use in adolescents presenting to a pediatric emergency department with chest pain. *J Toxicol Clin Toxicol* 1998;36:321.
Lawrence PR, Delaney AE. Chest pain in children and adolescents: most causes are benign. *Adv Nurse Pract* 2004;12:61.
Massin MM, Bourguignont A, Coremans C, et al. Chest pain in pediatric patients presenting to an emergency department or to a cardiac clinic. *Clin Pediatr (Phila)* 2004;43:863.
Owens TR. Chest pain in the adolescent. *Adolesc Med: State Art Rev* 2001;12:95.
Palmer KM, Selbst SM, Shaffer S, et al. Pediatric chest pain induced by tetracycline ingestion. *Pediatr Emerg Care* 1999;15:200.
Roodpeyma S, Sadeghian N. Acute pericarditis in childhood: a 10-year experience. *Pediatr Cardiol* 2000;21:363.
Sabri MR, Ghavanini AA, Haghighat M, et al. Chest pain in children and adolescents: epigastric tenderness as a guide to reduce unnecessary work-up. *Pediatr Cardiol* 2003;24:3.
Selbst SM. Consultation with the specialist: chest pain in children. *Pediatr Rev* 1997;18:169.

Taubman B, Vetter VL. Slipping rib syndrome as a cause of chest pain in children. *Clin Pediatr (Phila)* 1996;35:403.

Tunaoglu FS, Olgunturk R, Akcabay S, et al. Chest pain in children referred to a cardiology clinic. *Pediatr Cardiol* 1995; 16:69.

Varia I, Logue E, O'Connor C, et al. Randomized trial of sertraline in patients with unexplained chest pain of noncardiac origin. *Am Heart J* 2000;140:367.

Vichinsky EP, Neumayr LD, Earles AN, et al. National Acute Chest Syndrome Study Group. Causes and outcomes of the acute chest syndrome in sickle cell disease. *N Engl J Med* 2000;342:1855.

Zartner P, Raith W, Beitzke A. Acute chest pain in a young adult. *Cardiol Young* 2004;14:85.

Zirkin WM, Nadel ES, Brown DFM. Recurrent pleuritic chest pain. *J Emerg Med* 1999;17:329.

CHAPTER 38

Fibromyalgia Syndrome and Reflex Sympathetic Dystrophy

David M. Siegel

FIBROMYALGIA SYNDROME

Fibromyalgia syndrome (FS) is predominately a disorder of females, and is characterized by widespread pain, fatigue, poor sleep, and some or all of a variety of other complaints including recurrent headache, irritable bowel syndrome, dysmenorrhea, arthralgia, stiffness, irritable bladder syndrome, Raynaud phenomenon, paresthesias, and depression. Establishing the presence of FS can be challenging for the clinician and a significant number of patients will have had prolonged pain, fatigue, and other symptoms before diagnosis. Therefore, they have often acquired a significant degree of disability. In adolescents, this can manifest as a decline in school performance, increasing school absence, and withdrawal from usual activities.

Because the entity of FS has received widespread attention in the lay media, it is not rare for patients with varied somatic symptoms to incorrectly self-diagnose and somewhat insistently query their provider as to whether FS is present. It is therefore important for the clinician to have a working understanding of the diagnostic approach to FS to correctly identify those who do and do not have the condition. Once properly identified, it is equally important that an appropriate treatment strategy be implemented, which should result in a decrease in symptoms and return to and maintenance of a normal level of functioning and quality of life.

Descriptions of patients with widespread pain, tender points, and fatigue, in the absence of an alternative biomedical or psychiatric diagnosis, have appeared in the literature since the 1800s. These early reports used terms such as neurasthenia, muscular rheumatism, or soft tissue rheumatism as diagnostic labels for patients, many of whom we would now identify as having FS. The term *fibrositis* appeared in a paper by Gowers in 1904 and persisted until the 1980s when it was replaced by fibromyalgia, which was deemed more accurate given the lack of objective evidence for inflammation in the disorder Gowers (1904). Concurrent with this evolution in nomenclature was the landmark observation reported by Smythe and Moldofsky (1978) characterizing the sleep disturbance in FS (Smythe and Moldofsky, 1978). The diagnosis was further refined with the 1990 publication of major and minor diagnostic criteria by the American College of Rheumatology (ACR) (see subsequent text).

Prevalence

Prevalence of FS in a general population of adults has been estimated at 3.4% in women and 0.5% in men (Wolfe et al., 1995) whereas in adolescents the figure is likely to be lower (Buskila et al., 1993). In the North America Pediatric Rheumatology registry, 7.65% of a total of newly referred diagnoses were FS (Bowyer and Roettcher, 1996).

Diagnosis

The American College of Rheumatology 1990 Criteria for the Classification of Fibromyalgia

Because of the lack of standard diagnostic criteria and clarity regarding the number, location, and examination technique of tender points, a multicenter study was undertaken in which 558 adult patients (293 with FS, 265 controls) seen in rheumatology centers were enrolled. Various elements of the history, physical examination, and laboratory studies were analyzed as to their predictive and discriminating value in diagnosing FS. This ACR collaborative study (Wolfe et al., 1990), published in 1990, established the following two major criteria:

1. History of widespread pain has been present for at least 3 months. Pain is considered widespread when all of the following are present:
   a. Pain in both sides of the body
   b. Pain above and below the waist
   In addition, axial skeletal pain (cervical spine, anterior chest, thoracic spine, or low back pain) must be present. Low back pain is considered lower segment pain.
2. Pain, on digital palpation, must be present in at least 11 of the following 18 tender point sites:
   a. Occiput (2)—at the suboccipital muscle insertions.
   b. Low cervical (2)—at the anterior aspects of the intertransverse spaces at C5 to C7.
   c. Trapezius (2)—at the midpoint of the upper border.
   d. Supraspinatus (2)—at origins, above the scapula spine near the medial border.
   e. Second rib (2)—upper lateral to the second costochondral junction.
   f. Lateral epicondyle (2)—2 cm distal to the epicondyles.

g. Gluteal (2)—in upper outer quadrants of buttocks in anterior fold of muscle.

h. Greater trochanter (2)—posterior to the trochanteric prominence.

i. Knee (2)—at the medial fat pad proximal to the joint line.

Digital palpation should be performed with an approximate force of 4 kg. A tender point has to be markedly painful at palpation, not just "tender."

Subsequent work has suggested that in clinical setting, 11 tender points might represent an overly stringent threshold for establishing the diagnosis and proceeding with management, particularly in adolescents. In adolescents, we and others have maintained that in the presence of other consistent data, detecting fewer than 11 tender points does not exclude FS as a credible diagnosis.

Researchers have examined the concordance between the ACR criteria for fibromyalgia and clinician diagnosis, and between clinician diagnosis and diagnosis using a survey (Katz et al., 2006). Among the 206 patients, the clinician diagnosed fibromyalgia in 49.0%, whereas only 29.1% satisfied ACR criteria. They concluded that clinical diagnosis, diagnosis using ACR criteria, and diagnosis using the proposed survey were moderately concordant (72%–75%) and felt that all three methods had diagnostic utility.

History

1. Achiness: The typical adolescent with FS is a young woman who describes the gradual onset of diffuse achiness in the periarticular soft tissue, or in the joints themselves. There is no redness or warmth, but patients frequently describe a degree of muscle or joint swelling that is not perceived by the health professional.

2. Onset and precipitating events: Although a precipitating event (such as trauma or acute infection) can be reported, more commonly the onset is insidious.

3. Fatigue and exercise intolerance: With ongoing pain, a high percentage of patients report fatigue with everyday activity, and a progressive diminution in exercise tolerance, which is aggravated by the decline in aerobic activity that usually occurs.

4. Somatic complaints: Associated with the pain and fatigue are numerous somatic complaints including recurrent headache, abdominal pain with cramping and alternating diarrhea and constipation (irritable bowel syndrome), dysmenorrhea, joint stiffness, intermittent subjective swelling of hands and feet, Raynaud phenomenon, mood disturbance, and difficulty with concentration.

5. Family history: A study has found aggregation of FS in families (Arnold et al., 2004). This is consistent with mothers presenting to our clinic with their daughters and stating that the child has the same disease they have, that is, FS. The parent's diagnosis of the daughter is not always borne out by the physician's evaluation.

6. Quality of sleep (nonrestorative sleep): Although the above symptoms are frequently volunteered by the patient and parent(s), a key abnormality that warrants careful questioning and discussion by the provider is the quality of sleep and whether the adolescent feels tired much of the time. Delayed sleep initiation may be a problem, but the more telling finding concerns how one describes their state of restfulness on awakening. The adolescent with FS reports being tired in the morning.

Furthermore, if asked "How many hours of sleep do you need in order to feel rested and refreshed?" the FS patient will be at a loss for specifying a figure. "No matter how many hours of sleep I seem to get, I am always tired. Even if I nap during the day (and many of these individuals are engaged in quite a bit of purposeful, daytime sleeping) I am never able to regain any energy." This phenomenon is known as *nonrestorative sleep* and in our study was found in 98% of adolescents with FS (Siegel et al., 1998). More extensive questioning will uncover that the patient is quite restless during the night with multiple awakenings and descriptions of bed covers being significantly disheveled, or even entirely off the bed in the middle of the night or upon awakening in the morning. As found by Smythe and Moldofsky (Smythe and Moldofsky, 1978) and others, (Moldofsky, 2002) this restless, nonrestorative sleep pattern represents inadequate delta wave, or stage IV sleep because of intrusion upon by lighter alpha wave sleep. Eliciting a careful sleep description in an achy, tired teen is an essential part of the history.

7. Review of systems: Important negative elements in the review of systems include a lack of fever, weight loss, oral lesions, or joints with swelling, warmth, erythema, or limitation of motion.

Physical Examination

A comprehensive physical examination for FS should incorporate a systematic palpation of each of the 18 tender points (Fig. 38.1) as well as some control points. Proper technique involves identifying the cutaneous location and then applying 4 kg of pressure using the examiner's thumb or other finger. The physician can standardize her/his force of examination pressure by using a pinch strength meter to gauge one's technique (Baum, 1991). *The force required results in a degree of discomfort even in patients without the diagnosis. However, in those with FS, the examination experience is much more unpleasant and characterized by grimacing and withdrawal.* Typically, the patient is resistant to undergoing a repeat examination because of the magnitude of pain. The remainder of the physical examination is normal.

Laboratory and Imaging Studies

Laboratory and imaging studies in FS are consistently normal, and there are no diagnostic interventions that are absolutely confirmatory of the illness. In a patient with persistent symptoms suggestive of FS, and nothing found in the history or physical examination to suggest a competing condition, a judicious use of blood work consists of a complete blood count with differential, an erythrocyte sedimentation rate (and/or C-reactive protein) and, perhaps thyroid function studies. If depression is a comorbid concern, administration of a standardized metric such as the Beck Depression Inventory is a prudent step to better define the severity of affective disorder and the possible need for formal mental health consultation.

Treatment

Approaching the management of the adolescent with FS involves a focus on sleep quality, pain, exercise, and, when indicated, depression.

FIGURE 38.1 Locations of tender points in fibromyalgia.

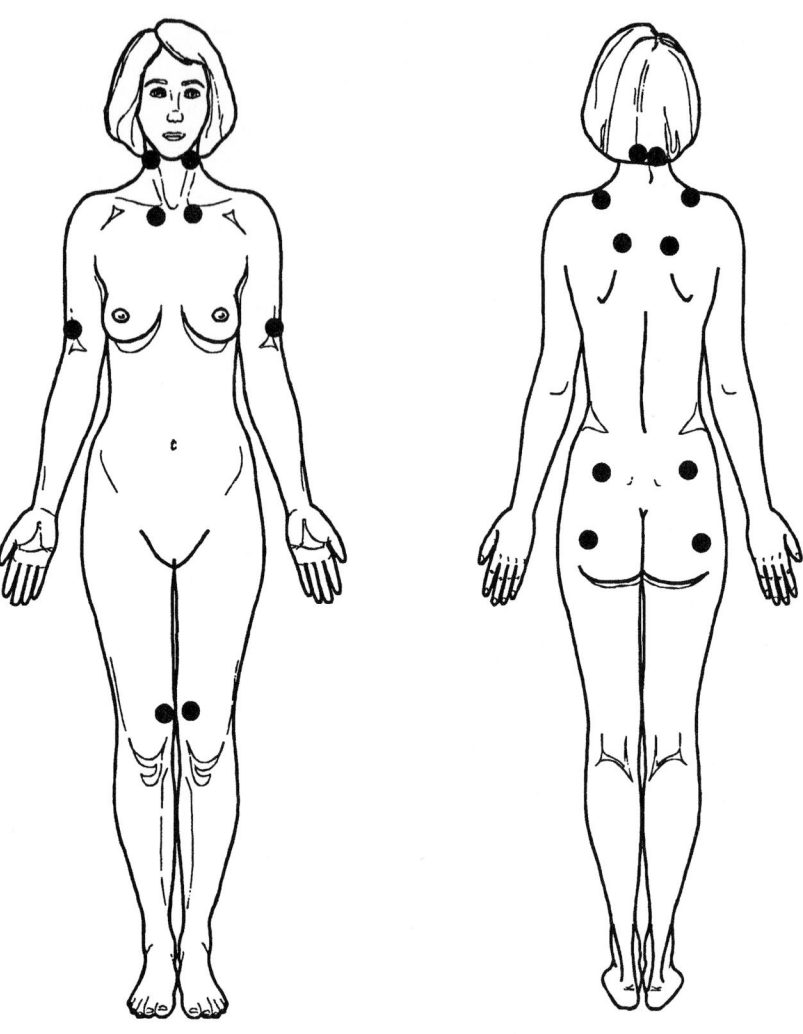

Sleep Interventions

1. Sleep hygiene: The poor, nonrestorative sleep pattern in FS is often the principle pathological process which, when adequately addressed, results in lessening of both pain and fatigue. The first priority is to establish proper sleep hygiene. This includes a consistent bedtime and morning wake-up time on both weekdays and weekends. We recommend a variation in the time when the adolescent retires at night and when she gets up in the morning of no more than $1\frac{1}{2}$ hours, regardless of the day of the week. We also strongly encourage avoidance of napping, as well as eliminating intake of caffeine, nicotine, alcohol, or stimulants.

2. Medications for sleep: Although sleep hygiene is necessary, it is not usually sufficient in the initial treatment of FS. Most patients will require medication, the effect of which is to facilitate stage IV sleep. The most commonly used preparations are tricyclic antidepressants given in low doses 1 to $1\frac{1}{2}$ hours before bedtime. Specifically, cyclobenzaprine at a dose of 10 to 20 mg nightly is often very effective in these patients, although some adolescents may require higher doses. In a meta-analysis of adults with FS, it was found that those taking cyclobenzaprine were three times as likely to report overall improvement and enhanced

sleep as compared with subjects treated with other medications (Tofferi et al., 2004). The initial benefit observed is a diminution in both nighttime awakening and disruption of bed covers. These changes occur before the patient reporting feeling more rested and refreshed in the morning. Usually, after 2 to 3 weeks of quieter, more restful sleep, an increase in energy begins to occur as well as a decrease in pain. If the quality of sleep is not changing within a couple of weeks, then upward titration of the dose in 5 to 10 mg increments is in order. Excessive morning grogginess can be a sign that the medication should be given earlier on the preceding evening.

If there is no clinical response to cyclobenzaprine, or adverse effects (such as morning sleepiness) preclude administration of a therapeutic dose, alternative medications include nortriptyline or doxepin. Other classes of drugs that have been studied and found to be variably successful include selective serotonin reuptake inhibitors (SSRIs) (Arnold et al., 2002), and serotonin/norepinephrine reuptake inhibitors (SNRIs) (Sayar et al., 2003). Although tramadol (a weak μ-opioid receptor) and sedative hypnotics (e.g., zolpidem tartrate) have been shown to be beneficial in FS, we discourage their use in adolescents because of the potential long-term complication of dependency. A combination of tramadol and acetaminophen (Ultracet) was found to be effective in adults with FS and may be safer than tramadol alone because of the lower dose (Bennett et al., 2005). Nonsteroidal antiinflammatory drugs and acetaminophen are not reliably helpful in these patients, but for the individual teen these analgesics might offer some interim relief while more definitive therapy takes hold.

3. Exercise: In addition to this important attention to correcting the sleep defect, regular moderate exercise has also been shown to improve the status of patients with FS, both in the physical and psychological realms (Mannerkorpi and Iversen, 2003). A low-intensity aerobic exercise routine, such as brisk walking for 20 to 30 minutes, three times a week is an example of appropriate physical activity to incorporate into the treatment plan for FS. Referral to a physical therapist, or to a gym with a definite prescribed program, may be necessary for those who are unable to initiate this level of activity on their own. In such instances, a more careful and graded exercise routine must be created. For the competitive athlete, or the adolescent who desires regular participation in high intensity exercise, it is important to design a schedule of *gradual* return to this more strenuous activity. Attempts to abruptly take on a demanding regimen of physical exertion in the patient with FS who has not yet established consistently restful sleep can very well result in deterioration and regression of their status. In fact, the physician may find herself/himself in the role of compelling the adolescent to hold back on aggressive exercise until it is clear that improved sleep, decreased pain, and restoration of adequate aerobic capacity have occurred.

4. Psychological support: In addition to these physical and pharmacological interventions, many of those with FS will benefit from some degree of psychological support and intervention. Obviously, if overt depression is present, appropriate mental health referral and treatment should take place. However, for some patients clinical depression is not the issue as much as it is distress and feeling discouraged and frustrated with the persistent fatigue and pain. This may be complicated by deterioration in school performance and/or disruption of peer relationships. In many families the presence of a teen with FS also introduces stress on siblings and parents. With all of the latter in mind, attention to the emotional and psychological burden of FS is an important priority. The adolescent care provider, pediatrician, or family physician can certainly assess these dimensions of the problem and undertake initial counseling for the patient and family as appropriate for her/his training background and level of expertise. Cognitive-behavioral therapy has been studied in FS and found to be a useful adjunct to treatment, as well (Williams, 2003). For some of these patients, formal mental health consultation will be necessary to fully address the psychological morbidity of the illness.

Evidence for Efficacy

Overall, the following evidence has been observed (Goldenberg et al., 2004):

1. Strong evidence for efficacy of amitriptyline and cyclobenzaprine to help with sleep. Other effective interventions have included increasing the aerobic exercise, cognitive-behavioral therapy, and multidisciplinary therapy.
2. Modest evidence for efficacy of tramadol, SSRIs, SNRIs, and pregabalin.
3. Weak evidence for efficacy of growth hormone, chiropractic, manual and massage therapy, electrotherapy, and ultrasonography.
4. No evidence for efficacy of opioids, corticosteroids, nonsteroidal antiinflammatory drugs, benzodiazepine and nonbenzodiazepine hypnotics, melatonin, calcitonin, thyroid hormone, guaifenesin, dehydroepiandrosterone, and magnesium. In addition, there is no efficacy for trigger/tender point injections (Goldenberg et al., 2004).

Prognosis

Generally, the adolescent with FS responds reasonably well to the above approach and over a period of weeks will become increasingly less symptomatic with regard to pain and fatigue. Restoring complete exercise tolerance may take longer than correction of fatigue and pain, depending on the duration of symptoms and degree of deconditioning at the onset of therapy. If recovery does not proceed, then reformulation of the treatment plan should be undertaken, and/or consideration of consultation with a pediatric rheumatologist. If new symptoms or signs appear that introduce the possibility of alternative diagnoses, then the clinician should readdress the correctness of the FS label. Whereas some of the popular information available concerning adults with FS might suggest a poor outcome, with teens we emphasize that early and prompt diagnosis, coupled with appropriate treatment, is an effective means to prevent chronic, pathological, behavioral and physical adaptations that might otherwise occur and that most adolescents with FS should be able to return to their previous, premorbid status (Buskila et al., 1995; Siegel et al., 1998).

REFLEX SYMPATHETIC DYSTROPHY

Reflex sympathetic dystrophy (RSD) (also known as neurovascular dystrophy, or more recently, complex regional pain syndrome, type I) is a noninflammatory musculoskeletal condition that includes a syndrome of pain, hyperesthesia, vasomotor disturbances, and eventually dystrophic changes. The pathophysiology of the disorder is not well understood but is thought to be related to abnormal activity in the sympathetic nervous system. Underrecognized in the pediatric age-groups, RSD is most common in adolescent girls but can occur in younger children and in either sex. Although the outlook is better in adolescents than in adults, RSD can produce long-term disability and eventually trophic changes, resulting in permanent damage to the extremity.

Predisposing Factors

1. Personality factors: Certain personality factors seem to predispose individuals to this syndrome. Characteristically, adolescents with RSD are overachievers. These are "perfect children from perfect families." Secondary gain (perhaps a respite from responsibilities) may be present.

2. Trauma: The classic case of RSD in adults follows a history of trauma or medical illness affecting the involved area. In contrast, RSD in children and adolescents is associated with such an insult in fewer than 50% of cases. When trauma has occurred it may be of any type (burn, contusion, fracture, laceration, and nerve injury), but it is often minor, such as a sprain, strain, or bruise. The typically trivial nature of the injury and the fact that it may antedate RSD symptoms by weeks (or longer) often results in the patient and family not immediately identifying or remembering the inciting event.
3. Neurological factors: These factors include multiple sclerosis, peripheral neuropathy, tumors, and cerebrovascular accidents, but occurring in only few adolescents with RSD.
4. Other precipitating factors: Local cold injury, revascularization of an ischemic injury or postoperative wound.

In summary, the precipitating factor in RSD is frequently trivial and the pain response is dramatically out of proportion to the injury.

Clinical Manifestations

Patients with RSD complain of severe pain, hyperesthesia, and inability to use the affected extremity. Most characteristic of the syndrome is exquisite tenderness to the lightest touch (known as *allodynia*). Many of these patients cannot tolerate so much as the weight of a bed sheet on the involved area. Objective changes (caused by vasomotor instability) include swelling, blotchiness or bluish discoloration, reduced skin temperature, and decreased pulses. Perspiration may be either decreased or increased in the involved area. Pain is present in 98% of cases, decreased motion in 75%, and vasomotor changes in 67%. Early symptoms include burning or aching pain, swelling, and hyperthermia or hypothermia. Diffuse osteoporosis due to disuse is a common sequel.

Laboratory Findings

1. Bone scan: A technetium bone scan may reveal reduced blood flow. A normal scan, however, does not rule out RSD (i.e., an abnormal scan is not required to diagnose RSD).
2. X-ray studies: In long-standing cases, there may be radiological signs of a macular osteoporosis (Sudeck atrophy), with patchy demineralization of the epiphyses and the short bones of the hands and feet (depending on the area affected).

Differential Diagnosis

Differential diagnosis and the features that distinguish RSD are as follows:

1. Chronic arterial insufficiency: Pulses are chronically diminished or absent (variable in RSD).
2. Raynaud disease: Episodic color changes (typically with a white to blue to red sequence) in the distal extremity, aggravated by cold (RSD is aggravated by exercise). Pain in Raynaud disease is restricted to the times of color change.
3. Phlebothrombosis: No associated hyperesthesia or vasomotor changes.

4. Rheumatic disorders such as systemic lupus erythematosus (RSD is usually associated with normal laboratory test results, including normal erythrocyte sedimentation rate, normal C-reactive protein, and a lack of significant elevation in autoimmune antibodies).
5. Localized infections (no fever or leukocytosis in RSD).

Treatment

Treatment outcome is improved if initiated early. The primary therapeutic aim should be the restoration of function, but a combination of pain relief and coping skills must also receive attention. The basic therapeutic approach is to employ a combination of physical therapy and psychological counseling

Treatment begins with discussing the diagnosis and its implications with the patient and parents in a clear, straightforward manner and placing greatest priority on immediate initiation of physical and, if indicated, occupational therapy. The fact that the prognosis is good with treatment should be emphasized and the importance of addressing the psychological dimension of the disease should be stressed. It may be useful to distinguish generally positive prognosis in adolescents from the frequently chronic course of RSD in adults. This is also the time to set the stage for the ongoing role of mental health care in the comprehensive management of RSD. Helping the family deal with the emotional aspects of the disease is crucial to the achievement of an excellent outcome. Although the prognosis for short-term improvement with physical therapy alone is good, without psychological intervention there is meaningful risk that RSD will recur or another pain amplification syndrome will develop.

1. Pain relief: In RSD, pain generally is not amenable to direct therapeutic intervention. Furthermore, experience has demonstrated that as function improves, pain tends to diminish. When the teen complains of pain, the practitioner should listen, acknowledge the validity of the patient's experience, and then move on to framing matters in terms of improvement in function. Narcotic analgesics, in particular, should not be used.
2. Physical therapy: Extremities should *not* be immobilized because this may very well worsen symptoms and increase risk of disuse atrophy and osteoporosis. Physical therapy fosters use of the involved extremity.
3. Psychological counseling and behavioral therapy: Behavioral therapy with psychological counseling is aimed at cultivating pain-coping strategies, helping the adolescent deal with underlying feelings and conflicts in ways that do not result in pain, as well as maximizing adherence to the physical therapy regimen. It should be emphasized to adolescents that the more they use the involved extremity, the quicker the extremity is going to get better; conversely, disuse will worsen the condition.
4. Medications
   a. Steroids and sympathetic blockers: The literature on adults with RSD reports that some patients benefit from corticosteroids, ganglionic blocking agents, and chemical sympathetic blockers. Our experience is that these modes of treatment generally produce short-lived or no benefit and may be associated with adverse effects. Furthermore, they may facilitate diverting the adolescent from dealing with underlying psychological issues. Except for the rare case in which

emotional factors are not implicated, these forms of therapy should therefore be avoided.

b. Nonsteroidal antiinflammatory drugs: These drugs usually have little effect in relieving the pain caused by RSD and long-term use is especially discouraged. The major emphasis should be on improving function. If normal functioning can be achieved, the pain will usually resolve or at least satisfactory coping strategies will develop.

c. Phenoxybenzamine: This adrenergic (α-receptor) blocker has been helpful in some of the more classic cases of RSD in adults, caused by obvious trauma. However, this is not an agent recommended for use in adolescents.

5. Hospitalization: In mild cases and even moderately severe cases, outpatient management will often suffice. In some centers, an outpatient program that provides 6 hours of exercises a day has produced good results. The practicalities of funding this approach can, of course, be challenging. With severe and long-standing symptoms, or failure of outpatient treatment, admission to an inpatient rehabilitation service may be necessary.

a. Admission: On admission, the diagnosis and its implications, both emotional and physical, are explained to the patient and family. This is the time to be very clear about the emotional factors involved in most adolescents with RSD. This is also the time that the "discharge goal" is established. A typical example of a "discharge goal" for the adolescent with lower extremity involvement might be to walk for a reasonable distance, wearing shoes and socks, with no more than a minimal limp. Prosthetic devices and aids, such as wheelchairs, crutches, and braces, are quickly withdrawn. Patients are permitted to receive mild analgesics, such as acetaminophen, if requested, but they are advised that drugs are not likely to provide major pain relief.

b. Weekly conferences: A weekly conference of multidisciplinary team members should be held to review the patient's progress and to set a series of objectives for the week. These objectives, usually exercises consisting of use of the involved extremity, must be quantifiable and sufficiently challenging so the teen will have to work diligently to accomplish them by the end of the week. At the same time, the objectives must be realistic and attainable. If the weekly objective is achieved earlier than the end of the week (e.g., on Friday), the teen may have a weekend pass. However, we attempt to avoid having the adolescent interpret not receiving a pass as punishment.

c. Role of the team members

- Physician: The physician sets the overall direction of the patient's medical management, is a central participant in determining the discharge goal, regularly examines the patient, and consistently communicates with the patient and her or his parents.
- Nurse: The primary nurse plays a key role in the day-to-day coordination of the patient's inhospital routine. These tasks include helping to schedule weekly team meetings, reinforcing and explaining or clarifying weekly objectives to the teen, and checking on the teen's progress in meeting these objectives. The nurse is responsible for reporting 24-hour daily nursing observations

of the patient's actions and interactions to the team members. Most important, the nurse has a special role to fulfill in establishing a trust relationship with the patient. This includes providing emotional support by encouraging the adolescent to talk about feelings and express anger in appropriate ways, listening to the teen's complaints of pain, and providing support to the family.

- Physical therapist: The physical therapist provides range-of-motion, strengthening, and weight-bearing exercises for the involved extremity. Desensitization techniques, such as vigorous toweling or immersion in contrast baths, are used. Atrophied muscles are strengthened and endurance is improved. Throughout this process, choices are permitted within limits (i.e., a win-win situation is set up in such a way that the teen attains her or his objectives while being allowed a certain amount of control over the treatment regimen). For example, the teen may be given the choice of vigorously toweling the involved extremity for a longer period or having the therapist do so for a shorter period. This fosters assertiveness and a shared responsibility in treatment and getting better. Throughout the process, the therapist uses a firm but nonpunitive approach.

- Occupational therapist (OT): In adolescents with RSD, upper extremity involvement is less common than lower extremity involvement. When the former is present, however, the OT provides tasks requiring hand and arm use in much the same way as the physical therapist does for the lower extremities. Adolescents with RSD are often overachievers. Clearly, being an overachiever carries with it a psychological "price." Therefore, the OT evaluates the teen's capabilities and the psychological costs involved in reaching his/her or the family's expectations. If these expectations are not appropriate, they need to be modified. The OT's role extends to facilitating age-appropriate activities and interactions. Occupational therapy provides opportunities for the teen to make choices and exercise age-appropriate independence, as well as to interact with other teens in a nonthreatening milieu.

- Mental health professional: The experience of this team member in dealing with RSD or other conditions characterized by chronic pain is crucial to the short-term outlook, but especially so to the long-term outlook. Her or his first task is to evaluate patient and family psychosocial dynamics. Studies have shown a high frequency of subtle family conflict, difficulty in expressing anger, and enmeshment with the mother. The father, on the other hand, is frequently viewed by teen and mother as powerful, but remote. Although the patient may be the family member with symptoms, ("the presenting patient" or "identified patient") RSD should be seen as a family disorder, and family therapy is highly desirable.

- The parents: The parents form a vital component of the therapeutic team. Without their active participation, recovery tends to be slower or may not occur, and relapses are more common. The mental health professional on the team uses a family systems perspective and facilitates parental involvement appropriately in that framework. Enmeshment between patient and parent (usually mother) is a common dynamic in these families and must be taken into account when determining the nature of parent participation.

The return to satisfactory functioning and a manageable (or absent) level of pain in these patients is usually fraught with patient and parent anxiety and resistance to treatment. Although there is a genuine desire to improve, aggressive physical therapy often strikes the family as counter intuitive ("My foot is exquisitely tender and painful and yet you tell me that the cure is for me to move, strengthen, and bear weight on that very part of my body that hurts the most?!!") Therefore, physicians and others on the team should expect major reluctance on the part of the patient to fully engage in treatment. Be cautious not to automatically frame this reluctance as oppositional or "noncompliance." Especially during this initial phase of therapy, it is rather essential that the team be consistent in its expectations and not waver from the therapeutic plan. By maintaining a supportive structure and a respectful but absolutely persistent adherence to the principles outlined in the preceding text, a gradual and substantial recovery is a realistic treatment outcome.

WEB SITES

For Teenagers and Parents

http://www.niams.nih.gov/hi/topics/fibromyalgia/fffibro .htm. NIH fact sheet on fibromyalgia.

http://www.familydoctor.org/handouts/061.html. Patient handout from American Academy of Family Physicians (AAFP) on fibromyalgia.

http://www.afsafund.org/. American Fibromyalgia Syndrome Association.

http://www.fmnetnews.com. Fibromyalgia Network.

http://www.angelfire.com/on/teenfms/main.html. Teen guide to fibromyalgia.

http://www.rheumatology.org. American College of Rheumatology.

http://www.ninds.nih.gov/disorders/reflex_sympathetic _dystrophy/reflex_sympathetic_dystrophy.htm. NIH facts sheet on RDS.

http://www.rsds.org. Reflex Sympathetic Dystrophy Syndrome Association of America.

http://www.arthritis.org/conditions/diseasecenter/rsds .asp. Question and answers on RSD from the Arthritis Foundation.

http://www.angelfire.com/wi/rsdhopeteens/. Teen site on RSD.

For Health Professionals

http://www.rsds.org/3/clinical_guidelines/index.html. Photo gallery of RSD patients.

REFERENCES AND ADDITIONAL READINGS

Fibromyalgia

Arnold LM, Hess EV, Hudson JI, et al. A randomized, placebo-controlled, double-blind, flexible-dose study of fluoxetine in the treatment of women with fibromyalgia. *Am J Med* 2002; 15:191.

Arnold LM, Hudson JI, Hess EV, et al. Family study of fibromyalgia. *Arthritis Rheum* 2004;50:944.

Baum J. Use of the pinch strength meter in tender point examination. *Arthritis Rheum* 1991;34:128.

Bennett RM. The rational management of fibromyalgia patients. *Rheum Dis Clin North Am* 2002;28:181.

Bennett RM, Schein J, Kosinski MR, et al. Impact of fibromyalgia pain on health-related quality of life before and after treatment with tramadol/acetaminophen. *Arthritis Rheum* 2005; 53:519.

Bowyer S, Roettcher P. Pediatric Rheumatology Database Research Group. Pediatric rheumatology clinic populations in the United States; results of a 3-year survey. *J Rheumatol* 1996;23:1968.

Buskila D, Neumann L, Hershman E, et al. Fibromyalgia syndrome in children—an outcome study. *J Rheumatol* 1995; 22:525.

Buskila D, Press J, Gedalia A, et al. Assessment of nonarticular tenderness and prevalence of fibromyalgia in children. *J Rheumatol* 1993;20:368.

Goldenberg DL, Burckhardt C, Crofford L. Management of fibromyalgia syndrome. *JAMA* 2004;292:2388.

Gowers WR. Lumbago: its lessons and analogues. *Br Med J* 1904; 1:117.

Katz RS, Wolfe F, Michaud K. Fibromyalgia diagnosis: a comparison of clinical, survey, and American College of Rheumatology criteria. *Arthritis Rheum* 2006;54:169.

Mannerkorpi K, Iversen MD. Physical exercise in fibromyalgia and related syndromes. *Best Pract Res Clin Rheumatol* 2003; 17:629.

Martin DP, Sletten CD, Williams BA, et al. Improvement in fibromyalgia symptoms with acupuncture: results of a randomized controlled trial. *Mayo Clin Proc* 2006;81: 749.

Moldofsky H. Management of sleep disorders in fibromyalgia. *Rheum Dis Clin North Am* 2002;28:353.

Sayar K, Aksu G, Ak I, et al. Venlafaxine treatment of fibromyalgia. *Ann Pharmacother* 2003;37:1561.

Siegel DM, Janeway D, Baum J. Fibromyalgia syndrome in children and adolescents: clinical features at presentation and status at follow-up. *Pediatrics* 1998;101:377.

Smythe HA, Moldofsky H. Two contributions to understanding the "fibrositis" syndrome. *Bull Rheum Dis* 1978;26:928.

Tofferi JK, Jackson JL, O'Malley PG. Treatment of fibromyalgia with cyclobenzaprine: a meta-analysis. *Arthritis Rheum* 2004; 51:9.

Williams DA. Psychological and behavorial therapies in fibromyalgia and related syndromes. *Best Pract Res Clin Rheumatol* 2003;17:649.

Wolfe F, Ross K, Anderson J. The prevalence and characteristics of fibromyalgia in the general population. *Arthritis Rheum* 1995;38:19.

Wolfe F, Smythe HA, Yunus MB, et al. The American College of Rheumatology 1990 criteria for the classification of fibromyalgia. *Arthritis Rheum* 1990;33:160.

Yousefi P, Coffey J. Clinical inquiries. For fibromyalgia, which treatments are the most effective? *J Fam Pract* 2005;54:1094.

Reflex Sympathetic Dystrophy

Bernstein BH, Singsen BH, Kent JT, et al. Reflex neurovascular dystrophy in childhood. *J Pediatr* 1978;93:211.

Cassidy JT. Progress in diagnosis and understanding chronic pain syndromes in children and adolescents. *Adolesc Med* 1998;9(1):101.

Cimaz R, Matucci-Cerinic M, Zulian F, et al. Reflex sympathetic dystrophy in children. *J Child Neurol* 1999;14(6):363.

Kozin E. Reflex sympathetic dystrophy syndrome: a review. *Clin Exp Rheumatol* 1992;10:401.

Lynch ME. Psychological aspects of reflex sympathetic dystrophy: a review of the adult and paediatric literature. *Pain* 1992;49:337.

Malleson PN, Al-Matar M, Petty RE. Idiopathic musculoskeletal pain syndromes in children. *J Rheumatol* 1992;19:1786.

Murray CS, Cohen A, Perkins T, et al. Morbidity in reflex sympathetic dystrophy. *Arch Dis Child* 2000;82(3):231.

Sherry DD, Weisman MA. Psychologic aspects of childhood reflex neurovascular dystrophy. *Pediatrics* 1988;81:572.

Silber TJ, Massoud M. Reflex sympathetic dystrophy syndrome in children and adolescents: report of 18 cases and review of the literature. *Am J Dis Child* 1988;142:1325.

Stanton RP, Malcolm JR, Wesdock KA, et al. Reflex sympathetic dystrophy in children: an orthopedic perspective. *Orthopedics* 1993;16(7):773.

Veldman PH, Reynen HM, Amtz IE, et al. Signs and symptoms of reflex sympathetic dystrophy: prospective study of 829 patients. *Lancet* 1993;342:101.

PART XI

Sexuality and Contraception

CHAPTER 39

Adolescent Sexuality

Martin M. Anderson and Lawrence S. Neinstein

Adolescents are sexual beings, a reality that many parents, health care providers, and adolescents themselves may not be comfortable addressing. Focusing solely on negative outcomes related to vaginal sexual intercourse such as pregnancy, human immunodeficiency virus (HIV), and other sexually transmitted diseases (STDs) ignores the fact that (a) all teenagers are sexual beings whether or not they are sexually active and (b) teens engage in sexual activities other than vaginal intercourse. Sexual behavior does not start during adolescence or adulthood, but with childhood sexual curiosity. There is a sudden upsurge of curiosity and interest in one's own body and that of peers during adolescence. Even very young adolescents are interested in "how things work" and are exposed to a wide range of sexual language and images through friends, family, school, and the media (television, movies, radio, videos, Internet). Understanding the sexual nature of adolescence is essential to developing the skills needed to answer teenagers' questions and to address their sexual feelings and problems. This chapter provides an overview of heterosexual adolescent sexuality and methods by which the professional can better assist adolescents in negotiating sexually related issues (see Chapter 40 for information relevant to gay, lesbian, bisexual, and transgender [GLBT] youth).

ADOLESCENT SEXUAL DEVELOPMENT

Preadolescence

Physical gender is established in utero and is based on chromosomes, gonads, and hormones. Gender identity (masculine, feminine) and sexual preference is established by early childhood. The exact timing is unknown. Characteristics of preadolescent sexual development include the following:

1. A low physical and mental investment in sexuality
2. Information gathering on the topic of sexuality (including facts and myths) from the media, friends, school, and family
3. Prepubertal appearance
4. Masturbation occurs as a normal behavior and provides a feeling of pleasure as opposed to being a response to a sexual feeling or urge.

Early Adolescence

Characteristics of sexual development in early adolescence include the following:

1. Initiation of puberty.
2. Extreme concern and curiosity exists about one's own body and that of peers.
3. Sexual fantasies are common and may serve as a source of guilt.
4. Masturbation in response to sexual feelings begins and may be accompanied by guilt.
5. Sexual activities are most often nonphysical. Early adolescents may be content with nonsexual interactions at school, during group activities, or at home (by telephone, e-mail, instant messaging, or chat rooms).

Middle Adolescence

Sexual development in middle adolescence is characterized by the following:

1. Full pubertal maturation is attained and menstruation has begun in females.
2. Sexual energy is at a high level, with more emphasis on physical contact.
3. Sexual behavior is of an exploratory, experimental nature.
4. Dating and noncoital sexual activities are common; casual relationships with noncoital contacts are prevalent.
5. Attention to the adverse consequences of sexual behavior is not fully developed.

Late Adolescence

Sexual development in late adolescence is characterized by the following:

1. Completion of puberty.
2. Sexual behavior becomes more expressive.
3. Intimate sharing relationships may develop.

As already outlined, sexuality is an important aspect of adolescent development. An understanding of issues related to adolescent identity and sexual development include:

1. How do I know I'm ready for sex?
2. What is important in a relationship?

3. How do I say no? Do I want to?
4. How do I deal with anger, rejection, and loneliness?
5. What is safe sex?
6. Am I gay or straight?

Adolescents are involved in sexual activity for a variety of reasons including:

1. Peer pressure
2. Experimentation
3. To experience feelings of pleasure, affection, and closeness
4. The expression of being grown up

NONCOITAL SEXUAL BEHAVIORS

There are more than 40 million adolescents between 10 and 19 years living in the United States. Data on rates of vaginal intercourse, pregnancy, and STDs are readily available. Data on noncoital sexual activities are more difficult to find. In 1996, Schuster et al. published one of the first papers on the sexual activity of virgins (no vaginal intercourse) (Schuster et al., 1996). This group studied male and female virgins attending an urban California high school. Thirty percent of males and females had engaged in mutual masturbation. Eleven percent of male virgins and 8% of female virgins had engaged in fellatio to the point of ejaculation. Cunnilingus was a sexual activity of 9% of males and 12% of female virgins (Table 39.1). This study compared nonsexual risk-taking behaviors of virgins with nonvirgins. The virgins who engaged in sexual activities had risk-taking behaviors that were closer to nonvirgins than to non–sexually active virgins. This data is supportive of the importance of asking about all sexual behaviors and not just focusing on vaginal intercourse (Table 39.2). Subsequently, there have been additional studies that have investigated sexual behaviors other than vaginal intercourse (Gates and Sonenstein, 2000; Mosher et al., 2005).

Oral Sex

Over the past several years there has been increased media attention regarding the prevalence of oral sex, giving the impression that it is of epidemic proportions. However, between 1988 and 2002 there did not appear to be any significant increase in males receiving oral sex from females (Gates and Sonenstein, 2000; Mosher et al., 2005). There are no comparable data for females over this time. The most recent data that includes both males and females is from the National Survey of Family Growth (NSFG) (Mosher et al., 2005) (Tables 39.3 and 39.4). This survey explored the sexual activities of 15- to 19-year olds. Forty-six percent of 15- to 17-year-old males were not sexually experienced whereas 36% had vaginal intercourse and 44% had oral sex. Twenty-one percent of 15- to 17-year-old male virgins (no vaginal intercourse) and 85% of nonvirgins had engaged in oral sex. The data for 15- to 17-year-old females indicated that 48.6% were not sexually experienced whereas 39% have had vaginal sex, 47% oral sex with a male, and 8% oral sex with a female. The

TABLE 39.1

Percentage of High School Virgins in Each Demographic Group who Engaged in Each Heterosexual Genital Sexual Activity during the Prior Year

Demographic Group	Number[a]	Activity %				
		Masturbation of Partner	Masturbation by Partner	Fellatio with Ejaculation	Cunnilingus	Anal Intercourse
Gender						
Male	385–387	30	31	11	9	1
Female	432–434	29	31	8	12	<0.5
Grade						
9th	255–260	25	27	7	7	1
10th	242–244	33	36	12	11	1
11th	176–178	30	30	8	10	0
12th	135–136	31	33	10	15	1
Race/ethnicity						
African-American	45–46	30	33	2	11	0
Asian and Pacific islander	104–106	16	16	4	10	0
Latino	190–192	24	24	7	7	1
White	403–407	36	39	13	12	1
Other/mixed	52	29[b]	37[b]	10[c]	13	2
Total number Males and Females	817–821	29	31	9[d]	10	1

[a]Covers the range of virgins in each demographic group who responded to each item.
Demographic groups differed significantly by chi-square test: [b]$p < 0.001$; [c]$p < 0.01$; [d]$p < 0.05$.
From Schuster MA, Bell RM, Kanouse DE. The sexual practices of adolescent virgins: genital sexual activities of high school students who have never had vaginal intercourse. *Am J Public Health* 1996;86:1570, with permission.

TABLE 39.2

Percentage of High School Students Who Used Illicit Substances and Engaged in Other Problem Behaviors during the Prior Year, by Category of Sexual Experience

	Virgins			All Students	
	No Sexual Activity[a] *(n = 496–502)*	*Masturbation with Partner[a]* *(n = 167–169)*	*Oral Sex* *(n = 110–113)*	*Virgins* *(n = 805–815)*	*Nonvirgins* *(n = 856–874)*
Illicit substances					
Drank beer, wine, liquor, or other alcoholic beverages (not counting religious ceremonies)	56	77	87[b]	64	88[b]
Smoked cigarettes	24	41	56[b]	32	59[b]
Used marijuana (pot, grass)	10	30	45[b]	19	57[b]
Other problem behaviors					
Skipped class or school without a good excuse	48	67	80[b]	56	78[b]
Stayed out late at night without parents' permission	35	58	63[b]	44	58[b]
Took something not belonging to you worth more than $50	8	17	27[b]	13	31[b]
Ran away from home for overnight or longer	3	8	9[c]	5	17[b]

The sample sizes reported in parentheses cover the range of respondents for each item in the left-hand column. The values for the three virgin categories do not add up to the values for all virgins because the response rate for the individual sexual acts was lower than that for virginity.

[a]The 'No Sexual Activity' category includes virgins who did not report engaging in heterosexual masturbation with a partner or oral sex during the previous year. The 'Masturbation with Partner' category includes virgins who reported engaging in heterosexual masturbation with a partner but not heterosexual oral sex during the previous year. The 'Oral Sex' category includes virgins who reported engaging in heterosexual fellatio with ejaculation or cunnilingus regardless of whether they had also engaged in heterosexual masturbation with a partner during the previous year.

Sexual experience groups differed significantly by chi-square test: [b]$p < 0.001$; [c]$p < 0.05$.

From Schuster MA, Bell RM, Kanouse DE. The sexual practices of adolescent virgins: genital sexual activities of high school students who have never had vaginal intercourse. *Am J Public Health* 1996;86:1570, with permission.

percentage of females engaging in oral sex differed between virgins and nonvirgins. Eighteen percent of virginal women between 15 and 17 years of age had oral sex with a male and 4.8% had oral sex with a female. Eighty percent of nonvirgin 15- to 17-year-old females reported oral sex with a male and 14% had oral sex with a female.

Adolescents believe that oral sex is significantly less risky than vaginal sex when considering health, social, and emotional consequences. It is less of a threat to their values and beliefs. However, oral sex is still more acceptable in dating than nondating relationships (Halpern-Felsher et al., 2005). The 2002 NSFG (Mosher et al., 2005) reported that 16.2% of males and 22% of females (Table 39.5) between 15 and 24 years of age who engaged in oral sex abstained from vaginal sex for moral or religious reasons; oral sex has a different religious or moral value than vaginal sex in their belief system.

Anal Sex

The 2002 NSFG reported that 8.1% of males had anal sex with a female and 3.9% had anal or oral sex with a male. In virgin males, the rate of anal sex with a female was 1%

and oral or anal sex with a male was 2.6%. For nonvirgin males, the rate of anal sex with a female was 20.7% and oral or anal sex with a male was 6.4%. In addition, 5.6% of females had anal sex with a male. For virgin females, the data did not reach statistical significance and for nonvirgins it was 28.6%.

Sexual Pressures

There is still much to learn about the full range of noncoital sexual behaviors of adolescents. The role that noncoital sexual behavior plays in the areas of pregnancy, STDs, and avoidance or protection of virginity is not completely understood.

COITAL SEXUAL BEHAVIORS

There are several sources of data on the rates of sexual intercourse in American adolescents. The four major surveys currently available are the following (see the Web sites for full data):

TABLE 39.3

Types of Sexual Contact for Males 15 to 19 Years Old Including Anal and Oral Sex

Characteristic	Number (in Thousands)	Any Opposite-Sex Sexual Contact	Opposite-Sex Sexual Contact Vaginal	Oral Any Oral	Oral Gave	Oral Received	Anal	Female Touched Penis	Any Oral or Anal Sex with a Male	No Sexual Contact with Another Person
Age										
15–19 years	10,208	63.9	49.1	55.2	38.8	51.5	11.2	52.4	4.5	35.4
15–17 years	5,748	53.2	36.3	44.0	28.2	40.3	8.1	42.7	3.9	46.1
15 years	1,930	43.2	25.1	35.1	15.5	30.3	4.6	35.4	2.2	55.9
16 years	1,998	53.3	37.5	42.0	27.0	39.4	7.3	43.2	3.1	46.3
17 years	1,820	63.5	46.9	55.7	43.2	51.9	12.9	50.1	6.6	35.6
18–19 years	4,460	77.7	65.5	69.5	52.4	66.0	15.2	65.0	5.1	21.6
18 years	2,392	74.4	62.4	65.4	50.5	61.7	15.1	59.2	4.3	24.6
19 years	2,067	81.6	68.9	74.2	54.6	70.9	15.3	71.6	6.0	18.0
Ever had vaginal intercourse with a female and age										
Yes	13,624	100.0	100.0	88.8	75.1	85.9	31.3	81.3	5.3	—
15–17 years	2,069	100.0	100.0	84.8	60.5	79.3	20.7	80.0	6.4	—
18–19 years	2,912	100.0	100.0	90.2	69.9	86.9	21.9	82.1	6.0	—
No	6,393	30.0	—	25.2	13.5	22.2	1.3	24.8	4.4	67.9
15–17 years	3,629	27.1	—	20.7	10.0	18.1	1.0	21.7	2.6	71.8
18–19 years	1,537	35.7	—	30.6	19.6	26.8	a	33.0	3.3	62.4

[a]Figure does not meet standards of reliability or precision.

Adapted from Mosher WD, Chandra A, Jones J. Centers for Disease Control and Prevention. Sexual behavior and selected health measures: men and women 15–44 years of age, United States, 2002. *Adv Data Vital Health Stat* 2005;362:1.

TABLE 39.4

Types of Sexual Contact for Women 15 to 19 Years Old Including Anal and Oral Sex

Characteristic	Number (in Thousands)	Any Opposite-Sex Sexual Contact	Opposite-Sex Sexual Contact					Any Oral or Anal Sex with a Male	No Sexual Contact with Another Person
			Vaginal	Any Oral	Oral		Anal		
					Gave	Received			
Age									
15–19 years	9,834	63.3	53.0	54.3	43.6	49.6	10.9	10.6	35.5
15–17 years	5,819	49.8	38.7	42.0	30.4	38.0	5.6	8.4	48.6
15 years	1,819	33.8	26.0	26.0	18.3	23.9	2.4	7.2	63.7
16 years	1,927	49.6	39.6	42.4	30.4	39.3	6.9	13.1	48.8
17 years	2,073	64.0	49.0	55.5	41.1	49.1	7.3	5.1	35.2
18–19 years	4,015	82.9	73.8	72.3	62.0	66.7	18.7	13.8	16.5
18 years	2,035	78.2	70.3	70.2	61.3	62.4	18.8	13.7	21.2
19 years	1,980	87.8	77.4	74.4	64.2	71.1	18.6	13.9	11.7
Ever had vaginal intercourse with a male and age									
Yes	13,782	100.0	100.0	87.4	77.6	83.4	28.6	15.6	—
15–17 years	2,251	100.0	100.0	80.1	60.6	74.5	13.9	14.1	—
18–19 years	2,953	100.0	100.0	85.6	75.8	78.7	25.2	17.4	—
No	5,858	24.1	—	24.3	17.9	21.1	0.8	4.8	73.0
15–17 years	3,563	18.1	—	18.0	11.4	14.9	a	4.8	79.2
18–19 years	1,049	35.3	—	35.3	26.2	33.0	a	3.7	62.5

[a]Figure does not meet standards of reliability or precision.
Adapted from Mosher WD, Chandra A, Jones J. Centers for Disease Control and Prevention. Sexual behavior and selected health measures: men and women 15–44 years of age, United States, 2002. *Adv Data Vital Health Stat* 2005;362:1.

TABLE 39.5

Main Reason for No Vaginal Intercourse among Males and Females 15 to 24 Years of Age

				Type of Sexual Contact		
Characteristic	Number in Thousands	Total	Vaginal Intercourse	Oral Sex, but No Vaginal Intercourse	No Vaginal Intercourse or Oral Sex, but Other Sexual Contact	No Opposite-Sex Sexual Contact
Male						
Against religion or morals	2,116	100	a	16.2 (2.8)	2.3 (0.9)	81.5 (2.8)
Don't want to get a female pregnant	1,178	100	a	30.2 (4.8)	11.9 (3.6)	58.0 (4.5)
Don't want to get an STD	569	100	a	23.4 (7.3)	6.4 (2.8)	70.2 (7.7)
Haven't found the right person yet	1,501	100	a	31.0 (4.7)	b	67.6 (4.7)
In a relationship, waiting for the right time	360	100	a	30.7 (10.4)	b	65.3 (10.8)
Other	492	100	a	13.7 (4.9)	b	83.7 (5.2)
Females						
Against religion or morals	2,497	100	a	21.8 (2.8)	c	78.2 (2.8)
Don't want to get pregnant	851	100	a	25.3 (4.8)	0	74.0 (4.8)
Don't want to get an STD	298	100	a	19.1 (6.6)	c	80.9 (6.6)
Haven't found the right person yet	1,100	100	a	26.5 (4.3)	c	73.5 (4.3)
In a relationship, waiting for the right time	357	100	a	37.0 (8.7)	c	63.0 (8.7)
Other	685	100	a	20.3 (7.6)	c	79.7 (7.6)

STD, sexually transmitted disease.

[a]Category not applicable.

[b]Figure does not meet standards of reliability or precision.

[c]Quantity zero.

Adapted from Mosher WD, Chandra A, Jones J. Centers for Disease Control and Prevention. Sexual behavior and selected health measures: men and women 15–44 years of age, United States, 2002. *Adv Data Vital Health Stat* 2005;362:1.

Youth Risk Behavior Survey (YRBS), http://www.cdc.gov/HealthyYouth/yrbs/index.htm;

National Survey of Family Growth (NSFG), http://www.cdc.gov/nchs/nsfg.htm;

National Longitudinal Study of Adolescent Health (Add Health), http://www.cpc.unc.edu/projects/addhealth;

National Survey of Adolescent Males (NSAM), http://www.nichd.nih.gov/about/cpr/dbs/res_national3.htm.

Although all four surveys collect information about sexual behavior, they differ in purpose, design, and implementation (Tables 39.3–39.7; Figs. 39.2–39.5).

The 2005 YRBS (http://www.cdc.gov/mmwr/preview/mmwrhtml/ss5505a1.htm) that surveyed "in-school" youth (Fig. 39.2) found that 47% of students in grades 9 to 12 had vaginal intercourse (48% male, 46% female). This increased from 34% (29% female, 39% male) in 9th grade to approximately 63% by their senior year (62% female, 64% male). Four percent of females and 9% of males in grades 9 to 12 started having sex before 13 years of age (Fig. 39.3). More than 20% of high school seniors had four or more partners (Fig. 39.4). The pregnancy rate for seniors (2003 survey, data not available in 2005) was 8%; 5% of male seniors revealed that they had fathered a pregnancy (Fig. 39.5).

The 2002 NSFG (http://www.cdc.gov/nchs/datawh/statab/pubd.htm-Sexual Activity) (Tables 39.3 and 39.4) surveyed both "in-and out-of school" youth and found that 39% of 15- to 17-year-old females and 36% of 15- to 17-year-old males had engaged in vaginal intercourse. By the time adolescents reached 17 years of age, 46.9% of males and 49% of females had vaginal intercourse and by 18 years, this increased to 62% for males and 70% for females.

Trends in Sexual Intercourse

To put adolescents' current sexual behavior into perspective, it helps to look at trends over time. Rates for sexual intercourse and its sequelae have been decreasing (Table 39.6). From 1991 to 2005, there has been a decrease in teens who had sexual intercourse and those who had four or more partners (Table 39.6). There was no change

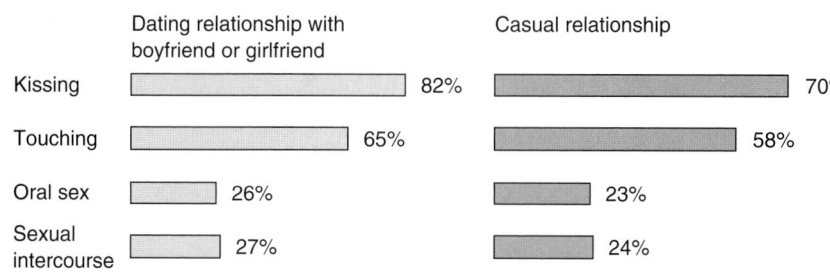

FIGURE 39.1 Defining relationships. Activities identified to be part of a relationship "almost always" or "most of the time." (From Kaiser Family Foundation. *Relationships: a series of national surveys of teens about sex.* www.kff.org/youthhivstds/3257 .index.cfm. 2003.)

in the percentage that had been sexually active within 3 months before the survey but there was a downward trend. Table 39.7 tabulates data from the 1997 and 2005 YRBS, the 1995 and 2002 NSFG, and the 1995 NSAM for males and females by ethnicity. It is important to note that each survey has different rates for sexual intercourse due to the different sampling methods and populations surveyed.

Protective and Risk-Promoting Factors

The Henry J. Kaiser Family Foundation and *Seventeen* magazine formed a public information partnership to provide young people with information and resources on sexual health issues. As part of this partnership, they regularly survey teens on their sexual lives. The Kaiser Family Foundation published the *National Survey of Adolescents and Young Adults: Sexual Health Knowledge, Attitudes and Experiences* in 2003 (Kaiser Family Foundation, 2003).

Oral sex was viewed by 24% (18% males, 31% females) of 15- to 17-year olds as a way to avoid vaginal intercourse.

Many of these teens agreed with the statement that "oral sex is not as big of a deal as sexual intercourse" (46% of all teens, 54% of males, and 38% of females). In fact, almost 40% (47% males, 30% females) of youth viewed oral sex as safer sex.

Kaiser Family Foundation also partnered with the *Seventeen* magazine and issued several reports under the heading of Sex Smarts (Web site www.kff.org). In October 2002, they released a report (http://www.kff.org/youthhivstds/3257-index.cfm) entitled "Relationships" (Fig. 39.1). In this report, both casual and dating relationships were common in 15- to 17-year olds. Twenty-six percent of the teens reported that oral sex was part of a dating relationship "almost always" or "most of the time;" 23% of teens surveyed reported that oral sex was part of a casual relationship.

Adolescents reported a number of reasons that influenced their decision not to have sex including worries about pregnancy (94%), concern about HIV/acquired immunodeficiency syndrome (AIDS) (92%), concerns about STDs (92%), feeling of being too young (91%), concerns about what their parents would think (91%), what they learned in sex education (89%), moral or religious values (84%), had not met the right person (83%), concerns about reputation (77%), partner is not ready (66%), and do not have access to birth control (59%) (Fig. 39.6). The major reasons that influenced their decision to have sex included curiosity (85%), partner wanted to (84%), felt like it was the right time (82%), ready to lose their virginity (80%), met the right person (76%), been with their partner for a long time (74%), hoped it would make relationship closer (70%), in love with their partner (69%), many of their friends had

TABLE 39.6

Trends in the Prevalence of Sexual Behaviors

1991	1993	1995	1997	1999	2001	2003	2005	Changes from 1991–2005[a]	Changes from 2003–2005[b]
Ever had sexual intercourse									
54.1 (±3.5)[c]	53 (±2.7)	53.1 (±4.5)	48.4 (±3.1)	49.9 (±3.7)	45.6 (±2.3)	46.7 (±2.6)	46.8 (±3.3)	Decreased, 1991–2005	No change
Had four or more sex partners during lifetime									
18.7 (±2.1)	18.7 (±2.0)	17.8 (±2.7)	16 (±1.4)	16.2 (±2.6)	14.2 (±1.2)	14.4 (±1.6)	14.3 (±1.5)	Decreased, 1991–2005	No change
Currently sexually active									
37.5 (±3.1)	37.5 (±2.1)	37.9 (±3.5)	34.8 (±2.2)	36.3 (±3.5)	33.4 (±2.0)	34.3 (±2.1)	33.9 (±2.5)	No change, 1991–2005	No change

[a]Based on linear and quadratic trend analyses using a logistic regression model controlling for sex, race/ethnicity, and grade.
[b]Based on T-test analyses.
[c]95% confidence interval.
Adapted from National Youth Risk Behavior Survey (YRBSS), 1991–2005.
(http://www.cdc.gov/yrbs/pdf/trends/2005_YRBS_sexual_behaviors.pdf)

TABLE 39.7

Percentage of High School Adolescents Aged 15 to 19 Years or Grade 9 to 12, Who Reported Ever Having Had Sexual Intercourse, by Gender and Survey, According to Race and Ethnicity

Survey, Year, and Comparison	Total	White	Black	Hispanic
FEMALE				
YRBS (9–12th grade)				
1997	48.4	44.7	67.2	48.1
2005	45.7	43.7	61.2	44.4
NSFG (15–19 years old)				
1995	36.5	34.3	45.4	47.8
2002	53.0	51.7	61.7	48.8
MALE				
YRBS				
1997	46.9	41.0	78.9	56.8
2005	47.9	42.2	74.6	57.6
NSAM				
1995	41.3	32.8	76.8	47.4
NSFG				
2002	48.9	44.5	65.6	56.0

YRBS, Youth Risk Behavior Survey; NSFG, National Survey of Family Growth; NSAM, National Survey of Adolescent Males.

Adapted from Mosher WD, Chandra A, Jones J. Centers for Disease Control and Prevention. Sexual behavior and selected health measures: men and women 15–44 years of age, United States, 2002. *Adv Data Vital Health Stat* 2005;362:1.

Santelli JS, Lindberg LD, Abma J, et al. Adolescent sexual behavior: estimates and trends from four nationally represented surveys. *Fam Plann Perspect* 2000;32:156.

Centers for Disease Control and Prevention. Youth risk behavior surveillance—United States, 2005. *MMWR* 2006;55:SS-5.

already done it (62%), wanted to get it over with (58%), ready to marry their partner (53%), and they were drinking or using drugs at the time (18%) (Fig. 39.7). In this survey, 29% (33% males, 23% females) of 15- to 17-year olds felt pressure to have sex. Sixty-three percent (66% males, 60% females) felt that waiting to have sex was nice but nobody really did. Almost 60% (59% males, 58% females) responded in the affirmative that there was pressure to have sex by a certain age and 39% (50% males, 27% females) agreed that "If you have been seeing someone for a while, it is expected that you will have sex."

Youth as young as 13 to 14 years old felt pressure to have sex. Forty-seven percent (40% males, 54% females) of 13- to 14-year olds felt pressure to have sex. Almost a one fourth (27% males, 18% females) agreed with the statement, "If you have been seeing someone for a while, it is expected that you will have sex." NSFG reported on the main reasons for not having sex among adolescents (both females and males) who had never had sexual intercourse (Fig. 39.8). The main reasons included it was against morals and religion beliefs, did not want to get pregnant (or partner pregnant), and had not found the right person. All of these were in the 20% to 35% range. Fear of STDs was given by <10% of adolescent males and females.

Some of the major protective factors associated with whether a teen had sexual intercourse included making a "virginity pledge" (especially for black and Hispanic males and white and black females), perceived personal and social costs to sex, and perceived costs of getting/making someone pregnant (Table 39.8). Virginity pledges are a commitment made by teenagers to refrain from sexual intercourse until marriage. Recent studies have raised questions about the effectiveness of virginity pledges in preventing adolescent sexual behavior. Bersamin et al. (2005) found that private rather than public pledges reduced the likelihood of sexual intercourse. Bruckner and Bearman (2005) found that teens who make virginity pledges start having sex at a later age, but have the same rates of STDs and are less likely to use condoms when they become sexually active. In addition, those who made a virginity pledge were more likely to substitute anal or oral sex for vaginal sex.

Social and Demographic Factors Associated with Sexual Activity

Sexual activity in teens is often described in terms of the traditional demographic factors of gender, race, socioeconomic status, and family structure. The richness of the Add Health study has allowed researchers to explore social factors beyond simple demographics. Blum et al. (2000a) analyzed the Add Health data, looking at several traditional as well as nontraditional variables in an attempt to predict sexual activity.

Race/ethnicity, income, and family structure explained only 9.7% of the difference between younger teens who have or have not had sexual intercourse and 2.9% of the difference for older teens. A more comprehensive picture of the social and demographic factors that affect a teen's choice of being or not being sexually active is described in Table 39.8. Considered jointly, these factors explain 25% to 34% of the difference between males who have and males who have not had sexual intercourse and 35% to 49% of the difference for females.

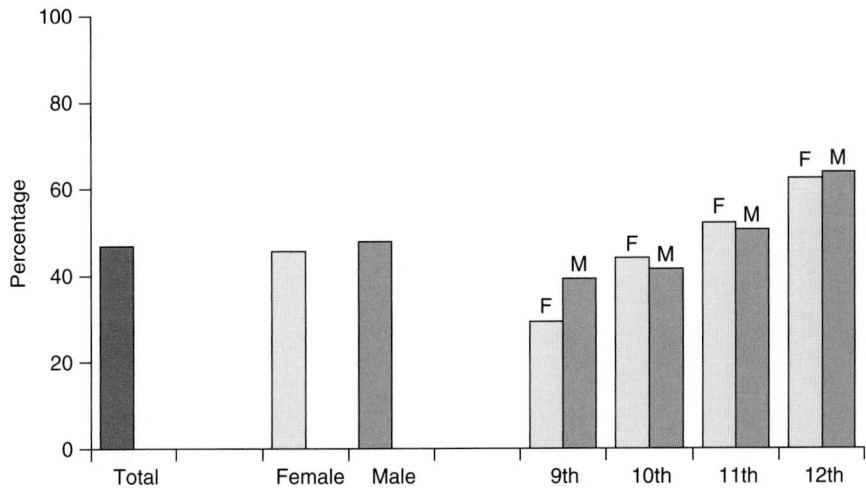

FIGURE 39.2 Percentage of high school students who had sexual intercourse, by sex and grade, 2005. Nationwide in 2005, 46.8% of high school students had had sexual intercourse during their life. Overall, the prevalence of having had sexual intercourse was higher among black than white and Hispanic students and higher among Hispanic than white students. (From the Centers for Disease Control and Prevention. Youth risk behavior surveillance–United States, 2005. *MMWR* 2006;55:SS-5.)

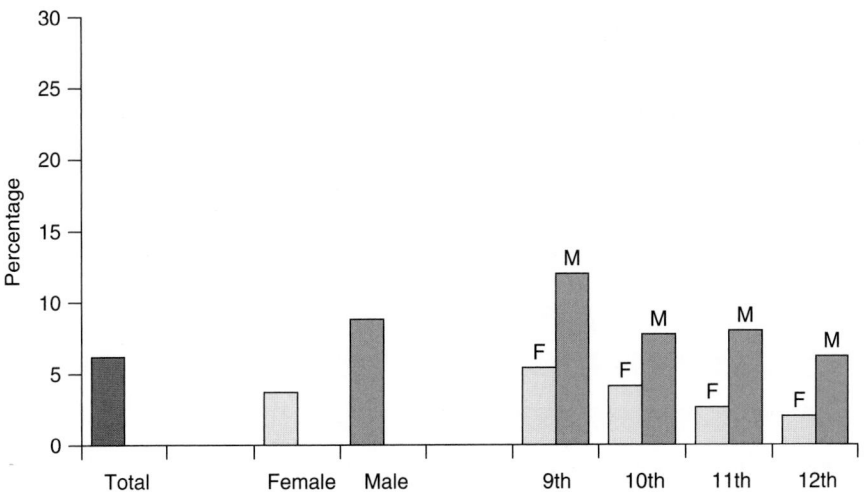

FIGURE 39.3 Percentage of high school students who engaged in their first sexual intercourse before age 13 years, by sex and grade, 2005. (From the Centers for Disease Control and Prevention. Youth risk behavior surveillance–United States, 2005. *MMWR* 2006;55:SS-5.)

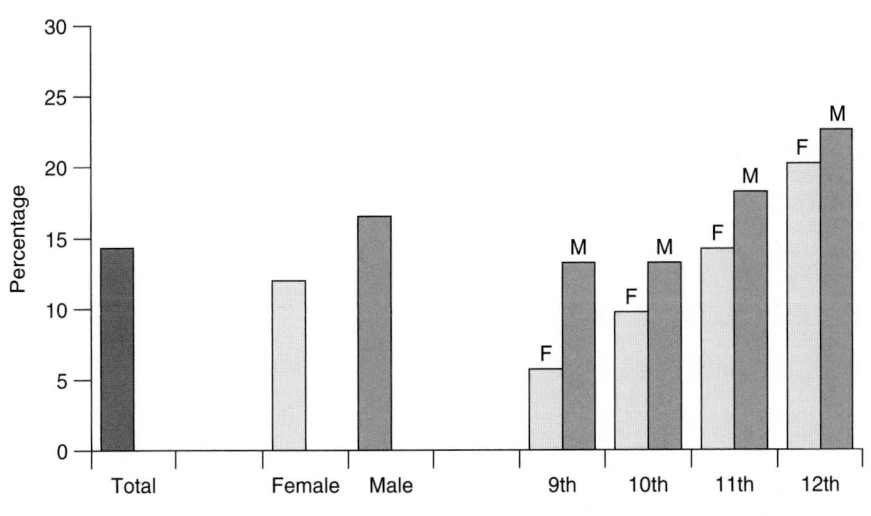

FIGURE 39.4 Percentage of high school students who have had four or more sex partners during their lifetime, by sex and grade, 2005. (From the Centers for Disease Control and Prevention. Youth risk behavior surveillance–United States, 2005. *MMWR* 2006;55:SS-5.)

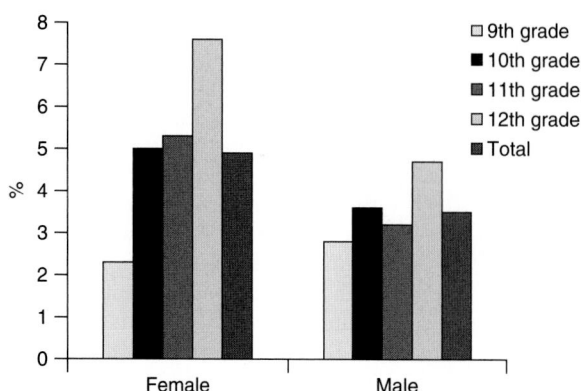

FIGURE 39.5 Percentage of high school students who have been pregnant or who have gotten someone pregnant, by sex and grade, 2003. (From the Centers for Disease Control and Prevention. Youth risk behavior surveillance—United States, 2004. *MMWR* 2004;53(2):1.)

Health Care Provider and Teen Communication about Sex

In a 2000 survey of 15,000 American high school students, only 43% of teenage females and 26% of teenage males discussed pregnancy or STDs with their physicians during routine examinations (Marchione, 2000).

The Commonwealth Fund (Schoen et al., 1997) published a survey that identified a gap between what adolescents believed doctors should discuss and what doctors actually discuss. Between 35% and 65% of boys thought doctors should discuss issues of physical or sexual abuse, pregnancy prevention, STD prevention, drinking and drugs, whereas <one third of doctors actually discussed these issues. More than 50% of girls wanted to discuss alcohol, drugs, STDs, and eating disorders. However, <30% of doctors discussed these issues (Figs. 39.9 and 39.10).

Age Difference Between Sexual Partners

Several states have enacted or started to enforce statutory rape laws because of a concern about adult men fathering babies of teenage females (Darroch et al., 1999; Donovan, 1997; Males and Chew, 1996).

The 2002 NSFG reported that 13% of females and 5% of males had a first sexual experience at 15 years or younger with an individual who was 3 or more years older (Fig. 39.11). The younger the teen was at first sexual intercourse, the more likely their partner was at least 3 years older (Fig. 39.12) (Manlove et al., 2005).

Although many teens have their first sexual intercourse with an older partner, 77% of these older male and female partners were still in their teens. Few relationships occur

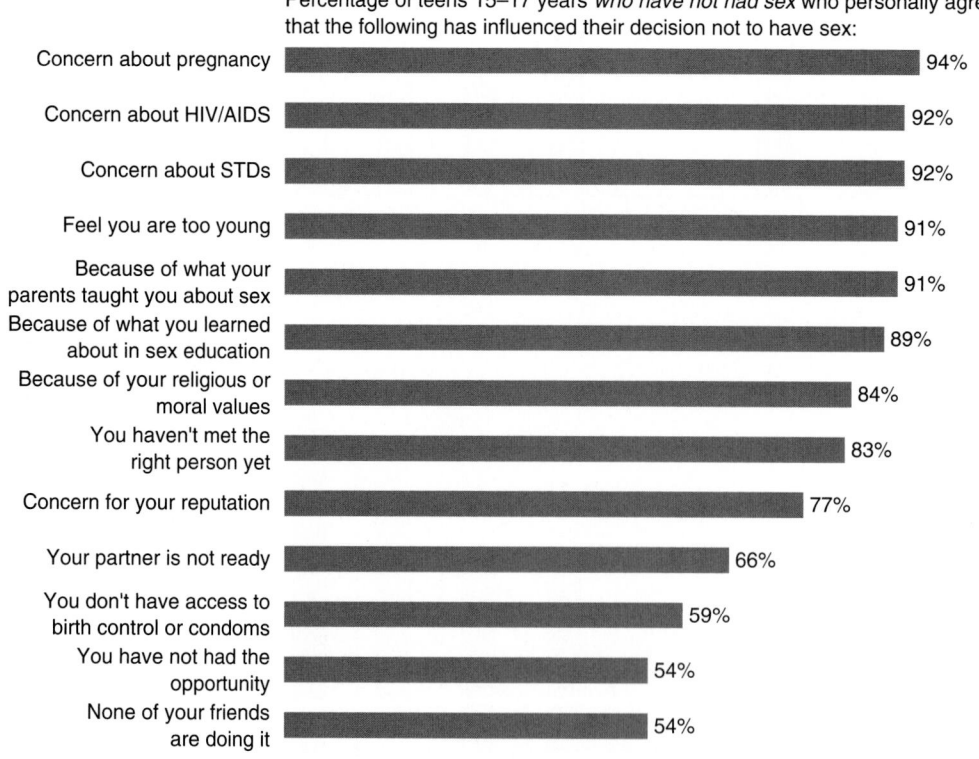

FIGURE 39.6 Reasons that have influenced teens (15 to 17 years old) regarding their decision not to have sex. HIV, human immunodeficiency virus; AIDS, acquired immunodeficiency syndrome; STD, sexually transmitted disease. (From Henry J. Kaiser Family Foundation and Seventeen. *Sex smarts: decision making about sex.* Henry J. Kaiser Family Foundation and Seventeen, http://www.kff.org/entpartnerships/3368-index.cfm. October, 2003.)

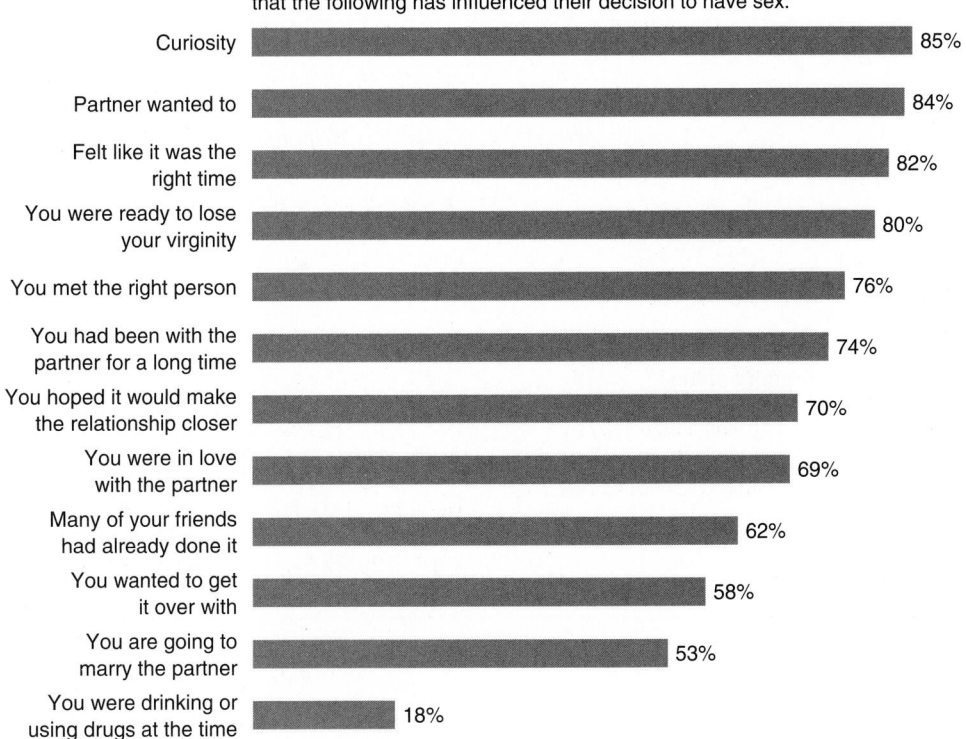

Percentage of teens 15–17 years *who have had sex* who personally agree that the following has influenced their decision to have sex:

Curiosity	85%
Partner wanted to	84%
Felt like it was the right time	82%
You were ready to lose your virginity	80%
You met the right person	76%
You had been with the partner for a long time	74%
You hoped it would make the relationship closer	70%
You were in love with the partner	69%
Many of your friends had already done it	62%
You wanted to get it over with	58%
You are going to marry the partner	53%
You were drinking or using drugs at the time	18%

FIGURE 39.7 Reasons that have influenced teens (15 to 17 years old) regarding their decision to have sex. (From Henry J. Kaiser Family Foundation and Seventeen. *Sex smarts: decision making about sex.* Henry J. Kaiser Family Foundation and Seventeen, http://www.kff.org/entpartnerships/3368-index.cfm. October, 2003.)

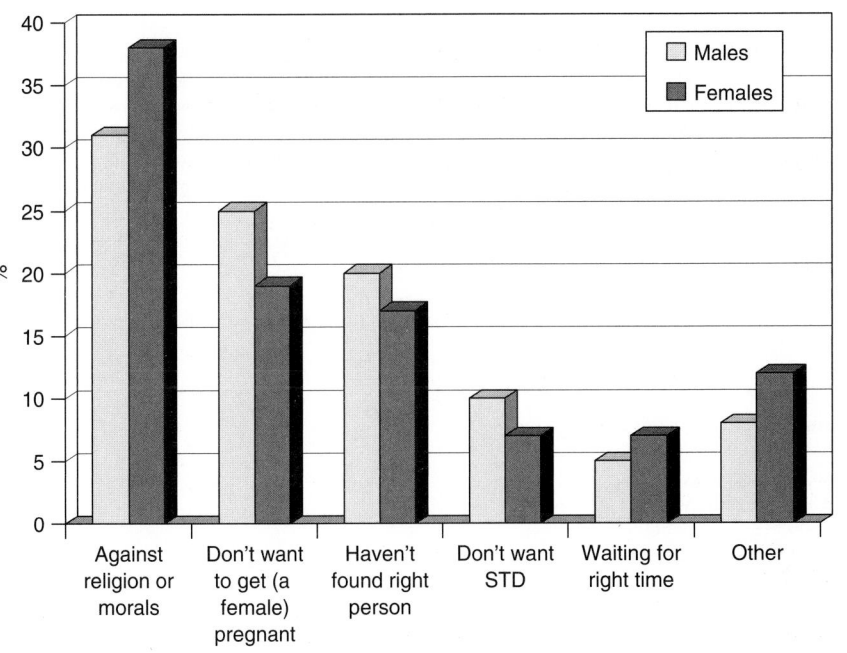

FIGURE 39.8 Main reasons for not having sex among adolescents who have never had sex: National Survey of Family Growth, 2002. (From Blum RW, Beuhring T, Rinehart PM. Protecting teens: beyond race, income and family structure, Center for Adolescent health, University of Minnesota, 200 Oaks Street SE, Suite 260, Minneapolis, MN., University of Minnesota Printing Services, Minneapolis, MN, 2000 with permission.)

TABLE 39.8

Factors Associated with Whether Youth had Sexual Intercourse[a]

	Males			Females		
	White[b]	Black	Hispanic	White[b]	Black	Hispanic
Individual sexual experience						
Opportunity						
Ever dated[c]					▲	
Ever kissed or necked[c]	▲	▲	▲			▲
Romantic relationship in 18 months before survey[c]	▲	▲	▲[e,f]	▲	▲	▲
Motivation						
Made public or written virginity pledge		○	○	○	○	
Perceived personal and social benefits to sex	▲[g]	▲[h]	▲[i]	▲		▲
Perceived personal and social costs to sex	○	○[j]	○[j]	○		○[k]
Perceived costs of getting/making someone pregnant	○[l]	○[l]		○[l]	○[l]	○[l]
Perceived (not actual) knowledge of birth control[d]	▲	▲		▲	▲	▲
Individual						
Ever repeated a grade[c]			▲[i]			
Frequent problems with school work						▲
Wants and expects to attend college			○			○
Religious beliefs						○[m]
Physical maturity						▲
Peer context						
Number of best friends who drink				▲	▲	
Prejudice among teens at school						▲
Family context						
Parents disapprove of youth having sex at this time in their life					○	○
Positive parent/family relationships					○	
Number of siblings					○	

[a]The following risk and protective factors were not associated with ever having had intercourse in any gender/ethnic subgroup: whether would keep child if became pregnant; frequency of religious activities or physical recreation; youth has bad temper; believes successes were earned; self-esteem; parent presence after school; parent presence at dinner; sets own curfew; frequency of parent drinking; family member suicide or attempt; joint decision making; whether Spanish was the primary language at home (Hispanic).

[b]The following were not consistently related to ever having had intercourse among white youths when their sample size was matched to the Hispanic and black sample sizes: ever dated; virginity pledge; ever repeated a grade; hobbies; college plans; parent-family relationship; extended family in the home (adults); friend's suicide or attempt; number of best friends who drink; worked 20+ hr/wk.

[c]Dichotomous (yes/no) variable. History of rape was asked only of girls.

[d]Extent of perceived knowledge of birth control was only weakly related to extent of actual knowledge regardless of grade or sexual experience.

[e]Risk is enhanced if the youth sees a benefit to sex.

[f]Risk is enhanced if the youth repeated a year.

[g]Risk is enhanced if the youth feels knowledgeable about birth control.

[h]Risk is enhanced if the youth sees few social costs.

[i]Risk is enhanced if the youth had a romantic relationship.

[j]Protection is enhanced if the youth sees risk of pregnancy.

[k]Protection is enhanced if the youth has strong religious belief.

[l]Protection is enhanced if the youth has good school attendance.

[m]Protection is enhanced if the youth sees many social costs.

▲ = Risk; ○ = Protection.

From Blum RW, Beuhring T, Rinehart PM. Protecting teens: beyond race, income, and family structure, Center for Adolescent Health, University of Minnesota, 200 Oaks Street SE, Suite 260, Minneapolis, MN, University of Minnesota Printing Services, Minneapolis, MN 2000.

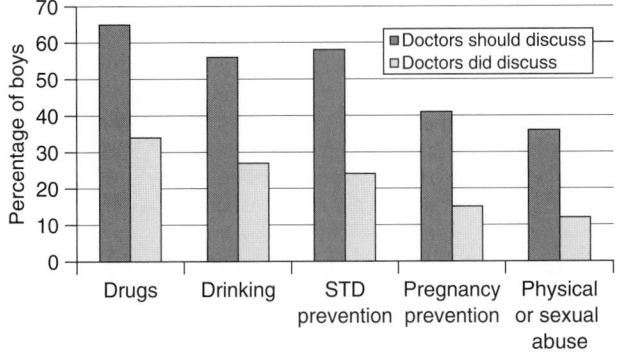

FIGURE 39.9 Boys' beliefs about what doctors should discuss and what doctors actually discuss. STD, sexually transmitted disease. Schoen C, Davis K, Collins KS, et al. *The commonwealth fund survey of the health of adolescent girls.* The Commonwealth Fund. Louis Harris and Associates, www.cmwf.org/publications/publications _show.htm?doc_id=221230. 1997.

when the adult partner is significantly older than the teen. The distribution of age differences between younger teens and older partners is shown in Figure 39.13.

Most young females who had sex with older males viewed these relationships as "going steady," whereas most young males having sexual intercourse with older females viewed these relationships as casual (Fig. 39.14).

Unwanted Sexual Experiences

Unfortunately, unwanted sexual experiences are very common. The earlier a woman has sex, the more likely it is unwanted (Fig. 39.15 and Table 39.9). During adolescence, intercourse was involuntary in 61% of females who were

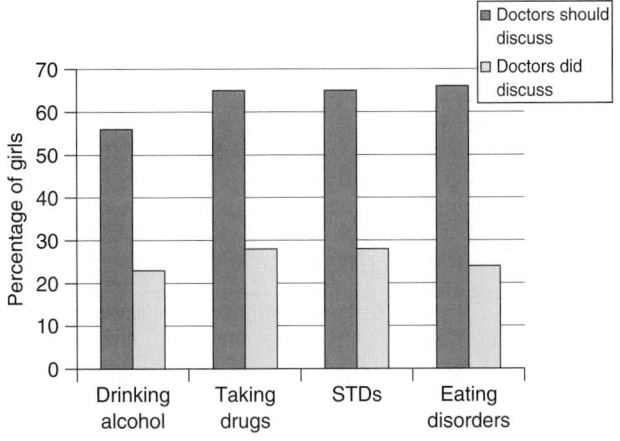

FIGURE 39.10 Girls' beliefs about what doctors should discuss and what doctors actually discuss. STD, sexually transmitted disease. (From Schoen C, Davis K, Collins KS, et al. *The commonwealth fund survey of the health of adolescent girls.* www.cmwf.org/publications/ publications_show.htm?doc_id=221230. 1997.)

13 years old and younger at the time of first intercourse (Table 39.9). Sex with an older male partner increases the likelihood it was forced (Fig. 39.15). In the NSFG, 15-year olds who had their first sexual intercourse with a male at least 3 years older were twice as likely to be forced to have intercourse as compared to other females who are younger than 18 years. One in five females who were 15 years or younger and having sex with a male at least 3 years older reported this experience as "voluntary and wanted" compared to one in three of all sexually active females who were younger than 18 years. Although not commonly reported, males do experience unwanted sexual intercourse. Of males younger than 15 years who had sex with an older woman (more than 3 years older), 22% stated it was unwanted as opposed to 8% of all sexually active males younger than 18 years (Fig. 39.16).

WHY IS ADOLESCENT SEXUALITY A CONCERN

Despite the fact that adolescent sexuality is part of normal development, it remains the focus of much attention and concern. The following are some explanations for this dichotomy:

1. Opposing views of sexuality: Inherent in the problem of adolescent sexuality are the often divergent attitudes expressed by adolescents, their parents, and the community. Predominant views among adolescents are that sex is justified as physical pleasure or as a new experience; it is an index of maturity; it reflects peer-group conformity; it represents a challenge to parents or to society; and it offers an escape from pressures. On the other hand, the adolescent's parents or the community often view sex among teenagers as ill advised, premature, risky, immoral, and frightening.
2. Menarche versus marriage: The age at menarche has decreased significantly over time with improved health and nutrition. In the 1400s, the age at menarche was close to the age at marriage, both of which were approximately 18 years of age. The current average age at menarche is approximately 12.6 years and marriage is put off until after education is completed or a career path is well established. This leaves a significant gap between the time from when teens are reproductively capable and when intercourse occurs within the bounds of marriage. It is no wonder that many teens and young adults find it difficult to delay sex until marriage. This, of course, excludes the GLBT youth who often do not have the legal option of marriage.
3. Difficulties in communication with parents: Numerous studies reveal that approximately two thirds or more of adolescents feel that they cannot communicate with their parents about sex. Many parents assume that their teenagers do not want to talk about sex. However, many adolescents wish they could talk with their parents about sex. This lack of communication or miscommunication perpetuates misunderstandings and lack of trust. Several studies have demonstrated a positive effect on sexual behavior secondary to parent–teen discussions (Dilorio et al., 1999; Whitaker et al., 1999; Parera and Suris, 2004).

FIGURE 39.11 Prevalence of sex between young teens and older individuals. (Source: National Survey of Family Growth, 2002.)

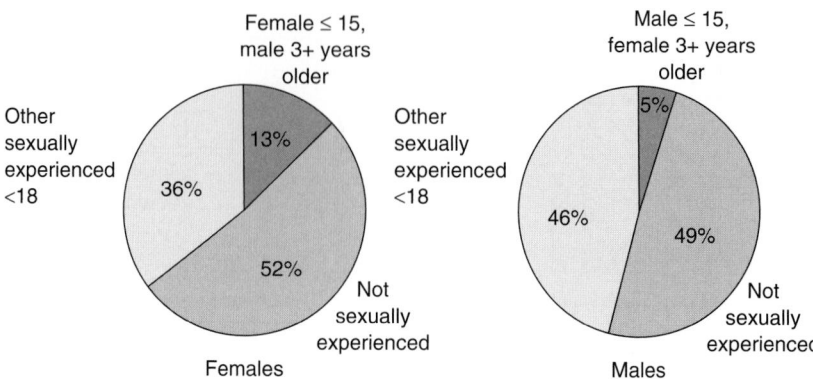

Females

Males

4. Media: The media (radio, printed media, movies, television, and the Internet) often depict unrealistic views of sexual behavior and its consequences. This can lead to confusion about what sexual behaviors are acceptable.
5. Peer pressure: Adolescents find increasing pressure from their peers to be sexual; a pressure that represents a formidable struggle for many adolescents.
6. Developmental stage: A typical characteristic of early and middle adolescent development (see Chapter 2) is a sense of immortality, with resultant risk-taking behavior. Adolescents often react without a full sense of the potential consequences of their actions. They are caught between the images of sex portrayed by the media, peer values, parental values, and their own developing values. Youth may therefore act impulsively, engaging in sexual activities without being psychologically and emotionally prepared for them. The resultant guilt that many adolescents feel might become a barrier to the development of healthy attitudes toward sex.
7. Sex education: Many sex education courses, if available, stress upon reproductive function and menstruation. More recently, sex education has focused federally funded abstinence-only education. Although it is important for teenagers to be informed about the mechanics of sexual relationships, they also need help in decision-making skills and in dealing with their feelings, fears,

and relationships. Unfortunately, many abstinence-only programs contain medically inaccurate information to frighten teens into not having sex.

American Medical Association, American Public Health Association, Institute of Medicine, Society for Adolescent Medicine and SIECUS, among others, support comprehensive sex education including education about abstinence and different methods of contraception (Klein, 2005; Committee on HIV Prevention Strategies, 2000; Society for Adolescent Medicine, 2006; SIECUS, 2004; Boostra, 2002).

RECOMMENDATIONS

Several suggestions to help adolescents deal better with their sexuality include the following:

1. Parent education
   a. Many parents are surprised (and even shocked) to learn that their teenagers are sexually active. Conversely, most adolescents do not think their parents actually have sex. Children need to learn and recognize their parents as sexual beings. It is not unusual for young children or adolescents to interrupt their parents during sex. Although this can be embarrassing for both parties, it can be an opportunity for parents and their children to have a conversation about sex and privacy.
      The preceding data on frequency and onset of early sexual activity raises the question of when parents should discuss sex with their children. If parents wait until adolescence, it may be too late. Sex is a topic that is often relegated to a one-time "birds and the bees" lecture. Rather than one big talk, parents should talk about sex throughout childhood and adolescence as they would about other aspects of life. These discussions may be hampered by a parent's discomfort with the subject or their personal experience of similar awkward discussions with their own parents. Most parents did not get adequate information about sexuality from their own parents and therefore have few role models to help them teach their own children about sex.
      • Infants and toddlers
        During this period, a child begins to comprehend gender differences. A first step in a child's sex education is using accurate anatomical terms to

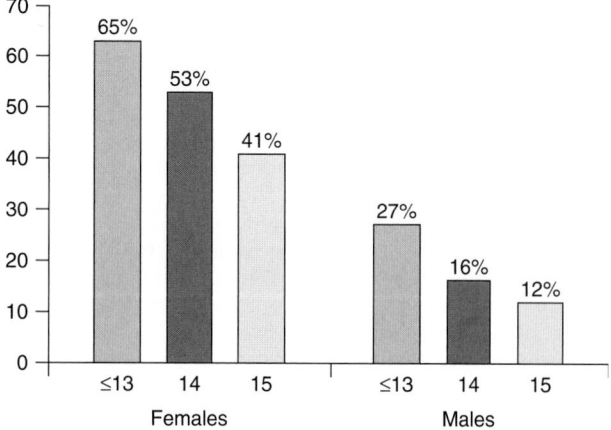

FIGURE 39.12 Percentage of young teens whose first sex was with an individual 3+ years older, by age at first sex. (Source: National Survey of Family Growth, 2002.)

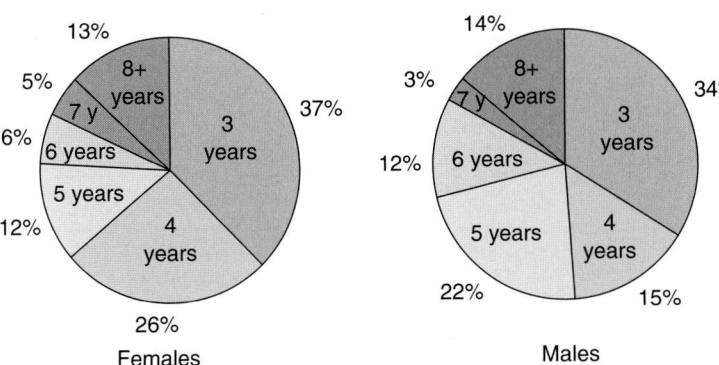

FIGURE 39.13 Distribution of age difference among young teens whose first sex was with an individual 3+ years older. (Source: National Survey of Family Growth, 2002.)

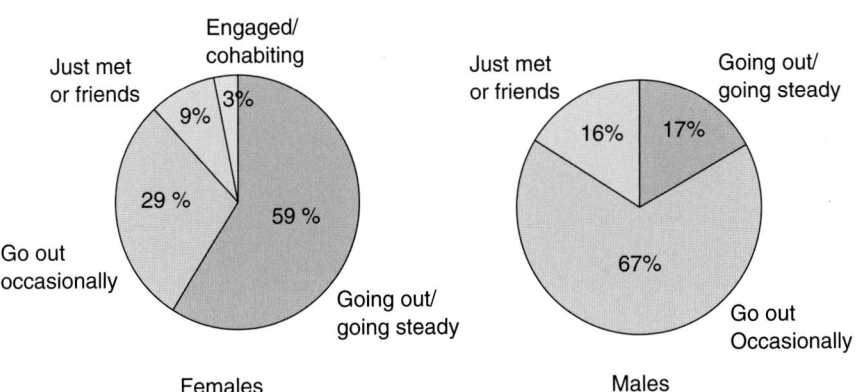

FIGURE 39.14 Self-reported relationship type at first sex among young teens whose first sex was with an individual 3+ years older. (Source: National Survey of Family Growth, 2002.)

TABLE 39.9

Percentage of Sexually Experienced U.S. Females Aged 19 Years and Younger with History of Involuntary Intercourse

Age at First Intercourse	Involuntary Intercourse Only (%)	Both Voluntary and Involuntary Intercourse (%)	Voluntary Intercourse Only (%)
13 and younger	61	13	26
14 and younger	42	17	40
15 and younger	26	14	60
16 and younger	10	14	76
17 and younger	5	13	82
18 and younger	3	12	85
19 and younger	1	14	85

From Alan Guttmacher Institute. *Sex and America's teenagers*. New York: Alan Guttmacher Institute, 1994, using data from Moore KA, Nord CW, Peterson JL. 1987 National survey of children. *Fam Plann Perspect* 1989;21:110, with permission.

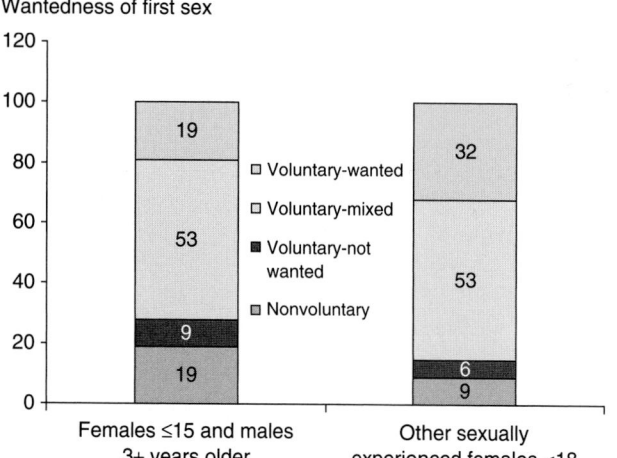

FIGURE 39.15 Wantedness of first sex among females who had sex before age 18. (Source: National Survey of Family Growth, 2002.)

name the parts of the body. Penises and vaginas should be named in the same matter-of-fact manner as ears, toes, elbows, or noses. It is important for parents to acknowledge that it is normal for toddlers to touch their own genitals. They can be taught that their genitals are private and not to be touched in public. Children can be taught this information in the same way they are educated to cover their mouths when they cough or not pick their noses in public.

- Preschoolers
At this age, children want to know where babies come from. The best approach is to answer questions with simple and honest answers as they arise. It is not advisable to put children off with "I'll tell you when you are older." Parents should take advantage of a child's environment which often presents common examples of sex and procreation—a family pet has a litter of puppies;

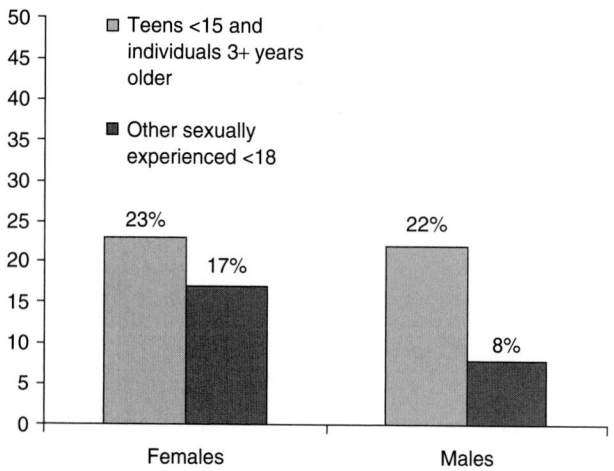

FIGURE 39.16 Percentage ever forced to have sexual intercourse among teens who had sex before age 18. (Source: National Survey of Family Growth, 2002.)

a teacher is pregnant; a younger sibling is born. Children should feel that it is acceptable to ask questions about sex. Children should also feel that sex is something natural that can be talked about within the family.

Sexual abuse of children is present in all societies. Children should be taught the difference between "good" and "bad" touches. A "good" touch is one that feels comfortable and safe. A "bad" touch is one that makes the child feel "uncomfortable" or "confused." It should be explained to a child that their body is their own and they have the right to say "no" to any touch that makes them feel uncomfortable. A child should also be encouraged to tell a trusted adult if they find themselves in an uncomfortable situation. Regardless, appropriate supervision is always needed.

- Elementary school–aged children
Children at this age are able to comprehend more complex explanations. They will often have questions about what they see on television or hear at school. In American households the television is on for an average of 7 hours a day; teenagers watch approximately 24 hours of television per week. In a year of prime television, there are more than 20,000 scenes of a sexual nature. Television watching and computer use should be supervised at this age. Screen time should be minimized. Parents can use television programs as the impetus for a discussion about sex.

School-aged children can begin to understand about germs, infections, and hygiene. This is an appropriate time to share information about AIDS (what it is, how it is transmitted, how to prevent). School-aged children need to understand that AIDS is not something you get from holding hands, sitting on a public toilet seat, or donating blood.

- Preteens
Onset of puberty is a time when parents should begin frank and open discussions with their adolescents about STDs and pregnancy. Masturbation occurs at all ages and in both males and females. During adolescence, it can be a source of guilt. There is no medical reason to proscribe this normal behavior. Parents should discuss masturbation, wet dreams, and menstruation. Children should be familiar with common terminology about sexuality such as "sexual intercourse" and "homosexuality." They should understand that feelings of physical attraction toward a member of the same sex are normal during puberty. They should know what intercourse is and that vaginal intercourse can result in pregnancy. They should also understand why preteens are not emotionally ready to have sexual intercourse. Sex can be discussed as a natural and wonderful experience to be shared with someone in a loving relationship. In many Western European countries sexuality is openly discussed from the early stages in a child's education. In these countries, the abortion and adolescent pregnancy rates are significantly lower than in the United States. There is no evidence that discussing sex makes children more likely to engage in it. At this age, preteens should have a good understanding of AIDS and STDs and should be taught that safe sex may help prevent their transmission.

- Teens

  In talking with a teenager, parents should openly express their opinions concerning the appropriate time for their child to become sexually active. Parents who believe that their teenager should delay initiation of sexual activities should do so in the context of their religious, moral, or ethical belief system. A teenager can begin to grasp the long-term consequences of their actions. Rules about dating and curfews should be openly discussed. Contraception and disease prevention should be reviewed.

Parents can help by walking their teens through various scenarios and role playing with them. For example, a parent might present their daughter with the following scenario:

"Your boyfriend invites you to come over and listen to a new CD with friends after school. When you arrive at his house, no one else is home. He sits on the couch with you and tells you how much he loves you. He becomes more "physical" than you are ready for. He wants to have sexual intercourse but you say "no." He becomes more forceful and angry."

Such a scenario allows the teenager to know that the parent understands the pressures the teen may be experiencing. It also reinforces that the parents are aware that there are situations in which saying "no" can be very difficult. Parents can help their adolescents negotiate difficult situations by building their child's confidence and self-esteem. This will help the teen to resist pressure from others.

Teens who are more physically developed or develop earlier than their peers may experience added pressure to engage in sexual behaviors before they are ready as their physical development may exceed their cognitive and emotional development.

Teenagers need to be somewhat rebellious in order to forge their own identities separate from that of their parents. Despite this, they usually assume a value system that is similar to their parents. Teenagers often admit that they really do want to know what their parents think. They long for appropriate guidance and limit setting. Sexual values should be taught along with other values. Sexually responsible behavior is part of the overall assumption of adult responsibility.

When asked, many adolescents would prefer their parents as counselors and sources of information about sex. If parents feel uncomfortable in this role, it is probably best to acknowledge this discomfort. Parents can admit that they are embarrassed to discuss these issues because of the way their parents talked to them about sex and that they do not want to make the same mistakes. The most important thing that teenagers need to know is that regardless of their "mistakes," their parents will still love them and try to help them.

b. Timing: Because sexuality begins in childhood, it is important to treat sexuality as a natural part of life from birth onward. Given this perspective, it is much less awkward to have discussions about sexuality as children grow up.

c. Education: Adolescents should be informed and knowledgeable with the help of parents, school, or community resources in the following areas:

- Basic reproductive anatomy and physiology
- Basic sexual functioning and alternatives to intercourse
- Discussion of common myths about sex and contraception; myths should be replaced by medically accurate information
- The consequences of sexual activities including pregnancy, STD, HIV, and parenthood
- Contraception
- The range of human relationships
- The components of decision making
- The importance of self-esteem and respecting one's choices
- Available resources to answer concerns, address questions, or tackle problems

d. Admit personal discomfort: Adolescents respect honesty and this approach will often allow for additional trust between the adolescent and the parent or counselor.

e. Resources: Be informed about available books, pamphlets, and other resources regarding adolescent sexuality. Some valuable references and organizations are listed at the end of the chapter and in Appendix II to this book.

f. Privacy: It is important to respect an adolescent's privacy and at the same time allow them the opportunity to comfortably discuss issues of sexuality without prying into details.

2. Community resources

a. Sex education: Schools need to incorporate a curriculum on sex education that, in addition to including facts, stresses concepts of sexual responsibility and sexual decision making.

b. Family-planning clinics: Increased availability of family-planning clinics that serve and are sensitive to the needs of adolescents is essential.

c. Professional education: It is crucial that health care providers continue to be educated regarding adolescent sexuality, resultant problems, and helpful resources.

3. Contraceptive technology: Development of continued safe, effective, easy-to-use contraception that would complement the adolescent's active lifestyle is needed. The birth control patch and ring are examples of this.

4. Sexual history: A sexual history should be taken of all patients. Providers should become comfortable obtaining a comprehensive sexual history. Chapter 3 includes a description of the HEADSS approach to psychosocial history taking. When taking a sexual history, confidentiality must be clearly stated with an explanation of the limits of confidential health care (e.g., sexual abuse and in some states, statutory rape). Teenagers should be informed that questions about sexual activity are asked of *all* patients. Acknowledge that the questions might be embarrassing but need to be asked in order to provide them with good health care. Make no assumptions about sexuality or sexual practices. Teens should be asked if they are "now having" or "have ever had" sexual contact, both noncoital and coital. Adolescents should also be asked if they have ever been forced to have sex. A brief sexual history should be obtained even during episodic care. A teen's symptom of abdominal pain or headaches could be the result of a prior history of sexual abuse or current relationship abuse (see Chapter 3 for more details).

5. Sexual health of adolescent with chronic illness: The sexual health of adolescents with chronic illness is often neglected. A study of teens with physical disabilities in the Add Health data reports that teens with disabilities have rates of sexual activity similar to teens without physical disabilities. They also found that adolescent females with physical disabilities consistently have higher odds of experiencing forced sex (Cheng and Udry, 2002). A review of studies on risk behaviors in teens with chronic illnesses found a substantial prevalence of sexual activity, but low level of knowledge and low prevalence of contraceptive use (Valencia and Cromer, 2000). The reader is referred to review articles by Gittes and Strickland (2005) for a discussion of the contraception options and dangers of pregnancy for chronically ill adolescents. The clinician should determine the patient's knowledge about sexuality and encourage discussion of sexual relationships, concerns about sexual performance, and ability to reproduce. Zeltzer et al. found that patients with cardiac disease were concerned about sexual activity and had fears of dying during intercourse (Zeltzer, 1980). Openly discussing sexual issues will make teenagers more comfortable about asking questions. Siecus has published a report on sexual education for teens with disabilities (Tepper, 2001).

WEB SITES

For Teenagers and Parents

www.noah-health.org/. Ask NOAH. New York Online Access to Health (NOAH). City University of New York, the Metropolitan New York Library Council, the New York Academy of Medicine, and the New York Public Library.

www.goaskalice.columbia.edu. Go Ask Alice is a source of general health and sex information maintained by Columbia University health educators. Most questions answered are submitted by high school and college-aged people.

www.itsyoursexlife.com. It's Your (Sex) Life is sponsored by the Kaiser Family Foundation. Provides sexual health information to young adults.

www.iwannaknow.org. This Web page is specifically designed for teenagers to find answers to their questions about their bodies, sex, and sexual feelings, and to provide them with "responsible educational information in a relaxed, safe, and fun environment."

http://healthfinder.gov/justforyou/. Just for You: Teens. healthfinderKIDS. HealthFinders Teen Page has multiple links to government-sponsored information for teens and providers.

http://www.ippfwhr.org/. International Planned Parenthood Federation (IPPF). An on-line guide about love and relationships developed by and for young people worldwide. Offers viewpoints on issues including sexual decision making, contraception, and relationships.

http://sxetc.org. Sex etc. is a teen-oriented newsletter from Rutgers University's Network for Family Life Education, produced by a teen editorial board with professional supervision. Topics include dating, relationships, sexuality, communication, and sexual health.

www.chebucto.ns.ca/Health/TeenHealth/. Teen Health, Dalhousie University. This site provides information to teens on a wide variety of reproductive health topics including healthy sexuality, sexual orientation, STDs, pregnancy, women's health, men's health, and sexual assault.

www.advocatesforyouth.org/CORNER.HTM. Teen Scene. Advocates for Youth. Provides a place for youth, particularly those involved in educating others about adolescent reproductive health issues, to connect with each other, share information, and describe experiences.

http://teensexuality.studentcenter.org. Teen Sexuality. The Student Center Network, 2000.

www.scarleteen.com. Advice, help and information about teen sexuality. This is a very sex positive site.

www.teenwire.com/index.asp. TeenWire is sponsored by the Planned Parenthood Federation of America. Provides teens with unbiased, uncensored sexuality and sexual health information.

www.unicef.org/voy. Voices of Youth. United Nations Children's Fund. Designed for youth worldwide as a venue to share ideas.

www.butyoudontlooksick.com/2006/03/breaking_the_ice _on_sex_intima.php

www.enablelink.org/abilities/archive.html?article=1663. Sexual Development in Teens with Disabilities

For Health Professionals

http://education.indiana.edu/cas/adol/adol.html. Adolescence Directory On-Line. Center for Adolescent Studies, Indiana University, 1996. Electronic guide to information on adolescent health issues.

http://www.ippfwhr.org. Adolescent Forum Listserv. IPPF/ Western Hemisphere Region (WHR) hosts an on-line newsletter that highlights adolescent sexual and reproductive health programs of IPPF/WHR affiliates and other organizations in the region.

http://www.nutrition.uio.no/ARHNe/. Adolescent Reproductive Health Network is a research network including several ongoing research programs and projects. It consists of 18 partner institutions in southern and eastern Africa, as well as in Europe involved in research and/or implementation of programs that target adolescent reproductive health and risk behaviors.

http://www.rho.org/html/adol_links.htm. Adolescent Reproductive Health Outlook. The reproductive health Web site produced by the Program for Appropriate Technology in Health is designed for reproductive health program managers and decision makers working in developing countries and low-resource settings.

http://www.agnr.umd.edu/users/nnfr/adolsex/home.html. Adolescent Sexuality. National Network for Family Resiliency (NNFR). The Adolescent Sexuality Special Interest Group of the NNFR seeks to promote research-based, educational programs that address adolescent sexuality.

http://www.advocatesforyouth.org/. Advocates for Youth provides information, training, and advocacy to youth-serving organizations. Advocates for Youth creates programs and promotes policies to help young people make informed and responsible decisions about their sexual and reproductive health.

http://www.agi-usa.org/index.html. The Alan Guttmacher Institute home page. The Alan Guttmacher Institute is a research, policy analysis, and public education organization dedicated to protecting the reproductive choices of men and women in the United States and throughout the world.

http://www.ashastd.org/ and www.iwannaknow.org/. American Social Health Association.

http://www.engenderhealth.org. Engender Health works to improve reproductive health services worldwide.

http://www.cedpa.org. Center for Development and Population Activities includes the following programs:

1. http://www.cedpa.org/trainprog/betterlife/betlife.htm. Better Life Options for Girls and Young Women. A global initiative to empower girls and young women to set goals, build skills, and improve self-esteem.

2. http://www.cedpa.org/trainprog/ppgyw.htm. Partnership Projects for Girls and Young Women, which focuses on community projects conducted by Egyptian nongovernmental organizations to help girls in upper Egypt strengthen their vocational and literacy skills and increase understanding of family life issues.

3. http://www.cedpa.org/trainprog/saharan/subsahaf.htm. Adolescent and Gender Project in sub-Saharan Africa. A multicountry initiative to protect and promote the rights of adolescents to reproductive health information and services, with shared responsibility among young women and young men.

http://www.positive.org/. Coalition for Positive Sexuality.

http://www.socio.com/data_arc/daappp_0.htm. The Data Archive on Adolescent Pregnancy and Pregnancy Prevention of the U.S. Office of Population Affairs is a repository for data on teenage sexual behavior including pregnancy, contraception, behavioral factors, and STDs. Data sets from more than 130 studies published since the late 1970s (many of them longitudinal) were selected as being among the best in the field by a national panel of experts. These data sets are briefly described and may be ordered on-line in several different formats.

http://ec.princeton.edu. Emergency Contraception Web site, a site maintained by the Office of Population Research at Princeton University, provides accurate information based on the medical literature about emergency contraception.

http://www.etr.org. ETR Associates develops health promotion products and services that emphasize sexuality and health education. Currently, they also have an adolescent pregnancy prevention Web site, called the Resource Center for Adolescent Pregnancy Prevention.

http://www.etr.org/recapp. Designed to provide health educators and program coordinators with practical tools and research on reducing sexual risk-taking behaviors among teens.

http://www.europeer.lu.se. Europeer: AIDS Peer Education is a collaborative effort of the department of community medicine, Lund University, Sweden and policy makers, professionals, and youth in 14 European Union countries, focusing on peer education. The site provides knowledge and guidance about the use of AIDS-peer-education with young people.

http://www.familycareintl.org. Family Care International is dedicated to improving women's sexual and reproductive health and rights in developing countries. Site includes publications and working papers, including case studies on adolescent reproductive health in eastern and southern Africa, and information on how to purchase video and text resources.

http://www.jsi.com/intl/seats. Family Planning Service Expansion and Technical Support Project is a program developing and expanding high quality, client-centered, sustainable family planning and reproductive health services in developing countries and enhancing access to these services. SEATS' Youth Initiative information (www.jsi.com/intl/seats/spcint/YOUTH.html) includes descriptions of eastern European and African programs.

http://www.pathfind.org/focus.htm. FOCUS on Young Adults. FOCUS is a Pathfinder International program in partnership with the Futures Groups International and Tulane University School of Public Health and Tropical Medicine. Its goal is to improve the health and well-being of young adults in developing countries.

http://www.kff.org/. The Henry J. Kaiser Family Foundation home page. You can sign up for daily e-mails regarding reproductive health. Has a wealth of information on teen behavior.

http://www.ippf.org. International Planned Parenthood Federation links family planning associations in more than 150 countries worldwide and provides information to a number of other sites.

http://www.jhuccp.org. Johns Hopkins University Center for Communications Programs is a rich source for family planning and reproductive health information. Includes a Media/Materials Clearinghouse; NetLinks, a showcase of on-line resources; PHOTOSHARE, an on-line database of international photos related to reproductive health; the full text of Population Reports (www.jhuccp.org/pr/index.stm); and Jim Shelton's Pearls (www.jhuccp.org/pearls/), which address various reproductive health issues.

http://healthfinder.gov/justforyou/. Just for You: Teens. HealthfinderKIDS. HealthFinders Teen Page has multiple links to government-sponsored information for teens and providers.

http://www.ppnyc.org/services/msci.html. Margaret Sanger Center International. The international arm of Planned Parenthood of New York City aims at developing multimedia education programs relating to sexual health in emerging democracies and expanding adolescent reproductive health services in clinics and community-based programs.

http://www.teenpregnancy.org. National Campaign to Prevent Teen Pregnancy. Information on organization's research, conferences, publications, and resources for parents, teens, and leaders of faith organizations.

http://www.cpc.unc.edu/. The National Longitudinal Study of Adolescent Health (1998) Web site regarding the Add Health Study data available and using the data.

http://www.girlshealth.gov/. The National Women's Health Information Center, Adolescent Health page. The Department of Health and Human Services Office on Women's Health. The page on adolescent health includes brief overviews of HIV/AIDS, STDs, eating disorders, nutrition, exercise, stress, and teen pregnancy in question-answer format.

http://www.piwh.org. Pacific Institute for Women's Health works to improve women's health through applied research, advocacy, community involvement, consultation and training. Information about their adolescent health programs in Africa at www.piwh.org/adolhlth_f.html.

http://www.paho.org. Pan American Health Organization (PAHO) addresses the health of adolescents and youth within the context of their social and economic environment, developing mechanisms to meet their needs. The adolescent health materials section (www.paho.org/english/hpp/hppadol.htm) includes an overview of general health and reproductive health issues. PAHO's Plan of Action for Health and Development of Adolescents and Youth in the Americas 1998–2001 is found at www.paho.org/english/hpp/downloads/planact.pdf.

http://www.plannedparenthood.org. Planned Parenthood Federation of America.

http://www.populationaction.org. Population Action International Web site includes policies and programs to slow population growth; advocates expansion of voluntary family planning and other reproductive health services; and includes search engine to find documents related to adolescent reproductive health.

http://www.popcouncil.org. The Population Council Organization conducts reproductive health research and policy work worldwide. Publications cover a range of reproductive health topics, including adolescent health. Abstracts of "Studies in Family Planning" are available on-line at www.popcouncil.org/publications/sfp/sfpabs .html.

http://www.arhp.org/rap/. Resources for Adolescent Providers. Information sharing network provides information on current clinical and social issues that affect adolescents and young adults. Links to sites for adolescents are provided on this site.

http://www.sxetc.org. Rutgers University's Network for Family Life Education. "Sex etc. Newsletter." Web site for teens.

http://www.siecus.org/index.html. Sexuality Information and Education Council of the United States develops, collects, and disseminates information, promotes comprehensive education about sexuality, and advocates the right of individuals to make responsible sexual choices.

http://www.who.int/dsa/cat98/adol8.htm. World Health Organization Publications. *Adolescent Health* (1991–2000).

REFERENCES AND ADDITIONAL READINGS

Alan Guttmacher Institute. *Teenage pregnancy: the problem that hasn't gone away*. New York: Alan Guttmacher Institute, 1981.

Alan Guttmacher Institute. *Sex and America's teenagers*. New York: Alan Guttmacher Institute, 1994.

American Academy of Pediatrics, Committee on Communications. Sexuality, contraception, and the media. *Pediatrics* 1995;95:298.

Bersamin MM, Walker S, Waiters ED, et al. Promising to wait: virginity pledges and adolescent sexual behavior. *J Adolesc Health* 2005;36:428.

Blum RW, Beuhring T, Rinehart PM. *Protecting teens: beyond race, income, and family structure*. Minnesota, Minneapolis: Center for Adolescent Health, University of Minnesota, Minneapolis, University of Minnesota Printing Service, 2000a.

Blum RW, Beuhring T, Shew M, et al. The effects of race/ethnicity, income, and family structure on adolescent risk behaviors. *Am J Public Health* 2000;90:1879.

Blum RW, Kelly A, Ireland M. Health-risk behaviors and protective factors among adolescents with mobility impairments and learning and emotional disabilities. *J Adolesc Health* 2001;28:48190.

Boostra H. Legislators craft alternative vision of sex education to counter abstinence-only drive. *Guttmacher Rep Public Policy* 2002;2:1.

Braverman PK, Strasburger VC. Adolescent sexuality: part 4. The practitioner's role. *Clin Pediatr (Phila)* 1994;33:100.

Britto MT, Garrett JM, Dugliss MA, et al. Risky behavior in teens with cystic fibrosis or sickle cell disease: a multicenter study. *Pediatrics* 1998;101:2506.

Brown RT. Adolescent sexuality at the dawn of the 21st century. *Adolesc Med* 2000;11:19.

Bruckner H, Bearman P. After the promise: the STD consequences of adolescent virginity pledges. *J Adolescent Health* 2006;36:271.

Butler N, Gilby R, McIntyre J, Rowntree C. Introducing sexuality. *A guide for presenting sexual issues to adolescent and young adults with developmental disabilities*. London, Ontario, Canada: 1995. Available from: Child and Parent Resource Institute, 600 Sanatorium Rd., London, OH N6H 3W7.

Caldirola D, Gemperle M, Guzinski G. Chronic pelvic pain as related to abdominal pain in childhood and to psychosocial disturbance in the family. In: Rizzi R, Visentini M, eds. *Pain: proceedings of the joint meeting of the european chapters of the international association for the study of pain*. Padua, Italy: Piccin/Butterworth, 1994:291.

Carroll G, Massarelli E, Opzoomer A. Adolescents with chronic disease–are they receiving comprehensive health care? *J Adolesc Health Care* 1983;4:261.

Centers for Disease Control and Prevention. Selected behaviors that increase risk for HIV infection, other sexually transmitted diseases, and unintended pregnancy among high school students–United States, 1991. *MMWR Morb Mortal Wkly Rep* 1992;41:945.

Centers for Disease Control and Prevention. Youth risk behavior surveillance–United States, 2005. *Morb Mortal Wkly Rep CDC Surveill Summ* 2006;55(SS05);1.

Cheng MM, Udry JR. Sexual behaviors of physically disabled adolescents in the United States. *J Adolescent Health* 2002; 31(1):48.

Choquet M, Du Pasquier FL, Manfredi R, et al. Sexual behavior among adolescents reporting chronic conditions: a French national survey. *J Adolesc Health* 1997;30:627.

Committee on HIV Prevention Strategies in the United States, Institute of Medicine. *No time to lose: getting more from HIV prevention*, Washington, DC: National Academy Press, 2000.

Darroch JE, Landry DJ, Oslak S. Age differences between sexual partners in the United States. *Fam Plann Perspect* 1999;31: 160.

Dilorio C, Kelley M, Hockenberry-Eaton M. Communication about sexual issues: mothers, fathers, and friends. *J Adolesc Health* 1999;24:282.

Donovan P. Can statutory rape laws be effective in preventing adolescent pregnancy? *Fam Plann Perspect* 1997;29:30.

Drossman DA, Leserman J, Nachman G. Sexual and physical abuse in women with functional or organic gastrointestinal disorders. *Ann Intern Med* 1990;113:828.

Elstein SG, Davis N. *Sexual relationships between adult males and young teen girls: exploring the legal and social issues*. Chicago: American Bar Association, 1997.

Enright R. *Caution: do not open until puberty! An introduction to sexuality for young adults with disabilities*. Ontario, Canada: Devinjer House, 1995.

Eyre SL, Read NW, Millstein SG. Adolescent sexual strategies. *J Adolescent Health* 1997;20:286.

Forrest JD, Singh S. The sexual and reproductive behavior of American women 1982–1988. *Fam Plann Perspect* 1990;22:206.

Frey MA, Guthrue B, Loveland-Cherry C, et al. Risky behavior and risk in adolescents with IDDM. *J Adolesc Health* 1997;20: 3845.

Gates GJ, Sonenstein FL. Heterosexual genital sexual activity among adolescent males: 1988 and 1995. *Fam Plann Perspect* 2000;32:295.

Gittes EB, Strickland JL. Contraceptive choices for chronically ill adolescents. *Adolesc Med Clin* 2005;16(3):635.

Gordon S, Scales P, Everly K. *The sexual adolescent: communicating with teenagers about sex.* Belmont, MA: Duxbury Press, 1979.

Grunbaum JA, Kann L, Kinchen S, et al. Youth risk behavior surveillance–United States, 2003. *MMWR Surveill Summ* 2004;53(2):1.

Haka-Ikse K, Mian M. Sexuality in children. *Pediatr Rev* 1993; 14:401.

Halpern-Flesher BL, Corell JL, Kropp RY, et al. Oral versus vaginal sex among adolescents: perceptions, attitudes and behavior. *Pediatrics* 2005;115:845.

Holt T, Greene L, Davis J. Kaiser Family Foundation. *National survey of adolescents and young adults: sexual health knowledge, attitudes and experiences.* Menlo Park, CA, Henry J. Kaiser Family Foundation, 2003.

Kaufman M. *Easy for you to say: Q & A's for teens living with chronic illness or disability.* Toronto, Ontario, Canada: Key Porter Books, 1995.

Klein JD. Committee on Adolescence. Adolescent pregnancy: current trends and issues. *Pediatrics* 2005;116(1):281.

Ku L, Sonenstein FL, Lindberg LD, et al. Understanding changes in sexual activity among young metropolitan men: 1979–1995. *Fam Plann Perspect* 1998;30:256.

Landry DJ, Forrest JD. How old are U.S. fathers? *Fam Plann Perspect* 1995;27:159.

Langdell JI. Adolescent sexual preoccupations. *Med Aspects Hum Sex* 1980;14:90.

Leitenberg H, Detzer MJ, Srebnik D. Gender differences in masturbation and the relation of masturbation experience in preadolescence and/or early adolescence to sexual behavior and sexual adjustment in young adulthood. *Arch Sex Behav* 1993;22:87.

Males M, Chew KSY. The ages of fathers in California adolescent births, 1993. *Am J Public Health* 1996;86:565.

Manlove J, Moore K, Liechty J, et al. *Sex between young teens and older individuals: a demographic portrait.* Child Trends Research Brief, September 2005.

Marchione M. Centers for Disease Control and Prevention National Center for HIV, STD, and TB Prevention. HIV/AIDS Information Center. Teens don't talk sex with physicians. *JAMA* Available at www.ama-assn.org/special/hiv/newsline/edc/120800g2.htm. Daily News Update: December 8, 2000.

Miller KS, Kotchick BA, Dorsey S, et al. Family communication about sex: what are parents saying and are their adolescents listening? *Fam Plann Perspect* 1998;30:218.

Miller KS, Levin ML, Whitaker DJ, et al. Patterns of condom use among adolescents: the impact of mother-adolescent communication. *Am J Public Health* 1998;88:1542.

Mosher WD, Chandra A, Jones J. Sexual behavior and selected health measures: men and women 15–44 years of age, United States, 2002. *Adv Data from Vital Health Stat* 2005;362:1.

National Adolescent Health Information Center. *Fact sheet on adolescent demographics.* San Francisco: National Adolescent Health Information Center, University of California, 2000.

Neinstein LS, Katz B. Contraceptive use in the chronically ill adolescent female. Part I. *J Adolesc Health Care* 1986;7:123.

Neinstein LS, Katz B. Contraceptive use in the chronically ill adolescent female. Part II. *J Adolesc Health Care* 1986;7:350.

Parera N, Suris JC. Having a good relationship with their mother: a protective factor against sexual risk behavior among adolescent females? *J Pediatr Adolesc Gynecol* 2004; 17:267.

Remafedi G. Sexually transmitted diseases in homosexual youth. In: Strasburger VC, Greydanus DE, eds. *The at-risk adolescent. adolescent medicine: state of the art reviews*, Vol. 1. 1990:565.

Remez L. Oral sex among adolescents: is it sex or is it abstinence? *Fam Plann Perspect* 2000;32(6):298–304.

Rew L. Sexual health promotion in adolescents with chronic health conditions. *Fam Community Health* 2006;29(1 Suppl): 61S.

Santelli JS, Brener ND, Lowry R, et al. Multiple sexual partners among U.S. adolescents and young adults. *Fam Plann Perspect* 1998;30:271.

Santelli JS, Lindberg LD, Abma J, et al. Adolescent sexual behavior: estimates and trends from four nationally represented surveys. *Fam Plann Perspect* 2000;32:156.

Schoen C, Davis K, Collins KS, et al. *The commonwealth fund survey of the health of adolescent girls.* The commonwealth fund. Louis Harris and Associates, Available at www.cmwf.org/publications/publications_show.htm?doc_id=221230. 1997.

Schoen C, Davis K, DesRoches C, et al. *The health of adolescent boys: commonwealth fund survey findings.* The Commonwealth Fund. Available at www.cmwf.org/publications/publications_show.htm?doc_id=221410. April 1998.

Schuster MA, Bell RM, Gberry SH, et al. Impact of a high school condom availability program on sexual attitudes and behaviors. *Fam Plann Perspect* 1998;30:67.

Schuster MA, Bell RM, Kanouse DE. The sexual practices of adolescent virgins: genital sexual activities of high school students who have never had vaginal intercourse. *Am J Public Health* 1996;86(11):1570.

Schuster MA, Bell RM, Petersen LP, et al. Communication between adolescents and physicians about sexual behavior and risk prevention. *Arch Pediatr Adolesc Med* 1996b; 150:906.

SIECUS. *SIECUS state profiles: a portrait of sexuality education and abstinence-only-until-marriage programs in the states.* New York: SIECUS, 2004.

Singh S, Darroch JE. Adolescent pregnancy and childbearing: levels and trends in developed countries. *Fam Plann Perspect* 2000;32:14.

Society for Adolescent Medicine. Abstinence-only education policies and programs: a position paper of the Society for Adolescent Medicine. *J Adolesc Health* 2006; 38(1):83.

Stout JW, Kirby D. The effects of sexuality education on adolescent sexual activity. *Pediatr Ann* 1993;22:120.

Suris JC, Parera N. Sex, drugs and chronic illness: health behaviours among chronically ill youth. *Eur J Public Health* 2005;15(5):484.

Suris JC, Resnick MD, Cassuto N, et al. Sexual behavior of adolescents with chronic disease and disability. *J Adolesc Health* 1996;19:12431.

Tepper MS. Becoming sexually able: education to help youth with disabilities. *SIECUS Rep* 2001;29(3):5.

US Department of Health and Human Services. *A decision-making approach to sex education: a curriculum guide and implementation manual for a model program with adolescents and parents.* Washington: US Government Printing Office, 1979.

Valencia LS, Cromer BA. Sexual activity and other high-risk behaviors in adolescents with chronic illness: a review. *J Pediatr Adolesc Gynecol* 2000;13:53.

Whitaker DJ, Miller KS, May DC, et al. Teenage partners' communication about sexual risk and condom use: the importance of parent-teenager discussions. *Fam Plann Perspect* 1999;31:117.

Zeltzer L, Kellerman J, Ellenberg L, et al. Psychologic effects of illness in adolescence. II. Impact of illness in adolescents–crucial issues and coping styles. *J Pediatr* 1980; 97(1):132.

CHAPTER 40

Gay, Lesbian, Bisexual and Transgender Adolescents

Eric Meininger and Gary Remafedi

HOMOSEXUALITY

Homosexuality is an emotionally charged issue. It is a difficult topic to deal with, not only for the adolescent but also for his or her family and practitioner. The health care provider should be equipped to address the concerns of adolescents with a clear homosexual orientation and the fears of others, including parents who are questioning their feelings. This chapter discusses homosexuality in the context of adolescent health. Important features of counseling homosexual teens and their parents are outlined.

General Considerations and Terminology

1. Sexual orientation: *Sexual orientation* refers to an individual's attractions to the same or opposite sex. Sexual orientation is not dichotomous, and individuals tend to fall along a continuum of sexual expression and desires rather than into exclusive categories. The phrase sexual preference implies choice and should not be used in reference to sexual orientation.
2. Gender identity: Sexual orientation should not be confused with *gender identity*. *Gender identity* relates to an individual's innate sense of maleness or femaleness. It is felt that gender identity develops in early childhood and normally is established by age 2.5 years (Yule, 2000).
3. Homosexuality: Although there is no absolute definition, *homosexuality* usually reflects "a persistent pattern of homosexual arousal accompanied by a persistent pattern of absent or weak heterosexual arousal" (Spitzer, 1981). Most homosexual individuals have a gender identity that is consistent with their biological sex.
4. Bisexuality: A *bisexual* person is attracted to both men and women. This does not preclude long-term relationships, nor does it imply promiscuity.

Complicating all of the definitions above is the fact that sexual identity, orientation, behavior, and attraction may all occur in ways that seem contradictory to some health care providers or others. Therefore, individuals may consider themselves to be heterosexual but engage in homosexual behaviors or vice versa.

Today, the term *gay* is usually applied to male homosexuals, but may also include lesbian females and bisexual and transgender individuals. The abbreviation GLBT is used to refer to these gay, lesbian, bisexual, and transgender populations collectively. *Lesbian* always refers to females. Youths who engage in sex with persons of the same gender usually identify as homosexual or bisexual, but sometimes as heterosexual, curious, or questioning.

Prevalence

Homosexuality has existed in all societies and cultures. Prevalence estimates vary according to the time, place, and different measures of homosexuality used in research. Although sexual orientation is thought to be determined before adolescence, its expression may be postponed until early adulthood or indefinitely, making it difficult to determine the actual prevalence of homosexuality during adolescence. Some adolescents who have had involuntary or coercive same-gender sex may experience confusion about their sexual orientation.

Although the prevalence, incidence, and acquisition patterns of homosexuality have been studied extensively, highly reliable data are difficult to find because of the lack of consistent clear definitions of homosexuality and the reluctance of some individuals to disclose sexual orientation information due to stigma.

1. Adolescent population: In a large, population-based study of 35,000 junior and senior high school students in Minnesota (Remafedi et al., 1992), greater than one fourth of 12-year-old students were unsure about their sexual orientation. By 18 years of age, the figure dropped to 5% and uncertainty gave way to heterosexual or homosexual identification. Reported homosexual attractions (4.5%) exceeded fantasies, the latter being more common in girls (3.1%) than in boys (2.2%). Overall, 1.1% of students described themselves as predominantly homosexual or bisexual. The prevalence of reported homosexual experiences remained constant among girls (0.9%), but increased from 0.4% to 2.8% in boys between the ages of 12 and 18 years. Childhood and adolescent sexual behavior is not necessarily predictive of an adolescent's sexual orientation. Only about a third of the teens who reported homosexual experience or fantasies identified themselves as homosexual or bisexual. A study by Garofalo et al. (1998), based on a question added to the Massachusetts Youth Risk Behavior Survey, found that 2.5% of youth self-identified as gay, lesbian, or bisexual.

2. Adult population: The National Health and Social Life Survey (NHSLS) of 1992 used several dimensions of sexuality including behavior, desire, and identification (Laumann and Gagnon, 1994). The prevalence of homosexual contact since puberty was approximately 10% of men and 5% of women and 5% and 4%, respectively, had had homosexual contact since age 18 years. The numbers have been questioned in this sample, secondary to sampling methods.

Etiology and Acquisition of Homosexual Identity

Significant evidence points to fundamental biological differences between heterosexual and homosexual persons. These findings have included:

1. Familial clustering: The clustering of homosexuality within some families has long been recognized. As compared to dizygotic twins, the greater concordance of homosexuality in monozygotic twins highlights the role of genetic constitution. Among identical twins, concordance rates for homosexuality are reported in the range of 48% to 66%. A chromosomal location has been identified that is thought to be involved in male homosexuality (Xq28), but a specific gene has not yet been identified. No clear patterns of inheritance have been established.
2. Hormonal differences: Although heterosexual and homosexual adults have comparable levels of circulating sex steroids, it has been proposed that perinatal hormones organize and activate key areas of the brain early in life. This might contribute to the eventual development of neuroanatomical and neuropsychological functional differences related to sexual orientation.
3. Brain structure: Genetic, hormonal, and other biological factors may influence behavior by their affect on the structure and functioning of the brain. In humans, brain regions thought to be involved in homosexuality include the interstitial nuclei of the anterior hypothalamus (designated INAH1, INAH2, INAH3, and INAH4), the supraoptic nucleus, the anterior commissure, and the corpus callosum. However, findings do vary among studies.
4. Animal models: Same-sex domestic and sexual relationships are a common occurrence not just in humans but in other animals.

Less well understood is the way that biology interacts with the environment and experience in shaping the expression of sexual orientation. Well-designed studies have not found differences in the familial and social backgrounds of homosexual and heterosexual men and women, nor any evidence that homosexuality is related to abnormal parenting, sexual abuse, and other traumatic events. However, environment can modulate the expression of fundamental biological predisposition by influencing the social behavior and visibility of homosexual persons.

Stages of Acquisition of Homosexual Identity

Troiden (1979, 1988) outlined the following four stages in the acquisition of homosexual identity:

1. Stage I: Sensitization. The child feels a sense of being different, without understanding the reason for these feelings. By early adolescence, there may be awareness of a different sexual orientation, including feelings and behaviors that would be considered homosexual.
2. Stage II: Identity confusion. The adolescent begins to identify behaviors and feelings that could be considered homosexual. The idea of homosexuality may conflict with the adolescent's previously held self-identity. Some adolescents seek counseling to repair or "cure" the feelings they are having. Adolescents may experience intense social isolation or feel that there is no one else like them.
3. Stage III: Identity assumption. The homosexual identity is adopted and, possibly, shared with others. This is a part of the process known as "coming out."
4. Stage IV: Commitment. The individual experiences satisfaction, self-acceptance, and an unwillingness to alter sexual identity.

A recent study (Smith et al., 2005a) found that gay and lesbian adolescents generally reported first awareness of same-sex attractions by 10 or 11 years of age, self-identification as homosexual at age 13 to 15 years, and first same-sex experiences near the time of self-identification. Self-identification usually precedes sexual debut with either male or female partners (Remafedi, 1994). Girls appear to "come out" later, in the context of a relationship; whereas boys appear to come out at a younger age, in the context of sexual encounters (Remafedi, 1994; D'Augelli, 2000).

Homophobia

The term *homophobia* was coined in 1967 to signify an irrationally negative attitude toward homosexuals (Weinberg, 1992). Greenberg (1988) found that two particularly prominent influences fostered homophobia in the United States—religious fundamentalism and heterosexism, the belief that heterosexuality is inherently morally superior to homosexuality. In interviews with gay, lesbian, and bisexual adolescents, D'Augelli (2000) found that 81% experienced verbal abuse; 38% had been threatened with physical harm; 15% reported a physical assault (6% with a weapon); and 16% reported a sexual assault. In the anonymous Minnesota school-based survey, gay, lesbian, and bisexual adolescents reported sexual abuse more than twice as often as the general adolescent population (Saewyc et al., 1998).

Health Concerns

Gay male, lesbian, and bisexual adolescents, like all teens, may face adverse medical consequences of either lifestyle changes, consequences of low self-esteem, or risky sexual behaviors. This is an overview of some specific issues that may arise in the care of homosexual adolescents.

Breast Cancer The risk of breast cancer and its complications among lesbians may be heightened by nulliparity, delayed pregnancy, alcohol use, obesity, and nonuse of screening services. This is an area of ongoing research.

Eating Disorders Gay males reported a significantly higher prevalence of poor body image, frequent dieting, binge eating, or purging than heterosexual males in a population-based survey of Minnesota schools (French et al., 1996).

Pregnancy and Parenthood In the 1987 Minnesota Adolescent Health Survey, lesbian or bisexual women were equally likely to have had intercourse with men, but more likely than their heterosexual peers to report a pregnancy (12% versus 5%) (Saewyc et al., 1999). Among sexually experienced adolescents, lesbian or bisexual women were also more likely to have engaged in prostitution during the previous year (9.7% versus 1.9%).

Runaway and Homelessness

Parental rejection, abandonment, and violence contribute to the disproportionately high numbers of GLBT teens in the homeless youth community. D'Augelli et al. (1998) found that 10% of mothers and 26% of fathers of GLBT adolescents in community centers rejected their children after they revealed their sexual orientation. With damaged self-esteem and few support networks, teens living on the streets may turn to prostitution, theft, or selling drugs as a means of survival.

School Problems

Adolescents facing a hostile school environment may exhibit declining school performance or school avoidance or dropout. Conversely, they may excel in schoolwork by concentrating on their studies in lieu of social and romantic relationships (Treadway and Yoakam, 1992). Russell et al. (2001) found that middle and high school students who identified having attraction to same or both sexes were more likely to have been in a fight that resulted in a need for medical treatment, and more likely to have witnessed violence than their peers.

Substance Abuse

State-wide surveys have found that GLBT adolescents are more likely to use tobacco than their heterosexual peers (Garofalo et al., 1999). They are also significantly more likely to initiate tobacco use at a younger age (48% GLBT youth versus 23% heterosexual Massachusetts youth used cigarettes before age 13 years). A recent study by Remafedi and Carol (2005) found the GLBT youths and professionals who interact with them recommend culturally specific approaches to tobacco prevention and cessation programs.

Rosario et al. (1997) reported rates of illicit substance use that were 6.4 times higher among lesbian or bisexual girls and 4.4 times higher among gay or bisexual boys than in national samples of heterosexual peers. Because adolescents are forced to cope with the stigma of their sexual orientation at a developmental point of limited skills and resources, they may turn to alcohol or other substances as a means to escape fear and to control emotional distress. Substance use may result in unsafe sexual practices leading to sexually transmitted diseases (STDs) or human immunodeficiency virus (HIV) infections. Methamphetamine use has been increasing, and there is a strong correlation between methamphetamine use and HIV (Purcell et al., 2005; Colfax et al., 2005).

Suicide

Rates of attempted suicide among homosexual youths have been found to be consistently higher than expected in the general population of adolescents, ranging from 20% to 42% (Remafedi, 1999). As compared to gender-matched heterosexual comparison groups, the risk of attempted and completed suicide appears to be especially accentuated in males. Suicide attempts often occur in proximity to "identity assumption" and may be associated with family conflict. Identified risk factors are young age at first awareness of homosexuality, experience of rejection based on sexual orientation, substance use, and perceived gender nonconformity. The severity of attempts is comparable with other adolescents. Two "psychological autopsy" studies have examined the sexual orientation of youths who had committed suicide with equivocal results.

HIV and Other STDs

The most common and serious sexually related conditions arise from unprotected penile-anal intercourse. The epithelial surfaces of the fragile rectal mucosa are easily damaged during sex, facilitating the transmission of pathogens. Rectal intercourse has been shown to be the most efficient route of infection by hepatitis B virus, cytomegalovirus, and HIV.

Oral-anal or digital-anal contact can transmit enteric pathogens such as the hepatitis A virus. Unprotected oral sex can also lead to oropharyngeal disease and gonococcal and nongonococcal urethritis for the insertive partner. Certain STDs, particularly ulcerative diseases such as syphilis and herpes simplex virus infection, can facilitate the spread of HIV.

Concordance between female sexual partners suggests that bacterial vaginosis is sexually transmitted among lesbians (Berger et al., 1995). Human papilloma virus (HPV) and *Trichomonas* infections may also be transmitted between women. Though possible, female-to-female sexual transmission of HIV is inefficient, and women who only engage in same-sex behavior are less likely than other youths to acquire STDs in general.

Men who have sex with other men (MSM) continue to be at great risk for HIV infection. In a study of HIV risk among 15-to 22-year-old MSM in seven U.S. cities from 1994 to 1998, Valleroy et al. (2000) interviewed and tested approximately 3,500 men who were recruited in public venues. Four out of ten (41%) reported unprotected anal intercourse (UAI) in the last 6 months (range 33% to 49% across cities), and the prevalence of HIV infection was 7.2% (range 2.2% to 12.1%). In a subsequent study of 23- to 29-year-old MSM in six U.S. cities from 1998 to 2000, Valleroy et al. (2001) found 46% of 2,401 men reported UAI in the last 6 months (range 41% to 53%) and HIV prevalence was 12.3% (range 4.7% to 18%). Altogether, 77% of the men found to be HIV seropositive from 1994 to 2000 did not know they were infected. In both of these studies, HIV prevalence was found to be higher in MSM of color than among white MSM.

Health Assessment

1. History: When evaluating adolescents for medical problems, the practitioner must elicit correct information about sexual practices. Begin by assuring the adolescent that all information will be kept in confidence (unless the adolescent poses a danger to him/herself or others). Explain that you will ask personal questions and that an honest response will help you give the best possible care. Ask questions in a nonjudgmental manner that maximizes the likelihood of an honest response. Inquiring about specific sexual practices will help determine the adolescent's risk for STDs and will direct laboratory studies. It also provides an opportunity to offer education regarding prevention of STDs and risk reduction. For those adolescents who are involved sexually, specific questions should include type of intercourse (penile-vaginal, orogenital, penile-anal, receptive or insertive, oral-anal), number of lifetime and recent

sexual partners, use of barrier methods, prior history of STDs, symptoms suggestive of STDs, and HIV status of adolescent or their partner(s).

2. STD screening: Not all homosexual adolescents need a full STD evaluation. If the history indicates that the teen is either not sexually active or scrupulously avoids risk, a simple physical examination may suffice. The reliability of the teen's history should be considered. If a question of veracity exists, it may be wise to offer more frequent follow-up appointments to establish a rapport and create an honest dialogue. Practitioners might routinely offer STD and HIV testing to high-risk populations such as incarcerated youth, youth in the sex industry, and institutionalized and homeless youth. Appropriate screening of the sexually active homosexual adolescent with risk factors identified during the sexual history might include a physical examination and laboratory testing for HIV, gonorrhea, chlamydia, syphilis, trichomonas, HPV infection, and other illnesses as indicated.

3. Specific sexually transmitted diseases or conditions: GLBT adolescents are at risk of contracting the same STDs as their heterosexual counterparts. A few specific conditions related to sexual practices that are more common among gay adolescents, such as rectal HPV infection from penile-anal intercourse or pharyngeal gonorrhea from oral-genital intercourse, are elaborated later in this chapter. For more detailed information please refer to the specific chapter on diagnosis and treatment of a particular STD.

   a. Enteric illnesses: Teenagers who engage in unprotected oral or anal sex run a higher risk of contracting various enteric pathogens. Male or female adolescents who engage in anal intercourse may experience local pain, bleeding, or skin lesions due to trauma, allergy to latex or lubricants, or STDs. Persistent gastrointestinal (GI) symptoms in adolescents who engage in anal intercourse should prompt a comprehensive history and physical examination. Pathogens include, but are not limited to, *Entamoeba histolytica, Giardia lamblia, Shigella, Neisseria gonorrhoeae, Treponema pallidum* (syphilis), *Chlamydia trachomatis*, HPV (warts), and herpes simplex virus.

      Diagnostic evaluation may include stool cultures for invasive bacteria and microscopic evaluation for ova and parasites. Tests for gonorrhea, chlamydia, and herpes should be obtained when proctitis is suggested by rectal discharge, tenesmus, or pain. Also consider anoscopy, anal Papanicolaou smear, and syphilis and HIV serologies.

   b. Chlamydia: Treatment for chlamydia is outlined in Chapter 62. However, clinicians should be aware of lymphogranuloma venereum (LGV), a systemic disease caused by *C. trachomatis* (serovars L1, L2, or L3) that occurs only rarely in the United States. As of September, 2004, the Netherlands saw a 19-fold increase in confirmed cases among MSM. Most cases were also coinfected with HIV. LGV should be considered in young MSM who have proctitis, proctocolitis, or painful inguinal lymphadenopathy as a presenting complaint (Centers for Disease Control and Prevention [CDC], 2004b).

   c. Gonorrhea: Gonococcal infections may be asymptomatic or associated with pharyngitis, urethritis, and proctitis. Treatment for gonorrhea is outlined in

Chapter 61. Clinicians should be aware of increasing fluoroquinolone-resistant *N. gonorrhoeae* (prevalence of 5% or more) in MSM. As of 2007, the CDC no longer recommends fluoroquinolones in treating any gonococcal infections.

   d. Syphilis: Since the mid 1990s, there has been growing concern about a resurgence of risky sexual behavior in MSM, possibly leading to an increase in HIV transmission. Reviews of sexual behavior data suggest that rates of UAI have been increasing among MSM. There have been outbreaks of syphilis (CDC, 2003) and gonorrhea among MSM in U.S. cities and increases in newly diagnosed HIV infections among MSM from 1999 to 2002 (Guenther-Grey et al., 2005).

      Detecting the primary lesion of syphilis at the anus, where it may not be seen or felt, can be difficult. Although generally painless, rectal syphilis can cause discomfort or may appear as an atypical lesion with shaggy borders, resembling carcinoma. Regular syphilis screening is recommended for sexually active MSM. There is evidence that coinfection with HIV may alter the course of syphilis. Syphilis in HIV-seropositive individuals may not respond to traditional therapy or may have an accelerated course. Evaluation and treatment for syphilis is outlined in Chapter 64.

   e. Hepatitis: Historically, there has been a higher prevalence of hepatitis B in the gay male community than in the general population. The American Academy of Pediatrics (AAP) recommends routine hepatitis B vaccination for all children. Hepatitis A can be transmitted by the fecal-oral route during orogenital and oral-anal sex. Because of this and the potential morbidity among infected adults, the hepatitis A vaccine series is recommended for all MSM. Hepatitis is discussed in more detail in Chapter 30.

   f. Cytomegalovirus infection: As many as 80% of homosexual males who engage in sex with multiple partners will acquire cytomegalovirus within a year (Mintz et al., 1983). This infection is largely asymptomatic but may lead to a severe mononucleosis-like illness, particularly in an immunosuppressed HIV-seropositive teen.

   g. HPV infection: Condyloma acuminatum (genital warts) can be found on the penis, vagina, or rectal area. Management of internal warts is complicated and should be carried out in consultation with an expert. Treatment for condyloma is outlined in Chapter 66. HPV is the cause of cervical dysplasia, which can be a risk factor for cervical cancer. It can also cause dysplasia in the anal or rectal mucosa increasing the risk for anal or rectal carcinoma. All sexually active female patients, whether they identify as heterosexual, bisexual, or lesbian, should be screened routinely with a Papanicolaou smear (guidelines can be found in Chapter 54). Anal Papanicolaou smears can also be used to screen for anal condyloma. The benefit of screening for anal carcinoma is an area of ongoing research. A vaccine for the prevention of HPV infections is now available for females between the ages of 9 and 26.

   h. Herpes simplex: Herpes simplex infections of the penis, vagina, mouth, or rectum can occur. Findings associated with herpes simplex proctitis include fever, difficulty with urination or defecation, sacral paresthesias, inguinal adenopathy, severe anorectal pain, tenesmus, constipation, perianal ulcerations, and the presence of diffuse ulcerations or vesicular or pustular lesions in the distal 5 cm of the rectum. Treatment of herpes simplex is outlined in Chapter 65.

  i. HIV infection: Acquired immunodeficiency syndrome (AIDS) and HIV are discussed further in Chapter 31. Because of limited social networks, meeting sexual partners through the Internet has become an increasingly popular and potentially risky behavior for MSM. Benotsch et al. (2002) found that one third of MSM met a sexual partner on-line. GLBT youth may be at particular risk for HIV exposure because of their relative inexperience and weaker position of power in negotiating drug use and condoms. Drug use (e.g., methamphetamines, marijuana, ecstasy, and others) has been shown to increase the likelihood of UAI in MSM. Recommend a barrier method of protection for all sexually active teens. Discuss Internet and drug usages with the adolescent and recommend the following safer sexual practices:

  • Abstain from sex or risky sexual practices such as anal intercourse.
  • Reduce numbers of sexual partners. Screen for Internet use as a means of meeting new partners.
  • Use condoms or barriers consistently during insertive and receptive oral, anal, and vaginal sex.
  • Use latex—not natural lambskin—condoms, because the latter have been shown to be potentially porous. Polyurethane condoms are an acceptable, albeit more expensive, alternative for teens with a sensitivity to latex.
  • Lubricants should be water-based products, rather than oil-based ones that can deteriorate condoms and contribute to pruritus ani.
  • Avoid sharing needles. If needles must be used, they should be clean, fresh from a sealed pack, or flushed with household bleach and then water.
  • Avoid substance use during sex. Brainstorm harm-reduction techniques to increase the likelihood of condom use during sex.

Counseling Issues

The AAP recognizes the physician's responsibility to provide health care for homosexual adolescents and for those young individuals struggling with issues of sexual expression. The removal of homosexuality from the American Psychiatric Association's (APA) *Diagnostic and Statistical Manual of Mental Disorders (DSM)* in 1973 signaled a change in our understanding and counseling of homosexual teens and their parents.

Given the opportunity to grow up in a supportive environment, most gay and lesbian adolescents are no more likely to experience serious mental health problems than the general adolescent population (Gonsiorek, 1988). Homophobia engenders guilt, shame, and psychological problems. Practitioners must also be prepared to counsel worried parents in their attempt to understand their child. If the health care provider is unable to accept homosexuality as healthy and normal, he or she should be prepared to refer the adolescent to an appropriate resource.

Counseling the Teen

1. Create an open environment in which the teen feels comfortable discussing issues of sexuality.
2. Do not minimize the adolescent's concerns regarding sexual orientation. Stating that "it's just a phase" may actually intensify the teen's confusion.
3. Discussing homosexuality with teens will not make them homosexual.
4. Assure the teen that homosexuality is a normal variation of sexual orientation and that sexual orientation is biologically driven.
5. Do not expect teens to define their sexual orientation prematurely. Sexual orientation unfolds during adolescence. Assuring them that questions about their sexual orientation will resolve over time may take some of the urgency out of the issue, "Am I, or am I not?" Remember, health care providers are not responsible for labeling, or even identifying youth who are nonheterosexual (American Academy of Pediatrics, 2004).
6. The position of the APA is that conversion therapy (i.e., attempts to repair or "cure" them of homosexuality) is not useful and may be damaging. In a review of outcomes, Haldeman (1991) found that attempts to replace homosexual fantasies with heterosexual ones were unsuccessful among men who had not experienced sexual attraction to women. Such attempts may contribute to guilt, low self-esteem, and psychological problems.
7. Irrespective of whether adolescents have resolved uncertainty about their sexual orientation, helping to prevent the spread of HIV/AIDS infection is of paramount importance. This is a prime reason to inquire about a teen's sexual practices.
8. Not all homosexual teens experience difficulties with their orientation. As with other healthy adolescents, well-adjusted homosexual individuals need sensitive and informed health care services. Some individuals will appreciate the opportunity to discuss their unique experiences or concerns as GLBT youth.

Counseling Concerned Parents

The following are some suggestions for helping families:

1. Help parents explore and address their feelings of anger, fear, shame, guilt, or grief.
2. Offer correct information about homosexuality.
3. Explain that not every emotional problem manifested by a teen is a result of his or her sexual orientation.
4. Challenge society's dichotomous belief that homosexuality is bad and that heterosexuality is good.
5. Explore religious beliefs and provide appropriate referrals. Affirming groups exist in most faiths and religious denominations.
6. Discuss HIV/AIDS prevention with parents. Some parents automatically associate homosexuality with illness.
7. Supplement counseling with referrals to support groups such as Parents and Friends of Lesbians and Gays (PFLAG). Another useful resource is the National Youth Advocacy Coalition (NYAC), which maintains a directory of local resources. The addresses of both organizations can be found in the Resources section of this chapter.
8. Finally, help parents understand that the adolescent who just "came out" is the same teen who sat before them before the disclosure. The adolescent's main need has been, is, and will always be love and acceptance.

TRANSGENDER ADOLESCENTS

If homosexuality is an emotionally charged issue, issues of gender identity are even more so. The available literature on transgender adolescents and gender identity is limited, but growing (Boehmer, 2002). This section discusses gender identity in the context of adolescent health, and highlights important points for counseling teens and their parents.

General Considerations and Terminology

The AAP (2004) defined *gender identity* as a person's innate sense of maleness or femaleness. A person whose assigned sex at birth does not match gender identity is *transgender*. *Transitioning* is the process of changing one's appearance to better reflect one's gender identity. A *transsexual* is someone who has done something—either medically, surgically, or merely cosmetically—to express the gender with which they identify. *Transgender* is a term that captures diverse individuals, including persons who have disclosed their gender identity to others, started mental health counseling, initiated medical hormone management, undergone sexual reassignment surgery (SRS), or some combination thereof. It is different from the paraphilia of cross-dressing or transvestitism (DSM 302.3), involving sexual pleasure from dressing or wearing clothes of the opposite gender. Although transgender individuals are typically identified by health professionals as male-to-female (conventionally, MTF) or female-to-male (FTM), affected youth may not even identify as transgender—but only as a male or a female.

Gender identity is inherently different from sexual orientation. However, from a sociocultural perspective, transgender persons often identify with GLBT communities. Some transgender individuals actually identify themselves as gay, lesbian, or bisexual (Clements-Nolle et al., 2001), although most have a heterosexual orientation—that is, opposite gender of their sex of conviction (Smith et al., 2005). Historically, individuals with ambiguous genitalia were not described as *transgender*, but as *intersex*. Some progressive organizations have started using the acronym GLBTI to acknowledge that intersexed persons may face similar challenges as others within the group.

Unlike homosexuality, which was removed from the Diagnostic and Statistical Manual as a mental illness, the diagnosis of gender identity disorder (GID) has persisted—hopefully, only to facilitate access to therapy and counseling specific to gender and transitioning issues, and to enable individuals to receive medical and surgical management of their gender identity. There are three diagnoses related to gender identity—Gender Identity Disorder of Childhood (DSM 302.6), Gender Identity Disorder of Adolescence and Adulthood (DSM 302.85), and Gender Identity Disorder, Not Otherwise Specified (NOS) (also DSM 302.6). Because most children with GID of childhood grow up to be homosexual (Zuger, 1984), experts have questioned the validity, utility, and ethicality of its diagnosis and treatment in children. A subset of children who experience conflict between their assigned sex and core gender identity (as opposed to gender role), may eventually identify as transgender. Medical treatment is rarely considered in prepubertal children with GID. Because adolescence is a period of identity development, there is some concern that a child with nonconforming gender role may be prematurely and/or erroneously considered transgender (Smith et al., 2002).

Prevalence

The most recent data from the Netherlands suggests that 1 in 11,900 males and 1 in 30,400 females (Harry Benjamin International Gender Dysphoria Association [HBIGDA], 2001) meet the criteria for GID. However, little is known about the actual prevalence of transgender individuals in populations. Transgender individuals may identify only as male or female, confounding epidemiological research. A measure of the success of the transition process is how well one feels authentic and comfortable with one's gender identity.

Etiology

Multiple studies have attempted to identify biological differences between transgender and nontransgender individuals. Except for intersexuality, variant gender identity is not necessarily associated with endocrinological disorders (Wilson, 2003), although some experts disagree.

Transphobia

Transgender youths are likely to experience homophobia because of widespread societal misunderstanding of gender identity. Like the term, homophobia, transphobia describes an individual and societal prejudice and stigma against transgender individuals, which likely contributes to some of the negative health outcomes that transgender youth experience.

Health Concerns

As a population with health disparities, transgender adolescents are at risk for multiple health problems.

Cancer Little is known about the risks of malignancy in transgender individuals. Health educators may not perceive someone who is MTF as a woman and may neglect to educate about breast self examination. Likewise, an FTM individual who has not had chest reconstruction, but who passes as a man, also may not receive appropriate instruction.

Pregnancy Transgender youth may be perceived to be at low risk for pregnancy. However, it is important to ask about sexual practices and the biological gender of partners. A gay-identified FTM who has intercourse with males is at risk for pregnancy; and it is important to discuss contraception with persons who might ovulate.

Smoking Transgender youth appear to have a higher prevalence of smoking compared with other adolescents (Cardona et al., 2005; Remafedi, *in press*). Some use tobacco to cope with the stress associated with a stigmatized identity. MTF youth may identify with glamorous women seen in advertisements. Alternatively, FTM teens may smoke to appear more masculine and to lower their voices (Cardona et al., 2005).

HIV Injection hormones are available illicitly. Silicone also may be injected to enhance features. Some youth, especially minors, may initiate self-treatment without medical supervision and share needles with friends. Because of employment discrimination, some young people turn to prostitution as a means to pay for therapy, hormones, or surgery (31% of adult FTM and 80% of adult MTF [Clements-Nolle et al., 2001]). For some, prostitution is related to stigma and is a validation of gender identity. Probably due to a combination of these factors, black transgender MTF youth have been identified as a subgroup with extraordinarily high rates of HIV, 63% in one study of Californians (Clements-Nolle et al., 2001).

Runaway and Homelessness For many of the same reasons as GLB youth, transgender youth have an increased likelihood of becoming homeless.

School Problems Transgender youth report high rates of verbal and physical abuse in school. One qualitative study in Philadelphia found that 96% of transgender youth reported being verbally harassed; 83% reported physical harassment; and 75% dropped out of school (Sausa, 2003).

Substance Abuse Substance abuse has been identified as a problem in the transgender adult community (Nemoto et al., 1999). No definitive studies of youth are available.

Suicide Transgender youth may be at an even greater risk of attempted suicide than GLB youth (Bockting et al., 2005). Clements-Noll et al. (2001) found that 62% of MTF and 55% of FTM transgender adults met the criteria for depression. Thirty-two percent of both populations had attempted suicide.

Hepatitis Transgender youth may be at an increased risk for hepatitis B and C if they are using injection hormones and sharing needles. One survey of MTF clients reported a high prevalence of hepatitis B in a pubic health STD clinic (Moriarty et al., 1998). MTF who have sex with men face the same risks as other MSM.

Mental Health Concerns

Teens who are dealing with the stress of gender dysphoria often lack resources for housing, medical care, and basic living expenses. The time delay between "coming out" as transgender and transitioning medically is a very unique stressor impacting upon their mental health. Age-related emotional immaturity can adversely impact identity formation and decision-making skills.

Counseling the Teen

1. Create an open environment where adolescents feel comfortable discussing issues that trouble them.
2. Do not make assumptions about names or pronouns. If unsure, ask which pronoun or name the young person prefers.
3. Do not trivialize concerns about gender identity. Acknowledging the adolescent's concerns can bring significant relief.
4. When youngsters express distress about gender identity, assure them that fluidity can be normal and that they do not need to find immediate resolution.
5. Puberty for transgender teens can be socially, emotionally, and physically stressful. It can feel as if the body is changing against one's will. Know the local resources for endocrinological treatment and mental health counseling and support.
6. Because of discomfort with certain body parts, both transgender individuals and their health care providers may avoid examining the breasts and genitals. Acknowledge the discomfort and remind the adolescent that it is important to continue comprehensive examinations.
7. Encourage adolescents to take advantage of professional resources. The Harry Benjamin Standards of Care (Harry Benjamin International Gender Dysphoria Association [HBIGDA], 2001), the most widely recognized approach to transgender management, encourage mental health evaluation and ongoing counseling as part of the medical and surgical transition.

Counseling Concerned Parents

1. Help parents explore and address their feelings of anger, fear, shame, guilt, or grief.
2. Reassure them that they did not cause gender confusion.
3. Offer support resources for parents to connect with other parents who have transgender children. PFLAG chapters are often good places to start.
4. Practitioners should be prepared to provide Web sites and printed resources for teens and their parents, and referrals for mental health assessment, diagnosis, and experienced counseling.

Medical and Surgical Management of the Transgender Teen

A discussion of the appropriate medical and surgical management of transgender youth is beyond the scope of this chapter. However, helpful references appear in the Resources section. The dilemma facing practitioners is to provide help with transitioning while avoiding irrevocable medical or surgical interventions that might cause regret. Young adolescents with a strong transgender identity may experience growing social anxiety or depression as their bodies rapidly change away from their gender conviction. In such situations, delaying treatment may have a deleterious impact on school performance, peer interactions, and romantic relationships. In addition, some of the normal physical transformations of puberty, such as breast development or deepening voice, may leave unerasable traces or may commit the young adult to future treatments that have potential morbidities. In such cases, some experts (Harry Benjamin International Gender Dysphoria Association [HBIGDA], 2001) recommend reversible interventions to delay the physical changes of puberty long enough to allow parents and adolescents to make an informed decision about treatment options. On the basis of a number of follow-up studies of adolescents and adults, unfavorable outcomes are related to starting sexual reassignment too late, rather than too early (Cohen-Kettenis and Gooren, 1999; Smith et al., 2001).

The authors would like to acknowledge the assistance provided by Walter Bockting, Ph.D., Janet Bystrom, MA, and Alex Nelson in the section on transgender adolescents.

RESOURCES

Federation of Parents and Friends of Lesbians and Gays (PFLAG)
1726 M St, NW, Suite 400
Washington, DC 20036
202-467-8180 Fax 202-467-8194 www.pflag.org.

A national organization of parent support groups organized in local chapters. A good resource of information and reading lists for parents. PFLAG's focus is advocacy, support, and education.

National Gay and Lesbian Task Force (NGLTF)
1325 Massachusetts Ave, NW, Suite 600, Washington, DC 20005
202-393-5177 Fax 202-393-2241 www.thetaskforce.org.

A national organization working for the civil rights of GLBT people. It has an extensive library of public policy summaries available on its Web site.

Bisexual Resource Center (BRC)
P.O. Box 1026, Boston, MA 02117
617-424-9595 www.biresource.org.

An organization providing information, programming, speakers, and a historical archive on bisexuality. The Web site has many links to bisexual resources across the Internet.

Gay and Lesbian National Help Center (GLNH)
800-246-PRIDE www.glnh.org.

An organization providing nationwide toll-free peer counseling, information, and referrals. The Web site includes a collection of resources arranged by region. The 800-246-PRIDE line is a national youth talk line providing peer counseling and information.

Advocates for Youth
2000 M Street, NW, Suite 750, Washington, DC 20036
202-419-3420 Fax 202-419-1448 www.youthresource.com.

An international advocacy group creating programs to help youth make responsible decisions about their sexual health. The Web site is youth oriented and has information forums on school, disabilities, HIV-seropositive youth, and youth of color.

National Youth Advocacy Coalition (NYAC)
1638 R Street, NW, Suite 300, Washington, DC 20009
202-319-7596 Fax 202-319-7365 www.nyacyouth.org.

National network and clearinghouse whose focus is advocacy in public policy. A good contact for up to date information on local resources and support. The Web site has a resource directory organized by region.

The World Professional Association for Transgender Health (WPATH)
1300 South Second Street, Suite 180, Minneapolis, MN 55454
612-624-9397 www.wpath.org.

A professional organization dedicated to advancing the understanding and treatment of GIDs.

BOOKS FOR TEENS, PARENTS, AND HEALTH CARE PROVIDERS

Age 6–12 Years

Harris RH. *It's perfectly normal.* Cambridge, MA: Candlewick, 1994. (Book about sexuality and growing up with a nonjudgmental section on homosexuality. Includes same-sex couples in its illustrations.)

Newman L. *Heather has two mommies.* Boston: Alyson, 1989. (A simple straightforward story of a little girl named Heather and her two lesbian mothers.)

Salat C. *Living in secret.* New York: Bantam, 1993. (Eleven-year-old Amelia runs away with her mother and her mother's lover when her father will not let them be together.)

Willhoite M. *Daddy's roommate.* Boston: Alyson, 1990. (A young boy describes his father's relationship with his roommate, Frank, and his healthy, affectionate relationship with these two men.)

Age 12 Years and Older

Bauer MD, ed. *Am I blue? Coming out from the silence.* New York: Harper Collins, 1994. (Collection of stories featuring gay characters by popular young adult writers.)

Beam J, ed. *In the life: a black gay anthology.* Boston: Alyson, 1986. (Writers and artists explore what it means to be doubly different—black and gay—in contemporary America.)

Howe J. *Totally Joe.* New York: Atheneum, 2005. (Written as a school assignment, 12-year-old Joe shares stories of his friends, family, and relationships in the context of being gay.)

Hutchins L, Kaahumanu L, eds. *Bi any other name: bisexual people speak out.* Boston: Alyson, 1991. (Anthology of prose, poetry, art, and essays by bisexual artists and writers.)

McClain LJ. *No big deal.* New York: Lodestar, 1994. (A thirteen-year-old girl is forced into action when her mother joins a campaign to get her favorite teacher fired because of rumors that he's gay.)

Nelson T. *Earthshine.* New York: Orchard, 1994. (Twelve-year-old Slim narrates the story of her life with her father and his lover during the last few months before the lover's death.)

Peters JA. *Luna.* New York: Time Warner Book Group, 2004. (Told by his brother, this is the story of a young man's struggle with gender identity, and his family's struggle to accept Luna for who she is.)

Sanchez A. *Rainbow boys.* New York: Simon and Schuster, 2001. (First in a series chronicling 3 gay high school friends and their adventures. Also *Rainbow High*, 2003, and *Rainbow Road*, 2005.)

Older Teens

Clark D. *Loving someone gay.* Berkeley, CA: Ten Speed Press, 1997. (Insight into the interaction of gay people with each other, their families, and their loved ones.)

Cowan T. *Gay men and women who enriched the world.* Boston: Alyson, 1996. (Biographies of 47 gay men and women who offered outstanding contributions in different fields.)

Feinberg L. *Stone butch blues: a novel.* Ithaca, NY: Firebrand Books, 1993. (A novel chronicling the life of a female to male transgender person in the context of the gay pride movement.)

Fricke A. *Reflections of a rock lobster.* Boston: Alyson Publishing, 1981. (Personal account written by a young man who made national headlines by bringing a male date to his high school prom.)

Heron A. *Two teenagers in twenty, writings by gay and lesbian youth.* Boston: Alyson Publications, 1994. (A collection of letters and essays contributed by gay and lesbian teens.)

Marcus E. *Is it a choice? Answers to the 300 most frequently asked questions about gays and lesbians.* San Francisco: HarperCollins, 1999. (Organized into 20 sections covering issues such as coming out, religion, aging, military, and education.)

Mastoon A. *Shared heart: portraits and stories celebrating lesbian, gay, and bisexual young people.* New York: William Morrow, 1997. (Photographic collection of gay, lesbian, bisexual, and transgender adolescents in the context of their families and schools.)

Reid J. *The best little boy in the world.* New York: Ballantine Books, 1976. (Humorous story about growing up gay in a straight world.)

Sarton M. *The education of Harriet Hatfield: a novel.* New York: WW Norton, 1989. (A story about an elderly woman who gradually comes out after her partner of 30 years dies.)

Parents

Boylan JF. *She's not there: a life in two genders.* New York: Broadway Books, 2003. (An articulate autobiography written by a MTF transgender college literature professor.)

Day FA. *Lesbian and gay voices: an annotated bibliography and guide to literature for children and young adults.* Westport, CO: Greenwood Press, 2000. (A resource compiled by a retired teacher of current literature for schools and parents.)

Fairchild B, Hayward N. *Now that you know: what every parent should know about homosexuality.* San Diego: Harcourt Brace, 1989. (A guide written by parents of gay children.)

Helminiak D. *What the Bible really says about homosexuality.* San Francisco: Alamo Square Press, 1995. (The author discusses research into those biblical texts that have been considered to relate to homosexuality.)

Professionals

Gonsiorek JC, ed. *A guide to psychotherapy with gay and lesbian clients.* Bingingham, NY: Harrington Park, 1990. (Affirmative psychotherapeutic models.)

Harbeck KM, ed. *Coming out of the classroom closet: gay and lesbian students, teachers, and curricula.* New York: Haworth Press, 1992. (A collection of research on homosexuality and education.)

Harry Benjamin Standards of care for gender identity disorder, 6th version. Available online at http://wpath.org/Documents2/socv6.pdf. (The definitive resource for transgender adolescents and adults.)

Ryan C, Futterman D. *Lesbian and gay youth: care and counseling.* New York: Columbia University Press, 1998. (Comprehensive guide on medical, psychological, and support needs of lesbian and gay youth. Recommended for medical providers, counselors, youth advocates, and parents.)

Tom Waddell Health Center protocols for hormonal reassignment of gender. Available online at http://www.dph.sf.ca.us/chn/HlthCtrs/HlthCtrDocs/TransGendprotocols.pdf. (An introduction to the risks, benefits, monitoring, and dosing of hormone therapy for transgender individuals.)

REFERENCES AND ADDITIONAL READINGS

American Psychiatric Association. *Diagnostic and statistical manual of mental disorders,* 4th ed. Washington, DC: American Psychiatric Association, 1994.

Bazemore PH, Wilson WH. *Homosexuality. eMedicine.* www.emedicine.com. Last accessed 9.25, 2006.

Benotsch EG, Kalichman S, Cage M. Men who have met sex partners via the Internet: prevalence, predictors, and implications for HIV prevention. *Arch Sex Behav* 2002;31:177.

Berger BJ, Kolton S, Zenilman J, et al. Bacterial vaginosis in lesbians: a sexually transmitted disease. *Clin Infect Dis* 1995; 21:1402.

Boehmer U. Twenty years of public health research: inclusion of lesbian, gay, bisexual, and transgender populations. *Am J Public Health* 2002;92:1125.

Cardona A, Hastings P, Zemsky B. *Creating an effective tobacco plan for Minnesota's gay, lesbian, bisexual and transgender communities.* Minneapolis, MN: Rainbow Health Initiative, 2005.

Centers for Disease Control and Prevention (CDC). Increases in fluoroquinolone-resistant Neisseria gonorrhoeae among men who have sex with men–United States, 2003, and revised recommendations for gonorrhea treatment, 2004. *MMWR Morb Mortal Wkly Rep* 2004a;53:335.

Centers for Disease Control and Prevention (CDC). Lymphogranuloma venereum among men who have sex with men—Netherlands, 2003–2004. *MMWR Morb Mortal Wkly Rep* 2004b;53:985.

Centers for Disease Control and Prevention (CDC). *Trends in reportable sexually transmitted diseases in the United States, 2003: national data on chlamydia, gonorrhea, and syphilis.* Retrieved from http://www.cdc.gov/std/stats/trends2003.htm, on 10/30/2005, 2005.

Centers for Disease Control and Prevention. Update to CDC's Sexually Transmitted Diseases Treatment Guidelines, 2006: Fluoroquinolones No Longer Recommended for Treatment of Gonorrhea. *MMWR* 2007;56(14),332. http://www.cdc.gov/std/default.htm (accessed 04/23/2007).

Clements-Nolle K, Marx R, Guzman R, et al. HIV prevalence, risk behaviors, health care use, and mental health status of transgender persons: implications for public health intervention. *Am J Public Health* 2001;91:915.

Cohen-Kettenis PT, Gooren LJG. Transexualism: a review of etiology, diagnosis and treatment. *J Psychosom Res* 1999; 46:315.

Colfax G, Coates TJ, Husnik MJ, et al. Longitudinal patterns of methamphetamine, popper (amyl nitrate), and cocaine use and high-risk sexual behavior among a cohort of San Francisco men who have sex with men. *J Urban Health* 2005; 82(1 Suppl 1):i62.

D'Augelli AR. *Sexual orientation milestones and adjustment among lesbian, gay, and bisexual youths from 14 to 21 years of age. Paper presented at the Seventh Biennial Conference of the European Association for Research on Adolescence.* Jena, Germany, June 3, 2000.

D'Augelli AR, Hershberger SL, Pilkington NW. Lesbian, gay, and bisexual youth and their families: disclosure of sexual orientation and its consequences. *Am J Orthopsychiatry* 1998; 68:361.

Frankowski, BL. American Academy of Pediatrics. The Committee on Adolescence. Sexual orientation and adolescents. *Pediatrics* 2004;113:1827.

French SA, Story M, Remafedi G, et al. Sexual orientation and prevalence of body dissatisfaction and eating disordered behaviors: a population-based study of adolescents. *Int J Eat Disord* 1996;19:119.

Garofalo R, Wolf RC, Kessel S, et al. The Association Between Health Risk Behaviors and Sexual Orientation Among a School-based Sample of Adolescents. *Pediatrics.* 1998;101:895.

Garofalo R, Wolf RC, Wissow LS, et al. Sexual orientation and risk of suicide attempts among a representative sample of youth. *Arch Pediatr Adolesc Med* 1999;153:487.

Gee R. Primary care health issues among men who have sex with men. *J Am Acad Nurse Pract* 2006;18:144.

Gonsiorek JC. Mental health issues of gay and lesbian adolescents. *J Adolesc Health Care* 1988;9:114.

Greenberg DE. *The construction of homosexuality.* Chicago: University of Chicago Press, 1988.

Guenther-Grey CA, Varnell S, Weiser JI, et al. Trends in sexual risk taking among urban young men who have sex with men (1999–2002). *J Natl Med Assoc* 2005;97:38S.

Haldeman DC. Sexual orientation conversion therapy for gay men and lesbians: a scientific examination. In: Gonsiorek JC, Weinrich JD, eds. *Homosexuality: research implications for public policy.* Newbury Park, CA: Sage Publications Inc, 1991:149.

Harry Benjamin International Gender Dysphoria Association (HBIGDA). Standards of care for gender identity disorders, sixth version. *J Psychol Human Sex* 2001;13:1.

James WH. Biological and psychosocial determinants of male and female human sexual orientation. *J Biosoc Sci* 2005; 37:555.

Knight D. Health care screening for men who have sex with men. *Am Fam Physician* 2004;69:2149.

Laumann EO, Gagnon JH. *The social organization of sexuality: sexual practices in the United States.* Chicago, Ill: University of Chicago Press, 1994.

Mintz L, Drew L, Miner RC, et al. Cytomegalovirus infections in homosexual men: an epidemiological study. *Ann Intern Med* 1983;99:326.

Moriarty HJ, Thiagalingam A, Hill PD. Audit of service to a minority client group: male to female transsexuals. *Int J STD AIDS* 1998;9:238.

Mravcak SA. Primary care for lesbians and bisexual women. *Am Fam Physician* 2006;74:279.

Nemoto T, Luke D, Mamo L, et al. HIV risk behaviours among male-to-female transgenders in comparison with homosexual or bisexual males and heterosexual females. *AIDS Care* 1999;11:297.

Purcell DW, Moss S, Remien RH, et al. Illicit substance use, sexual risk, and HIV-positive gay and bisexual men: differences by serostatus of casual partners. *AIDS* 2005;19:S37.

Remafedi G. Predictors of unprotected intercourse among gay and bisexual youth: knowledge, beliefs, and behavior. *Pediatrics* 1994;94:163.

Remafedi G. Sexual orientation and youth suicide. *JAMA* 1999; 282:1291.

Remafedi G, Carol H. Preventing tobacco use among lesbian, gay, bisexual, and transgender youths. *Nicotine Tob Res* 2005; 7:249.

Remafedi G. Lesbian, gay, bisexual, and transgender youths: Who smokes, and why? *Nicotine Tob Res* 2007;9 (Suppl 1): S65–71.

Remafedi G, Resnick M, Blum R, et al. Demography of sexual orientation in adolescents. *Pediatrics* 1992;89:714.

Rosario M, Hunter J, Gwadz M. Exploration of substance use among lesbian, gay, and bisexual youth: prevalence and correlates. *J Adolesc Res* 1997;12:454.

Russell ST, Franz BT, Driscoll AK. Same-sex romantic attraction and experiences of violence in adolescence. *Am J Public Health* 2001;91:903.

Saewyc E, Bearinger L, Blum R, et al. Sexual intercourse, abuse, and pregnancy among adolescent women: does sexual orientation make a difference? *Fam Plann Perspect* 1999;31:127.

Saewyc EM, Bearinger LH, Heinz PA, et al. Gender differences in health and risk behaviors among bisexual and homosexual adolescents. *J Adolesc Health* 1998;23:181.

Sausa LA. *The HIV prevention and educational needs of trans youth.* (University Microfilms No. AAT-3087465). Unpublished doctoral dissertation, University of Pennsylvania, 2003.

Smith YLS, Cohen L, Cohen-Kettenis PT. Postoperative psychological functioning of adolescent transsexuals: a Rorschach study. *Arch Sex Behav* 2002;31:255.

Smith SD, Dermer SB, Astramovich RL. Working with non-heterosexual youth to understand sexual identity development, at-risk behaviors, and implications for health care professionals. *Psychol Rep* 2005a;96:651.

Smith YLS, Van Goozen SHM, Cohen-Kettanis PT. Adolescents with gender identity disorder who were accepted or rejected for sex reassignment surgery: a prospective follow-up study. *J Am Acad Child Adolesc Psychiatry* 2001;40:472.

Smith YLS, Van Goozen SHM, Kuiper AJ, et al. Sex reassignment: outcomes and predictors of treatment for adolescent and adult transsexuals. *Psychol Med* 2005b;35:89.

Spitzer RL. The diagnostic status of homosexuality in DSM-III: a reformulation of the issues. *Am J Psychiatry* 1981;138:210.

Treadway L, Yoakam J. Creating a safer school environment for lesbian and gay students. *J Sch Health* 1992;62:352.

Troiden RR. Becoming homosexual: a model of gay identity acquisition. *Psychiatry* 1979;42:362.

Troiden RR. Homosexual identity development. *J Adolesc Health Care* 1988;9:105.

Valleroy L, MacKellar D, Karon J, et al. HIV prevalence and associated risks in young men who have sex with men. *JAMA* 2000;284:198.

Valleroy L, Secura G, MacKellar D, et al. *High HIV and risk behavior prevalence among 23- to 29- year-old men who have sex with men in 6 US cities. 8th Conference on Retroviruses and Opportunistic Infections.* Chicago, IL. 2001. Abstract 211.

Weinberg GH. *Society and the healthy homosexual.* New York: St. Martin's Press, 1992.

Wilson JD. Hormones and sexual behavior. *Endocrinologist* 2003;13:208.

Yule W. *Developmental psychology through infancy, childhood, and adolescence.* In: Gelder MG, Lopez-Ibor JJ, Andreasen N, eds. New Oxford Textbook of Psychiatry. Vol 1. Oxford University Press; 2000:257–267.

Zuger B. Early effeminate behavior in boys: outcome and significance for homosexuality. *J Nerv Ment Dis* 1984;172:90.

CHAPTER 41

Teenage Pregnancy

Joanne E. Cox

Teen pregnancy, despite consistent declines over the last decade, remains an important medical, social, and public health issue in adolescent health. This chapter discusses the epidemiology of adolescent pregnancy, contributing factors, prevention interventions, the management of the pregnant or parenting adolescent, and the outcomes associated with adolescent pregnancy and parenting. Teen pregnancy presents challenges to adolescent health practitioners at multiple levels in the United States.

EPIDEMIOLOGY OF ADOLESCENT PREGNANCY

1. Teenage pregnancies: There are approximately 800,000 pregnancies/year in females aged 15 to 19 with more than 60% of these pregnancies occurring in 18- to 19-year-old females. Of all births in the United States, approximately 13% are in adolescents, and approximately 31% of all nonmarital births are in teens (a reduction from 50% in 1970). Approximately 51% of adolescent pregnancies result in a live birth, 35% end with an abortion, and 14% end with a miscarriage or stillbirth. Eighty percent of teen pregnancies are unintentional. In females younger than 20 years, 34% will become pregnant at least once. Among all 15- to 19-year olds in the United States, approximately 10% become pregnant each year, and among those who have had intercourse, approximately 19% become pregnant each year. For younger 10- to 14-year-old females, there are approximately 15,000 pregnancies/year (Abma et al., 2004).

2. Pregnancy and birth rate trends: The United States has set a national goal of decreasing the rate of teenage pregnancies to 43 pregnancies per 1,000 females of ages 15 to 17 years by 2010. In 2000, the teen pregnancy rate for 15- to 17-year-old females was 48.2. From 1990 to 2004, the birth rate for females aged 15 to 19 decreased 33%, from 62 per 1,000 females to 41.6. For 15- to 17-year olds the birth rate decreased from 38.6 in 1991 to 22.1 in 2004 (Martin et al., 2005; Forum on Child and Family Statistics, 2006) (Fig. 41.1). Likewise, the induced abortion rate which peaked in 1983 at 30.7 decreased to 14.5 by 2000. During the 1960s and 1970s, there was a consistent downward trend in births to teen females that was followed by a temporary surge in teen pregnancies

during the mid-1980s (Fig. 41.1). The largest decline in the birthrate since 1970 was in women aged 18 to 19 years (28%), compared with a 19% decline for adolescents aged 15 to 17 years. These declines in teen pregnancies and births have occurred across all 50 states (Ventura et al., 2004).

In 2003, the birth rate per 1,000 females aged 10 to 14 years was 0.6 live births, less than one half that of 1990 (1.4 per 1,000) and the lowest level since 1946 with 6,661 females aged 10 to 14 years giving birth in 2003. This is a 45% decline for births in this age-group since 1990. Approximately two fifths of the pregnancies among 10- to 14-year olds in 2000 ended in a live birth, two fifths ended in induced abortion, and approximately one in six ended in miscarriage (Martin et al., 2005; Menacker et al., 2004).

The decline in teen pregnancy is due to both increasing use of effective contraception and decreased sexual activity. Analysis of 1991–2001 national data showed a 53% decline in adolescent sexual experience and a 46% increase in use of contraceptives. Both can be

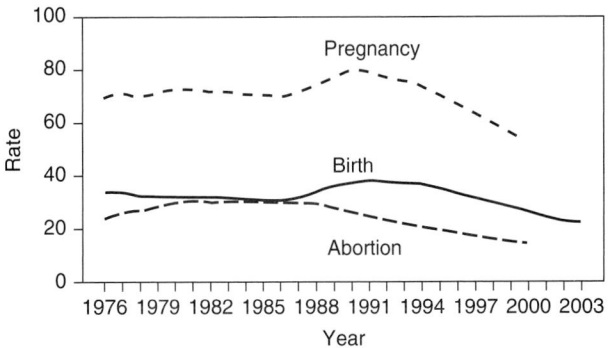

* Per 1,000 females

FIGURE 41.1 Pregnancy, birth, and abortion rates for teenagers 15 to 17 years old. (From National Campaign to Prevent Teen Pregnancy. *Fact sheet: recent trends in teen pregnancy, sexual activity, and contraceptive use.* Washington, DC: National Campaign to Prevent Teen Pregnancy, 2004. Available at: www.teenpregnancy.org/resources/reading/pdf/rectrend.pdf. Accessed June 19, 2005.)

attributed to interventions and changing social customs that have emphasized abstinence or safe sex (Flanigan, 2001; Santelli et al., 2004). The positive economic climate of the 1990s was also a major contributor to declining pregnancy rates as impoverished teens had more hope for future personal opportunities by remaining in school and working (Centers for Disease Control and Prevention, 2005).

3. Ethnicity: There are major differences in birth rates by race/ethnicity, with black and Hispanic females disproportionately experiencing pregnancy compared with whites (Table 41.1). The largest decline since 1991 by race was for black women. The birth rate for black teens aged 15 to 19 fell 45% from 1991 to 2003 although Hispanic teen birth rates declined 21% between 1991 and 2003. The rates of both Hispanics and blacks, however, remain higher than for other groups. Hispanic females are most likely to experience birth before the age of 20 (24% versus 8% among non-Hispanic whites) (Alan Guttmacher Institute, 2004).

4. Geography: Pregnancy rates vary considerably from state to state. In 2003, North Dakota had the lowest teen pregnancy rate (15–19-year olds) of 42 per 1,000 compared to the highest rate in Nevada of 113 per 1,000. Because of state variability in abortion rates, there is a different distribution of teen births rates which range from a low of 18.1 per 1,000 in New Hampshire to a high of 62.9 per 1,000 in Texas. The National Campaign to Prevent Teen Pregnancy has an excellent analysis of teen pregnancy by age, race, and state available at www.teenpregnancy.org.

5. Repeat pregnancy: Of 561,330 births to teens aged 15 to 19 years in 2003, 453,826 were first births and 107,512 were subsequent births. The rate of second births was 4.0 and the rate of third births was 0.5. Repeat pregnancy accounted for 11% of the births to females aged 15 to 17 years and 26% of births to females aged 18 to 19 years. Overall, 27.5% of teen mothers by age 20 had a repeat pregnancy in 1993 compared with 23.5% in 2002 (Martin et al., 2005; Centers for Disease Control and Prevention, 2005).

6. Prenatal care: In 2003, 70.2% of teens aged 15 to 19 years began prenatal care in the first trimester compared with only 49% of those younger than 15 years. Adequate prenatal care was lowest in non-Hispanic black teens and was directly proportional to age (Martin et al., 2005).

7. Income levels: Teens who give birth more often come from families that have a low income (83%) than are teens who have abortions (61%) or teens overall (38%).

FACTORS CONTRIBUTING TO ADOLESCENT PREGNANCY

1. High rates of sexual activity: According to the 2005 Youth Risk Behavior Survey (YRBS) (Centers for Disease Control and Prevention, 2006), 47% of U.S. high school students had engaged in intercourse representing a 13% decline since 1991. One third of high school students had had sex in the last 3 months, which suggests that a significant proportion of teens are currently having intercourse. Males are slightly more likely to be sexually experienced than females, and sexual activity increases with high school grade. For high school males, ever sexually active decreased from 55% in 1995 to 48% in 2005. Among never-married females, for those aged 15 to 17, there was a significant decline in the percentage of sexually experienced; whereas, for those aged 18 to 19 there was no significant change. African-American teens have the highest rates of early sexual activity, followed by Latin and white teens (Table 41.2) (Abma et al., 2004).

In 2005, approximately 91% of males and 83% of females used contraception at their last (most recent) sex. Approximately three out of four teens used a method of contraception at their first intercourse. The condom was the most popular method at first intercourse, with 55% of females and 70% of males using this method at their most recent intercourse (Center for Disease Control and Prevention, 2006). Contraceptive use increases sharply with increasing age at first sex for females. However, only 45% of adolescent males report always using condoms, and condom use actually decreases with age when comparing males 15 to 17 years old with males 18 to 19 years old. Females report less frequent use of condoms during intercourse than males which may in part be due to the fact that many adolescent females are sexually active with older partners (Kaplan et al., 2001). For females, there are sharp differences in contraceptive use by ethnicity. In 2002, 36% of Latino girls used contraception at most recent intercourse, compared with 57% of African-American girls and 72% of white teens (Terry-Humen et al., 2006).

2. Physical and sexual abuse: Abusive relationships are common features in the lives of adolescent mothers. Nearly half of teen mothers have reported previous sexual abuse or previous coercive sexual experiences (Boyer and Fine, 1992). Another study indicates that 25% of pregnant adolescents give a positive history of abuse in the year before the pregnancy, and 50% of that group will continue to experience abuse during the pregnancy (Kenney et al., 1997; Parker et al., 1994). Sexual victimization may increase risk of pregnancy. Hillis et al. (2004) showed a direct relationship between childhood adverse events and teen pregnancy.

3. Economic concerns: Adolescents who live in poverty face many obstacles that may increase their risk of pregnancy. In one study, 60% of teen mothers lived in families with incomes at or below the poverty level at the time of the birth, and one third of them dropped out of high school before becoming pregnant (Moore et al., 2001). Some researchers hypothesize that living in an impoverished environment leads teenagers to have low perceptions of their life choices and options, leading to a low perceived cost of teenage motherhood. This lack of hope for the present and future translates into overall risky behavior and lack of attention for the consequences. Also, a baby can represent success and hope for the future for teens who have faced economic and educational obstacles (Young et al., 2004).

4. Cultural values: Early initiation of sexual activity is not unusual if other family members have a prior history of becoming pregnant during adolescence (Furstenberg et al., 1987). Teen parents often have mothers, sisters, or brothers who were themselves teen parents (East and

TABLE 41.1

Teen Pregnancies, Births, Abortions, and Miscarriages and Stillbirths by Ethnicity and State

State	Pregnancies[a]			Births			Abortions[a]			Miscarriages and Stillbirths[a]		
	Non-Hispanic White	Black	Hispanic	Non-Hispanic White	Black	Hispanic	Non-Hispanic White	Black	Hispanic	Non-Hispanic White	Black	Hispanic
U.S. total	**346,980**	**235,650**	**204,980**	**204,056**	**118,954**	**129,469**	**92,830**	**84,460**	**45,110**	**50,090**	**32,240**	**30,400**
Alabama	7,310	6,600	390	4,976	4,380	305	1,210	1,220	20	1,120	1,000	60
Alaska	u	u	u	483	80	83	u	u	u	u	u	u
Arizona	6,670	930	9,480	3,732	559	6,585	1,990	240	1,440	950	140	1,460
Arkansas	5,470	2,890	460	3,942	1,992	358	670	460	30	860	440	70
California	u	u	u	10,279	5,406	36,919	u	u	u	u	u	u
Colorado	6,190	850	4,810	3,258	594	3,539	2,070	120	520	860	130	760
Connecticut	u	u	u	1,108	851	1,249	u	u	u	u	u	u
Delaware	1,160	1,120	240	589	577	158	420	390	40	160	150	40
District of Columbia	u	u	150	10	926	126	u	u	u	u	u	u
Florida	11,510	12,890	u	10,311	9,255	5,481	2,180	2,760	160	1,740	1,920	420
Georgia	u	u	2,580	7,593	8,213	2,004	u	u	u	u	u	u
Hawaii	470	130	u	164	57	414	250	50	100	60	20	90
Idaho	2,590	30	670	1,724	18	517	480	10	40	390	b	110
Illinois	u	u	u	7,063	7,647	5,832	u	u	u	u	u	u
Indiana	(11,600)	3,240	1,020	7,858	2,045	851	(1,970)	720	u	(1,770)	480	u
Iowa	(4,930)	410	410	3,061	272	344	(1,140)	70	u	(730)	60	u
Kansas	4,640	1,030	1,100	3,070	629	832	860	250	100	700	150	180
Kentucky	(8,740)	1,530	u	6,472	1,075	194	(890)	210	b	(1,380)	240	40
Louisiana	(6,350)	9,030	200	4,422	6,546	170	(950)	1,070	u	(980)	1,420	b
Maine	2,110	40	u	1,205	20	14	610	10	10	300	10	u
Maryland	u	8,840	640	2,645	3,934	533	u	3,740	u	u	1,160	u
Massachusetts	u	u	u	2,543	1,009	1,727	u	u	u	u	u	u
Michigan	u	u	u	7,204	4,545	1,152	u	u	u	u	u	u
Minnesota	5,580	1,400	920	3,280	779	660	1,500	420	120	810	200	140
Mississippi	4,280	7,140	110	3,075	4,796	80	540	1,260	10	670	1,090	20
Missouri	9,920	4,230	550	6,782	2,541	407	1,620	1,070	60	1,520	620	90
Montana	(1,530)	10	u	854	10	61	(460)	b	u	(220)	b	u

(continued)

TABLE 41.1

(Continued)

State	Pregnancies[a]			Births			Abortions[a]			Miscarriages and stillbirths[a]		
	Non-Hispanic White	Black	Hispanic	Non-Hispanic White	Black	Hispanic	Non-Hispanic White	Black	Hispanic	Non-Hispanic White	Black	Hispanic
Nebraska	u	u	u	1,615	293	404	u	u	u	u	u	u
Nevada	u	u	u	1,518	445	1,658	u	u	u	u	u	u
New Hampshire	u	u	u	854	18	53	u	u	u	u	u	u
New Jersey	5,310	10,090	5,640	1,961	3,259	3,000	2,690	5,620	1,860	660	1,210	790
New Mexico	1,790	190	4,460	1,001	103	2,976	540	60	810	250	30	680
New York	18,300	22,890	14,660	6,010	7,325	7,251	10,080	12,820	5,410	2,210	2,750	1,990
North Carolina	u	9,400	u	7,229	5,621	1,996	u	2,420	u	u	1,370	b
North Dakota	770	10	u	472	9	20	180	b	10	110	b	b
Ohio	19,550	8,760	1,130	12,432	5,127	787	4,210	2,370	170	2,910	1,260	170
Oklahoma	u	1,560	u	4,619	1,076	813	u	240	u	u	240	u
Oregon	6,560	460	1,760	3,423	198	1,209	2,230	200	290	910	60	270
Pennsylvania	13,710	8,510	2,340	8,066	4,218	1,665	3,660	3,130	310	1,980	1,160	360
Rhode Island	u	340	u	540	170	385	u	120	u	u	50	u
South Carolina	5,970	6,200	470	3,738	4,217	361	1,350	1,040	30	880	950	80
South Dakota	1,030	20	60	698	14	41	180	10	10	160	b	10
Tennessee	10,540	5,680	690	7,224	3,631	536	1,700	1,210	50	1,620	850	110
Texas	23,910	12,660	42,430	14,811	8,065	30,924	5,580	2,710	4,840	3,520	1,880	6,670
Utah	4,010	90	1,270	2,924	55	962	460	20	100	630	10	200
Vermont	930	10	u	501	2	3	300	10	b	130	b	b
Virginia	u	6,880	u	4,656	3,987	864	u	1,900	u	u	990	u
Washington	u	u	u	4,806	536	1,968	u	u	u	u	u	u
West Virginia	(3,780)	250	u	2,663	161	5	(530)	50	u	(590)	40	u
Wisconsin	6,560	2,640	1,210	3,960	1,656	867	1,640	590	150	960	390	190
Wyoming	u	10	u	632	12	126	‡	‡	u	u	u	u

From Guttmacher Institute. *U.S. teenage pregnancy statistics, National and state trends and trends by race and ethnicity.* New York: Guttmacher Institute, 2006. <http://www.guttmacher.org/pubs/2006/09/12/USTPstats.pdf>. Accessed November 13, 2005.

u = unavailable.

Numbers of pregnancies include estimates of the numbers of miscarriages and stillbirths. Numbers of pregnancies and abortions in parentheses include abortions obtained by Hispanic women; in these states ≤10% of births to white women aged 15–19 years were to Hispanics. Even though abortions have been tabulated according to state of residence where possible, in states with parental notification or consent requirements for minors, the number of abortions and pregnancies may be too low because minors have traveled to other states for abortion services.

[a] Rounded to the nearest 10.

[b] <5 abortions.

TABLE 41.2

Reported Sexual Activity by Age and Race for Adolescents Aged 15 to 19 Years

Race	Sexually Experienced (%)
White	
Total surveyed	45.1
15- to 17-year-old teens	44.7
Black	
Total surveyed	71.2
15- to 17-year-old teens	67.2
Latinos	
Total surveyed	54.1
15- to 17-year-old teens	48.1

From Santelli JS, Lindberg LD, Abma J, et al. Adolescent sexual behavior: estimates and trends from four nationally representative surveys. *Fam Plann Perspect* 2000;32:156, with permission.

Jacobson, 2001; Cox et al., 1995b). In this regard, many adolescents live in communities familiar with adolescent parenthood, so they are less likely to postpone sexual intercourse. Adolescents who live in families with little parental support, little restriction of risky behaviors, and poorly defined goals are more likely to become sexually active and are more likely to become adolescent parents. Other cultural factors that may play a role in an adolescent's decision to become pregnant include peer pressure, early dating, and lack of religious affiliation.

5. Psychological factors: Although psychological factors, such as depression, may have some influence on an adolescent's decision to become pregnant, the role of psychological and behavioral antecedents is unclear. Other risky behaviors may be associated with sexual activity. The YRBS revealed that overall 23% of adolescents used alcohol or drugs when having sex (Centers for Disease Control and Prevention, 2006).

6. Early puberty: Since the turn of the century, the average age at onset of menarche has decreased approximately 3 months per decade from approximately 16 to 17 years in the late 19th century to 12.4 years at present (Jaskiewicz and McAnarney, 1994). This earlier physical maturation has widened the gap between reproductive capacity and cognitive and emotional maturation and has increased the risk of unintended pregnancy in this age-group.

7. Developmental issues: Many developmental characteristics of adolescents, particularly of younger teens, interfere with decision making regarding sexual activity and the successful use of contraceptives. These include a limited ability to plan for the future or to foresee the consequences of their actions and a sense of personal invulnerability (Weinberger et al., 2005).

8. Barriers to contraceptive use: Many environmental, social, and psychological barriers interfere with decision making regarding sexual activity and contraception among teens. Significant obstacles to successful contraception include the following:
   a. Inaccurate information: Many teens have misinformation regarding conception and reproduction. Among other myths, many mistakenly believe that they are too young to become pregnant or that

pregnancy cannot occur the first time they have intercourse.
   b. Accessibility: Many young people want to prevent pregnancy but are unable to because of following factors:
      • They lack information regarding available methods.
      • They do not know about their legal rights to health care.
      • They do not know where to obtain contraceptives.
      • They have concerns regarding confidentiality.
      • They have concerns regarding cost.
      • Services are not readily accessible.
   c. Contraceptive acceptability: Teens may seek out contraceptive services but often have the following reservations:
      • Fearful of specific methods and perceived side effects (particularly the possibility of cancer and weight gain they assume to be associated with oral contraceptives)
      • Concerned about contraceptive use affecting their future fertility
      • Embarrassed over the acquisition or use of the method
      • Concerned that the method might interfere with pleasure
   d. Partner issues: Many young people are interested in contraception but are often unable to discuss contraception with their partners or their partners refuse to use available methods. Females with significantly older male partners are much less likely to use contraception at last intercourse.
   e. Intended pregnancy: Some young women do not protect themselves from pregnancy because of a desire to have a baby. This desire may emerge from the following needs:
      • To solidify their relationship with their partner or please their partner
      • Have someone to love and take care of
      • Change their status in their family or assert their independence
      • To escape from an abusive home environment by creating their own new family
      • To establish their fertility
   f. Provider problems: Acquiring contraceptive services can be difficult for young people because of the following:
      • Clinicians may not address sexuality and contraceptive use with their adolescent patients, who may be too embarrassed to initiate the discussion.
      • Some providers are unwilling to prescribe contraceptives for their patients without parental knowledge or consent.
      • Some providers are overtly judgmental about sexual activity among their young patients, which discourages discussion of sexual involvement and prohibits dispensing of appropriate education and birth control methods.

TEEN PREGNANCY PREVENTION INTERVENTIONS

Both primary (first pregnancy) and secondary (repeat pregnancy) interventions have been created and evaluated. The program designs are varied and may be developed by parents, schools, physicians, religious groups, social agencies, and government departments. Successful programs include elements of abstinence promotion, contraceptive information/availability, sexual education, education/school completion strategies, job training, and other youth development strategies such as volunteerism, and involvement in arts or sports. Research strongly supports a two-pronged approach to primary prevention by using methods to delay sexual initiation and by providing contraceptive education and availability if necessary. No research exists that links contraceptive education with increased sexual activity (Kirby, 2001).

EVALUATION AND MANAGEMENT OF THE PREGNANT ADOLESCENT

When an adolescent presents to a health care facility for reproductive health services or advice, it is important to provide an environment that is welcoming and comfortable for young people. The providers in such facilities must be comfortable with adolescents, and familiar with the common presentations and the initial management of adolescent pregnancy.

Role of the Practitioner

Pregnancy in an adolescent can be a crisis for the teen and her family. The provider is in a unique position to offer guidance and support during this time. This health issue requires the provider to give balanced attention to the pregnant adolescent's medical issues and her counseling needs. The teen should be granted confidentiality as they discuss choices and plans. It is vital that the practitioner be familiar with their state's laws on adolescent confidentiality as they vary considerably from state to state (English and Kenney, 2003). In ideal circumstances, the adolescent's family and her partner need to be considered as a plan is formulated to manage the pregnancy. However, the practitioner must ascertain whether there has been sexual coercion, history of physical abuse, or potential for abuse. The practitioner's intervention is recommended in the following:

1. Diagnosis of pregnancy and facilitated decision making
2. Open, nonjudgmental service planning
3. Management of pregnancy, if the teen chooses to continue the pregnancy
4. Preparation for parenthood, if the teen chooses to raise the child
5. Referrals for subspecialty services, as needed
6. Support if the teen chooses adoption
7. Family planning and safe-sex education

Open, nonjudgmental service planning is critical. Despite a provider's personal preferences, the provider needs to counsel the adolescent about her options or refer to a provider who is comfortable with counseling pregnant adolescents. Appropriate referrals for care should be made for adolescents needing services that are not available within the provider's own health program. Timely referrals are important, because some of the choices are only available during the early weeks of the pregnancy.

Common Presentations of Pregnancy in Adolescents

Adolescents may present with various complaints that may suggest early pregnancy. The most frequent objective concern is a missed or an abnormal menstrual period. Others may report abdominal pain, fatigue, breast tenderness, vomiting, or appetite changes. Adolescents with such concerns should be questioned about sexual activity, contraceptive use, and desire for a pregnancy test. Adolescents may need extra time to discuss their concerns and any fears that they may have about a possible pregnancy. A flexible approach can allow adolescents to make healthy decisions for their particular situation.

Pregnancy Tests

The development of very sensitive and specific pregnancy tests has significantly facilitated the diagnosis of early pregnancy. Pregnancy tests measure levels of human chorionic gonadotropin (hCG), a glycoprotein that is secreted by invasive cytotrophoblast cells in early pregnancy and implantation. The most sensitive pregnancy test is a radioimmunoassay (RIA) that detects serum levels of the β subunit of hCG as low as 7 mIU/mL. Most urine pregnancy tests will detect hCG when levels exceed 25 mIU/mL, thereby giving a positive test result around the first missed menstrual period. The ease of use, low cost, and high degree of accuracy make the urine pregnancy test an essential component of any adolescent health program.

1. hCG levels during pregnancy: It is important for the practitioner to remember that hCG levels change significantly during the course of pregnancy and that the results must be interpreted on the basis of the particular test used (sensitivity and specificity). Serum hCG is detectable 8 days after conception in approximately 5% of women and by day 11 in >98% of women. At 4 weeks of gestation, serum hCG doubling times are approximately 2.2 days, but only every 3.5 days by 9 weeks of gestation. Levels peak at 10 to 12 weeks of gestation and then decline rapidly until a slower rise begins at 22 weeks of gestation, which continues until term.
   a. Abnormally elevated levels can indicate either a multiple-gestation pregnancy or a molar pregnancy. Anticonvulsants, phenothiazine, and promethazine may increase serum hCG levels.
   b. Abnormally low levels can indicate a spontaneous abortion or ectopic pregnancy. Low levels may also indicate delayed ovulation or implantation. Diuretics and promethazine can decrease hCG levels.
2. hCG levels after pregnancy: Levels gradually decrease after a delivery or abortion and the initial decrease is quite rapid. After 2 weeks, the serum hCG level should be <1% of the level when the pregnancy was terminated.
   a. Term delivery: Levels should drop to <50 mIU/mL by 2 weeks—undetectable by 3 to 4 weeks.
   b. First-trimester abortion: Initial hCG levels are much higher. If the abortion is at 8 to 10 weeks and initial hCG levels are >150,000 mIU, then levels at 2 weeks can be 1,500 mIU/mL and detectable for 8 to 9 weeks.
3. Types of pregnancy kits
   a. Immunometric tests: These tests are based on enzyme-linked immunosorbent assay (ELISA) techniques that identify two different antibodies for hCG, making these tests specific for the β subunit of hCG.

There is no cross-reactivity with other hormones. The urine test kits usually provide accurate qualitative response within 5 to 15 minutes and measure hCG levels as low as 5 to 50 mIU/mL. This can provide positive test results as soon as 10 days after fertilization. These are the most common tests used in most family planning, teen clinics, and women's health clinics. Examples of such tests include Hybritech ICON II, Abbott TestPack +Plus hCG COMBO, Quidel Quick-Vue Semi-Q hCG Combo Test, and Quadratech Q-b HS Dipstrip Check-4 Pregnancy Test.

b. Home pregnancy testing (HPT): HPTs are popular because they are convenient, quick, and very confidential. Seventeen percent of college women report that they have used a urine home test at least once. The actual accuracy of home tests is not ideal. HPTs are commonly used in the week after the missed menstrual period. During this period of pregnancy, urine hCG values are extremely variable and can range from 12 mIU/mL to >2,500 mIU/mL. This variability continues through the fifth week, when values range from 13 mIU/mL to >6,000 mIU/mL. A percentage of urine hCG values during the fourth and fifth weeks are below the sensitivities of detection for common HPTs (range 25–100 mIU/mL). Problems with technique and following instructions may cause inaccurate results. A common error is to perform the home test too early. Therefore, it is important not to make clinical decisions based on a home pregnancy test result (Cole et al., 2004).

c. Quantitative β-hCG RIA: This highly sensitive test for specific levels of serum hCG takes 4 hours to complete and is positive 10 to 18 days postconception. However, it has no advantage over the immunometric urine tests for the regular clinical setting. The serum test is expensive. The major use is in identifying an abnormal pregnancy such as ectopic pregnancy, trophoblastic disease, or threatened miscarriage by checking either the doubling time or hCG disappearance over time.

4. False-positive and false-negative results
   a. False-negative hCG test results most often involve urine and are due to misreading or interpretation of color changes. Reasons for a negative test result may include an hCG concentration below the sensitivity threshold of the specific test being used, a miscalculation of last menstrual period (LMP), delayed ovulation, or delayed menses from early pregnancy loss. Elevated lipid and immunoglobulin levels, and low serum protein levels can interfere with the serum test.
   b. False-positive test results with immunometric tests are very rare but can also occur with laboratory error. Very rarely, pregnancy test results are positive due to hCG production from a nonpregnancy source such as tumors of the ovaries, breast, and pancreas. For this reason, clinical correlation with the laboratory finding is essential. Should the laboratory result be inconsistent with the clinical presentation, it is imperative that the provider verify the pregnancy test, using the more sensitive tests available (Braunstein, 2002).

5. The physical examination is also an essential element of the evaluation of the pregnant adolescent. Although the pregnancy test will determine whether the adolescent is pregnant, the pelvic examination will help determine the gestational age of the fetus and will identify any problems that may require immediate attention.

6. Uterine enlargement: Uterine enlargement usually indicates the following:
   a. 8 weeks of gestation: Uterine enlargement detected
   b. 12 weeks of gestation: Uterus palpated at symphysis pubis
   c. 20 weeks of gestation: Fundal height at umbilicus. At this point in the pregnancy, fetal movements should be detected, and fetal heart sounds should be audible by Doppler study.

7. Other signs
   a. Softening of the cervix
   b. Discoloration of the cervix (it may appear purple or hyperemic)
   c. Uterine softness

   Should vaginal bleeding be present or abdominal pain be elicited, it suggests pregnancy complications, such as a threatened abortion or an ectopic pregnancy.

Ascertaining the Gestational Age

Most adolescents will want to know the gestational age of the fetus. Providers should be careful to determine the LMP that was normal. This can be accomplished by asking careful questions of the adolescent regarding their cycles, including any lighter than normal cycles that may represent implantation. Those having regular cycles lasting approximately 28 days are best able to predict the gestational age, which is calculated by counting the weeks since the LMP. A pregnancy wheel can be very helpful for calculating gestational age by dates.

The expected date of delivery (also called the expected date of confinement) can be obtained from the pregnancy wheel or is estimated using the Nägele rule. Add 7 days to the first day of the LMP, subtract 3 months from the month of the LMP, and add 1 year to the calculated date. Physical findings can also be used to estimate gestational age by size as indicated earlier. An ultrasonography will also predict gestational age, although this test has a margin of error of 1 week. If the uterus is smaller than expected by menstrual dates, considerations include error in pregnancy test, ectopic pregnancy, incomplete or missed spontaneous abortion, and fertilization that occurred later than dates suggest. If the uterus is larger than expected, considerations include twins, uterine fibroids, uterine anomaly, hydatidiform mole, or fertilization that occurred earlier than dates suggested.

ALTERNATIVES FOR PREGNANT ADOLESCENTS AND PREGNANCY COUNSELING

Counseling the pregnant adolescent about her pregnancy options is perhaps the most important aspect of early pregnancy management. Providers who offer pregnancy tests should be prepared to provide such counseling and medical assessment including pelvic examination for confirmation of gestational age of the fetus, sexually transmitted disease (STD) screening, and multivitamins prescription with folate supplementation.

Critical elements of counseling the pregnant adolescent include the following:

1. An assessment of the adolescent's expectations and desires regarding the possible pregnancy. It is to initiate

this discussion in a private setting, when the provider is alone with the adolescent patient. Some adolescents are very anxious and emotional, whereas others are calm and have begun to formulate a plan for a possible pregnancy. A preliminary assessment of any stressors or safety concerns is useful while counseling the adolescent about her test results. A private discussion allows the provider to offer counseling without distractions, and it permits the provider to consider the adolescent independent of others who are involved with the pregnancy (Klein et al., 2005).

2. Support of the partner or concerned adult: The adolescent may be accompanied by a partner or by a concerned adult. In such instances, a provider should offer the patient the choice of including this person during a part of the pregnancy counseling session. If the pregnancy test result is positive, adolescents should be encouraged to seek the support of elders (e.g., parents, grandparents, or other trusted adult). These adults will likely form a "core of support" for the adolescent, should she elect to carry the pregnancy to term or decide to terminate the pregnancy. The adolescent's partner may also share in the decision-making process. It is vital, however, to screen the adolescent for safety in both their relationship and family domains.

3. Confidentiality: Adolescents are entitled to confidentiality, although family members sometimes disagree. Adolescents should be reminded that any discussions (in a health facility) remain confidential, unless the adolescent wishes to inform or include others. This allows the adolescent to make her own choices regarding disclosure of the pregnancy. Occasionally, there are mental health concerns, such as the threat of suicide or homicide, or there is a threat of abuse. In such cases, it will be necessary to share information about the pregnancy with other health professionals and with the adolescent's adult caretakers (parents or guardians). The practitioners should familiarize themselves with the medical confidentiality laws of their state particularly in regard to statutory rape, parental consent for termination, and guidelines for judicial bypass (English and Kenney, 2003).

4. Nonjudgmental approach: The provider needs to give the opportunity for open discussion when counseling an adolescent about a positive pregnancy test result. The provider should allow the adolescent to express her wishes for this pregnancy, without imposing the provider's personal values on the teenager. A provider who is nonjudgmental will enhance the adolescent's ability to identify the pregnancy option that is most appropriate for the adolescent. Appropriate referrals should be available from the provider that will assist the adolescent in achieving her desired pregnancy outcome.

5. Presenting options: The adolescent needs to consider many options for this pregnancy, which include the following:
   a. Carrying the pregnancy to term and assuming parental responsibility
   b. Family-centered care for the adolescent and her new baby, thereby sharing child-care responsibility among the baby's extended family
   c. Placing the baby with adoptive parents after the baby is born
   d. Terminating the pregnancy (e.g., induced abortion)

Adolescents Assuming Parental Responsibility

This is the most common outcome for pregnant adolescents, yet it is, in many respects, the most difficult commitment to fulfill, because it requires the adolescent to assume long-term responsibility for a baby. A comprehensive care program that is designed to address the health and social needs of pregnant adolescents will offer the adolescent the best opportunity for a good outcome. Essential elements for adolescent-focused prenatal programs include a complement of medical, psychological, social, and educational services; staff knowledgeable in adolescent health; services that are culturally sensitive; continuity of care through the postpartum period; and linkages to mother-infant programs (Cox et al., 2005).

Family-Centered Care for the Adolescent and the Newborn

Because adolescents are rarely able to assume independence after the birth of a baby, the adolescent's family (or community) will usually offer support to the young mother and her child. This allows the adolescent more flexibility and more options for personal development; however, it requires that she abdicate a significant amount of parental responsibility to other family members. Arrangements are unpredictable but may provide (financial and social) stability for the adolescent and the baby. Providers who care for the adolescent parent will need to be linked to community-based services for extended families. Specialized adolescent health services are an essential component of these health programs that reach out to adolescent parents. Such programs offer counseling, health awareness, and parenting classes, in addition to medical care and family planning (Woods et al., 2003). However, long-term continuous relationships with caring providers are essential to positive outcomes (Klerman, 2004).

Adoption after Delivery

Most adolescents who continue their pregnancy intend to raise their baby, although few will express an interest in placing their child in a home with adoptive parents. Few adolescents consider this option at the time that the pregnancy test is obtained, although it is important that the pregnant adolescent be counseled about this option. In most states and the District of Columbia, mothers who are minors may legally place their child for adoption without parental involvement. Fewer than 10% of the babies born to unmarried teens are placed in adoptive homes. Unmarried teen mothers who place their children for adoption are more likely to be white, have higher socioeconomic status and educational aspirations, and be from suburban residences (Mosher and Bachrach, 1996).

Terminating the Pregnancy

Unintended pregnancies account for >90% of pregnancies in 15- to 19-year-olds. Adolescents represent 19% of the approximately 1.3 million abortions that occur each year in the United States. More than half of unintended adolescent pregnancies end in induced or spontaneous abortion compared with 35% of adult pregnancies. The rate of abortions in the United States has consistently declined across all age-groups since 1990 with a 24% decline in adolescents younger than 20 years.

There are many possible explanations for this trend, such as a decline in the availability and accessibility of abortions nationwide. A recent study showed lower abortion rates in low-density population areas when compared to high-density urban areas (Barbieri, 2004). Abortion is a service that is frequently offered in free-standing clinics that are separate from the more traditional, primary health care programs. Therefore, a referral to another facility is generally required for this procedure. Some adolescents lack the skills to negotiate health services in a health facility that is new to them. This may result in a delay in obtaining an abortion, or the adolescent may fail to have the abortion because she is not timely with her preparations (Cates et al., 2000; Jones et al., 2002).

Providers of patients who seek an abortion should be aware that careful follow-up and psychological support is needed while the adolescent explores this option. Providers need to be open minded and respectful of the adolescent's wishes in such circumstances. Adolescents will also need the support of loved ones who are familiar with the adolescent, such as a parent, an older sibling, or other adult relative. Sixty-one percent of minors who have abortions do so with at least one parent having knowledge of the abortion. Most parents appear to support their daughter's decision to have an abortion (Henshaw and Kost, 1992).

Health care providers should be aware of their state's laws governing adolescents who seek abortion services. Many states require that parents of adolescents play an active role in securing an abortion for their daughter. Careful attention to legal considerations, including the rights of parents, will be important as the provider advocates for the adolescent. Any financial barriers that may interfere with the adolescent's ability to obtain the abortion should also be reviewed.

Adolescents who are certain about their decision to terminate the pregnancy should be encouraged to do so in the early stages of the pregnancy. This will minimize both the complications and the costs of the procedure. Most induced abortions are frequently performed within 8 weeks of conception. Delays will increase the cost, both financial and psychological, for the adolescent and her family.

After a teen has decided to end her pregnancy, she may need help in selecting the best method. There are more options for those who have earlier terminations but adolescents may delay abortion until later than 15 weeks. Methods in the first 12 weeks include vacuum aspiration, curettage, and medical terminations with either methotrexate-misoprostol or mifepristone-misoprostol. Between 12 and 24 weeks, methods include dilation and evacuation, amnioinfusion, and uterotonic/hypertonic techniques. Most teens have a first-trimester abortion and decide between a medical or surgical method.

Choice of Medical versus Surgical Early Abortion Methods

Medical Method

Advantages of the medical method are that it avoids surgery and anesthesia, is less painful, may be easier emotionally, provides the girl with more control, is a more private process, and has less risk of infection.

Disadvantages include bleeding, cramping and nausea, more waiting and uncertainty, extra clinic visit, limited to pregnancies up to 7 to 9 weeks, and risk of methotrexate-induced birth defects if abortion is incomplete.

Types of Medical Methods

First trimester Two new methods in United States include (1) mifepristone (RU-486) with misoprostol or (2) methotrexate with misoprostol.

1. Mifepristone-misoprostol: Mifepristone is a progesterone antagonist that is an effective abortifacient. The efficacy increases with the addition of a prostaglandin analog such as misoprostol. The earlier in pregnancy that these are used, the higher the efficacy. In women with pregnancies <7 weeks, approximately 95% have a complete abortion. This decreases to approximately 80% in the ninth week. Bleeding and cramping are common with the method, because the drugs' actions are to induce uterine cramping and bleeding. The technique involves at least three visits:
   First visit: Mifepristone 600 mg
   Two days later: Misoprostol dose. Some abortions are complete before this visit. If not, two 200-µg tablets are given orally. In those who have not aborted, two thirds occur within 4 hours of the prostaglandin administration.
   Two weeks later: Checkup to ensure completed abortion. Complications include incomplete abortion and heavy bleeding. There are also infection risks. A recent study reported four deaths from toxic shock syndrome and *Clostridium sordellii* following medical abortion (Fischer et al., 2005).
2. Methotrexate and misoprostol: Methotrexate is a cytotoxic drug that is lethal to trophoblastic tissue and is an abortive agent. When used with misoprostol, the combination is approximately 95% successful in terminating early pregnancies. These regimens involve off-label use of the drug. Several protocols have been developed and all involve at least two clinic visits. Similar to the mifepristone technique, the first visit involves administration of methotrexate. The misoprostol is sometimes given for self-administration at home or at a return visit. There is then a follow-up visit to confirm the termination of pregnancy. Complications include incomplete abortion, infection, and heavy bleeding.

Any clinic or clinician contemplating medical terminations of pregnancy must have availability of both ultrasound dating of pregnancies and surgical backup for incomplete abortions.

Surgical Method

Advantages to using the surgical method are—quicker (one visit); more certain; teen can be less involved; can be done under general anesthesia; and continuation of pregnancy is rare.

Disadvantages include invasiveness (need for local or general anesthesia) and small risk of uterine or cervical injury or infection.

Types of Surgical Methods

In the United States, surgical methods are the most common method of termination of pregnancy.

1. Vacuum aspiration
   a. The most widely used and standard first-trimester surgical method

  b. Relatively simple technique requiring small cervical dilation
  c. May be performed with local anesthesia
  d. Can be done in an office for up to 14 weeks' gestation.
2. Dilation and evacuation
  a. Most common second-trimester method of abortion.
  b. Requires more dilation than the aspiration method. Laminaria or other osmotic dilators are often inserted before the procedure to gradually dilate the cervix. This may be a 1- to 2-day procedure.
  c. Is commonly used for procedures between 13 and 16 weeks, although many clinicians use this procedure up through 20-plus weeks.
  d. Paracervical or general anesthesia is used before evacuating the uterus.

Second trimester Medical techniques for second-trimester abortions include hypertonic saline instillation, hypertonic urea instillation, and prostaglandin E_2 suppository insertion. These techniques account for less than 1% of all abortions in the United States. Most have been replaced by dilation and evacuation procedures, which are faster, safer, and less expensive.

Abortion Risks and Complications
Short-term
1. Infection (up to 3%): This can be minimized by prior diagnosis and treatment of gonorrhea and chlamydia, as well as by the use of prophylactic antibiotics. Infection due to retained products of conception requires antibiotic treatment and an additional procedure.
2. Intrauterine blood clots (<1%)
3. Cervical or uterine trauma: Women younger than 17 years have an increased risk of cervical injury. Use of laminaria and skillful technique lowers the risk.
4. Bleeding (0.03%–1%)
5. Failed abortion (0.5%–1%)

The mortality rate is <1 per 100,000 abortions.

Long-term Postabortion Complications
1. Medical: Data relating to long-term complications of abortion do not show major risks. First-trimester abortion with vacuum aspiration does not appear to affect fertility rates or cause future spontaneous abortions.
2. Psychological: Although some studies report that teens may consider abortion to be a stressful experience, these symptoms are often short lived and can be mitigated with support before, during, and after the procedure (Biro et al., 1986). In a prospective study of 360 black teenage women from urban family planning clinics, Zabin et al. (1989) found that those adolescents having a therapeutic abortion were more likely to remain in school and were better off economically than those continuing their pregnancy or those having a negative pregnancy test result. Those teens terminating their pregnancy experienced no greater levels of stress or anxiety and were no more likely to have psychological problems 2 years later. The teens obtaining an abortion were also less likely to experience a subsequent pregnancy than either of the other two groups.

MEDICAL MANAGEMENT OF THE PREGNANT ADOLESCENT

Pregnant adolescents, because of increased maternal and fetal risks, require special prenatal management. Prenatal care is a major factor predicting a positive outcome for a teen birth. In 2003, 6.4% of all teens received late or no prenatal care (Martin et al., 2005). Factors associated with adequate teen prenatal care are increased age, a longer interpregnancy interval, partner/social support, and participation in a specialized adolescent pregnancy program. These programs often include a multidisciplinary team of medicine, social work, nursing, and nutrition. Practitioners should note that teens are at risk for inadequate care, so they should make special efforts to ensure early linkages with prenatal providers. Following is a brief guide for the practitioner in important areas of prenatal care for the adolescent patient.

1. Initial evaluation: Should include a thorough history, including both a family history of chronic illness and a personal medical history. A drug history for tobacco, alcohol, and substance use is important. A thorough and sensitive discussion regarding the pregnant teen's and her partner's risk for human immunodeficiency virus (HIV) infection should be initiated. Because of young people's reluctance to disclose sensitive information during an initial visit, practitioners should continue to assess a teen's risk status throughout her pregnancy. A complete physical examination and pelvic examination should be performed. Laboratory evaluation should include the following:
   a. Complete blood cell count
   b. Urinalysis
   c. Blood type and group
   d. Screening syphilis serology
   e. Sickle cell test in black patients
   f. Test for Tay-Sachs disease for Mediterranean or Jewish heritage
   g. Rubella titer
   h. Pap smear if they have been sexually active for 3 years
   i. Gonococcal and Chlamydia test
   j. Hepatitis B serology
   k. HIV antibody counseling and testing
2. Topics to be covered on successive visits
   a. Physiology of pregnancy
   b. Maternal nutrition
   c. Substance abuse
   d. STDs and HIV infection
   e. Discussion and referral to a prepared childbirth class
   f. Childbirth
   g. Breast feeding and infant nutrition
   h. Infant care and infant development
   i. Contraception and sexuality
   j. Postdelivery care needs
3. Nutrition
   a. Ideal weight gain should be 25 to 40 lb.
   b. See Chapter 6 for specific changes in daily requirements during pregnancy.
   c. The teen should be advised against dieting during pregnancy.
   d. A prenatal vitamin supplement should be prescribed.
   e. Additional iron is required if iron deficiency is diagnosed.

f. Adolescents consuming <1,000 mg/day of calcium should be given a calcium supplement.

4. Prenatal visits: Pregnant adolescents should have visits every 2 to 4 weeks, through the seventh month. Visits are every 2 weeks in the eighth month, and weekly thereafter.

5. Psychosocial aspects: It is essential to consider that the pregnant teenager's acceptance of the pregnancy and her relationship with her parents or the father of the child may change during the course of the pregnancy. Several studies have demonstrated increased risk for domestic violence during teen pregnancy. It is important to monitor the teen's psychosocial needs and to intervene appropriately.

6. Substance abuse: Because of the serious consequences of substance use for both mother and infant, a thorough assessment of drug use history and current practices is necessary at pregnancy diagnosis and throughout the prenatal period. One large epidemiological study found that adolescents were more likely than adult women to stop alcohol and drug use once pregnancy was confirmed. The following is a list of common substances and their effects during pregnancy.

a. Alcohol: Fetal alcohol syndrome including prenatal and postnatal growth retardation; facial dysmorphogenesis (microcephaly, short palpebral fissures, cleft palate, and micrognathia); abnormalities of the central nervous system (CNS); and increased risk of cardiac defects, joint abnormalities, hepatic fibrosis, mental retardation, and learning difficulties

b. Amphetamines: May cause malformations

c. Cocaine: Increased risk of spontaneous abortion and premature delivery; neurobehavioral deficits in the newborn; increased prevalence of abruptio placentae; increased risk of genital and urinary tract defects including prune belly syndrome, hypospadias, and hydronephrosis

d. Heroin: Intrauterine growth retardation; neonatal abstinence syndrome (infant irritability, tremor, convulsions, or poor feeding due to heroin withdrawal); increased risk of hepatitis, HIV, and other infections in the mother

e. Lysergic acid diethylamide: Increased risk of congenital abnormalities including hydrocephalus, spina bifida, and myelomeningocele

f. Marijuana: Questionable increased risk of birth defects

g. Nicotine: Impaired growth; increased risk of spontaneous abortion

7. Medications and pregnancy: Medication should be avoided when possible during pregnancy. The following is a list of commonly used drugs and their effects during pregnancy.

a. Adrenocortical steroids: Low incidence of cleft palate suspected

b. Amphetamines: May cause malformations

c. Angiotensin-converting enzyme inhibitors: Prolonged renal failure in neonates, decreased skull ossification, renal tubular dysgenesis

d. Anticholinergic drugs: Neonatal meconium ileus

e. Antacids: May cause malformations; avoid in early pregnancy

f. Antibiotics
   • Acyclovir: Safety unknown; use only under strong indications
   • Aminoglycosides: Possible eighth nerve toxicity in fetus
   • Cephalosporins: Probably safe
   • Clindamycin: None known; caution advised
   • Erythromycin: Considered safe
   • Erythromycin estolate: Risk of cholestatic hepatitis in mother; avoid during pregnancy
   • Isoniazid: Embryotoxic in animals; caution advised
   • Metronidazole: May affect chromosomes; avoid during pregnancy if possible, particularly in first trimester
   • Penicillins: Considered safe
   • Sulfonamides: Hemolysis in newborns with glucose-6-phosphate dehydrogenase deficiency and increased risk of kernicterus in newborns; avoid at term
   • Tetracycline: Congenital limb abnormalities, cataracts, decreased bone growth, discoloration of fetal teeth; avoid during pregnancy
   • Trimethoprim: Folate antagonist; avoid during pregnancy

g. Anticonvulsants
   • Carbamazepine (Tegretol): Neural tube defects, questionable association with facial dysmorphism, hypoplasia of fingers or toenails, bifida and congenital heart disease
   • Diazepam (Valium): Possible risk of cleft lip without cleft palate
   • Ethosuximide (Zarontin): Low teratogenic potential
   • Phenobarbital: Possible increase in learning difficulties
   • Phenytoin (Dilantin): Developmental disturbances appear less than previously reported and anomalies may be genetically linked to epilepsy; hypertelorism and digital hypoplasia reported in higher frequency with use of phenytoin; other problems are more questionable, including intrauterine growth retardation, mental retardation, and developmental delay; craniofacial abnormalities including depressed nasal bridge, ptosis, inner epicanthal folds, and ocular hypertelorism; limb abnormalities (digital and limb hypoplasia); cardiac defects; and hernias
   • Valproic acid: Teratogenic in rodents; increased risk of spina bifida if used in first trimester. It also appears that valproate may be related to a significant amount of mental retardation in children born to mothers using the medications during pregnancy as well as other pregnancy complications.

h. Antidepressants: The American Academy of Pediatrics' Committee on Drugs recommends careful assessment of the indications for use of psychoactive drugs during pregnancy. Specifically, selective serotonin uptake inhibitors (Prozac, Effexor, Wellbutrin) may be associated with a small increased risk for minor anatomical abnormalities. However, rapid withdrawal can have negative consequences physically and psychologically (Kulig, 2005).

i. Antihistamines
   • Fexofenadine has not been adequately studied in pregnant women.
   • Diphenhydramine and cetirizine are class B drugs with no known complications during pregnancy.

j. Antithyroid drugs: Fetal and neonatal goiter and hypothyroidism, aplasia cutis (with methimazole)

k. Aspirin: Association with hydrocephalus, congenital heart disease, and hip dislocation; conflicting reports

l. Albuterol: No current evidence of abnormalities

m. Hypoglycemic drugs: Neonatal hypoglycemia

n. Lithium: Ebstein anomaly

o. Misoprostol: Moebius sequence

p. Nonsteroidal antiinflammatory drugs: Constriction of the ductus arteriosus, necrotizing enterocolitis

q. Phenothiazines: Cleft palate, hypospadias, microcephaly, syndactyly, cardiac malformations, club foot

r. Retinoic acid: Severe teratogenic effects causing craniofacial, cardiac, and thymic malformations

s. Warfarin: Skeletal and CNS defects, Dandy-Walker syndrome

8. The chronically ill adolescent: Pregnancy in chronically ill adolescents presents specific challenges and requires coordination with their specialty care providers. Each illness is associated with specific risks.

9. HIV disease: Practitioners should offer HIV counseling and testing to all pregnant teens. Education regarding the risks of perinatal transmission should also be provided. Pregnant women infected with HIV should be referred for appropriate treatment and supportive services. Some women found to be infected may choose to terminate their pregnancy once their HIV status is known. Others will want access to specialized care designed to manage their infection and reduce their risk of perinatal transmission. Because of the risks of HIV transmission through breast milk, breast feeding is not recommended for HIV-infected mothers.

10. Battering: Battering often starts or becomes worse during pregnancy. Prenatal risk assessment should include specific questions regarding family and partner violence. Practitioners must be knowledgeable about domestic violence–reporting laws in their state and should be familiar with community resources.

MEDICAL COMPLICATIONS OF PREGNANCY IN ADOLESCENCE

Adolescents are not at a higher risk of developing complications during early pregnancy.

1. Spontaneous abortion: As with adults, a spontaneous abortion may occur in 20% of pregnancies. A spontaneous abortion occurring in the first 20 weeks of pregnancy usually results from abnormal chromosomal development in the fetus or abnormalities of the pelvic structure in the adolescent.

   Abdominal cramping and vaginal bleeding characterize the early stages of a miscarriage, or a spontaneous abortion. The term threatened abortion refers to pregnancies complicated by bleeding and cramping, but the cervix remains long and closed. Should the condition progress, the pregnancy is nonviable and an abortion is considered "inevitable." Physical changes include a widening of the cervical os and an increase in the bleeding and cramping. A "complete abortion" occurs when all the products of conception have passed. A sonogram will confirm the absence of the fetus, and physical examination will show that cervical os is closed. If the

miscarriage is considered an incomplete abortion, a dilation and evacuation procedure will be necessary to prevent blood loss and infection.

2. Ectopic pregnancy: Abdominal cramping and bleeding also suggest an ectopic, or extrauterine, pregnancy. An ectopic pregnancy occurs in only 2% of all pregnancies (see Chapter 56).

3. Hydatidiform mole, or gestational trophoblastic disease, may occur in 1 of 1,000 pregnancies each year. Although adolescents commonly experience vaginal bleeding and abdominal cramping with a problem pregnancy, those with a hydatidiform mole usually have severe and profuse bleeding. The uterus is larger than expected given the estimated gestational age of the fetus, and the hCG levels are very high. The hCG levels are often >100,000 mIU/mL. Ultrasonogram of the uterus demonstrates the characteristic cluster of grapes appearance of the mass.

An immediate procedure is needed to terminate a molar pregnancy. Treatment with dilation and suction is the treatment of choice, although the procedure is complicated because it places the patient at increased risk for severe hemorrhage. Close follow-up of the hCG level is required to ensure that the tumor has been adequately removed. The hCG level should remain <2 mIU/mL for 1 year. If the hCG level remains elevated, it suggests that the tumor has not been sufficiently removed; if the hCG level rises, it suggests the tumor has recurred. If the patient has persistent or recurrent disease, she should use a reliable method of contraception for the year after the diagnosis of trophoblastic disease.

OTHER CONSEQUENCES OF ADOLESCENT PREGNANCY

Child Outcomes

For teens older than 15 years, pregnancies do not have increased risk of adverse outcomes if they receive adequate prenatal care. However, for teens younger than 15 years, there are increased risks, independent of prenatal care, for prematurity, low birth weight, and mortality. Factors associated with pregnancy outcome are variations in prenatal care, nutritional status, prepregnancy weight, STD exposure, smoking, and substance use. Owing to these factors, adolescents are at doubled risk for low infant birth weight and tripled risk for neonatal death.

The children of teen mothers face significant challenges with risks of developmental delay, behavioral problems, school failure, mental health problems, and high-risk behaviors during adolescence. Sons are at increased risk for incarceration and teen fatherhood and daughters are at increased risk for pregnancy; thereby, continuing family cycles of teen pregnancy.

Growth and Development

Although some recent studies have suggested small potential decreases in hip bone mineralization and ultimate height in the very young pregnant adolescents, no definitive data suggest that adolescent pregnancy adversely affects growth and development. Young adolescents (e.g., those younger than 15 years) may not fully understand the long-term implications of childbirth, particularly in the early stages of the pregnancy.

Education

Fifty percent of adolescent mothers complete high school by 18 years of age, compared with 97% of adolescents who do not get pregnant before finishing high school. By age 35 to 39 years, 70% of adolescent mothers have high school degrees. Factors linked to higher educational attainment for adolescent mothers are race (blacks do better than whites), growing up in a smaller family, the presence of reading materials in the home, mother's employment, and higher parental educational level (Barnett et al., 2004).

Socioeconomic Issues

Teen parenthood is associated with socioeconomic disadvantage. Teen mothers are more likely to end up on welfare (80% receive assistance at some point in time). An estimated 50% of funds of the Temporary Assistance for Needy Families (TANF) budget is expended on families in which the mother was a teenager when her first child was born. As teenage mothers get older however, many move off public assistance. A recent follow-up study of teenage mothers found that a substantial majority finished high school, found regular employment, and achieved economic independence albeit with lower incomes than women who delayed childbearing into adulthood (Klerman, 2004).

Subsequent Childbirth

Repeat pregnancy is often targeted by adolescent parenting interventions because short interpregnancy intervals are associated with adverse pregnancy, neonatal, and child outcomes. The rate of second births to adolescent mothers has declined over the last decade. However, within 2 years, 10% to 40% of teen mothers become pregnant again. Protective factors against repeat adolescent pregnancy are older maternal age (>16 years), participation in a specialized adolescent parent program, use of effective contraception, school attendance, new sex partner, and avoidance of interpersonal violence (Klerman, 2004).

Male Adolescents as Fathers

Young fathers rarely receive the same degree of attention and support that is offered to adolescent mothers. Fathers may not be included in decisions regarding pregnancy options, they may not participate in prenatal or childbirth classes, and they may not establish a long-term supportive relationship with the mother of the child.

Whenever possible, the provider should attempt to discuss reproductive health issues with their male patients who are sexually active. This is easily done during health maintenance visits, but it should also be done during visits for evaluation of STDs. Asking the male patient about whether he has fathered a child is reasonable when he indicates that he is sexually active. Supportive counseling should be available to male adolescents who are actively involved with babies they have fathered and to male adolescents who have pregnant girlfriends (Anda et al., 2002).

WEB SITES

For Teenagers and Parents

http://www.teenpregnancy.org/. National Campaign to Prevent Teenage Pregnancy, contains a teen sub-site and youth online network.

http://www.siecus.org/pubs/fact/fact0010.html. Fact sheet from SIECUS on teenage pregnancy.

http://www.teenwire.com. On teen pregnancy.

http://www.plannedparenthood.org. General home page of Planned Parenthood that also includes information in Spanish.

http://www.noah-health.org/. Information on pregnancy from NOAH-Health has many other health issues, and available in Spanish.

For Health Professionals

http://www.cdc.gov/reproductivehealth/unintendedpregnancy/. CDC site on teenage pregnancy.

http://www.urban.org/family/invmales.html. From the Urban Institute: Involving males in preventing teen pregnancy.

http://aspe.hhs.gov/hsp/teenp/intro.htm. Department of Health and Human Services (DHHS), a national strategy to prevent teen pregnancy.

http://aspe.hhs.gov/hsp/teenp/. Annual report from the DHHS on teenage pregnancy.

http://www.hhs.gov/opa/titlexx/oapp.html. The DHHS Office of Adolescent Pregnancy Programs.

http://arhp.org. Web site of the American Association of Reproductive Health Professionals.

http://www.agi-usa.org/sections/adolescnts/php. Alan Guttmacher Institute (AGI) site with many pages on teenage pregnancy.

http://www.agi-usa.org/pubs/. AGI area on teen pregnancy.

http://www.guttmacher.org/pubs/state_pregnancy_trends.pdf. AGI pregnancy trends with state-by-state analysis.

http://www.agi-usa.org/pubs/or_teen_preg_decline.html. AGI on why teenage pregnancy rates are declining.

http://www.agi-usa.org/pubs/or_teen_preg_survey.html. AGI study on teenagers' pregnancy intentions and decisions.

http://www.socio.com/. The Data Archive on Adolescent Pregnancy and Pregnancy Prevention (DAAPPP). The DAAPPP was established by the U.S. Office of Population Affairs in 1982 as the repository for the best social science data on the incidence, prevalence, antecedents, and consequences of teenage pregnancy and family planning.

http://www.childtrends.org. Excellent research briefs and facts in at-a-glance sections.

http://www.nlm.nih.gov/medlineplus/teenagepregnancy.html. Excellent index of timely information, a bilingual site from the National Institutes of Health.

REFERENCES AND ADDITIONAL READINGS

Abma JC, Martinez GM, Mosher WD, et al. Teenagers in the United States: sexual activity, contraceptive use, and childbearing, 2002. National Center for Health Statistics. *Vital Health Stat* 2004:23(24):1.

Alan Guttmacher Institute. *Sex and America's teenagers.* New York: Alan Guttmacher Institute, 1994.

Alan Guttmacher Institute. *Why is teenage pregnancy declining? The roles of abstinence, sexual activity and contraceptive use. Occasional report.* New York, NY: Alan Guttmacher Institute, Available at: www.guttmacher.org/pubs/or_teen_preg_decline.pdf. Accessed November 13, 2005. 1999.

Alan Guttmacher Institute. *Teen pregnancy: trends and lessons learned.* Available at: www.guttmacher.org/pubs/tgr/05/1/gr050107. Accessed November 13, 2005. 2002.

Alan Guttmacher Institute. *U.S. teenage pregnancy statistics: overall trends by race and ethnicity and state-by-state information, 2004.* Accessed June 19, www.guttmacher.org/pubs/state_pregnancy_trends.pdf. 2005.

Alexander CS, Greyer B. Adolescent pregnancy occurrence and consequences. *Pediatr Ann* 1993;22:2.

American Academy of Pediatrics. Committee on adolescence adolescent pregnancy current trends and issues: 1998. *Pediatrics* 1999;103:516.

Anda RF, Chapman DP, Felitti VJ, et al. Adverse childhood experiences and risk of paternity in teen pregnancy. *Obstet Gynecol* 2002;100(1):37.

Bacon JL. Adolescent sexuality and pregnancy. *Curr Opin Obstet Gynecol* 2000;12:345.

Barbieri RL. Population density and teen pregnancy. *Obstet Gynecol* 2004;104(4):741.

Barnett B, Arroyo C, Devoe M, et al. Reduced school dropout rates among adolescent mothers receiving school-based prenatal care. *Arch Pediatr Adolesc Med* 2004;158(3):262.

Berenson AB, Wiemann C. Contraceptive use among adolescent mothers at 6 months. *J Adolesc Health* 1997;89:999.

Biro FM, Wildey IS, Hillard PJ, et al. Acute and long term consequences of adolescents who choose abortion. *Pediatr Ann* 1986;15:667.

Boggess S, Bradner C. Trends in adolescent males' abortion attitudes, 1988–1995: differences by race and ethnicity. *Fam Plann Perspect* 2000;32:118.

Boyer D, Fine D. Sexual abuse as a factor in adolescent pregnancy and child maltreatment. *Fam Plann Perspect* 1992; 24:4.

Braunstein GD. False-positive serum human chorionic gonadotropin results: Causes, characteristics, and recognition. *Am J Obstet Gynecol* 2002;187(1):217.

Cassell C, Santelli J, Gilbert BC, et al. Mobilizing communities: an overview coalition partnership programs for the prevention of teen pregnancy. *J Adolesc Health* 2005;37:S3.

Cates W, Grimes DA, Schulz KF. Abortion surveillance at CDC. *Am J Prev Med* 2000;19(Suppl 1):12.

Centers for Disease Control and Prevention. Health risk behaviors among adolescents who do and do not attend school—U.S., 1992. *MMWR Morb Mortal Wkly Rep* 1994; 43(8):129.

Centers for Disease Control and Prevention. Abortion surveillance: preliminary data—United States, 1992. *JAMA* 1995; 273:371.

Centers for Disease Control and Prevention. National and state-specific pregnancy rates among adolescents—United States, 1995–1997. *MMWR Morb Mortal Wkly Rep* 2000;49:605.

Centers for Disease Control and Prevention. Effect of revised population counts on county-level hispanic teen birthrates—United States, 1999. *MMWR Morb Mortal Wkly Rep* 2004;53(40);946.

Centers for Disease Control and Prevention. Trends from 1976–2003 in pregnancy, birth and abortion rates in teens 15–17 years, source. *MMWR Morb Mortal Wkly Rep* 2005; 54(04);100.

Centers for Disease Control and Prevention. Youth risk behavior surveillance—United States, 2003. *MMWR Morb Mortal Wkly Rep* 2006;55(SS-5):1.

Cheyne KL. Adolescent pregnancy prevention. *Curr Opin Pediatr* 1999;11:594.

Cole LA, Khanlian SA, Sutton JM, et al. Accuracy of home pregnancy tests at the time of missed menses. *Am J Obstet Gynecol* 2004;190(1):100.

Corcoran J. Ecological factors associated with adolescent pregnancy: a review of the literature. *Adolescence* 1999;34:603.

Cox JE, Bevill L, Forsyth J, et al. Youth preferences for prenatal and parenting teen services. *J Pediatr Adolesc Gynecol* 2005; 18:167.

Cox JE, Bithoney WG. Fathers of children born to adolescent mothers: predictors of contact with their children at 2 years. *Arch Pediatr Adolesc Med* 1995a;149:962.

Cox J, DuRant RH, Emans SJ, et al. Early parenthood for the sisters of adolescent mothers: a proposed conceptual model of decision-making. *Adolesc Pediatr Gynecol* 1995b;8:188.

Covington D, Churchill M, Wright B. Factors affecting number of prenatal care visits during second pregnancy among adolescents having rapid repeat births. *J Adolesc Health* 1994; 15:536.

Darroch JE, Landry DJ, Oslak S. Age difference between sexual partners in the United States. *Fam Plann Perspect* 1999; 31(4):160.

Davies S, Byrn F, Cole LA. Human chorionic gonadotropin testing for early pregnancy viability and complications. *Clin Lab Med* 2003;23(2):257.

Davies SL, DiClemente RJ, Wingood GM, et al. Relationship characteristics and sexual practices of African American adolescent girls who desire pregnancy. *Health Educ Behav* 2004;31(4 Suppl):85S.

Duncan GJ, Hoffman SD. Teenage welfare receipt and subsequent dependence among black adolescent mothers. *Fam Plann Perspect* 1990;22:16.

East P, Jacobson L. The younger siblings of teenage mothers: a follow-up of their pregnancy risk. *Dev Psychol* 2001;37(2): 254.

English A, Kenney KE. *State minor consent laws: a summary,* 2nd ed. Chapel Hill, NC: Center for Adolescent Health and the Law, 2003.

Fischer M, Bhatnagar J, Guarner J, et al. Fatal toxic shock syndrome associated with Clostridium sordellii after medical abortion. *N Engl J Med* 2005;253:2352.

Flanagan PJ, McGrath MM, Meyer EC, et al. Adolescent development and transitions to motherhood. *Pediatrics* 1995;96:273.

Flanigan C. *What's behind the good news: the decline in teen pregnancy rates during the 1990s.* Washington, DC: The National Campaign to Prevent Teen Pregnancy, 2001.

Forum on Child and Family Statistics. *America's children in brief: key national indicators of well-being 2006.* http://childstats.gov. Assessed August 4, 2006.

Foster HW. Taming the tempest of teen pregnancy. *Am J Obstet Gynecol* 1999;181(suppl):S28.

Foster HW, Bond T. Teen pregnancy—problems and approaches: panel presentations. *Am J Obstet Gynecol* 1999;181(suppl):S32.

Franklin C, Corcoran J. Preventing adolescent pregnancy: a review of programs and practices. *Soc Work* 2000;45:40.

Fraser AM, Brockert LE, Ward RH. Association of young maternal age with adverse reproductive outcomes. *N Engl J Med* 1995;332:1113.

Furstenberg FF, Brooks-Gunn J, Morgan SP. Adolescent mothers and their children in later life. *Fam Plann Perspect* 1987; 19:142.

Geary FH, Wingate CB. Domestic violence and physical abuse of women: the Grady Memorial Hospital experience. *Am J Obstet Gynecol* 1999;181:S17.

Glei D. Measuring contraceptive use patterns among teenage and adult women. *Fam Plann Perspect* 1999;31(2):73.

Goldenberg RL, Klerman LV. Adolescent pregnancy—another look. *N Engl J Med* 1995;332:1161.

Gottlieb BJ. Abortion—1995. *N Engl J Med* 1995;332:532.

Grimes DA. Adolescent pregnancy prevention programs. *Contracep Rep* 1994;5:4.

Grogger J, Bronars S. The socioeconomic consequences of teenage childbearing: findings from a natural experiment. *Fam Plann Perspect* 1993;25:156.

Gutierrez Y, King JC. Nutrition during teenage pregnancy. *Pediatr Ann* 1993;22:2.

Hamilton BE, Martin JA, Sutton PD. *Births, preliminary data 2002*. National Vital Statistics Reports, 2003:51.

Hardy JB, Duggan AK, Masnyk K, et al. Fathers of children born to young urban mother. *Fam Plann Perspect* 1989; 21:159.

Hatcher RA, Trussell J, Stewart F, et al. *Contraceptive technology*, 18th ed. New York: Ardent Media, 2004.

Hausknecht RU. Methotrexate and misoprostol to terminate early pregnancy. *N Engl J Med* 1995;333:537.

Henshaw SK. *U.S. teenage pregnancy statistics with comparative statistics for women aged 20–24*. New York: The Alan Guttmacher Institute, 2003.

Henshaw SK, Kost K. Parental involvement in minors' abortion decisions. *Fam Plann Perspect* 1992;24:196.

Hillis SD, Anda RF, Dube SR, et al. The association between adverse childhood experiences and adolescent pregnancy, long-term psychosocial consequences, and fetal death. *Pediatrics* 2004;113(2):320.

Hoffman SD. Teenage childbearing is not so bad after all: or is it? A review of the new literature. *Fam Plann Perspect* 1998; 30:236.

Hughes ME, Furstenberg FF, Teitler JO. The impact of an increase in family planning services on the teenage population of Philadelphia. *Fam Plann Perspect* 1995;27:60.

Jacoby M, Gorenflo D, Black E, et al. Rapid repeat pregnancy and experiences of interpersonal violence among low-income adolescents. *Am J Prev Med* 1999;16:318.

Jaskiewicz JA, McAnarney ER. Pregnancy during adolescence. *Pediatr Rev* 1994;15:32.

Jones RK, Darroch JE, Henshaw SK. Patterns in the socioeconomic characteristics of women obtaining abortions in 2000–2001. *Perspect Sex Reprod Health* 2002;34(5):226.

Kalmuss DS, Namerow PB. Subsequent childbearing among teenage mothers: the determinants of a closely spaced second birth. *Fam Plann Perspect* 1994;26:149.

Kaplan DW, Feinstein RA, Fisher MM, et al. Condom use by adolescents. *Pediatrics* 2001;107(6):1463.

Kaunitz AM, Grimes DA, Kaunitz KK. A physician's guide to adoption. *JAMA* 1987;258:3537.

Kenney JW, Reinholtz C, Angelini PJ. Ethnic differences in childhood and adolescent sexual abuse and teenage pregnancy. *J Adolesc Health* 1997;21:3.

Kirby D. Reflections on two decades of research on teen sexual behavior and pregnancy. *J Sch Health* 1999;69:89.

Kirby D. *Emerging answers: research findings on programs to reduce teen pregnancy (summary)*. Washington, DC: National Campaign to Prevent Teen Pregnancy, 2001.

Kirby DB, Baumler E, Coyle KK, et al. The "Safer Choices" intervention: its impact on the sexual behaviors of different subgroups of high school students. *J Adolesc Health* 2004; 35(6):442.

Klein JD. Adolescent pregnancy: current trends and issues. *Pediatrics* 2005;103:516.

Klerman LV. *Another chance: preventing additional births to teen mothers*. Washington, DC: National Organization to Prevent Teen Pregnancy, 2004.

Koren G, Pastuszak A, Ito S. Drugs in pregnancy. *N Engl J Med* 1998;338:1128.

Kulig JW. Committee on Substance Abuse. Tobacco, alcohol, and other drugs: the role of the pediatrician in prevention, identification, and management of substance abuse. *Pediatrics* 2005;115(3):816.

Landry DJ, Forrest JD. How old are U.S. fathers? *Fam Plann Perspect* 1995;27:159.

Leland NL, Petersen DJ, Braddock M, et al. Variations in pregnancy outcomes by race among 10–14-year-old mothers in the United States. *Public Health Rep* 1995;110:53.

Lemus JF. Ectopic pregnancy: an update. *Curr Opin Obstet Gynecol* 2000;12:369.

Lindberg LD, Sonenstein FL, Martinez G. Age differences between minors who give birth and their adult partners. *Fam Plann Perspect* 1997;29:61.

Lugaila TA. *Marital status and living arrangements: March 1997 (update)*. Current population reports, P20–506, US Bureau of the Census. Washington, DC: US Department of Commerce, 1998.

Manlove J, Terry E, Gitelson L, et al. Explaining demographic trends in teenage fertility, 1980–1995. *Fam Plann Perspect* 2000;32:166.

Marianne E. East, Patricia, and Felice. *Adolescent pregnancy and parenting: findings from a racially diverse sample*. Mahwah, NJ: Lawrence Erlbaum Associates, 1996.

Marsiglio W. Adolescent fathers in the U.S.: their initial living arrangements, marital experience, and educational outcomes. *Fam Plann Perspect* 1987;19:247.

Martin JA, Hamilton BE, Sutton PD, et al. *Births: final data for 2003. National vital statistics reports*, Vol. 54, No. 2, Hyattsville, MD: National Center for Health Statistics, 2005.

Maynard, RA, ed. *Kids having kids: a robin hood foundation special report on the costs of adolescent childbearing*. New York: Robin Hood Foundation, 1996.

Menacker F, Martin JA, MacDorman MF, et al. Births to 10–14 year-old mothers, 1990–2002: trends and health outcomes. *Natl Vital Stat Rep* 2004;53(7):1.

Moore MR, Chase-Lansdale PL. Sexual intercourse and pregnancy among African American adolescent girls in high poverty neighborhoods: the role of family and perceived community involvement. *J Marriage Fam* 2001;63:1146.

Mosher WD, Bachrach CA. Understanding U.S. fertility: continuity and change in the National Survey of Family Growth, 1988–1995. *Fam Plann Perspect* 1996;28:4.

National Campaign to Prevent Teen Pregnancy. *Fact sheet: recent trends in teen pregnancy, sexual activity, and contraceptive use*. Washington, DC: National Campaign to Prevent Teen Pregnancy, Available at: www.teenpregnancy.org/resources/reading/pdf/rectrend.pdf, accessed June 19, 2005. 2004.

Neinstein LSN. *Issues in reproductive management*. New York: Thieme Medical Publisher, 1994.

Ness RB, Grisso JA, Hirschinger N, et al. Cocaine and tobacco use and the risk of spontaneous abortion. *N Engl J Med* 1999; 340:333.

Nitz K. Adolescent pregnancy prevention: a review of interventions and programs. *Clin Psychol Rev* 1999;19:457.

Parker B, McFarlane J, Soeken K. Abuse during pregnancy: effects on maternal complications and birth weight in adult and teenage women. *Obstet Gynecol* 1994;84:323.

Pastuszak A, Schick-Boschetto B, Zuber C, et al. Pregnancy outcome following first-trimester exposure to fluoxetine (Prozac). *JAMA* 1993;269(17):2246.

Peplow PV. RU486 combined with PGE1 analog in voluntary termination of early pregnancy: a comparison of recent findings with gemeprost or misoprostol. *Contraception* 1994; 50:69.

Polaneczky M, O'Connor K. Pregnancy in the adolescent patient: screening, diagnosis, and initial management. *Pediatr Clin North Am* 1999;46:649.

Resnick MD, Bearman PS, Blum RW, et al. Protecting adolescents from harm: findings from the National Longitudinal Study on Adolescent Health. *JAMA* 1997;278:823.

Richardson KK. Adolescent pregnancy and substance use. *J Obstet Gynecol Neonatal Nurs* 1999;28:623.

Santelli JS, Abma J, Ventura S, et al. Can changes in sexual behaviors among high school students explain the decline in teen pregnancy rates in the 1990s? *J Adolesc Health* 2004; 35:80.

Satin AJ, Leveno KJ, Sherman ML, et al. Maternal youth and pregnancy outcomes: middle school versus high school age groups compared with women beyond the teen years. *Am J Obstet Gynecol* 1994;171:184.

Singh S, Darroch JE. Adolescent pregnancy and childbearing: levels and trends in developed countries. *Fam Plann Perspect* 2000;32:14.

Sonenstein FL, Ku LC, Lindberg LD, et al. Changes in sexual behavior and condom use among teenage males: 1988 to 1995. *Am J Public Health* 1998;88:956.

Stevens-Simon C, Sheeder J. Paradoxical adolescent reproductive decisions. *J Pediatr Adolesc Gynecol* 2004;17(1):29.

Terry-Humen E, Manlove J. *Cottinghams. Trends and recent estimates: sexual activity among US teen.* Child Trends Research Brief, http://www.childtrends.org/Files/SexualActivityRB.pdf. Assessed August 4, 2006. 2006.

Ventura SJ, Abma JC, Mosher WD, et al. Estimated pregnancy rates for the United States, 1990–2000: an update. *Natl Vital Stat Rep* 2004;52(23):1.

Ventura SJ, Freedman MA. Teenage childbearing in the United States, 1960–1997. *Am J Prev Med* 2000;19:18.

Weinberger DR, Elvevag B, Giedd JN. *The adolescent brain: a work in progress.* Washington, DC: The National Campaign to Prevent Teen Pregnancy, 2005.

Woods ER, Obeidallah-Davis D, Sherry MK, et al. The parenting project for teen mothers: the impact of a nurturing curriculum on adolescent parenting skills and life hassles. *Ambul Pediatr* 2003;3:240.

Wolfe B, Perozek M. Teen children's health and health care use. In: Maynard RA, ed., *Kids having kids: economic costs and social consequences.* Washington DC: The Urban Institute Press, 1996, 181–206.

Young T, Turner J, Denny G, et al. Examining external and internal poverty as antecedents of teen pregnancy. *Am J Health Behav* 2004;28(4):361.

Zabin LS, Hirsch MB, Emerson MR. When urban adolescents choose abortion: effects on education, psychological status, and subsequent pregnancy. *Fam Plann Perspect* 1989;21: 248.

Zabin LS, Sedivy V, Emerson MR. Subsequent risk of childbearing among adolescents with a negative pregnancy test. *Fam Plann Perspect* 1994;26:212.

CHAPTER 42

Contraception

Anita L. Nelson and Lawrence S. Neinstein

CURRENT TRENDS

Today, adolescence can last for up to a decade—the longest period in human history. Onset of puberty occurs much earlier in life and the assumption of adult roles is delayed until the 20s. During this decade, teens undergo tremendous physical and intellectual changes, and transfer from adult to peer group identification on their way to developing their own individual moral values and mature personal identities. An important element in this process is the emergence of sexual identity, behaviors, and attributes. Teens are profoundly affected by social conditions, peer pressures, and the media images, which when combined with their proclivity for experimentation and their sense of invulnerability, has resulted in risk-taking behaviors in all arenas, including reproductive health. Sexual activity, abortion, and birth rates among teens increased in the 1960s and 1970s, but those rates started to decline early in the 1990s, partially in response to the acquired immunodeficiency syndrome (AIDS) epidemic. Between 2001 and 2004, those rates were stable. Contraceptive use has increased dramatically to decrease adolescent pregnancy rates.

Sexual Activity

Despite this progress, significant adolescent sexual activity and risk-taking behaviors remain. The 2005 Centers for Disease Control and Prevention (CDC) Youth Risk Behavior Survey found that 46.8% of high school students had had sexual intercourse during their lifetimes and 33.9% of students had sexual intercourse during the 3 months preceding the survey (Centers for Disease Control and Prevention, 2006). These rates are about the same as in 2003 and slightly higher than the ones reported in their 2001 survey. Prevalence of sexual activity was higher among male students than female students. Sexual debut can occur at an early age; 6.2% of students had sexual intercourse before age 13, although this percentage has declined since 1999. Quite naturally, sexual experience increases with age. Almost one third (29.3%) of 9th grade female adolescents had had intercourse; this rate rose to 62.4% for 12th grade female adolescents. Adolescents also tend to have multiple partners over time, generally in a series of monogamous relationships, 14.3% of high school students reported having had four or more

partners in their lifetime (Centers for Disease Control and Prevention, 2006).

As concerning as these estimates are, it must be remembered that they *underestimate* adolescent sexual activity for several reasons. They exclude the sexual activity of teens who are not enrolled in school. To capture information about a broader sample of adolescents, data for 15- to 19-year olds is available from the 2002 National Survey of Family Growth (NSFG) (Mosher et al., 2005). In that survey, 26% of 15-year-old female adolescents had had sexual intercourse as had 77% of 18-year olds. Male adolescents reported lower rates (25% of 15 year olds; 62% of 18 year olds), which reflects the influence of older men having sex with adolescent females (Abma et al., 2004). Most 15- to 19-year olds (54.9% of men and 57.1% of women) had had at least one partner in the last year; more than 20% had had two or more partners.

In addition, many of the surveys do not ask about noncoital sexual practices, such as same-sex practices, heterosexual anal intercourse, or oral-genital sexual pleasuring. Although these practices do not result in pregnancy, they may expose the young person to sexually transmitted diseases (STDs) (see Chapters 60–67). Oral sex among teens aged 15 to 19 is more common than vaginal intercourse. Of the male and female adolescents aged 15 to 19 in the NSFG, 49% reported having vaginal intercourse, 55.1% reported heterosexual oral sex. More than one in five teens aged 15 to 19, who have not had vaginal intercourse, report that they have had oral sex. Fewer than 10% of teens report using a condom the last time they had oral sex. Interestingly, both males and females aged 15 to 17 reported receiving oral sex at higher rates (40.3% and 38%) than giving it (Mosher et al., 2005). Halpern-Felsher et al. (2005) demonstrated that oral sex is a reality among young adolescents, and that most of them do not believe that it is either dangerous to their health or inconsistent with their moral values. Heterosexual anal intercourse was reported by approximately 11% of teens. Same-sex sexual contact was reported by 4.5% of male teens and 10.6% of female teens (Mosher et al., 2005).

Additional insights into teen sexual activity are available from other surveys. The National Campaign to Prevent Teen Pregnancy reported that more than 1 in 10 young women who first had sexual intercourse before age 15 described it as nonvoluntary and many more described it as unwanted (Albert et al., 2003). A Kaiser Foundation survey of 15- to 17-year olds who had "had sex," 51% said that when they had sex for the first time, it was because they "met the right person," 45% said it was because "the other person wanted to," 32% said it was because they were "just curious," 28% said it was because they "hoped it would make the relationship closer," and 16% said it was because "many of their friends already had" (Sex Smarts, 2000). Cohen et al. (2002) reported that more than 70% of high school students said they had had sex in their parents' home or the home of their partner; more than half of acts occurred during week days. Pittman et al. (2005) reported that "doing nothing" was the immediate antecedent activity for sexual intercourse.

Pregnancy Rates

There was a 28% reduction in U.S. adolescent pregnancy rates between 1991 and 2004. Adolescent pregnancy rates are now the lowest they have been in the last 30 years. The elective abortion rate peaked in 1983 at 30.7/1,000 and steadily declined by more than half to 14.5/1,000 by 2000 (QuickStats, 2005). The birth rate in 15 to 19 old females declined 33% from its peak of 61.8/1,000 women in 1991 to 41.2/1,000 in 2004. Birth rates among younger teens 15 to 17 years of age declined the most and were 22.1/1,000, down by 42.7% from 1991 to 2004 (Hamilton et al., 2005). The NSFG data shows that the probability of a U.S. woman giving birth by age 20 is 13%. There are some other disturbing factors behind those numbers. Half of births to teen mothers involve men aged 20 to 24 and an additional one sixth of those fathers are older than 25 years (Males, 2004). The National Center for Health Statistics (NCHS) found that >80% of new adolescent mothers were unmarried in 2004 (Hamilton et al., 2005).

Despite the recent reduction in pregnancy-related rates, teen pregnancy rates in the United States are still much higher than those rates in other developed countries whose teens are generally as sexually active as their American counterparts (Darroch et al., 2001). Only the Russian Federation and Bulgaria have comparable pregnancy rates, but their teen birth rates are lower than in the United States. The primary difference in pregnancy rates is attributable to lack of contraceptive use by U.S. teens. Decreases in pregnancy rates are vitally important to the long-term well-being of teens. The impact of pregnancy on the teen can be ascertained by her actions and her attitudes. Estimates are that 78% of teen pregnancies are unintended (Abma et al., 2004), and 28% are electively terminated (Henshaw, 2004). Of those pregnancies that are continued to delivery, 57% are categorized by the young mother herself as mistakes, whereas only 22% of births are intended.

Contraceptive Usage

The recent decline in adolescent pregnancies is due both to decrease in sexual experience of adolescents (53% of decline) and to more effective contraception use (47% of decline) (Santelli et al., 2004). Between 1991 and 2001, the percentage of young women in high school who had ever had sexual intercourse declined from 51% to 43%, but it rose to 45.3% by 2003. Sexual activity among those who were sexually experienced did not change, but effective contraceptive use did. This is reflected in the fact that from 1991 to 2001, there was a notable decrease on the weight-average contraceptive failure rates (WACFRs) for teens. This decrease was due to a decline in the use of less

effective methods such as withdrawal (which decreased from 20% to 13%) and no method (which decreased from 17% to 13%) and an increase in the use of condoms (from 40% to 51%) (Santelli et al., 2004). Other important changes are notable. Ever use of birth control pills increased from 52% to 61% between 1995 and 2002. Of women who had intercourse in the last 3 months, 83% reported using a method with their most recent episode (Abma et al. 2004). Injectable contraception use increased among sexually experienced women from 10% to 21% between 1995 and 2002. Importantly, dual method use (condom and hormonal method) more than doubled from 1995 to 2002 (8% to 20%) (Abma et al., 2004). However, these changes were not seen in every group. Among whites, there was no decrease in the WACFR, but the WACFR did decline from 1991 to 2001, by 20% among blacks, and by 24% among Hispanics (Santelli et al., 2004).

Condoms are the most popular method at first intercourse. Approximately 67% of women and 71% of men reported using this method with first coitus. However, 26% of 15- to 19-year olds still report not using any method with first coitus. Women who are older at sexual debut are more likely to report condom use at first intercourse than are younger women (Abma et al., 2004).

Contraceptive use patterns are complex. Analysis has shown that contraceptive use was more likely in female teens who had waited a longer time between the start of a relationship and first sex with that partner, had discussed contraception before first having sex, or used dual contraceptive methods. On the other hand, contraception was less likely to be used (or used consistently) if the women had taken a virginity pledge, had an older partner, had a number of close friends who knew her partner, or reportedly had a relationship that was not romantic but had those trappings (Manlove et al., 2003). Studies have shown that women who use contraception at first intercourse have significantly lower birth rates as teens, suggesting more consistent long-term teen use of contraception (Abma et al., 2004).

Contraceptive Education

One interesting study asked public high school students *where* they would like to obtain information about contraception. Men were more likely than women to prefer receiving information from parents (23% versus 18%) and health education classes (16% versus 7.5%), whereas women were more likely than men to prefer a clinical setting (51% versus 27%) (Hacker et al., 2000). Understanding the differences in teen preferences can help providers meet the educational needs of adolescents. Also, appreciating the adverse impact that prior sexual abuse can have on the survivor's future use of contraception highlights the need to identify these women and provide special counseling (Saewyc et al., 2004).

One opportunity that is often overlooked in teaching adolescents is teaching their *parents*. Studies have shown that parent–teenager discussions where the parent was open, skilled, and comfortable with the discussion were associated with better teen-partner communications and ultimately better teen condom use. On the other hand, poor teen-parent discussions were negatively associated with condom use (Whitaker et al., 1999). This may be particularly important in one-parent households (Oman et al., 2005).

Since 1996, the Federal government has invested more than a billion dollars in abstinence-only, school-based programs, which has decreased access to comprehensive contraceptive information and services. Analysis of prototype abstinence-only programs developed in the earlier 1990s demonstrated no long-term beneficial impact (Kirby et al., 1997; Cagampang et al., 1997). Currently, no official analysis of the current federally funded programs has been reported, although the quality of these programs has been found to vary considerably (Wilson et al., 2005). According to the report "Abstinence Education Evaluation Phase 5 Technical Report" from the Texas Health Department, the number of adolescents who had had sexual intercourse did not change or actually increased after they had received abstinence-only education (Tanne, 2005).

A preliminary analysis of virginity pledge programs has been published. Despite the obvious influence on outcomes of selection bias (those who choose to pledge versus those who do not pledge), it has been reported that those who took pledges delayed their sexual debut by 12 to 18 months and married earlier. However, STD rates for virginity pledge-takers did not differ from nonpledgers, in part because pledge-takers were *less* likely to use condoms at sexual debut. In addition, pledgers were more likely to say that they had had oral or anal intercourse but not vaginal intercourse (Bruckner and Bearman, 2005). The all-or-nothing approach required by the abstinence-only programs may create barriers to knowledge and loss of protection for teens.

CONTRACEPTIVE OPTIONS

The list of contraceptive options available in the United States has both expanded and retracted over the last decade. Table 42.1 lists the currently available methods and those expected to be approved shortly. Oral contraceptive (OC) pills and condoms are still the most frequently used methods, but new hormonal delivery systems such as transdermal patches and vaginal rings have been

TABLE 42.1

Contraceptive Options

Category	Brand Name	Duration of Use
Intrauterine contraceptives		
Copper T-380A IUD	ParaGard	10 years
Levonorgestrel-releasing IUS	Mirena	5 years
Injections		
DMPA-IM	Depo-Provera	11–13 weeks
DMPA-SQ	depo-subQ provera 104	12–14 weeks
Implants	Implanon	3 years
Combined hormonal vaginal ring	NuvaRing	21 days
Combined hormonal transdermal patch	Ortho Evra	7 days
Combined hormonal pills	Multiple	1 day
Progestin-only pills	Multiple	1 day
Male condoms	Wide array	Single use
Female condoms	Reality	Single use
Cervical barriers	Diaphragms	24 hours
	Today sponge	Single episode
	Lea's Shield	48 hours
	FemCap	24 hours
Spermicides	Foams	Single episode
	Suppositories	Single episode
	Films	Single episode
	Today sponge	Single episode
Periodic abstinence and fertility awareness	Rhythm method	
	Billings method	
	Basal body temperature method	
	Standard Days Method	
	Symptomothermal method	
Withdrawal ("pulling out")	None	

IUD, intrauterine device; IUS, intrauterine system.

introduced to add convenience in use and, hopefully, to increase efficacy. The once-a-month combined hormonal injection was introduced but then removed from the market due to production problems and low sales.

Oral Contraceptive Pills

New pill formulations with lower doses of estrogen, different progestins, different pill utilization patterns, and new noncontraceptive benefits have been introduced. The first nonandrogenic progestin (drospirenone) is now available in two different formulations. More pills with lower doses of ethinyl estradiol (20 and 25 µg) are available. New patterns of utilization are also available. Three low-dose pill formulations reduce the number of placebo pills in their 28-day packet to minimize estrogen-withdrawal symptoms. Extended cycle use of pills with U.S. Food and Drug Administration (FDA)-approved products and off-label use of other pill formations, patches, and rings reduces the number of episodes of withdrawal bleeding women have each year. Although eliminating withdrawal bleeds offers significant health and quality-of-life benefits to female adolescents, careful counseling of teens is needed so that they can understand the safety of not bleeding with use of hormonal contraception use compared with the concerns that amenorrhea raises without hormone use. Each of these issues is discussed at greater length in Chapter 43.

Implants and Injectable Contraceptives

During the late 1990s, the implantable contraceptive system (Norplant-6) was withdrawn from the market. However, Implanon was approved by the FDA in July 2006. This is a single rod system, which greatly simplifies insertion and removal procedures. The injectable progestin-only method (depot medroxyprogesterone acetate [DMPA], Depo-Provera) made a significant contribution to teen contraception in the 1990s and early 2000s. A new formulation of DMPA with different buffers has been introduced with the name depo-subQ provera 104. This formulation reduces the injection dose from 150 mg to 104 mg while maintaining an intermediate term (12–14 weeks) efficacy and replacing intramuscular injections with subcutaneous shots. Subcutaneous injections offer the potential for self injection to streamline access. It is also approved for the treatment of symptomatic endometriosis. Concerns about the possible adverse effects that DMPA-induced hypoestrogenemia may have on adolescent bone mineralization have prompted a new black box warning on both formulations. This is discussed at greater length in Chapter 47.

Intrauterine Devices

Changes in labeling for the copper intrauterine device (IUD) have made it a more attractive option for female adolescents. There is no longer a recommendation that the copper IUD candidate be parous or be in a stable, mutually monogamous relationship with no history of pelvic inflammatory disease (PID). The levonorgestrel IUD retains the more restrictive labeling, but offers candidates significant reduction in menstrual blood loss.

Condoms

Male condoms have been greatly improved to encourage more consistent and successful utilization. The quality of condoms as a whole has increased in the last decade. Two polyurethane condoms are available for couples with latex allergy. New condom features such as ribs, scents, vibrating rings, different sizes, and different shapes have attempted to appeal to potential users. The snugger fit condom addresses the needs of younger men who have not completed all their secondary sexual growth. Extra large condoms with additional room at the tip have answered the needs of men who are well endowed. Simplified packaging, which eliminates the chance that the condom will be incorrectly unrolled, increases the chance that every use will be more successful. Spermicide coating has been removed from many condoms because the spermicide added no benefit for contraception or STD risk reduction, but it did increase cost. Condoms are now being marketed directly to women, which it is hoped will increase access. Adolescents should be told that condoms reduce the transmission of human immunodeficiency virus (HIV) and that correct and consistent use of condoms is a key component of safer sex practices.

Female Barrier Methods

Female barrier methods have also changed. Diaphragms may reemerge in the near future as a delivery system for microbicides. The female condom is available, but not as frequently utilized as the male condom because it is more expensive, more complicated to use, and less effective than the male condom. The latex cervical cap (Prentif Cervical Cap) is no longer available in the United States. However, the vaginal contraceptive sponge (Today), a cervical "shield" (Lea's Shield), and a silicone cervical cap (FemCap) have been introduced to be used with spermicide. See Chapter 45 on barrier methods.

Fertility Awareness Methods

Fertility awareness methods such as periodic abstinence and periodic use of contraception are less reliable for adolescents because of their irregular cycles. However, for women with well-established cycles lasting 26 to 32 days, the Standard Days Method with a ring of color-coded beads ("CycleBeads") to help the couple identify at-risk days has greatly simplified the introduction and use of these methods. Other sexual practices, such as withdrawal, are quite prevalent with adolescents. If patients are going to rely on withdrawal, they should be carefully counseled on correct coital positioning and other techniques to make the method more effective as a contraceptive method.

Emergency Contraception

One of the most important new products to be introduced in recent years is emergency contraceptives (ECs). The first FDA-approved EC, with estrogen and progestin (Preven), is no longer available. It has been replaced by the only other FDA-approved product (Plan B), a levonorgestrel-only EC. Plan B is safe and can be used by virtually every adolescent female in need. There are only three contraindications—pregnancy, because there is no benefit (EC is not an abortifacient); unexplained abnormal uterine bleeding (until pregnancy is ruled out); and allergies to any of the ingredients. EC provides a back-up in case the couple's primary method did not function or was not correctly used. Because EC works most effectively if taken as soon as possible after unprotected coitus, the optimal strategy is to provide EC by advance prescription. Advise the patient to fill the prescription and keep the product readily available (see Chapter 46). Plan B has been approved for behind-the-counter availability for people age 18 and over with government identification.

SELECTING A CONTRACEPTIVE METHOD

Age alone should not limit contraceptive choices for young individuals (Faculty of Family Planning and Reproductive Health Care Clinical Effectiveness Unit, 2004). Female adolescents need to be provided an overview of all methods of contraception. A brief description of how each method is used, how well it works to prevent pregnancy, what noncontraceptive benefits may accrue, and what side effects and health risks are possible with its use are necessary for informed consent and for long-term contraceptive continuation.

To help clinicians effectively counsel women and help them work with their patients to select optimal methods, the concept of "contraceptive fit" has been developed (Farrington, 2001). This approach recognizes that the best method for any one woman is the method with the greatest pregnancy protection that she will use consistently. There are four dimensions to the contraceptive fit model:

1. Safety: What medical contraindications does she have?
   A patient's medical conditions may exclude some methods. For example, clinicians should not prescribe estrogen-containing methods to an adolescent woman with severe hypertension or breast cancer. Similarly, women taking medications that have significant drug–drug interactions with some contraceptives may not be offered those methods. Women with Chlamydia cervicitis are not IUD candidates.
2. The woman's reproductive stage: How soon does she want to become pregnant? How important is it to her to prevent pregnancy?
   This question helps providers establish the concept that pregnancy should be planned and prepared for and also helps highlight or diminish the attractiveness of long-acting methods. The typical use failure rates are helpful in identifying methods that best meet the patient's needs in this dimension.
3. Her lifestyle: What challenges does she have in using contraceptives?
   Adolescent lifestyle can be quite hectic and certainly are the most variable of any age-group.
   • A new mother, especially an adolescent mother, may be overwhelmed by all the pressures and demands of child care. Convenience in the contraception may be critically important.
   • An adolescent who has not disclosed her sexual activity to adult authority figures may need to use very discrete and private contraceptive methods.
   • A woman who travels across different time zones or works different shifts may be confused about when to take daily methods. Longer acting methods may be needed.

Episodic sexual activity patterns may discourage a woman from using methods that require daily administration, especially during weeks or months when she is not having coitus.

A young adolescent female may not be able to negotiate with her partner about sexual activities or the use of condoms (Stone and Ingham, 2002).
4. The patient's own preferences: What has she heard from her friends and from the media?
   Although modifiable with education, this element may be the most critical one in the equation to ensure an adolescent's commitment to using her contraceptive method. Women who are concerned about using "synthetic hormones" or those who believe that pills make them gain weight will be far less likely to be successful OC users. Those women who recognize that the pills are responsible for the fact that their menses are less painful and more predictable are apt to be more consistent pill users. For female adolescents who rely strongly on their peers for advice, it is helpful to have teen success stories with which they can relate.

IMPORTANT PROPERTIES OF CONTRACEPTIVES FOR FEMALE ADOLESCENTS

Although female adolescents differ in their understanding of, commitment to, and need for contraception, there are some important features of different contraceptives that are particularly important for teen women.

Convenience

It may be quite challenging for teens to use contraceptive methods correctly and consistently. Not only is sexual activity often unplanned and "spontaneous," but it is also often episodic. Methods that require little forethought and/or preparation are most likely to be more successfully utilized. Injections, implants, and intrauterine contraceptives all share this property. Among the combined hormonal methods, the once-a-month contraceptive vaginal ring is most convenient, followed by the once-a-week patch. Teens, generally, more successfully utilize these longer acting methods than OC pills, which require daily dosing (Audet et al., 2001).

Effectiveness

Adolescent utilization of contraceptives is generally less consistent than that of older women, but because adult utilization is so suboptimal, typical use failure rates for female adolescents are very similar to that of adults (Trussell, 2004) (Table 42.2). The discrepancies seen between the failure rate with correct and consistent use and the failure rates with typical use are greatest with methods that require action at the time of coitus (condoms) or regular administration (OCs). Since pregnancy prevention is very critical in this age-group, it is important to select methods with higher effective rates (IUDs, implants, and injections) and/or methods that may not be as inherently effective but are appealing to the teen (see following text). Mistakes do happen and passion does occasionally overwhelm good

TABLE 42.2

Typical Use Failure Rates—Percentage of Women Experiencing an Unintended Pregnancy within the First Year of Use

Method	Correct and Consistent Use[a]	Typical Use[b]
No method[c]	85	85
Implanon	0.05	0.05
Intrauterine contraceptives		
Copper T-380A (Paraguard)	0.6	0.8
LNG-IUS (Mirena)	0.2	0.2
DMPA (SQ and IM)	0.3	3
Nuvaring	0.3	No data available
Evra Patch	0.3	No data available
Combined pill and minipill	0.3	8
Male condoms	2	15
Diaphragms[d]	6	16
Female condoms	5	21
Periodic abstinence		25
Withdrawal	4	27
Spermicides[e]	18	29
Sponge		
Parous women	20	32
Nulliparous women	9	16

LNG-IUS, levonorgestrel intrauterine system.

Modified from Hatcher RA, Trussell J, Nelson AL. Contraceptive technology, 19th ed. New York: Ardent Media, 2007.

[a] Among typical couples who initiate use of a method (not necessarily for the first time), the percentage who experience an accidental pregnancy during the first year if they do not stop use for any other reason. Estimates of the probability of pregnancy during the first year of typical use for spermicides, withdrawal, periodic abstinence, the diaphragm, the male condom, the pill, and Depo-Provera are taken from the 1995 National Survey of Family Growth corrected for underreporting of abortion.

[b] Among couples who initiate use of a method (not necessarily for the first time) and who use it perfectly (both consistently and correctly), the percentage who experience an accidental pregnancy during the first year if they do not stop use for any other reason.

[c] The percentages becoming pregnant in "typical use" and "correct and consistent use" are based on data from populations where contraception is not used and from women who cease using contraception in order to become pregnant. Among such populations, about 89% become pregnant within 1 year. This estimate was lowered slightly (to 85%) to represent the percentage who would become pregnant within 1 year among women now relying on reversible methods of contraception if they abandoned contraception altogether.

[d] With spermicidal cream or jelly.

[e] Foams, creams, gels, vaginal suppositories, and vaginal film.

judgment, so emergency contraception should be provided by advance prescription to every sexually active female adolescent and to each of those who may be contemplating sexual activity.

Sexually Transmitted Disease Risk Reduction

Adolescents are more likely to acquire STDs than other age-groups because of both their intrinsic biological vulnerability and their more risky sexual practices. Careful counseling about the risks attendant with the decision to become sexually active is an important element in providing contraceptive education. For adolescents who are sexually active, pregnancy protection should not be sacrificed for the sake of STD risk reduction. Adolescents who are at risk for pregnancy *and* for STDs should be

offered methods to minimize each risk. The most effective method of contraception that she will use should be combined with male condoms (or to some extent, female condoms) to reduce the risk of many STDs, especially those transmitted by body fluids. Reassuring information has been presented indicating that none of the hormonal methods of contraception increases the risk of HIV infection (Morrison et al., 2005).

Maximize Noncontraceptive Benefits

Hormonal contraceptives can provide important health benefits and improve a young woman's quality of life in addition to providing birth control. Some birth control pills can be used to treat acne, reduce hirsutism, regulate menses (for those who want predictable bleeding), or eliminate or minimize menses (for women who suffer from dysmenorrhea, catamenial seizures, menstrual migraine, premenstrual syndrome [PMS], or premenstrual dysphoric disorder [PMDD]). Hormonal contraceptives can also reduce menstrual blood loss, which may be particularly important to women with anemia or clotting disorders. Women with active lifestyles (athletes) and those with other hypoestrogenemic conditions (eating disorders) may benefit from both menstrual control and restoration of normal estrogen levels with potential beneficial effects on the skeleton. Women who have polycystic ovary syndrome (PCOS) benefit from the progestin in hormonal contraceptives to offset the unopposed estrogen exposure induced by their condition. All women benefit from long-term health improvement, such as the reduction in the risk of ovarian and endometrial cancers. New designs of condoms may enhance sexual pleasure as well as reduce the risk of acquiring and transmitting STDs.

Minimize Side Effects

The importance of side effects cannot be overstated. Foster et al. (2004) found that 9% of women in California who were at risk for unintended pregnancy used no method of contraception, mostly for method-related reasons, such as a concern about side effects. There are two strategies for reducing the impact that side effects have on contraceptive continuation rates. The first is to select a method with few side effects. The second is to counsel intensively about potential side effects before initiation and to respond promptly to any complaints of "nuisance" side effects, if they arise. In order to anticipate what side effects might cause an individual teen to stop using contraceptives, it is often instructive to ask her what problems she has heard about the method and what concerns she herself might have. Teens are very image conscious and generally live in the present. Therefore, if the patient notices any complexion changes or weight gain, she will often blame the contraceptive and discontinue its use. The need for adherence to a daily administration is more challenging for teens than it is for adults. Research has demonstrated the effectiveness targeted counseling can have on continuation rates. Working with a group of low-literacy Mexican women who were very worried about amenorrhea, Canto De Cetina et al. (2001) showed that structured counseling about the impact the injection had on menses decreased the discontinuation rates from 43% to 19%.

Flexibility in Contraceptive Initiation and Use

Beyond selecting a method with the adolescent, clinicians can enhance the young woman's success with the method by being flexible in its use. Each of the following Chapters (Chapters 43–47) gives more detailed examples of these practices, which although relatively new, have been shown to be safe and to reduce barriers to contraceptive use. The following principles and practices are especially important for teens:

1. No pelvic examination is needed before initiating any contraceptive method except intrauterine contraceptives, diaphragms, and, perhaps, vaginal rings (if ring use is to be demonstrated).

2. No cervical cytological testing (Pap smear) is needed before the initiation of any method in an asymptomatic woman. Even a history of an abnormal pap smear does not preclude use of any hormonal or barrier methods of contraception. Urine testing can be done to screen for STDs.

3. Immediate initiation of contraceptive methods should be offered. Beyond the traditional barrier methods, examples of this include the Quick Start of birth control pills, contraceptive vaginal rings, contraceptive transdermal patches, DMPA, and copper IUDs. Each of these methods can be started on any day of a woman's cycle if it is relatively certain she is not pregnant. Back-up methods for 7 to 9 days are needed after Quick Start of various methods. In addition, it is prudent to provide emergency contraception with Quick Start. Quick Start protocols should also be applied to women who have lapses in their contraceptive use, such as women who return late for reinjection of DMPA or for pill refills.

4. Extended cycle use of combined hormonal contraceptives (pills, patches, and rings) can add health benefits and improve young women's quality of life, although the patch may be associated with higher estrogen levels.

5. Identify opportunities to provide contraception. One group of high-risk women is women who come for pregnancy testing and have negative results. Those who are not seeking pregnancy, may be maximally attentive and motivated to embrace changes in their methods. Investing time with them and acting immediately to provide them with effective contraceptives can make a tremendous difference (Zabin et al., 1996).

6. If possible, provide condoms in generous quantities. Give specific instructions for use and storage.

CHALLENGES FACING CLINICIANS

There are few issues in medicine that excite as much controversy as provision of contraceptive and reproductive health services to adolescents. In many jurisdictions, there are legal restrictions on the services that can be provided to the teen patient based only on the teen's request. Only 21 States and the District of Columbia explicitly allow all minors to consent for contraceptive services. Another 25 require prior pregnancy, high school graduation, parental consent, or other conditions (Guttmacher Institute, 2005). Even when there are no legal requirements for parental involvement, there is a challenge in many practices to preserve patient confidentiality in the face of inquiring parents, itemized billing, and indiscrete insurance companies.

The presence of the mother in the examination room may limit the clinician's access to complete information from her daughter. Regardless of whether or not a pelvic exam is needed that day, it is important to have a mother excused from the room for at least a few moments to permit private conversation with the patient.

Teens have short attention spans. A call from them or a request for an appointment requires immediate response. It can be challenging to arrange a busy office practice to accommodate these urgent calls. Having someone on staff who is sensitive to teen issues and capable of effectively communicating with them can be very valuable to a practice. American College of Obstetricians and Gynecologists (ACOG) has produced a script that can be used by staff to answer common adolescent-related telephone questions (American College of Obstetricians and Gynecologists, 2003). When interacting with teens, reflective, open-ended questioning is more effective than direct, closed questions. Reflective questions, such as "If you had a friend who was thinking about having sex with her boyfriend, what would you want her to know?" can reveal much about your patient's knowledge base and attitude.

Clinicians have even greater challenges reaching young men with important contraceptive and STD risk-reducing messages and methods. Historically, the woman has been used as the proxy to carry condoms to the man. Although providing the young woman with barriers and supplies is unquestionably important (she *is* the one at risk for pregnancy), young men also need one-on-one education and medical counseling about their risks, responsibilities, and choices. Just more than one third of young men aged 18 to 19 reported that they had talked to a parent about contraception before they turned age 18 (Abma et al., 2004). Because many young men get no information at school or from their parents and may receive inaccurate information from their peers, access to medically accurate information may be only available in the confines of the medical office or as part of community outreach efforts in which medical professionals participate.

CHALLENGES FACING TEENS

Adolescent patients are confronted with several challenges in accessing contraceptive services. These barriers can be classified into the following groups of concerns:

Access to Low-Cost, Appropriate Medical Services

Adolescents often have limited financial resources. Even low-cost medical services can be prohibitively expensive for them. Lack of familiarity with large managed care systems can functionally limit access. Once in a system, teens must find providers to address their issues. Adolescents often wish to discuss issues of sexuality and contraception with their providers, but are reluctant to introduce the subjects when they are with their clinicians. This reluctance, together with the provider's hesitancy, results in a wide discrepancy between what teens want to discuss and what they do discuss with their primary health care physicians (Malus et al., 1987).

Access to Confidential Services

A randomized, controlled trial has clearly shown that teens are more willing to communicate with and seek health care from physicians who ensure confidentiality (Ford et al., 1997). Most (60%) teen women seeking sexual health services in one recent study reported that a parent or guardian was aware that they were in a family planning clinic. However, of the 40% of teens whose adult figures were not aware of their attending, more than 70% said they would not use the clinic for prescription contraception if parental notification were mandatory (Jones et al., 2005). The study also showed that lack of access to prescriptions would not reduce teen sexual activity, but would likely increase rates of adolescent pregnancies and STDs. Unfortunately, studies have shown that 17% to 37%

of private physicians are unwilling to or do not provide reproductive health services to minors without parental consent (Jones et al., 2005), which may reflect state laws.

Access to Age-Appropriate Teen Services

Modern media profoundly affect adolescents' attitudes toward sex, as well as their communication and learning styles. Estimates are that the average teen witnesses 14,000 instances of sexual behavior on television each year, and that in <10% of those sexual encounters is there any mention of contraception or STDs. These exposures may not increase the accuracy of teens' understanding of sexuality and its risks, but they increase the teen's curiosity and expectations and may significantly influence behavior.

Television and videos have also transformed adolescent learning styles. Attention spans have been constricted to the 40-second sound bite. In the age of MTV, written handouts may have very limited educational benefit. If written materials are used, they must be corrected for age-appropriate literacy and for short reader attention spans. ACOG suggests that written materials be pocket sized. Furthermore, because some adolescents may not have confided to their parents that they are sexually active, written materials found in their possession might be incriminating. Videotapes or DVDs played in the office before the patient–provider interaction are quite helpful, as are individual counseling sessions with office staff trained in dealing with teens. Peer counselors are also effective adjuncts in outreach programs and in practice settings. Web sites can provide the teen more private and conveniently timed access to information.

Most adolescents do not get out of school until late in the afternoon, and they may have difficulty keeping appointments during the office hours of most practices. This may be particularly true if they have limited access to transportation and are trying to maintain privacy. Late afternoon or early evening office hours or weekend availability can enhance adolescent access to services. Privacy needs may also limit the times and ways in which the teen can interact with a health care provider. The adolescent who calls from a pay phone or cell phone to ask about a contraceptive side effect during her lunch break cannot be put on hold or called back later when the provider is between patients. One successful arrangement is to identify someone on the staff to answer such calls and then arrange the staff person's lunch hour around most teens' schedules.

Access to Broader Community-Based Programs

Each of the access issues listed previously is relevant at the individual provider level. To make even more impact on adolescent pregnancy rates and teenage sex activity, political, community, educational, and religious institutions require modification and involvement (Brindis, 1999). Demonstration projects have shown that broader, multicomponent, community-based programs are needed (Paine-Andrews et al., 1999). A comprehensive community-based program in South Carolina that involved media, local clergy, and schools and emphasized on decision making, communication skills, self-esteem enhancement, and human reproduction caused the pregnancy rates for 14- to 17-year-old adolescent females to fall from 67 to 25 per 1,000 (Koo et al., 1994). After the removal of key providers and support elements of that program, the pregnancy rate rose again.

Other programs using peer counseling in schools and nurse practitioner counselors in off-campus sites have also been successful, but a coordinated effort that focuses on the root causes of teen sexuality and other risk-taking behaviors has even more leverage. Often girls have unprotected sex because of a secret desire to keep a boyfriend (by becoming pregnant), to have someone of her own to love, or to act out against a parent (Dodson, 1996).

The practitioner must be aware of whether his or her own office or clinic hours and setup are conducive to adolescent health care needs. In addition, the practitioner should become familiar with sources of referral for services such as contraception, STD treatment, and elective abortion. Finally, because virtually all studies show that parent–teenager communication is important to improving contraceptive use (Whitaker et al., 1999), clinicians (particularly pediatricians) can advise parents of small children about how to discuss sexuality issues with their children.

CONTRACEPTIVE CONSIDERATIONS IN ADOLESCENTS WITH COMMON ILLNESSES OR DISABILITIES

As many as 10% to 20% of all children and adolescents experience illness or disability by age 20. The standard used to evaluate the safety of contraception in any individual situation is that the risks of using the method must be less than the risks presented by pregnancy. For women with serious medical problems, pregnancy may be very hazardous. Therefore, it may be reasonable to accept higher risks with birth control with these women than would be acceptable for healthier women. Some methods may be absolutely contraindicated in women. The appropriateness of use of any method must be evaluated considering how important pregnancy prevention is and what are the woman's other options.

The World Health Organization (WHO) Medical Eligibility Guidelines represent a consensus of contraceptive experts based on current research. The guidelines are not intended to be a basis for individual risk recommendations, but to provide national family planning organizations with recommendations upon which to base their protocols. Their recommendations are rated on a scale of 1 to 4 (Table 42.3).

It should be noted that the WHO rated category 1 ("no restriction on use") includes all methods of reversible contraception for women with the following medical conditions—gestational diabetes, benign breast conditions, family history of breast cancer, varicose veins, nonmigraine headaches, benign ovarian tumors, past PID with subsequent pregnancy, viral hepatitis carrier, simple thyroid goiter, hypothyroidism, hyperthyroidism, pelvic tuberculosis, epilepsy, schistosomiasis (except with severe fibrosis of the liver), taking antibiotics (except rifampin or griseofulvin), more than 21 days after childbirth, or after first-trimester abortion. WHO rated as category 2 ("advantages generally outweigh theoretical or proven risks") the use of estrogen-containing hormonal methods in the following situations—smoking at less than age 35, uncomplicated valvular heart disease, superficial thrombophlebitis, major

surgery without prolonged immobilization, and breastfeeding 6 months or more after delivery. In these conditions, all other methods can be used without restriction (WHO category 1). Similarly, progestin-only pills carry a unique WHO 2 rating for past ectopic pregnancy and intrauterine contraceptives are uniquely identified as WHO 2 rating for past PID without subsequent pregnancy, vaginitis without cervicitis, uterine fibroids, thalassemia, anemia, nulliparity, severe dysmenorrhea, endometriosis, uterine abnormalities not disturbing cavity, and immediately following second-trimester abortion.

Initiating intrauterine contraceptives carries a WHO category 3 rating (theoretical or proven risks generally outweigh the advantages) for those with ovarian cancer, increased risk for STDs, HIV infection, AIDs, and benign trophoblastic disease. All other methods are rated WHO category 1 for this condition. The use of estrogen-containing hormonal methods is uniquely rated as WHO category 3 for nonbreastfeeding women less than 21 days postpartum or breastfeeding women between 6 weeks and 6 months postpartum, whereas all others are rated WHO category 1.

On the other hand, WHO rates as category 4 ("should not use") estrogen-containing hormonal contraceptives for women who are having major surgery with prolonged immobility or leg surgery, but has no restriction on the use of all other methods (WHO category 1) in these situations. Use of intrauterine contraceptives is rated WHO category 4 while all other methods are rated as WHO category 1 in the following situations—current STDs or PID, distorted uterine cavity, pelvic tuberculosis, endometrial cancer, malignant trophoblastic disease, and immediately after septic abortion. Lactational amenorrhea was contraindicated (WHO category 4) with mood altering medications or other medications that are contraindicated for use in breastfeeding.

Conditions which involve considerations for more than one method are listed on Table 42.4. Additional conditions, which may be encountered in adolescent patients, are discussed subsequently.

Pulmonary Disease

Asthma All methods of contraception may be used by women with asthma. Historically, theoretical concern was raised about estrogen increasing mucus production and/or progesterone increasing mucus viscosity. However, clinical studies have failed to find any consistent association between OC use and the severity or frequency of asthma attacks. If theophylline is used in treatment of asthma, there can be notable drug–drug interactions. Both the estrogen and the theophylline levels may decrease and require higher dosing. It should be noted that current labeling of the levonorgestrel intrauterine system (LNG-IUS) recommends against its use in women who are immunosuppressed by chronic steroid use.

Cystic Fibrosis In a similar vein, the concern that exists with hormonal methods in individuals with cystic fibrosis involves the effect of progesterone on mucus. Progesterone causes thick cervical mucus, and this same effect could lead to thick bronchial mucus. A preliminary study Fitzpatrick et al. (1984) suggested that OCs containing <50 µg ethinyl estradiol doses may not exacerbate pulmonary disease. Stead et al. (1987) studied the pharmacokinetics

TABLE 42.3

WHO Categories for Temporary Methods

WHO Category 1   *Can use* the method. *No restriction on use.*

WHO Category 2   *Can use* the method. *Advantages generally outweigh theoretical or proven risks.* Category 2 conditions could be considered in choosing a method. If the client chooses the method, longer than usual follow-up may be needed.

WHO Category 3   *Should not use* the method unless a doctor or nurse makes a clinical judgment that the client can safely use it. *Theoretical or proven risks usually outweigh the advantages* of the method. Method of last choice, for which regular monitoring will be needed.

WHO Category 4   *Should not use* the method. Condition represents an *unacceptable health risk* if method is used.

---

of sex steroids in women with cystic fibrosis using OCs and found that women with cystic fibrosis receive contraceptive protection similar to that achieved by healthy women. However, hormonal contraceptives should be used with extreme caution in teens with cystic fibrosis until further studies indicate that they are safe in such patients. If used, lower dose formulations would be preferred.

Inflammatory Bowel Disease

If disease is active and malabsorption of steroid sex hormone is possible, OC use is not appropriate (Faculty of Family Planning and Reproductive Health Care, Clinical Effectiveness Unit, 2003). Nonoral hormonal delivery systems (implants, injections, patches, and rings) bypass the enteric absorption problems and can, therefore, be used. In teens with stable, quiescent inflammatory bowel disease, OCs can be used with caution with close monitoring for possible impact on disease activity.

Diabetes

Adolescents with diabetes mellitus are a particularly important group. Fennoy (1989) found that they were at higher risk than expected to become pregnant at a time when their glucose control was often at its worst. Adolescents are also less likely to have developed vascular complications than older diabetic patients and may be the best candidates to use low-dose hormonal methods. Implants may be attractive because of their limited impact on glucose and lipid profiles. Progestin injections have more notably deleterious effects on glucose control and lipid profiles, necessitating careful consideration of benefits and risks. All women with diabetes using hormonal methods of birth control require ongoing glucose monitoring. They also need counseling to plan and prepare for any pregnancies, because preconceptional glucose control has profound impact on pregnancy outcomes.

Hematological Disorders

Iron Deficiency Anemia Hormonal methods of birth control can be helpful for patients with iron deficiency anemia because they tend to limit menstrual flow. Long-term use of progestin injections and LNG-IUS usually results in amenorrhea, which is extremely attractive to patients with anemia. Extended cycle with combined hormone methods reduces menstrual blood loss.

Initiation of copper-bearing IUDs should be discouraged in the face of severe anemia.

Hemorrhagic Disorders Hormonal methods of birth control are excellent choices for patients with hemorrhagic disorders that are intrinsic or medication induced. Hormonal contraceptives tend to diminish the menorrhagia experienced by many women with coagulation disorders by limiting or eliminating menstrual flow (Neinstein, 1994). Combination hormonal contraceptives, as well as progestin injections also suppress ovulation and decrease the ever-present risk of hemorrhage with extrusion of the follicle.

Psychiatric Disease and Mental Retardation

Adolescents with psychiatric conditions frequently have their family planning needs overlooked. Sometimes, their sexuality is seen as acting out or a manifestation of their underlying disease. Once recognized as having contraceptive needs, these patients may have difficulty in providing informed consent or in effectively using a contraceptive method. Many mentally ill patients have dual diagnoses, such as substance abuse and mental illness (often depression) or epilepsy. Barrier methods provide needed reduction in the risk of acquiring an STD, but they may not be consistently used. IUDs are often not appropriate because these patients can be at high risk for PID. Hormonal methods may be preferable with the following caveats:

1. Patients with severe depression, especially with suicidal ideation, are not current candidates for hormonal methods. Others with more mild disease may be considered for hormonal methods.
2. Women who are also being treated for convulsive disorders must have that problem factored into method selection. Those using medications, which induce hepatic clearance of hormones may require higher doses. Injections and IUDs provide robust coverage, but implants are associated with higher failure rates.
3. Institutionalized patients and those who are in supervised living settings may benefit from daily OCs. However, those whose living arrangements are less secure (e.g., homeless persons) may not be able to comply with a daily regimen and will benefit from long-acting agents.

TABLE 42.4

Selected Conditions with Multiple Ratings for Contraceptive Methods

Condition	COC	P/R	POP	DMPA NET-EN	LNG/ETG Implants	Cu-IUD	LNG-IUD
Cardiovascular disease							
Multiple risk factors for arterial cardiovascular disease (such as older age, smoking, diabetes, and hypertension)	3/4	3/4	2	3	2	1	2
Hypertension							
1. Adequately controlled hypertension, where blood pressure CAN be evaluated	3	3	1	2	1	1	1
2. Elevated blood pressure levels (properly taken measurements)							
a. Systolic 140–159 or diastolic 90–99 mm Hg	3	3	1	2	1	1	1
b. Systolic >160 mm Hg or diastolic >100 mm Hg	4	4	2	3	2	1	2
3. Vascular disease	4	4	2	3	2	1	2
Deep venous thrombosis (DVT)/pulmonary embolism (PE)							
1. History of DVT/PE	4	4	2	2	2	1	2
2. Current DVT/PE	4	4	3	3	3	1	3
3. Family history (first-degree relatives)	2	2	1	1	1	1	1
4. Major surgery							
a. With prolonged immobilization	4	4	2	2	2	1	2
b. Without prolonged immobilization	2	2	1	1	1	1	1
Known thrombogenic mutations (e.g., factor V Leiden; prothrombin mutation; protein S, protein C, and antithrombin deficiencies)	4	4	2	2	2	1	2
Superficial thrombophlebitis	2	2	1	1	1	1	
Current and history of ischemic heart disease	4	4	I 2 / C 3	3	I 2 / C 3	1	I 2 / C 3
Stroke (history of cerebrovascular accident)	4	4	I 2 / C 3	3	I 2 / C 3	1	2
Known hyperlipidemias (screening is NOT necessary for safe use of contraceptive methods)	2/3	2/3	2	2	2	1	2
Valvular heart disease							
1. Uncomplicated	2	2	1	1	1	1	1
2. Complicated (pulmonary hypertension, atrial fibrillation, history of subacute bacterial endocarditis)	4	4	1	1	1	2	2
Neurological conditions							
Headaches	I / C	I / C	I / C	I / C	I / C		I / C
1. Non-migrainous (mild or severe)	1 / 2	1 / 2	1 / 1	1 / 1	1 / 1	1	1 / 1
2. Migraine							
a. Without aura (age <35)	2 / 3	2 / 3	1 / 2	2 / 2	2 / 2	1	2 / 2
b. With aura (at any age)	4 / 4	4 / 4	2 / 3	2 / 3	2 / 3	1	2 / 3
Reproductive tract infections and disorders							
Unexplained vaginal bleeding (suspicious for serious condition)						I / C	I / C
Before evaluation	2	2	2	3	3	4 / 2	4 / 2

(continued)

TABLE 42.4

(Continued)

Condition	COC	P/R	POP	DMPA NET-EN	LNG/ETG Implants	Cu-IUD I	Cu-IUD C	LNG-IUD I	LNG-IUD C
Cervical cancer (awaiting treatment)	2	2	1	2	2	4	2	4	2
Breast cancer									
1. Current	4	4	4	4	4	1		4	
2. Past and no evidence of current disease for 5 years	3	3	3	3	3	1		3	
Endometrial cancer	1	1	1	1	1	4	2	4	2
Ovarian cancer	1	1	1	1	1	3	2	3	2
Current pelvic inflammatory disease (PID)	1	1	1	1	1	4	2	4	2
Sexually transmitted diseases (STDs)									
1. Current purulent cervicitis or chlamydial infection or gonorrhoea	1	1	1	1	1	4	2	4	2
2. Increased risk of STDs	1	1	1	1	1	2/3	2	2/3	2
AIDS	1	1	1	1	1	3	2	3	2
Endocrine conditions									
Diabetes									
1. Nephropathy/retinopathy/neuropathy	3/4	3/4	2	3	2	1		2	
2. Other vascular disease or diabetes of >20 years' duration	3/4	3/4	2	3	2	1		2	
Gastrointestinal conditions									
Current symptomatic gall-bladder disease	3	3	2	2	2	1		2	
Past history of COC-related cholestasis	3	3	2	2	2	1		2	
Active viral hepatitis	4	4	3	3	3	1		3	
Cirrhosis									
1. Mild (compensated)	3	3	2	2	2	1		2	
2. Severe (decompensated)	4	4	3	3	3	1		3	
Liver tumor									
1. Benign (adenoma)	4	4	3	3	3	1		3	
2. Malignant (hepatoma)	4	4	3	3	3	1		3	
Drug interactions									
Drugs which affect liver enzymes									
1. Rifampicin	3	3	3	2	3	1		1	
2. Certain anticonvulsants (phenytoin, carbamazepine, barbiturates, primidone, topiramate, oxcarbazepine)	3	3	3	2	3	1		1	
Antibiotics (excluding rifampicin)									
1. Griseofulvin	2	2	2	1	2	1		1	
2. Other antibiotics	1	1	1	1	1	1		1	
Antiretroviral therapy	2	2	2	2	2	2/3	2	2/3	2

COC, combined oral contraceptives; P/R, Patch/Ring; POP, progestin-only pills; DMPA/NET-EN, depot medroxyprogesterone acetate/norethisterone enantate; LNG/ENG implant, levonorgestrel/etonogestrel implants; Cu-IUD, copper intrauterine device; LNG-IUD, levonorgestrel intrauterine device; LNG-IUD, levonorgestrel intrauterine device; AIDS, acquired immunodeficiency syndrome; I, initiation; C, continuation. Modified from: Medical eligibility criteria for contraceptive use - 3rd edition, World Health Organization, Geneva, 2004.

Mentally retarded adolescents also require special considerations because often they are quite curious and uninhibited. Many are vulnerable to exploitation. Sex education is often neglected in these patients. The provider faces both legal questions and practical problems in trying to assess patients' understanding of methods and their ability to apply the selected method effectively. Mental retardation, by itself, usually does not constitute a medical contraindication to use of hormonal contraceptives, but studies show that long-term compliance with OCs in noncontrolled environments is very low. In one study of mentally retarded female adolescents (Chamberlain et al., 1984), the 1-year continuation rate with OCs was only 32%. Satisfaction was highest with injectable contraception. Implants require patient cooperation for insertion and removal under local anesthesia; severely retarded patients may not be able to comply. Injections offer effective intermediate-term contraception, and the progestin injections usually offer the additional benefit of ultimate amenorrhea. Barrier methods and natural family planning (NFP) have no adverse effects on women who are mentally retarded, but the severely impaired patient may not be capable of understanding how to use the methods.

Connective Tissue Disease

Systemic Lupus Erythematosus Systemic lupus erythematosus (SLE) has been closely related to hormones. The strong bias in the female-to-male ratio and the relative frequency of flares during pregnancy raise concerns for the use of estrogen-containing hormonal contraceptives. Two recent studies suggested that the incidence of adverse events were similar among women with SLE, irrespective of the type of contraceptive they were using (Sanchez-Guerrero et al., 2005), and that OCs do not increase the risk of flare among women with SLE whose disease was stable (Petri et al., 2005). It would appear reasonable to consider the use of combined OCs for those women with inactive or moderately active, stable disease. Progestin-only methods appear safe in most women with lupus; in studies to date, there have been no significant differences in numbers of episodes of active SLE flares in progestin users versus controls. Labeling for the LNG-IUS indicates that its use is not recommended if the SLE patient is immunocompromised by her condition or by corticosteroid use, but copper-bearing IUDs are allowed. Barrier methods have the least number of side effects and offer STD risk reduction; however, they have high failure rates, and pregnancy can pose serious hazards to the woman with SLE. NFP similarly has no direct adverse effects but is associated with significantly higher failure rates.

Rheumatoid Arthritis Hormonal contraceptive methods are excellent choices for women with rheumatoid arthritis. Some studies have suggested that OCs may reduce the risk of developing this disease, but there is little evidence they reduce the severity of preexisting disease. Copper IUDs may be used by affected women who are able to check monthly for strings, but the LNG-IUS may not be appropriate for those using steroids or other immunosuppressive therapy. Barrier methods are not contraindicated, but female barrier methods may not be appropriate for women with severe disabilities of their hands and hips.

Renal Disease

Hemodialysis Most adolescents with chronic renal failure are infertile due to hypothalamic-pituitary dysfunction. During dialysis therapy, however, some women resume normal ovulatory function. For sexually active adolescents with menstrual function, contraception is an important issue. The major contraindications to OC use in these adolescents are hypertension and thromboembolic problems. Serum concentrations of progestin from injections in patients undergoing hemodialysis are maintained within therapeutic levels. Intrauterine contraceptive may be contraindicated either because of anemia and/or immunocompromise associated with renal failure. Barrier methods are not contraindicated, but may be associated with unacceptably high failure rates. NFP methods are difficult to use in the face of irregular menstruation.

Transplantation Ovulation and fertility often return within 6 months of successful renal transplantation. Information regarding OC use in an adolescent with a renal transplant is very limited. In teens with no significant hypertension, low-dose, estrogen-containing methods could be used with extreme caution. Progestin-only methods are good choices, except the LNG-IUS because the women are immunosuppressed to prevent graft rejection. Other methods may be used as outlined earlier.

SUMMARY

Comprehensive contraceptive education is the healthiest approach to providing reproductive health care to adolescents. Recognizing that human beings are sexual beings is the starting point for cultivating a long-term commitment to sexual health in adolescents. Encouraging abstinence is one important message, but helping teens assume responsible adult roles in protecting themselves and their partner's current health and well-being as well as their fertility is also important. Parents benefit if they can learn accurate information and skills in order to feel comfortable when discussing this important dimension of human life with their children. Health care providers can work directly with adolescents to provide them all the information they need; they can work through the parents to help families and they can work in their communities to advocate adolescent rights to accurate information and reproductive health services.

WEB SITES

For Teenagers and Parents

http://www.engenderhealth.org. Engender Health International site with basic information on contraception.

http://www.itsyoursexlife.com/. Henry J. Kaiser Family Foundation site provides sexual health information for young adults and their parents.

http://www.sxetc.org/. This online teen newsletter examines love, sex, relationships, and health.

http://www.teenwire.com/. This teen site from the Planned Parenthood Federation of America provides information and news about teen sexuality, sexual health, and relationships.

http://www.youngwomenshealth.org/. The Center for Young Women's Health site, sponsored by Children's Hospital in Boston, provides information on health issues that affect teenage girls and young women.

http://www.reproline.jhu.edu/english/1fp/1methods/ 1methods.htm. Reproductive Health Online: On methods.

http://www.reproline.jhu.edu/english/1fp/1special/ 1special.htm. Reproductive Health Online: On special circumstances.

For Health Professionals

http://www.acog.org/. Information and resources from the American College of Obstetricians and Gynecologists.

http://www.agi-usa.org/index.html. Information and resources from the Alan Guttmacher Institute, a nonprofit organization focused on reproductive health research, policy analysis, and public education.

http://www.arhp.org/. Information and resources from the Association of Reproductive Health Professionals, an interdisciplinary organization that fosters research and advocacy to promote reproductive health.

http://www.conrad.org/. Contraceptive Research and Development Program site provides general information on birth control methods, updates on ongoing research projects, and provides information on contraceptive technology workshops.

http://www.fhi.org/. Family Health International's site provides information on AIDS/HIV, STDs, family planning, reproductive health, and women's studies.

http://www.kff.org/. Henry J. Kaiser Family Foundation site provides information on Adolescent Sexual Health.

http://www.ncbi.nlm.nih.gov/PubMed/. National Library of Medicine search service to access the 9 million citations in MEDLINE and other related databases, with links to participating online journals.

http://www.reproline.jhu.edu/. The Reproductive Health Online site, which is based at The Johns Hopkins University, provides information on family planning and selected reproductive health issues.

http://www.teenpregnancy.org. The National Campaign to Prevent Teen Pregnancy provides comprehensive information about teen pregnancy rates as well as public policy and programmatic recommendations.

REFERENCES AND ADDITIONAL READINGS

Abma JC, Martinez GM, Mosher WD, et al. Teenagers in the United States: sexual activity, contraceptive use, and childbearing, 2002. *Vital Health Stat 23* 2004;(24):1.

Albert B, Brown S, Flanigan C, eds. *14 and younger: the sexual behavior of young adolescents.* Washington, DC: National Campaign to Prevent Teen Pregnancy, 2003.

American College of Obstetricians and Gynecologists. *Tool kit for teen care: suggested responses to common adolescent-related telephone questions.* Washington, DC: American College of Obstetricians and Gynecologists, 2003.

Audet MC, Moreau M, Koltun WD, et al. ORTHO EVRA/EVRA 004 Study Group. Evaluation of contraceptive efficacy and cycle control of a transdermal contraceptive patch vs. an oral contraceptive: a randomized controlled trial. *JAMA* 2001;285(18):2347.

Bermas BL. Oral contraceptives in systemic lupus erythematosus—a tough pill to swallow? *N Engl J Med* 2005;353:2602.

Brindis C. Building for the future: adolescent pregnancy prevention. *J Am Med Womens Assoc* 1999;54:129.

Bruckner H, Bearman P. After the promise: the STD consequences of adolescent virginity pledges. *J Adolesc Health* 2005;36(4):271.

Cagampang HH, Barth RP, Korpi M, et al. Education now and babies later (ENABL): life history of a campaign to postpone sexual involvement. *Fam Plann Perspect.* 1997;29(3):109.

Canto De Cetina TE, Canto P, Ordonez Luna M. Effect of counseling to improve compliance in Mexican women receiving depot-medroxyprogesterone acetate. *Contraception* 2001;63(3):143.

Centers for Disease Control and Prevention. Youth risk behavior surveillance, United States, 2005. Surveillance Summaries June 9, 2006. *MMWR Morb Mortal Wkly Report;* 2006;55(SS-5).

Chamberlain A, Rauh J, Passer A, et al. Issues in fertility control for mentally retarded female adolescents. I. Sexual activity, sexual abuse, and contraception. *Pediatrics* 1984;73(4):445.

Cohen DA, Farley TA, Taylor SN, et al. When and where do youths have sex? The potential role of adult supervision. *Pediatrics* 2002;110(6):e66.

Darroch JE, Singh S, Frost JJ. Differences in teenage pregnancy rates among five developed countries: the roles of sexual activity and contraceptive use. *Fam Plann Perspect* 2001;33(6):244.

Dodson L. *We could be your daughters.* Cambridge, MA: Radcliffe Public Policy Institute, 1996.

Faculty of Family Planning and Reproductive Health Care, Clinical Effectiveness Unit. FFPRHC guidance (October 2003): first prescription of combined oral contraception. *J Fam Plann Reprod Health Care* 2003;29(4):209.

Faculty of Family Planning and Reproductive Health Care Clinical Effectiveness Unit. FFPRHC guidance (October 2004) contraceptive choices for young people. *J Fam Plann Reprod Health Care* 2004;30(4):237; quiz 251.

Farrington A. Today's contraceptive options: finding the right fit. *Health Sex* 2001;6(3):4. Accessed 11/27/05 at http://www.arhp.org/files/H&Sndic2001.pdf.

Fennoy I. Contraception and the adolescent diabetic. *Health Educ.* 1989;20:21.

Fitzpatrick SB, Stokes DC, Rosenstein BJ, et al. Use of oral contraceptives in women with cystic fibrosis. *Chest* 1984;86(6):863.

Ford CA, Millstein SG, Halpern-Felsher BL, et al. Influence of physician confidentiality assurances on adolescents' willingness to disclose information and seek future health care. A randomized controlled trial. *JAMA* 1997;278(12):1029.

Foster DG, Bley J, Mikanda J, et al. Contraceptive use and risk of unintended pregnancy in California. *Contraception* 2004;70(1):31.

Grunbaum JA, Kann L, Kinchen S, et al. Youth risk behavior surveillance—United States, 2003. *MMWR Surveill Summ* 2004;53(2):1.

Guttmacher Institute. *Minors' access to contraceptive services as of November 1, 2005. State policies in brief.* New York: Guttmacher Institute, Accessed 11/27/05 at http://www.agi-usa.org/statecenter/spibs/spib_MACS.pdf. 2005.

Hacker KA, Amare Y, Strunk N, et al. Listening to youth: teen perspectives on pregnancy prevention. *J Adolesc Health* 2000;26(4):279.

Halpern-Felsher BL, Cornell JL, Kropp RY, Oral versus vaginal sex among adolescents: perceptions, attitudes, and behavior. *Pediatrics* 2005;115(4):845.

Hamilton BE, Ventura SJ, Martin JA, et al. *Preliminary births for 2004. Health E-Stats.* National Center for Health Statistics. Released October 28, 2005. Accessed 11/27/05 at http://www.cdc.gov/nchs/products/pubs/pubd/hestats/prelim_births/prelim_births04.htm. 2005.

Henshaw SK. *U.S. teenage pregnancy statistics with comparative statistics for women aged 20–24.* New York: Guttmacher Institute, Accessed 11/27/05 at http://www.agi-usa.org/pubs/teen_stats.html. 2004.

Jones RK, Purcell A, Singh S, et al. Adolescents' reports of parental knowledge of adolescents' use of sexual health services and their reactions to mandated parental notification for prescription contraception. *JAMA* 2005;293(3):340.

Kirby D, Korpi M, Barth RP, et al. The impact of the postponing sexual involvement curriculum among youths in California. *Fam Plann Perspect* 1997;29(3):100.

Koo HP, Dunterman GH, George C, et al. Reducing adolescent pregnancy through a school- and community-based intervention: Denmore SC, revisited. *Fam Plann Perspect* 1994;26:206.

Males M. *Teens and older partners. ReCAPP.* 2004 May-June. Accessed 11/27/05 at http://www.etr.org/recapp/research/AuthoredPapOlderPrtnrs0504.htm. 2005.

Malus M, LaChance PA, Lamy L, et al. Priorities in adolescent health care: the teenager's viewpoint. *J Fam Pract* 1987;25(2):159.

Manlove J, Ryan S, Franzetta K. Patterns of contraceptive use within teenagers' first sexual relationships. *Perspect Sex Reprod Health* 2003;35(6):246.

Morrison CS, Richardson BA, Celentano DD, et al. Prospective clinical trials designed to assess the use of hormonal contraceptives and risk of HIV acquisition. *J Acquir Immune Defic Syndr* 2005;38(Suppl 1):S17.

Mosher WD, Chandra A, Jones J. Sexual behavior and selected health measures: men and women 15–44 years of age, United States, 2002. *Adv Data* 2005;15;(362):1.

Neinstein LS. *Issues in reproductive management.* New York: Thieme Medical Publishers, 1994.

Oman RF, Vesely SF, Aspy CB. Youth assets and sexual risk behavior: the importance of assets for youth residing in one-parent households. *Perspect Sex Reprod Health* 2005; 37(1):25.

Paine-Andrews A, Harris KJ, Fisher JL, et al. Effects of a replication of a multicomponent model for preventing adolescent pregnancy in three Kansas communities. *Fam Plann Perspect* 1999;31(4):182.

Petri M, Kim MY, Kalunian KC, et al. Combined oral contraceptives in women with systemic lupus erythematosus. *N Engl J Med* 2005;353:2550.

Pittman S, Tita AT, Barratt MS, et al. Seasonality and immediate antecedents of sexual intercourse in adolescents. *J Reprod Med* 2005;50(3):193.

QuickStats from the National Center for Health Statistics. Pregnancy, birth and abortion rates for teenagers aged 15–17 years—United States, 1976–2003. *JAMA* 2005;293:1722.

Saewyc EM, Magee LL, Pettingell SE. Teenage pregnancy and associated risk behaviors among sexually abused adolescents. *Perspect Sex Reprod Health* 2004;36(3):98.

Sanchez-Guerrero J, Uribe AG, Jimenez-Santana L, et al. A trial of contraceptive methods in women with systemic lupus erythematosus. *N Engl J Med* 2005;353:2539.

Santelli JS, Abma J, Ventura S, et al. Can changes in sexual behaviors among high school students explain the decline in teen pregnancy rates in the 1990s? *J Adolesc Health* 2004;35(2):80.

Forman G. *Sex smarts: decision making.* Menlo Park, CA: Henry Kaiser Family Foundation and Seventeen Magazine, September 2000.

Smith BL, Martin JA, Ventura SJ. Births and deaths: preliminary data for July 1997–June 1998. *Natl Vital Stat Rep* 1999;47:1.

Stead RJ, Grimmer SF, Rogers SM, et al. Pharmacokinetics of contraceptive steroids in patients with cystic fibrosis. *Thorax* 1987;42(1):59.

Stone N, Ingham R. Factors affecting British teenagers' contraceptive use at first intercourse: the importance of partner communication. *Perspect Sex Reprod Health* 2002;34(4):191.

Tanne JH. Abstinence only programmes do not change sexual behaviour, Texas study shows. *Br Med J* 2005;330(7487):326.

Trussell J. The essentials of contraception: efficacy, safety and personal considerations. In: Hatcher RA, Trussell J, Stewart F, et al. *Contraceptive technology*, 18th ed. New York: Ardent Media, 2004:226.

Whitaker DJ, Miller KS, May DC, et al. Teenage partners' communication about sexual risk and condom use: the importance of parent-teenager discussions. *Fam Plann Perspect* 1999;31(3):117.

Wilson KL, Goodson P, Pruitt BE, et al. A review of 21 curricula for abstinence-only-until-marriage programs. *J Sch Health* 2005;75(3):90.

Zabin LS, Emerson MR, Ringers PA, et al. Adolescents with negative pregnancy test results. An accessible at-risk group. *JAMA* 1996;275(2):113.

CHAPTER 43

Combination Hormonal Contraceptives

Anita L. Nelson and Lawrence S. Neinstein

Combination hormonal contraceptives are agents that include both estrogen and progestin. In general, the progestin component provides contraception (primarily by thickening cervical mucus and suppressing ovulation) and the estrogen component provides cycle control. Currently, several forms of combination hormonal contraception are available in the United States—oral contraceptive (OC) pills, contraceptive transdermal patches, and contraceptive vaginal rings. Progestin-only pills are also discussed in this chapter.

ORAL CONTRACEPTIVES

OCs are the most widely used method of reversible birth control in the United States. With >45 years of successful use, considerable professional confidence has developed in the safety and efficacy of OCs, and a growing appreciation is building among health care providers for the extensive noncontraceptive benefits that pills offer. However, public understanding of these issues lags considerably. Until recently, most Americans could not name a single noncontraceptive benefit of the pill. Today, many women are at least aware of the acne treatment and cycle control benefits, but many women remain concerned about the safety of the pill. These public (mis)perceptions directly influence patient compliance and continuation rates.

Efficacy

The first-year failure rate in typical use for combined OCs has been calculated to be 8%, which is virtually the same as the progestin-only OCs (Trussell, 2004). Because the failure rates observed in clinical trials are generally observed to be <1%, much of the real world failure has been attributed to incorrect pill-taking habits. The lack of daily use of pills has been substantiated by a telephone survey by Oakley et al. (1991), who found that among new start OC users, only 13% reported having taken the pill correctly for 9 months. Often, women are not even aware of their incorrect pill-taking habits. Potter et al. (1996) compared patients' diaries with records generated by computer chips built into the pill packaging, which recorded the time and date the pill

was removed from its pack. In the first cycle, nearly 60% of patients' diaries reported that the patient had missed no pills at all, whereas the electronic device reported that only one third of women had reported perfect use. By the third cycle, the electronic device reported that >50% of women had missed more than two pills during that cycle.

Body Weight and Efficacy Recent studies have suggested a connection between heavier body weight and increased failure rates with OCs. Comparing women in the highest quartile of weight (>70.5 kg) with the lower-weight women, Holt et al. (2002) found that the failure rates in heavier women were 1.2 to 4.5 times higher. In Holt's initial analysis, there was evidence that this increased pregnancy rate was even higher with lower-dose formulations. However, the author's later analysis did not report any dose-related pregnancy risk, although the second article confirmed the higher failure rates with greater body weight (Holt et al., 2005). It is not clear what the underlying cause of such a trend might be. Is it that taller women have a larger volume of distribution? Could it be that heavier women have more adipose tissue, which produces more estrogen to keep the cervical mucus favorable? Finally, are there other nonbiologic features that may explain the higher failure rates? A retrospective analysis of the 1997 National Health Interview Survey and the 1995 National Survey of Family Growth found that the increase in pregnancy rates seen in women with body mass indexes (BMIs) >30 was no longer statistically significant after adjustments were made for age, marital status, education, poverty, ethnic/race parity, and dual method use (Brunner and Hogue, 2005). More research is needed to answer this question. In the interim, clinicians may need to put this issue into perspective. Heavier women have a demonstrated increased risk for thrombotic complications with higher-dose pills. Their known risk for thrombosis outweighs the evidence currently available, suggesting the need for higher-dose pills to prevent pregnancy. However, it is appropriate to counsel heavier women that they may be at higher risk for pregnancy than are slender women to encourage more careful taking of pills and weight loss.

Changes in pill packets and new delivery systems have been designed to enhance successful use of hormonal contraception.

Current Formulations

The doses of the sex steroids in OCs have been dramatically reduced since the 1960 introduction of norethynodrel (Enovid), which contained 9.85 mg of progestin and 150 µg of estrogen. All pills with >50 µg of estrogen have been removed from the U.S. market. The hormones used in combination birth control pills include an estrogen component and a progestin component:

1. Estrogen component: All combination OCs contain one of two synthetic estrogens, mestranol or ethinyl estradiol (EE). These two estrogens differ by a methyl group at the C3 site. Mestranol is biologically inactive. It must be hepatically cleaved into EE; 50 µg of mestranol is approximately equivalent to 35 to 40 µg of EE. Most combination pills currently prescribed contain 30 to 35 µg of EE, although formulations with 20 or 25 µg of EE are increasing in popularity. Formulations with 50 µg of EE are reserved for use with other medications that induce hepatic enzymes.
2. Progestin component: All pills in the United States currently have one of eight synthetic progestins. Seven (norethindrone, norethindrone acetate, ethynodiol diacetate, norgestrel, levonorgestrel, norgestimate, and desogestrel) are derived from an androgen precursor. Therefore, these progestins have both progestational and androgenic metabolic effects. In many instances, the latter can be interpreted as antiestrogenic. The eighth progestin, drosperinone, is a derivative of spironolactone and has progestational, antiandrogenic, and antimineralocorticoid properties.

An extensive array of formulations has evolved over the years in an attempt to meet the needs of women with individual sensitivities to particular sex hormone combinations and strengths. Table 43.1 lists the names, components, and doses of the branded pills currently available. Generic formulations of most of the branded pills are also used frequently to reduce contraceptive costs and are listed in Table 43.1.

Packaging Most packs are for a single cycle. Some include only the active pills (generally 21), whereas others add additional (generally nonactive) pills to make a total of 28 pills in the pack. Active pills are packaged in one of three patterns:

1. Monophasic packets: Each of the active pills has the same dose of estrogen and progestin.
2. Multiphasic packets (biphasic or triphasic): The active pills vary the dose of the estrogen and progestin components throughout the active pill cycle. In most cases, the progestin progressively increases in dose; however, a few formulations hold the dose of progestin constant and increase the estrogen dose over the cycle. Some formulations vary both hormone doses.
3. Progestin-only or minipill packets: Each pill contains a small dose of a progestin. No estrogen is included in the pills. There are no placebo pills.

Pill-Free Intervals The placebo pills have been the focus of much recent innovation in pills. Some formulations add iron supplements to the placebo pills. The 7-day pill-free interval has been recognized to be excessively long with modern low-dose formulations (Mishell, 2005). The early, higher-dose pills required 5 days for serum hormone levels to drop low enough to permit the endometrium to start sloughing; with modern formulations endometrial support is lost within 2 days of taking the last active pill. Ovarian follicular recruitment with the low-dose formulations also begins much earlier during the pill-free week. As a result, breakthrough ovulation may be more likely with low-dose pills, especially if a woman misses any of the first pills in her next pill packet. In addition, patients have more time to develop estrogen-deficiency symptoms during the 7 days of placebo pills. To reduce the 7-day hormone-free interval, one formulation (Mircette) replaced the last five placebo pills with five pills containing 10 µg of EE. Two newer formulations (Yaz and Loestrin 24 Fe) include 24 active low-dose pills and either four placebo pills (Yaz) or four pills with ferrous sulfate (Loestrin 24 Fe) in their 28-day pill packet.

The most profound change in pill packaging and in pill-utilization patterns is the elimination or at least minimization of the number of withdrawal bleeding episodes a pill user experiences each year. Monthly withdrawal bleeding was critical to the acceptance of Enovid in 1960. Women wanted monthly reassurances that they were not pregnant. This was important because OCs were new and because the high-dose pills often caused symptoms that were suggestive of pregnancy, such as nausea, vomiting, and breast tenderness. In 1960, there were no rapid, early pregnancy tests, so the monthly withdrawal bleeding functioned as a home pregnancy test. The withdrawal bleed also signaled that "everything was still working" to women who might have been skeptical about how the pills might adversely impact their reproductive systems. When menstruation-like monthly withdrawal bleeding was built into the pill, it improved women's menses in two ways: OC withdrawal bleeding was generally shorter and lighter than the woman's usual spontaneous menstrual flow, and it was entirely predictable. For the first time, women could plan their lives and activities around their menses rather than having the menses interrupt their lives.

Extended Cycle Pills Currently, we recognize that the placebo pill–induced withdrawal bleeding is not medically necessary and that it causes measurable suffering. Elimination of the pill-free interval also reduces breakthrough ovulation (Archer et al., 2005; Pierson et al., 2005). Extended cycle use of hormonal contraceptives is clearly the wave of the future for most women. Although extended cycle use of any monophasic formulation is possible, the available FDA-approved extended cycle OCs (EE and levonorgestrel [Seasonale and Seasonique]) allow easier patient education and utilization, which is very important for young women. Many insurance plans allow women only one pack of pills/month; extended cycle packages require fewer return trips for refills and less negotiation with pharmacists in months that last >28 days. Seasonale has 84 pills containing 30 µg EE with 0.15 mg levonorgestrel followed by 7 placebo pills. To reduce second cycle spotting, the seven placebo pills are replaced with 10 µg EE tablets in Seasonique. Lybrel was approved in May 2007 and includes 365 active pills per year. Other formulations with lower-dose pills (20 µg EE) in 84/7 configurations.

Drug Interactions

Drugs that induce hepatic enzymes can decrease serum concentrations of the estrogen or progestin components of

TABLE 43.1

Estrogen-Containing Contraceptive Formulations Currently Available in the United States

Progestin-only pills

Major Brand Name	Companies	Progestin (21 pills)	Inactive Pills	Other Names	Companies
Ortho Micronor	O	Norethindrone 0.35 mg	7	Camila	B
				Errin	B
				Jolivette	W
				Nor-QD	W
				Nora-BE	W

Mestranol, 50 μg—Monophasic Oral Contraceptives

Major Brand Name	Companies	Progestin (21 pills)	Inactive Pills	Other Names	Companies
Norinyl 1 + 50 21-d	W	Norethindrone, 1 mg	0	Necon 1/50 21	W
				Norethin[a] 1/50M-21	W
Ortho-Novum 1/50–28	O	Norethindrone, 1 mg	7	Necon 1/50 28	W
				Norethin[a] 1/50M-28	W
				Norinyl 1 + 50 28-d	W

EE, 50 μg—Monophasic Oral Contraceptives

Major Brand Name	Companies	Progestin (21 pills)	Inactive Pills	Other Names	Companies
Demulen 1/50–21	S	Ethynodiol diacetate, 1 mg	0	Zovia 1/50E-21	W
Demulen 1/50–28	S	Ethynodiol diacetate, 1 mg	7	Zovia 1/50E-28	W
Ogestrel 0.5/50–21	W	Norgestrel, 0.5 mg	0	—	
Ogestrel 0.5/50–28	W	Norgestrel, 0.5 mg	7	—	
Ovcon 50	V	Norethindrone, 1 mg	7	—	

EE, 35 μg—Monophasic Oral Contraceptives

Major Brand Name	Companies	Progestin (21 pills)	Inactive Pills	Other Names	Companies
Balziva-21	B	Norethindrone, 0.4 mg	0	—	
Demulen 1/35–21	S	Ethynodiol diacetate, 1 mg	0	Zovia 1/35E-21	W
Demulen 1/35–28	S	Ethynodiol diacetate, 1 mg	7	Kelnor	B
				Zovia 1/35E-28	W
Modicon 28	O	Norethindrone, 0.5 mg	7	Brevicon	W
				Necon 0.5/35 28	W
				Nortrel 0.5/35–28	B
Norinyl 1 + 35 21-d	W	Norethindrone, 1 mg	0	Necon 1/35 21	W
				Norethin[a] 1/35E-21	W
				Nortrel 1/35–21	B
Nortrel 0.5/35–21	B	Norethindrone, 0.5 mg	0	Necon 0.5/35 21	W
Ortho-Cyclen-28	J	Norgestimate, 0.25 mg	7	MonoNessa	W
				Previfem	A
				Sprintec	B
Ortho-Novum 1/35–28	O	Norethindrone, 1 mg	7	Necon 1/35 28	W
				Norethin[a] 1/35E-28	W
				Norinyl 1 + 35 28-d	W
				Nortrel 1/35–28	B
Ovcon 35	V	Norethindrone, 0.4 mg	7	Balziva-28	
				Ovcon 35 chewable	

TABLE 43.1

(Continued)

EE, 30 µg—Monophasic Oral Contraceptives

Major Brand Name	Companies	Progestin (21 pills)	Inactive Pills +	Other Names	Companies
Nordette	D	Levonorgestrel, 0.150 mg	7	Levlin 28	C
				Levora 0.15/30–28	W
				Portia	B
Loestrin 21 1.5/30	B	Norethindrone, 1.5 mg	0	Junel 1.5/30	B
				Microgestin 1.5/30	W
Loestrin FE 1.5/30	B	Norethindrone, 1.5 mg	75-mg ferrous fumarate (7)	Junel FE 1.5/30	B
				Microgestin Fe 1.5/30	W
Low-Ogestrel-21	W	Norgestrel, 0.300 mg	0	Cryselle	D
Lo/Ovral-28	Z	Norgestrel, 0.300 mg	7	Cryselle	D
				Low-Ogestrel	W
Ortho-Cept	O	Desogestrel, 0.150 mg	7	Apri	B
				Desogen	N
				Reclipsen	W
Seasonale	D	Levonorgestrel, 0.150 mg (84 pills)	7	—	
Seasonique	D	Levonorgestrel, 0.150 mg (84 pills)	7 EE,10 µg	—	
Yasmin		Drospirenone, 3.0 mg	7	—	

EE, 20 µg—Monophasic Oral Contraceptives

Major Brand Name	Companies	Progestin (21 pills)	Inactive Pills +	Other Names	Companies
Alesse	Z	Levonorgestrel, 0.1 mg	7	Aviane	D
				Lessina	B
				Levlite	C
				Lutera	W
Loestrin 21 1/20	B	Norethindrone, 1 mg	0	Junel 1/20	B
				Microgestin 1/20	W
Loestrin FE 1/20	B	Norethindrone, 1 mg	75-mg ferrous fumarate (7)	Junel FE 1/20	B
				Microgestin Fe 1/20	W
Mircette	N	Desogestrel, 0.150 mg	2 + EE, 10 µg (5)	Kariva	B
Lybrel (taken continuously 365 days/year)	W	Levonorgestrel, 0.90 mg	None	None	

EE, 20 µg—Monophasic Oral Contraceptives 24-d active pill formulation

Major Brand Name	Companies	Progestin (24 pills)	Inactive Pills +	Other Names	Companies
Yaz	C	Drospirenone 3 mg	4		
Loestrin 24 Fe	V	Norethindrone 1 mg	75 mg ferrous fumarate (4)		

EE, 35 µg—Biphasic Oral Contraceptives

Major Brand Name	Companies	Progestin (pills)	Inactive Pills	Other Names	Companies
Necon 10/11–21	W	Norethindrone, 0.5 (10) Norethindrone, 1.0 mg (11)	0	Gencept[a] 10/11–21	B
Ortho-Novum 10/11–28	O	Norethindrone, 0.5 (10)	7	Gencept[a] 10/11–28	B
		Norethindrone, 1.0 mg (11)		Necon 10/11–28	W

(continued)

TABLE 43.1

(Continued)

EE, 35 µg—Triphasic Oral Contraceptives

Major Brand Name	Companies	Progestin (pills)	Inactive Pills	Other Names	Companies
Ortho-Novum 7/7/7–28	O	Norethindrone, 0.50 mg (7)	7	Necon 7/7/7	W
		0.75 mg (7)		Nortrel 7/7/7	B
		1.00 mg (7)			
Ortho Tri-Cyclen 28	J	Norgestimate, 0.180 mg (7)	7	Tri-Previfem	A
		0.215 mg (7)		Tri-Sprintec	B
		0.250 mg (7)		TriNessa	W
Tri-Norinyl-28	W	Norethindrone, 0.50 mg (7)	7	Aranelle	B
		1.00 mg (9)		Leena	W
		0.50 mg (5)			

EE, 20/30/35 µg—Triphasic Oral Contraceptives

Brand name	Companies	Estrogen (pills)	Progestin (pills)	Inactive Pills +	Other Names	Companies
Estrostep 21	V	EE, 20 µg (5), 30 µg (7), 35 µg (9)	Norethindrone, 1 mg (5)	0		
			1 mg (7)			
			1 mg (9)			
Estrostep FE	V	EE, 20 µg (5), 30 µg (7), 35 µg (9)	Norethindrone, 1 mg (5)	75-mg ferrous fumarate (7)		
			1 mg (7)			
			1 mg (9)			

EE, 30/40/30 µg—Triphasic Oral Contraceptives

Brand name	Companies	Estrogen (pills)	Progestin (pills)	Inactive	Other Names	Companies
Triphasil-28	Z	EE, 30 µg (6), 40 µg (5), 30 µg (10)	Levonorgestrel, 0.050 mg (6)	7	Enpresse	D
			0.075 mg (5)		Tri-Levlen 28	C
			0.125 mg (10)		Trivora-28	W

EE, 25 µg—Triphasic Oral Contraceptives

Major Brand Name	Companies	Progestin (pills)	Inactive Pills	Other Names	Companies
Cyclessa	N	Desogestrel, 0.100 mg (7)	7	Velivet	B
		0.125 mg (7)			
		0.150 mg (7)			
Ortho Tri-Cyclen Lo	O	Norgestimate, 0.180 mg (7)	7		
		0.215 mg (7)			
		0.250 mg (7)			

O, Ortho-McNeil Pharm; B, Barr; W, Watson Labs; EE, ethinyl estradiol; S, GD Searle LLC; V, Warner-Chilcott; J, Johnson RW; A, Andrx Pharms; D, Duramed Pharms (Barr); C, Berlex; Z, Wyeth Pharms Inc.; N, Organon USA Inc; Y, Wyeth-Ayerst.

[a]Trademark abandoned.

combination hormonal contraceptives and increase failure rates (see Table 43.2).

Anticonvulsants Anticonvulsants are the most common class of drugs known to have this effect. These drugs are of particular concern because they are also teratogens. The anticonvulsants that increase hepatic clearance include barbiturates (phenobarbitol and primidone), phenytoin, carbamazepine, felbamate, topiramate, and vigabatrin and are all known to decrease serum steroid levels in women taking OCs. Instead, women using these agents may be better served by using progestin injections or intrauterine contraceptives. If OCs are desired, low-dose formulations (<35 µg EE) or progestin-only pills should not be prescribed for women using these anticonvulsants. The 35-µg EE formulations should be used with caution. If a 3-month trial of 35-µg EE pills coupled with condoms yields continued breakthrough bleeding, a 50-µg EE formulation may be necessary. It should be recognized that no published data support the enhanced contraceptive efficacy of higher-dose (50 µg EE) pills (ACOG Committee on Practice Bulletins-Gynecology, 2006). Clinicians should avoid the use of 50-µg mestranol-containing pills in this situation, as 50 µg of mestranol converts to substantially lower levels (35–40 µg) of EE. There are also no data about the effectiveness of nonoral delivery systems of combination hormonal contraceptives used with these drugs. The transdermal method may be attractive, as the total estrogen delivery is higher than with 35 µg pills, but no specific studies of efficacy have been published. It is advisable to shorten or eliminate the hormone-free interval when any of the combination hormonal contraceptives are used in women taking any of these anticonvulsants. Not all anticonvulsants impact liver metabolism; valproic acid, gabapentin, lamotrigine, and tiagabim do not affect sex steroid levels.

Antibiotics Contrary to popular belief and, in some cases, product labeling, there are only two antiinfective agents that decrease steroid levels in women taking combination OCs. These drugs are rifampin and griseofulvin. Isoniazid increases hepatic transaminase levels and may mask markers of an estrogen-induced hepatoma. Other more common antiinfective agents that do NOT decrease steroid levels in women taking combination OCs include tetracycline (Murphy et al., 1991), doxycycline (Neely et al., 1991), ampicillin (Joshi et al., 1980; Friedman et al., 1980), metronidazole (Joshi et al., 1980), and quinalones (Maggiolo et al., 1991; Back et al., 1991; Csemiczky et al., 1996). Routine use of backup methods with these antibiotics is not warranted (World Health Organization, Department of Reproductive Health and Research, 2005).

St. John's Wort Studies have suggested that St. John's wort, which is sold over-the-counter to treat mild-to-moderate depression, may halve the circulating levels of sex steroids. One placebo-controlled study found that unscheduled bleeding was significantly higher in OC users who took St. John's wort; large follicles (≥30 mm) were seen at higher rates in St. John's wort users (40% versus 6%); and ovulation was detected in up to five times as many women if they used St. John's wort (Murphy et al., 2005).

Other Interactions Some antiretroviral drugs induce hepatic enzymes and lower circulating steroid levels,

whereas others decrease such activity and raise the steroid levels. Tobacco use also increases metabolism of sex steroids.

Mechanisms of Action

1. Thickening of cervical mucus: The progestin component produces thick, viscous, scant cervical mucus that blocks sperm penetration into the upper genital tract. This is the single most important mechanism of action common to all hormonal methods of contraception.
2. Inhibition of ovulation: The progestin-only pill contains such a low dose of progestin that ovulation is inhibited in only 40% to 60% of cycles. Combination pills, however, contain higher doses of progestin and suppress ovulation in 95% to 98% of cycles by inhibiting the surge in luteinizing hormone (LH). With combination pills, levels of follicle-stimulating hormone (FSH) are decreased by estrogen to 70% of normal; LH levels are only 20% of those found in women who are not taking OCs.
3. Endometrial changes: The presence of a progestin early in the cycle induces a thin endometrium with atrophic glands and minimal glycogen stores, which is not conducive to implantation. However, the contribution these endometrial changes make to contraceptive efficacy is undoubtedly minimal, because fertilization is so profoundly prevented by ovulation suppression and impenetrable cervical mucus.
4. Slowed tubal motility: The progestin in the pill slows tubal motility and disrupts the carefully orchestrated sequence of events necessary for successful fertilization and implantation. Again, the role that this theoretical mechanism plays in providing contraception is minor, because the ectopic pregnancy rates are significantly reduced by all combination hormonal methods.

Work-up Needed for Pill Initiation

A complete medical history is needed to identify any contraindications requiring further evaluation (see subsequent text). Blood pressure measurement is prudent before starting estrogen-containing contraceptives. Breast examination may also be needed. No other examinations are needed before initiating OCs (Stewart et al., 2001; World Health Organization, Department of Reproductive Health and Research, 2005). Having determined that the young woman wants to use birth control pills and is a good candidate, the next questions that arise are how to initiate the pills, how many packs to dispense, and when to schedule a return visit.

Pill Initiation

Quick Start/Same-Day Start The quick start or same-day start of birth control pills is the most attractive protocol to use with adolescent women. Teens are often in acute need for immediate contraception. Studies have shown that up to 25% of teens given prescriptions to start their pills with their next menses never start them (Westhoff et al., 2003). The most common reasons for not starting pills include interval pregnancy, change in method, confusion about pill instructions, and fear about possible side effects. Virtually all of these barriers can be overcome by immediate initiation of the pills. If the clinician is reasonably certain that a woman is not pregnant, she should be told to

TABLE 43.2

Drug Interactions

Drugs that decrease contraceptive hormonal levels and/or efficacy

- Anticonvulsants that decrease ethinyl estradiol (EE) and progestins
  - Barbiturates (including phenobarbital and primidone)
  - Carbamazepine
  - Felbamate
  - Oxcarbazepine
  - Phenytoin
  - Topiramate
  - Vigabatrin (Listed on ACOG Committee on Practice Bulletins-Gynecology, 2000, but research and FFPRHC find no impact)
- Antibiotics/antifungals that reduce EE and progestins
  - Rifabutin
  - Rifampicin
  - Griseofulvin (pregnancies documented)
- Antiretrovirals that reduce EE and progestins
  - Protease inhibitors
    - Amprenavir
    - Atazanavir
    - Nelfinavir
    - Lopanavir
    - Saquinavir
    - Ritonavir
  - Nonnucleoside reverse transcription inhibitors
    - Efavirenz
    - Nevirapine
- Other agents that induce liver enzymes
  - Lansoprazole (no reduction in EE)
  - Tacrolimus (no published evidence of decreased efficacy)
  - Bosentan (no published evidence of decreased efficacy, but potent teratogen requiring monthly pregnancy testing)
  - Modafinil

Drugs whose effects may be altered by use of combination hormonal contraceptives

	Decreased clinical effect
• All antihypertensives	Hypotensive effect may be antagonized
• Antidiabetics	Hypoglycemic effects maybe antagonized
• Anticoagulants: *Phenidione, Warfarin*	Anticoagulant effect reduced[a]
• Tricyclic antidepressants	Antidepressant effects of tricyclics may be reduced, but side effects may increase because serum concentration increased. No evidence identified
	Increased clinical effect
• Immunosuppressants: *Cyclosporin*	Serum levels increased; potential toxicity
• Corticosteroid	Serum levels increased; no significant clinical effect
• Bronchodilators: *Theophylline*	Serum levels increased; potential toxicity[a]
• Dopaminergics: *Ropinirole*	Serum levels increased; no significant clinical effect
• Potassium-sparing diuretics	Drospirenone may lead to hyperkalemia[a]

FFPRHC, Faculty of Family Planning and Reproductive Health Care
[a]Measuring serum levels after contraceptive initiation may be appropriate.
Adapted from ACOG Committee on Practice Bulletins-Gynecology. ACOG practice bulletin. The use of hormonal contraception in women with coexisting medical conditions. Number 18, July 2000. *Int J Gynaecol Obstet* 2001;75(1):93.
Faculty of Family Planning and Reproductive Health Care Clinical Effectiveness Unit. FFPRHC Guidance (April 2005). Drug interactions with hormonal contraception. *J Fam Plann Reprod Health Care* 2005;31(2):139.

start taking her pills the same day (starting with the first one in the pack) and to abstain from intercourse or to use condoms for the next 7 days. If she has had unprotected sexual intercourse within the previous 5 days, administer two levonorgestrel emergency contraceptive pills immediately and have her start the first pill in her pack the next day. Sensitive urine pregnancy testing may be performed if there is anything in her history that raises suspicion of an ongoing pregnancy. The patient should be advised that her next menses will be delayed and will start with the placebo pills. If she fails to have a withdrawal bleed or has any symptoms of pregnancy, she should have pregnancy testing done as soon as possible. There is no concern that birth control pills are teratogenic, but early diagnosis of pregnancy is always important (Ahn, 2005).

Reassuringly, clinical studies that compared women who used quick start with those who used conventional start of OCs found no increase in the number of days of unscheduled spotting, or bleeding. In fact, the only significant difference between the two groups was that many more of the quick start users (72%) were on the pill 3 months later than were the conventional start users (56%) (Lara-Torre and Schroeder, 2002; Westhoff et al., 2003).

Quick Start in Women with Irregular Menses For women who do not have regular menses, the same quick start initiation rules apply. For example, if a woman is amenorrheic, she can start OCs at any time if it is reasonably certain that she is not pregnant. She will need to abstain or to use the backup method for 7 days. If a patient has just had an abortion (spontaneous or elective), she can start using OCs immediately; no backup method is necessary. If a woman is switching from another method, she can start pills immediately. There is no need to wait for menses. She will need to use a backup method for 7 days if there has been any interruption in her prior protection (e.g., >13 weeks since her last depot medroxyprogesterone acetate [DMPA] injection, late for restart of patches, etc.). In each of these circumstances, the need for emergency contraception (EC) should be evaluated.

First Day Start If quick start of OCs is not possible, then the first day start is acceptable. With this protocol, the patient is given an interval method (condoms) to use until the *first* day of her next menses, when she should start her pills. No backup method is needed after a first day start. The patient may need to align the pills in her pack to correspond to her pill-taking day.

Sunday Start The least attractive pill initiation protocol is the Sunday start. The most significant drawback for the Sunday start is that if a patient needs last-minute refills, she may have difficulty getting in touch with her provider during the weekend. Furthermore, as a Sunday start represents a start on cycle day 1 to 6, instructions for backup methods can be unduly complex, confusing, and are often ignored. However, sometimes the pill packets require a Sunday start.

Condoms All teens should be given condoms and taught how to use them, even if they select OCs. This is important because teens need dual methods to help reduce the risk of sexually transmitted diseases. In addition, many will decide to discontinue the pill before they return for their scheduled follow-up visit (Rosenberg et al., 1995). If those young women are knowledgeable about condom use and have a supply of condoms available, they may be less likely to have unprotected intercourse. Because many women will forget to take all their pills, providing a prescription for EC in advance of need is an important part of OC initiation. At the time of pill initiation, be sure to review with the patient when she is to take her pills, where she plans to store them, what she should do about missed pills, and how she plans to remember to take her pills.

When OCs are initiated, two other practical and somewhat interrelated issues arise: How many cycles to dispense/prescribe, and how soon to see the patient in follow-up.

Prescription Length and Follow-up Appointments For adult women, the World Health Organization (WHO) recommends that a year's requirement of OCs be given to reduce barriers to access (World Health Organization, Department of Reproductive Health and Research, 2005). However, adolescent women have relatively high rates of brand switching and method switching. Pills that are generously dispensed to a woman cannot be recalled and used by other patients if she changes methods or formulations. For that reason, clinics often limit initial users to three packs. Insurance companies may limit dispensing even more stringently for other reasons: To guarantee that a woman is still under their plan at the time she uses her pills, that she will not switch brands or methods, and that she pays a full co-pay for each pack of pills. In adolescents, the OC discontinuation rate is high and teenaged girls often think of new questions as they use their pills. For these reasons, the traditional 3-month follow-up visit is still important for new-start adolescents. In some situations, it may be advisable to see the teen in 1 month and again at 3 months after pill initiation.

Noncontraceptive Benefits Important to Adolescent Women

Decreased Menstrual Discomfort Cyclically administered combination OCs significantly reduce monthly menstrual blood loss, the number of days of bleeding, and dysmenorrhea. Mittelschmerz is eliminated in most women because ovulation is inhibited in all but a very small percentage of cycles. Women with anovulatory cycles or dysfunctional uterine bleeding—common problems in adolescents—achieve predictable, controlled cycles with the use of OCs. Women who are taking medications that increase menstrual blood loss (e.g., anticonvulsants, anticoagulants) benefit from these impacts of OC use. Women who have bleeding disorders also benefit from suppression of ovulation, which reduces their risk of internal hemorrhage each month.

Dysmenorrhea is a particularly important problem faced by adolescent girls (see Chapter 50). Dysmenorrhea inflicts considerable suffering and compromises the young woman's productive potential. Painful menses is the single greatest reason why women younger than 25 years miss days at school and work (Davis et al., 2000). OCs significantly reduce dysmenorrhea, even when given in traditional cyclic manner. In a placebo-controlled study of teenaged girls with moderate-to-severe menorrhea, the mean overall pain scores decreased significantly in OC users by 3 months (Davis et al., 2005).

Premenstrual tension syndrome may be reduced by the cyclic use of combination OCs. One formulation (Yaz) has been proved to be an effective treatment for premenstrual dysphoric disorder (Yonkers et al., 2005).

More creative applications of birth control pills, such as extended use of monophasic active pills ("bicycling," "tricycling," or continuous use), can provide even more benefits to women who have dysmenorrhea or exacerbations of their medical problems during menses. For example, women who have menstrual-related migraine headaches, catamenial seizures, or asthma exacerbations with menses can eliminate those problems by eliminating the placebo pills and avoiding hormone withdrawal. The first FDA-approved product for this was Seasonale. Other variations are expected soon. Flexibility in pill use can allow women to control more routinely when they have their menses. Health care providers frequently use OCs to avoid onset of menses while a patient is on her honeymoon; these same techniques can prevent menses from interfering with other important events in young women's lives.

Improvement in Acne, Hirsutism, and Other Androgen Excess Problems

The FDA has approved 3 brands of oral contraceptives for the treatment of mild-to-moderate cystic acne in women desiring to use oral contraceptives (Ortho Tri-Cyclen, Estrostep and Yaz). By reducing ovarian production of androgens and reducing circulating levels of free testosterone (through increased hepatic production of sex hormone–binding globulin [SHBG]), these OCs reduce the number of lesions and their intensity. Maximal beneficial effects in the clinical trials were seen at 6 months, which might encourage longer-term use. Hair shaft diameter is smaller in OC users, although this beneficial impact of OCs on hirsutism may take 12 months to become clinically apparent.

Treatment of Hypothalamic Hypoestrogenism

Many adolescents have eating disorders (e.g., anorexia nervosa, bulimia), excessive exercise programs, and/or stresses that suppress gonadotrophin production and create a hypoestrogenic state (see Chapters 33 and 52). The lack of estrogen in a teen can compromise bone mineral density accumulation and put her at risk for osteoporosis and fracture at an early age (Gordon and Nelson, 2003). Although it is important to deal with the underlying problems that cause hypoestrogenism, it may also be important to supply adequate estrogen to promote bone health. In most circumstances, the physiological doses of estrogen used to prevent bone loss in postmenopausal women are not adequate to build bone density in adolescent girls. Birth control pills have been the mainstay of therapy in treating women with the athletic triad (Hergenroeder et al., 1997). However, the skeletal benefits of estrogen continue to be debated among different patient groups (Liu and Lebrun, 2006). In addition, because menses may compromise athletic performance, many coaches oppose OC use unless the pills can be used in extended cyclic manner to maintain amenorrhea.

Reduce the Risk of Ovarian and Endometrial Carcinoma

OCs are the only medical intervention with strong evidence that they reduce the risk of developing ovarian cancer later in life. Women who have used OCs for at least 1 year reduce their risk of developing epithelial ovarian cancer by 40%. Long-term users (>10 years) enjoy an 80% reduction in risk. This effect endures for >15 years after the last pill. Ovarian cancer protection is most clearly demonstrated when the pill is taken by young women, just as childbearing and breast-feeding reduce ovarian cancer risk only if they occur before 30 years of age. A case–control study suggested that carriers of the BRCA1 genetic mutation also experience a reduction in ovarian cancer with OC use (Narod et al., 1998). Two mechanisms have been postulated to explain this risk reduction—the inhibition of "incessant ovulation" and increased follicular cell apoptosis.

OC use at any time during the reproductive years significantly reduces a woman's risk of developing any of the three major histological forms of endometrial carcinoma by providing progestin. This protection increases with longer duration of use; women who use OCs for 12 years reduce their risk of endometrial carcinoma by 72%. This protection endures 19 years beyond the last pill use (Schlesselman, 1995). Women with anovulatory cycles achieve the greatest risk reduction.

Other Health Benefits

Anemia is reduced because menstrual blood loss is diminished by OC use. This can benefit women with sickle cell disease and those with iron deficiency anemia. The thickened cervical mucus induced by OCs can block migration of bacteria into the upper genital tract, which reduces a woman's risk of acquiring gonococcal-related pelvic inflammatory disease. Long-term OC use has also been associated with a reduction in benign breast changes.

Metabolic Impacts

Both estrogen and progestin have important metabolic effects, with which clinicians should be familiar (Fig. 43.1). In many formulations, the estrogen-induced metabolic impacts may be partially cancelled by the androgenicity of the progestin acting as an antiestrogen. This is why different pills with the same dose of estrogen, but with different progestins or different doses of the same progestin, may have different estrogenic impacts. In general, the second-generation progestins (norgestrel and levonorgestrel) have greater androgenicity than do the first-generation progestins (norethindrone compounds) or the third-generation progestins (norgestimate and desogestrel). The newest progestin, drosperinone, has *anti*androgenic activity itself, and it allows full expression of the estrogen's impact. By the same logic, the androgen-induced metabolic impacts are partially canceled by the estrogen component of the pill. The net metabolic impact of each formulation differs. These differences may be helpful in selecting formulations for women with different medical problems or side effects.

Coagulation Factors

Factors associated with the extrinsic clotting pathway (fibrinogen and factors I, V, VII, VIII, and X) are uniformly increased by estrogen-containing birth control pills in proportion to their estrogen dose. The percutaneous delivery system may have different dose-dependent impacts on coagulation factors than seen with OCs. Most women balance their increases in clotting factors by inducing compensatory increases in their fibrinolytic and anticoagulation factors. However, some women are genetically unable to compensate. The clinical

	Ethinyl Estradiol	Progestins
Protein	↑ Globulins	None
Carbohydrate	↓ Insulin response	↓ Insulin resistance:
		↑ Insulin
		↓ Glucose tolerance
Lipids	↑ HDL cholesterol	↓ HDL cholesterol
	↓ LDL cholesterol	↑ LDL cholesterol
	↑ Triglycerides	
Electrolytes	↑ Na retention	↑ Na retention

FIGURE 43.1   Metabolic effects of oral contraceptives. HDL, high-density lipoprotein; LDL, low-density lipoprotein; Na, sodium.

significance of these changes is discussed later in the section Thromboembolism.

Binding Globulins Estrogen increases hepatic synthesis of carrier proteins such as albumin, SHBG, thyroxine-binding globulin (TBG), and corticosteroid-binding globulin (CBG). These increases can affect the interpretation of some laboratory tests (such as total thyroxine), but do not affect measures of unbound hormones (such as FT_4). Increased levels of SHBG bind free testosterone and reduce androgen-induced changes such as hirsutism and acne (see earlier discussion).

Angiotensin The estrogen component of the combination birth control pill increases angiotensin by increasing hepatic production of its precursor. Angiotensin can cause reversible hypertension in vulnerable patients. However, angiotensin sensitivity is difficult to predict. The pill also activates adrenal production of aldosterone, which causes fluid retention and contributes to higher blood pressure. A history of pregnancy-induced hypertension is not predictive nor is an increased risk for the development of increased blood pressure with OC use. However, women who have experienced hypertension with OC use in the past face at least a 10% risk of recurrence if rechallenged with estrogen-containing contraceptives.

Lipid Metabolism Triglyceride levels are increased by approximately 20% to 30% with exogenous estrogen use. However, estrogen-induced triglycerides are composed of remnants that are not generally conducive to plaque formation. Triglycerides may pose a problem if a patient has baseline elevated triglyceride concentrations near a range predisposing to pancreatitis (>500). Estrogen also increases total cholesterol, high-density lipoprotein (HDL) cholesterol, while decreasing low-density lipoprotein (LDL) cholesterol. The androgenic component of the progestin has the opposite effect. The net impact on lipids, therefore, varies with different formulations. The third-generation progestins, designed to have greater selectivity for progestin receptors, have less androgenic impacts.

In combination with estrogen they cause no significant changes in LDL. The drosperinone-containing pills have antiandrogenic effects and have the most notable impacts on reducing LDL and raising HDL. First-generation progestins at lower doses also have minimal impacts on lipid metabolism. The second-generation progestins and higher doses of the first-generation progestins have a slightly adverse impact on HDL/LDL ratio. The clinical significance of this impact has been questioned by experiments showing that OC usage in female monkeys was accompanied by a decrease in coronary artery plaque formation despite adverse lipid impacts (Clarkson et al., 1990). However, until human data are more firmly established, patients with dyslipidemia should be closely monitored when they use combination hormonal methods.

Glucose Metabolism Both estrogen and progesterone have been implicated in influencing glucose metabolism—estrogen may suppress insulin production and progesterone can increase peripheral insulin resistance. With higher hormonal doses, older formulations of birth control pills were noted to cause deterioration in glucose tolerance. Most studies have found that modern pill formulations with lower hormonal doses cause no impairment in glucose tolerance in euglycemic women, but some minor impact of insulin resistance remains (Godsland and Crook, 1994). Even in high-risk patients, however, this is not clinically significant. In a prospective study of women with a history of gestational diabetes who used low-dose OC pills, Kjos et al. (1998) reported no acceleration in the development of glucose intolerance or overt diabetes compared with similar women using nonhormonal contraceptives. OC use in women with overt diabetes rarely changes insulin requirements and has been shown not to increase the risk of diabetic nephropathy or retinopathy.

Contraindications

Medical complications that are considered to be contraindications for estrogen-containing contraceptive use on the basis of current scientific evidence are listed in Table 43.3

TABLE 43.3

Absolute Contraindications to Estrogen-Containing Contraceptives

On Label	WHO Category 4
Exclusive breast-feeding	Breast-feeding ≤6 wk
History of thromboembolism	Current or history of DVT/PE
History of thrombophilia	Known thrombogenic mutation
Coronary artery disease	Current or history of ischemic heart disease
Cerebral vascular disease	Stroke (history of CVA)
Known or suspected cancer of the breast	Current breast cancer
Hepatic tumor (benign or malignant)	Liver tumors (benign or malignant)
History of cholestatic jaundice or jaundice with prior pill use	—
Known or suspected cancer of the endometrium or other estrogen-sensitive neoplasm	—
Unexplained abnormal vaginal bleeding	—
Known or suspected pregnancy	—
postpartum (<3 wk)	—
	Age ≥35 years and smoking ≥15 cigarettes/d
	$BP_S > 160$ or $BP_D > 100$
	Hypertension with vascular disease
	Major surgery with prolonged immobilization
	Complicated vascular heart disease
	Migraine headaches with aura
	Active viral hepatitis
	Severe cirrhosis

WHO, World Health Organization; DVT/PE, deep vein thrombosis/pulmonary embolism; CVA, cerebral vascular accident; BP_S, systolic blood pressure; BP_D, diastolic blood pressure.

as WHO category 4. The contraindications from product labeling are also listed in that table. Apart from the different categories used for the major problems, there are some profound differences between the two lists. For example, endometrial cancer is listed as an absolute contraindication to OC use on product labeling, but is rated by WHO as category 1 (no restriction on use). Similarly, a history of cholestatic jaundice is a contraindication on the labeling, but has been found to be only a relative contraindication by recent scientific evidence (WHO category 2). These differences underscore the need to be familiar with more than product labeling when addressing an individual woman's contraceptive needs. The full WHO list is in Table 42.3.

Health Issues and Risks with Combination Hormonal Contraceptive Use

A summary of the serious side effects traditionally associated with combination hormonal contraceptive use is provided in Table 43.4, with estimates of both relative risk (RR) and absolute risk. These estimates are based on a mixture of newer and older formulations, as well as different age-groups. More specific information about selected issues is provided in the following paragraphs.

Thromboembolism Estrogen-containing combination hormonal contraceptives increase hepatic production of extrinsic clotting factors. Some women, such as those with anticardiolipin antibodies or factor V_{Leiden} mutation, are unable to compensate for this increase in clotting factors and may be subject to a substantially increased risk for thromboembolic events. The overall RR of thrombosis is between 2.6 and 4.0; the absolute incidence of venous thrombosis is 15 to 30 per 100,000 women-years for most of the low-dose OC formulations. The first-year RRs of venous thromboembolism are even higher, but these rates are still lower than the incidence of venous thromboembolism in healthy pregnant women (approximately 60 per 100,000).

Reports in the mid-1990s that third-generation progestins (desogestrel and gestodene) may have had more profound thrombotic impacts (three 1995 articles from the WHO [World Health Organization Collaborative Study of Cardiovascular Disease and Steroid Hormone Contraception, 1995a, b, c]) were questioned by later analysis, which controlled for selection bias (Lewis, 1999). The fact that the rates of thromboembolism in the United Kingdom *increased* after the market share of the third-generation OC formulations *decreased* from 40% to 5%, suggests the lack of increased risk with third-generation progestins. Labeling reflects the uncertainty of the data.

However, the controversy highlighted the need to identify women at risk of venous thromboembolism when taking OCs, not only on the basis of a personal history of prior thromboembolic events but also by inquiring about family history. Suspect histories are those with multiple family members who experienced multiple unexplained clots, generally at an early age. Routine laboratory screening of all potential OC candidates for coagulopathies is inappropriate because it is clearly not cost effective and because

TABLE 43.4

Serious Side Effects Associated with Oral Contraceptive Use

Adverse Effects	Relative Risk	Absolute Risk
Cholelithiasis	2×	1:1,250
Myocardial infarction (smokers aged >35 yr)	3×	1:5,000
Thrombophlebitis	3×	1:10,000
Thromboembolism	4×	1:30,000
Stroke	3×	1:30,000
Hepatic adenoma	500×	1:50,000
Mild hypertension	2–3×	<1:20

Courtesy of Paul Brenner, M.D., University of Southern California.

current testing cannot identify all at-risk women. Screening of high-risk women should be considered. The recommendation to stop estrogen-containing contraceptives 1 month before scheduled surgery has been tempered to reflect modern surgical practices. OC use may not need to be interrupted if a low-risk patient is not expected to require prolonged postoperative bed rest; higher-risk women and low-risk women undergoing high-risk procedures should respect the 30-day rule before elective surgery.

Studies with low-dose formulations have detected no overall increased risk of hemorrhagic or ischemic stroke in healthy young women using OC, but one study did find that women who reported a history of migraine headaches doubled their risk of stroke with OC use (Schwartz et al., 1998). Analysis of the Transnational Research Group study concluded that the attributable risk of occlusive stroke for healthy OC users is very small and is overwhelmed by other risk factors, such as hypertension and smoking (Heinemann et al., 1998).

Cardiovascular Disease Low-dose OCs (<50 μg EE) do not increase the risk of myocardial infarction (MI) in healthy, nonsmoking women. OCs do not increase plaque formation in adolescents; researchers reported a decrease in intima-media thickness in new-start OC users (Kapella et al., 2005). There are clearly identified groups of at-risk women. Smokers at all ages have increased risks for cardiovascular disease when they use OCs. In the study by Dunn et al. (1999), the adjusted odds ratio for MI in OC users who smoked 20 or more cigarettes/day was 12.5 (95% confidence interval [CI], 7.3 to 21.5). Schwingl et al. (1999) estimated that the attributable risk of death from cardiovascular disease resulting from OC use is 0.06 per 100,000 nonsmokers aged 15 to 34 years. In smokers, this risk rises to 1.73 per 100,000. However, the absolute risk of death with OC use in smokers is less than the risk of death during pregnancy until women are 35 to 40 years old. Smoking cessation should always be promoted in teens, but they do not need to avoid pill use if they continue to smoke. Selection of a low-androgenic formulation may be prudent for smokers (Straneva et al., 2000), as would shortening the pill-free interval, as smokers metabolize estrogen more rapidly.

Hypertension Up to 3% of OC users experience increased blood pressure while using birth control pills. Estrogen is responsible for much of this risk. OCs also stimulate adrenal production of aldosterone, which can lead to rise in blood pressure induced by fluid retention. The increases in both diastolic and systolic measures are usually reversible within 3 months of pill cessation. If the hypertension does not spontaneously resolve, then other etiologies must be considered. The need for initial therapy depends on the severity of the hypertension.

Liver and Gallbladder Effects A doubling of the risk of gallstones has been suggested by several prospective and retrospective studies. Although the increase in risk was more impressive with higher-dose pills, it may still be seen with the lower-dose formulations. Cholelithiasis is due to increased cholesterol saturation and biliary stasis. The risk appears to be concentrated in a few short-term users who may be prone to gallbladder disease.

Cholestatic jaundice is very rare, but it has been reported as a result of using estrogen-containing contraceptives.

Pruritus similar to that seen in pregnancy may develop with usage of estrogen-containing contraceptives.

Impact of Combination Hormonal Contraceptive Use on Neoplasia The single largest concern women voice about OC use is the risk of cancer. Almost one third of all women believe that OCs cause cancer, but only a small minority is aware that OC use decreases the incidence of ovarian and endometrial cancer. A few of the more pertinent neoplasms in adolescents are discussed here.

Leiomyoma Historically, there has been concern that OC use might stimulate growth of leiomyomas (fibroids), because they are known to be estrogen-sensitive tumors. Chiaffarino et al. (1999) found in a case–control study of 843 women with fibroids that the risk for current users of OCs was lower than for those who had never used OCs (RR, 0.3; 95% CI, 0.2 to 0.6). The risk of uterine fibroids decreases with duration of OC use. Marshall et al. (1998) also reported a reduction in risk of fibroids in current OC users; however, he noted a higher risk (RR, 1.26; 95% CI, 1.05 to 1.51) for development of clinically diagnosed fibroids in nurses who started using OCs at age 13 to 16 years, compared with never-users. This modest risk should not deter OC use by adolescents, because this association may reflect an earlier age of menarche, which is itself a risk factor for fibroids.

Women who have existing fibroids are often successfully prescribed OCs to reduce their menorrhagia.

Cervical Cancer OC use for >5 years causes a slight increase in the risk of cervical dysplasia. However, the risk for squamous cell carcinoma does not appear to be affected by OC use. The risk of adenocarcinoma of the cervix may be increased, although this has not yet been conclusively demonstrated. OC users do not require any more intensive or more frequent Pap smears than their relevant risk factors (e.g., age, number of sexual partners, exposure to human papillomavirus, smoking) would routinely dictate.

Breast Cancer In contrast to the obvious benefits OCs have in reducing the risks of endometrial and ovarian cancer, the impact of OCs on breast cancer has been more controversial. In humans, there is no evidence that either estrogen or progestin can initiate the development of abnormal mitotic figures in normal breast cells. However, breast cancer cells do divide more rapidly in the presence of estrogen.

Epidemiological studies of present and past OC users have presented conflicting results, but virtually all the risk ratios for breast cancer calculated in these studies show either no increased risk or a small and temporary increased risk, especially with low-dose formulations.

The Cancer and Steroid Hormone (CASH) study of the Centers for Disease Control and Prevention (CDC) found no overall increase in breast cancer with OC use (Centers for Disease Control and Prevention, 1983), but in young women who used the pill, the risk of development of breast cancer by the age 35 years was raised by 2 to 3 cases per 100,000 women (Centers for Disease Control and Prevention, 1984). Importantly, these researchers investigated several high-risk groups and found that OC use was not associated with an increased incidence of breast cancer in the following important subgroups (a) women with a family history of breast cancer, (b) women with and without benign breast disease, and (c) women who started using OCs before their first pregnancy.

The Collaborative Group on Hormonal Factors in Breast Cancer (1996) meta-analysis of 54 studies from 23 countries reported that current users and women who had used OCs within the previous 10 years had a slightly increased risk of developing breast cancer (RR, 1.24; 95% CI, 1.15 to 1.33). Women who started OC use before 20 years of age had an even higher increase in risk when they were current or recent users. However, the magnitude of this increased risk was minimal; the estimated excess numbers of cancers diagnosed up to 10 years after stopping use was 0.5 per 10,000 women. The risk was reversible; no group displayed any increased risk 10 years after stopping OCs. No duration of usage effect was seen. More importantly, the increase in breast cancer was concentrated in the development of localized disease; in fact, the meta-analysis demonstrated that the risk of metastatic breast cancer with lower-dose pills was *not* increased among current or recent OC users.

Marchbanks et al. (2002) studied women aged 35 to 64 years and found no increased risk of breast cancer in current or past OC users. No increased risk was seen in women with family history of breast cancer or in women who used pills early in their reproductive lives. Norman et al. (2003) reported the results of a population-based case–control study of 1,847 postmenopausal women with invasive breast cancer and 1,932 normal controls and found

that OC users were not at increased risk for invasive breast cancer. The risk of breast cancer was highest in women using postmenopausal hormone therapies, who had never used OCs.

On the basis of all these studies, it is not appropriate to deny any adolescent girl hormonal contraceptives even if she has fibrocystic breast changes or a family history of breast cancer. A strong family history of breast cancer, including (at a minimum) one affected first-degree relative is at most, a relative contraindication for the use of modern, low-dose pills. Only a personal history of breast cancer is a contraindication.

Side Effects

As described earlier, the sex hormones in OCs have various degrees of progestogenic, estrogenic, antiestrogenic, and androgenic activities. These differences are important to understand, especially when responding to a patient's concerns about side effects. The impacts of the relative potencies of different formulations vary from individual to individual.

Prospective, double-blind, placebo-controlled studies that were conducted to evaluate the role of the triphasic, norgestimate-containing birth control pills in treating acne provided a unique opportunity to evaluate the incidence of side effects with modern low-dose pills (Redmond et al., 1999). In the 6-month study period, the placebo group had the same incidence of headache, nausea, mastalgia, and other side effects, generally attributed to OCs, as the OC group did. Even the incidence of excessive weight gain was identical. The lack of attributable weight gain with OC use had earlier been demonstrated by Reubinoff et al. (1995), who also reported that users of low-dose OCs did not change body composition or fat distribution.

Some women have particular sensitivity to sex steroids. They may experience side effects either as a result of the pharmacological doses of hormone or because of hormonal imbalances. Many side effects are temporally self-limited and resolve spontaneously in the first few cycles, but sometimes women require a change of pill formulation. When these side effects arise, it is important to analyze them by their constituent hormonal effects (see Table 43.5) to select pills that meet the patient's needs.

Management of Common Side Effects

Breakthrough Bleeding Typically, 20% to 25% of women experience unscheduled spotting or bleeding at some time during the first three cycles. The incidence of breakthrough bleeding with the more recent ultra–low-dose (20 µg) formulations containing levonorgestrel or desogestrel is roughly comparable to that of 30- to 35-µg pills, although an earlier 20-µg formulation containing low-dose norethindrone did have higher rates of unscheduled bleeding (DelConte et al., 1999; Rosenberg et al., 1999; Sulak et al., 1999). Other causes of vaginal spotting or bleeding must be considered in adolescent girls. Chlamydial cervicitis is a common cause of postcoital bleeding in teens. Inconsistent pill use also commonly causes breakthrough bleeding or spotting. Smokers have notably more challenges with breakthrough bleeding, especially with low-dose pills.

Treatment for persistent spotting or bleeding due to OCs in the face of appropriate pill use depends on the timing of those events within the woman's cycle. For women who have unscheduled spotting and/or bleeding at the

TABLE 43.5

Impact of Hormones on Side Effects

Estrogen-Related	Progestin-Related	
	Progestogenic	Androgenic
Nausea and vomiting	Fatigue	Noncyclic weight gain
Edema, leg cramps	Depression	Oily skin
Bloating	Bloating	Hirsutism
Cervical ectropion	Mastalgia	Acne
Visual changes or vascular headaches	Increased breast size	Increased appetite
Telangiectasia	Venous dilation, pelvic congestion	Decrease in libido
Cyclic weight gain	Oligomenorrhea, amenorrhea, vaginal spotting	Decreased breast size
Irritability		
Clear vaginal discharge	Cholestatic jaundice	
Cystic breast changes	Pruritus	
Chloasma, hyperpigmentation		
Hypermenorrhea (menorrhagia)		

end of their active pills, use a formulation with higher progesterone activity to support the endometrium during those days. Triphasic formulations, which progressively increase progestin dose, are particularly helpful in this situation. If the unscheduled spotting and/or bleeding occurs with the early pills, consider using formulations with higher doses of estrogen in the early pills, or those with lower progestin levels. This will allow the estrogen in the pills to induce endometrial proliferation and cover the denuded, bleeding areas left by menstrual shedding. Spotting and bleeding that occurs sporadically throughout the cycle is highly suspicious for inconsistent pill use, smoking, or drug–drug interactions. However, for women who do not have those problems but are still spotting, shortening the pill-free interval can reduce the frequency of that bleeding, especially if lower-dose formulations are being used.

Acne and Hirsutism These symptoms are caused by free androgens. In order to cope, switch to a formulation with a higher estrogen content, which will increase SHBG and reduce the level of unbound testosterone, and/or switch to a formulation with a less androgenic progestin.

Chloasma or Melasma These symptoms are caused by estrogen stimulation of melanocytes. In this situation, it would be prudent to decrease (or eliminate) estrogen content and advise the use of sunscreen and hats.

Weight Gain Explore other causes of weight gain before attributing it to pill use. If the weight gain is concentrated in a woman's breast, hips, and thighs, decrease the estrogen content of her pills. If the gain is accompanied by bloating and fluid retention, switch to a lower dose pill or to a drosperinone-containing formulation. If the weight gain is slowly progressive (and not due to other factors), change to a less androgenic formulation.

Headaches Rule out serious problems, such as hypertension and new-onset or worsening migraines, which would require OC cessation. Reduce the dose of estrogen or change to a progestin-only method. If the headache occurs only before or during menses (menstrual or migraine), shorten or eliminate the pill-free interval.

Nausea Have the patient take her pill at night. Reduce the estrogen dose if the first maneuver is not successful or if it will interfere with successful pill taking.

Mastalgia Breast tenderness is usually self-limited, but if the problem persists, reduce the estrogen dose of the pill.

Coping with Missed Pills The WHO has developed advice to be given to women when they miss OCs. The advice differs depending upon how many pills are missed, the strength of her formulation, and when in the cycle the pills are missed. The recommendations are summarized in Figure 43.2.

Because this may be somewhat complicated for a patient to remember, it may be prudent to simplify the instructions to cover two situations: One missed pill versus more than one missed pill. If one pill is missed, have her take it as soon as possible and take the current day's pill within 12 hours. If more than one pill is missed, then have her take two pills today, resume daily pill taking tomorrow, and use condoms for 7 days. If she has had intercourse in the 5 days before the missed pills, she should use EC in place of her two pills today (see Chapter 46).

Increasing Adolescent Compliance

Adolescent compliance with contraceptive methods is often suboptimal; however, adult compliance is also far from perfect. Studies of high-risk teenaged mothers found a 50% discontinuation rate by 12 months (Berenson and Wiemann, 1995). Many factors contribute to noncompliance. The desire of teens for independence and seeming invincibility decreases their motivation to use contraception. The unpredictability and frequent disruptions in their

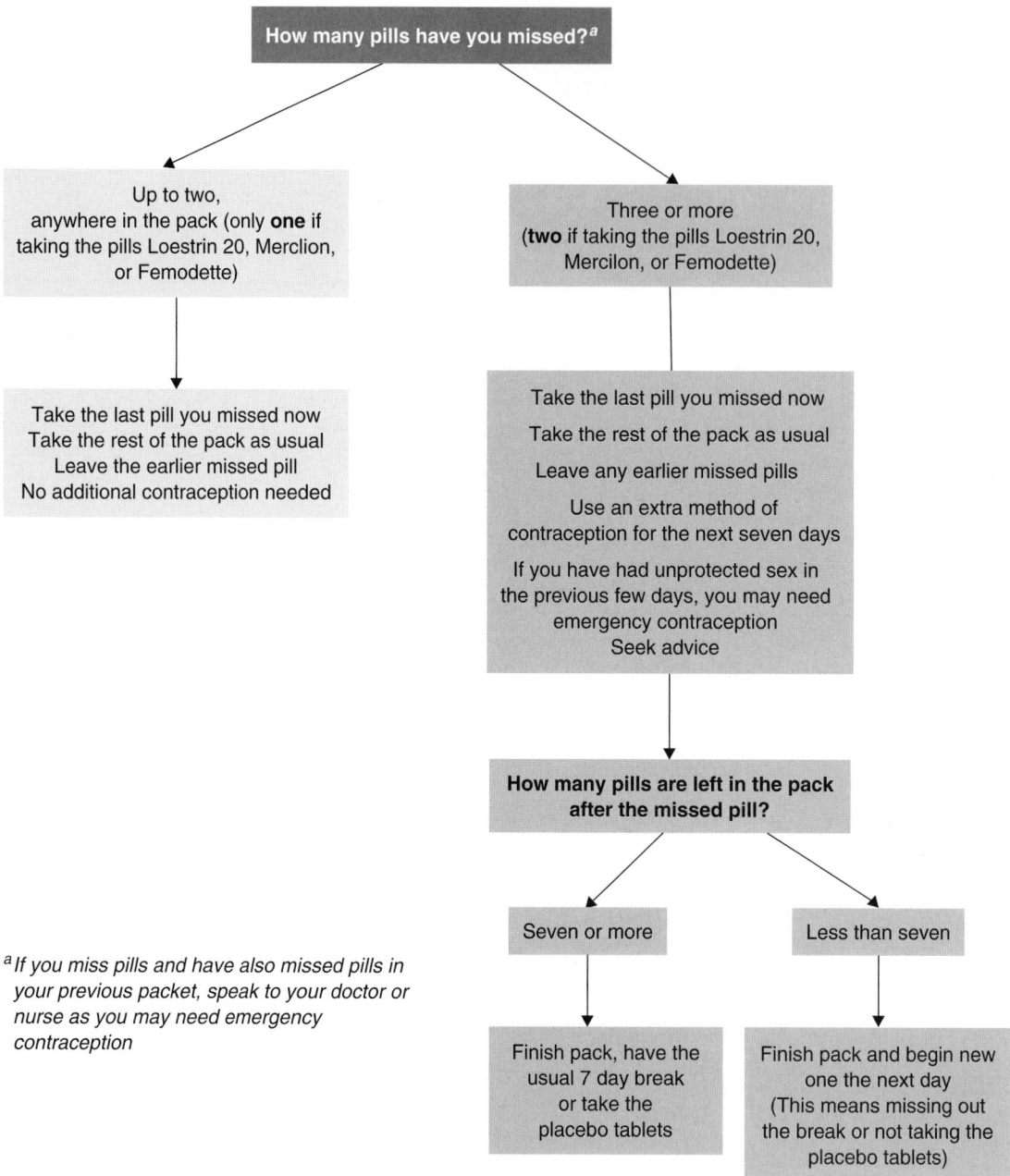

FIGURE 43.2 Handling missed oral contraceptive pills. (Adapted from Family Planning Association. *How many Pills have you missed? Contraception and Sexual Health Guide.* London: Family Planning Association.)

relationships often cause them to stop using contraception. Many adolescents receive incorrect information from sex education teachers in American schools (Davis, 1994); this misinformation about OCs affects the effectiveness of the method and also reduces compliance.

To enhance compliance, experts have suggested several measures:

1. Emphasize the noncontraceptive benefits of OCs. Robinson et al. (1992) found that adolescent girls who experienced reduction in dysmenorrhea with OC use were eight times more likely to be consistent OC users.

2. Demonstrate concretely how to use the pills.
3. Have the patient discuss her concerns about pill use explicitly so that they can be addressed. Widespread myths about the dangers of OCs abound and can magnify the significance of a minor side effect in the mind of a young user.
4. Help the teen plan for crucial logistics, such as where to store the pills (school lockers don't work on weekends!) and how to remember to take the pills each day (placing them next to makeup or an earring holder may work better in the real world than placing them near the tube of toothpaste).

5. Start the pills immediately if pregnancy can be ruled out, to simplify instructions, and use a barrier method as backup for first cycle.
6. Shorten the pill-free interval. Start each new pack of pills on the first day of menses. Or eliminate the pill-free interval for several packs ("bicycling," "recycling," or "combination continuous use").
7. If the patient is unable to take daily pills use a longer-acting product, such as the contraceptive patch or vaginal ring (see subsequent text).

Special considerations in adolescents:

1. When to start
   a. Young users: Ideally, a teen would have at least three to six regular periods after menarche before starting the pill. However, if a young menarchal teen is sexually active, the risks of pregnancy exceed those of taking hormonal contraceptives; there is no evidence that the early use of OCs leads to premature epiphyseal closure or to any disruption in the maturation of the hypothalamic-pituitary-ovarian axis.
   b. After pregnancy: After a first-trimester therapeutic abortion or miscarriage, the pill should be started immediately to prevent ovulation. After a pregnancy, a 3- to 4-week delay should be allowed before starting OCs, because of the risk of thromboembolism. However, progestin-only methods can be initiated immediately.
2. If the teen has very irregular cycles, she should be informed that her cycles are likely to be regular while she is using the pills, but will return to their usual, irregular intervals when the pills are stopped. However, there is no evidence that the teen's fertility rate will be any lower after she discontinues the pills than if she had never used them.
3. Initial examination
   a. History: Menstrual history, past history, risk factors for sexually transmitted diseases (STDs), history of problems that suggest any contraindications for use of the pill, and sexual and family histories.
   b. Physical examination: The optimal examination would include weight and blood pressure measurements, thyroid examination, breast examination, abdominal examination, and pelvic examination. However, only a blood pressure measurement and a breast examination are required to start hormonal contraceptives. The pelvic examination may be deferred for 3 to 6 months at least (Stewart et al., 2001). This is particularly the case for women who are being prescribed OCs for noncontraceptive benefits and who may not be sexually active.
   c. Laboratory tests: Screening for *Chlamydia* is recommended for every sexually active teen. This can be performed using a urine specimen. It is not needed before prescribing pills.
   d. Education: Counseling is the most critical component of the visit.
4. Follow-up
   a. It is preferable to see the teenager at 1 month and again at 3 months after starting the pill, and then every 6 months. The visit after 1 month is important, especially in younger teens, because of their high rate of pill discontinuation during the first months.
   b. Check blood pressure at 3 months and then as indicated for well-adolescent care.
   c. Perform a breast and pelvic examination as indicated every 12 months for routine care. Pap smears should start 3 years after sexual debut. Screening for *Chlamydia* is required at least annually for sexually active women younger than 26 years.

PROGESTIN-ONLY PILLS

Progestin-only pills have traditionally been reserved for use by breast-feeding women. However, their potential is much greater than that niche. Virtually every woman may be a candidate from a medical standpoint for use of progestin-only pills. The only condition that the WHO rates as category 4 (do not use) for progestin-only pills is current breast cancer. Because the dose of progestin is significantly lower in progestin-only pills than it is in combination OCs, success requires consistent use. The progestin-only pill must be taken at the same time each day. The progestin-only pill works primarily by thickening cervical mucus to prevent sperm entry into the upper reproductive tract. Ovulation is suppressed in 40% to 60% of cycles. There are no placebo pills; a woman takes one active pill a day, even if she is menstruating. The most common side effect from progestin-only pills is unscheduled spotting and bleeding or amenorrhea, just as is seen with other progestin-only methods. Whenever estrogen is contraindicated or undesired (e.g., with melasma), the progestin-only pill is an excellent option. Table 43.1 lists the progestin-only pills available in the United States.

TRANSDERMAL CONTRACEPTIVE PATCH

The Ortho Evra transdermal contraceptive system is composed of a 20 cm^2 tan-colored thin patch containing EE and 17-diacetyl norgestimate. This patch was very popular with adolescent girls because its once-a-week use is more convenient compared with the daily dosing requirement of OCs. The patch can be worn anywhere on the woman's trunk (except the breasts) or on her upper arms. Women should be cautioned to avoid placing it on areas subjected to friction from undergarments or waistbands. With current fashions, many women have abandoned the attempt to hide the patch and wear it as a fashion statement.

The efficacy of the patch is at least equivalent to that of standard birth control pills for women weighing <90 kg. For women weighing >90 kg, the risk of pregnancy is higher. In the clinical trials, >30% of the pregnancies occurred in the 3% of the study population who weighed >198 pounds (Zieman et al., 2002).

In clinical studies, it was shown that at every age-group, more patch users reported correct and consistent use of their method than did pill users. This difference was greatest among the adolescent girls in the study; 87.7% of 18- and 19-year-old girls in the patch arm used their patches correctly and consistently during the 1-year trial compared with 67.7% of the 18- and 19-year olds who used OCs (Creasy et al., 2000).

The first patch should be applied during the first 5 days of a woman's cycle. Each patch is to remain in place for 7 days, at which time another patch is applied at a different site. The third patch replaces the second patch at a different site 7 days later. After the last patch has been in place for 7 days, product labeling instructs the patient to remove it and use no patch for the following week, during which time she should start her withdrawal bleeding. It is important to give guidance to patients about what to do if things go wrong.

- If the patch detaches, she should attempt to reattach it using its own adhesive; never anchor the patch in place with tape. If the patch will not reattach, have the patient place a new patch at a different site and replace that patch on her next regularly scheduled "change day" or modify her change day to the current day. If the patch was detached for <24 hours, no further action is needed. If it was detached for longer than 24 hours, she should use a backup method for 7 days and consider whether she needs EC (see Chapter 46).
- If she is late in changing her patch, she should change it as soon as possible. If she is late by 2 days or less, no further action is necessary. If she is >2 days late, she should replace the patch and use a backup method for 7 days and consider whether she needs EC (see Chapter 46).

Patch initiation guidelines should also be flexible. Women switching from pills to patches should place their first patch on the first day of their withdrawal bleeding; they should not wait until they complete their pill pack. The patch should be started immediately after a first trimester pregnancy loss or after intrauterine contraception is removed or 13 weeks after the last DMPA injection. Remember, it takes 2 days to achieve therapeutic hormonal levels, so a backup method should be recommended if the patient is at risk.

The safety and efficacy of quick start of the contraceptive patch has been demonstrated. However, compared with quick start with OCs, quick start with the patch did not increase short-term continuation rates (Murthy et al., 2005). Extended cycle use of the patch has also been reported (Stewart et al., 2005 OBGYN 1389–96). Women using extended cycles had less frequent, but more prolonged, scheduled bleeding episodes than did women using the patch cyclically. There is a slight increase over time of serum levels of estrogen with extended cycle use of the contraceptive patch.

The patch has virtually the same contraindications, precautions, and side effects as combination OCs. One exception is that transdermal administration does not require gastrointestinal (GI) absorption, so that conditions which limit GI absorption, such as diarrhea associated with irritable bowel syndrome (IBS), do not present any problems with patch use. It is not known what the efficacy of the patch is when used by women taking anticonvulsants or other liver enzyme–inducing drugs. Patches cannot be applied to irritated skin surfaces. Women with sunburn, psoriasis, or rashes should not apply the contraceptive patch over affected areas. The patch will not attach or may detach if oils or moisturizers, sun tan lotions, or other skin products coat the area. However, baby oil is very helpful in removing the remnants of adhesive that may stick to the skin after the patch has been removed. Women using the patch are more likely to report first-cycle mastalgia than OC users, but by the second month the frequency of the problem drops to <10%, which is comparable to pill users.

The progestin in the patch is a derivative of norgestimate, which is the low androgen progestin in Ortho Tri-Cyclen. The peak levels of serum estrogen achieved with the patch are only two thirds as high as the daily peak of estrogen from 35-μg EE pills. However, because the patch maintains the same level of hormones in the bloodstream 24 hours/day, the total daily estrogen exposure is 60% higher than with a 35-μg EE pill and 3.4 times higher than the vaginal ring. Product labeling acknowledges the higher estrogen exposure, but it also states that the clinical significance of this higher dose is not known. The reason that higher doses of estrogen from the patch may not have the same thrombotic and other metabolic impacts as higher dose pills is that the percutaneous route of administration bypasses the pill's first pass effect. With the patch, the liver is not exposed to estrogen that does not appear in the bloodstream. With oral drugs, serum levels reflect only a fraction of the drug exposure of the liver, because much of the initial drug that is absorbed is conjugated in the liver and excreted back into the intestine by way of the gallbladder. More than 5 million women in the United States have used the patch; to date, there has been no convincing evidence of any increased risk of thrombosis, but the *U.S. Food and Drug Administration (FDA) now requires that Ortho Evra packaging contain a warning about this potential serious complication.* Epidemiological studies focusing on the question of thrombosis have provided conflicting answers about the risk of thromboembolism with patch use.

VAGINAL CONTRACEPTIVE RINGS

1. Metabolism and efficacy: NuvaRing contraceptive vaginal ring is a soft, flexible ring with an outer diameter of 54 mm and a cross section diameter of 4 mm. The ring is impregnated with EE and etonogestrel (a metabolite of desogestrel). The ring produces total daily serum EE levels <50% of those seen with a 30-μg EE pill (van den Heuvel et al., 2005). The ring is placed in a woman's vagina, where it releases a constant amount of contraceptive hormones. The ring is placed inside the vaginal fornix within the first 5 cycle days and remains in place for 21 days, at which time it is removed and placed in its resealable pouch and discarded. The woman places a new ring 7 days later. Efficacy is at least comparable to that of OCs. Little data is available about efficacy in heavier women. In meta-analysis of existing clinical trials, which studied 3,259 women, none of the 41 ring users who weighed at least 89.9 kg became pregnant (Westhoff, 2005).
2. Advantages: The ring has many features that are very attractive for adolescent women. It is a once-a-month, self-administered method with no telltale external evidence of its use. Cycle control is impressive; tested against the best modern pill for cycle control (Nordette), ring users had fewer days of unscheduled spotting and bleeding than pill users (Bjarnadottir et al., 2002). There are no published studies on the efficacy of the vaginal ring in women using hepatic enzyme–inducing medications, such as St. John's wort or anticonvulsants. Because the ring releases estrogen directly into the vagina, it increases vaginal lubrication and has been reported to reduce recurrences of bacterial vaginosis. Women who need vaginal therapies, such as antifungal agents or spermicides, may use them without fear of adversely affecting vaginal ring efficacy.
3. Contraindications: The vaginal ring has the same contraindications as the transdermal patch except that there are no concerns about dermatologic conditions.

Pelvic support is needed for the ring. The greatest barrier to acceptance of the vaginal ring is its placement and removal. Placement can be facilitated by loading the ring into an emptied tampon inserter with blunt opening. Have the woman place the tampon inserter into the vault and press the ring out. Once the ring is inside the vagina, it can rest against the vaginal wall in any location, and its movement within the vault causes no problems. In the clinical trials, the vast majority of male partners did not notice any adverse effects from the ring on their sexual satisfaction. If a woman's partner does complain, she can remove the ring and place it in its foil pouch until coitus is over. She must not leave the ring out of her vagina for >3 hours in any 24-hour period. Removal of the ring only requires that the woman introduce a finger into her vagina, locate the ring with her fingertip, and withdraw it from her vagina. If the ring is located high in the vault, it may help to have the woman squat slightly to remove it.

4. Quick start and extended cycle use: Clinical trials have now been published validating the safety of quick start for the vaginal ring (Westhoff et al., 2005) and extended cycle use of NuvaRing (Miller et al., 2005). In the extended cycle study, some women changed rings every 3 weeks for up to a year without having a scheduled withdrawal bleed. Shorter interval cycles (2 and 4 months) were associated with less breakthrough bleeding. There is no evidence of accumulation of the contraceptive hormones with extended cycle use of the vaginal ring.

5. Other formulations: Another estrogen-progestin ring that is to be used in 3-week cycles with 1 week out for up to 1 year is now undergoing clinical trials. Progestin-only vaginal rings are under development to provide the benefits of 1- to 3-month duration vaginal rings without estrogen's side effects or contraindications. At the time of this writing, none is available in the United States.

WEB SITES

For Teenagers and Parents

http://www.advocatesforyouth.org/youth/health/contraceptives/pill.htm. Advocates for Youth information on OCs with links to other contraceptive choices.
http://www.sex-ed101.com/oral.html. Sex Education 101 Web site on OCs and other contraceptives.
http://www.teenwire.com/index.asp. Teenwire from Planned Parenthood with information about reproductive health including contraception.
http://www.fhi.org/en/RH/FAQs/COC_faq.htm. Frequently Asked Questions sheet on combined OCs from Family Health International.
http://www.orthowomenshealth.com/birthcontrol/options/pills.html. Information from the Ortho Women's Health Web site.

For Health Professionals

http://www.arhp.org/healthcareproviders/resources/contraceptionresources/. Association of Reproductive Health Professionals.

REFERENCES AND ADDITIONAL READINGS

ACOG Committee on Practice Bulletins-Gynecology. ACOG practice bulletin. No. 73: Use of hormonal contraception in women with coexisting medical conditions. Obstet Gynecol. 2006;107(6):1453.
Ahn HK. Poster presented at Teratology Society. Reported in www.obgynnews.com. Sept 15, 2005. Accessed 12/25/05 at http://download.journals.elsevierhealth.com/pdfs/journals/0029-7437/PIIS0029743705710090.pdf. 2005.
Archer DF, Kovalevsky G, Ballagh S, et al. Effect on ovarian activity of a continuous-use regimen of oral levonorgestrel/ethinyl estradiol. Abstract O-57. Fertil Steril 2005;84(Suppl 1):S24.
Back DJ, Tjia J, Martin C, et al. The lack of interaction between temafloxacin and combined oral contraceptive steroids. Contraception 1991;43(4):317.
Becker WJ. Use of oral contraceptives in patients with migraine. Neurology 1999;53(Suppl 1):S19.
Berenson AB, Wiemann CM. Use of levonorgestrel implants versus oral contraceptives in adolescence: a case-control study. Am J Obstet Gynecol 1995;172:1128.
Bjarnadottir RI, Tuppurainen M, Killick SR. Comparison of cycle control with a combined contraceptive vaginal ring and oral levonorgestrel/ethinyl estradiol. Am J Obstet Gynecol 2002;186(3):389.
Brunner LR, Hogue CJ. The role of body weight in oral contraceptive failure: results from the 1995 national survey of family growth. Ann Epidemiol 2005;15(7):492.
Castelli WP. Cardiovascular disease: pathogenesis, epidemiology, and risk among users of oral contraceptives who smoke. Am J Obstet Gynecol 1999;180:S349.
Centers for Disease Control and Prevention. Cancer and steroid hormone study. Long-term oral contraceptive use and the risk of breast cancer. JAMA 1983;249:1591.
Centers for Disease Control and Prevention. OC use and the risk of breast cancer in young women. MMWR Morb Mortal Wkly Rep 1984;22:353.
Chiaffarino F, Parazzini F, La Vecchia C, et al. Use of oral contraceptives and uterine fibroids: results from a case-control study. Br J Obstet Gynaecol 1999;106:857.
Clarkson TB, Shively CA, Morgan TM, et al. Oral contraceptives and coronary artery atherosclerosis of cynomolgus monkeys. Obstet Gynecol 1990;75:217.
The Collaborative Group on Hormonal Factors in Breast Cancer. Breast cancer and hormonal contraceptives: collaborative reanalysis of individual data on 53 297 women with breast cancer and 100 239 women without breast cancer from 54 epidemiological studies. Lancet 1996;347:1713.
Creasy G, Hall N, Shangold G. Patient adherence with the contraceptive patch dosing schedule versus oral contraceptives. Obstet Gynecol 2000;95(4 Suppl 1):S60.
Csemiczky G, Alvendal C, Landgren BM. Risk for ovulation in women taking a low-dose oral contraceptive (Microgynon) when receiving antibacterial treatment with a fluoroquinolone (ofloxacin). Adv Contracept 1996;12(2):101.
Davis AJ. The role of hormonal contraception in adolescents. Am J Obstet Gynecol 1994;170:1581.
Davis A, Lippman J, Godwin A, et al. Triphasic norgestimate/ethinyl estradiol oral contraceptive for the treatment of dysfunctional uterine bleeding. Obstet Gynecol 2000;95(4 Suppl 1):S84.

Davis AR, Westhoff C, O'Connell K, et al. Oral contraceptives for dysmenorrhea in adolescent girls: a randomized trial. *Obstet Gynecol* 2005;106(1):97.

DelConte A, Loffer F, Grubb GS, et al. Cycle control with oral contraceptives containing 20 micrograms of ethinyl estradiol: a multicenter, randomized comparison of levonorgestrel/ethinyl estradiol (100 micrograms/20 micrograms) and norethindrone/ethinyl estradiol (1,000 micrograms/20 micrograms). *Contraception* 1999;59:187.

Dunn N, Thorogood M, Faragher B, et al. Oral contraceptives and myocardial infarction: results of the MICA case-control study. *BMJ* 1999;318:1579.

Edelman A, Gallo MF, Nichols MD, et al. Continuous versus cyclic use of combined oral contraceptives for contraception: systematic Cochrane review of randomized controlled trials. *Hum Reprod* 2006;21(3):573.

Emans SJ, Grace E, Woods ER, et al. Adolescent compliance with the use of oral contraceptives. *JAMA* 1987;257:3377.

Friedman CI, Huneke AL, Kim MH, et al. The effect of ampicillin on oral contraceptive effectiveness. *Obstet Gynecol* 1980;55:33.

Godsland IF, Crook D. Update on the metabolic effects of steroidal contraceptives and their relationship to cardiovascular disease risk. *Am J Obstet Gynecol* 1994;170:1528.

Gordon CM, Nelson LM. Amenorrhea and bone health in adolescents and young women. *Curr Opin Obstet Gynecol* 2003; 15:377.

Grabrick DM, Hartmann LC, Cerhan JR, et al. Risk of breast cancer with oral contraceptive use in women with a family history of breast cancer. *JAMA* 2000;284:1791.

Halpern V, Grimes DA, Lopez L, et al. Strategies to improve adherence and acceptability of hormonal methods for contraception. *Cochrane Database Syst Rev* 2006;(1):CD004317.

Heinemann LA, Lewis MA, Spitzer WO, et al. Thromboembolic stroke in young women: a European case-control study on oral contraceptives. Transnational Research Group on Oral Contraceptives and the Health of Young Women. *Contraception* 1998;57:29.

Hergenroeder AC, Smith EO, Shypailo R, et al. Bone mineral changes in young women with hypothalamic amenorrhea treated with oral contraceptives, medroxyprogesterone, or placebo over 12 months. *Am J Obstet Gynecol* 1997;176:1017.

van den Heuvel MW, van Bragt AJ, Alnabawy AK, et al. Comparison of ethinylestradiol pharmacokinetics in three hormonal contraceptive formulations: the vaginal ring, the transdermal patch and an oral contraceptive. *Contraception* 2005; 72(3):168.

Holt VL, Cushing-Haugen KL, Daling JR. Body weight and risk of oral contraceptive failure. *Obstet Gynecol* 2002;99(5 Pt 1):820.

Holt VL, Scholes D, Wicklund KG, et al. Body mass index, weight, and oral contraceptive failure risk. *Obstet Gynecol* 2005; 105(1):46.

Joshi JV, Joshi UM, Sankholi GM, et al. A study of interaction of low-dose combination oral contraceptive with Ampicillin and Metronidazole. *Contraception* 1980;22(6):643.

Kapella JG, Binder C, Shingler KC, et al. *Hormonal contraceptives and intima-media thickness of common carotid artery in adolescent girls. Presented at Society for Adolescent Medicine Meeting.* Century City, CA: April 1, 2005.

Kjos SL, Peters RK, Xiang A, et al. Contraception and the risk of type 2 diabetes mellitus in Latina women with prior gestational diabetes mellitus. *JAMA* 1998;280:533.

Kripke C. Cyclic vs. continuous or extended-cycle combined contraceptives. *Am Fam Phy* 2006;73(5):804.

Lara-Torre E, Schroeder B. Adolescent compliance and side effects with Quick Start initiation of oral contraceptive pills. *Contraception* 2002;66(2):81.

Lewis MA. The transnational study on oral contraceptives and the health of young women: methods, results, new analyses and the healthy user effect. *Hum Reprod Update* 1999;5:707.

Liu SL, Lebrun CM. Effect of oral contraceptives and hormone replacement therapy on bone mineral density in premenopausal and perimenopausal women: a systematic review. *Br J Sports Med* 2006;40:11.

Maggiolo F, Puricelli G, Dottorini M, et al. The effect of ciprofloxacin on oral contraceptive steroid treatments. *Drugs Exp Clin Res* 1991;17(9):451.

Marchbanks PA, McDonald JA, Wilson HG, et al. Oral contraceptives and the risk of breast cancer. *N Engl J Med* 2002; 346(26):2025.

Marshall LM, Spiegelman D, Goldman MB, et al. A prospective study of reproductive factors and oral contraceptive use in relation to the risk of uterine leiomyomata. *Fertil Steril* 1998; 70:432.

Miller L, Verhoeven CH, Hout J. Extended regimens of the contraceptive vaginal ring: a randomized trial. *Obstet Gynecol* 2005;106(3):473.

Mishell DR Jr. Rationale for decreasing the number of days of the hormone-free interval with use of low-dose oral contraceptive formulations. *Contraception* 2005;71(4):304.

Murphy PA, Kern SE, Stanczyk FZ, et al. Interaction of St. John's Wort with oral contraceptives: effects on the pharmacokinetics of norethindrone and ethinyl estradiol, ovarian activity and breakthrough bleeding. *Contraception* 2005; 71(6):402.

Murphy AA, Zacur HA, Charache P, et al. The effect of tetracycline on levels of oral contraceptives. *Am J Obstet Gynecol* 1991;164:28.

Murthy AS, Creinin MD, Harwood B, et al. Same-day initiation of the transdermal hormonal delivery system (contraceptive patch) versus traditional initiation methods. *Contraception* 2005;72(5):333.

Narod SA, Risch H, Moslehi R, et al. Hereditary Ovarian Cancer Clinical Study Group. Oral contraceptives and the risk of hereditary ovarian cancer. *N Engl J Med* 1998;339:424.

Neely JL, Abate M, Swinker MR, et al. The effect of doxycycline on serum levels of ethinyl estradiol, norethindrone, and endogenous progesterone. *Obstet Gynecol* 1991;77(3): 416.

Norman SA, Berlin JA, Weber AL, et al. Combined effect of oral contraceptive use and hormone replacement therapy on breast cancer risk in postmenopausal women. *Cancer Causes Control* 2003;14(10):933.

Oakley D, Sereika S, Bogue EL. Oral contraceptive pill use after an initial visit to a family planning clinic. *Fam Plann Perspect* 1991;23:150.

Pierson RA, Birtch RL, Olatunbosun OA. Ovarian follicular dynamics during conventional versus continuous oral contraceptive use. Abstract O-58. *Fertil Steril* 2005;84(Suppl 1): S24.

Pons JE. Hormonal contraception compliance in teenagers. *Pediatr Endo Rev* 2006;(3 Suppl 1):164.

Potter L, Oakley D, de Leon-Wong E, et al. Measuring compliance among oral contraceptive users. *Fam Plann Perspect* 1996;28:154.

Redmond G, Godwin AJ, Olson W, et al. Use of placebo controls in an oral contraceptive trial: methodological issues and adverse event incidence. *Contraception* 1999;60:81.

Reubinoff BE, Gurbstein A, Meirow D, et al. Effects of low-dose estrogen oral contraceptives on weight, body composition, and fat distribution in young women. *Fertil Steril* 1995;63:516.

Robinson JC, Plichta S, Weisman CS, et al. Dysmenorrhea and use of oral contraceptives in adolescent women attending a family planning clinic. *Am J Obstet Gynecol* 1992;166:578.

Rosenberg MJ, Meyers A, Roy V. Efficacy, cycle control, and side effects of low- and lower-dose oral contraceptives: a randomized trial of 20 micrograms and 35 micrograms estrogen preparations. *Contraception* 1999;60:321.

Rosenberg MJ, Waugh MS, Long S. Unintended pregnancies and use, misuse and discontinuation of oral contraceptives. *J Reprod Med* 1995;40(5):355.

Sarkar NN. The combined contraceptive vaginal device (NuvaRing): a comprehensive review. *Eur J Contracept Reprod Health Care* 2005;10(2):73.

Schlesselman JJ. Net effect of oral contraceptive use on the risk of cancer in women in the United States. *Obstet Gynecol* 1995;85:793.

Schwartz SM, Petitti DB, Siscovick DS, et al. Stroke and use of low-dose oral contraceptives in young women: a pooled analysis of two U.S. studies. *Stroke* 1998;29:2277.

Schwingl PJ, Ory HW, Visness CM. Estimates of the risk of cardiovascular death attributable to low-dose oral contraceptives in the United States. *Am J Obstet Gynecol* 1999;180:241.

Sidney S, Siscovick DS, Petitti DB, et al. Myocardial infarction and use of low-dose oral contraceptives: a pooled analysis of 2 U.S. studies. *Circulation* 1998;98:1058.

Stewart FH, Harper CC, Ellertson CE, et al. Clinical breast and pelvic examination requirements for hormonal contraception: current practice vs. evidence. *JAMA* 2001;285:2232.

Stewart FH, Kaunitz AM, Laguardia KD, et al. Extended use of transdermal norelgestromin/ethinyl estradiol: a randomized trial. *Obstet Gynecol* 2005;105(6):1389.

Straneva P, Hinderliter A, Wells E, et al. Smoking, oral contraceptives, and cardiovascular reactivity to stress. *Obstet Gynecol* 2000;95:78.

Sucato GS, Gerschultz KL. Extended cycle hormonal contraception in adolescents. *Cur Opin Obstetr Gynecol* 2005;17(5):461.

Sulak P, Lippman J, Siu C, et al. Clinical comparison of triphasic norgestimate/35 micrograms ethinyl estradiol and monophasic norethindrone acetate/20 micrograms ethinyl estradiol: cycle control, lipid effects, and user satisfaction. *Contraception* 1999;59:161.

Trussell J. The essentials of contraception: efficacy, safety, and personal considerations. In: Hatcher RA, Trussell J, Stewart F, et al. eds. *Contraceptive technology*, 18th ed. New York: Ardent Media, 2004:226.

Westhoff C. *Higher body weight does not affect NuvaRing®'s efficacy. Poster Presented at the 53rd Annual Meeting of the American College of Obstetricians and Gynecologists.* San Francisco, CA: May 7–11, 2005.

Westhoff C, Morroni C, Kerns J, et al. Bleeding patterns after immediate vs. conventional oral contraceptive initiation: a randomized, controlled trial. *Fertil Steril* 2003;79(2):322.

Westhoff C, Osborne LM, Schafer JE, et al. Bleeding patterns after immediate initiation of an oral compared with a vaginal hormonal contraceptive. *Obstet Gynecol* 2005;106(1):89.

World Health Organization Collaborative Study of Cardiovascular Disease and Steroid Hormone Contraception. Venous thromboembolic disease and combined oral contraceptives: results of international multicentre case-control study. *Lancet* 1995a;346:1575.

World Health Organization Collaborative Study of Cardiovascular Disease and Steroid Hormone Contraception. Effect of different progestagens in low-oestrogen oral contraceptives on venous thromboembolic disease. *Lancet* 1995b;346:1582.

World Health Organization Collaborative Study of Cardiovascular Disease and Steroid Hormone Contraception. Risk of idiopathic cardiovascular death and nonfatal venous thromboembolism in women using oral contraceptives with differing progestagen components. *Lancet* 1995c;346:1589.

World Health Organization, Department of Reproductive Health and Research. *Selected practice recommendations for contraceptive use*, 2nd ed. Geneva, Switzerland: World Health Organization, Accessed 12/22/05 at http://www.who.int/reproductive-health/publications/spr/index.htm. 2005.

Yonkers KA, Brown C, Pearlstein TB, et al. Efficacy of a new low-dose oral contraceptive with drospirenone in premenstrual dysphoric disorder. *Obstet Gynecol* 2005;106(3):492.

Zieman M, Guillebaud J, Weisberg E, et al. Contraceptive efficacy and cycle control with the Ortho Evra/Evra transdermal system: the analysis of pooled data. *Fertil Steril* 2002;77 (2 Suppl 2):S13.

CHAPTER 44

Intrauterine Contraception

Patricia A. Lohr

Intrauterine contraception (IUC) is the most effective form of reversible birth control available yet it remains tremendously underutilized. Among women aged 15 to 44 only 1.3% use IUC (Mosher et al., 2004). In comparison, 18% of women in Scandinavian countries, 20% of Mexican women, and 40% of women in China choose IUC (Hubacher et al., 2001; Trieman et al., 1995). The low usage of IUC in the United States can be attributed to a lack of knowledge and unfavorable attitudes toward IUC (Forrest, 1996; Stanwood and Bradley, 2005), as well as widespread misperceptions about associated risks of genital tract infection and subsequent infertility. The latter raises concerns about recommending IUC to adolescents, which is reflected in the percentage of 15- to 19-year olds in the United States who use IUC (0.1%). Current thinking regarding recommendations for potential IUC candidates is evolving as more research becomes available on the use of IUC in nulliparous women, including adolescents, and as the relationship between IUC and pelvic inflammatory disease (PID) is better understood. Given the continued high rate of unintended pregnancies and abortions among adolescents, IUC represents a method that, if appropriately utilized, could substantially aid in their reduction (Wildemeersch, 2001).

Two IUCs are currently available in the United States—the copper-bearing T-380A intrauterine contraceptive device (IUD) and the levonorgestrel-releasing intrauterine contraceptive system (IUS). They share efficacy but differ in their side effects and labeling recommendations.

Candidates for IUC are multiparous and nulliparous women who desire long-term reversible contraception. IUC offers effectiveness and convenience comparable to sterilization and is considerably more cost-effective. Estimates are that every copper T-380A IUD used for 5 years saves the health care system $14,122 (Trussell et al., 1995). It is important to note that IUC candidates need *not* have completed their families; IUC is an excellent interval method. The IUS may also be an ideal method for young women with menstrual problems such as menorrhagia or dysmenorrhea. IUC may also be ideal for women with medical problems such as diabetes or hypertension. Selection of which IUC to use should be individualized to maximize the benefits achieved.

Most women are candidates for IUC, however there are restrictions, some of which are device specific. In general, the following conditions contraindicate IUC use (American College of Obstetricians and Gynecologists, 2005):

1. Pregnancy or suspicion of pregnancy
2. PID (current or within the last 3 months)
3. Acute and/or purulent cervicitis
4. Puerperal or postabortion sepsis (current or within the last 3 months)
5. Undiagnosed abnormal vaginal bleeding
6. Malignancy of the genital tract
7. Uterine abnormalities that distort the cavity in a way that is incompatible with insertion
8. Allergy to any component of the IUD or Wilson disease (for copper-containing IUDs)

Nulliparity has never been a contraindication to IUC; however, nulliparous women require careful counseling. The woman needs to understand that her fertility is untested, and that she may experience difficulty conceiving after removal that is not related to IUC. In addition, the expulsion rate for nulliparous women may be higher than for parous women. Counseling should include the signs and symptoms, indicating that the woman may be expelling the device.

COMMON MISCONCEPTIONS ABOUT INTRAUTERINE CONTRACEPTION

Issues Regarding Pelvic Infection

Studies in the 1970s and 1980s linked Dalkon shield use to an increased risk of PID. Over time, the long-term consequences of PID, such as ectopic pregnancy, infertility, and pelvic pain were also observed in women who had used the Dalkon shield. Because the Dalkon shield dominated the IUC market in those days, all IUCs were initially implicated. Further analysis, however, revealed that there were methodological flaws in many early observational studies (Grimes, 2000). The design of the device, the user, and the insertion technique are the most important factors to consider when assessing the risk of PID with IUC.

The Dalkon shield had a polyfilament tail that allowed pathogens from the vagina to ascend into the upper genital tract by a wicking action (Tatum et al., 1975). Modern

IUCs, which have monofilament tails, do not facilitate such infection (Ebi et al., 1996). IUC users who were at risk for STDs were found to be more likely to have upper tract involvement, but monogamous IUC users faced no increase in their long-term risk for PID (Cramer et al., 1985; Daling et al., 1985). It is important to note that there is a transient increase in infection immediately after insertion. This risk is generally limited to the first 20 days of use and results from endometrial contamination during IUC insertion (Farley et al., 1992).

The risk of PID with contemporary IUC is extremely rare (1 in 1,000) (Skjeldestat et al., 1996; Walsh et al., 1998). However, the potential for infection underscores the need to carefully evaluate the patient for possible cervicitis and to meticulously use sterile insertion techniques. Routine antibiotic prophylaxis for insertion is not warranted (Grimes and Schulz, 1999). The American Heart Association does not recommend spontaneous bacterial endocarditis prophylaxis at the time of IUC insertion or removal in the absence of infection (Dajani et al., 1997).

Actinomyces israelii is a gram-positive anaerobic bacterium normally found in the human gastrointestinal tract and is likely a component of female genital tract flora (Persson and Holmberg, 1984). Colonization with *Actinomyces* appears to increase with duration of IUC use (Evans, 1993). However, the correlation between finding *Actinomyces* on a Pap smear in an asymptomatic IC user and the development of pelvic actinomycosis, a very rare but serious condition, is unclear (Lippes, 1999). Management of asymptomatic users of IUC with *Actinomyces* on Pap test should be based on clinical judgment and includes expectant management, oral antibiotics, removal of the IUD, or both antibiotic use and IUD removal (American College of Obstetricians and Gynecologists, 2005).

Issues Regarding Ectopic Pregnancy

Both the copper T-380A IUD and the levonorgestrel IUS reduce a woman's risk of ectopic pregnancy compared with the risk faced by a woman not using birth control (Sivin, 1991; Sivin and Stern, 1994). The copper T-380A IUD and the levonorgestrel IUS have an ectopic pregnancy rate of 0 to 0.5 per 1,000 woman-years, compared with an ectopic pregnancy rate of 3.25 to 5.25 per 1,000 woman-years among women who do not use contraception. This protection is so dramatic that women with prior ectopic pregnancies are candidates for IUC, although product labeling of the levonorgestrel IUS discourages use in women with history of or risk factors for ectopic pregnancies.

Issues Regarding Fertility

IUC is a rapidly reversible birth control method and, as such, is an excellent contraceptive choice for appropriate candidates to use to space their children. In prospective controlled studies of copper IUD users, the fertility of women after IUD removal was shown to be comparable with that in the general population; within 48 months of IUD removal 91.5% of the nulligravid women and 95.7% of the gravid women had conceived. Wilson found that there was no difference in the first-year rates of fertility, ectopic pregnancy, miscarriage, or preterm delivery for women who asked to have IUDs removed in order to conceive compared with women who had IUDs removed because of complications (Wilson, 1989). Similar percentages of women discontinuing the levonorgestrel IUS were found to be pregnant when followed up for 1 year (Sivin et al., 1992).

Although implicated as a cause of tubal infertility in early studies, a more recent, large case–control study comparing nulligravid women with primary infertility with and without tubal occlusion and primigravid controls found no increased risk of tubal infertility among previous users of IUC (Hubacher et al., 2001). The only significant association was between antichlamydial antibodies and infertility.

Issues Regarding Mechanism of Action

The mechanisms of action for the various IUCs differ, and the details of each are described separately in later sections. However, it is important to note that *IUC does not work by causing an abortion*. Serial determinations of beta human chorionic gonadotropin (β-hCG) concentration obtained from users of IUC over several months failed to show the anticipated initial rise and fall characteristic of postimplantation (pregnancy) interruption (Segal et al., 1985). Interference with implantation is also highly unlikely, although a "hostile endometrial environment" is often offered as a mechanism of action. This hypothesis has been rejected because intrauterine flushing experiments failed to yield blastocysts. The most compelling direct experimental support for the contraceptive (prefertilization) action of IUC comes from tubal flushing/salpingectomy specimens, obtained from dozens of women undergoing sterilization procedures who had timed periovulatory intercourse. In the control group, 50% of the women not using contraception were found to have normally dividing fertilized ova indicative of successful fertilization. *None* of the IUC users had any normally dividing ova, which demonstrates the profound contraceptive action of IUC (Alvarez et al., 1988).

Lack of Knowledge about Intrauterine Contraception

A recent study of young pregnant women (age 14–25 years) revealed that only 50% had heard of IUC. Even those who had heard of it were not aware of its safety (71%) or efficacy (58%). Younger women were less likely to have information about IUC, highlighting the importance of teaching women about this highly effective method of contraception (Stanwood and Bradley, 2005).

TYPES OF INTRAUTERINE CONTRACEPTIVE DEVICES

Two different designs of IUC are currently available in the United States—the copper T-380A IUD (ParaGard T-380A) and the levonorgestrel IUS (Mirena). Each provides effective and safe birth control, but each has sufficiently different individual characteristics to warrant separate discussion.

ParaGard Copper T-380A Intrauterine Device

Description of Device The copper T-380A IUD is composed of a flexible T-shaped polyethylene frame whose vertical stem is wrapped with a copper wire coil and whose horizontal arms are each encased in a collar of solid copper. The copper surface area totals 380 mm^2. Monofilament strings are threaded through the bulb at the end of the stem. The stem contains barium sulfate to render it radiopaque. The U.S. Food and Drug Administration (FDA) has approved the copper T-380A IUD for 10 years of continuous use, but long-term studies show that it is quite effective for 12 years (UN Development Programme/United Nations Population Fund/World Health Organization/World Bank, Special Programme of Research, Development and Research Training in Human Reproduction, 1997). Insertion is relatively easy, but require training.

Candidates for IUD Use In 2005, the FDA approved revisions to the prescribing label to explicitly include nulliparous women, women who are not in mutually monogamous relationships, and those with past history of PID. The list of potential users was also broadened to include women who are immunosuppressed (acquired immunodeficiency syndrome (AIDS), chemotherapy, corticosteroids). Current vaginitis and an abnormal Pap smear that is not suggestive of cervical or endometrial carcinoma were also removed as contraindications to use.

The IUD has traditionally been inserted during menses to exclude the possibility of pregnancy; however, it can be inserted at any time in the cycle if the patient is not pregnant. In fact, early expulsion rates can be halved if insertion is delayed until the end of menses (White et al., 1980). The use of local paracervical or intracervical anesthesia may be helpful in decreasing pain when insertions are performed in nulliparous women. Immediate insertion after an uncomplicated first trimester abortion is safe and effective (Grimes et al., 2004) although the practice is not common in the United States. Analysis shows that immediate postabortal insertion is estimated to result in 13 fewer pregnancies per 1,000 women compared to delayed insertion (Reeves et al., 2005). A new IUD can be placed immediately after the prior one has been removed if the patient is still an appropriate candidate. The labeling allows up to 10 years of use, but studies show that it is effective for at least 12 years (UN Development Programme/United Nations Population Fund/World Health Organization/World Bank, Special Programme of Research, Development and Research Training in Human Reproduction, 1997).

Effectiveness The typical first-year failure rate of the copper T-380A IUD is 0.8% (Trussell, 2004), the 10- and the 12-year cumulative failure rates are 2.7% and 2.2%, respectively (UN Development Programme/United Nations Population Fund/World Health Organization/World Bank, Special Programme of Research, Development and Research Training in Human Reproduction, 1997). The failure rate of the IUC is lower than the typical first-year failure rate with oral contraceptives, Depo Provera, the contraceptive ring, and contraceptive patch. It is also lower than the 10-year failure rates of many interval sterilization techniques used in young women (Peterson et al., 1996).

Mechanisms of Action The copper released from the IUD interferes with sperm transport and capacitation (Zipper et al., 1971). Forward motility of sperm is markedly impaired and sperm head-tail disconnection is frequently observed (WHO Scientific Group, 1987). The inflammatory reaction in the endometrium induced by the foreign body is spermicidal (Sagiroglu, 1971). Copper ions that spread into the fallopian tubes also inhibit acrosomal enzyme activation. Without the acrosomal enzymes, the sperms are unable to penetrate the zona pellucida. Ova fertilizability is also reduced due to increased prostaglandin peritoneal levels, probably induced by copper. The best overall description of the mechanism of action of the copper T-380A IUD is that it is a "functional spermicide."

Contraindications The copper T-380A IUD should not be inserted if any of the previously listed contraindications exist (see page 615) or if the patient has (a) Wilson disease or known allergy to copper or (b) a uterine cavity <6 cm or >9 cm on uterine sounding.

Relative Contraindications
1. Anemia
2. Menorrhagia
3. Severe dysmenorrhea

Advantages
1. Extremely effective form of contraception
2. Decreased risk of ectopic pregnancy
3. Convenient; does not require daily, weekly, or quarterly method adherence
4. Private: The IUD is not generally detectable by parents and is often unnoticed by the partner
5. Rapidly reversible after removal
6. Can be used as emergency contraception if inserted within 5 days of unprotected intercourse (Cheng et al., 2004)

Disadvantages
1. Available only through medical providers: Professional assistance is required for insertion and removal
2. Provides no protection against STDs
3. *Actinomyces* colonization appears to increase with duration of IUD use
4. Side effects (discussed later)
5. Relatively high initial cost, which may not be covered by insurance. However, programs have been introduced that assist with reimbursement, payment plans, and financial support for low-income women.

Side Effects
1. Increased menstrual bleeding and cramping: The copper T-380A IUD typically increases menstrual blood loss by approximately 35%, and dysmenorrhea can result. These side effects are common reasons for discontinuation, particularly among nulliparas, and women should be thoroughly counseled on their occurrence before IUD insertion. Prophylactic ibuprofen taken during the menstrual cycle does not appear to have any benefit in reducing early removals due to bleeding and/or pain (Hubacher et al., 2005). An isolated episode of increased or untimely bleeding or cramping may indicate partial expulsion or failure and requires prompt medical evaluation.
2. IUD expulsion: First-year expulsion rates range from 2% to 10%, with an average of 6%. In a randomized trial comparing different types of copper IUDs in nulliparous women, the expulsion rate among those who received the copper T-380 A IUD was 3.3% at 1 year (Otero-Flores et al., 2003). All of the expulsions occurred within the first 3 months of use, highlighting the importance of

counseling about the signs and symptoms of expulsion in the initial months after insertion.

3. Perforation or embedment: The partial or total uterine perforation is a rare event with the copper T-380A IUD (1 in 1,000). Rates are increased in a woman whose uterus is not fully involuted after delivery, who is lactating, or whose uterus is markedly averted or immobile. The most important predictive variable, however, is the experience of the inserter. Embedment of the copper T-380A IUD in the endometrium or myometrium can make removal difficult. Removal of an adherent IUD generally can be accomplished with alligator forceps in an office setting, but a more deeply embedded IUD may require hysteroscope-guided or surgical removal.

Mirena Intrauterine System (Levonorgestrel Intrauterine System)

Description of Device The levonorgestrel IUS is composed of a flexible T-shaped frame with a steroid reservoir surrounding its vertical stem. The reservoir consists of a cylinder made of a mixture of levonorgestrel and polydimethylsiloxane, which releases 20 μg of levonorgestrel per day. The polymer is mixed with barium sulfate, which renders it radiopaque. The unit is also visible ultrasonographically, but its appearance is subtler than that of the copper T-380A IUD. The levonorgestrel IUS has two monofilament tail strings, which are threaded through a bulb at the base of the T. With its arms open, the levonorgestrel IUS measures 32 mm in both the horizontal and vertical directions. The levonorgestrel IUS is approved for 5 years of use. It is recommended that insertion be performed during the first 5 days of menses to ensure that the levonorgestrel IUS will provide adequate first-cycle protection. The insertion technique for the levonorgestrel IUS is quite straightforward, but it differs significantly from that of other such devices and requires training.

Efficacy The typical and perfect first-year failure rates for the levonorgestrel IUS are both 0.1% (Trussell, 2004). The cumulative 5-year failure rate found in various studies has ranged from 0.5% to 1.1%.

Mechanisms of Action The levonorgestrel IUS prevents pregnancy primarily by exerting a very potent, continuous progestin effect on the cervical mucus to render it impenetrable to sperm. The IUS induces inflammatory changes in the endometrium, which are spermicidal. The progestin produces a thin, atrophic endometrium and slows tubal motility. The clinical significance of these last two progestin effects is not yet known. Systemic progestin levels are not sufficiently elevated to consistently suppress ovulation.

Contraindications In addition to the general contraindications for IUC (see page 615), the levonorgestrel IUS is not intended for use in women who have allergic reactions to any of its ingredients. Menorrhagia is not a contraindication to the use of levonorgestrel IUS, because the levonorgestrel IUS significantly reduces monthly menstrual blood loss. In fact, in 98 of the 100 countries that have approved the levonorgestrel IUS, it is used to treat menorrhagia as a labeled indication (Irvine et al., 1998). Dysmenorrhea can also be reduced with the use of the levonorgestrel IUS and appears to be superior to combined oral contraceptives in reducing painful menstruation (Suhonon et al., 2004).

Advantages The advantages are similar to those of the copper T-380A IUD, except that the levonorgestrel IUS reduces menstrual loss and dysmenorrhea (Ronnerdag and Odlind, 1999; Suhonen et al., 2004). The levonorgestrel IUS may lower the risk of PID, but the data are not conclusive (Grimes, 2000). One small study found that levonorgestrel IUS users had an 85% lower incidence of Pap smears showing *Actinomyces*-like organisms, compared with users of a copper IUD (Merki-Feld et al., 2000).

Disadvantages The disadvantages are similar to those of the copper T-380A IUD. The levonorgestrel IUS cannot be used as a form of emergency contraception.

Side Effects

1. Bleeding irregularities: Initially, most levonorgestrel IUS users experience unpredictable spotting or bleeding, which usually resolves within 3 to 6 months and is replaced by either complete amenorrhea or significant oligomenorrhea due to endometrial atrophy. Although the absence of menses may be considered a benefit for women who have menorrhagia or dysmenorrhea, many young women perceive bleeding irregularities, including amenorrhea, as undesirable side effects. In a survey of 328 adolescents, 74% said they would stop using a contraceptive that caused irregular menses, and 65% would stop using a method that caused amenorrhea (Gold and Coupey, 1998). The issue of bleeding irregularities must, therefore, be discussed in detail to avoid early discontinuation of the method.
2. IUS expulsion: The expulsion rate in the first 1 to 2 years of use is approximately 4%, and the cumulative 5-year rate is approximately 11% (Sivin et al., 1991). In a study of the levonorgestrel IUS in nulliparous women, only 1 expulsion occurred out of 92 insertions (Suhonen et al., 2004).
3. Pain at insertion: Discomfort at the time of insertion of the levonorgestrel IUS appears to be higher in nulliparous women as compared with insertion of the copper IUD (Suhonen et al., 2004). This may be due to the larger diameter of the insertion tube. Cervical dilation or the use of local anesthetic has been described to reduce discomfort.
4. Ovarian cysts: Enlarged ovarian follicles are seen more frequently with the levonorgestrel IUS because the locally increased progestin concentration slows follicular atresia. These cysts typically resolve within 2 weeks and are not an indication for intervention (Bahamondes et al., 2003).
5. Progestin effects: Other systemic progestin effects (breast tenderness, acne, headaches) have been reported by levonorgestrel IUS users, although the circulating levels of the progestin are much lower than with oral contraceptives.

USE IN ADOLESCENTS

Although the teen birth rate in the United States is declining, teen pregnancy remains higher in the United States than in any other industrialized country and the vast majority of these pregnancies are unintended (Abma et al., 2004). The reduction in the number of adolescent pregnancies has been attributed in large part to the use of long-acting contraceptive methods that circumvent inconsistent use by avoiding daily method adherence. Adolescents who experience a pregnancy are at particularly high risk of unintended repeat pregnancy (Maynard and Rangaranhan, 1994). The need for highly effective, safe, long-acting birth control for adolescents at risk of pregnancy can be met by IUC for select teens.

The use of IUC in adolescents and nulliparous women is not new. Early studies on interval and immediate postabortal insertion of IUC in adolescents found high continuation and low complication rates (Goldman et al., 1979; Edwards et al., 1974; Roy et al., 1974). Recent data on the levonorgestrel IUS suggest that it is a very acceptable method (Otero-Flores et al., 2003; Suhonen et al., 2004). Diaz et al. (1993) compared the clinical performance of 995 parous adolescents using a copper T-380A IUD with a cohort of paired controls 10 years older of the same parity. Although the rates for pregnancy, expulsion, and removal were higher in adolescents, the ranges were within those reported in the literature for IUC. Removals due to infection were few, and the rate was not significantly different from that for older women. Overall, the performance was similar or better than other reversible methods in this age-group. Therefore, in the appropriate adolescent or young adult, IUC should be considered along with other methods. Selection of the appropriate device should be tailored to individual needs.

PREGNANCY WITH INTRAUTERINE CONTRACEPTION IN PLACE

Pregnancies in current users of IUC are rare. The location of the pregnancy should be determined as early as possible, because 8% of pregnancies that occur with the copper T-380A IUD and 50% of pregnancies with the levonorgestrel IUS are ectopic. It is recommended that the device be removed in the first trimester of an intrauterine gestation if the strings are visible in the vagina because of the risk of spontaneous or septic abortion. Although the loss rate may be higher if IUC is retained, no IUC-related deaths among pregnant women in the United States have been reported. First trimester removal reduces the risk of spontaneous abortion by approximately 50%. Late in pregnancy, the strings are rarely visible unless the placenta is low-lying, and there is no demonstrated benefit to IUC removal at this time. If the strings are not visible, it is prudent to obtain an ultrasound study, because the most common reason for pregnancy is a previously undetected expulsion. If the device is present, there is no reason to remove it. The risk of birth defects is not increased, but the patient should be alerted to signs and symptoms of preterm labor, because an increased risk of premature birth has been demonstrated. If a teen elects to abort the pregnancy, the device can be removed at the time of the procedure.

FUTURE DEVELOPMENTS

Several smaller copper IUDs as well as a "frameless" IUD specifically designed for nulliparous women have been studied in Europe, Asia, and Latin America. These devices appear to have lower expulsion rates and greater acceptability than the copper T-380A IUD (Duenas et al., 1996; Otero-Flores et al., 2003; Wildemeersch et al., 2003). A small intracervical levonorgestrel-releasing device has also been developed and appears to be equal in efficacy to the levonorgestrel IUS (Pakarinen and Luukkainen, 2005).

GUIDELINES FOR PATIENTS

The following is a suggested format for informing teens about IUC.

1. What is IUC?
   IUC is a small plastic device that is placed in the uterus (womb).
2. How is IUC placed?
   IUC is inserted in the doctor's office. It does not require surgery but sometimes a local anesthetic is used to numb the cervix (the opening to the uterus) and make inserting IUC more comfortable.
3. How does IUC work?
   IUC appears to work primarily by preventing fertilization of an egg by sperm. The copper in the ParaGard IUD probably has an antisperm effect, and the hormones in the medicated IUS blocks sperm from entering the womb.
4. Are there different types of IUC?
   In the United States currently, there are two types of IUC available. One contains copper, and the other contains the hormone levonorgestrel. Both are shaped like the letter T and are approximately 11/4 in. tall. Each has a thread or "tail" on the end, which allows the woman to check that the device is in place and also makes removal easier. The copper IUD is effective for up to 12 years. The levonorgestrel IUS can be used for up to 5 years.
5. How effective is IUC?
   IUC is the most effective form of reversible birth control. Both the copper T380-A IUD and the levonorgestrel IUS are more than 99% effective at preventing pregnancy in the first year of use.
6. Are there side effects?
   With the copper T-380A IUD, the most common side effects are increased menstrual flow and cramps, which may be reduced by use of an over-the-counter pain medication such as ibuprofen. These side effects lessen after the first few months. With the levonorgestrel IUS, irregular spotting and bleeding are common in the first 3 to 6 months, but after that a woman's periods decrease dramatically and may stop altogether. Absence of a period is not dangerous and does not mean that the blood is "building up inside." Rather, the lining of the uterus is so thin that there is very little or no tissue to be shed each month.
7. Is IUC safe?
   IUC is safe when used in the appropriate individuals. IUC should be used in women who are in relationships that do not put them at risk for STDs.
8. What are the benefits of IUC?
   IUC is a safe, effective, easy-to-use, and cost-effective form of contraception. There is no need to remember to use the method every day or with every act of sex.

Remember

1. IUC does not protect against STDs. If you may be at risk for STDs and have IUC, use a latex or polyurethane condom to help protect yourself against infection.
2. If you ever have fever, pelvic pain, severe cramping, heavy vaginal bleeding, or a foul-smelling vaginal discharge contact your clinician immediately. These may be signs of a serious infection or pregnancy or a warning that your IUC may be coming out.
3. If you have any symptoms of pregnancy, contact your provider immediately.
4. Do not remove IUC yourself or tug on the strings.
5. If you have any problems or questions, call your provider.

WEB SITES

For Teenagers and Parents

http://www.plannedparenthood.org/pp2/portal/files/portal/medicalinfo/birthcontrol/pub-contraception-iud.xml. Planned Parenthood site on IUDs.

http://www.aafp.org/afp/981200ap/981200c.html. American Academy of Family Physicians handout on IUDs.

http://kidshealth.org/teen/sexual_health/contraception/contraception_iud.html. Teen site with explanation of IUDs.

For Health Care Providers

http://www.paragard.com/. Ortho-McNeil site for ParaGard T-380A IUD. In addition to educational materials, the Web site also includes information for providers and patients on assistance with reimbursement.

http://www.mirena.com/. Berlex site for Mirena.

https://www.arhp.org/healthcareproviders/cme/onlinecme/IUDCP/TOC.cfm. Association of Reproductive Health Professionals Web site for the 2004 "New Developments in Intrauterine Contraception" educational program.

http://www.aafp.org/afp/20050101/95.html. American Academy of Family Physicians, Insertion and Removal of IUDs.

http://www.archfoundation.com/. The ARCH foundation is a not-for-profit foundation established to assist low-income women who do not have insurance coverage for the Mirena® IUS.

REFERENCES AND ADDITIONAL READINGS

Abma JC, Martinez GM, Mosher WD, et al. *Teenagers in the United States: sexual activity, contraceptive use and childbearing, 2002. Vital Health Statistics, National Center for Health Statistics* 2004; 23.

Alvarez R, Brache V, Fernandez F, et al. New insights on the mode of action of intrauterine devices in women. *Fertil Steril* 1988;49:768.

American College of Obstetricians and Gynecologists. Intrauterine device. ACOG practice bulletin no. 59. *Obstet Gynecol* 2005;105:223.

Bahamondes L, Hidalgo M, Petta CA, et al. Enlarged ovarian follicles in users of a levonorgestrel-releasing intrauterine system and contraceptive implant. *J Reprod Med* 2003;48:637.

Bromham DR. Intrauterine contraceptive devices: a reappraisal. *Br Med Bull* 1993;49:100.

Cheng L, Gulmezoglu AM, Van Oel CJ, et al. Cochrane Fertility Regulation Group. Interventions for emergency contraception. *Cochrane Database Syst Rev* 2004;4.

Contracept Technol Update. Third-generation IUDs have fewer complications. 1992;(February):23.

Cramer DW, Schiff I, Schoenbaum SC, et al. Tubal infertility and the intrauterine device. *N Engl J Med* 1985;12:941.

Dajani AS, Taubert KA, Wilson W, et al. Prevention of bacterial endocarditis. Recommendations by the American Heart Association. *JAMA* 1997;277:1794.

Daling JR, Weiss NS, Metch BJ, et al. Primary tubal infertility in relation to the use of an intrauterine device. *N Engl J Med* 1985;312:937.

Dardano KL, Burkman RT. The intrauterine contraceptive device: an often-forgotten and maligned method of contraception. *Am J Obstet Gynecol* 1999;181:1.

Diaz J, Neto AMP, Bahamondes L, et al. Performance of the Copper T 200 in parous adolescents: are copper IUDs suitable for these women? *Contraception* 1993;48:23.

Duenas JL, Albert A, Carrasco F. Intrauterine contraception in nulligravid vs parous women. *Contraception* 1996;53:23.

Ebi KL, Piziali RL, Rosenberg M, et al. Evidence against tailstrings increasing the rate of pelvic inflammatory disease among IUD users. *Contraception* 1996;53:25.

Edwards LE, McCreary MK, Hakanson EY. A comparison of intrauterine contraceptive devices and oral contraceptives in the nullipara. *Am J Obstet Gynecol* 1974;120:470.

Evans DT. *Actinomyces israelii* in the female genital tract: a review. *Genitourin Med* 1993;69:54.

Farley TM, Rosenberg MS, Rowe PJ, et al. Intrauterine devices and pelvic inflammatory disease: an international perspective. *Lancet* 1992;339:785.

Farr G, Rivera R. Interactions between intrauterine contraceptive device use and breast-feeding status at time of intrauterine contraceptive device insertion: analysis of Tcu-380A acceptors in developing countries. *Am J Obstet Gynecol* 1992;167:144.

Forrest JD. U.S. women's perceptions of and attitudes about the IUD. *Obstet Gynecol Surv* 1996;51:S30.

Fortney JA, Feldblum PJ, Raymond EG. Intrauterine devices: the optimal long-term contraceptive method? *J Reprod Med* 1999;44:269.

Franks AL, Beral V, Cates W, et al. Contraception and ectopic pregnancy rates. *Am J Obstet Gynecol* 1990;163:1120.

Gold MA, Coupey SM. Young women's attitudes toward injectable and implantable contraceptives. *J Pediatr Adolesc Gynecol* 1998;11:17.

Goldman JA, Dekel A, Reichman J. Immediate postabortion intrauterine contraception in nulliparous adolescents. *Isr J Med Sci* 1979;15:522.

Grimes DA. Intrauterine device and upper genital tract infection. *Lancet* 2000;356:1013.

Grimes DA, Schulz KF. Prophylactic antibiotics for intrauterine device insertion: a metaanalysis of the randomized controlled trials. *Contraception* 1999;60:57.

Grimes D, Schulz K, Stanwood N. Immediate postabortal insertion of intrauterine devices. *Cochrane Database Syst Rev* 2004;(4):CD001777.

Heartwell SE, Schlesselman S. Risk of uterine perforation among users of intrauterine devices. *Obstet Gynecol* 1983;61:31.

Hubacher D, Lara-Ricalde R, Taylor DJ, et al. Use of copper intrauterine devices and the risk of tubal infertility among nulligravid women. *N Engl J Med* 2001;345:561.

Hubacher D, Reyes V, Lillo S, et al. Preventing copper intrauterine device removals due to side effects among first-time users: randomized trial to study the effect of prophylactic ibuprofen. *Hum Reprod.* 2006;21(6):1467.

Irvine GA, Campbell-Brown MB, Lumsden MA, et al. Randomised comparative trial of the levonorgestrel intrauterine system and norethisterone for treatment of idiopathic menorrhagia. *Br J Obstet Gynaecol* 1998;105:592.

Kulig JW, Raugh JL, Burket RL, et al. Experience with the Copper 7 intrauterine device in an adolescent population. *J Pediatr* 1980;96:746.

Lee NC, Rubino GL, Borueki R. The intrauterine device and pelvic inflammatory disease revisited: new results for the women's health study. *Obstet Gynecol* 1988;72:1.

Lippes J. Pelvic actinomycosis: a review and preliminary look at prevalence. *Am J Obstet Gynecol* 1999;180:265.

Maynard R, Rangaranhan A. Contraceptive use and repeat pregnancies among welfare-dependent teenage mothers. *Fam Plann Perspect* 1994;26:198.

Merki-Feld GS, Lebeda E, Hogg B, et al. The incidence of actinomyces-like organisms in papanicolaou-stained smears of copper and levonorgestrel intrauterine devices. *Contraception* 2000;61:365.

Mishell DR Jr. Intrauterine devices: mechanisms of action, safety, and efficacy. *Contraception* 1998;58:45S.

Mishell D Jr, Roy S. Copper intrauterine contraceptive device event rates following insertion 4 to 8 weeks postpartum. *Am J Obstet Gynecol* 1982;143:29.

Mosher WD, Martinez GM, Chandra A, et al. *Use of contraception and use of family planning services in the United States, 1982–2002. Advance Data from Vital and Health Statistics,* 2004; 350.

Newton J. The current status of intra-uterine contraceptive devices and systems. *Br J Fam Plann* 2000;26:14.

Ortiz ME, Croyatto HB. The mode of action of IUDs. *Contraception* 1987;36:37.

Otero-Flores JB, Guerrero-Carreno FJ, Vazquez-Estrada LA. A comparative randomized study of three different IUDs in nulliparous Mexican women. *Contraception* 2003;67:273.

Pakarinen P, Luukkainen T. Five years' experience with a small intracervical/intrauterine levonorgestrel-releasing device. *Contraception* 2005;72(5):342.

Persson E, Holmberg K. A longitudinal study of actinomyces israelii in the female genital tract. *Acta Obstet Gynecol Scand* 1984;63:207.

Peterson HB, Xia Z, Hughes JM, et al. The risk of pregnancy after tubal sterilization: findings from the U.S. Collaborative Review of Sterilization. *Am J Obstet Gynecol* 1996;174:1161.

Reeves MG, Smith KJ, Creinin MD. Decision analysis of immediate vs. delayed insertion of intrauterine devices after abortion to prevent pregnancy. *Contraception* 2005;72:237.

Ronnerdag M, Odlind V. Health effects of long-term use of the intrauterine levonorgestrel-releasing system: a follow-up study over 12 years of continuous use. *Acta Obstet Gynecol Scand* 1999;78:716.

Roy S, Cooper D, Mishell DR Jr. Experience with three different models of the Copper T intrauterine contraceptive device in nulliparous women. *Am J Obstet Gynecol* 1974;119:414.

Sagiroglu N. Phagocytosis of spermatozoa in the uterine cavity of woman using intrauterine device. *Int J Fertil* 1971;16:1.

Segal SJ, Alvarez-Sanchez F, Adejuwon CA, et al. Absence of chorionic gonadotropin in sera of women who use intrauterine devices. *Fertil Steril* 1985;44:214.

Sivin I. IUDs are contraceptives, not abortifacients: a comment on research and belief. *Stud Fam Plann* 1989;20:355.

Sivin I. Dose- and age-dependent ectopic pregnancy risks with intrauterine contraception. *Obstet Gynecol* 1991;78:291.

Sivin I, Schmidt E. Effectiveness of IUDs: a review. *Contraception* 1987;36:55.

Sivin I, Stern J. International Committee for Contraception Research. Health during prolonged use of levonorgestrel 20 micrograms/d and the copper TCu 380Ag intrauterine contraceptive device: a multicenter study. *Fertil Steril* 1994;61:70.

Sivin I, Stern J, Coutinho E, et al. Prolonged intrauterine contraception; a seven year randomized study of the levonorgestrel 20 mcg/day (LNg 20) and the copper T380 Ag IUDs. *Contraception* 1991;44:474.

Sivin I, Stern J, Diaz S, et al. Rates and outcomes of planned pregnancy after use of Norplant capsules, Norplant II rods, or levonorgestrel-releasing or copper TCu 380Ag intrauterine contraceptive devices. *Am J Obstet Gynecol* 1992;166:1208.

Skjeldestad F, Bran H. Fertility after complicated and non-complicated use of IUDs: a controlled prospective study. *Adv Contracept* 1988;4:179.

Skjeldestad FE, Halvorsen LE, Kahn H, et al. IUD users in Norway are at low risk for *C. trachomatis* infection. *Contraception* 1996;54:209.

Stanwood NL, Bradley KA. Young pregnant women's knowledge of modern intrauterine devices. *Obstet Gynecol.* 2006;108(6):1417.

Suhonen A, Haukkamaa M, Jakobsson T, et al. Clinical performance of a levonorgestrel-releasing intrauterine system and oral contraceptives in young nulliparous women: a comparative study. *Contraception* 2004;69:407.

Tatum HJ. Clinical aspects of intrauterine contraception: 1976. *Contraception* 1977;28:16.

Tatum HJ, Schmidt FH, Phillips D, et al. The Dalkon Shield controversy: structural and bacteriological studies of IUD tails. *JAMA* 1975;231:711.

Trieman K, Liskin L, Kols A, et al. *IUDs—an update. Population Reports, Series B, No. 5.* Baltimore: Johns Hopkins School of Public Health Population Information Program, 1995:23.

Trussell J. Contraceptive failure in the United States. *Contraception* 2004;70:89.

Trussell J, Leveque A, Koenig JD, et al. Economic value of contraception: a comparison of 15 methods. *Am J Public Health* 1995;85:494.

UN Development Programme/United Nations Population Fund/ World Health Organization/World Bank, Special Programme of Research, Development and Research Training in Human Reproduction. Long-term reversible contraception: twelve years of experience with the TCu380A and TCu220C. *Contraception* 1997;56:341.

Walsh T, Grimes D, Frezieres R, et al. Randomised controlled trial of prophylactic antibiotics before insertion of intrauterine devices. IUD Study Group. *Lancet* 1998;351:1005.

White MK, Ory HW, Rooks JB, et al. Intrauterine device termination rates and the menstrual cycle day of insertion. *Obstet Gynecol* 1980;55:220.

Wildemeersch D. Taking up the challenge: can effective long-term intrauterine contraceptive methods radically reduce the number of unintended pregnancies? *J Fam Plann Reprod Health Care* 2001;27:121.

Wildemeersch D, Batar I, Affandi B, et al. The 'frameless' intrauterine system for long-term reversible contraception: a review of 15 years of clinical experience. *J Obstet Gynaecol Res* 2003;29:164.

Wilson JC. A prospective New Zealand study of fertility after removal of copper intrauterine contraceptive devices for contraception and because of complications: a four year study. *Am J Obstet Gynecol* 1989;160:391.

World Health Organization. *Medical eligibility criteria for contraceptive use*, 3rd ed. Geneva: World Health Organization, 2004.

WHO Scientific Group. *Mechanisms of action, safety and efficacy of intrauterine devices*. WHO Technical Report 753. Geneva: World Health Organization, 1987.

Zhang J, Chi I-C, Feldblum PJ, et al. Risk factors for Copper T IUD expulsion: an epidemiologic analysis. *Contraception* 1992;46:427.

Zipper JA, Tatum HJ, Medel M, et al. Contraception through the use of intrauterine metals. I. Copper as an adjunct to the "T" device. The endouterine copper "T". *Am J Obstet Gynecol* 1971;109:771.

CHAPTER 45

Barrier Contraceptives and Spermicides

Patricia A. Lohr

Spermicides are agents that kill sperms whereas barrier contraceptives block their movement toward the upper genital tract. Barrier contraceptives are available in a wide variety of designs, including the male and female condom, diaphragm, cervical cap, cervical shield, and sponge. Vaginal spermicides come in many forms such as foam, gel, cream, suppository, and film. In general, barrier methods and spermicides have higher failure rates but fewer systemic side effects than other modern contraceptive methods. Barrier methods also offer some reduction in the risk of sexually transmitted diseasesSTDs). Many barrier contraceptives and all spermicides are available over the counter and improve adolescent access to birth control. The high typical-use failure rates of barrier methods and spermicides can be considerably lowered if they are used more consistently or in combination with other contraceptive methods.

MALE CONDOMS

Condoms (Fig. 45.1) are the oldest method of male contraception and the second most popular reversible form of birth control in the United States (Mosher et al., 2004). Since the mid-1980s, condom use among teenage males has been increasing. The most recent data from the 2002 National Survey of Family Growth (NSFG) shows a continuation in this trend; 71% of teenage males reported condom use at sexual debut and an equal percentage reported condom use during the last episode of sexual intercourse (Abma et al., 2004). Trends differed by ethnicity and gender. Non-Hispanic black teens were more likely than other groups to report condom use at first sex, and Hispanic males were more likely to report no contraceptive use. Female teens report lower rates of male condom use than male teens; however, the number using condoms is also increasing. The percentage of female teenagers using a condom during their most recent sexual activity increased from 38% in 1995 to 54% in 2002.

Consistent condom utilization remains a problem for teenagers. In 1998, fewer than half (45%) of sexually experienced adolescent men used condoms consistently (Sonenstein et al., 1998). According to the 2002 NSFG data, the percentage of teenage males who reported using a condom every time they had intercourse over the preceeding 12-month period was only 37% (Abma et al., 2004).

Condoms are very cost-effective for episodic intercourse, which is often found among teens. For long-term use, however, the condom's higher failure rate drives its overall cost much higher.

The human immunodeficiency virus (HIV) epidemic has heightened public awareness and acceptance of condoms. A significant degree of STD protection is afforded by latex and polyurethane condoms, which are impermeable to *Chlamydia trachomatis, Neisseria gonorrhoeae*, herpes simplex virus, cytomegalovirus, hepatitis B virus, and human papillomavirus (HPV). Millions of women use condoms in conjunction with other methods (e.g., sterilization, birth control pills, or spermicides) to capture this STD risk reduction benefit. Seventeen percent of adolescents combine the male condom with a female method of contraception for STD risk reduction and/or enhanced contraceptive efficacy (Sonenstein et al., 1998; Abma et al., 2004).

Uses of Male Condoms

Contraceptive Uses
1. As a primary method of birth control, alone or in conjunction with a spermicide, a female barrier, hormonal method or intrauterine contraception
2. As a backup method of contraception after a late start with a hormonal method (e.g., oral contraceptives, injections) or whenever two or more combined oral contraceptive pills or one progestin-only pill have been missed
3. As a barrier contraceptive, used as part of the fertility awareness method (FAM) of contraception during vulnerable days of the woman's cycle

Noncontraceptive Uses
1. To reduce transmission of STDs
2. To blunt sensation, to treat premature ejaculation
3. To reduce cervical antisperm antibody titers in women with associated infertility
4. To reduce allergic reaction in women with sensitivity to sperm

Types of Male Condoms

The more than 100 brands of condoms available in the United States provide a wide range of choices in size, shape, thickness, lubricant, and design features intended

The male condom is a sheath of plastic or rubber that fits snugly over the erect penis. It blocks the man's sperm from entering the woman's body. It also covers the penis to help protect the man and the woman from getting sexually transmitted infections from each other. The male condom can be used with other contraceptives. It can be used with other birth control methods such as birth control pills, shots, implants, spermicide and diaphragms. It should not be used with the female condom. On average, if 100 couples use condoms for a year, 12 will become pregnant. Correct and more consistent use can reduce the risk of pregnancy even more.

♦ Use a condom every time you have sex. Keep a few handy.

♦ Put the condom on before there is any genital contact.

♦ Open the package carefully.

♦ Unroll the condom all the way to the base of the penis.

♦ Squeeze the air out of the top of the condom to make room for the ejaculate.

♦ Make sure your partner is well lubricated. Use spermicide or water-based or silicon-based lubricants. Do *not* use petroleum-based lubricants with latex condoms.

♦ If the condom tears or starts to slip off during sex, grasp the rim of the condom against the penis and withdraw the penis. The man should wash his hands and his penis. The woman should wash her hands and her labia (do *not* douche). If spermicide is available, the woman should insert spermicide into her vagina according to product directions. She should also use emergency contraception as soon as possible. If the couple wants to have sex again, use a new condom.

♦ Right after ejaculation, while the penis is still firm, the rim of the condom could be gently pressed against the penis as it is removed from the vagina.

♦ Check the used condom for any breaks or tears. If breaks or tears are noticed follow instructions above regarding spermicide and emergency contraception. Tie up the end and throw it away.

FIGURE 45.1   The male condom—patient information sheet.

to enhance sensation and utilization. Three materials are used in manufacturing condoms: latex, lamb cecum (used to make natural membrane or "skin" condoms), and polyurethane. Condoms made from other synthetic materials are in development and testing. Latex condoms dominate the market (99%), whereas natural membrane and polyurethane condoms account for <1%. Condoms are available in several sizes, but most condoms are 170 mm long and 50 mm wide. The thickness ranges from 0.03 to 0.10 mm. Condom shapes vary (straight-sided, baggy, or contoured), as do their textures (smooth or ribbed).

One experimental nonlatex design, the eZ·on condom, is a baggy sheath that is slipped on like a sock rather than rolled on. Condoms are lubricated by a wide range of materials such as silicones, spermicides, and water-based gels. Other features that are intended to make condoms more pleasurable to use include an array of colors, scents, and tastes.

Some latex condoms are available with a spermicidal coating of nonoxynol-9. Spermicides may provide lubrication, but they do not contribute to STD risk reduction (Roddy et al., 1998) and existing data is very limited to support an added improvement in preventing pregnancy.

DOs and DON'Ts:

Do use a new condom each time you have sex	Don't reuse a condom
Do use a condom made of latex or polyurethane	Don't use lambskin or fake plastic condoms
Do change your condom if you have oral or anal sex before you have intercourse	Don't use the same condom for different sex practices or different sex partners
Do check the expiration date of the condom	Don't use a condom after the expiration date
Do place the condom before the penis touches her genitals	Don't let the penis touch her genitals before the condom goes on
Do use water-based lubricants if needed, such as spermicide, K-Y jelly	Don't use the petroleum-based products, such as Vaseline, oils, vaginal creams for infection treatment
Do hold the condom rim against the penis and pull them out together before the penis starts to soften or after ejaculation	Don't let the penis become soft inside her vagina – the condom can fall off
Do check the condom for tears, then tie it off and throw it away	Don't ever wash the condom and recycle it
Do keep emergency contraception and spermicide ready in case something happens and the condom does not work well	Don't wait until you need it, because emergency contraception works better the sooner you use it

FIGURE 45.1   (*Continued*)

Spermicides may cause genital irritation, potentially leading to increased STDs and urinary tract infections (Handley et al., 2002). The spermicidal coating also drastically reduces the shelf life of latex condoms, from an average of 5 to 2 years. The current recommendations of the Centers for Disease Control and Prevention state that use of nonoxynol-9 lubricated condoms is preferable to not using a condom. However, given the option, use of condoms with nonoxynol-9 is not advocated because of their increased cost, shorter shelf life, association urinary tract infections in young women, and lack of apparent benefit when compared with other lubricated condoms (Workowski and Levine, 2002).

Polyurethane male condoms are nonbiodegradable and require less fastidious handling before use. They are not susceptible to damage by petroleum-based lubricants, lack the latex allergens, and do not have the unexpected taste or smell, occasionally associated with latex condoms, during oral-genital contact. Polyurethane itself is a stronger material than latex, but it lacks elasticity. With the exception of the experimental eZ·on condom, pregnancy rates in clinical trials were not higher in polyurethane condom users, but the slippage and breakage rates for the polyurethane condoms were four to eight times higher than for a standard latex condom (Frezieres et al., 1998; Steiner et al., 2003). The higher breakage and slippage rates of polyurethane condoms may diminish some of their protective effect against STDs. Polyurethane male condoms may best be reserved for couples who cannot tolerate latex products.

Natural "skin" condoms afford almost equal pregnancy protection as latex or polyurethane condoms, but do not reduce STD risks. They are also significantly more expensive which may be a barrier to use by teens.

Mechanism of Action

Condoms are sheaths made of latex (rubber-based), polyurethane, or processed lamb cecum which fit over the penis and block transmission of semen.

Effectiveness

The male condom is the most effective barrier method available for pregnancy protection. The first-year failure rate for typical use of the latex male condom is 15%, and the failure rate for correct and consistent use is 2% (Trussell, 2004). Comparative trials of latex versus nonlatex condoms have confirmed higher breakage and slippage rates for nonlatex condoms during intercourse or withdrawal, but similar pregnancy rates (Gallo et al., 2003). Both latex and nonlatex condoms appear to have similar efficacy in preventing STDs. The most critical variable in predicting efficacy is consistent use, followed closely by proper technique. Condom quality has also improved dramatically in recent years. Research described in *Consumer Reports* found that 7 of 37 condom models failed routine testing in 1995, but by 1999 only 2 of 30 models failed those tests (Consumer's Union, 1995, 1999). The self-proclaimed "strength" and "contour" of the condom did not influence test scores.

Improving Condom Success

Dozens of excellent studies have been conducted to identify factors that predict consistent use of barrier methods, variables that would predict poor use, and ways to design interventions that might improve utilization. Most of this research has focused on the male condom. Given the vital role that barriers play in slowing the spread of STDs, answers to these questions are desperately needed. Unfortunately, studies show that solutions will not be easy to achieve.

There are profound differences in condom use by gender, with female adolescents reporting far less use of condoms than male adolescents (Brown et al., 1992; Ku et al., 1994; Abma et al., 2004). This may be due to the fact that female teens most commonly have older sexual partners and condom use by males tends to decrease with increasing age. Adolescent males appear to have greater knowledge about condom use and efficacy than females and may feel more comfortable obtaining condoms (Leland and Barth, 1992). Self-esteem may also play a role. Adolescent African-American females with higher self-esteem were found to be more likely to have positive attitudes toward condom use, feel more efficacious and less fearful about negotiating condom use, and perceived fewer barriers to using condoms (Salazar et al., 2005).

Many teens have misperceptions about condoms. Among 16,677 teens surveyed, approximately one third believed that condoms work just as well when Vaseline is used

with them, and approximately one fifth believed that natural membrane condoms provide better protection against HIV than the latex condom (Crosby and Yarber, 2001). In addition, perception of knowledge about condoms among teens is not always associated with actual knowledge or use. In a longitudinal study of 404 virginal male adolescents who became sexually active during the study, those with low objective but high-perceived knowledge were approximately 3 times less likely to report using a condom at first intercourse (Rock et al., 2005).

Adolescents remain at high risk of STDs, particularly minority youth and young men who have sex with men (Centers for Disease Control and Prevention, 2003; Lightfoot et al., 2005). Youth who identify as bisexual appear to be at extremely high risk due to higher frequencies of multiple sexual partners, STDs, unprotected intercourse, and injection drug use (Goodenow et al., 2002). A perceived risk of STD or HIV infection is associated with higher condom use and also with intention to use condoms in the future (Brown et al., 1992; Donald et al., 1994; Orr and Langefeld, 1993). However, several studies show that many adolescents who are clearly at increased risk for STDs have little appreciation of their vulnerability (Rosenthal et al., 1994; O'Donnell et al., 1995). Teens with a history of a STD also do not appear to apply the factual knowledge gained from the prior experience to alter sexual behaviors, thereby providing an additional challenge to educational prevention efforts (DiClemente et al., 2002).

A common finding of virtually all studies is that condom use is increased when adolescents believe that their peers use condoms. Other factors that increase condom use are when teens believe that condoms can prevent STDs, when teens feel that they can talk to their partner about risks, when they have easy access to a supply of condoms, know how to use a condom, and carry condoms with them (Joffe and Radius, 1993; Schuster et al., 1998; Dilorio et al., 2001). Condom use is decreased when risky sexual behavior is just one of a cluster of risky health behaviors (e.g., smoking, substance abuse) or other lifestyle risks (e.g., violence). Substantial societal changes apparently are needed to address these issues. Putting condoms in open containers may be necessary to provide adolescent access to condoms, but it is clearly not sufficient to ensure their use.

For individual success in clinical practice, providers should be aware of condom misuse (Wood and Buckle, 1994) and should do the following:

1. Teach the patient how best to use condoms (Fig. 45.1)
   a. Plan where to store condoms for ready access, privacy, and condom safety.
   b. Incorporate condom placement into the lovemaking process—when the penis is still somewhat flaccid, if possible, but certainly before any genital contact. The preejaculatory semen contains few sperm, but STD spread may occur early. Furthermore, a teen's ability to delay sexual activity to place the condom is markedly diminished after genital contact. Inexperienced youth benefit greatly from the opportunity to practice placing condoms on models or even over two fingers during office visits.
   c. Open the packaging carefully. Avoid using sharp objects. Any foil edges shearing across the condom may tear the latex. Between 24% and 65% of latex condom breakages occur before intercourse.

d. Correctly place the condom. Judge which way the condom will unroll. Allow some slack at the top of condoms that have no reservoir tip; fit more snugly those with ejaculatory reservoirs once erection is complete. Squeeze the air out of the reservoir areas. Completely unroll the full length of the condom.

e. Change condoms if different body orifices are penetrated. In particular, if a condom is used during anal or oral sex, it must be removed and replaced before vaginal penetration.

f. Use only water-based lubricants or spermicides to reduce vaginal friction against the latex condom. Lubricant should be applied only to the external surface of the condom or to the vaginal area; lubricant should not be placed on the penis or on the inner surface of the condom, because that practice increases problems with slippage and breakage. Avoid petroleum-based products such as Vaseline, baby oils, and lotions. All vaginal antifungal treatments and some of the vaginal products for treatment of bacterial vaginosis also contain petroleum-based ingredients. Petroleum can react with the latex in seconds and undermine the strength of the condom; within 1 minute, microscopic tears may develop and become large enough to permit the passage of virus.

g. After ejaculation, firmly grasp the rim of the condom at the base of the penis and carefully withdraw the unit while the penis is still firm. Any delays in removal can result in spillage and loss of protection.

h. Inspect the condom for signs of breakage or spillage.

i. Be prepared with fast-acting spermicide should the condom break or spill.

j. Use emergency contraception as needed (see Chapter 46).

2. Be responsive to patient complaints and apprehension

a. For the young woman who is unsure that her partner will use condoms, role-play different scenarios with her until she believes she has the ability to discuss the issue with her partner and persuade him to use condoms. The same techniques are helpful to reduce STD risk for the receptive partner when men have sex with men.

b. If the male partner complains of constriction or blunted sensation, recommend one of the following strategies:
   - Try a larger condom size.
   - Try a different condom style. Condoms with reservoirs at the side are available; these reduce glans pressure and purportedly enhance stimulation. Ribbed condoms are also designed to increase sensation.
   - Advise the couple to place a second, larger condom over the first one after the outer surface of the first condom has been well lubricated. The friction between the condoms may enhance penile sensation. It also reduces the impact of breakage problems.

Advantages

1. Readily available: Condoms may be purchased in drug stores, by mail order on-line or through catalogs, and vending machines, or obtained in family planning or school clinics without prescription.

2. Relatively inexpensive: Sometimes they are even available free from clinics. Male condoms cost $0.30 to $1.50 each. Frequent use raises the direct (out-of-pocket) costs and indirect (pregnancy-related) costs because of their moderately high failure rates.

3. Portable: Condoms can easily be carried in a purse or other vehicle to be available whenever the need arises.

4. Male participation: Although women purchase more than half of condoms, the sheaths are still used by men; men definitely benefit from detailed instructions.

5. Visible proof of protection: Couples can get reasonably accurate feedback that protection was offered by observing the ejaculate contained in the condom.

6. Significant reduction in risk of STDs, including HIV infection and cervical dysplasia: Transmission of bacterial STDs, such as chlamydia and gonorrhea, is markedly reduced by effective condom use (Cates and Holmes, 1996; Cates, 1997; d'Oro et al., 1994; Rosenberg et al., 1992). The impact that condom use has on the transmission of viral STDs depends on the site of infection. Studies consistently demonstrate that condoms provide important protection against HIV transmission. A meta-analysis of 25 studies of serodiscordant heterosexual couples found that condoms reduced transmission by 87% (range, 60%-90%). Consistent users had annual HIV seroconversion rates of 0.9%, compared with 6.8% for those who never used condoms (Davis and Weller, 1999). Consistent condom use also accelerates the regression of cervical and penile HPV-associated lesions and accelerates clearance of genital HPV infection in women (Holmes et al., 2004).

Disadvantages

1. Requires placement with each act of intercourse
2. May interrupt lovemaking
3. Requires cooperation of male partner
4. Carries a higher pregnancy rate than hormonal contraceptive methods or intrauterine contraception
5. May diminish the pleasure of intercourse
   a. May blunt sensation for man; less "natural"
   b. May result in less vigorous intercourse due to fear that the condom may slip or break
   c. Requires prompt withdrawal after ejaculation, which may not permit sexual satisfaction of partner
   d. May increase vaginal irritation in women, especially those with inadequate lubrication
6. Side effects (see subsequent text)

Side Effects of Male Condoms

Latex allergies are becoming more common in the United States; estimates are that latex allergies are found in 2% to 4% of couples using condoms. Among latex-exposed workers, the average may be as high as 18%. This number may be lower in the teen population with less previous exposure to latex. Polyurethane condoms are strongly recommended for latex-allergic couples, because the transition from mild reactions to anaphylaxis can develop rapidly. Some authors have suggested that the unsensitized partner could still use a latex condom if it is covered by a plastic condom. This strategy may reduce topical irritation, but the latex powder is a potent allergen and can induce severe, even life-threatening allergic reactions.

Future Developments

Condoms made of newer, nonlatex plastic materials, such as Tactylon, are in clinical trials and may be able to reduce the slippage and breakage problems associated with polyurethane (Callahan et al., 2000). A deproteinized latex condom (Manix Crystal) is available in France and other European countries and appears to be a safe alternative for latex-allergic individuals (Levy et al., 2001). Male condoms with new shapes (cap condoms) and different sized condoms (including snugger fit and custom-sized condoms) are increasingly available. The Unisex Condom, which can be used by either partner, is available in Canada and can be purchased through on-line condom distribution sites.

FEMALE CONDOMS

The only female condom currently available in the United States is the FC Female Condom (formerly known as the *Reality condom*; Fig. 45.2). The device is a thin polyurethane sheath measuring 17 cm in length and 7.8 cm in width. It contains flexible polyurethane rings at each end. The inner ring is loose within the sheath. At the time of insertion, the inner ring is pivoted parallel to the axis of the vagina and is used to introduce the device through the introitus to the vault, just as a diaphragm is placed. After insertion, the inner ring is rotated at the top of the vault to stabilize the device during intercourse. The outer ring, which is fixed to the base of the device, remains outside the vagina. The female condom provides a barrier along the length of vagina and partially covers the introitus. It is lined internally with a silicone-based "dry" lubricant and may be combined with vaginal spermicides. The female condom should never be used with the latex male condom, because each device can compromise the integrity of the other.

Far fewer adolescents use the female condom than the male condom; only 1.7% report ever using the female condom (Abma et al., 2004). As with the male condom, adolescents appear to use the female condom inconsistently, often choosing to use a male condom instead—even when supplied with female condoms (Marshall et al., 2002). Among female teens with experience using the female condom, more than half found it to be an acceptable method and a very low percentage (4%) reported that they did not use the female condom because of embarrassment.

Efficacy

The female condom underwent 6-month clinical efficacy trials, during which time a 12.5% failure rate was observed in typical use in the United States. This rate has been annualized to a typical first-year failure rate of 21% (Trussell, 2004). Perfect-use rates are considerably lower (5%), reflecting perhaps the difficulty users experienced with this method. The female condom is impermeable to HIV and comparative studies of male and female condoms have found similar protection against STDs (Drew et al., 1990; French et al., 2003).

Advantages and Disadvantages

The female condom is available over the counter in single-size disposable units (Fig. 45.2); they are considerably more expensive than the male condom. The female condom causes no known adverse physical side effects. The polyurethane is not sensitive to petroleum-based products. However, its use may be challenging; even users who are experienced with diaphragm insertion may find the female condom difficult to insert. The package instructions say that correct placement may be difficult in the first or second attempt because of the device's lubrication. The female condom may be inserted up to 8 hours before intercourse to permit a relaxed insertion. The consumer is warned not to tear the sheath with fingernails or other sharp objects. During intercourse, the penis should be manually guided into the device. The couple is to remain attentive throughout coitus to the position of the outer ring to ensure that it does not ride up or get pushed into the vagina. The male partner must avoid excessive friction between his penis and the device, which could increase the breakage rate or cause inversion of the device on withdrawal. Additional lubrication applied within the condom can help reduce this risk and also reduces the noise the device may make during intercourse.

The relative complexity of the device and its low typical efficacy rate make the female condom a second choice after the male latex or polyurethane condom. However, the female condom may make an important contribution for women whose partners refuse to use male condoms. For adolescents, extensive education and hands-on practice may be needed to ensure correct use of the female condom. Emergency contraception should be offered in advance to all female condom users.

Future Developments

Female condoms made of latex (which is less expensive than polyurethane) are currently in development and testing. Models available in other countries include the Reddy female condom, which is latex and uses a soft, polyurethane sponge to hold it in place inside the vagina, and the Natural Sensation Panty Condom that is shaped and worn like a woman's panty with a built-in condom.

DIAPHRAGM

The diaphragm (Fig. 45.3) is a dome-shaped latex device which, when introduced into the vagina, extends from the posterior fornix to the anterior vaginal wall to completely cover the cervix. The semirigid outer ring stabilizes the device in the upper vagina, and the dome holds spermicide directly against the cervix. As a mechanical barrier alone, the diaphragm has an unacceptably high failure rate; it is intended for use with contraceptive gel. The diaphragm must be professionally fitted and is available only by prescription.

Although not a commonly used method of contraception, there is a renewed interest in the diaphragm and other female barrier contraceptives that shield the cervix as a result of research indicating that they may be protective against the acquisition of HIV and other STDs (Moench et al., 2001). In addition, intensive research is being done to develop a vaginal microbicide (a topical product that protects against acquisition of HIV and other STDs) that may be used in conjunction with a diaphragm or similar vaginal device.

The Female Condom

What is the female condom?

The female condom is a thin, soft, loose-fitting pouch with two flexible rings at either end. One ring helps hold the device in place inside the woman's vagina over the end of the womb (cervix), while the other ring rests outside the vagina.

Outer ring lies against the labia (lips of the vulva)

Inner ring is used for insertion; helps hold female condom in place

How does it work?

The female condom is made of polyurethane, a type of plastic. The plastic condom covers the inside of the vagina, cervix, and area around the opening to the vagina. The device acts as a barrier to help prevent pregnancy and the transmission of germs that can cause sexually transmitted diseases (STDs), including human immunodeficiency virus (HIV) and acquired immunodeficiency syndrome (AIDS). The device can be inserted by the woman up to 8 hours before sex.

How to insert the female condom

1. Find a comfortable position. You may want to stand up with one foot on a chair, squat with knees apart, or lie down with legs bent and knees apart.
2. Hold the female condom with the open end hanging down. Squeeze the inner ring with your thumb and middle finger.
3. Holding the inner ring squeezed together, insert the ring into the vagina and push the inner ring and pouch into the vagina past the pubic bone.
4. When properly inserted, the outer ring will hang down slightly outside the vagina. During intercourse, when the penis enters the vagina, the slack will lessen.

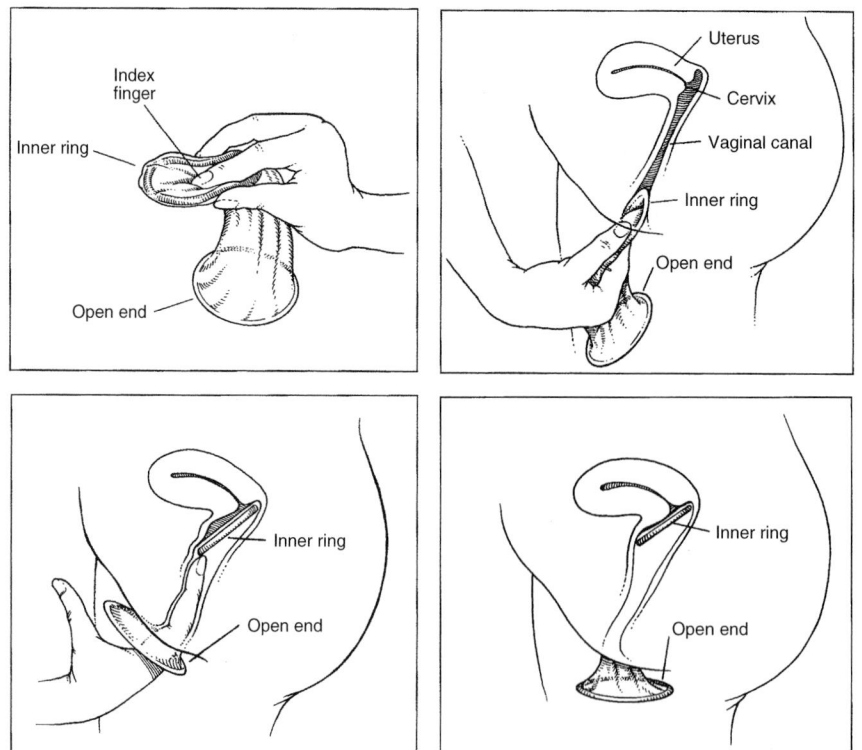

FIGURE 45.2   The female condom.

Remember:

The female condom may be hard to hold or slippery at first. Before you use one for the first time during sex, practice inserting one to get used to it. Take your time. Be sure to insert the condom straight into the vagina without twisting the pouch.

During Sex

1. It's helpful to use your hand to guide the penis into the vagina inside the female condom.
2. The ring may move from side to side or up and down during intercourse. This is OK.
3. If the female condom seems to be sticking to and moving with the penis rather than resting in the vagina, stop and add more lubricant to the inside of the device (near the outer ring) or to the penis.

How to remove the female condom after intercourse

1. Squeeze and twist the outer ring to close it.
2. Pull the female condom out gently.
3. Throw the condom away in the garbage. Do not flush down the toilet.
4. Do not wash out and use again.

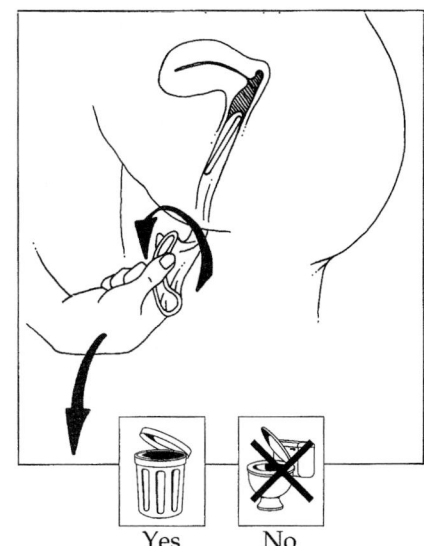

Yes   No

Special Reminders

- Use a new female condom with every act of intercourse.
- Use it every time you have intercourse.
- Read and follow the directions carefully.
- Do not use a male and female condom at the same time.
- Be careful not to tear the condom with fingernails or sharp objects.
- Use enough lubricant.

Latex condoms for men are highly effective at preventing STDs, including HIV infection (AIDS), if used properly. If your partner refuses to use a male latex condom, use a female condom to help protect yourself and your partner.

FIGURE 45.2   *(Continued)*

Types of Diaphragm

Diaphragms are available in sizes ranging from 50 to 105 mm in 5-mm increments and in four styles, which vary primarily by the construction of the rim or the seal.

1. Arcing spring rim: A very sturdy rim that folds for insertion but springs open to stabilize the device's position within the vagina. It is designed for universal use, but is uniquely good for vaginas with limited muscle tone. There are two versions—one that folds only in one direction and another that is flexible in all directions. This latter design is the most popular style because of its ease of introduction. Most diaphragms currently used in the United States are versions of the arcing spring rim.
2. Coil-spring rim: Sturdier rim that folds flat for insertion with no arc. It is suitable for a woman with average muscle tone and pubic arch angle. A plastic diaphragm introducer may be used, if needed.
3. Flat-spring rim: Thin, delicate rim with gentle spring action that is more comfortable for women with firm

vaginal wall tone. A plastic diaphragm introducer may be used.
4. Wide-seal rim: Has a flexible flange attached to the inner edge of the rim to hold spermicide in place and to maintain a better seal. It has very limited availability and can be obtained only by direct order with arcing spring . and coil-spring rims.

Contraindications to Use

1. History of toxic shock syndrome
2. Allergy to latex or spermicidal agents
3. Recent pregnancy, before renormalization of anatomy
4. Inability of patient to correctly insert and remove diaphragm

Effectiveness

The typical-use failure rate varies between 16% and 18%. The failure use with correct and consistent use is estimated

Diaphragm Patient Information and Instructions

The diaphragm is a shallow, dome-shaped cup made of soft rubber. It is inserted into the vagina and placed securely over the cervix. It must be used with spermicidal cream or jelly. The diaphragm prevents pregnancy by providing a barrier between the sperm and uterus.

Instructions to patients

Check diaphragm for tears or holes by holding it up to a bright light and stretching the rubber slightly. Always use with contraceptive cream or jelly. Hold the diaphragm with the dome down and squeeze a tablespoon of cream or jelly into the dome and spread it around the dome and onto the rim with your finger.

To insert your diaphragm, stand with one foot propped up (i.e., on the toilet seat), squat, or lie on your back. Press the edges of the diaphragm together with one hand. With your other hand, spread the lips of your vagina and insert the diaphragm into your vagina. Push the diaphragm downward and back along the back wall of your vagina as far as it will go. Then tuck the front rim of the diaphragm up along the roof of your vagina behind the pubic bone.

Check the placement of your diaphragm by sweeping your index finger across the diaphragm to make sure the cervix is completely covered by the soft rubber dome and that the front rim of the diaphragm is snugly in place behind your pubic bone. (The cervix will feel like the tip of your nose.) When properly placed, the diaphragm will neither cause discomfort nor interfere with sex. The diaphragm and contraceptive cream or jelly can be inserted up to 6 hours before intercourse. If 6 hours have passed since insertion and the time intercourse occurs, put another applicator full of jelly or cream into your vagina without removing the diaphragm.

FIGURE 45.3   Sample instruction sheet for diaphragms. (Courtesy of Teenage Health Center, Children's Hospital of Los Angeles, Los Angeles, California.)

to be 6%. Women who are more successful users of diaphragms are usually older, are comfortable touching their genitals, and are able to anticipate coitus. However, adolescents certainly can be taught to use diaphragms effectively (Fig. 45.3).

Tips to Improve Success of Method

1. Correct fitting of device (see later discussion)
2. Detailed, hands-on instruction for patient education (see later discussion)
3. Careful monitoring of diaphragm between uses to identify any defects (see later discussion)
4. Careful selection of patient
   a. Offer only to motivated woman willing to touch her genitals and to use the device with *every* act of intercourse
   b. Avoid offering to a woman with a markedly anteverted or retroverted uterus (diaphragm tends to dislodge)
   c. Discourage coital positions that compromise stability of diaphragm, particularly the female superior position

A new application of spermicidal cream or jelly is necessary with each additional act of intercourse. Do not remove the diaphragm. Use the plastic applicator to insert the jelly or cream in front of the diaphragm.

The diaphragm must be left in place for 6 to 8 hours after the last time you have intercourse, but never leave the diaphragm in place for more than 24 hours. Do not douche.

To remove the diaphragm

To remove the diaphragm, place your index finger behind the front rim of the diaphragm and pull down and out. Sometimes squatting and pushing with your abdominal muscles (i.e., bearing down as though you were having a bowel movement), helps to hook your finger behind the diaphragm. After use, the diaphragm should be washed with soap and water, rinsed thoroughly, and dried with a towel. Store it in its plastic container. You may dust it with cornstarch. Do not use talcum, perfumed powder, Vaseline, baby oil, or contraceptive foam, as they may damage the diaphragm. Inspect the diaphragm (especially around the rim) for holes or defects.

Side effects

Occasionally, the spermicidal cream or jelly has been found to be irritating. Changing to another brand should resolve the problem. Some patients have reported bladder symptoms or urinary tract infections with use of the diaphragm. Rare cases of toxic shock syndrome have been reported in users of the diaphragm. Contact your physician if you have:

- Fever above 38.3° C (101 °F)
- Diarrhea
- Vomiting
- Muscle aches
- Rash (sunburnlike)

FIGURE 45.3   (*Continued*)

Correct Fitting of Diaphragm

A diaphragm must be fitted properly to be effective. The diagonal length of the vaginal canal from the posterior aspect of the symphysis pubis to the posterior vaginal fornix is measured during the bimanual examination. The second and third fingers are inserted deeply into the vagina until the tip of the middle finger touches the posterior vaginal wall; then the point at which the index finger touches the symphysis pubis is marked with the thumb. The hand is withdrawn and the diaphragm is placed on the tip of the third finger with the opposite rim in front of the thumb to measure the correct size. This is a first approximation, which requires reconfirmation through actual fitting. The diaphragm is inserted and checked. Then the next larger size is fitted. The correct size is one size smaller than the first one perceived by the patient. For example, starting at size 60 and increasing the sizes until the patient perceives pressure with a size 70 would suggest that a size 65 would be appropriate for her. This is confirmed by examining the patient with the diaphragm in place. The diaphragm should touch the lateral vaginal walls, cover the cervix, and fit snugly between the posterior vaginal fornix and behind the symphysis pubis. A diaphragm that is too large may buckle and permit sperm to bypass the diaphragm. A diaphragm that is too small may slip out of place. The health care provider should appreciate that the adolescent may be tense during initial fitting, causing the fitting of a smaller diaphragm than would be required if the adolescent were relaxed.

Patient Education

Patient education programs should include the following.

1. Demonstration of insertion and removal techniques: After being shown how to place the diaphragm, the teen should insert and remove it at least once in the office and have the placement checked by the provider.
2. Detailed guidance about use of spermicide
   a. Coat the inner surface of the diaphragm with spermicidal gel. One application is effective for up to 6 hours.
   b. Add additional spermicide with the applicator if intercourse is delayed beyond 6 hours or if additional acts of coitus are anticipated. Additional doses must be placed into the vagina; the diaphragm should not be removed to add spermicide.
   c. Apply an extra dose immediately if the diaphragm is dislodged during intercourse, and consider using emergency contraception.
3. Removal instructions
   a. Wait at least 6 hours after the last episode of coitus to remove the device.
   b. Remove before 24 hours of use to reduce the risk of toxic shock syndrome.
4. Concrete instructions about cleaning and storage of device: Recommend washing device in soap and water, then soaking it in an alcohol solution (70% isopropanol or 80% ethanol) for at least 20 minutes after each application. Coat the device with cornstarch or another agent to prevent contamination or cracking, and store it in a dry container.
5. Return for refitting of the diaphragm every 1 to 2 years, after every pregnancy, and after any 10% to 20% change in body weight.

Advantages

1. The most effective of the female barrier methods available today
2. Reduced risks of STDs, including HIV
3. May be placed in anticipation of coitus

Disadvantages

1. Requires professional sizing and is available only by prescription
2. Requires motivation and extensive education for proper use
3. Requires preparation and access to supplies; therefore, it may limit spontaneity and may not meet the impulsive needs of the adolescent
4. May be considered messy, especially for multiple acts of intercourse

5. Not an acceptable method if either partner is allergic to spermicide or latex
6. There is a small risk of toxic shock syndrome associated with poorly timed or prolonged use
7. The diaphragm increases the risk of cystitis by increasing the count of enteric organisms within the vagina

Future Developments

The SILCS intravaginal barrier is a one-size-fits-all diaphragm made of silicone that is entering phase II clinical trials. It is designed to be easier to use and intended for sale over the counter. The BufferGel Duet is a disposable, one-size-fits-all diaphragm made of dipped polyurethane that is in development. It will be marketed with prefilled BufferGel, a candidate microbicide and contraceptive.

CERVICAL CAP AND CERVICAL SHIELD

The cervical cap and the cervical shield are cup-shaped devices made of silicone or latex, designed to cover the cervix and protect it from semen. Both are used with spermicide and provide contraceptive protection over multiple acts of intercourse for up to 48 hours without device removal. Each can be placed hours before coitus. The position should be reconfirmed before each coital act. The cap and the shield must be removed 48 hours after placement to reduce problems with odor and the possibility of toxic shock syndrome.

The U.S. Food and Drug Administration (FDA) approved a silicone cervical cap, the FemCap, in 2003. It is shaped like a sailor's hat with a dome, rim, brim, and removal strap (Fig. 45.4). The brim has a short side and long side, with the long side worn to the back of the vagina. The underside of the dome forms a bowl that covers the cervix. The brim forms a seal against the vaginal wall to hold the device in place. A small amount of spermicide is used in the bowl, spread on the outer brim, and placed in the groove between the dome and the brim. The FemCap comes in three sizes determined by the diameter of the inner rim. The smallest rim diameter (22 mm) is intended for nulliparous women, the medium (26 mm) cap is intended for women who have

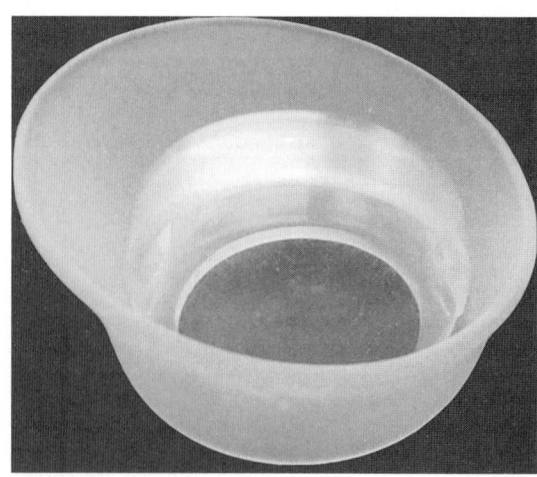

FIGURE 45.4   The FemCap. (Courtesy of FemCap, Inc., and Alfred Shihata, MD.)

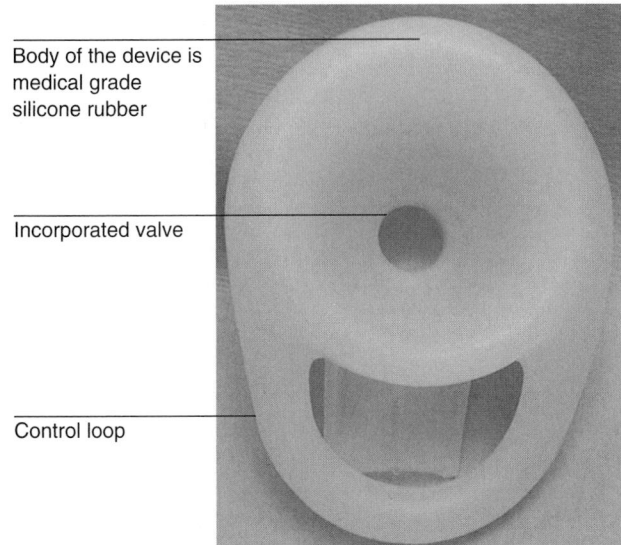

Body of the device is medical grade silicone rubber

Incorporated valve

Control loop

FIGURE 45.5   The Lea's Shield.

been pregnant but have not had a vaginal delivery, and the largest (30 mm) is for women who have had a full-term vaginal delivery. Although the sizing of the FemCap is determined by obstetric history, a clinician visit is required as the device can only be obtained with a prescription.

Lea's Shield is a reusable silicone cervical barrier that is held in place by its volume rather than its diameter (Fig. 45.5). The FDA approved it for use in 2002. The shield is oval in shape with a bowl that covers the cervix and fills the posterior fornix of the vagina, an anterior loop to aid in insertion and withdrawal, and a flat, tubular flutter valve leading from the inner surface of the bowl through to the convex side. This one-way valve prevents trapping of air between the cervix and the device after insertion and is intended to allow for egress of menstrual and other cervical secretions. Like the FemCap, the shield is held in place by the vaginal muscles rather than through suction. It is designed as a one-size-fits-all device but requires a clinician visit as it can only be obtained by prescription. The shield can be used with or without spermicide, although the addition of spermicide increases its contraceptive efficacy.

Contraindications for the cervical cap and shield include all those mentioned for the diaphragm. Cervical caps are not intended for use during menses. The shield may be used during menstruation, although none of the efficacy or safety trials included women who were menstruating.

Efficacy

The FemCap has been compared in a randomized trial with the diaphragm but was not found to be equivalent in efficacy (Mauck et al., 1999). Overall, the 6-month typical-use failure rate for the cap was 13.5% compared with 7.9% for diaphragm users. The differences between nulliparous and parous women in the FemCap group were not statistically significant (9.5% and 15.8%, $p = 0.12$). Extrapolating the 6-month unadjusted failure rate to 12 months gives a probability of 22.8 pregnancies per 100 women for the cap.

A 6-month efficacy trial of the Lea's Shield found a typical-use pregnancy rate of 8.7 per 100 women among those who used the device with spermicide (Mauck et al., 1996). There were no pregnancies among nulliparous women in this trial. The unadjusted typical-use failure rate for parous women was 11 per 100 women.

Fitting the Cervical Cap

Neither the FemCap nor Lea's Shield requires formal fitting, although a clinician visit is recommended to assure proper application and comfort with the devices.

Patient Education

Insertion of the FemCap
1. Apply approximately $\frac{1}{4}$ teaspoon of spermicide in the bowl, spread a thin layer over the outer brim, and insert $\frac{1}{2}$ teaspoon between the brim and the dome.
2. Gently squeeze the cup and insert it into the vagina with the bowl facing upward and the longer brim entering first.
3. Push the cap down toward the rectum and back as far as it can go.
4. Check to make sure that the cap completely covers the cervix.

Removal of the FemCap
1. To remove the cap, squat and bear down.
2. Push the tip of a finger against the dome cap to break the suction.
3. Grasp the removal strap with the tip of your finger and gently remove the device.
4. Wash the cap thoroughly with a mild soap then rinse it with tap water. Allow the cap to air dry or gently pat it dry with a clean, soft towel and store.

Insertion of Lea's Shield
1. Apply a small amount of spermicide in the bowl of the device.
2. Gently squeeze the shield and insert into the vaginal bowl-first as high as it will go.
3. Check to make sure that the entire cervix is covered by the bowl.

Removal of Lea's Shield
1. Insert a finger into the vagina, grasp and twist the control loop to break the suction and gently remove.
2. The shield should be washed thoroughly with mild liquid soap for approximately 2 minutes, dried, and then stored.

Advantages

1. Effective for up to 48 hours; additional doses of spermicide are not required for multiple acts of intercourse
2. May be placed early and is usually not detected by the partner
3. May offer some reduction of STD risk, especially for cervical and upper genital tract infections

Disadvantages

1. Requires a clinician visit to obtain a prescription
2. Requires training in placement, removal, cleaning, and storage
3. Replacement every 1 to 3 years; and refitting for the FemCap is needed after pregnancy
4. May be difficult to insert or remove for some women

CONTRACEPTIVE SPONGE

After the introduction of the vaginal contraceptive sponge in 1983, it quickly became the leading female-controlled nonprescription contraceptive method. The manufacturer of sponges in the United States discontinued its production in early 1995 because the FDA found possible contamination along the production line, although the product was not compromised. The contraceptive sponge (Today Sponge) was brought back to the U.S. market in 2005.

The contraceptive sponge is made of pliable polyurethane foam that contains 1 gm of nonoxynol-9. A concave depression, or "dimple," on one side fits against the cervix, and a woven polyester loop on the other side can be grasped for removal. After it is moistened with water, it is inserted into the vagina and is effective immediately. The sponge protects against pregnancy for 24 hours without the need to add spermicidal cream or jelly, regardless of the number of acts of intercourse. After intercourse the sponge must be left in place for 6 hours before is removed and discarded. Wearing the sponge for longer than 24 hours in not recommended because of the possible risk of toxic shock syndrome.

The sponge comes in one size and does not require fitting by a physician. It is relatively inexpensive ($10 for a package of three sponges) although the cost may be prohibitive for some adolescents. It is available without a prescription, can be inserted well before the onset of sexual activity, and is easy to use, making the contraceptive sponge well suited for adolescents.

Mechanism of Action

The primary contraceptive action of the sponge is provided by the spermicidal activity of nonoxynol-9, which is impregnated in the polyurethane foam. The sponge releases 125 to 150 mg of nonoxynol-9 slowly over a 24-hour period. The sponge also traps and absorbs semen and acts as a physical barrier between sperm and the cervical os.

Efficacy

The contraceptive sponge has different failure rates depending on the consistency of use and possibly parity. Overall, the typical-use failure rate of 16% in nulliparous women compared with 32% in parous women. Perfect-use rates are 9% and 20%, respectively (Trussell, 2004). Observational data have suggested that parity may be less of a factor than motivation to use the sponge consistently when determining contraceptive efficacy of the sponge (Edelman and North, 1987).

Patient Education

Insertion

1. Remove the sponge from its package and hold it with the "dimple" side facing up and the loop hanging down
2. Moisten with approximately 2 tablespoons of water and squeeze the sponge a few times until it becomes sudsy
3. Fold the sides of the sponge upward with a finger on each side to support it
4. While in a standing, lying, or squatting position gently introduce the sponge into the vagina and using one or two fingers push the sponge upward as far as it will go
5. Check the position of the sponge by running a finger around the edge of the sponge to make sure that the cervix is covered

Removal

1. Wait 6 hours after the last act of intercourse before removing the sponge
2. Insert one finger into the vagina until the loop is felt
3. If the loop cannot be felt, bear down, lie on your back on the bed with your knees up against your chest, squat down in a low position, or sit on the toilet and tilt your pelvis forward (so that the small of your back is rounded) to bring the sponge closer to the vaginal opening
4. Hook one finger into the loop then gently and slowly pull the sponge out
5. Check to make sure the sponge is intact; if it is torn remove all pieces from the vagina
6. Discard sponge

Contraindications

1. History of toxic shock syndrome
2. Allergy or sensitivity to polyurethane foam, nonoxynol-9, or metabisulfite (the preservative used in the sponge; women or partners with an allergy to sulfa should consult with a health care provider)
3. The sponge is not recommended for use during menstruation

Advantages

1. Lack of hormonal side effects or medical contraindications
2. Allows for spontaneity after insertion; can be used over repeated acts of intercourse
3. Available without a prescription or fitting by health care personnel; one size fits all
4. Female-controlled method; does not require partner participation
5. May be more comfortable to wear than other barrier methods such as the diaphragm
6. Easy to use and not "messy"

Disadvantages

1. Relatively high failure rate
2. Teen must be comfortable touching genitals in order to insert device
3. Spermicide may cause vaginal, vulvar, or penile irritation
4. Sponge can become discolored or malodorous in the presence of vaginitis
5. Can be difficult to remove

Side Effects

Approximately 4% of users will experience a sensitivity reaction to the sponge that can lead to itching, burning, redness, or a rash. Although this may be due to nonoxynol-9, other components of the sponge such as the preservative may be the source of the sensitivity reaction.

Future Developments

Two contraceptive sponges, Protectaid and Pharmatex, are available in Canada and Europe and may eventually be brought to the United States. Clinical trials of an additional contraceptive sponge, Avert, are planned.

VAGINAL SPERMICIDES

Vaginal spermicides are available in a wide array of delivery systems (Table 45.1). Spermicides can be used alone or in combination with barrier methods. They can play an important role in contraception for the adolescent, because they require neither a prescription nor a pelvic examination and are free from systemic side effects.

Spermicides have been shown to have bactericidal and virucidal activity in vitro, but clinical data in vivo have failed to demonstrate any reduction in the risk of STD acquisition. Several studies of spermicide use in high-risk women have found that nonoxynol-9 does not reduce the risk of HIV or other STD transmission. There is no clear evidence that the risk of seroconversion is increased by the use of spermicides, although one case–control study of commercial sex workers in Africa found that multiple uses daily (>3.5) may increase the risk of HIV transmission (World Health Organization, 2002). Eleven percent of heterosexual adolescent males report experience with anal intercourse (Gates and Sonenstein, 2000). Although little has been documented about lubricant use among heterosexual couples who practice anal intercourse, a large proportion of men who have sex with men use lubricants during rectal intercourse, and 41% choose products that contain nonoxynol-9 (Gross et al., 1998). Lavage and biopsy studies of rectal epithelium exposed to nonoxynol-9 have demonstrated rapid epithelial sloughing with exposure of the underlying submucosa (Phillips et al., 2004). Because this damage may increase the risk of transmission of STDs, including HIV, the use of nonoxynol-9–containing products during anal intercourse should be discouraged.

Types of Spermicides

The various spermicidal preparations differ in their onset and duration of action and mode of application. Table 45.1 displays the more commonly used types of spermicidal products as well as the differences in the concentration of nonoxynol-9 in each formulation. In general, each agent is active for approximately 1 hour unless used with a diaphragm, cap, or shield. Foam, which is the most commonly used agent, is instantly effective. Suppositories and film require 10 to 15 minutes to melt and distribute over the cervix. Each type of suppository comes with complete and appropriate patient instructions for use. Encourage patients to choose a spermicidal agent with a use pattern that will work well for them.

Nonoxynol-9 is the active agent in all spermicides available in the United States. In other countries, agents such as octoxynol and benzalkonium chloride are also available as spermicides. However, benzalkonium has been shown to be irritating to vaginal epithelial cells and to reduce lactobacillus counts (Patton et al., 1999).

Efficacy

Typical first-year failure rates for spermicides used alone are estimated to be as high as 29% (Trussell, 2004). A randomized trial comparing three spermicidal gels containing different doses of nonoxynol-9 (52.5 mg, 100 mg, and 150 mg) with a spermicidal film and suppository (both containing 100 mg of nonoxynol-9) found 6-month failure rates that ranged from 10% to 22% (Raymond et al., 2004). The pregnancy risk was statistically higher in the gel containing 52.5 mg of nonoxynol-9, but there was no difference between any of the formulations containing 100 mg of nonoxynol-9. Correct and consistent use of spermicidal agents is estimated to reduce the pregnancy rate to 18%. In the trial described, perfect-use probabilities ranged from 5.1% to 15.7%. When used in conjunction with other methods, such as barriers and emergency contraception, the pregnancy rate drops.

Mechanism of Action

The components of spermicidal agents include an inert base (foam, cream, or jelly), which holds the spermicidal agent and blocks sperm from entering the cervical os. Spermicides destroy sperm by breaking down the outer cell membrane.

TABLE 45.1

Vaginal Spermicides

Base of Carrier	Onset of Action (min)	Duration of Action (min)	Concentration (%)
Aerosol foams	Immediate	60	8–12
Creams and gels[a]	Immediate	60	2–5
Suppositories and tablets	10–15	60	2.3–5.6
Film	15	60	28

[a]Creams and gels are usually used in conjunction with diaphragms or cervical caps but may be used as single agents.
Data from Hatcher RA, Trussell J, Stewart F, et al. *Contraceptive technology*, 17th rev. ed. New York: Ardent Media, 1998:358.

Contraindications

1. Allergy or sensitivity to spermicidal agents or to the ingredients in the base
2. Inability to use due to vaginal abnormalities or inability to master the insertion technique

Advantages

1. No proven systemic side effects
2. Readily available without prescription
3. A fairly convenient, easy-to-learn method for teenagers
4. May be used by women with or without involvement of partner
5. May provide lubrication
6. May be useful as a backup method for other contraceptives

Disadvantages

1. Relatively high failure rate
2. Considered messy by some teenagers (some forms)
3. Must be used only a short time before intercourse is started
4. Requires 10 to 15 minutes for activation (some formulations)
5. Requires that woman be comfortable with touching her genitals
6. Unpleasant taste if oral-genital sex is involved
7. May cause a local allergic reaction

Future Developments

The need for vaginal agents that are contraceptive and protective against HIV and other STDs is increasingly compelling. Much of current research and development activity is centered on developing an agent with these properties.

WEB SITES

For Teenagers and Parents

Condoms
http://www.plannedparenthood.org/birth-control-pregnancy/birth-control/condom.htm. Planned Parenthood information sheet on condoms.
http://kidshealth.org/teen/sexual_health/contraception/contraception.html. Teen oriented Web site with information on condoms and other birth control methods.
http://www.condomania.com/. Information site and selection site for different types of condoms.
http://www.siecus.org/pubs/fact/fact0011.html. Siecus information sheet on condoms.
http://www.youngwomenshealth.org/femalebarrier1.html. Information from Boston Children's Hospital on female condoms.

Diaphragms, Cervical Caps, Cervical Shields
http://www.plannedparenthood.org/utah/diaphragm.htm. Planned Parenthood information sheet on diaphragms.

http://www.mayoclinic.com/health/birth-control/BI99999/PAGE=BI00009. Information sheet on diaphragms, cervical caps, and cervical shields from the Mayo Foundation for Medical Education and Research.
http://www.femcap.com/index.htm. Product Web site for the FemCap.
http://www.leasshield.com/index.htm. Product Web site for Lea's Shield®.

Contraceptive Sponge
http://www.mayoclinic.com/health/birth-control/BI99999/PAGE=BI00011. Information about the contraceptive sponge from the Mayo Foundation for Medical Education and Research.
http://www.todayssponge.com/. Product Web site with user and purchasing information.

Spermicides
http://www.sex-ed101.com/spermx.html. Sex Education 101 site with information on spermicides and many other issues.
http://www.fhi.org/en/. Family Health International Frequently Asked Questions on spermicides.

For Health Professionals

http://www.reproline.jhu.edu/english/1fp/1methods/1condom/condom.htm. Web site with presentation slides on condoms.
http://www.cervicalbarriers.org/. Informative Web site of The Cervical Barrier Advancement Society.

REFERENCES AND ADDITIONAL READINGS

Abma JC, Martinez GM, Mosher WD, et al. *Teenagers in the United States: sexual activity, contraceptive use and childbearing, 2002*. Vital Health Statistics, National Center for Health Statistics, 2004:23.

ACOG Committee Opinion. *Condom availability for adolescents.* Washington, DC: American College of Gynecologists and Obstetricians, 1995:154.

American Academy of Pediatrics. Condom availability for youth. *Pediatrics* 1995;95:281.

Brown LK, DiClemente RJ, Park T. Predictors of condom use in sexually active adolescents. *J Adolesc Health* 1992;13:651.

Callahan M, Mauck C, Taylor D, et al. Comparative evaluation of three Tactylon condoms and a latex condom during vaginal intercourse: breakage and slippage. *Contraception* 2000;61:205.

Cates WC Jr. How much do condoms protect against sexually transmitted diseases. *Int Plann Parenthood Fed Bull* 1997;31:2.

Cates WC Jr, Holmes KK. Re: condom efficacy against gonorrhea and nongonococcal urethritis. *Am J Epidemiol* 1996;15:143.

Centers for Disease Control and Prevention. Trends in HIV-related sexual risk behaviors among high school students—selected U.S. cities, 1991–1997. *JAMA* 1999;282:228.

Centers for Disease Control and Prevention. *Centers for Disease Control and Prevention: sexually transmitted disease surveillance, 2003.* Atlanta, GA, U.S. Department of Health and Human Services, Centers for Disease Control and Prevention, 2003.

Consumer's Union. How reliable are condoms? *Consum Rep* 1995;60:320.

Consumer's Union. Condoms get better: tests of 30 models show far fewer failures than in past years. *Consum Rep* 1999; 64:46.

Crosby RA, Yarber WL. Perceived versus actual knowledge about correct condom use among U.S. adolescents: results from a national study. *J Adolesc Health Care* 2001;28:415.

Davis KR, Weller SC. The effectiveness of condoms in reducing heterosexual transmission of HIV. *Fam Plann Perspect* 1999; 31:272.

DiIorio C, Dudley WN, Kelly M, et al. Social cognitive correlates of sexual experience and condom use among 13- through 15-year old adolescents. *J Adolesc Health Care* 2001;29:208.

DiClemente RJ, Wingood GM, Sionean C, et al. Association of adolescents' history of sexually transmitted disease (STD) and their current high-risk behavior and STD status: a case for intensifying clinic-based prevention efforts. *Sex Transm Dis* 2002;29:503.

Donald M, Lucke J, Dunne M, et al. Determinants of condom use by Australian secondary school students. *J Adolesc Health* 1994;15:503.

Drew WL, Blair M, Miner RC, et al. Evaluation of the virus permeability of a new condom for women. *Sex Transm Dis* 1990;17:110.

Edelman DA, North BB. Parity and the effectiveness of the Today contraceptive sponge. *Adv Contracept* 1987;3:327.

French PP, Latka M, Gollub EL, et al. Use-effectiveness of the female versus male condom in preventing sexually transmitted disease in women. *Sex Transm Dis* 2003;30:433.

Frezieres RG, Walsh TL, Nelson AL, et al. Breakage and acceptability of a polyurethane condom: a randomized controlled study. *Fam Plann Perspect* 1998;30:73.

Gallo MF, Grimes DA, Schulz KF. Nonlatex vs. latex male condoms for contraception: a systematic review of randomized controlled trials. *Contraception* 2003;68:319.

Gallo MF, Grimes DA, Schulz KF. Cervical cap versus diaphragm for contraception. *Cochrane Database Syst Rev.* 2002;(4):CD003551.

Gates GJ, Sonenstein FL. Heterosexual genital sexual activity among adolescent males: 1988 and 1995. *Fam Plann Perspect* 2000;32:295.

Goodenow C, Netherland J, Szalacha L. Related risk among adolescent males who have sex with males, females, or both: evidence from a statewide survey. *Am J Public Health* 2002; 92:203.

Gross SP, Buchbinder C, Celum P, et al. Rectal microbicides for U.S. gay men. Are clinical trials needed? Are they feasible? *Sex Transm Dis* 1998;25:296.

Handley MA, Reingold AL, Shiboski S, et al. Incidence of acute urinary tract infection in young women and use of male condoms with and without nonoxynol-9 spermicides. *Epidemiology* 2002;13:431.

Holmes KK, Levine R, Weaver M. Effectiveness of condoms in preventing sexually transmitted infections. *Bull World Health Organ* 2004;82:454.

Hufford D. Adolescents and condom use. *Arch Pediatr Adolesc Med* 1994;148:879.

Joffe A. Adolescents and condom use. *Am J Dis Child* 1993; 147:746.

Joffe A, Radius SM. Self-efficacy and intent to use condoms among entering college freshmen. *J Adolesc Health* 1993; 14:262.

Ku L, Sonenstein FL, Pleck JH. The dynamics of young men's condom use during and across relationships. *Fam Plann Perspect* 1994;26:246.

Leland NL, Barth RP. Gender differences in knowledge, intentions, and behaviors concerning pregnancy and sexually transmitted disease prevention among adolescents. *J Adolesc Health* 1992;13:589.

Levy DA, Moudiki P, Laynadier F. Deproteinised condoms are well tolerated by latex allergic patients. *Sex Transm Infect* 2001;77:202.

Lightfoot M, Song J, Rotherman-Borus MJ, et al. The influence of partner type and risk status on the sexual behavior of young men who have sex with men living with HIV/AIDS. *J Acquir Immune Defic Syndr* 2005;38:61.

Marshall S, Giblin P, Simpson P. at al Adolescent girls' perception and experiences with the reality female condom. *J Adolesc Health Care* 2002;31:5.

Mauck C, Callahan M, Wiener DH, et al. A comparitive study of the safety and efficacy of FemCap®, a new vaginal barrier contraceptive, and the Ortho All-Flex® diaphragm. *Contraception* 1999;60:71.

Mauck C, Glover LH, Miller E, et al. Lea's Shield®: a study of a the safety and efficacy of a new vaginal barrier contraceptive used with and without spermicide. *Contraception* 1996;53:239.

Moench TR, Chipato T, Padian N. Preventing disease by protecting the cervix: the unexplored promise of internal vaginal barrier devices. *AIDS* 2001;15:1595.

Mosher WD, Martinez GM, Chandra A, et al. *Use of contraception and use of family planning services in the United States, 1982–2002.* Advance Data from Vital and Health Statistics, 2004;350.

O'Donnell L, Doval AS, Duran R, et al. Predictors of condom acquisition after an STD clinic visit. *Fam Plann Perspect* 1995; 27:29.

d'Oro LC, Parazzini F, Naldi L, et al. Barrier methods of contraception, spermicides, and sexually transmitted diseases: a review. *Genitourin Med* 1994;70:410.

Orr DP, Langefeld CD. Factors associated with condom use by sexually active male adolescents at risk for sexually transmitted disease. *Pediatrics* 1993;91:873.

Patton DL, Kidder GG, Sweeney YC, et al. Effects of multiple applications of benzalkonium chloride and nonoxynol 9 on the vaginal epithelium in the pigtailed macaque (*Macaca nemestrina*). *Am J Obstet Gynecol* 1999;180:1080.

Phillips DM, Sudol KM, Taylor CL, et al. Lubricants containing N-9 may enhance rectal transmission of HIV and other STDs. *Contraception* 2004;70:107.

Raymond EG, Chen PL, Luoto J. Contraceptive effectiveness and safety of five nonoxynol-9 spermicides: a randomized trial. *Obstet Gynecol* 2004;103:430.

Rock EM, Ireland M, Resnick MD, et al. A rose by any other name? Objective knowledge, perceived knowledge, and adolescent male condom use. *Pediatrics* 2005;115: 667.

Roddy RE, Cordero M, Ryan KA, et al. A randomized controlled trial comparing nonoxynol-9 lubricated condoms with silicone lubricated condoms for prophylaxis. *Sex Transm Infect* 1998;74:116.

Rosenberg MJ, Davidson AJ, Chen JH, et al. Barrier contraceptives and sexually transmitted diseases in women: a comparison of female-dependent methods and condoms. *Am J Public Health* 1992;82:669.

Rosenthal SL, Biro FM, Succop PA, et al. Reasons for condom utilization among high-risk adolescent girls. *Clin Pediatr (Phila)* 1994;33:706.

Salazar LF, Crosby RA, DiClemente RJ, et al. Self-esteem and theoretical mediators of safer sex among African American female adolescents: implications for sexual risk reduction interventions. *Health Educ Behav* 2005;32:413.

Santelli JS, Lindberg LD, Abma J, et al. Adolescent sexual behavior: estimates and trends from four nationally representative surveys. *Fam Plann Perspect* 2000;32:156.

Schuster MA, Bell RM, Berry SH, et al. Impact of a high school condom availability program on sexual attitudes and behaviors. *Fam Plann Perspect* 1998;30(2):67.

Sonenstein FL, Ku L, Lindberg LD, et al. Changes in sexual behavior and condom use among teenaged males: 1988 to 1995. *Am J Public Health* 1998;88:956.

Steiner MJ, Dominik R, Rountree R, et al. Contraceptive effectiveness of a polyurethane condom and a latex condom: a randomized controlled trial. *Obstet Gynecol* 2003;101: 539.

Trussell J. Contraceptive failure in the United States. *Contraception* 2004;70:89.

Workowski KA, Levine WC. Sexually transmitted disease treatment guidelines–2002. *MMWR Recomm Rep* 2002;51 (RR-6):1.

World Health Organization. WHO/CONRAD technical consultation on nonoxynol-9, World Health Organization, Geneva, 9–10 October 2001: summary report. *Reprod Health Matters* 2002;10:175.

Wood VD, Buckle RA. Condom misuse among adolescents. *J Natl Med Assoc* 1994;86:39.

CHAPTER 46

Emergency Contraception

Lisa M. Johnson and Melanie A. Gold

Emergency contraception (EC) has a tremendous potential to reduce the numbers of unplanned pregnancies and to decrease the need for abortion in women of all ages. It has been estimated that, with proper use, EC could prevent 1.7 million unplanned pregnancies and 800,000 abortions each year (Glasier and Baird 1998). EC use among women of all ages has increased from 17,000/year in 1995 to 634,000/year in 2002 and it remains an important pregnancy prevention measure because unprotected or poorly protected intercourse occurs at a higher rate from unanticipated intercourse (e.g., impulse, date, or rape), lack of perceived need for protection, and/or incorrect or inconsistent contraceptive use.

EMERGENCY CONTRACEPTION METHODS

Three types of EC are available in the United States. The first two are hormonal methods that should be started within 120 hours (5 days) of exposure. The Yuzpe regimen, which has been available for >25 years, entails two doses of at least 100 µg ethinyl estradiol and 0.5 mg levonorgestrel (or 1.0 mg norgestrel) taken 12 hours apart. The progestin-only method entails either two single doses of 0.75 mg levonorgestrel (or 1.5 mg norgestrel) taken 12 hours apart or a single dose of 1.5 mg of levonorgestrel. The third method is insertion of a copper intrauterine device (IUD) within 5 days of unprotected intercourse.

The Yuzpe regimen, introduced in 1974, was the most commonly used EC method. Table 46.1 lists combination oral contraceptives that can be used to make up the Yuzpe regimen and their appropriate doses. In 1998, the U.S. Food and Drug Administration (FDA) approved the first dedicated EC product (Preven emergency contraceptive kit) using the Yuzpe regimen. Preven was taken off the market in 2004 when rights to the product were acquired by the company that makes the only current dedicated EC product (Plan B).

In 1999, the FDA approved a dedicated progestin-only product (Plan B), which contains two tablets each containing 0.75 mg of levonorgestrel. The FDA-approved instructions for Plan B are to take a single tablet as soon as possible after unprotected intercourse (up to 72 hours after coitus) and to take the second single tablet 12 hours later. More recently, von Hertzen et al. (2002) found that levonorgestrel could be given as a single dose of two tablets taken up to 120 hours after unprotected intercourse without causing any increase in side effects or decrease in efficacy. *A progestin-only EC product should be used whenever possible because it is the current product of choice.*

The progestin-only method of EC has several advantages over the Yuzpe method (Ho and Kwan, 1993; Task Force on Postovulatory Methods of Fertility Regulation, 1998). The efficacy of the progestin-only method is superior to that of the Yuzpe method (Table 46.2). Virtually every nonpregnant woman is eligible to use it, and side effects (especially gastrointestinal complaints such as

TABLE 46.1

Hormonal Emergency Contraception Regimens: Two Doses 12 Hours Apart

Brand	Manufacturer	Tablets/Dose
Progestin-only emergency contraceptive pills		
Plan B	Barr	1 white tablet[a]
Combination emergency contraceptive pills (Yuzpe regimen)		
Ogestrel	Watson	2 white tablets
Alesse	Wyeth-Ayerst	5 pink tablets
Aviane	Barr	5 orange tablets
Lessina	Barr	5 orange tablets
Levlite	Berlex	5 pink tablets
Levlen	Berlex	4 light-orange tablets
Levora	Watson	4 white tablets
Lo/Ovral	Wyeth-Ayerst	4 white tablets
Low-Ogestrel	Watson	4 white tablets
Nordette	Wyeth-Ayerst	4 light-orange tablets
Seasonale	Barr	4 pink tablets
Tri-Levlen	Berlex	4 light-yellow tablets
Triphasil	Wyeth-Ayerst	4 light-yellow tablets
Trivora	Watson	4 pink tablets

[a]Preferable to give both doses (two tablets) at once and can be given up to 120 hr after unprotected intercourse.

TABLE 46.2

Comparative Efficacy of Combination Emergency Contraception (EC) Pills versus Progestin-Only EC Pills versus Copper Intrauterine Device Used for EC

EC Method	Combination EC Pills	Progestin-Only EC Pills	Copper IUD
Number of women	1,000	1,000	1,000
Number of pregnancies without EC	80	80	80
Number of pregnancies with EC	20	10	1
Percentage reduction	75%	89%	99%

EC, emergency contraception; IUD, intrauterine device.

nausea and vomiting) occur significantly less often with the progestin-only method as compared to the Yuzpe regimen (Table 46.3).

The third type of EC, the T-380A copper IUD (or Para-Gard), can be inserted up to 5 days after unprotected coitus and provides the best pregnancy protection. Although the copper IUD is more effective than the hormonal options for EC, it is rarely used for EC in female adolescents or among women who may be at risk for having a sexually transmitted infection (see Chapter 44 on IUD in adolescents). The copper IUD is also very expensive for single use for EC. Therefore, its use in the United States for this indication has been quite limited.

Several large studies conducted outside the United States found that when mifepristone is used for EC it is more effective than the Yuzpe regimen and equally effective as the progestin-only regimen (Ashok et al., 2002). There are very few side effects with low dose mifepristone used for EC; one study found the incidence of nausea was 1% (Ashok et al., 2004). When mifepristone is used for EC there is more of a delay in the timing of the next menstrual period than with other hormonal EC regimens. However, mifepristone is only available in the United States for use in medical abortions and off label use for EC is rare. Furthermore, studies have shown that 1/60th of the dose of mifepristone

used for abortion (600 mg) is needed for EC (10 mg). No such 10 mg preparation is available in the United States, although mifepristone is used for EC in other parts of the world (Task Force on Postovulatory Methods of Fertility Regulation, 1999).

EFFICACY

The expected pregnancy rate per single act of unprotected intercourse is estimated to be 8%. Efficacy for EC can be expressed in two ways—the observed pregnancy rate or the percentage reduction in the expected number of pregnancies (Table 46.2). For example, the single-use failure rate for the Yuzpe regimen is a little more than 3.2%, which represents a 75% reduction in expected pregnancies. Levonorgestrel alone is more effective, with a failure rate of only 1.1% (when compared with the Yuzpe regimen), which is an 89% reduction in the expected number of pregnancies (Lancet, 1998). The copper IUD is the most effective EC method currently available; its failure rate is 0.1%, which is a 99% reduction in the expected number of pregnancies. The estimates of overall efficacy for the Yuzpe regimen were calculated from a wide range of results observed in different

TABLE 46.3

Side Effects of Yuzpe Regimen versus Levonorgestrel (World Health Organization, 1998)

Side Effect	% with Symptom (95% CI)		p
	Yuzpe (n = 979)	Levonorgestrel (n = 977)	
Nausea	50.5 (47.3–53.6)	23.1 (20.5–25.9)	<0.01
Vomiting	18.8 (16.4–21.4)	5.6 (4.3–7.3)	<0.01
Dizziness	16.7 (14.4–19.1)	11.2 (9.3–13.3)	<0.01
Fatigue	28.5 (25.7–31.4)	16.9 (14.6–19.4)	<0.01
Headache	20.2 (17.8–22.9)	16.8 (14.5–19.3)	0.06
Breast tenderness	12.1 (10.1–14.3)	10.8 (8.9–12.9)	0.40
Low abdominal pain	20.9 (18.4–23.6)	17.6 (15.3–20.1)	0.07
All other adverse effects[a]	16.7 (14.4–19.1)	13.5 (11.4–15.8)	0.06

CI, confidence interval.
Based on women for whom full information was available.
[a]Mostly diarrhoea and some irregular bleeding or spotting.

TABLE 46.4

Comparative Efficacy (Reduction in Pregnancy Rate) of Combination Emergency Contraceptive (EC) Pills versus Progestin-Only EC Pills over Various Time Periods

Time (hr)	Combination EC Pills (Yuzpe)	Progestin-Only EC Pills
<24 hr	77%	95%
25–48 hr	36%	85%
49–72 hr	31%	58%

clinical trials. One trial found a 56% reduction in expected pregnancy rates with the Yuzpe regimen, while another found 89% (Trussell et al., 1999). In part, this variation may have reflected the inclusion of women who were already pregnant at the time they were treated. A recent, large-scale World Health Organization (WHO) trial demonstrated that the effectiveness of hormonal EC depends on how soon it is initiated after intercourse (Piaggio et al., 1999; Task Force on Postovulatory Methods of Fertility Regulation, 1998) (Table 46.4), although earlier studies did not show such a temporal relationship (Trussell et al., 1996). In the WHO study, when hormonal EC was started within the first 12 hours, the pregnancy rate was 0.5% (a 94% reduction), but if the first dose was delayed until 60 to 72 hours after the exposure, the pregnancy rate was 4% (a 50% reduction). The 72-hour limit is expandable to 120 hours, but there is controversy over whether later use is associated with diminished protection. Some studies show no impact in efficacy based on timing whereas others do show a decline in efficacy with later use. In a 2003 study, 675 women using the Yuzpe regimen within 72 hours of unprotected intercourse were compared with 111 women using the Yuzpe regimen between 72 hours to 120 hours after unprotected intercourse; no statistically significant difference was found in failure rate between the two groups (Ellerston et al., 2003). However, the observation that earlier use of EC may be more efficacious has influenced prescribing patterns and led to the approval for behind-the-counter availability for people age 18 and over with government identification.

MECHANISMS OF ACTION

Hormonal methods of EC (Yuzpe or progestin-only) are approved by the FDA as *contraceptives*. This classification is supported by the observations (a) that most conceptions occur when intercourse precedes ovulation and (b) that EC with oral contraceptives is more effective when administered early after coitus. The primary action of the hormonal methods of EC appears to be delaying or inhibiting ovulation, but new analysis suggests that other mechanisms may be important (Trussell and Raymond, 1999). Studies have found that levonorgestrel and the Yuzpe regimen suppress or delay the luteinizing hormone (LH) peak and inhibit follicle rupture (Croxatto et al., 2003; Marions et al., 2004). EC may also alter tubal motility, production of progesterone by the corpus luteum, and the composition of the endometrium to block implantation (Glasier, 1997).

Although it may not always be clear whether oral EC is working by delaying ovulation or impeding implantation, EC does not work as an abortifacient. EC taken after a pregnancy has been established to have no effect; it will not cause a miscarriage, and it will not increase the risk of fetal malformations (Raman-Wilms et al., 1995; Blumenthal and McIntosh, 1996). EC is contraindicated in pregnancy because it is ineffective once implantation of a fertilized egg has occurred.

The mechanisms of action for the copper IUD as a postcoital method have not been well elucidated. It is unclear how important the copper ions are to the copper IUD's contraceptive effect when used as an EC (Rivera et al., 1999). Because sperm can live in the cervical canal for up to 5 days before fertilization, the spermicidal action of the copper IUD could be important. The presence of a foreign body (the IUD) may alter the endometrium and prevent implantation.

INDICATIONS

EC is indicated any time a woman of reproductive age wishes to lower her risk of becoming pregnant following unprotected intercourse (e.g., following sexual assault or unplanned intercourse.) EC is also indicated after inadequately protected sexual intercourse from failure or misuse of a contraceptive method (Table 46.5).

CONTRAINDICATIONS

Yuzpe Method

The FDA labeling for combination oral contraceptives used for EC includes the same contraindications as when combination oral contraceptives are taken on a daily basis (see Chapter 43). However, approximately four decades of use has shown that such stringent restrictions for a single use of the Yuzpe regimen are not necessary. Current pregnancy, allergy, and acute current migraine with neurological deficits are the only absolute contraindications to prescribing the Yuzpe regimen. A history of previous thrombosis should not be a contraindication to a single course of the Yuzpe regimen (Webb and Tabemer, 1993), although, if available, progestin-only pills would be preferable for medicolegal reasons in addition to being more effective and having fewer side effects compared with the Yuzpe regimen. The risk of a clot for a patient with prior history of deep vein thrombosis (DVT) or pulmonary embolism (PE) remains higher in pregnancy than for a single course of the Yuzpe regimen.

Progestin-Only Method

The three contraindications for progestin-only oral contraceptives including Plan B are:

1. Pregnancy
2. Hypersensitivity to any component of product
3. Undiagnosed abnormal genital bleeding

However, in an adolescent who is having abnormal genital bleeding, as long as pregnancy is ruled out, EC can

TABLE 46.5

Indications for Using Emergency Contraception

Method	Reason for Failure
Anytime sex is unprotected	Nothing used, sexual assault
Condom	Breaks or slips
Combination oral contraceptive pills (COCs)	Started the pill within the last 7 d (but not during menses), and did not use a back up or back up failed
	Missed two or more pills in a row during the first 3 wk of any pack of pills
	More than 2 d late in starting a new pack of pills after 7 d of placebo pills
Progestin-only oral contraceptive pills (POPs)	Started the pill within the past 2 d (but not during menses), and did not use a back up or back up failed
	Missed 1 or more pills in any row of the pack
	More than 1 d late in starting a new pack of pills
Transdermal patch (Ortho-Evra) (Ortho-McNeil, Raritan, NJ)	Started the patch within the past 7 d (but not during menses), and did not use a back up or back up failed
	Patch off >24 hr during patch-on wk
	Left patch on for >9 d straight
	>2 d late in putting new patch on after patch-off wk
Vaginal contraceptive ring (NuvaRing) (Organon, Roseland, NJ)	Started the ring within the past 7 d (but not during menses), and did not use a back up or back up failed
	Taken out for >3 hr during ring-in wk
	Left in >5 wk in a row
	>2 d late in putting new ring in after ring-out wk
Depot medroxyprogesterone acetate injection (Depo-Provera) (Pfizer, New York, NY)	Started Depo-Provera within the last 14 d (but not within 5 d of menses), and did not use a back up or back up failed
	More than 13 wk since got last Depo-Provera shot
Diaphragm or cervical cap	Slipped during intercourse
	Removed too early after intercourse (<6 h)
Withdrawal	Did not wipe off tip of penis before vaginal penetration
	Ejaculation occurred while penis was inside the vagina
Spermicide	Put in more than an hour before intercourse
	Dose not repeated before subsequent episodes of intercourse
	Any time used without another back up (like a condom)

be given. The progestin-only method is preferred for breast-feeding women because the estrogen in the Yuzpe regimen has the potential to decrease breast milk production.

Copper Intrauterine Device Method

The copper IUD for long-term has several contraindications (see Chapter 44 on IUDs). Because short-term use cannot be ensured, these same contraindications have been applied to the use of the copper IUD for EC.

SIDE EFFECTS

Side effects of the Yuzpe regimen and progestin-only EC are largely hormone related and can last for 2 to 3 days. The most common side effects are gastrointestinal. With the Yuzpe method, 30% to 66% of women report nausea, and 12% to 22% have vomiting. Gastrointestinal complaints can be reduced by routinely giving a long-acting antiemetic over-the-counter (OTC) agent such as meclizine 50 mg 1 hour before the first EC dose. Raymond et al. (2000) found that meclizine can halve the risk of nausea and vomiting, but most women experience drowsiness. The progestin-only method has a lower incidence of gastrointestinal side effects; only 23% of women report nausea, 6% vomiting, and 5% report diarrhea, therefore antiemetics are not routinely offered when prescribing progestin-only EC.

Other hormone-related side effects include breast tenderness, headache, abdominal bloating, fatigue, and dizziness. Among women who took the Yuzpe regimen, 10% had vaginal spotting at some point before the next menses which usually lasted 1 to 2 days. There was no difference in spotting rates between women who became pregnant following EC use and those who did not. Women who took EC in the first half of the menstrual cycle (before day 12) were more likely to have their next period earlier than expected (by >3 days) (Webb et al., 2004). Depending on when in the cycle EC is used, the timing and flow of the next menses may be altered. However, 98% of women should have menstrual bleeding within 3 weeks of EC use; if an EC user has not started menses 3 weeks after EC use, she should get a pregnancy test. Some adolescent health care providers recommend a pregnancy test 14 days after EC use, regardless of menses.

MANAGEMENT ISSUES

1. Advance prescription: Until recently, EC was administered primarily on an as-needed basis after unprotected intercourse. However, the most effective way to provide EC is in advance of need. Advance provision of EC may increase immediate use and enhance efficacy. Glasier and Baird (1998) found that women who had EC available at home were 74% more likely to use it than those who had to obtain EC on demand at a clinic. Raine et al. (2000) found that those who had EC in advance tripled their use of it. Gold et al. (2004b) found that adolescents 15 to 20 years old were nearly twice as likely to use EC if they had it in advance and they used EC sooner after unprotected intercourse compared with the control group. In seven of the eight advance provision studies to date, female adolescents and adults who got advance provision of EC did not have higher rates of unprotected intercourse and did not reduce their use of ongoing contraception compared with those in the control groups (Glasier and Baird, 1998; Lovvorn et al., 2000; Ellertson et al., 2001; Jackson et al., 2003; Lo et al., 2004; Gold et al., 2004b; Raine et al., 2005).
2. Education: EC should be discussed during routine office visits with both male and female adolescents who want to avoid pregnancy (Gold et al., 2004a).
3. Assessment: A woman who presents for EC after unprotected intercourse needs minimal assessment. It is prudent to record her last menstrual period, the number and timing of any previous acts of intercourse (protected or not) during the cycle, any symptoms of pregnancy, prior experience with EC or birth control pills, and any contraindications to EC that she may have. No physical examination is needed. Patients can be rescheduled for routine gynecological care such as a Pap smear or sexually transmitted disease (STD) testing if they are asymptomatic for a current STD. No laboratory tests are mandatory, although some providers do a sensitive urine pregnancy test in the office if there is any question about whether the patient might already be pregnant. Many practitioners prescribe EC for patients after telephone triage. To date, pharmacists in several states can provide EC without a prescription. In Alaska, Hawaii, and Washington State pharmacists have collaborative practice agreements, specifically for EC. In California, Maine, and New Mexico pharmacists have independent prescribing authority for EC. Other states, including Massachusetts, have recently passed legislation in favor of similar pharmacist agreements.
4. Multiple doses: Women who present with multiple episodes of unprotected intercourse can be provided EC for their last coital exposure if they are not pregnant. In addition, there is no absolute limit to the number of times EC can be used within one cycle or within a particular time frame, if there is need. However, women

who are using EC frequently should be advised that other birth control methods are more effective in the long run.
5. Dosing by timing in cycle when coitus occurred: Because of variations in menstrual cycle length and the long life span of sperm, unprotected intercourse at any time in the cycle may warrant EC protection.
6. EC is a standard of care: Courts have ruled that EC is a community standard of care for women who have been exposed to potential unintended pregnancy (especially for sexual assault victims) (Brownfield v. Daniel Freeman Marina Hospital, 1989). Other authorities, such as the American College of Obstetricians and Gynecologists (2005), have reconfirmed that postcoital contraception is standard of care. Likewise, the Society for Adolescent Medicine and the American Academy of Pediatrics have published statements confirming that EC is a standard of care for adolescents (Gold et al., 2004a; AAP EC Policy Statement, http://www.aap.org).
7. Contraception after EC: Ongoing methods of birth control may be started or restarted immediately after using EC. Daily use of oral contraceptives, the Ortho-Evra patch or the NuvaRing can be started the same day that either the Yuzpe regimen or Plan B is taken or can be started 24 hours later. Patients should be prescribed a single cycle of contraception and asked to return 2 weeks after their EC dose for a urine pregnancy test and for subsequent supply of contraception. Depot medroxyprogesterone acetate (DMPA or Depo-Provera) can be administered the same day EC is taken if the patient understands and accepts the uncertainty of the impact her contraceptive will have on her next menses, and if she agrees to return for routine pregnancy testing in 10 to 14 days. Appropriate backup methods should be provided for the first cycle. Women who have a copper IUD inserted are provided with both EC and ongoing contraceptive protection.

MANAGEMENT OF SIDE EFFECTS

1. Nausea and vomiting
   a. Symptoms can be reduced by using progestin-only EC such as Plan B or by prescribing a long-acting antiemetic 1 hour before starting the Yuzpe method (Raymond et al., 2000).
   b. The nausea and vomiting do not result from gastric irritation but rather from central nervous system stimulation. Therefore, the first dose of EC should be repeated only if the vomiting occurs within 30 to 60 minutes of ingestion of the first dose. Most experts also recommend repeat administration of the second dose if the patient vomits it within 30 minutes, although the importance of the second dose has recently been questioned (Ellertson et al., 2003).
2. Change in menstrual flow: Approximately 13% of women experienced heavier flow and the same percentage had lighter flow after EC use. Most have their next menses at the expected time or a few days early or late (Task Force on Postovulatory Methods of Fertility Regulation, 1998).
3. Amenorrhea: A woman who does not menstruate within 21 days of taking EC should be tested for pregnancy. If she is pregnant, she should be reassured that taking EC will not adversely affect her fetus or the pregnancy. If she is not pregnant, watchful waiting for return to normal cycling is appropriate for up to 3 months, but contraception should be offered.

ACCESS ISSUES

1. Provider issues: EC is remarkably cost-effective. Routine advance prescription of EC to women who rely upon male condoms as their only contraceptive saves the health system $263 per user in managed care systems and $99 in public sector settings (Trussell et al., 1997). Nevertheless, EC remains underutilized in the United States. Studies show that obstetrician-gynecologists, emergency room physicians, and general practitioners are very aware of EC, and most feel comfortable prescribing it. However, the average number of prescriptions written each year by the most actively prescribing doctors is only approximately 5.5 (Delbanco et al., 1997). Most physicians prescribe EC only for victims of sexual assault. A Kaiser survey in 1999 found that 83% of obstetrician-gynecologists prescribed EC in the past year, but 52% had written only one to five prescriptions for it within the last year, whereas 37% of family practitioners prescribed EC in the last year, with more than half prescribing it only one to five times. Only 17% of family practitioners and 31% of obstetrician-gynecologists had written six or more prescriptions for EC in the preceding 12 months (Henry J. Kaiser Family Foundation, 2000). A survey of pediatricians found that knowledge deficits, not attitude-related variables, were associated with low EC use and counseling (Sills et al., 2000). Gold et al. (1997) found that 88% of adolescent health experts said they would prescribe EC to teens, but 12% were concerned that doing so would encourage contraceptive risk taking; 29% believed that repeated EC use could pose a health threat; and 56% would not prescribe EC in advance of need. More recently, Rowlands et al. (2000) found that 5% of 14- to 29-year olds in Britain received EC each year, and only 4% reported using it more than twice in any year.

2. Patient issues: Many physicians justify under-prescribing EC by noting that women do not ask for it. This reflects that, until recently, few women knew that EC was available. Surveys of adult American women found that only 40% were aware of EC and even fewer adolescents (25%) had ever heard about it (Delbanco et al., 1997; Delbanco et al., 1998). However, awareness is rising. In 2002, Aiken et al., compared the awareness, attitudes, and perceived barriers to using EC among a sample of young women from 1996 with a different sample of women from 2002. Between 1996 and 2002, the percentage of participants reporting that they ever heard of EC grew from 44% to 73% (Aiken et al., 2005). Public service campaigns and articles in teen and women's magazines have highlighted the availability of EC. Special episodes of popular television shows (e.g., "ER," "Law & Order: Special Victims Unit") and MTV have featured the use and availability of EC.

3. Pharmacy issues: Pharmacies in many areas of the country refuse to carry EC because of their confusion about its mechanisms of action (Cohen, 1999). Some states have passed "conscience clauses" that provide a legal basis for this refusal practice. Other pharmacists and pharmacy chains claim that their decisions are based on economic factors—that the demand for EC is too low to justify the cost of the shelf space. The need for advance prescriptions is particularly critical in these settings. It may take a patient several days

to locate a pharmacy with Plan B—hours that may decrease efficacy. If a patient presents after unprotected intercourse for EC and it is known that she may encounter problems filling a prescription for Plan B, it may be prudent to use one of the standard Yuzpe regimens (Table 46.1), with prescription instructions to "take as directed," while providing the patient with specific EC instructions.

Patients can learn the names and addresses of local providers of EC by accessing the EC hotline, either by telephone at 1-888-NOT-2-LATE (Trussell et al., 1998) or on the Internet at http://www.NOT-2-LATE.com/. Physicians and clinics can contact these same hotlines to join the network of EC providers.

Some European countries and recently Canada have allowed levonorgestrel EC to be sold as an OTC medication. After a 3 year delay, the FDA approved OTC sales of Plan B in August 2006 to individuals ages 18 years and older. However, Plan B remains prescribtion-only status for female adolescents ages 17 years and under. There is ongoing lobbying of the FDA to extend OTC access of Plan B to adolescents under the age of 18.

WEB SITES

For Teenagers and Parents

EC Web site from Office of Population Research with list of providers, information, news, EC availability by country, and references: http://ec.princeton.edu/ or http://www.NOT-2-LATE.com

EC information from the Planned Parenthood Federation of America: http://www.plannedparenthood.org/ec/

Duke University Student Health Center information site on EC: http://healthydevil.studentaffairs.duke.edu/health_info/emergency%20contraception.html

Duke University Student Health Center information site on Sexual Health: http:healthydevil.studentaffairs.duke.edu/health_info/

Women's Capital Corporation Web site for Plan B: http://www.go2planb.com/

Boston Children's Hospital website with EC information: www.youngwomenshealth.org/emergencycontraception.html

For Health Professionals

American Academy of Pediatrics Policy Statement on EC, Fact Sheet for Parents and Adolescents, and Speaking Points for Pediatricians: http://www.aap.org (Policy Statement and Fact Sheet)

http://www.aap.org/moc (Speaking Points for Pediatricians at AAP member center)

Information about EC and directory of providers on the internet: http://www.NOT-2-LATE.com

http://ec.princeton.edu

Toll-free telephone information about EC and provider referrals 1-888-NOT-2-LATE (English and Spanish instructions)

Information about enrolling as a provider in the U.S. directory http://ec.princeton.edu/questions/ecsignup.html

EC and other information about contraception: http://www.managingcontraception.com

EC information from the Planned Parenthood Federation of America http://www.plannedparenthood.org/ec/

Article from *Hospital Practice* on EC: http://www.hosppract.com/issues/1998/08/stewart.htm.

Sites to download PowerPoint presentation on EC from Association of Reproductive Health Professionals: http://www.arhp.org/files/clinical.ppt and http://www.arhp.org/file/strategy.ppt

REFERENCES AND ADDITIONAL READINGS

Aiken AM, Gold MA, Parker AM. Changes in young women's awareness, attitudes, and perceived barriers to using emergency contraception. *J Pediatr Adolesc Gynecol* 2005;18(1):25.

American College of Obstetricians and Gynecologists. ACOG practice bulletin: clinical management guidelines for obstetricians-gynecologists: emergency contraception. No. 69, December 2005. (Replaces No. 25, March 2001). *Obstet Gynecol* 2005;106(6):1443.

Ashok PW, Hamoda H, Flett GM, et al. Mifepristone versus the Yuzpe regimen (PC4) for emergency contraception. *Int J Gynaecol Obstet* 2004;87(2):188.

Ashok PW, Stalder C, Wagaarachchi PT, et al. A randomised study comparing a low dose of mifepristone and the Yuzpe regimen for emergency contraception. *Br J Obstet Gynaecol* 2002;109(5):553.

Blumenthal P, McIntosh N. Emergency contraception. In: Oliveras E, ed. *Pocket guide for family planning service providers*, 3rd ed. Baltimore: JHPIEGO Corporation, 1996:65.

Brownfield v. Daniel Freeman Marina Hospital. *No. B032109. Court of Appeals of California, Second Appellate District, Division Four, 208 Cal. App. 3d 405; 1989 Cal. App. LEXIS 157;256 Cal. Rptr. 240.* March 2, 1989.

Cohen SA. Objections, confusion among pharmacists threaten access to emergency contraception. *Guttmacher Rep Public Policy* 1999;2:1.

Conard LE, Gold MA. Emergency contraception update: providing emergency contraception in the pediatrician's office. *Contemp Pediatr* 2006;23(2):49.

Croxatto HB, Oritz ME, Müller AL. Mechanisms of action of emergency contraception. *Steroids* 2003;68:1095.

Delbanco SF, Mauldon J, Smith MD. Little knowledge and limited practice: emergency contraceptive pills, the public, and the obstetrician-gynecologist. *Obstet Gynecol* 1997;89:1006.

Delbanco SF, Parker ML, McIntosh M, et al. Missed opportunities: teenagers and emergency contraception. *Arch Pediatr Adolesc Med* 1998;152:727.

Ellertson C, Ambardekar S, Hedley A, et al. Emergency contraception: randomized comparison of advance provision and information only. *Obstet Gynecol* 2001;98(4):570.

Ellertson C, Webb A, Blanchard K, et al. Modifying the Yuzpe regimen of emergency contraception: a multicenter randomized controlled trial. *Obstet Gynecol* 2003;101(6):1160.

Glasier A. Emergency postcoital contraception. *N Engl J Med* 1997;337:1058.

Glasier A, Baird D. The effects of self-administering emergency contraception. *N Engl J Med* 1998;339:1.

Gold MA, Schein A, Coupey SM. Emergency contraception: a national survey of adolescent health experts. *Fam Plann Perspect* 1997;29:15.

Gold MA, Sucato G, Conard LE, et al. Provision of emergency contraception to adolescents: position paper of the Society for Adolescent Medicine. *J Adolesc Health* 2004a;35:66.

Gold MA, Wolford JE, Smith KA, et al. The effects of advance provision of emergency contraception on adolescent women's sexual and contraceptive behaviors. *J Pediatr Adolesc Gynecol* 2004b;17:87.

Henry J. Kaiser Family Foundation. *National survey of health care providers on emergency contraception, 2000.* Menlo Park, CA: Kaiser Family Foundation, 2000.

von Hertzen H, Piaggio G, Ding J, et al. Low dose mifepristone and two regimens of levonorgestrel for emergency contraception: a WHO multicentre randomized trial. *Lancet* 2002; 360:1803–1810.

Ho PC, Kwan MS. A prospective randomized comparison of levonorgestrel with the Yuzpe regimen in post-coital contraception. *Hum Reprod* 1993;8:389.

Jackson RA, Schwarz EB, Freedman L, et al. Advance supply of emergency contraception: effect on use and usual contraception—a randomized trial. *Obstet Gynecol* 2003;102(1):8.

Lo SST, Fan SYS, Ho PC, et al. Effect of advanced provision of emergency contraception on women's contraceptive behaviour: a randomized controlled trial. *Hum Reprod* 2004; 19(10):2404.

Lovvorn A, Nerquaye-Tetteh J, Glover EK, et al. Provision of emergency contraceptive pills to spermicide users in Ghana. *Contraception* 2000;61:287.

Marions L, Cekan SZ, Bygdeman M, et al. Effect of emergency contraception with levonorgestrel or mifepristone on ovarian function. *Contraception* 2004;69:373.

Piaggio G, von Hertzen H, Grimes DA, et al. Task Force on Postovulatory Methods of Fertility Regulation. Timing of emergency contraception with levonorgestrel or the Yuzpe regimen. *Lancet* 1999;353:721.

Raine T, Harper C, Leon K, et al. Emergency contraception: advance provision in a young, high-risk clinic population. *Obstet Gynecol* 2000;96:1.

Raine TR, Harper CC, Rocca CH, et al. Direct access to emergency contraception through pharmacies and effect on contraception and STDs: a randomized controlled trial. *JAMA* 2005;293:54.

Raman-Wilms L, Tseng AL, Wighardt S, et al. Fetal genital effects of first-trimester sex hormone exposure: a meta-analysis. *Obstet Gynecol* 1995;85:141.

Raymond EG, Creinin MD, Barnhart KT, et al. Meclizine for prevention of nausea associated with use of emergency contraceptive pills: a randomized trial. *Obstet Gynecol* 2000; 95:271.

Rivera R, Yacobson I, Grimes D. The mechanism of action of hormonal contraceptives and intrauterine contraceptive devices. *Am J Obstet Gynecol* 1999;181:1263.

Rowlands S, Devalia H, Lawrenson R, et al. Repeated use of hormonal emergency contraception by younger women in the UK. *Br J Fam Plann* 2000;26:138.

Sills MR, Chamberlain JM, Teach SJ. The associations among pediatricians' knowledge, attitudes, and practices regarding emergency contraception. *Pediatrics* 2000;105:954.

Task Force on Postovulatory Methods of Fertility Regulation. Randomised controlled trial of levonorgestrel versus the Yuzpe regimen of combined oral contraceptives for emergency contraception. *Lancet* 1998;352:428.

Task Force on Postovulatory Methods of Fertility Regulation. Comparison of three single doses of mifepristone as emergency contraception: a randomised trial. *Lancet* 1999; 353:697.

Trussell J, Bull J, Koenig J, et al. Call 1-888-NOT-2-LATE: promoting emergency contraception in the United States. *J Am Med Womens Assoc* 1998;53:247.

Trussell J, Ellertson C, Rodriguez G. The Yuzpe regimen of emergency contraception: how long after the morning after? *Obstet Gynecol* 1996;88:150.

Trussell J, Koenig J, Ellertson C, et al. Preventing unintended pregnancy: the cost-effectiveness of three methods of emergency contraception. *Am J Public Health* 1997;87: 932.

Trussell J, Raymond EG. Statistical evidence about the mechanism of action of the Yuzpe regimen of emergency contraception. *Obstet Gynecol* 1999;93:872.

Trussell J, Rodriguez G, Ellertson C. Updated estimates of the effectiveness of the Yuzpe regimen of emergency contraception. *Contraception* 1999;59:147.

Webb A, Shochet T, Bigrigg A, et al. Effect of hormonal emergency contraception on bleeding patterns. *Contraception* 2004;69:133.

Webb A, Tabemer D. Clotting factors after emergency contraception. *Adv Contracept* 1993;9:75.

Wilcox AJ, Dunson D, Baird DD. The timing of the "fertile window" in the menstrual cycle: day specific estimates from a prospective study. *Br Med J* 2000;321:1259.

Yuzpe AA, Lancee WJ. Ethinylestradiol and Dl-norgestrel as a postcoital contraceptive. *Fertil Steril* 1977;9:932.

CHAPTER 47

Long-Acting Progestins

Anita L. Nelson

Long-acting progestin contraceptives have many features that make them particularly attractive to female adolescents. They are in the top tier of efficacy, are long lasting, safe, and convenient. Because they contain no estrogen, progestins may be used by women with contraindications to that hormone, including history of thrombosis. Long-acting progestin contraceptives are available in three different delivery systems—injections, implants, and intrauterine contraceptives. The levonorgestrel intrauterine system (LNG-IUS) is discussed in Chapter 44. The injections are currently available in two different formulations. The levonorgestrel-releasing (LNG) implants have not been available in the United States since 1998. However, the single-rod etonogestrel-releasing (ENG) implant was approved by the U.S. Food and Drug Administration (FDA) in July 2006 and is becoming increasingly available in the U.S.

INJECTABLE PROGESTINS

Today, there are two different formulations of depot medroxyprogesterone acetate (DMPA) available in the United States—the traditional 150 mg formulation (Depo-Provera, Pfizer Inc., Kalamazoo MI), which is injected intramuscularly every 11 to 13 weeks (DMPA-IM) and a newer formulation with different buffers (depo-subQ provera 104, Pfizer Inc., New York, NY), which is administered subcutaneously every 12 to 14 weeks (DMPA-SC). The two formulations have very similar labeling and side effect profiles.

Efficacy

The failure rate with correct and consistent use of the DMPA-IM is 0.3%. However, recalculation of typical-use failure rates to reflect potential late returns for reinjection yields a typical-use failure rate of 3% (Trussell, 2004). O'Dell et al. (1998) compared DMPA and oral contraceptives (OCs) in postpartum female adolescents and found that the DMPA users had median duration of use of 8.1 months compared to 5.4 months for OC users. More importantly, the repeat pregnancy rates by 15 months were lower in the DMPA users (15%) as compared to OC users (36%).

In clinical trials involving 16,023 women-cycles of DMPA-SC use, there were no pregnancies (Jain et al., 2004b).

Importantly, patient weight did not influence efficacy. The clinical trials included women with body mass indices (BMIs) that ranged from 18.2 to 46.7 kg/m^2. Typical-use failure rates are not yet available.

Mechanisms of Action

DMPA is a contraceptive agent; that is, it prevents fertilization. DMPA has two primary contraceptive mechanisms of action. DMPA thickens cervical mucus to prevent sperm entry into the upper genital track and it suppresses gonadotropin levels, especially at midcycle, which blocks ovulation (Jain et al., 2004a). The progestin also alters the endometrial lining, which has profound impacts on bleeding patterns, but has not been demonstrated to affect efficacy. Similarly, progestin may also affect tubal motility, but the clinical relevance of that observation is not known. There were no ectopic pregnancies in recent clinical trials with DMPA-SC (Jain et al., 2004b).

Drug Interactions

Aminoglutethimide increases hepatic clearance of DMPA and, if administered concomitantly with DMPA, may significantly depress serum concentrations of medroxyprogesterone acetate. Some antiretroviral medications impact cytochrome P-450 activity, but have not been reported to affect DMPA efficacy. Anticonvulsants do not detract from the contraceptive protection afforded by DMPA.

Contraindications

The list of medical contraindications is limited. From labeling, the following conditions are listed as contraindications:

Contraindications	Comments
Known or suspected pregnancy	No clinical benefit offered
Undiagnosed vaginal bleeding	May delay diagnosis of pathology
Known or suspected malignancy of breast	Receptor positive cancers can respond to progestin

Contraindications	Comments
Active thrombophlebitis, or current or past history of thromboembolic disorders or cerebral vascular disease	No evidence progestin impacts coagulation factors
Significant liver disease	Hepatic clearance needed
Allergy to medroxyprogesterone acetate (MPA) or its ingredients	Rare

World Health Organization (WHO) has even fewer medical contraindications for DMPA use. The only condition that is rated by WHO as category 4 (should not use) is current breast cancer. Conditions with WHO categories 3 or 4 ratings are listed in Table 47.1.

Administration

Labeling for both DMPA products advises that injections in women with regular cycles should be administered in the first 5 days of a normal menstrual cycle. It also states that women who are switching from other contraceptive methods should be given the first dose in a manner that ensures continuous contraceptive coverage. According to labeling, breast-feeding women wait 6 weeks after delivery for their first injection. Reinjections for DMPA-IM are to be scheduled in 11 to 13 weeks; reinjections for DMPA-SC are to be in 12 to 14 weeks. Avoid massaging the injection site after injection because early massage increases the surface area of the drug, allows faster absorption, and results in shorter effective life.

For female adolescents, these recommendations for injection can be too restrictive. Often teens are in immediate need of contraception. Female adolescents often follow a "start–stop" pattern of DMPA use (Polaneczky and Liblanc, 1998). After one or two injections, teens may discontinue DMPA use or switch to another method such as patches, OCs, or condoms, although quite frequently they return later for at least another injection of DMPA. In part, this intermittent pattern of use reflects the dynamics of adolescent sexual activity and relationships. However, in part it reflects the young woman's coping with side effects (see subsequent text).

Whatever the pattern of use is over time, it is important to be ready to administer the injections in response to the young woman's needs. Because of these needs, the WHO advises that women can have their first DMPA injection within the first 7 days of menses without the need for back-up contraceptives (World Health Organization, 2005). WHO guidelines also state that a woman can have a DMPA injection at any other time in the cycle if it is reasonably certain that she is not pregnant. If she is beyond the first 7 days of her cycle, she should abstain from intercourse or use an additional contraceptive method for 7 days after her off-label injection time. Petta et al. (1998) demonstrated that cervical mucus becomes impenetrable within 7 days of injection at any time in the cycle. If there has been recent unprotected intercourse, WHO also suggests that emergency contraception be offered. Reassuringly, Borgatta et al. (2002) found no fetal anomalies with intrauterine exposure to DMPA.

One algorithm used to expedite DMPA start/restart (Quick Start or Same-day Start) is outlined in Figure 47.1. The Quick Start or Same-day Start DMPA injection has been shown to save 46% of women a return visit for injection (Balkus and Miller, 2005). The pregnancy rate among the same-day starters was <1% (1 of 104); there is no known harm done by early intrauterine exposure to DMPA.

In a second study, researchers offered Quick Start OCs as a bridge to DMPA injection, which was done at the time of the OC-withdrawal bleeding. They reported that 86% of the women were satisfied with this bridge (Morroni et al., 2004). This underscores the need for immediate effective contraception.

Advantages

1. Extremely effective: Pregnancy protection is excellent, although that feature is not highly prized by teens themselves. Only 15% of those interviewed cited that as a reason for selecting DMPA (Harel et al., 1995).
2. Private: With DMPA there is no external evidence of contraceptive use (no pill packs or condoms to hide), but itemized insurance bills or changes in needs for sanitary protection may raise adult suspicions.
3. Convenient and low maintenance: Many studies have found that this feature is "most important" or "likely important" to 89.3% of teens surveyed (Harel et al., 1995). This same survey found that the most important reason teens continued to use DMPA was that "they didn't have to take the pill every day" (54%), and the second reason was that it was "easier to take" than their previous method (16%). Most teens were not concerned about the need for return to health care providers for reinjection.
4. Cost-effective without high initial cost: Because payment for DMPA is almost "pay as you use it," DMPA can initially be more affordable than implants or intrauterine contraceptives.
5. Intermediate-term method with built-in grace period.
6. No estrogen contraindications or side effects.
7. Frequent amenorrhea with long-term use: This is helpful for busy women, athletes, patients with anemia, those with human immunodeficiency virus (HIV) infection, those with coagulopathies or renal failure, those taking anticoagulants, and mentally challenged women.
8. Reduced incidence of painful sickle cell crises (de Abood et al., 1997).
9. Decreased risk of endometrial and, perhaps, epithelial ovarian cancer.
10. May be used off label by breast-feeding women after delivery (Halderman and Nelson, 2002). Providing convenient and reliable contraception to teen mothers can make a significant contribution in reducing the rate of repeat pregnancies.
11. Thick cervical mucus and amenorrhea: This limits the incidence of pelvic inflammatory disease in patients with cervicitis.
12. DMPA-SC is also used to treat symptomatic endometriosis (Crosignani et al., 2005).

Metabolic Impacts

Because there is no estrogen component, DMPA causes no alterations in coagulation factors, angiotensinogen, or hepatic globulin production. Blood pressure (BP)

TABLE 47.1

World Health Organization 2004 Medical Eligibility Criteria for Contraceptive Use

WHO Categories:

1. *A condition for which there is no restriction for the use of the contraceptive method*
2. *A condition where the advantages of using the method generally outweigh the theoretical or proven risks*
3. *A condition where the theoretical or proven risks usually outweigh the advantages of using the method*
4. *A condition which represents an unacceptable health risk if the contraceptive method is used*

Conditions with Category 3 and/or Category 4	*Category*			*Clarifications/Evidence*
	DMPA	*LNG/ENG Implant*		
Breast-feeding <6 wk postpartum	3	3		Clarification: There is concern that the neonate may be at risk of exposure to steroid hormones during the first 6 wk postpartum. However, in many settings pregnancy morbidity and mortality risks are high, and access to services is limited. In such settings, POCs may be one of the few types of methods widely available and accessible to breast-feeding women immediately postpartum. Evidence: Studies have shown that among breast-feeding women <6 wk postpartum, progestogen-only contraceptives did not affect breast-feeding performance, and infant health and growth. However, there are no data evaluating the effects of progestogen exposure through breast milk on brain and liver development.
Multiple risk factors for arterial cardiovascular disease (such as older age, smoking, diabetes, and hypertension)	3	2		Clarification: When multiple major risk factors exist, risk of cardiovascular disease may increase substantially. The effects of DMPA may persist for some time after discontinuation.
Hypertension • Elevated blood pressure levels (properly taken measurements) systolic >160 mm Hg or diastolic >100 mm Hg • Vascular disease	3	2		Evidence: Limited evidence suggests that among women with hypertension, those who used progestogen-only injectables had a small increased risk of cardiovascular events compared with women who did not use these methods.
Deep venous thrombosis (DVT)/Pulmonary embolism (PE) Current DVT/PE	3	3		
Current and history of ischemic heart disease	3	I 2	C 3	
Stroke (history of cerebrovascular accident)	3	I 2	C 3	
Headaches	I	C	I	C
Migraine with aura, at any age	2	3	2	3

(continued)

TABLE 47.1

(Continued)

Conditions with Category 3 and/or Category 4	Category DMPA	Category LNG/ENG Implant	Clarifications/Evidence
Unexplained vaginal bleeding (suspicious for serious underlying condition) Before evaluation	3	3	Clarification: If pregnancy or an underlying pathological condition (such as pelvic malignancy) is suspected, it must be evaluated and the category adjusted after evaluation.
Breast disease Breast cancer • Current	4	4	
• Past and no evidence of current disease for 5 years	3	3	
Diabetes • Nephropathy/retinopathy/ neuropathy • Other vascular disease or diabetes of >20 years' duration	3	2	
Viral hepatitis Active	3	3	
Cirrhosis Severe (decompensated)	3	3	
Liver tumors	3	3	
Drugs which affect liver enzymes • Rifampicin • Certain anticonvulsants (phenytoin, carbamazepine, barbiturates, primidone, topiramate, oxcarbazepine)	2	3	Clarification: Although the interaction of rifampicin or certain anticonvulsants with LNG/ENG implants is not harmful to women, it is likely to reduce the effectiveness of LNG/ENG implants. Use of other contraceptives should be encouraged for women who are long-term users of any of these drugs. Evidence: Use of certain anticonvulsants decreased the contraceptive effectiveness of POCs.

I, initiation; C, continuation; POCs, progestogen-only contraceptives; DMPA, depot medroxyprogesterone acetate; LNG, levonorgestrel-releasing; ENG, etonogestrel-releasing.

measurements are unchanged with DMPA (World Health Organization Expanded Programme of Research, Development and Research Training in Human Reproduction Task Force on Long-Acting Systemic Agents for Regulation of Fertility, 1983). However, the serum levels of progestin with the injections are higher than is seen with the implants or intrauterine contraceptives. DMPA has greater impact on glucose tolerance, insulin levels, and lipid profiles. For healthy subjects, the changes in glucose tolerance are not clinically significant (Liew et al., 1985). Teens with glucose intolerance or overt diabetes must be monitored closely when using the DMPA injections. However, because glucose and insulin levels are increased during DMPA use. DMPA can lower total cholesterol (TC) and triglycerides; it has a negligible impact on low-density lipoprotein cholesterol (LDL-C) and high-density lipoprotein cholesterol (HDL-C) (Deslypere et al., 1985).

Disadvantages

1. Side effects (see later discussion).
2. Must continue to remind patients of the need for safer sex practices and provide a method to reduce the risks of sexually transmitted infections (STDs).
3. Requires medical intervention (unless self injection of subcutaneous DMPA becomes available). A hotline is available 24 hours a day, 7 days a week in English and Spanish to answer patient's questions and to remind patients about appointments for reinjection (1-866-554 DEPO (3376)).

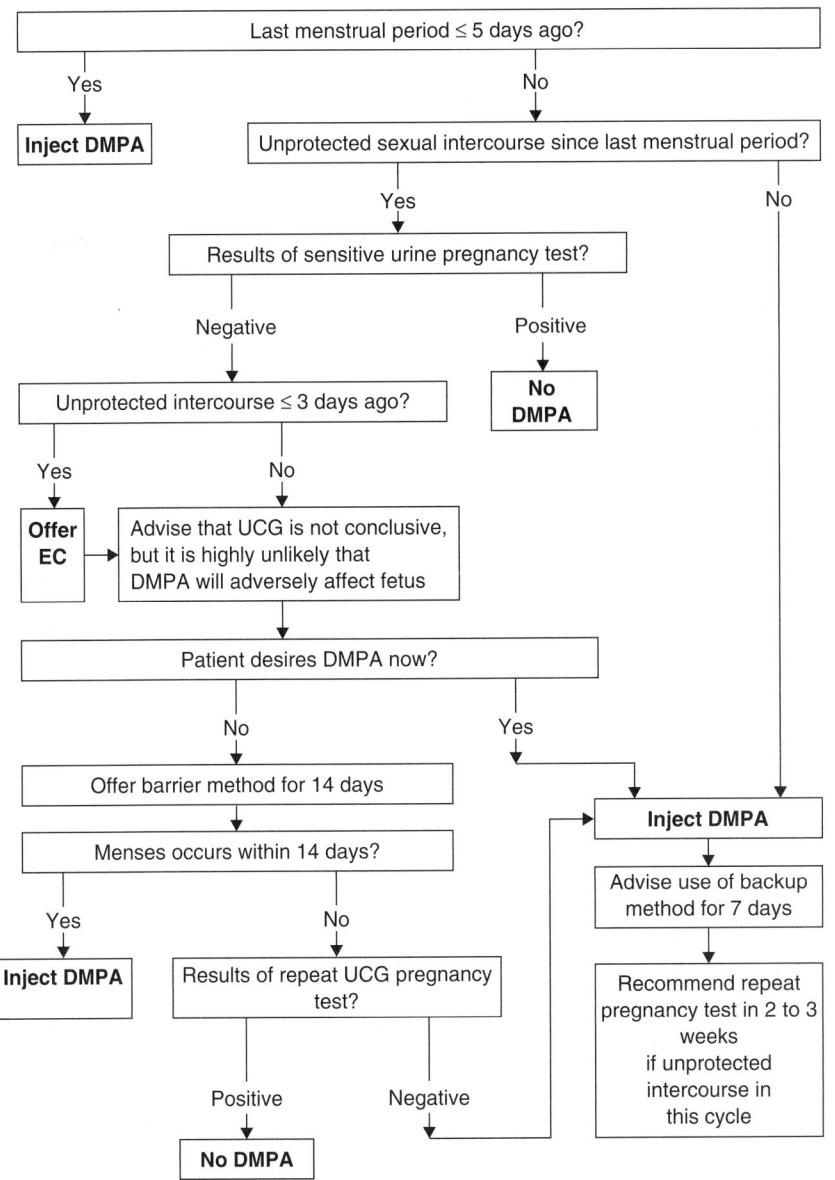

FIGURE 47.1 Quick Start DMPA. Initial injection or late reinjection (>13 weeks since last injection) of DMPA. DMPA, depot medroxyprogesterone acetate; EC, emergency contraception; UCG, urinary chorionic gonadotropin. (From Nelson AL, Haatcher RA, Zieman M, et al. *A pocket guide to managing contraception,* 3rd ed. Tiger, GA: Bridging the Gap Foundation, 2002:117.)

4. Delays return to fertility: Average delay is 10 months after last injection but there is considerable variation in that estimate. Higher BMIs are associated with slower return to fertility.
5. Immediate anaphylactic reactions (extremely rare).

Side Effects

1. Menstrual changes: Missed menstrual periods and amenorrhea become more common over time with DMPA. After the first year of use, approximately 50% of DMPA users are amenorrheic, and after 2 years that number rises to 75%. With the initial 1 to 3 injections, many women experience significant unscheduled menstrual spotting, and bleeding. Early reinjection (at 6 weeks) did not alter the bleeding episodes, onset of bleeding, or total days of bleeding after the second injection (Harel et al., 1995). Similarly, the practice of giving a 300-mg dose initially is *not* recommended, because the risk of developing other side effects is proportionately increased. Although there are no studies of effective interventions, clinicians often advise short courses of nonsteroidal antiinflammatory drugs (NSAIDs) (e.g., ibuprofen 800 mg orally 3 times a day for 3 days) or low-dose estrogen supplementation to reduce immediate bleeding irregularities. Research is now underway to understand the impacts progestin-only methods have on the endometrium and its underlying vascular supply in order to develop more targeted therapies to deal with the unscheduled spotting and bleeding.

2. Bone mineral density (BMD) changes: Controlled cross-sectional studies of older, long-term DMPA users found that, although the BMD of DMPA users was statistically significantly lower than that of controls, BMD measurements normalized after women stopped using DMPA. Former users of DMPA have BMD measurements identical to that of never users (Orr-Walker et al., 1998; Petitti et al., 2000). For women who have completed bone

formulation, DMPA may create temporary, probably reversible decreases in bone mineralization, akin to the changes seen during pregnancy and lactation.

The impact that DMPA may have on decreasing BMD through suppression of estrogen is a critical issue for teens, because most lifetime bone mineralization occurs during adolescence. Several studies have demonstrated that many female adolescents using DMPA not only fail to increase their BMD as expected but they may also experience bone loss, such that their BMD measurements on DMPA are lower than they were at baseline. One recent study has demonstrated that adolescent DMPA users had 4% to 7% decrease in BMD compared to unprotected controls. Partial recovery of BMD was seen in many women in short-term follow-up after DMPA discontinuation.

The FDA issued a black box warning for both formulations of DMPA advising "Women who use Depo-Provera Contraceptive Injection may lose significant BMD. Bone loss is greater with increasing duration of use and may not be completely reversible. It is unknown if use of Depo-Provera Contraceptive Injection during adolescence or early adulthood, a critical period of bone accretion, will reduce peak bone mass and increase the risk for osteoporotic fractures in later life. Depo-Provera Contraceptive Injection should be used as a long-term birth control method (e.g., >2 years) only if other birth control methods are inadequate." The labeling also advises that if prolonged use is contemplated, the patient's BMD should be evaluated.

Unfortunately, this recommendation has led to some confusion in female adolescents. Using the T-score, which compares the teen's BMD to the peak BMD of a healthy 20- to 30-year-old woman, will predictably demonstrate "osteopenia" or "osteoporosis." Younger women have not yet reached their peak bone mass. The California Office of Family Planning sent clinicians' recommendations that "Bone mineral density screening should not be recommended to a client for the sole purpose of evaluating appropriateness of DMPA usage" (Office of Family Planning, 2005). If there is to be a dual-energy x-ray absorptiometry (DXA) evaluation, it is important to focus on the Z-score, which compares the patient's BMD to that of age-matched controls to see if the patient has any bone-related concerns that should be considered when deciding to continue DMPA use beyond 2 years.

An alternative approach to use when evaluating female adolescents for prolonged DMPA use is to determine if the young woman has other underlying risks for low BMD, such as family history of osteoporosis, heavy cigarette smoking, corticosteroid use, eating disorders, or excessive exercise patterns. For women without additional risk factors for low BMD, many experts believe that the 2-year restriction appears unwarranted (Dialogues in Contraception Editorial Board, 2005). All adolescents, whether they use DMPA or not, should be advised to consume at least 1,300 mg calcium and adequate vitamin D (minimum of 200–400 IU) to ensure maximal bone accretion. O'Brien et al. (2003) have demonstrated that higher calcium intake by adolescent women, even in pregnancy, protects against trabecular bone loss. For women with additional risk factors for low BMD, possible health risks associated with prolonged DMPA use should be balanced against the patient's ability and likelihood of effectively using alternative effective means of contraception. Some experts have recommended measuring a woman's follicle-stimulating hormone (FSH) or estradiol level just before reinjection to determine if DMPA use has induced hypoestrogenemia. If not, her risks of BMD loss is likely minimal (Beksinska et al., 2005). The addition of estrogen supplements is protective of bone in adolescent girls who receive DMPA for contraception (Cromer et al., 2005) and may be a prudent option for women who do not have contraindications to that hormone. In 20 women with endometriosis, the use of DMPA-SC was shown to have significantly less impact on BMD than leuprolide (Crosignani et al., 2005).

3. Hypoestrogenic symptoms: Most users of DMPA maintain adequate estradiol levels in the follicular range. However, in a small percentage of users, ovarian hormonal production is more profoundly suppressed and estradiol levels can fall into the postmenopausal range. These patients may complain of dry vagina, dyspareunia (Miller et al., 2000), and even hot flashes. Once other causes have been excluded, these symptoms respond well to physiological estrogen supplementation or to a change in method (e.g., vaginal contraceptive ring).

4. Weight changes: Despite widespread belief that DMPA use increases weight, clinical trials do not consistently support any attributable risk for weight gain. Complicating the analysis is the fact that U.S. women gain an average of >2 lb/year regardless of the contraceptive method used. Female adolescents gain even more weight. Furthermore, individual weight changes vary considerably.

Uncontrolled studies conducted in the late 1960s and in the 1970s showed that women who used DMPA had a mean weight increase of 5 lb during the first year, 8.1 lb by 2 years, and 13.8 lb by 4 years (Schwallie and Assenzo, 1974). Moore et al. (1995) monitored women who used OCs, DMPA, or implants for 1 year and found no significant weight gain in any group; the average weight gain with DMPA use was +0.1 lb. Cromer et al. (1994) did not note weight gain in teens with DMPA use, but Harel et al. (1996) found DMPA-associated weight gain, which persisted for 6 months after discontinuance. Risser et al. (1999) reported weight gains of 3 to 4.5 lb while using DMPA; heavier teens had greater gains. The only double blind, placebo-controlled study of this issue was for a short term, but found no weight changes in DMPA users compared to either baseline weight or to placebo control (Pelkman et al., 2001). Importantly, DMPA users had no change in their appetite or basal metabolic rates. There may be subgroups of women who are more susceptible to weight gain with DMPA use; Templeman et al. (2000) reported a 9.8 lb (±10.5 lb) weight gain. Given that obesity is a growing major public health problem in the United States, ongoing evaluation of and education about weight is a part of quality health care. However, theoretical concerns about potential adverse impacts that DMPA could have on her weight in the absence of a patient's personal experience should not preclude the use of injectable contraception.

5. Breast tenderness: Mastalgia is reported in 15% to 20% of women starting DMPA, but this side effect usually decreases rapidly.

6. Mood disturbances: Although there is no consistent evidence that DMPA use causes psychological side

effects, such as nervousness, insomnia, somnolence, fatigue, dizziness, and depression, labeling mentions these as possible side effects. Many patients with chronic depression tolerate DMPA, but use in those cases must be individualized (Kaunitz, 1999). West-hoff (1996) reported that community epidemiological survey depression scores after DMPA did not change compared with baseline scores, but Civic et al. (2000) reported an increased likelihood that DMPA users would report depressive symptoms, compared with nonusers.

7. Headaches: Progestin may increase headaches by increasing fluid retention, but no placebo-controlled study results are available.

8. Other changes: Acne, alopecia, hirsutism, fluid retention, changes in libido, changes in cervical secretions, nausea, cholestatic jaundice, and local skin reaction to injection have been reported but have seldom been serious enough to warrant a change in method.

Summary

DMPA-IM and DMPA-SC are attractive contraceptive options for female adolescents. They provide top-tier efficacy, are low in maintenance, and are safe. The side effect profile and the need for periodic reinjection pose challenges for long-term continuation. Adolescents at risk for STDs need to use dual methods (male condoms) to meet all their reproductive needs.

ETONOGESTREL-RELEASING IMPLANT

Subdermal implants provide long-acting, extremely effective, rapidly reversible contraception that requires little user effort. Progestin-only implants avoid estrogen side effects and can be used by virtually every woman. There are only a few medical conditions that were rated 3 (risks usually outweigh advantages) or 4 (unacceptable health risk) for implant use in the WHO 2004 medical eligibility criteria for contraceptive use; they are listed in Table 47.1.

Clinical experience with the LNG implant (Norplant 6 Contraceptive System, Wyeth, Philadelphia, PA) suggested new properties and features that would be important for the next generation of implants. These features included a single-rod system (to simplify insertion and removal), release of hormones sufficient to inhibit ovulation (to increase acceptance of the method), a duration of action of at least 2 to 3 years (for effective birth spacing), and a smaller diameter implant (to allow for use of an injection system for insertion). These features have been incorporated into the ENG implant.

The ENG implant (Implanon, NV Organon, Oss, the Netherlands) is available in more than 30 countries, including the United Kingdom, Chile, Australia, Indonesia, and 10 European countries. It has been used by more than 2 million women worldwide since 1999.

Description of System

The ENG implant is a single-rod contraceptive implant made of a core and a membrane. The core consists of steroid microcrystals containing 68 mg etonogestrel (3-ketodesogestrel) imbedded in a rod of ethylene vinyl acetate (EVA) copolymer. This core is covered by a thin EVA copolymer membrane measuring 0.06 mm. The implant is 40 mm long and has an external diameter of 2 mm. ENG (the biologically active metabolite of desogestrel) has no demonstrated estrogenic, antiinflammatory, or mineralo-corticoid activity, but it does have weak androgenic and anabolic activity and strong antiestrogenic activity. The relative binding affinity of ENG to progesterone receptors in rat uterine activity is 10 times greater than that of progesterone (Jordan, 2002). The implant provides contraceptive protection at least for 3 years. The ENG implant comes individually packaged in the needle of a sterile, disposable, specifically designed inserter for subdermal placement.

Mechanisms of Action

The ENG-implant was developed specifically to inhibit ovulation. It acts as a contraceptive to prevent fertilization by providing sustained release of a relatively low dose of contraceptive hormone. Dose finding studies concluded that a release rate of 25 to 30 µg ENG per day, resulting in serum levels of 90 pg/mL, would be needed to inhibit ovulation (Wenzel et al., 1998). No ovulation was found in any test cycle during the first 2 years of ENG implant use. Ovulation was first seen at 30 months; two women (3.1% of subjects) ovulated at least once from 30 to 36 months of use (Makarainen et al., 1998; Davies et al., 1993). With those exceptions, gonadotropin studies showed a consistent prevention of luteinizing hormone (LH) surges. The progestins also make the cervical mucus viscous and impenetrable by sperm, so fertilization does not take place (Meirik et al., 2003; Croxatto, 2002).

However, in contrast to DMPA, ENG implant use does not cause hypoestrogenemia. There was interindividual variability, but no consistently high or low estradiol (E_2) levels were seen; 95% of the measures were more than 110 pmol/L. Although ovulation is inhibited effectively, by year 1, FSH and estradiol serum levels were consistent with follicular development in most subjects (Makarainen et al., 1998).

ENG impacts on the endometrium are measurable. The mean value of the endometrial stripe determined by transvaginal ultrasound was 4 mm. Endometrial biopsies did not show atrophy but showed inactive or weakly proliferative endometrium (Jordan, 2002). Sperm transport in the uterus and fallopian tubes also was slowed. However, because both ovulation suppression and cervical mucus viscosity prevented the union of gametes, these impacts on the endometrium and the tube may be superfluous (Glasier, 2002).

There is no accumulation of ENG over time. The average half-life ($t_{1/2}$) elimination of ENG is approximately 25 hours, which is much lower than the 42 hours found with the LNG implant system. However, ENG is lipophilic, so women with higher BMIs are expected to have greater volumes of distribution and longer $t_{1/2}$ elimination (40 hours in heavier women versus 20 hours in lighter women) (Wenzl et al., 1998). The variation in half-lives of elimination and the variation in serum concentrations of hormones are much smaller with ENG implant than with the LNG implants (Makarainen et al., 1998). Etonogestrel is bound mainly to albumin, in contrast to levonorgestrel binding to sex hormone binding globulin, which is more sensitive to circulating estradiol levels (Wenzl et al., 1998).

Contraceptive Efficacy

The core data set includes 1,716 women from more than a dozen representative countries, who were treated for 53,530 cycles. No pregnancies were seen in ENG-implant users, resulting in a Pearl index of 0.0 (0.00–0.09). Additional studies in the United States and China raised the total number of woman-cycles, all without any pregnancies. Efficacy in heavier women was not so well studied. Only 365 women who weighed ≥70 kg were reported in the literature. However, none of these women experienced any pregnancies (Newton and Newton, 2003).

After more than 200,000 ENG implant devices had been placed in Australia, Harrison-Woolrych et al. (2005) analyzed the 218 pregnancies reported with ENG-implant use. Researchers could not determine cause in 45 cases, but of the remaining 173 women the greatest single reason for "failure" of the device (84 women; 48.6%) was that the clinician had never actually inserted the rod. The second most frequent cause of implant "failure" (46 women; 26.6%) was that the patient was already pregnant before insertion. Only 13 pregnancies were attributed to product failure. Therefore, the failure rate was <1/1,000. Many of these problems have been corrected in Australia (Wenck and Johnston, 2004). The lessons learned from these postmarketing experiences in Australia have been incorporated into the training. U.S. clinicians are being given information about patient selection and thorough training in insertion and removal techniques.

Drug Interactions

Serum ENG levels are quite low. Concomitant use with other drugs that enhance cytochrome P-450 activity reduces implant efficacy. WHO lists anticonvulsants and other drugs as a category 3 for this reason (World Health Organization, 2004) (Table 47.1).

Return to Fertility

In four studies involving 32 women, return to ovulation after implant removal was studied by ultrasound or serum progesterone concentrations for up to 3 months; 30 of 32 (94%) women demonstrated return to fertility, usually within 3 weeks of removal (Davies et al., 1993). Because return to ovulation is rapid after implant removal, women desiring continued pregnancy prevention should begin another method immediately or have a new rod inserted through the incision made for removal (Cherry, 2002).

Continuation Rates

Continuation rates in the clinical trials varied considerably by country. Overall 81.8% of women continued to use the ENG implant for up to 24 months (Edwards and Moore, 1999). In Europe and Canada, continuation rates were 70% during the study. In Southeast Asia, continuation rates were 99%.

Since its introduction into mainstream use in Britain, Smith and Reuter (2002) have reported that in three clinical services in that country, the 6-month continuation rates ranged between 84% and 88%, and the 12-month continuation rates were 67% to 78%. Smith and Reuter (2002) found that intolerance of side effects and a change of mind about wanting contraception were leading reasons for requesting removal. Recent U.S. continuation rates were similar to the British experience; 67% continued for 1 to 2 years.

Breast-feeding Women

In an open, comparative, nonrandomized trial of breast-feeding women 6 weeks postpartum, the effects of the ENG implant on 42 women were contrasted with those seen in 38 women using a nonmedicated intrauterine device (IUD). The volume of breast milk production and the quality of milk content (total fat, total protein, and lactose) were not affected by the use of the ENG implant. The timing and quantity of supplementary feedings did not differ between the groups. There were no statistically significant differences in the growth parameters in the infants (Reinprayoon et al., 2000). However, the authors agreed with the WHO recommendation that insertion of ENG implant be delayed until the infant is 6 weeks old, because the risk of pregnancy is low during the first 3 weeks postpartum and because of the absence of knowledge about the impact on the newborn's central nervous system during its rapid early extrauterine development period (World Health Organization, 2004; Reinprayoon et al., 2000; Diaz, 2002).

Insertion

The ENG implant comes packaged in a preloaded, sterile, disposable inserter. Clinicians must be trained and maintain their competency in the appropriate insertion and removal techniques. Insertion of ENG implant is fundamentally different from the techniques used for LNG implant. ENG implant should be inserted during the first 5 days of a woman's menstrual cycle. An area is identified on the medial aspect of the nondominant upper arm, 6 to 8 cm above the elbow, in the sulcus between the biceps and the triceps. The skin is cleansed with an antiseptic agent. A small amount (<0.5 cc) of local anesthetic with lidocaine is infused. The needle of the syringe with the implant loaded in is introduced directly under the skin and advanced in the subdermal layer while tenting the skin until the needle hub is at the level of the skin. The obturator is rotated 90 degrees, moving the plunger into position. Stabilizing the base, the needle is smoothly retracted, leaving the implant behind. The implant remains invisible for most women, but it is easy to palpate. It is important to palpate the area immediately after the removal of the insertion needle to confirm implant placement. Pressure is applied to the skin incision site for hemostasis. A steristrip is placed to close the incision. Routine precautions should be provided for postinsertion care.

In clinical trials, the time for insertion from the skin entry to complete insertion was 1 minute. It should be noted that this does not include the time for preparation or anesthetic injection and onset of action.

There was a low complication rate with insertion in the clinical studies; only 10 out of 1,710 (0.6%) women reported complications. The most common were bleeding at insertion site or failure of the insertion device. No expulsions occurred, but 1% of women complained of pain at the insertion site at some time during the trial (Edwards and Moore, 1999).

Removal

Removal of ENG implants is distinctly more straightforward than the removal of the LNG capsules for several reasons. First, the single-rod system requires the removal of only one implant, not six. Secondly, the ENG rod is stiffer than the LNG capsules and is easier to palpate for localization at the time of removal. With LNG capsules insertion, the position of previous capsules could be disturbed by the placement of later ones—the so-called "U-ing" of capsules where the advancing trocar could catch the edge of a previously inserted implant and displace it upward in the arm. The single-rod system does not have the potential for those complications. And finally, the EVA capsule of the ENG rod induces less fibrous formation around the rod than did the silastic LNG capsules.

The digital extrusion or "pop out" technique is encouraged for removal. In the "pop out" technique, the rod is first palpated, and the area is cleansed. Approximately 0.5 to 1.0 cc of local anesthetic is infused beneath the distal tip of the rod. A 2 mm incision parallel to the rod is made at the distal tip of the implant. Then pressure is applied at the proximal end, pushing the rod toward the incision until it pops out, at which time it can be grasped with fingers or forceps (Darney et al., 1992). Instrument removal with noncrushing clamps also may be utilized. In clinical studies, the ENG implant was removed in less than 5 minutes in most women.

It should be noted that because there is no free drug inside the capsule, a broken capsule is not associated with spillage of medication as it might have been with the LNG capsules. Although the ENG rod is firmer and stiffer than the LNG capsules, it is possible that the rod may be placed so deeply that it is not palpable. ENG is not easily visualized with plain film x-rays. Lantz et al. (1997) have demonstrated that nonpalpable ENG rod implants can be best visualized under ultrasound guidance, indirectly by identifying the posterior acoustic shadow cast by the implant.

Capsule Fracture

The ENG rod is very robust. There are only two case reports of fractures of the capsule in situ. In one case, the fracture occurred after a "rough and tumble" with the subject's 7-year-old son (Pickard and Bacon, 2002). In the second case, no cause for the broken capsule was identified (Agrawal and Robinson, 2003).

Advantages

1. Extremely effective: No pregnancies were reported in clinical trials. Rates in clinical practice are only 1 in 1,000 users.
2. Private: Implants are not generally visible, but the same factors that compromise DMPA privacy occur with implants.
3. Convenient and low maintenance: One office insertion procedure provides up to 3 years of contraceptive protection.
4. Cost-effective.
5. No estrogen contraindications or side effects.

Metabolic Impacts

Bone Mineral Density
There has been concern that ovarian suppression with DMPA may be associated with bone loss secondary to estrogen deficiency. However, Makarainen et al. found that no woman using ENG implant had consistently low estradiol concentrations (Makarienen et al., 1998). In an open, prospective, comparative 2-year study of 44 ENG implant users and 29 nonmedicated IUD users, Beerthuizen et al. (2000) found that estradiol levels were not significantly suppressed at any point. Importantly, the changes from baseline BMD measurements in implant users were not different from those in the IUD group. Even the ENG implant users with amenorrhea had no deleterious impact on their BMD. Although the authors did not analyze their findings by age, they concluded that their study demonstrated that ENG implant use would be safe in young women who had not achieved maximum bone density.

Carbohydrate Metabolism
Comparative trials of ENG implant versus LNG implant by Biswas et al. (2001) in 80 healthy volunteers, aged 18 to 40, for 24 months revealed a slight increase in insulin resistance with use of both implants. Fasting glucose levels with ENG implant remained stable throughout the study period. Fasting insulin levels had large interindividual variations at all times; however, at 24 months, a statistically significant increase was seen with ENG implant. The 2-hour oral glucose tolerance test demonstrated small increases over baseline glucose levels only after 24 months of use (12%), but 2-hour insulin levels were elevated consistently. Area under-the-curve analysis revealed statistically significant increases in glucose (30%–60%) and insulin levels (50%) by 6 months. Fasting Hb A_{Ic} levels were also increased throughout the study period. Although each of these changes was statistically significant, it should be noted that virtually all the values remained in the normal range. No glucose intolerance or diabetes was induced.

Lipid Impacts
Biswas et al. (2003) followed up 80 healthy volunteers randomized to use ENG implant or LNG implant for 2 years. At the end of the study, ENG implant users had slight decreases in TC (8.9%), HDL-C (5.8%), and LDL-C (5.9%), but there were no significant differences in their HDL/TC ratios or HDL/LDL ratios, indicating that the ENG implant implants are unlikely to contribute directly to any increased cardiovascular risk. However, the atherogenic risk ratio of apolipoprotein A-I (Apo A-I) to Apo B worsened, both because Apo A-I initially dropped (0.3%) and because Apo B increased by 25%.

Coagulation Factors and Other Hepatic Effects
Because initial international studies indicated that levonorgestrel-containing OCs were associated with less thrombosis than desogestrel-containing pills, Egberg et al. (1998) conducted a randomized comparative trial of LNG and ENG implants in 56 women. They measured the impact each implant system had on hemostasis (coagulation times and factors for coagulation, anticoagulants, and fibrinosis). In general, statistically significant changes to antithrombotic tendencies were seen in activated partial thromboplastin time (APTT), antithrombin III (AT-III) activity, protein C activity, and protein S free antigen, as well as plasminogen. They also monitored potential prothrombotic changes seen in factor VII activity, D-dimer antigen, and α_2-antiplasmin activity. However, in a parallel study, the use of two baseline measurements for each subject showed that the change seen in the different parameters with the

implants generally were not greater than the differences between the two baseline values. Both implants had similar small effects on the hemostatic system; the authors concluded that they were not suggestive of a tendency toward thrombosis. The same investigators studied liver function with the two implant systems and found that total bilirubin and γ-glutamyl transferase increased, whereas alanine aminotransferase and aspartate aminotransferase levels decreased. Total bilirubin increased with ENG implant. The clinical implications of this mild increase in healthy subjects are probably not significant, but the implications of such a rise for women with hepatic compromise are not known (Dorflinger, 2002).

Disadvantages

1. Side effects (see subsequent text).
2. Provides no protection against STDs. Dual methods are needed for at-risk couples.
3. Requires medical intervention, including insertion and removal procedures performed by trained clinicians.
4. Expensive, with large up-front costs.

Side Effects

Changes in Bleeding Patterns

Menstrual bleeding changes are to be expected with progestin-only methods. There was no consistency or predictable trends in the bleeding patterns seen in individual women using ENG implants. Amenorrhea rates start low (<20%) at 3 months, but by 6 months approximately 20% of users had no menses, and, for the rest of the study, approximately 30% to 40% of women were amenorrheic. Amenorrhea occurred at any constant estradiol level, either early or late follicular levels (Makarainen et al., 1998). The incidence of infrequent bleeding (<3 bleeding episodes/90 days) decreased in the first 3 months. Frequent bleeding (>5 bleeding/spotting episodes in the 90-day period) was relatively unchanged in early use and decreased for the remainder of the study. Prolonged bleeding (at least one episode lasting at least 14 days) was relatively common in the first 3 months but decreased over time. Hemoglobin levels of women studied were relatively unchanged. Importantly, the bleeding patterns were unpredictable. A woman who initially experienced amenorrhea could later report frequent or prolonged bleeding. Normal menses returns within 3 months of removal of capsules in almost all subjects (Zheng et al., 1999).

Weight Changes

Weight increase was reported as an adverse event by 6.4% of all ENG implant users in the clinical trial. In the clinical trials, weight gain was the reason for discontinuation in 1.5% of users. It is also the side effect that is most difficult to interpret. What proportion of the observed gains were attributed to ENG implant, and which resulted from natural gains? The observations reported included the following:

- Within 3 months of insertion, 36.4% of women gained at least 1 kg, and approximately 10% had gained at least 3 kg.
- At the end of a year, more than half of women (53.5%) gained at least 1 kg, and 21.9% were at least 3 kg heavier than baseline.

- At the end of 2 years, 64.4% of study completers had documented gains of at least 1 kg, and 36.9% had at least 3 kg weight increase.
- Lighter women (<50 kg) were more likely to gain weight than those whose baseline weight was >50 kg (Edwards and Moore, 1999).

Headaches

Although headache has been the most frequent complaint of users of implantable contraception (Brache et al., 2002), in the clinical trials with ENG implant, the frequency of women complaining of headache was generally not excessive. In the comparative trial, 21% of the ENG implant users complained of headaches, but only 4.7% of women discontinued the method for this reason (Edwards and Moore, 1999). It should also be remembered that in the randomized, double-blinded, 6-month trial of low-dose OCs for acne therapy, 20.5% of placebo users reported headaches compared to 18.4% of OC users (Redmond et al., 1997).

Acne

Acne was the most frequently reported drug-related adverse event in the ENG implant clinical trials. Slightly more than 15% of the women reported acne as an adverse event, but only 1% of users had the implants removed because of this problem.

Mood Changes, Nervousness, and Depression

There are no estimates of risks attributable for these mood problems. In the clinical trials, ENG implant users reported rates of nervousness that varied between 1% and 1.2% in all study sites except Chile, where 30% of women complained of this problem. Requests for removal for each of these complaints ranged from 0% to 2% (Brache et al., 2002).

Blood Pressure

Significant BP increases were defined as BP_S >140 mm Hg or increased by 20 mm Hg over baseline or last visit reading or BP_D >90 mm Hg or increased by 10 mm Hg over baseline or last visit reading. Such increases were observed in 0.7% of women (10/1,640) at any time during the 24 months of the studies. In comparative studies, 0.6% of ENG implant users and 0.7% of LNG implant users had significant increases.

Ovarian Cysts

Progestins are known to slow atresia of ovarian cysts. In the large clinical trials, ovarian cysts were found on physical examination in 2% to 3% of implant users. In Chile, 9% of ENG implant users were found at some time to have such cysts (Brache et al., 2002). In asymptomatic women, no action was needed.

Summary

Clinical experience has demonstrated that the ENG contraceptive implant provides unsurpassed contraceptive efficacy, working primarily by ovulation suppression and thickened cervical mucus to prevent fertilization. This is achieved with very low levels of progestin and has very little metabolic impact in part because ovarian production of estradiol continues in the follicular range. Overall continuation rates with this method have been encouraging. Return to fertility is very rapid. Medical contraindications are rare, so virtually any woman can be offered this implant. The bleeding patterns with ENG implant are generally better than with previous generations of implants, but they are still unpredictable. Unscheduled bleeding can be disruptive for a woman. Therefore, careful patient counseling is imperative and may help reduce discontinuations for menstrual changes. Weight changes may be less well tolerated, but other side effects, such as headaches and acne, rarely cause patient discontinuation. Both the insertion and removal procedures have been greatly simplified and are more easily accomplished in a busy office practice. However, specific training is required.

WEB SITES

For Teenagers and Parents

http://kidshealth.org/teen/sexual_health/contraception/contraception_depo.html. Teen site with information about DMPA-IM.
http://www.depoprovera.com/. Pfizer site on DMPA-IM.
http://www.depo-subqprovera104.com/. Pfizer site on DMPA-SC.
http://www.plannedparenthood.org/pp2/portal/files/portal/medicalinfo/birthcontrol/pub-depo-provera.xml. Planned Parenthood information about DMPA-IM.
http://familydoctor.org/016.xml. AAFP information about DMPA-IM.
http://www.youngwomenshealth.org/femalehormone1.html. Children's Hospital Boston Web site on contraception including DMPA-IM.
http://www.cfoc.org/411AboutSex/birthcontrol/. Campaign For Our Children teen site with information about many contraceptives including DMPA-IM.

For Health Professionals

http://www.depoprovera.com/. Pfizer site on DMPA-IM.
http://www.depo-subqprovera104.com/. Pfizer site on DMPA-SC.
http://www.organon.com/products/gynecology/contraception/implanon.asp. Organon site for ENG implant (not yet approved in the United States).

Telephone Hotlines for Health Providers

DMPA hotline: 1-866-554-DEPO (3376)

REFERENCES AND ADDITIONAL READINGS

de Abood M, de Castillo Z, Guerro F, et al. Effect of depo-provera or microgynon on the painful crises of sickle cell anemia patients. *Contraception* 1997;56:313.
Agrawal A, Robinson C. Spontaneous snapping of an implanon in two halves in situ. *J Fam Plann Reprod Health Care* 2003;29:238.
Balkus J, Miller L. Same-day administration of depot-medroxyprogesterone acetate injection: a retrospective chart review. *Contraception* 2005;71(5):395.
Beerthuizen R, van Beek A, Massai R, et al. Bone mineral density during long-term use of the progestagen contraceptive implant Implanon compared to a non-hormonal method of contraception. *Hum Reprod* 2000;15:118.
Beksinska ME, Smit JA, Kleinschmidt I, et al. Bone mineral density in women aged 40–49 years using depot-medroxyprogesterone acetate, norethisterone enanthate or combined oral contraceptives for contraception. *Contraception* 2005;71:170.
Biswas A, Viegas OA, Coeling Bennink HJ, et al. Implanon contraceptive implants: effects on carbohydrate metabolism. *Contraception* 2001;63:137.
Biswas A, Viegas OA, Roy AC. Effect of Implanon and Norplant subdermal contraceptive implants on serum lipids–a randomized comparative study. *Contraception* 2003;68:189.
Borgatta L, Murthy A, Chuang C, et al. Pregnancies diagnosed during Depo-Provera use. *Contraception* 2002;66:169.
Brache V, Faundes A, Alvarez F, et al. Nonmenstrual adverse events during use of implantable contraceptives for women: data from clinical trials. *Contraception* 2002;65:63.
Cherry S. Implanon. The new alternative. *Aust Fam Physician* 2002;31:897.
Civic D, Scholes D, Ichikawa L, et al. Depressive symptoms in users and non-users of depot medroxyprogesterone acetate. *Contraception* 2000;61:385.
Cromer BA, Smith RD, Blair JM, et al. A prospective study of adolescents who choose among levonorgestrel implant (Norplant), medroxyprogesterone acetate (Depo-Provera), or the combined oral contraceptive pill as contraception. *Pediatrics*. 1994;94(5):687.
Cromer BA, Harel Z. Prescribing long-acting progestin-only contraceptives to adolescents. *Contemp Ob Gyn* 1997;43:145.
Cromer BA, Lazebnik R, Rome E, et al. Double-blinded randomized controlled trial of estrogen supplementation in adolescent girls who receive depot medroxyprogesterone acetate for contraception. *Am J Obstet Gynecol* 2005;192:42.
Crosignani PG, Luciano A, Ray A, et al. Subcutaneous depot medroxyprogesterone acetate versus leuprolide acetate in the treatment of endometriosis-associated pain. *Hum Reprod* 2006;21(1):248.
Croxatto HB. Mechanisms that explain the contraceptive action of progestin implants for women. *Contraception* 2002;65:21.
Croxatto HB, Urbancsek J, Massai R, et al. Implanon Study Group. A multicentre efficacy and safety study of the single contraceptive implant Implanon. *Hum Reprod* 1999;14(4):976.
Darney PD, Klaisle C, Walker DM. The "pop-out" method of Norplant removal. *Adv Contracept* 1992;8:188.
Davies GC, Feng LX, Newton JR, et al. Release characteristics, ovarian activity and menstrual bleeding pattern with a single contraceptive implant releasing 3-ketodesogestrel. *Contraception* 1993;47:251.
Deslypere JP, Thiery M, Vermeulen A. Effect of hormonal contraception on plasma lipids. *Contraception* 1985;31:633.
Dialogues in Contraception Editorial Board. Dialogues. *Contraception* 2005;9(1):7.
Diaz S. Contraceptive implants and lactation. *Contraception* 2002;65:39.
Dorflinger LJ. Metabolic effects of implantable steroid contraceptives for women. *Contraception* 2002;65:47.
Edwards JE, Moore A. Implanon. A review of clinical studies. *Br J Fam Plann* 1999;24(4 Suppl):3.
Egberg N, van Beek A, Gunnervik C, et al. Effects on the hemostatic system and liver function in relation to Implanon

and Norplant. A prospective randomized clinical trial. *Contraception* 1998;58:93.

Glasier A. Implantable contraceptives for women: effectiveness, discontinuation rates, return of fertility, and outcome of pregnancies. *Contraception* 2002;65:29.

Gold MA. Contraception update: implantable and injectable methods. *Pediatr Ann* 1995;24:203.

Halderman LD, Nelson AL. Impact of early postpartum administration of progestin-only hormonal contraceptives compared with nonhormonal contraceptives on short-term breast-feeding patterns. *Am J Obstet Gynecol* 2002;186:1250.

Harel Z, Biro FM, Kollar LM. Depo-Provera in adolescents: effects of early second injection or prior oral contraception. *J Adolesc Health* 1995;16:379.

Harel Z, Biro FM, Kollar LM, et al. Adolescents' reasons for and experience after discontinuation of the long-acting contraceptives Depo-Provera and Norplant. *J Adolesc Health* 1996;19:118.

Harrison-Woolrych M, Hill R. Unintended pregnancies with the etonogestrel implant (Implanon): a case series from post-marketing experience in Australia. *Contraception* 2005;71:306.

Hellerstedt WL, Story M. Adolescent satisfaction with postpartum contraception and body weight concerns. *J Adolesc Health* 1998;22:446.

Hubacher D, Goco N, Gonzalez B, et al. Factors affecting continuation rates of DMPA. *Contraception* 1999;60:345.

Jain J, Dutton C, Nicosia A, et al. Pharmacokinetics, ovulation suppression and return to ovulation following a lower dose subcutaneous formulation of Depo-Provera. *Contraception* 2004a;70:11.

Jain J, Jakimiuk AJ, Bode FR, et al. Contraceptive efficacy and safety of DMPA-SC. *Contraception* 2004b;70:269.

Jordan A. Toxicology of progestogens of implantable contraceptives for women. *Contraception* 2002;65:3.

Kaunitz AM. Long-acting hormonal contraception: assessing impact on bone density, weight, and mood. *Int J Fertil Womens Med* 1999;44:110.

Lantz A, Nosher JL, Pasquale S, et al. Ultrasound characteristics of subdermally implanted Implanon contraceptive rods. *Contraception* 1997;56:323.

Liew DFM, Ng CSA, Yong YM, et al. Long-term effects of Depo-Provera on carbohydrate and lipid metabolism. *Contraception* 1985;31:51.

Lim SW, Rieder J, Coupey SM, et al. Depot medroxyprogesterone acetate use in inner-city, minority adolescents: continuation rates and characteristics of long-term users. *Arch Pediatr Adolesc Med* 1999;153:1068.

Makarainen L, van Beek A, Tuomivaara L, et al. Ovarian function during the use of a single contraceptive implant: Implanon compared with Norplant. *Fertil Steril* 1998;69:714.

Matson SC, Henderson KA, McGrath GJ. Physical findings and symptoms of depot medroxyprogesterone acetate use in adolescent females. *J Pediatr Adolesc Gynecol* 1997;10:18.

Meirik O. Implantable contraceptives for women. *Contraception* 2002;65:1.

Meirik O, Fraser IS, d'Arcangues C. WHO Consultation on Implantable Contraceptives for Women. Implantable contraceptives for women. *Hum Reprod Update* 2003;9:49.

Miller L, Patton DL, Meier A, et al. Depomedroxyprogesterone-induced hypoestrogenism and changes in vaginal flora and epithelium. *Obstet Gynecol* 2000;96:431.

Mishell DR Jr, Kharma KM, Thomeycroft IH, et al. Estrogenic activity in women receiving an injectable progesterone for contraception. *Am J Obstet Gynecol* 1972;113:372.

Moore LL, Valuck R, McDougall C, et al. A comparative study of one-year weight gain among users of medroxyprogesterone acetate, levonorgestrel implants, and oral contraceptives. *Contraception* 1995;52:215.

Morroni C, Grams M, Tiezzi L, et al. Immediate monthly combination contraception to facilitate initiation of the depot medroxyprogesterone acetate contraceptive injection. *Contraception* 2004;70:19.

Newton J, Newton P. Implanon: the single-rod subdermal contraceptive implant. *J Drug Eval* 2003;1:177.

O'Brien KO, Nathanson MS, Mancini J, et al. Calcium absorption is significantly higher in adolescents during pregnancy than in the early postpartum period. *Am J Clin Nutr* 2003;78:1188.

O'Dell CM, Forke DM, Polaneczky MM, et al. Depot medroxyprogesterone acetate or oral contraception in postpartum adolescents. *Obstet Gynecol* 1998;91:609.

Office of Family Planning. Depo-provera and bone density. *Family PACT Clinical Practice Committee.* Sacramento CA: California Department of Health Services, 2005.

Orr-Walker BJ, Evans MC, Ames RW, et al. The effect of past use of the injectable contraceptive depot medroxyprogesterone acetate on bone mineral density in normal post-menopausal women. *Clin Endocrinol (Oxf)* 1998;49:615.

Paul C, Skegg DC, Williams S. Depot medroxyprogesterone acetate: patterns of use and reasons for discontinuation. *Contraception* 1997;56:209.

Pelkman CL, Chow M, Heinbach RA, et al. Short-term effects of a progestational contraceptive drug on food intake, resting energy expenditure, and body weight in young women. *Am J Clin Nutr* 2001;73:19.

Petitti DB, Piaggio G, Mehta S, et al. Steroid hormone contraception and bone mineral density: a cross-sectional study in an international population. The WHO Study of Hormonal Contraception and Bone Health. *Obstet Gynecol* 2000;95:736.

Petta CA, Faundes A, Dunson TR, et al. Timing of onset of contraceptive effectiveness in Depo-Provera users: part I. Changes in cervical mucus. *Fertil Steril* 1998;69:252.

Pickard S, Bacon L. Persistent vaginal bleeding in a patient with a broken Implanon. *J Fam Plann Reprod Health Care* 2002;28:207.

Pinkston-Koenigs LM, Miller NH. The contraceptive use of Depo-Provera in U.S. adolescents. *J Adolesc Health* 1995;16:347.

Polaneczky M, Liblanc M. Long-term depot medroxyprogesterone acetate (Depo-Provera) use in inner-city adolescents. *J Adolesc Health* 1998;23:81.

Rahimy MH, Cromie MA, Hopkins NK, et al. Lunelle monthly contraceptive injection (medroxyprogesterone acetate and estradiol cypionate injectable suspension): effects of body weight and injection sites on pharmacokinetics. *Contraception* 1999;60:201.

Redmond GP, Olson WH, Lippman JS, et al. Norgestimate and ethinyl estradiol in the treatment of acne vulgaris: a randomized, placebo-controlled trial. *Obstet Gynecol* 1997;89:615.

Reinprayoon D, Taneepanichskul S, Bunyavejchevin S, et al. Effects of the etonogestrel-releasing contraceptive implant (Implanon) on parameters of breastfeeding compared to those of an intrauterine device. *Contraception* 2000;62:239.

Risser WL, Gefter LR, Barratt MS, et al. Weight change in adolescents who used hormonal contraception. *J Adolesc Health* 1999;24:433.

Sangi-Haghpeykar H, Poindexter AN III, Bateman L, et al. Experiences of injectable contraceptive users in an urban setting. *Obstet Gynecol* 1996;88:227.

Schwallie PC, Assenzo JR. The effect of depo-medroxyprogesterone acetate on pituitary and ovarian function, and the return of fertility following its discontinuation: a review. *Contraception* 1974;10:181.

Smith A, Reuter S. An assessment of the use of Implanon in three community services. *J Fam Plann Reprod Health Care* 2002; 28:193.

Taneepanichskul S, Reinprayoon D, Khaosaad P. Comparative study of weight change between long-term DMPA and IUD acceptors. *Contraception* 1998;58:149.

Templeman C, Boyd H, Hertweck SP. Depomedroxyprogesterone acetate use and weight gain among adolescents. *J Pediatr Adolesc Gynecol* 2000;13:45.

Trussell J. Contraceptive efficacy. In: Hatcher RA, Trussell J, Stewart F, et al. eds. *Contraceptive technology*, 18th ed. New York: Ardent Media, 2004:773.

Wenck BC, Johnston PJ. Implanon and medical indemnity: a case study of risk management using the Australian standard. *Med J Aust* 2004;181:117.

Wenzl R, van Beek A, Schnabel P, et al. Pharmacokinetics of etonogestrel released from the contraceptive implant Implanon. *Contraception* 1998;58:283.

Westfall JM, Main DS, Barnard L. Continuation rates among injectable contraceptive users. *Fam Plann Perspect* 1996;28:275.

Westhoff C. Depot medroxyprogesterone acetate contraception: metabolic parameters and mood changes. *J Reprod Med* 1996;41(5 Suppl):401.

Westhoff C, Wieland D, Tiezzi L. Depression in users of depomedroxyprogesterone acetate. *Contraception* 1995;51:351.

World Health Organization, Department of Reproductive Health and Research. *Medical eligibility criteria for contraceptive use*, 3rd ed. Geneva: World Health Organization, 2004.

World Health Organization, Department of Reproductive Health and Research. *Selected practice recommendations for contraceptive use*, 2nd ed. Geneva: World Health Organization, 2005.

World Health Organization Expanded Programme of Research, Development and Research Training in Human Reproduction Task Force on Long-Acting Systemic Agents for Regulation of Fertility. Multinational comparative clinical evaluation of two long-acting injectable contraceptive steroids: norethisterone enanthate and medroxyprogesterone acetate. *Contraception* 1983;28:1.

Zheng SR, Zheng HM, Qian SZ, et al. A randomized multicenter study comparing the efficacy and bleeding pattern of a single-rod (Implanon) and a six-capsule (Norplant) hormonal contraceptive implant. *Contraception* 1999;60:1.

PART XII

Adolescent Gynecology

CHAPTER 48

Gynecological Examination of the Adolescent Female

Merrill Weitzel and Jean S. Emans

A gynecological examination is an essential component of the health care of adolescent girls. This is especially important because the first pelvic examination can influence an adolescent's attitudes about reproductive health care for the rest of her life. Most adolescents are apprehensive about the examination of their genitalia, especially during a first examination. A sensitive approach to the adolescent's concerns and needs can aid in creating a positive and instructive experience.

OFFICE SETTING

The office setting is particularly important in creating a positive atmosphere for the adolescent girl. To create such an atmosphere a clinician should do the following:

1. Provide an office setting that is a comfortable and friendly. Support staff should be welcoming. A special seating area for teens with appropriate reading material is optimal. Privacy is a fundamental component for teens. An assessment of office procedures—such as weighing patients in the examination room, not in hallways—is key to meeting the needs of teens for privacy. Teens who wish to contact the office by telephone should have easy access to staff to schedule appointments and ask questions.
2. Special appointment times can be reserved for teens. Late afternoon or evening appointments may be more convenient for teens than morning times.
3. Practices limited to adolescents can have posters and pamphlets directed at the concerns of teens, such as smoking cessation, healthy nutrition, sexual decision-making, "how to say no," birth control, sexually transmitted diseases (STDs), and human immunodeficiency virus (HIV) infection. Practices with patients of a wider age range usually opt for neutral decors but can still have pamphlets and materials displayed in areas "especially for teens" within the examination room. Computer "hot spots" with pertinent Web sites posted may be helpful.
4. Parents of adolescent patients should be included as much as possible in the history gathering and medical plan. However, the adolescent's need for medical privacy and confidentiality should be respected. An explicit statement (and in some practices a written statement) about confidentiality should be included early in the discussion because it will encourage more open discussion about risk behaviors. The limits of confidentiality (conditions that are life threatening or that require reporting by law) should also be discussed with the patient and her family.
5. During part of the gynecological assessment, the adolescent should be interviewed privately in a comfortable environment about risk behaviors and health-promoting behaviors. If at all possible, she should be fully clothed and seated eye-to-eye with the examiner for the first visit. Reassure her that what she communicates, regarding her reproductive health will be kept confidential. She should be made aware that the results of the examination will not be discussed with her parents or others without her permission but that you will encourage her to share her health concerns, medications prescribed, and management plans with her parents or caretakers.
6. Be aware of the fears and worries of the adolescent about the pelvic examination. These fears may be expressed as anxiety or occasionally as hostility. Ask the patient about her feelings concerning the examination and the worries or questions that she may have regarding her body. Many teens are worried about pain, discomfort, or embarrassment ("It will hurt" or "The doctor will judge me"), and need to be reassured about the tempo of the examination. The adolescent needs to feel in control of the tempo of each part of the examination.
7. Listening to rather than lecturing the adolescent is essential. The examination can be a critical time for health education and for helping the teen to value and protect her body. A virginal teen may be concerned about whether the examination will alter her hymen and should be reassured that the small speculum that is used was designed for girls who have not had intercourse. Girls who have used tampons are generally more comfortable with their bodies and can be particularly reassured as to the ease of the examination. Dispelling myths and respecting cultural preferences about pelvic examinations is important.
8. During each step of the examination, it is important to reassure the teen of her normality, as appropriate. The question, "Am I normal?" may be an underlying reason for any teen's visit. Other concerns may be "Do I have a STD?" or "Are my labia too big?"

INDICATIONS FOR GYNECOLOGICAL EXAMINATIONS

The indications for a complete or modified pelvic examination in an adolescent vary with the patient's complaint. For example, a 13-year-old girl who is not sexually active and who has a white vaginal discharge may be evaluated by obtaining one or two saline-moistened cotton-tipped applicator samples of the discharge and by examining the samples under the microscope for physiological discharge or *Candida* vaginitis. In contrast, a 16-year-old, sexually active girl who has had lower abdominal pain for 2 days and has a vaginal discharge deserves a complete pelvic examination. It is also important for clinicians to assess whether the answer can be obtained by the use of urine-based STD screening for *Chlamydia trachomatis* and/or *Neisseria gonorrhea* or by pelvic ultrasonography. For example, a girl with primary amenorrhea may be willing to allow only an external genital inspection; the internal genital structures can then be assessed by transabdominal ultrasonography.

Most professional organizations suggest that cervical cancer screening be initiated at 21 years of age or 3 years after the onset of sexual activity, whichever occurs first. Girls receiving episodic care or who are immunosuppressed (e.g., HIV infection) should be screened earlier. The American College of Obstetricians and Gynecologists recommends annual Pap tests in women younger than 30 years after initiation of screening. An adolescent who is not sexually active can begin routine gynecological care whenever she feels comfortable, with the hope that by the age of 18 to 21 years she will have initiated routine care. However, the age of 18 to 21 years should be seen as a general guideline, and the wishes and background of the patient should be respected. It should be stressed that adolescents should have routine health guidance initiated before becoming sexually active. The American College of Obstetricians and Gynecologists recommends that the first visit for health guidance, screening, and preventive services should take place approximately at 13 to 15 years of age. It is an ideal time to provide education about preventive care needs, including the need for STD testing in sexually active females. Providers should separate the provision of contraceptive services and STD screening from requirements of cervical cancer screening. Pelvic examinations should not be a barrier to the prescription of oral contraception and other effective hormonal methods. In addition, patients and parents need to understand that there is still a need for preventive health care other than Pap testing. It is important for patients (and their parents) to realize that a pelvic examination and a Pap test are not the same. Most importantly, the first pelvic examination should be an educational and positive experience. Indications for modified or complete pelvic examinations therefore include the following:

1. Sexually active (vaginal intercourse) (within 3 years)
2. Symptoms of vaginal or uterine infection
3. Menstrual disorders including amenorrhea, dysfunctional uterine bleeding, severe dysmenorrhea, or mild-to-moderate dysmenorrhea unresponsive to therapy
4. Undiagnosed lower abdominal pain
5. Sexual assault (modified to collect the appropriate information and samples)
6. Suspected pelvic mass
7. Request by the adolescent

OBTAINING THE HISTORY

The history should include a gynecological assessment, general health history, review of systems, and information on risk behaviors. The HEADSS framework can be used; it focuses on *H*ome, *E*ducation/career plans, *A*ctivities, *D*rugs/alcohol/tobacco, *D*epression, *S*uicidality, *S*exuality, and *S*afety. These questions can be asked through a clinical interview, a written questionnaire, or a computer-aided questionnaire. Most of the visit should be devoted to seeing the teenager alone, because her presenting complaint is often different from her parents' concerns. However, it is essential to understand the concerns and the family history of the parent or parents. Mothers often attribute symptoms of their daughters to diagnoses that they themselves have had, such as ovarian cysts or other gynecological problems within the family. Although some medical conditions (e.g., polycystic ovary syndrome, endometriosis) clearly can occur within families, many other conditions are not related to the complaint that brings the teen to the clinician.

It is essential to know what the parent told the patient regarding the reason for the visit and whether the examination was explained. If the parent discussed the examination with the patient, it is important to gather information on how it was explained. Some patients are told, "Don't worry, you don't need an examination," and others are told about the full speculum examination when potentially they only need one or two cotton-tipped applicator samples. It is also important to know what and how the parent has explained about menstrual periods, sexuality, and other issues to the young adolescent.

The younger teen may feel more comfortable if most of the history is obtained with parent or parents in the room. A few moments of privacy are all that is needed to obtain pertinent negatives about risk behaviors. It is often best to begin the interview by asking the adolescent why they have come to the office for an evaluation that day. It is imperative to address the chief complaint and to relate the gynecological examination (modified or complete) to that concern. Reasons for the visit may include pelvic pain, vaginal discharge, a menstrual disorder, or a possible pregnancy. A presenting complaint such as irregular menses may actually lead to a diagnosis of pregnancy; in such cases, the patient may be denying the possibility of pregnancy, or a menstrual complaint may be the only way for her to access medical care. Dysmenorrhea may mask a "hidden agenda" for obtaining oral contraceptives. The sexual history should be part of the structured questioning: "Have you ever had sexual intercourse?" "How old were you when you first had sex?" "Tell me about your partners." "Are you sexually active with men? Women? Both?" "How many partners have you had?" "Have you ever been pregnant?" "Have you ever had a STD?" "Have you ever been forced to have sexual intercourse?" "Have you ever used condoms?" "If yes, how often?" It is important that these questions be preceded by the comment, "I ask all my patients these questions."

The history should include the following:

1. Menstrual history
   a. Age at menarche
   b. Duration of menses and interval between periods; intermenstrual staining
   c. Amount of flow and any recent changes in amount of flow (this is often best accomplished by asking

whether the patient uses tampons or pads and how often during the day she needs to change).
  d. Date of last menstrual period
  e. Dysmenorrhea—if present, severity and extent of missed school or activities
  f. Premenstrual symptoms
2. History and type of vaginal discharge
3. Sexual history
  a. Relationships, sexual contact, number and age of partners (men, women, or both), age at first sexual intercourse
  b. Contraceptive methods used: Condoms ever? Frequency of use? ("all the time?" "never miss?") Use at last intercourse? Previous use of hormonal contraceptive—benefits, problems
  c. Prior STDs: Gonorrhea, chlamydia, syphilis, herpes, warts, HIV, pelvic inflammatory disease
  d. Prior pregnancies (number and outcome of each—abortion, term, ectopic, miscarriage), and fertility concerns. Trying to get pregnant now?
  e. Pap smear screening: Ever had a Pap test? When was the last Pap performed? Ever had an abnormal Pap smear? Colposcopy?
  f. If the patient is sexually active, ask whether her partner treats her well and whether she has ever been in a situation where she felt unsafe, felt coerced to have sex, or was hit or slapped
4. Family history
  a. Family history of gynecological problems (e.g., polycystic ovary syndrome, endometriosis)
  b. Blood clotting disorders or stroke
  c. Breast cancer or gynecological cancer (cervical, ovarian, uterine)

GYNECOLOGICAL EXAMINATION EQUIPMENT

Materials needed for the gynecological examination include the following:

1. Examination table with ankle supports: Oven mittens or other cloth holders placed over the metal supports increase foot comfort
2. Gowns, sheets
3. Light source (speculum light or lamp)
4. Specula: Metal—Pederson or Huffman (also sometimes called a *Huffman-Graves speculum*)—or plastic (medium and small), with or without self-contained light source
5. Gonorrhea culture medium or nonculture gonorrhea test (can also be done on urine)
6. *Chlamydia* screening tests (e.g., NAATS) (can also be done on urine)
7. Spatula and cytobrush (or cytobroom) for Pap test
8. Cotton swabs and either tubes or slides for wet mounts
9. Ten percent potassium hydroxide (KOH) and saline for wet mounts, pH paper
10. Pap slide containers and fixative, or kits for ThinPrep or other Pap systems
11. Water-soluble lubricating jelly
12. Warm water source
13. Nonsterile gloves
14. Handheld mirror (use is optional and up to the patient)
15. Tissues
16. Tampons and sanitary napkins
17. Rapid pregnancy test kits

PELVIC EXAMINATION

A pelvic examination is generally performed annually for sexually active adolescents starting approximately three years after the initiation of sexual intercourse. The adolescent should be made to feel that she is in control and can stop the examination at any point to ask questions or, if need be, stop the examination entirely. A handheld mirror to permit viewing of her genitalia is helpful for some adolescents. The clinician should acknowledge that adolescent girls may feel nervous, particularly at the first examination. Explain that it takes only 2 or 3 minutes to perform the examination. Adolescents should be given the choice of whether to have their mother or another person (e.g., sister, aunt) stay in the room as support. The young adolescent may request that her mother stay with her during the pelvic examination; most older patients prefer that their mothers stay in the waiting room. The patient's wishes should be respected. Generally, male providers use a female chaperone for pelvic examinations. Female providers in some settings always use chaperones, and in other settings the use is considered optional. Many patients actually prefer to have only the provider in the room.

Before the examination begins, it is helpful to explain to the teen, while she is still fully clothed and seated, the various parts of the examination—general physical examination, inspection of the genitalia, speculum examination, and bimanual examination, indicating the reasons why each part is important for evaluating her medical complaint. It is also good, both in the early discussion and during the examination to talk about feelings related to the examination and ways to relax and feel in control, such as the use of imagery, deep breathing and other relaxation techniques, a mirror, a step-by-step format, or distraction from a family member. She should also be reassured that adequate drapes will be used. Each step is then explained again as the actual examination is done.

The steps are as follows:

1. Make sure that the patient has emptied her bladder before the examination.
2. Ask the patient to undress completely and put on a gown.
3. Perform a general examination including inspection of the skin (acne, hirsutism, acanthosis nigricans); palpation of the thyroid gland; and examination of the breasts, heart, abdomen, and inguinal area for lymphadenopathy.
4. Have the patient lie supine on the examination table, feet resting either in or on the ankle supports. Instruct the patient to slide her buttocks to the edge of the table. Elevating the head of the table 30 degrees is optional; it can provide the adolescent an increased sense of control and can make sliding down easier. The foot of the examination table should be turned away from a doorway. The drape or sheet should be positioned so that eye contact can be maintained with the patient.
5. Ask the patient to touch her knees to your hands, which are held out to the side. Do not try to pry her legs apart.
6. Inspect the external genitalia (Fig. 48.1).
  a. Note pubic hair distribution and sexual maturity rating (Tanner stage).
  b. Assess for signs of erythema, inflammation, nevi, warts, or other lesions over the perineum, thighs, mons, labia, and perianal region. After informing the patient that you are about to do so, place the palms of both hands adjacent to the labia majora and gently

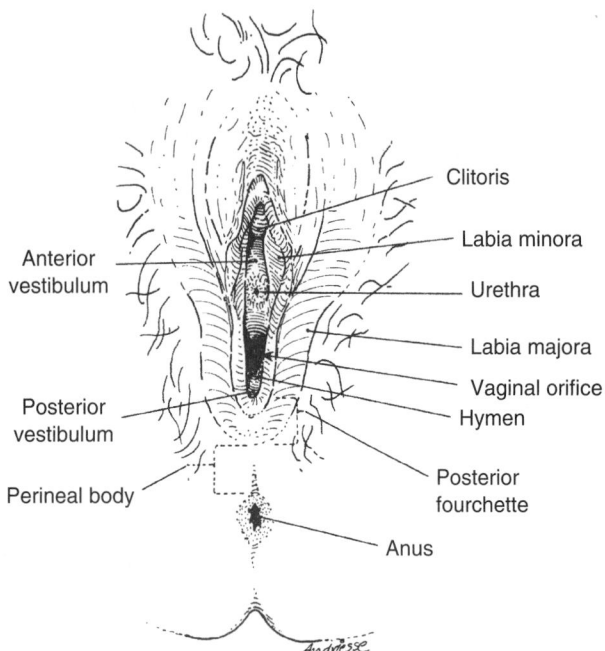

FIGURE 48.1 External genitalia of the pubertal female. (Reproduced from Emans SJ, Laufer MR, Goldstein DP. *Pediatric* and *adolescent gynecology*, 5th ed. Philadelphia: Lippincott Williams & Wilkins; 2005, with permission.)

separate them to examine the external structures. Check the size of the clitoris, which is typically 2 to 4 mm wide; a width of 5 to 10 mm is considered a possible sign of virilization, and >10 mm indicates definite virilization.

- Skene glands: These are two small glands located just inside the urethra. They are usually not visible.
- Bartholin glands: These are two small mucus-secreting glands located just outside the hymeneal ring at the 5 and 7 o'clock positions. They can become enlarged, infected, or both.

c. The hymen should be carefully inspected for estrogen effect (light pink, thickened), for congenital anomalies (septate, imperforate, microperforate), and for transections that might result from consensual or nonconsensual sexual intercourse. For girls who are being evaluated for prior sexual abuse or assault, a saline-moistened cotton-tipped applicator can be used to run the edge of the hymen to look for transections. With gentle retraction, the anterior vagina may be visible and again the estrogen effect can be observed—pink mucosa, white vaginal secretions.

d. Obtaining samples: For patients who need a vaginal smear done to assess estrogenization (amenorrhea) or who need wet mounts obtained to evaluate vaginal discharge, saline-moistened or dry cotton-tipped applicators can be used to obtain samples (see later discussion). This may be all that is needed to assess the particular gynecological complaint.

7. Speculum examination: The correct size of speculum should be selected, and the speculum should be warmed, if possible, before insertion. It should not be lubricated with anything other than water if a Pap test or other

samples are to be taken (Fig. 48.2). If the hymeneal opening is small, a Huffman (Huffman-Graves) speculum ($\frac{1}{2} \times 4\frac{1}{2}$ in.) is used to visualize the cervix. For the sexually active teen, a Pederson speculum ($\frac{7}{8} \times 4\frac{1}{2}$ in.) or occasionally a Graves speculum ($\frac{3}{8} \times 3\frac{3}{4}$ in.) is appropriate. A plastic speculum with an attached light source is also useful for facilitating the examination. Some examiners believe it is helpful to remove the speculum from its package and show it to the patient. Other experts believe that the value of showing the adolescent the speculum in advance is limited and that the adolescent may become more fearful of the examination. If you choose to show the adolescent the speculum, explain that although the speculum is long it is the exact length of the vagina and allows visualization of the cervix, which is the opening of the uterus located at the end of the vagina. In the virginal teenager a one-finger, gloved (water-moistened) examination demonstrates the size of the hymeneal opening and the location of the cervix and allows subsequent easy insertion of the speculum. To avoid surprising the patient during the speculum examination, touch the speculum to the thigh first and tell the patient that you are going to place the cool speculum into the vagina. The speculum should be inserted posteriorly in a downward direction to avoid the urethra (Fig. 48.3). Applying pressure to the inner thigh at the same time the speculum is inserted into the vagina may be helpful.

a. Observe the vaginal walls for signs of estrogenization, inflammation, or lesions.

b. Inspect the cervix. The stratified squamous epithelium of the external os is usually a dull pink color. There is often a more erythematous area of columnar epithelium surrounding the cervical os, called a *cervical ectropion*. The junction between the two types of mucosa is called the *squamocolumnar junction*, and it is particularly important that this area be sampled during the Pap test screening. This ectropion may persist throughout the adolescent years, especially in hormonal contraceptive users. Mucopurulent discharge from the cervix characterizes cervicitis, typical of infections with *N. gonorrhea, C. trachomatis,* and herpes virus. Small, pinpoint hemorrhagic spots on the cervix, so-called "strawberry" cervix, can occur rarely with *Trichomonas* infections. The cervix should be examined for any lesions or polyps. Any abnormal growth on the cervix should be referred for further evaluation and colposcopy.

c. To assess signs and symptoms of vaginitis, swabs for wet mounts and pH can be obtained from the vagina and then placed in one or two drops of saline on one slide (for *Trichomonas*, white cells, or "clue cells") and in one drop of 10% KOH (for pseudohyphae) on another slide. A swab should also be applied to pH paper; a pH <4.5 suggests normal physiological discharge or *Candida* infection, and a pH >4.5 suggests bacterial vaginosis or *Trichomonas* infection.

d. If indicated, obtain a Pap test of the cervix. This should include at least a 360-degree rotation of the spatula in contact with the cervix, with care taken to sample the "transition zone" or squamocolumnar junction. Nylon cytobrushes are also commonly used in addition to the spatula, thereby ensuring the collection of cells from the endocervical canal.

e. Endocervical tests for STDs: Tests for gonorrhea and chlamydia include nucleic acid amplification tests

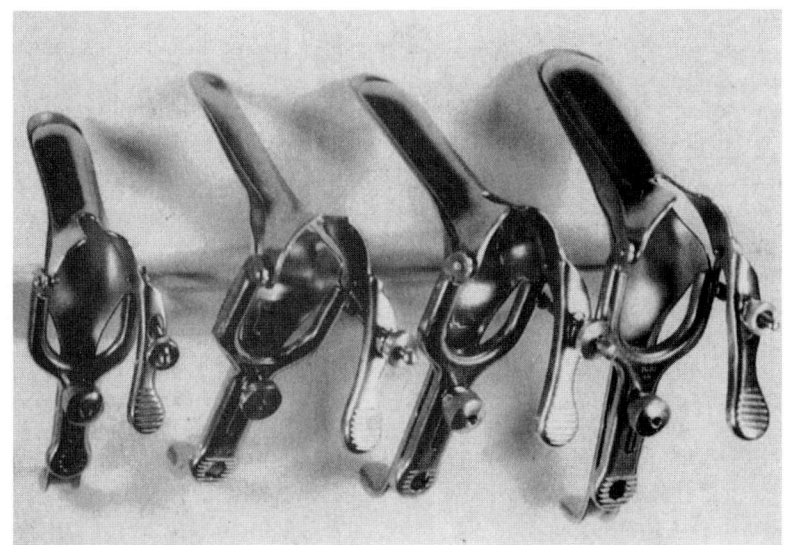

FIGURE 48.2 Types of specula *(left to right)*: infant, Huffman, Pederson, and Graves. (Reproduced from Emans SJ, Laufer MR, Goldstein DP. *Pediatric and adolescent gynecology,* 5th ed. Philadelphia: Lippincott Williams & Wilkins; 2005, with permission.)

(NAATs), DNA probes, immunoassays, and cultures. Endocervical *Chlamydia* NAAT screening has higher sensitivity than urine screening, but urine screening is an excellent option if a pelvic examination is not being performed. The speculum is removed after the samples for STD tests are obtained.

8. Bimanual examination: The bimanual vaginal–abdominal examination involves the insertion of one or two gloved, lubricated fingers into the vagina while the other hand is placed on the abdomen. If this is her first bimanual examination, it is worthwhile to have the patient practice relaxing her abdominal muscles first: "Take a few deep breaths and blow it out." Once her abdomen is relaxed, the bimanual examination can begin. Remind the patient

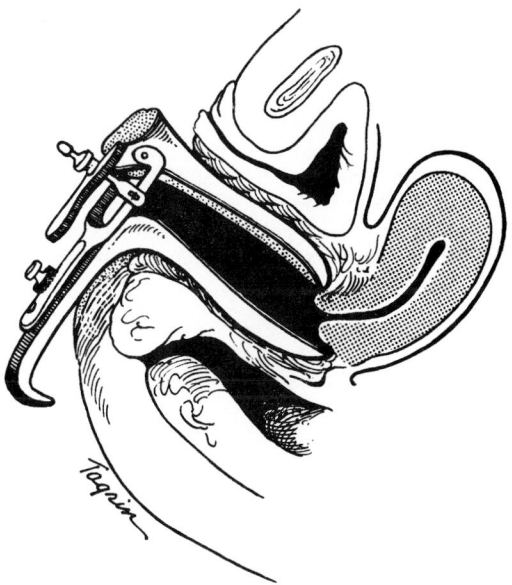

FIGURE 48.3 Speculum examination of the cervix. (From Clarke-Pearson D, Dawood M. *Green's gynecology: essentials of clinical practice,* 4th ed. Boston: Little, Brown and Company; 1990, with permission.)

that you will be examining her uterus and ovaries and to communicate any feelings of discomfort she may be experiencing during the examination. If it is not comfortable for the patient to tolerate a vaginal–abdominal examination or there are cultural preferences, then a rectal–abdominal examination, in the lithotomy position, usually will yield the needed information.

a. Palpation of the vagina and cervix: Check for lesions along the side walls and on the cervix and any tenderness on cervical motion.

b. Palpation of the uterus: Assess the size, the position of the uterus, and any masses or tenderness. Pushing backward on the cervix causes the uterus to move anteriorly, allowing for its palpation with the abdominal hand.

c. Gently explore the posterior fornix and the rectouterine pouch (pouch of Douglas) for masses, fullness, and tenderness.

d. Palpation of the adnexa: Assess for any masses, tenderness, or abnormalities of the ovaries or the adnexal area. To palpate these structures, insert the examining fingers into each lateral fornix, positioning them slightly posteriorly and high. Sweep the abdominal examining hand downward over the internal fingers. Normal ovaries are usually <3 cm long and are rubbery.

If there is a history of significant pelvic pain or an adnexal mass is felt, a rectovaginal–abdominal examination can help complete the evaluation of the adnexa or uterus and the rectum, anus, and posterior cul-de-sac. A rectovaginal–abdominal examination is performed with the index finger in the vagina, the middle finger in the rectum, and the other hand on the abdomen. The examination permits evaluation of the uterosacral ligaments and cul-de-sac as well as the mobility of the uterus. It is important to inform the patient that she may experience an urge to defecate: "You may feel like you are having a bowel movement, but you won't go. Your brain is just giving you a different message." The rectovaginal septum should be thin and pliable, and the pelvic floor should be free of masses and tenderness. On indication, stool retrieved can be tested for occult blood.

9. At the completion of the examination, offer the patient a box of tissues to be used to remove the lubrication from her perineum after you leave the room. Some patients may require assistance in sliding up the table before taking their feet out of the ankle supports. Instruct the patient to dress fully and return to the office for a discussion of your findings and plan. Before the practitioner leaves the room, the patient should be in a sitting position and draped.

During the postexamination discussion, the patient should be congratulated for her cooperation, and the importance of the findings of the examination (positive or negative), should be discussed in relation to her chief complaint. All questions should be answered, and any therapy and further tests required should be outlined. This is an important time for discussion of the adolescent's concerns about normal anatomy and physiology, contraception (including emergency contraception), and sexuality. Reinforce the positive experience of sharing her information with you as a demonstration of her ability to think about her sexual health and be responsible. During this discussion with the adolescent, it is important for the examiner to listen carefully, remembering that teenagers may not communicate all their concerns initially. At the conclusion of the discussion, the parent or partner can be invited to join the health care provider and the teenager. The parent can be informed of the results of the examination and the treatment plan. Any confidential information that is revealed to the parent should have been previously agreed upon with the teenager, so as to maintain trust. Parents should be encouraged to ask questions and to voice concerns.

Helping a teen through her first gynecological visit sets the stage for reproductive health care for a lifetime. The gynecological visit is an ideal opportunity to provide education, listen to concerns, assess medical and psychosocial complaints, and promote a healthy future. The examination also allows the clinician an opportunity to impart to the teenager a positive attitude toward her body and to stress the importance of health maintenance.

WEB SITES

For Teenagers and Parents

http://www.youngwomenshealth.org/pelvicinfo.html. Information about your first pelvic examination from Boston Children's Hospital.

http://www.goaskalice.columbia.edu/0643.html. From Columbia University for college students and older teens. Questions and answers about reproductive health and specifically here about pelvic examination.

http://www.sa.psu.edu/uhs/womenshealth/pelvicexam.cfm. From Penn State University Health Service, information about pelvic examination and Pap smears.

www.cdc.gov/std/hpv. Centers for Disease Control about sexually transmitted diseases and HPV.

http://teenadvice.about.com/cs/girlstuff/ht/pelvicexamht.htm. A Web site on the first pelvic examination developed in collaboration with The New York Times.

REFERENCES AND ADDITIONAL READINGS

American College of Obstetricians and Gynecologists. Cervical cancer screening in adolescents. ACOG Committee Opinion No. 300. *Obstet Gynecol* 2004;104(4):885.

Emans SJ, Laufer MR, Goldstein DP. *Pediatric and adolescent gynecology*, 5th ed. Philadelphia: Lippincott Williams & Wilkins; 2005.

Emans SJ, Woods ER, Allred EN, et al. Hymenal findings in adolescent women: impact of tampon use and consensual sexual activity. *J Pediatr* 1994;125:153.

Ford CA, Millstein SG, Halpern-Feilsher BL, et al. Influence of physician confidentiality assurances on adolescents' willingness to disclose information and seek future health care. *JAMA* 1997;278:1029.

Gray SH, Walzer TB. New strategies for cervical cancer screening in adolescents. *Curr Opin Pediatr* 2004;16:344.

Kahn J, Chiou V, Allen J, et al. Beliefs about Pap smears and compliance with Pap smear follow-up in adolescents. *Arch Pediatr Adolesc Med* 1999;153:1046.

Larsen SB, Kragstrup J. Experiences of the first pelvic examination in a random sample of Danish teenagers. *Acta Obstet Gynecol Scand* 1995;74:137.

Millstein SG, Adler NE, Irwin CE Jr. Sources of anxiety about pelvic examinations among adolescent females. *J Adolesc Health Care* 1984;5:105.

Saslow D, Runowicz CD, Solomon D, et al. American Cancer Society guideline for the early detection of cervical neoplasia and cancer. *CA Cancer J Clin* 2002;52:342.

Thrall JS, McCloskey L, Ettner SL, et al. Confidentiality and adolescents' use of providers for health information and for pelvic examinations. *Arch Pediatr Adolesc Med* 2000;154:885.

CHAPTER 49

Normal Menstrual Physiology

Sari L. Kives and Judith A. Lacy

This chapter reviews normal menstrual physiology and the next several chapters discuss common abnormalities of menstrual function in adolescents.

The development of the menstrual cycle depends on the maturation of the hypothalamic-pituitary-ovarian axis that occurs during puberty. For cyclic menses to occur, there must be a coordinated sequence of events, beginning with the hypothalamic secretion of gonadotropin-releasing hormone (GnRH). In response to GnRH, the pituitary secretes follicle-stimulating hormone (FSH) and luteinizing hormone (LH), and the ovaries secrete, estrogen, progesterone, activin, and inhibins. Ultimately, the endometrium of the uterus responds to estrogen and progesterone with stimulation and endometrial growth, as well as withdrawal. This process culminates in menses.

The menstrual cycle is under the influence of both positive and negative feedback mechanisms. In the beginning of the menstrual cycle, low levels of estradiol perpetuate a positive feedback mechanism and subsequently stimulate secretion of FSH and LH. At higher levels, estradiol and progesterone create a negative feedback effect and suppress FSH and LH, thereby preventing further follicular recruitment. Although the gonadotropins act synergistically, FSH primarily affects follicular growth and LH mainly stimulates ovarian steroid biosynthesis.

Although the trigger for menarche is unknown, hypothesized mechanisms for the onset of menses include the following:

1. A progressive decrease in the sensitivity of the hypothalamus to gonadal steroids made possible by the following:
   a. A decrease in the negative feedback settings of the hypothalamus to estradiol and testosterone, resulting in higher levels of LH and FSH.
   b. The rise in LH and FSH may be secondary to a central biological clock, altering GnRH response and unrelated to feedback sensitivity to gonadal steroid secretion.
   c. A rise in LH secretion: During early puberty LH spikes occur only at night, in a pulsatile manner. In late puberty and adulthood, pulsatile LH secretion occurs throughout the day and night.
2. An increase in the pulsatile secretion of GnRH, both in amplitude and in frequency, leading to an increase in sex steroid secretion. Ultimately, the development of a positive feedback system allows critical levels of estradiol to trigger pulsatile secretion of GnRH and subsequently that of LH.
3. A critical body composition or percentage of body fat. There is evidence to suggest that menarche occurs at approximately 17% body fat. The maintenance or restoration of menstruation is thought to require a minimum of 22% body fat (Frisch and McArthur, 1974).

In the United States, menarche occurs in girls at an average age of approximately 12.7 years, with a range (2 standard deviations) of 11 to 15 years. In approximately two thirds of girls, menarche occurs at sexual maturity rating (SMR) 4 (Tanner pubertal stage 4).

Menarche occurs approximately 3.3 years after the start of the growth spurt, approximately 2 years after thelarche, and approximately 1.1 years after the peak height velocity. The earlier the onset of puberty (secondary sexual characteristics) the longer is the interval until the onset of menses. Additionally, females who have a late menarche will also experience a longer duration of anovulatory cycles (Emans, 2005). Menarche is followed by approximately 5 to 7 years of increasing regularity as the cycles shorten to reach the usual reproductive pattern. The greatest variability in cycle length occurs in the immediate years following the onset of menarche and those preceding the menopause (Silberstein and Merriam, 2000).

DEFINITION OF MENSTRUAL CYCLE

A menstrual cycle is defined as that period of time from the first day of menstrual period to the first day of the next menstrual flow. On the basis of current understanding, the menstrual cycle may be described by the response of the pituitary (i.e., FSH and LH levels), the ovary (follicular, ovulatory, and luteal phases), and the endometrium (proliferative and secretory phases) (Fig. 49.1).

FSH and LH are secreted in a pulsatile manner, with frequency varying between 1 and 2 hours in the follicular and luteal phases, respectively. The pulsatile spikes are higher in amplitude during the luteal phase. The pulsatile secretion of FSH and LH are secondary to the pulsatile secretion of GnRH from the hypothalamus. The pulsatile release of GnRH can be modulated by estradiol and progesterone feedback. Neurotransmitters (i.e., dopamine, norepinephrine) and endorphins (opioids) also play a role

FIGURE 49.1 Normal menstrual cycle. LH, luteinizing hormone; FSH, follicle-stimulating hormone. (Reproduced from Neinstein LS. Menstrual disorders. *Semin Fam Med* 1981;2:184.)

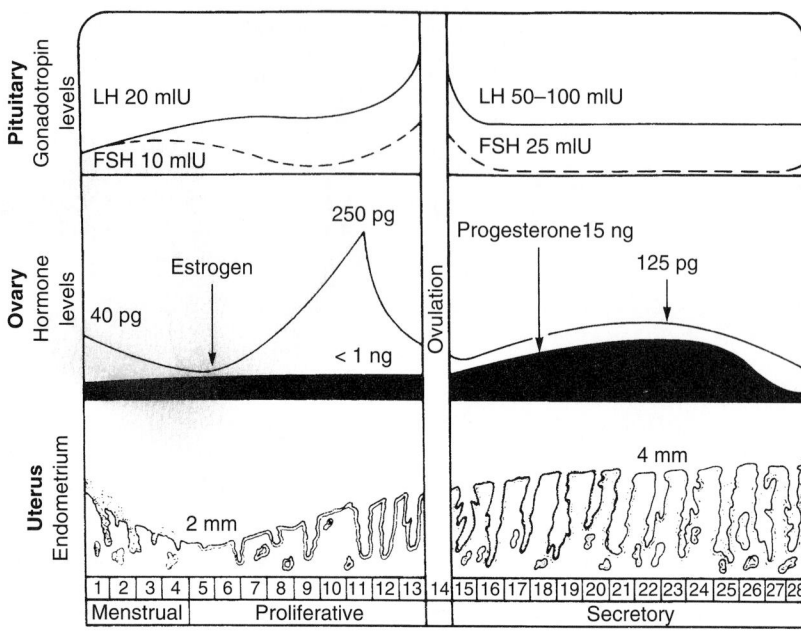

in modulating GnRH secretion. Menstrual irregularities that occur with weight loss, stress, exercise, and drugs may be secondary to the effect of these compounds on the hypothalamus.

The physiological mechanisms of the menstrual cycle can be divided into three descriptive phases—the follicular phase, the ovulatory phase, and the luteal phase.

Follicular Phase

The duration of the follicular phase is usually 14 days, but the length is highly variable (range 7 to 22 days). This phase begins with the onset of menses and ends with ovulation. The duration of the follicular phase is the major determinant of menstrual cycle length.

1. During the end of the prior menstrual cycle, corpus luteum involution occurs, with resulting decreasing levels of estradiol and progesterone. The low levels stimulate the hypothalamic release of GnRH, which in turn increases the pituitary's release of FSH and LH.
2. FSH stimulates the recruitment of ovarian follicles.
3. At present, it is believed that LH stimulates ovarian theca cells to produce androgens, which are then converted to estrogens in the granulosa cells of the ovary under the influence of FSH (Fig. 49.2). Estradiol increases FSH binding to granulosa cell receptors, leading to amplification of the FSH effect, allowing one follicle to predominate.
4. Under the influence of estrogen, the proliferative phase of the endometrium occurs. The binding of estradiol to its receptor sites on the endometrium results in the production of growth factors that stimulate marked proliferation within the glandular and stromal compartments of the endometrium. The height of the endometrium increases from approximately 1 mm at the time of menstruation to 5 mm at the time of ovulation. The major effect of estrogen on the endometrium is that of growth. Estrogen also increases the number of estrogen and progesterone receptors in endometrial cells.

5. Estrogen causes maturation of vaginal basal cells into superficial squamous epithelial cells and the formation of watery vaginal mucus, which can be strung out (spinnbarkeit) or dried, forming a ferning pattern.
6. In response to rising estradiol levels in the middle and late follicular phase, FSH release begins to fall.

Ovulatory Phase

1. A preovulatory estradiol surge leads to a midcycle LH surge which initiates ovulation approximately 10 to 16 hours after the LH surge. An estradiol level of approximately 200 pg/mL or higher for at least 2 days is

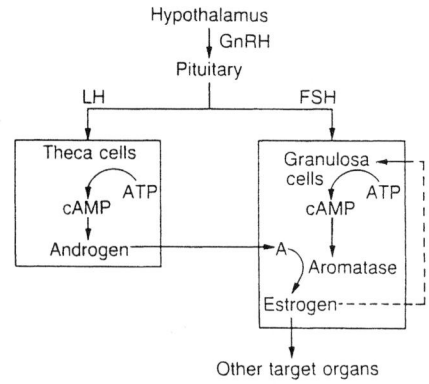

FIGURE 49.2 Two-cell two-gonadotropin hypothesis of gonadal steroid synthesis. GnRH, gonadotropin-releasing hormone; LH, luteinizing hormone; FSH, follicle-stimulating hormone; ATP, adenosine triphosphate; cAMP, cyclic adenosine monophosphate. (Adapted from Hylka VW, Dizerega GS. Reproductive hormones and their mechanisms of action. In: Michell DR, Davajan VC, Lobo RC, eds. *Infertility, contraception, and reproductive endocrinology.* Boston: Blackwell Science; 1991.)

needed to induce ovulation. A small preovulatory rise in progesterone is required to induce the FSH surge.
2. A mature follicle releases an oocyte and becomes a functioning corpus luteum.
3. At this stage there are copious, clear vaginal secretions, with maximum spinnbarkeit and a positive fern test result.

Luteal Phase

The luteal phase begins with ovulation and ends with the menstrual flow. This phase is more constant, lasting approximately 14 ± 2 days, reflecting the life of the corpus luteum.

1. The corpus luteum produces large amounts of progesterone, as well as increased levels of estrogen. Granulosa cells are exposed to low-density lipoprotein (LDL) cholesterol as a result of the invasion of blood vessels into the collapsed follicle. LDL acts as a substrate for progesterone synthesis. A progesterone serum level of >3 ng/mL is a presumptive evidence of ovulation. Rising levels of estrogen and progesterone lead to falling levels of FSH and LH.
2. Progesterone antagonizes the action of estrogen by reducing estrogen receptor sites and increasing conversion of estradiol to estrone, a less potent estrogen. Progesterone halts the growth of the endometrium and stimulates differentiation into a secretory endometrium. The secretory phase is characterized histologically by increased tortuosity of glands and spiraling of blood vessels. Secretory activity is maximal, and stromal edema occurs. The secretory endometrium is prepared for implantation.
3. Local progesterone produced by the corpus luteum suppresses follicular development in the ipsilateral ovary so that ovulation in the following month usually occurs in the contralateral ovary.
4. The cervical mucus becomes thick during the luteal phase, owing to the influence of progesterone, and no ferning or spinnbarkeit occurs.
5. Unless there is fertilization with subsequent production of human chorionic gonadotropin, the corpus luteum involutes after approximately 10 to 12 days. Sloughing of the endometrium occurs secondary to a loss both of estrogen and of supportive progesterone. Local prostaglandins cause vasoconstriction and uterine contractions.
6. The decreased levels of estrogen and progesterone lead to increased levels of FSH and LH, providing the positive feedback loop required to initiate another menstrual cycle.

CONCLUSION

Menarche is that time in the female life cycle denoting the beginning of menses and the commencement of orderly cyclic hormonal changes. Normal menstrual cycles require an orchestrated sequence of events to occur between the hypothalamus, pituitary, ovaries, and the endometrium. Abnormal menstrual cycles are not uncommon and require appropriate clinical assessment and evaluation to determine etiology. Common menstrual disorders experienced by adolescents, including dysmenorrhea, dysfunctional uterine bleeding, and amenorrhea will be discussed in the following chapters.

WEB SITES

http://www.fda.gov/fdac/reprints/ots_mens.html. U.S. Food and Drug Administration Web site for teenagers, abridged from *FDA Consumer,* December, 1993. Provides general information on menstruation for teens.

http://www.youngwomenshealth.org/menstrual.html. Boston Children's Hospital site, guide to puberty and menses.

REFERENCES AND ADDITIONAL READINGS

Emans SJ. Endocrine abnormalities and hirsutism. In: Emans SJ, Laufer MR, Goldstein DP, eds. *Pediatric and adolescent gynecology.* Philadelphia: Lippincott Williams & Wilkins; 2005.

Filicori M, Santoro N, Merriam GR, et al. Characteristics of the physiological pattern of episodic gonadotropin secretion throughout the human menstrual cycle. *J Clin Endocrinol Metab* 1986;6:1136.

Frisch RE, McArthur JW. Menstrual cycles: fatness as a determinant of minimum weight necessary for their maintenance or onset. *Science* 1974;53:384.

Fritz MA, Speroff L. The endocrinology of the menstrual cycle: the interaction of the folliculogenesis and neuroendocrine mechanisms. *Fertil Steril* 1982;38:509.

Gobelsmann U. The menstrual cycle. In: Mishell DR Jr, Davajan V, eds. *Infertility, contraception, and reproductive endocrinology.* Oradell, NJ: Medical Economics Books; 1986.

Gobelsmann U, Mishell DR. The menstrual cycle. In: Mishell DR Jr, Davajan V, Lobo A, eds. *Infertility, contraception, and reproductive endocrinology,* 3rd ed. Boston: Blackwell Science; 1991.

Hermann-Giddens ME, Slora EJ, Wasserman RC, et al. Secondary sexual characteristics and menses in young girls seen in office practice: a study from the pediatric research in office settings network. *Pediatrics* 1997;99:505.

Iglesias EA, Coupey SM. Menstrual cycle abnormalities: diagnosis and management. Female reproductive health; adolescent medicine. *State Art Rev* 1999;10:255–273.

Lobo RA, Paulson RJ, Mishell DR Jr, et al., eds. *Textbook of infertility, contraception, and reproductive endocrinology,* 4th ed. Malden, MA: Blackwell Science; 1997.

Mandel D, Zimlichman E, Mimouni FB, et al. Age at menarche and body mass index: a population study. *J Pediatr Endocrinol* 2004;17:1507.

Neinstein LS. Menstrual disorders. *Semin Fam Med* 1981;2:184.

Neinstein LS. Menstrual problems in adolescents. *Med Clin North Am* 1990;74:1181.

Rosenfield RL, Barnes RB. Menstrual disorders in adolescence. *Endocrinol Metab Clin North Am* 1993;22:491.

Silberstein SD, Merriam GR. Physiology of the menstrual cycle. *Cephalalgia* 2000;20:148.

Speroff L, Glass RH, Kase NG, eds. *Clinical gynecologic endocrinology and infertility,* 6th ed. Baltimore: Williams & Wilkins; 1999.

Vuorento T, Huhtaniemi I. Daily levels of salivary progesterone during menstrual cycle in adolescent girls. *Fertil Steril* 1992; 58:685.

CHAPTER 50

Dysmenorrhea and Premenstrual Syndrome

Paula K. Braverman

More than 50% of female adolescents experience menstrual dysfunction, including dysfunctional uterine bleeding, amenorrhea, dysmenorrhea, and the premenstrual syndrome. Many of the problems are minor, including mild dysmenorrhea and minor variations in cycle length or amount of flow. However, the dysfunction can become more severe when amenorrhea, debilitating dysmenorrhea, or severe dysfunctional bleeding occurs. This chapter and the next several chapters deal with the evaluation of common adolescent menstrual dysfunctions. Dysmenorrhea, the most prevalent of these, is considered first.

DYSMENORRHEA

The term *primary dysmenorrhea* refers to pain associated with the menstrual flow, with no evidence of organic pelvic disease. *Secondary dysmenorrhea* refers to pain associated with menses secondary to organic disease such as endometriosis, outflow tract obstruction, or pelvic inflammatory disease.

Etiology

Psychological Factors Psychosocial factors may play a role in dysmenorrhea.

1. One study of college students found an association between dysmenorrhea and anxiety, depression, and a loss of social support networks (Alonso and Coe, 2001).
2. A study of adolescents taking naproxen therapy for dysmenorrhea found that those with more severe symptoms had lower self-concept (DuRant et al., 1985).

Myometrial Factors Pain is caused by myometrial contractions induced by prostaglandins from the secretory endometrium.

1. Uterine pressure during menses can exceed contraction pressures found during labor.
2. In patients with dysmenorrhea, contractions have been noted to have high frequency, amplitude, and resting tone.
3. When comparing more severe primary dysmenorrhea to mild symptoms, there may be higher intrauterine pressure and more vasoconstriction in smaller branches

of the uterine artery (Alvin and Litt, 1982; Dmitrovic et al., 2003).

Prostaglandins Prostaglandins are formed in the secretory endometrium. Phospholipids from cell membranes are converted into arachidonic acid, the fatty acid precursor for prostaglandin synthesis. Prostaglandin E_2 (PGE_2) and $PGF_{2\alpha}$ are the key prostaglandins involved in dysmenorrhea, although $PGF_{2\alpha}$ is considered the most important. They are formed through the cyclooxygenase pathway, which also produces thromboxanes and prostacyclin. $PGF_{2\alpha}$ induces myometrial contractions, vasoconstriction, and ischemia and mediates pain sensation, whereas PGE_2 causes vasodilation and platelet disaggregation. There are two enzymes in the cyclooxygenase system. The COX-1 enzyme has homeostatic functions including gastrointestinal mucosal integrity, renal and platelet function, and vascular hemostasis. COX-2 is induced by inflammation. It has been noted that:

1. Locally, prostaglandins cause uterine contractions, but they enter the systemic circulation and cause associated symptoms such as headache, nausea, vomiting, backache, diarrhea, dizziness, and fatigue.
2. Exogenous injection of PGE_2 and $PGF_{2\alpha}$ produce myometrial contractions and pain similar to dysmenorrhea, although PGE_2 also inhibit contractions in the nonpregnant uterus.
3. Anovulatory cycles are associated with lower prostaglandin levels in the menstrual fluid and usually no dysmenorrhea. Because many cycles in the first 2 years after menarche are anovulatory, many adolescents do not experience dysmenorrhea from the outset. Rather it occurs more frequently 1 to 3 years after menarche.
4. Patients with dysmenorrhea have higher levels of prostaglandins in the endometrium.
5. Most of the prostaglandins are released in the first 48 hours of menstruation, correlating with the most severe symptoms.
6. Prostaglandin inhibitors decrease dysmenorrhea.

From this evidence it has been presumed that primary dysmenorrhea is related to prostaglandins released during menses, which seems to be increased during ovulatory cycles. It is postulated that women with dysmenorrhea may be more sensitive to prostaglandins. Prostaglandin levels have also been shown to be locally elevated in cases of secondary dysmenorrhea such as endometriosis (Koike et al., 1992).

Epidemiology

Dysmenorrhea is the greatest single cause of lost work and school hours in females, with >140 million hours lost per year (Ylikorkala and Dawood, 1978). Various studies worldwide have shown the following:

1. Forty-three percent to 93% of all postpubescent females have some degree of dysmenorrhea; between 5% and 42% of these females describe the pain as severe and are incapacitated for 1 to 3 days per month.
2. Reports of school absence increase with more severe symptoms.
3. Ethnicity and cultural factors may also influence responses to pain.
    a. In a study utilizing a cross-sectional national probability sample of 12- to 17-year olds from the National Center for Health Statistics, black adolescents in the United States were more likely to miss school because of dysmenorrhea (23.6%) than whites (12.3%) despite having the same rates of dysmenorrhea (Klein and Litt, 1981).
    b. A more recent study of 706 Hispanic adolescents surveyed in a high school showed that they were even more likely to report missing school (38%) (Banikarim et al., 2000).

The prevalence of dysmenorrhea increases with age and pubertal stage.

1. In the study by Klein and Litt (1981), the prevalence of dysmenorrhea rose from 39% of 12-year-old girls to 72% of 17-year-old girls and 38% at SMR 3 to 66% at SMR 5 (Klein and Litt, 1981).
2. Pedron-Nuevo et al. (1998) found rates of 52.1% for those younger than 15 years and 63.8% for those 15- to 19-years old.
3. Teperi and Rimpela (1989) found dysmenorrhea among 48% of 12-year-old postmenarchal girls and among 79% of 18-year olds.

Clinical Manifestations

Primary dysmenorrhea usually begins within 1 to 3 years of menarche and is associated with the establishment of ovulatory cycles. Although the pain usually begins within a few hours of starting menses, it may also start several days before the onset of menses. Local symptoms include pain that is spasmodic in nature and is strongest in the lower abdomen, with radiation to the back and anterior aspects of the thighs. In most cases, the pain resolves within 24 to 48 hours but sometimes the symptoms may persist further into the menstrual cycle. Associated systemic symptoms can include nausea or vomiting, fatigue, mood change, dizziness, diarrhea, backache, and headache.

It may be useful to grade dysmenorrhea as follows:

1. Grade I: Mild dysmenorrhea that does not interfere with the adolescent's participation in everyday activity
2. Grade II: Moderate dysmenorrhea that may interfere in the adolescent's participation in some activities; minimal, if any, systemic symptoms
3. Grade III: Severe discomfort; adolescent restricted from activities for several days; often associated with systemic symptoms

Differential Diagnosis

Gynecological Causes

1. Endometriosis: Endometriosis is characterized by the presence of endometrial glands and stroma outside of the uterus. These implants are commonly located in various locations throughout the pelvis. This condition is not as rare in adolescents as previously thought. In addition to being the most common pathological condition in adolescents with chronic pelvic pain (Laufer and Goldstein, 2005), it is considered a progressive disease that increases in prevalence and severity with age (American College of Obstetrics and Gynecology, 2005). Endometriosis has been diagnosed as follows:
    a. By laparoscopy in 19% to 73% of adolescents being evaluated for chronic pelvic pain
    b. In premenarchal girls at the initial stages of puberty and as young as age 8 (Laufer et al., 2003).
    c. By laparoscopy in 50% to 70% of adolescents with chronic pelvic pain not responsive to oral contraceptive pills (OCP) and nonsteroidal antiinflammatory drugs (NSAIDs).
    The symptoms of endometriosis in adolescents include chronic pelvic pain, which may be cyclic or acyclic. Cyclic pain alone is found in only 9.4% of adolescents (American College of Obstetrics and Gynecology, 2005). This is in contrast to adults who are more likely to have cyclic pain. Other associated symptoms can include dyspareunia; irregular menses; bowel symptoms such as rectal pain, nausea, constipation, diarrhea, and pain on defecation; and urinary symptoms such as dysuria, urgency, and frequency.
    On examination, a tender or nodular cul-de-sac or tender uterosacral ligaments may be found. However, adolescents may not have the classic thickened nodular sacrouterine ligaments. Ovarian endometriomas are not usually found before the mid-twenties. Goldstein et al. (1980) found pelvic tenderness in 76% of adolescents with endometriosis whereas Reese et al. (1996) found diffuse tenderness in 95% of patients and localized tenderness in 77.6%.
    Endometriosis should by considered in patients with dysmenorrhea who do not respond to a combination of OCP and NSAID, as well as those with associated bowel or urinary function symptoms. This diagnosis is also more common when there is a positive family history for endometriosis.
2. Pelvic inflammatory disease
3. Benign uterine tumors: Fibroids
4. Intrauterine device
5. Anatomical abnormalities: Congenital obstructive müllerian malformations, outflow obstruction. Obstructive müllerian abnormalities predispose the patient to endometriosis.
6. Pelvic adhesions
7. Ovarian cyst or mass

Nongynecological Causes

1. Gastrointestinal disorders: Inflammatory bowel disease, irritable bowel syndrome, constipation, lactose intolerance

2. Musculoskeletal pain: Inflammatory process, trauma, tumor
3. Genitourinary abnormalities: Cystitis, ureteral obstruction, calculi
4. Psychogenic disorders: History of abuse, trauma, psychogenic complaints

Diagnosis

History

1. Menstrual history: Primary dysmenorrhea usually starts 1 to 3 years after menarche, most commonly begins between the ages of 14 and 15 years, and peaks at age 17 or 18. It usually decreases during the twenties and thirties. Secondary dysmenorrhea should be considered if the pain starts with the onset of menarche or after the age of 20 years. Adolescents should be asked about the degree of pain and the amount of impairment in school and other activities. Any previous use of therapeutic modalities and their effectiveness should be ascertained.
2. Prior sexually transmitted diseases and sexual history: This information helps to eliminate infection as a cause.
3. Gastrointestinal and genitourinary systems history: This information helps to eliminate gastrointestinal or genitourinary problems (e.g., cystitis, irritable bowel syndrome) as a cause of pain.
4. Musculoskeletal history: This reveals bone or joint problems including trauma or possible tumor.
5. Psychosocial history: Evaluate for stressors, substance abuse, and sexual abuse. Cigarette smoking, especially heavy smoking, has been found to be associated with dysmenorrhea (Hornsby et al., 1998).

Physical Examination

Examine the pelvis for evidence of endometriosis, endometritis, fibroids, uterine or cervical abnormalities, or adnexal masses and tenderness. However, if the teen is not sexually active and the history is typical for dysmenorrhea, a pelvic examination is indicated only if the symptoms do not respond to standard medical therapy. Examination limited to a cotton swab inserted into the vagina can help rule out a hymenal abnormality or vaginal septum without performing a speculum examination. The musculoskeletal examination should focus on range of motion of the hips and spine to assess for tenderness and limitation in motion.

Laboratory Tests

A complete blood count and a determination of the erythrocyte sedimentation rate should be done if pelvic inflammatory disease or inflammatory bowel disease is suspected. Sexually active adolescents should be tested for sexually transmitted diseases and pregnancy. A urinalysis and urine culture will help diagnose urinary tract problems. If a müllerian abnormality is suspected, ultrasonography or magnetic resonance imaging will define the anatomy. If evaluation of the genitourinary, gastrointestinal, and musculoskeletal systems fail to reveal a cause of the pain and if the pain is severe and intractable despite treatment with antiprostaglandins and oral contraceptives, laparoscopy should be considered.

Therapy

The two most effective treatments for primary dysmenorrhea are with NSAIDs and oral contraceptives.

Education The patient should be educated and reassured that the problem is physiological and can be helped. The importance of education has been demonstrated repeatedly in studies demonstrating that adolescents have a knowledge deficit about available treatment modalities and how to use them most effectively (Johnson, 1988; Wilson and Keye, 1989; Campbell and McGrath, 1997; Hillen et al., 1999).

Nonsteroidal Antiinflammatory Drugs NSAIDs are the primary modality of therapy; 80% of dysmenorrhea can be relieved with these medications. Because much of primary dysmenorrhea is secondary to prostaglandin-mediated uterine hyperactivity, prostaglandin inhibitors can alleviate menstrual cramps and associated systemic symptoms. Many NSAIDs have been found effective in alleviating menstrual cramps. They are divided into two classes—carboxylic acids and enolic acids. Carboxylic acids are more widely used and are divided into four subgroups: (a) salicylic acids (aspirin), (b) acetic acids (indomethacin), and the two most useful subgroups—(c) propionic acids such as ibuprofen (Motrin), naproxen (Naprosyn), and naproxen sodium (Anaprox), and the (d) fenamates such as mefenamic acid (Ponstel). Of the propionic acids, naproxen sodium may have a shorter onset of action because it is more rapidly absorbed. Mefenamic acid has an additional mechanism of action: It competes with prostaglandin-binding sites and antagonizes existing prostaglandins in addition to inhibiting prostaglandin synthesis. Some of these drugs and their typical doses are as follows:

Drug (Trade Name)	Initial Dose (mg)	Following Dose (mg)
Propionic acids		
Ibuprofen (Motrin)	400	400 q4–6h
Naproxen (Naprosyn)	500	250 q6–8h
Naproxen sodium (Anaprox)	550	275 q6–8h
Fenamates		
Mefenamic acid (Ponstel)	500	250 q6h

Over-the-counter ibuprofen is available in preparations such as Advil and Nuprin. Naproxen is available as Aleve. Because these over-the-counter medications come in lower doses than the prescription formulations, a larger number of tablets may be needed for effectiveness. The medications should be started either as soon as possible when the symptoms of dysmenorrhea occur or to coincide with the first sign of menstruation. It is not necessary to start before the onset of menses. Usually, these medications are needed only for 1 to 3 days. After one of the NSAIDs is started, it should be tried for two or three menstrual cycles before being judged ineffective. At that time, a trial of a different prostaglandin inhibitor should be performed with a minimum trial of at least 6 months for this mode of therapy.

With the outlined doses used for short periods, side effects are usually minimal, but they include the following in more than 1% of patients:

1. Gastrointestinal: Nausea, epigastric pain, vomiting, constipation
2. Central nervous system (CNS): Dizziness, headache
3. Skin: Rash
4. Cardiovascular: Edema, palpitations
5. Other: Tinnitus

The NSAIDs discussed in the preceding text inhibit both the COX-1 and COX-2 enzymes. However, selective COX-2 inhibitors will have less gastrointestinal side effects and may also be preferred in patients with coagulation disorders related to platelet function. Multiple studies have evaluated various drugs in this class and have found that they are equivalent to naproxen in relieving dysmenorrhea symptoms. Because of recent drug recalls, the only COX-2 inhibitor available at the time of this printing is celecoxib. The dosing is 400 mg as a loading dose followed by 200 mg every 12 hours (Harel, 2005). These medications are more expensive, potentially more toxic and not necessarily superior in efficacy to less expensive, nonselective NSAIDs.

Hormonal Therapies If the patient wishes contraception or the pain is severe and not responsive to NSAIDs, oral contraceptives can be tried. The maximal effect may not become apparent for several months.

1. Combined oral contraceptives inhibit ovulation and lead to an atrophic decidualized endometrium resulting in decreased menstrual flow and prostaglandin release.
2. Oral contraceptives decrease symptoms in >90% of patients with primary dysmenorrhea.
3. OCPs are also useful to treat endometriosis because they decrease endometrial proliferation and thereby decrease total local prostaglandin production.

A 2001 Cochrane review (Proctor et al., 2001) conducted a meta-analysis of randomized clinical trials and concluded that OCPs with older first and second generation progestins and higher hormone doses than current OCPs were more effective than placebo for primary dysmenorrhea. However, they commented on the small size of the studies and poor quality. Two more recent studies address this knowledge deficit:

1. A randomized, double-blind, placebo-controlled study of a low-dose OCP containing 20 µg of ethinyl estradiol and 150 µg of desogestrel has shown a significant decrease in primary dysmenorrhea (Hendrix and Alexander, 2002).
2. A randomized, double-blind, placebo-controlled study in 76 adolescents with moderate to severe dysmenorrhea showed that a modern low-dose OCP containing 20 µg of ethinyl estradiol and 100 µg of levonorgestrel was more effective than placebo (Davis et al., 2005).

If cyclic hormonal contraception is ineffective then continuous combination hormonal therapy can be tried. Monophasic OCPs can be used by skipping the placebo pills. An extended cycling OCP, Seasonale, is currently available as a 91-pill regimen containing 84 hormonal pills before the week of placebo with 30 µg of ethinyl estradiol and 150 µg of levonorgestrel. Extended cycling may be particularly helpful in endometriosis (American College of Obstetrics and Gynecology, 2005; Vercellini et al., 2003a; Sulak et al., 2002). Theoretically, the contraceptive patch and vaginal ring could be used in the same manner. However, one study showed that cycling with OCPs provided better relief of dysmenorrhea than cycling with the patch (Audet et al., 2001). Injectable depot medroxyprogesterone acetate has also been effective.

Other Hormonal Modalities

1. Gonadotropin-releasing hormone (GnRH) agonists with utilization of add-back therapy to prevent side effects related to hypoestrogenic state (including bone loss) have been tried in severe cases of endometriosis unresponsive to other modalities. Caution should be utilized in patients younger than 16 years because of concerns about compromised bone density accrual (American College of Obstetrics and Gynecology, 2005).
2. Danazol is equivalent to GnRH agonists, but it less utilized because of androgenic side effects (American College of Obstetrics and Gynecology, 2005).
3. Levonorgestrel-releasing intrauterine system has been effective for dysmenorrhea and endometriosis. The current brand marketed is Mirena (Baldaszti et al., 2003; Vercellini et al., 2003b).

Other Nonhormonal Modalities
Likely to be beneficial

1. Vitamin B_1 (Proctor and Farquhar, 2004)
2. Magnesium (Proctor and Farquhar, 2004)
3. Vitamin E (Proctor and Farquhar, 2004)
4. Transcutaneous nerve stimulation (Dawood and Ramos, 1990; Kaplan et al., 1997; Proctor and Farquhar, 2004)

Unclear benefit

5. Dietary supplementation with ω-3 fatty acids (Harel et al., 1996; Proctor and Farquhar, 2004)
6. Acupuncture (Helms, 1987; National Institutes of Health, 1998; Proctor and Farquhar, 2004)

PREMENSTRUAL SYNDROME

The term *premenstrual syndrome* (PMS) is used to describe an array of predictable physical, cognitive, affective, and behavioral symptoms that occur cyclically during the luteal phase of the menstrual cycle and resolve quickly at or near the onset of menstruation. It is characterized by a broad spectrum of symptoms and until recently had confusing definitions. The etiology of PMS is currently unknown, but there is some evidence that reduced serotonergic function during the luteal phase and alterations in the γ aminobutyric acid (GABA) receptor complex response, may be responsible, among other mechanisms (Johnson, 2004; Freeman et al., 2004).

In the mid 1980s, more specific criteria were defined, and studies evaluating both the pathophysiology and treatment modalities were designed according to strict scientific standards. Evidence is accumulating that PMS is not a single condition but a set of interrelated symptom complexes, with multiple phenotypes of subtypes, and pathophysiological events that begin with ovulation (Johnson, 2004; Halbreich, 2004).

In the mental health field, criteria have been developed to define a syndrome called *premenstrual dysphoric disorder* (PMDD) as a distinct clinical entity. Although the PMS and PMDD overlap, in PMDD the focus is more on problems with mood and symptoms are more severe. There is a higher level of dysfunction before the onset of menses. Both Johnson (2004); Speroff and Fritz (2005) conclude that it is not useful to differentiate PMS from PMDD, and agree that there is a broad spectrum of severity. Johnson suggests characterizing PMDD as severe PMS with impairment.

Epidemiology

The exact prevalence is unknown, but estimates are that up to 85% of menstruating women have some degree of symptoms before menses, and that 3% to 8% are so severely afflicted that daily activities are hindered. This smaller subset of women meet criteria for PMDD (Chakmakjian, 1983; Singh et al., 1998; American College of Obstetrics and Gynecology, 2000; Grady-Weliky, 2003). As noted by Johnson (2004), approximately 50% of women have only a few mild symptoms for several days during the luteal phase and probably should not be diagnosed as having PMS. Some selected studies in adolescents have shown the following:

1. In one longitudinal study of 384 15-year-old adolescent girls, Raja et al. (1992) found a 14% prevalence of PMS symptoms.
2. In a survey study of 207 adolescents, 89% reported at least one PMS symptom that the teens considered moderately severe, 59% reported at least one symptom considered severe, and 43% had at least one symptom considered extreme (Fisher et al., 1989).
3. A more recent study of 10- to 17-year-old menstruating females attending an Adolescent Outpatient Clinic found that 61.4% had PMS symptoms, with 49.5% having mild symptoms, 37.1% reporting moderate symptoms, and 13.4% with severe symptoms; 71% with dysmenorrhea also had PMS (Derman et al., 2004).

Risk Factors

Risk factors for PMS include advancing age (beyond 30 years) and genetic factors. Some studies suggest that women whose mothers report PMS are more likely to develop PMS (70%, versus 37% of daughters of unaffected mothers) (Van der Akker et al., 1987; Dalton, 1987). In addition, concordance rates for PMS are significantly higher in monozygotic twins (93%) compared with dizygotic twins (44%) (Dalton, 1987). There are no significant differences in personality profile or level of stress in women with PMS compared with asymptomatic women. However, women with PMS may not handle stress as well. One recent article prospectively evaluating a community cohort of 1,488 women aged 14 to 24 over a 42-month period found that traumatic events such as a physical threat, childhood sexual abuse, and severe accidents increased the odds of developing PMDD (Perkonigg et al., 2004).

Pathophysiology

The exact mechanism of PMS is unknown, but is probably the result of an interaction between sex steroids and central neurotransmitters (Mortola, 1998).

1. Alterations in neurotransmitters: Endorphins, GABA, and serotonin have been implicated (Steiner and Pearlstein, 2000).
   a. There is inconsistent evidence for differences (e.g., a drop) in circulating endorphins in symptomatic patients.
   b. Women with PMS and PMDD have reduced GABA receptor sensitivity and reduced plasma GABA during the luteal phase.
   c. Serotonergic dysregulation is the most plausible theory, although not all women respond to selective serotonin reuptake inhibitors (SSRIs), implying that other factors must be involved (Halbreich, 2004).
2. Hormonal factors: Women with PMS/PMDD are felt to be more sensitive to normal cyclical hormonal fluctuations.
   a. The levels of sex steroids, estrogen, progesterone, and testosterone are normal, but women with PMS may be more vulnerable to normal fluctuations. This vulnerability may be in part related to serotonin (Steiner and Pearlstein, 2000). Further evidence for the lack of abnormal hormonal changes in the luteal phase comes from the following:
      • In a study utilizing the progesterone-antagonist mifepristone to induce menses, there was no relationship between the induction of menses and the timing or severity of PMS symptoms (Schmidt et al., 1991).
      • A placebo-controlled study of women with PMS who had ovarian suppression with a GnRH agonist were found to have recurrence of PMS symptoms when given estrogen and progesterone compared to a lack of mood change in the placebo group (Schmidt et al., 1998). These data strongly suggest an abnormal response to normal hormonal changes.
   b. Other hormones: There is no proof of a relationship between PMS and prolactin, growth hormone, thyroid hormone, adrenal activity, luteinizing hormone (LH), follicle-stimulating hormone (FSH), antidiuretic hormone, insulin, aldosterone, renin-angiotensin, or cortisol.
3. Vitamin deficiencies: Zinc, vitamin A, vitamin E, thiamine, magnesium, and pyridoxine (vitamin B_6) have been implicated, but not documented. No significant differences have been found, and the data show inconsistent scientific evidence.

Clinical Manifestations

More than 150 symptoms have been described in literature, ranging from mild symptoms to those severe enough to interfere with normal activities.

1. Emotional symptoms
   a. Irritability
   b. Depression
   c. Fatigue or lethargy
   d. Anger/argumentative
   e. Insomnia or hypersomnia
   f. Mood lability
   g. Anxiety
   h. Poor concentration
   i. Confusion
   j. Tearfulness
   k. Social withdrawal
2. Physical symptoms
   a. Headaches
   b. Swelling: Legs or breasts/breast tenderness
   c. Increased appetite

d. Food cravings
e. Weight gain
f. Sense of abdominal bloating
g. Fatigue
h. Muscle and joint aches and pain
i. Hot flashes

Diagnosis

The diagnosis relies on the history of cyclic symptoms. No specific physical findings or laboratory tests have proved useful. Although there are no universally accepted specific diagnostic criteria among the various sources defining PMS including the World Health Organization's International Classification of Diseases, ACOG, the National Institute of Mental Health, and the *Diagnostic and Statistical Manual of Mental Disorders*, (Halbreich, 2004), three important findings are usually needed to make a diagnosis of PMS:

1. Symptoms must occur in the luteal phase and resolve within a few days of onset of menstruation. Symptoms should not be present in the follicular phase.
2. The symptoms must be documented over several menstrual cycles and not caused by other physical or psychological problems.
3. Symptoms must be recurrent and severe enough to disrupt normal activities.

A calendar such as the one shown in Figure 50.1 can be helpful in the diagnosis and in monitoring teens after the start of any therapy. Prospective recording should be done for at least 2 to 3 months to document that symptoms are occurring cyclically in the luteal phase. Other assessment tools include the Self-Assessment Disk (Magos and Studd, 1988), the Premenstrual Assessment Form (Halbreich et al., 1982), Calendar of Premenstrual Experience (COPE) (Mortola et al., 1990), the Prospective Record of the Impact and Severity of Menstrual Symptoms (PRISM) (Reid, 1985), Premenstrual Syndrome Diary (Thys-Jacobs et al., 1995), Daily Record of Severity of Problems (Endicott and Harrison, 1990), and the Penn Daily Symptom Rating (Freeman et al., 1996).

The National Institute of Mental Health (NIMH) criteria require a change of 30% in intensity of symptoms, as measured with the use of an instrument, comparing days 5 through 10 of the cycle with the 6 days before menses. These changes must be documented for at least two consecutive cycles (American College of Obstetrics and Gynecology, 2000).

The *Diagnostic and Statistical Manual of Mental Health Disorders*, 4th edition text revision (American Psychiatric Association, 2000) lists similar criteria for PMDD (Table 50.1). It is important to remember that the symptoms cannot represent exacerbation of an existing disorder such as major depression, anxiety disorders, panic, dysthymic disorder, or personality disorder, but they may be superimposed on one of these psychiatric disorders. Women may have psychiatric disorders that become exacerbated during menstruation (menstrual magnification). Certain medical disorders can also become worse during menses, including seizures, migraine headaches, irritable bowel syndrome, asthma, and allergies.

Therapy

No single treatment is universally accepted as effective. Studies have yielded conflicting results with most therapies, and most trials have not been well controlled. Treatments include the following:

1. Lifestyle changes: Although lifestyle changes have not been definitively proved in controlled studies, establishing good exercise and stress management practices can improve overall feelings of well being.
   a. Education: The teen should be educated regarding menstrual physiology and the relationship of changing hormones to symptoms. A small study of college students with PMS demonstrated a decrease in perimenstrual symptoms with a health promotion intervention in a peer group setting that positively reframed menstrual cycle perceptions (Morse, 1999).
   b. Stress management: The teen can be taught or referred for techniques to manage stress (e.g., biofeedback, self-hypnosis, relaxation exercises). If symptoms of stress are more significant, psychological counseling including cognitive-behavioral therapy or group therapy may be helpful (Girman et al., 2003; Johnson, 2004). Studies have demonstrated improvement in PMS with cognitive-behavior therapy (Kirkby, 1994; Christensen and Oei, 1995; Blake et al., 1998).
   c. Exercise: Regular aerobic exercise has been reported to help some women with PMS (Prior et al., 1987; Steege and Blumenthal, 1993; Scully et al., 1998).
2. *Vitamin, mineral supplementation, herbal preparations, and dietary manipulation*: There have been some positive outcomes for these complementary and alternative therapies. However, although some show promise, more research needs to be carried out to recommend definitively any of these therapies (American College of Obstetrics and Gynecology, 2000; Pearlstein and Steiner, 2000; Stevinson and Ernst, 2001; Girman et al., 2003; Johnson, 2004).
   a. Calcium (1,200 mg/day) in the form of calcium carbonate was reported to reduce physical and emotional symptoms in a well-designed, multi-center study (Thys-Jacobs et al., 1998; American College of Obstetrics and Gynecology, 2000; Girman et al., 2003; Johnson, 2004). Further evidence for a role for calcium was found in a recent case–control study, nested in the Nurses' Health Study II, which prospectively evaluated women initially free from PMS and followed them up three times between 1991 and 1999. The results showed that high intake of calcium and vitamin D was associated with a reduced risk of developing PMS (Bertone-Johnson et al., 2005).
   b. Magnesium (200 to 400 mg/day) has been noted to reduce negative mood and to reduce water retention and appears to be more effective than placebo in some studies. The mechanism of action is not fully understood and usage not well studied (Facchinetti et al., 1991; Walker et al., 1998; American College of Obstetrics and Gynecology, 2000; Girman et al., 2003).
   c. Pyridoxine (vitamin B_6) has been used extensively in the past, particularly in treating the emotional symptomatology of PMS. However, a review of the literature yields conflicting results, and this vitamin is considered to be of limited benefit. The other concern is that peripheral neuropathy can develop with doses >100 mg/day (Wyatt et al., 1999; American College of

Premenstrual Changes

Name: _____

Rate each of the following words or phrases according to how you feel today. Each item should be rated on a 5-point scale. The numbers refer to the following: 0 = not at all; 1 = a little; 2 = moderately; 3 = quite a bit; 4 = extremely. For each item, write the number in the box for the response that best describes your feeling or behavior today. The best time of day to complete this questionnaire is early evening. Grading of menses: 0 = none; 1 = slight spotting; 2 = moderate; 3 = heavy; 4 = heavy and clots.

Day of cycle	1	2	3	4	5	6	7	8	9	10	11	12	13	14	15	16	17	18	19	20	21	22	23	24	25	26	27	28	29	30
Menstruation																														
Angry																														
Unable to concentrate																														
Fatigue																														
Anxious, tense																														
Constipation																														
Confused																														
Nervous																														
Avoiding social activities																														
Tender or painful breasts																														
Bad temper																														
Headaches																														
Craving for foods																														
Swelling of breasts, ankles, or abdomen																														

FIGURE 50.1 Premenstrual symptom calendar.

TABLE 50.1

Diagnosis of Premenstrual Dysphoric Disorder (DSM-IV-TR Criteria)

I. In most menstrual cycles in the last year at least 5 of these symptoms (including at least one of the symptoms in category A) were present for most of the time 1 wk before menses, began to remit within a few days after the onset of the follicular phase (menses), and were absent in the week after menses.
   A. 1. Markedly depressed mood, feelings of hopelessness or self-deprecating thoughts
      2. Marked anxiety, tension
      3. Marked affective lability (i.e., feeling suddenly sad or tearful)
      4. Persistent and marked anger or irritability or increased interpersonal conflicts
   B. Other symptoms
      1. Decreased interest in usual activities such as friends and hobbies
      2. Subjective sense of difficulty in concentrating
      3. Lethargy, easy fatigability, or marked lack of energy
      4. Marked change in appetite, overeating, or specific food cravings
      5. Hypersomnia or insomnia
      6. A subjective sense of being overwhelmed or out of control
      7. Other physical symptoms (e.g., breast tenderness, bloating, weight gain, headache, joint or muscle pain)
II. The symptoms markedly interfere with work, school, usual activities, or relationships with others.
III. Symptoms are not merely an exacerbation of another disorder, such as major depressive disorder, panic disorder, dysthymic disorder, or a personality disorder (although it may be superimposed on any of these disorders).
IV. Criteria I, II, and III are confirmed by prospective daily ratings for at least two consecutive symptomatic menstrual cycles.

Adapted from American Psychiatric Association. *Diagnostic and statistical manual of mental disorders text revision*, 4th ed. Washington, DC: American Psychiatric Press, 2000.

Obstetrics and Gynecology, 2000; Girman et al., 2003; Johnson, 2004).

d. Vitamin E (400 IU/day) was found to improve somatic and affective symptoms. However, there is limited evidence of its effectiveness (London et al., 1987; American College of Obstetrics and Gynecology, 2000; Stevinson and Ernst, 2001).

e. *Vitex agnus-castus* (chasteberry) has been found to be superior to placebo in reducing PMS symptoms in some studies. Long-term randomized trials are needed. Chasteberry extracts can potentially affect gonadotropins, as well as estrogen, progesterone, and prolactin. It may also have agonistic effects at dopamine receptors. It should be avoided in pregnancy and breast-feeding (Berger et al., 2000; Schellenberg, 2001; Stevinson and Ernst, 2001; Atmaca et al., 2003; Girman et al., 2003; Johnson, 2004).

f. *Ginkgo biloba* (ginkgo leaf extract) has been shown to improve breast tenderness, fluid retention, and mood in a placebo-controlled study. The dose is 80 mg twice a day from day 16 of the menstrual cycle through day 5 of menses. Ginkgo inhibits platelet activating factor and may increase bleeding risks. It also interacts with the CYP 450 enzymes and may not be appropriate for individuals on certain medications. Finally, there is concern about increasing the risk of seizures (Girman et al., 2003; Johnson, 2004).

g. Carbohydrate supplements: Mood and carbohydrate food craving improved in randomized trials evaluating the intake of simple and complex carbohydrates. Carbohydrates may increase tryptophan, which is a precursor to serotonin (Sayegh et al., 1995; Stevinson and Ernst, 2001; Johnson, 2004).

h. Other dietary recommendations: Recommendations have been made based on observations that included eliminating high-sodium foods and caffeine, as well as consuming a low-fat, high-fiber diet, and eliminating refined and processed carbohydrates. However, these have not been adequately studied to date to assess efficacy for PMS (Girman et al., 2003; Johnson, 2004).

i. Primrose oil: This method does not appear to be effective.

3. Suppression of ovulation: Because PMS appears to be a cyclic disorder of menses occurring in the luteal phase, suppression of ovulation has been used as a therapy.

a. Combination oral contraceptives: Some authorities consider OCPs to be first-line medications. However, data on their effectiveness is mixed. Symptoms in some individuals with PMS worsen with use of oral contraceptives (Joffe et al., 2003). A newer double-blind placebo-controlled study of an OCP containing drospirenone and 30 μg of ethinyl estradiol was conducted for PMDD (Freeman et al., 2001). Drospirenone has spironolactone antimineralocorticoid and antiandrogenic properties. Statistically significant improvement with this OCP was limited to appetite, acne, and food cravings. However, a more recent multi-center, double-blind, randomized study using 24/4 formulation OCP containing drospirenone and 20 μg of ethinyl estradiol demonstrated improvement in both mood and physical symptom scores in subjects with PMDD.

Possible reasons for efficacy of this new formulation include the lower estrogen dose, as well as improved follicular suppression. The maintenance of a more stable hormonal environment due to the longer number of days on hormone may also be helpful (e.g., 24 rather than 21 days) (Yonkers et al., 2005). The current thinking is that OCP should be considered if the symptoms are primarily physical and not mood related because they appear to be better for the physical symptoms. However, the 24/4 formulation OCP appears to be effective for both types of symptoms.

- Medroxyprogesterone acetate (Depo-Provera) is an alternative contraceptive to suppress ovulation.
- Continuous hormonal therapy with combined hormonal contraceptives can also be considered to suppress cyclic changes and endogenous sex hormone variability (Johnson, 2004; Speroff and Fritz, 2005; Laufer and Goldstein, 2005).

b. GnRH: Most studies have shown benefit from the use of GnRH, but the hypoestrogenic effects with loss of bone density is concerning, especially for adolescents, and therefore limit its use. GnRH with add-back therapy with estrogen and progesterone can be considered when other modalities have failed (Freeman et al., 1997; American College of Obstetrics and Gynecology, 2000; Johnson, 2004; Laufer and Goldstein, 2005). However, add-back regimens may cause a recurrence in PMS/PMDD symptoms. Some have used progestin-only add-back therapy with norethindrone (Johnson, 2004).

c. Bilateral salpingo-oophorectomy would not be considered in adolescents.

4. Natural progesterones: Double-blind, crossover, placebo-controlled trials of vaginal suppositories and oral micronized progesterone have failed to show any benefit.

5. Medications to suppress symptoms
a. Prostaglandin inhibitors: NSAIDs have been used to treat PMS, particularly for the physical symptoms. These have included naproxen sodium, naproxen, or mefenamic acid during the luteal phase. Therapy is stopped after menses begins.

b. Spironolactone, 100 mg/day on days 15 through 28, has been shown to have some positive effects on somatic and affective symptoms, but the results are not conclusive. Spironolactone may be helpful in patients with breast tenderness, bloating, or weight gain from fluid retention (Grady-Weliky, 2003; Johnson, 2004; Laufer and Goldstein, 2005). Other diuretics are not effective (Wang et al., 1995; American College of Obstetrics and Gynecology, 2000).

6. SSRIs: SSRIs are the drugs of choice and first-line therapy for severe PMS/PMDD (Dimmock et al., 2000). Placebo-controlled studies have shown that they are effective for severe PMS and PMDD and improve both physical symptoms and mood (Wyatt et al., 2005). Fluoxetine, sertraline, paroxetine, citalopram, and escitalopram are all effective (Freeman, 2004; Freeman et al., 2005). Venlafaxine inhibits both serotonin and norepinephrine uptake and has been effective for PMDD (Freeman et al., 2001; Freeman, 2004; Johnson, 2004).

a. Studies have shown that using these drugs intermittently only during the luteal phase (i.e., 14 days before onset of menses) rather than continuously is equally effective for symptom reduction.

b. Unlike treatment for depression, symptoms improve within 24 to 48 hours of initiating therapy and there are no reports of discontinuation symptoms when SSRIs are used intermittently for PMDD.

c. Low doses are usually effective (Table 50.2).

d. The most common adverse effects include insomnia, gastrointestinal disturbances, and fatigue. Other side effects include dizziness, sweating, and sexual function disturbances, but these medications are usually well tolerated (Wyatt et al., 2005).

7. Medications to suppress psychological symptoms: Studies have shown some positive effects on somatic and affective symptoms. Suggested therapies have included anxiolytics and other antidepressants such as benzodiazepines (especially alprazolam), clomipramine, and buspirone. These medications can be given in the luteal phase rather than continuously (Smith et al., 1987; Harrison et al., 1990; Freeman et al., 1995; Landen et al., 2001).

a. Buspirone is a partial serotonin receptor agonist.

b. Clomipramine, a tricyclic antidepressant is a nonselective inhibitor of serotonin reuptake.

c. Alprazolam affects the GABA receptor complex.

None of these medications would be recommended for routine use in adolescents, but only for use in selected adolescents with severe symptoms unresponsive to other treatment modalities.

TABLE 50.2

Doses of Commonly Used Medications for Premenstrual Dysphoric Disorder

Name of Drug	Dose	Schedule
Fluoxetine	20 mg/d	Intermittent
Sertraline	50–100 mg/d	Intermittent
Citalopram	20–30 mg/d	Intermittent
Paroxetine	20–30 mg/d	Intermittent
Escitalopram	10–20 mg/d	Intermittent[a]
Venlafaxine	50–200 mg/d	Continuous[b]
Clopramine	50–77 mg/d	Intermittent
Alprazolam	1.25–2.25 mg/d	Intermittent
Buspirone	5–30 mg twice a d	Intermittent

[a] Preliminary study Freeman EW, Sondheimer SJ, Sammel MD, et al. A preliminary study of luteal phase versus symptom-onset dosing with escitalopram for premenstrual dysphoric disorder. *J Clin Psychiatry* 2005;66:789.

[b] Intermittent dosing with just preliminary data, Cohen LS, Soares CN, Lyster A, et al. Efficacy and tolerability of premenstrual use of venlafaxine (flexible dose) in the treatment of premenstrual dysphoric disorder. *J Clin Psychopharmacol* 2004;24:540; Freeman EW, Rickels K, Yonkers KA, et al. Venlafaxine in the treatment of premenstrual dysphoric disorder. *Obstet Gynecol* 2001;98:737.

Adapted from Grady-Weliky TA. Premenstrual dysphoric disorder. *N Engl J Med* 2003;348:433; Johnson SR. Premenstrual syndrome, premenstrual dysphoric disorder, and beyond: a clinical primer for practitioners. *Obstet Gynecol* 2004;104:845; Freeman EW, Rickels K, Sondheimer SJ, et al. Continuous or intermittent dosing with sertraline for patients with severe premenstrual syndrome or premenstrual dysphoric disorder. *Am J Psychiatry* 2004;161:343.

Summary: Steps in the Treatment of Symptoms of Premenstrual Syndrome

The following successive steps were outlined in an American College of Obstetrics and Gynecology (2000) and in a recent review by Johnson (2004):

Step 1: a. If mild/moderate symptoms: Supportive therapy with good nutrition, complex carbohydrates, aerobic exercise, calcium supplements, and possibly magnesium or chasteberry fruit.
b. If physical symptoms predominate: Spironolactone, NSAIDs, or hormonal suppression with OCPs or medroxyprogesterone acetate.
Step 2: When mood symptoms predominate: SSRI therapy. An anxiolytic can be used for specific symptoms not relieved by the SSRI medication.
Step 3: If not responsive to steps 1 or 2: GnRH agonists.

WEB SITES

For Teenagers and Parents

http://kidshealth.org/teen/sexual_health/girls/menstruation.html. Teen site on dysmenorrhea.
http://www.aafp.org/afp/990800ap/489.html. American Academy of Family Physicians (AAFP) article on primary dysmenorrhea.
http://www.obgyn.upenn.edu/mudd/PMSarticle.html. Information on PMS from University of Pennsylvania Obstetrics and Gynecology Department.
http://www.youngwomenshealth.org/menstrual.html. Information from Children's Hospital Boston on dysmenorrhea and PMS.
http://www.nlm.nih.gov/medlineplus/ency/article/001505.htm. Medical encyclopedia from the U.S. National Library of Medicine and National Institutes of Health. Information on PMS and dysmenorrhea.

For Health Professionals

http://www.emedicine.com/emerg/topic156.htm. E-medicine site on dysmenorrhea.
http://vh.org/navigation/vh/topics/menstruation.html. Information from the University of Iowa on dysmenorrhea and PMS.

REFERENCES AND ADDITIONAL READINGS

Alonso C, Coe CL. Disruptions of social relationships accentuate the association between emotional distress and menstrual pain in young women. *Health Psychol* 2001;20:411.
Alvin PE, Litt IF. Current status of the etiology and management of dysmenorrhea in adolescence. *Pediatrics* 1982;70:516.
American College of Obstetrics and Gynecology. *ACOG practice bulletin: premenstrual syndrome.* Washington, DC: ACOG, 2000:15.
American College of Obstetrics and Gynecology. ACOG Committee on Adolescent Health Care. Committee opinion No 310. Endometriosis in adolescents. *Obstet Gynecol* 2005;105:921.
American Psychiatric Association. *Diagnostic and statistical manual of mental disorders,* 4th ed. DSM-IV-Text Revision. R.R. Washington, DC: American Psychiatric Association, 2000.
Anderson FD, Hait H, Seasonale-301 Study Group. A multicenter, randomized study of an extended cycle oral contraceptive. *Contraception* 2003;68:89.
Atmaca M, Kumru S, Tezcan E. Fluoxetine versus *Vitex agnus castus* extract in the treatment of premenstrual dysphoric disorder. *Human Psychopharmacol Clin Exp* 2003;18:191.
Attaran M, Gidwani GP. Adolescent endometriosis. *Obstet Gynecol Clin North Am* 2003;30:379.
Audet M-C, Moreau M, Koltun WD, et al. Evaluation of contraceptive efficacy and cycle control of a transdermal contraceptive patch vs. an oral contraceptive. *JAMA* 2001;285:2347.
Baldaszti E, Wimmer-Puchinger B, Loschke K. Acceptability of the long-term contraceptive levonorgestrel-releasing intrauterine system (Mirena): a 3-year follow-up. *Contraception* 2003;67:87.
Banikarim C, Chacko MR, Kelder SH. Prevalence and impact of dysmenorrhea on Hispanic female adolescents. *Arch Pediatr Adolesc Med* 2000;154:1226.
Berger D, Schaffner W, Schrader E, et al. Efficacy of *Vitex agnus castus* L.extract Ze 440 in patients with pre-menstrual syndrome (PMS). *Arch Gynecol Obstet* 2000;264:150.
Bertone-Johnson ER, Hankinson SE, Bendich A, et al. Calcium and vitamin D intake and the risk of incident premenstrual syndrome. *Arch Int Med* 2005;165:1246.
Blake F, Salkovskis P, Gath D, et al. Cognitive therapy for premenstrual syndrome: a controlled trial. *J Psychosom Res* 1998;45:307.
Campbell MA, McGrath PJ. Use of medication by adolescents for the management of menstrual discomfort. *Arch Pediatr Adolesc Med* 1997;151:905.
Chakmakjian ZH. A critical assessment of therapy for the premenstrual tension syndrome. *J Reprod Med* 1983;28:532.
Chan WY, Dawood MY, Fucih F. Prostaglandins in primary dysmenorrhea. Comparison of prophylactic and nonprophylactic treatment with ibuprofen and use of oral contraceptives. *Am J Med* 1981;70:535.
Christensen AP, Oei TP. The efficacy of cognitive behaviour therapy in treating premenstrual dysphoric changes. *J Affect Disord* 1995;33:57.
Cohen LS, Soares CN, Lyster A, et al. Efficacy and tolerability of premenstrual use of venlafaxine (flexible dose) in the treatment of premenstrual dysphoric disorder. *J Clin Psychopharmacol* 2004;24:540.
Dalton K, Dalton ME, Guthrie K. Incidence of premenstrual syndrome in twins. *Br Med J* 1987;295:1027.
Daniels SE, Talwalker S, Torri S, et al. Valdecoxib, a cyclooxygenase-2-specific inhibitor, is effective in treating primary dysmenorrhea. *Obstet Gynecol* 2002;100:350.
Davis AR, Westhoff C. Primary dysmenorrhea in adolescent girls and treatment with oral contraceptives. *J Pediatr Adolesc Gynecol* 2001;14:3.
Davis AR, Westhoff C, O'Connell K, et al. Oral contraceptives for dysmenorrhea in adolescent girls. A randomized trial. *Obstet Gynecol* 2005;106:97.
Dawood MY, Ramos J. Transcutaneous electrical nerve stimulation (TENS) for the treatment of primary dysmenorrhea: a randomized crossover comparison with placebo, TENS, ibuprofen. *Obstet Gynecol* 1990;75:656.
Derman O, Kanbur NO, Tokur TE, et al. Premenstrual syndrome and associated symptoms in adolescent girls. *Eur J Obstet Gynecol Reprod Biol* 2004;116:201.

Diegoli MS, da Fonseca MA, Diegoli CA, et al. A double-blind trial of four medications to treat severe premenstrual syndrome. *Int J Gynaecol Obstet* 1998;62:63.

Di Girolamo G, Gimeno MA, Faletti A, et al. Menstrual prostaglandin and dysmenorrhea: modulation by non-steroidal antiinflammatory drugs. *Medicina (B Aires)* 1999;59:259.

Dimmock PW, Wyatt KM, Jones PW, et al. Efficacy of selective serotonin-reuptake inhibitors in premenstrual syndrome: a systematic review. *Lancet* 2000;356:1131.

Dmitrovic R, Peter B, Cvitkovic-Kuzmic A, et al. Severity of symptoms in primary dysmenorrhea-a doppler study. *Eur J Obstet Gynecol Reprod Biol* 2003;107:191.

DuRant RH, Jay S, Shoffitt T, et al. Factors influencing adolescents' responses to regimens of naproxen for dysmenorrhea. *Am J Dis Child* 1985;139:489.

Emans SJ, Laufer MR, Goldstein DP. *Pediatric and adolescent gynecology*, 5th ed. Philadelphia: Lippincott Williams &Wilkins, 2005.

Endicott J, Harrison W. *Daily rating of severity of problem form*. New York: Department of Research Assessment and Training, New York State Psychiatric Institute, 1990.

Facchinetti F, Borella P, Sauces G, et al. Oral magnesium successfully relieves premenstrual mood changes. *Obstet Gynecol* 1991;78:177.

Facchinetti F, Genazzani AD, Martignoni E, et al. Neuroendocrine changes in luteal function in patients with premenstrual syndrome. *J Clin Endocrinol Metab* 1993;76:1123.

Fisher M, Trieller K, Napolitano B. Premenstrual syndrome in adolescents. *J Adolesc Health Care* 1989;10:369.

Freeman EW. Luteal phase administration of agents for the treatment of premenstrual dysphoric disorder. *CNS Drugs* 2004;18:453.

Freeman EW, DeRubeis RJ, Rickels K. Reliability and validity of a daily diary for premenstrual syndrome. *Psychiatry Res* 1996;65:97.

Freeman EW, Kroll R, Rapkin A, et al. Evaluation of a unique oral contraceptive in the treatment of premenstrual dysphoric disorder. *J Womens Health Gender-Based Med* 2001;10:561.

Freeman EW, Rickels K, Sondheimer SJ, Ineffectiveness of progesterone suppository treatment for premenstrual syndrome. *JAMA* 1990;264:349.

Freeman EW, Rickels K, Sondheimer SJ. Premenstrual symptoms and dysmenorrhea in relation to emotional distress factors in adolescents. *J Psychosom Obstet Gynaecol* 1993;14:41.

Freeman EW, Rickels K, Sondheimer SJ, et al. A double-blind trial of oral progesterone, alprazolam, and placebo in treatment of severe premenstrual syndrome. *JAMA* 1995;274:51.

Freeman EW, Rickels K, Sondheimer SJ, et al. Differential response to antidepressants in women with premenstrual syndrome/premenstrual dysphoric disorder: a randomized controlled trial. *Arch Gen Psychiatry* 1999;56:932.

Freeman EW, Rickels K, Sondheimer SJ, et al. Continuous or intermittent dosing with sertraline for patients with severe premenstrual syndrome or premenstrual dysphoric disorder. *Am J Psychiatry* 2004;161:343.

Freeman EW, Rickels K, Yonkers KA, et al. Venlafaxine in the treatment of premenstrual dysphoric disorder. *Obstet Gynecol* 2001;98:737.

Freeman EW, Sondheimer SJ, Rickels K. Gonadotropin-releasing hormone agonist in treatment of premenstrual symptoms with and without ongoing dysphoria: a controlled study. *Psychopharmacol Bull* 1997;33:303.

Freeman EW, Sondheimer SJ, Sammel MD, et al. A preliminary study of luteal phase versus symptom-onset dosing with escitalopram for premenstrual dysphoric disorder. *J Clin Psychiatry* 2005;66:789.

Girman A, Lee R, Kigler B. An integrative medicine approach to premenstrual syndrome. *Am J Obstet Gynecol* 2003;188:S56.

Goldstein DP, deCholnoky C, Emans SJ. Adolescent endometriosis. *J Adolesc Health Care* 1980;1:37.

Grady-Weliky TA. Premenstrual dysphoric disorder. *N Engl J Med* 2003;348:433.

Halbreich U. The diagnosis of premenstrual syndromes and premenstrual dysphoric disorder-clinical procedures and research perspectives. *Gynecol Endocrinol* 2004;19:320.

Halbreich U, Endicott J, Schact S, et al. The diversity of premenstrual changes as reflected in the premenstrual assessment form. *Acta Psychiatr Scand* 1982;65:46.

Harel Z. Cyclooxygenase-2 specific inhibitors in the treatment of dysmenorrhea. *J Pediatr Adolesc Gynecol* 2004;17:75.

Harel Z. Approach to the adolescent girl as she transits from irregular to regular menstrual cycles. *J Pediatr Adolesc Gynecol* 2005;18:193.

Harel Z, Biro FM, Kottenhahn RK, et al. Supplementation with omega-3-polyunsaturated fatty acids in the management of dysmenorrhea in adolescents. *Am J Obstet Gynecol* 1996;174:1335.

Harlow SD, Park M. A longitudinal study of risk factors for the occurrence, duration, and severity of menstrual cramps in a cohort of college women. *Br J Obstet Gynecol* 1996;103:1134.

Harrison WM, Endicott J, Nee J. Treatment of premenstrual dysphoria with alprazolam. A controlled study. *Arch Gen Psychiatry* 1990;47:270.

Helms JM. Acupuncture for the management of primary dysmenorrhea. *Obstet Gynecol* 1987;69:S1.

Hendrix SL, Alexander NJ. Primary dysmenorrhea treatment with a desogestrel-containing low-dose oral contraceptive. *Contraception* 2002;66:393.

Henzl MR, Ortega-Herrera E, Rodriguez C, et al. Anaprox in dysmenorrhea: reduction of pain and intrauterine pressure. *Am J Obstet Gynecol* 1979;135:455.

Hillen TI, Grbavac SL, Johnston PJ, et al. Primary dysmenorrhea in young western Australian women: prevalence, impact, and knowledge in treatment. *J Adolesc Health* 1999;25:40.

Hornsby PP, Wilcox AJ, Weinburg CR. Cigarette smoking and disturbance of menstrual function. *Epidemiology* 1998;9:193.

Jamieson DJ, Steege JF. The prevalence of dysmenorrhea, dysparuenia, pelvic pain, and irritable bowel syndrome in primary care practices. *Obstet Gynecol* 1996;87:55.

Joffe H, Cohen LS, Harlow BL. Impact of oral contraceptive pill use on premenstrual mood: predictors of improvement and deterioration. *Am J Obstet Gynecol* 2003;189:1523.

Johnson J. Level of knowledge among adolescent girls regarding effective treatment for dysmenorrhea. *J Adolesc Health Care* 1988;9:398.

Johnson SR. Premenstrual syndrome, premenstrual dysphoric disorder, and beyond: a clinical primer for practitioners. *Obstet Gynecol* 2004;104:845.

Kaplan B, Rabinerson D, Lurie S, et al. Clinical evaluation of a new model of a transcutaneous electrical nerve stimulation device for the management of primary dysmenorrheal. *Gynecol Obstet Invest* 1997;44:255.

Kendall KE, Schnurr PP. The effects of vitamin B6 supplementation on premenstrual symptoms. *Obstet Gynecol* 1987;70:145.

Kirkby RJ. Changes in premenstrual symptoms and irrational thinking following cognitive-behavioral coping skills training. *J Consult Clin Psychol* 1994;62:1026.

Klein JR, Litt IF. Epidemiology of adolescent dysmenorrhea. *Pediatrics* 1981;68:661.

Koike H, Egawa H, Ohtsuka T, et al. Correlation between dysmenorrheic severity and prostaglandin production in women with endometriosis. *Prostaglandins Leukot Essent Fatty Acids* 1992;46:133.

Landen M, Eriksson O, Sundblad C, et al. Compounds with affinity for serotonergic receptors in the treatment of premenstrual dysphoria: a comparison of busprione, nefazodone and placebo. *Psychopharmacology* 2001;155:292.

Laufer MR, Goitein L, Bush M, et al. Prevalence of endometriosis in adolescent girls with chronic pelvic pain not responding to conventional therapy. *J Pediatr Adolesc Gynecol* 1997;10:199.

Laufer MR, Goldstein DP. Gynecologic pain: dysmenorrhea, acute and chronic pelvic pain, endometriosis and premenstrual syndrome. In: Emans SJ, Laufer MR, Goldstein DP, eds. *Pediatric and adolescent gynecology*, 5th ed. Philadelphia: Lippincott Williams & Wilkins, 2005:417.

Laufer MR, Sanfilippo J, Rose G. Adolescent endometriosis: diagnosis and treatment approaches. *J Pediatr Adolesc Gynecol* 2003;16:S3.

Ling FW. Recognizing and treating premenstrual dysphoric disorder in the obstetric, gynecologic, and primary care practices. *J Clin Psychiatry* 2000;61(Suppl 12):9.

London RS, Murphy L, Kitowski KE, et al. Efficacy of alpha-tocopherol in the treatment of premenstrual syndrome. *J Reprod Med* 1987;32:400.

Lumsden MA, Baird DT. Intra-uterine pressure in dysmenorrhea. *Acta Obstet Gynecol Scand* 1985;64:183.

Lundstrom V, Green K. Endogenous levels of prostaglandin $F_{2\alpha}$ and its main metabolites in plasma and endometrium of normal and dysmenorrheic women. *Am J Obstet Gynecol* 1978;130:640.

Magos JAL, Studd JW. A simple method for the diagnosis of premenstrual syndrome by use of a self-assessment disk. *Am J Obstet Gynecol* 1988;158:1024.

Marjoribanks H, Proctor ML, Farquhar C. Nonsteroidal anti-inflammatory drugs for primary dysmenorrhea. *Cochrane Database Syst Rev* 2003;(4):CD001751. DOI:10.1002/14651858.CD001751.

Miller LM, Hughes JP. Continuous combination oral contraceptive pills to eliminate withdrawal bleeding: a randomized trial. *Obstet Gynecol* 2003;101:653.

Moore J, Kennedy S, Prentice A. Modern combined oral contraceptives for pain associated with endometriosis. *Cochrane Database Syst Rev* 1007;(4):CD001019. DOI:10.1002/14651858.CD001019.

Morrison BW, Daniels SE, Kotey P, et al. Rofecoxib, a specific cyclooxygenase-2 inhibitor, in primary dysmenorrhea: a randomized controlled trial. *Obstet Gynecol* 1999;94:504.

Morse G. Positively reframing perceptions of the menstrual cycle among women with premenstrual syndrome. *J Obstet Gynecol Neonatal Nursing* 1999;28:165.

Mortola JF. A risk-benefit appraisal of drugs used in the management of premenstrual syndrome. *Drug Saf* 1994;10:160.

Mortola JF. Premenstrual syndrome-pathophysiologic considerations. *N Engl J Med* 1998;338:256.

Mortola JF, Girton L, Beck L, et al. Diagnosis of premenstrual syndrome by a simple, prospective, and reliable instrument: the calendar of premenstrual experiences. *Obstet Gynecol* 1990;76:302.

National Institutes of Health. NIH consensus conference: acupuncture. *JAMA* 1998;280:1518.

Owen PR. Prostaglandin synthetase inhibitors in the treatment of primary dysmenorrhea. *Am J Obstet Gynecol* 1984;148:96.

Pearlstein T, Steiner M. Non-antidepressant treatment of premenstrual syndrome. *J Clin Psychiatry* 2000;61(suppl):22.

Pearlstein TB, Stone A, Lund SA, et al. Comparison of fluoxetine, buproprion, and placebo in the treatment of premenstrual dysphoric disorder. *J Clin Psychopharmacol* 1997;17:261.

Pedron-Nuevo N, Gonzalez-Unzaga LN, De Celis-Carrillo R, et al. Incidence of dysmenorrhea and associated symptoms in women aged 13–24 years. *Ginecol Obstet Mex* 1998;66:492.

Perkonigg A, Yonkers KA, Pfister H, et al. Risk factors for premenstrual dysphonic disorder in a community sample of young women: the role of traumatic events and posttraumatic stress disorder. *J Clin Psychiatry* 2004;65:1314.

Prior JC, Vigna Y, Sciarretta D, et al. Conditioning exercise decreases premenstrual symptoms: a prospective controlled 6-month trial. *Fertil Steril* 1987;47:402.

Proctor M, Farquhar C. Dysmenorrhea. *Clin Evid* 2004;12:2524.

Proctor ML, Murphy PA. Herbal and dietary therapies for primary and secondary dysmenorrhoea. *Cochrane Database Syst Rev* 2001;(2):CD002124. DOI: 10.1002/14652858. CD002124.

Proctor ML, Roberts H, Farquhar CM. Combined oral contraceptive pill (OCP) as treatment for primary dysmenorrhea. *Cochrane Database Syst Rev* 2001;(2):CD002120. DOI:10.1002/14651858.CD002120.

Raja SN, Feehan M, Stanton WR, et al. Prevalence and correlates of the premenstrual syndrome in adolescence. *J Am Acad Child Adolesc Psychiatry* 1992;31:783.

Reese KA, Reddy S, Rock JA. Endometriosis in an adolescent population: the Emory experience. *J Pediatr Adolesc Gynecol* 1996;9:125.

Reid RL. Premenstrual syndrome. *Curr Probl Obstet Gynecol Fertil* 1985;8:1.

Robinson JC, Plichta S, Weisman CS, et al. Dysmenorrhea and use of oral contraceptives in adolescent women attending a family planning clinic. *Am J Obstet Gynecol* 1992;166:578.

Romano S, Judge R, Dillon J, et al. The role of fluoxetine in the treatment of premenstrual dysphoric disorder. *Clin Ther* 1999;21:615.

Ruoff G, Lema M. Strategies in pain management: new and potential indications for COX-2 specific inhibitors. *J Pain Symptom Manage* 2003;25:S21.

Sayegh R, Schiff I, Wurtman J, et al. The effect of a carbohydrate-rich beverage on mood, appetite, and cognitive function in women with premenstrual syndrome. *Obstet Gynecol* 1995;86:520.

Schellenberg R. Treatment for the premenstrual syndrome with agnus castus fruit extract: prospective, randomized, placebo controlled study. *Br Med J* 2001;322:134.

Schmidt PJ, Nieman LK, Danaceau MA, et al. Differential behavioral effects of gondal steroids in women with and in those without premenstrual syndrome. *N Engl J Med* 1998;338:209.

Schmidt PJ, Neiman LK, Grober GN, et al. Lack of effect of induced menses on symptoms in women with premenstrual syndrome. *N Engl J Med* 1991;324:1174.

Schroeder B, Sanfilippo JS. Dysmenorrhea and pelvic pain in adolescents. *Pediatr Clin North Am* 1999;46:555.

Scully D, Kremer J, Meade MM, et al. Physical exercise and psychological well being: a critical review. *Br J Sports Med* 1998;32:111.

Shapiro SS. Treatment of dysmenorrhoea and premenstrual syndrome with non-steroidal anti-inflammatory drugs. *Drugs* 1988;36:475.

Singh BB, Berman BM, Simpson RL, et al. Incidence of premenstrual syndrome and remedy usage: a national probability sample study. *Altern Ther Health Med* 1998;4:75.

Smith S, Rinehart JS, Ruddock VE. Treatment of premenstrual syndrome with alprozolam: results of a double-blind, placebo-controlled, randomized crossover clinical trial. *Obstet Gynecol* 1987;70:37.

Speroff L, Fritz MA. *Clinical gynecologic endocrinology and infertility*, 7th ed. Philadelphia: Lippincott Williams & Wilkins, 2005.

Steege JF, Blumenthal JA. The effects of aerobic exercise on premenstrual symptoms in middle-aged women: a preliminary study. *J Psychosom Res* 1993;37:127.

Steiner M, Pearlstein T. Premenstrual dysphoria and the serotonin system: pathophysiology and treatment. *J Clin Psychiatry* 2000;61(Suppl 12):17.

Steiner M, Steinberg S, Stewart D, et al. Fluoxetine in the treatment of premenstrual dysphoria. *N Engl J Med* 1995;332:1529.

Stevinson C, Ernst E. Complementary/alternative therapies for premenstrual syndrome: a systematic review of randomized controlled trials. *Am J Obstet Gynecol* 2001;185:227.

Sucato GS, Gold MA. Extended cycling of oral contraceptive pills for adolescents. *J Pediatr Adolesc Gynecol* 2002; 15:325.

Sulak PJ, Kuehl TJ, Ortiz M, et al. Acceptance of altering the standard 21 day/7-day oral contraceptive regimen to delay menses and reduce hormone withdrawal symptoms. *Am J Obstet Gynecol* 2002;186:1142.

Surrey ES, Hornstein MD. Prolonged GnRH agonist and add-back therapy for symptomatic endometriosis: long-term follow up. *Obstet Gynecol* 2002;99:709.

Teperi J, Rimpela M. Menstrual pain, health and behaviour in girls. *Soc Sci Med* 1989;29:163.

Thys-Jacobs S, Alvir JM, Fratarcangelo P. Comparative analysis of three PMS assessment instruments-the identification of premenstrual syndrome with core symptoms. *Psycopharmacol Bull* 1995;31:389.

Thys-Jacobs S, Starky P, Bernstein D, et al. Premenstrual Syndrome Study Group. Calcium carbonate and the premenstrual syndrome: effects on premenstrual and menstrual symptoms. *Am J Obstet Gynecol* 1998;179:444.

Van der Akker OB, Stein GS, Neil MC, et al. Genetic and environmental variation in 2 British twin samples. *Acta Genet Med Gemellol (Roma)* 1987;36:541.

Vercellini P, Frontino G, De Giorgi O, et al. Continuous use of an oral contraceptive for endometriosis-associated recurrent dysmenorrhea that does not respond to a cyclic pill regimen. *Fertil Steril* 2003a;80:560.

Vercellini P, Frontino G, De Giorgi O, et al. Comparison of a levonorgestrel-releasing intrauterine device versus expectant management after conservative surgery for symptomatic endometriosis: a pilot study. *Fertil Steril* 2003b;80: 305.

Vicdan K, Kukner S, Dabakoglu T, et al. Demographic and epidemiologic features of female adolescents in Turkey. *J Adolesc Health* 1996;18:54.

Walker AF, De Souza MC, Vickers MF, et al. Magnesium supplementation alleviates premenstrual symptoms of fluid retention. *J Womens Health* 1998;7:1157.

Wang M, Hammarback S, Lindhe BA, et al. Treatment of premenstrual syndrome by spironolactone: a double-blind placebo controlled study. *Acta Obstet Gynecol Scand* 1995;74: 803.

Weaver AL. Rofecoxib: clinical pharmacology and clinical experience. *Clin Ther* 2001;23:1323.

Widholm O. Dysmenorrhea during adolescence. *Acta Obstet Gynecol Scand Suppl* 1979;87:61.

Widholm O, Kantero RL. A statistical analysis of the menstrual patterns of 8,000 Finnish girls and their mothers. *Acta Obstet Gynecol Scand* 1971;14(suppl):1.

Wilson CA, Keye WR. A survey of adolescent dysmenorrhea and premenstrual symptom frequency. *J Adolesc Health Care* 1989;10:317.

Wyatt KM, Dimmock PW, Jones PW, et al. Efficacy of vitamin B6 in the treatment of premenstrual syndrome: systematic review. *Br Med J* 1999;318:1375.

Wyatt KM, Dimmock PW, O'Brien PMS. Selective serotonin reuptake inhibitors for premenstrual syndrome. *Cochrane Database Syst Rev* 2005;(3):CD001396. DOI:10.1002/14651858.CD001396.

Ylikorkala O, Dawood MY. New concepts in dysmenorrhea. *Am J Obstet Gynecol* 1978;130:833.

Yonkers KA, Brown C, Pearlstein TB, et al. Efficacy of a new low-dose oral contraceptive with drosperionone in premenstrual dysphoric disorder. *Obstet Gynecol* 2005;106:492.

Zhang WY, Li Wan Po A. Efficacy of minor analgesics in primary dysmenorrhoea:a systematic review. *Br J Obstet Gynecol* 1998;105:780.

CHAPTER 51

Dysfunctional Uterine Bleeding

Laurie A. P. Mitan and Gail B. Slap

Dysfunctional uterine bleeding (DUB) is a common menstrual problem during adolescence. When severe, it can result in life-threatening anemia. Even when mild, it is usually both a concern and a nuisance for the adolescent. By definition, DUB is irregular and/or prolonged vaginal bleeding due to endometrial sloughing in the absence of structural pathology. In adolescents, anovulation secondary to physiological immaturity explains most cases of irregular bleeding. Although structural pathology accounts for <10% of abnormal uterine bleeding during adolescence, it must be excluded before the diagnosis of DUB can be established.

DEFINITIONS

1. Normal menstrual cycles during adolescence are 21 to 40 days long, with 2 to 8 days of bleeding and 20 to 80 mL blood loss per cycle.
2. Ovulatory cycles are characterized by a follicular phase ending with ovulation and a luteal phase ending with menstruation. During the follicular phase, rising serum levels of follicle-stimulating hormone (FSH) stimulate ovarian follicular maturation and estrogen production. The rising serum estrogen levels stimulate endometrial proliferation and progressive thickening. A preovulatory surge in estrogen is followed by a surge in luteinizing hormone (LH), which triggers ovulation. During the luteal phase, the residual follicle converts to a corpus luteum that produces increasing levels of progesterone and estrogen. The progesterone stabilizes the thickened endometrium and stops further proliferation. In the absence of fertilization, the corpus luteum involutes, estrogen and progesterone levels fall, and the endometrium sloughs, resulting in menstrual bleeding.

   Up to 80% of menstrual cycles are anovulatory in the first year after menarche. Cycles become ovulatory at an average of 20 months after menarche.
3. DUB during adolescence is abnormal endometrial sloughing in the absence of structural pathology or anomaly, usually due to anovulation.
4. Menorrhagia is prolonged or heavy uterine bleeding that occurs at regular intervals.
5. Metrorrhagia is uterine bleeding that occurs at irregular intervals.
6. Menometrorrhagia is prolonged or heavy uterine bleeding that occurs at irregular intervals.
7. Oligomenorrhea is uterine bleeding that occurs at prolonged intervals of 41 days to 3 months but is of normal flow, duration, and quantity.

DIFFERENTIAL DIAGNOSIS

An estimated 10% of adolescents managed as outpatients for abnormal bleeding, compared with 25% of those requiring hospitalization, have an identifiable structural, infectious, or clotting abnormality. Among adolescents hospitalized with hemorrhage at menarche resulting in a hemoglobin level <10 g/dL, 50% have a systemic bleeding disorder (Claessens and Cowell, 1981).

The differential diagnosis of abnormal bleeding is quite different in the adolescent than the adult. Uterine fibroids and endometrial malignancy lead the differential diagnosis in the adult but are rare in the adolescent. Conversely, congenital anomalies of the outflow tract may be subclinical until menarche, but rarely remain unrecognized until adulthood. Apart from DUB, the differential diagnosis of abnormal bleeding during adolescence includes the following conditions:

1. Pregnancy-related causes: Ectopic pregnancy; spontaneous, threatened, or incomplete abortion; placental polyp; hydatidiform mole
2. Local pathology: Foreign body in the vagina (e.g., retained tampon) or uterus (e.g., intrauterine device); cervicitis or endometritis due to a sexually transmitted disease (STD) or instrumentation; laceration or other trauma; polyp of the cervix or uterus; congenital anomaly of the outflow tract; premalignant or malignant lesion of the cervix or uterus
3. Bleeding diathesis: Idiopathic thrombocytopenic purpura; von Willebrand disease; abnormal platelet function due to drugs (e.g., aspirin) or systemic illness (e.g., renal failure); bone marrow suppression (e.g., chemotherapy) or infiltration (e.g., leukemia); coagulopathy due to inherited clotting factor deficiency, systemic illness (e.g., liver failure), or anticoagulant therapy (e.g., warfarin)
4. Hormonal causes: Anovulatory bleeding

   Anovulatory causes usually relate to one of three hormonal imbalance conditions:
   a. Estrogen breakthrough bleeding: This occurs when excess estrogen stimulates the endometrium to proliferate in an undifferentiated manner. With inadequate

progesterone levels to provide support to the endometrium, portions of the lining will slough at irregular intervals. In addition, the vasoconstriction mediated through progesterone and prostaglandin levels does not occur, often resulting in profuse bleeding.

b. Estrogen withdrawal bleeding: This bleeding results from a sudden decrease in estrogen levels. This could occur after stopping exogenous estrogen therapy or just before ovulation in the normal menstrual cycle. This type of withdrawal bleeding is usually self-limited.

c. Progesterone breakthrough bleeding: This occurs when the ratio of progesterone to estrogen is high, such as with progesterone-only contraceptive methods. In these individuals, the endometrium becomes atrophic and more prone to frequent, irregular bleeding.

Hormonally mediated DUB therefore tends to be less associated with dysmenorrhea than normal menses following ovulation or abnormal bleeding due to a structural or infectious problem. The most common causes of hormonally mediated DUB (anovulatory bleeding) during adolescence are the following:

1. Gynecological immaturity: Immaturity of the hypothalamic-pituitary-ovarian axis is the leading cause of DUB during adolescence. After menarche, anovulation is associated with 50% to 80% of bleeding episodes during the first 2 years, 30% to 55% during years 2 to 4, and 20% during years 4 to 5. The likelihood of anovulatory bleeding increases with menarcheal age. More than 50% of bleeding episodes are anovulatory for 1 year when menarche occurs before age 12 years, for 3 years when menarche occurs at age 12 to 13 years, and for 4 years when menarche occurs after age 13 years. Despite these high rates of anovulation, the negative feedback of estrogen on the hypothalamic-pituitary axis protects most adolescents from DUB. Even when ovulation does not occur, gonadotropin levels decrease in response to increasing estrogen levels. Estrogen production then declines before the endometrium becomes excessively thickened, and withdrawal bleeding occurs. Most anovulatory cycles therefore tend to be fairly regular, and the bleeding tends to be limited in duration and quantity.

2. Defective corpus luteum: DUB can occur in an ovulatory cycle with early involution of the corpus luteum and inadequate progesterone production.

3. Hormonal contraception or replacement therapy: Exogenous estrogen and/or progestins, whether intended for contraception or replacement therapy, may cause anovulation and irregular bleeding. If a uterus is present, unopposed estrogen is associated with an increased risk for endometrial carcinoma. In any postpubertal patient with a uterus, the regimen therefore should include both estrogen and a progestin administered cyclically or in a fixed daily dose. Among patients using hormonal contraception, irregular bleeding is more common with progestin-only than combined estrogen-progestin methods.

4. Hypothyroidism or hyperthyroidism: Although either condition may cause DUB, hypothyroidism is more commonly associated with menorrhagia than hyperthyroidism.

5. Polycystic ovary syndrome (PCOS): See Chapter 52.

6. Late-onset congenital adrenal hyperplasia (e.g., partial 21-hydroxylase deficiency): See Chapter 58.

7. Hypothalamic hypogonadism: Eating disorders, weight loss from other causes, excessive exercise, and emotional or physical stress typically present with amenorrhea or oligomenorrhea rather than DUB. However, there may be intermittent ovulatory cycles with withdrawal bleeding or sufficient endogenous estrogen to produce breakthrough bleeding over time.

EVALUATION

The evaluation of any patient with bleeding begins with an assessment of hemodynamic stability. The next objective is to determine the site of the bleeding (e.g., gastrointestinal, urinary, vaginal, cervical, or uterine). Once the bleeding is found to be uterine, the evaluation focuses on determination of its cause.

History

Part of the history should be obtained from the adolescent and, if possible, the parent or guardian. The sexual history should be obtained from the adolescent alone unless she makes it clear that she is comfortable discussing it with the parent present.

1. Menstrual history: Age at menarche, cycle regularity, cycle duration, flow duration, change in cycle or flow, change in number of saturated pads or tampons, dysmenorrhea, pelvic pain between menses, change in pain associated with menses

2. Sexual history: Age at coitarche, use of condoms, contraception, pregnancies, deliveries, miscarriages, abortions, past STDs, past pelvic inflammatory disease (PID), number of partners, recent new partner, vaginal discharge, known exposure to a partner with an STD

3. History of systemic illness

4. Endocrine history: Symptoms suggestive of hypothyroidism (e.g., fatigue, weight gain, dry skin), hyperthyroidism (e.g., palpitations, increased appetite, weight loss), or hyperandrogenism (e.g., hirsutism, acne, weight gain); use of hormonal contraception or exogenous hormones

5. Family history: PCOS, bleeding diathesis

6. Review of systems: Fatigue, lightheadedness, rapid heart beat, palpitations, gum bleeding, epistaxis, significant weight changes, stress

Physical Examination

1. Vital signs: Blood pressure and heart rate in supine, sitting, and standing positions to detect orthostatic changes; height, weight, and body mass index (BMI)

2. Sexual maturity ratings: Breasts and pubic hair

3. Skin, hair, and mucosa: Scalp hair thinning or dryness, hirsutism, acanthosis nigricans, acne, petechiae, purpura, ecchymoses, gum bleeding, epistaxis

4. Thyroid: Enlargement, tenderness, nodules

5. Breasts: Galactorrhea

6. Lymph nodes: Lymphadenopathy

7. Abdomen: Hepatosplenomegaly, palpable uterus, mass

8. Pelvic examination: Essential in all sexually active adolescents; also indicated if the history suggests structural pathology as the cause of the bleeding; can be deferred in the adolescent with suspected anovulatory DUB, who has never had sexual intercourse

Laboratory Tests

Laboratory testing may not be necessary in the adolescent with mild anovulatory DUB associated with physiological immaturity. Depending on the history and physical examination results, other patients may require the following laboratory evaluation:

1. Pregnancy test: A urine test for β-human chorionic gonadotropin (β-hCG) should be done in all patients if there is any question of past sexual intercourse. If the urine test result is positive, a quantitative serum test for β-hCG should be performed. In these cases of possible ectopic pregnancies, an ultrasound and gynecology referral should strongly be considered.
2. Complete blood cell count: Unless the bleeding is mild and of recent onset, all patients should have hemoglobin, hematocrit, and platelet count evaluation. A white blood cell count with differential is helpful if PID is suspected.
3. STD screening: Endocervical tests for gonorrheal and chlamydial infections are indicated for all adolescents who have ever had sexual intercourse.
4. Erythrocyte sedimentation rate: May help support a diagnosis of PID or underlying systemic illness.
5. Thyroid function tests for all patients with moderate to severe menorrhagia.
6. Prothrombin time, partial thromboplastin time, and PFA-100 as a preliminary screen for a bleeding disorder. The PFA-100 has a negative predictive value of 91% for von Willebrand disease and common platelet function disorders (Buyukasik et al., 2002). Anemia decreases the performance of the PFA-100 and concomitant use of estrogens can falsely elevate von Willebrand factor levels. Patients with moderate to severe anemia, personal history of bleeding in addition to menorrhagia, or family history of significant bleeding should be evaluated with more specific diagnostic tests such as von Willebrand factor antigen and ristocetin cofactor activity. Hematology consultation may be necessary.
7. Liver function tests and blood urea nitrogen are required if there is evidence of abnormal clotting factors or platelet function.
8. Antinuclear antibody: Preliminary screen for autoimmune disease.
9. LH, FSH, testosterone (total and free), and dehydroepiandrosterone sulfate levels, if PCOS is suspected (see Chapter 52).
10. Pelvic ultrasonography: Transabdominal ultrasonography performed through a full bladder is essential in the virginal patient with possible structural pathology who cannot tolerate a pelvic examination. Transabdominal and transvaginal ultrasonography is indicated if the pregnancy test is positive or if a mass is palpated on pelvic examination.
11. Endometrial aspirate and/or biopsy are rarely indicated in adolescents.

THERAPY

The severity and cause of the bleeding guide its management. Severe bleeding with hemodynamic instability, regardless of cause, requires immediate intervention with intravenous fluids and/or blood transfusion. Adolescents without underlying cardiovascular disease usually respond quickly to intravenous fluids and supplemental iron therapy, without the need for transfusion. Severe anemia that developed over months or years of abnormal bleeding is better tolerated than the same level of anemia that developed over hours or days of acute bleeding. Bleeding secondary to pregnancy, infection, or structural pathology requires prompt treatment of the underlying condition. Bleeding secondary to a systemic problem, such as a clotting abnormality or thyroid dysfunction, may require short-term hormonal therapy identical to that for anovulatory bleeding until the systemic problem is brought under control.

Anovulatory Dysfunctional Uterine Bleeding

The approach to anovulatory DUB depends on bleeding severity, hemoglobin and/or hematocrit value, hemodynamic tolerance, and emotional tolerance. It can generally be divided into the following categories:

1. Light to moderate flow, hemoglobin level of at least 12 g/dL: Reassurance, multivitamin with iron, menstrual calendar, reevaluation within 3 months.
2. Moderate flow, hemoglobin level of 10 to 12 g/dL: Begin a 35-μg combined oral contraceptive pill to be taken every 6 to 12 hours for 24 to 48 hours until the bleeding stops, along with an antiemetic if necessary for nausea and vomiting. Oral supplemental iron therapy should be initiated as early as possible but may not be tolerated during the first 2 days of high-dose hormonal therapy. Nonsteroidal antiinflammatory drugs (NSAIDs) can be used as adjunctive therapy, along with the oral contraceptive to decrease both bleeding and, when present, dysmenorrhea. Taper the oral contraceptive to one pill daily by day 5. Begin a new 28-day pill packet and inform the patient that a withdrawal bleed is likely during the week of placebo pills. Continue the combined oral contraceptive for 3 to 6 months.

   Medroxyprogesterone acetate (Provera) has been used alone by some providers, although it does not appear to be as effective and leads to breakthrough bleeding.
3. Heavy flow, hemoglobin level <10 g/dL: If the patient is hemodynamically stable, reliable, and able to tolerate the oral contraceptive, management is as stated earlier. Otherwise, hospitalization is indicated until the bleeding stops on the previously described regimen. A 50-μg combined oral contraceptive every 6 hours may be necessary to control the bleeding in some patients. If the bleeding does not slow within two doses of the 50-μg pill, add conjugated estrogen intravenously (25 mg every 6 hours for a maximum of six doses). Then taper the oral contraceptive to one pill daily by day 7. If the bleeding does not stop within six doses of intravenous estrogen plus the combined oral contraceptive, cervical dilation with endometrial curettage is usually necessary.

Dysfunctional Uterine Bleeding Secondary to Hormonal Contraception

1. Persistent bleeding on a 20-μg combined oral contraceptive pill usually stops when a higher-dose estrogen (e.g., 30–35 μg) pill is prescribed.
2. Persistent bleeding on a 30 to 35-μg pill requires either a 50-μg pill for one cycle or the addition of conjugated estrogen at 0.625 mg daily to the 35-μg pill for one cycle.

3. Persistent bleeding on progesterone-only contraceptives can be managed with the short-term addition of conjugated estrogen (1.25–2.50 mg daily for 5–7 days) and/or NSAIDs. Although this will stop the bleeding, the likelihood of subsequent spotting is also increased because of the estrogen-induced endometrial proliferation.

Bleeding Diatheses

Iatrogenic DUB is common in patients receiving chemotherapeutic or other interventions that alter bone marrow production, platelet function, or clotting factor synthesis. The management of DUB in these patients attempts to decrease menstrual frequency or induce endometrial atrophy. Options are as follows:

1. Combined oral contraceptive pill (21-day packet), one pill daily continuously. The pill should be discontinued for 1 week every 3 months to allow a withdrawal bleed and thereby prevent excessive endometrial proliferation.
2. Depot medroxyprogesterone (DMPA), 150 mg intramuscularly every 12 weeks. Would consider potential deleterious skeletal effects associated with long-term (>2 year) use of this agent (see Chapter 47).
3. Progesterone, 10 mg orally daily for an unlimited number of months.
4. Gonadotropin-releasing hormone analog (e.g., leuprolide acetate). Owing to its hypoestrogenemic side effects, this option should be used for no more than 6 months. It is an excellent choice for prophylactic use in conditions associated with short-term thrombocytopenia, such as bone marrow transplantation, and should be started at least 2 weeks before onset of thrombocytopenia (Ghalie et al., 1993).

WEB SITES

For Teenagers and Parents

www.youngwomenshealth.org. From Children's Hospital Boston.
www.healthfinder.gov. Government health information finder.
www.kidshealth.org., From Nemours Foundation.
www.nlm.nih.gov, The National Library of Medicine health information site.
http://www.womenshealthchannel.com/dub/index.shtml. From the Women's Health Channel.

For Health Professionals

www.acog.org. American College of Obstetricians and Gynecologists (ACOG).
www.naspag.org, North American Society for Pediatric and Adolescent Gynecology (NASPAG)

http://www.sh.lsuhsc.edu/fammed/OutpatientManual/DUB.htm. From the Family Practice Program, Louisiana State University Health Sciences Center
http://www.aafp.org/afp/991001ap/1371.html. From the American Academy of Family Physicians. Patient information handout provided by link within.

REFERENCES AND ADDITIONAL READINGS

Bayer SR, DeCherney AH. Clinical manifestations and treatment of dysfunctional uterine bleeding. *JAMA* 1993;14:1823.

Bevan JA, Maloney KW, Hillery CA, et al. Bleeding disorders: a common cause of menorrhagia in adolescents. *J Pediatr* 2001;138(6):856.

Bravender T, Emans SJ. Menstrual disorders. Dysfunctional uterine bleeding. *Pediatr Clin North Am* 1999;46(3):545.

Buyukasik Y, Karakus S, Goker H, et al. Rational use of the PFA-100 device for screening of platelet function disorders and von Willebrand disease. *Blood Coagul Fibrinolysis* 2002;13:349.

Chiusolo P, Salutari P, Sica S, et al. Luteinizing hormone-releasing hormone analogue: leuprorelin acetate for the prevention of menstrual bleeding in premenopausal women undergoing stem cell transplantation. *Bone Marrow Transplant* 1998;21:821.

Claessens EA, Cowell CA. Acute adolescent menorrhagia. *Am J Obstet Gynecol* 1981;139:277.

Cowan BD, Morrison JC. Management of abnormal genital bleeding in girls and women. *N Engl J Med* 1991;324:1710.

Emans SJ. Dysfunctional uterine bleeding. In: Emans SJ, Laufer MR, Goldstein DP, eds. *Pediatric and adolescent gynecology*, 5th ed. Philadelphia: Lippincott, Williams & Wilkins; 2005,270.

Ghalie R, Porter C, Radwanska E, et al. Prevention of hypermenorrhea with leuprolide in premenopausal women undergoing bone marrow transplantation. *Am J Hematol* 1993;42:350.

Iglesias EA, Coupey SM. Menstrual cycle abnormalities: diagnosis and management. *Adolesc Med* 1999;10:255.

Minjarez DA, Bradshaw KD. Abnormal uterine bleeding in adolescents. *Obstet Gynecol Clin North Am* 2000;27:63.

Mitan LAP, Slap GB. Adolescent menstrual disorders: update. *Med Clin North Am* 2000;84:851.

Ragni MV, Bontempo FA, Hassett AC. von Willebrand disease and bleeding in women. *Haemophilia* 1999;5:313.

Shaw RW. Assessment of medical treatments for menorrhagia. *Br J Obstet Gynaecol* 1994;101(Suppl 11):15.

Shwayder JM. Pathophysiology of abnormal uterine bleeding. *Obstet Gynecol Clin North Am* 2000;27:219.

Winikoff R, Amesse C, James A, et al. The role of haemophilia treatment centres in providing services to women with bleeding disorders. *Haemophilia* 2004;10(Suppl 4):196.

CHAPTER 52

Menstrual Disorders: Amenorrhea and the Polycystic Ovary Syndrome

Amy Fleischman, Catherine M. Gordon, and Lawrence S. Neinstein

AMENORRHEA

Definition

Amenorrhea is defined by a variety of diagnostic criteria. However, strict adherence to these criteria can potentially lead to improper management. Chronological age and developmental stage, in association with clinical data, must be integrated into the criteria for establishing a diagnosis of amenorrhea. Such guidelines are listed in this chapter. The need for evaluation can be determined by the number of criteria that are present.

A brief review of normal development is essential in determining abnormalities of the menstrual cycle.

- For the American adolescent, the average age at menarche is 12.7 years, with a two standard deviation range of 11 to 15 months. Although there have been some reports of a trend toward younger ages for pubertal initiation, the average age at menarche seems to have remained stable.
- Ninety-five percent to 97% of females reach menarche by age 16 years and 98% by 18 years.
- There is an average of 2 years between the start of thelarche, the first sign of puberty, and the onset of menarche.
- The onset of menarche is fairly constant in adolescent development, with approximately two thirds of females reaching menarche at a Tanner sexual maturity rating (SMR) of 4. Menarche occurs at SMR 2 in 5% of girls, SMR 3 in 25%, and not until SMR 5 in 10%.
- Ninety-five percent of teens have attained menarche 1 year after attaining SMR 5.

1. Primary amenorrhea
   a. No episodes of spontaneous uterine bleeding by the age of 14 years with secondary sexual characteristics absent.
   b. No episodes of spontaneous uterine bleeding by age 16 years regardless of normal secondary sexual characteristics (chronological criteria).
   c. No episodes of spontaneous uterine bleeding, despite having attained SMR 5 for at least 1 year or despite the onset of breast development 4 years previously (developmental criteria).
   d. No episodes of spontaneous uterine bleeding by age 14 years in any individual with clinical stigmata of or genotype consistent with Turner syndrome.

2. Secondary amenorrhea: After previous uterine bleeding, no subsequent menses for 6 months or a length of time equal to three previous cycles.

Etiology

1. Primary amenorrhea without secondary sexual characteristics (absent breast development), but with normal genitalia (uterus and vagina)
   a. Genetic or enzymatic defects causing gonadal (ovarian) failure (hypergonadotropic hypogonadism): Approximately 30% of primary amenorrhea cases are secondary to a genetic cause. The most common disorders are as follows:
      - Turner syndrome, Turner mosaicism or related genotypes (45,X; 45,XX/X; or 45,XY/X: Stigmata are variable in mosaicism, but classically include short stature (height usually <60 in.); streaked gonads; sexual infantilism; and somatic anomalies (webbed neck, short fourth metacarpal, cubitus valgus, coarctation of the aorta).
      - Structurally abnormal X chromosome: Phenotype varies. Long-arm deletion commonly causes normal stature, no somatic abnormalities, streaked gonads, and sexual infantilism. Short-arm deletion defects lead to a phenotype similar to that of Turner syndrome.
      - Mosaicism: X/XX. Eighty percent of such individuals are short, 66% have some somatic anomaly, and 20% have spontaneous menses. The characteristics for X/XXX and X/XX/XXX individuals are similar to those for X/XX individuals.
      - Pure gonadal dysgenesis (46,XX or 46,XX/XY with streaked gonads): Stigmata include normal stature, streaked gonads, sexual infantilism, and usually no somatic abnormalities. Etiologies can include autoimmunity, and enzymatic or genetic abnormalities. The etiology may be important in directing further evaluation and in counseling families. For example, a fragile X premutation in a female carrier can cause ovarian failure while future generations in the family would be at risk for severe mental retardation in males. Evidence of autoimmunity, such as ovarian and/or adrenal antibodies, suggests the need to evaluate adrenal status

and consider clinical evidence of other autoimmune phenomenons, such as hypothyroidism, hypoparathyroidism, or type 1 diabetes.
- 17α-hydroxylase deficiency with 46,XX karyotype: These individuals have normal stature, sexual infantilism, hypertension, and hypokalemia. Their laboratory test results show an elevated progesterone (>3 ng/mL), low 17α-hydroxyprogesterone (<0.2 ng/mL), and elevated serum deoxycorticosterone level.
b. Isolated pituitary gonadotropin insufficiency: Very rare. Kallmann syndrome should be considered and can be associated with anosmia.
c. Hypothalamic failure secondary to inadequate gonadotropin-releasing hormone (GnRH) release.
2. Primary amenorrhea with normal breast development, but absent uterus
   a. Complete androgen insensitivity (formerly testicular feminization): In these XY-karyotype individuals, the Wolffian ducts fail to develop and external female genitalia are present in the absence of a response to testosterone stimulation. The underlying defect is a mutation in the androgen receptor, rendering it insensitive to testosterone's actions. Because müllerian inhibitory factor (MIF) continues to be secreted by the Sertoli cells of the male gonads, the müllerian ducts regress, and there is lack of formation of internal female genitalia. Internally, the teen has normal male gonads and fibrous müllerian remnants. At puberty, the low levels of endogenous gonadal and adrenal estrogens, unopposed by androgens, result in breast development. Because of the end-organ insensitivity to androgens, the teen develops sparse or absent pubic and axillary hair. In summary, manifestations include the following:
      - 46,XY karyotype
      - Female phenotype in the case of complete androgen insensitivity (genital ambiguity often presents in incomplete forms)
      - Testes present in abdomen, pelvis, or inguinal canal
      - Lack of axillary and pubic hair
      - Normal breast development
      - Blind vaginal pouch with absence of ovaries, uterus, and fallopian tubes
      - Normal or elevated male testosterone concentrations
   b. Congenital absence of uterus
      - 46,XX karyotype
      - Ovaries are present: These adolescents may experience cyclic breast and mood changes
      - Normal secondary sexual characteristics
      - Uterus absent or rudimentary cords
      - Absent or blind vaginal pouch
      - Normal female testosterone concentration
      - May have associated renal, skeletal, or other congenital anomalies
3. Primary amenorrhea with no breast development and no uterus:
   This condition is extremely rare. The individual usually has a male karyotype, elevated gonadotropin levels, and testosterone values that are either equal to or less than the level in a healthy female. These individuals produce enough MIF to inhibit development of female internal genital structures, but not enough testosterone to develop male internal and external genitalia. The causes include the following:

a. 17,20-Lyase deficiency
b. Agonadism, including no internal sex organs
c. 17α-Hydroxylase deficiency with 46,XY karyotype: Manifestations include sexual infantilism, absent uterus, and hypertension.
4. Primary and secondary amenorrhea with normal secondary sexual characteristics (breast development) and normal genitalia (uterus and vagina)
   a. Hypothalamic causes
      - Idiopathic: Usually associated with a normal response of luteinizing hormone (LH) and follicle-stimulating hormone (FSH) to GnRH. The disorder is probably secondary to a subtle defect in GnRH secretion. Unstimulated levels of FSH and LH are typically within the low-normal reference range.
      - Medications and drugs: Particularly phenothiazines, oral, injectable or transdermal contraceptives, glucocorticoids, and heroin.
      - Other endocrinopathies: Hyperthyroidism or hypothyroidism, and cortisol excess
      - Stress: Common in adolescents and may relate to family, school, or peer problems, or to a fear of pregnancy
      - Exercise: Athletes, particularly runners, gymnasts, competitive divers, figure skaters, and ballet dancers, have higher rates of amenorrhea and higher rates of disordered eating (female athlete triad includes a combination of disordered eating, amenorrhea, and decreased bone density). Sports that may place athletes at higher risk for this condition include those that emphasize leanness, such as dance or gymnastics, or those that use weight classification, such as martial arts. The prevalence of secondary amenorrhea in adult athletes ranges from 3.4% to 66% depending on the sport studied (American Academy of Pediatrics, Committee on Sports Medicine and Fitness, 2000). As many as 18% of female recreational runners, 50% of competitive runners training 80 m/week, and 47% to 79% of ballet dancers may be amenorrheic (Goodman and Warren, 2005; Eliakim and Beyth, 2003; Calabrese et al., 1983; Cumming and Rebar, 1983). The prevalence of secondary amenorrhea in the teen athlete is unknown.
        The pulsatile nature of LH, and thereby normal menstrual function, appears to be dependent on energy availability (caloric intake minus energy expenditure). Low energy availability appears to result in a hypometabolic state that can include the metabolic alterations, hypoglycemia, hypoinsulinemia, euthyroid sick syndrome (low total triiodothyronine [T_3]), hypercortisolemia, and suppression of the total secretion and amplitude of the diurnal rhythm of leptin (American Academy of Pediatrics, Committee on Sports Medicine and Fitness, 2000; Laughlin and Yen, 1997). Leptin, a hormone secreted by fat tissue, has been shown to be a permissive factor in menstruation, likely due to its correlation with adequate fat mass (Welt et al., 2004). Although both amenorrheic athletes and regularly menstruating athletes have reduced LH pulsatile secretions and reduced 24-hour mean leptin levels, amenorrheic runners have more extreme suppression and disorganization of LH pulsatility. The level of energy availability needed to maintain normal reproductive function is not known. Exercise-induced

menstrual dysfunction may also relate to elevated dopamine or endorphin levels altering GnRH/LH secretion. Constantini and Warren (1995) report on amenorrhea in swimmers. Results from their study suggest that female competitive swimmers are vulnerable to delayed puberty and menstrual irregularities, but the associated hormonal profile is different from that described in dancers and runners. Their study suggests a different mechanism for reproductive dysfunction in swimmers that is associated with mild hyperandrogenism, rather than with hypoestrogenism. Predisposing factors to exercise-induced amenorrhea include the following:
 – Training intensity
 – Weight loss
 – Changes in percentage of body fat
 – Nulliparity
 – Menstrual dysfunction before exercise
 – Years of intense training before the onset of menarche

Low levels of estradiol (E_2) may be present, which has been implicated as the cause of bone loss, placing these young women at increased risk of stress fractures. The condition may be reversible with weight gain or with lessening of the intensity of exercise; however, there is also evidence that this loss of bone density might be partially irreversible despite resumption of menses, estrogen replacement, or calcium supplementation. There are many questions about exercise-induced amenorrhea that remain unanswered, especially related to whether estrogen replacement therapy is beneficial in minimizing skeletal loss in this population.

- Weight loss: This group includes adolescents with simple weight loss and those with anorexia nervosa (see Chapter 33). In both patients with anorexia nervosa and patients with simple weight loss, the mechanism of amenorrhea appears to be hypothalamic derangement. This derangement appears to be more severe in adolescents with anorexia nervosa. The E_2 levels in patients with weight loss and anorexia nervosa can vary from low to normal. Consequently, such individuals may or may not respond to progesterone withdrawal with uterine bleeding. The teens with amenorrhea and severe weight loss also are at risk for decreased bone density.
- Chronic illnesses: Certain chronic illnesses can affect the hypothalamic-pituitary axis. Examples include cystic fibrosis (Moshang and Holsclaw, 1980; Neinstein et al., 1983) and chronic renal disease (Mooradian and Morley, 1984).
- Hypothalamic failure
  – Idiopathic
  – Lesions: rare, include craniopharyngioma, tuberculous granuloma, or meningoencephalitis
- Polycystic ovary syndrome (PCOS): Many researchers believe PCOS to be primarily a hypothalamic disorder. More than half of affected individuals have an LH : FSH ratio >3, with an LH level >10 mIU and often >25 mIU (see "PCOS" section)

b. Pituitary causes
- Nonneoplastic lesions resulting in hypopituitarism: Sheehan syndrome (pregnancy related), Simmonds disease (nonpregnancy related), aneurysm, or empty sella syndrome
- Tumors: Adenoma or carcinoma
- Idiopathic
- Infiltrative: Hemochromatosis

c. Ovarian causes
Premature ovarian failure: Menopause occurring at younger than 35 years. This is often associated with autoantibodies directed against ovarian tissue and may be found in association with thyroid and adrenal autoantibodies. This can also occur in some individuals who received chemotherapy and/or radiation therapy for cancer as children or adolescents (Byrne et al., 1987, 1992; Shalet, 1980; Stillman et al., 1981; Waxman, 1983).

d. Uterine causes: Uterine synechiae (Asherman syndrome)

e. Pregnancy

Diagnosis

The evaluation of amenorrhea can be done with a thorough history, physical examination, and performance of several laboratory tests in a logical sequence. Too often, adolescents are subjected to an expensive "shotgun" approach to evaluation. It is essential to rule out the diagnosis of pregnancy before conducting an extensive evaluation.

History
History should include the following:

1. Systemic diseases: Diseases associated with secondary amenorrhea should include anorexia nervosa, inflammatory bowel disease, diabetes mellitus, and pituitary adenoma. A history of thyroid dysfunction is particularly important, because even mild thyroid dysfunction can lead to menstrual abnormalities.
2. Family history, including ages of parental growth and development, mother's and sister's ages at onset of menarche, as well as a family history of any thyroid disease, diabetes mellitus, eating disorders, or menstrual problems.
3. Past medical history including childhood development.
4. Pubertal growth and development, including breast and pubic hair development, and the presence of a growth spurt.
5. Emotional status.
6. Medications: Including illicit drugs (heroin and methadone are strongly correlated with menstrual dysfunction).
7. Nutritional status and recent weight changes.
8. Exercise history, particularly for sports that might predispose to amenorrhea.
9. Sexual history, contraception, and symptoms of pregnancy.
10. Menstrual history.
11. History of androgen excess suggesting PCOS, or another ovarian or adrenal abnormality.

Physical Examination
The physical examination should include the following:

1. Check for signs of systemic disease or malnutrition.
2. Evaluate for SMR: This is important for evaluating progress in secondary sexual characteristics, because

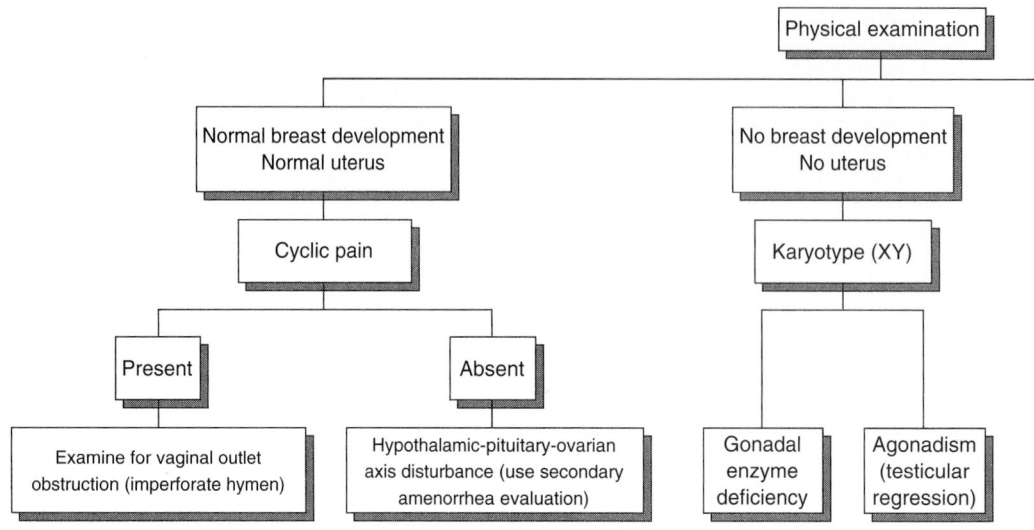

FIGURE 52.1 The evaluation of primary amenorrhea.

most adolescents are not menarcheal until SMR 4, and 95% are menarcheal by 1 year after SMR 5.

3. Check height and weight.
4. Check for signs of androgen excess such as acne or hirsutism.
5. Check for signs of thyroid dysfunction.
6. Check for signs of insulin resistance such as acanthosis nigricans, hyperpigmented velvety skin changes on neck, axillae, or other intertriginous areas.
7. Check for signs of gonadal dysgenesis: Webbed neck, low-set ears, broad shield-like chest, short fourth metacarpal, and increased carrying angle of the arms.
8. Test for anosmia in females with primary amenorrhea to evaluate for Kallmann syndrome.
9. Breast examination: Check for galactorrhea.
10. Pelvic examination: Search for a stenotic cervix, vaginal agenesis, imperforate hymen, transverse vaginal septum, absent uterus, or pregnancy. An external genital examination is a critical component of the workup. A full pelvic examination may not be necessary if the teen is not sexually active, and the history or physical examination has revealed the cause of amenorrhea.

Laboratory Evaluation

The laboratory evaluation for adolescents can be done on the following basis:

- Primary and secondary amenorrhea with normal secondary sexual characteristics and normal genitalia
- Primary amenorrhea and absent secondary sexual characteristics or absent uterus or vagina

Figures 52.1 and 52.2 review the evaluation of primary and secondary amenorrhea.

1. Evaluation for primary and secondary amenorrhea with normal secondary sexual characteristics:
   a. If evidence of galactorrhea or androgen excess is present, the adolescent should be evaluated, as described in Chapters 57 and 58, respectively.
   b. Pregnancy should always be considered and ruled out.
   c. Diabetes mellitus and hypothyroidism should be considered and if clinically indicated, should be ruled out with measurements of blood sugar or thyroid function tests.
   d. Uterine synechiae, or Asherman syndrome, should be considered if there is a history of dilation and curettage or endometritis. This condition may cause partial or total obliteration of the uterine cavity. If this problem is suggested by the history, a gynecological referral for evaluation by hysteroscopy or hysterosalpingography is indicated.

If the results of the aforementioned evaluation are negative, the work-up should proceed as follows (Fig. 52.2):

Administer progesterone withdrawal test or "challenge": A positive response correlates with circulating E_2 levels adequate to prime the endometrium. A positive response (ranges from minimal brown staining to normal menstrual flow) indicates a serum E_2 level >40 pg/mL.

- A *positive response to progesterone* indicates the presence of adequate estrogen levels, as seen with either hypothalamic-pituitary dysfunction or PCOS.
  – Prolactin level should be measured, because this is the most sensitive test for pituitary microadenomas. Rarely, a patient who responds to progesterone withdrawal can have a microadenoma.
  – In addition, thyroid-stimulating hormone and T_4 should be measured to rule out the possibility of either primary or central hypothyroidism.
  – LH or LH : FSH ratios have been used in the past to evaluate for PCOS. However, these values lack sensitivity and specificity.
- If there is *no response to progesterone*, then either hypothalamic-pituitary dysfunction or ovarian failure is likely. A high FSH level indicates ovarian failure, whereas a normal or low FSH level suggests a hypothalamic-pituitary disturbance. If ovarian failure is suspected, a karyotype, antiovarian antibodies, and screening for autoimmune endocrinopathies should be considered. If hypothalamic-pituitary failure is suspected, a magnetic resonance imaging (MRI), visual fields, and pituitary stimulation tests should be considered.

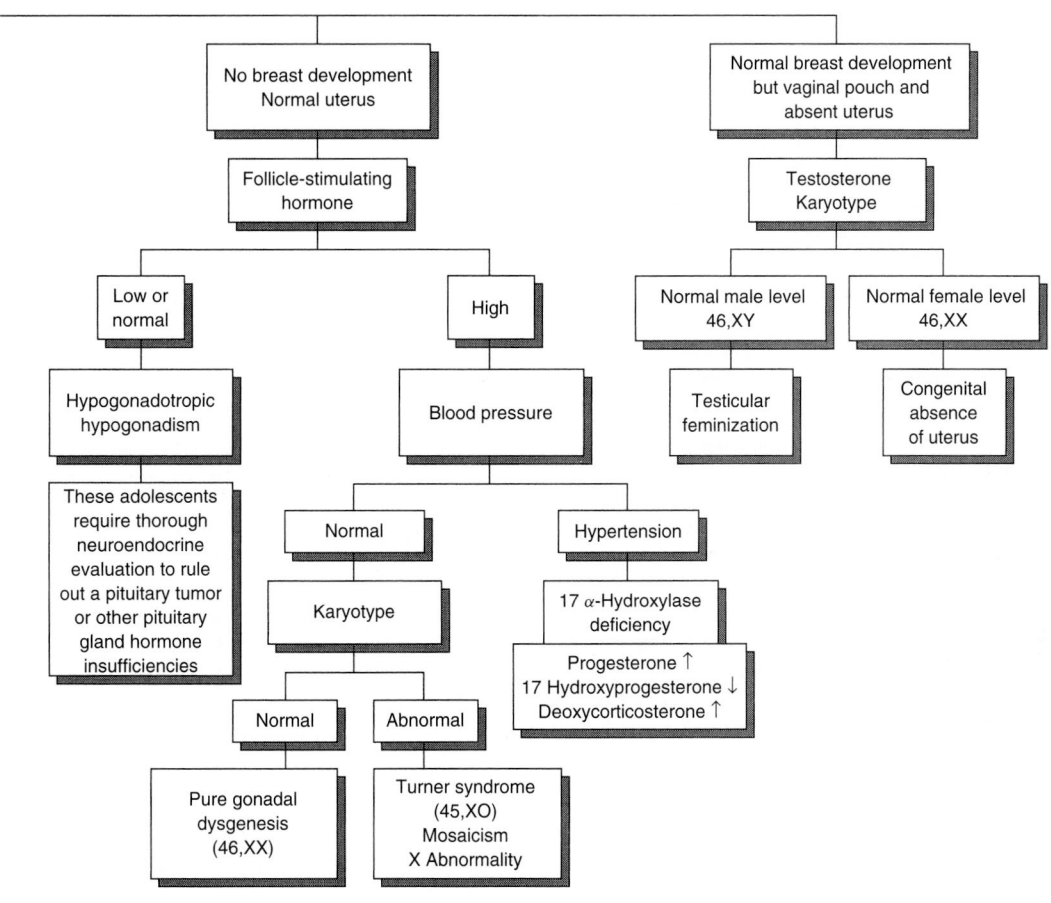

FIGURE 52.1   *(Continued)*

- Individuals with weight loss, anorexia nervosa, heavy substance abuse, or heavy exercise may or may not respond to progesterone withdrawal. If they do not experience bleeding within 10 to 14 days of discontinuing the progesterone, it is indicative of low E_2 levels.

If the teen has a normal prolactin level, she would not require an MRI unless otherwise indicated on the history and physical examination. However, a prolactin test would be indicated every 6 to 12 months if there are no spontaneous menses. An MRI should always be considered in a female patient with a history of headaches or visual changes.

2. Evaluation for primary amenorrhea with either absent uterus or absent secondary sexual characteristics (Fig. 52.1):

a. A physical examination will divide the teens into three groups:
- Absent uterus, normal breasts
- Absent breasts, normal uterus
- Absent breasts, absent uterus

In general, breast development should be at least at stage SMR 4 to be considered indicative of full gonadal function. A breast stage of SMR 2 or SMR 3 may indicate adrenal function alone without gonadal function.

b. If the examination reveals normal breast development, but an absent uterus and blind vaginal pouch, a karyotype and a test for serum testosterone concentrations are indicated.
- XX karyotype plus female testosterone concentration: Congenital absence of uterus
- XY karyotype plus male testosterone concentration: Androgen insensitivity

c. If the examination reveals absent secondary sexual characteristics, but a normal uterus, an FSH test is ordered.
- A low or normal FSH level suggests a hypothalamic or pituitary abnormality, and a careful neuroendocrine evaluation is in order.
- A high FSH level and a blood pressure within the reference range suggest a genetic disorder or gonadal dysgenesis. A karyotype should be ordered.
- A high FSH level and hypertension suggest 17α-hydroxylase deficiency. This is confirmed by an elevated progesterone level (>3 ng/mL), low 17α-hydroxyprogesterone level (<0.2 ng/mL), and an elevated serum deoxycorticosterone level.

d. The absence of both breast development and uterus or vagina is very rare. These findings suggest gonadal failure and the presence of MIF secretion from a testis. This could arise from anorchia occurring after MIF activity was present or an enzyme block, such as a 17,20-lyase defect. The evaluation should include LH, FSH, progesterone, and 17-hydroxyprogesterone measurements, and a karyotype.

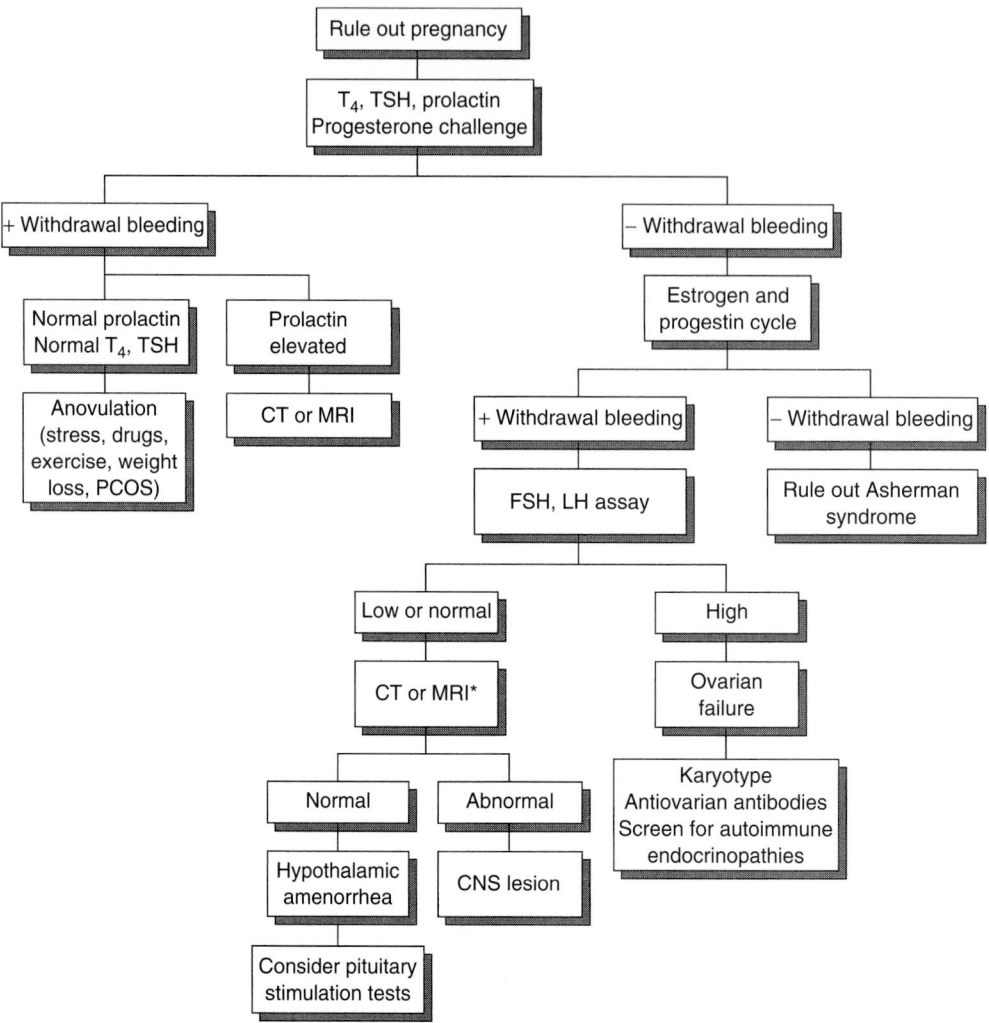

FIGURE 52.2   The evaluation of secondary amenorrhea. TSH, thyroid-stimulating hormone; PCOS, polycystic ovary syndrome; CT, computed tomography; MRI, magnetic resonance imaging; FSH, follicle-stimulating hormone; LH, luteinizing hormone; CNS, central nervous system.

Treatment

Primary Amenorrhea

Hypothalamic Hypogonadotropic Hypogonadism (Hypothalamic Failure) Therapy should begin with estrogen therapy (0.3 mg/day or less if the adolescent is short to avoid premature epiphyseal closure). A transdermal patch can be used to start at 0.025 mg/day of estradiol, or half of the 0.3 mg-Premarin pill can be utilized. Patients with normal height can receive up to 0.625 mg/day of conjugated estrogen (Premarin) or 0.1 mg of estradiol via transdermal patch. High doses of estrogen and premature introduction of progesterone should be avoided early to prevent abnormal breast development manifested by increased subareolar breast development and abnormal contours.

A typical maintenance schedule would be 0.625 to 1.25 mg/day of conjugated estrogens on days 1 through 25 of each month or twice-weekly estrogen patch application of 0.1 mg of estradiol, with 10 mg of medroxyprogesterone acetate (Provera) on days 12 through 25. The progestin is added to induce withdrawal bleeding and thereby avoid endometrial hyperplasia. This schedule can be repeated each month. The dose of estrogen may range from 0.625 to 2.5 mg/day, depending on the individual and the estrogen response, but usually does not exceed 1.25 mg/day of conjugated estrogens. GnRH will probably be used for these conditions when a more easily tolerated delivery system is available. If pregnancy is desired, pulsatile GnRH is an option.

Pituitary Defect Hormonal therapy, as outlined.

Genetic Abnormalities Leading to Gonadal Defects Hormonal therapy, as already outlined. If a Y chromosome is present in an XX-karyotyped individual, gonadal removal is necessary because of the risk of gonadoblastoma development. If a 46,XX karyotype is present, then the gonadal tissue should be visualized to assess whether more than a streaked gonad is present. It is important to start hormonal replacement therapy in early adolescence. With complete gonadal dysgenesis, these individuals are universally sterile. However, with an intact uterus, the individual could be able to bear children after donor oocyte implantation and hormonal support.

Enzyme Defects For 17α-hydroxylase deficiency, both glucocorticoid and estrogen-progesterone replacement are needed and removal of gonads is needed if Y chromosome is present. For 17,20-lyase deficiency, prescribe estrogen–progesterone replacement; remove gonads if Y chromosome is present.

Androgen Insensitivity

1. Gonadal removal: All intraabdominal gonads associated with a Y chromosome have a relatively high potential for malignancy and should be removed. The appropriate timing for removal should be individualized for each patient.
2. After the testes are removed, maintenance estrogen therapy is needed.
3. The adolescent should be informed that she may require vaginoplasty to have normal sexual function.
4. The adolescent should be informed that she cannot become pregnant.
5. Counseling: The adolescent should be informed that she has an abnormal sex chromosome. She may require extra reassurance and counseling regarding her identity and concerns about infertility and sexual function.

Congenital Absence of the Uterus Because these adolescents have normal-functioning ovaries, they do not require hormonal replacement therapy. They may require a vaginoplasty for normal sexual function and an MRI or intravenous pyelogram to rule out renal anomalies. These adolescents must be informed that they cannot become pregnant; therefore, they may require additional support and counseling regarding their identity and body image.

Primary and Secondary Amenorrhea with Normal Secondary Sexual Characteristics
1. PCOS
   a. Medroxyprogesterone acetate (10 mg) should be given for 10 days every 1 to 2 months to induce withdrawal bleeding, or estrogen and progestins can be given as oral contraceptive pills with or without spironolactone.
   b. Insulin-sensitizing agents should be considered, particularly in adolescent girls with clinical (acanthosis nigricans) or biochemical evidence of hyperinsulinism.
   c. When pregnancy is desired, referral for use of clomiphene citrate and/or insulin-sensitizing agents, such as metformin can be recommended.
2. Hypothalamic-pituitary dysfunction
   a. Alleviate the precipitating cause, if known.
   b. Hormonal therapy with progestins to induce uterine bleeding every 1 to 2 months is recommended.
3. Hypothalamic-pituitary failure
   a. The cause must be evaluated and corrected if possible.
   b. Replacement therapy with cyclic conjugated estrogens and progestins, as outlined earlier for hypothalamic failure, is recommended.
   c. If the adolescent or young adult desires pregnancy, refer her to an infertility clinic.

4. Ovarian failure
   a. These adolescents also require cyclic estrogen and progestin therapy.
   b. These adolescents are generally sterile and should be counseled regarding this aspect.
5. Uterine synechiae: This problem requires referral to a gynecologist for possible transhysteroscopic lysis of the adhesions.

Amenorrhea Associated with Weight Loss
In young women with amenorrhea associated with weight loss, bone mineral density (BMD) loss can occur soon after amenorrhea develops. Treatment to prevent BMD loss or to promote bone accretion should probably start after 6 months of amenorrhea (Hergenroeder, 1995). The efficacy of estrogen replacement therapy in this setting is an area of debate. Estrogen likely has beneficial effects on bone and other tissues, but other supplemental therapies may also be warranted. Experimental therapies, such as low-dose androgen supplementation (dehydroepiandrosterone [DHEA] or testosterone), insulin-like growth factor 1 (IGF-1) or growth hormone, and bisphosphonates are gaining further support in the literature (Gordon, 1999; Gordon et al., 2002; Grinspoon et al., 2002; Miller et al., 2005; Golden et al., 2005). Most adolescents who recover from anorexia nervosa at a young age (younger than 15 years) can have normal total-body BMD, but regional (lumbar spine and femoral neck) BMD may remain low (Hergenroeder, 1995). The longer the duration of anorexia nervosa and/or weight loss, the less likely the BMD will return to normal values.

The Female Athlete Triad

Female children and adolescents who participate regularly in athletics may develop the female athlete triad, which includes disordered eating, menstrual dysfunction (typically amenorrhea), and decreased BMD (Goodman and Warren, 2005).

1. Disordered eating: Physically active female adolescents and young adults may develop an energy deficit of calories that may either be unintentional, related to increased demands of training, or intentional in an attempt to lose weight or body fat for enhanced performance or appearance. Disordered eating behaviors may include restricting food intake, bingeing and/or purging by vomiting, laxative use, diuretics, and diet pills. These individuals may also develop compulsive exercise behaviors. Disordered eating behaviors may impair athletic performance, increase risk of injury, and increase the risk of menstrual dysfunction and loss of BMD.
2. Menstrual dysfunction: Menstrual dysfunction in athletes may include primary amenorrhea, secondary amenorrhea, oligomenorrhea, and luteal phase deficiency. Menstrual dysfunction is more common in athletes than in the general population. Athletes, particularly runners, gymnasts, and dancers, with secondary amenorrhea may fall into either the hypothalamic-pituitary dysfunction or the hypothalamic-pituitary failure category.
3. Decreased BMD: There is evidence to suggest that athletes with amenorrhea have low levels of estrogen and may be at risk for osteoporosis and stress fractures (Cann et al., 1984; Drinkwater et al., 1986; Marcus et al., 1985). Some studies suggest that when amenorrhea

persists for 6 months with bone loss, the bone mass may never be regained, whereas other studies indicate a 20% increase in bone mass when weight is gained. Baer (1993) compared reproductive function in ten amenorrheic and eumenorrheic adolescent female runners and seven untrained controls. Amenorrheic subjects were found to run more miles per day and consume fewer calories per day compared with eumenorrheic subjects. Mean levels of fasting plasma E_2, LH, FSH, free T_4, and T_3 were significantly lower in amenorrheic patients compared with eumenorrheic patients and the control subjects. In addition, those who were amenorrheic indicated that they were very concerned about their weight and fearful of gaining fat mass. Other studies have indicated that the change in bone density may also relate to the type of athletics performed—with gymnastic exercises, for example, yielding a stronger bone mass. One recent Scandinavian study demonstrated that most women who exercise regularly at moderate levels are not at significant risk for athletic amenorrhea with its accompanied decrease in BMD. Summary considerations for athletes with amenorrhea include the following (Hergenroeder, 1995):

a. Most bone mineralization in female adolescents occurs by the middle of the second decade of life.
b. Premature bone demineralization occurs in young women with hypothalamic dysfunction that manifests as either amenorrhea or oligomenorrhea in the setting of participation in athletics or dance, and eating disorders.
c. Regular menses and fertility should return with a decrease in the intensity of activity. An adolescent with significant menstrual dysfunction attributed to exercise should be encouraged to increase her caloric intake and modify excessive exercise activity.
d. Calcium intake should be increased to 1,500 mg/day in these young women.
e. Hormonal therapy: If the teen does not respond to progesterone withdrawal or has a documented low circulating E_2 level, estrogen and progesterone replacement therapy should be considered, particularly in amenorrheic athletes who show no signs of gaining weight or reducing activity after 6 months. These individuals may require higher doses of estrogen than replacement doses (1.25 mg/day of conjugated estrogen [Premarin], rather than 0.625 mg/day). However, controversy still exists regarding the beneficial effects on BMD in amenorrheic athletes, particularly those who are underweight. Conjugated estrogen, in doses that improve BMD in postmenopausal women and in combination with medroxyprogesterone, has not been shown to improve BMD in young women with anorexia nervosa (Klibanski et al., 1995). The role of oral medroxyprogesterone (10 mg/day, 10 days/month) in improving BMD in teenage girls with hypothalamic amenorrhea or oligomenorrhea also remains unclear, but preliminary data suggest that it may have negative effects on BMD (Hergenroeder et al., 1997). Some authorities have advocated the use of combination oral contraceptive pills in young women with hypothalamic amenorrhea. In addition, androgens, growth hormone, IGF-1 and bisphosphonates are the being used in clinical trials (Gordon, 1999; Gordon et al., 2002; Grinspoon et al., 2002; Miller et al., 2005; Golden et al., 2005).

f. The practitioner should evaluate these individuals, as outlined previously, to eliminate the possibility of pregnancy, thyroid dysfunction, prolactinoma, or a disorder of androgen excess. It should not be assumed that amenorrhea is simply secondary to exercise.

POLYCYSTIC OVARY SYNDROME

Definition

PCOS is a disorder of the hypothalamic-pituitary-ovarian system, giving rise to temporary or persistent anovulation and androgen excess. The syndrome was originally described in 1935 by Stein and Leventhal as amenorrhea, hirsutism, and obesity associated with enlarged cystic ovaries. For many years, there was an emphasis on the morphological changes in the ovary. However, enlarged polycystic ovaries may occur in healthy women and in women with other conditions such as Cushing syndrome and congenital adrenal hyperplasia (CAH). In addition, women with other classic features of PCOS may have ovaries of normal size. A 1990 U.S. NIH consensus conference identified key features for the diagnosis of PCOS—hyperandrogenism, menstrual dysfunction, clinical evidence of hyperandrogenism, and the exclusion of CAH. Probable criteria for PCOS included insulin resistance and perimenarchal onset.

The 2003 Rotterdam consensus workshop defined PCOS more broadly, recognizing ovarian dysfunction as the primary component, without mandatory anovulation. The revised definition included two of the three following criteria with the exclusion of other etiologies of hyperandrogenism:

- Oligo and/or anovulation
- Clinical and/or biochemical signs of hyperandrogenism
- Polycystic ovaries by ultrasonography

The consensus definitions are broad, allowing for a clinical and biochemical diagnosis of a wide spectrum of phenotypes. Diagnosis is particularly important because PCOS is now believed to increase metabolic and cardiovascular risks, which is linked to insulin resistance and compounded by obesity. Insulin resistance and its associated risks are also present in nonobese women with PCOS. PCOS is one of the most common endocrine disorders, affecting approximately 5% to 10% of premenopausal women and is the most common cause of hyperandrogenism in women and girls.

Etiology

Endocrine Findings PCOS is characterized by menstrual irregularities ranging from amenorrhea or oligomenorrhea, to dysfunctional uterine bleeding. An androgen-excess state is present, leading to hirsutism and acne with rare mild virilization. The changes in gonadotropins and steroid hormones that cause these manifestations are as follows:

1. Inappropriate gonadotropin secretion (IGS) characterized by the following:
   a. Elevated serum LH level (>21 mIU/mL)
   b. Reference-range or low FSH level
   c. Exaggerated response of LH, not FSH, to GnRH
   d. LH : FSH ratio often >3

e. Elevated bioactive LH (generally a research tool, but even more sensitive for PCOS than an elevated immunoreactive LH level)
2. Steroid hormones
   a. Estrone (E_1): Significantly elevated serum levels
   b. E_2: Reference-range level of total E_2, but elevated unbound or free E_2 level
   c. Androstenedione and dehydroepiandrosterone sulfate (DHEAS): Elevated serum levels
   d. Testosterone: Often minimally elevated serum levels are seen, with elevated free (unbound) testosterone
3. Source of excess androgens: The source may be secretion from the ovaries, the adrenal gland, or both, in women with a primary diagnosis of PCOS. Two other sources contribute to androgen excess:
   a. Androstenedione is converted peripherally in adipose tissue to testosterone.
   b. There is a decrease in binding of testosterone to sex hormone-binding globulin (SHBG). Healthy females have approximately 96% of their testosterone bound to SHBG, where it is inactive, whereas patients with PCOS have only 92% of their testosterone bound; therefore, there is a larger percentage of free and active testosterone in patients with PCOS.

Pathophysiology The exact initiating cause of PCOS is not known but may be related to the following:

1. Abnormal hypothalamic-pituitary function
2. Abnormal ovarian function
3. Abnormal adrenal androgen metabolism
4. Insulin resistance: Insulin resistance may exist in both obese and lean women with PCOS and may promote the hyperandrogenic state

Factors leading to the development of PCOS include the following:

1. Insulin resistance at the time of puberty contributing to a relative hyperinsulinemic state
2. Insulin and IGF-1 have mitogenic effects on the ovaries, causing theca cell hyperplasia, which leads to excessive androgen production. Hyperinsulinemia has been directly correlated with a decrease in hepatic production of insulin-like growth factor–binding protein 1 (IGFBP1). The decrease in bound IGF-1 results in an increase in free IGF-1. The increase in IGF-1 and the decrease in IGFBP1 have both been found to correlate with increases in adrenal and ovarian androgens, resulting in the clinical presentation of premature adrenarche and PCOS (Ibanez et al., 1997; Silfen et al., 2002). Therefore, both high IGF-1 levels and low IGFBP1 levels may correlate with early insulin resistance and be pathophysiologically and clinically linked to the progression to PCOS and insulin resistance.
3. The increased ovarian androgen levels cause follicular atresia, impairing E_2 production.
4. The E_1 levels are elevated due to increased conversion of androstenedione to E_1 in adipose cells, which leads to suppression of FSH and tonic stimulation of LH, which further aggravate theca cell stimulation.
5. The combination of theca cell hyperplasia and arrested follicular maturation constitutes the typical histological features of PCOS.
6. Because not all adolescents ultimately develop PCOS, it is thought that there is a genetic factor involved. Genetic studies of family clusters have shown a high

incidence of affected relatives (Legro, 1995). A dominant mode of inheritance seems most likely, but the type and degree of expression may vary within the same family. The syndrome may be transmitted through paternal or maternal sides of a family. Both the insulin-receptor genes and the LH β-subunit gene have been mapped to chromosome 19. However, chromosomal studies of patients with PCOS have shown no consistent abnormality.

Gulekli et al. (1993) compared adolescent girls with PCOS and adult women with PCOS and found that clinical manifestations and hormonal changes were similar. In addition, the rates of insulin resistance and glucose intolerance found in adolescent girls with PCOS are similar to the rates in adult women, of up to 30% (Palmert et al., 2002).

Valproate can also induce menstrual disturbances, polycystic ovaries, and hyperandrogenism (Isojarvi et al., 1993). In a study of 238 women with epilepsy, Isojarvi et al. found 43% of the women using valproate had polycystic ovaries. In those women using valproate before reaching age 20 years, 80% had polycystic ovaries or hyperandrogenism.

Clinical Consequences

PCOS can present with many symptoms. Table 52.1 indicates the prevalence of various signs and symptoms associated with PCOS.

1. Anovulation: Anovulation is a key feature. Usually, the anovulation in PCOS is chronic and presents as either oligomenorrhea or amenorrhea of perimenarcheal onset. Some women who report normal menses may be anovulatory. Few women with PCOS have ovulatory function.
2. Polycystic ovaries: The ovaries in patients with PCOS are usually enlarged, pearly white, sclerotic with multiple (20 to 100) cystic follicles. Normally, follicles develop to approximately 19 to 20 mm and then ovulation occurs. In women with PCOS, multiple follicles develop, but only to approximately 9 to 10 mm in size. Histologically, the ovaries have the same number of primordial follicles, but the number of atretic follicles is doubled. Also, there is an absence of corpora lutea. The polycystic ovary is a sign, not a disease entity on its own. The typical histological changes of the polycystic ovary can be seen in ovaries of any size. A sonographic spectrum exists within patients with PCOS, and polycystic ovaries on ultrasound are not by themselves sufficient for diagnosis of PCOS.
3. Hyperandrogenism/hirsutism: Hyperandrogenism is a key feature of PCOS. Hyperandrogenism in PCOS is primarily ovarian in origin, although adrenal androgens may contribute. The development of hirsutism depends not only on the concentration of androgens in the blood but also on the genetic sensitivity of the hair follicles to androgens. Clinical hirsutism may not occur in all women with PCOS, but women with PCOS have elevated blood androgen levels.
4. Obesity: Originally, obesity was regarded as a classic feature, but its presence is extremely variable and not mandatory for diagnosis. Approximately 40% to 50% of women with PCOS are obese. Obesity in women with PCOS is usually of the android type, with increased

TABLE 52.1

Prevalance of Major Clinical Features of Polycystic Ovary Syndrome

	Goldzieher and Axelrod (1963)[a]	Balen et al. (1995)[b]	Carmina and Lobo (1996)[c]
No. of patients	1,079	1,741	240
Amenorrhea	51%	19.2%	16%
Oligomenorrhea	NR	47%	64%
Polymenorrhea	NR	2.7%	4%
Normal menses	12%	29.7%	15%
Hirsutism	69%	66.2%	70%
Acne	NR	34.7%	11.2%
Obesity	41%	38.4%	43.7%
Acanthosis nigricans	—	2.5%	2.1%

[a]Compilation of data from 187 published studies. Polycystic ovary syndrome (PCOS) was diagnosed on the basis of clinical data and the laparoscopic diagnosis of polycystic ovaries.

[b]Patients were diagnosed on the basis of ultrasonographic findings alone.

[c]PCOS was diagnosed on the basis of hyperandrogenic chronic anovulation (unpublished data).

From Lobo RA. Polycystic ovary syndrome. In: Lobo RA, Mishell DR, Shoupe D, et al. eds. *Infertility, contraception and reproductive endocrinology.* Malden, MA: Blackwell Science, 1997, with permission.

waist-hip ratios. The obesity with PCOS also worsens insulin resistance and increases cardiovascular risks. In obese women, weight loss may improve and/or cure the signs and symptoms of PCOS.

5. Infertility: Although infertility is usually not of concern to the adolescent patient, the risk is significantly elevated due to anovulation.

6. Cancer risk: There is an increased risk for cancer of the endometrium due to prolonged unopposed estrogen stimulation of the endometrial lining from chronic anovulation. There may also be an increased risk of breast cancer associated with chronic anovulation during the reproductive years. The risk of endometrial cancer is increased threefold, and there may also be an increased risk of breast cancer in these women.

7. Elevated lipoprotein profile: The abnormalities in women with PCOS include elevated levels of cholesterol, triglycerides, and low-density lipoprotein cholesterol (LDL-C) and lower levels of high-density lipoprotein cholesterol (HDL-C) and apolipoprotein A-1. Although hyperandrogenism plays some role in these changes, hyperinsulinemia (insulin resistance) and increased inflammatory cytokines probably have a larger effect.

8. Insulin resistance and hyperinsulinemia: Both are well-recognized features of PCOS and associated with many of the late complications of PCOS (Lobo and Carmina, 2000). Approximately 50% of women with PCOS are insulin resistant. Although insulin resistance is associated with obesity, it can also be found in normal-weight women with PCOS. The cause-effect relationship between insulin and androgens in PCOS is still controversial and is under investigation. It has also been suggested that anovulation is a major factor associated with insulin resistance in women with PCOS. The exact pathogenesis of insulin resistance is not clear and may be related to excessive serine phosphorylation of the insulin receptor or downstream insulin signaling effects.

9. Impaired glucose tolerance and diabetes: Women with PCOS are at increased risk for impaired glucose tolerance and overt type 2 diabetes mellitus because of the insulin resistance. One study found that 31% of obese, reproductive-age women with PCOS had impaired glucose tolerance and 7.5% had overt diabetes (Legro et al., 1999). Even in the nonobese women with PCOS, 10.3% had impaired glucose tolerance and 1.5% had diabetes, three times the rate in the general population. Adolescents with PCOS have been found to be similarly at risk for insulin resistance and diabetes (Palmert et al., 2002).

10. Cardiovascular disease: Because of the prevalence of the risk factors listed previously, women with PCOS may be at long-term risk for increased cardiovascular disease. Adult women with PCOS have an estimated sevenfold risk of myocardial infarction (Lobo and Carmina, 2000). In addition, these young women can also have increased levels of plasminogen-activator inhibitor 1 (PAI-1), which inhibits fibrinolysis and is a risk factor for myocardial infarction (Ehrmann et al., 1997).

Differential Diagnosis

1. Familial hirsutism and/or increased sensitivity to normal androgen levels.

2. Androgen-producing ovarian and adrenal tumors: For further discussion, see Chapter 58 on hirsutism and virilism.

3. Cushing syndrome: Potential influence of Cushing syndrome is usually excluded by history and physical examination, and if needed, a 24-hour urine collection for free cortisol and an overnight dexamethasone suppression test can be done.

4. CAH: A mild 21-hydroxylase deficiency can mimic PCOS. The diagnosis of CAH is based on elevated morning serum 17-hydroxyprogesterone level, particularly after a 0.25-mg single-dose injection of adrenocorticotropic hormone.

5. Stromal hyperthecosis: Stromal hyperthecosis probably represents a disorder related to PCOS. However, in this disorder, the testosterone levels are higher and may be as high as those in patients with androgen-producing tumors. These patients may be not only hirsute but also virilized. The history is one of slow-onset progression of symptoms and signs. Ovarian vein catheterization shows increased, but equal amounts, of testosterone from each ovary.

Diagnosis

Criteria for the diagnosis of PCOS include the following:

1. Irregular menses: Chronic anovulation with a perimenarcheal onset of menstrual irregularities.
2. Hyperandrogenism with or without skin manifestations: Biochemical or clinical evidence of androgen excess. Serum testosterone level is the best marker for ovarian causes of hyperandrogenism and DHEAS is the best marker of adrenal sources.
3. Absence of other androgen disorders (adrenal hyperplasia or tumor).

The following are not needed for diagnosis but are supportive evidence of the diagnosis:

1. Polycystic ovaries on ultrasonography (not required for diagnosis but extremely prevalent).
2. Increased body weight: Body mass index (BMI) >30 kg/m^2 in adults or $>$85th percentile in children.
3. Elevated LH and FSH levels: Although LH and FSH levels have been used widely, the sensitivity and specificity of these hormones are low.
4. Prolactin: Most individuals with PCOS have reference-range levels of prolactin, although 20% have mildly elevated levels (Luciano et al., 1984). Prolactin may augment adrenal androgen secretion in this subset of patients.

Therapy

Infertility Infertility is usually not a concern in the adolescent patient. However, when fertility is desired, clomiphene citrate and/or metformin therapy may be used to stimulate ovulation. The use of exogenous gonadotropins is also found in research and clinical practice.

Hirsutism
1. Cosmetic methods, including shaving, waxing, or electrolysis.
2. Oral contraceptives have some utility in 60% to 100% of women, but 6 to 12 months are required before noticeable differences are seen. Combination pills that contain low androgenic progestins such as norethindrone, norgestimate, or desogestrel should be used. Pills with antiandrogenic components (Yasmin) can also be considered (Guido et al., 2004).
   Oral contraceptives work in the following manner:
   a. Suppressing LH production and thereby reducing ovarian androgen production
   b. Increasing the binding capacity of SHBG and thereby decreasing free testosterone production
   c. Decreasing adrenal androgen production
   d. Decreasing 5α-reductase activity

In addition to oral contraceptives, antiandrogens such as spironolactone can be used (see Chapter 50). The combination of low-dose oral contraceptives and spironolactone is very effective. Antiandrogen therapies have been used as primary and secondary therapeutics in the treatment of PCOS. Results have been conflicting as to the contribution to improving insulin resistance (Dunaif et al., 1990; Moghetti et al., 2000). Antiandrogens include spironolactone and cyproterone acetate which interfere with steroidogenesis. These medications are most often used in combination with estrogen or combined estrogen/progestin therapy (Yasmin). Although, spironolactone has some effect in ameliorating the clinical effects of hyperandrogenism, when used without additional hormonal therapy irregular menstrual bleeding is common.

Menstrual Irregularities The patient with amenorrhea or oligomenorrhea can receive medroxyprogesterone acetate (Provera) (10 mg daily for 10 days every 6 to 12 weeks) for withdrawal bleeding. However, the monthly use of medroxyprogesterone acetate has no significant effect on androgen production by the ovaries, so it is not helpful if hirsutism is present.

Obesity Obesity may be a major focus of preventive health care for women with PCOS to lower associated cardiovascular risks and insulin resistance. Lifestyle modification with dietary and activity interventions should be the initial intervention in obese women with PCOS. However, weight loss is difficult to achieve. Older adolescents and young adults with morbid obesity (BMI >40 kg/m^2 or BMI >35 kg/m^2 and secondary complications, such as hypertension, sleep apnea, cardiovascular disease, and PCOS) may be candidates for medication use and/or surgical therapy.

Metabolic Changes Because of the potential for abnormal glucose tolerance (insulin resistance) and hyperlipidemia, it can be important to evaluate these factors in adolescents with PCOS and to consider therapeutic interventions. The use of insulin-sensitizing medications in the treatment of PCOS has recently become an area of great interest. Many clinicians and scientists favor the treatment of insulin resistance in women with PCOS because these women are at increased risk for the development of type 2 diabetes and cardiovascular disease. In addition, the reduction of hyperandrogenism by hormonal therapy does not correct the hyperinsulinism (Nestler, 1997). The use of insulin-sensitizing agents such as metformin may reduce the risk of hyperinsulinism, type 2 diabetes, and the metabolic syndrome (Knowler et al., 2002; Morin-Papunen et al., 2003). In addition, the reduction in hyperinsulinism has been shown to induce ovulation and regulation of menstrual cycling (Velazquez et al., 1994; Fleming et al., 2002; Baillargeon et al., 2003). Studies have shown that the use of metformin in young adolescents with PCOS may regulate menstrual cycling and reduce the clinical hyperandrogenic effects. In addition, metformin may be able to prevent the development of the PCOS phenotype in young girls with premature adrenarche (Morin-Papunen et al., 2000; Glueck et al., 2001; Ibanez et al., 2004). These remain areas of active research.

Women with PCOS should have their cholesterol, triglycerides, and both LDL-C and HDL-C measured, although there is no consensus at what age this should be done and how often the tests should be rechecked if the results are normal. In addition, these women should be checked and followed for impaired glucose tolerance and diabetes. The screening evaluation for abnormal glucose metabolism is an area of continued debate. The current American Diabetes Association recommendations for pediatric diabetes screening include the evaluation of a fasting blood sugar every 2 years, beginning at age 10 years or puberty, in all children who are overweight, as defined by a BMI of greater that the 85th percentile for age and sex, weight for height >85th percentile, or weight >120% of ideal for height plus any two of the designated risk factors:

- Family history of type 2 diabetes in a first- or second-degree relative
- High-risk race/ethnicity (American Indian, African-American, Hispanic, Asian/Pacific Islander)
- Signs of insulin resistance or conditions associated with insulin resistance (acanthosis nigricans, hypertension, dyslipidemia, PCOS) (American Diabetes Association, 2000).

PCOS is listed as a condition associated with insulin resistance, and therefore, the diagnosis of PCOS in an adolescent who is obese and has a family history of diabetes or a high-risk ethnicity meets the criteria for a fasting blood glucose screening. However, there is growing evidence that lean adolescents with PCOS may also be at risk for insulin resistance and that both lean and obese girls with PCOS may benefit from oral glucose tolerance testing (oral glucose challenge of 1.75 g/kg up to a maximum of 75 g) (Palmert et al., 2002). The absence of obesity and acanthosis nigricans does not rule out insulin resistance in the presence of clinical hyperandrogenism. Diagnosis and continued monitoring of these individuals may reduce the risk of metabolic and cardiovascular disease. Reduction in insulin resistance is important, and diet and exercise are critical first-line steps. Insulin-sensitizing medications may prove beneficial, but a consensus regarding guidelines for their usage has not been reached to date for adolescents with PCOS.

WEB SITES

For Teenagers and Parents

http://www.youngwomenshealth.org/. Children's Hospital Boston Adolescent and Young Adult Program Web site.

http://www.goaskalice.columbia.edu/0814.html. Go Ask Alice site for missed periods.

http://www.nlm.nih.gov/medlineplus/ency/article/001218 .htm. National Library of Medicine on amenorrhea.

http://www.turner-syndrome-us.org. The Turner's Syndrome Society of the United States. This Web site provides information and allows young women to exchange information.

http://www.medhelp.org/ais/. Androgen Insensitivity Syndrome Support Group. This site contains medical information about androgen insensitivity, support group contacts, newsletters, and personal accounts of people with androgen insensitivity syndrome.

Polycystic Ovary Syndrome Web Sites

http://www.pcosupport.org/. The PCOS Association's Web site includes facts and figures on PCOS, as well as on-line support.

http://www.pcosupport.org/living/teen/. The PCO Teenlist home page is dedicated to teenagers with PCOS. Includes a chat room and bulletin board so teens can share their thoughts on the disease.

http://www.obgyn.net/pcos/pcos.asp. PCOS Pavilion.

REFERENCES AND ADDITIONAL READINGS

Adashi EY, Resnick CE, Ricciarella E, et al. Granulosa cell-derived insulin-like growth factor (IGF) binding proteins are inhibitory to IGF-I hormonal action: evidence derived from the use of a truncated IGF-I analog. *J Clin Invest* 1992;90:1593.

American Academy of Pediatrics, Committee on Sports Medicine and Fitness. Medical concerns in the female athlete. *Pediatrics* 2000;106:610.

American Diabetes Association. Type 2 diabetes in children and adolescents. American Diabetes Association. *Pediatrics* 2000;105:671.

Bachrach LK, Katzman DK, Litt IF, et al. Recovery from osteopenia in adolescent girls with anorexia nervosa. *J Clin Endocrinol Metab* 1991;72:602.

Baer JT. Endocrine parameters in amenorrheic and eumenorrheic adolescent female runners. *Int J Sports Med* 1993;14:191.

Baer JT, Taper LJ, Gwazdauskas FG, et al. Hormonal and metabolic factors affecting bone mineral density in adolescent amenorrheic and eumenorrheic female runners. *J Sports Med Phys Fitness* 1992;32:51.

Balen AH, Conway GS, Kaltsas G, et al. Polycystic ovary syndrome: the spectrum of the disorder in 1741 patients. *Hum Reprod* 1995;10;2107.

Baillargeon JP, Iuorno MJ, Nestler JE. Insulin sensitizers for polycystic ovary syndrome. *Clin Obstet Gynecol* 2003;46:325.

Brooks-Gunn J, Warren MP, Hamilton LH. The relation of eating problems and amenorrhea in ballet dancers. *Med Sci Sports Exerc* 1987;19:41.

Bullen BA, Skrinar GS, Beitins IZ, et al. Induction of menstrual disorders by strenuous exercise in untrained women. *N Engl J Med* 1985;312:1349.

Byrne J, Fears TR, Gail MH, et al. Early menopause in long-term survivors of cancer during adolescence. *Am J Obstet Gynecol* 1992;1666:788.

Byrne J, Mulvihill JJ, Myers MH, et al. Effects of treatment on fertility in long-term survivors of childhood and adolescent cancer. *N Engl J Med* 1987;317:1315.

Calabrese LH, Kirkendall DT. Nutritional and medical considerations in dancers. *Clin Sports Med* 1983;2:539.

Cann CE, Martin MC, Genant HK, et al. Decreased spinal mineral content in amenorrheic women. *JAMA* 1984;251:626.

Carmina E, Lobo RA. Polycystic ovary syndrome (PCOS): arguably the most common endocrinopathy is associated with significant morbidity in women. *J Clin Endocrinol Metab* 1999;84:1897.

Carpenter SE. Psychosocial menstrual disorders: stress, exercise, and diet's effect on the menstrual cycle. *Curr Opin Obstet Gynecol* 1994;6:536.

Constantini NW, Warren MP. Menstrual dysfunction in swimmers: a distinct entity. *J Clin Endocrinol Metab* 1995;80:2740.

Copeland PM, Sacks NR, Herzog DB. Longitudinal follow-up of amenorrhea in eating disorders. *Psychosom Med* 1995;57:121.

Cumming DC, Strich G, Brunsting L. Amenorrheic joggers differ in hormone profile. *Obstet Gynecol News* 1982;17:12.

Cumming DC, Rebar RW. Exercise and reproductive function in women. *Am J Ind Med* 1983;4:113.

Davajan V. Primary amenorrhea. In: Mishell DR Jr, Davagan V, Lobo A, eds. *Infertility, contraception, and reproductive endocrinology*, 3rd ed. Boston: Blackwell Science, 1991.

Davajan V. Secondary amenorrhea. In: Mishell DR Jr, Davagan V, Lobo A, eds. *Infertility, contraception, and reproductive endocrinology*, 3rd ed. Boston: Blackwell Science, 1991.

Devereaux MD, Parr GR, Lachmann SM, et al. The diagnosis of stress fractures in athletes. *JAMA* 1984;252:531.

Drinkwater BL, Nilson K, Chesnut CH III, et al. Bone mineral content of amenorrheic and eumenorrheic athletes. *N Engl J Med* 1984;311:277.

Drinkwater BL, Nilson K, Ott S, et al. Bone mineral density after resumption of menses in amenorrheic athletes. *JAMA* 1986;256:380.

Dueck CA, Manore MM, Matt KS. Role of energy balance in athletic menstrual dysfunction. *Int J Sport Nutr* 1996;6:165.

Dunaif A. Insulin resistance and ovarian dysfunction. In: Moller DE, ed. *Insulin resistance*. New York: John Wiley and Sons, 1993:301.

Dunaif A, Graf M, Mandeli J, et al. Characterization of groups of hyperandrogenic women with acanthosis nigricans, impaired glucose tolerance, and/or hyperinsulinemia. *J Clin Endocrinol Metab* 1987;65:499.

Dunaif A, Green G, Futterweit W, et al. Suppression of hyperandrogenism does not improve peripheral or hepatic insulin resistance in the polycystic ovary syndrome. *J Clin Endocrinol Metab* 1990;70:699.

Dunaif A, Seqal KR, Shelley DR, et al. Evidence for distinctive and intrinsic defects in insulin action in polycystic ovary syndrome. *Diabetes* 1992;41:1257.

Ehren EM, Mahour GH, Isaacs H Jr. Benign and malignant ovarian tumors in children and adolescents: a review of 63 cases. *Am J Surg* 1984;147:339.

Ehrmann DA. Polycystic ovary syndrome. *N Engl J Med* 2005;352:1223.

Ehrmann DA, Schneider DJ, Sobel BE, et al. Troglitazone improves defects in insulin action, insulin secretion, ovarian steroidogenesis and fibrinolysis in women with polycystic ovary syndrome. *J Clin Endocrinol* 1997;82:2108.

Eliakim A, Beyth Y. Exercise training, menstrual irregularities and bone development in children and adolescents. *J Pediatr Adolesc Gynecol* 2003;16:201.

Emans SJ. The athletic adolescent with amenorrhea. *Pediatr Ann* 1984;13:605.

Emans SJ, Grace E, Hoffer FA, et al. Estrogen deficiency in adolescents and young adults: impact on bone mineral content and effects of estrogen replacement therapy. *Obstet Gynecol* 1990;76:585.

Evangelia Z, Erasmia K, Dimitrios L. Treatment options of polycystic ovary syndrome in adolescence. *Pediatr Endo Rev* 2006;3(Suppl 1):208.

Fagan KM. Pharmacologic management of athletic amenorrhea. *Clin Sports Med* 1998;17:327.

Fleming R, Hopkinson ZE, Wallace AM, et al. Ovarian function and metabolic factors in women with oligomenorrhea treated with metformin in a randomized double blind placebo-controlled trial. *J Clin Endocrinol Metab* 2002;87:569.

Franks S. Polycystic ovary syndrome. *N Engl J Med* 1995;333:853.

Frisch RE, Wyshak G, Vincent L. Delayed menarche and amenorrhea in ballet dancers. *N Engl J Med* 1980;303:17.

Goldzieher JW, Axelrod LR, Clinical and Biochemical Features of Polycystic Ovarian Disease. *Fertil Steril* 1963;14:631.

Guido M, Romualdi D, Giuliani M, et al. Drospirenone for the treatment of hirsute women with polycystic ovary syndrome: a clinical, endocrinological, metabolic pilot study. *J Clin Endocrinol Metab* 2004;89:2817.

Goswami D, Conway GS. Premature ovarian failure. *Hum Reprod Update* 2005;11:391.

Guido M, Romualdi D, Giuliani M, et al. Drospirenone for the treatment of hirsute women with polycystic ovary syndrome: a clinical, endocrinological, metabolic pilot study. *J Clin Endocrinol Metab* 2004;89:2817.

Glueck CJ, Wang P, Fontaine R, et al. Metformin to restore normal menses in oligo-amenorrheic teenage girls with polycystic ovary syndrome (PCOS). *J Adolesc Health* 2001;29:160.

Golden NH, Iglesias EA, Jacobson MS, et al. Alendronate for the treatment of osteopenia in anorexia nervosa: randomized, double-blind, placebo-controlled trial. *J Clin Endocrinol Metab* 2005;90:3179.

Goodman LR, Warren MP. The female athlete and menstrual function. *Curr Opin Obstet Gynecol* 2005;17:466.

Gordon CM. Menstrual disorders in adolescents: excess androgens and the polycystic ovary syndrome. *Pediatr Clin North Am* 1999;46:519.

Gordon CM. Bone density issues in the adolescent gynecology patient. *J Pediatr Adolesc Gynecol* 2000;13:157.

Gordon CM, Grace E, Emans SJ, et al. Effects of oral dehydroepiandrosterone on bone density in young women with anorexia nervosa: a randomized trial. *J Clin Endocrinol Metab* 2002;87:4935.

Greene JW. Exercise-induced menstrual irregularities. *Compr Ther* 1993;19:116.

Griffin JE, Edwards C, Madden JD, et al. Congenital absence of the vagina: clinical review. *Ann Intern Med* 1976;85:224.

Grinspoon S, Thomas L, Miller K, et al. Effects of recombinant human IGF-I and oral contraceptive administration on bone density in anorexia nervosa. *J Clin Endocrinol Metab* 2002;87:2883.

Grimes DA, Godwin AL, Rubin A, et al. Ovulation and follicular development associated with three low-dose oral contraceptives: a randomized controlled trial. *Obstet Gynecol* 1994;83(1):29.

Gulekli B, Turhan NO, Senoz S, et al. Endocrinological, ultrasonographic, and clinical findings in adolescent and adult polycystic ovary patients: a comparative study. *Gynecol Endocrinol* 1993;7:273.

Hergenroeder AC. Bone mineralization, hypothalamic amenorrhea, and sex steroid therapy in female adolescents and young adults. *J Pediatr* 1995;126:683.

Hergenroeder AC, Smith EO, Shypailo R, et al. Bone mineral changes in young women with hypothalamic amenorrhea treated with oral contraceptives, medroxyprogesterone or placebo over 12 months. *Am J Obstet Metab Gynecol* 1997;176:1017.

Hintz RL. New approaches to growth failure in Turner syndrome. *Adolesc Pediatr Gynecol* 1989;2:172.

Hobart JA, Smucker DR. The female athlete triad. *Am Fam Physician* 2000;61:3357.

Holt VL, et al. Functional ovarian cysts in relation to the use of monophasic and triphasic oral contraceptives. *Obstet Gynecol* 1992;79:529.

Huffman JW, Dewhurst CJ, Capraro UJ, eds. Ovarian tumors in children and adolescents. In: *The gynecology of children and adolescence*, 2nd ed. Philadelphia: WB Saunders, 1981.

Ibanez L, Potau N, Zampolli M, et al. Hyperinsulinemia and decreased insulin-like growth factor-binding protein-1 are common features in prepubertal and pubertal girls with a history of premature pubarche. *J Clin Endocrinol Metab* 1997; 82:2283.

Ibanez L, Valls C, Marcos MV, et al. Insulin sensitization for girls with precocious pubarche and with risk for polycystic ovary syndrome: effects of prepubertal initiation and postpubertal discontinuation of metformin treatment. *J Clin Endocrinol Metab* 2004;89:4331.

Ibanez L, de Zegher F. Flutamide-metformin plus ethinylestradiol-drospirenone for lipolysis and antiatherogenesis in young women with ovarian hyperandrogenism: the key role of metformin at the start and after more than one year of therapy. *J Clin Endocrinol Metab* 2005; 90:39.

Iglesias EA, Coupey SM. Menstrual cycle abnormalities: diagnosis and management. *Female Reprod Health Adolesc Med State Art Rev* 1999;10:255.

Imai A, Furui T, Tamaya T. Gynecologic tumors and symptoms in childhood and adolescence: 10-years' experience. *Int J Gynaecol Obstet* 1994;5:227.

Isojarvi JIT, Laatikainen TJ, Pakarinen AJ, et al. Polycystic ovaries and hyperandrogenism in women taking valproate for epilepsy. *N Engl J Med* 1993;329:1383.

Jacobs HS. Polycystic ovary syndrome: etiology and management. *Curr Opin Obstet Gynecol* 1995;7:203.

Jansen RP. Ovulation and the polycystic ovary syndrome. *Aust N Z J Obstet Gynaecol* 1994;34:277.

Johnson C, Powers PS, Dick R. Athletes and eating disorders: the National Collegiate Athletic Association study. *Int J Eat Disord* 1999;26:179.

Jonnavithula S, Warren MP, Fox RP, et al. Bone density is compromised in amenorrheic women despite return of menses: a 2-year study. *Obstet Gynecol* 1993;81:669.

Kahn JA, Gordon CM. Polycystic ovary syndrome. *Adolesc Med* 1999;10:321.

Klibanski A, Biller BM, Schoenfeld DA, et al. The effects of estrogen administration on trabecular bone loss in young women with anorexia nervosa. *J Clin Endocrinol Metab* 1995; 80:898.

Knowler WC, Barrett-Connor E, Fowler SE, et al. Reduction in the incidence of type 2 diabetes with lifestyle intervention or metformin. *N Engl J Med* 2002;346:393.

Lane DE. Polycystic ovary syndrome and its differential diagnosis. *Obstet Gynecol Surv* 2006;61:125.

Lanes SF, Birmann B, Walker AM, et al. Oral contraceptive type and functional ovarian cysts. *Am J Obstet Gynecol* 1992; 166:95.

Laughlin GA, Yen SS. Nutritional and endocrine-metabolic aberrations in amenorrheic athletes. *J Clin Endocrinol Metab* 1996;81:4301.

Laughlin GA, Yen SS. Hypoleptinemia in women athletes: absence of a diurnal rhythm with amenorrhea. *J Clin Endocrinol Metab* 1997;82:318.

Legro RS. The genetics of polycystic ovary syndrome. *Am J Med* 1995;98:9S.

Legro RS, Kunselman AR, Dodson WC, et al. Prevalence and predictors of risk for type 2 diabetes mellitus and impaired glucose tolerance in polycystic ovary syndrome: a prospective, controlled study in 254 affected women. *J Clin Endocrinol Metab* 1999;84:165.

Lindberg JS, Fears WB, Hunt MM, et al. Exercise-induced amenorrhea and bone density. *Ann Intern Med* 1984;101:647.

Lindberg JS, Powell MR, Hunt MM, et al. Increased vertebral bone mineral in response to reduced exercise in amenorrheic runners. *West J Med* 1987;146:39.

Lint VS, Auletta F, Kathpalia S. Gonadal function in women with chronic renal failure: a study of the hypothalamic-pituitary axis. *Proc Clin Dial Transplant Forum (Washington)* 1977;7:39.

Lobo RA. Polycystic ovary syndrome. In: Mishell DR Jr, Davajan V, eds. *Infertility, contraception, and reproductive endocrinology*. Oradell, NJ: Medical Economics Books, 1986.

Lobo RA, Carmina E. The importance of diagnosing the polycystic ovary syndrome. *Ann Intern Med* 2000;132:989.

Luciano AA, Chapler FK, Sherman BM. Hyperprolactinemia in polycystic ovary syndrome. *Fertil Steril* 1984;41:719.

Lutter JM, Cushman S. Menstrual patterns in female runners. *Phys Sportsmed* 1982;10:60.

Mantzoros CS. Recombinant human leptin in women with hypothalamic amenorrhea. *N Engl J Med* 2004;351:987.

McGowan L. Adnexal masses: a visual guide. *Female Patient* 1989;14:48.

McKenna TJ. Pathogenesis and treatment of polycystic ovary syndrome. *N Engl J Med* 1988;318:558.

Marcus R, Cann C, Madvig P, et al. Menstrual function and bone mass in elite women distance runners. *Ann Intern Med* 1985;102:158.

Marshall LA. Clinical evaluation of amenorrhea in active and athletic women. *Clin Sports Med* 1994;13:371.

Master-Hunter T, Heiman DL. Amenorrhea: evaluation and treatment. *Am Fam Physician* 2006;73:1374.

Micklesfield LK, Lambert EV, Fataar AB. Bone mineral density in mature, premenopausal ultramarathon runners. *Med Sci Sports Exerc* 1995;27:688.

Miller KK, Grieco KA, Klibanski A. Testosterone administration in women with anorexia nervosa. *J Clin Endocrinol Metab* 2005;90:1428.

Moghetti P, Castello R, Negri C, et al. Metformin effects on clinical features, endocrine and metabolic profiles, and insulin sensitivity in polycystic ovary syndrome: a randomized, double-blind, placebo-controlled 6-month trial, followed by open, long-term clinical evaluation. *J Clin Endocrinol Metab* 2000;85:139.

Mooradian AD, Morley JE. Endocrine dysfunction in chronic renal failure. *Arch Intern Med* 1984;144:351.

Morin-Papunen L, Rautio K, Ruokonen A, et al. Metformin reduces serum C-reactive protein levels in women with polycystic ovary syndrome. *J Clin Endocrinol Metab* 2003;88:4649.

Morin-Papunen LC, Vauhkonen I, Koivunen RM, et al. Endocrine and metabolic effects of metformin versus ethinyl estradiol-cyproterone acetate in obese women with polycystic ovary syndrome: a randomized study. *J Clin Endocrinol Metab* 2000; 85:3161.

Moshang T, Holsclaw DS. Menarchal determinants in cystic fibrosis. *Am J Dis Child* 1980;134:1139.

Nader S. Polycystic ovary syndrome and the androgen-insulin connection. *Am J Obstet Gynecol* 1991;165:346.

Neinstein LS. Menstrual dysfunction in pathophysiologic states. *West J Med* 1985;143:476.

Neinstein LS. Menstrual problems in adolescents. *Med Clin North Am* 1990;74:1181.

Neinstein LS, Castle GE. Congenital absence of the vagina. *Am J Dis Child* 1983;137:669.

Neinstein LS, Stewart D, Wang CI, et al. Menstrual dysfunction in cystic fibrosis. *J Adolesc Health Care* 1983;4:153.

Nestler JE. Role of hyperinsulinemia in the pathogenesis of the polycystic ovary syndrome, and its clinical implications. *Semin Reprod Endocrinol* 1997;15(2):111.

Okano H, Mizunuma H, Soda M. Effects of exercise and amenorrhea on bone mineral density in teenage runners. *Endocrinol Jpn* 1995;42:271.

Olson BR. Exercise-induced amenorrhea. *Am Fam Physician* 1989;39:213.

Otis CL, Drinkwater B, Johnson M, et al. American College of Sports Medicine position stand. The female athlete triad. *Med Sci Sports Exerc* 1997;29:i.

Palmert MR, Gordon CM, Kartashov AI, et al. Screening for abnormal glucose tolerance in adolescents with polycystic ovary syndrome. *J Clin Endocrinol Metab* 2002;87:1017.

Pasloff ES, Slap GB, Pertschuk MJ, et al. A longitudinal study of metacarpal bone morphometry in anorexia nervosa. *Clin Orthop* 1992;278:217.

Patterson DE. Menstrual dysfunction in athletes: assessment and treatment. *Pediatr Nurs* 1995;21:310.

Pletcher JR, Slap GB. Menstrual disorders. Amenorrhea. *Pediatr Clin North Am* 1999;46:505.

Polaneczky MM, Slap GB. Menstrual disorders in the adolescent: amenorrhea. *Pediatr Rev* 1992;13:43.

Porcu E, Venturoli S, Prato LD, et al. Frequency and treatment of ovarian cysts in adolescence. *Arch Gynecol Obstet* 1994; 255:69.

Poretsky L, Piper B. Insulin resistance, hypersecretion of LH, and a dual-defect hypothesis for the pathogenesis of polycystic ovarian syndrome. *Obstet Gynecol* 1994;84(4):613.

Puffer JC. Athletic amenorrhea and its influence on skeletal integrity. *Bull Rheum Dis* 1994;43:5.

Putukian M. The female athlete triad. *Clin Sports Med* 1998; 17:675.

Rencken ML, Chesnut CH III, Drinkwater BL. Bone density at multiple skeletal sites in amenorrheic athletes. *JAMA* 1996;276:238.

Richardson GS, Scully RE, Niktui N, et al. Common epithelial cancers of the ovary (two parts). *N Engl J Med* 1985;312: 415.

Rodin A, Thakkar H, Taylor N, et al. Hyperandrogenism in polycystic ovary syndrome. *N Engl J Med* 1994;330:460.

The Rotterdam E/A. Revised 2003 consensus on diagnostic criteria and long-term health risks related to polycystic ovary syndrome (PCOS). *Hum Reprod.* 2004;19:41.

Russell JB, Mitchell D, Musey PI, et al. The relationship of exercise to anovulatory cycles in female athletes: hormonal and physical characteristics. *Obstet Gynecol* 1984a;63:452.

Sanborn CF, Horea M, Siemers BJ, et al. Disordered eating and the female athlete triad. *Clin Sports Med* 2000;19:199.

Schwartz B, Rebar RW, Yen SSC. Amenorrhea and long distance running. *Fertil Steril* 1980;34:306.

Seino S, Seino M, Bell GI. Human insulin-receptor gene. *Diabetes* 1990;39:129.

Shalet SM. Effects of cancer chemotherapy on gonadal function of patients. *Cancer Treat Rev* 1980;7:141.

Shangold MM. How I manage exercise-related menstrual disturbances. *Phys Sportsmed* 1986;14:113.

Siegel ML, Surratt IT. Pediatric gynecologic imaging. *Obstet Gynecol Clin North Am* 1992;19:103.

Silfen ME, Manibo AM, Ferin M, et al. Elevated free IGF-I levels in prepubertal Hispanic girls with premature adrenarche: relationship with hyperandrogenism and insulin sensitivity. *J Clin Endocrinol Metab* 2002;87:398.

Singh KB. Menstrual disorders in college students. *Am J Obstet Gynecol* 1981;140:299.

Solomon CG. The epidemiology of polycystic ovary syndrome: prevalence and associated disease risks. *Endocrinol Metab Clin North Am* 1999;28:247.

Spanos WJ. Preoperative hormonal therapy of cystic adnexal masses. *Am J Obstet Gynecol* 1973;116:551.

Speroff L, Glass RH, Kase NG. Amenorrhea. In: Speroff L, Glass, RH, Kase NG, eds. *Clinical gynecologic endocrinology and infertility,* 4th ed. Baltimore: Williams & Wilkins, 1989:165.

Speroff L, Shangold MM, Dale E. Impact of exercise on menstruation and reproduction. *Contrib Gynecol Obstet* 1982; 19:54.

Stager JM, Ritchie-Flanagan B, Robertshaw D. Reversibility of amenorrhea in athletes. *N Engl J Med* 1984;310:51.

Stillman RJ, Schinfeld JS, Schiff I. Ovarian failure in long term survivors of childhood malignancy. *Am J Obstet Gynecol* 1981; 139:62.

Trent ME, Rich M, Austin SB, et al. Quality of life in adolescent girls with polycystic ovary syndrome. *Arch Pediatr Adolesc Med* 2002;156:556.

Trent ME, Rich M, Austin SB, et al. Fertility concerns and sexual behavior in adolescent girls with polycystic ovary syndrome: implications for quality of life. *J Pediatr Adolesc Gynecol* 2003;16(1):33.

Tweedy A. Polycystic ovary syndrome. *J Am Acad Nurse Pract* 2000;12:101.

Velazquez EM, Mendoza S, Hamer T, Sosa F and Glueck CJ. Metformin therapy in polycystic ovary syndrome reduces hyperinsulinemia, insulin resistance, hyperandrogenemia, and systolic blood pressure, while facilitating normal menses and pregnancy. *Metabolism* 1994;43:647.

Vigersky RM, Andersen AE, Thompson RN, et al. Hypothalamic dysfunction in secondary amenorrhea associated with simple weight loss. *N Engl J Med* 1977;297:1141.

Warren MP. The effects of exercise on pubertal progression and reproductive function in girls. *J Clin Endocrinol Metab* 1980;51:1150.

Warren MP, Jewelewicz R, Dyrenfurth I, et al. The significance of weight loss in the evaluation of pituitary response to LH-RH in women with secondary amenorrhea. *J Clin Endocrinol Metab* 1975;40:601.

Warren-Ulanch J, Arslanian S. Treatment of PCOS in adolescence. *Best Pract Res Clin Endocrinol Metab* 2006;20:311.

Watson RE, Bouknight R, Alguire PC. Hirsutism: evaluation and management. *J Gen Intern Med* 1995;10:283.

Waxman J. Chemotherapy and the adult gonad: a review. *J R Soc Med* 1983;76:144.

Welt CK, Chan JL, Bullen J, et al. Recombinant human leptin in women with hypothalamic amenorrhea. *N Engl J Med* 2004;35:987.

West RV. The female athlete: the triad of disordered eating, amenorrhea and osteoporosis. *Sports Med* 1998;26:63.

Winer-Muram MT, Emerson DE, Muram D, et al. The sonographic features of the peripubertal ovaries. *Adolesc Pediatr Gynecol* 1989;2:160.

Yurth EE. Female athlete triad. *West J Med* 1995;162:149.

CHAPTER 53

Pelvic Masses

Paula J. Adams Hillard

A pelvic mass can be identified during a routine screening examination, or it can be discovered during an evaluation for abdominopelvic pain or abnormal bleeding. The list of likely diagnoses of a pelvic mass for prepubertal and adolescent females is different than that for older women, although there may be some overlap (Hillard, 2002). For example, an imperforate hymen causing severe cyclic abdominal pain and a large pelvic mass are more likely to present in a 14-year-old girl than in a 34-year-old woman. Germ cell tumors of the ovary are more common in teens than epithelial carcinoma. Uterine masses such as uterine fibroids are not common in adolescents but are quite common among adult women. Table 53.1 lists a number of conditions that may be diagnosed as a pelvic mass in women of reproductive age.

CONGENITAL ANOMALIES

Anatomical genital anomalies are rare, but they can have profound implications for future reproductive capability in teens (Spence, 1998). Many of these can present as pelvic masses.

Uterine Defects: Incomplete Fusion

The uterus is formed by fusion of paramesonephric ducts in the midline. If lateral fusion is incomplete, then a uterine didelphys may form with two separate uterine halves (each with its own cervix, corpus-attached fallopian tube and ovary, and possibly vaginal canal). This diagnosis may be suspected when menstrual flow cannot be controlled with a tampon. On examination, one of the two uteri may be mistaken for an adnexal mass. If uterine fusion is partial, there may be a bicornuate uterus or blind uterine horn. If functional endometrium is present within this obstructed horn, severe cyclic pain can occur (Kim and Laufer, 1994). The diagnosis can be suggested on the basis of a screening pelvic ultrasound examination. If a developmental anomaly is suspected on ultrasound examination, magnetic resonance imaging (MRI) is the best technique for clarifying genital anomalies, although laparoscopy may be required to delineate anatomical structures adequately (Economy et al., 2002). If fusion is complete but the resorption of the midline is incomplete, a

septate uterus can result. Renal and skeletal anomalies are common in conjunction with uterine fusion defects.

Vaginal Defects: Incomplete Fusion

The vagina also forms in two parts, and defects typically occur as a result of failure of longitudinal fusion or

TABLE 53.1
Conditions Diagnosed as a Pelvic Mass in Women of Reproductive Age
Full urinary bladder
Urachal cyst
Sharply anteflexed or retroflexed uterus
Pregnancy (with or without concomitant leiomyomas)
Intrauterine
Tubal
Abdominal
Ovarian or adnexal masses
Functional cysts
Inflammatory masses
Tuboovarian complex
Diverticular abscess
Appendiceal abscess
Matted bowel and omentum
Peritoneal cyst
Stool in sigmoid
Neoplastic tumors
Benign
Malignant
Paraovarian or paratubal cysts
Intraligamentous myomas
Less common conditions that must be excluded
Pelvic kidney
Carcinoma of the colon, rectum, appendix
Carcinoma of the fallopian tube
Retroperitoneal tumors (anterior sacral meningocele)
Uterine sarcoma or other malignant tumors

706

canalization. The upper approximate three fourths form from the inferior portion of the fused paramesonephric ducts and the lower one fourth from the sinovaginal bulbs. The lowest portion of these bulbs fills with a solid core of tissue called the *vaginal plate*. If the upper and lower vaginal portions do not fuse, then a transverse vaginal septum forms. Similarly, if the solid core of tissue at the junction of the vaginal plate and the urogenital sinus do not canalize completely, the woman can have an imperforate hymen or vaginal agenesis. If a uterus with functional endometrium is present along with a transverse vaginal septum or imperforate hymen, menstrual fluid accumulates within the patent portion of the vagina (hematocolpos) and within the uterus (hematometra), which then presents as a "pelvic mass"(Kim and Laufer, 1994).

Uterovaginal Agenesis

Women with uterovaginal agenesis—Mayer-Rokitansky-Küster-Hauser syndrome—may have uterine remnants that may or may not contain functioning endometrium that can cause pain and a mass that is diagnosed with ultrasonography or MRI.

Müllerian Duct Remnants

Another class of anatomical congenital anomalies that can create pelvic masses arises from remnants of the mesonephric/müllerian duct system or mesovarium that should have degenerated in utero in the presence of antimüllerian hormone. At least 25% of women have small remnants of these systems. These remnants can present in the lateral adnexa as paraovarian cysts or paratubal cysts. They are often multiple and can vary in size from <1 cm to 20 cm. Along the lateral wall of the vagina or uterus, these remnants present as Gartner duct cysts. These müllerian remnants are rarely symptomatic; however, torsion can occur, and persistent larger masses may be confused with an ovarian neoplasm.

Urachal Cysts and Pelvic Kidneys

Urachal cysts, although rare, can be found along the midline above the bladder and can be confused with other pelvic masses. A pelvic kidney must also be included in the differential diagnosis, particularly in a young woman who has not undergone previous pelvic or renal imaging. Any other structure in the pelvis, such as a full bladder or hard stool in the bowel, can be confused with a pelvic mass.

PREGNANCY PRESENTING AS PELVIC MASS

The possibility of an intrauterine pregnancy enlarging the uterus or an ectopic pregnancy (see Chapter 56) causing an adnexal mass must be considered in the differential diagnosis of every young woman with secondary sexual characteristics. A sensitive urine pregnancy test can reliably rule out a clinically significant pregnancy. However, in many instances the test is not ordered because the provider does not consider it likely that the young woman has been sexually active. Adolescents

may be unwilling or unable to disclose their history of sexual activity for a variety of reasons—they may fear disappointing their parents or the clinician; they may have insufficient knowledge or awareness of pregnancy-related symptoms; they may deny the possibility of pregnancy; the clinician may not have established or discussed provisions of confidentiality; or the question may not have been asked in a sensitive manner in a private setting. Currently, it is recognized that both sexual abuse and early consensual sexual activity occur at surprisingly high rates. If pregnancy testing is a routine order, then its use in any individual case does not require justification. The consequences of missing a pregnancy-related cause of pain, bleeding, or asymptomatic pelvic mass justify routine pregnancy testing in all young women presenting with pain, amenorrhea, abnormal bleeding, or a pelvic mass (Adams Hillard and Deitch, 2005).

INFECTION AS A CAUSE OF A PELVIC MASS

As the rates of sexually transmitted diseases (particularly chlamydia) have increased among adolescents, the incidence of upper track involvement with salpingitis or pelvic abscess (tuboovarian abscess [TOA]) has also increased (see Chapter 63). The U.S. Centers for Disease Control and Prevention (CDC) estimates that adolescents have the highest age-specific rates for chlamydia and gonorrhea, and therefore high rates of pelvic inflammatory disease (PID) (Centers for Disease Control and Prevention, 2002). Gonococcal PID has classic signs and symptoms and is relatively easy to diagnose clinically. However, chlamydia PID is more subtle in its presentation. Usually, *Chlamydia trachomatis* elaborates a heat shock protein that silently destroys the cilia lining the fallopian tube with only minimal symptomology. If the tissues become secondarily infected with enteric organisms, a clinically apparent salpingitis can develop. In the acute stage, pelvic infection is often accompanied by fever, cervical discharge, motion tenderness, and possibly adnexal masses (pyosalpinges or TOAs). After resolution of the acute infection, the tubes may remain dilated and filled with fluid (hydrosalpinges), particularly if their fimbriae have been sealed. Treated pelvic abscesses may also cause palpable masses due to adhesions—pelvic scarring with matting or agglutination of bowel, ovary, fallopian tube, and other structures. Other infectious causes of pelvic masses include an appendiceal abscess or (rarely in young girls) diverticulitis or Meckel diverticulum.

ADNEXAL TORSION

Adnexal torsion involves the acute rotation of adnexal structures. Torsion of the normal adnexa can occur, particularly in prepubertal girls; however, torsion is more likely to occur when an adnexal mass—a benign ovarian neoplasm, functional ovarian cyst, or a paratubal cyst—rotates around its vascular pedicle. Once rotated, the venous flow to the mass is obstructed while arterial flow continues, inflating the mass until arterial flow is compressed. The adnexal structures become edematous and ultimately gangrenous.

Clinical Manifestations

Women usually experience bouts of intense pelvic pain, which may be accompanied by nausea and vomiting. Findings on examination include peritoneal signs with rebound tenderness.

Diagnosis

Typical findings on ultrasound examination with Doppler flow studies include the presence of a mass, edema, adnexal asymmetry, and absent venous and/or arterial flow; unfortunately, these findings are neither perfectly sensitive nor specific, and clinical judgment must be used, including a high index of suspicion (Breech and Hillard, 2005). Spiraling or whirlpool configuration of the vessels may be seen and is a more specific finding. Consultation with a gynecologist is essential, as adnexal torsion is a surgical emergency.

Treatment

Treatment consists of untwisting the adnexae, even if hemorrhage and apparent necrosis are present. This can usually be performed laparoscopically. Excision of the cyst can be delayed and performed as an interval procedure once edema has resolved. Attempts to remove the cyst acutely may fail because of the marked edema that is typically present. Every attempt should be made to preserve the involved ovary.

UTERINE NEOPLASMS

In adolescent women, uterine neoplasms are quite rare. Leiomyomas (fibroids) develop within the wall of the uterus (intramural myomas) and later extend toward the endometrium (submucosal myomas) or toward the external surface of the myometrium (subserosal myomas). Although fibroids are extremely common in adult women, occurring in up to 50% of women older than 35, they are rare in adolescents. Although fibroids are frequently asymptomatic in adults, adolescents presenting with abnormal bleeding or pelvic pain may have demonstrable fibroids palpable on examination or demonstrated on pelvic ultrasonography.

BENIGN OVARIAN MASSES

Benign ovarian masses include *functional ovarian cysts, endometriomas, and benign ovarian neoplasms.* Whenever an ovarian mass is diagnosed in an adolescent female or prepubertal child, every effort must be made to preserve the reproductive function in that female in order to ensure future childbearing—whether the mass is physiological or neoplastic, benign or malignant (Kozlowski, 1999). Table 53.2 lists benign ovarian tumors. Figure 53.1 provides a plan for management of pelvic masses in premenarchal and adolescent girls.

Physiological (Functional) Ovarian Cysts

Functional ovarian cysts include *follicular cysts, corpus luteum cysts(CLCs), and theca lutein cysts.* All are benign

TABLE 53.2

Benign Ovarian Tumors

Functional
  Follicular
  Corpus luteum
  Theca lutein
Inflammatory
  Tuboovarian abscess or complex
Neoplastic
  Germ cell
  Benign cystic teratoma
  Other and mixed
Epithelial
  Serous cystadenoma
  Mucinous cystadenoma
  Fibroma
  Cystadenofibroma
  Brenner tumor
  Mixed tumor
Other
  Endometrioma

and usually do not cause symptoms or require surgical management. Cigarette smoking has been associated with an increased risk of functional cysts (Holt et al., 1994). Functional cysts result from expansion of the cavity of a preovulatory follicle (follicular cyst) or corpus luteum (CLCs), and are associated with the disordered function of the pituitary-ovarian axis. The incidence of functional ovarian cysts in adolescents is not well established, but most are asymptomatic, and they are frequently an incidental finding on pelvic imaging. One study, in which adolescents were followed up for 1 year with monthly serial ultrasound studies, found ovarian cysts in 12% of those observed (Porcu et al., 1994). Theca lutein cysts—the least common type of functional cyst—result from human chorionic gonadotropin (hCG) stimulation, producing bilateral follicular cystic ovarian enlargement. They occur in patients with gestational trophoblastic disease (molar pregnancies and choriocarcinoma) and multiple pregnancies and regress with the removal of the pregnancy-associated hCG production.

1. Follicular cysts: The most common type of functional ovarian cyst is a follicular cyst. Follicular cysts range in size from 3 to 15 cm in diameter, but rarely exceed 8 cm. Follicular cysts can be seen in prepubertal girls, and management depends on symptoms, patient age, menarchal status, cyst size and character, as well as associated medical conditions (Helmrath et al., 1998). They do not usually cause any symptoms, and may be an incidental finding on ultrasonography or other imaging studies. Torsion (see previous discussion) or rupture may occasionally occur, causing pain. In adolescents, follicular cysts usually resolve spontaneously in 4 to 8 weeks unless the patient is taking progestins (e.g., Mirena IUS, depot medroxyprogesterone acetate [DMPA]), which can slow follicular atresia and require a longer time for resolution. In general, conservative management of cysts smaller than 8 cm in a premenopausal woman is recommended for up to 8 weeks (Christensen et al., 2002;

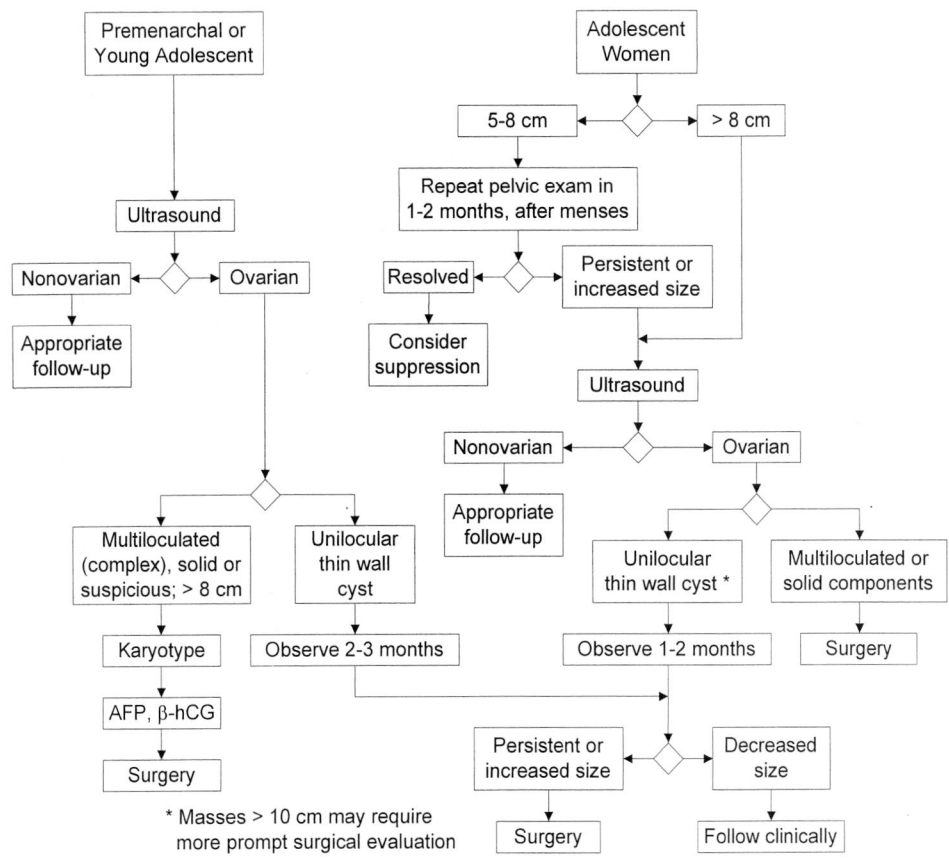

FIGURE 53.1   Management of pelvic masses in premenarchal and adolescent girls. AFP, α-fetoprotein; hCG, human chorionic gonadotropin.

Kanizsai et al., 1998). Persistent ovarian masses are more likely to be neoplastic and should prompt a referral for consideration of surgical excision (Spanos, 1973). Decisions about whether surgical excision of ovarian masses is required are best made by gynecological surgeons who have experience with adolescent and pediatric patients. Decisions about the type of surgical intervention are guided by the suspicion of malignancy; in general, benign-appearing masses can usually be managed using operative laparoscopy, while masses suspicious for malignancy require laparotomy (Mane and Penketh 1999; Parker and Berek 1994).

2. Corpus luteum cysts: CLCs are a variant of the normal corpus luteum. By definition, CLCs exceed 3 cm in diameter, but they can reach larger dimensions. They may be associated with delayed menses. CLCs are less common than follicular cysts but are clinically more significant because they can be associated with acute pain (due to bleeding into the enclosed cystic space) or rupture, leading to acute hemoperitoneum. This can be a surgical emergency if the patient is anticoagulated. A cyst may rupture during intercourse late in the cycle (days 21 to 26); although rarely, rupture can also follow pelvic examination, strenuous exercise, or trauma. Pain can occur in the absence of trauma. Patients presenting with pain and an adnexal mass on ultrasound examination may require gynecological consultation to differentiate an unruptured CLC, which should be managed medically, from a mass with an acute surgical emergency such

as torsion, hemoperitoneum, or appendicitis. Typical ultrasonographic findings include a mixed echogenic adnexal mass. Doppler flow ultrasonographic studies can suggest the possibility of torsion.

Because oral contraceptives suppress ovulation and follicular development, they reduce the risk of CLCs and follicular cysts in a dose-dependant manner (Grimes et al., 1994). DMPA also reduces the risk of functional ovarian cyst formation. Administration of oral contraceptives to induce cyst regression is no more effective than an observation period with no hormonal therapy, although it will suppress the development of subsequent functional cysts (Steinkampf et al., 1990).

3. Polycystic ovary syndrome (PCOS):   PCOS (see Chapter 52) is common in adults, occurring in 5% to 10% of adult women. This condition is increasingly being recognized as having the onset of symptoms during adolescence. Moderate to severe acne, abnormal menses (including both irregular or frequent menses and oligo- or amenorrhea), and obesity that had previously been ascribed to "normal adolescence" should now be recognized as presenting symptoms of PCOS. Newly described diagnostic criteria, include two of the following three:
   a. Oligo- or anovulation
   b. Clinical or biochemical evidence of hyperandrogenism
   c. Ultrasonographic demonstration of polycystic appearing ovaries along with the exclusion of other causes of hyperandrogenism

Although transvaginal ultrasonography is useful in demonstrating these findings—multiple (>10–12) small follicles <1 cm in diameter—this technique may be problematic in young or virginal adolescents. In addition, studies have suggested that up to 25% of women may have such ovarian morphology without the other diagnostic criteria. The volume of the ovary may be increased by a factor of 2 to 3, not only by the presence of these follicles but also by an increase in the ovarian stroma; this ovarian enlargement may be unilateral or bilateral. Although PCOS does not cause pain and this is not a condition that requires surgical management when the ultrasonographic characteristics are noted, clinical evaluation is appropriate to minimize the morbidity and improve quality of life. The lifelong metabolic implications of the condition should prompt management with lifestyle modification. Oral contraceptives and/or insulin-sensitizing agents can be helpful in management.

Endometriomas and Endometriosis

Definition

Endometriosis is a condition in which ectopic endometrium is present outside of the uterus. The presence of ovarian endometriosis can result in the formation of an ovarian endometrioma. There is a broad range of ultrasound appearances of endometriomas—diffuse, low level internal echoes occur in most endometriomas, and hyperechoic wall foci and multilocularity also suggest the diagnosis of an endometrioma.

Epidemiology

Endometriosis has historically been considered to be a condition affecting adult women; however, it is receiving increasing recognition as a cause of pelvic pain in adolescents (American College of Obstetricians and Gynecologists, 2005). Although the prevalence of endometriosis in adolescents is not well established, there is a familial incidence, and endometriosis can be demonstrated in up to 40% to 50% of adolescents undergoing laparoscopy because of chronic pelvic pain unresponsive to the use of hormonal manipulation, such as oral contraceptives and nonsteroidal anti-inflammatory drugs (NSAIDS). Endometriomas are also rare in adolescents, who typically have early stage or mild disease.

Clinical Manifestations

- The presenting symptoms include worsening dysmenorrhea, premenstrual or acyclic pelvic pain, and deep dyspareunia.
- On pelvic examination, findings of diffuse or localized tenderness, particularly in the cul-de-sac posterior to the uterus, diminished uterine motility (a result of adhesion formation particularly between the uterus and the sigmoid), cervical motion tenderness (from adhesions), and possibly an ovarian mass (endometrioma) are suggestive of endometriosis.
- Adolescents rarely have the "classic" finding of uterosacral nodularity.

Diagnosis

Because laparoscopy is indicated for diagnosing and managing suspected endometriosis in adolescents, adolescents with pelvic pain or dysmenorrhea that is unresponsive to NSAIDS and oral contraceptives should be referred to a gynecologist for consideration of surgical confirmation before medical therapy.

Benign Ovarian Neoplasms

The ultrasonographic characteristics of an ovarian mass will dictate the management. Adolescents with persistent cystic ovarian masses on ultrasonography following 6 to 8 weeks of observation may have an ovarian neoplasm and should be referred to a gynecologist for surgical management. Because benign cystic teratomas (dermoid cysts) are the most common ovarian neoplasm in adolescents, an adolescent with an ultrasonogram showing characteristics suspicious of this tumor should also be referred for gynecological surgical evaluation. Solid masses of any size are suspicious for a malignant tumor, and should lead to prompt referral.

Benign Germ Cell Tumors Benign cystic teratomas (dermoid cysts) are the most common benign ovarian neoplasm of adolescent and reproductive years (Koonings et al., 1989). Dermoid cysts are composed of all three germ cell layers. They are generally thick-walled cysts and may be filled with sebaceous material, hair; they may also contain cartilage, teeth, or other tissues such as thyroid. These embryological elements produce characteristic findings on ultrasonography that can suggest the likelihood of a benign cystic teratoma (Patel et al., 1998). Malignant transformation occurs in less than 2% of dermoid cysts in women of all ages and is rare in adolescents. Dermoid cysts vary in size from millimeters to quite large, but the vast majority is smaller than 10 cm. On examination, they are unilateral (only 10% are bilateral), very mobile, anteriorly positioned (fat floats), nontender adnexal masses. Benign cystic teratomas are usually asymptomatic. The risk of torsion with dermoid cysts is approximately 15%, and it occurs more frequently with ovarian tumors in general, perhaps because of the high fat content of most dermoid cysts, allowing them to float within the abdominal and pelvic cavity (Templeman et al., 2000a). An ovarian cystectomy is almost always possible, even if it appears that only a small amount of ovarian tissue remains. Preserving a small amount of ovarian cortex in a young patient with a benign lesion is preferable to the loss of the entire ovary (Templeman et al., 2000b). Laparoscopic cystectomy is usually possible, and intraoperative spill of tumor contents is rarely a cause of complications (Lin et al., 1995). Laparoscopy results in lower operative morbidity, as well as less postoperative pain and analgesic requirements, and a shorter hospital stay and recovery period when compared with laparotomy (Yuen et al., 1997). Adolescents with ultrasonography suggesting a dermoid should be referred to a gynecological surgeon skilled in laparoscopic surgery, who appreciates the importance of ovarian conservation.

Benign Epithelial Neoplasia Serous or mucinous cystadenomas account for 10% to 20% of benign ovarian neoplasms in female adolescents. These tumors are multiloculated, fluid-filled cystic masses. Serous cystadenomas may not be recognized as a neoplasm; cyst aspiration without removal of the entire cyst (including multiple loculated areas and cyst wall) may result in recurrence. Benign mucinous cystadenomas have smooth, lobulated surfaces with multiloculations filled with viscous mucoid material; these masses can reach very large dimensions. Surgical removal of these adenomas is necessary for tissue diagnosis and to prevent symptoms from an enlarging mass or torsion.

Sex Cord-Stromal Tumors Overall, these tumors are relatively rare, but they occur with higher prevalence in premenarchal girls than in adolescents or adults, and comprise 10% to 20% of childhood ovarian tumors. They may be hormonally active. Granulosa cell tumors and theca cell tumors produce estrogen whereas Sertoli-Leydig cell tumors produce androgens with or without estrogen. As a result of this sex-steroid production, sex cord-stromal tumors can cause precocious puberty, menstrual abnormalities, endometrial hyperplasia or carcinoma, or hirsutism, acne, and virilization. These signs should prompt pelvic imaging for diagnosis. Pure granulosa cell tumors are highly malignant, whereas mixed tumors behave less aggressively. Prognosis is excellent with unilateral salpingo-oophorectomy and appropriate surgical staging for the 95% of tumors that are unilateral.

MALIGNANT OVARIAN MASSES

Ovarian cancer is rare in adolescents and younger girls. Only slightly more than 1% of all ovarian cancers occur in women younger than 20 (Young et al., 2003). Ultrasound features of an ovarian mass that are a cause of concern for malignancy include solid consistency, large size, complex appearance (not entirely cystic), internal loculations, internal or external excrescences, and ascites (Stepanian and Cohn, 2004). Efforts to preserve fertility are important considerations in the management of ovarian malignancies in adolescents.

Malignant Germ Cell Tumors

In women younger than 20 years, one half to two thirds of all ovarian tumors are of germ cell origin and one third of those tumors are malignant. Malignant germ cell tumors include dysgerminoma, mixed germ cell tumor, endodermal sinus tumor, immature teratoma, embryonal tumor, choriocarcinoma, and polyembryoma. Because some ovarian neoplasms secrete protein tumor markers, including α-fetoprotein (AFP), hCG, carcinoembryonic antigen (CEA), lactate dehydrogenase (LDH), and others, measurement of these substances can be considered in making a diagnosis of an ovarian tumor and in following up malignant tumors for recurrence and clinical response (Kawai et al., 1992). CA-125 is a tumor marker for epithelial ovarian cancer, and while useful in evaluating adnexal masses in postmenopausal women it is not very specific, and in adolescents and premenopausal women it may be elevated with endometriosis, PID, pregnancy, Crohn disease, and other abdominal malignancies. Decisions about whether to obtain tumor markers before surgery should be made in consultation with a gynecologist or gynecological oncologist. Measurement of estradiol and testosterone can be helpful in evaluating and following up hormonally active tumors.

Dysgerminomas comprise 50% of all ovarian germ cell malignancies. They represent abnormal proliferations of the undifferentiated germ cell. Five percent to 10% of these tumors occur in phenotypically female patients with gonadal dysgenesis (e.g., pure gonadal dysgenesis—46, XY; mixed gonadal dysgenesis 45X/46/XY;

or complete androgen insensitivity syndrome—46, XY). Dysgerminomas have also been reported in girls with Turner syndrome. Because the presence of a Y chromosome or antigen is associated with a high risk of malignancy, bilateral gonadectomy is recommended. With androgen insensitivity syndrome, the risk of malignancy is low before puberty, and therefore the gonads should be removed after pubertal development is complete. Dysgerminomas are more likely to be bilateral than other germ cell tumors.

Immature teratomas represent 10% to 20% of all ovarian malignancies in women younger than 20 years. Approximately half of all pure immature teratomas occur in adolescent females. Premenarchal and younger age is associated with a greater risk of an immature malignant teratoma (Azizkhan and Caty 1996). Immature teratomas contain elements that resemble tissues derived from the embryo that do not mature. The amount of immature neural tissue is most predictive of lethality. Surgical staging and histological grade determine survival rates. Surgery alone is curative for most children and adolescents with completely resected ovarian immature teratoma (Cushing et al., 1999).

Endodermal sinus tumors ("yolk sac tumors") of the ovary are rare. Most (70%) patients present with abdominal or pelvic pain, and these tumors have an aggressive clinical course, and therefore chemotherapy is indicated (Stepanian and Cohn 2004). Most of these tumors secrete tumor markers such as α-fetoprotein (AFP).

Malignant Epithelial Tumors

Although these tumor types are the most common type of ovarian malignancy in adult women, they rarely develop in adolescents (Richardson et al., 1985). Included in this group of neoplasias are serous cystadenocarcinoma, mucinous cystadenocarcinoma, and endometrial cystadenocarcinoma. In adolescents, approximately 7% of epithelial tumors will be borderline malignancies, which can be managed with conservative surgery (unilateral salpingo-oophorectomy), careful assessment of the contralateral ovary, and appropriate staging procedures. Often, the borderline characteristics are diagnosed on permanent section pathological examination of a mass that was initially felt to be benign. Consultation and management in conjunction with a gynecological oncologist is appropriate in this situation, as recurrences may occur many years later. Less than 5% of ovarian epithelial tumors in adolescents are invasive malignancies. In these patients, appropriate surgical staging, cytoreductive surgery, and chemotherapy are required, as in adults; conservative management in early stage disease may allow the preservation of fertility. These patients require ongoing management by a gynecological oncologist.

Genetic Risk of Epithelial Ovarian Cancers

Approximately 5% of ovarian cancer before 70 years of age is associated with the genetic mutations in the breast cancer gene 1 (BRCA-1). Presence of this gene confers an increased risk of ovarian and breast cancer. Families with multiple family members with breast and/or ovarian cancer should be offered referral to specific familial cancer centers, which are present in many medical centers around the country. Decision making around these issues is challenging, and clinicians must balance providing information to families and adolescent patients, facilitating decision making, and minimizing family members' anxiety. Although the optimal age at which genetic testing should be performed has not been well established, many clinicians recommend offering counseling and testing in young adulthood (Laufer and Goldstein, 2005).

Other Carcinomas

In young women, the more common metastatic lesions of the ovary include lymphomas and leukemias.

Minimizing the Risks of Ovarian Masses and Malignancies

Oral contraceptive pills minimize the risks of functional ovarian masses in a dose-dependent manner (Grimes et al., 1994). Because they consistently prevent ovulation, CLCs are minimized. Ultra-low-dose estrogen-containing oral contraceptive pills as well as oral contraceptives containing higher doses of estrogen may not prevent follicular cysts.

Adolescents who have had an oophorectomy, an ovarian cystectomy, or an ovarian neoplasm may particularly benefit from the use of oral contraceptive pills to minimize the risks of developing a subsequent functional cyst (Muram et al., 1990). Oral contraceptives minimize the risks that a functional cyst will leave a sole-remaining ovary vulnerable to surgical extirpation. In adolescents with a previous malignancy who are being monitored for recurrence, the development of a functional cyst will almost invariably lead to patient and parental anxiety, additional diagnostic testing, and even potential surgical exploration. Therefore, suppression of ovarian functional cysts can be particularly beneficial.

Combination oral contraceptives are associated with a 30% to 60% reduction in the risk of epithelial ovarian malignancies (Grimes and Economy, 1995). Preventing ovarian cancer is seldom a motivating factor for adolescents, although when combined with the contraceptive and other noncontraceptive benefits of oral contraceptives, such as decreased acne, dysmenorrhea, menorrhagia, and ovarian cysts, this benefit may provide additional motivation for ongoing oral contraceptive use to teens and their families.

WEB SITES

For Teenagers and Parents

http://www.nlm.nih.gov/medlineplus/ency/article/001504 .htm. National Institutes of Health site with references and links on ovarian cysts.

http://familydoctor.org/handouts/279.html. American Academy of Family Physicians handout on ovarian cysts.

http://www.4women.gov/faq/ovarian_cysts.pdf. The National Women's Health Information Center. U.S. Department of Health and Human Services, Office on Women's Health.

http://www.goaskalice.columbia.edu/0724.html. Go Ask Alice information on ovarian cysts from the Columbia University Student Health Center.

For Health Professionals

http://www.emedicine.com/emerg/topic352.htm. E-medicine site about ovarian cysts.

REFERENCES AND ADDITIONAL READINGS

Adams Hillard PJ, Deitch HR. Menstrual disorders in the college age female. *Pediatr Clin North Am* 2005;52:179.

American College of Obstetricians and Gynecologists. ACOG Committee Opinion #310: endometriosis in adolescents. *Obstet Gynecol* 2005;105:921.

Azizkhan RG, Caty MG. Teratomas in childhood. *Curr Opin Pediatr* 1996;8:287.

Breech LL, Hillard PJ. Adnexal torsion in pediatric and adolescent girls. *Curr Opin Obstet Gynecol* 2005;17:483.

Centers for Disease Control and Prevention. Sexually transmitted diseases treatment guidelines 2002. *MMWR Recomm Rep* 2002;51:1.

Christensen JT, Boldsen JL, Westergaard JG. Functional ovarian cysts in premenopausal and gynecologically healthy women. *Contraception* 2002;66:153.

Cushing B, Giller R, Ablin A, et al. Surgical resection alone is effective treatment for ovarian immature teratoma in children and adolescents: a report of the pediatric oncology group and the children's cancer group. *Am J Obstet Gynecol* 1999; 181:353.

Economy KE, Barnewolt C, Laufer MR. A comparison of MRI and laparoscopy in detecting pelvic structures in cases of vaginal agenesis. *J Pediatr Adolesc Gynecol* 2002;15:101.

Grimes DA, Economy KE. Primary prevention of gynecologic cancers. *Am J Obstet Gynecol* 1995;172:227.

Grimes DA, Godwin AJ, Rubin A, et al. Ovulation and follicular development associated with three low-dose oral contraceptives: a randomized controlled trial. *Obstet Gynecol* 1994;83:29.

Helmrath MA, Shin CE, Warner BW. Ovarian cysts in the pediatric population. *Semin Pediatr Surg* 1998;7:19.

Hillard PA. Benign diseases of the female reproductive tract: symptoms and signs. In: Berek JS, Adashi EY, Hillard PA, eds. *Novak's gynecology*, 13th ed. Philadelphia, PA: Lippincott Williams & Wilkins; 2002:351.

Holt VL, Daling JR, McKnight B, et al. Cigarette smoking and functional ovarian cysts. *Am J Epidemiol* 1994;139:781.

Kanizsai B, Orley J, Szigetvari I, et al. Ovarian cysts in children and adolescents: their occurrence, behavior, and management. *J Pediatr Adolesc Gynecol* 1998;11:85.

Kawai M, Kano T, Kikkawa F, et al. Seven tumor markers in benign and malignant germ cell tumors of the ovary. *Gynecol Oncol* 1992;45:248.

Kim HH, Laufer MR. Developmental abnormalities of the female reproductive tract. *Curr Opin Obstet Gynecol* 1994;6: 518.

Koonings PP, Campbell K, Mishell DR Jr, et al. Relative frequency of primary ovarian neoplasms: a 10-year review. *Obstet Gynecol* 1989;74:921

Kozlowski KJ. Ovarian masses. *Adolesc Med* 1999;10:337.

Laufer MR, Goldstein DP. Benign and malignant ovarian masses. In: *Pediatric and adolescent gynecology*, 5th ed. Philadelphia, PA: Lippincott Williams & Wilkins; 2005:685.

Lin P, Falcone T, Tulandi T. Excision of ovarian dermoid cyst by laparoscopy and by laparotomy. *Am J Obstet Gynecol* 1995; 173:769.

Mane S, Penketh R. Laparoscopic management of benign ovarian disease. *Semin Laparosc Surg* 1999;6:104.

Muram D, Gale CL, Thompson E. Functional ovarian cysts in patients cured of ovarian neoplasms. *Obstet Gynecol* 1990; 75:680.

Parker WH, Berek JS. Laparoscopic management of the adnexal mass. *Obstet Gynecol Clin North Am* 1994;21:79.

Patel MD, Feldstein VA, Lipson SD, et al. Cystic teratomas of the ovary: diagnostic value of sonography. *AJR Am J Roentgenol* 1998;171:1061.

Porcu E, Venturoli S, Dal Prato L, et al. Frequency and treatment of ovarian cysts in adolescence. *Arch Gynecol Obstet* 1994;255:69.

Richardson GS, Scully RE, Nikrui N, et al. Common epithelial cancer of the ovary (2). *N Engl J Med* 1985;312:415.

Spanos WJ. Preoperative hormonal therapy of cystic adnexal masses. *Am J Obstet Gynecol* 1973;116:551.

Spence JE. Vaginal and uterine anomalies in the pediatric and adolescent patient. *J Pediatr Adolesc Gynecol* 1998;11:3.

Steinkampf MP, Hammond KR, Blackwell RE. Hormonal treatment of functional ovarian cysts: a randomized, prospective study. *Fertil Steril* 1990;54:775.

Stepanian M, Cohn DE. Gynecologic malignancies in adolescents. *Adolesc Med Clin* 2004;15:549.

Templeman C, Fallat ME, Blinchevsky A, et al. Noninflammatory ovarian masses in girls and young women. *Obstet Gynecol* 2000a;96:229.

Templeman CL, Fallat ME, Lam AM, et al. Managing mature cystic teratomas of the ovary. *Obstet Gynecol Surv* 2000b;55: 738.

Young JL Jr, Cheng Wu X, Roffers SD, et al. Ovarian cancer in children and young adults in the United States, 1992–1997. *Cancer* 2003;97:2694

Yuen PM, Yu KM, Yip SK, et al. A randomized prospective study of laparoscopy and laparotomy in the management of benign ovarian masses. *Am J Obstet Gynecol* 1997;177: 109.

CHAPTER 54

Pap Smears and Abnormal Cervical Cytology

Anna-Barbara Moscicki

PREVALENCE OF ABNORMAL CYTOLOGY

Several large studies have shown that approximately 3% to 14% of females younger than 19 years have abnormal cervical cytology (Bjorge et al., 1995; Mount and Papillo, 1999; Sadeghi et al., 1984). Fortunately, most of these abnormal cytologies are primarily low-grade squamous intraepithelial lesions (LSILs), which are considered as benign changes due to human papillomavirus (HPV) infection. These rates are consistent with the high rates of HPV infection reported in this age-group, which range from 20% to 57% (Moscicki et al., 1990, 1999; Rosenfeld et al., 1989, Winer et al., 2003) with approximately 50% of adolescents acquiring an HPV infection within 5 years of starting sexual activity. Although rates of high-grade squamous intraepithelial lesions (HSILs), considered true pre-cancer lesions, are substantially lower than those of LSILs in adolescents, recent studies suggest that these rates are higher than previously reported. In 1981, Sadeghi et al. (1984) performed an analysis of more than 194,000 Papanicolaou (Pap) smears in adolescents aged 15 to 19 years. Using the World Health Organization's cytological classification, they found a combined rate for cervical intraepithelial neoplasia (CIN) grades 1 and 2 of 18/1,000 smears, and for carcinoma in situ, 1/1,000. In comparison, Mount et al. (1999) examined more than 10,000 Pap smears from young women and found that 14% of the smear results from females aged 15 to 19 years were considered abnormal, with 7% having LSIL and 0.7% having HSIL. Interestingly, the rate of HSIL in the 15- to 19-year-old group was similar to that reported in comparable smear tests from women aged 20 to 29 years (0.8%) and higher than that for women aged 30 to 39 years (0.5%). These rates reported for adolescents are likely underestimates because they only reflect women who enter the health care system. In a nationwide organized cervical screening program, Bjorge et al. (1995) reported a 0.2% incidence rate for HSIL among 20,000 smears of adolescents aged 15 to 19 years. However, the LSIL rate was highest for this age-group. Because of this disproportionate rate between LSIL and HSIL in adolescents, most adolescents with abnormal cytology are unnecessarily referred for colposcopy.

VULNERABILITY OF THE CERVIX TO HUMAN PAPILLOMAVIRUS

The characteristic histological changes of the cervix associated with HPV infections generally occur within the transformation zone (T-zone). It is useful to review the formation of this zone and the natural history of HPV in understanding abnormal cervical changes.

During embryological development, the müllerian ducts give rise to the fallopian tubes, uterus, and vagina. These structures in the fetus are lined by immature cuboidal epithelium (which becomes columnar epithelium) from the uterus to the hymenal ring. The urogenital sinus epithelium grows up the vaginal vault and replaces the native epithelium up to the ectocervix with squamous epithelium. This replacement is usually incomplete, creating an abrupt squamocolumnar junction (SCJ) on the ectocervix. Squamous metaplasia is a process during which undifferentiated columnar cells transform themselves into squamous epithelium. However, the process is relatively quiescent until puberty, resulting in little changes to the SCJ during childhood. The area of columnar epithelium seen on the ectocervix is referred to as *ectopy*.

With puberty the pH level of the vagina drops. This is associated with glycogen production by squamous cells induced by rising levels of estrogen. The glycogen provides a source of carbohydrate for the vaginal flora. Vaginal bacteria proliferate, and the lactobacilli convert glycogen to lactic acids, resulting in a lowered pH level. This new acidic environment most likely contributes to the augmentation of the squamous metaplastic process, resulting in relatively rapid replacement of columnar epithelium by squamous epithelium.

Transformation Zone (T-zone)

Location With conversion of the columnar epithelium to squamous epithelium, a T-zone is created. The T-zone is a relatively fluid area of definition, because it represents the area between the original SCJ and the current SCJ. By a woman's late 20 s and early 30 s, most have had substantial replacement of their columnar epithelium, resulting in little to no visible ectopy. Although squamous metaplasia continues, it is now found well inside the endocervical canal.

Native squamous epithelium appears as smooth, pink, and featureless epithelium. In general, it covers the vagina and a portion of ectocervix. Native columnar epithelium is a single-layer, mucus-producing, tall epithelium extending between the endometrium and into the T-zone. This area has an irregular surface with long papillae and deep clefts, often referred to as having a "grapelike" appearance. The physiological T-zone has a combination of columnar and squamous epithelium features, as well as several unique features, which are dependent on the stage of development. In early stages, the zone is predominantly covered with columnar epithelium and discrete patches where the fusion of the villi causes a loss of translucency and the villi assume a ground glass appearance. Later, successive villi are fused and the intervening spaces are filled. Eventually the papillary structures are lost, and the new surface takes on a less translucent, vascular, pearly tongue appearance. Because the conversion of columnar epithelium to squamous epithelium occurs in often disjointed or fragmented segments, the examiner can often see small glands that are predominantly lined with columnar or metaplastic epithelium. When these gland openings become completely closed by squamous epithelium, the mucus-secreting epithelium may continue to produce mucus. If that mucus becomes inspissated, the gland dilates and a nabothian cyst results. Nabothian cysts eventually self-destruct from the pressure of the inspissated mucus.

Vulnerability of the T-Zone The T-zone is the area of the cervix most prone to the development of squamous intraepithelial lesions (SILs) and invasive squamous cell cancers. The vulnerability of the T-zone is most likely related to the process of squamous metaplasia and its vulnerability to HPV and SIL development (Moscicki et al., 1999). This association reflects the natural life cycle of HPV and its dependence on host cell proliferation and differentiation, both characteristics of squamous metaplasia. Initial HPV infections are thought to occur by invasion of cells of the basal epithelium. Disruption of the epithelium by inflammation or trauma may cause an increased risk for infection with HPV. Differentiation of these basal cells to well-differentiated squamous epithelial cells supports HPV replication by allowing expression of certain viral proteins at different layers of differentiation. The expression of the oncogenic proteins E_6 and E_7 in turn causes histological changes, which include abnormal cell proliferation, and the appearance of abnormal mitotic figures, both features of SIL. Features that are mild in nature and restricted to the basal and parabasal areas are referred to as LSIL. When these features become more extensive and extend into the upper half of the epithelium, the changes are referred to as HSIL. These changes coincide with increased expression of the oncogenes E_6 and E_7. Consequently, both LSIL and HSIL are pathological changes due to HPV infection.

CERVICAL DYSPLASIA

Impact of Cofactors

HPV infection is clearly the causative factor for cervical SIL. However, because rates of HPV are 4 to 10 times more common than SIL, and 100 to 700 times more common than invasive cancers, it is assumed that HPV is necessary but not sufficient for the development of these lesions. In the case of cancer, numerous molecular events are most likely needed. Although HPV infection is clearly one of the first steps, most HPV infections are quickly eliminated by the host's immune response. Lack of an adequate immune response results in persistence of HPV infection, and in turn, HPV persistence is a strong risk for the development of HSIL (Ho et al., 1995; Moscicki et al., 1998, Ylitalo et al., 2000). HPV persistence is a common problem among persons with immunodeficiencies including human immunodeficiency virus (HIV) infection (Moscicki et al., 2004a; Sun et al., 1997). Other factors associated with HSIL and cancer development include tobacco exposure. Even when adjusted for numbers of sex partners, women who smoke have a higher risk of developing cervical SIL and invasive cancers than nonsmokers (Haverkos et al., 2003). This relationship appears to be dose related, because women who are heavier smokers for a longer time have the highest risk for developing SIL and cancers. Other risk factors implicated include herpes simplex virus (HSV) and *Chlamydia Trachomatis* infections, multiparity, and history of prolonged oral contraceptive use (Smith et al., 2003, 2004).

Cervical Screening Tests

Three U.S. organizations have established guidelines for the initiation and frequency of cervical cancer screening (Table 54.1). Current recommendations for Pap smear testing are that women should start having Pap smears within 3 years of becoming sexually active or at age 21 years (American College of Obstetricians and Gynecologists, 2004; Saslow et al., 2002). After a patient has had three consecutive annual tests whose results are read as normal, she may be screened at 1- to 3-year intervals, depending on risk behavior (i.e., multiple partners), older partners, and a high rate of sexually transmitted diseases (STDs) (ACOG, 2006; American Medical Association, 1997). STD screening is generally performed at least annually for sexually active adolescents. The pelvic examination is generally included in this screening at least every 1 to 2 years starting 3 years after the initiation of sexual intercourse, and following the first three consecutive annual Pap smears. The recommendation to wait for Pap smears is recent because many groups recommended screening once sexual activity ensued. Waiting has raised anxiety among health care providers because the first Pap smear was considered an opportune time to discuss anatomy, birth control, and risk behaviors. The new guidelines continue to support this, but do not recommend starting a chain of events with triage and referral for abnormal cytology when most (93%) lesions in this age-group will regress (Moscicki et al., 2004).

TABLE 54.1

Current Guidelines for Initiation and Frequency of Cervical Cancer Screening: Select U.S. Organizations

Criteria	American Cancer Society (2002)	American College of Obstetricians and Gynecologists (2003)	U.S. Preventative Services Task Force (2003)
Beginning screening	Approximately 3 y after onset of vaginal intercourse, but no later than age 21 y	Approximately 3 y after initiation of sexual intercourse, but no later than age 21 y	Within 3 y of onset of sexual activity or age 21 y, whichever comes first
Screening interval			
Conventional cytology	Annual	Annual	At least every 3 y
Liquid-based cytology	Biennial	No separate recommendation	Insufficient evidence to recommend for or against
Women aged ≥30 y with three consecutive, normal cytology test results	Every 2 to 3 y[a]	Every 2 to 3 y[b]	No separate recommendation
Cytology with concurrent HPV DNA testing[c]	Not more often than every 3 y If HPV DNA negative, cytology normal	Not more often than every 3 y if HPV DNA negative, cytology normal	Insufficient evidence to recommend for or against

HPV, human papillomavirus.

[a]Exceptions: women who are immunocompromised (due to organ transplantation, chemotherapy, chronic corticosteroid treatment) are infected with human immunodeficiency virus (HIV), and/or have a history of in utero diethylstilbestrol exposure.

[b]Exceptions: women who are immunocompromised, are infected with HIV, have a history of in utero diethylstilbestrol exposure, and/or have a history of cervical intraepithelial neoplasia 2 or 3.

[c]only for women age 30 y or older

Reproduced with permission from the American Medical Association. A 21-year-old woman with atypical squamous cells of undetermined significance. *JAMA* 2005;294:2210.

Most cytologists in the United States have adopted the Bethesda reporting system and now provide more descriptive reports of their findings after screening of the specimen for adequacy and correct preparation. Smear tests that are considered inadequate or with missing endocervical cells should be repeated. A summary of the Bethesda system findings is found in Figure 54.1.

Liquid Cytology Sample preparation may contribute to the poor sensitivity of the Pap smears; that is, most Pap smears are difficult to read because of obscuring cells, drying artifact, and cell distortion. Liquid cytology has been devised, whereby exfoliated cells are placed immediately into a liquid fixative rather than smeared onto a slide. The fixative solution is transported to the laboratory, where monolayers are prepared using a company's processor. The cells are transferred from the filter onto a glass slide for routine Pap staining. An advantage is clearer images of the cells because the samples are depleted of blood and inflammatory cells that can obscure the readings. Because the agreement rate between conventional smears and liquid cytology is more than 90%, and the cost of liquid cytology smears is sometimes substantially more than that of conventional smears, the cost-effectiveness of using liquid cytology is in question. One advantage may be that the cells preserved in the liquid fixative can be used for ancillary studies such as reflex HPV testing (see subsequent text). Another advantage is that liquid cytology appears to pick up more abnormalities; hence screening intervals may be increased to every 2 years if liquid cytology is used (Saslow et al., 2002). The American

Cancer Society has recommended biennial testing using this method (Table 54.1).

The follow-up evaluation required for benign Pap smear findings not associated with neoplastic changes is shown in Table 54.2. Current triage practices for abnormal Pap smear changes in adults followed by recommendations for adolescents are outlined in the following sections.

Recommendations for Adult Women

1. Atypical squamous cells of undetermined significance (ASCUS)
   a. Alternative one: One option is to repeat the Pap smear within 4 to 6 months. If the Pap smear results remain positive for ASCUS or worsen, the patients should be referred for colposcopy. If the second Pap smear result is normal, another Pap smear should be obtained within 6 months. After two consecutive smears, the patient may return to routine screening. A diagnosis of ASCUS that cannot rule out HSIL should be treated as HSIL.
   b. Alternative two: An alternative to repeat cytology is HPV DNA testing. HPV testing is best performed in the situation of reflex testing. This currently refers to using a liquid cytological method in which the sample obtained for cytology is also adequate to test for the presence of high-risk HPV DNA at a later date. In these situations, the reference laboratory would automatically run an HPV DNA test for high-risk types if an ASCUS result was present on cytology. Studies show that HPV testing is more sensitive for

BETHESDA SYSTEM 2001

SPECIMEN TYPE: *Indicate conventional smear (Pap smear) vs. liquid-based vs. other*

SPECIMEN ADEQUACY
- ❑ Satisfactory for evaluation (*describe presence or absence of endocervical/transformation zone component and any other quality indicators, e.g., partially obscuring blood, inflammation, etc.*)
- ❑ Unsatisfactory for evaluation . . . (*specify reason*)
  - ❑ Specimen rejected/not processed (*specify reason*)
  - ❑ Specimen processed and examined, but unsatisfactory for evaluation of epithelial abnormality because of (*specify reason*)

GENERAL CATEGORIZATION (*optional*)
- ❑ Negative for intraepithelial lesion or malignancy
- ❑ Epithelial cell abnormality: See Interpretation/Result (*specify 'squamous' or 'glandular' as appropriate*)
- ❑ Other: See Interpretation/Result (*e.g., endometrial cells in a woman ≥ 40 years of age*)

AUTOMATED REVIEW
If case examined by automated device, specify device and result.

ANCILLARY TESTING
Provide a brief description of the test methods and report the result so that it is easily understood by the clinician.

INTERPRETATION/RESULT
NEGATIVE FOR INTRAEPITHELIAL LESION OR MALIGNANCY (*when there is no cellular evidence of neoplasia, state this in the General Categorization above and/or in the Interpretation/Result section of the report, whether or not there are organisms or other non-neoplastic findings*)

ORGANISMS:
- ➢ *Trichomonas vaginalis*
- ➢ Fungal organisms morphologically consistent with *Candida* sp
- ➢ Shift in flora suggestive of bacterial vaginosis
- ➢ Bacteria morphologically consistent with *Actinomyces* sp
- ➢ Cellular changes consistent with Herpes simplex virus

OTHER NON-NEOPLASTIC FINDINGS (*Optional to report; list not inclusive*):
- ➢ Reactive cellular changes associated with
  - inflammation (includes typical repair)
  - radiation
  - intrauterine contraceptive device (IUD)
- ➢ Glandular cells status post hysterectomy
- ➢ Atrophy

OTHER
- ➢ Endometrial cells (*in a woman ≥ 40 years of age*) (*Specify if 'negative for squamous intraepithelial lesion'*)

FIGURE 54.1 Summary of Bethesda system findings. (From Solomon D, Davey D, Kurman R, et al. The 2001 Bethesda system: terminology for reporting results of cervical cytology. *JAMA* 2002;287;(16):2114, with permission.)

EPITHELIAL CELL ABNORMALITIES

SQUAMOUS CELL

➢ Atypical squamous cells
- of undetermined significance (ASCUS)
- cannot exclude HSIL (ASC-H)

➢ Low grade squamous intraepithelial lesion (LSIL)
encompassing: HPV/mild dysplasia/CIN 1

➢ High grade squamous intraepithelial lesion (HSIL)
encompassing: moderate and severe dysplasia, CIS/CIN 2 and CIN 3
- with features suspicious for invasion (*if invasion is suspected*)

➢ Squamous cell carcinoma

GLANDULAR CELL

➢ Atypical
- endocervical cells (NOS *or specify in comments*)
- endometrial cells (NOS *or specify in comments*)
- glandular cells (NOS *or specify in comments*)

➢ Atypical
- endocervical cells, favor neoplastic
- glandular cells, favor neoplastic

➢ Endocervical adenocarcinoma in situ

➢ Adenocarcinoma
- endocervical
- endometrial
- extrauterine
- not otherwise specified (NOS)

OTHER MALIGNANT NEOPLASMS: (*specify*)

EDUCATIONAL NOTES AND SUGGESTIONS (*optional*)

Suggestions should be concise and consistent with clinical follow-up guidelines published by professional organizations (references to relevant publications may be included).

FIGURE 54.1 (*Continued*)

TABLE 54.2

Follow-up Evaluation Recommendations for Abnormal Pap Smear Findings

Pap Smear Finding	Recommendation
Insufficient quantity	Repeat Pap smears in 2–3 mo
Poor specimen	Repeat Pap smears in 2–3 mo
Air-drying artifact	Repeat Pap smears in 2–3 mo
No endocervical cells	No need to repeat Pap smear if patient has had normal test results previously and is in compliant with therapy; if not, repeat in 2–3 mo
Endometrial cells	Normal if near menses or while using oral contraceptives or intrauterine devices; otherwise, recall and evaluate endometritis
Trichomoniasis	Recall patient, perform sexually transmitted disease evaluation, and treat patient and partner
Yeast	Review chart; if no symptoms, no need to follow-up
Inflammation	Consider recent coitus, infection
Reactive, reparative changes	Identify irritant, if possible; essentially normal

the detection of HSIL than repeat cytology (Manos et al., 1999). This triage works best in women aged 21 years and older. HPV testing in adolescents (see subsequent text) is not recommended. Currently, Hybrid Capture II HPV Test (Digene Diagnostics, Gaithersburg, MD) is the only U.S. Food and Drug Administration-approved commercially available test kit for clinical high-risk DNA detection in the United States. ASCUS with a positive result for high-risk HPV DNA test should be referred for colposcopy in the nonadolescent age-group.

2. LSIL: This category includes evidence of HPV infection referred to as *koilocytosis* and CIN 1 lesions merged together to reflect the technical difficulties in artificially distinguishing between them and to reflect the fact that very few of these lesions have any progressive or oncogenic potential.

The original intent of the developers of the Bethesda system was to permit more conservative management of patients with low-grade lesions. However, as many as 25% to 30% of patients with LSIL on Pap smears actually harbor more advanced disease, including HSIL and rarely invasive cancer. Currently, it is recommended that all LSIL in adult women be referred for colposcopy. HPV testing for triage in patients with LSIL is not recommended (Atypical Squamous Cells of Undetermined Significance/Low-Grade Squamous Intraepithelial Lesions Triage Study [ALTS] Group, 2000).

3. HSIL: This category includes moderate and severe dysplasia and carcinoma in situ. HSIL requires colposcopic evaluation with directed biopsies and endocervical evaluation

4. HPV testing as primary screening in women 30 years or older (Fig. 54.2)   Natural history studies have shown that HPV DNA detection in older women commonly reflects a persistent HPV infection, which is in contrast to HPV DNA detection in adolescents and young women where it is predominantly transient. This distinction has been modeled into screening strategies for older women. It is now recommended that women 30 years

and older have both high-risk HPV DNA testing and cytology for primary cervical cancer screening. The high negative predictive value of HPV DNA testing allows a greater interval for repeat testing in women who are HPV DNA negative and have normal cytology. Recommended options for the use of the FDA-approved HPV DNA test for colposcopy triage in patients with abnormal cytology are as follows (Fig. 54.2):

a. Cytology normal, HPV test negative: Repeat cytology and HPV test in 3 years.
b. Cytology normal, HPV test positive: Repeat cytology and HPV test 6 to 12 months later.

Triage on the basis of cytology results using this dual screening method in women older than 30 with ASCUS, LSIL, and HSIL is the same as the preceding recommendations 1 to 3. The major purpose of this dual screening is to allow a longer screening interval in those at low risk (negative cytology and HPV screening) and a more intense follow-up for those with HPV positive test despite negative cytology.

Special Considerations for Triage of Cytology in Adolescents

The rate of invasive cancers among adolescents is extremely low, whereas a LSIL diagnosis is at its highest. The common nature of LSIL in adolescents is not surprising given the high rate of HPV infections in this group. Fortunately, LSIL and HPV are mostly transient in this age-group, with more than 90% of HPV infections and LSIL showing regression in adolescents and young women within 3 years (Moscicki et al., 2004a). For this reason, triage for ASCUS and LSIL differ for adolescents (defined as <21 years of age) than adult women. The following are recommendations by the author and other experts in adolescent health care, but are always subject to the latest consensus recommendations available at the American Society for Colposcopy and Cervical Pathology Web site: http://www.asccp.org/consensus.shtml. The major consensus recommendations have been based on consensus reports from 2001, ACOG committee opinion and expert opinion.

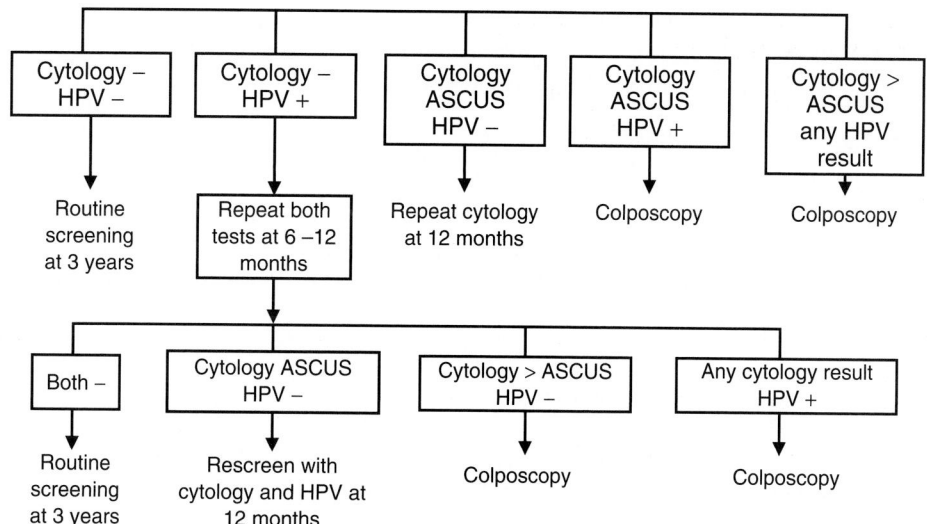

FIGURE 54.2 Algorithm for human papilloma virus (HPV) DNA testing and cytology as primary screening in women aged 30 years and older. ASCUS, atypical squamous cells of undetermined significance.

1. *HPV testing in triage or follow-up for ASCUS or LSIL is not recommended in this age-group.* Detection of HPV in adolescents is reflective of a transient infection, whereas in adult women, HPV detection most likely reflects a persistent infection which is a strong risk for HSIL development. These data support the use of HPV in triage for ASCUS in adult women and its use in primary screening in women 30 years or older, but not in adolescents.

2. *ASCUS and LSIL are both treated with identical follow-up strategies that include follow-up with cytology alone for up to 2 years.* It is recommended that patients with ASCUS/LSIL can be followed up with repeat cytology at 12-month intervals for 2 years, without immediate referral for colposcopy. During the 2 years of follow-up, a threshold of HSIL or greater is recommended before referral for colposcopy. After 2 years, a threshold of ASCUS or greater is recommended before referral for colposcopy. These guidelines do not include HIV infected adolescents because progression to HSIL is common (Moscicki et al., 2004b).

Therapy for Cervical Dysplasia

The colposcopically directed biopsy and the endocervical test results determine the extent of the lesion and direct the therapy. The principle in developing a treatment plan is that cervical dysplasia, specifically HSIL, is treated to prevent progression to cancer. If the lesions are confined to the ectocervix, a wide range of treatment options is available (Table 54.3).

One practice to be avoided, particularly in adolescents, is to combine the diagnostic and treatment steps by performing colposcopic examination to rule out invasion and excising the T-zone by a loop electrocautery excision procedure (LEEP) without biopsy confirmation. This practice is inappropriate and expensive. Approximately 90% of such referred adolescents have no HSIL found on the specimen on undergoing an LEEP, and the cost exceeds the benefit for patients without dysplasia with regard to side effects

(Sadler et al., 2004). As can be seen in Table 54.3, each of the major treatment modalities has minimal adverse impacts when used once. However, because recurrent lesions may develop and require further treatment, the cumulative effects of multiple treatments (particularly LEEP) must be considered. A recent meta-analysis showed that excisional therapy has a higher rate of premature labor and low birth weight (Kyrgiou et al., 2006). Hillard et al. (1991) reported another complication of treatment of cervical dysplasia related to cryotherapy in a group of 67 adolescents. Nine percent developed pelvic inflammatory disease (PID) within 1 month of treatment, and 2 teens developed cervical stenosis and hematometra. In general, screening for STDs before cryotherapy or LEEP is recommended to avoid the complications of PID. Because of the benign nature of histological CIN 1 in all ages, it is recommended that CIN 1 be observed and not treated. Observation of CIN 2 in compliant adolescents is also allowed. (www.asccp.org and American College of Obstetricians-Gynecologists ACOG Committee Opinion, 2006).

All women with dysplasia who smoke should be encouraged to stop smoking. Advise them that continued tobacco use increases susceptibility to cancer. Condom use has been shown to enhance LSIL regression, so condom use should be encouraged (Hogewoning et al., 2003).

After treatment, patients require repeat cytology or colposcopy and cytology at 4 to 6 months until three consecutive normal Pap smears are reported. The patient then can return to normal screening, including annual Pap smears for 3 years, then if all results remain normal, every 3 years. Follow-up with HPV testing at 6 months is also considered optional. The patient can return to normal screening after a single HPV negative test (www.asccp.org).

Conflicting information exists for associations between cervical cancer and HSV and *C. Trachomatis* infections, prolonged oral contraceptive use (>5–8 years), and multiparity (>6 children) (Smith et al., 2003, 2004, Lehtinen et al., 2002). It is currently not recommended to screen male partners of women with abnormal Pap smears for HPV infections

TABLE 54.3

Cervical Dysplasia Treatment Regimen Response Rates

	Cryotherapy	LEEP
Response rate		
Single (%)	80	95
Repeated (%)	95	95
Advantages	Simple office-based procedure	SCJ on ectocervix
	Inexpensive	Can tailor to lesion
	Only mildly painful	Provides specimen for pathology
Disadvantages	Watery vaginal discharge for 4–6 wk	Expensive
		More painful
	May not be as effective for large lesions or those that extend well onto the ectocervix	Bleeding complications
		Premature rupture of membrane in future
	New SCJ on endocervix	
	No specimen for pathology	
	Stenosis	

LEEP, loop electrocautery excision procedure; SCJ, squamocolumnar junction.

because few studies have demonstrated HPV disease in this group.

Recommendations for treatment of cervical lesions change over time and differ based on the patient's age and other risk factors. Clinicians involved in the treatment of cervical lesions should refer to the American Society for Colposcopy and Cervical Pathology Web site where consensus recommendations are updated as they become available: http://www.asccp.org/consensus.html.

Vaccination The latest intervention for prevention of HPV infection is the HPV vaccine. One vaccine was approved in 2006 for types 6/11/16/18 and another vaccine is under approval process for types 16/18. These vaccines have the potential to significantly alter the prevalence of HPV infections in women (see Chapter 66).

WEB SITES

For Teenagers and Parents

http://www.ashastd.org. American Social Health Association: Learn about STDs/HPV.

http://www.youngwomenshealth.org/abpap.html. Center for Young Women's Health information sheet for teens on abnormal Pap smears.

http://www.familydoctor.org/handouts/223.html. American Academy of Family Physicians handout.

http://www.nccc-online.org/. National Cervical Cancer Coalition site.

http://www.4woman.gov/faq/pap.htm. National Women's Health information center frequently asked questions sheet.

http://www.asccp.org. American Society for Colposcopy and Cervical Pathology: Patient Education.

For Health Professionals

http://www.asccp.org. American Society for Colposcopy and Cervical Pathology: Practice Recommendations.

http://www.asct.com/. American Society for Cytotechnologists.

http://www.ascp.org/general/pub_resources/papsmear/questions.asp. American Society of Clinical Pathologists.

http://www.bethesda2001.cancer.gov/terminology.html. Bethesda 2001 classifications.

REFERENCES AND ADDITIONAL READINGS

Adimora AA, Quinlivan EG. Papillomavirus infection: recent findings on progression to cervical cancer. *Postgrad Med* 1995;98:109.

American College of Obstetricians-Gynecologists ACOG Committee Opinion. Evaluation and management of abnormal cervical cytology and histology in the adolescent. *Obstet Gynecol* 2006;107:963.

American College of Obstetricians and Gynecologists. *ACOG guidelines for women's health care*. Washington: American College of Obstetricians and Gynecologists; 1996.

American Family Physician. NIH releases consensus statement on cervical cancer. *Am Fam Physician* 1996;54:2310.

American Medical Association. *Guidelines for adolescent preventive services*. Chicago, IL: American Medical Association; 1997.

Atypical Squamous Cells of Undetermined Significance/Low-Grade Squamous Intraepithelial Lesions Triage Study (ALTS) Group. Human papillomavirus testing for triage of women with cytologic evidence of low-grade squamous intraepithelial lesions: baseline data from a randomized trial. *J Natl Cancer Inst* 2000;92:397.

Becker TM. Genital warts—a Sexually Transmitted Disease (STD) epidemic. *Colposc Gynecol Laser Surg* 1984;1:193.

Beckmann A, Daling JR, Sherman KJ, et al. Human papillomavirus infection and anal cancer. *Int J Cancer* 1989;43:1042.

Bjorge T, Gunbjorud AB, Langmark F, et al. Cervical mass screening in Norway—510,000 smears a year. *Cancer Detect Prev* 1994;18:463.

Campion MJ, McCance DJ, Cuzick J, et al. Progressive potential of mild cervical atypia: prospective cytological, colposcopic, and virological study. *Lancet* 1986;2:237.

Campion MJ, Singer A, McCance DJ, et al. Subclinical penile human papillomavirus infection in consorts of women with cervical neoplasia: a due to the high-risk male. *Colposc Gynecol Laser Surg* 1987;3:11.

Centers for Disease Control and Prevention, Department of Health and Human Services. Guidelines for treatment of sexually transmitted diseases, cervical cancer screening for women who attend STD clinics or have a history of STDs. *MMWR Morb Mortal Wkly Rep* 1998;47:95.

Chuang T, Perry HO, Kurland LT, et al. Condylomata acuminatum in Rochester, Minn., 1950–1979. *Arch Dermatol* 1984; 120:476.

Davis AL, Emans SJ. Human papillomavirus infection in the pediatric and adolescent patient. *J Pediatr* 1989;115:1.

Eron LJ, Judson F, Tucker S, et al. Interferon therapy for condylomata acuminata. *N Engl J Med* 1986;315:1059.

Evander M, Edlund K, Gustafsson A, et al. Human papillomavirus infection is transient in young women: a population-based cohort study. *J Infect Dis* 1995;171:1026.

Ferenczy A, Mitae M, Nagai N, et al. Latent papillomavirus and recurring genital warts. *N Engl J Med* 1986;313:1059.

Ferenczy A. Epidemiology and clinical pathophysiology of condylomata acuminata. *Am J Obstet Gynecol* 1995;172:1331.

Ferenczy A, Choukroun D, Falcone T, et al. The effect of cervical loop electrosurgical excision on subsequent pregnancy outcome: North American experience. *Am J Obstet Gynecol* 1995;172(4):1246.

Haverkos HW, Soon G, Steckley SL, et al. Cigarette smoking and cervical cancer: Part I: a meta-analysis. *Biomed Pharmacother* 2003;57:67–77.

Hillard PA, Biro FM, Wildey L. Complications of cervical cryotherapy in adolescents. *J Reprod Med* 1991;36:711.

Ho GYF, Birman R, Beardsley L, et al. Natural history of cervicovaginal papillomavirus infection in young women. *N Engl J Med* 1998;338:423.

Ho GY, Burk KD, Klein S, et al. Persistent genital human papillomavirus infection as a risk factor for persistent cervical dysplasia. *J Natl Cancer Inst* 1995;87:1365.

Hogewoning CJ, Bleeker MC, van den Brule AJ, et al. Condom use promotes regression of cervical intraepithelial neoplasia and clearance of human papillomavirus: a randomized clinical trial. *Int J Cancer* 2003;107:811.

Johnstone JD, McGoogan E, Smart GE, et al. A population-based, controlled study of the relation between HIV infection and cervical neoplasia. *Br J Obstet Gynaecol* 1994;101:986.

Kiviat NB, Koutsky LA, Critchlow CW, et al. Prevalence and cytologic manifestations of human papilloma virus HPV types 6, 11, 16, 18, 31, 33, 35, 42, 44, 45, 51, 52 and 56 among 500 consecutive women. *Int J Gynecol Pathol* 1992;11:197.

Korkolopoulou P, Kolokythas C, Kittas C, et al. Correlation of colposcopy and histology in cervical biopsies positive for CIN and/or HPV infection. *Eur J Gynaecol Oncol* 1992;13:502.

Kyrgiou M, Koliopoulos G, Martin-Hirsch P, et al. Obstetric outcomes after conservative treatment for intraepithelial or early invasive cervical lesions: systematic review and meta-analysis. *Lancet* 2006;367:489.

Lehtinen M, Koskela P, Jellum E, et al. Herpes simplex virus and risk of cervical cancer: a longitudinal, nested case-control in the Nordic countries. *Am J Epidemiol* 2002;156:687.

Lonky NM, Navarre GL, Saunders S, et al. Low-grade Papanicolaou smears and the Bethesda system: a prospective cytohistopathologic analysis. *Obstet Gynecol* 1995;85:716.

Lynch PD. Condylomata acuminata. *Clin Obstet Gynecol* 1985; 28:142.

Manos MM, Kinney WK, Hurley LB, et al. Identifying women with cervical neoplasia: using human papillomavirus DNA testing for equivocal Papanicolaou results. *JAMA* 1999;281:1605.

Maymon R, Bekerman A, Werchow M, et al. Clinical and subclinical condyloma: rates among male sexual partners of women with genital human papillomavirus infection. *J Reprod Med* 1995;40:31.

McLachlin CM. Pathology of human papillomavirus in the female genital tract. *Curr Opin Obstet Gynecol* 1995;7:24.

Moscicki AB. Cervical cytology testing in teens. *Curr Opin Obstet Gynecol* 2005;17:471.

Moscicki AB, Ellenberg JH, Farhat S, et al. HPV persistence in HIV infected and uninfected adolescent girls: risk factors and differences by phylogenetic types. *J Infect Dis* 2004a;190:37.

Moscicki AB, Ellenberg JH, Crowley-Nowick P, et al. Risk of high-grade squamous intraepithelial lesion in HIV-infected adolescents. *J Infect Dis* 2004b;190:1413.

Moscicki AB, Grubbs-Burt V, Kanowitz S, et al. The significance of squamous metaplasia in the development of low grade squamous intra-epithelial lesions in young women. *Cancer* 1999;85:1139.

Moscicki AB, Palefsky J, Gonzales J, et al. Human papillomavirus infection in sexually active adolescent females: prevalence and risk factors. *Pediatr Res* 1990;28:507.

Moscicki AB, Palefsky JM, Gonzales J, et al. The association between human papillomavirus deoxyribonucleic acid status and the results of cytologic rescreening tests in young, sexually active women. *Am J Obstet Gynecol* 1991;165:67.

Moscicki AB, Shiboski S, Broering J, et al. The natural history of human papillomavirus infection as measured by repeated DNA testing in adolescent and young women. *J Pediatr* 1998; 132:277.

Moscicki AB, Shiboski S, Hills NK, et al. Regression of low-grade squamous intra-epithelial lesions in young women. *Lancet* 2004;364:1678.

Mount SL, Papillo JL. A study of 10,296 pediatric and adolescent Papanicolaou smear diagnoses in northern New England. *Pediatrics* 1999;103:539.

Quek SC, Mould T, Canfell K, et al. The Polarprobe—emerging technology for cervical cancer screening. *Ann Acad Med Singapore* 1998;5:717.

Reid R, Greenberg M, Jenson AB, et al. Sexually transmitted papilloma viral infections: the anatomic distribution and pathologic grade of neoplastic lesions associated with different viral types. *Am J Obstet Gynecol* 1987;156:212.

Reid R, Herschman BR, Crum CP, et al. Genital warts and cervical cancer: the tissue basis of colposcopic change. *Am J Obstet Gynecol* 1984;149:293.

Rosenfeld WD, Vermund SH, Wentz SJ, et al. High prevalence rate of human papillomavirus infection and association with abnormal Papanicolaou smears in sexually active adolescents. *Am J Dis Child* 1989;143:1443–1447.

Sadeghi SB, Hsieh EW, Gunn SW. Prevalence of cervical intraepithelial neoplasia in sexually active teenagers and young adults. *Am J Obstet Gynecol* 1984;148:726.

Sadler L, Saftlas A, Wang W, et al. Treatment for cervical intraepithelial neoplasia and risk of preterm delivery. *JAMA* 2004;291:2100.

Saslow D, Runowicz CD, Solomon D, et al. American Cancer Society guideline for the early detection of cervical neoplasia and cancer. *CA Cancer J Clin* 2002;52(6):342.

Sawaya GF. A 21-year-old woman with atypical squamous cells of undetermined significance. *JAMA* 2005;294:2210.

Sherman ME, Kurman RJ. The role of exfoliative cytology and histopathology in screening and triage. *Obstet Gynecol Clin North Am* 1996;23:641.

Shew ML, Fortenberry JD, Miles P. Interval between menarche and first sexual intercourse, related to risk of human papillomavirus infection. *J Pediatr* 1994;125:661.

Sidawy MK, Tabbara SO. Reactive change and atypical squamous cells of undetermined significance in Papanicolaou smears: a cytohistologic correlation. *Diagn Cytopathol* 1993;9:423.

Singer A. The cervical epithelium during puberty and adolescents. In: Gordon JA, Singer A, eds. *The cervix*. Philadelphia: WB Saunders; 1978:88.

Smith JS, Bosetti C, Munoz N, et al. Chlamydia trachomatis and invasive cervical cancer: a pooled analysis of the IARC multicentric case-control study. *Int J Cancer* 2004;111(3):431.

Smith JS, Green J, Berrington de Gonzalez A, et al. Cervical cancer and use of hormonal contraceptives: a systematic review. *Lancet* 2003;361(9364):1159.

Sun XW, Kuhn L, Ellerbrock TV, et al. Human papillomavirus infection in women infected with the human immunodeficiency virus. *N Engl J Med* 1997;337:1343.

Vermund SH, Kelley KF, Klein RS, et al. High risk of human papillomavirus infection and cervical squamous intraepithelial lesions among women with symptomatic human immunodeficiency virus infection. *Am J Obstet Gynecol* 1991;165:392.

Widra EA, Dookhan D, Jordan A, et al. Evaluation of the atypical cytologic smear: validity of the 1991 Bethesda system. *J Reprod Med* 1994;39(9):682.

Winer RL, Lee SK, Hughes JP, et al. Genital human papillomavirus infection: incidence and risk factors in a cohort of female university students. *Am J Epidemiol* 2003;157:218.

Wright TC Jr, Cox JT, Massad LS, et al. 2001 Consensus guidelines for the management of women with cervical cytological abnormalities. *JAMA* 2002;287(16):2120.

Wright JD, Davila RM, Pinto KR, et al. Cervical dysplasia in adolescents. *Obstet Gynecol* 2005;106(1):115.

Wright TC Jr, Gagnon S, Richart RM, et al. Treatment of cervical intraepithelial neoplasia using the loop electrosurgical excision procedure. *Obstet Gynecol* 1992;79:173.

Ylitalo N, Josefsson A, Melbye M, et al. A prospective study showing long-term infection with human papillomavirus 16 before the development of cervical carcinoma in situ. *Cancer Res* 2000;60:6027.

CHAPTER 55

Vaginitis and Vaginosis

Loris Y. Hwang and Mary-Ann B. Shafer

VAGINA: NORMAL STATE

The vagina is a dynamic ecosystem extending from the vulva to the cervix uteri. Embryologically, the upper four fifth of the vagina is derived from the müllerian ducts and the lower one fifth from the urogenital sinus. The vagina is lined with epithelial cells that are estrogen dependent. Before puberty and after menopause, the cells are thin, leading to heightened susceptibility to infection. During puberty, there is an involution of the squamocolumnar junction such that squamous epithelial cells gradually replace the columnar epithelial cells that line the ectocervix during childhood.

Vaginal Flora Before the onset of puberty, the vagina is colonized with various bacterial species ranging from fecal flora to skin flora, resulting in a vaginal pH of >4.7. After puberty, the estrogen-stimulated epithelial cells produce more glycogen, and lactobacilli become predominant, comprising >95% of the normal flora. Metabolism of glycogen to lactic acid by the lactobacilli contributes to the lowering of the vaginal pH to <4.5 and helps to maintain a vaginal environment that appears to protect the individual from colonization by more pathogenic organisms. Some lactobacilli also produce hydrogen peroxide, a potential microbicide.

Vaginal Secretions Vaginal secretions are a normal result of the changing hormonal milieu of the menstrual cycle. Six to 12 months before menarche, there may be a physiological increase in secretions arising from the adnexa, uterus, cervix, or vaginal epithelium itself. These secretions may be copious but are not associated with odor or pruritus.

Changes during the menstrual cycle include the following:

1. After menses, there is little secretion.
2. As estrogen levels increase, a cloudy, sticky, white secretion develops.
3. Just before ovulation, the cervical secretions become clear and profuse.
4. After ovulation, progesterone stimulates a thick and sticky cervical secretion.
5. Before menses, a watery cervical secretion develops again.

These normal, odorless secretions are composed primarily of mucus, with occasional squamous cells from the vaginal wall.

Defense Mechanisms of the Vagina Normal defense mechanisms in the postpubertal teen include the following:

1. Acid pH level of 3.8 to 4.4
2. Protective thick epithelium
3. Estrogen support
4. Physiological mucous secretion

VULVOVAGINITIS IN PREPUBERTAL FEMALES

Vulvar skin in prepubertal girls is more susceptible to irritation because of the lack of "estrogenization" and the absence of protective labial hair and fat. The hypoestrogenic vaginal mucosa is also thin and has an alkaline pH. Most vulvovaginitis in this group is related to poor hygiene, obesity, tight clothing, or nonabsorbent underpants. Usually, the organisms involved are either normal flora (i.e., lactobacilli, diphtheroids, streptococci, and *Staphylococcus epidermidis*) or gram-negative enteric organisms (i.e., *Escherichia* coli). Current evidence suggests that patients should be counseled regarding hygienic measures, and antibiotics should be prescribed only if a single or predominant organism is identified by culture of secretions (Joishy et al., 2005). All sexually transmitted diseases (STDs) can also be associated with vaginitis in prepubertal females. *Neisseria gonorrhoeae* and *Chlamydia trachomatis* in prepubertal females infect the vagina and not the cervix. Therefore, vaginal cultures are sufficient. The identification of sexually transmissible agents in prepubertal children beyond the neonatal period suggests sexual abuse (Centers for Disease Control and Prevention, 2002). The significance of the identification of a sexually transmitted agent in such children as evidence of possible child sexual abuse varies by pathogen. Postnatally acquired gonorrhea; syphilis; and nontransfusion, nonperinatally acquired human immunodeficiency virus (HIV) are usually diagnostic of sexual abuse. Sexual abuse should be suspected in the presence of genital herpes, as well.

VULVOVAGINITIS AND VAGINOSIS IN PUBERTAL FEMALES: GENERAL APPROACH

Prevalence

The three most common types of vaginitis are vulvovaginal candidiasis (VVC) (20%–25%), trichomoniasis (15%–20%), and bacterial vaginosis (BV) (40%–45%). (BV is not a true "vaginitis" as it does not cause a major inflammatory reaction of the vaginal mucosa, but from a clinical standpoint is included here.) The prevalence of VVC, trichomoniasis, and BV is not well-known because these entities are not reportable, but it is estimated that approximately 75% of women experience VVC during their lifetime, with most first episodes occurring during adolescence. Patients may notice a change in vaginal discharge, and vulvar irritation, itching, vaginal odor, dyspareunia, and/or dysuria. Other causes of discharge include birth control pills (estrogen effect), stress (psychophysiological), chemical irritants, foreign bodies (i.e., tampons), trauma, allergies, and poor hygiene. To the patient, vaginal discharge secondary to cervicitis from *N. gonorrhoeae* or *C. trachomatis* can be indistinguishable from discharge secondary to vaginitis.

Evaluation

History
The history in an adolescent with vaginitis should include questions regarding the following:

1. Type, duration, and extent of symptoms
2. Location of any pain: Vulva, introitus, or deep vagina. Internal pain may occur with either urinary tract infection or vaginitis, whereas external pain with urination is usually associated with vaginitis
3. Relationship of symptoms to the menstrual cycle
4. Sexual activity: Frequency, type, number of sexual partners, and recent changes in partners
5. Previous STDs
6. Contraceptive history
7. Changes in diet, exercise, stress, and medications including antibiotics, steroids, use of spray deodorants, soaps, lubricants, or douches
8. Family history of diabetes mellitus

Physical Examination
The physical examination in a teen with vaginitis includes the following:

1. Inspection of color, texture, origin (vaginal or cervical), adherence, and odor of the vaginal discharge
2. Inspection of the perineum, vulva, vagina, and cervix for erythema, swelling, lesions, atrophy, and signs of trauma
3. Palpation of the introitus for tenderness
4. Palpation of the uterus and adnexa for tenderness or masses
5. Inspection for foreign bodies, such as forgotten tampon

Laboratory Evaluation
The office evaluation should include the following:

1. pH value of vaginal secretions: The normal pH value of the vagina is <4.5 (3.8–4.4). The pH should be sampled from the anterior vaginal fornix or lateral vaginal wall.

Cervical mucus should not be used (typical pH ~7.0) as sample.
2. Saline wet mount preparation for microscopic evaluation: A drop of saline is placed on a glass slide and then the swab of vaginal discharge is applied to the saline area. Alternatively, the swab of vaginal discharge is placed in a test tube together with 0.5 to 1 mL of saline and then the suspension is swabbed onto a glass slide. A coverslip is applied. Microscopic examination under dry high-power must look for the following:
   a. White blood cells (WBCs): The normal wet prep should have <5 to 10 WBCs per high-power field or ≤1 WBC per epithelial cell.
   b. Presence of trichomonads, may be motile: Motility of trichomonads decreases with time (Kingston et al., 2003), therefore immediate inspection of the sample is advised. Preservation of the sample at a temperature as close to body temperature as possible until time of viewing may also help preserve motility.
   c. Type of background bacterial flora: Normal long lactobacilli versus pleomorphic coccobacilli.
   d. Presence of "clue cells": Epithelial cells with indistinct borders, intracellular debris, and covered with bacteria.
3. Potassium hydroxide (KOH) 10% preparation for microscopic evaluation: A swab of vaginal discharge is applied to a glass slide and a drop of KOH 10% solution is added.
   a. Amine or "whiff test": Presence of a fishy, amine odor on addition of the KOH solution, before application of cover slip
   b. Microscopic examination under dry high-power: Presence of pseudohyphae or budding yeast forms
4. Testing for *C. trachomatis* and *N. gonorrhoeae*: To rule out endocervical infection that is causing the discharge.

   Other laboratory tests as indicated include:

1. Gram stain of vaginal or cervical secretions
2. Urinalysis and urine culture
3. Pregnancy test
4. Culture systems (InPouch TV) and polymerase chain reaction (PCR) tests for *Trichomonas vaginalis*
5. Amine/pH test cards to assist in the diagnosis of BV

VULVOVAGINAL CANDIDIASIS

VVC is a common form of vaginitis in girls. A major issue in diagnosis is distinguishing true infection from nonpathogenic colonization.

Etiology

VVC is usually caused by *Candida albicans* (85%–90% of clinical cases) and occasionally by other *Candida* sp, *Torulopsis* sp, or other yeasts. *C. albicans* has greater adherence to vaginal epithelium than the other species of *Candida*.

Epidemiology

1. Prevalence: The overall prevalence of VVC is unknown, but there appears to be increased incidence in the second decade of life and on initiation of sexual activity.

Candida species is isolated from 20% of healthy asymptomatic females presumably indicating a commensal relationship of the candidal species with other vaginal flora. However, an estimated 75% of women experience at least one episode of VVC during their lifetime, and 40% to 45% will have two or more episodes (Centers for Disease Control and Prevention, 2006).

2. Transmission: Although VVC is usually not sexually acquired or transmitted, evidence exists that sexual contact plays a role in transmission in some patients. Approximately 20% of male partners have asymptomatic penile colonization. Symptomatic male partners might present with balanitis.

3. Predisposing factors:
   a. Immunosuppressive states: Diabetes mellitus, HIV infection, or therapy with steroids or immunosuppressive agents
   b. Estrogen exposure (enhances adherence of *Candida* organisms to vaginal epithelium) including pregnancy and estrogen-containing oral contraceptives. While oral contraceptives have been suspected as a predisposing factor, epidemiological study results are conflicting.
   c. Antibiotic therapy: Often reported by some women, but studies do not show an association (Glover and Larsen, 2003; Wilton et al., 2003)
   d. Behavioral factors: Orogenital sex, douching
   e. Innate host factors: Genetic predispositions, decreased local vaginal immune responses (i.e., nonsecretors of Lewis antigens, impaired *Candida* antigen-specific immunity)

Clinical Manifestations

1. VVC is usually accompanied by intense burning, vulvar pruritus, erythema, vaginal discharge, soreness, and external dysuria that may worsen before the onset of menses, but these symptoms are nonspecific
2. Occasional dysuria or dyspareunia
3. Discharge
   a. Onset: May worsen before menses
   b. Consistency: Usually described as thick, curd-like, "cottage cheese" appearance
   c. Color: Milky, white
   d. Odor: Usually none
4. Often accompanied by a history of risk factors as described in the preceding text
5. Examination reveals the following:
   a. Normal or erythematous vulva, fissures, excoriations, satellite lesions including skin folds and thighs, especially in obese females
   b. Vulvar edema
   c. Thick, white, cheesy, adherent discharge

Diagnosis

1. A wet prep with saline or KOH shows budding yeast with pseudohyphae. Yeast is more readily visualized with the use of KOH, which lyses epithelial cells. The KOH prep has a sensitivity of 40% to 80%.
2. The pH range is usually <4.5 (normal range).
3. On gram stains, yeast cells appear as gram-positive oval masses, and pseudohyphae appear as long gram-positive tubes. Gram stain sensitivity is 70% to 100%.
4. Rapid in-office tests for *Candida* antigens in vaginal discharge are commercially available, but their use in the clinical setting has not been well studied. They are not currently recommended.
5. Cultures may be useful in cases of recurrent VVC, but are not used for routine diagnosis because asymptomatic colonization is common.
6. The diagnosis can be made in the presence of signs and symptoms of vaginitis with evidence of yeast on wet prep or KOH prep. VVC is further classified as "uncomplicated," with sporadic/infrequent episodes, mild-to-moderate symptoms, *C. albicans* species, non-immunocompromised women; or "complicated," with recurrent VVC (four or more episodes in 12 months), severe symptoms, non-albicans species, immunocompromised women or pregnant women. Women who have the presence of yeast on laboratory testing but are asymptomatic should not be treated.

Therapy

1. Regimens for uncomplicated cases in nonpregnant patients:
   a. Topical, intravaginal agents: Short-course topical formulations (i.e., single dose and regimens of 1–3 days) effectively treat uncomplicated VVC, and topical azoles are more effective than nystatin (Centers for Disease Control and Prevention, 2006). Azoles have a clinical cure rate of 80% to 95%, whereas nystatin agents have a cure rate of 70% to 90%. Relief of symptoms and negative cultures are seen in 80% to 90% of patients who complete therapy. If symptoms are more consistent with vaginitis than vulvitis, suppositories are superior to creams with increased cure rates (Carr et al., 1998). Regimens recommended by the Centers for Disease Control and Prevention (CDC) are listed below (Centers for Disease Control and Prevention, 2006). Self-medication with over-the-counter (OTC) formulations is common, but a recent study indicates that self-diagnosis is unreliable, even in women who have had prior diagnoses of VVC (Ferris et al., 2002). The creams and suppositories listed here are oil-based, and may weaken a latex condom or diaphragm.
      - Butoconazole 2% cream (Mycelex-3 OTC) 5 g intravaginally for 3 days or Butoconazole 2% cream sustained release, single intravaginal application, or
      - Clotrimazole 1% cream (Gyne-Lotrimin 7, Mycelex-7 OTC), 5 g intravaginally for 7 to 14 days, or
      - Clotrimazole 100-mg vaginal tablet (Gyne-Lotrimin 7, Mycelex-7 OTC) for 7 days, or
      - Clotrimazole 100-mg vaginal tablet, two tablets for 3 days, or
      - Miconazole 2% cream (Monistat-7 OTC), 5 g intravaginally for 7 days, or
      - Miconazole 200-mg vaginal suppository (Monistat-3 OTC), one suppository for 3 days, or
      - Miconazole 100-mg vaginal suppository (Monistat-7 OTC), one suppository for 7 days, or
      - Miconazole 1,200 mg vaginal suppository, one suppository for 1 day, or
      - Nystatin 100,000-unit (U) vaginal tablet for 14 days, or
      - Tioconazole 6.5% ointment (Monistat 1-day OTC), 5 g intravaginally in a single application, or
      - Terconazole 0.4% cream (Terazol 7), 5 g intravaginally for 7 days, or

- Terconazole 0.8% cream (Terazol 3), 5 g intravaginally for 3 days, or
- Terconazole 80-mg suppository (Terazol 3), one suppository for 3 days
  b. Oral agent: Fluconazole 150-mg oral tablet, one tablet in a single dose
  c. Patients often prefer single-dose oral therapy over intravaginal therapy because of convenience and ease of use. Treatment choice should take into account patient preference, the severity of disease, the history of recurrent vaginitis, and the existence of any immunosuppressive state (see subsequent text).
2. Management of sex partners: Because VVC is not considered an STD, partners are not routinely treated unless the male partner has symptoms and signs of balanitis. Partner treatment may be considered in cases of recurrent VVC.
3. Side effects to therapy: Topical azole medications do not usually cause systemic side effects, but occasional problems with local irritation or burning can occur. Oral azole agents can cause nausea, abdominal pain, headaches, and rarely an elevation in liver enzymes. Assessment for drug interactions should be performed before oral agents are prescribed.
4. Follow-up: Follow-up is not necessary for individuals who become asymptomatic after treatment. If symptoms occur four or more times in a year (recurrent VVC), an evaluation should be performed for the predisposing conditions listed earlier.
5. Pregnancy: Topical azole medications can be used during pregnancy, but oral agents should be avoided. Seven-day therapy is preferred during pregnancy. Several treatments have been approved for use during pregnancy, including topical butoconazole, clotrimazole, miconazole, and terconazole.
6. Severe VVC, or immunocompromised host: Cases with severe symptoms and signs have lower clinical cure rates with short-course medications. Treatment with either 7 to 14 days of topical azoles or fluconazole 150 mg once and then again in 3 days is advised.
7. HIV infection: Treatment of VVC in adolescents with HIV infection does not differ from treatment in those without HIV infection. However, cases of clinically severe VVC may be treated as discussed in the preceding text. Prompt treatment of VVC in HIV-infected patients is especially advised because of potential for increased transmission of HIV to their sexual partners in these cases. HIV should be considered in cases of recurrent VVC, although routine HIV screening in adolescents with otherwise low risk for HIV is not routinely recommended because recurrent VVC often occurs in immunocompetent adolescents as well.
8. Recurrent VVC (four or more episodes per year) is seen in <5% of women.
   a. Eliminate or reduce risk factors
      - Minimize the estrogen dose in oral contraceptives
      - Avoid broad-spectrum antibiotics
      - Minimize steroid use
      - Improve control of diabetes
      - Avoid constricting clothing, and wear cotton underwear
      - Avoid douching and vaginal sprays
   b. Obtain vaginal cultures and treat accordingly
      - Individual episodes caused by *C. albicans* usually respond well to the typical short courses of topical or oral azole regimens as above for uncomplicated

VVC, but some experts recommend longer courses, that is, 7 to 14 days of topical treatment, or fluconazole 150 mg PO once and repeated in 3 days (Centers for Disease Control and Prevention, 2006).
   - Non-*albicans Candida* species appear to respond to boric acid 600 mg gelatin capsule PO once daily for 14 days, or flucytosine vaginal cream 5 g once nightly (Sobel et al., 2003).
   c. Partner treatment: Routine treatment of all sex partners has not been shown to clearly benefit women with recurrent VVC. However, examination and treatment of partners with candidal balanitis is warranted.
   d. Consider HIV testing if other risk factors are present, as discussed in the preceding text.
   e. Long-term maintenance regimens: Several studies have shown decreased recurrences with maintenance regimens, although 30% to 50% of women experience recurrence after medication is discontinued. Regimens have included the following:
      - Fluconazole 150 mg PO once each week for 6 months
      - Clotrimazole 500-mg vaginal tablet each week for 6 months
      - Itraconazole 400 mg PO once monthly, or 100 mg PO once daily for 6 months
      - Ketoconazole 100 mg PO once daily for 6 months. Oral ketoconazole has a risk of mild reversible hepatitis of 5% to 10% and a risk of serious, potentially life-threatening hepatitis of 1 in 15,000. Ketoconazole should therefore be reserved only for resistant, recurrent VVC. Patients require monitoring for hepatotoxicity.
      - For non-*albicans Candida* species, a maintenance regimen of flucytosine vaginal cream 5 g once nightly for 6 to 8 weeks may be helpful (Sobel et al., 2003).

TRICHOMONIASIS

Etiology

T. vaginalis infection of the vaginal epithelium is caused by protozoa with four anterior flagella and one posterior flagellum.

Epidemiology

1. Prevalence: *T. vaginalis* is not a reportable STD, but is estimated to be one of the most common treatable STDs, with an estimated 5 million cases annually in the United States and as many as 180 million cases worldwide (Cates, 1999). The peak prevalence rates are between the ages of 16 and 35 years. Prevalence in adolescent females is 10% to 20%, depending on the population examined and diagnostic test used.
2. Transmission: The organism is almost always sexually transmitted. Because the organism can survive for approximately 1.5 hours on a wet sponge and up to 24 hours on a wet cloth, transmission can possibly occur through sharing of washcloths, communal bathing, or during routine child care.
3. Incubation period: 4 to 28 days.

4. Sites of colonization: Trichomonads can infect sites in addition to the vagina, for example the urethra (82.5% of cases) and periurethral glands (98% of cases).
5. Predisposing factors: Multiple sex partners, lower socioeconomic status, prior history of STDs, inconsistent condom use.

Clinical Manifestations

1. Up to 25% to 50% of females are asymptomatic. Nonspecific symptoms include pruritus, dysuria, dyspareunia, lower abdominal pain, and postcoital bleeding. Most males are asymptomatic.
2. Discharge (50% of cases)
   a. Onset: Any time during the menstrual cycle
   b. Consistency: Classically diffuse, bubbly or frothy
   c. Color: Yellow or greenish
   d. Odor: Only 10% of women complain of malodorous discharge
3. Examination
   a. Edema and excoriation of the external genitalia
   b. Frothy, foul-smelling vaginal discharge
   c. Erythematous, edematous, and granular vaginal walls
   d. Cervicitis ("strawberry cervix"): May have erosions or petechiae of the cervix (colpitis macularis), seen only in 2% of cases
   e. Bartholinitis
   f. Urethritis
   g. Rarely, abdominal tenderness and symptoms that may be consistent with pelvic inflammatory disease (PID)
4. Complications: Trichomoniasis does not cause disseminated disease. However, emerging evidence now links trichomonas infection to sequelae such as increased HIV acquisition and transmission, perinatal morbidity, infertility, and cervical cancer. It is postulated that identification and treatment of *T. vaginalis* infection would substantially decrease HIV acquisition (Sorvillo et al., 2001).

Diagnosis

1. Wet prep: At least 10 microscopic fields are examined for the presence of trichomonads which appear as flagellated pear-shaped motile organisms similar in size to polymorphonuclear leukocytes. This is the most frequently used diagnostic method due to its low cost, ready availability, and immediate results. However, the sensitivity is 60% to 70% at best and is dependent on the examiner technique and number of organisms viewable in the sample. The slide must also be viewed as soon as possible because the motility of the trichomonads decreases with time (Kingston et al., 2003). Preservation of the sample at a temperature as close to body temperature as possible until time of viewing may also help preserve motility.
2. KOH prep: Malodorous whiff is noted
3. pH: Usually >4.5
4. Gram stains: More time consuming and lower sensitivity than wet preps
5. Cultures: Culture is the most sensitive and specific commercially available method of diagnosis. In women in whom trichomoniasis is suspected but not confirmed by microscopy, vaginal secretions should be cultured for *T. vaginalis* (Centers for Disease Control and Prevention,

2006). Cultures are more time consuming, expensive, and less readily available than wet preps, but require lower concentrations of organisms for diagnosis and can be useful in cases of treatment failure or recurrence of symptoms. Broth culture of a vaginal sample has traditionally been considered to be the gold standard for diagnosis, although newer techniques appear to have better sensitivity, as discussed in the subsequent text.
6. Rapid point-of-care tests: There are two U.S. Food and Drug Administration-approved methods for rapid testing of vaginal samples (Centers for Disease Control and Prevention, 2006). The OSOM Trichomonas Rapid Test yields results in 10 minutes, and the Affirm VP III yields results in 45 minutes. Sensitivity is >83% and specificity is >97%, compared to culture. These tests are more sensitive than the wet prep, but are more expensive, and false positives occur in low prevalence populations (Briselden and Hillier, 1994; DeMeo et al., 1996; Huppert et al., 2005).
7. DNA-based techniques: PCR tests have not been FDA-approved, are expensive, and have limited availability through commercial laboratories. Compared to reference standards that incorporate both culture and PCR, wet prep and culture demonstrate sensitivities of only 36% and 70% respectively whereas PCR demonstrates sensitivity of 97% (Madico et al., 1998). The specificity is 98%.
8. Papanicolaou smear: Trichomonads are seen in Pap smears, but Pap smears are unreliable for the routine diagnosis of *T. vaginalis* infection. The sensitivity to detect *T. vaginalis* by Pap smear is only approximately 50% when compared against culture. The sensitivity is even lower in populations in which rates of trichomonal infections are <20% (Wiese et al., 2000).
9. Urine sediment: Trichomonads are occasionally seen in the urinary sediment. Microscopic examination of urine sediments in conjunction with wet preps has been shown to increase sensitivity (Blake et al., 1999). Urinary samples can be useful in males in whom urethral secretions are difficult to obtain.

Therapy

1. Regimens for nonpregnant patients (Centers for Disease Control and Prevention, 2006)
   a. Recommended: Metronidazole 2 g PO in a single dose, or Tinidazole 2 g orally in a single dose.
   b. Alternative: Metronidazole 500 mg PO twice a day for 7 days.
   c. Both regimens of metronidazole have a cure rate of 90% to 95%. The single-dose regimen is preferred to increase compliance. Treatment of asymptomatic girls is advisable.
   d. Intravaginal metronidazole gel has not been shown to be effective (<50%) and therefore is not recommended.
   e. Revised CDC treatment guidelines now include recommendations for the use of tinidazole (Centers for Disease Control and Prevention, 2006). Randomized controlled trials comparing single 2 g doses of metronidazole and tinidazole suggest that tinidazole is equivalent to, or superior to, metronidazole in achieving parasitological cure and resolution of symptoms (Forna and Gulmezoglu, 2003).
2. Side effects of therapy: Oral metronidazole can cause nausea, vomiting, and a metallic taste. Disulfiram-like

effects occur if alcohol is ingested. All patients should be advised to avoid alcohol during treatment and until 24 hours after completion of metronidazole.

3. Management of sex partners: Routine treatment of partners is recommended. Patients should also avoid sexual contact until the patient and all partners have completed medications and are asymptomatic.

4. Allergy: Patients with allergy to nitroimidazole should receive desensitization because no alternative medication classes are effective for *T. vaginalis*.

5. Follow-up: Follow-up is not necessary for individuals who become asymptomatic after treatment.

6. Treatment failure: If failure occurs with either regimen, the adolescent should be retreated with metronidazole 500 mg twice daily for 7 days. If failure occurs again, the teen can be treated with metronidazole 2 g PO daily for 3 to 5 days. Some *T. vaginalis* strains demonstrate decreased susceptibility to medications, but high-level resistance is rare. Any suspicions of resistance to metronidazole should be reported to the CDC for discussion of further susceptibility, testing, and recommendations (Centers for Disease Control and Prevention, 2006).

7. Pregnancy: Published data have *not* shown an association between teratogenicity and metronidazole during pregnancy; it is safe to be used during all stages of pregnancy (Medical Letter, 1999). Recommended treatment includes 2 g of metronidazole PO in one dose.

8. HIV infection: Same treatment regimens as above.

BACTERIAL VAGINOSIS

Bacterial vaginosis (BV), also known as *Gardnerella* vaginitis, "clue cell" vaginitis, *Haemophilus* vaginitis, or *Corynebacterium* vaginitis, is not a true vaginitis as it is not characterized by a marked inflammatory response at the vaginal mucosa. The current term BV was adopted to reflect the syndrome that is characterized by the presence of diverse bacteria without signs of vaginal mucosal inflammation. It is the most frequent cause of abnormal vaginal discharge and odor in postpubertal females.

Etiology

The syndrome consists of the replacement of normal lactobacilli in the vagina with *Gardnerella vaginalis*, anaerobic bacteria (i.e., *Bacteroides* sp, *Mobiluncus* sp), and *Mycoplasma hominis*. In most females without BV, the dominant vaginal organism is *Lactobacillus* sp (>95% of all vaginal organisms), whereas in females with BV, lactobacilli are often not found or found with decreased bacterial counts (100-fold to 1,000-fold decrease).

As discussed earlier, lactobacilli help maintain an acid pH level that prevents the growth of *G. vaginalis* and anaerobic bacteria. In BV, there is loss of lactobacilli, an elevated pH level, and high concentrations of *G. vaginalis*, anaerobes such as *Bacteroides* and *Mobiluncus* sp, and genital mycoplasmas. The sequence of this disruption is not well understood.

Epidemiology

1. Prevalence: BV is the most common cause of abnormal vaginal discharge. However, BV is not a reportable disease, and prevalence varies widely (10% to 50%), depending on the population sampled.

2. Transmission: The mechanism of transmission of BV is unresolved. Sexual transmission is suggested by the age and sexual experience of the infected patients (Shafer et al., 1985), and by the isolation of the organism from the urethras in 70% to 90% of male partners. Although rarely isolated from nonsexually active individuals, it is not an exclusive STD (Yen et al., 2003). *G. vaginalis*, *Mobiluncus* sp, and *M. hominis* have been isolated from the rectum of females with BV and indicate a potential source of autoinfection (Catlin, 1992).

3. Predisposing factors: BV is more common in women who have new sex partners, female sex partners, or multiple sex partners in the last 6 months, women who douche, and African-American women. Nansel et al. (2006), in a 1-year longitudinal study of 3,614 women, found that psychosocial stress was associated with increase in overall prevalence and incidence of BV.

Clinical Manifestations

1. Symptoms can include vaginal pruritus and vaginal discharge. Up to 50% of cases are asymptomatic.

2. Vaginal discharge
   a. Onset: May be more noticeable after vaginal intercourse or after menses
   b. Consistency: Thin, homogeneous
   c. Color: Grayish white
   d. Odor: Often patients note a "fishy" odor, particularly in the presence of semen. The combination of *G. vaginalis* and anaerobes produces organic acids and several amines. In the presence of an elevated vaginal pH level, these products volatilize to the malodorous compounds of putrescine and cadaverine. Trimethylamine may also contribute to the odor.

3. Examination
   a. Thin gray-white discharge, adhering to the vaginal walls
   b. Usually no vulvar or vaginal wall changes
   c. Possibly a pungent "fishy" odor

4. Complications: There is growing evidence that BV is linked to serious sequelae including PID, increased HIV acquisition and transmission, infertility, and postsurgical/postabortal infection. Obstetric complications include chorioamnionitis, premature rupture of membranes, preterm labor, and postpartum endometritis.

Diagnosis

Variations of the Amsel criteria are commonly used for the clinical diagnosis of BV. *Three* of the following four clinical symptoms and signs are required:

1. The presence of a homogeneous, white, noninflammatory discharge that smoothly coats the vaginal walls.

2. The presence of "clue cells" (epithelial cells that appear granular and stippled with indistinct cell borders due to adherence of bacteria and cellular debris between cells) on wet prep examination. Clue cells should comprise at least 20% of the epithelial cells examined.

3. The vaginal pH level is >4.5.

4. The vaginal discharge has a positive result on whiff test, a fishy odor before or after the addition of 10% KOH.

TABLE 55.1

Nugent Scoring System for Gram-Stained Vaginal Smears

Score	Lactobacilli Morphotypes per Oil Immersion Field	Gardnerella Morphotypes per Oil Immersion Field	Curved Bacteria (Mobiluncus) per Oil Immersion Field
0	>30	0	0
1	5–30	<1	<1–4
2	1–4	1–4	>5
3	<1	5–30	
4	0	>30	

Final Total Score	Conclusion
0–3	Normal flora
4–6	Intermediate flora
7–10	Bacterial vaginosis

Gram stain is also sometimes available as a diagnostic tool and is indicative of BV if the relative concentration of bacterial types shows the characteristic altered flora. Gram stains are classified according to the Nugent criteria, which designate a score of 0 to 10 based on the proportion of bacterial morphotypes, with a score of more than 7 considered as BV (Nugent et al., 1991). Table 55.1 outlines the Nugent scoring system. Culture is currently not recommended as a diagnostic test because of its questionable specificity. Finally, a number of newer commercial probe tests that detect vaginal pathogens including *G. vaginalis* DNA are under study.

Therapy

1. All women with symptomatic BV should be treated, regardless of pregnancy status. The primary goal of treatment is to relieve symptoms and signs. Screening and treatment of asymptomatic women found to have BV before surgical procedures or other intervention is also recommended by many experts. Treatment of BV with metronidazole has been shown to reduce postabortion PID rates.
2. Regimens for nonpregnant patients (Centers for Disease Control and Prevention, 2006)
   a. Recommended
      * Metronidazole 500 mg PO twice daily for 7 days, or
      * Clindamycin cream 2% one full applicator (5 g) intravaginally each night for 7 days, or
      * Metronidazole gel 0.75% one full applicator (5 g) intravaginally twice daily for 5 days

      Cure rates for these recommended regimens are comparable (75%–85%). All patients treated with metronidazole should be advised to avoid alcohol during treatment and until 24 hours after completion of medication. (See "side effects" in the "Trichomoniasis" section in the preceding text.) Clindamycin cream may weaken latex condoms but offers the advantage of lack of systemic side effects.
   b. Alternative (Centers for Disease Control and Prevention, 2006)
      * Clindamycin 300 mg PO twice daily for 7 days
      * Clindamycin ovules 100 g intravaginally once at bedtime for 3 days

      Metronidazole 2 g single-dose therapy has the lowest efficacy for BV and is no longer a recommended or alternative regimen (Centers for Disease Control and Prevention, 2006). The FDA has also approved the use of metronidazole extended release 750 mg PO once daily for 7 days, and metronidazole gel 0.75% intravaginally once daily for 5 days, but efficacy data are not published.
3. Patients should be advised to avoid douching and reduce the number of sex partners.
4. Management of sex partners: Treatment of male partners is not routinely recommended because it does not alter the female patient's response rate or the rate of recurrence. However, female sex partners should be evaluated and treated if BV is found.
5. Follow-up: Follow-up is not necessary if the patient becomes asymptomatic. Adolescents with recurrent or persistent infections should be reevaluated for other infections.
6. Recurrent BV: Recurrence occurs in 20% to 30% of cases within 3 months. The cause of recurrence is poorly understood and management is controversial. Studies have not shown exogenous lactobacillus and yogurt therapies to be effective. Maintenance regimens are under study.
7. Pregnancy
   a. All symptomatic pregnant women in any trimester should be treated. Recommended regimens for pregnant women are as follows (Centers for Disease Control and Prevention, 2006):
      * Metronidazole 500 mg orally twice a day for 7 days
      * Metronidazole 250 mg PO three times daily for 7 days, or
      * Clindamycin 300 mg PO twice a day for 7 days
   b. Optimal screening and treatment of asymptomatic pregnant women is unclear. Because BV is associated with adverse pregnancy outcomes, asymptomatic pregnant women at high risk (i.e., those with history of premature delivery) may be screened during early second trimester. Screening of asymptomatic pregnant women at low risk is not recommended.
8. HIV infection: Same treatment regimens as above.

OTHER CAUSES OF VAGINAL DISCHARGE

1. Physiological discharge: A normal overall increase in vaginal secretions occurs 6 to 12 months before menarche. Vaginal and cervical secretions also vary depending on the hormonal state—estrogen induces a more profuse discharge, whereas progesterone induces a thicker discharge. At the time of ovulation or just before menses, vaginal secretions tend to increase. Physiological discharge is characterized by:
   a. Lack of offensive odor
   b. Lack of pruritus or burning
   c. Lack of vulvar, vaginal, or cervical erythema
   d. Possible brown stain on the underwear
   e. Lack of polymorphonuclear leukocytes on wet mount

TABLE 55.2

Vaginal Discharge in the Adolescent

Condition	Signs and Symptoms	Diagnosis	Treatment
Physiological discharge	Clear gray discharge No offensive odor No burning or itching	Wet prep: Epithelial cells with no or few polymorphonuclear cells; no pathogens	Reassurance and explanation
Vulvovaginal candidiasis (VVC)	Curd-like discharge Intense burning, pruritus Usually no odor Often associated vulvitis	KOH: Budding yeast and pseudohyphae	Numerous acceptable regimens listed in text
Trichomoniasis	Pruritus Malodorous, frothy, yellow-green discharge Dysuria Rarely, abdominal pain	Wet prep: Pear-shaped organism with motile flagella	Metronidazole: 2 g single dose or 500 mg b.i.d. for 7 days Treat and evaluate partner
Bacterial vaginosis	Homogenous, malodorous, gray-white discharge Usually mild or no pruritus or burning	Wet prep: Epithelial cells covered with gram-negative rods Few polymorphonuclear leukocytes pH >4.5	Metronidazole: 500 mg b.i.d. for 7 days, or metronidazole gel 0.75% one applicator b.i.d. for 5 days, or clindamycin cream 2% one applicator (5 g) intravaginally for 7 days Alternative regimens listed in text Evaluate female partners and treat accordingly
N. gonorrhoeae infection	Majority asymptomatic Gray-white cervical discharge	Culture Gram stain can be used, but a negative smear must be confirmed by culture	Ceftriaxone 125 mg IM once, or cefixime 400 mg once; plus azithromycin 1 g orally once, or doxycycline 100 mg orally b.i.d. for 7 days
C. trachomatis infection	Majority asymptomatic Yellowish cervical discharge Cervicitis	Nucleic acid amplification test or culture Exclusion of other organisms in a girl with cervicitis	Azithromycin 1 g once, or doxycycline 100 mg PO b.i.d. for 7 days
Retained tampon	Malodorous discharge Local discomfort	History and physical examination History of exposure to deodorant spray or scented tampons	Removal of tampon
Irritant vaginitis	Vaginal discharge, erythema	Other agents listed in text	Cessation of irritant agent

2. Extravaginal disease: Extravaginal lesions may cause staining of the underwear, leading to the perception of a discharge. These lesions include the following:
   a. Perineal lesions: Herpes, syphilis, intertrigo
   b. Bartholin gland abscess
   c. Proctitis
   d. Bleeding hemorrhoids
3. *Enterobius vermicularis*: Pinworms
4. Irritant vaginitis: Vaginal discharge can result from irritation associated with agents such as chemical douches, vaginal deodorants, vaginal sprays, tampons or pads, colored or perfumed toilet paper, bubble bath, laundry detergents, fabric softeners, swimming pools or hot tubs, powders, soaps, spermicides, or medications used by male partners that remain on the penis.
5. Foreign bodies: Vaginal discharge may be caused by items such as forgotten tampons, intrauterine devices (uterine discharge), and objects for masturbation.
6. Vulvodynia or vulvar vestibulitis: Clinical manifestations include pain with penetration during intercourse and small inflamed areas at 5 and 7 o'clock positions on the perineum that are exquisitely tender to touch. The vaginal examination results (including pH, flora, and wet prep) are normal. A course of topical steroids may be helpful.
7. *N. gonorrhoeae*: See Chapter 61. Gonorrhea generally infects the endocervix and not the vaginal walls. Most females are asymptomatic, although approximately 25% experience a foul-smelling cervical discharge that may be perceived as vaginal discharge.

8. *C. trachomatis*: See Chapter 62. Cervical infections are common, and cervical discharge may be perceived as vaginal discharge.

Table 55.2 outlines the treatment of vaginitis in adolescents.

WEB SITES

For Teenagers and Parents

http://kidshealth.org/teen/sexual_health/. Teen-oriented Web site from the Nemours Foundation, including information on STDs and vaginitis.

http://www.nichd.nih.gov/health/topics/vaginitis.cfm. Vaginitis information from the National Institutes of Health.

http://www.health.state.mn.us/divs/idepc/diseases/vaginitis/. Vaginitis information from the Minnesota Department of Health, includes patient handouts in various languages (pdf files).

http://www.mayoclinic.com/invoke.cfm?id=DS00255. Vaginitis information from the Mayo Clinic.

http://www.ashastd.org/learn/learn_vag_trich.cfm. American Social Health Association Web site on vaginal infections and other STDs.

http://www.mckinley.uiuc.edu/Handouts/vaginal_discharge.html. Information on vaginal discharge from the University of Illinois student health center.

For Health Professionals

http://www.cdc.gov/nchstp/dstd/Whats_New.htm. Updates from the CDC regarding STDs.

http://www2a.cdc.gov/stdtraining/self-study/default.asp. Self-study modules from the CDC that include vaginitis and STD topics.

http://www.emedicine.com/EMERG/topic631.htm. E-medicine site on vaginitis.

http://www.aafp.org/afp/20041201/2125.html. American Academy of Family Physicians article on vaginitis, includes patient handouts.

REFERENCES AND ADDITIONAL READINGS

Ament LA, Whalen E. Sexually transmitted diseases in pregnancy: diagnosis, impact, and intervention. *J Obstet Gynecol Neonatal Nurs* 1996;25:657.

Amsel R, Totten PA, Spiegel CA, et al. Nonspecific vaginitis: diagnostic criteria and microbial and epidemiologic associations. *Am J Med* 1983;74:14.

Anderson MR, Klink K, Cohrssen A. Evaluation of vaginal complaints. *JAMA* 2004;29:1368.

Augenbraun M, Bachmann L, Wallace T, et al. Compliance with doxycycline therapy in sexually transmitted diseases clinics. *Sex Transm Dis* 1998;25:1.

Blake D, Duggan A, Joffe A. Use of spun urine to enhance detection of *Trichomonas vaginalis* in adolescent women. *Arch Pediatr Adolesc Med* 1999;153:1222.

Briselden AM, Hillier SL. Evaluation of affirm VP microbial identification test for gardnerella vaginalis and Trichomonas vaginalis. *J Clin Microbiol* 1994;32:148.

Burtin P, Taddio A, Ariburnu O, et al. Safety of metronidazole in pregnancy: a metaanalysis. *Am J Obstet Gynecol* 1995;172:525.

Caliendo AM, Jordan JA, Green AM, et al. Real-time PCR improves detection of Trichomonas vaginalis infection compared with culture using self-collected vaginal swabs. *Infect Dis Obstet Gynecol* 2005;13:145.

Carey JC, Klebanoff MA, Hauth JC, et al. National Institute of Child Health and Human Development Network of Maternal-Fetal Medicine Units. Metronidazole to prevent preterm delivery in pregnant women with asymptomatic bacterial vaginosis. *N Engl J Med* 2000;342:534.

Carr P, Felenstein D, Friedman R. Evaluation and management of vaginitis. *J Gen Intern Med Clin Rev* 1998;13:335.

Cates W Jr. Estimates of the incidence and prevalence of sexually transmitted diseases in the United States. American Social Health Association Panel. *Sex Transm Dis* 1999;26(4 Suppl):S2.

Catlin BW. Gardnerella vaginalis: characteristics, clinical considerations, and controversies. *Clin Microbiol Rev* 1992;5(3):213.

Centers for Disease Control and Prevention, Division of STD Prevention. *Sexually transmitted disease surveillance, 2003.* Atlanta: Department of Health and Human Services, 2004.

Centers for Disease Control and Prevention. *Sexually transmitted diseases: treatment guidelines, 2002.* MMWR 2002:51 (RR-6):1.

Centers for Disease Control and Prevention. Workowski KA, Berman SM. Sexually transmitted diseases treatment guidelines, 2006. *MMWR Recomm Rep* 2006;4;55(RR-11):1.

Chernesky MA. Nucleic acid tests for the diagnosis of sexually transmitted diseases. *Fems Immunol Med Microbiol* 1999;24:437.

Ciemins EL, Flood J, Kent CK, et al. Reexamining the prevalence of *Chlamydia trachomatis* infection among gay men with urethritis: implications for STD policy and HIV prevention activities. *Sex Transm Dis* 2000;27:249.

Cohen CR, Plummer FA, Mugo N, et al. Increased interleukin-10 in the endocervical secretions of women with non-ulcerative sexually transmitted diseases: a mechanism for enhanced HIV-1 transmission? *AIDS* 1999;13:327.

DeMeo LR, Draper DL, McGregor JA, et al. Evaluation of a deoxyribonucleic acid probe for the detection of Trichomonas vaginalis in vaginal secretions. *Am J Obstet Gynecol* 1996;174:1339.

Dun E. Antifungal resistance in yeast vaginitis. *Yale J Biol Med* 2000;72:281.

Farrington PF. Pediatric vulvo-vaginitis. *Clin Obstet Gynecol* 1997;40:135.

Ferrer J. Vaginal candidosis: epidemiological and etiological factors. *Int J Gynaecol Obstet* 2000;71(Suppl 1):S21.

Ferris DG, Nyirjesy P, Sobel JD, et al. Over-the-counter antifungal drug misuse associated with patient-diagnosed vulvovaginal candidiasis. *Obstet Gynecol* 2002;99:419.

Fiori PL, Rapelli P, Addis MF. The flagellated parasite *Trichomonas vaginalis:* new insights into cryopathogenicity mechanisms. *Microbes Infect* 1999;1:149.

Forna F, Gulmezoglu AM. Interventions for treating trichomoniasis in women. *Cochrane Database Syst Rev* 2003;(2):CD000218.

Forsum U, Hallen A, Larsson PG. Bacterial vaginosis–a laboratory and clinical diagnostics enigma. *Apmis* 2005;113:153.

Forsum U, Holst E, Larsson PG, et al. Bacterial vaginosis–a microbiological and immunological enigma. *Apmis* 2005;113:81.

Gardner HL. *Haemophilus vaginalis* after twenty-five years. *Am J Obstet Gynecol* 1980;137:385.

Glover DD, Larsen B. Relationship of fungal vaginitis therapy to prior antibiotic exposure. *Infect Dis Obstet Gynecol* 2003; 11:157.

Hammerschlag MR. Sexually transmitted diseases in sexually abused children: medical and legal implications. *Sex Transm Infect* 1998;74:167.

Heine RP, Wisenfeld HC, Sweet RL, et al. PCR Analysis of distal vaginal specimens less invasive strategy for the detection of trichomonas. *Clin Infect Dis* 1997;24:985.

Hillier S, Holmes KK. Bacterial vaginosis. In: Holmes KK, Mardh PA, Sparling PF, et al. eds. *Sexually transmitted diseases*, 3rd ed. New York: McGraw-Hill, 1999.

Holmes KK, Stamm WE. Lower genital tract infection in women. In: Holmes KK, Mardh PA, Sparling PF, et al. eds. *Sexually transmitted diseases*, 3rd ed. New York: McGraw-Hill, 1999.

Huppert JS, Batteiger BE, Braslins P, et al. Use of an immunochromatographic assay for rapid detection of Trichomonas vaginalis in vaginal specimens. *J Clin Microbiol* 2005;43:684.

Hwang L, Shafer MA. Chlamydia trachomatis infection in adolescents. *Adv Pediatr* 2004;51:379.

Joishy M, Ashtekar CS, Jain A, et al. Do we need to treat vulvovaginitis in prepubertal girls? *Br Med J* 2005;330:186.

Kingston MA, Bansal D, Carlin EM. 'Shelf life' of Trichomonas vaginalis. *Int J STD AIDS* 2003;14:28.

Krieger JN, Alderete JF. *Trichomonas vaginalis* and *Trichomoniasis*. In: Holmes KK, Mardh PA, Sparling PF, et al. eds. *Sexually transmitted diseases*, 3rd ed. New York: McGraw-Hill, 1999.

Krohn MA, Hillier SL, Nugent RP, et al. Vaginal Infection and Prematurity Study Group. The genital flora of women with intraamniotic infection. *J Infect Dis* 1995;171:1475.

Larsen B. Vaginal flora in health and disease. *Clin Obstet Gynecol* 1993;36:107.

Madico G, Quinn TC, Rompalo A, et al. Diagnosis of Trichomonas vaginalis infection by PCR using vaginal swab samples. *J Clin Microbiol* 1998;36:3205.

Mardh PA. The vaginal ecosystem. *Am J Obstet Gynecol* 1991; 165:1163.

McGregor JA, French JI. Bacterial vaginosis in pregnancy. *Obstet Gynecol Surv* 2000;55:S1.

Medical Letter. Drugs for sexually transmitted infections. *Med Lett* 1999;41:1062.

Merchant J, Oh K, Klerman L. Douching: a problem for adolescent girls and young women. *Arch Pediatr Adolesc Med* 1999;153:834.

Metzger GD. Laboratory diagnosis of vaginal infections. *Clin Lab Sci* 1998;11:47.

Mitchell H. Vaginal discharge–causes, diagnosis, and treatment. *Br Med J* 2004;328:1306.

Nansel TR, Riggs MA, Yu KF, et al. The association of psychosocial stress and bacterial vaginosis in a longitudinal cohort. *Am J Obstet Gynecol* 2006;194:381.

Nugent RP, Krohn MA, Hillier SL. Reliability of diagnosing bacterial vaginosis is improved by a standardized method of gram stain interpretation. *J Clin Microbiol* 1991;29:297.

Nyirjesy P. Vaginitis in the adolescent patient. *Pediatr Clin North Am* 1999;46:733.

Nyirjesy P, Sobel JD. Vulvovaginal candidiasis. *Obstet Gynecol Clin North Am* 2003;30:671.

Ohlemeyer CC, Hornberger LL, Lynch DA, et al. Diagnosis of *Trichomonas vaginalis* in adolescent females. In Pouch TV culture versus wet-mount. *J Adolesc Health* 1998;22:205.

Peipert JF, Montagno AB, Cooper AS, et al. Bacterial vaginosis as a risk factor for upper genital tract infection. *Am J Obstet Gynecol* 1997;177:1184.

Petrin D, Delgaty K, Bhatt R, et al. Clinical and microbiological aspects of *Trichomonas vaginalis*. *Clin Microbiol Rev* 1998; 11:300.

Plummer PA, Simonsen JN, Cameron DW, et al. Co-factors in male-female sexual transmission of human immunodeficiency virus type 1. *J Infect Dis* 1991;163:233.

Shafer MA, Sweet RL, Ohm-Smith MS, et al. Microbiology of the lower genital tract in postmenarchal adolescent girls: differences by sexual activity, contraception, and presence of nonspecific vaginitis. *J Pediatr* 1985;107:974.

Sobel JD. Vulvovaginal candidiasis. In: Holmes KK, Mardh PA, Sparling PF, et al. eds. *Sexually transmitted diseases*, 3rd ed. New York: McGraw-Hill, 1999.

Sobel JD. What's new in bacterial vaginosis and trichomoniasis? *Infect Dis Clin North Am* 2005;19:387.

Sobel JD, Brooker D, Stein GE, et al. Fluconazole Vaginitis Study Group. Single oral dose fluconazole compared with conventional clotrimazole topical therapy of *Candida vaginitis*. *Am J Obstet Gynecol* 1995;172:1263.

Sobel JD, Chaim W, Nagappan V, et al. Treatment of vaginitis caused by Candida glabrata: use of topical boric acid and flucytosine. *Am J Obstet Gynecol* 2003;189:1297.

Sobel JD, Wiesenfeld HC, Martens M, et al. Maintenance Fluconazole therapy for recurrent vulvovaginal candidiasis. *N Engl J Med* 2004;351:876.

Sorvillo F, Smith L, Kerndt P, et al. Trichomonas vaginalis, HIV, and African-Americans. *Emerg Infect Dis* 2001;7:927.

Spinillo A, Pizzoli G, Colonna L, et al. Epidemiologic characteristics of women with idiopathic recurrent vulvovaginal candidiasis. *Obstet Gynecol* 1993;81:721.

Sweet RL. Role of bacterial vaginosis in pelvic inflammatory disease. *Clin Infect Dis* 1995;20(Suppl 2):S271.

Sweet RL. The enigmatic cervix. *Dermatol Clin* 1998;16:739.

Swygard H, Sena AC, Hobbs MM, et al. Trichomoniasis: clinical manifestations, diagnosis and management. *Sex Transm Infect* 2004;80:91.

Syed TS, Braverman PK. Vaginitis in adolescents. *Adolesc Med Clin* 2004;15:235.

Van Der Pol B, Williams JA, Orr DP, et al. Prevalence, incidence, natural history, and response to treatment of Trichomonas vaginalis infection among adolescent women. *J Inf Dis* 2005; 192:2039.

Vermillion ST, Holmes MM, Soper DE. Adolescents and sexually transmissible diseases. *Obstet Gynecol Clin North Am* 2000;27:163.

Weinstock H, Berman S, Cates W Jr. Sexually transmitted diseases among American youth: incidence and prevalence estimates, 2000. *Perspect Sex Reprod Health* 2004;36:6.

Wiese W, Patel SR, Patel SC, et al. A meta-analysis of the Papanicolaou smear and wet mount for diagnosis of vaginal trichomoniasis. *Am J Med* 2000;108:301.

Wilton L, Kollarova M, Heeley E, et al. Relative risk of vaginal candidiasis after use of antibiotics compared with antidepressants in women: postmarketing surveillance data in England. *Drug Saf* 2003;26:589.

Yen S, Shafer MA, Moncada J, et al. Bacterial vaginosis in sexually experienced and non-sexually experienced young women entering the military. *Obstet Gynecol* 2003;102 (5 Pt 1):927.

CHAPTER 56

Ectopic Pregnancy

Melissa D. Mirosh and Mary Anne Jamieson

ECTOPIC PREGNANCY

Ectopic pregnancy in the adolescent population is fortunately uncommon. Teens usually have not had sufficient time to establish enough exposures to infection or other intraabdominal pathologies to acquire tubal damage and then conceive with resultant ectopic pregnancy. However, in managing ectopic pregnancies in teens, one must remember that access to care may be limited before or after the diagnosis, confidentiality must be respected, future fertility should be protected, and reliable and acceptable contraception should be offered and encouraged during and after treatment.

Ectopic pregnancy should be a consideration when any pregnant adolescent presents for an office visit with new onset of abnormal uterine vaginal bleeding or abdominal/pelvic pain.

Incidence and Prevalence

The risk of ectopic pregnancy in United States is approximately 19 per 1,000 pregnancies, which has remained stable for several years (MMWR, 1995). This is only an approximation because there are many miscarriages, abortions, and medically treated ectopic pregnancies that are not reported.

1. Trends: From 1991 to 1999, ectopic pregnancies were responsible for 6% of all pregnancy-related deaths in the United States, of which 93% were due to hemorrhage (Chang et al., 2003). This represents an overall decrease of 13% since 1992, most likely due to increased detection of early pregnancy. The risk of death from ectopic pregnancy in the United Kingdom fell from 16 to 4 per 10,000 ectopic pregnancies during the nearly 30 years spanning 1973 to 2002 (Lewis, 2004), although mortality still remains high in developing countries (Igberase et al., 2005).
2. Ectopic pregnancy occurs throughout the reproductive age spectrum. A review from California found a low rate of 12.5 per 1,000 reported pregnancies in women aged 15 to 19 to a high rate of 42.5 per 1,000 pregnancies in women aged 40 to 49 (Van Den Eeden et al., 2005).
3. Ectopic pregnancies occur more frequently in black women (8%) than in white women (4%). This demographic trend is also seen with respect to overall maternal mortality. This discrepancy is unexplained at present, although it is consistent with the higher sexually transmitted disease (STD) rate and lower socioeconomic status seen in the black population in United States (Anderson et al., 2004; Centers for Disease Control and Prevention, CDC, 2006; MMWR, 1995).
4. Location: Ectopic pregnancies occur almost exclusively in the oviduct (95.5%), while 1.3% are abdominal, and approximately 3% are cervical or ovarian. Within the tube itself, most ectopic pregnancies (70%) are located in the ampullary region, 12% are isthmic, 11% are fimbrial, and 2.4% are interstitial (Bouyer et al., 2002).

Etiology and Risk Factors

There are many factors associated with an increased risk of developing an ectopic pregnancy. (Table 56.1)

1. Tubal abnormalities: The most common predisposing factor for adolescents is a previous episode of pelvic inflammatory disease (PID). This is more likely in females with a previous chlamydial infection because Chlamydia infections tend to be less symptomatic than gonorrhea and therefore may go untreated for longer, causing significant pelvic organ damage. The resulting salpingitis is responsible for approximately 45% of initial ectopic pregnancies (Westrom et al., 1981). Scarring of the tubes impairs the ability of the tube to permit normal motility within its lumen. Histopathological study of excised tubes previously involved with PID has shown multiple pockets and tortuous pathways that may also trap embryos (Green and Kott, 1989). Other tubal pathology associated with ectopic pregnancy includes damage or adhesions from previous pelvic surgery (previous tubal surgery for an ectopic pregnancy, ruptured appendix, trauma, inflammatory bowel disease, endometriosis, tubal ligation, or tubal reanastomosis). Adhesions outside the tube to nearby structures such as bowel or other pelvic organs may also cause distortion of the tube. Diethylstilbestrol (DES) exposure (extremely unlikely in this generation of adolescents) and other reproductive congenital anomalies may contribute to abnormal anatomy as well.
2. Tubal pregnancy with the intrauterine contraceptive devicentrauterine Contraceptive Device (IUD): The IUD has long been erroneously associated with an increased risk of ectopic pregnancy. In fact, the absolute

TABLE 56.1

Risk Factors for Ectopic Pregnancy

	Adjusted OR (95% CI)	OR (95% CI)
Previous tubal surgery	4.0 (2.6–6.1)	4.7–21.0
Infertility (risk increases with length of infertility)	2.1–2.7	2.5–21.0
Previous genital infection confirmed	3.4 (2.4–5.0)	2.5–3.7
Previous miscarriage	3.0 (>2)	—
Previous induced abortion	2.8 (1.1–7.2)	—
Past or ever smoker	1.5 (1.1–2.2)	2.5 (1.8–3.4)
Current smoker (risk increases with amount smoked per day)	1.7–3.9	2.3–2.5
Age 40 years and older	2.9 (1.4–6.1)	—
Intrauterine device use (>2 years)	2.9 (1.4–6.3)	4.2–45.0
Previous intrauterine device	2.4 (1.2–4.9)	—
Sterilization[a]	—	9.3 (4.9–18.0)
Previous ectopic pregnancy	—	8.3 (6.0–11.5)
Documented tubal pathology	3.7 (1.2–4.8)	2.5–3.5
More than one sexual partner	—	2.1–2.5
Diethylstilboestrol exposure	—	5.6 (2.4–13.0)

OR, odds ratio; CI, confidence interval.
From Farquhar CM. Ectopic pregnancy. *Lancet* 2005;366(9485):583.

risk of ectopic pregnancy is significantly reduced in women with an IUD compared with women who use no method of contraception. The current copper IUDs are no longer considered to increase the absolute risk of ectopic pregnancy (Xiong et al., 1995). However, if a patient becomes pregnant with an IUD in situ, the chance that the fetus will implant outside of the uterus is 15% to 20% (Weir, 2003). Progestin-releasing IUDs are associated with an even lower pregnancy rate than nonhormonal IUDs and thereby further reduce the chance of an ectopic pregnancy when compared with sexually active women who are not using contraception (French et al., 2004).
3. Other factors: Other factors that increase the risk of ectopic pregnancy include smoking, infertility, in vitro fertilization, and prior ectopic pregnancy. In the adolescent population, smoking is the most common risk factor.

Differential Diagnosis

The differential diagnosis of ectopic pregnancy and those teens presenting with acute abdominal or pelvic pain is best divided into obstetrical, gynecological, and nongynecological categories.

1. Obstetrical
   a. Normal intrauterine pregnancy
   b. Hemorrhagic corpus luteum
   c. Spontaneous or threatened abortion
2. Gynecological
   a. Ovarian torsion
   b. Hemorrhagic ovarian cyst
   c. Symptomatic or ruptured ovarian cyst
   d. Pelvic inflammatory disease
3. Nongynecological
   a. Appendicitis
   b. Renal colic
   c. Inflammatory bowel disease
   d. Gastroenteritis
   e. Severe constipation

Clinical Presentation

The range of symptoms depends on the integrity of the teen's fallopian tube and can range from mild cramping and vaginal spotting to frank hemorrhagic shock. However, the classic triad of vaginal bleeding, delayed menses, and severe lower abdominal pain is associated with tubal rupture and is now a fairly infrequent presentation, because early diagnosis is more routine. In general, there are two distinctly different constellations of signs and symptoms that are expressed by women with ectopic pregnancies, each of which dictates different action plans.

Acute Presentation: Classic, Ruptured Ectopic Pregnancy

1. Symptoms: The patient who presents with an acutely ruptured ectopic pregnancy would typically exhibit the following symptoms:
   a. Sudden onset of extreme, sharp, or stabbing unilateral pelvic pain, as well as shoulder pain. The shoulder pain is referred pain resulting from subdiaphragmatic irritation caused by hemoperitoneum.
   b. Dizziness, lightheadedness, or loss of consciousness from acute intraperitoneal hemorrhage leading to hypotension.
   c. Abnormal menses: The patient may have missed her menses and/or experienced several days of abnormal vaginal spotting or bleeding, as well as vague pelvic pain before the onset of her acute symptoms. Teens often have irregular bleeding, and may not have noticed any difference from their "routine" menstrual pattern.

d. Pregnancy symptoms: The patient may also have noticed nausea, vomiting, breast tenderness, or other symptoms of early pregnancy.

Statistically, the teen who presents with a ruptured ectopic pregnancy is more likely to have had a previous pregnancy and therefore usually does not suspect a problem (Saxon et al., 1997). Generally, gestational age at the time of active symptom development varies by the implantation site. For example, ampullary implantations are more likely to rupture at 6 to 8 weeks of gestation, but cornual implantations may not rupture until near the end of the first trimester.

2. Classic signs of a ruptured ectopic pregnancy:
   a. Vital signs: the patient may be in shock with rapid thready pulse, hypotension, and change in mental status.
   b. Abdomen will be tender to palpation, possibly even rigid, with marked rebound tenderness.
   c. Bimanual examination: Cervical motion tenderness is apparent with a slightly enlarged and globular uterus. Often a pelvic mass is not palpable, either because of guarding or because the rupture has eliminated the bulging mass in the fallopian tube.
3. Laboratory tests: Laboratory testing requirements are minimal and are necessary only to prepare for surgery and to rule out other pathologies.
   a. Pregnancy testing: Sensitive urine pregnancy test results should be positive. A baseline quantitative serum β-human chorionic gonadotropin (β-hCG) will allow monitoring of pregnancy resolution.
   b. The "Three C's of hemorrhage:"
      • Complete blood cell (CBC) count—including hemoglobin and hematocrit.
      • Crossmatch—blood group and screen to prepare for possible transfusion as well as Rh typing to determine the need for Rh immunoglobulin.
      • Coagulation factors—if the blood loss has been significant, patients may have evidence of disseminated intravascular coagulation (DIC) and consideration should be given to appropriate laboratory testing.
   c. Ultrasonography: If the patient is hemodynamically unstable, an ultrasonography is not indicated and should not delay a patient from getting into surgery. If an ultrasonography is performed, however, the most remarkable finding will be free fluid and clots in the pelvis; blood may fill the entire abdominal cavity. If there is a positive pregnancy test result, a corpus luteum cyst may be seen and the endometrium may be thickened with decidual material. In fact, a hemorrhagic corpus luteum cyst is the other main consideration in the differential diagnosis. The presence of an intrauterine pregnancy essentially rules out ectopic pregnancy in an adolescent because heterotopic pregnancy is extremely rare without assisted reproductive technologies. It is not necessary to visualize the pregnancy in the tube, although the absence of a uterine pregnancy seen on ultrasonography is not diagnostic of an ectopic pregnancy. In the context of an acute and unstable presentation, the final diagnosis will usually be confirmed at the time of surgery.
4. Therapy:
   a. Fluids: The patient requires intravenous access in the form of at least one (preferably two) large-bore intravenous line(s). Fluid resuscitation should start immediately. Blood transfusion may be started if clinically indicated (and with informed consent whenever possible), but surgery should not be delayed by the need to give the patient a transfusion to some arbitrary hemoglobin level; the patient may be losing blood internally at a rate faster than can be replaced by transfusion.
   b. Emergency surgery is required: At surgery, every effort should be made in an adolescent to preserve the fallopian tube if possible, performing a salpingostomy as opposed to salpingectomy. If a hemorrhagic corpus luteum is determined to be the cause of the bleeding then every effort should be made to preserve the ovary. If an oophorectomy is required, progesterone supplementation should be instituted until 10- to 12-weeks gestation if the patient wishes to continue the pregnancy.
   c. The patient's Rh status must be confirmed and Rh immunoglobulin given if she is Rh negative.

Subacute Presentations: Probable Ectopic Pregnancy and Possible Ectopic Pregnancy

A woman with a positive pregnancy test result who presents with cramping, abnormal vaginal spotting or bleeding, and lower abdominal/adnexal pain should be suspected of having an ectopic pregnancy, particularly if the diagnosis is supported by physical findings of cervical motion tenderness, a closed cervix, adnexal tenderness, and (possibly) an adnexal mass. Women who present in early pregnancy with complaints of vaginal spotting or bleeding and cramping without those suspicious physical findings must also be evaluated to rule out an ectopic pregnancy, although their diagnosis is more likely to be threatened abortion. The workup and treatment depend on the woman's risk factors and her pregnancy intentions.

The initial diagnosis of a clinically suspected ectopic pregnancy in the hemodynamically stable patient begins with a complete history and physical examination, lab work, and transvaginal ultrasound imaging. If the patient has a regular menstrual cycle, her last menstrual period may be helpful in establishing correct pregnancy dates. Other history that may assist in establishing gestational age includes the date of the first positive pregnancy test result and findings from any previous ultrasonography. The reason for established gestational age is that some authors have recommended using this as a starting point for the diagnostic work-up. In this approach, the first step in the evaluation is an ultrasonography if the gestational age is at least 6 weeks. However, the last menstrual period is often not a reliable or secure data point, particularly in adolescents who may have irregular cycles or imprecise recollections of their menstrual dates. Mol et al. (1998) reviewed 354 patients evaluated for ectopic pregnancy and found that gestational age did not discriminate between intrauterine and ectopic pregnancy. Quantitative β-hCG levels have more reproducibility and, therefore, are used as the basis of most management protocols. The lab work should include CBC count (for white blood cell [WBC], hemoglobin [Hgb], and hematocrit), blood typing, and screening to determine Rh status, and a serum quantitative β-hCG. The adolescent patient may need an explanation for the role of transvaginal ultrasonography as she may be hesitant to have a probe inserted vaginally.

Laboratory and Imaging Evaluation

The properties and limitations of each diagnostic test should be recognized to appropriately use each of them in the workup.

1. β-hCG: Typically, β-hCG levels will double every 2 days in a normal first trimester intrauterine gestation. Only 15% of normal pregnancies will fail to have this appropriate increase in β-hCG levels. The smallest increase over 48 hours that can still be associated with a continuing intrauterine pregnancy is 53% (Barnhart et al., 2004). If β-hCG measurements are unchanged or increasing abnormally, the pregnancy is nonviable; it may be an abnormal intrauterine pregnancy (destined to abort), or it may be an ectopic pregnancy. Pregnancies that have inappropriately low β-hCG levels are more likely to be ectopic. Serial β-hCG measurements can be extremely helpful in determining the fate of these pregnancies.
2. Ultrasonography: Ultrasound studies at appropriate β-hCG levels are usually diagnostic, and often the definitive method of pregnancy dating in adolescents. Although ectopic pregnancies can have characteristic appearances on ultrasonography (Frates and Laing, 1995), ultrasound is not used to visualize the tubal pregnancy, but to identify a pregnancy within the uterine cavity. There is still debate over what β-hCG cutoff should be used as the discriminatory level (the lowest concentration of β-hCG that is associated with a visible normal intrauterine gestation), but this level is generally considered to be above 1,500 to 2,000 IU/L when using a transvaginal ultrasound probe. Above this level of serum β-hCG, a normal intrauterine gestational sac should be seen (Condous et al., 2005; Mehta et al., 1997). Although an intrauterine pregnancy may be detected at lower levels, the possibility that the pregnancy in question is intrauterine cannot be excluded until the β-hCG levels reach the discriminatory range. If no intrauterine gestation is seen, then an ectopic pregnancy should be strongly suspected. One must also keep in mind that multiple gestation pregnancies will not be visible until the β-hCG concentration is above 2,000 IU/L (Mol et al., 1998). If transabdominal scanning is the only method available, the β-hCG cutoff should be 6,500 IU/L (Kadar et al., 1994).

Outpatient Follow-up—Using Serial β-hCG Levels:

1. Declining β-hCG levels: If the β-hCG levels are declining by 50% to 66% every 3 days, it is likely that the patient has experienced a complete resolution of the pregnancy. The β-hCG levels must be followed up until they are undetectable (based on local laboratory values).
2. Increasing β-hCG levels: If the β-hCG levels are increasing by at least 66% every 2 to 3 days, they should be followed up in a mildly symptomatic patient until they reach the discriminatory zone and the diagnosis can be made ultrasonographically. If the patient becomes increasingly symptomatic before reaching the discriminatory zone, laparoscopic investigation may be considered. It is useful to discuss with the patient whether the pregnancy is wanted. A dilation and curettage (D&C) can be performed at the time of laparoscopy if the pregnancy is discovered to be intrauterine. If the pregnancy is wanted, consider delaying insertion of the uterine manipulator until an ectopic gestation is confirmed.
3. Abnormally changing β-hCG levels: If the β-hCG levels are declining or rising at an inappropriate rate, the pregnancy (either intrauterine or ectopic) is likely nonviable.
   a. If her β-hCG levels are above the discriminatory level, an ultrasonography should be obtained to localize the pregnancy. If it is not within the endometrial cavity, the pregnancy is presumed to be ectopic.
   b. If her β-hCG levels are less than the discriminatory range, it is important to assess the patient's desire for pregnancy. If she does not wish to continue with the pregnancy, the presence of an abnormal uterine pregnancy can be ruled out by performing a D&C. A β-hCG level, obtained 12 to 24 hours after the procedure, should be compared with a preprocedure level (Lipscomb et al., 2000). If levels drop by 50% in that time, an ectopic pregnancy can be ruled out. If time allows, the histopathology from the D&C specimen will usually confirm trophoblastic tissue and villi. Otherwise, the asymptomatic patient who is well-informed and compliant can be followed up expectantly until the β-hCG levels either fall, plateau, or reach the discriminatory zone and the ultrasonography can be performed. At this point, decisions about laparoscopy, D&C, and conservative or medical therapy can be made.
   c. Methotrexate may be therapeutic for both abnormal intrauterine pregnancies and ectopic pregnancies. Therefore, some investigators have suggested forgoing the D&C and immediately using the methotrexate therapy (see later discussion) to treat the abnormal pregnancy (Tulandi and Saleh, 1999). Misoprostol can be used orally or intravaginally for treatment of an abnormal intrauterine pregnancy.

Other Diagnostic Modalities

1. Serum progesterone levels: A meta-analysis done by Mol et al., in 1998 looked at the use of a single serum progesterone level for diagnosing ectopic pregnancy. A progesterone level <5 ng/mL is associated with a failing pregnancy (in any location) whereas levels >25 ng/mL are diagnostic of normal intrauterine pregnancies in 98% of cases. Most women presenting with a possible ectopic pregnancy had progesterone levels that fell within this range, therefore it did not appear to be helpful in determining either the potential for viability or the location of the pregnancy (Mol et al., 1998).
2. Culdocentesis to determine if there is blood in the cul-de-sac is rarely used today. It has been replaced by ultrasonic imaging.

Management

Issues Unique to Adolescents

1. Access to care and follow-up: There are several factors in the evaluation and treatment of ectopic pregnancy that are unique to, or should be emphasized in, adolescents. These patients may present later in gestation because of denial of pregnancy or fear of consequences. They may have trouble accessing the medical system, or be unable to seek help due to lack of transportation or money. Once in your office, establishing an accurate history is often difficult as menstrual cycles can be irregular and teens may be poor historians.

2. Confidentiality and consent for treatment: One must be aware of the local legislation with respect to informed consent for minors. Fortunately, in most states and provinces, health care providers can use clinical judgment and provide medical care to an adolescent who understands the nature of the diagnosis and/or treatment, without necessarily involving a parent or guardian. Teens may have a particular need for confidentiality and this must be respected. On the other hand, health care providers should make every effort to negotiate with the teen to involve a parent or a guardian in such an important issue as the diagnosis and treatment of an ectopic pregnancy.

Approaches to Management

In the adolescent with an ectopic pregnancy, treatment should generally be fertility-sparing and should take into account that adolescents may have difficulty complying with follow-up recommendations.

1. Surgical approach: Most women diagnosed with an ectopic pregnancy will be treated surgically through laparoscopy or laparotomy. Open surgery is the method of choice for hemodynamically unstable patients, surgeons with little laparoscopic experience, or both. Some surgeons may consider laparoscopic treatment of their hemodynamically unstable patients, depending on their surgical experience and available equipment (Sagiv et al., 2001). A recent Cochrane review concluded that although the laparoscopic route was less successful than a laparotomy for complete resolution of trophoblastic tissue, it remains the cornerstone of treatment in hemodynamically stable patients owing to its decreased operative time, hospital stay, and recovery times (Hajenius et al., 2000). Finally, laparoscopy has also been shown to have equivalent success when compared with laparotomy in obese patients (Hsu et al., 2004).

    Conservative or radical treatment? The most common surgical procedures are salpingostomy and salpingectomy. Unfortunately, there are no randomized controlled studies that directly compare the two. In theory, the benefit of removing the affected tube is an almost guaranteed resolution of the ectopic pregnancy, while treating conservatively preserves the potential for fertility with that tube (which is crucial in adolescents). Five nonrandomized studies have been published that observed the outcomes of conservative versus radical therapy (Bangsgaard et al., 2003; Bouyer et al., 2000; Job-Spira et al., 1996; Mol et al., 1998; Silva et al., 1993). Three of them showed a significant difference in future fertility, but the two more recent studies have implied that conservative surgery may be advantageous with respect to subsequent fertility (Bangsgaard et al., 2003; Bouyer et al., 2000). A randomized controlled trial will likely be needed to complete the debate. Two studies have confirmed that it is not necessary to close the tubal defect after salpingostomy (Fujishita et al., 2004; Tulandi and Saleh, 1999).

    There are some patients in whom salpingectomy is the preferred method of treatment. These would include cases of intractable hemorrhage, three recurrent ectopic pregnancies in the same tube, or in women who have completed childbearing. The latter two scenarios seldom occur in the adolescent. One aspect to consider before removing the affected tube is the state of the contralateral tube. If the patient wishes to conserve her chances for spontaneous conception, the unaffected tube must appear normal. If it is abnormal or damaged, salpingostomy for the ectopic pregnancy would be recommended.

2. Medical therapy: Early diagnosis of ectopic pregnancy using laboratory tests and sensitive imaging techniques has significantly reduced the mortality and morbidity of this condition. It has also enabled the use of outpatient medical therapy in lieu of surgical intervention, which in time has reduced hospitalization costs and surgical complications.

    Methotrexate: Methotrexate has become an established method of treatment for patients diagnosed with an unruptured ectopic pregnancy. The main advantage of medical therapy over surgical therapy is that it is less invasive and less expensive.

    a. Modality of action: Methotrexate is a folic acid antagonist and therefore exerts its effect on rapidly dividing cells. The medication disrupts cytotrophoblast syncytialization and blunts β-hCG production, thereby decreasing support for progesterone secretion by the corpus luteum (Creinin et al., 1998).

    b. Success rate: Meta-analysis of outpatient methotrexate treatment for appropriate candidates demonstrated a cure rate of 92% (Slaughter and Grimes, 1995). At least 85% of those women successfully completed therapy, although 5% to 16% required a second dose of methotrexate (Henry and Gentry, 1994). Only 2.7% required three or more doses. Failure rates are higher with higher initial β-hCG levels. One study found that the failure rate was 32% when the presenting β-hCG levels were more than 15,000, but was 6% when the pretreatment β-hCG level was less than 10,000 (Lipscomb et al., 1999).

    There are no randomized controlled trials comparing single dose to multi-dose treatment. However a meta-analysis found that although a multi-dose regimen is more successful (92.7% versus 88.1%), the overall success of medically treating an ectopic pregnancy with any method of methotrexate is 89% (Barnhart et al., 2003). Often one dose is sufficient (Lipscomb et al., 1998). One study reviewed a group of 55 adolescents who had successfully used the single-dose method and were able to follow the strict follow-up protocols. In this group of teens, the success rate of methotrexate for ectopic pregnancy resolution was 85% (McCord et al., 1996).

    Efforts to determine factors that argue favorably for methotrexate therapy identified an initial β-hCG level of <4,000 and lack of fetal cardiac activity as strong predictors of success. Indicators predictive of failure included visible extrauterine yolk sac on ultrasonography and previous ectopic pregnancy (Lipscomb et al., 2004). Patients must be counseled about the possibility of treatment failure (and possible tubal rupture) and the signs and symptoms that may indicate complications and necessitate return to hospital. Because it is common for abdominal pain to occur as the ectopic pregnancy resolves 24 to 48 hours after administration of methotrexate, the differentiation of "normal" from "abnormal" pain can be challenging and may result in additional emergency room visits for reassessment and reassurance.

TABLE 56.2

Methotrexate Therapy for Ectopic Pregnancy—Exclusion Criteria

Patient characteristics:
  Hemodynamically unstable
  Unable to comply with follow-up visit schedule or to return if complications develop
  Immunocompromised (white blood cell count <3,000)
  Anemia (Hemoglobin <8 g/dL)
  Active pulmonary disease
  Renal compromise (creatinine clearance >1.3 mg/dL)
  Hepatic compromise (elevated liver function test results; aspartate aminotransferase >50 IU/L)
  Hematological dysfunction
  Thrombocytopenia
β-hCG characteristics:
  Most institutions exclude levels >10,000 mIU/ng
Ultrasonography findings:
  Gestational sac (maximum density of entire mass) >3.5–4.0 cm[a]
  Fetal cardiac motion[a]
  Excessive fluid in cul-de-sac consistent with hemorrhage

[a]Relative contraindication.

Gazvani et al., examined the addition of mifepristone to any outpatient regimen of methotrexate and found no benefit (Gazvani et al., 1998).

  c. Dose: The dose used for treating ectopic pregnancy, usually 50 mg/m^2, is much lower than that used for cancer chemotherapy. Many different regimens of methotrexate delivery have been employed for treatment of ectopic pregnancy, including oral, intramuscular, and local injection (under laparoscopic or ultrasound guidance). Tables 56.2 and 56.3 list exclusion criteria and logarithm for using methotrexate.

  d. Side effects: Because the doses are so much lower than chemotherapy, the common side effects of methotrexate at higher dosages including nausea, vomiting, stomatitis, and diarrhea are rarely seen with the doses used to treat ectopic pregnancies. Rarely, a reversible leukopenia or transient hair loss may be seen.

Other medical modalities: Other medical interventions have included injecting the embryo with methotrexate, hypertonic saline, or prostaglandins. Although successful, these methods are more cumbersome and invasive compared to oral or intramuscular methotrexate, and therefore are much less frequently used (Hajenius et al., 2000; Yao et al., 1996).

  3. Treatment of unusual ectopic pregnancy sites: As mentioned previously, ectopic pregnancies are rarely located outside the fallopian tubes. There are a number of individual case reports documenting surgical and medical management of pregnancies located on ovaries, surgical scars, omentum, and the cervix. The method of treatment for pregnancies in these sites is usually systemic or local methotrexate under ultrasound guidance (Doubilet et al., 2004), as treating them surgically would be technically difficult or dangerous due to uncontrollable bleeding or poor surgical access.

TABLE 56.3

Systemic Methotrexate Treatment Algorithm

Treatment Day	Investigation/Management
1	Patient eligible for methotrexate therapy
	Labs: Quantitative β-hCG, renal function tests, liver function tests, CBC count, blood type and screen
	Methotrexate administered in 50 mg/m^2 dose intramuscularly
	Patient care instructions including anticipated symptoms and analgesia
4	Labs: Quantitative β-hCG
7	Labs: Quantitative β-hCG, renal and liver function tests, CBC count
	Compare β-hCG levels from day 4 and 7: If the decline in value is $\geq$15%, continue to monitor β-hCG until they resolve. If the decline is <15%, a second methotrexate dose is needed
	Consider surgical treatment if the patient becomes hemodynamically unstable, has increasing pain and/or falling hematocrit, or if there is an ineffective response to methotrexate

hCG, human chorionic gonadotropin; CBC, complete blood cell.

4. Expectant management: Expectant management is reasonable for a certain subset of women presenting with ectopic pregnancy. These patients are asymptomatic and generally have a β-hCG level below 1,000 IU/L (Trio et al., 1995). They also need to be reliable, as losing a woman to follow-up could be disastrous. Under these circumstances, Pisarska showed that 68% of women had complete resolution of their ectopic pregnancy without intervention (Pisarska et al., 1998). Patients who have spontaneous resolution of their ectopic pregnancies also tend to have a good chance of return to normal fertility. Rantala et al., found that 93% of their study patients had patent tubes on a subsequent hysterosalpingogram and did not have an increased rate of second ectopic pregnancy when compared to the general population (Rantala and Makinen, 1997). Unfortunately, the need to carefully assess these patients over the course of several weeks, especially if they develop pain, may result in the need for repeated clinical visits. Adolescents should be considered on an individual basis as candidates for conservative management because for many teens the follow-up and surveillance requirements will be too compliance demanding.

Follow-up

Surgical

Complete resolution of the ectopic pregnancy must be documented because residual trophoblastic tissue proliferation can cause clinical problems. Overall, with salpingostomy, almost 5% of women undergoing laparotomy and 8% to 15% of women who are treated laparoscopically will develop persistent trophoblastic tissue (Seifer et al., 1993). In this situation, it is prudent to ensure that the β-hCG levels return to normal, and another pregnancy should be prevented until that time. β-hCG levels should be measured 6 days postoperatively. If the sixth day value is greater than 15% of the baseline value obtained at the time of surgery, persistent disease is presumed. Some have suggested that postoperative day 1 determinations replace the more delayed follow-up measurements; if day 1 serum β-hCG levels are decreased by 50%, there is an 85% probability that persistent trophoblastic tissue will not occur, and that the patient has been adequately treated (Spandorfer et al., 1997). Expression of ectopic tissue from the end of the fallopian tube (i.e., milking the tube) has been associated with residual disease in up to 25% of cases. Careful postoperative monitoring in these cases is critical.

Nonsurgical

Obviously, women treated with methotrexate or expectant management will require weekly (or more frequent) quantitative β-hCG determinations until the levels of that hormone become undetectable. Table 56.4 outlines specific guidelines for following up a patient treated with methotrexate.

Persistent Disease If persistent disease is diagnosed, further treatment is necessary. If surgical treatment was used initially, methotrexate should probably be used as second line as long as the patient is not continuing to bleed from the ectopic pregnancy. If methotrexate was used initially, options include surgical treatment or repeat methotrexate (Graczykowski and Mishell, 1997). Very occasionally, expectant management can be considered but would again require a well-informed, compliant patient.

Contraception It is important to provide your patient effective contraception during her recovery period, not only to prevent a second pregnancy from complicating the β-hCG results, but also to allow the tubal tissue time to heal, thereby presumably reducing the risk of a second ectopic pregnancy in rapid succession. Waiting until the β-hCG levels "zero out" before starting contraception puts a woman in jeopardy for pregnancy because ovulation often precedes complete β-hCG clearance. Assuming the

TABLE 56.4

Systemic Methotrexate Follow-up Instructions

To patients:
    Avoid sexual intercourse (may rupture ectopic pregnancy)
    Avoid sun exposure (photosensitivity reaction possible)
    Avoid consuming gas-producing foods—leeks, beans, corn, cabbage (abdominal bloating may worsen)
    No alcohol
    No ibuprofen, naproxen, aspirin, or other nonsteroidal antiinflammatory agents
    No penicillin
    No prenatal vitamins or folate supplements
    Return to clinic in 4 days for repeat tests of the pregnancy hormone β-human chorionic gonadotropin
    Be aware that in the next few days, you may experience sharp abdominal pain and some cramping. This discomfort should be self-limited, but if you feel dizzy or weak, or if the pain does not resolve, have someone take you to the emergency room immediately. There is a small chance that the pregnancy could rupture through the tube and you would need immediate surgery
    Your next period may be particularly heavy
To providers:
    No need for vaginal examination
    No need for transvaginal ultrasonography unless patient experiences acute clinical deterioration

adolescent is not seeking to conceive, every effort should be made to offer and provide reliable and acceptable contraception to the teen who has had a failed pregnancy (intrauterine or ectopic) or any pregnancy for that matter.

Rh Considerations Unsensitized Rh-negative women should be given an appropriate dose of Rh immunoglobulin (50–120 μg if gestational age <12 weeks; 300 μg if >12 weeks) promptly (ACOG, 1999; Fung Kee Fung et al., 2003). Although very occasionally the blood type of the "father" is used to determine whether an Rh-negative woman receives immunoglobulin, it is always prudent to treat the Rh-negative adolescent anyway, because of the uncertainty that may exist with respect to paternity.

Fertility after Treatment of Ectopic Pregnancy

Several studies have looked at ectopic pregnancy recurrence rates and the rates of subsequent intrauterine gestations. On an average, ectopic pregnancies recur in 10% of patients (Bouyer et al., 2002; Pouly et al., 1991). In women seeking pregnancy, reproductive success varies between 50% and 88% within 2 years of the initial ectopic pregnancy (Bangsgaard et al., 2003; Bouyer et al., 2002; Fernandez et al., 1998).

There is no consensus in the literature about the preferred method of surgical treatment with respect to subsequent fertility (Hajenius et al., 2000). Two recent studies suggest that conservative (tube sparing) surgery may lead to a higher intrauterine conception rate than radical (salpingectomy) surgery (Bangsgaard et al., 2003; Fernandez et al., 1998).

Studies looking at fertility after medical treatment of an ectopic pregnancy are also reassuring. Gervaise et al., showed that 64 of 81 women had spontaneous intrauterine pregnancies after local or systemic methotrexate (Gervaise et al., 2004). Fifty-two of these were intrauterine (with 12 spontaneous abortions), and 12 (18%) were recurrent ectopic pregnancies.

Regardless of the method of treatment, adolescent patients who have had only one ectopic pregnancy can be reassured that their chances of having an intrauterine pregnancy in the future are excellent. The method of treatment can therefore be tailored to the needs of the individual patient.

WEB SITES

For Teenagers and Parents

http://www.rxmed.com/b.main/b1.illness/b1.illness.html. RxMed Web site providing basic information on ectopic pregnancy.

For Health Professionals

http://emedicine.com/emerg/topic478.htm. eMedicine Web site on ectopic pregnancy.
http://www.aafp.org/afp/20051101/1719ph.html. American Academy of Family Physicians article on ectopic pregnancy.

http://www2.mc.duke.edu/depts/obgyn/ivf/ectopic.htm. Information on ectopic pregnancy from Duke University.
http://www.cmaj.ca/cgi/content/full/173/8/905. Review article on diagnosis and management of ectopic pregnancy from the Canadian Medical Association Journal.

REFERENCES AND ADDITIONAL READINGS

American College of Obstetrics and Gynecology. ACOG Practice Bulletin. Prevention of Rh D alloimmunization. Clinical management guidelines for obstetrician-gynecologists. *Int J Gynaecol Obstet* 1999;66:63.

Anderson FW, Hogan JG, Ansbacher R. Sudden death: ectopic pregnancy mortality. *Obstet Gynecol* 2004;103:1218.

Bangsgaard N, Lund CO, Ottesen B, et al. Improved fertility following conservative surgical treatment of ectopic pregnancy. *Br J Obstet Gynaecol* 2003;110(8):765.

Barnhart KT, Gosman G, Ashby R, et al. The medical management of ectopic pregnancy: a meta-analysis comparing "single dose" and "multidose" regimens. *Obstet Gynecol* 2003; 101:778.

Barnhart K, Sammel MD, Chung K, et al. Decline of serum human chorionic gonadotropin and spontaneous complete abortion: defining the normal curve. *Obstet Gynecol* 2004;104: 975.

Bouyer J, Coste J, Fernandez H, et al. Sites of ectopic pregnancy: a 10 year population-based study of 1800 cases. *Hum Reprod* 2002;17:3224.

Bouyer J, Job-Spira N, Pouly JL, et al. Fertility following radical, conservative-surgical or medical treatment for tubal pregnancy: a population-based study. *Br J Obstet Gynaecol* 2000;107:714.

Centers for Disease Control and Prevention; Workowski KA, Berman SM. Sexually transmitted diseases treatment guidelines, 2006. *MMWR Recomm Rep* 2006;4;55(RR-11):1.

Chang SC, O'Brien KO, Nathanson MS, et al. Characteristics and risk factors for adverse birth outcomes in pregnant black adolescents. *J Pediatr* 2003;143:250.

Condous G, Okaro E, Khalid A, et al. The accuracy of transvaginal ultrasonography for the diagnosis of ectopic pregnancy prior to surgery. *Hum Reprod* 2005;20:1404.

Creinin MD, Stewart-Akers AM, DeLoia JA. Methotrexate effects on trophoblast and the corpus luteum in early pregnancy. *Am J Obstet Gynecol* 1998;179:604–9.

Doubilet PM, Benson CB, Frates MC, et al. Sonographically guided minimally invasive treatment of unusual ectopic pregnancies. *J Ultrasound Med* 2004;23:359.

Fernandez H, Yves Vincent SC, Pauthier S, et al. Randomized trial of conservative laparoscopic treatment and methotrexate administration in ectopic pregnancy and subsequent fertility. *Hum Reprod* 1998;13:3239.

Frates MC and Laing FC. Sonographic evaluation of ectopic pregnancy: an update. *AJR Am J Roentgenol* 1995;165:251.

French R, Van Vliet H, Cowan F, et al. Hormonally impregnated intrauterine systems (IUSs) versus other forms of reversible contraceptives as effective methods of preventing pregnancy. *Cochrane Database Syst Rev* 2004;(3)CD001776.

Fujishita A, Masuzaki H, Khan KN, et al. Laparoscopic salpingotomy for tubal pregnancy: comparison of linear salpingotomy with and without suturing. *Hum Reprod* 2004;19: 1195.

Fung Kee Fung K, Eason E, Crane J, et al. Prevention of Rh alloimmunization. *J Obstet Gynaecol Can* 2003;25:765.

Gazvani MR, Baruah DN, Alfirevic Z, et al. Mifepristone in combination with methotrexate for the medical treatment of tubal pregnancy: a randomized, controlled trial. *Hum Reprod* 1998;13:1987.

Gervaise A, Masson L, de Tayrac R, et al. Reproductive outcome after methotrexate treatment of tubal pregnancies. *Fertil Steril* 2004;82:304.

Graczykowski JW, Mishell DR Jr. Methotrexate prophylaxis for persistent ectopic pregnancy after conservative treatment by salpingostomy. *Obstet Gynecol* 1997;89:118.

Green LK, Kott ML. Histopathologic findings in ectopic tubal pregnancy. *Int J Gynecol Pathol* 1989;8:255.

Hajenius PJ, Mol BW, Bossuyt PM, et al. Interventions for tubal ectopic pregnancy. *Cochrane Database Syst Rev* 2000;(2)CD000324.

Henry MA, Gentry WL. Success rates of methotrexate in ectopic pregnancy? *Fertil Steril* 1998;70:595.

Hsu S, Mitwally MF, Aly A, et al. Laparoscopic management of tubal ectopic pregnancy in obese women. *Fertil Steril* 2004;81:198.

Igberase GO, Ebeigbe PN, Igbekoyi OF, et al. Ectopic pregnancy: an 11-year review in a tertiary centre in the Niger Delta. *Trop Doct* 2005;35:175.

Job-Spira N, Bouyer J, Pouly JL, et al. Fertility after ectopic pregnancy: first results of a population-based cohort study in france. *Hum Reprod* 1996;11:99.

Jolly MC, Sebire N, Harris J, et al. Obstetric risks of pregnancy in women less than 18 years old. *Obstet Gynecol* 2000;96:962.

Kadar N, Bohrer M, Kemmann E, et al. The discriminatory human chorionic gonadotropin zone for endovaginal sonography: a prospective, randomized study. *Fertil Seril* 1994;61:1016.

Lewis G. RCOG. *Why Mothers Die 2000–2002*. London: RCOG Press, 2004.

Lipscomb GH, Bran D, McCord ML, et al. Analysis of three hundred fifteen ectopic pregnancies treated with single-dose methotrexate. *Am J Obstet Gynecol* 1998;178:1354.

Lipscomb GH, Givens VA, Meyer NL, et al. Previous ectopic pregnancy as a predictor of failure of systemic methotrexate therapy. *Fertil Steril* 2004;81:1221.

Lipscomb GH, Stovall TG, Ling FW. Nonsurgical treatment of ectopic pregnancy. *N Engl J Med* 2000;343:1325.

Lipscomb GH, McCord ML, Stovall TG, et al. Predictors of success of methotrexate treatment in women with tubal ectopic pregnancies. *N Engl J Med.* 1999;341:1974.

McCord ML, Muram D, Lipscomb GH, et al. Methotrexate therapy for ectopic pregnancy in adolescents. *J Pediatr Adolesc Gynecol* 1996;9:71.

Mehta TS, Levine D, Beckwith B. Treatment of ectopic pregnancy: is a human chorionic gonadotropin level of 2,000 mIU/mL a reasonable threshold? *Radiology* 1997;205:569.

MMWR. Ectopic pregnancy–United States, 1990–1992. *MMWR Morb Mortal Wkly Rep* 1995;44:46.

Mol BW, Hajenius PJ, Engelsbel S, et al. Serum human chorionic gonadotropin measurement in the diagnosis of ectopic pregnancy when transvaginal sonography is inconclusive. *Fertil Steril* 1998;70:972.

Mol BW, Lijmer JG, Ankum WM, et al. The accuracy of single serum progesterone measurement in the diagnosis of ectopic pregnancy: a meta-analysis. *Hum Reprod* 1998;13:3220.

Mol BW, Matthijsse HC, Tinga DJ, et al. Fertility after conservative and radical surgery for tubal pregnancy. *Hum Reprod* 1998;13:1804.

Murray H. Baakdah H. Bardell T, et al. Diagnosis and treatment of ectopic pregnancy. *CMAJ Canadian Med Assoc J* 2005;173(8):905.

Pisarska MD, Carson SA, Buster JE. Ectopic pregnancy. *Lancet* 1998;351:1115.

Pouly JL, Chapron C, Manhes H, et al. Multifactorial analysis of fertility after conservative laparoscopic treatment of ectopic pregnancy in a series of 223 patients. *Fertil Steril* 1991;56:453.

Ramakrishnan K, Scheid DC. Ectopic pregnancy: expectant management of immediate surgery? *J Fam Pract* 2006;55(6):517.

Ramakrishnan K, Scheid DC. Ectopic pregnancy: forget the "classic presentation" if you want to catch it sooner. *J Fam Pract* 2006;55(5):388.

Rantala M, Makinen J. Tubal patency and fertility outcome after expectant management of ectopic pregnancy. *Fertil Steril* 1997;68:1043.

Sagiv R, Debby A, Sadan O, et al. Laparoscopic surgery for extrauterine pregnancy in hemodynamically unstable patients. *J Am Assoc Gynecol Laparosc* 2001;8:529.

Saxon D, Falcone T, Mascha EJ, et al. A study of ruptured tubal ectopic pregnancy. *Obstet Gynecol* 1997;90:46.

Seeber BE, Barnhart KT. Suspected ectopic pregnancy. *Obstet Gynecol* 2006;107(2 Pt 1):399.

Seifer DB, Gutmann JN, Grant WD, et al. Comparison of persistent ectopic pregnancy after laparoscopic salpingostomy versus salpingostomy at laparotomy for ectopic pregnancy. *Obstet Gynecol* 1993;81:378.

Silva PD, Schaper AM, Rooney B. Reproductive outcome after 143 laparoscopic procedures for ectopic pregnancy. *Obstet Gynecol* 1993;81:710.

Slaughter JL, and Grimes DA. Methotrexate therapy. Nonsurgical management of ectopic pregnancy. *West J Med* 1995;162:225.

Spandorfer SD, Sawin SW, Benjamin I, et al. Postoperative day 1 serum human chorionic gonadotropin level as a predictor of persistent ectopic pregnancy after conservative surgical management. *Fertil Steril* 1997;68:430.

Trio D, Strobelt N, Picciolo C, et al. Prognostic factors for successful expectant management of ectopic pregnancy. *Fertil Steril* 1995;63:469.

Tulandi T, Saleh A. Surgical management of ectopic pregnancy. *Clin Obstet Gynecol* 1999;42:31.

Van Den Eeden SK, Shan J, Bruce C, et al. Ectopic pregnancy rate and treatment utilization in a large managed care organization. *Obstet Gynecol* 2005;105:1052.

Weir E. Preventing pregnancy: a fresh look at the IUD. *Can Med Assoc J* 2003;169:585.

Westrom L, Bengtsson LP, Mardh PA. Incidence, trends, and risks of ectopic pregnancy in a population of women. *Br Med J (Clin Res Ed)* 1981;282:15.

Xiong X, Buekens P, Wollast E. IUD use and the risk of ectopic pregnancy: a meta-analysis of case-control studies. *Contraception* 1995;52:23.

Yao M, Tulandi T, Falcone T. Treatment of ectopic pregnancy by systemic methotrexate, transvaginal methotrexate, and operative laparoscopy. *Int J Fertil Menopausal Stud* 1996;41(5):470.

Zhang J, Meikle S, Trumble A. Severe maternal morbidity associated with hypertensive disorders in pregnancy in the United States. *Hypertens Pregnancy* 2003;22:203.

CHAPTER 57

Galactorrhea

Sandra Loeb Salsberg and Norman P. Spack

Galactorrhea is the discharge of milk or a milk-like fluid from the breast in the absence of parturition or beyond 6 months postpartum in a nonbreastfeeding woman. It is usually bilateral, may occur intermittently or persistently, and may be spontaneous or expressed. Fluid that is yellow, green, purulent, serosanguineous, or bloody is suggestive of local breast disease and will not be included in this discussion.

Prolactin secretion is necessary for normal lactation. During pregnancy, prolactin concentrations rise and stimulate the mammary gland to produce colostrum. Elevated prolactin levels are a major cause of galactorrhea in women, but rarely cause galactorrhea in men. Male mammary tissue, unexposed to high levels of estrogen and progesterone, is less sensitive to the lactogenic effects of prolactin.

REGULATION OF PROLACTIN SECRETION

Prolactin is secreted by the lactotrophs of the anterior pituitary under the neuroendocrine control of hypothalamic prolactin-releasing factors (PRFs) and prolactin-inhibiting factors (PIFs) (Fig. 57.1).

1. Dopamine is the predominant regulator of prolactin release. It traverses the hypothalamic-pituitary portal vasculature and binds to lactotrophs, where it *inhibits* prolactin secretion.
2. Transection or compression of the pituitary stalk *increases* prolactin secretion by interfering with dopaminergic pathways.
3. Prolactin secretion is increased by stress, suckling, sleep, and intercourse.

DIFFERENTIAL DIAGNOSIS

The most common etiologies of galactorrhea are medication-induced and prolactinomas.

1. Associated with hyperprolactinemia
   a. Medications (Table 57.1)
   b. Hypothalamic and infundibular lesions (which inhibit dopamine release increase prolactin through hyperplasia of lactotrophs)
   - Space-occupying lesions (e.g., craniopharyngiomas, meningiomas) and infiltrative disorders (e.g., lymphocytic hypophysitis, sarcoidosis, Langerhans cell histiocytosis, and tuberculosis)
   - Damage to the infundibulum from surgery or head trauma
   c. Pituitary
   - Prolactinomas are benign anterior pituitary neoplasms that secrete prolactin through hyperplasia of lactotrophs
     – Microprolactinomas are <10 mm in diameter
     – Macroprolactinomas are >10 mm in diameter
   - Primary hypothyroidism: Thyrotropin-releasing hormone (TRH) stimulates lactotroph activity
   - Acromegaly: Lactotrophs and somatotrophs have common precursor cells. Prolactin can be directly secreted from a GH-secreting tumor
   - Cushing Disease: Prolactin can also be cosecreted along with adrenocorticotropic hormone (ACTH)
   - Empty Sella Syndrome: Retained lactotrophs have lost dopaminergic inhibition
   d. Idiopathic: 10% of these patients have a prolactinoma that is too small to be visualized on magnetic resonance imaging (MRI)
   e. Extracranial

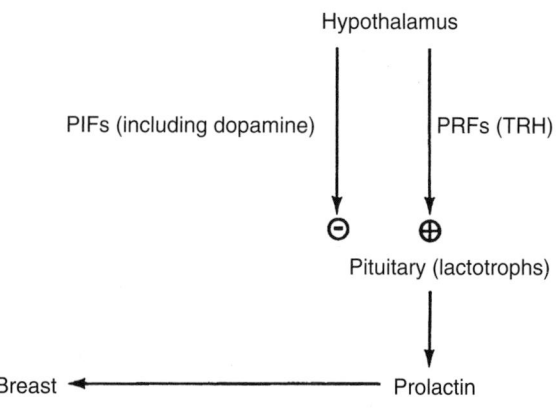

FIGURE 57.1 Schema of prolactin control. PIF, prolactin-inhibiting factors; PRF, prolactin-releasing factors; TRH, thyrotropin-releasing hormone.

TABLE 57.1

Medications Causing Hyperprolactinemia

Antipsychotics	Antihypertensive Agents
Risperidone	Verapamil
Butyrophenones (haloperidol)	α-Methyldopa
Benzamines	Reserpine
Sulpiride	
Thioxanthenes	Gastrointestinal Medications
Phenothiazines	Metoclopramide
	Domperidone
Antidepressants	
Tricyclic antidepressants	Others
Monoamine oxidase inhibitors	Opiates
Elective serotonin reuptake inhibitors	Estrogens

- Neurogenic: Stimulation of the spinal cord (directly or by intercostal nerves) inhibits release of dopamine
  - Chest wall including Surgery, burns, Herpes zoster and Breast stimulation from suckling, self-manipulation, sexual activity, or nipple piercing.
  - Spinal cord injury
- Renal failure: Decreased clearance of prolactin
- Cirrhosis: Decreased dopamine synthesis
- Adrenal insufficiency: Lack of glucocorticoid increases prolactin gene transcription

2. Associated with normal prolactin levels
   a. Women with an unexplained hypersensitivity to prolactin
   b. Acromegaly: growth hormone (GH) is homologous to prolactin and is a potent lactogen

DIAGNOSIS

Given that most of the etiologies of galactorrhea are mediated by elevations in prolactin, the work-up should start with a carefully drawn serum prolactin level.

1. Prolactin is secreted in a pulsatile manner and is augmented by stress, eating, and breast stimulation. Levels should be drawn in the morning in a fasting, nonexercised state without prior breast manipulation (including tight-fitting clothes or physical examination). If results are abnormal, the tests must be repeated.
2. Level of prolactin elevation may be helpful in predicting diagnosis.
   Normal is <25 ng/mL in females and <20 ng/mL in males.
   25 to 150 ng/mL suggests nonprolactin-secreting tumor or dysfunction in dopaminergic pathway.
   150 to 250 ng/mL is indicative of microprolactinoma.
   >250 ng/mL is indicative of macroprolactinoma.
3. Pregnancy, hypothyroidism, estrogen use, and renal failure should always be evaluated first with a blood test for TSH, pregnancy, blood urea nitrogen (BUN), and creatinine.

4. With persistent prolactin elevation, an evaluation should attempt to identify a pharmacological cause. If possible, the offending drug should be changed or discontinued. If prolactin levels fail to decrease by 2 weeks, an intracranial mass should be considered.
   a. Exogenous estrogen (e.g., high-estrogen–content birth control pills) has been linked to mild hyperprolactinemia and galactorrhea. However, oral contraceptive pills that are currently on the market are no longer thought to cause prolactinomas.
   b. Galactorrhea is a common side effect of risperidone and the older antipsychotic agents (see Table 57.1). It occurs less frequently with the atypical antipsychotic agents, such as, clozapine, olanzapine, aripiprazole, quetiapine, and ziprasidone. A trial of one of these drugs is recommended.
5. Any patient with persistent hyperprolactinemia with no known underlying etiology, or prolactin >200 ng/mL, requires an MRI with contrast to evaluate for an intracranial lesion

PROLACTINOMAS

1. Microadenomas, which do not cause any local symptoms have <10% chance of increasing in size, and a 7% risk of progressing to macroprolactinomas. The decision to treat should be based on severity of symptoms and the woman's desire to conceive. Regardless of treatment, serum prolactin levels should be followed closely and an MRI repeated if the prolactin levels increase.
2. If estrogen levels are within the reference range, menses are unaltered, and galactorrhea is tolerable, treatment is not necessary.
3. For restoration of gonadal function and prevention of decreased bone mass, treatment should start with either a dopamine agonist (see "Specific Therapeutic Options and Monitoring" section) or estrogen replacement.
4. If a patient wishes to conceive, initial treatment should be with bromocriptine. Barrier contraceptive should be used until two normal menstrual cycles have occurred, and bromocriptine should be discontinued after the first missed menstrual cycle.
5. Macroadenomas have a significant potential for growth. They can be associated with visual field defects, headaches, neurological deficits, and their compressive mass may lead to the loss of anterior pituitary function.
6. Because of the increased risk of progression, initial treatment with dopamine agonists is recommended. MRI should be done annually or with any increase in symptoms or serum prolactin level.
7. There is a 26% chance of enlargement during pregnancy.
   a. Bromocriptine should be used to induce ovulation, but should be stopped when pregnancy is confirmed.
   b. With suprasellar expansion of the adenoma, tumor debulking should be considered before pregnancy, with postoperative bromocriptine to induce ovulation.
   c. Visual fields and serum prolactin should be evaluated throughout the pregnancy. An MRI is necessary when prolactin increases, there is a loss of visual fields, or headaches ensue. With enlargement, bromocriptine should be restarted.

SPECIFIC THERAPEUTIC OPTIONS AND MONITORING

1. Dopamine agonists decrease prolactin secretion and synthesis.
   a. Bromocriptine
      - Outcome: Between 80% and 90% of patients with microprolactinomas will improve (restoration of menses or normoprolactinemia). In patients with macroprolactinomas, 80% will have a reduction in tumor size, and 80% to 90% will have improved visual fields. Bromocriptine improves, but may not normalize, bone density in amenorrheic and oligomenorrheic patients with osteopenia.
      - Dosing: Bromocriptine has a short half-life and multiple daily doses are necessary to maintain therapeutic levels. Therapy may be started at 1.25 mg at bedtime, and increased to 2.5 to 5 mg twice a day.
      - Side effects: Nausea, vomiting, and dizziness are intolerable in 12% of patients.
      - Pregnancy risk: When bromocriptine is used to restore fertility, and stopped when pregnancy is confirmed, there is no increased risk of spontaneous abortions, ectopic pregnancies, or congenital malformations.
   b. Cabergoline
      - Outcome: Cabergoline has consistently been shown to be as effective as bromocriptine, and may be effective in patients resistant to bromocriptine. It is the drug of choice in large tumors invading vital spaces (cavernous sinus) or compressing optic nerves, where fast-action is required.
      - Dosing: Cabergoline has a long half-life and is given at a dose of 0.5 to 1 mg, 1 to 2 times a week.
      - Side effects: Only 3% of patients are unable to tolerate the drug because of side effects. However, it is considerably more expensive than bromocriptine.
      - Pregnancy risk: Experience is much more limited than for bromocriptine. Although there are no known detrimental fetal effects, current recommendations are to discontinue the drug 1 month before attempting conception.
   c. Pergolide is a dopamine agonist approved in the United States for the treatment of Parkinson disease. It is used outside the United States for treatment of hyperprolactinemia.
2. Transsphenoidal surgery is rarely required, and reserved for patients who are resistant to or intolerant of dopamine-receptor agonists or have invasive macroprolactinomas with compromised vision. Prolactin levels normalize in approximately 70% of patients who have been operated on for microprolactinomas, and in 30% with macroprolactinomas. However, the recurrence risk is 20% to 50%.
3. Radiation has been used rarely in patients with aggressive tumors that do not respond to dopamine agonists or surgery.
4. It is important to evaluate estrogen status in young women with hyperprolactinemia because of the known risk of low bone density associated with the accompanying hypoestrogenic amenorrhea (e.g., using a vaginal smear or progestin challenge). Bone density appears to improve with therapy, but does not return to normal. Fracture risk also appears to be increased in adult patients even before a diagnosis of a prolactinoma is confirmed. Therefore, a baseline bone density measurement should be considered in teenage girls with hyperprolactinemia and amenorrhea.

WEB SITES

For Teenagers and Parents

http://massgeneral.org/pituitary/htm Program's Web site containing patient information on prolactinomas.
http://familydoctor.org/673.xml. American Academy of Family Physicians Web site about galactorrhea.
http://endocrine.niddk.nih.gov/pubs/prolact.htm. National Institutes of Health site on prolactinomas.
http://patients.uptodate.com/topic.asp?file=endo_hor/8753. Up To Date Web site on prolactinomas.
http://www.merck.com/mmhe/sec13/ch162/ch162f.html. Merck manual's website on galactorrhea.

For Health Professionals

http://www.postgradmed.com/issues/2000/06_00/whitman.htm. Web site for physicians on the evaluation of galactorrhea.
http://www.emedicine.com/med/topic1915.htm. E-medicine article discussing prolactinomas.
http://www.mayoclinic.com/health/galactorrhea/DS00761,
http://www.mayoclinic.com/health/prolactinoma/DS00532. Web sites on prolactinoma and galactorrhea from the Mayo Clinic.

REFERENCES AND ADDITIONAL READINGS

Alvarez-Tutor E, Forga-Llenas L, Rodriguez-Erdozain R, et al. Persistent increase of prolactin after oral contraceptive treatment. Alterations in dopaminergic regulation as possible etiology. *Arch Gynecol Obstet* 1999;263:45.
Bankowski B, Zacur HA. Dopamine agonist therapy for hyperprolactinemia. *Clin Obstet Gynecol* 2003;46:349.
Benjamin F. Normal lactation and galactorrhea. *Clin Obstet Gynecol* 1994;37:887.
Biller BM. Diagnostic evaluation of hyperprolactinemia. *J Reprod Med* 1999;44:1095.
Biller BM, Luciano A, Crosignani PG, et al. Guidelines for the diagnosis and treatment of hyperprolactinemia. *J Reprod Med* 1999;44:1075.
Colao A, Loche S, Cappa M, et al. Prolactinomas in children and adolescents. Clinical presentation and long-term follow-up. *J Clin Endocrinol Metab* 1998;83:2777.
Galli-Tsinopoulou A, Nousia-Arvanitakis S, Mitsiakos G, et al. Osteopenia in children and adolescents with hyperprolactinemia. *J Pediatr Endocrinol Metab* 2000;13:439.
Jaquet P. Medical therapy of prolactinomas. *Acta Endocrinol* 1993;129(Suppl 1):31.
Kane LA, Leinung MC, Scheithauer BW, et al. Pituitary adenomas in childhood and adolescence. *J Clin Endocrinol Metab* 1994;79:1135.

Katz E, Adashi EY. Hyperprolactinemia disorders. *Clin Obstet Gynecol* 1990;33:622.

Klibanski A, Biller BMK, Rosenthal DI, et al. Effects of prolactin and estrogen deficiency in amenorrheic bone loss. *J Clin Endocrinol Metab* 1988;67:124.

Klibanski A, Greenspan SL. Increase in bone mass after treatment of hyperprolactinemic amenorrhea. *N Engl J Med* 1986;315:542.

Klibanski A, Zervas NT. Diagnosis and management of hormone-secreting pituitary adenomas. *N Engl J Med* 1991; 324:822.

Leung AKC, Pacaud D. Diagnosis and management of galactorrhea. *Am Acad Fam Physicians* 2004;70(3):543.

Losa M, Mortini P, Barzaghi R, et al. Surgical treatment of prolactin-secreting pituitray adenoma: early results and long-term outcome. *J Clin Endocrinol Metab* 2002;87:3190.

Luciano AA. Clinical presentation of hyperprolactinemia. *J Reprod Med* 1999;44:1085.

McCutcheon IE. Management of individual tumor syndromes. Pituitary neoplasia. *Endocrinol Metab Clin North Am* 1994;23:37.

Modest GA, Fangman JJW. Nipple piercing and hyperprolactinoma. *N Engl J Med* 2002;347:1626.

Molitch ME. Disorders of pituitary secretion. *Endocrinol Metab Clin North Am* 2001;30:585.

Molitch ME. Prolactinoma. In: Melmed S, ed. *The pituitary.* 2002:455.

Molitch ME. Medical management of prolactin-secreting pituitary adenomas. *Pituitary* 2003;5:55.

Molitch MA. Medication-induced hyperprolactinemia. *Mayo Clin Proc* 2005;80(8):1050.

Olive D. Indications for hyperprolactinemia therapy. *J Reprod Med* 1999;44:1091.

Rohn RD. Benign galactorrhea/breast discharge in adolescent males probably due to breast self-manipulation. *J Adolesc Health Care* 1984;5:210.

Scamoni C, Balzarini C, Crivelli G, et al. Treatment and long-term follow-up results of prolactin secreting pituitary adenomas. *J Neurosurg Sci* 1991;35:9.

Schelechte JA. Prolactinoma. *N Engl J Med* 2003;349:2035.

Schlechte J, Walkner L, Kathol M. A longitudinal analysis of premenopausal bone loss in healthy women and women with hyperprolactinemia. *J Clin Endocrinol Metab* 1992;75:698.

Taler SJ, Coulam CB, Annegers JE, et al. Case-control study of galactorrhea and its relationship to the use of oral contraceptives. *Obstet Gynecol* 1985;65:665.

Tyson D, Reggiardo D, Sklar C, et al. Prolactin-secreting macroadenomas in adolescents. Response to bromocriptine therapy. *Am J Dis Child* 1993;147:1057.

Vestegaard P, Jorgensen JO, Hagen C, et al. Fracture risk is increased in patients with GH deficiency or untreated prolactinomas—a case control study. *Clin Endocrinol (Oxf)* 2002;56:159.

Webster J, Piscitelli G, Polli A, et al. A Comparison of cabergoline and bromocriptine in the treatment of hyperprolactinemic amenorrhea. *N Engl J Med* 1994;331:904.

Whitman-Elia GF, Windham NQ. Galactorrhea may be clue to serious problems. Patients deserve a thorough work-up [Review]. *Postgrad Med* 2000;107:165.

Wudarsky M, Nicolson R, Hamburger SD, et al. Elevated prolactin in pediatric patients on typical and atypical antipsychotics. *J Child Adolesc Psychopharmacol* 1999;9: 239.

Yarkony GM, Novick AK, Roth EJ, et al. Galactorrhea: a complication of spinal cord injury. *Arch Phys Med Rehabil* 1992;73:878.

CHAPTER 58

Hirsutism and Virilization

Catherine M. Gordon and Lawrence S. Neinstein

Hirsutism is defined as increased growth of terminal (long, coarse, and pigmented) hair in a young woman, more than is cosmetically acceptable in a certain culture. The condition commonly refers to an increase in length and coarseness of the hair, in a male pattern, including predominantly midline hair of the upper lip, chin, cheeks, inner thighs, lower back, and periareolar, sternal, abdominal, and intergluteal regions. Virilization implies the development of male secondary sexual characteristics in a woman, and may include a deepened voice, increased libido, increased muscle mass, clitoromegaly (>5-mm diameter), temporal balding, and acne. Decreased breast tissue, oligomenorrhea, or amenorrhea may also accompany these physical signs.

Hypertrichosis implies the predominance of excessive vellus hair on the body, particularly the forehead, forearms, and lower legs.

Androgen excess, or hyperandrogenism, results in appearance changes in a young woman and can be associated with abnormal menstrual patterns, infertility, and metabolic disturbances that include decreased high-density lipoprotein cholesterol level, insulin resistance, decreased sex hormone–binding globulin (SHBG), and alterations in the balance between thromboxane and α_2-prostacyclin (Haseltine et al., 1994). Polycystic ovary syndrome (PCOS), a common cause of hyperandrogenism, can increase a patient's risks for developing obesity, type 2 diabetes mellitus, and cardiovascular disease (Gordon, 1999; Ehrmann, 2005; Pfeifer, 2005). These young women can also have increased levels of plasminogen-activator inhibitor-1, which inhibits fibrinolysis and is a risk factor for myocardial infarction (Ehrmann et al., 1997).

Androgen disorders must be evaluated, particularly in female adolescents, because appropriate interventions are now available. The evaluation does not require complicated, expensive procedures; and if untreated, the hyperandrogenism will persist and can lead to excess morbidity and psychosocial dysfunction (Trent et al., 2002). It is also important to delineate the etiology of the hyperandrogenism so that an appropriate management plan can be developed around a specific diagnosis (e.g., PCOS and late-onset congenital adrenal hyperplasia).

HAIR PHYSIOLOGY

Hair grows from follicles that develop at 8 weeks of gestation. All hair follicles are developed in utero, and no new follicles develop during life. The concentration of hair follicles per unit area of skin is similar in males and females, but differs between races and ethnic groups. Whites have a greater concentration than Asians, and Mediterranean individuals have a greater concentration than those of Nordic descent. Hair grows in cycles according to the following phases:

1. Anagen phase: Growing phase
2. Catagen phase: Rapid involution phase
3. Telogen phase: Resting phase

Hair length is determined by the duration of the growing phase. Factors influencing hair growth include the following:

1. Androgens: Androgens initiate hair growth and increase hair diameter and pigmentation. These changes occur secondary to dihydrotestosterone (DHT) conversion of vellus hair to terminal hair. Once hair growth is established, the pattern may continue despite androgen withdrawal, albeit at a slower rate. Once the androgen level is reduced, there may be a lag time of 6 to 9 months before a significant change is noticed, as old terminal hairs fall out and are replaced by new vellus hairs.
2. Estrogens: Estrogens retard initiation and the rate of hair growth, and may prolong the anagen phase.

The effects of sex hormones and other factors on hair development and distribution can be more easily understood by considering the pilosebaceous unit (Fig. 58.1). The clinical manifestations of androgen excess vary depending on end-organ sensitivity to androgens, as is shown. Hirsutism can result either from overproduction or increased sensitivity of hair follicles to androgens (Azziz, 2003). Terminal hair growth is stimulated by the increased conversion of testosterone to DHT from excess 5α-reductase within this unit or the presence of more numerous hair follicles.

ANDROGEN PHYSIOLOGY

Androgens are synthesized from the ovary or adrenals from steroidogenic pathways within each gland (Fig. 58.2).

1. Circulating androgenic steroids in females
   a. 17-Ketosteroids (17-KSs)
      • Dehydroepiandrosterone sulfate (DHEAS)

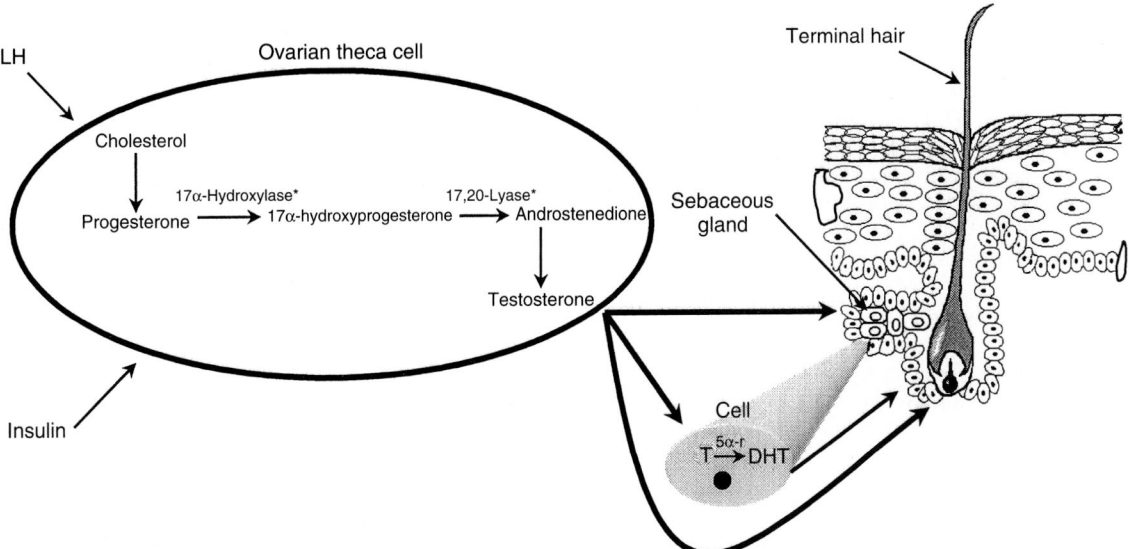

FIGURE 58.1   Effect of ovarian androgens on the pilosebaceous unit. Within the ovarian theca cell, insulin and luteinizing hormone (LH) may stimulate cytochrome P-450c17α activity, resulting in increased 17α-hydroxylase and 17,20-lyase activity, as denoted by *asterisks* above. These two enzymes comprise the P-450c17α complex. Ovarian testosterone, along with dihydrotestosterone (DHT) from 5α-reductase within the pilosebaceous unit, stimulates the androgen receptors at the hair follicle and sebaceous glands. Hirsutism and acne can result. (From Gordon CM. Menstrual disorders in adolescents: excess androgens and the polycystic ovary syndrome. *Pediatr Clin North Am* 1999;46:519–543, with permission.)

- Dehydroepiandrosterone (DHEA)
- Androstenedione
b. 17β-Hydroxysteroids
- Testosterone
- DHT
- Androstenediol
- 3β-Androstenediol

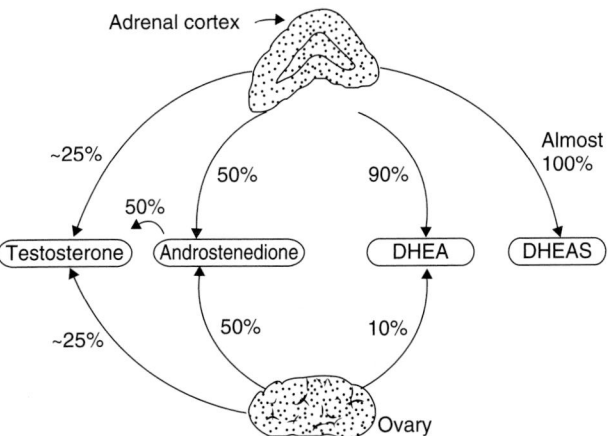

FIGURE 58.2   Sources of androgens in women. DHEA, dehydroepiandrosterone; DHEAS, dehydroepiandrosterone sulfate. (From Emans SJ. Androgen abnormalities in the adolescent girl. In: *Pediatric and adolescent gynecology*, 5th ed. Philadelphia: Lippincott Williams & Wilkins; 2005:301, with permission.)

2. Metabolism: Androgens originate in the adrenal gland and ovaries, either through direct secretion or peripheral conversion of precursors (Fig. 58.2). DHEAS, DHEA, and androstenedione, which are mainly produced in the adrenal gland, exert their androgenic activity after peripheral conversion to testosterone or its metabolites.
   a. Adrenal: Androgens are by-products of cortisol synthesis (Fig. 58.3).
      - 17-KSs: Most of the 17-KSs are generated from adrenal sources. This includes a daily secretion of 7 mg of DHEAS (90% of total daily secretion), 5.5 mg of DHEA, and 1.8 mg of androstenedione (50% of total daily secretion). All of these compounds have low androgenic activity because they are precursors of testosterone.
      - Testosterone: Twenty-five percent is derived from adrenal secretion, or a total of 0.06 mg/day is secreted from the adrenal gland. Testosterone is a potent androgen, although the most potent androgen is DHT, formed after conversion by 5α-reductase.
   b. Ovarian: Androgens from the ovary are metabolized as intermediates in the production of estrogen and progesterone. Androgenic hormones secreted by the ovary include the following (Fig. 58.2):
      - Testosterone: Approximately 25% of total daily secretion (0.06 mg/day)
      - Androstenedione: Approximately 50% of total daily secretion (1.7 mg/day)
   c. Peripheral conversion: Approximately 50% of testosterone is derived from peripheral conversion of androstenedione in liver, fat, and skin cells.

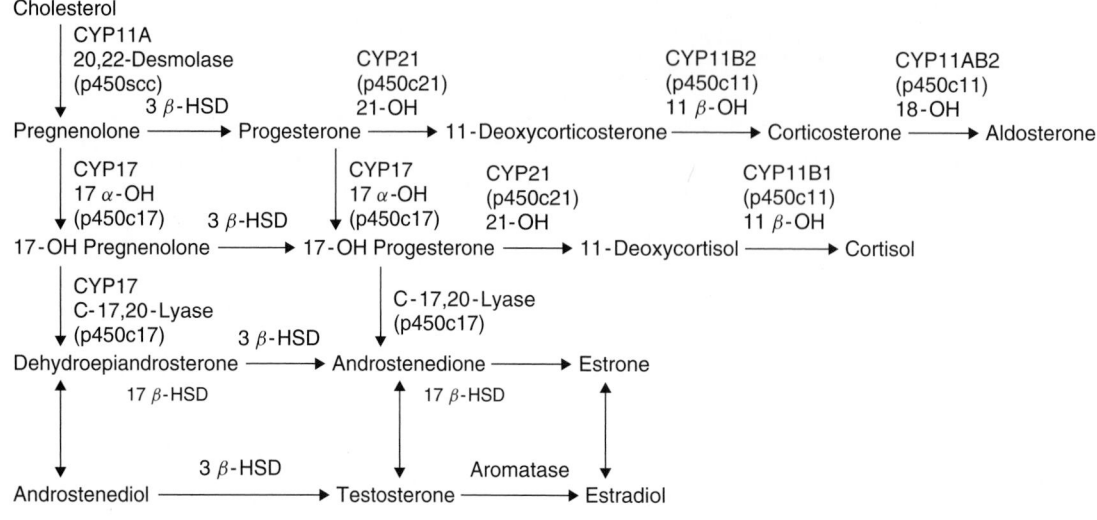

FIGURE 58.3 Major pathways of steroid biosynthesis. 21-OH, 21-hydroxylase; 11β-OH, 11β-hydroxylase; 18-OH, 18-hydroxylase; 3β-HSD, 3β-hydroxysteroid dehydrogenase; 17β-HSD, 17β-hydroxysteroid dehydrogenase (17-ketosteroid reductase); 17β-OH, 17-β hydroxylase; C-17,20 lyase also termed 17,20 desmolase. (From: Emans SJ. Androgen abnormalities in the adolescent girl. In: *Pediatric and adolescent gynecology*, 5th ed. Philadelphia: Lippincott Williams & Wilkins; 2005:312, with permission.)

d. Testosterone is 95.5% bound to SHBG in females; only the free portion is active. During pregnancy, approximately 99% is bound. In healthy males, 92.8% of testosterone is bound.

DIFFERENTIAL DIAGNOSIS

The relative prevalence of hirsutism is presented in Table 58.1 (Curran et al., 2005), with data obtained from an original sample of more than 1,000 women (Azziz et al., 2004). Note that PCOS is the most common cause of androgen excess and one of the most common endocrine abnormalities in female adolescents and young women.

1. Idiopathic hirsutism: As the pathophysiology behind specific causes of hyperandrogenism is better delineated, the percentage of hirsute women with idiopathic hirsutism has continued to fall. This diagnosis represents between 4% and 15% of hirsute women (Azziz, 2003; Curran et al., 2005).
2. Ovarian causes
   a. PCOS or functional ovarian hyperandrogenism (see Chapter 52), with or without insulin resistance
   b. Tumor: Sertoli-Leydig cell tumor, lipoid cell tumor, hilar cell tumor
   c. Pregnancy: Luteoma
3. Adrenal causes
   a. Congenital adrenal hyperplasia: 21-hydroxylase or 11-hydroxylase deficiency, classic or nonclassic, late onset
   b. Tumors: Adenomas and carcinomas
   c. Cushing syndrome
4. Nonandrogenic causes of hirsutism
   a. Genetic: Racial, familial
   b. Physiological: Pregnancy, puberty, postmenopausal
   c. Endocrine: Hypothyroidism, acromegaly

d. Porphyria
e. Hamartomas
f. Drug-induced: Drugs that cause hirsutism by increasing androgenic activity include testosterone, DHEAS, danazol, corticotropin, high-dose corticosteroids, metyrapone, phenothiazine derivatives, anabolic steroids, androgenic progestin, and acetazolamide. Nonandrogenic drugs that can cause hirsutism include cyclosporine, phenytoin, diazoxide, triamterene-hydrochlorothiazide, minoxidil, hexachlorobenzene, penicillamine and psoralens, and minoxidil. Valproate is also associated with menstrual disturbances and hyperandrogenism (Isojarvi et al., 1993).
g. Central nervous system lesions: Multiple sclerosis, encephalitis
h. Congenital lesions: Hurler syndrome, de Lange syndrome

DIAGNOSIS

Indications for Evaluation

1. Rapid onset of signs and symptoms
2. Virilization
3. Onset of hirsutism or virilism that is not peripubertal
4. Symptoms suggesting Cushing syndrome (e.g., weight gain, weakness, or hypertension)

Consider hyperandrogenism in any female with premature pubarche, severe acne, hirsutism, or androgenetic alopecia. Girls with premature pubarche are at higher risk to develop PCOS and metabolic syndrome during adolescence (Ibanez et al., 2000). Insulin resistance can accompany the clinical picture with the potential to alter lipid profiles and glucose.

TABLE 58.1

Differential Diagnosis of Clinically Apparent Androgen Excess

Diagnosis	Sample (%)	Key History/Examination Findings	Additional Testing
Polycystic ovary syndrome (PCOS)	82.0	±Irregular menses, slow-onset hirsutism, obesity, infertility, diabetes, hypertension, family history of PCOS, diabetes	Fasting glucose, insulin and lipid profile, blood pressure (BP), ultrasonography positive for multiple ovarian cysts
Hyperandrogenism with hirsutism, normal ovulation	6.8	Regular menses, acne, hirsutism without detectable endocrine cause	Elevated androgen levels and normal serum progesterone in luteal phase
Idiopathic hirsutism	4.7	Regular menses, hirsutism, possible overactive 5 α-reductase activity in skin and hair follicle	Normal androgen levels, normal serum progesterone in luteal phase
Hyperandrogenic insulin-resistant acanthosis nigricans (HAIR-AN)	3.1	Brown velvety patches of skin (acanthosis nigricans), obesity, hypertension, hyperlipidemia, strong family history of diabetes	Fasting glucose and lipid profile, BP, fasting insulin level >80 μIU/mL or insulin level >300 on 3-hr glucose tolerance test
21-Hydroxylase nonclassic adrenal hyperplasia (late-onset CAH)	1.6	Severe hirsutism or virilization, strong family history of CAH, short stature, signs of defeminization, more common in Ashkenazi Jews and Eastern European decent	17-HP level before and after ACTH stimulation test >10 ng/dL, CYP21 genotyping
21-Hydroxylase nondeficient congenital adrenal hyperplasia	0.7	See late-onset CAH Congenital virilization	17-HP levels >30 ng/dL
Hypothyroidism	0.7	Fatigue, weight gain, history of thyroid ablation and untreated hypothyroidism, amenorrhea	TSH
Hyperprolactinemia	0.3	Amenorrhea, galactorrhea, infertility	Prolactin
Androgenic secreting neoplasm	0.2	Pelvic masses, rapid-onset hirsutism or virilization	Pelvic ultrasonography or abdomen/pelvic CT scan
Cushing syndrome	0	Hypertension, buffalo hump, purple striae, truncal obesity	Elevated BP, positive dexamethasone suppression test

ACTH, adrenocorticotropic hormone; TSH, thyroid-stimulating hormone; CT, computed tomography.
The causes of clinically apparent hyperandrogenism were evaluated in 1,281 consecutive patients presenting to a university endocrinology clinic (Azziz et al., 2004). The investigators excluded 408 women because of the inability to assess hormonal or ovulatory status. Of the remaining 873 women, 75.5% had hirsutism and 77.8%, hyperandrogenemia. The majority had PCOS, as shown.
Adapted from Curran DR, Moore C. What is the best approach to the evaluation of hirsutism? *J Fam Prac* 2005;54:465, with permission.

History

1. Menstrual history, evaluating for amenorrhea or oligomenorrhea
2. Drug history
3. Ethnic background and family history of hirsutism, irregular menses, infertility, miscarriages, type 2 diabetes mellitus
4. Rapidity of androgenizing or virilizing symptoms and signs: Most women with an androgen-producing ovarian or adrenal tumor have rapid onset of virilization.

Physical Examination

1. Extent of hirsutism: Grading systems are available that enable a clinician to quantitate the degree of hirsutism in a patient. One method is illustrated and discussed by Hatch et al. (1981), based on grading the nine areas of the body from 1 to 4. The Ferriman-Gallwey hirsutism scoring system (Ferriman and Gallwey, 1961) is another frequently used system that enables clinicians to quantify the extent of hirsutism by circling an individual's appearance on a flow sheet and recording the total score on the patient's chart. These scores can be helpful for making comparative assessments between visits and for appraising the efficacy of a particular therapy. Some terminal hair on the lower abdomen, face, and around the areola is normal, but hair on the upper back, shoulders, sternum, and upper abdomen suggests more marked androgen activity.
2. Stigmata of Cushing syndrome (e.g., truncal obesity, striae, posterior fat pad)

3. Signs of virilization: Check clitoral diameter or index. A clitoral diameter >5 mm is abnormal and is a measurement that can be easily followed up. The clitoral index is the product of the vertical and horizontal dimensions of the glans. The normal range is 9 to 35 mm^2; a clitoral index >100 mm^2 suggests a serious underlying disorder.
4. Presence of ovarian or adrenal masses.
5. Evidence of insulin resistance (e.g., acanthosis nigricans, as is seen in patients with PCOS).

Laboratory Evaluation

The goals of the laboratory evaluation include demonstrating androgen excess and locating the source of the excess.

1. Measuring androgen excess
   a. Plasma testosterone is the most important measurement, although this is a subject of debate in the diagnostic work-up of these patients. Levels >150 to 200 ng/dL suggest significant hyperandrogenism and potentially, severe disease.
   b. Other important indicators
      - DHEAS: Levels >700 µg/dL suggest significant adrenal androgen production. An adrenal tumor must be ruled out. Rarely, PCOS, congenital adrenal hyperplasia, or an ovarian tumor will result in levels this high.
      - 17-Hydroxyprogesterone (17-OHP): This hormone should only be measured in the morning (ideally between 7 and 9 a.m.). This is characteristically elevated in patients with congenital adrenal hyperplasia due to 21-hydroxylase deficiency. One can also measure 11-deoxycortisol in the morning to rule out 11-hydroxylase deficiency.
      - Free testosterone: Free testosterone may be elevated in the presence of normal total testosterone. However, free testosterone will be elevated in the presence of hirsutism, so it is not a specific test. Total testosterone tests are less expensive and may be sufficient to point the diagnosis toward an ovarian cause.
   c. 17-KS: This is a nonspecific test, because some 17-KSs are nonandrogenic and the potent 17β-hydroxysteroids are not measured.
   d. If the teen has either amenorrhea or oligomenorrhea, prolactin and thyroid-stimulating hormone should be measured and a pregnancy test performed.

      Overall, in most individuals minimal laboratory testing is necessary because of the complete response to combination oral contraceptives, with or without spironolactone. This includes a total testosterone determination to eliminate the rare individual with a testosterone-secreting tumor. A baseline early morning level of 17-OHP is useful. DHEAS is also usually measured, but in many instances, a moderate increase is found in women with anovulation who have no adrenal disease.
2. Locating the source of androgen excess
   a. If male levels of testosterone are obtained or a mass is felt on examination, perform an ultrasonography or computed tomography (CT) scan of adrenal glands and ovaries. Markedly elevated serum testosterone and DHEAS levels suggest an adrenal tumor and the need for a CT scan, whereas markedly elevated serum testosterone and normal DHEAS levels suggest an ovarian source and the need for ultrasonography of the ovaries.
   b. If any of the androgens' levels are elevated or signs suggest hypercortisolism, perform a dexamethasone suppression test.
      - An ovarian source is suggested by cortisol suppression, but a lack of androgen suppression. An ultrasonography of the ovaries is helpful in this instance.
      - Both adrenogenital syndrome and idiopathic hirsutism are suggested by suppression of cortisol and androgens after dexamethasone administration.
      - Cushing syndrome or an adrenal tumor is suggested by lack of cortisol suppression.
      Indicators of suppression after dexamethasone (0.5 mg q.i.d. for 5 to 7 days)
         – Free testosterone level <8 pg/mL
         – Total testosterone level <58 ng/dL
         – Free plasma 17β-hydroxysteroid level <42 pg/mL
         – Decrease in DHEAS level of at least 50%
   c. If 17-OHP level is elevated, perform an adrenocorticotropic hormone (ACTH) stimulation test. This is helpful in differentiating normal and idiopathic hirsute females from those with late-onset congenital adrenal hyperplasia due to incomplete 21-hydroxylase deficiency.

      To perform the test measure a baseline 17-OHP and repeat a serum level 60 minutes after 0.25 mg of ACTH is administered intravenously. In a positive result, there is an increase in the serum level to >30 ng/mL, whereas in normal or idiopathic hirsute females, the levels are usually <5 ng/mL. This test can also be used to rule out less common forms of late-onset congenital adrenal hyperplasia due to 11-hydroxylase or 3β-hydroxysteroid dehydrogenase deficiency.
3. Specific diagnoses
   a. Idiopathic hirsutism: These women generally ovulate regularly and have normal levels of androgens. 5α-reductase activity in the skin and follicle appears to be overactive in these young women, leading to hirsutism in the face of normal androgen (Azziz, 2003). The definitive underlying mechanism remains to be identified, with the following other possible causes of androgen excess:
      - Altered gonadotropin secretory patterns
      - Exaggerated adrenal androgen secretion
      - Increased prolactin levels, augmenting adrenal androgen secretion
      - Alteration of SHBG (decreased SHBG level, resulting in mild elevation of free testosterone level)
      - Obesity
      - Hyperinsulinism
   b. Ovarian tumors
      - Palpable adnexal mass
      - Testosterone level >200 ng/mL
      - Nonsuppression of androgens after dexamethasone
   c. PCOS or functional ovarian hyperandrogenism (see Chapter 52)
      - Hirsutism, infertility, menstrual irregularities, obesity
      - Elevations in androgen levels (free and/or total testosterone; 50% or more may also have an elevated DHEAS level)
      - Increase in luteinizing hormone (LH) level and LH: follicle stimulating hormone (FSH) ratio. LH and FSH have been suggested as markers for PCOS

with a high LH and low-normal FSH level (ratio >3:1), but this test is neither sensitive nor specific, because only approximately 50% of patients with PCOS exhibit these abnormalities.
- Adolescent girls with severe acne: High incidence of PCOS

d. Congenital adrenal hyperplasia: Elevated 17-OHP, with large increase after ACTH administration is diagnostic of incomplete 21-hydroxylase deficiency. This condition is often recognized during adolescence with presentation similar to PCOS syndrome. Elevated 11-deoxycortisol or DHEAS and 17-hydroxypregnenolone levels are found in 11-hydroxylase and 3β-hydroxysteroid dehydrogenase deficiencies.

e. Adrenal tumors
- Androgen-secreting tumors: Rare and associated with rapid defeminization
- Adrenal mass: Palpable in many individuals
- Elevated 17-KS, DHEAS, and DHEA levels
- Subnormal suppression with dexamethasone administration
- Mass on ultrasonography, intravenous pyelogram, or CT scan

f. Drug-induced hirsutism: The cause of nonandrogen drug-induced hirsutism is not well understood. The pattern is not restricted to androgen-dependent areas, and the hair is usually vellus in nature.

g. Anabolic steroid abuse

h. Hyperandrogenic insulin-resistant acanthosis nigricans (HAIR-AN) syndrome: This includes the following characteristic features: *h*yper *a*ndrogenism, *i*nsulin *r*esistance, and *a*canthosis *n*igricans. This syndrome may lead to the clinical and metabolic features of PCOS, as well as myocardial hypertrophy. Insulin receptor mutations, circulating antibodies to the insulin receptor, and postreceptor signaling defects have been described in variants of this syndrome. These individuals have fasting basal insulin levels of >80 μU/mL compared with reference-range levels of approximately 7 to 8 μU/mL, as well as peaks of >1,000 μU/mL compared with approximately 60 μU/mL in healthy individuals.

THERAPY

1. Tumor: Remove the androgen source
2. Drug-induced: Stop medication
3. Congenital adrenal hyperplasia: Replace cortisol and suppressive adrenal androgen precursors with oral hydrocortisone or prednisone. In rare instances, use low-dose dexamethasone (0.25 mg q.d.). Oral contraceptives may also be used to regulate menstrual bleeding and provide contraception.
4. Functional ovarian hyperandrogenism (e.g., PCOS): Multi-faceted treatment directed at individual problems (e.g., hirsutism, menstrual irregularity, insulin resistance, hyperlipidemia, obesity)
5. Specific therapies (hyperandrogenism)
a. Hirsutism
- Cosmetic approaches: Standard treatments include camouflaging with heavy make-up, bleaching, and removal with physical methods such as rubbing, cutting, shaving, plucking, or waxing. Chemical depilatories are designed to use on specific body locations. Most of these methods last from hours to days. Electrolysis or thermodestruction of the hair follicle retards regrowth for days to weeks and can permanently remove hair. Electrolysis can be expensive, time-consuming, and uncomfortable. Photothermodestruction with a laser is a new hair-removal technique. It is expensive but can offer long periods between regrowth and can lead to permanent hair loss. All of these methods can cause skin irritation, folliculitis, and pigment abnormalities.
- Topical therapy: Eflornithine hydrochloride 13.9% cream has been approved by the U.S. Food and Drug Administration (FDA) for the treatment of unwanted facial hair. The agent is an irreversible inhibitor of L-ornithine decarboxylase, an enzyme that is important in controlling hair growth and proliferation. The agent slows and miniaturizes hairs that are present. Side effects are mild, including rash and stinging, and occur in <10% of patients (Balfour and McClellan, 2001).
- Weight loss: Weight loss in obese girls with PCOS and hirsutism can reduce hirsutism. Weight loss reduces insulin resistance and therefore insulin levels, thereby reducing testosterone secretion.
- Estrogen/progestins: Oral contraceptives work in 60% to 100% of hirsute girls. Medical therapy is slow and requires 6 to 12 months before physical changes are evident. Lag time occurs because of the delay before terminal hair falls out and is replaced by thinner less-pigmented hair. Combination pills that contain low androgenic progestins, such as norethindrone or norgestimate, are optimally used. Oral contraceptives also provide contraception for women who are on other antiandrogenic medications that may be teratogenic. Combinations of oral contraceptives and antiandrogenic medications may enhance therapeutic effectiveness and prolong remission. A new estroprogestinic preparation is available containing the antimineralocorticoid progestin drospirenone and 30-μg ethinyl estradiol. In one study, hirsutism improved from the 6th cycle onward (Guido, 2004). All oral contraceptives decrease androgen production in the following ways:
  - Lowering LH levels, thus decreasing androgen production
  - Increasing SHBG, thereby lowering free androgens
  - Decreasing adrenal androgen production
  - Decreasing 5α-reductase activity
  The above is an off-label use of oral contraceptives.
- Antiandrogenic agents: Antiandrogenic agents include drugs that block androgen cytochrome P-450 receptors, resulting in decreased testosterone, DHT, and DHEAS levels; and drugs that inhibit 5α-reductase, reducing conversion of testosterone to DHT. Spironolactone and cyproterone acetate (investigational) have been used. Spironolactone works primarily by competing at the androgen receptor peripherally, and also inhibits 5α-reductase. The starting dose is usually 50 mg/day and is typically effective between approximately 75 and 200 mg/day. The medication can be increased by 25 mg every 1 to 2 weeks. However, the maximal response is not seen for 6 months to 1 year. Side effects are minimal but can include dry mouth,

diuresis, fatigue, and menstrual spotting, and hyperkalemia on laboratory evaluation. The drug is contraindicated during pregnancy, because it can lead to feminization of the male fetus. Therefore, an oral contraceptive should be prescribed simultaneously. In Europe, flutamide (a nonsteroidal antiandrogen) and 5α-reductase inhibitors (such as finasteride) have been used, but reports of severe hepatotoxicity prohibit its use in teenagers.
- Combination therapy: The combination of low-dose oral contraceptives and spironolactone is very effective.
- Future directions: Therapies will probably include more widespread use of insulin-sensitizing agents, inhibitors of the enzyme 5α-reductase, and long-acting gonadotropin-releasing hormone (GnRH) agonists. The efficacy of insulin-sensitizing agents (e.g., metformin) in patients with PCOS is an area of intensive research, and efficacy and safety data from adolescent studies to date have been encouraging (Arslanian et al., 2002). One study of women showed effective treatment of moderate to severe hirsutism after 12 months of metformin (Harborne, et al., 2003). GnRH agonists are alternative agents for patients with PCOS, but should be reserved for severe cases of hyperandrogenism, because they are fraught with adverse side effects. Carr et al. (1995) compared the use of oral contraceptives alone, GnRH agonists alone, or the two in combination. They found that by 6 months, measurements of hirsutism were not different between the groups. GnRH agonists alone had a negative impact on bone density. For this reason, GnRH agonists are used only rarely in young women with PCOS.
b. Menstrual abnormality
- Cyclic progestin
- Combined oral contraceptives
c. Infertility (referral to infertility specialist)
- Clomiphene citrate
- Dexamethasone
- Human chorionic gonadotropin
- Insulin-sensitizing agents plus/minus clomiphene citrate (their use in adolescents is currently experimental

WEB SITES

For Teenagers and Parents

http://www.obgyn.net/pcos/articles/hairissue_article.htm. OB-GYN net handout on hirsutism.

http://www.pcosupport.org. PCOS Association Web site includes facts and figures on PCOS, as well as on-line support.

http://www.obgyn.net/pcos/pcos.asp. PCOS Pavilion.

http://www.pcosupport.org/proteen. PCO Teenlist home page is dedicated to teenagers with PCOS. Includes a chat room and bulletin board so teens can share their thoughts on the disease.

http://www.noah-health.org/en/endocrine/endocrine/hirsutism.html. New York On-line Access to Health list of resources for hirsutism information.

http://www.hormone.org/Public/polycystic.cfm. A helpful overview of PCOS, including treatment options. Developed by the professional organization, The Endocrine Society.

http://www.youngwomenshealth.org/pcosinfo.html. A teen-friendly Web site developed at Children's Hospital Boston that is written using terminology that adolescents can easily understand.

For Health Professionals

http://www.postgradmed.com/issues/2000/06_00/bergfeld.htm. Postgraduate Medicine symposium on hirsutism.

REFERENCES AND ADDITIONAL READINGS

Alonso LC, Rosenfield RL. Molecular genetic and endocrine mechanisms of hair growth. *Horm Res* 2003;60:1.

American College of Obstetricians and Gynecologists. Hyperandrogenic chronic anovulation [Technical Bulletin, no 202, February 1995]. Committee on Technical Bulletins of the American College of Obstetricians and Gynecologists. *Int J Gynaecol Obstet* 1995;49:201.

Arslanian SA, Lewy V, Danadian K, et al. Metformin therapy in obese adolescents with polycystic ovary syndrome and impaired glucose response. *J Clin Endocrinol Metab* 2002; 87:1555.

Azziz R. The evaluation and management of hirsutism. *Obstet Gynecol* 2003;101:995.

Azziz R, Sanchez A, Knochenhauer ES, et al. Androgen excess in women: experience with over 1000 consecutive patients. *J Clin Endocrinol Metab* 2004;89:453.

Balfour JA, McClellan K. Topical eflornithine. *Am J Clin Dermatol* 2001;2:197.

Barth JH. How hairy are hirsute women? *Clin Endocrinol* 1997; 47:255.

Bergfeld WF. Hirsutism in women. Effective therapy that is safe for long-term use. *Postgrad Med* 2000;107:93.

Burkman RT Jr. The role of oral contraceptives in the treatment of hyperandrogenic disorders. *Am J Med* 1995;98:130S.

Carr BR. Disorders of the ovary and female reproductive tract. In: Wilson JD, Foster DW, eds. *Williams textbook of endocrinology*, 8th ed. Philadelphia: WB Saunders; 1992.

Carr BR, Breslau NA, Givens C, et al. Oral contraceptive pills, gonadotropin-releasing hormone agonists, or use in combination for treatment of hirsutism: a clinical research center study. *J Clin Endocrinol Metab* 1995;80:1169.

Chetkowski RJ, DeFrazid J, Shamonki L, et al. The incidence of late-onset congenital adrenal hyperplasia due to 21-hydroxylase deficiency among hirsute women. *J Clin Endocrinol Metab* 1984;58:595.

Chang RJ. A practical approach to the diagnosis of polycystic ovary syndrome. *Am J Obstet Gynecol* 2004;191:713.

Curran DR, Moore C, Huber T. Clinical inquiries. What is the best approach to the evaluation of hirsutism? *J Fam Pract* 2005;54:465.

Ehrmann DA. Polycystic ovary syndrome. *N Engl J Med* 2005;352(12):1223.

Ehrmann D, Schneider DJ, Sobel BE, et al. Troglitazone improves defects in insulin action, insulin secretion, ovarian steroidogenesis and fibrinolysis in women with polycystic ovary syndrome. *J Clin Endocrinol Metab* 1997;82:2108.

Emans SJ. Androgen abnormalities in the adolescent girl. In: Emans SJ, Laufer MR, Goldstein DP, eds. *Pediatric and adolescent gynecology.* Philadelphia: Lippincott Williams & Wilkins; 2005.

Ferriman D, Gallwey JD. Clinical assessment of body hair growth in women. *J Clin Endocrinol Metab* 1961;21:1440.

Gordon CM. Menstrual disorders in adolescents: excess androgens and the polycystic ovary syndrome. *Pediatr Clin North Am* 1999;46:519.

Guido M, Romualdi D, Giuliani M, et al. Drospirenone for the treatment of hirsute women with polycystic ovary syndrome: a clinical, endocrinological, metabolic pilot study. *J Clin Endocrinol Metab* 2004;89(6):2817.

Hammond MG, Talbert LM, Groff TR. Hyperandrogenism. *Postgrad Med* 1986;79:107.

Harborne L, Fleming R, Lyall H, et al. Metformin or antiandrogen in the treatment of hirsutism in polycystic syndrome. *J Clin Endocrinol Metab* 2003;88:4116.

Haseltine F, Wentz AC, Redmond GP, et al. Androgens and women's health: NICHD conference. *Clinician* 1994;12:3.

Hatch R, Rosenfield RL, Kim MH, et al. Hirsutism: implications, etiology, and management. *Am J Obstet Gynecol* 1981;140:815.

Herter LD, Magalhaes JA, Spritzer PM. Association of ovarian volume and serum LH levels in adolescent patients with menstrual disorders and/or hirsutism. *Braz J Med Biol Res* 1993;26:1041.

van Hooff MH, Voorhorst FJ, Kaptein MB, et al. Polycystic ovaries in adolescents and the relationship with menstrual cycle patterns, luteinizing hormone, androgens, and insulin. *Fertil Steril* 2000;74:49.

Hunter MH, Carek PJ. Evaluation and treatment of women with hirsutism. *Am Fam Physician* 2003;67:2565.

Huppert J, Chiodi M, Hillard PJ. Clinical and metabolic findings in adolescent females with hyperandrogenism. *J Pediatr Adolesc Gynecol* 2004;17:103.

Ibanez L, Dimartino-Nardi J, Potau N, et al. Premature adrenarche—normal variant or forerunner of adult disease. *Endocr Rev* 2000;21(6):671.

Isojarvi JI, Laatikainen TJ, Pakarinen AJ. Polycystic ovaries and hyperandrogenism in women taking valproate for epilepsy. *N Engl J Med* 1993;329:1383.

Jahanfar S, Eden JA. Idiopathic hirsutism or polycystic ovary syndrome. *Aust N Z J Obstet Gynaecol* 1993;33:414.

Kahn JA, Gordon CM. Polycystic ovary syndrome. *Adolesc Med* 1999;10:321.

Kustin J, Rebar RW. Hirsutism in young adolescent girls. *Pediatr Ann* 1986;15:522.

Lobo RA, Goebelsman V. Adult manifestation of congenital adrenal hyperplasia due to incomplete 21-hydroxylase deficiency mimicking polycystic ovarian disease. *Am J Obstet Gynecol* 1980;138:720.

Lucky AW. Hormonal correlates of acne and hirsutism. *Am J Med* 1995;98(Suppl 1A):89S.

Marshburn PB, Carr BR. Hirsutism and virilization. A systematic approach to benign and potentially serious causes. *Postgrad Med* 1995;97:99.

Morris DV. Hirsutism. *Clin Obstet Gynecol* 1985;12:649.

Nestler JE, Jakubowizc DJ. Decreases in ovarian cytochrome P450c17α activity and serum free testosterone after reduction of insulin secretion in polycystic ovary syndrome. *N Engl J Med* 1996;335:617.

Neithardt AB, Barnes RB. The diagnosis and management of hirsutism. *Semin Reprod Med* 2003;21:285.

Pfeifer SM. Polycystic ovary syndrome in adolescent girls. *Semin Pediatr Surg* 2005;14:111.

Plouffe L Jr. Disorders of excessive hair growth in the adolescent. *Obstet Gynecol Clin North Am* 2000;27:79.

Redmond GP. Androgenic disorders of women: diagnostic and therapeutic decision making. *Am J Med* 1995;98:1205.

Richards RN, Meharg GE. Electrolysis: observations from 13 years and 140,000 hours of experience. *J Am Acad Dermatol* 1995;33:662.

Rittmaster RS. Clinical relevance of testosterone and dihydrotestosterone metabolism in women. *Am J Med* 1995a;98:17S.

Rittmaster RS. Clinical review 73: medical treatment of androgen-dependent hirsutism. *J Clin Endocrinol Metab* 1995b;80:2559.

Rosenfield RI, Lucky AW. Acne, hirsutism, and alopecia in adolescent girls. Clinical expressions of androgen excess. *Endocrinol Metab Clin North Am* 1993;22:507.

Sane K, Pescovitz OH. The clitoral index: a determination of clitoral size in normal girls and girls with abnormal sexual development. *J Pediatr* 1992;120:265.

Trent ME, Rich M, Austin SB, et al. Quality of life in girls with polycystic ovary syndrome. *Arch Pediatr Adolesc Med* 2002;156:556.

Vetr M, Sobek A. Low dose spironolactone in the treatment of female hyperandrogenemia and hirsutism. *Acta Univ Palacki Olomuc Fac Med* 1993;135:55.

Wild RA. Obesity lipids, cardiovascular risk, and androgen excess. *Am J Med* 1995;98:275.

Wild RA, Demers LM, Applebaum-Bowden D, et al. Hirsutism: metabolic effects of two commonly used oral contraceptives and spironolactone. *Contraception* 1991;44:113.

CHAPTER 59

Breast Disorders

Heather R. Macdonald

Adolescence is a time of significant physiological and psychological changes for young adults. Many of these changes center around a patient's developing reproductive capability. Although serious breast disorders are rare in this age-group, breast complaints and anxieties regarding normal development are common. To identify breast pathology, and reassure patients concerned about normal breast development, health care providers must understand normal breast development and its variations, common breast complaints, and warning signs of serious disease. Equally important is sensitivity to the complex emotions these physical changes can illicit in a teenage patient. In the course of evaluating and treating a breast complaint or disorder, her or his feelings and anxieties should be addressed. Table 59.1 lists common breast complaints in adolescence.

NORMAL DEVELOPMENT

Breast tissue begins as ectoderm-derived mammary bands apparent in embryos 4 mm in length (Rebar, 1999). By 4 weeks of embryonic life or 7 mm in embryonic length, breast tissue has coalesced into a ridge (*mammary crest* or *milk line*) running from the axilla to inguinal region along each ventrolateral side of the body wall. The thoracic part of this ridge thickens to form the primordial mammary buds by 10 to 12 mm in embryonic length as the caudal ridges regress. By the 6 to 12 weeks, the nipple and areola form over the breast buds.

Breast development remains quiescent until the fifth gestational month when the primitive mammary bud forms 15 to 25 secondary buds that will eventually develop into the ductal system of the mature breast, with each duct opening separately into the nipple. As the secondary buds elongate to form cords and then lumen within cords, two types of epithelial cells become evident—a secretory inner layer and myoepithelial outer layer. By the time of birth, these epithelial ducts will have undergone limited proliferation, likely due to maternal hormones in the fetal circulation as pregnancy reaches term. Breast glands in newborns are still rudimentary, but can respond to high maternal prolactin levels at birth and secrete "witch's milk," a natural phenomenon. Parents should be discouraged from expressing the milky discharge as repeated stimulation encourages production

and delays resolution. The discharge and associated breast enlargement is self-limiting, if left alone.

Common breast complaints in adolescents are outlined in Table 59.1. Occasionally, a prepubertal boy or girl can present with a breast "mass." Physical examination finds a soft mobile nodule behind one or both areolas, and no signs of pubertal initiation. This prepubertal breast enlargement is not a cause for concern and resolves spontaneously. Excisional biopsy of these masses is not indicated because removal of the child's breast bud will prevent normal breast development. The child may be monitored for signs of precocious puberty, but no other further action should be taken.

Until puberty, male and female breast development is equivalent. Puberty is a complex endocrinological event involving multiple hormones and varying classes of receptors. At puberty, a different hormonal milieu develops in boys and girls. Figures 1.5 and 1.10 demonstrate the stages of breast development as described by Tanner. The first sign of puberty is accelerated growth followed by thelarche, the onset of secondary breast development. Normal and abnormal pubertal development including breast development is discussed in Chapters 1 and 8.

Anatomy

The milk-producing alveolus, or terminal duct, is the primary unit of the breast and it drains through a branching duct system to the nipple. Each lobule consists

TABLE 59.1

Common Breast Complaints in Adolescents

Congenital Anomalies	Disorders of Development	Benign Breast Disease
Polythelia	Asymmetry	Mastalgia
Polymastia	Macromastia	Nipple discharge
Supernumerary breast	Hypoplasia	Mastitis
Amastia	Tuberous breast deformity	Abscess
Inverted nipple	Gynecomastia	Mass

of approximately 10 to 100 alveoli and the lobules drain into lactiferous ducts that merge to form a sinus beneath the nipple. The stroma, consisting of fibrous tissue, surrounds and supports the lobules and ducts. Other structures in the breast are lymphatics, fat tissue, and nerves. Most benign breast diseases and almost all breast cancers begin within the terminal duct lobular unit. In pubertal females, circulating estrogens, estradiol in particular, stimulate duct development whereas progesterone influences lobular and alveolar development.

Women of reproductive age tend to have breasts that have a nodular texture representing the glandular units or lobules of the breast. During each menstrual cycle, these units undergo proliferative changes under hormonal stimulation. This nodularity can increase, particularly with lobular enlargement and edema that may occur toward the end of menstrual cycles. This process may vary from a feeling of breast fullness to distinct masses suggestive of a pathological process.

CONGENITAL ANOMALIES

Aberrant Breast Tissue

Failure of the primordial milk crest to regress leads to the persistence of breast tissue along the milk line and occurs in 2% to 6% of women (Graydanus et al., 1989). *Polythelia*, or accessory nipple, is the most common congenital breast anomaly in males or females. *Polymastia*, or the presence of accessory breast tissue along the milk line, is differentiated from a *supernumerary breast*, or the presence of a nipple and underlying breast tissue. All three terms describe aberrant breast tissue found most often along the milk line, although aberrant tissue has been reported in other locations. Isolated case reports exist of carcinoma found in accessory breast tissue (Smith and Greening, 1972). Previous association between accessory breast tissue and renal anomalies were likely overstated. Larger studies show that 10% to 15% of patients with supernumerary breast tissue will have major structural renal anomalies if two or more other phenotypic anomalies are present (Hersh et al., 1987). Isolated accessory nipples with or without breast tissue do not appear to be associated with other congenital anomalies.

Patients with aberrant breast tissue usually present with complaints of a soft tissue mass along the primordial milk line. Work-up includes ultrasonography and biopsy if clinical examination does not definitively make the diagnosis. Excision is unnecessary unless the mass is increasing in size or the patient has cosmetic concerns. These masses may grow with pregnancy and lactation.

Absence of Breast Tissue (Amastia and Athelia)

Complete involution of the mammary ridge leads to *amastia*, or absence of breast tissue. This rare abnormality is usually unilateral. *Poland syndrome* presents with amastia, ipsilateral rib anomalies, webbed fingers, and radial nerve palsies. Amastia can be extremely disturbing to an adolescent, but can be surgically corrected, in one or staged surgeries. Tragically, a common cause of amastia is iatrogenic. In an adolescent who presents with failed breast development on one side and a surgical history of a breast biopsy as a young child for a breast mass, the breast biopsy removed a normal asymmetric breast bud. This child should be referred to a plastic surgeon for reconstruction of her breast. Athelia is the absence of the nipple on one or both sides. Surgical correction is an option for this condition.

Nipple Inversion

Nipple inversion is common in newborns and usually resolves within a few days of birth. Patients with persistent nipple inversion from birth should be reassured that this is a normal variant and poses no other problem than cosmetic. Surgery to correct the inversion is only indicated for chronic infection as surgical correction of nipple inversion is rarely successful.

DISORDERS OF DEVELOPMENT

Breast Asymmetry

Extremes of normal variants of breast development can present as disorders. It is normal for some female adolescents and women to exhibit a moderate amount of breast asymmetry. It is also normal for one breast to develop at a slightly different rate than the other breast. If the physical examination reveals breast asymmetry with normal breast tissue and no dominant masses, the appropriate treatment is reassurance. If the adolescent is pubertal, 75% of breast asymmetry will resolve completely by adulthood (Graydanus et al., 1989). However, if the asymmetry is marked and causes psychological distress for the patient it can be addressed with plastic surgery. In the discussion with the patient and her family, the health care provider must be sensitive to the adolescent's desire to be "normal" and not appear different than her peers. What may seem like a trivial issue to an adult may provoke shame and embarrassment in an adolescent. Breast asymmetry may also be caused by a large mass that distorts the normal breast tissue, such as a giant fibroadenoma; these masses are typically evident during a routine breast examination. Pseudoasymmetry is also a possibility, resulting from deformities of the rib cage such as a pectus excavatum.

Macromastia

Another extreme of normal development that presents in adolescence is *macromastia*, its further extreme *gigantomastia*, or *virginal/juvenile hypertrophy*. In patients with juvenile hypertrophy, pendulous breasts can reach 30 to 50 lb. This disorder may be unilateral or bilateral.

1. Etiology: The cause of juvenile hypertrophy is not well understood, but may represent an abnormal response of the breast to normal hormonal stimulation, especially by estrogen. Eighty percent of macromastia and gigantomastia present in adolescence, and are strongly associated with family history and obesity (Corriveau and Jacobs, 1990). There has been no evidence linking elevated hormone levels to excessive breast volume.
2. Clinical manifestations: While adult patients usually present with physical complaints of back and shoulder

pain and limited activity, adolescent concerns tend to focus more on self image, and social and athletic limitations (Losee et al., 2004).

3. Treatment: No definite therapeutic guidelines have been developed. Although it is preferable to delay surgery until the breasts have fully matured, this may not be practical in some adolescents if their breast size is unbearable.

 a. Surgical options: Once an underlying mass or tumor has been ruled out by physical examination with breast ultrasonography and biopsy if necessary, management for this problem is reassurance and plastic surgery if desired. Standard treatment is a reduction mastopexy. Owing to the risk of recurrence after surgery, some physicians have recommended subcutaneous mastectomy with reconstruction. Patients should be referred to plastic surgeons with experience in treating teens, and who are sensitive to the teens' particular body image concerns.

 b. Psychological approaches: Teen girls with excessive breast volume are at risk for a secondary eating disorder, a dysfunctional attempt to achieve more "normal" body proportions (Kreipe et al., 1997; Losee et al., 2004). Girls who present with macromastia or gigantomastia should be evaluated carefully for a distorted body image or eating disorder and treated appropriately. Studies have shown that reduction mammaplasty may play an important role in treating these psychiatric disorders by helping these girls achieve more acceptable breast size (Kreipe et al., 1997) and improving quality of life (Blomqvist et al. 2004).

 c. Hormonal manipulation: Hormonal treatment has been attempted in these patients using medroxyprogesterone, dydrogesterone, or danazol. Teratogenic and carcinogenic effects have been a concern with these medications.

 d. Combination of medications and surgery: Postoperative treatment with dydrogesterone has been used to prevent recurrences.

Breast Hypoplasia

Breast hypoplasia may also present in adolescence. Underlying causes include iatrogenic injury as previously mentioned, trauma, malnutrition, or it may be an idiopathic condition. Hypoplasia may occur with aggressive weight loss or athletic activity. Teens with breast hypoplasia should be carefully screened for eating disorders, as breast underdevelopment may be a presenting symptom of anorexia or bulimia in a girl with low self-esteem. Other disorders in the differential diagnosis include premature ovarian failure, androgen excess (from tumor or exogenous anabolic steroid use), and chronic diseases—like diabetes mellitus, inflammatory bowel disease and others—that lead to weight loss. Work-up consists of a careful physical examination to document the condition as well as search for underlying causes listed in the preceding text. Treatment is targeted at the underlying primary disorder. Idiopathic breast hypoplasia can be addressed by a plastic surgeon.

Tuberous Breast Deformity

A rare disorder of breast development is *tuberous breast deformity*. Teens present with long narrow ptotic breasts that appear to be an overdevelopment of the nipple-areolar complex with an underdevelopment of the breast mound. Treatment of choice is plastic surgery; reassurance is also an option in this condition for the milder cases.

BENIGN BREAST DISEASE

Mastalgia

Moderate to severe breast pain can be a distressing problem to a patient and is not uncommon in teens. It must be distinguished from physiological tenderness and swelling that occurs with most women's menses, due to proliferative lobular changes induced by hormonal stimulation. *Mastalgia* can be cyclic pain, worse immediately before menses, or noncyclic pain, *mastodynia*. Pathophysiology is unknown. Pain charts will assist the patient in characterizing the nature and timing of her breast pain. A thorough physical examination, with imaging and biopsy studies if any abnormalities are found, is indicated to rule out underlying pathology. Other causes of breast pain include breast pathology, costochondritis, rib fracture, and gastritis. Once the diagnosis of mastalgia or mastodynia has been made by exclusion, treatment includes analgesics (nonsteroidal antiinflammatory drugs [NSAIDs]), good bra support (both night and day if needed), and reassurance that the pain is not a symptom of a more serious illness. Most breast pain resolves spontaneously within 3 to 6 months. Medication used to treat severe pain in adults, bromocriptine and tamoxifen, have not been studied in teens. Evening primrose oil has shown minimal symptom relief (Hindle, 1999) but may take months to show an effect.

Nipple Discharge

Nipple discharge can be caused by endocrine disorders, as well as breast pathology. High serum prolactin levels can be due to prolactinoma-induced galactorrhea (see Chapter 57), a bilateral milky discharge. Review of systems should include menstrual irregularities and headaches. In addition to a breast examination, the patient should undergo visual field testing. Prolactinomas can impinge on the optic nerve, causing visual field defects. Work-up for a suspected prolactinoma includes measurement of serum prolactin levels and magnetic resonance imaging (MRI) of the brain. If identified, many patients can be treated medically with bromocriptine, or be surgically resected.

 Galactorrhea can also occur during pregnancy, post-abortion, and post-partum. Medications can induce galactorrhea as well. If no underlying cause is identified, the diagnosis of physiological galactorrhea is made by exclusion. Patients should be reassured that they have no underlying breast pathology and counseled to reduce stimulation to the breast. The condition is usually self-limiting.

 Nonmilky discharges usually indicate an underlying breast or nipple problem. Physical examination may reveal a local contact dermatitis of the nipple that can give rise to serous, purulent, or bloody discharge. Culprits include soap, clothes, clothing detergent, or lotion used by the patient. Treatment is identification and discontinuation of the offending agent, with topical steroid cream for symptom relief.

 Purulent discharge indicates infection. It should be cultured and the patient treated with the appropriate antibiotics and warm compresses. If the infection fails to respond to antibiotic therapy, incision and drainage may be indicated.

Serous or bloody discharge from a single duct may be due to an intraductal papilloma and should be examined by ductogram. Any abnormality found should be excised. Cytological analysis has not been shown to be cost effective in teens. Usually, serous discharge is a self-limiting condition and may be related to fibrocystic change. Again, patients should be counseled to limit stimulation of the breast. Bloody nipple discharge, although a matter of concern in adults, is usually not related to underlying carcinoma in teens due to the extremely low incidence of breast cancer in this population. Again, intraductal papilloma and duct ectasia are more common causes.

Intraductal Papilloma

This is a pathology rarely seen in teens. It can present either as a diffuse thickening of the breast or a nipple discharge, usually bloody. It represents a focal hyperplasia of the ductal epithelium invaginating into the duct on a vascular stalk. Disruption of this stalk leads to bloody discharge. If the proliferation of duct epithelium grows large enough it creates a palpable mass. This is an infrequent finding in an adolescent, although a palpable mass associated with a bloody nipple discharge has a 95% probability of being an intraductal papilloma, even in teens. Treatment is surgical excision.

Montgomery Tubercles

Discharge may be associated with *Montgomery* or *Morgagni* tubercles. These are enlarged sebaceous glands around the areola associated with lactiferous ducts. They present as soft papules that may enlarge with pregnancy and lactation, and elicit an episodic thin clear or brown discharge. Breast examination may reveal a soft mass beneath the areola. This condition resolves spontaneously within several months.

Breast Infection

Mastitis or breast abscesses present with an acute history of a red inflamed breast.

1. Predisposing conditions include pregnancy, lactation, history of recent cessation of breast-feeding, preexisting cyst, and breast trauma.
2. Patients may or may not present with constitutional symptoms of malaise or fever. Physical examination reveals an edematous erythematous breast. Purulent discharge may or may not be identified. Any drainage or discharge should be sent for culture and sensitivity.
3. Treatment is as follows:
   a. Treatment for mastitis without abscess is antibiotics and warm compresses, begun as soon as the condition is clinically suspected.
   b. Antibiotic therapy should be targeted at the most likely pathogen, skin flora including *Staphylococcus aureus*. Occasionally, streptococci or hemophilus species are found at culture. Dicloxacillin or cephalexin provides adequate coverage of skin pathogens. For penicillin allergic–patients, clindamycin provides good abscess penetration.
   c. Breast-feeding: If patients are breast-feeding, expression of milk from the affected side should continue to prevent milk stasis. Infants can continue breast-feeding from the affected side.
   d. Persistent infection: Patients should be re-examined within several days to confirm response to therapy. Persistent infection despite antibiotic therapy should be evaluated with ultrasonography for an underlying abscess.
   e. Abscess: Any area of fluctuance on physical examination implies an underlying abscess. Drainage can be attempted in the office with a large-bore needle. Injecting a solution of normal saline with lidocaine into the abscess will serve two functions—pain relief and dilution of viscous purulent material, making aspiration easier. If needle aspiration is unsuccessful or if the abscess reaccumulates, the patient should be referred for incision and drainage. Incisions should be as small as possible to limit resulting distortion. Material obtained at aspiration or incision and drainage should be cultured.
   f. Surgery: Infections that fail to respond to adequate antibiotic therapy should also be referred for surgical management. These patients should be screened for underlying immunosuppressive disease that may interfere with their ability to clear the infection, like diabetes mellitus or human immunodeficiency virus (HIV) infection.

BREAST MASSES

The presence of a dominant breast mass in a female patient of any age causes concern, but in adolescence, breast masses are overwhelmingly benign (Table 59.2). Surgical studies show that 86% of excisional biopsies are fibroadenomas (68%), and fibrocystic changes (18%) or other benign findings such as cysts and mastitis. Malignancies comprised less than 1% of excisional biopsies performed. A review of the adolescent literature in 1994 found 0.89% of breast masses excised to be primary adenocarcinoma (Neinstein, 1994). Therefore, in addition to appropriately establishing the cause of a dominant mass, practitioners must reassure patients and their parents that it is very unlikely they have a malignant disease.

Work-up of a Breast Mass

Every breast mass that feels benign should be confirmed with imaging and biopsy. Physical examination is not sensitive enough to differentiate benign from malignant lesions (Chateil et al., 1998; Garcia et al., 2000; Hays et al., 1997). Mammography is of low yield in adolescents and young women as the breast density of these patients obscures pathological findings on mammogram (Williams et al., 1986). A targeted ultrasonography is a noninvasive nonpainful way to characterize a mass. However, a retrospective series of breast ultrasonograms in adolescent girls with metastatic malignancies in their breasts, found that malignant lesions had at least one benign characteristic on ultrasound evaluation (Chateil et al., 1998; Hays et al., 1997).

Although excisional biopsy was commonly performed previously, current management of breast disease seeks to establish a diagnosis without surgical excision, saving patients with benign lesions from an unnecessary surgery (Pacinda and Ramzy, 1998). This is achieved by

TABLE 59.2

Breast Masses in Adolescence

Benign Breast Masses—Common	Benign Breast Masses—Rare	Malignant Breast Masses—Extremely Rare
Fibroadenoma	Intraductal papilloma	Adenocarcinoma
Cyst	Juvenile papillomatosis	Cystosarcoma
Abscess	Tubular/lactational adenoma	Rhabdomyosarcoma
	Cystosarcoma phyllodes (benign)	Angiosarcoma
		Lymphoma
		Cystosarcoma phyllodes (malignant)
		Adenocarcinoma

either core needle biopsy or fine needle aspiration (FNA). For younger patients, FNA is a less painful way to obtain diagnosis, and is cost effective and quick. Studies of FNA in pediatric and adult patients have shown 99% correlation between excisional histology and the diagnostic triad of concordant physical examination, biopsy, and imaging (Silverman et al., 1991; Eisenhut et al., 1996; Vetto et al., 1996). (For further detail see "Breast Imaging" and "Breast Biopsy" sections.)

Fibroadenomas

Fibroadenomas are well-circumscribed fibroepithelial lesions. Grossly, they appear as uniformly smooth or nodule white or tan lesions, sharply demarcated from surrounding tissue. They do not form a true capsule, but rather a pseudocapsule of compressed normal breast tissue pushed aside as the lesion grows. If the lesion outgrows its blood supply and becomes infarcted it could have a hemorrhagic appearance. Histologically, fibroadenomas show both an epithelial and stromal component. Ducts are usually compressed giving a classic branching or fern-like appearance. Components of fibrocystic change, epithelial hyperplasia, sclerosing adenosis, and other complex changes within a fibroadenoma are called *complex fibroadenomas* (Dehner et al., 1999). A complex fibroadenoma is a benign lesion, although data suggest they may confer an elevated risk of primary breast cancer in later life (Dupont et al., 1994). A *cellular fibroadenoma* includes epithelial hyperplasia with complex architecture and cellular stroma, and is a benign finding that does not elevate future breast cancer risk. A fibroadenoma that grows to 8 cm has been called *giant fibroadenoma*, a distinction that is only clinical and carries no difference in histology or management (Dehner et al., 1999). Giant fibroadenomas occur more frequently in teens than in adults and more frequently in African-Americans.

1. Prevalence: Common fibroadenomas are the most common breast tumor found in adolescents in surgical reports, comprising 60% to 90% of benign breast lesions. Most adolescents with this condition are older than 14 years, with a large increase in prevalence in 15- and 16-year olds. The condition has been reported to be twice as common in African-Americans. There is no evidence of progression to cancer.
2. Clinical manifestations: On physical examination, they feel like a round or oval firm mass distinct from the rest of the breast. They can be multiple and bilateral.

3. Diagnosis: Usually, the diagnosis can be made with a combination of clinical examination, ultrasonography and FNA, and core biopsy or excisional biopsy. On ultrasonography, fibroadenomas appear as hypoechoic lesions with smooth round distinct borders, and are wider than tall.
4. Management: Once the diagnosis of fibroadenoma is confirmed, management of the mass is expectant with careful observation, physical examination, and ultrasonography every 6 months, or surgical excision. Patients who desire expectant management should be advised that their lesion might shrink and regress, or may grow, especially with subsequent pregnancy. For small fibroadenomas, <3 centimeters, minimally invasive surgical techniques allow patients to have their lesion removed with less anesthesia exposure and scarring. Under ultrasound guidance and using a large-bore needle, core biopsies of the lesion are taken until is has been removed. Alternatively, a small fibroadenoma can be cryoablated as an outpatient procedure.

Giant fibroadenomas may distort the affected breast and should the patient desire removal, simple surgical excision should be performed, sparing as much normal compressed breast tissue as possible. Preoperatively, consideration should be given to plastic surgical assistance to correct the resulting deformity. Some patients benefit from a staged surgery, with plastic surgical correction delayed until the normal compressed breast tissue has a chance to recover.

Cysts

A dominant breast mass may also be a simple cyst. The incidence of cysts is underrepresented in series of excisional adolescent breast biopsies because their management rarely requires surgery. Patients with breast cysts can present with multiple breast masses, or increasing size or tenderness of a mass associated with menses. Physical examination reveals a firm, well-circumscribed mass distinct from the surrounding breast. Ultrasonography reveals a round, well-demarcated hypoechoic structure with increased shine through transmission because of its fluid content. Cysts are easily treated with FNA of fluid and resolution of the mass. If fluid is yellow, green, or brown it can be discarded. Bloody fluid should be sent for cytology and should raise concern regarding malignancy. Any persistent solid mass after FNA expression of fluid implies a complex cyst, a more concerning lesion, and the patient should be referred for image-guided core biopsy. Patients should be warned that simple cysts can recur and can easily be reaspirated. Symptomatic cysts that recur after multiple aspirations should be referred for simple excision.

Fibrocystic Changes

Patients with symptomatic fibrocystic change complain of multiple masses or nodularity, with pain increasing with menses. If surgical excision is performed, histology reveals proliferative changes of ducts and lobules, duct dilatation and elongation, and terminal duct cyst formation (Vorherr, 1986).

1. Although the true prevalence of fibrocystic changes in adolescents is unknown, they are likely very common in women in the reproductive–age-group. The prevalence increases even during the third and fourth decade of life.
2. Pathophysiology is unknown but this probably represents changes associated with effects of estrogen and progesterone on breast tissue.
3. Clinical manifestations: On physical examination, nodularity is apparent, most commonly in the upper outer quadrant of one or both breasts. Masses may not be as mobile and distinct from surrounding breast as fibroadenomas or cysts. Symptoms, particularly tenderness are more common a week before menstruation and are often relieved by menstruation.
4. Ultrasonography fails to reveal a single underlying mass; it may show areas of increased fibrous tissue or microcysts.
5. Treatment: Treatment in adolescents includes mild analgesics, well supporting bras and a trial of oral contraceptives for those with more severe symptoms. Symptoms in teens are rarely severe and aggressive measures used in adults, such as oral danazol or tamoxifen, have not been studied in teens. A previously suggested correlation between caffeine intake and breast symptomatology has not been validated in larger studies.

Tubular and Lactating Adenoma

Additional histologies that can be found rarely at biopsy of a solitary mass in an adolescent are tubular and lactating adenomas. Tubular adenomas are a well-circumscribed collection of uniform tubular structures spaced closely together (Dehner et al., 1999). A lactating adenoma adds generalized lactational changes and hyperplastic lobules. Both are rare benign findings that do not require further management.

Juvenile Papillomatosis

This lesion presents as a unilateral solitary painless breast mass clinically consistent with a fibroadenoma. Fifty percent of patients with this diagnosis are younger than 20 years (Rosen and Kimmel, 1990). Grossly, it is a firm well-circumscribed mass with multiple cysts separated by fibrous septa. On histological inspection, simple cysts with cuboidal epithelial cells, papillary ductal hyperplasia, and apocrine metaplasia are found in varying proportions. Epithelial hyperplasia may exhibit papillary, micropapillary, and cribriform architecture. Some cysts may be filled with foamy macrophages and secretions. Fibrocystic changes are also seen, including lobular hyperplasia, sclerosing adenosis, and fibroadenomatoid hyperplasia.

The clinical significance of this lesion involves the controversy over its inclusion as a preneoplastic lesion. The initial study that identified this entity noted that 50% of patients with juvenile papillomatosis had a history of breast cancer in a first-degree relative (Rosen and Kimmel, 1990). Seven older patients in this series had concurrent breast cancer. Local recurrence after diagnosis does occur (Dehner et al., 1999). For these reasons, treatment is wide surgical excision and close clinical follow-up.

BREAST MALIGNANCY

Prevalence

Primary breast cancer is a rare phenomenon in adolescents. One 25-year survey of a tertiary children's hospital identified 18 patients with breast cancer, 16 females and 2 males (Rogers et al., 1994). Of these 18 tumors identified, 13 were metastatic disease, 2 were primary breast malignancy, and 3 were secondary malignancy. Breast carcinoma, so common a disease in older age, is extremely rare in adolescents. Neinstein's review of 1,791 breast excisions found five primary adenocarcinomas in teens (Neinstein, 1994). Dehner et al., found only 1 case of breast carcinoma in a review of 134 cases of breast pathology in patients through 20 years of age. History of prior radiotherapy to the chest may be a predisposing factor. Rogers et al., found three cases of breast carcinoma diagnosed in adulthood as secondary malignancies in patients with a history of Hodgkin lymphoma as teens (Rogers et al., 1994). The more common primary breast malignancies found in teens are rhabdomyosarcoma, angiosarcoma or cystosarcoma phyllodes, or lymphoma. Tumors that metastasize to the breast include rhabdomyosarcoma, lymphoma, and neuroblastoma.

History

Whenever possible the history should be taken with the patient dressed. She may feel more comfortable answering sensitive questions (e.g., her gynecological history or about illicit drug use), without the added vulnerability of being undressed.

1. History of symptoms: A detailed history of symptoms can give important clues to a patient's underlying diagnosis. For example, a pain chart can reveal cyclic or constant pain.
2. Change in size of mass: Masses that change in size with menstrual cycles may be cysts; those that do not are more likely solid masses. Sudden increase in growth is a concerning sign.
3. Medication history: Recent initiation of medication could explain mastodynia or nipple discharge. Although there have been obvious benefits of oral contraceptives in the risk of endometrial and ovarian cancer, their impact on breast cancer has been more controversial. Almost all epidemiological studies of present and past oral contraceptive users demonstrate risk ratios whose confidence intervals cluster around 1.0 or include 1.0 indicating no statistically significant increased risk. Some studies have indicated a slight increased risk in selected subgroups. Both the Centers for Disease

Control and Prevention (CDC) Cancer and Steroid Hormone Study and a World Health Organization study of 5,000 women found no increased risk of breast cancer with duration of use. Overall, there is no conclusive evidence that oral contraceptives increase a woman's risk of breast cancer. See Chapter 43 for a more in-depth discussion.

4. History of trauma: Also important is a history of trauma; this may not only explain breast complaints, but also alert a clinician to a serious underlying social problem and other potential injuries.

5. Past medical history: Past medical history may identify factors that increase the risk of malignancy. Chest wall radiation, for example for lymphoma, increases the risk of subsequent breast cancer (Rogers et al., 1994). Patients with a history of malignancy that can metastasize to the breast (lymphoma, rhabdomyosarcoma) should raise concern. Any patient with a history of cancer must be followed up carefully for evidence of recurrence, including breast cancer recurrence.

6. Family history: Risk factors for malignancy should be queried of each patient although most patients with cancer have no identifiable risk factors (Cady et al., 1998). First-degree family members affected by cancer increase a patient's risk; the age of these family members should be carefully documented. Screening for breast disease should begin 10 years before the age at which the youngest close relative was diagnosed. Patients with strong family histories of breast cancer, especially if bilateral disease or in conjunction with ovarian or endometrial cancer, should be referred for genetic counseling. Estimates of breast cancer risk show as much as an eightfold increase if the disease developed before menopause or was bilateral (Cady et al., 1998). Genetic testing may be indicated in the affected family member.

7. Genetics: At least eight candidate-susceptibility genes have been identified. Probably the most important that lead to striking family clusters of breast cancer are mutations of BRCA1 and BRCA2, accounting for almost 80% of hereditary breast cancer and approximately 5% to 6% of all breast cancers (Greene, 1997; Calederon-Margalit and Paltiel, 2004; Evans et al., 2005). Although these mutations are rare in the general population (5–50 per 100,000), they may occur in approximately 1% of all Jewish women of Ashkenazic descent (Evans et al., 2005). Routine screening of BRCA1 is not warranted because of the difficulty in evaluating the multiple mutations, social discrimination issues such as insurance, and the lack of appropriate preventive strategies. However, genetic testing for cancer risk is likely to change dramatically in the coming years. Elger and Harding (2000) discuss testing for BRCA1 in the adolescent population, and the importance of making distinctions between testing children and adolescents. Samuel and Ollila (2005) review the difficult decisions faced by young women who carry a BRCA mutation regarding radiological screening and potential prophylactic surgery.

BREAST SELF-EXAMINATION

The question regarding instruction of breast self-examination engenders controversy. Breast self-examination has a sensitivity of only 30% in detecting breast disease. As sensitivity improves over time as patients learn what is normal in their own breasts, specificity decreases (O'Malley and Fetcher, 1987). Breast self-examination has not been shown to improve survival in breast cancer (O'Malley and Fetcher, 1987). Indeed, it has been shown to increase anxiety and depression in patients who believe they find an abnormality (Baxter, 2001; Ellman et al., 1993). Gaskie and Nashelsky, 2005 report that although breast self-examination has little impact on breast cancer mortality, careful clinical breast examination can affect breast cancer mortality rates. In young women, in whom malignant disease is rare, examinations are more likely to discover clinically insignificant benign disease than malignancy. However, there is benefit to breast self-examination in that it establishes a life-long habit of patients investing in their own breast health. Current recommendations from the American Cancer Society as listed on their Web site for the general public defers any recommendations for or against breast self-examination saying: "Women should be told about the benefits and limitations of breast self-examination." The World Health Organization does not recommend teaching women younger than 20 years to do breast self-examination (World Health Organization, 1983).

PHYSICAL EXAMINATION OF THE BREAST

A thorough and careful breast examination is essential to the evaluation of any breast complaint. In the adolescent patient, a clinician must be sensitive to her feelings of embarrassment or modesty. Before the examination begins, she should be informed of its components and given the opportunity to be accompanied by a parent or friend. If she declines, a chaperone should accompany the examiner, especially if he is male. A discussion of what changes she can expect during breast development, with an emphasis on the wide range of what is normal, may reduce her anxiety of the examination.

The optimal time for a breast examination is within a week of completion of menses, when the breast is most quiescent and least tender. If an examination is indeterminant, repeating it at a different point in her menstrual cycle may be informative. Inspection is an important and often overlooked first step in the examination. This should be performed with arms outstretched, overhead, and resting at the waist to allow the clinician to see possible distortion in various positions, as well as dermatological conditions affecting the breasts. Attention should also be paid to comparing the two breasts for symmetry.

Palpation

Palpation should be performed both sitting and standing, especially in large-breasted patients. It does not matter with which technique the palpation is performed as long as it is thorough and systematic, covering each breast from the clavicle to inframammary fold, and from sternum to mid-axillary line. Studies show time spent on examination correlates best with detection (Fletcher et al., 1985). Uncovering only the breast being examined may help the patient feel more comfortable.

Palpation should include the axillae and supraclavicular fossa. These areas are best assessed while the patient is sitting. If she rests her upper arm on the arm of the examiner and relaxes her shoulder, deep palpation of the axilla can be performed with minimal discomfort.

The examiner can examine the breast in one of the following several ways:

1. Spokes of a wheel: In this method, the examiner uses a pattern similar to the spokes of a wheel. Starting with the tail of the breast in the axilla, the examiner moves in a straight line to the nipple. Using straight lines from the outer boundary of the breast to the nipple, the examiner can work around the whole breast.
2. Concentric circles: A second method involves covering the breast in either concentric circles or a spiral pattern around the breast.
3. Vertical strips: A third method involves covering the breast by examining vertical strips. In a study by Atkins et al. (1991) this was found to be the most effective method.

Whichever method is used, the entire anterior chest wall should be palpated, applying varying degrees of pressure with the pads of the second, third, and fourth fingers and rotating in small dime-sized circles. Particular attention should be given to the nipple and areolar areas, as 15% of breast cancers are located here. The areola should be compressed to elicit nipple discharge. Notation of nipple discharge if elicited should include its color, from which and how many ducts it appeared, and palpation of which quadrant of the breast elicited it. Using the analogy of a clock face to describe the offending duct or quadrant of breast from which it is elicited is the most reproducible way to locate the source of discharge. The examiner should also palpate for supraclavicular, infraclavicular, and axillary nodes. Occasionally, using talc in palpating the breast may be helpful.

If breast masses are appreciated, they too should be described with careful attention to their location. Only dominant masses with texture distinct from the surrounding tissue should be identified as masses; areas of increased nodularity without discrete masses should be identified as such. This distinction is important as one condition implies underlying pathology whereas the other is often a variant of normal. Notation should be made of the mobility and firmness of a mass, as well as tenderness.

When examining a patient complaining of an ill-defined or deep mass, or nipple discharge not elicited by the examiner, lotion, gel, soap, or lubrication on the examiners fingers can assist in deep or repeated palpation with less discomfort to the patient.

Once the examiner has completed their examination, it is useful to ask the patient to pinpoint the location of the complaint that brought her into the office. This will allow the examiner to form an independent opinion of the normality or abnormality of her examination, and then address her specific concern. Likewise, it is useful to begin the examination on the unaffected side, to gain an appreciation of what her normal breast tissue feels like, before evaluating an area of suspected pathology.

BREAST IMAGING

Breast imaging is indicated any time a clinician appreciates an abnormality on physical examination. Physical examination alone is not enough to rule out malignancy, despite its rarity in this age-group.

Mammography

Mammography is an excellent screening tool for breasts that are primarily fatty replaced. As the developing breast is more fibroglandular than fatty, mammography is not as sensitive as it is in an older population (Chateil et al., 1998). Another study found that mammograms failed to identify 75% of palpable masses in women younger than 30 (Williams et al., 1986). The problem is mass and calcifications, the two most important findings on mammography, appear white. Glandular tissue also appears white. In a young patient this means a white lesion on a white background. Fatty tissue is grey; in older women white lesions on a grey background are easier to see.

Ultrasonography

Ultrasonography is ideally suited to evaluating masses in the adolescent population as it is superior to mammography in characterizing lesions in fibroglandular breasts (Garcia et al., 2000). Ultrasonography is superior in characterizing masses and can distinguish a cystic mass from a solid one. It cannot distinguish a benign solid mass from a malignant one. The hallmarks of benign lesions in adult patients—smooth regular borders, multiple masses, and homogeneous solid masses—can also be seen in metastatic lesions to juvenile breasts (Chateil et al., 1998). Abscesses carry the same characteristics of malignant adult lesions—irregular borders, heterogeneous contents.

Breast Biopsy

Because of the limitations of physical examination and imaging, careful consideration should be given in obtaining a biopsy of any palpable mass. A FNA of the mass obtains important histological evidence without causing much discomfort to the patient. If an aspiration obtains nonbloody cyst fluid, the lesion can be diagnosed and treated with the same diagnostic test—it is a benign cyst. Cytology on the cyst fluid is not indicated unless it is bloody. If the cyst fails to resolve, but leaves a palpable mass, it needs to be biopsied.

If FNA reveals a solid mass, a smear of cells obtained can characterize the mass. FNA has been demonstrated to have a sensitivity of 90% and specificity of 100% in pediatric patients when diagnosing carcinoma (Silverman et al., 1991). If any doubt remains regarding the benign nature of a mass, despite a reassuring FNA, further tissue must be obtained for diagnosis. Previously, excisional biopsies were performed to diagnose and excise the lesion. However, the value of achieving a diagnosis through a minimally invasive core biopsy has merit—it can save a patient a surgery and a scar or breast deformity in a cosmetically sensitive area if the results are benign. If the results show metastatic disease, this procedure could save a patient an unnecessary surgery. If the results show primary breast cancer, like cystosarcoma, this allows for appropriate preoperative planning of one definitive surgery for the patient.

Once cytological or core biopsy results have been obtained, all three pieces of the diagnostic triad must be reviewed—physical examination, imaging, and biopsy. If all three concur the mass is benign, the health care provider can be 99% certain the mass is truly benign (Hindle, 1999). The patient may then safely decline further intervention.

She should be followed up with serial examinations and ultrasonograms, every 6 months to a year, to establish stability of the lesion. Any sudden growth should raise suspicion of malignant transformation. If any one piece of the diagnostic triad is not in concordance, the lesion must be excised.

Management Management of these tumors depends on the underlying primary disease. Primary breast carcinoma and breast lymphoma in teens should be treated as it is in adults.

Specific Breast Mass Lesions

Cystosarcoma Phyllodes Cystosarcoma phyllodes are tumors more commonly found in the fourth and fifth decades of life, and can be benign or malignant. They are the most common breast sarcoma of adolescence (Rogers et al., 1994). They comprise 1% of breast neoplasms and 2.5% of fibroepithelial lesions (Rajan et al., 1998). Features that indicate malignant transformation include invasive tumor border, high stromal cell mitotic counts, cytological atypia, and necrosis. They are further divided into low and high grade. A series of 45 lesions in patients aged 10 to 24 found 34 benign lesions and 11 malignancies (Rajan et al., 1998). Treatment of cystosarcoma phyllodes and other primary breast sarcomas is wide local resection with achievement of negative margins being the surgical goal. Recent evidence shows teens may have less aggressive tumors and lower recurrence rates than adults (Rajan et al., 1998). These tumors do not metastasize to axillary lymph nodes, so no axillary procedure is indicated. The most common sites of metastases are lung and bone, so metastatic work-up should focus on these areas.

Rhabdomyosarcoma Patients with a breast biopsy showing rhabdomyosarcoma should be screened for occult primary disease outside the breast. Metastatic rhabdomyosarcoma is more common than primary breast rhabdomyosarcoma. Isolated primary breast sarcoma should be resected aggressively as negative surgical margins are the only factors proved to influence survival (Pandey et al., 2004). Mastectomy is indicated only if the tumor-to-breast ratio does not favor breast conservation. Metastatic rhabdomyosarcoma to the breast carries an exceedingly poor prognosis as it frequently is a hallmark of widely disseminated disease (Hays et al., 1997). Treatment is chemotherapy.

SUMMARY

As adolescence is a period of rapid and complex physical and psychological change, breast complaints in this age-group commonly center around discomfort (mastalgia), developmental variations (asymmetry), or developmental anomalies (hypo- or hyperplasia). It is the health care provider's role to reassure patients and their families regarding the spectrum of normal development, while appropriately intervening when developmental anomalies occur. Clinicians should not hesitate to involve mental health experts and plastic surgeons, when appropriate. Masses in this age-group are uncommon; malignant masses are thankfully rare. Persistent masses require evaluation. The physical examination, fine needle biopsy, and ultrasound imaging provide diagnostic information in a minimally invasive manner.

WEB SITES

For Teenagers and Parents

http://www.puberty101.com. A Web site with general information about puberty, including breast size and normal breast development.

http://www.youngwomenshealth.org. Section on breast health among glossary of terms; from Children's Hospital Boston Web site.

http://www.womenshealth.about.com. Contains a section on teen breast complaints, as well as provides question and answers.

http://www.goaskalice.Columbia.edu. Frank answers to common and uncommon teen questions from the Health Services at Columbia University, including those on breast health.

http://www.wdxcyber.com. Written by obstetrician-gynecologists. Has a breast section, written more specifically for general women's health, rather than adolescents. Advice from the Women's Diagnostic Cyber.

http://www.teenshealth.com. Detailed discussions regarding plastic surgery in teens, including excellent breast section.

For Health Professionals

http://www.cdc.gov/cancer/NBCCEDP. The CDC Women's Health page.

http://www.acog.org. Web site of the American College of Obstetrics and Gynecology.

REFERENCES AND ADDITIONAL READINGS

Atkins E, Soloman LJ, Worden JK, Foster RS, Jr. Relative effectiveness of methods of breast self-examination. *J Behav Med* 1991;14(4):357.

Baxter N. Preventative health care, 2001 update: should women be routinely taught breast self-exam to screen for breast cancer. *CMAJ* 2001;164:1837.

Blomqvist L, Brandberg Y. Three-year follow up on clinical symptoms and health-related quality of life after reduction mammoplasty. *Plast Reconstr Surg* 2004;114(1):49.

Cady B, Steele GD Jr, Morrow M, et al. Evaluation of common breast problems: guidance for primary care givers. *CA Cancer J Clin* 1998;48:49.

Calederon-Margalit R, Paltiel O. Prevention of breast cancer in women who carry BRCA1 or BRCA2 mutations: a critical review of the literature. *Int J Cancer* 2004;112:357.

Chateil J, Arboucalot F, Perel Y. Breast metastases in adolescent girls: US findings. *Pediatr Radiol* 1998;28:832.

Corriveau S, Jacobs JS. Macromastia in adolescence. *Clin Plast Surg* 1990;17:151.

Dehner LP, Hill DA, Deschryver K. Pathology of the breast in children, adolescents, and young adults. *Semin Diagn Pathol* 1999;16(3):235.

Dupont WD, Page DL, Fritz FP. Long-term risk of breast cancer in women with fibroadenoma. *N Engl J Med* 1994;331:10.

Eisenhut CC, King DE, Nelson WA, et al. Fine-needle biopsy of pediatric lesions: a three-year study in an outpatient biopsy clinic. *Diagn Cytopathol* 1996;14:43.

Elger BS, Harding TW. Testing asolescents for a hereditary breast cancer (BRCA1): respecting their autonomy is in their best interest. *Arch Pediatr Adolesc Med* 2000 Feb;154(2):113.

Ellman R, Moss SM, Coleman D, et al. Breast self-examination programmes in the trial of early detection of breast cancer: 10 year findings. *Br J Cancer* 1993;68:208.

Evans JP, Skrzynia C, Susswein L, et al. Genetics and the young woman with breast cancer. *Breast Dis* 2005–2006;23:17.

Fletcher SW, O'Malley MS, Bruce LA. Physician's abilities to detect lumps in silicone breast models. *JAMA* 1985;253:2224.

Garcia CJ, Espinoza A, Dinamarca V. Breast US in children and adolescents. *Radio Graphics* 2000;20:1605.

Gaskie S, Nashelsky J. Clinical inquiries. Are breast self-exams or clinical exams effective for screening breast cancer? *J Fam Pract* 2005;54(9):803.

Graydanus DE, Matytsina L, Gains M. Breast disorders in children and adolescents. *Prim Care* 2006;33:455.

Graydanus DE, Parks DS, Farrell EG. Breast disorders in children and adolescents. *Pediatr Clin North Am* 1989;36:601.

Greene MH. Genetics of breast cancer. *Mayo Clin Proc* 1997;72(1):54.

Grenader T, Peretx T, Lifchitz M, et al. BRCA1 and BRCA2 germline mutations and oral contraceptives: to use of not to use. *Breast* 2005;14:264.

Hays DM, Donaldson SS, Shimada H, et al. Primary and metastatic rhabdomyosarcoma in the breast: neoplasms of adolescent females, a report from the intergroup rhabdomyosarcoma study. *Med Pediatr Oncol* 1997;29:181.

Hersh JH, Bloom AS, Cromer AO, et al. Does a supernumerary nipple/renal field defect exist? *Am J Dis Child* 1987;141:989.

Hindle WH. *Breast Care*. New York, NY: Springer; 1999.

Kreipe RE, Lewand AG, Dukarm CP, et al. Outcome for patients with bulimia and breast hypertrophy after reduction mammaplasty. *Arch Pediatr Adolesc Med* 1997;151:176.

Losee JE, Jiang S, Long DA, et al. Macromastia as an etiologic factor in bulimia nervosa. *Ann Plast Surg* 2004;52(5):452.

Neinstein LS. Review of breast masses in adolescents. *Adolesc Pediatr Gynecol* 1994;7:119.

O'Malley MS, Fetcher SW. Screening for breast cancer with breast self-examination. *JAMA* 1987;257:2196.

Pacinda SJ, Ramzy I. Fine needle aspiration of breast masses. *J Adolesc Health* 1998;23:3.

Pandey M, Matthew A, Abraham EK, et al. Primary sarcoma of the breast. *J Surg Oncol* 2004;87:121.

Parent A, Teilmann G, Juul A, et al. The timing of normal puberty and the age limits of sexual precocity: variations around the world, secular trends, and changes after migration. *Endocr Rev* 2003;24(5):668.

Rajan PB, Cranor ML, Peter P. Cystosarcoma phyllodes in adolescent girls and young women: a study of 45 patients. *Am J Surg Pathol* 1998;22(1):64.

Rogers DA, Lobe TE, Rao BN, et al. Breast malignancy in children. *J Pediatr Surg* 1994;29(1):48.

Rebar RW. The breast and the physiology of lactation. In: Creasey RK, Resnik R, eds. *Maternal fetal medicine*, 4th ed. Philadelphia, PA: WB Saunders; 1999:106.

Rosen PP, Kimmel M. Juvenile papillomatosis of the breast. A follow-up study of 41 patients having biopsies before 1979. *Am J Clin Pathol* 1990;93:599.

Samuel JC, Ollila DW. Prophylaxis and screening options: recommendations for young women with BRCA mutations. *Breast Dis* 2005–2006;23:31.

Silverman JF, Gurley AM, Holbrook CT, et al. Pediatric fine needle aspiration biopsy. *Am J Clin Pathol* 1991;95:653.

Smith GMR, Greening WP. Carcinoma of aberrant breast tissue: a report of 3 cases. *Br J Surg* 1972;59:89.

Traggi C. Disorders of pubertal development. *Best Pract Res Clin Obstet Gynaecol* 2003;17(1):41.

Vetto J, Pommier R, Schmidt W. Diagnosis of palpable breast lesions in younger women by the modified triple test is accurate and cost effective. *Arch Surg* 1996;131:967.

Vorherr H. Fibrocystic breast disease, pathophysiology, pathomorphology, clinical picture and management. *Am J Obstet Gynecol* 1986;154:161.

Williams SM, Kaplan PA, Peterson JC, et al. Mammography in women under age 30: is there clinical benefit. *Radiology* 1986; 161:49.

World Health Organization. *Self-examination in the early detection of breast cancer: a report on a consultation on self-examination in breast cancer early detection programmes.* Geneva: World Health Organization; 1983.

PART XIII

Sexually Transmitted Diseases

CHAPTER 60

Overview of Sexually Transmitted Diseases

J. Dennis Fortenberry and Lawrence S. Neinstein

From a clinical and public health perspective, sexually transmitted diseases (STDs) are one of the visible tracks marking the occasionally obscure developmental trails of sexuality through adolescence. Sexual activity itself occupies an uncomfortable, ambiguous position among the health challenges of adolescence—development of healthy sexuality balanced against the fear and stigma associated with STDs and their genuine threats to health.

The key clinical considerations include direct attention to issues of sexuality within the adolescent's developmental path, attention to behaviors that increase or reduce risk of acquiring an STD, immunization, screening by physical examination and laboratory testing, treatment of identified infections, and counseling for partner treatment and prevention of infections. Annual attention to these issues is recommended and some experts suggest even more frequent risk-reduction counseling and STD screening, particularly in teens with prior infections or in those involved in higher risk sexual behaviors. STD screening provides an opportunity to discuss risk of human immunodeficiency virus (HIV) testing and prevention.

STDs are associated with significant disease burden among adolescents. In 2005, 15- to 19-year-old female adolescents had the highest gonorrhea and chlamydia rates of any age-group. Gonorrhea rates among male and female adolescents have slowly declined during the last decade. Chlamydia rates are typically 6% to 18% among female adolescents, although rates decrease when aggressive screening and treatment policies are implemented. *Trichomonas vaginalis* rates are up to 14% in female adolescents and 3% to 5% in asymptomatic males. Serological studies show positivity rates for herpes simplex virus (HSV) of up to 30% for some groups of adolescents; most do not have symptomatic infection. HSV type 1 is now a common cause of genital herpes among adolescents and young adults. Evidence for human papillomavirus (HPV) infection may be seen in up to one third of some clinical samples. A vaccine for some HPV types (types 6, 11, 16, 18) is now commercially available.

The elevated STD risk in adolescents is almost certainly multifactorial in origin. Developmental susceptibility of the reproductive tract of female adolescents, the substantial rates of sex partner infections, and inconsistent or incorrect condom use are potential contributors. Socioenvironmental risks such as high endemic STD rates, sexual and physical abuse, social chaos, poverty, drug trafficking and use, and inadequate health care access also contribute and may be more powerful explanations of STD risk than developmental or individual behaviors.

Diagnostic possibilities for many STDs, particularly gonorrhea and chlamydia, have been revolutionized by nucleic acid amplification (NAATs) and hybrid capture (HC) techniques. NAATs and HC techniques have superior sensitivity and specificity compared with culture or other diagnostic tests such as direct fluorescent antibody (DFA) or DNA probe tests. NAATs and HC also allow use of urine and vaginal specimens, in addition to cervical or urethral specimens. Higher initial costs, compared with other tests, may be offset by reductions in morbidity.

In view of the fact that most adolescents complain of a particular set of symptoms and not a specific organism, a list of presenting symptoms for the STDs is also included (Table 60.1). As a broad overview, the Appendix to this chapter summarizes the clinical features and treatments of many of the well-known STDs. The remaining chapters in Section XIII focus on individual STDs in more detail.

TABLE 60.1

Sexually Transmitted Diseases by Presenting Symptom

1. Urethral discharge/dysuria
   a. *Neisseria gonorrhoeae*
   b. *Chlamydia trachomatis*
   c. *Ureaplasma urealyticum*
   d. Herpes genitalis
   e. *Trichomonas vaginalis*
2. Vaginal discharge
   Vaginal site of infection:
     a. *Candida* species
     b. *T. vaginalis*
     c. Bacterial vaginosis
   Cervical site of infection:
     a. *N. gonorrhoeae*
     b. *C. trachomatis*
     c. Herpes genitalis

(continued)

TABLE 60.1

(Continued)

3. Genital ulcer/lymphadenopathy
   a. Herpes genitalis
   b. *Treponema pallidum*
   c. *Haemophilus ducreyi*
   d. *C. trachomatis* (LGV types)
   e. *Calymmatobacterium granulomatis*
4. Genital growths
   a. Human papillomavirus (genital warts)
   b. Molluscum contagiosum
   c. Condyloma latum (secondary syphilis)
5. Abdominal/pelvic pain
   a. Pelvic inflammatory disease
6. Anorectal pain/discharge/bleeding
   a. *N. gonorrhoeae*
   b. *C. trachomatis*
   c. *Shigella* species
   d. *Campylobacter* species
   e. *Entamoeba histolytica*
   f. *Giardia lamblia*
7. Epididymitis
   a. *N. gonorrhoeae*
   b. *C. trachomatis*
   c. Coliform/enteric bacteria
8. Hepatitis
   a. Hepatitis A and B virus
   b. Cytomegalovirus
   c. *T. pallidum*
9. Arthralgia/arthritis
   a. *N. gonorrhoeae*
   b. Hepatitis B virus
10. Pruritus
    a. *Pthirus pubis*
    b. *Sarcoptes scabiei*
    c. *T. pallidum*
11. Flu-like or mononucleosis syndrome
    a. Cytomegalovirus
    b. Herpes genitalis
    c. Hepatitis A and B virus
    d. Human immunodeficiency virus

WEB SITES

For Teenagers and Parents

http://www.iwannaknow.org. The American Social Health Association Web site designed specifically for teens. Sexuality and STD prevention are directly and explicitly addressed.

http://www.scarleteen.com/index.html. A teen-friendly, accurate and up-to-date site targeted at young women.

http://www.niaid.nih.gov/publications/stds.htm. National Institute of Allergy and Infectious Diseases fact sheet on STDs.

http://www.cdc.gov/women/. Centers for Disease Control and Prevention (CDC) women's health home page on STDs.

For Health Professionals

http://www.cdc.gov/STD/treatment/. The CDC Web site with recent statistics and treatment guidelines.

http://www.ashastd.org. The American Social Health Association home page. Lots of information and hotline access.

http://www.cdc.gov/std/training/. CDC site with a variety of training resources related to STDs.

APPENDIX 60.1

Sexually Transmitted Diseases Summary

Note: Adapted from the Centers for Disease Control and Prevention, Department of Health and Human Services. 2006 guidelines for treatment of sexually transmitted diseases. *MMWR Morb Mortal Wkly Rep* 2006;55(RR-11), with permission. For a copy of this publication, write to CDC, Technical Information Services, Atlanta, GA 30333. Copies, updates, downloadable PDA versions and slide show summaries are available on-line, at http://www.cdc.gov/STD/treatment/.

NONGONOCOCCAL URETHRITIS

Etiological Agents

Chlamydia trachomatis (15%–55%)
Ureaplasma urealyticum (10%–40%)
Mycoplasma genitalium (5%–15%)
Trichomonas vaginalis (2%–5%)
HSV on occasion

TYPICAL CLINICAL PRESENTATION

Men usually have dysuria, frequency, and mucoid-to-purulent urethral discharge. Some men have asymptomatic infections.

Urethral discharge associated with nongonococcal urethritis (NGU) tends to occur 1 to 5 weeks after infection; NGU produces less discharge and dysuria than gonococcal urethritis.

However, no symptoms or signs reliably distinguish gonococcal urethritis from NGU or among various etiological causes of NGU.

PRESUMPTIVE DIAGNOSIS

(Warrants full treatment and follow-up.)
Mucopurulent or purulent discharge.

Absence of gram-negative intracellular diplococci and ≥5 polymorphonuclear (PMN) leukocytes/oil immersion field on a smear of an intraurethral swab specimen.

Positive leukocyte esterase test (LET) results on first-void urine or microscopic examination of first-void urine demonstrating ≥10 PMN leukocytes/high-power field. Positive LET results should always be confirmed with a Gram stain of a urethral swab specimen and/or gonorrhea and chlamydia testing.

Asymptomatic men with negative gonorrhea test results are presumed to have NGU if they have ≥5 PMN/oil immersion field on an intraurethral smear.

DEFINITIVE DIAGNOSIS

An agent etiologically associated with NGU is recovered from the male urethra. Specific diagnostic tests for organisms other than *Neisseria gonorrhoeae* and *C. trachomatis* are not indicated in the evaluation of males with urethritis.

Note: Coinfection by multiple organisms is common.

THERAPY

Recommended Regimen: Azithromycin 1 g PO in a single dose, OR

Doxycycline 100 mg PO b.i.d. for 7 days.

Alternative Regimens: Erythromycin base 500 mg PO q.i.d. for 7 days, OR

Erythromycin ethylsuccinate 800 mg PO q.i.d. for 7 days, OR

Ofloxacin 300 mg PO b.i.d. for 7 days, OR

Levofloxacin 500 mg PO once a day for 7 days.

COMPLICATIONS AND SEQUELAE

Urethral strictures

Prostatitis

Epididymitis

Reiter syndrome

Chlamydial NGU may be transmitted to female sex partners, resulting in mucopurulent endocervicitis, pelvic inflammatory disease (PID), and other adverse outcomes. (See entries related to these conditions in the succeeding pages.) Now that quinolones are not recommended for gonorrhea treatment, testing with culture or NAAT for gonorrhea is essential when treating Chlamydia or NGU.

OTHER CONSIDERATIONS

Follow-up: Regimens for persistent/recurrent urethritis have not been rigorously evaluated. Noncompliant patients and those with reexposure to untreated partners should be re-treated with the initial regimen. Azithromycin is more active against *M. genitalium* infections. Patients with objective evidence of persistent/recurrent urethritis should be evaluated for *T. vaginalis* infection. A recommended treatment for persistent/recurrent urethritis is as follows:

Metronidazole 2.0 g PO in a single dose, OR

Tinidazole 2.0 g PO in a single dose, PLUS

Azithromycin 1.0 g PO (if not used in initial treatment)

Management of Sex Partners: Sex partners should be referred for evaluation and treatment.

HIV Infection: Patients with HIV infection should receive the same treatment as patients without HIV.

EPIDIDYMITIS

Etiological Agents

C. trachomatis
Neisseria gonorrhoeae
Coliform/enteric bacteria

TYPICAL CLINICAL PRESENTATION

Scrotal, inguinal, or flank pain and scrotal swelling. Subacute onset is typical, but acute symptoms are not uncommon. Most patients with epididymitis associated with sexually transmitted organisms have accompanying dysuria, urethral discharge, or both.

PRESUMPTIVE DIAGNOSIS

Requires ruling out testicular torsion. Gram stain of urethral secretions may show PMN leukocytes and gram-negative intracellular diplococci. Urinalysis is often positive for white blood cells (WBCs).

DEFINITIVE DIAGNOSIS

Definitive bacterial diagnosis may be made after ruling out testicular torsion. Positive Chlamydia test result (culture, direct immunofluorescence assay, DNA probe, or NAAT) or a positive gonorrhea test result (gram stain, culture, DNA probe, or NAAT). Rarely, epididymal aspiration is used to establish a diagnosis before surgery.

THERAPY

For epididymitis most likely caused by gonococcal or chlamydial infection:

Ceftriaxone 250 mg IM in single dose, PLUS

Doxycycline 100 mg PO b.i.d. for 10 days.

For epididymitis most likely caused by coliform/enteric organisms, or for patients allergic to cephalosporins or tetracyclines:

Ofloxacin 300 mg PO b.i.d. for 10 days, OR

Levofloxacin 500 mg PO once a day for 10 days.

COMPLICATIONS AND SEQUELAE

Testicular/scrotal abscess

Testicular infarction

Chronic epididymitis

Infertility

OTHER CONSIDERATIONS

Follow-up: Failure to improve within 3 days requires reevaluation.

Management of Sex Partners: Sex partners should be managed as appropriate for the identified STD. Partners of presumptively treated patients should be notified, evaluated, and treated for infections identified or suspected in the index patient.

HIV Infection: Patients with HIV infection should receive the same treatment as patients without HIV infection. Fungal and mycobacterial causes are more common among immunosuppressed patients and should be considered if initial treatment fails.

MUCOPURULENT CERVICITIS
Etiological Agents
N. gonorrhoeae
C. trachomatis

In most cases, neither of these organisms are isolated.

TYPICAL CLINICAL PRESENTATION

Most patients are asymptomatic. Symptomatic patients may complain of yellow vaginal discharge or abnormal vaginal bleeding (e.g., after coitus).

PRESUMPTIVE DIAGNOSIS

Mucopurulent cervicitis (MPC) is not a sensitive and specific predictor of infection by *C. trachomatis* or *N. gonorrhoeae*.

The presence of yellow mucopurulent endocervical discharge or the finding of yellow discharge on a white cotton-tipped swab of endocervical secretions suggests infection.

The presence of increased numbers of PMN leukocytes on a Gram stain of endocervical mucus is not standardized and has low predictive value. This evaluation is not recommended.

DEFINITIVE DIAGNOSIS

Definitive diagnosis is made by a positive Chlamydia test result (culture, direct immunofluorescence assay [DFA], DNA probe, or NAAT) or a positive gonorrhea test result (culture, DNA probe, or NAAT).

THERAPY

Treatment is based on the results of Chlamydia and gonorrhea testing. If the patient is unreliable or in an area of high likelihood of gonorrhea or chlamydial infection, treat presumptively with coverage for both gonorrhea and Chlamydia.

COMPLICATIONS AND SEQUELAE

Complications are those associated with etiological microbiological agents.

OTHER CONSIDERATIONS

Follow-up: Follow-up should be appropriate for identified sexually transmitted organisms.

Management of Sex Partners: Sex partners should be managed as appropriate for the identified STD. Partners of presumptively treated patients should be notified, evaluated, and treated for infections identified or suspected in the index patient.

HIV Infection: Patients with HIV infection should receive the same treatment as patients without HIV infection.

GONORRHEA
Etiological Agent
N. gonorrhoeae

TYPICAL CLINICAL PRESENTATION

When symptomatic, men complain of dysuria, urinary frequency, and purulent urethral discharge. Variable degrees of edema and erythema of the urethral meatus are often present.

Many infections in women are asymptomatic. Symptoms in women include abnormal vaginal discharge, intermenstrual bleeding, menorrhagia, or dysuria.

Symptoms of rectal gonococcal infection include mild anal pruritus, painless mucopurulent discharge, and mild bleeding. Symptoms of severe proctitis sometimes occur.

Pharyngeal infections are usually asymptomatic.

PRESUMPTIVE DIAGNOSIS

(Warrants full treatment and follow-up.)

Identification of typical gram-negative intracellular diplococci on smear of urethral discharge (men) or endocervical mucus (women). Gram stain is insufficiently sensitive for diagnosis in women and should be supplemented (if used) by culture, DNA probe, or NAAT confirmation.

DEFINITIVE DIAGNOSIS

Growth on selective medium, demonstrating typical colonial morphology, positive oxidase reaction, and typical Gram stain morphology. Nucleic acid probes and NAATs are highly sensitive and specific for the diagnosis of gonorrhea. Tests based on several methods are U.S. Food and Drug Administration (FDA)-approved and commercially available. Approved specimen sources include urethral and cervical discharge/mucus and urine. Urine is generally less sensitive for diagnosis of gonococcal infections in women. Provider and self-obtained vaginal swabs show high sensitivity and specificity in research settings, but are FDA-approved specimen sources for only one of the commercially available tests. False-positive tests may be due to other nonpathogenic bacterial species and should be considered when screening patients with low probability of infection.

THERAPY

Uncomplicated Urogenital or Anorectal Gonococcal Infections (see Other Considerations):
Ceftriaxone 125 mg IM at one time.

Cefixime 400 mg PO in a single dose.

Treatment for coinfection by *C. trachomatis* should be added unless appropriate diagnostic test results are negative for Chlamydia.

Uncomplicated Pharyngeal Infections (see Other Considerations):
Ceftriaxone 125 mg IM at one time, OR

Concomitant treatment for pharyngeal chlamydial infection is recommended, although coinfection is unusual.

Alternative Regimens: Spectinomycin 2 g IM a single dose (for potential shortage see Other Considerations) Injectable cephalosporin regimens such as ceftizoxime (500 mg IM in a single dose), cefotaxime (500 mg IM in a single dose), cefotetan (1 g IM in a single dose), and cefoxitin (2 g IM in a single dose).

Azithromycin 2 g orally is effective against uncomplicated gonococcal infection but is expensive and causes gastrointestinal distress and therefore is not recommended for treatment of gonorrhea. Azithromycin 1 g orally is not recommended because of concerns regarding the possible rapid emergence of antimicrobial resistance.

COMPLICATIONS AND SEQUELAE

Ten percent to 20% of women develop PID and are at risk for its sequelae (see following entry).

Men are at risk for epididymitis, sterility, urethral stricture, and infertility. Newborns are at risk for ophthalmia neonatorum, scalp abscess at the site of fetal monitors, rhinitis, pneumonia, or anorectal infections.

All infected, untreated persons are at risk for disseminated gonococcal infection (includes septicemia, arthritis, dermatitis, meningitis, and endocarditis).

GONORRHEA
(Continued)

OTHER CONSIDERATIONS

Because of rising quinolone resistance among gonococci, fluoroquinolones are no longer recommended for treatment of gonococcal infections and associated conditions such as pelvic inflammatory disease.

Note on spectinomycin shortage (http://www.cdc.gov/std/specshortage.htm): With the possible discontinuation of spectinomycin in the United States, patients allergic to cephalosporins may need desensitization treatment by a specialist. Two grams of azithromycin is an approved regimen, but is not recommended due to the gastrointestinal distress, and there is no data documenting the safety and efficacy in pregnant women. If used, patients should be observed for at least 30 minutes after ingestion to monitor tolerance.

Pregnant Women: Should not be treated with tetracycline or quinolones.

Follow-up: No test of cure is needed for patients with uncomplicated gonorrhea who are treated with one of the regimens in these guidelines. Treatment failures are most likely due to reinfection.

Management of Sex Partners: Sex partners should be referred for evaluation and treatment. Sexual intercourse should be avoided until the patient and partner are cured.

HIV Infection: Patients with HIV infection should receive the same treatment as patients without HIV infection.

CHLAMYDIA
Etiological Agent
C. trachomatis

TYPICAL CLINICAL PRESENTATION

Many patients are asymptomatic. Symptomatic women complain of dysuria or abnormal vaginal discharge. Symptomatic men usually have dysuria, urinary frequency, and a mucopurulent urethral discharge.

PRESUMPTIVE DIAGNOSIS

(Warrants full treatment and follow-up.)

Women: Sexual contact with a partner with diagnosed nongonococcal or chlamydial urethritis. MPC is sometimes used as presumptive diagnosis of cervical chlamydial infection.

Men: Sexual contact with partners with urogenital chlamydial infection. NGU (i.e., typical clinical symptoms and ≥5 PMN leukocytes/oil immersion field on a smear of an intraurethral swab specimen).

DEFINITIVE DIAGNOSIS

Definitive diagnosis is made with a positive Chlamydia test result (culture, DFA, nucleic acid probe or NAAT).

THERAPY

Recommended Regimens:

Azithromycin 1 g PO in a single dose, OR

Doxycycline 100 mg PO b.i.d. for 7 days.

Alternative Regimens:

Ofloxacin 300 mg PO b.i.d. for 7 days, OR

Levofloxacin 500 mg PO once a day for 7 days, OR

Erythromycin base 500 mg PO q.i.d. for 7 days, OR

Erythromycin ethylsuccinate 800 mg PO q.i.d. for 7 days.

COMPLICATIONS AND SEQUELAE

Ascending infections may lead to symptomatic or asymptomatic endometritis and salpingitis and subsequent infertility. Ascending infection during pregnancy may lead to adverse obstetric outcomes, conjunctivitis, or pneumonia in the infant, and to puerperal infection.

OTHER CONSIDERATIONS

Pregnant Women: Doxycycline, ofloxacin, and levofloxacin are contraindicated for use during pregnancy. Azithromycin is a Class B drug, so its safety for pregnant and lactating women is not known. However, there is now extensive clinical experience with azithromycin treatment during pregnancy.

Recommended Regimen for Pregnant Women:

Azithromycin 1.0 g PO as a single oral dose, OR

Amoxicillin 500 mg PO t.i.d. for 7 days.

Alternative Regimens:

Erythromycin base 500 mg PO q.i.d., for 7 days, OR

Erythromycin base 250 mg PO q.i.d. for 14 days, OR

Erythromycin ethylsuccinate 800 mg PO q.i.d. for 7 days, OR

Erythromycin ethylsuccinate 400 mg PO q.i.d for 14 days

Follow-up: No need for retesting after completing treatment with doxycycline or azithromycin. Retesting at 3 weeks after completion of therapy may be useful for pregnant women because none of the regimens are highly efficacious and the erythromycin side effects may prevent compliance. Reinfection is common in women with *C. trachomatis* and rescreening in 3 to 4 months after treatment is recommended, particularly in adolescents.

Management of Sex Partners: Sex partners should be referred for evaluation and treatment.

HIV Infection: Patients with HIV infection should receive the same treatment as patients without HIV infection.

PELVIC INFLAMMATORY DISEASE
Etiological Agents

In most cases, sexually transmitted organisms, especially *N. gonorrhoeae* and *C. trachomatis,* are implicated. However, other microorganisms that can be part of vaginal flora, such as anaerobes, *Gardnerella vaginalis, Haemophilus influenzae,* enteric gram-negative rods, and *Streptococcus agalactiae* can cause PID. *Mycoplasma hominis* and *U. urealyticum* may also play a role.

TYPICAL CLINICAL PRESENTATION

The spectrum of PID includes any combination of endometritis, salpingitis, tuboovarian abscess (TOA), and pelvic peritonitis. The patient may present with pain and tenderness involving the lower abdomen, cervix, uterus, and adnexa. Fever, chills, elevated WBC count, and elevated erythrocyte sedimentation rate (ESR) are often absent.

PRESUMPTIVE DIAGNOSIS

The clinical diagnosis of PID is difficult because of the wide variation in symptoms and signs. No combination of symptoms, signs, or laboratory findings is both sensitive and specific for PID. Because delay in treatment increases the potential for damage to the reproductive health of the woman with PID, a low threshold for the diagnosis of PID is necessary.

Minimum Criteria:

- Adnexal tenderness, OR
- Uterine tenderness, OR
- Cervical motion tenderness

Empirical treatment of PID should be initiated in sexually active young women and others at risk for STDs if the minimum criteria are present and no other cause(s) for the illness can be identified. Although PID occurs during pregnancy, patients with positive pregnancy tests require careful evaluation for ectopic pregnancy as a cause for pelvic pain.

Additional Criteria: Additional criteria may increase the specificity of the diagnosis. The likelihood of PID is reduced if all of these criteria are normal or negative.

Routine Criteria:

- Oral temperature >38.3°C
- Abnormal cervical or vaginal discharge
- Presence of WBCs on saline microscopy of vaginal secretions
- Elevated ESR
- Elevated C-reactive protein
- Laboratory documentation of cervical infection with *N. gonorrhoeae* or *C. trachomatis*
  If the cervical discharge appears normal and no WBCs are observed on the wet prep of vaginal fluid, the diagnosis of PID is unlikely, and another diagnosis should be explored.

Elaborate Criteria:

- Histopathological evidence of endometritis on endometrial biopsy
- TOA on sonography
- Laparoscopic abnormalities consistent with PID

DEFINITIVE DIAGNOSIS

Direct visualization of inflamed (edema, hyperemia, or tubal exudate) fallopian tube at laparoscopy or laparotomy makes the diagnosis of PID definitive. A culture of tubal exudate establishes the etiology.

THERAPY

Some experts recommend that all patients with PID be hospitalized to initiate parenteral antibiotics. Hospitalization of patients with PID is particularly recommended in the following circumstances:

1. The diagnosis is uncertain; and surgical emergencies such as appendicitis and ectopic pregnancy cannot be excluded.
2. A pelvic abscess is suspected.
3. The patient is pregnant.
4. The patient has HIV infection.
5. Severe illness or nausea and vomiting preclude outpatient management.
6. The patient is unable to follow or tolerate an outpatient regimen.
7. The patient has failed to respond to outpatient therapy.
8. Clinical follow-up within 72 hours of starting antibiotic treatment cannot be arranged.

ORAL TREATMENT

Little information is available from clinical trials on intermediate and long-term outcomes using outpatient regimens. If patients do not respond within 72 hours to outpatient regimens, they should be hospitalized to confirm diagnosis and receive parenteral treatment.

Ceftriaxone 250 mg IM once, OR

Cefoxitin 2 g IM, plus probenecid 1 g concurrently, OR

Other parenteral third-generation cephalosporin such as ceftizoxime or cefotaxime, PLUS

Doxycycline 100 mg orally twice a day for 14 days

WITH or WITHOUT

Metronidazole 500 mg PO b.i.d. for 14 days.

PELVIC INFLAMMATORY DISEASE
(Continued)

PARENTERAL TREATMENT

Regimen A:

Cefoxitin 2 g IV q6h, OR cefotetan 2 g IV q12h, PLUS

Doxycycline 100 mg IV or PO q12h.

Oral and IV doxycycline have similar bioavailability. Oral administration should be used when possible because of pain of IV administration.

Regimen B:

Clindamycin 900 mg IV q8h, PLUS

Gentamicin loading dose IV or IM 2 mg/kg of body weight, followed by a maintenance dose, 1.5 mg/kg q8h.

These regimens should be continued for at least 48 hours after the patient demonstrates improvement. Thereafter, doxycycline (100 mg PO b.i.d.) or clindamycin (450 mg PO q.i.d.) should be continued for 14 days. When TOA is present, many health care providers use clindamycin for continued therapy, rather than doxycycline, because clindamycin provides more effective anaerobic coverage.

Alternative Parenteral Regimens: Few data support the use of other parenteral regimens, but the following regimen has been investigated in at least one clinical trial:

Ampicillin/sulbactam 3 g IV q6h PLUS

Doxycycline 100 mg IV or PO q12h.

COMPLICATIONS AND SEQUELAE

Life-threatening complications include ectopic pregnancy and pelvic abscess. Other complications are involuntary infertility, recurrent PID, chronic PID, chronic abdominal pain, pelvic adhesions, premature hysterectomy, and depression.

OTHER CONSIDERATIONS

Pregnant Women: Should be treated as inpatients.

Follow-up: Hospitalized patients should show substantial clinical improvement within 3 to 5 days or require further diagnostic workup. Patients treated as outpatients should be followed up for 72 hours and after significant clinical improvement. Some experts recommend retesting for *N. gonorrhoeae* and *C. trachomatis* 4 to 6 weeks after completing therapy.

Management of Sex Partners: Sex partners should be referred for evaluation and treatment. Treatment should include coverage for both *N. gonorrhoeae* and *C. trachomatis* infections. Sexual intercourse should be avoided until the patient and partner are cured.

HIV Infection: Patients with HIV infection should be managed aggressively, including hospitalization.

VAGINITIS
Etiological Agent

The three diseases most frequently associated with vaginal discharge are the following:

- Bacterial vaginosis (sometimes incorrectly called nonspecific vaginitis or *G. vaginalis*-associated vaginitis). Clinical syndrome resulting from replacement of normal vaginal flora with anaerobic bacteria, *G. vaginalis,* and *M. hominis.*
- Trichomoniasis *(T. vaginalis)*
- Candidiasis (vulvovaginal candidiasis[VVC]) usually caused by *Candida albicans*

Other vaginitides (vaginitis caused by other infectious, chemical, allergenic, and physical agents).

TYPICAL CLINICAL PRESENTATION

Presentations vary from no signs or symptoms to erythema, edema, and pruritus of the external genitalia. Excessive or malodorous discharge is a common finding. Symptoms and clinical findings do not reliably distinguish among etiologies.

Male sex partners may develop urethritis, balanitis, or cutaneous lesions on penis.

PRESUMPTIVE DIAGNOSIS

(Warrants full treatment and follow-up.)

The diagnosis of vaginitis is made by vaginal pH and microscopic examination of fresh samples of the discharge.

T. vaginalis **Vaginitis:** Small, punctate cervical hemorrhages called *colpitis macularis* or *strawberry cervix* are highly specific for the diagnosis of vaginal trichomoniasis. However, this finding is present on routine speculum examination in fewer than 5% of women. Vaginal pH level is almost always >4.5 and wet mount examination often shows many WBCs.

Bacterial Vaginosis: The clinical criteria include three of the following:

- A homogenous gray or white noninflammatory discharge that adheres to vaginal walls
- Vaginal pH level >4.5
- A fishy odor from vaginal fluid before or after addition of 10% potassium hydroxide (KOH)
- Presence of "clue cells" on microscopic examination

Vulvovaginal Candidiasis: The presumptive criteria are the typical symptoms of vaginitis or vulvitis and microscopic identification of yeast forms (budding cells or hyphae) in Gram stain or KOH wet mount preparation of vaginal discharge.

DEFINITIVE DIAGNOSIS

T. vaginalis **Vaginitis:** A vaginal culture, or commercially available test (e.g., detection of *T. vaginalis* DNA or rapid antigen tests) is positive for *T. vaginalis,* OR

Typical motile trichomonads are identified in a saline wet mount of vaginal discharge (only 60%–70%

sensitive). NAATs are currently under development but are commercially unavailable.

Bacterial Vaginosis: Gram stain demonstration of few or no lactobacilli, with a predominance of gram-variable rods (likely representing *G. vaginalis*) plus other organisms resembling gram-negative *Bacteroides* sp, anaerobic gram-positive cocci, or curved rods.

Vulvovaginal Candidiasis: Culture may be useful when signs and symptoms are suggestive but when the fungus cannot be identified by direct microscopy. Therapy of apparent treatment failures is best guided by culture.

THERAPY
T. vaginalis **Vaginitis:**

Recommended regimen:

Metronidazole 2 g PO in a single dose, OR

Tinidazole 2 g PO in a single dose.

Alternative regimen:

Metronidazole 500 mg b.i.d. for 7 days.

Both regimens have cure rates of approximately 95%. Metronidazole resistance is reported, but its prevalence is not known. Tinidazole has a longer half-life and reaches higher concentrations in genital fluids and may be useful if metronidazole resistance is suspected. Metronidazole gel is associated with unacceptably high failure rates.

Bacterial Vaginosis:

Recommended Regimen:

Metronidazole 500 mg PO b.i.d. for 7 days, OR

Clindamycin cream 2% one applicator (5 g) intravaginally at bedtime for 7 days, OR

Metronidazole gel 0.75% one applicator (5 g) intravaginally q.d. for 5 days.

Alternative Regimens:

Clindamycin 300 mg PO b.i.d. for 7 days OR

Clindamycin ovules 100 mg intravaginally once at bedtime for 3 days.

VAGINITIS
(Continued)

Vulvovaginal Candidiasis:

Intravaginal Agents:

Clotrimazole, miconazole nitrate, terconazole, or butoconazole creams or vaginal tablets are recommended. Regimens range from 1 to 14 days of treatment. Several are available for over-the-counter purchase. Some contain oils that may weaken latex condoms.

Oral Agent:

Fluconazole 150-mg tablet in a single dose.

COMPLICATIONS AND SEQUELAE

Secondary excoriations are common.

Recurrent infections are common.

Bacterial vaginosis and trichomoniasis are associated with infectious complications of pregnancy, such as chorioamnionitis and puerperal infection, and with polymicrobial upper genital tract infections in nonpregnant women, such as endometritis and salpingitis. Intravaginal preparations are not recommended during pregnancy.

VVC in pregnancy increases the risk of neonatal oral thrush.

OTHER CONSIDERATIONS
Pregnant Women

Metronidazole may be used during pregnancy in a single dose of 2 g.

Clindamycin vaginal cream should be avoided during pregnancy.

VVC should be treated with topical azole therapies during pregnancy. Many experts recommend 7 days of therapy.

Follow-up:

Bacterial vaginosis: No follow-up visits are necessary.

Trichomoniasis: Follow-up is unnecessary for patients who become asymptomatic after treatment.

Vulvovaginal candidiasis: Follow-up is unnecessary for patients who respond to therapy.

Management of Sex Partners

Bacterial Vaginosis: Treatment of partners is not recommended.

Trichomoniasis: Sex partners should be treated and sexual contact should be avoided until the patient and partner are cured.

Vulvovaginal candidiasis: Treatment of sex partners is not routinely warranted unless male sex partner has balanitis.

HIV Infection: Bacterial vaginosis, trichomoniasis, and VVC: Patients with HIV infection should be managed in the same manner as patients without HIV infection.

CONDYLOMATA ACUMINATA (GENITAL WARTS)
Etiological Agent
Human papillomavirus

More than 130 types have been identified and more than 25 types infect the genital tract. Certain types (usually 6 and 11) cause exophytic benign genital and anal warts. Other types (e.g., 16, 18, 31, 33, and 35 among others) are associated with several types of anogenital carcinomas.

TYPICAL CLINICAL PRESENTATION

Condylomata acuminata present as single or multiple soft, fleshy, papillary or sessile, painless growths around the anus, vulvovaginal area, penis, urethra, or perineum.

PRESUMPTIVE DIAGNOSIS

(Warrants full treatment and follow-up.)

A diagnosis is made on the basis of the typical clinical presentation.

Colposcopy may also aid in the diagnosis of certain cervical lesions.

Condylomata lata can be excluded by dark-field microscopy or a serological test for syphilis.

DEFINITIVE DIAGNOSIS

A biopsy, although usually unnecessary, can make a definitive diagnosis. Atypical lesions, in which neoplasia is a consideration, should be biopsied before initiating therapy.

A Papanicolaou (Pap) smear of cervical lesions shows typical cytological changes of koilocytosis. Direct DNA immunofluorescence staining techniques can diagnose certain types of HPV.

A HC test for detection of high-risk HPV types is now FDA-approved for triage of atypical squamous cells of undetermined significance (ASCUS). Women with ASCUS by Pap smear and a positive HC test result can be further evaluated by colposcopy. The role of HPV screening among women with low-grade squamous intraepithelial lesions is under investigation. Routine HPV screening, for women or for men, is not recommended.

THERAPY

The goal of therapy is removal of exophytic warts and alleviation of signs and symptoms, not the eradication of HPV.

External Genital Warts

Patient Applied:

Podofilox 0.5% solution or gel: Apply to visible warts b.i.d. for 3 days, followed by 4 days without therapy.

Repeat as necessary up to four cycles. Total area treated should not exceed 10 cm^2 and total volume should not exceed 0.5 mL/day.

Imiquimod 5% cream: Apply to visible warts at bedtime, three times per week. Treatment area should be washed with soap and water 6 to 10 hours after application.

Provider Applied:

Cryotherapy with liquid nitrogen or cryoprobe: For vaginal warts, do not use cryoprobe (to avoid perforations), OR

Podophyllin 10% to 25% in compound tincture of benzoin: Wash off in 1 to 4 hours to reduce irritation, OR

Trichloroacetic acid (TCA) or bichloracetic acid 80% to 90%: Weekly for maximum of 6 weeks, OR

Electrodesiccation or electrocautery.

Cervical Warts: Cervical dysplasia must be excluded before treatment is begun. Management is complicated and should be carried out in consultation with an expert.

Vaginal Warts: Cryotherapy with liquid nitrogen, TCA, or podophyllin. Podophyllin treatments should be limited to ≤2 cm^2 and the treated area should be dry before speculum removal.

Anal or Oral Warts: Cryotherapy with liquid nitrogen or TCA or surgical removal.

COMPLICATIONS AND SEQUELAE

Lesions may enlarge and produce tissue destruction. Giant condyloma, although histologically benign, may stimulate carcinoma. Cervical lesions are associated with neoplasia.

In pregnancy, warts enlarge, are extremely vascular, and may obstruct the birth canal, necessitating cesarean section delivery.

CONDYLOMATA ACUMINATA (GENITAL WARTS)
(Continued)

OTHER CONSIDERATIONS

Prevention/Immunization: An effective vaccine against four HPV types (6, 11, 16, 18) is available for females 9 to 26 years of age (see Chapter 66).

Pregnancy: Use of podophyllin and podofilox are contraindicated. The safety of imiquimod during pregnancy is not established.

Follow-up: Not necessary after warts have responded to therapy. Annual cytological screening is recommended for women with or without genital warts.

Management of Sex Partners: Routine referral of partners for examination and treatment is not recommended. Partners may wish to be treated for clinical lesions. Reinfection from a partner is unusual. Use of condoms reduces (but does not eliminate) transmission to uninfected partners, and may shorten the duration of viral persistence.

HIV Infection: Patients with HIV may not respond to therapy for HPV, as well as persons without HIV. Cervical dysplasia may progress more rapidly among HIV-infected persons.

HERPES GENITALIS
Etiological Agents
HSV types 1 and 2

TYPICAL CLINICAL PRESENTATION

Single or multiple vesicles appear anywhere on the genitalia. Vesicles spontaneously rupture to form shallow ulcers that may be very painful. Lesions resolve spontaneously without scarring. The first occurrence is termed initial infection (mean duration, 12 days). Subsequent, usually milder, occurrences are termed recurrent infections (mean duration, 4–5 days). The interval between clinical episodes is termed latency. Viral shedding occurs intermittently and unpredictably during latency.

DIAGNOSIS

(Warrants full treatment and follow-up.)

Clinical diagnosis of genital herpes is both insensitive and nonspecific. However, when typical genital lesions are present or a pattern of recurrence has developed, herpes infection is likely. Classic, painful multiple vesicular or ulcerative lesions are often not seen in many infected individuals. While approximately 50% of first-episode cases of genital herpes are caused by HIV-1, most cases of recurrent genital herpes are caused by HSV-2. Therefore, the type of HSV could influence prognosis and counseling. Therefore, the clinical diagnosis of genital herpes should be confirmed by laboratory testing. Both virological and type-specific serological tests for HSV should be available in clinical settings that provide care for individuals.

Virological Tests: Cell culture is the preferred virological test but the sensitivity of culture is low, especially in recurrent lesions. Polymerase chain reaction (PCR) assays for HSV DNA are more sensitive but are not yet FDA-cleared for genital specimens. Viral culture isolates should be typed for HSV-1 or HSV-2.

Type-Specific Serological Tests:
Accurate type-specific HSV serological assays should be used and are based on the HSV-specific glycoprotein G2 (HSV-2) and G1 (HSV-1). The newer type-specific glycoprotein G (gG)-based assays should be requested. HSV-2 positivity generally implies a genital infection whereas HSV-1 positivity is difficult to interpret because most are related to oral infections. Sensitivities range from 80% to 98% for HSV-2 antibody and >96% for specificity. These tests might be useful in:

* Recurrent genital symptoms or atypical symptoms with negative HSV cultures
* A clinical diagnosis of genital herpes without laboratory confirmation
* A partner with genital herpes

THERAPY
First Clinical Episode of Genital Herpes:

Acyclovir 400 mg PO t.i.d. for 7 to 10 days, OR

Acyclovir 200 mg PO 5 times daily for 7 to 10 days, OR

Famciclovir 250 mg PO t.i.d. for 7 to 10 days, OR

Valacyclovir 1 g PO b.i.d. for 7 to 10 days.

Treatment may be extended if healing is incomplete after 10 days of therapy.

First Clinical Episode of Herpes Proctitis:

Acyclovir 400 mg PO 5 times a day for 10 days or until clinical resolution is attained.

Famciclovir and valacyclovir may also be effective, but clinical experience is lacking.

Episodic Treatment of Recurrent Episodes of Genital Herpes and Herpes Proctitis: When treatment is started during prodrome or within 1 day of onset of lesions, many patients experience shortened duration of symptoms.

Acyclovir 400 mg PO t.i.d. for 5 days, OR

Acyclovir 800 mg PO b.i.d. for 5 days, OR

Acyclovir 800 mg t.i.d. for 2 days, OR

Famciclovir 125 mg PO b.i.d. for 5 days, OR

Famciclovir 1,000 mg PO twice daily for 1 day OR

Valacyclovir 500 mg PO b.i.d. for 3 days, OR

Valacyclovir 1.0 g PO once a day for 5 days.

Daily Suppressive Therapy of Genital Herpes and Herpes Proctitis: Daily suppressive therapy can reduce frequency of HSV recurrences by at least 75% with patients with six or more recurrences per year. Suppressive therapy reduces viral shedding and reduces risk of transmission to partners.

Acyclovir 400 mg PO b.i.d., OR

Famciclovir 250 mg PO b.i.d., OR

Valacyclovir 500 mg PO once a day, OR

Valacyclovir 1.0 g PO once a day

COMPLICATIONS AND SEQUELAE

Neuralgia, meningitis, ascending myelitis, urethral strictures, and lymphatic suppuration may occur.

Neonates: Virus from an active genital infection may be transmitted during vaginal delivery, causing neonatal herpes infection, which has a high case fatality rate, and many survivors have ocular or neurological sequelae.

HERPES GENITALIS
(Continued)

OTHER CONSIDERATIONS

Pregnant Women: The safety of systemic acyclovir, valacyclovir, and famciclovir during pregnancy has not been established. Available data do not indicate increased risk of birth defects among women receiving acyclovir during the first trimester.

Counseling: Counseling of infected persons and their sex partners is critical. All persons with genital HSV should be strongly encouraged to inform their current and future sex partners that they have genital herpes. Individuals need to be aware of asymptomatic shedding, about potential decreased risk of transmission through use of antivirals, the protective effects of condoms, the possibility of acquisition by partners even if partners do not develop symptoms, and the risk of neonatal transmission.

Management of Sex Partners: Patients should abstain from sexual activity while lesions are present. Sexual transmission of HSV can occur during periods without evidence of lesions. The use of condoms should be encouraged during all sexual contact. Sex partners may require evaluation and counseling.

HIV Infection: HSV lesions are common among HIV-infected patients. Intermittent or suppressive therapy with oral acyclovir may be required.

SYPHILIS
Etiological Agent
Treponema pallidum

TYPICAL CLINICAL PRESENTATION

Primary: The classic chancre is painless, indurated, and located at the site of exposure. Genital chancres are often accompanied by tender inguinal lymphadenopathy.

Secondary: Patients may have a macular, maculopapular, or papulosquamous skin rash. Other signs include mucous patches and condylomata lata.

Tertiary: Patients have cardiac, neurological, ophthalmic, auditory, or gummatous lesions.

Latent: Patients are without clinical signs.

PRESUMPTIVE DIAGNOSIS

(Warrants full treatment and follow-up.)

Presumptive diagnosis relies on both nontreponemal serological tests for syphilis (STS) (e.g., Venereal Disease Research Laboratories or rapid plasma reagin) and treponemal tests (fluorescent treponemal antibody-absorption, *T. pallidum* particle agglutination (TP-PA), and enzyme immunoassays). Nontreponemal test antibody titers usually correlate with disease activity, and decline with therapy.

Primary: Patients have typical lesions and either a newly positive STS or STS titer at least fourfold greater than the last, or syphilis exposure within 90 days of lesion onset.

Secondary: Patients have the typical clinical presentation and a strongly reactive STS.

Latent: Patients have serological evidence of untreated syphilis without clinical signs.

HIV-infected patients: When clinical findings indicate presence of syphilis but serological test results are negative, alternative tests, such as biopsy, dark-field examination, and DFA staining of lesion material, should be employed.

DEFINITIVE DIAGNOSIS

Demonstration of characteristic spirochetes with dark-field microscopy of serous transudate from genital lesions. DFA of material from a chancre, regional lymph node, or other lesion.

THERAPY
Primary and Secondary Syphilis:

Penicillin G benzathine 2.4 million units IM in a single dose

For penicillin-allergic patients
Doxycycline 100 mg PO b.i.d. for 2 weeks, OR

Tetracycline 500 mg PO q.i.d. for 2 weeks.

Ceftriaxone 1 g IM or IV daily for 8 to 10 days.

Note: The optimal dose and duration of treatment have not been established. Some penicillin-allergic patients are also allergic to ceftriaxone.

Azithromycin 2.0 g PO in a single oral dose.

Note: Some areas have noted rapid emergence of resistant *T. pallidum* strains, suggesting need for careful clinical and serological follow-up if this regimen is used.

Latent Syphilis:
Early latent (<1 year) syphilis: Penicillin G benzathine, 2.4 million units IM in a single dose.

Late latent (>1 year) syphilis or latent syphilis of unknown duration: Penicillin G benzathine, 7.2 million units total, administered as three doses of 2.4 million units IM each at 1-week intervals.

Late Syphilis:
Patients with gumma or cardiovascular syphilis but not neurosyphilis: Penicillin G benzathine, 7.2 million units total, administered as three doses of 2.4 million units IM at 1-week intervals.

Neurosyphilis:
Recommended regimen: Aqueous crystalline penicillin G, 18 to 24 million units daily, administered as 3 to 4 million units IV q4h for 10 to 14 days.

Alternative regimen: 2.4 million units procaine penicillin IM daily, plus probenecid 500 mg PO q.i.d., both for 10 to 14 days.

COMPLICATIONS AND SEQUELAE

Both late syphilis and congenital syphilis are complications, because they are preventable with prompt diagnosis and treatment of early syphilis. Sequelae of late syphilis include neurological complications (general paresis, tabes dorsalis, and focal neurological signs), cardiovascular syphilis (thoracic aortic aneurysm, aortic insufficiency), and localized gumma formation.

Syphilis

(Continued)

OTHER CONSIDERATIONS

Pregnant Women: Pregnant women should receive the same therapy as listed earlier, except that tetracycline, doxycycline, and erythromycin should not be used. Pregnant women with a history of penicillin allergy should be skin tested, desensitized if allergy is documented, and then treated with penicillin.

Follow-up: Patients should be reexamined clinically and serologically at 3 and 6 months for primary and secondary syphilis and at 6 and 12 months for latent syphilis. STS results become negative or reactive only in low titers (<1:8) in most successfully treated patients.

Management of Sex Partners: Persons exposed to a patient with primary, secondary, or early latent syphilis within 90 days should be treated presumptively. Those exposed >90 days should be treated presumptively if serological tests are not available immediately or follow-up is uncertain. Partners considered at risk are those exposed within 3 months plus duration of symptoms for primary syphilis, within 6 months plus duration of symptoms for secondary syphilis, and within 1 year for early latent syphilis.

HIV Infection: Unusual serological response may occur in HIV-infected persons. Penicillin regimens should be used whenever possible. Some authorities recommend cerebrospinal fluid examination or treatment with a regimen appropriate for neurosyphilis for all patients coinfected with syphilis and HIV. Patients should be followed up clinically and serologically at 1, 2, 3, 6, 9, and 12 months after therapy.

CHANCROID

Etiological Agent

Haemophilus ducreyi

A gram-negative bacillus with rounded ends, commonly observed in small clusters along strands of mucus. On culture, the organism tends to form straight or tangled chains.

TYPICAL CLINICAL PRESENTATION

Usually a single (but sometimes multiple), superficial, painful ulcer surrounded by an erythematous halo. Ulcers may also be necrotic or severely erosive with ragged serpiginous borders. Accompanying adenopathy is usually unilateral. A characteristic inguinal bubo occurs in 25% to 60% of cases.

PRESUMPTIVE DIAGNOSIS

(Warrants full treatment and follow-up.)

Chancroid is the third most common sexually transmitted cause of genital ulcer in the United States, although it is far less frequently seen than genital herpes or primary syphilis. Presumptive diagnosis depends on a clinically consistent lesion, a negative dark-field examination of lesion fluid, and absence of serological evidence of syphilis.

DEFINITIVE DIAGNOSIS

Culture identification of *H. ducreyi*. No FDA-cleared PCR test of *H. ducreyi* is available in the United States, but such testing can be performed by clinical laboratories that have developed their own PCR test and conducted a Clinical Laboratory Improvement Amendments (CLIA) verification study.

THERAPY

Recommended Regimens:

Azithromycin 1 g PO in a single dose, OR

Ceftriaxone 250 mg IM in a single dose, OR

Ciprofloxacin 500 mg PO b.i.d. for 3 days, OR

Erythromycin base 500 mg PO t.i.d. for 7 days.

COMPLICATIONS AND SEQUELAE

Systemic spread is not known to occur.

Lesions may become secondarily infected and necrotic.

Bubo may rupture and suppurate, resulting in fistulae.

Ulcers on the prepuce may cause paraphimosis or phimosis.

OTHER CONSIDERATIONS

Pregnant Women: Safety of azithromycin during pregnancy has not been established. Ciprofloxacin is contraindicated during pregnancy.

Follow-up: Successfully treated ulcers clinically improve by 7 days after institution of therapy. If the condition does not improve, the clinician should consider whether antimicrobials were taken as prescribed; the *H. ducreyi* is resistant to the prescribed antimicrobial; the diagnosis is correct; there is a coinfection with another STD; or the patient is infected with HIV.

Management of Sex Partners: Partners who had contact within 10 days before the onset of symptoms should be examined and treated.

HIV Infection: Patients with HIV infections should be closely monitored and may require longer courses of therapy.

LYMPHOGRANULOMA VENEREUM
Etiological Agent
C. trachomatis

An obligate intracellular organism of serovars L1, L2, or L3.

TYPICAL CLINICAL PRESENTATION

The primary lesion of lymphogranuloma venereum (LGV) is a 2- to 3-mm painless vesicle or nonindurated ulcer at the site of inoculation. Patients commonly fail to notice this primary lesion. Regional adenopathy, typically unilateral, follows a week to a month later and is the most common clinical presentation.

Sensation of stiffness and aching in the groin, followed by swelling of the inguinal region, may be the first indications of infection in most patients. Adenopathy may subside spontaneously or proceed to the formation of abscesses that rupture to produce draining sinuses or fistulae.

PRESUMPTIVE DIAGNOSIS

(Warrants full treatment and follow-up.)

The LGV complement-fixation test result is typically positive, with titers of 1:64 or higher. Cross-reactions due to other chlamydial infections may be misleading. Because the sequelae of LGV are serious and preventable, treatment should be provided pending laboratory confirmation.

DEFINITIVE DIAGNOSIS

A definitive diagnosis requires isolation of *C. trachomatis* from an appropriate specimen and confirmation of the isolate as an LGV immunotype. However, such laboratory diagnostic capabilities are not widely available.

THERAPY

Recommended regimen:
Doxycycline 100 mg PO b.i.d. for 21 days.

Alternative regimen:
Erythromycin 500 mg PO q.i.d. for 21 days.

COMPLICATIONS AND SEQUELAE

Dissemination may occur with nephropathy, hepatomegaly, or phlebitis.

Large polypoid swellings of the vulva, anal margin, or rectal mucosa may occur.

The most common severe morbidity results from rectal involvement; perianal abscess and rectovaginal or other fistulae are early consequences, and rectal stricture may develop 1 to 10 years after infection.

OTHER CONSIDERATIONS

Pregnant Women: Pregnant patients should be treated with the erythromycin regimen.

Follow-up: Patients should be followed up clinically until signs and symptoms have resolved.

Management of Sex Partners: Persons having had sexual contact with a patient who has LGV within 30 days before onset of the patient's symptoms should be examined and treated.

HIV Infection: Patients with HIV infection are managed in the same manner as patients without HIV infection.

MOLLUSCUM CONTAGIOSUM

Etiological Agent

Molluscum contagiosum virus

The largest DNA virus of the poxvirus group.

TYPICAL CLINICAL PRESENTATION

Both sexual and nonsexual transmission modes are likely. Lesions are 1 to 5 mm, smooth, rounded, shiny, firm, and flesh-colored to pearly white papules with umbilicated centers. They are most commonly seen on the trunk and anogenital. Itching or tenderness is occasionally noted but most patients are asymptomatic. Extensive skin involvement is seen in immunocompromised hosts, particularly in those with advanced HIV disease. Dissemination does not occur.

PRESUMPTIVE DIAGNOSIS

(Warrants full treatment and follow-up.)

Usually diagnosed on the basis of the typical clinical presentation.

DEFINITIVE DIAGNOSIS

Microscopic examination of lesions or lesion material reveals the pathognomonic molluscum inclusion bodies.

THERAPY

Lesions resolve spontaneously; most within 2 months. However, they may be removed by curettage after cryoanesthesia.

Caustic chemicals (podophyllin, TCA, silver nitrate) and cryotherapy (liquid nitrogen) have been used successfully. Self-applied podophyllotoxin may also be effective. Recurrence is reported in 15% to 35% of cases.

COMPLICATIONS AND SEQUELAE

Secondary infection, usually with *Staphylococcus*, occurs.

Lesions rarely attain a size >10 mm in diameter.

OTHER CONSIDERATIONS

Pregnant Women: Podophyllin should be avoided during pregnancy.

Follow-up: Patients should return for evaluation 1 month after treatment so any new lesions can be removed.

Management of Sex Partners: Sex partners should be examined.

HIV Infection: Patients with HIV infection should be managed in the same manner as patients without HIV infection.

PEDICULOSIS PUBIS
Etiological Agent
Pthirus pubis (pubic or crab louse)

A grayish ectoparasite that is 1 to 4 mm long with segmented tarsi and claws for clinging to hairs.

TYPICAL CLINICAL PRESENTATION

Symptoms range from slight discomfort to intolerable itching. Erythematous papules, nits, or adult lice clinging to pubic, perineal, or perianal hairs are present and often noticed by patients.

PRESUMPTIVE DIAGNOSIS

(Warrants full treatment and follow-up.)

A presumptive diagnosis is made when a patient with a history of recent exposure to pubic lice has pruritic, erythematous macules, papules, or secondary excoriations in the genital area.

DEFINITIVE DIAGNOSIS

A definitive diagnosis is made by finding lice or nits attached to genital hairs.

THERAPY

Recommended Regimens:
Permethrin 1% creme rinse applied to affected areas and washed off after 10 minutes, OR

Pyrethrins with piperonyl butoxide applied to the infested area and washed off after 10 minutes.

Alternative Regimens
Malathion 0.5% lotion applied for 8 to 12 hours and then thoroughly washed off, OR

Ivermectin 250 µg/kg by mouth, repeated in 2 weeks.

Owing to increased risk of neurotoxicity, lindane should be used only if other treatments are not tolerated or have failed.

The recommended regimens should not be applied to the eyes. Involvement of the eyelashes should be treated by applying occlusive ophthalmic ointment to the eyelid margins b.i.d. for 10 days.

Clothing and linen should be disinfected by washing them in hot water, by dry cleaning them, or by removing them from human exposure for at least 72 hours.

COMPLICATIONS AND SEQUELAE

Secondary excoriations; lymphadenitis; pyoderma

OTHER CONSIDERATIONS

Pregnant Women: Lindane is contraindicated in pregnant or lactating women.

Follow-up: Patients should be evaluated after 1 week if symptoms persist. If lice are found or if eggs are observed at the hair-skin junction, re-treatment may be necessary. Increasing resistance of lice to permethrin is reported in some studies and may account for treatment failures.

Management of Sex Partners: Sex partners within the last month should be treated.

HIV Infection: Patients with HIV infection are managed in the same manner as patients without HIV infection.

SCABIES

Etiological Agent

Sarcoptes scabiei

The female organism is 0.3 to 0.4 mm; the male is somewhat smaller. The female burrows under the skin to deposit eggs.

TYPICAL CLINICAL PRESENTATION

Symptoms include itching, often worse at night, and the presence of erythematous, papular eruptions. Excoriations and secondary infections are common. Reddish-brown nodules are caused by hypersensitivity and develop 1 or more months after infection has occurred. The primary lesion is the burrow. When not obliterated by excoriations, burrows are usually seen on the fingers, penis, and wrists.

PRESUMPTIVE DIAGNOSIS

(Warrants full treatment and follow-up.)

The diagnosis is often made on clinical grounds alone. Exposure to a person with scabies within the previous 2 months supports the diagnosis.

DEFINITIVE DIAGNOSIS

Definitive diagnosis is made by microscopic identification of the mite or its eggs, larvae, or feces in scrapings from an elevated papule or burrow.

THERAPY

Recommended Regimen: Permethrin cream 5% applied to all areas of the body from the neck down and washed off after 8 to 14 hours, OR

Ivermectin 200 µg/kg orally, repeated in 2 weeks.

Alternative Regimens: Lindane (1%) 1 oz of lotion or 30 g of cream applied thinly to all areas of the body from the neck down and washed off thoroughly after 8 hours.

Lindane should not be used after a bath and should not be used by persons with extensive dermatitis, pregnant or lactating women, and children younger than 2 years. Not recommended for pregnant or lactating women, or infants and young children. Lindane should be used only if other treatments fail or are not tolerated.

COMPLICATIONS AND SEQUELAE

Secondary bacterial infection occurs, particularly with nephritogenic strains of streptococci. Norwegian or crusted scabies (with up to 2 million adult mites in the crusts) is a risk for patients with neurological defects and for the immunologically compromised.

OTHER CONSIDERATIONS

Pregnant Women: Lindane is contraindicated in pregnant or lactating women.

Follow-up: Pruritus may persist for several weeks. Re-treatment should be considered in patients who are symptomatic after 1 week, particularly if live mites are observed.

Management of Sex Partners: Sex partners and close personal or household contacts within the last month should be examined and treated.

HIV Infection: Patients with HIV infection are managed in the same manner as patients without HIV infection.

HEPATITIS B
Etiological Agent

Hepatitis B virus (HBV)

A DNA virus with multiple antigenic components.

Sexual transmission accounts for an estimated one third to two thirds of the estimated 200,000 to 300,000 new HBV infections that occur annually in the United States.

TYPICAL CLINICAL PRESENTATION

Hepatitis B is clinically indistinguishable from other forms of hepatitis. Most infections are clinically inapparent. Clinical symptoms and signs include various combinations of anorexia, malaise, nausea, vomiting, abdominal pain, and jaundice. Skin rashes, arthralgias, and arthritis can also occur.

PRESUMPTIVE DIAGNOSIS

(Warrants full treatment and follow-up.)

HBV infection is clinically indistinguishable from other forms of viral hepatitis and many times from hepatitis caused by toxins or drugs. The diagnosis should be considered in a symptomatic patient with symptoms suggestive of an acute viral illness and with an occupational exposure or sexual history that places the patient in a high-risk group.

Groups at high risk of acquiring infection include immigrants or refugees from areas of high HBV endemicity, patients in institutions for the mentally retarded, persons with multiple sex partners, users of illicit parenteral drugs, men who have sex with men, household contacts of HBV carriers, and patients of hemodialysis units.

DEFINITIVE DIAGNOSIS

Serodiagnosis of HBV infection is the only method for clinicians to reach a definitive diagnosis. A positive result for hepatitis B surface antigen (HBsAg) indicates active infection with HBV, either acute hepatitis B or the chronic carrier state. Hepatitis B e antigen (HBeAg) correlates with infectivity. Antibody to HBsAg (anti-HBs) usually indicates past infection with present immunity.

THERAPY

No specific therapy is available for the various types of acute hepatitis, whether sexually transmitted or not. Vaccination for hepatitis B is recommended for:

- All infants
- All unvaccinated children and adolescents through age 18

- All previously unvaccinated adults at increased risk for infection such as those with multiple sex partners within the past 6 months, intravenous drug users, men and women diagnosed as having recently acquired another STD, and residents of correctional or long-term care facilities
- In addition, immunoprophylaxis of infants born to HBsAg-positive mothers or infants born to mothers with unknown HBsAg status

For immunization recommendations, refer to Chapter 30.

COMPLICATIONS AND SEQUELAE

Long-term sequelae include chronic persistent and chronic active hepatitis, cirrhosis, hepatocellular carcinoma, hepatic failure, and death. Rarely, the course may be fulminant with hepatic failure, resulting in early death. Infectious chronic carriers may be completely asymptomatic.

OTHER CONSIDERATIONS

Oral contraceptives are contraindicated for women with active hepatitis.

Pregnant Women: Pregnancy is not a contraindication to HBV or hepatitis B immune globulin (HBIG) vaccine administration.

Management of Sex Partners: Susceptible persons who have been exposed to HBV through sexual contact with a person who has acute or chronic HBV infection should receive postexposure prophylaxis. This should include 0.06 mL/kg of HBIG in a single IM dose within 14 days of their last exposure. This should be followed with the standard three-dose immunization series with HBV vaccine.

HIV Infection: Patients with HIV infection who have HBV are more likely to develop a chronic HBV state. HIV infection may also impair the response to HBV vaccine. HIV-infected persons should be tested for anti-HBs 1 to 2 months after the third vaccine and those who have not responded should be revaccinated with one or more doses.

ENTERIC INFECTIONS
Etiological Agent

Proctitis: N. gonorrhoeae, C. trachomatis, T. pallidum, and *HSV.*
Proctocolitis: Campylobacter sp. *Shigella* sp. *Entamoeba histolytica, and rarely C. trachomatis.*
Enteritis: Giardia lamblia. Among HIV-infected patients, others include cytomegalovirus (CMV), Mycobacterium avium-intracellulare, Salmonella sp, *Cryptosporidium, microsporidia,* and *Isospora.*

These are particularly common among persons who participate in anal intercourse (proctitis) or whose sexual practices include oral-fecal contact (enteritis).

TYPICAL CLINICAL PRESENTATION

Infections are frequently asymptomatic or minimally symptomatic. Symptoms include the following:

Proctitis: Anorectal pain, tenesmus, and rectal discharge.

Proctocolitis: Symptoms of proctitis plus diarrhea or abdominal cramps.

Enteritis: Diarrhea and abdominal cramping.

PRESUMPTIVE DIAGNOSIS

(Warrants full treatment and follow-up.)

The typical clinical findings suggest enteric infection. Examination of a fresh stool specimen can be helpful. The finding of WBCs on direct microscopy of a suspension of fresh stool or the finding of occult or grossly bloody stools supports the diagnosis.

DEFINITIVE DIAGNOSIS

Definitive diagnostic tests vary according to the agent and site of infection involved.

THERAPY

Treatment of proctitis and enteritis should be based on etiological diagnosis. Some asymptomatic infected individuals for whom anal-oral contact is a sexual practice should be treated in accordance with recommendations for symptomatic individuals, as should persons whose work or social situation is associated with a likelihood of infection transmission (e.g., food handlers, hospital workers, day-care center employees). Until laboratory test results are available, persons with acute proctitis who have recently practiced receptive anal intercourse and have either anorectal pus on examination or PMN leukocytes on a Gram stain should receive treatment for anogenital gonorrhea and doxycycline (100 mg PO b.i.d. for 7 days).

COMPLICATIONS AND SEQUELAE

Complications and sequelae vary with the disease agent, health of the host, therapy, and other factors. Spontaneous cures are common. Morbidity may be severe, requiring hospitalization and intravenous hydration. Infections may become systemic (such as gram-negative septicemia) or distantly localized (amebic hepatic cyst). Some infections may be rarely fatal (hepatitis A, disseminated bacterial disease).

OTHER CONSIDERATIONS

Follow-up: Follow-up should be based on severity of clinical symptoms and specific etiological agent involved.

Management of Sex Partners: Sex partners should be evaluated for any diseases diagnosed in the index patient.

HIV Infection: Patients with HIV infection should be managed in the same manner as patients without HIV infection. HIV-infected patients are at risk for infections not commonly found in non-HIV–infected patients.

HUMAN IMMUNODEFICIENCY VIRUS INFECTIONS AND ACQUIRED IMMUNODEFICIENCY SYNDROME
Etiological Agent
HIV-1 or HIV-2

HIV-1 and HIV-2 are members of one of seven genera of retroviruses.

TYPICAL CLINICAL PRESENTATION

The range of symptoms associated with HIV infection extends from an acute illness shortly after infection to the full clinical syndrome of acquired immunodeficiency syndrome (AIDS). Acute HIV infection includes a mononucleosis-like syndrome consisting of headache, myalgia, sore throat, rash, diarrhea, fever, and lymphadenopathy. The acute HIV retroviral syndrome is reported 1 to 3 weeks after initial infection and resolves within a few weeks. This is a period of high levels of viral replication and viremia, with great potential for transmission. A latent or asymptomatic stage, lasting from a year to a decade or more, often follows. Disease progression appears inevitable, with ongoing destruction of the host immune system, followed by wasting and weight loss, symptoms specific to opportunistic infections (e.g., shortness of breath and cough from *Pneumocystis carinii* pneumonia [PCP] infection), or purple to bluish skin lesions associated with Kaposi sarcoma. Virtually all organ systems are affected by advanced HIV disease.

PRESUMPTIVE DIAGNOSIS

Presumptive diagnosis of HIV infection is made usually by clinical evidence, supported by tests for antibodies to HIV infection. Screening tests are based on enzyme immunoassay, with positive results confirmed by immunoblot (Western blot). Rapid serological tests are now available that provide results within 15 to 30 minutes, although these tests always require confirmation by immunoblot. Screening may also be done with whole blood, saliva, or urine. These tests increase the ease of screening, but their results should be confirmed by immunoblot. Clinicians and patients should keep in mind that the median time between infection and confirmed seropositivity is 3 months and may be as long as 6 months. Retesting is recommended when suspicion is high, particularly when the clinical presentation is consistent with the acute HIV syndrome.

DEFINITIVE DIAGNOSIS

Currently, isolation of the virus from body fluids is the most highly specific means to make a definitive diagnosis of HIV infection. Only very few research laboratories have the technology to perform viral isolation. Results from reactive enzyme immunoassay tests, confirmed by immunoblot (Western blots) or other confirmatory tests, are considered diagnostic. Indeterminate test results are usually resolved by retesting, combined with examination of the pattern of the indeterminate Western blot and a careful risk-assessment interview.

THERAPY

To date, no treatments eradicate either HIV-1 or HIV-2. A number of antiretroviral drugs are used to limit viral replication, restore immunocompetence, and delay onset of AIDS-related illness.

Acute Retroviral Syndrome

Immediate initiation of antiretroviral treatments improves prognosis of HIV-related infection. The optimal regimen is not known. Single-drug therapy with zidovudine may be effective, but many experts recommend two nucleoside reverse-transcriptase inhibitors and a protease inhibitor. Antiretroviral therapy is central to the treatment of HIV disease. Three classes of antiretroviral agents are available and are typically used in combination. Therapy can be monitored with highly sensitive viral load assays. Tuberculin skin testing, review of vaccination status, provision of pneumococcal and influenza vaccines, and STS are all important aspects of comprehensive therapy. PCP prophylaxis with trimethoprim-sulfamethoxazole, dapsone, or aerosolized pentamidine should be instituted for adolescents and adults with <200 CD4$^+$ T cells/mL, or after an initial episode of PCP. Prophylaxis should be continued for the lifetime of the patient. Prophylaxis for individuals seropositive for *Toxoplasma gondii* and CD4$^+$ counts <100 T cells/mL includes trimethoprim-sulfamethoxazole, or dapsone with pyrimethamine.

COMPLICATIONS AND SEQUELAE

Most people with HIV will eventually have symptoms related to the infection. Aggressive antiretroviral therapy improves disease-free survival, but relapse is expected when therapy is stopped. In many HIV-infected persons it may be years, even decades, before there is a development of AIDS-related condition.

OTHER CONSIDERATIONS

Management of Sex Partners: Sex partners should be notified either by their partners or through a referral to health department partner-notification programs. Partners should receive counseling and testing.

CHAPTER 61

Gonorrhea

Margaret J. Blythe

Gonorrhea is one of the most important sexually transmitted diseases (STDs) in adolescents because of its high incidence and potential for serious complications.

ETIOLOGY

Gonorrhea is an STD caused by *Neisseria gonorrhoeae,* which has the following characteristics:

1. The organisms are small, gram-negative cocci, kidney shaped and arranged in pairs (diplococci) with long axes in parallel.
2. The organisms are typically intracellular and usually located within or associated with polymorphonuclear (PMN) leukocytes.
3. The organisms grow optimally at 36°C to 37°C, with a moist environment enriched with 10% carbon dioxide in media containing blood or serum to ensure growth. *N. gonorrhoeae* is an oxidase-positive diplococcus, which can be differentiated from other *Neisseria* species by its use or nonuse of different carbohydrates.
4. As a human pathogen, the organism cannot live outside its host, and is easily killed by drying, soap and water, and other antiseptic agents.
5. Gonococci are killed by PMN cells, but when phagocytosed by macrophages, survive and replicate. Surrounded by macrophages' intracellular organelles, and granules, the cocci multiply within them and as such are not recognized by host's PMN cells.
6. Gonococci have the ability to turn off or vary the expression of cell surface components; this antigenic variation of surface proteins is thought to be a means of escape from host-specific antibody detection.
7. Cell envelope of the gonococci is composed of three parts—outer membrane, a peptidoglycan layer, and cytoplasmic membrane.
8. Pili are hair-like appendages which attach to the cell membrane. Pili from different strains are diverse with the ability of the same bacteria to "antigenically" vary the composition of its pili. There are pilated and nonpilated strains of gonococci.
9. Three proteins associated with the cell membrane and surface of the gonococci characterize the bacteria with regard to its virulence and association with clinical presentation and disease. These are protein I (PI), protein II (PII) (opacity-associated protein [Opa]), and protein III (PIII).
10. Types of organisms: There are >70 different strains of *Neisseria. N. gonorrhoeae* species have been differentiated by several characteristics:
    a. Presence or absence of pili
    b. Opaque or transparent colonies
    c. Auxotyping
    d. Serotyping
    e. Molecular methods: Molecular methods were first used to characterize the plasmids associated with antibiotic resistance. Nucleic acid amplification techniques (NAATs) such as polymerase chain reaction (PCR) are now available to analyze entire gonococcus chromosome. The method is currently being used to determine the Opa-typing of different gonococci to study sexual networks.

EPIDEMIOLOGY

Incidence

1. Gonorrhea is the second most frequently reportable disease in the United States after *Chlamydia trachomatis* infections. Approximately 339,583 cases were reported in 2005, with reported cases thought to represent less than 50% of all cases. Rates of gonorrhea declined by 73.8% between 1975 and 1998 to 122.4 per 100,000, but then increased by 7.8% in 1998. Since 1998, the rates have continued to decline with the most recent rate from 2005 reported at 115.6 cases per 100,000, only a slight increase from the 113.5 per 100,000 reported in 2004, which was the lowest rate ever reported by the Centers for Disease Control and Prevention (CDC) (Table 61.1) (Weinstock, 2004; Centers for Disease Control and Prevention, 2004).
2. The incidence remains high in some groups as defined by age, race/ethnicity, geography, or sexual risk behavior (Centers for Disease Control and Prevention, 2004).
   a. Age: Adolescents (ages 15–19 years) and young adults (ages 20–24 years) continue to be at highest risk in 2004 for acquiring this disease with the peak incidence occurring in men aged 20 to 24 years (430.6 per 100,000), and in female adolescents aged 15 to 19 years (610.9 per 100,000). Approximately 60% of all reported cases

TABLE 61.1

Cases and Incidence of Gonorrhea in the United States, 1975–2004

	1975	1985	1998	2000	2001	2002	2003	2004	2005
Cases	999,937	911,419	356,492	363,136	361,705	351,852	335,104	330,132	339,593
Incidence per 100,000	467.7	383.0	129.2	128.7	126.8	122.0	115.2	113.5	115.6

Adapted from Centers for Disease Control and Prevention Division of STD Prevention. Department of Health and Human Services, with permission. Centers for Disease Control and Prevention. STD Surveillance 2004. National Profile (http://www.cdc.gov/STD/stats/tables/table1.htm).

occur in men and women between ages 15 and 24 years and 80% between ages 15 and 29 years.

b. Ethnicity: Rates vary dramatically among adolescents from different racial/ethnic backgrounds and practice settings. Incidence in African-Americans, Hispanics, and Native Americans, is disproportionately high compared with whites and Asians. The gonorrhea rate among African-Americans declined from 2003 to 2005, falling 4.5% (from 655.8 to 626.4); however, African-Americans remained the group most heavily affected by gonorrhea. Reported rates of gonorrhea in African-Americans were 18 times greater than those of whites in 2005, down from 20 times in 2003. Rates increased 27.2% among American-Indians/Alaska Natives from 2003 to 2005 (from 103.5 to 131.7). Rates increased 7.3% in these two years among Latinos to 74.8 per 100,000, and 8% among whites to 35.2 per 100,000. Rates increased between 2003 and 2005 for Asians/Pacific Islanders from 22.8 to 25.9 (Centers for disease Control and Prevention, 2004 and http://www.cdc.gov/std/stats/trends2005.htm#trendsgonorrhe)

c. Geography: The highest reported rates of gonorrhea are in the Southeastern region of United States. In 2005, rates among parts of the United States varied - South, 143.9 per 100,000; Midwest, 142.5 per 100,000; Northeast, 74.7; West 71.8 per 100,000. However, in contrast to declines in the other areas of the country, gonorrhea rates in the West have increased steadily in recent years (35.4% between 2001 and 2005).

d. Gender: The male-to-female ratio of reported gonorrhea infection approaches 1:1. In 2004, the *N. gonorrhoeae* rate for women was 116.5 per 100,000 compared with men, 110 per 100,000.

e. Risk factors: Risk factors for acquiring gonorrhea include:
   • Multiple or new sex partners
   • Inconsistent, incorrect or no condom use
   • Belonging to a minority group
   • Living in an urban area where prevalence of gonorrhea is high
   • Being adolescent (especially female)
   • Having a lower socioeconomic status
   • Using drugs including alcohol
   • Exchanging sex for drugs or money
   • Men who have sex with men (MSM)

3. Approximately the same number of cases of gonorrhea is reported in the age-groups of 15 to 19 years and 20 to 24 years, when combining cases in males and females. However, almost twice as many individuals are sexually active in the 20- to 24-year-old age-group as

in the 15- to 19-year-old age-group. When corrected for this difference, the incidence in sexually active 15- to 19-year-olds is twice that of 20- to 24-year-olds.

4. The reasons for the high incidence in 15- to 19-year-old adolescents include psychosocial and biological factors.

a. Psychosocial factors
   • Increased number of sexual partners, increased frequency of sexual intercourse, and decreased age at first intercourse.
   • Low rates of consistent and appropriate use of condoms and other barrier methods (Crosby et al., 2005; Paz-Bailey et al., 2005).
   • Lack of accessible clinical services providing confidential services for adolescents.
   • Lack of screening by health care providers in health care settings (Chacko et al., 2004).

b. Biological factors
   • More columnar epithelial cells exposed on the ectocervix of teens referred to as cervical ectopy. *N. gonorrhoeae* preferentially infects these cells.
   • High percentage of infections, asymptomatic particularly in females.

Prevalence

1. The prevalence rates vary and depend on rates of "routine screening" for gonorrhea. Public health clinics and therefore the populations that attend such clinics as minorities are more likely screened and reported (Centers for Disease Control and Prevention, 2004).

a. National sample: The overall *prevalence* of gonococcal infection in a nationally representative sample of 14,322 young adults aged 18 to 26 years was 0.43% with little variation between males (0.44%) and females (0.42%) and among the different ages studied. Substantial variation occurred by race/ethnicity with the lowest prevalence noted for white men and women (0.07%) and highest for black men and women (2.36%) (Miller et al., 2004).

b. STD clinics: Males, range 8% to 25%.
   For 32,595 men with 45,390 visits to STD clinics at each of three cities, range of gonorrhea positive cultures varied from 8.1% in Seattle, to 20.8% in Indianapolis, and 24% in New Orleans (Kohl et al., 2004). In 2004, as in prior years, a higher proportion of male gonorrhea cases (42.7%) were reported from STD clinics than female cases (17.9%).

c. Family planning clinics in the United States serving 15- to 24-year-old females: In 2004, median rate was 0.88% (range 0.1%–4.2%). One study of family planning clinics in Missouri indicated an overall prevalence for gonorrhea of 0.7% for 31,762 women aged 15 to 24 years and 4% for chlamydia. The gonorrhea rate was 4% for blacks and 0.4% for whites; the chlamydia rate was 9% for black women and for white, 4%. Independent predictors of gonorrhea in both races were presence of symptoms, recent sexual contact with a partner who had STD symptoms, and *Chlamydia* infection (Einwalter et al., 2005).

d. Job Corps: In 2004, the female median rate was 2.4%, (range 0.0%–6.4%) and in males the median rate was 3.7% (range 1.0%–5.7%) from different states.

e. University and college student health centers: <1% to 2% positive for gonorrhea.

f. Juvenile detention facilities: In 2004, in males the median gonorrhea prevalence rate was 0.8% (range 0%–18.2%) compared to 4.5% in females (range 0%–16.6%). In another study, the prevalence of gonorrhea was 5.1% in 33,619 adolescent females and 1.3% in 98,296 adolescent males. This compared to chlamydia rates of 15.6% in the adolescent females and 5.9% in the males. Of females with gonorrhea, 54% were coinfected with *Chlamydia*, and 51% of males with gonorrhea were coinfected with *Chlamydia* (Kahn et al., 2005). At a study at three juvenile facilities, approximately 93% of adolescent males testing positive for gonorrhea were asymptomatic. This compared to 97% of those testing positive for chlamydial infections (Mertz et al., 2002).

g. Adolescent clinics: Approximately 3% to 9% of teens are positive for gonorrhea. Similar rates were found for teens attending adolescent clinics when comparing cervical cultures (9.4%) with urine specimens using NAATs (9.1%) (Xu et al., 1998; Jones et al., 2000).

h. Urban emergency departments (EDs): One percent to 7% (Aledort et al., 2005).

i. Correlation with drug use: Thirty-two percent of female adolescents with gonorrhea in San Francisco had received money or drugs in exchange for sex (Schwarcz et al., 1992).

Host

Humans are the only natural host for *N. gonorrhoeae.*

Transmission

Transmission is virtually exclusively through oral, vaginal, or anal sexual contact. The exception is gonococcal ophthalmia, which usually occurs in newborns but has been reported in physicians, laboratory technicians, and the general adult population presumably when direct contact of the organism with the eye through hand transmission has occurred.

PATHOPHYSIOLOGY

N. gonorrhoeae causes disease by direct invasion and spread on mucosal and glandular structures lined by columnar or cuboidal, noncornified epithelium.

Virulence

The virulence of the infection may be related to certain characteristics of the organism.

1. Pili: Pili increase adhesion of gonococci to tissues, are associated with small colonies and increased virulence. Pili also decrease the ability of neutrophils to ingest and kill the organism. Nonpilated organisms have advantages once past mucosal entry.

2. Colony morphology: Cells with protein II or Opa have "opaque" colony morphology, whereas strains without Opa are "transparent." Opaque colonies have increased adherence to host cells and are more often found in specimens from males with gonococcal urethritis and in cervical isolates obtained from females. Transparent colonies appear to represent the invasive form of *N. gonorrhoeae*. The other proteins in the outer membrane are protein I and protein III.

3. Auxotype: This is determined by the nutritional or specific growth requirements of the organism including amino acids, nucleic acid bases such as purines and pyrimidines, as well as vitamins.

4. Other virulence factors
   a. Lipo-oligosacchride (LOS): As the major protein in the outer membrane of gram-negative bacteria, LOS with potent endotoxic activity serves as the target protein for much of the bactericidal antibody produced.
   b. Other possible molecular mechanisms: Immunoglobulin A_1 (IgA_1) protease and iron-regulated proteins.

Clinical Manifestations

Clinical manifestations of *N. gonorrhoeae* are similar to those caused by *C. trachomatis,* and both *C. trachomatis* and *N. gonorrhoeae* occur frequently together in the same individual. Susceptible sites are usually mucosal columnar epithelial areas. The spectrum of gonococcal infections includes the following:

1. Asymptomatic infections:
   a. Urethral/cervical infections may persist for months if untreated.
   b. In women, asymptomatic rates range from 25% to 90% of the infections.
   c. Estimates suggest that less than 10% of infections in males are asymptomatic, but studies of adolescent males in juvenile detention facilities report high rates of asymptomatic males (Pack et al., 2000).
   d. More than half of men with rectal infections are asymptomatic.
   e. Because symptomatic individuals seek treatment and most asymptomatic individuals do not, asymptomatic individuals remain untreated, infected, and spread infection.
   f. Asymptomatic infections can involve the following:
      • Urethra: male and female
      • Endocervix
      • Rectum
      • Pharynx

2. Symptomatic uncomplicated infections may result in the following:
   a. Urethritis
   b. Cervicitis
   c. Proctitis
   d. Pharyngitis
   e. Bartholinitis
   f. Conjunctivitis

3. Local complications include the following:
   a. Pelvic inflammatory disease
   b. Epididymitis
   c. Bartholin gland abscess
   d. Penile edema
   e. Periurethral abscess: Abscess of bulbourethral glands (Cowper glands) or sebaceous glands of the prepuce or foreskin (Tyson glands)
   f. Prostatitis
   g. Perihepatitis: Complication of salpingitis (Fitz-Hugh-Curtis Syndrome)
   h. Seminal vesiculitis
4. Systemic complications might include the following:
   a. Disseminated gonococcal infection (DGI)
   b. Arthritis-dermatitis syndromes
   c. Gonococcal meningitis
   d. Gonococcal endocarditis

Genitourinary Infections The most common clinical manifestation of gonorrhea is a genitourinary infection.

Males
1. Urethritis
   a. Incubation period: Ranges from 1 to 14 days with most men symptomatic 2 to 5 days after exposure
   b. Symptoms: Dysuria, meatal pruritus
   c. Clinical findings: Profuse purulent urethral discharge (25% scanty, minimally purulent discharge)
2. Infection can spread and cause epididymitis, prostatitis, seminal vesiculitis, and infection of Cowper and Tyson glands.
   a. Epididymitis: Ten percent to 30% of *untreated* men develop this complication, which is manifested by the following:
      • Urethral discharge and dysuria
      • Scrotal pain and tenderness, usually unilateral
      • Scrotal swelling and erythema
      • Pain in the inguinal area and flank pain in severe cases
      • Pain, tenderness, or swelling of the lower pole of the epididymis, which can spread to the head of the epididymis
      • Swelling and pain of spermatic cord
   b. Prostatitis: Prostatitis is a rare complication of gonorrhea. Signs and symptoms include the following:
      • May be asymptomatic
      • Chills, fever, malaise, myalgia
      • Rectal pain and discomfort
      • Lower back pain
      • Lower abdominal pain, suprapubic discomfort
      • Dysuria, urinary frequency, and occasionally acute urinary retention
3. Risk of infection: Risk of infection is approximately 20% to 50% for a male after a single exposure through vaginal intercourse with an infected female (McMillian, 2002).

Females
Signs and symptoms are less specific in females than in males. Often the teen may complain of vaginal discharge, dysuria, or frequency. The incubation period is more variable than in males, but symptoms usually appear within 10 days of exposure. Common local problems include the following:

1. Endocervicitis
   a. Increased vaginal discharge, often purulent
   b. Dyspareunia
   c. Erythema, edema, and friability of cervix resulting in spotting
   d. Risk of infection: Estimated at 60% to 90% for a female after single exposure to an infected male
2. Urethritis
   a. Dysuria
   b. Urinary frequency
   c. Exudate from urethra or periurethral glands (Skene gland)
   d. Suprapubic pain
3. Bartholinitis: Purulent exudate from Bartholin gland
4. Bartholin gland abscess: Labial pain and swelling. The most common complication in females apart from pelvic inflammatory disease (PID) is abscess of the Bartholin gland.
5. Spread of infection can extend into the following areas:
   a. Endometritis: Recent data suggests that one in four women infected with *C. trachomatis* or *N. gonorrhoeae* and 15% of women with bacterial vaginosis have histological endometritis, in the absence of signs or symptoms of acute PID (Wiesenfeld et al., 2002).
   b. Fallopian tubes: PID (see Chapter 63) occurs in as many as 10% to 20% of females with acute urogenital gonorrhea. Strains causing PID have different auxotypes, different patterns of antibiotic resistance, and are often "transparent" colonies. Patients with gonococcal-associated PID compared to chlamydial-associated PID or nongonococcal, nonchlamydial–associated PID may be more ill and febrile at clinical presentation with the onset on symptoms within 7 days of the menstrual cycle (Wiesenfeld et al., 2005).
   c. Upper abdomen: Perihepatitis (Fitz-Hugh-Curtis syndrome): Presents as right-upper-quadrant pain.
   d. Ovary: Tuboovarian abscess.

Extragenital Sites
1. Pharyngitis
   a. Pharyngeal involvement is usually asymptomatic in >90% of infected individuals.
   b. Pharyngitis may be manifested by a sore throat 3 to 7 days after exposure and occasionally with fever and cervical adenopathy.
   c. Positive pharyngeal cultures may be found in 3% to 7% of heterosexual males, 10% to 20% of heterosexual females, and 10% to 25% of homosexual males with genital gonorrhea, with the pharynx as the sole site of infection estimated in <5% of individuals. Fellatio is a more effective mode of transmission than cunnilingus. Pharyngeal infection may be a significant cause of urethral gonorrhea in MSM.
   d. Spontaneous elimination of the organism can occur in 12 weeks.
   e. Significance of infection: Infected individuals may be at risk for dissemination of gonorrhea.
2. Rectal gonorrhea
   a. Prevalence rates: Rectal cultures may be positive in 35% to 50% of females with genital infection. Most anorectal infections in females are asymptomatic and are thought related to infected perineal secretions. In one study, anorectal gonococcal infections in MSM were associated with distinct auxotype/serovar classes (Geisler et al., 2002).
   b. Rectal gonorrhea can produce the following symptoms of distal proctitis:
      • Mucopurulent anal discharge
      • Rectal bleeding

- Anorectal pain or *pruritus ani*
- Tenesmus
- Constipation

c. Proctoscopic examination may show a normal appearance or patchy, generalized erythema of rectal mucosa or purulent exudate, erythema, edema, friability, or other inflammatory changes of the rectal mucosa.

d. The differential diagnosis for infections involving the first 5 to 10 cm of the rectum causing proctitis is chlamydia, herpes, (cytomegalovirus [CMV] infection, and syphilis. Inflammation extending more than 15 cm and causing proctocolitis is usually caused by Shigella, *Campylobacter, Entamoeba histolytica,* or Salmonella. Other diagnoses to consider are ulcerative colitis and Crohn disease.

3. Conjunctivitis is usually severe with high risk of sequelae

Disseminated Disease

Less than 1% of individuals with gonorrhea develop disseminated disease (DGI) characterized by fever, rash, arthritis, or arthralgia. Certain strains of *N. gonorrhoeae* are more likely to disseminate. These strains tend to cause asymptomatic urogenital infection or pharyngeal infections and are more resistant to complement-mediated bacterial activity in serum. DGI is more common in females with a 4:1 ratio of female:male. Recurrent bacteremia has been described in individuals with deficiency of 6th, 7th, and/or 8th components of complement (Young and McMillan, 2002). Other risk factors for dissemination include immune-altering disease states such as lupus erythematosus.

Arthritis-Dermatitis Syndrome

1. Purulent arthritis: Purulent arthritis is the most common systemic complication of *N. gonorrhoeae* and usually occurs within 1 month of exposure. Approximately 25% to 50% of patients complain of pain in a single joint. The knee is the most common site of purulent gonococcal arthritis but may involve the wrist, metacarpophalangeal joints, and ankle. Monoarticular septic arthritis may present without preceding dermatitis or tenosynovitis.

2. Migratory polyarthralgias/arthritis: Others have migratory polyarthralgia or asymmetrical polyarticular arthritis involving the knees, wrists, small joints of hands, ankles, and elbows with not enough fluid to aspirate. Knees are the most frequently involved joints, but all joints including the hip and shoulder have been affected. Sacroiliac, temporomandibular, and sternoclavicular joints are rarely involved.

3. Tenosynovitis: Tenosynovitis may affect the hands and fingers but less likely the lower extremities, involving the extensor and flexor tendons and sheaths of the hands and feet.

4. Fever, chills, and leukocytosis are common but 40% are afebrile.

5. Approximately 90% will have a skin rash:
   a. Variable presentations:
      - *Hemorrhagic lesions* presenting as purpura and necrotic centers
      - *Vesiculopapular lesions* on an erythematous base
   b. All lesions begin as *erythematous papules* with hemorrhagic lesions most often on palms and soles while others progress from papules, to vesicles, to pustules.

c. Frequently painful, asymmetrical lesions over extremities near the joints, palms, soles of feet and occasionally on trunk and rarely on face.

6. Diagnosis:
   a. Positive blood cultures in 20% to 30% of patients, but cultures should be done in the first few days of the illness.
   b. Joint cultures are rarely positive with polyarticular presentation. For monoarticular presentation, the affected joint's synovial fluid will appear turbid, with predominance of PMN cells and low glucose. Positive cultures result in less than 50% of cases and are associated with negative blood cultures. PCR has been used on joint fluid to make the diagnosis.
   c. Gram stain results and cultures are usually negative from skin, but immunofluorescent stains if available on biopsy specimens of skin identify gonorrhea in more than half the specimens in studies.
   d. Elevated peripheral white counts occur in the majority and elevation of sedimentation rate in most. Elevated liver enzymes occur in 50% of cases.
   e. Gonococci have been found on the mucosal surfaces of cervix and pharynx 80% of the time despite negative blood, skin, and joint fluid cultures.

7. Differential diagnosis of gonococcal arthritis
   a. Infections: Meningococcemia, bacteremias, endocarditis, infectious arthritis, and infectious tenosynovitis
   b. Seronegative arthritides: Reiter syndrome, ankylosing spondylitis, psoriatic arthritis, rheumatoid arthritis, rheumatic fever, Lyme disease, bacterial endocarditis
   c. Lupus erythematosus
   d. Allergic reaction to drugs

Sexually Acquired Reactive Arthritis (Reiter Syndrome)

See Chapter 62 on *Chlamydia* infections. Table 61.2 compares gonococcal arthritis and acute Reiter syndrome.

Other Sites of Dissemination

1. Perihepatitis: Most often a complication of salpingitis, found rarely in men. Presentation usually involves pain in right upper quadrant and occasionally right shoulder suggesting irritation of right side of diaphragm.
2. Mild hepatitis: Found in up to 50% of patients, but not usually clinically suspected and usually follows bacteremia of DGI.
3. Gonococcal meningitis: Rare complication that can be clinically indistinguishable from other meningococcal infections.
4. Rare cardiac manifestations: Myopericarditis, heart block, endocarditis.
5. Other: Osteomyelitis, pneumonia.

DIAGNOSIS

Gonococcal Urethritis: Males

1. Gram-negative intracellular diplococci on smear of urethral exudates:
   a. If positive, sufficient for diagnosis of gonorrhea.
   b. Sensitivity and specificity of Gram stains for infected male urethra is 90% to 95% and 95% to 100%

TABLE 61.2

Comparison of Acute Gonococcal Arthritis and Acute Reiter Syndrome

Characteristic	Acute Gonococcal Arthritis (%)	Acute Reiter Syndrome (%)
Back pain	0	20
Urethritis	28	76
Migratory arthralgias	83	10
Chills	33	0
Temperature >39.4°C	27	39
Skin lesions	Isolated papules and pustules on extremities and trunk	Circinate balanitis; keratoderma of shaft of penis. Asymptomatic oral macular lesions on palate, buccal mucosa.
Sacroiliac involvement	3	30
Wrist involvement	67	30
Heel involvement	7	67
Antigen HLA-B27	Usually negative	>90 positive

respectively if symptomatic and 50% to 70% and 95% to 100% if asymptomatic.

2. If Gram stain result is negative or not done or urethral exudate not present, culture a specimen from anterior urethra:
   a. Use a sterile calcium alginate urethral swab inoculating a modified Thayer-Martin medium culture plate (chocolate [blood] agar), which has antibiotics added to suppress other organisms that "normally" colonize the sites.
   b. Cultures obtained from other sites normally colonized by other organisms (i.e., rectum, pharynx, or endocervix) should be cultured on selective medium (Thayer-Martin) as well.
   c. Cultures obtained from sterile areas (i.e., blood, spinal fluid, or synovial fluid) can be plated onto nonselective, chocolate agar.
   d. Organisms have to be inoculated directly on medium, transported in warm 36°C to 37°C environment with 5% to 10% carbon dioxide.
   e. Growth of oxidase-positive, gram-negative diplococci on selective media is sufficient evidence for a diagnosis.
   f. Carbohydrate tests to discriminate types of Neisseria show that N. gonorrhoeae metabolize only glucose and not other sugars such as lactose, maltose, sucrose, and/or fructose as do other Neisseria species. Culture sensitivity is 92.7% in symptomatic males and 46.2% in asymptomatic men but 100% specific (Martin et al., 2000).

3. NAATs are used to diagnose male urethral infections (Table 61.3).
   a. In symptomatic patients: Sensitivities of NAATs are 96.5% to 100%, specificities, 95% to 98.8% (Martin et al., 2000; Wheeler et al., 2005; Chernesky et al., 2005).
   b. In asymptomatic patients: Sensitivities of NAATs are 73.1% to 98.1%, specificities, 97.5% to 99% (Martin et al., 2000; Wheeler et al., 2005; Chernesky et al., 2005).

4. An alternative to urethral swab would be urine testing with NAATs:
   a. All methods—PCR, transcriptional mediated amplification (TMA), and strand displacement amplification (SDA)—have been FDA approved for chlamydia and gonorrhea screening on both male and female urine except PCR for gonorrhea on female urine.
   b. Although urethral culture for gonorrhea is less expensive than NAATs, many males prefer urine testing.
   c. In symptomatic male patients: Sensitivities of NAATs using urine are 98.2% to 99.9%, specificities 98.2% to 99.9% (Martin et al., 2000; Chernesky et al., 2005; Cook et al., 2005).
   d. In asymptomatic male patients: Sensitivities of NAATs using urine are 42.3% to 98.2%, specificities 98% to 99.9% (Martin et al., 2000; Chernesky et al., 2005; Cook et al., 2005).
   e. Urethral gonorrhea culture in asymptomatic males also has a relatively poor sensitivity (46.2%).
   f. Although testing with urine (42.3%) did not perform as well as urethral swab (73.1%) for PCR in asymptomatic males, it may be easier to get cooperation collecting a urine sample rather than a urethral specimen.

5. The homosexual male adolescent should also have cultures obtained from the rectum and pharynx to assess those sites, because NAAT methods are not approved for those sites.

6. In asymptomatic males, the urinary leukocyte esterase dipstick test (LET) on first-catch urine, in certain situations, can be a valuable screening technique.
   a. In low-prevalence settings (<5%), LET has poor positive predictive value but has a high negative predictive value.
   b. As a cost-saving measure, LET may be used to screen with any positive test sent for a specific diagnosis by NAAT.

Gonococcal Endocervicitis: Females

1. Cultures should be obtained from the endocervical canal and inoculated on Thayer-Martin medium to diagnose gonorrhea:
   a. Do not use a lubricant during the pelvic examination, because this may be toxic to the organism.
   b. Place a swab in the cervical os for 20 to 30 seconds and rotate. For screening purposes, only endocervical cultures are recommended. A single culture is 80% to 95% sensitive in detecting gonorrhea.
   c. If anorectal sex has occurred, a separate swab can be used in the anal canal. Approximately 5% of females

TABLE 61.3

Comparison of Nucleic Acid Amplification Tests (NAATS) for *Neisseria gonorrhoeae*

	PCR	SDA	TMA	Culture
Test	COBAS Amplicor	Probe Tec	Aptima	
Company	Roche	Becton Dickinson	Gen Probe	
Gender/site				
Male/urethra				
Sensitivity	97.3%–99.0%[a]	98.5%–100%	73.1%–98.1%	80%–95%[b]
Specificity	98.8%–99.9%	91.9%–100%	95.9%–97.5%	100%
Male/urine				Not available
Sensitivity	94.1%–100%[c]	97.9%	95.2%	
Specificity	99.2%–99.9%	92.5%–100%	98.2%	
Female/cervix				
Sensitivity	92.4%–100%	95.6%–99.6%	83.7%–96.1%	76.6%–84.8%
Specificity	99.5%	99.3%–99.6%	98.1%–99.6%	100.0%
Female/urine[d]				Not available
Sensitivity	64.8%–94.4%	98.5%–100%	86.5%–97.4%	
Specificity	95.9%–99.5%	99.3%–99.6%	99.1%–99.5%	
Vaginal swab			FDA approved	Not available

PCR, polymerase chain reaction: COBAS Amplicor (Roche); TMA, transcriptional mediated amplification: Aptima Combo (Gen Probe); Aptima Ct and Aptima *N. gonorrhoeae* (Gen Probe); SDA, strand displacement amplification: Probe Tec (Becton Dickinson).

[a]Asymptomatic, 73.1%.
[b]Asymptomatic, 46.2%.
[c]Asymptomatic, 42.3%.
[d]All sites for all tests FDA approved except for female urine *N. gonorrhoeae* PCR; only TMA FDA approved for vaginal swabs (Martin et al., 2000; Wheeler et al., 2005; Chernesky et al., 2005; Crotchfelt et al., 1997; Cook et al., 2005; Cosentino et al., 2003; Schachter et al., 2003).

have positive culture from this site only. The swab can be inserted approximately 2 cm, avoiding fecal mass, and moved side to side for 20 to 30 seconds.

    d. Gram stain smears from the endocervix are not recommended. Such smears are only 50% to 70% sensitive in uncomplicated endocervical infection.

2. Newer diagnostic methods (e.g., NAATs)

    a. PCR, TMA, and SDA tests can be used on *endocervical specimens* for both chlamydia and gonorrhea (Martin et al., 2000; Crotchfelt et al., 1997; Gaydos et al., 2003; Van der Pol et al., 2001) (Table 61.3).

    b. PCR, TMA, and SDA tests are approved for first-void *urine specimens* in females for chlamydia, and TMA and SDA are approved for gonorrhea but not PCR (Martin et al., 2000; Crotchfelt et al., 1997; Gaydos et al., 2003; Van der Pol et al., 2001) (Table 61.3).

    c. PCR* and SDA tests on *vaginal swabs* show similar or superior results to cervical specimens. SDA was recently FDA approved for vaginal samples (Wiesenfeld et al., 1996; Black et al., 2002; Cosentino et al., 2003; Schachter et al., 2003).

    Note: *Cross-reacts with other nonpathogenic *Neisseria* species found in the vagina.

    d. Summary and limitations of NAATs testing for chlamydia and gonorrhea:

      • For each of the three commercially available nucleic acid tests for *C. trachomatis*, the sensitivity and specificity of urine and endocervical samples for women as well as urine and urethral samples for men were nearly identical.

• Sensitivity and specificity of the PCR urine to detect *N. gonorrhoeae* in women were significantly lower than cervical samples, but did not appear different for SDA and TMA (Cook et al., 2005).

• Results of sensitivity and specificity testing for gonorrhea in symptomatic men comparing urine and urethral samples were similar.

• Specificities were high (from 98%–100%). However, if specificity is closer to 98% then screening in low-prevalence populations could result in almost one third of positives to be falsely positive (Cook et al., 2005).

• Inhibitors of enzyme amplification can prevent assays from providing a positive result leading to decreased sensitivity. For PCR and TMA, rates of inhibition vary from 5% to 20% whereas SDA did not seem to be affected (Cook et al., 2005).

Anorectal Gonorrhea

Positive cultures from the rectum are required for diagnosis of anorectal gonorrhea. The nucleic acid assays have not been adequately studied for this site. Gram stains are not suitable as anal swabs are only 40% to 60% sensitive and 95% to 100% specific.

Gonococcal Pharyngitis

1. Diagnosis requires a positive culture from the pharynx. As with anal infection, nucleic acid detection techniques

are not considered appropriate and Gram stains are not appropriate.

2. Several studies have indicated that routine pharyngeal screening in adolescents is not cost-effective (Brown et al., 1989; Roochvarg and Lovchik, 1991).

Systemic Infection

1. Positive cultures from the urethra, endocervix, pharynx, rectum, and conjunctiva, or positive NAATs from urethra and/or endocervix/vagina.
2. Positive cultures from skin lesions, synovial fluid, or blood.

THERAPY

Treatment of gonorrhea should take into account that strains of *N. gonorrhoeae* resistant to traditional treatment are rising, that chlamydial infections often coexist with gonorrhea, and that serious complications can arise from both gonococcal and chlamydial infections.

Resistance

The incidence of isolates of *N. gonorrhoeae* resistant to antibiotics has increased dramatically since the early 1980s. The 2004 report on surveillance of antibiotics used to treat *N. gonorrhoeae* is available (Centers for Disease Control and Prevention, 2004) and included the following information:

1. Plasmid mediated
   a. Penicillin: Penicillinase-producing *N. gonorrhoeae* (PPNG)
   b. Tetracycline: Tetracycline-resistant *N. gonorrhoeae* (TRNG)
   c. Penicillin and tetracycline: Plasmid-mediated penicillin and tetracycline-resistant *N. gonorrhoeae* (PPNG/TRNG)
2. Chromosomally mediated resistant *N. gonorrhoeae*
   a. Penicillin (chromosomally mediated penicillin-resistant *N. gonorrhoeae*): PenR
   b. Tetracycline (chromosomally mediated tetracycline-resistant *N. gonorrhoeae*): TetR
   c. Penicillin and tetracycline (chromosomally mediated penicillin- and tetracycline-resistant *N. gonorrhoeae*): CMRNG
   d. Ciprofloxacin (intermediate resistance and resistance)
   e. Spectinomycin
   f. Ceftriaxone (decreased susceptibility)
   g. Cefixime (decreased susceptibility)
   h. Azithromycin (susceptibility)

In 1986, the Gonococcal Isolate Surveillance Project (GISP) was established to monitor trends in antimicrobial susceptibilities of strains of *N. gonorrhoeae* in the United States. In 1976, PPNG was recognized in the United States and TRNG since 1985. In 1983, a mechanism of resistance involving multiple chromosomal mutations was identified that caused alterations in the cell membrane to antibiotics and changes in antibiotic-binding proteins. Data from the GISP showed that in 2004, 15.9% of isolates were resistant to either penicillin or tetracycline or both. A shift in type of resistance has evolved over the last decade from plasmid to chromosomal with the most recent data showing 0.6%

PPNG, 3.4% TRNG, 0.5% PPNG-TRNG, 1.1% PenR, 6.1% TetR, and 4.3% CMRNG.

In 2004, all isolates were susceptible to spectinomycin, ceftriaxone, and cefixime. In 2003, 4.1% of the isolates demonstrated resistance to ciprofloxacin and in 2004, 6.8%. This is in comparison to 0.4% in 2000. Most of the "resistant" samples were from California. In 2004, Honolulu, Hawaii, continues to experience a high percentage of gonorrhea samples resistant to ciprofloxacin (22.8%) up from 13.3% in 2003. Other West-coast cities have experienced high rates of resistance. Resistance to ciprofloxacin increased from 7.2% in 2002 to 15% in 2003 and 23.8% in 2004 in MSM; whereas it increased from 0.9% in 2002 to 1.5% in 2003 and 2.9% in 2004 in heterosexuals.

Therefore the recommendation as of April 13th, 2007 in the CDC update to the 2006 STD Guidelines is to no longer use fluoroquinolones for the treatment of gonococcal infections and associated conditions such as pelvic inflammatory disease.

In 2004, 57 samples (0.9%) demonstrated decreased susceptibility to azithromycin compared to 26 (0.4%) in 2003.

Coinfection

1. Household sample 18- to 26-year-olds: 0.3% of the population had both gonorrhea and chlamydia. For those with gonorrhea, 70% had chlamydia. For those with chlamydia, 7.9% had gonorrhea (Miller et al., 2004).
2. In an STD population, the prevalence of chlamydia in those with diagnosed or contact of gonorrhea was 20% for men and 42% for women. Among patients with gonorrhea, the chlamydia prevalence was higher among men younger than 25 years than older (27% versus 13%) and also among women younger than 25 years than older (54% versus 20%) (Lyss et al., 2003).
3. Of females in juvenile detention facilities with gonorrhea, 54% were coinfected with *Chlamydia*, and 51% of males with gonorrhea were coinfected with *Chlamydia* (Kahn et al., 2005).
4. Another study of family planning attendees indicated approximately 40% of those with gonorrhea were also infected with *Chlamydia* (Einwalter et al., 2005).

Treatment Recommendations

Guidelines from Centers for Disease Control and Prevention, 2006.

1. Uncomplicated urethral, endocervical, or rectal infections in adolescents and adults:
   a. Recommended regimens
      • Cefixime 400 mg PO in a single dose
        OR
      • Ceftriaxone 125 mg IM at one time
        PLUS
        A regimen effective against possible coinfection with *C. trachomatis* such as azithromycin (1 g PO in a single dose) OR doxycycline (100 mg PO b.i.d. for 7 days)
        – Each of these regimens appears to cure >97% of anal and genital infections.
        – Cefixime has the advantage of a one-time oral dose, but availability is uncertain. The serum levels are not as high as with ceftriaxone or

as sustained and therefore not recommended for oral infections. Its effectiveness against incubating syphilis is not known.
- 125 mg of ceftriaxone appears to be as effective as 250 mg, and no ceftriaxone-resistant strains of *N. gonorrhoeae* have been reported.
  b. Alternative regimens
  - Spectinomycin (2 g IM in a single dose): Disadvantages include the expense, injectable use only, and ineffectiveness against syphilis.
  - Injectable cephalosporins are ceftizoxime (500 mg IM in a single dose), cefotaxime (500 mg IM in a single dose), cefotetan (1 g IM in a single dose), and cefoxitin (2 g IM with 1 g of probenecid in a single dose). None offers any significant advantage compared with ceftriaxone.
  - Oral cephalosporins other than cefixime (400 mg): These include cefuroxime axetil (1 g PO in a single dose) and cefpodoxime (1 g PO in a single dose). These appear to have less antigonococcal activity than cefixime (400 mg).

  These regimens should be followed with a therapy that treats chlamydia. Although, azithromycin (2 g as a single dose) is effective for uncomplicated gonococcal infection, the expense and gastrointestinal side effects make it difficult to use. The 1-g dose is not considered effective.
2. Treatment of sex partners
  a. All adolescents exposed to gonorrhea should be examined, cultured, and treated presumptively, as should sex partner(s) of patients diagnosed with gonorrhea.
  b. Treatment should be given for both chlamydia and gonorrhea, if chlamydia was not ruled out.
  c. Teens should be instructed to avoid sexual intercourse until they and their partners are cured.
  d. No sexual intercourse for 7 days after one-dose treatment and no longer having symptoms
     OR
     No sexual intercourse until 7 days of therapy completed and no longer having symptoms.
  e. Expedited partner therapy (EPT): EPT refers to the practice of treating sex partners of persons with STDs without an intervening medical evaluation or professional prevention counseling. One study of 2,751 patients demonstrated reduced levels of recurrent gonorrhea with EPT compared to standard management (3% versus 11%; RR = 0.32 [0.13–0.77]) (Golden et al., 2005). In another study in an STD clinical setting, many partners of identified patients with infection had infections different from or in addition to those infections identified in the index patient (Khan et al., 2005). A recent CDC communication addressed the legal concerns and safety/benefits of EPT (Centers for Disease Control and Prevention, 2005).
3. Follow-up
   Routine follow-up cultures are not needed for persons treated for *uncomplicated* gonorrhea. Adolescents should be told to return for an examination if symptoms or signs persist after therapy. Most treatment failures are due to reinfection.
4. Pharyngeal gonococcal infection
   Gonococcal infection of the pharynx may be more difficult to eradicate than urogenital and anorectal sites. Few regimens have consistent cure rates >90%.

Recommended regimens include the following:
Ceftriaxone 125 mg IM in a single dose
PLUS treatment for chlamydia
Azithromycin 1 g PO in a single dose
OR
Doxycycline 100 mg PO b.i.d. for 7 days
   Cefixime or any other oral cephalosporin or spectinomycin IM is not considered effective enough for pharyngeal infection. Only ceftriaxone should be used to treat MSM and heterosexuals with history of recent foreign travel or partners' travel.
5. Treatment of gonorrhea in pregnant adolescents
   Pregnant adolescents should be screened for gonorrhea, chlamydia, and syphilis at the first prenatal care visit, with tests repeated in the third trimester. Tetracyclines (i.e. doxycline) should be avoided during pregnancy. *N. gonorrhoeae* infection should be treated with one of the recommended cephalosporin regimens. Spectinomycin (2 g IM) can be used as an alternative, but may be difficult to obtain.
   Recommended regimens to cover potential *Chlamydia* coinfection include:
Azithromycin 1 g orally, single dose
OR
Amoxicillin 500 mg orally three times daily for 7 days
   Alternative Regimens
Erythromycin base 500 mg orally four times a day for 7 days
OR
Erythromycin base 250 mg orally four times a day for 14 days
OR
Erythromycin ethylsuccinate 800 mg orally four times a day for 7 days
OR
Erythromycin ethylsuccinate 400 mg orally four times a day for 14 days
   Note: Erythromycin estolate is contraindicated during pregnancy because of drug-related hepatotoxicity
6. Human immunodeficiency virus (HIV) infection
   Teens infected with HIV and *N. gonorrhoeae* should receive the same treatment as those not infected with HIV.
7. Acute salpingitis
   See Chapters 60 and 63 for discussion and treatment of PID.
8. Acute epididymitis
  a. Ceftriaxone 250 mg IM once
     PLUS
     Doxycycline 100 mg b.i.d. for 10 days
9. Disseminated gonococcal infection
   Hospitalization for intravenous treatment is recommended for initial therapy.
   Recommended regimen
     a. Ceftriaxone 1 g IM or IV every 24 hours
   Alternative regimens
     a. Cefotaxime 1 g IV every 8 hours
        OR
     b. Ceftizoxime 1 g IV every 8 hours
        OR
     c. Spectinomycin 2 g IM every 12 hours
   All of the preceding regimens should be continued for 24 to 48 hours after improvement begins, at which time therapy may be switched to the following regimen to complete at least 1 week of antimicrobial therapy.

a. Cefixime[†]400 mg orally twice daily
   OR
b. b. Cefixime suspension 500 mg twice daily orally (25 cc twice daily)
   OR
c. Cefpodoxime 400 mg orally twice daily

[†]The tablet formulation of cefixime is currently not available in the United States

10. Meningitis and endocarditis

    These serious complications require high-dose intravenous therapy with an antibiotic effective against the causative strain. The recommended initial regimen is 1 to 2 g of ceftriaxone IV every 12 hours. Although optimal duration is not known, most authorities treat gonococcal meningitis for 10 to 14 days and endocarditis for at least 4 weeks.

11. Gonococcal ophthalmia

    For adolescents and children weighing >20 kg, the treatment includes ceftriaxone (1 g IM once), and eye irrigation with buffered ophthalmic solution should be performed once to help clear the discharge followed by careful eye examination, including slit-lamp examination. For neonates and infants, 25 to 50 mg/kg IV or IM in a single dose not to exceed 125 mg. Simultaneous infection with *C. trachomatis* should be considered and appropriate treatment given if the individual does not respond to antibiotics.

12. Doses in adolescents

    Adolescents weighing >45 kg should be treated with the adult doses, as already outlined. Adolescents who weigh <45 kg should be treated as follows:

    a. For *uncomplicated gonococcal vulvovaginitis, cervicitis, urethritis, pharyngitis, and proctitis*
       - Ceftriaxone (125 mg IM once)
         OR
       - Spectinomycin (40 mg/kg of body weight IM [maximum 2 g] once)
         PLUS
       - Doxycycline (100 mg b.i.d. for 7 days) in addition to the previously described regimen (if 8 years or older and >45 kg)
         OR
       - Azithromycin (20 mg/kg [maximum 1 g] once)
    b. For *bacteremia or arthritis*
       - Ceftriaxone (50 mg/kg as a single dose [maximum 1 g] IV/IM for 7 days)
    c. For *meningitis*
       - Ceftriaxone (50 mg/kg as a single daily dose [maximum 2 g] IV/IM for 10 to 14 days)

    Adolescents with documented gonorrhea but no history of sexual activity should be carefully evaluated for sexual abuse.

Prevention

Male Latex Condoms

Used consistently and correctly, male latex condoms are effective in preventing the sexual transmission of HIV infection and can reduce the risk for other STDs (i.e., gonorrhea, chlamydia, and trichomonas). Generally, studies evaluating the effectiveness of male condoms to protect from gonorrhea infection have been supportive, including a "dose response protection" (Holmes et al., 2004;

Sanchez et al., 2003; Crosby et al., 2003; Ahmed et al., 2001; Warner et al., 2004,2005). Condom failure usually results from not only inconsistent but incorrect use (e.g., condom breakage) (Crosby et al., 2005; Paz-Bailey et al., 2005).

PUBLIC HEALTH ISSUES

1. High prevalence rates of gonorrhea in adolescents, particularly among minority youth, as compared with other age-groups
2. Poor screening rates for infection by clinicians in health care settings (Chacko et al., 2004)
3. High prevalence in certain groups—urban populations; young men who have sex with men; teens and young adults; street involved and substance-abusing youth; and youth in detention centers
4. High coinfection rates with other STDs, particularly *C. trachomatis* infections
5. Rapid emergence of multiple types of antibiotic resistance to gonorrhea
6. Large number of asymptomatic gonococcal infections in both females and males

WEB SITES

For Teenagers and Parents

http://www.cdc.gov/std/Gonorrhea/STDFact-gonorrhea.htm CDC fact sheet on gonorrhea (Accessed 09/04/05).

http://www.niaid.nih.gov/factsheets/stdgon.htm. National Institutes of Health (NIH) fact sheet on gonorrhea. (Accessed 09/04/05).

http://www.plannedparenthood.org/. Planned parenthood website with STD information (Accessed 05/02/07).

http://kidshealth.org/teen/infections/stds/std_gonorrhea.html Teen health site information sheet on gonorrhea. (Accessed 09/04/05)

http://www.iwannaknow.org/. American Social Health Web Site for Teen Sexual Health (Accessed 09/04/05).

http://www.youngwomenshealth.org/gonorrhea.html. The Center for Young Women's Health. Children's Hospital of Boston (Accessed 09/04/05).

For Health Professionals

http://www.cdc.gov/std/stats/gonorrhea.htm Centers for Disease Control and Prevention. STD Surveillance 2004. National Profile (Accessed 12/02/05).

http://www2a.cdc.gov/stdtraining/self-study/gonorrhea.asp Web-based training course designed to guide clinicians in the diagnosis, treatment, and prevention of gonorrhea, based on STD curriculum developed by the National Network of STD/HIV Prevention Training Centers (Accessed 12/05/05).

http://www.ahrq.gov/clinic/uspstf/uspsgono.htm. U.S. Preventive Services Task Force report on Screening for Gonorrhea (Accessed 12/02/05).

http://www2a.cdc.gov/stdclinic/PowerPoint/Gonorrhea.ppt. CDC PowerPoint slides on gonorrhea and other STDs (Accessed 12/02/05).

http://www.cdc.gov/std/stats/ CDC Power Point slides on gonorrhea (Accessed 11/28/05). Centers for Disease Control and Prevention found at Centers for Disease Control and Prevention. Sexually transmitted diseases treatment guidelines 2006. *MMWR* 2006;55(RR-11): 42. http://www.cdc.gov/std/treatment (Accessed 04/21/07) Updated recommended treatment regimens for gonococcal infections and associated conditions - United States, April 2007 MMWR 2007; 56 (14): 332. http://www.cdc.gov/std/treatment/2006/updated-regimens.htm

REFERENCES AND ADDITIONAL READINGS

Ahmed S, Lutalo T, Wawer M, et al. HIV prevalence associated with condom use: a population study in rakai, uganda. *AIDS* 2001;15:2171.

Aledort JE, Hook EW III, Weinstein MC, et al. The cost effectiveness of gonorrhea screening in urban emergency departments. *Sex Transm Dis* 2005;32:425.

Black CM, Marroazzo J, Johnson RE, et al. Head-to head multicenter comparison of DNA probe and nucleic acid amplification tests for Chlamydia trachomatis infections in women performed with an improved reference standard. *J Clin Microbiol* 2002;40:3757.

Brown RT, Lossick JG, Mosure DJ, et al. Pharyngeal gonorrhea screening in adolescents: is it necessary. *Pediatrics* 1989;84:623.

Centers for Disease Control and Prevention found at Centers for Disease Control and Prevention. Sexually transmitted diseases treatment guidelines 2006. *MMWR* 2006;55(RR-11):42–49. http://www.cdc.gov/std/treatment (Accessed 04/12/07).

Centers for Disease Control and Prevention. *Trends in reportable sexually transmitted diseases in the United States*, 2003. National Data on Chlamydia, Gonorrhea and Syphilis. http://www.cdc.gov/std/stats/2003SurveillanceSummary.pdf (Accessed 12/02/05).

Centers for Disease Control and Prevention. *Sexually transmitted disease surveillance 2003 supplement: Gonococcal Isolate Surveillance Project (GISP) annual report—2003.* Atlanta, GA: U.S. Department of Health and Human Services; November 2004.

http://www.cdc.gov/std/gisp2003/GISP2003.pdf (Accessed 12/02/05)

Center for Disease Control and Prevention. STD Surveillance 2004. Trends in reportable sexually transmitted diseases in the United States. http://www.cdc.gov/std/stats/) (Accessed 12/18/05).

Centers for Disease Control and Prevention. *Expedited partner treatment.* 2005.

Centers for Disease Control and Prevention. STD Surveillance 2004. National Profile. http://www.cdc.gov/std/stats/gonorrhea.htm (Accessed 12/02/05)

Chacko MR, Wiemann CM, Smith PB. Chlamydia and gonorrhea screening in asymptomatic young women. *J Pediatr Adolesc Gynecol* 2004;17:169.

Chernesky MA, Martin DH, Hook EW, et al. Ability of new APTIMA CT and APTIMA GC assays to detect Chlamydia trachomatis and neisseria gonorrhoeae in male urine and urethral swabs. *J Clin Microbiol* 2005;43:127.

Cook RL, Hutchinson SL, Ostergaard L, et al. Systematic review: non-invasive testing for Chlamydia trachomatis and Neisseria gonorrhoeae. *Ann Intern Med* 2005;142:914.

Cosentino La, Landers DV, Hillier SL. Detection of Chlamydia trachomatis and Neisseria gonorrhoeae by strand displacement amplification and relevance of the amplification control for use with vaginal swab specimens. *J Clin Microbiol* 2003;41:3592.

Crosby RA, DiClemente RJ, Wingood GM, et al. Value of consistent condom use: a study of sexually transmitted disease prevention among African American adolescent females. *Am J Public Health* 2003;93:901.

Crosby RA, DiClemente RJ, Wingood GM, et al. Condom failure among adolescents: implications for STD prevention. *J Adolesc Health* 2005;36:534.

Crotchfelt KA, Pare B, Gaydos C, et al. Detection of Chlamydia trachomatis by the Gen Probe Amplified Chlamydia trachomatis Assay (AMP CT) in urine specimens from men and women and endocervical specimens. *J Clin Microbiol* 1997;36:391.

Einwalter LA, Ritchie JM, Ault KA, et al. Gonorrhea and Chlamydia infection among women visiting family planning clinics: racial variation in prevalence and predictors. *Perspect Sex Reprod Health* 2005;37:135.

Emans SJ, Laufer MR, Goldstein DP, eds. *Pediatric and adolescent gynecology*, 5th ed. Philadelphia: Lippincott–Raven Publishers; 2004.

Gaydos CA, Quinn TC, Willis D, et al. Performance of the APTIMA Combo2 assay for detection of Chlamydia trachomatis and Neisseria gonorrhoeae in female urine and endocervical swab specimens. *J Clin Microbiol* 2003;41:304.

Geisler WM, Whittington WL, Suchland RJ, et al. Epidemiology of anorectal Chlamydial and gonococcal infections among men having sex with men in seattle: utilizing serovar and auxotype strain typing. *Sex Transm Dis* 2002;29:189.

Golden MR, Whittington WL, Handsfield HH, et al. Effect of expedited treatment of sex partners on recurrent or persistent gonorrhea or Chlamydial infection. *N Engl J Med* 2005;352:676.

Holmes KK, Levine R, Weaver M. Effectiveness of condoms in preventing sexually transmitted infections. *Bull WHO* 2004;82:454.

Joffe A, Blythe M. Handbook of adolescent medicine. *State Art Rev Adolesc Med* 2003;14:345.

Jones CA, Knaup RC, Hayes M, et al. Urine screening for gonococcal and Chlamydial infections at community-based organizations in a high-morbidity area. *Sex Transm Dis* 2000;27:146.

Kahn RH, Mosure DJ, Blank S, et al. Jail STD Prevalence Monitoring Project. Chlamydia trachomatis and Neisseria gonorrhoeae prevalence and coinfection in adolescents entering selected US juvenile detention centers, 1997–2002. *Sex Transm Dis* 2005; 32:255.

Khan A, Fortenberry JD, Temkit MH, et al. Gender differences in sexual behaviors in response to genitourinary symptoms. *Sex Transm Dis* 2005;32:260.

Kohl KS, Sternberg MR, Markowitz LE, et al. Screening of males for Chlamydia trachomatis and Neisseria gonorrhoeae infections at STD clinics in three US cities—Indianapolis, New Orleans, Seattle. *Int J STD AIDS* 2004;15:822.

Lyss SB, Kamb ML, Peterman TA, et al. Project Respect Study Group. Chlamydia trachomatis among patients infected with and treated for Neisseria gonorrhoeae in sexually transmitted disease clinics in the united states. *Ann Intern Med* 2003; 139:178.

Martin DH, Cammarata C, Van Der Pol B, et al. Multicenter evaluation of Amplicor and automated Cobas Amplicor CT/NG tests for *Neisseria gonorrhoeae*. *J Clin Microbiol* 2000; 38:3544.

McMillan A. Sexually acquired reactive arthritis. In: McMillan A, Young H, Ogilvie MM, et al., eds. *Clinical practice in sexually transmissible infections*. Edinburgh: WB Saunders; 2002:379.

Mertz KJ, Voigt RA, Hutchins K, et al. Jail STD Prevalence Monitoring Group. Findings from STD screening of adolescents and adults entering corrections facilities: implications for STD control strategies. *Sex Transm Dis* 2002;29:834.

Miller WC, Ford CA, Morris M, et al. Prevalence of Chlamydial and gonococcal infections among young adults in the united states. *JAMA* 2004;291:2229.

Pack RP, DiClemente RJ, Hook EW III, et al. High prevalence of asymptomatic STDs in incarcerated minority male youth: a case for screening. *Sex Transm Dis* 2000; 27:175.

Paz-Bailey G, Koumans EH, Sternberg M, et al. The effect of correct and consistent condom use on Chlamydial and gonocccocal infection among urban adolescents. *Arch Pediatr Adolesc Med* 2005;159:536.

Peter NG, Clark LR, Jaeger JR. Fitz-Hugh-Curtis syndrome: a diagnosis to consider in women with right upper quadrant pain. *Cleve Clin J Med* 2004;71:233.

Rice PA. Gonococcal arthritis (disseminated gonococcal infection). *Infect Dis Clin North Am* 2005;19:853.

Roochvarg LB, Lovchik JC. Screening for pharyngeal gonorrhea in adolescents. A reexamination. *J Adolesc Health* 1991; 12:269.

Sanchez J, Campos PE, Courtois B, et al. Prevention of sexually transmitted diseases (STDs) in female sex workers: prospective evaluation of condom promotion and strengthened STD services. *Sex Transm Dis* 2003;30:273.

Schachter J, McCormack WM, Chernesky MA, et al. Vaginal swabs are appropriate specimens for diagnosis of genital tract infection with *Chlamydia trachomatis*. *J Clin Microbiol* 2003;41:3784.

Schwarcz SK, Bolan GA, Fullilove M, et al. Crack cocaine and the exchange of sex for money or drugs. Risk factors for gonorrhea among black adolescents in San Francisco. *Sex Transm Dis* 1992;19:7–13.

Spigarelli MG, Biro FM. Sexually transmitted disease testing: evaluation of diagnostic tests and methods. *Adolesc Med Clin* 2004;15:287.

Van Der Pol B, Ferrero DV, Buck-Barrington L, et al. Multicenter evaluation of BDProbeTec ET system for detection of Chlamydia trachomatis and Neisseria gonorrhoeae in urine specimens, female endocervical swabs, and male urethral swabs. *J Clin Microbiol* 2001;39:1008.

Vickerman P, Peeling RW, Watts C, et al. Detection of gonococcal infection : pros and cons of a rapid test. *Mol Diagn* 2005;9:175.

Warner L, Newman DR, Austin HD, et al. Project Respect Study Group. Condom effectiveness for reducing transmission of gonorrhea and Chlamydia: the importance of assessing partner infection status. *Am J Epidemiol* 2004;159: 242.

Warner L, Macaluso M, Sustin HD, et al. Application for the case cross-over design to reduce unmeasured confounding in studies of condom effectiveness. *Am J Epidemiol* 2005; 162:765.

Warner L, Stone KM, Macaluso M, et al. Condom use and risk of gonorrhea and Chlamydia: a systematic review of design and measurement factors assessed in epidemiologic studies. *Sex Transm Dis* 2006;33:36.

Weinstock H, Berman S, Cates W. Sexually transmitted diseases among American youth: incidence and prevalence estimates, 2000. *Perspect Sex Reprod Health* 2004;36:6.

Wheeler HL, Skinner CJ, Khunda A, et al. Molecular testing (strand displacement assay) for identification of urethral gonorrhoea in men: can it replace culture as the gold standard. *Int J STD AIDS* 2005;16:430.

Wiesenfeld HC, Heine RP, Rideout A, et al. The vaginal introitus: a novel site for Chlamydia trachomatis testing in women. *Am J Obstet Gynecol* 1996;174:1542.

Wiesenfeld HC, Hillier SL, Krohn MA, et al. Lower genital tract infection and endometritis: insight into subclinical pelvic inflammatory disease. *Obstet Gynecol* 2002;100:456.

Wiesenfeld HC, Sweet RL, Ness RB, et al. Comparison of acute and subclinical pelvic inflammatory disease. *Sex Transm Dis* 2005;32:400.

Xu K, Glanton V, Johnson SR, et al. Detection of Neisseria gonorrhoeae by ligase chain reaction testing of urine among adolescent women with and without Chlamydia trachomatis infection. *Sex Transm Dis* 1998;25:533.

Young H, McMillan A. Gonorrhea. In: McMillan A, Young H, Ogilvie MM, et al., eds. *Clinical practice in sexually transmissible infections*. Edinburgh: WB Saunders; 2002:313.

CHAPTER 62

Chlamydia Trachomatis

Catherine A. Miller and Mary-Ann B. Shafer

Genital infections caused by *Chlamydia trachomatis* represent the most prevalent bacterial sexually transmitted disease (STD) in the United States and the most frequently reported infectious disease. An estimated 3 million new cases occur annually, with most identified among patients younger than 25 years. Chlamydial infections and their sequelae have a large impact on health care expenditures, resulting in more than $2 billion in health care costs per year in the United States alone (Eng and Butler, 1997). Chlamydial infections pose a major public health threat because of associated harmful sequelae in females; the most serious of these include pelvic inflammatory disease (PID), ectopic pregnancy, and infertility.

ETIOLOGY

The genus *Chlamydia* is divided into four species: *Chlamydia psittaci, C. pecorum, C. pneumoniae,* and *C. trachomatis.*

1. *C. psittaci* is responsible for zoonosis and psittacosis, an infection contracted by humans from infected birds, and characterized by interstitial pneumonitis.
2. *C. pecorum* affects domestic animals.
3. *C. pneumoniae* causes pneumonia, pharyngitis, and bronchitis and most recently has been associated with possible etiological factors in coronary artery disease. Epidemiological studies have revealed that *C. pneumoniae* is a relatively common cause of infection in school-aged children, and it is probably the most common cause of community-acquired pneumonia in this age-group.
4. *C. trachomatis* is associated with a spectrum of diseases. This species contains 18 serologically distinct variants known as *serovars.* Chlamydial genital disease and neonatal disease (pneumonia and conjunctivitis) are caused by serovars B, D, E, F, G, H, I, J, and K. Table 62.1 outlines the major serovars of *C. trachomatis.* This chapter focuses on nonlymphogranuloma venereum (non-LGV), non–trachoma-causing serovars of *C. trachomatis.*

DEVELOPMENTAL CYCLE AND PATHOGENESIS

1. Developmental cycle (Fig. 62.1):
   a. *C. trachomatis* exhibits a unique developmental cycle lasting between 48 and 72 hours.
   b. The cycle is characterized by transformation between two morphologically distinct infectious and reproductive forms (Schachter, 1999).
   c. The extracellular infectious form, the elementary body, attaches to a susceptible epithelial cell and is ingested.
   d. Susceptible host cells seem to have a specific receptor that facilitates attachment to *C. trachomatis* and facilitates its ingestion. The trachoma serovars responsible for human genital infections may have a very specific attachment site, which may help explain its restricted host range.
   e. Once within an endocytotic vesicle, the elementary body reorganizes into the replicating form, the reticulate body. As the reticulate body divides, it fills the endosome with its progeny.
   f. After 48 hours, multiplication ceases and the reticulate bodies transform to new infectious elementary bodies. The elementary bodies are then released from the cell by cytolysis or by a process of extrusion of the entire inclusion, which often results in the destruction of the host cell.
2. Affinity for columnar epithelium: Of particular importance to the young female adolescent, *C. trachomatis* has a predilection for columnar epithelium commonly found in the cervix of young women. This tissue involutes into the endocervical canal with age.
3. Immune response: The signs and symptoms associated with infection are mainly secondary to tissue destruction and the body's immunopathogenic response to the infection.
   a. Major outer membrane protein (MOMP): A very important component in the immune response is the presence of this *C. trachomatis* membrane protein that can induce both a neutralizing antibody and a T-cell mediated immune response. Antibody to MOMP neutralizes chlamydial infectivity both in cellular and animal models. However, the MOMP gene appears capable of frequently developing variants and this mechanism may serve as a type of escape from the neutralizing antibodies mounted by the host. The ability of these polymorphisms to actually protect *C. trachomatis* from inactivation by the host is not known but would have an important impact on the design and development of future potential vaccines.
   b. Heat shock protein: Another important protein is the *C. trachomatis* heat shock protein (cHSP60),

TABLE 62.1

Serovars of *C. trachomatis*

Species	Serovar	Disease
C. trachomatis	L1, L2, L3	Lymphogranuloma venereum
C. trachomatis	A, B, Ba, C	Hyperendemic blinding trachoma
C. trachomatis	D, E, F, G, H, I, J, K	Inclusion conjunctivitis, nongonococcal urethritis, cervicitis, proctitis, salpingitis, epididymitis, pneumonia of newborns

which is 50% homologous to human HSP60. This homology could potentially cause cross-reactive immune responses with healthy human tissues and could help explain the apparent tissue immune-mediated destruction associated with *C. trachomatis* infections, such as the scarring of the fallopian tubes as a result of PID.

EPIDEMIOLOGY

C. trachomatis is the most common reported bacterial STD in the United States, with more than 900,000 infections reported to the Centers for Disease Control and Prevention (CDC) in 2005. Because many *C. trachomatis* infections are asymptomatic and go undiagnosed, it is estimated that the actual infection rate may be approximately 3 times the reported number, which translates into approximately 3 million Americans infected with chlamydia annually (Centers for Disease Control and Prevention, 2004). Adolescent females ages 15 to 19 had the highest rates of reported *C. trachomatis* infection in 2004. In men, although rates are much lower than in women, the highest rates were among 20- to 24 year-olds (see Fig. 62.2 for age- and sex-specific rates). Increased testing in females may help explain their higher infection rates. Prevalence rates of *C. trachomatis* among select adolescent populations are reviewed in Table 62.2.

Overall, national rates reported by the CDC in 2005 are as follows:

1. From 50 states and the District of Columbia, 976,445 *C. trachomatis* infections were reported to CDC during 2005

FIGURE 62.1 Life cycle of *C. trachomatis*. (Courtesy of California STD/HIV Prevention Training Center.)

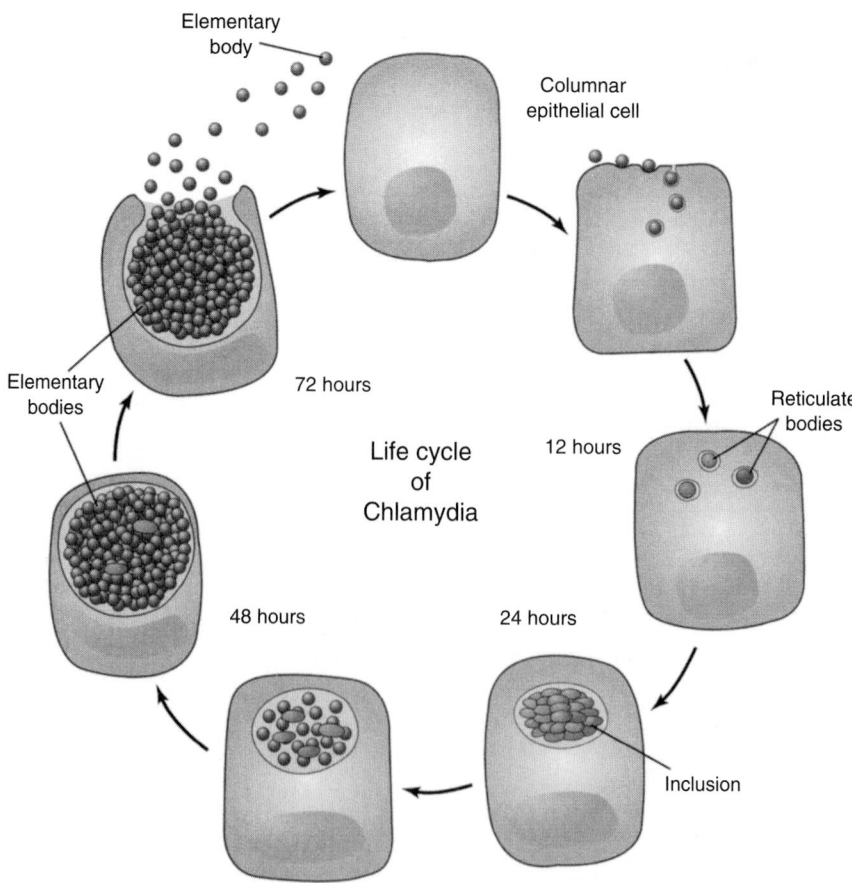

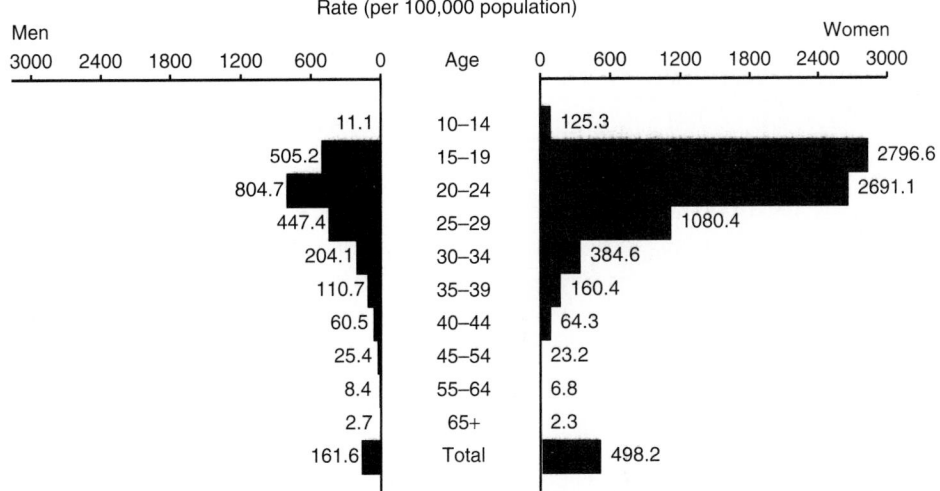

Rate (per 100,000 population)

Men							Age		Women					
3000	2400	1800	1200	600	0			0	600	1200	1800	2400	3000	
					11.1		10–14	125.3						
			505.2				15–19						2796.6	
		804.7					20–24					2691.1		
			447.4				25–29				1080.4			
				204.1			30–34		384.6					
				110.7			35–39	160.4						
				60.5			40–44	64.3						
				25.4			45–54	23.2						
				8.4			55–64	6.8						
				2.7			65+	2.3						
				161.6			Total		498.2					

FIGURE 62.2   *C. trachomatis*—United States age- and sex-specific rates: Centers for Disease Control and Prevention, STD Surveillance, National Profile, 2005: http://www.cdc.gov/std/stats/natprointro.htm (Figure 7 in the CDC report.)

2. Overall rate in the United States (2005): 332.5 cases per 100,000 population, an increase of 5.1% since 2004.
   a. 496.5 per 100,000 women
   b. 161.5 per 100,000 men
   c. 2,796.6 per 100,000 females aged 15 to 19 years
   d. 505.2 per 100,000 males aged 15 to 19 years
   e. 1,247 per 100,000 African Americans, more than eight times higher than the rate among whites (152.1 per 100,000)
3. Median chlamydia test positivity was 6.3% (3.2%–16.3%) in women aged 15 to 24 years screened during visits to selected family planning clinics in all states and outlying areas in 2004.
4. National household sample prevalence: A national household sample was reported in 2004 of more than 14,000 young adults aged 18 to 26 (Miller et al., 2004). The overall prevalence was 4.19% with the following rates by gender and race:

Race	Males	Females
African-American	11.1%	13.95%
Latino	7.24%	4.42%
White	1.38%	2.52%
Asian-American	1.14%	3.31%

There was only a small difference in rates based on age with the highest percentage in those aged 20 to 21 (4.7%). In addition, the highest prevalence was in the South (5.4%) versus the Midwest (3.95%), West (3.2%), and Northeast (2.4%). In this sample 0.3% had both chlamydia and gonorrhea infections, with 70% of those with gonorrhea also having chlamydia and 8% of those with chlamydia also having gonorrhea.

5. Since 1996, there has been a 57% increase in chlamydia positivity from 4.9% to 7.7% among women aged 15 to 24 years in the family planning clinics screening programs in Health and Human Services Region X.
6. The overall trend in the 15- to 19-year-old age-group has been an increase in the chlamydia infection rates from 1,318.6 per 100,000 in 2000 to 1621.0 per 100,000 in 2005. A contributing factor in this overall 16% increase in positivity may be the expansion of screening programs to populations with higher prevalence of disease in some regions.

7. The Midwest had the overall highest infection rates in 2002 to 2005. The Northeast had the lowest infection rates.

Risk Factors

C. trachomatis infection is associated with a number of factors including younger age, presence of cervical ectopy, female gender, prior history of STDs, new sexual partner, multiple sexual partners, living in a community with a high background prevalence, oral contraceptive use, douching, nonwhite race/ethnicity (African-American predominance), unmarried, and young age at sexual debut (Burstein et al., 2001; Williams et al., 2003; Berman and Hein, 1999; Boyer et al., 1999; Baeten et al., 2001; Scholes et al., 1998; Marrazzo et al., 1997; Orr et al., 1994; Stamm, 1999a,b).

Transmission

1. *C. trachomatis* can be transmitted during vaginal, anal, or oral sex. An infected mother can also pass infection to her baby during vaginal childbirth.
2. Sixty percent to 75% of females with male sex partners who have *C. trachomatis* urethritis test positive for *C. trachomatis* infection (Lycke et al., 1980; Quinn et al., 1996).
3. Twenty-five percent to 50% of male sex partners of females with a mucopurulent cervicitis (MPC) or PID test positive for *C. trachomatis* infection.
4. Male to female transmission may be more efficient. Reasons may include increased pathogen contact time in females and more efficient infection of the female endocervix compared to the male urethra (Bolan et al., 1999).
5. However, transmission data among partnerships using the newer nucleic acid amplification technology (NAATs) suggest that the male-to-female and

TABLE 62.2

Adolescent *C. trachomatis* Prevalence Rates by Population and Type of Testing

Population	Test	CT (+) Rate (%)	n/N	Author	Year
FEMALES					
a. Teen detention, school, and community clinics	LCR urine	8.5	424/4,968	Marrazzo et al.	1997
b. Teen clinic	PCR urine	14.9	47/315	Oh et al.	1997
c. Teen clinic	PCR cervix	20.7	86/415	Beck-Sague et al.	1998
d. School-based clinic	PCR cervix LCR urine	15.7	64/408	Gaydos et al.	1998
e. STD, family planning, school-based clinic	PCR urine PCR cervix	24	771/3,202	Burstein et al.	1998
f. Detention clinic	LCR urine	28.3	13/46	Oh et al.	1998
g. Army recruits	LCR urine	9.2	1,215/13,204	Gaydos et al.	1998
h. Community outreach clinic	LCR urine	12.9	8/62	Rietmeijer et al.	1998
i. Teen clinic	PCR cervix	27	70/260	Bunnell et al.	1999
j. School-based clinic	LCR urine	11.5	286/2,497	Cohen et al.	1999
k. Emergency department	LCR urine	9.9 (females and males)	28/282	Embling et al.	2000
l. Marine recruits	LCR cervix, urine, vagina	11	193/1,756	Shafer et al.	2000
m. National job training program	EIA probe urine	9.2	413/4,488	Lifson et al.	2001
n. High school–based clinic	LCR urine	3.9	11/283	Kent et al.	2002
o. Health maintenance organization	SDA urine	5.8	23/393	Shafer et al.	2002
p. Sports-related school-based clinic	LCR urine	6.5	13/200	Nsuami et al.	2003
q. Marine recruits	LCR urine, cervix, vagina	11.6	207/1,786	Shafer et al.	2003
r. Army recruits	LCR urine	9.5	2,189/23,010	Gaydos et al.	2003
Population	Test	CT (+) Rate (%)	n/N	Author	Year
MALES					
a. Teen, detention school and community clinics	LCR urine	5.3	275/5,150	Marrazzo et al.	1997
b. Detention clinic	LCR urine	8.8	19/217	Oh et al.	1998
c. Community outreach	LCR urine	10.7	17/159	Rietmeijer et al.	1998
d. Enlisted military, nonclinic-based screening	LCR urine	3.4	21/618	Brodine et al.	1998
e. Health maintenance organization teen clinic	LCR urine	2.11	3/118	Boyer et al.	1999
f. School-based clinic	LCR urine	6.2	143/2,308	Cohen et al.	1999
g. Emergency department	LCR urine	9.9 (males and females)	28/282	Embling et al.	2000
h. Detention clinic	LCR urine	14.4	41/284	Pack et al.	2000
i. High school-based clinic	LCR urine	0.8	3/381	Kent et al.	2002
j. Correctional facility clinic	LCR urine	2.8–8.9 range	Not reported	Mertz et al.	2002
k. Sports related school-based clinic	LCR urine	2.8	12/436	Nsuami et al.	2003
l. Health maintenance organization	SDA urine	4.0	27/711	Tebb et al.	2004

CT, *Chlamydia trachomatis*; LCR, ligase chain reaction; PCR, polymerase chain reaction; STD, sexually transmitted disease; EIA, enzyme immunoassay; SDA, strand displacement amplification.

female-to-male transmission after multiple sexual encounters may actually be equivalent (Quinn et al., 1996).

6. Recent data suggest that correct and consistent condom use is protective against *C. trachomatis* transmission (Paz-Bailey et al., 2005; Sayegh et al., 2005).

CLINICAL MANIFESTATIONS

The clinical manifestations of *C. trachomatis* are similar to those of *Neisseria gonorrhoeae* (Table 62.3). Both organisms preferentially infect columnar or transitional epithelium of the urethra, with extension to the epididymis; the endocervix, with extension to the endometrium, salpinx, and peritoneum; and the rectum. Both organisms can invade deeper tissue, causing extensive subepithelial inflammation, epithelial ulceration, scarring, and PID. PID is responsible for most of the acute illness and long-term economic cost related to chlamydial infections. Most infections caused by *C. trachomatis* are asymptomatic or have few or no symptoms, unlike *N. gonorrhoeae* infections. An estimated 70% to 90% of *C. trachomatis* endocervical infections have no symptoms (Brunham and Peeling, 1994).

Male Infections

Studies of infected male patients have historically been limited to those who were largely adult symptomatic clients attending STD clinics and who were diagnosed with nongonococcal urethritis (NGU). Complications other than urethritis, epididymitis, proctitis, and Reiter syndrome are unusual in males. However, there is some evidence, although still controversial, that *C. trachomatis* infection may affect male fertility (Eley et al., 2005).

Urethritis

1. Urethritis is the most common problem associated with *C. trachomatis* in males.
2. *C. trachomatis* causes approximately 40% to 60% of NGU in males.
3. *C. trachomatis* urethral infection is more often asymptomatic than gonococcal urethral infection, and when symptoms occur they are milder with chlamydial urethritis. However, most males with asymptomatic chlamydial urethral infection have a persistent inflammatory response shown by urethral leukocytosis.
4. Urethritis caused by *C. trachomatis* is associated with the finding of more than 4 polymorphonuclear (PMN) leukocytes per high-power field (HPF) on Gram stains of urethral secretions and/or white blood cells (WBCs) on a first-void urine specimen.
5. There is a 7- to 21-day incubation period from infection to development of symptoms.

Epididymitis

1. *C. trachomatis* and *N. gonorrhoeae* infections are responsible for most of the epididymitis cases among men younger than 35 years. In particular, *C. trachomatis* is responsible for 70% of cases in adolescent and young men.
2. The pathogenesis of chlamydial epididymitis is unclear.
3. Chlamydial urethritis often accompanies the epididymitis among sexually active young males.
4. Males with epididymitis usually complain of unilateral testicular pain and tenderness, and a hydrocele or swelling of the epididymis is usually present. Onset is usually gradual but can be sudden (see Chapter 28 for further description of the workup for scrotal pain).
5. Complaints of dysuria are present in less than half of men with epididymitis.

Prostatitis Despite continued study, the role of *C. trachomatis* in causing nonbacterial prostatitis remains

TABLE 62.3

Comparison of Clinical Manifestations of *C. trachomatis* and *N. gonorrhoeae*

	Resulting Clinical Syndrome	
Site of Infection	Neisseria gonorrhoeae	Chlamydia trachomatis
Males		
Urethra	Urethritis	Nongonococcal urethritis
Epididymis	Epididymitis	Epididymitis
Rectum	Proctitis	Proctitis
Conjunctiva	Conjunctivitis	Conjunctivitis
Systemic	Disseminated gonococcal infection: Arthritis-dermatitis syndrome	Reiter syndrome
Females		
Urethra	Acute urethral syndrome	Acute urethral syndrome
Bartholin gland	Bartholinitis	Bartholinitis
Cervix	Cervicitis	Cervicitis
Fallopian tube	Salpingitis	Salpingitis
Conjunctiva	Conjunctivitis	Conjunctivitis
Liver capsule	Perihepatitis	Perihepatitis
Systemic	Disseminated gonococcal infection: Arthritis-dermatitis syndrome	Reiter syndrome

controversial. Although definitive studies are lacking, *C. trachomatis* has been isolated from prostatic secretions and prostatic biopsies from some patients with prostatitis.

Proctitis Most of the information about *C. trachomatis* and proctitis is derived from studies of homosexual men. Either the lymphogranuloma venereum (LGV) strains or the genital strains D through K are responsible for the development of proctitis. The LGV strains can produce a primary ulcerative proctitis and a histopathological picture of giant cell formation and granulomas similar to those seen in acute Crohn disease, whereas the non-LGV immunotypes produce more mild disease, from no symptoms present to rectal bleeding, diarrhea, and rectal discharge.

Female Infections

Cervicitis
1. Approximately 70% of women infected with *C. trachomatis* are asymptomatic, others have mild symptoms such as vaginal discharge, vaginal spotting, mild abdominal pain, or dysuria. On examination, the cervix may appear normal or exhibit "hypertrophic" ectopy that appears edematous, and may bleed easily when touched by a swab. There may be a mucopurulent discharge from the cervical os.
2. Ectopy is not synonymous with the inflammatory reaction of the cervix to infection or cervicitis. Ectopy, the presence of columnar epithelial cells on the ectocervix, is a common and normal finding of the developing adolescent cervix. It occurs in 60% to 80% of adolescent cervices. Ectopy is also associated with birth control use. It may be that more adolescents use birth control pills than older adults, birth control pills slow the maturation and involution of the columnar epithelia into the endocervical canal, or birth control pills actually do stimulate the formation of ectopy. However, *C. trachomatis* infection is greater in young women with ectopy than in those without ectopy.
3. Chlamydial and gonococcal cervicitis are associated with the finding of more than 30 PMN leukocytes/HPF on Gram stains of cervical secretions.
4. Although the presence of MPC has been related to both *C. trachomatis* and *N. gonorrhoeae* infections, in most cases of MPC neither organism is identified on testing. The reverse is also true: in most cases of documented chlamydial and gonococcal cervical infection, MPC is not found on examination.

Urethritis
1. Screening studies in STD clinics suggest that more than 50% of women infected with *C. trachomatis* have coinfections at both the urethra and endocervix (Stamm, 1999a,b). Women with *C. trachomatis* isolated from both the cervix and the urethra were more likely to complain of dysuria than women with cervical infection alone.
2. The acute urethral syndrome of chlamydial urethritis is characterized by the finding of "sterile" pyuria for urine pathogens in the face of symptoms of dysuria and frequency in sexually active young women.

Pelvic Inflammatory Disease
See Chapter 63 on PID.

1. Infections can ascend through the cervical os causing endometriosis and infection of the fallopian tubes. When the infection extends to the ovaries and peritoneal cavity it can result in abscess formation.
2. The risk for a 15-year-old female to develop PID is ten times the risk for a 24-year-old young woman.
3. *C. trachomatis* has been associated with 20% to 50% of the PID cases in the United States.
4. It is estimated that 10% to 40% of females with untreated chlamydial infections develop PID (Cates and Wasserheit, 1991).
5. The spectrum of PID associated with *C. trachomatis* infection ranges from acute, severe disease to asymptomatic or "silent" disease.
6. Women with a history of PID can experience serious reproductive sequelae, including infertility, ectopic pregnancy, and chronic pelvic pain. Two studies of *C. trachomatis* and PID in infertile female patients demonstrated PID as the cause of the infertility in half the patients and found that antichlamydial antibody was strongly associated with a tubal problem associated with infertility (Jones et al., 1982a; Kelver and Nagamani, 1989). Many of these females denied a past history of salpingitis. Undetected or "silent" cases of salpingitis may also be a contributor to ectopic pregnancies.

Perihepatitis (Fitz-Hugh-Curtis Syndrome) This syndrome can occur in up to 25% of those individuals with PID and may be associated with chlamydial (70% of cases) and gonococcal salpingitis. Signs and symptoms include right-upper-quadrant pain and tenderness, fever, nausea, and vomiting. Women may also have signs of PID. Although usually related to STD infections in females, perihepatitis has been described in males in rare cases.

Pregnancy-Related Chlamydial Infections
1. *C. trachomatis* infections during pregnancy have been associated with adverse outcomes such as spontaneous miscarriage and premature delivery. Infected women can develop PID after vaginal delivery or after therapeutic abortion.
2. Two thirds of infants born to infected mothers become colonized during delivery. Conjunctivitis develops in 18% to 50% of colonized infants, and symptoms peak in the first 5 to 14 days of life.
3. Pneumonia develops in 10% to 20% of colonized infants. Approximately 50% of infants with pneumonia will have concurrent conjunctivitis (Darville, 1998).

Other Infections and Complications, Male and Female

Pharyngeal Colonization *C. trachomatis* is isolated from the pharynx but causes few problems. It is present in 3.7% of males and 3.2% of females at risk of genital infection (Jones et al., 1985). In a study by Neinstein and Inderlied (1986), the organism was only isolated in 1 of 100 adolescents examined using older, less-accurate tests.

Conjunctivitis Direct contact with infectious secretions during sexual activity or from autoinoculation can result in conjunctivitis. Of patients with urogenital infections, approximately 1% have a concurrent ophthalmologic infection. Symptoms usually include unilateral eye discharge, hyperemia, and pain.

Cardiac Complications Rare cardiac complications include endocarditis (Dimmitt et al., 1985; Jones et al., 1982b) and myocarditis.

Reiter Syndrome Reiter syndrome, or reactive arthritis, is a disease characterized by a prolonged immune response focused mainly on the skin and joints. The syndrome of conjunctivitis, dermatitis, urethritis, and arthritis occurs most frequently after a bacterial infection of the genital tract or gastrointestinal tract. The common organisms implicated in Reiter syndrome are *C. trachomatis* (post–genital tract infection), and *Salmonella enteritidis* and *S. typhimurium* in the postdysenteric form. Most individuals who develop Reiter syndrome are HLA-B27 positive and it occurs more commonly in males. *C. trachomatis* infection can also be associated with an arthritis or reactive tenosynovitis without the other characteristics of Reiter syndrome.

DIFFERENTIAL DIAGNOSIS

The differential diagnosis of a reproductive-related problem is dependent on the symptom complex of the patient (e.g., urethritis, cervicitis, epididymitis, or PID). The reader is also directed to the chapters in this book dealing with these individual problems.

Females

Although most cases of *C. trachomatis* in female patients are asymptomatic, a common problem in those with chlamydial infection is MPC or urethritis, which can also be caused by the following:

1. Infections from *N. gonorrhoeae, Trichomonas vaginalis,* herpes simplex, human papillomavirus, and other organisms such as *Escherichia coli*
2. Intrauterine device (IUD)
3. Allergic reaction to contraceptive foam, gel, or film
4. Idiopathic disease, such as local irritation due to feminine hygiene products, perfumes, or sexual activity

Males

The most common problem in males is urethritis, which can also be caused by the following:

1. Infections such as *N. gonorrhoeae, Ureaplasma urealyticum, T. vaginalis,* human papillomavirus and herpes simplex
2. Allergic reaction to contraceptive foam, gel, or film
3. Idiopathic disease (see earlier description)

In males presenting with symptoms of acute epididymitis or orchitis, it is important to consider the following in the differential diagnosis:

1. Most epididymitis infections that affect sexually active adolescents and young adults are associated with urethritis due to *C. trachomatis* (most frequent), *N. gonorrhoeae,* and gram-positive cocci.

2. In young postpubertal men, coliform and *Pseudomonas aeruginosa* are less common.
3. Gram-negative enteric organisms occur more frequently in men older than 35 years.
4. In homosexual males, epididymitis may also be caused by sexually transmitted organisms such as *E. coli* among the insertive partners involved in anal intercourse.
5. It must be remembered that another common cause of an acute painful scrotal swelling in the sexually active male adolescent is torsion of the spermatic cord, which is a surgical emergency. Therefore, the workup for torsion and an infectious etiology must be done in concert and must be done with urgency. The diagnosis is based on a dual diagnostic workup for infection and torsion.

DIAGNOSIS

The introduction of NAATs for the diagnosis of *C. trachomatis* infections now provides readily available, highly sensitive, inexpensive, and noninvasive screening tests. In comparison to the former cell culture testing, which required cervical or urethral sampling, the newer testing technology allows noninvasive sampling of first-void urine and self-administered vaginal swabs to collect specimens. The focus for testing has broadened from testing symptomatic individuals to also screening at-risk asymptomatic individuals. The noninvasive testing is preferred by patients and also allows for testing in nontraditional, nonclinical sites, potentially leading to earlier detection and screening of populations not utilizing clinics.

Clinical Clues

C. trachomatis infections should be suspected in all sexually active adolescents, particularly those with multiple partners or signs and symptoms of genitourinary infection including urethritis, cervicitis, epididymitis, or PID. This includes female patients with an edematous friable cervix, mucopurulent endocervical discharge, and WBCs on the wet mount or patients with a urethritis with Gram stains or cultures not consistent with gonococcal infection. In asymptomatic male patients, the urinary leukocyte esterase dipstick test (LET) on a first-catch urine sample is a good screening test for further evaluation for *C. trachomatis* or *N. gonorrhoeae*. It must be emphasized that approximately 75% of females and 50% of males with chlamydia are asymptomatic. By treating only presumptive symptomatic cases, a large proportion of infected teenagers will be missed.

Collection of Specimens

Correct specimen collection and handling are essential for all testing methods. As *C. trachomatis* is an obligate intracellular organism infecting columnar epithelium, the presence of columnar epithelial cells has been associated with increased sensitivity in most studies evaluating various screening tests. The preferred method of collection is dictated by the particular test manufacturer's directives.

Collection Sites
Endocervix
If a pelvic examination is performed, the endocervix can be used as the site for specimen collection. Before

obtaining a specimen, a large swab should be used to remove secretions and discharge from the cervical os. After cleaning the cervix, the physician inserts a small swab approximately 1 cm into the os and rotates it several times to collect the specimen. All types of chlamydial testing techniques can be applied to the cervix.

Urethra

This is the main site of infection in the male patient but is also a site of infection in females either alone or in conjunction with an endocervical infection. The urogenital swab should be gently inserted into the urethra, in males 2 to 3 cm and in females 1 to 2 cm. All types of *C. trachomatis* tests have been applied successfully to urethral specimens. Urethral swabs for chlamydial testing are being replaced by the noninvasive urine sampling.

Urine

Noninvasive urine-based testing is becoming widely used to screen adolescent males and females for chlamydial infection. To optimize the urine sample—first-void "dirty" sample (first 15–20 mL of micturition) should be used, and if possible, specimen collection should be delayed until more than 1 hour after prior urination.

Vagina

The U.S. Food and Drug Administration (FDA) recently approved the transcription-mediated amplification assay for chlamydial testing of vaginal samples (Cook et al., 2005).

Recent studies of other types of assays have also shown that results obtained with vaginal specimens are identical if not superior to the results obtained with cervical specimens. Vaginal swabs can be accurately self-collected by patients and do not require a pelvic examination.

Other Sites

For conjunctival samples, culture is preferred because of high sensitivity and specificity. Enzyme immunoassay (EIA), nucleic acid probe, and direct fluorescent antibody (DFA) tests are also FDA cleared for use with conjunctival specimens. Rectal specimens have not proved to be amenable to NAATs because of inhibitors present in rectal specimens. Culture isolation is acceptable for detecting *C. trachomatis* in rectal or pharyngeal swab specimens. DFA can also be performed on rectal or pharyngeal swab specimens.

Laboratory Diagnosis

It must be remembered that a lower prevalence rate, particularly less than 5%, increases the potential for a false-positive test result among the nonculture testing techniques. Testing technologies are summarized in Table 62.4.

Chlamydia-Specific Tests

1. Cell culture: Cultures can be taken from endocervical, urethral, rectal, conjunctival, and nasopharyngeal sites.

TABLE 62.4

Comparison of *C. trachomatis* Testing Technologies

	Test Types	Preferred Test	Collection Site	Sensitivity	Specificity
Nucleic acid amplification technology (NAAT)	Ligase chain reaction (LCR) Polymerase chain reaction (PCR) Transcription-mediated amplification (TMA) Strand displacement amplification (SDA)	Yes	Male and female urine, endocervical and urethral swabs Vaginal swab (TMA)	80%–90%	>98%
Cell culture		No	Endocervical, urethral, rectal, conjunctival, nasopharyngeal	60%–80%	>99%
Direct fluorescent antibody (DFA)		No	Endocervical, urethral, rectal, conjunctival, nasopharyngeal	65%–75%	97%–99%
Enzyme immunoassay (EIA)		No	Endocervical, urethral, conjunctival	60%–75%	97%–99%
Nucleic acid probe	DNA probe hybridization Hybrid capture with signal amplification	No	Endocervical, urethral, conjunctival	65%–75%	98/99%

From Centers for Disease Control and Prevention: Screening Tests To Detect *Chlamydia trachomatis* and *Neisseria gonorrhoeae* Infections–2002. MMWR 2002:51.

California STD/HIV Prevention Training Center: Sexually transmitted chlamydial infections: A primary care clinician's guide to diagnosis, treatment and prevention, http://www.stdhivtraining.org/pdf/chlamydia_screen.pdf, Dec 2003.

The CDC recommends culture as one option for legal evidence collection in sexual assault cases (Centers for Disease Control and Prevention, 2006). See discussion regarding testing in sexual assault cases in subsequent section Testing after Sexual Assault.

2. DFA or EIA: These tests were the first generation of specific nonculture tests. Although the test performances were slightly poorer than culture in the best laboratories, the DFA and EIA tests can be applied to urine.
3. Nucleic acid probes: The first-generation nonamplified nucleic acid probes included the nucleic hybridization tests. The performance of these nonamplified nucleic acid probes is not significantly better than that of DFA, EIA, and culture.
4. NAATs: The amplified nucleic acid tests have revolutionized chlamydial screening because they have increased sensitivity and can be applied to noninvasive specimens such as urine in both male and female patients. Differing in their approach to amplification of nucleic acid, examples of such tests applied to C. trachomatis detection include ligase chain reaction (LCR), polymerase chain reaction (PCR), transcription-mediated amplification (TMA), and strand displacement amplification (SDA).

Nonspecific Tests

1. Urinary LET: A nonspecific, but inexpensive test that can be used as a first step to screen asymptomatic males. An LET reading of at least 1+ is suggestive of infection (sensitivity 70%, specificity 80%, and positive predictive value (PPV) 23% for C. trachomatis infection in asymptomatic men ≤25 years of age) (Marrazzo et al., 2001). Further definitive testing should be done, when possible, if the LET is positive.
2. Cytology: Cytological specimens are unsatisfactory to detect chlamydial infection.
3. Serology: There is no use for the application of serology in acute genital infection with C. trachomatis. Previous chlamydial infection frequently elicits long-lasting antibodies that cannot be easily distinguished from the antibodies produced in a current infection. Epidemiological studies linking the presence of antibody to tubal factor infertility and most recently to possibly cervical cancer have been of some clinical usefulness.

Who Should Be Tested for Chlamydial Infection?

The approach recommended by the CDC and most professional health services and policy organizations (e.g., the American Academy of Pediatrics, the American Medical Association, Health Plan Employer Data and Information Set [HEDIS], American College of Obstetricians and Gynecologists, among others) is that all sexually active adolescent females aged 25 and younger should be screened for C. trachomatis at least once a year, with some calling for more frequent screening. National guidelines do not yet specify a screening recommendation for adolescent males, but screening programs for males are currently being explored, and are particularly useful in settings with high prevalence. In addition to the obvious teenage male or female who has genitourinary symptoms, adolescents on the street, in detention, who are paid for sex, who use intravenous drugs, who are pregnant, who

are victims of sexual assault, who have chosen to have a therapeutic abortion, who have had prior STDs, who have new and multiple partners, and who do not use barrier contraception consistently should be considered for screening.

Testing after Sexual Assault

Testing for C. trachomatis, with culture or FDA-cleared NAATs, should be performed from specimens collected from any site of penetration or attempted penetration (Centers for Disease Control and Prevention, 2006). Testing should be repeated within 1 to 2 weeks of the assault unless prophylactic treatment was provided at the time of the initial testing.

TREATMENT

Principles of Chlamydial Treatment

Treatment guidelines and recommendations were derived from the 2006 CDC guidelines. The following general principles can help guide the treatment of C. trachomatis in adolescents and young adults:

- Emergence of resistance to current regimens is not a problem, which is unlike that found with gonococcal infections.
- Most single-dose regimens for treatment of gonorrhea do not eradicate concomitant chlamydial infections.
- Coinfection with C. trachomatis often occurs among patients who have gonococcal infection, and therefore presumptive treatment of such patients for C. trachomatis infection is appropriate.
- Dispensing medications for chlamydial infection on site and directly observing the first dose can help maximize compliance with treatment.
- Sexual abstinence for 7 days is needed to ensure effective treatment and reduce reinfection between partners.
- Single-dose oral azithromycin, or a 7-day course of amoxicillin, is now the recommended regimen for treatment of pregnant women.
- Urine-based NAATs have rendered much empirical treatment unnecessary, except in select cases in which the risk is very high and likelihood of follow-up is very low.

Empirical Treatment

Definitive testing and subsequent appropriate disease-specific treatment should be the rule regarding chlamydial treatment. Empirical treatment is reserved for the following specific situations in the adolescent client:

- Urethritis: Presence of urethritis should be documented if possible. "Documentation" would include the presence of mucopurulent urethral discharge, Gram stain consistent with chlamydial or gonococcal infection, positive LET results on first-catch urine sample, or ≥10 WBCs/HPF on first-catch urine. If none of these documentation criteria are present, treatment can be deferred and further testing for N. gonorrhoeae and C. trachomatis can be done with close follow-up. Empirical treatment without documentation of urethritis should be limited to symptomatic patients at high risk for infection (new or multiple sex partners, and unprotected sex) who are unlikely to return for follow-up evaluation.

- Mucopurulent cervicitis: Empirical treatment should be initiated if there is mucopurulence on examination in adolescents at increased risk for infection (new or multiple sex partners, and unprotected sex), if follow-up is unlikely, or a relatively insensitive diagnostic test (not a NAAT) is used.
- Pelvic inflammatory disease: Empirical treatment should be initiated in sexually active young women and other women at risk for STDs if the following minimum criteria for PID are present and no other cause for the illness can be identified—uterine/adnexal tenderness or cervical motion tenderness.

Uncomplicated Urethral, Cervical, or Rectal Infection

Recommended Regimens
Uncomplicated urethral, endocervical, or rectal infection in adults and adolescents should be treated with one of the following:

1. Azithromycin 1 g orally in a single dose, OR
2. Doxycycline 100 mg orally b.i.d. for 7 days

Alternative Regimens
Alternative regimens are as follows:

1. Erythromycin base 500 mg by mouth q.i.d. for 7 days, OR
2. Erythromycin ethylsuccinate 800 mg by mouth q.i.d. for 7 days, OR
3. Ofloxacin 300 mg orally b.i.d. for 7 days, OR
4. Levofloxacin 500 mg orally once a day for 7 days

The results of clinical trials indicate that azithromycin and doxycycline are equally efficacious (microbial cure rates of 97% and 98% respectively). However, azithromycin has the advantage of single-dose administration and the price is becoming competitive with other traditionally cheaper regimes. In addition, because of higher compliance with azithromycin it might be more cost-effective as it enables the provision of a single dose of directly observed therapy. Ofloxacin is also very effective but may be more expensive and should not be used during pregnancy. Nonpregnant adolescents who weigh >45 kg can be treated with adult doses of quinolones. Now that quinolones are not recommended for gonorrhea treatment, testing with culture or NAAT for gonorrhea is essential when treating Chlamydia. Erythromycin is less efficacious and has more gastrointestinal toxicity, but is inexpensive and can be used during pregnancy.

Follow-up
When taken as directed, azithromycin or alternative regimens are highly effective (>95%). If one of these regimens is used, posttreatment tests of cure are not recommended unless symptoms persist, reinfection is suspected, therapeutic compliance is in question, or the patient is pregnant. Posttreatment testing 3 weeks after completion of treatment should be considered if erythromycin is used. Retesting before 3 weeks after completion of therapy can lead to false-positive results. Patients with positive posttreatment test results should be re-treated with one of the preceding regimens, because resistant chlamydiae have not been described. Partners should also be re-treated.

Adolescents with chlamydial infections appear to be twice as likely to have a recurrent chlamydial infection as compared with young women. Because of the concern about increased tissue damage with increased numbers of infections in female patients, health care providers should consider advising all women with chlamydial infection to be screened for reinfection 3 to 4 months after treatment. Providers are also strongly encouraged to rescreen all women treated for chlamydial infection whenever they next present for care within the following 12 months.

Sex Partners
All sex partners should be referred for evaluation and treatment. The exact time intervals for exposure have not been well evaluated. The CDC recommends that sex partners should be evaluated, tested, and treated if they had sexual contact with the patient during the 60 days preceding onset of symptoms in the patient or diagnosis of *C. trachomatis*. The most recent sex partner should be treated even if the time interval is more than 60 days. Sex partners of mothers with infected newborns should also be evaluated and treated.

Delivery of antibiotic therapy by heterosexual female or male patients to their partners might be an option if there is concern that partners will not seek evaluation and treatment. Written information for female partners regarding the importance of seeking evaluation for PID should be given with patient-delivered partner therapy. Because of the high risk for coexisting infections in males engaging in sex with males, patient-delivered partner therapy is not recommended in this patient population.

Patients should avoid sexual contact until they and their partners are treated and are assumed cured—7 days after completing single-dose treatment or following a 7-day antibiotic course.

Pregnant Patients
Recommended Regimen During Pregnancy
1. Azithromycin 1 g PO in a single oral dose, OR
2. Amoxicillin 500 mg PO t.i.d. for 7 days

Alternative Regimens
1. Erythromycin base 500 mg orally q.i.d. for 7 days, OR
2. Erythromycin base 250 mg orally q.i.d. for 14 days, OR
3. Erythromycin ethylsuccinate 800 mg q.i.d. for 7 days, OR
4. Erythromycin ethylsuccinate 400 mg q.i.d. for 14 days

Doxycycline, ofloxacin, levofloxacin, and erythromycin estolate are contraindicated during pregnancy. Three weeks after completion of therapy, repeat testing is recommended for all pregnant women.

Human Immunodeficiency Virus Infection
Adolescents with human immunodeficiency virus (HIV) and chlamydial infections should receive the same treatments listed for those without HIV infection.

Pelvic Inflammatory Disease

Because many cases of PID are caused by more than one organism, treatment regimens must include broad coverage. Evaluation and treatment of PID are discussed in detail in Chapter 63.

Acute Epididymitis

Regimen of Choice
1. Ceftriaxone 250 mg intramuscularly once AND
2. Doxycycline 100 mg orally b.i.d. for 10 days

Bed rest and elevation of the scrotum are also recommended.

Alternative Regimen
For acute epididymitis most likely caused by enteric organisms or for patients allergic to cephalosporins and/or tetracyclines:

1. Ofloxacin 300 mg orally b.i.d. for 10 days (can be used in nonpregnant adolescents who weigh >45 kg and young adults older than 18 years) OR
2. Levofloxacin 500 mg orally once daily for 10 days

These regimens are similar in HIV-infected teens. However, in immunocompromised adolescents fungal and mycobacterial causes are more common. Those teens who fail to respond within 3 days require close reevaluation of the diagnosis and therapy.

Sex Partners
Sex partners should be examined for an STD and treated with a regimen effective against uncomplicated gonococcal and chlamydial infections. Both partners should avoid sexual contact until therapy is completed and both individuals are asymptomatic.

PREVENTION

1. Goals
   a. To prevent overt and "silent" chlamydial PID and its sequelae
   b. To prevent perinatal and postpartum infections
   c. To prevent adverse consequences of chlamydial infections at other anatomical sites
   d. To prevent recurrence of infection in young women that is linked to increased upper reproductive tract tissue damage
2. Prevention strategies
   a. Primary prevention
      Behavioral changes include reduction of the number of sex partners, delaying age at first intercourse, and the use of condoms. *C. trachomatis* is often neglected in discussions of HIV risk and sexual behaviors. Information about *C. trachomatis* should be incorporated into educational materials and discussions regarding risk behaviors. Specific areas to cover include the following:
      • *C. trachomatis* infection is the most common reported STD, particularly among adolescents and young adults
      • Adverse consequences of chlamydial infection in self, current, and future partners (e.g., PID and infertility, question of link to cervical cancer in women)
      • Symptoms and signs of infection in self and partner (and other STDs)
      • Asymptomatic or "silent" infection, particularly the link to undetected PID

      • Need for discussion with and treatment of sex partners
      • Referrals and services available in the community for testing and treatment of partners
      • Discussion of the link between substance use (particularly alcohol and marijuana), poor decision making, and acquisition of STDs including *C. trachomatis* infections.
   b. Secondary prevention
      • Screen females to identify and treat asymptomatic chlamydial infections at least once a year and more often if risky behaviors are identified.
      • Implementation of system-wide screening programs in large health maintenance organizations has been shown to be feasible and effective in significantly increasing the *C. trachomatis* screening rates (Shafer et al., 2002).
      • Rescreening: Retest of index-positive cases 3 to 4 months after treatment.
         A high prevalence of *C. trachomatis* infection is found in women who have had chlamydial infection in the preceding several months. Most posttreatment infections result from reinfection, often occurring because patient's sex partners were not treated or because the patient resumed sex among a network of persons with a high prevalence of infection. Repeat infection confers an elevated risk of PID and other complications when compared with initial infection.
      • Track and treat all positive clients and their partners.
      • Recognize *C. trachomatis*-associated syndromes such as MPC and treat as appropriate.
3. Target populations
   a. Sexually active adolescents and young adults
      • Female patients: It is recommended to screen sexually active adolescents and females younger than 25 years for *C. trachomatis* at least annually. With the advent of urine-based testing, the goal should be to screen for *C. trachomatis* first and perform a pelvic examination only when necessary—not just for chlamydial screening purposes.
      • Males patients: The urinary LET has been shown to be a useful "first step" among lower risk sexually active male adolescents and young adult males. If positive, it is more efficacious to perform a more definitive *C. trachomatis* screening test such as a NAAT.
   b. Pregnant women, including those who will have an induced abortion
   c. Adolescents, particularly females, in detention facilities or attending an STD clinic

WEB SITES

For Teenagers and Parents

http://www.cdc.gov/std/Chlamydia/STDFact-Chlamydia.htm. CDC fact sheet on chlamydia.
http://www.niaid.nih.gov/factsheets/stdclam.htm. National Institutes of Health (NIH) fact sheet on chlamydia.
http://www.plannedparenthood.org/sexual-health/std/chlamydia.htm. Planned Parenthood frequently asked questions sheet on chlamydia.

http://www.kidshealth.org/teen/infections/stds/std
_chlamydia.html. Teen health site information sheet on
chlamydia.

http://www.4woman.gov/faq/stdchlam.htm.   National
Women's Health Information Center facts about
Chlamydia.

http://www.youngwomenshealth.org/chlamydia.html.
Health information for teens from the Center for Young
Women's Health, Children's Hospital Boston.

For Health Professionals

http://www.emedicine.com/emerg/topic925.htm.
E-medicine article on chlamydia.

http://www.cdc.gov/std/chlamydia/. CDC link to chlamydia
facts, 2003 surveillance statistics, and treatment guidelines.

REFERENCES AND ADDITIONAL READINGS

Antilla T, Saikku P, Koskela P, et al. Serotypes of *Chlamydia trachomatis* and risk for development of cervical squamous cell carcinoma. *JAMA* 2001;285:47.

Bachmann LH, Richey CM, Waites K, et al. Patterns of *Chlamydia trachomatis* testing and follow-up at a university hospital medical center. *Sex Transm Dis* 1999;26:496.

Baeten JM, Nyange PM, Tichardson BA, et al. Hormonal contraception and risk of sexually transmitted disease acquisition: results from a prospective study. *Am J Obstet Gynecol* 2001;185:380.

Barnhart KT, Sondheimer SJ. Contraception choice and sexually transmitted disease. *Curr Opin Obstet Gynecol* 1993;5:823.

Beck-Sague CM, Farshy CE, Jackson TK, et al. Detection of *Chlamydia trachomatis* cervical infection by urine tests among adolescents clinics. *J Adolesc Health* 1998;22:197.

Berman SM, Hein K. Adolescents and STDs. In: Holmes KK, Sparling PF, March PA, et al., eds. *Sexually transmitted diseases*, 3rd ed. New York: McGraw-Hill; 1999.

Black CM. Current methods of laboratory diagnosis of *Chlamydia trachomatis* infections. *Clin Microbiol Rev* 1997;10(1):160.

Bolan G, Ehrhardt AA, Wasserheit JN. Gender perspectives and STDs. In: Holmes KK, Sparling PF, March PA, et al., eds. *Sexually transmitted diseases*, 3rd ed. New York: McGraw-Hill; 1999.

Bowden FJ. Reappraising the value of urine leukocyte esterase testing in the age of nucleic acid amplification. *Sex Transm Dis* 1998;25(6):322.

Boyer CB, Shafer MA, Teitle E, et al. Sexually transmitted diseases in a health maintenance organization teen clinic. *Arch Pediatr Adolesc Med* 1999;153:838.

Boyer CB, Shafer MA, Wibbelsman CJ, et al. Associations of sociodemographic, psychosocial, and behavioral factors with sexual risk and sexually transmitted diseases in teen clinic patients. *J Adolesc Health* 2000;27:102.

Brodine SK, Shafer MA, Shaffer RA, et al. Asymptomatic sexually transmitted disease prevalence in four military populations: application of DNA amplification assays for chlamydia and gonorrhea screening. *J Infect Dis* 1998;178:1202.

Brunham RC, Peeling RW. *Chlamydia trachomatis* antigens: role in immunity and pathogenesis. *Infect Agents Dis* 1994;3:218.

Brunham RC, Zhang DJ, Yang X, et al. The potential for vaccine development against chlamydial infection and disease. *J Infect Dis* 2000;181(Suppl 3):S538.

Bull SS, Jones CA, Granberry-Owens D, et al. Acceptability and feasibility of urine screening for Chlamydia and gonorrhea in community organizations: perspectives from Denver and St. Louis. *Am J Public Health* 2000;90:285.

Bunnell RE, Dahlberg L, Rolfs R, et al. High prevalence and incidence of sexually transmitted diseases in urban adolescent females despite moderate risk behaviors. *J Infect Dis* 1999;180:1624.

Burstein GR, Gaydos CA, Diener-West M, et al. Incident *Chlamydia trachomatis* infections among inner-city adolescent females. *JAMA* 1998;280:521.

Burstein GR, Zenilman JM. Nongonococcal urethritis—a new paradigm. *Clin Infect Dis* 1999;28(Suppl 1):S66.

Burstein GR, Zenilman JM, Gaydos CA, et al. Predictors of repeat Chlamydia trachomatis infections diagnosed by DNA amplification testing among inner city females. *Sex Transm Infect* 2001;77(1):26.

Bush MR, Rosa C. Azithromycin and erythromycin in the treatment of cervical chlamydial infection during pregnancy. *Obstet Gynecol* 1994;84:81.

California STD/HIV Prevention Training Center. *Sexually transmitted chlamydial infections: A primary care clinician's guide to diagnosis, treatment and prevention*, http://www.stdhivtraining.org/pdf/chlamydia_screen.pdf, Dec 2003, accessed Aug 30, 2005.

Cates W. The epidemiology and control of sexually transmitted diseases in adolescents. *Adolesc Med State Art Rev* 1990;1:409.

Cates W, Wasserheit JN. Genital chlamydial infections: epidemiology and reproductive sequelae. *Am J Obstet Gynecol* 1991;164:1771.

Centers for Disease Control and Prevention. Screening tests to detect *Chlamydia trachomatis* and *Neisseria gonorrhoeae* infections 2002. *MMWR* 2002;51(RR-15):1.

Centers for Disease Control and Prevention. Sexually transmitted disease surveillance 2003 supplement. *Chlamydia prevalence monitoring project*. Atlanta, GA: U.S. Department of Health and Human Services, Centers for Disease Control and Prevention; October 2004.

Centers for Disease Control and Prevention. *Sexually transmitted disease surveillance, 2004*. Atlanta, GA: U.S. Department of Health and Human Services; September 2005.

Centers for Disease Control and Prevention. *STD Surveillance 2005*, http://www.cdc.gov/std/stats/toc2005.htm.

Centers for Disease Control and Prevention. Sexually transmitted diseases treatment guidelines, 2006. *MMWR* 2006;55(RR-11):40.

Chernesky MA. Nucleic acid tests for the diagnosis of sexually transmitted diseases. *FEMS Immunol Med Microbiol* 1999;24:437.

Cohen DA, Nsuami M, Martin DH, et al. Repeated school-based screening for sexually transmitted diseases: a feasible strategy for reaching adolescents. *Pediatrics* 1999;104:1281.

Cook RL, Hutchison SL, Ostergaard L, et al. Systematic review: noninvasive testing for Chlamydia trachomatis and Neisseria gonorrhoeae. *Ann Intern Med* 2005;142:914.

Darville T. Chlamydia. *Pediatr Rev* 1998;19:85.

Debattista J, Timms P, Allan J. Immunopathogenesis of Chlamydia trachomatis infections in women. *Fertil Steril* 2003;79:1273.

Dimmitt SR, Pearman JW, Woolard KV. Chlamydial endocarditis. *Aust N Z J Med* 1985;15:340.

Eley A, Pacey AA, Galdiero M, et al. Can Chlamydia trachomatis directly damage your sperm. *Lancet Infect Dis* 2005;5(1):53.

Embling ML, Monroe KW, Oh MK, et al. Opportunistic urine chain reaction screening for sexually transmitted diseases in adolescents seeking care in an urban emergency department. *Ann Emerg Med* 2000;36:28.

Eng TR, Butler WT, eds. *The hidden epidemic: confronting sexually transmitted diseases.* Washington, DC: Institute of Medicine; 1997.

Fortenberry JD, Brizendine EJ, Katz BP, et al. Subsequent sexually transmitted infections among adolescent women with genital infection due to *Chlamydia trachomatis, Neisseria gonorrhoeae,* or *Trichomonas vaginalis. Sex Transm Dis* 1999; 26:26.

Gaston JS. Immunological basis of *Chlamydia* induced reactive arthritis. *Sex Transm Infect* 2000;76:156.

Gaydos CA, Crotchfelt KA, Howell MR, et al. Molecular amplification assays to detect chlamydial infections in urine specimens from high school female students and to monitor the persistence of chlamydial DNA after therapy. *J Infect Dis* 1998;177:417.

Gaydos CA, Howell MR, Quinn TC, et al. Sustained high prevalence of Chlamydia trachomatis infections in female army recruits. *Sex Transm Dis* 2003;30(7):539.

Genc M, Ruusuvaara L, Mardh PA. An economic evaluation of screening for *Chlamydia trachomatis* in adolescent males. *JAMA* 1993;270:2057.

Guaschino S, De Seta F. Update on *Chlamydia trachomatis. Ann N Y Acad Sci* 2000;900:293.

Haddon L, Heason J, Fay T, et al. Managing STDs identified after testing outside genitourinary medicine departments: one model of care. *Sex Transm Infect* 1998;74:256.

Hammerschlag MR. Sexually transmitted diseases in sexually abused children: medical and legal implications. *Sex Transm Infect* 1998;74:167.

Hillis SD, Nakashima A, March Banks PA, et al. Risk factors for recurrent *Chlamydia trachomatis* infections in women. *Am J Obstet Gynecol* 1994;170(3):801.

Holder DW, Woods ER. *Chlamydia trachomatis* screening in the adolescent population. *Curr Opin Pediatr* 1997;9:317.

Hook EW, Smith K, Mullen C, et al. Diagnosis of genitourinary *Chlamydia trachomatis* infections by using the ligase chain reaction on patient-obtained vaginal swabs. *J Clin Microbiol* 1997;35:2133.

Hu D, Hook EW III, Goldie SJ. Screening for *Chlamydia trachomatis* in women 15 to 29 years of age: a cost-effectiveness analysis. *Ann Intern Med* 2004;141:501.

Hwang L, Shafer MA. Chlamydia trachomatis infection in adolescents. *Adv Pediatr* 2004;51:379.

Hwang LY, Tebb KP, Shafer MA, et al. Examination of the treatment and follow-up care for adolescents who test positive for Chlamydia trachomatis infection. *Arch Pediatr Adolesc Med* 2005;159:1162.

Jones RB, Ardery BR, Hui SL, et al. Correlation between serum antichlamydial antibodies and tubal factor as a cause of infertility. *Fertil Steril* 1982a;38:553.

Jones RB, Priest JB, Kuo CC. Subacute chlamydial endocarditis. *JAMA* 1982b;247:655.

Jones RB, Rabinovitch RA, Katz BP, et al. *Chlamydia trachomatis* in the pharynx and rectum of heterosexual patients at risk for genital infection. *Ann Intern Med* 1985;102:757.

Kacena KA, Quinn SB, Howell MR, et al. Pooling urine samples for ligase chain reaction screening for genital *Chlamydia trachomatis* infection in asymptomatic women. *J Clin Microbiol* 1998;36:481.

Kelver ME, Nagamani M. Chlamydial serology in women with tubal infertility. *Int J Fertil* 1989;34:42.

Kent CK, Branzuela A, Fischer L, et al. Chlamydia and gonorrhea screening in San Francisco high schools. *Sex Transm Dis* 2002;29:373.

Lifson AR, Halcon LL, Hannan P, et al. Screening for sexually transmitted infections among economically disadvantaged youth in a national job training program. *J Adolesc Health* 2001;28:190.

Lycke E, Lowhagen GB, Hallhagen G, et al. The transmission of genital Chlamydia trachomatis infection is less than that of genital Neisseria gonorrhoeae infection. *Sex Transm Dis* 1980;7:6.

Marrazzo JM, White CL, Krekeler B, et al. Community-based urine screening for *Chlamydia trachomatis* with a ligase chain reaction assay. *Ann Intern Med* 1997;127:796.

Marrazzo JM, Whittington WL, Celum CL, et al. Urine-based screening for *Chlamydia trachomatis* in men attending sexually transmitted disease clinics. *Sex Transm Dis* 2001;28:219.

Martin DH, Mroczkowski IF, Dalu AZ, et al. A controlled trial of a single dose of azithromycin for the treatment of chlamydial urethritis and cervicitis. *N Engl J Med* 1992;327:921.

McNagny SE, Parker RM, Zenilman JM, et al. Urinary leukocyte esterase test: a screening method for the detection of asymptomatic chlamydial and gonococcal infections in men. *J Infect Dis* 1992;165:573.

Mertz KJ, Boigt RA, Hutchins K, et al. Findings from STD screening of adolescents and adults enteringcorrections facilities: implications for STD control strategies. *Sex Transm Dis* 2002;29:834.

Miller WC, Ford CA, Morris M. Prevalence of chlamydial and gonococcal infections among young adults in the United States. *JAMA* 2004;291:2229.

Miller WC, Zenilman JM. Epidemiology of chlamydial infection, gonorrhea, and trichomoniasis in the United States–2005. *Infect Dis Clin North Am* 2005;19:281.

Neinstein LS, Inderlied C. Low prevalence of *Chlamydia trachomatis* in the oropharynx of adolescents. *Pediatr Infect Dis J* 1986;5:660.

Newhall WJ, Johnson RE, DeLisle S, et al. Head-to-head evaluation of five Chlamydia tests relative to a quality-assured culture standard. *J Clin Microbiol* 1999;37:681.

Nsuami M, Elie M, Brooks BN, et al. Screening for sexually transmitted diseases during preparticipation sports examination of high school adolescents. *J Adolesc Health* 2003;32:336.

Oh MK, Cloud GA, Fleenor M, et al. Risk for gonococcal and chlamydial cervicitis in adolescent females: incidence and recurrence in a prospective cohort study. *J Adolesc Health* 1996;18:270.

Oh MK, Richey CM, Pate MS, et al. High prevalence of *Chlamydia trachomatis* infections in adolescent females not having pelvic examinations: utility of PCR-based urine screening in urban adolescent clinic setting. *J Adolesc Health* 1997;21:80.

Oh MK, Smith KR, O'Cain M, et al. Urine-based screening of adolescents in detention to guide treatment for gonococcal and chlamydial infections: translating research into intervention. *Arch Pediatr Adolesc Med* 1998;152:52.

Olshen E, Shrier LA. Diagnostic tests for chlamydial and gonorrheal infections. *Semin Pediatr Infect Dis* 2005;16:192.

Orr P, Sherman E, Beanchard J, et al. Epidemiology of infection due to *Chlamydia trachomatis* in Manitoba, Canada. *Clin Infect Dis* 1994;19:8.

Pack RP, Diclemente RJ, Hook EW, et al. High prevalence of asymptomatic STDs in incarcerated minority male youth: a case for screening. *Sex Transm Dis* 2000;27:175.

Paz-Bailey G, Koumans EH, Markowitz LE, et al. The effect of correct and consistent condom use on chlamydial and gonococcal infection among urban adolescents. *Arch Pediatr Adolesc Med* 2005;159(6):536.

Polaneczy M, Quigley C, Pollock L, et al. Use of self-collected vaginal specimens for detection of *Chlamydia trachomatis* infection. *Obstet Gynecol* 1998;91:375.

Quinn TC, Gaydos C, Shepherd M, et al. Epidemiologic and microbiologic correlates of *Chlamydia trachomatis* infection in sexual partnerships. *JAMA* 1996;276:1737.

Reitmeijer CA, Bull SS, Ortiz CG, et al. Patterns of general health care and STD services use among high-risk youth in Denver participating in community-based urine Chlamydia screening. *Sex Transm Dis* 1998;25:457.

Sanders JW, Hook EW, III, Welsh LE, et al. Evaluation of an enzyme immunoassay for detection of *Chlamydia trachomatis* in urine of asymptomatic men. *J Clin Microbiol* 1994; 32:24.

Sayegh MA, Fortenberry JD, Anderson J, et al. Relationship quality, coital frequency, and condom use as predicators of incident genital Chlamydia trachomatis infection among adolescent women. *J Adolesc Health* 2005;37(2):163.

Schachter J. DFA, EIA, PCR, LCR and other technologies: what tests should be used for diagnosis of Chlamydia infections. *Immunol Invest* 1997;26:157.

Schachter J. Biology of *Chlamydia trachomatis*. In: Holmes KK, Sparling PF, March PA, et al., eds. *Sexually transmitted diseases*, 3rd ed. New York: McGraw-Hill; 1999:391.

Schachter J, McCormack WM, Chernesky MA, et al. Vaginal swabs are appropriate specimens for diagnosis of genital tract infection with *Chlamydia trachomatis*. *J Clin Microbiol* 2003;41:3784.

Schillinger JA, Dunne EF, Markowitz LE, et al. Prevalence of Chlamydia trachomatis infection among men screened in 4 U.S. cities. *Sex Transm Dis* 2005;32(2):74.

Scholes D, Stergachis A, Heidrich FE, et al. Prevention of pelvic inflammatory disease by screening for cervical chlamydial infection. *N Engl J Med* 1996;34:21.

Scholes D, Stergachis A, Ichikawa LE, et al. Vaginal douching as a risk factor for cervical Chlamydia trachomatis infection. *Obstet Gynecol* 1998;91:993.

Shafer MA, Schachter J, Moscicki AB, et al. Urinary leukocyte esterase screening test for asymptomatic chlamydial and gonococcal infections in males. *JAMA* 1989;262:2562.

Shafer MA, Schachter J, Moncada J, et al. Evaluation of urine-based screening strategies to detect *Chlamydia trachomatis* among sexually active asymptomatic young males. *JAMA* 1993;270:2065.

Shafer MA, Tebb KP, Pantell RH, et al. Effect of a clinical practice improvement Intervention on chlamydial screening among adolescent girls. *JAMA* 2002;288:2846.

Shafer MA, Boyer CB, Pang F, et al. Comparison of 3 specimen collection techniques—endocervical and self-administered vaginal swab to screen for *C. trachomatis* (CT) and *N. gonorrhoeae* (GC) by NAATs in women Marine recruits. In: Saikku P, ed. *Proceedings of the IV european Chlamydia congress, Chlamydia 2000, Helsinki, Finland; August 2000*. Finland: Universitas Helsingiensis; 2000:138.

Shafer MA, Pantell R, Schachter J. Is the routine pelvic examination needed with the advent of urine-based screening for sexually transmitted diseases. *Arch Pediatr Adolesc Med* 1999;153:119.

Shafer MA, Moncada J, Boyer CB, et al. Comparing first-void urine specimens, self-collected vaginal swabs, and endocervical specimens to detect Chlamydia trachomatis and Neisseria gonorrhoeae by a nucleic acid amplification test. *J Clin Microbiol* 2003;41:4395.

Shepard MK, Jones RB. Recovery of *Chlamydia trachomatis* from endometrial and fallopian tube biopsies in women with infertility of tubal origin. *Fertil Steril* 1989;52:232.

Stamm WE. *Chlamydia trachomatis* infections of the adult. In: Holmes KK, Sparling PF, March PA, et al., eds. *Sexually transmitted diseases*, 3rd ed. New York: McGraw-Hill; 1999a.

Stamm WE. *Chlamydia trachomatis* infections: progress and problems. *J Infect Dis* 1999b;179(Suppl 2):S380.

Stamm WE, Guinan ME, Johnson C. Effect of treatment regimens for *Neisseria gonorrhoeae* on simultaneous infections with *Chlamydia trachomatis*. *N Engl J Med* 1984;310:545.

Stamm WE, Hicks CB, Martin DH, et al. Azithromycin for empirical treatment of the nongonococcal urethritis syndrome in men: a randomized double-blind study. *JAMA* 1995;274:545.

Stary A, Schuh E, Kerschbaumer M, et al. Performance of transcription-mediated amplification and ligase chain reaction assays for detection of chlamydial infection in urogenital samples obtained by invasive and noninvasive methods. *J Clin Microbiol* 1998;36:2666.

Sweet RL, Landers DV, Walker C, et al. *Chlamydia trachomatis* infection and pregnancy outcome. *Am J Obstet Gynecol* 1987; 156:824.

Tebb KP, Shafer MA, Wibbelsman CJ, et al. To screen or not to screen: prevalence of C. Trachomatis among sexually active asymptomatic male adolescents attending health maintenance pediatric visits. *J Adolesc Health* 2004;34:166.

Vermillion ST, Holmes MM, Soper DE. Adolescents and sexually transmitted diseases. *Adolesc Gynecol* 2000;27:163.

Viscidi RP, Bobo L, Hook EW, et al. Transmission of *Chlamydia trachomatis* among sex partners assessed by polymerase chain reaction. *J Infect Dis* 1993;168:488.

Williams H, Tabrizi SN, Lee W, et al. Adolescence and other risk factors for Chlamydia trachomatis genitourinary infection in women in Melbourne, Australia. *Sex Transm Infect* 2003; 79:31.

Wisenfeld HC, Heine RP, Rideout A, et al. The vaginal introitus: a novel site for *Chlamydia trachomatis* testing in women. *Am J Obstet Gynecol* 1996;174:1542.

Witkin SS, Jeremias J, Toth M, et al. Detection of *Chlamydia trachomatis* by the polymerase chain reaction in the cervices of women with acute salpingitis. *Am J Obstet Gynecol* 1993;168: 1438.

Wood VD, Shoroye A. Sexually transmitted disease among adolescents in the juvenile justice system of the District of Columbia. *J Natl Med Assoc* 1993;85:435.

CHAPTER 63

Pelvic Inflammatory Disease

Lydia A. Shrier

Pelvic inflammatory disease (PID) is an ascending polymicrobial infection of the female upper genital tract and includes endometritis, parametritis, salpingitis, oophoritis, tuboovarian abscess (TOA), peritonitis, and perihepatitis. *Neisseria gonorrhoeae* and *Chlamydia trachomatis* are usually the causative agents of PID, but vaginal and enteric microorganisms also contribute to its pathogenesis. Approximately 20% of women with PID experience at least one long-term consequence, such as chronic pelvic pain, ectopic pregnancy, or infertility. Intervention efforts aimed at preventing PID during adolescence focus on primary prevention of all sexually transmitted diseases (STDs) and secondary prevention through aggressive screening for and early treatment of gonorrhea and chlamydial infection. The rates of U.S. cases of gonorrhea, chlamydial infection, and hospitalization for PID decreased during the 1990s. Although it is likely that the overall rate of PID decreased, there has also been a shift in the management of most cases of PID from the inpatient to the outpatient setting.

ETIOLOGY

Risk Factors

1. Age: Adolescents account for 33% of all cases of PID, and women younger than 25 years account for 70% of cases. Both biological and behavioral factors explain the tenfold increased risk of PID and threefold increased risk of gonococcal or chlamydial infection among sexually active adolescents compared with that of adults.
   a. Cervical ectropion: The erythematous ring around the cervical os that is commonly seen on speculum examination of adolescents, represents the transitional zone between the columnar and squamous epithelium. Cells in this zone are highly susceptible to STDs. During childhood, the transitional zone is located in the distal vagina. By adulthood, it usually recedes into the more protected environment of the endocervical canal.
   b. Cervical secretory immunoglobulin A: The levels are lower during adolescence than adulthood owing to the lower prevalence of past exposure to immunogenic factors.
   c. Cervicitis with *N. gonorrhoeae* or *C. trachomatis*: Female adolescents have the highest rates of chlamydial infection of any age–sex group. Chlamydial infection is frequently asymptomatic and therefore can evolve into PID without prior symptoms prompting the infected young woman to seek early treatment. Adolescents with a gonococcal or chlamydial infection of the endocervix may have a 30% increased risk of PID.
   d. Sexual and other health risk behaviors: Adolescents frequently engage in behaviors associated with increased rates of STDs and PID including unprotected intercourse, frequent intercourse, multiple sex partners, intercourse during menses, smoking, alcohol and other drug use, and douching.
   e. Age at first intercourse: Risk for STDs is inversely related to adolescent age at coitarche.
2. Previous PID: A history of previous PID increases the risk of subsequent PID 2.3 times. At least one in five females with PID will experience a subsequent episode.
3. Race: Nonwhite adolescents are 2.5 times more likely to develop PID than white adolescents.
4. Contraceptive methods
   a. Condom: Inconsistent condom use is associated with a two to three time increased risk of PID.
   b. Spermicide: Nonoxynol-9 promotes cell wall destruction of *N. gonorrhoeae* and *C. trachomatis.*
   c. Oral contraceptives: Oral contraceptive use may decrease the risk of PID by thickening the cervical mucus and by decreasing cervical dilation, uterine contraction, and blood flow during menses. However, oral contraceptives have been associated with an increased risk of chlamydial infection and not all studies have found that oral contraceptives reduce the risk of PID.
   d. Intrauterine device (IUD): Women who have an STD at the time of IUD insertion have a greater, although still low risk of PID than women who are free of infection. The use of the more recently developed IUDs appear to carry a far lower risk of PID than the earlier systems. The risk is concentrated in the first 3 weeks after insertion of the IUD and then declines rapidly. Overall, the current risk of PID with IUDs is rare (1 in 1,000). There is no evidence that IUDs should be removed in women with acute PID. IUDs may be associated with increased risk of failed conservative treatment and need for surgical treatment of PID (Viberga et al 2006).

5. Bacterial vaginosis (BV):   BV may facilitate ascension of organisms pathogenic for PID to the upper genital tract. BV has been associated with PID after first-trimester therapeutic abortion, as well as third-trimester preterm delivery. However, longitudinal studies have not consistently supported an association between BV and PID.
6. Menses: Menses may be associated with an increased risk of ascending infection because of the loss of the cervical mucus plug, shedding of the endometrium, presence of menstrual blood (a good culture medium), and/or occurrence of myometrial contractions resulting in reflux of blood into the fallopian tubes.

Microbiology

PID is a polymicrobial infection that usually begins with a sexually transmitted organism such as *N. gonorrhoeae* or *C. trachomatis* but involves other organisms as well, such as anaerobes. Organisms isolated from the upper genital tract of women with PID include the following:

1. *N. gonorrhoeae:* Twenty-five percent to 50% of women with PID have evidence of upper tract gonococcal infection, and of these, 40% also have evidence of chlamydial infection. The likelihood of positive endocervical test results for gonorrhea is three times higher among women with PID who present within the first 24 hours of symptoms than among women who present after 48 hours.
2. *C. trachomatis:* Ten percent to 43% of women with PID are reported to have evidence of upper tract chlamydial infection. However, because laboratory testing for *C. trachomatis* has improved dramatically over the last decade, it is likely that the rates are higher than those previously reported.
3. *Bacteroides* species and other anaerobes: Fifty percent of women with PID have evidence of upper tract infection with anaerobic organisms.
4. *Escherichia coli, Streptococcus* species, and other facultative bacteria
5. *Mycoplasma hominis* and *Ureaplasma urealyticum*

Pathogenesis

1. After lower tract infection with *N. gonorrhoeae* or *C. trachomatis,* the normal vaginal lactobacilli are supplanted by anaerobes, facultative bacteria, and genital mycoplasmas.
2. Inflammatory disruption of the cervical barrier facilitates ascension of the inciting sexually transmitted pathogens and other microorganisms from the vagina into the normally sterile uterus. Plasma cell infiltration of the endometrium is the hallmark of PID.
3. Decreased tubal motility secondary to inflammation results in collection of fluid (hydrosalpinx) or pus (pyosalpinx) within the tube.
4. Spillage of infected contents from the tubal fimbriae into the peritoneal cavity may result in the following:
   a. Peritonitis
   b. Perihepatitis (Fitz-Hugh-Curtis syndrome): Infected material tracks along the paracolic gutter. Inflammation of the hepatic capsule and diaphragm causes right-upper-quadrant (RUQ) pain and referred right subscapular pain. Liver function study results are normal or minimally elevated and nonspecific markers of

inflammation, such as the erythrocyte sedimentation rate (ESR) or C-reactive protein (CRP) may be higher than is typically seen in mild, uncomplicated PID.
   c. TOA: TOA develops if resolution of the upper tract infection is delayed or if previous tubal scarring occludes the tube. The abscess can form in the tube or between the tube and ovary. Estimates of TOA formation range from 7% to 19% of women with PID.
   d. Adhesions: As PID resolves, scar tissue may form in the tube, between the tube and ovary, or in the peritoneal cavity. Adhesions are the cause of subsequent infertility, ectopic pregnancy, and chronic pain.

PRESENTING SIGNS AND SYMPTOMS

Classically, PID presents with lower abdominal or pelvic pain, abnormal vaginal and/or cervical discharge, and fever and chills, with leukocytosis and increased ESR. However, this constellation of signs and symptoms is seen in approximately one in five laparoscopically verified cases of PID. Subclinical infection likely accounts for most cases of PID; more than 70% of women with infertility from bilateral tubal occlusion have serum antibodies to *C. trachomatis* and approximately 60% do not report a history of PID.

1. Pelvic or abdominal pain: More than 80% of adolescents with PID present with pelvic or abdominal pain and 50% to 75% of those with pain present within 7 days of menses. The pain of PID is constant, cramping, and exacerbated by walking and intercourse.
2. Abnormal vaginal bleeding: The endometritis of PID is associated with irregular, prolonged, and/or heavy vaginal bleeding in 35% of patients with PID. Unlike with anovulation, the most common cause of irregular bleeding during adolescence, bleeding due to PID is painful.
3. Vaginal discharge: Cervicitis and/or vaginitis cause an abnormal discharge in approximately 50% of patients with PID.
4. Gastrointestinal (GI) symptoms: Peritonitis may cause an ileus with anorexia, nausea, or vomiting. Severe vomiting is not common in PID and should suggest a careful exploration of another GI problem.

Other history, signs, and symptoms compatible with a diagnosis of PID include dysuria or urinary frequency, dyspareunia, onset of symptoms within 1 week of menses, and a sexual partner with recent urethritis.

Findings on Physical Examination

1. Vital signs: Temperature higher than 38°C is present in 40% of patients with laparoscopically verified PID. Tachycardia secondary to the pain and fever is common.
2. Abdomen: Tenderness to palpation of the lower abdomen, with or without rebound and guarding.
3. Pelvic examination
   a. Abnormal vaginal or cervical discharge
   b. Friable, inflamed cervix
   c. Cervical motion tenderness (present in >80% of patients with PID)
   d. Adnexal tenderness (unilateral or bilateral)
   e. Palpation of an adnexal mass (5% to 60%)
   f. Uterine tenderness (common)

Laboratory and Radiological Evaluation

No single test is diagnostic of PID. The following laboratory and radiological tests should be considered in the evaluation of suspected PID.

1. White blood cell (WBC) count: Elevated in 30% to 67% of patients with PID.
2. ESR (or CRP): An ESR of >15 mm/hour is found in 75% to 80% of patients with PID.
3. Saline wet mount of vaginal secretions: Most women with PID have either mucopurulent cervical discharge or WBCs on microscopic examination of a saline wet mount of vaginal secretions (90.9% sensitive, 26.3% specific for PID). The absence of any leukocytes in the secretions suggests a diagnosis other than PID (negative predictive value is 94.5%).
4. Microbiological tests: Presumptive diagnosis and treatment of PID should not await microbiological test results. Positive results for *N. gonorrhoeae* or *C. trachomatis* infection support but do not confirm the diagnosis of PID and negative results do not eliminate the diagnosis.
   a. Specimens should be collected and sent to the laboratory before initiating antibiotic therapy.
   b. Because a pelvic examination is required for the diagnosis of PID, endocervical, rather than vaginal or urine specimens, are preferred.
   c. The specimens should be examined for *N. gonorrhoeae* and *C. trachomatis,* but not for anaerobes, mycoplasmas, or enteric organisms that normally colonize the vagina.
   d. The preferred test for *N. gonorrhoeae* in patients with suspected PID is either endocervical cell culture or a nucleic acid amplification test (NAAT), such as polymerase chain reaction (PCR), transcription-mediated amplification (TMA), or strand displacement amplification (SDA).
   e. The preferred test for *C. trachomatis* in patients with suspected PID is a NAAT.
5. Urinalysis and urine culture: To evaluate for possible urinary tract infection/pyelonephritis.
6. Urine pregnancy test. If positive, an ectopic pregnancy must be considered.
7. Human immunodeficiency virus (HIV) testing: All patients with STDs should be offered HIV counseling and testing.
8. Pelvic ultrasonography: Used if the clinician cannot adequately assess the adnexa, palpate an adnexal mass, or questions the presence of an ectopic pregnancy or TOA. Ultrasonography (especially if performed transvaginally) can be useful in narrowing the differential diagnosis, but is a relatively insensitive test for PID.
9. Laparoscopy: Indicated diagnostically in the patient whose pain does not respond to antibiotic therapy and therapeutically in the patient with a persistent TOA.

DIAGNOSIS

Timely and accurate diagnosis of PID is essential in preventing sequelae. Depending on the criteria used and the epidemiological characteristics of the patient population, the positive predictive value of a clinical diagnosis of PID, using laparoscopic diagnosis as the gold standard, ranges from 65% to 90%. The differential diagnosis is broad (Table 63.1).

The Centers for Disease Control and Prevention (CDC) has made recommendations on the use of minimum and elaborate criteria for the diagnosis of PID (Table 63.2). These recommendations for diagnosing PID are intended to help health care providers recognize when PID should be suspected and when additional information is needed to increase diagnostic certainty. PID should be considered as a likely diagnosis in any woman with pelvic tenderness and signs or symptoms of lower genital tract inflammation. Empirical treatment should be initiated in young women at risk for STDs if any of the minimum criteria is present and no other cause(s) for the illness can be identified.

The CDC urges that clinicians maintain a low threshold for the diagnosis and empirical treatment of PID. However, because incorrect diagnosis and management can cause unnecessary morbidity, more elaborate diagnostic criteria may be used to enhance the specificity of the minimum criteria.

TABLE 63.1

Differential Diagnosis of Pelvic Inflammatory Disease

Gastrointestinal
  Appendicitis
  Cholecystitis
  Cholelithiasis
  Constipation
  Diverticulitis
  Gastroenteritis
  Hernia
  Inflammatory bowel disease
  Irritable bowel syndrome
Gynecological
  Corpus luteum cyst
  Dysmenorrhea
  Ectopic pregnancy
  Endometriosis
  Mittelschmerz
  Ovarian
    Cyst
    Torsion
    Tumor
  Pregnancy
    Ectopic
    Spontaneous, septic, or threatened abortion
    Postabortion endometritis
Urological
  Cystitis
  Nephrolithiasis
  Pyelonephritis
  Urethritis
Musculoskeletal
Rheumatologic/autoimmune
Psychiatric

TABLE 63.2

Centers for Disease Control and Prevention Diagnostic Criteria for Pelvic Inflammatory Disease

Minimum criteria (initiate treatment in females at risk for STDs and complaining of lower abdominal pain when one or more clinical sign is present and no other diagnosis is apparent)
  Cervical motion tenderness, OR
  Uterine tenderness, OR
  Adnexal tenderness
Additional criteria (support a diagnosis of PID)
  Oral temperature >101°F (>38.3°C)
  Abnormal cervical or vaginal mucopurulent discharge
  Presence of abundant numbers of white blood cells on saline microscopy of vaginal secretions
  Elevated erythrocyte sedimentation rate
  Elevated C-reactive protein level
  Laboratory documentation of cervical infection with *N. gonorrhoeae* or *C. trachomatis*
Definitive criteria (warranted in selected cases)
  Endometrial biopsy with histopathological evidence of endometritis
  Transvaginal sonography or magnetic resonance imaging techniques showing thickened, fluid-filled tubes with or without free pelvic fluid or tuboovarian complex, or Doppler studies suggesting pelvic infection (e.g., tubal hyperemia)
  Laparoscopic abnormalities consistent with PID

THERAPY

PID requires treatment with broad-spectrum antibiotics as soon as a presumptive diagnosis is made. CDC-recommended treatment regimens for PID are summarized in Tables 63.3 and 63.4. Fluoroquinolones are no longer recommended for the treatment of PID due to increased prevalence of gonococcal resistance.

CDC criteria for hospitalization are as follows:

1. Surgical emergencies such as appendicitis cannot be excluded
2. Pregnancy
3. Poor response to oral antimicrobial therapy
4. Inability to follow or tolerate an outpatient oral regimen
5. Severe illness, nausea and vomiting, or high fever
6. TOA (at least 24-hours inpatient followed by outpatient antimicrobial therapy for a total of at least 10 days)
7. Immunodeficiency (e.g., HIV infection with low CD4 counts, immunosuppressive therapy)

Other reasons to consider hospitalization in the adolescent with suspected PID include age <15 years, abortion or other gynecological surgery procedure within previous 14 days, a history of a previous episode of PID, and other extenuating medical or social circumstances that may preclude receipt of appropriate treatment as an outpatient.

Among women with mild-to-moderate PID, there does not appear to be any difference in reproductive outcomes between inpatient and outpatient treatment. Whether treatment is provided is an inpatient or outpatient setting, the following general recommendations should be considered:

1. Patients should be educated about the importance of completing a full 14-day course of antibiotics. The duration of treatment does not depend on the result of any laboratory test.
2. All sex partners within the preceding 60 days require treatment for *C. trachomatis* and *N. gonorrhoeae* infections, regardless of patient or partner microbiological test results.
3. The use of nonsteroidal antiinflammatory drugs is recommended to treat abdominal pain or cramping.
4. In the setting of TOA, clindamycin or metronidazole with doxycycline is used as continued therapy for expanded anaerobic coverage.

TABLE 63.3

CDC-Recommended Parenteral Antibiotic Regimens for Pelvic Inflammatory Disease

A. Cefotetan 2 g IV every 12 hr *or* cefoxitin 2 g IV every 6 hr, *plus* doxycycline 100 mg PO or IV every 12 hr
B. Clindamycin 900 mg IV every 8 hr *plus* gentamicin loading dose IV *or* IM (2 mg/kg of body weight), followed by a maintenance dose (1.5 mg/kg) every 8 hr (single daily dosing may be substituted)
C. Alternatives
  Ampicillin/sulbactam 3 g IV every 6 hr *plus* doxycycline 100 mg PO *or* IV every 12 hr
  Parenteral therapy can be discontinued 24 hours after clinical improvement. Therapy should be continued with doxycycline 100 mg PO twice a day *or* clindamycin 450 mg PO four times a day to complete a total of 14 days of therapy

TABLE 63.4

CDC-Recommended Oral Regimens for Pelvic Inflammatory Disease

Ceftriaxone 250 mg IM in a single dose *or*
Cefoxitin 2 g IM and probenecid 1 g PO concurrently in a single dose *or* another
    parenteral third-generation cephalosporin (e.g., ceftizoxime or cefotaxime), *plus* doxycycline 100 mg PO
    twice a day for 14 days *with or without* metronidazole 500 mg PO twice a day for 14 days

5. Single-dose azithromycin (used for treatment of chlamydial cervicitis or urethritis) has not been shown to be effective for the treatment of PID.

If a parenteral regimen is used, the following points should be considered:

1. Patients who do not improve clinically within 72 hours require further evaluation and possibly surgical intervention.
2. Intravenous doxycycline should be avoided because of pain and venous sclerosis with infusion.
3. Cephalosporins other than cefotetan or cefoxitin are less active against anaerobes and are not recommended.

Adolescents with PID who are treated as outpatients, should have a follow-up examination within 72 hours to document defervescence and improvement in pain. If the baseline *C. trachomatis* and/or *N. gonorrhoeae* tests are positive, repeated screening for reinfection is warranted 4 to 6 weeks after the completion of therapy.

CONSEQUENCES

1. Recurrence: Reported rates vary from 12% to 33%. Risk is inversely correlated with treatment of sexual contacts.
2. TOA: May occur in as many as one third of women hospitalized with salpingitis. Antibiotic therapy is effective in 42% to 92% of cases. Surgical therapy is indicated for rupture or ultrasound evidence of increasing size or nonresponse.
3. Infertility: One episode of PID is associated with a 13% to 21% risk; two episodes, a 35% risk; and three or more episodes, a 55% to 75% risk. It is important to counsel an adolescent who has had PID about the risk of infertility. If the risk of possible infertility is overemphasized, the adolescent may assume that she is unable to conceive or may not use effective contraception in an effort to test her fertility.
4. Ectopic pregnancy: PID is the single most common predisposing factor for ectopic pregnancy. One episode of PID increases the risk of ectopic pregnancy six- to tenfold.
5. Chronic abdominal and/or pelvic pain: Dysmenorrhea and dyspareunia occur in up to 18% of women after one episode of PID.

PREVENTION

1. Primary prevention involves education about STD prevention and aggressive screening of all sexually active adolescents.
   a. Education about the signs and symptoms of STDs, the consequences of STDs, and behaviors that increase or decrease the risk should begin early.
   b. Communities must prioritize the establishment and maintenance of comprehensive STD control strategies that include health promotion, as well as confidential clinical service.
2. Secondary prevention focuses on those adolescents with a history of PID.
   a. Counseling should begin with the initiation of antibiotic therapy. If the adolescent is hospitalized, the inpatient stay provides an important opportunity for intense education and discussion.
   b. Sex partners should be included in secondary counseling and education.
   c. Prevention continues after treatment, with the promotion of secondary abstinence or safer sexual behaviors.

ACKNOWLEDGMENTS

Dr. Shrier is supported in part by grant #1 R21 MH072533-01A1 (Shrier) from the National Institute of Mental Health, National Institutes of Health, and Leadership Education in Adolescent Health grant #5 T71 MC 00009 from the Maternal and Child Health Bureau, Health Resources and Services Administration.

WEB SITES

For Teenagers and Parents

http://www.youngwomenshealth.org/pid.html. The Center for Young Women's Health of Children's Hospital Boston handout, available in English and Spanish.
http://www.mckinley.uiuc.edu/health-info/womenhlt/pid.html. University of Illinois Health Center handout.
http://womenshealth.gov/faq/stdpids.htm. The National Women's Health Information Center Web site.
http://www.engenderhealth.org/wh/inf/dpid.html. Engender Health worldwide women's health Web site.
http://www.cdc.gov/std/PID/STDFact-PID.htm. CDC patient information sheet, available in English and Spanish.

For Health Professionals

http://www.cdc.gov/mmwr/preview/mmwrhtml/rr5511a1.htm. Sexually Transmitted Diseases Treatment Guidelines 2006 from the CDC.
http://www.emedicine.com/med/topic1774.htm. eMedicine Web site.
http://edcenter.med.cornell.edu/CUMC_PathNotes/Female_Genital_Tract/FGT_2.html. Cornell University teaching slides on female genital tract.

REFERENCES AND ADDITIONAL READINGS

Barrett S, Taylor C. A review on pelvic inflammatory disease. *Int J STD AIDS* 2005;16:715.

Benaim J, Pulaski M, Coupey SM. Adolescent girls and pelvic inflammatory disease: experience and practices of emergency department pediatricians. *Arch Pediatr Adolesc Med* 1998;152:449.

Centers for Disease Control and Prevention. Sexually transmitted diseases treatment guidelines 2006. *MMWR* 2006;55(No. RR-116):56.

Centers for Disease Control and Prevention. Screening tests to detect *Chlamydia trachomatis* and *Neisseria gonorrhoeae* infections—2002. *MMWR Morb Mortal Wkly Rep* 2002;51 (RR-15):1.

Cohen CR, Brunham RC. Pathogenesis of Chlamydia induced pelvic inflammatory disease. *Sex Transm Infect* 1999;75:21.

Crossman SH. The challenge of pelvic inflammatory disease. *Am Fam Physician* 2006;73:859.

Eschenbach DA, Buchanan HM, Pollock M, et al. Polymicrobial etiology of acute pelvic inflammatory disease. *N Engl J Med* 1973;293:166.

Eschenbach DA, Wolner-Hanssen P, Hawes SE, et al. Acute pelvic inflammatory disease: associations of clinical and laboratory findings with laparoscopic findings. *Obstet Gynecol* 1997;89:184.

Gaitan H, Angel E, Diaz R, et al. Accuracy of five different diagnostic techniques in mild-to-moderate pelvic inflammatory disease. *Infect Dis Obstet Gynecol* 2002;10:171.

Grodstein F, Rothman KJ. Epidemiology of pelvic inflammatory disease. *Epidemiology* 1994;5:234.

Haggerty CL, Ness RB. Epidemiology, pathogenesis and treatment of pelvic inflammatory disease. *Expert Rev Anticancer Ther* 2006;4:235.

Heinonen PK, Miettinen A. Laparoscopic study on the microbiology and severity of acute pelvic inflammatory disease. *Eur J Obstet Gynecol Reprod Biol* 1994;57:85.

Hillier SL, Kiviat NB, Hawes SE, et al. Role of bacterial vaginosis-associated microorganisms in endometritis. *Am J Obstet Gynecol* 1996;175:435.

Jossens MO, Schachter J, Sweet RL. Risk factors associated with pelvic inflammatory disease of differing microbial etiologies. *Obstet Gynecol* 1994;83:989.

McCormack WM. Pelvic inflammatory disease. *N Engl J Med* 1994;330:115.

McNeeley SG, Hendrix SL, Mazzoni MM, et al. Medically sound, cost-effective treatment for pelvic inflammatory disease and tuboovarian abscess. *Am J Obstet Gynecol* 1998;178:1272.

Mohlajee AP, Curtis KM, Peterson HV. Does insertion and use of an intrauterine device increase the risk of pelvic inflammatory disease among women with sexually transmitted infection? A systematic review. *Contraception* 2006;73:145.

Molander P, Cacciatore B, Sjoberg J, et al. Laparoscopic management of suspected acute pelvic inflammatory disease. *J Am Assoc Gynecol Laparosc* 2000;7:107.

Munday PE. Pelvic inflammatory disease—an evidence-based approach to diagnosis [Review]. *J Infect* 2000;40:31.

Ness RB, Soper DE, Holley RL, et al. The PID Evaluation and Clinical Health (PEACH) study investigators. Douching and endometritis: Results from the PID Evaluation and Clinical Health (PEACH) study. *Sex Transm Dis* 2001;28:240.

Ness RB, Soper DE, Holley RL, et al. The PID Evaluation and Clinical Health (PEACH) study investigators. Hormonal and barrier contraception and risk of upper genital tract disease in the PID Evaluation and Clinical Health (PEACH) study. *Am J Obstet Gynecol*. 2001;185:121.

Ness RB, Soper DE, Holley RL, et al. The PID Evaluation and Clinical Health (PEACH) study investigators. Effectiveness of inpatient and outpatient treatment strategies for women with pelvic inflammatory disease: results from the Pelvic Inflammatory Disease Evaluation and Clinical Health (PEACH) Randomized Trial.[Comment]. *Am J Obstet Gynecol* 2002; 186:929.

Ness RB, Soper DE, Holley RL, et al. The PID Evaluation and Clinical Health (PEACH) study investigators. Bacterial vaginosis and risk of pelvic inflammatory disease. *Obstet Gynecol* 2004;104:761.

Ness RB, Smith KJ, Chang CC, et al. Gynecologic Infection Follow-Through, GIFT, Investigators. Prediction of pelvic inflammatory disease among young, single, sexually active women. *Sex Transm Dis* 2006;33:13.

Peipert JF, Ness RB, Blume J, et al. The Pelvic Inflammatory Disease Evaluation Clinical Health (PEACH) Study Investigators. Clinical predictors of endometritis in women with symptoms and signs of pelvic inflammatory disease. *Am J Obstet Gynecol* 2001;184:856.

Safrin S, Schachter J, Dahrouge D, et al. Long-term sequelae of acute pelvic inflammatory disease. A retrospective cohort study. *Am J Obstet Gynecol* 1992;166:1300.

Scholes D, Daling JR, Stergachis A, et al. Vaginal douching as a risk factor for acute pelvic inflammatory disease. *Obstet Gynecol* 1993;81:601.

Scholes D, Stergachis A, Heidrich FE, et al. Prevention of pelvic inflammatory disease by screening for cervical chlamydial infection. *N Engl J Med* 1996;334:1362.

Shrier LA. Bacterial sexually transmitted infections: gonorrhea, chlamydia, pelvic inflammatory disease, and syphilis. In: Emans SJ, Laufer MR, Goldstein DP, eds. *Pediatric and adolescent gynecology*, 5th ed. Philadelphia: Lippincott Williams & Wilkins; 2005:565.

Shrier LA, Moszczenski SA, Emans SJ, et al. Three years of a clinical practice guideline for uncomplicated pelvic inflammatory disease in adolescents. *J Adolesc Health* 2000;27:57.

Simms I, Stephenson JM. Pelvic inflammatory disease epidemiology: what do we know and what do we need to know [Review]. *Sex Transm Infect* 2000;76:80.

Slap GB, Forke CM, Cnaan A, et al. Recognition of tubo-ovarian abscess in adolescents with pelvic inflammatory disease. *J Adolesc Health* 1996;18:397.

Sweet RL. The role of bacterial vaginosis in pelvic inflammatory disease. *Clin Infect Dis* 1995;20(Suppl 2):S271.

Trent M, Ellen JM, Walker A. Pelvic inflammatory disease in adolescents: care delivery in pediatric ambulatory settings. *Pediatr Emerg Care* 2005;21:431.

Viberga I, Odlind V, Lazdane G, et al. Microbiology profile in women with pelvic inflammatory disease in relation to IUD use. *Infect Dis Obstet Gynecol* 2005;13:183.

Viberga I, Odlind V, Berglund L. The impact of age and intrauterine contraception on the clinical course of pelvic inflammatory disease. *Gynecol Obstet Invest* 2006;6:65.

Washington AE, Cates W Jr, Wasserheit JN. Preventing pelvic inflammatory disease. *JAMA* 1991;266:2574.

Wiesenfeld HC, Hillier SL, Krohn MA, et al. Lower genital tract infection and endometritis: insight into subclinical pelvic inflammatory disease. *Obstet Gynecol* 2002;100:456.

Wiesenfeld HC, Sweet RL, Ness RB, et al. Comparison of acute and subclinical pelvic inflammatory disease. *Sex Transm Dis* 2005;32:400.

Westrom L, Eschenbach D. Pelvic inflammatory disease. In: Holmes K, et al., eds. *Sexually transmitted diseases*, 3rd ed. New York: McGraw-Hill; 1999:783.

CHAPTER 64

Syphilis

J. Dennis Fortenberry and Lawrence S. Neinstein

Syphilis is a chronic systemic infection transmitted by sexual contact. Teens are most likely to present with either signs or symptoms of a primary infection, that is, ulcer at the infection site or a secondary infection manifested by symptoms such as skin rash, lymphadenopathy, fever, or mucocutaneous lesions.

ETIOLOGY

The agent causing syphilis is *Treponema pallidum,* a motile, spiral microorganism 6 to 20 μm in length and 0.10 to 0.18 μm in diameter. The organisms do not stain well and are best visualized by dark-field microscopy. *T. pallidum* does not grow in artificial media.

Most infections are contracted during sexual contact, including kissing and sexual intercourse. Rare cases are caused by direct contact with infectious cutaneous or mucous membrane lesions. Rashes are not infectious if the skin is intact. Other modes of transmission include congenital and transfusion-related transmission. The estimated rate of transmission after sexual exposure to a person with a chancre is 30%. The risk of transmission persists during the first 4 years of untreated syphilis.

EPIDEMIOLOGY

1. Incidence: Syphilis incidence shows a cyclical waxing and waning, with peaks at intervals of approximately 7 to 10 years. The incidence decreased during most of the 20th century especially after the discovery and use of penicillin in the 1940s. There was an increase in the mid-1980s due to increases in IV drug use, crack cocaine, and multiple sexual partners. The rates peaked in 1990 at 53.8 cases per 100,000 and these were 18 per 100,000 for 15- to 19- year-old males and 42 per 100,000 for teenage females. Rates fell throughout the 1990s, secondary to aggressive screening and use of condoms. However, from 2003 to 2004 there was an increase of 8% in the cases of primary and secondary syphilis to a rate of 2.7 cases per 100,000. There were 8,724 cases reported of primary and secondary syphilis in 2005.
2. Geographical concentration: Syphilis shows substantial geographical concentration, with more than 50% of primary and secondary cases reported from fewer than 1% of U.S. counties. The southeastern part of the United States bears an especially heavy burden of syphilis.
3. Race: Non-Hispanic blacks are at higher risk for syphilis than non-Hispanic whites. This ratio was 44 times higher in 1997 and declined to 8 times higher in 2002.
4. Sex: Male-to-female ratios of primary and secondary syphilis have increased in recent years to 3:1 after falling until 1994.
5. Age: Highest infection rates occur in young adults aged 20 to 29 years. Adolescents participating in commercial sex work, in cocaine and crack cocaine distribution or use, or in other social or sexual networks are important foci in localized outbreaks.

PATHOGENESIS

T. pallidum enters the body through minute abrasions in the skin and through exposure to sera of moist, mucocutaneous lesions. The infection is spread through lymphatics and blood vessels. The spirochetes cause cellular infiltrates, granuloma formation, and an obliterative endarteritis. This can lead to necrosis, with resultant ulcerations and erosions. In later stages, tissue hypersensitivity becomes prominent and can lead to gummas. Syphilitic lesions heal by scar formation so that in tertiary lesions scarring is considerable.

CLINICAL MANIFESTATIONS

Primary Syphilis

Syphilis should be considered in the differential diagnosis of any ulcerating lesion of the anogenital or oral areas. Less frequently affected areas are breasts and fingers. After an incubation period of 9 to 90 days with an average of 21 days, the primary lesions appear. Syphilis is characterized by a chancre at the point of inoculation. Characteristics of the syphilitic chancre are as follows:

1. Location
   a. Ninety-five percent are on the external genitalia.
   b. Single lesions are typical but multiple lesions are common.

c. Lesions may also appear as "kissing lesions," chancres that touch each other across a fold of skin.

d. Other primary sites include the cervix, mouth, anus, lips, face, breast, and fingers.

2. Size: 1 to 2 cm.

3. Chancre: Starts as a painless papule eroding to an indurated, painless ulcer. The ulcer typically has a punched out, clean appearance, with slightly elevated, firm margins.

4. Regional lymphadenopathy accompanies the lesion. The nodes are firm, nonsuppurative, and bilateral and may be painless.

5. Healing: The chancre heals in 3 to 6 weeks.

The primary infection may manifest with an inconspicuous lesion, particularly in women. Infection may occur with no papule or ulcer at all, particularly in previously infected patients.

Secondary Syphilis

Approximately 6 to 8 weeks (maximum, 6 months) after exposure and 4 to 10 weeks after the onset of the chancre, the manifestations of secondary syphilis appear. During this stage, *T. pallidum* can be identified in lesions and body fluids. The signs and symptoms of secondary syphilis usually disappear after weeks or months. Up to 25% of patients with untreated secondary syphilis develop relapses of secondary disease, with approximately one fourth of these having multiple relapses. Secondary syphilis lesions are infectious if the lesions are open (e.g., on mucous membranes, in intertriginous areas). Signs and symptoms of secondary syphilis include the following:

1. General skin eruption: Most common manifestation, affecting 90% of individuals with secondary syphilis
   a. Eruption involves the trunk and extremities with a predilection for palms and soles. The lesions on the palms and soles may be scaly and hyperkeratotic, and they may be the last to clear.
   b. Eruption involves skin as well as mucous membranes.
   c. Eruption tends to follow the lines of cleavage.
   d. Eruption is bilateral and symmetrical.
   e. Individual lesions are sharply demarcated, 0.5 to 2.0 cm in diameter with a reddish-brown hue.
   f. Eruption is most commonly macular, papular, or papulosquamous. Less common are follicular rashes. Vesicular and pustular rashes are rare.
   g. Lesions are typically nonpruritic, but pruritus is not infrequent.
   h. Eruption may last a few weeks to 12 months.
   i. Variety: Almost any type of rash can occur with syphilis, including acneform lesions, herpetiform lesions, and lesions similar to psoriasis. Lesions in intertriginous areas may erode and fissure, especially in the nasolabial folds and near the corners of the mouth. In warm, moist areas, hypertrophic granulomatous lesions (condylomata lata) may occur. These lesions usually occur near the area of the original chancre and have a broad, flat appearance.

2. General or regional lymphadenopathy (~70%)
   a. Nonpainful nodes
   b. Rubbery, hard feeling; discrete; with no suppuration
   c. Occasional hepatosplenomegaly

3. Flu-like syndrome (~50%)
   a. Sore throat and malaise most common
   b. Headaches
   c. Lacrimation
   d. Nasal discharge
   e. Arthralgias and myalgias
   f. Weight loss
   g. Fever

4. Syphilis alopecia (uncommon): Moth-eaten—appearing alopecia of the scalp and eyebrows

5. Other rare manifestations
   a. Arthritis or bursitis
   b. Hepatitis
   c. Iritis and anterior uveitis
   d. Glomerulonephritis

Latent Syphilis

Latent syphilis, neurosyphilis, and tertiary syphilis are unusual in adolescents. Readers should consult with more detailed references if these entities are suspected.

The *early latent period* is defined as the first year of infection. Early syphilis includes primary, secondary, and early latent syphilis. The *late latent stage* refers to the period after this first year unless late (tertiary) syphilis occurs. Latent syphilis is characterized by the following:

1. Absence of clinical signs and symptoms of syphilis
2. Repeated positive serological test results (Venereal Disease Research Laboratory [VDRL] and fluorescent treponemal antibody absorption [FTA-ABS]) for syphilis
3. Negative results from serological tests of the spinal fluid

Neurosyphilis

Neurosyphilis develops in 10% to 20% of patients with untreated syphilis but is uncommon in adolescents. Neurological involvement may become evident within 2 years of the initial infection. Most cases of neurosyphilis in adolescents are asymptomatic or manifest as acute syphilitic meningitis. Meningovascular syphilis is rare.

1. Asymptomatic neurosyphilis: Characterized by abnormal cerebrospinal fluid (CSF), including pleocytosis, elevated protein, and positive CSF-VDRL

2. Acute syphilitic meningitis
   a. Usually occurs during secondary syphilis or the early latent period
   b. Common symptoms: Fever, headache, photophobia, and meningismus
   c. Cranial nerve palsies (40%)
   d. Less frequent symptoms: Confusion, delirium, and seizures
   e. CSF: Increased protein, lymphocytic pleocytosis, and sometimes lowered glucose

3. Meningovascular syphilis
   a. Rare in adolescents (occurs 5 to 12 years after initial infection)
   b. Symptoms and signs from a syphilitic endarteritis producing local areas of infarction
   c. Symptoms: Headache, dizziness, mood changes, and memory loss
   d. Signs: Hemiparesis, hemiplegia, aphasia
   e. Other signs of parenchymal nervous system damage: Argyll-Robertson pupils (accommodation, but no response to light); injury to the posterior column of the spinal cord, causing tabes dorsalis

Late Syphilis

Signs and symptoms of late syphilis may occur 2 to 10 years after initial exposure in untreated or inadequately treated patients. This includes individuals with gummas and cardiovascular syphilis but not neurosyphilis. Late syphilis has not been reported in adolescents.

Cardiovascular syphilis usually occurs 10 to 30 years after exposure.

Gummas are granulomatous lesions of late syphilis that involve skin, soft tissue, viscera, or bones. They are usually few in number, asymmetrical, indolent, and not contagious.

Congenital Syphilis

The fetus becomes susceptible to infection after the fourth month of gestation. Therefore, adequate treatment of the mother before the 16th week of gestation prevents infection of the fetus. The risk of infection of the fetus during untreated early maternal syphilis is approximately 80% to 95%. Approximately 25% of infants infected in utero die before birth, and 25% die shortly after birth, if untreated. The remainder develop either early or late lesions.

1. Early congenital syphilis lesions (lesions occurring during the first 2 years of life and usually by 3 months of age)
   a. Vesicular and vesiculobullous eruptions
   b. Superficial desquamation
   c. Rhinitis
   d. Hepatosplenomegaly
   e. Hemolytic anemia, thrombocytopenia
   f. Skeletal involvement: Osteochondritis with periarticular swelling
   g. Neurosyphilis
   h. Ocular: Glaucoma, uveitis, and chorioretinitis
   i. Nephropathy: Uncommon
2. Late congenital syphilis: This type of syphilis corresponds to tertiary syphilis in adults. In 60% of cases the infection remains latent, and in the rest the lesions can be divided into the following categories:
   a. Inflammatory or hypersensitivity lesions
   b. Gummas
   c. Neurosyphilis
   d. Interstitial keratitis
   e. Clutton joints: Symmetrical, painless swelling of knees
   f. Palatal deformations
   g. Paroxysmal cold hemoglobinuria
3. Unique stigmata
   a. Hutchinson incisors: Centrally notched, screwdriver-shaped upper incisors
   b. Abnormal facies: Saddlenose, frontal bossing
   c. Eighth nerve deafness
   d. Scaphoid scapulas
   e. Hutchinson triad: Malformed incisors, eighth nerve deafness, and interstitial keratitis

DIFFERENTIAL DIAGNOSIS

Primary Syphilis

Sexually Transmitted Causes of Genital Ulcers
The most common sexually transmitted genital ulcers in the United States are herpes, syphilis, and chancroid, in that order. Lymphogranuloma venereum and donovanosis (granuloma inguinale) are rare in the United States.

1. Herpes simplex: Usually painful, multiple lesions beginning as vesicles on an erythematous base. Primary lesions are usually bilateral, extensive, and associated with tender adenopathy, and recurrent lesions are usually unilateral without significant adenopathy. The vesicles break down into ulcers with nonindurated borders.
2. Chancroid: Usually painful lesions with a deep purulent base and often erythematous borders. Local lymph nodes are often fluctuant and tender.
3. Lymphogranuloma venereum: The primary lesion may be a nonindurated, herpetiform ulcer that heals rapidly. Many patients present with advanced disease including fever and massive regional adenopathy.
4. Granuloma inguinale (donovanosis): Nontender, fleshy, beefy-red ulcers that bleed easily.

Nonsexually Transmitted Causes of Genital Ulcers
The most common nonsexually transmitted cause is trauma.

1. Traumatic lesions: There should be a history of appearance of the lesion at the time of the trauma. However, many patients attribute genital ulcers to trauma without a specific history of injury.
2. Fixed drug reaction: There may be history of a similar lesion after prior drug exposure. Lesions may start as reddish plaque and become hyperpigmented, edematous, or eroded.
3. Candida balanitis.
4. Behçet syndrome: Not limited to genital area.
5. Psoriasis, if excoriated.
6. Lichen planus, if excoriated.
7. Erythema multiforme, if excoriated.
8. Cancer: Extremely rare in adolescents.

Secondary Syphilis

1. Psoriasis
2. Pityriasis rosea
3. Drug eruptions
4. Tinea versicolor
5. Alopecia areata
6. Lichen planus
7. Viremia
8. Lupus erythematosus
9. Scabies
10. Pediculosis
11. Rosacea
12. Infectious mononucleosis
13. Keratoderma blennorrhagica
14. Condyloma acuminatum

Although the clinical history and appearance of these conditions can often separate them from secondary syphilis, a VDRL or rapid plasma reagin (RPR) test should be performed whenever doubt exists.

DIAGNOSIS

Syphilis screening is an important element of routine health care for sexually experienced adolescents. Adolescents should also be screened during pregnancy or when diagnosed with other sexually transmitted infections. However, as the prevalence falls in certain lower-risk groups, such as college students, the criteria for screening syphilis serology will have to be reevaluated.

Laboratory Findings

Dark-Field Examination   The dark-field examination is essential in evaluating moist ulcers and lesions such as a chancre or condyloma lata. Technique is as follows:

1. Clean lesion with saline and gauze.
2. Abrade gently with dry gauze. Avoid inducing bleeding, which makes dark-field examination more difficult.
3. Squeeze lesion (with gloves) to express serous transudate.
4. Place a drop of transudate on a slide.
5. Place a drop of saline on transudate and cover with a cover slip.
6. Examine under dark-field microscope.
7. For internal lesions, a bacteriological loop can be used to transfer the fluid to a slide.
8. For lymph node aspirations: Clean the skin, inject 0.2 mL or less of sterile saline, and aspirate the node. Place the fluid on a slide.

Direct Fluorescent Antibody   Specimens from primary lesions can also be sent to reference laboratories or some state health departments for direct fluorescent antibody (DFA) staining. These specimens can be collected as described previously; however, saline should not be added to the slides, and they should be allowed to air-dry.

Both dark-field microscopy and DFA staining are very specific except for oral specimens, but sensitivity depends on many factors, including collection technique, age of lesions, and experience of laboratory personnel.

Serological Tests

1. Nontreponemal antibody tests: Tests for a nonspecific anticardiolipin antibody that forms in response to surface lipids on the treponeme
   a. Types
      * Agglutination: RPR
      * Flocculation: VDRL
   b. Use: Nontreponemal tests should be used for screening and to monitor treatment success. Nontreponemal test titers correlate with disease activity and fall after treatment. Positive nontreponemal tests should be titered out to the highest point, and monitored over time. A fourfold change in titer, equivalent to a change of two dilutions (e.g., from 1:8 to 1:32 or 1:16 to 1:4), demonstrates a substantial change if the same serological test is used.
2. Specific treponemal antibody tests
   a. Types
      * Immunofluorescence: FTA-ABS is used to confirm a positive result from RPR or VDRL.
      * Microhemagglutination: The *T. pallidum* particle agglutination (TP-PA) test has replaced the FTA-ABS test in many laboratories as the specific treponemal test to confirm a positive result from VDRL.
      * Enzyme-linked immunosorbent assay (ELISA)—used by some blood banks for donor screening.

   b. Use: Treponemal tests are specific and sensitive, but because of their expense and more difficult technical requirement, they are typically used to confirm positive results from a screening test. Once an individual tests positive on treponemal tests, he or she usually remains positive for life. Titers are unrelated to disease activity or treatment. Treponemal antibody titers therefore should not be quantitated but recorded as reactive, nonreactive, or minimally reactive. A minimally reactive test result may represent a false-positive finding, and the test should be repeated.
3. Sensitivity
   a. The sensitivity of nontreponemal tests (RPR and VDRL) in primary syphilis ranges from 60% to 90% depending on the duration of infection and the population under study. Results are positive at the following times:

Onset of primary chancre	Approximately 25% of individuals are positive
2 wk after chancre appearance	50% are positive
3 wk after chancre appearance	75% are positive
4 wk after chancre appearance	100% are positive

   b. Treponemal tests (TP-PA and FTA-ABS) are positive in 80% to 100% of primary syphilis. Sensitivity of nontreponemal and treponemal tests approaches 100% in secondary syphilis.
4. False-positive serology test results: Approximately 20% to 40% of all positive nontreponemal test results are false-positive, as shown by a nonreactive treponemal test. Most false-positive nontreponemal test results show a low titer (dilution <1:8), and the probability of a false-positive finding decreases with increasing titer. The causes of false-positive test results include the following:
   a. Acute infection: Viral infections, chlamydial infections, Lyme disease, *Mycoplasma* infections, nonsyphilitic spirochetal infections, and various bacterial, fungal, and protozoal infections
   b. Autoimmune diseases
   c. Narcotic addiction
   d. Aging
   e. Hashimoto thyroiditis
   f. Sarcoidosis
   g. Lymphoma
   h. Leprosy
   i. Cirrhosis of the liver
   j. Human immunodeficiency virus (HIV) infection: Can lead to unusually high, unusually low, or fluctuating titers
   k. False-positive findings can occasionally arise in treponemal tests. However, most of these are reported as borderline and not positive.
5. Tests most commonly used
   a. RPR (screening and quantitative measurement of clinical activity)
   b. VDRL (quantitative measurement to assess clinical activity and response to therapy or qualitative test for screening)
   c. TP-PA or FTA-ABS (to confirm diagnosis in a patient with a positive result from VDRL or RPR)

d. Other tests under development are based on polymerase chain reaction (PCR), or enzyme-linked immunospot testing for treponeme-specific antibody–secreting cells. Clinical experience with these tests is limited, and they have not replaced existing modes of screening and confirmation.

Diagnosis by Stage

Primary Syphilis
1. Definitive diagnosis of early syphilis requires a positive result on dark-field examination or DFA test of lesion transudate or tissue.
2. Presumptive diagnosis relies on a positive nontreponemal test result (VDRL or RPR) with a high titer (1:8 or higher) or rising titer (two or more than two dilutions) *and* a positive treponemal test result (e.g., FTA-ABS or TP-PA).

Adolescents with a positive dark-field examination should be treated, as should those with a typical lesion and a positive serological test result. Sexual partners (within the previous 90 days, even if asymptomatic and seronegative) of persons with documented infection should also be treated. If the initial serological test result is negative, it should be repeated 1 week, 1 month, and 3 months later in suspected cases. An FTA-ABS or TP-PA test should be used to confirm a positive nontreponemal test result.

Lumbar puncture is not recommended for routine evaluation of primary syphilis unless clinical signs and symptoms of neurological involvement are present. The role of lumbar puncture in the care of HIV-infected persons with primary syphilis is controversial. Most experts would reserve lumbar puncture for the evaluation of apparent treatment failures.

Secondary Syphilis
1. Dark-field examination of material from lesions or lymph nodes
2. VDRL or RPR

An adolescent should be treated if the dark-field examination result is positive or if the patient has typical findings of secondary syphilis and a positive result from VDRL or RPR. Positive nontreponemal test results should be confirmed with an FTA-ABS or TP-PA test.

Neurosyphilis
The standard test is the CSF-VDRL. It is a specific but not a sensitive test for active neurosyphilis. On the other hand, the FTA-ABS is sensitive but not specific for neurosyphilis. Serum antibody may diffuse into the CSF and may not be reflective of active central nervous system (CNS) disease. However, a nonreactive FTA-ABS probably indicates the absence of active neurosyphilis. Pleocytosis in the CSF is another good indicator of active disease.

1. CNS invasion by treponemes occurs in 30% to 40% of patients with primary or secondary syphilis. However, this may not be an accurate predictor of poor neurological outcome. A spinal tap is not indicated in patients with early syphilis.
2. Indications for CSF examination can include latent syphilis of unknown duration if:
   a. Neurological or ophthalmological signs or symptoms are present

b. Treatment failure
c. Serum nontreponemal test titer is greater than or equal to 1:32 unless duration of infection is known to be <1 year
d. Nonpenicillin therapy is planned unless duration of infection is known to be <1 year
e. HIV infection

Evaluation of neurosyphilis should be done in consultation with an expert in this area. There are no perfect tests for evaluating neurosyphilis. The cell count is usually elevated in the presence of neurosyphilis and is an excellent marker for assessing treatment. The VDRL is the standard and most specific test on spinal fluid, but it has a sensitivity of only 60% to 70%. Although the FTA-ABS is highly sensitive, the false-positive rate may be 6% or greater because of transfer of antibodies across the blood–brain barrier. Some experts order both tests. If the FTA-ABS result is negative, the likelihood of neurosyphilis is very small.

Syphilis in Pregnancy All pregnant adolescents should be screened early in pregnancy. Seropositive subjects should be considered infected unless a prior history documents recent treatment and serological titers have appropriately declined. Screening should be repeated in the third trimester and again at delivery in areas or populations with a high prevalence of syphilis. A woman delivering a stillborn infant after 20 weeks' gestation should also be tested for syphilis.

Syphilis and Human Immunodeficiency Virus Ulcerative lesions such as syphilitic chancres increase the risk of transmission of HIV. There is also evidence that infection with HIV may alter the serological response to syphilis. There have been reports of patients who were coinfected with HIV and syphilis and had unusual serological responses. Many of these reports involved higher than expected serological titers, but false-negative serological test results have also been reported. Most treponemal and nontreponemal serological tests for syphilis are accurate for most individuals with both syphilis and HIV infection. If serological tests are not consistent with clinical findings, alternative tests, such as biopsy and DFA staining of lesion material, should be considered. HIV-infected individuals with neurological symptoms or failure to respond to antibiotic treatment should be evaluated for neurosyphilis.

Latent Syphilis A RPR/VDRL and a FTA-ABS test should be done. The FTA-ABS is essential in latent and late syphilis because the nontreponemal tests are only approximately 70% sensitive in these states. The adolescent should be treated if the FTA-ABS result is positive and there is no documentation of appropriate prior treatment. A decision about a lumbar puncture in these instances should be done in consultation with an expert in this area.

THERAPY

Penicillin is the optimal antibiotic for syphilis treatment and the dosage and length depends on the state of syphilis. For individuals in these categories with a history of penicillin allergy, skin testing and desensitization, if indicated, are recommended.

Fewer data are available on nonpenicillin regimens. Adolescents treated for gonorrhea or chlamydia with ceftriaxone, doxycycline, and azithromycin are probably covered for incubating syphilis. If a different antibiotic regimen is used to treat gonorrhea or chlamydia, the teen should have a second serological test for syphilis in 3 months.

Primary and Secondary Syphilis

1. Benzathine penicillin G: The total recommended dose is a single injection of 2.4 million units intramuscularly (IM).
2. Penicillin-allergic nonpregnant patients:
   a. Doxycycline 100 mg orally two times a day for 14 days, or
   b. Tetracycline 500 mg orally four times a day for 14 days is recommended.
   c. Ceftriaxone is effective for treatment of early syphilis but the optimal dose and duration have not been defined.
   d. Azithromycin 2 g as a single oral dose. However, treatment failure due to acquired azithromycin resistance of *T. pallidum* has been reported in several geographical areas. This treatment should be considered only if other options are not available and careful follow-up can be assured.
   e. Use of any of these therapies in HIV-infected persons has not been well studied.
   f. For those who cannot tolerate one of the above therapies referral for desensitization to penicillin is indicated.
   g. Pregnancy: Pregnant patients who are allergic to penicillin should be desensitized and treated with penicillin.
3. Other considerations
   a. All patients with syphilis should be tested for HIV. For high-risk patients or in high-prevalence areas, patients with primary syphilis should be retested for HIV after 3 months.
   b. Those individuals with signs or symptoms that suggest neurological or ophthalmic disease should be evaluated by CSF analysis or slit-lamp examination, respectively. Routine lumbar puncture is not recommended for individuals with primary or secondary syphilis unless clinical signs and symptoms suggest neurological involvement or if patients fail to respond to antibiotic treatment.
4. Follow-up
   a. Infected individuals should be reexamined clinically, and serological test results should be rechecked at 3 and 6 months. Quantitative nontreponemal tests should be used for follow-up, because the FTA-ABS and TP-PA results usually remain positive throughout the individual's life. If signs or symptoms persist or nontreponemal antibody titers have not decreased fourfold by 6 months, the patient should have a CSF examination and HIV test and be re-treated. Most individuals with primary syphilis are seronegative by 3 to 12 months, and 75% to 95% of individuals with secondary syphilis are seronegative by 1 year. The drop in titers for primary and secondary syphilis applies only to first episodes of primary or secondary syphilis; those with reinfections have less predictable serological drops.

   b. Individuals are at risk for treatment failure if their nontreponemal titers have not declined fourfold by 3 months after treatment for primary or secondary syphilis. HIV testing should be performed at 3 months in these individuals. Re-treatment should probably include three weekly injections of benzathine penicillin G 2.4 million units IM unless neurosyphilis is present.

Latent Syphilis

Latent syphilis is defined as disease characterized by seroreactivity without other evidence of disease. If acquired in the preceding year this is classified as early latent syphilis. These individuals can be classified as early latent, if during the year before evaluation they had:

• Seroconversion or fourfold or greater increase in titer of a nontreponemal test
• Unequivocal symptoms of primary or secondary syphilis
• A sex partner with documented primary, secondary, or early latent syphilis; or
• Reactive nontreponemal and treponemal tests from possible exposure within the previous 12 months

Late latent syphilis identifies a disease duration of 1 year or longer. The term *latent syphilis of unknown duration* is used when the timing of the initial infection cannot be established.

There are two regimens for patients who are not allergic to penicillin and who have normal findings on CSF examinations:

1. Early latent syphilis: Benzathine penicillin G 2.4 million units IM in a single dose
2. Late latent syphilis or latent syphilis of unknown duration: Benzathine penicillin G 7.2 million units total administered as three doses of 2.4 million units IM each at 1-week intervals
3. Penicillin-allergic patients: No clinical data exist that adequately document the efficacy of drugs other than penicillin for syphilis of more than 1 year duration. CSF examinations should be performed before therapy with these regimens. Suggested regimens are doxycycline 100 mg orally two times a day, or tetracycline 500 mg orally four times a day. Either is given for 14 days for individuals with early latent syphilis or 28 days for other individuals. If the CSF examination shows any evidence of neurosyphilis, the patient should be treated for neurosyphilis.
4. Other considerations
   a. All individuals with latent syphilis should be evaluated for tertiary disease including neurosyphilis, aortitis, iritis, and gummas.
   b. All patients with syphilis should be tested for HIV.
5. Follow-up
   a. Quantitative nontreponemal serological titers should be done at 6, 12, and 24 months after treatment. If titers increase fourfold or initial high titers (1:32 or greater) fail to decrease fourfold (two dilutions) within 12 to 24 months, or if signs or symptoms of syphilis occur, the individual should be evaluated for neurosyphilis and re-treated appropriately.
   b. Approximately 75% of the patients with early latent disease (duration 4 years or less) become seronegative by 5 years; the remaining 25% have positive serology for life.

Late Syphilis

The term *late syphilis* describes patients with gumma disease or cardiovascular involvement but not neurosyphilis. Late syphilis should not occur in adolescents and young adults.

Neurosyphilis

Neurosyphilis can occur during any stage of syphilis. Patients with syphilitic eye involvement should be treated with regimens covering neurosyphilis. Individuals with neurological symptoms should have a CSF examination.

1. Recommended regimen for neurosyphilis or syphilitic eye disease in individuals not allergic to penicillin: Aqueous crystalline penicillin G 18 to 24 million units daily administered as 3 to 4 million units intravenously (IV) every 4 hours for 10 to 14 days.
    a. Alternative regimen if compliance is a problem: Procaine penicillin G IM 2.4 million units daily, plus probenecid 500 mg orally four times a day, both for 10 to 14 days.
    b. Some experts add benzathine penicillin G 2.4 million units IM after completion of either of these two regimens.
2. Penicillin-allergic patients: Patients should be desensitized to penicillin, if necessary, and treated with penicillin. No alternatives have been adequately evaluated. Some specialists recommend ceftriaxone 2 g daily IM or IV for 10 to 14 days.
3. Follow-up: If the initial CSF examination showed an increased cell count, the examination should be repeated every 6 months until the cell count is normal. If the count has not decreased at 6 months or is not normal by 2 years, re-treatment should be strongly considered.

Syphilis in Pregnancy

All pregnant women should receive penicillin doses appropriate for their stage of syphilis. Although penicillin is effective in preventing transmission to the fetus and in treating infections in the fetus, the exact optimal penicillin regimens have not been adequately studied. Treatment in pregnancy should be the penicillin regimen appropriate for the stage of syphilis. Some experts recommend additional therapy, such as a second dose of benzathine penicillin G 2.4 million units IM given 1 week after the first dose for women who have primary, secondary, or early latent syphilis. During the second half of pregnancy, syphilis treatment may be adjusted by sonographic fetal evaluation for congenital syphilis. Tetracycline should not be used, because it is contraindicated in pregnancy. Erythromycin has a high risk of failure to cure the fetus. Therefore, pregnant women with a history of an allergy to penicillin should be skin tested and either treated or desensitized. A Jarisch-Herxheimer reaction during the second half of pregnancy can induce premature labor or fetal distress.

Treatment of Sex Partners

1. Persons exposed to an individual with primary, secondary, or early latent syphilis within the preceding 90 days should be treated presumptively. These individuals might be infected even if they are seronegative. If exposure occurred more than 90 days before examination, the individual should be treated presumptively if serological test results are not immediately available and follow-up is uncertain.
2. Partners should be notified and treated if the affected patient has syphilis of unknown duration and high nontreponemal serological test titers (1 : 32 or greater).
3. Sex partners of patients with late syphilis should be evaluated both clinically and serologically for syphilis.
4. Identification of at-risk sex partners: Time periods used to determine partners at risk are as follows:
    a. Three months plus duration of symptoms for primary syphilis
    b. Six months plus duration of symptoms for secondary syphilis
    c. One year for early latent syphilis

Human Immunodeficiency Virus-Infected Individuals

Among HIV-positive individuals, there have been reports of higher rates of neurological complications and treatment failures with traditional regimens for syphilis. There have also been cases of rapid progress of syphilis into secondary and tertiary stages in HIV-positive patients. However, no treatment regimens have yet been demonstrated to be more effective in treating HIV-infected individuals than those used in patients without HIV infection. HIV-positive patients with syphilis require careful evaluation for late and unusual manifestations of syphilis, including CSF evaluation. These patients require careful follow-up after therapy.

1. Penicillin regimens should be used whenever possible. Skin testing and desensitization can be used as appropriate.
2. Primary and secondary syphilis in HIV-infected patients: The Centers for Disease Control and Prevention (CDC) recommends no change in therapy for early syphilis in HIV-infected patients. Some experts recommend adding multiple doses of benzathine penicillin G, similar to the dosages used to treat late syphilis.
    a. Because of the confusing CSF findings and difficulty in definitively diagnosing neurosyphilis, some authorities recommend CSF examination of all individuals who are HIV infected, with treatment altered accordingly.
    b. Follow-up: HIV-infected adolescents should have follow-up serological testing at 3, 6, 9, 12, and 24 months. Those individuals with treatment failure should have a CSF examination and be re-treated similarly to those who are not HIV infected. If the CSF is normal, most experts would re-treat with benzathine penicillin G 7.2 million units as three weekly doses of 2.4 million units each.
3. Latent syphilis
    a. Patients with HIV and latent syphilis should have a CSF examination before treatment begins.
    b. Treatment in those individuals with normal CSF should include benzathine penicillin G 7.2 million units (as three weekly doses of 2.4 million units each). Those with abnormal findings on CSF examination should be treated and managed as patients with neurosyphilis.

Jarisch-Herxheimer Reaction

A remarkable reaction occurs within 2 hours of treatment in 50% of patients with primary syphilis, in 90% of those with secondary syphilis, and in 25% of those with early latent syphilis. The reaction consists of the following:

1. Fever and chills
2. Myalgias
3. Headache
4. Elevated neutrophil count
5. Tachycardia

The duration of symptoms is 12 to 24 hours, and treatment is reassurance, bed rest, and aspirin. The reaction can induce transient uterine contractions in pregnant women.

WEB SITES

For Teenagers and Parents

http://www.cdc.gov/std/Syphilis/STDFact-Syphilis.htm. CDC site on syphilis.

http://www.drkoop.com/ency/93/001327.html. Dr. Koop's site on syphilis.

http://www.iwannaknow.org. The American Social Health Association Web site designed specifically for teens. Sexuality and STD prevention are directly and explicitly addressed on general STD topics.

http://kidshealth.org/parent/infections/bacterial_viral/syphilis.html. Kids health site on syphilis.

For Health Professionals

http://www.cdc.gov/STD/treatment/. The CDC Web site with recent statistics and treatment guidelines.

http://www.ashastd.org. The American Social Health Association home page—lots of information and hotline access.

http://www.niaid.nih.gov/factsheets/stdsyph.htm. National Institute of Allergy and Infectious Diseases fact sheet from National Institutes of Health.

http://emedicine.com/ped/topic2193.htm. E-medicine site on syphilis.

REFERENCES AND ADDITIONAL READINGS

Alexander JM, Sheffield JS, Sanchez PJ, et al. Efficacy of treatment for syphilis in pregnancy. *Obstet Gynecol* 1999; 93:5.

Augenbraun M, Rolfs R, Johnson R, et al. Treponemal specific tests for the serodiagnosis of syphilis. *Sex Transm Dis* 1998; 25:549.

Beltrami JF, Cohen DA, Hamrick JT, et al. Rapid screening and treatment for sexually transmitted diseases in arrestees: a feasible control measure. *Am J Public Health* 1997;87: 1423.

Birnbaum NR, Goldschmidt RH, Buffett WO. Resolving the common clinical dilemmas of syphilis. *Am Fam Physician* 1999; 59:2233.

Centers for Disease Control and Prevention. Guidelines for treatment of sexually transmitted diseases. *MMWR* 2006; 55(RR–11):22.

Colletti JE, Giudice EL. Syphilis screening in a high-risk, inner-city adolescent population. *Am J Emerg Med* 2005;23: 225.

Doroshenko A Sherrard J Pollard AJ. Syphilis in pregnancy and the neonatal period. *Int J STD AIDS* 2006;17(4):221–227.

Ellen JM, Langer LM, Zimmerman RS, et al. The link between the use of crack cocaine and the sexually transmitted diseases of a clinic population: a comparison of adolescents with adults. *Sex Transm Dis* 1996;23:511.

Genç M, Ledger WJ. Syphilis in pregnancy. *Sex Transm Infect* 2000;76:73.

Ghanem KG, Erbelding EJ, Cheng WW, et al. Doxycycline compared with benzathine penicillin for the treatment of early syphilis. *Clin Infect Dis* 2006;42(6):e45–e49.

Holmes KK, Levine R, Weaver M. Effectiveness of condoms for prevention of sexually transmitted infections. *Bull WHO* 2004;82:454.

Joyanes P, Borobio MV, Arquez JM, et al. The association of false-positive rapid plasma reagin results and HIV infection. *Sex Transm Dis* 1998;25:569.

Kamb ML, Fishbein M, Douglas JM Jr, et al., Project RESPECT Study Group. Efficacy of risk-reduction counseling to prevent human immunodeficiency virus and sexually transmitted diseases: a randomized controlled trial. *JAMA* 1998;280: 1161.

Klausner JD, Wolf W, Fischer-Ponce L, et al. Tracing a syphilis outbreak through cyberspace. *JAMA* 2000;284:447.

Lukehart SA, Godornes C, Molini BJ, et al. Macrolide resistance in Treponema pallidum in the United States and Ireland. *N Engl J Med* 2004;351:154.

Marra CM. Neurosyphilis. *Curr Neurol Neurosci Rep* 2004;4:435.

Marra CM, Maxwell CL, Tantalo L, et al. Normalization of cerebrospinal fluid abnormalities after neurosyphilis therapy: Does HIV status matter? *Clin Infect Dis* 2004;38: 1001.

Musher DM. Early syphilis in the adult. In: Holmes KK, Sparling PF, Mardh PA, et al., eds. *Sexually transmitted diseases*, 3rd ed. New York: McGraw-Hill; 1999.

Myles TD, Elam G, Park-Hwang E, et al. The Jarisch-Herxheimer reaction and fetal monitoring changes in pregnant women treated for syphilis. *Obstet Gynecol* 1998;92:859.

Peeling RW, Hook EW III. The pathogenesis of syphilis: the great mimicker, revisited. *J Pathol* 2006;208(2):224–232.

Peterman TA, Heffelfinger JD, Swint EB, et al. The changing epidemiology of syphilis. *Sex Transm Dis* 2005;32 (Suppl 10):S4.

Peterman TA, Zaidi AA, Lieb S, et al. Incubating syphilis in patients treated for gonorrhea: a comparison of treatment regimens. *J Infect Dis* 1994;170:689.

Radolf JD, Sanchez PJ, Schulz KF, et al. Congenital syphilis. In: Holmes KK, Sparling PF, Mardh PA, et al., eds. *Sexually transmitted diseases*, 3rd ed. New York: McGraw-Hill; 1999.

Riedner G, Rusizoka M, Todd J, et al. Single-dose azithromycin versus penicillin G benzathine for the treatment of early syphilis. *N Engl J Med* 2005;353(12):1236–1244.

Sparling PE. Natural history of syphilis. In: Holmes KK, Sparling PF, Mardh PA, et al., eds. *Sexually transmitted diseases*, 3rd ed. New York: McGraw-Hill; 1999.

Stamm LV. Biology of *Treponema pallidum*. In: Holmes KK, Sparling PF, Mardh PA, et al., eds. *Sexually transmitted diseases*, 3rd ed. New York: McGraw-Hill; 1999.

Weiss HA, Thomas SL, Munabi SK, et al. Male circumcision and risk of syphilis, chancroid, and genital herpes: a systematic review and meta-analysis. *Sex Transm Infect* 2005;82(2): 101–109.

Young F. Syphilis: still with us, so watch out! *J Fam Health Care* 2006;16:77.

Zhou P, Gu Z, Xu J, et al. A study evaluating ceftriaxone as a treatment agent for primary and secondary syphilis in pregnancy. *Sex Transm Dis* 2005;32(8):495–498.

CHAPTER 65

Herpes Genitalis

Gale R. Burstein and Kimberly A. Workowski

Genital herpes is a chronic lifelong viral disease. Herpes genitalis lesions are caused by a large DNA virus, herpes simplex virus (HSV), with two serotypes, herpes simplex type 1 (HSV-1) and herpes simplex type 2 (HSV-2). Although HSV-1 is becoming more prominent as a cause of first-episode genital herpes, most cases of recurrent genital herpes are caused by HSV-2. These viruses have the ability to become latent and recur. Although the herpes genitalis prevalence has increased dramatically over the last 30 years, over the last decade the HSV-2 infection has declined. On the basis of serological studies, genital HSV-2 infection has affected at least 50 million persons in the United States. Most persons infected with HSV-2 have not been diagnosed. Many such persons have mild or unrecognized infections but shed virus intermittently in the genital tract. Most genital herpes infections are transmitted by persons unaware that they have the infection or who are asymptomatic when transmission occurs.

EPIDEMIOLOGY

Incidence and Prevalence

1. HSV infections are the most common cause of genital ulcerative disease in the United States and one of the most common sexually transmitted diseases (STDs). However, most people who have serological evidence of infection are asymptomatic. The National Health and Nutrition Examination Survey III (NHANES III) conducted between 1988 and 1994 estimated that 22% of the U.S. population older than 12 years is seropositive for HSV-2, yet only 9% of those testing HSV-2-positive reported a history of genital ulcerative disease (Fleming et al., 1997).
2. The incidence of new HSV-2 infections among the seronegative population increased sharply during the 1970s and 1980s. From 1970 to 1985, the annual incidence of HSV-2 infection increased by 82% (Armstrong et al., 2001). However, the U.S. age-adjusted HSV-2 prevalence has decreased from 21.0% (95% CI, 19.1–23.1) in the NHANES III conducted between 1988 and 1994 to 17.0% (95% CI: 15.8–18.3) in the NHANES conducted between 1999 and 2004 (Xu et al., 2006). This represents a 19% decrease in prevalence.
3. HSV-2 prevalence varies by age, gender, and race.

   a. Age: The prevalence of infection increases rapidly after puberty, reaching a peak in the third decade of life. Approximately 1.6% (95% CI, 1.3–2.0) of adolescents aged 14 to 19 years are infected with HSV-2 (a 72% decrease observed from the 1999 to 2004 NHANES compared to NHANES III data) and 10.6% (95% CI, 8.9–12.5) of 20- to 29-year-olds are HSV-2 seropositive (a 38% decrease observed from the 1999–2004 NHANES compared to NHANES III data) (Xu et al., 2006).

   b. Ethnicity: NHANES in 1999 to 2004 estimated overall HSV-2 seroprevalence rates to be higher among blacks (41.7%; 95% CI, 38.5–45.1) than whites (13%; 95% CI, 21.0–14.1) (Xu et al., 2006).

   c. Gender: NHANES in 1999 to 2004 estimated overall HSV-2 seroprevalence rates to be higher among females (22.8%; 95% CI, 21.2–24.4) than among males (11.2%; 95% CI, 9.9–12.6). Differences in HSV-2 prevalence rates by gender may reflect that females are more than 5 to 6 times susceptible to acquire an incident HSV-2 infection following exposure as compared to males (Wald et al., 2001).
4. Up to 50% of first-episode cases of genital herpes are caused by HSV-1. However, an estimated 96% of recurrent symptomatic genital infections are caused by HSV-2 and 4% by HSV-1 (Solomon et al., 2003).

Recurrent Episodes

1. Symptomatic recurrent episodes are more likely following primary HSV-2 infection as compared to HSV-1. In a cohort study, 180 days following a primary genital herpes episode, only 40% of HSV-1 infected patients but 90% of 123 HSV-2 infected patients experienced a symptomatic recurrence (Reeves et al., 1981). Identification of the type of infecting strain may have some prognostic importance to the individual and may be useful in counseling.
2. Asymptomatic viral shedding is more frequent following initial infection with HSV-2 than for HSV-1. In a cohort study of 110 HSV-infected females followed up with daily genital specimens for a median of 105 days, subclinical viral shedding was detected in 29% of 14 HSV-1 infected females, in 55% of HSV-2 infected females, and in 52% of females coinfected with HSV-1 and HSV-2 (Wald et al., 1995). Shedding occurred for a longer duration

in HSV-2 infected females (2% of days) compared to HSV-1 infected females (0.7% of days).

Transmission

1. Mode of transmission: Transmission is through sexual contact, either genital–genital or oral–genital, and by mucosal contact with infected secretions.
2. Reservoir: Humans are the sole known reservoir of infection.
3. Risk of transmission
   a. Gender: Females are at greater risk of HSV acquisition compared to men. Among 528 monogamous couples discordant for HSV-2 infection (261 male and 267 female susceptible to HSV-2 infection), 9.7% of females versus 1.5% of males acquired HSV-2, at a rate of 8.9/10,000 episodes of sex in females and 1.5/10,000 episodes of sex in males (Wald et al., 2001).
   b. Asymptomatic versus symptomatic: Although viral shedding is highest while genital lesions are present, most sexual transmission of HSV-2 occurs on days without genital lesions in the source partner. In a 7-week study of 69 immunocompetent persons with genital HSV-2 infection who provided daily genital mucosal swabs for HSV detection, HSV-2 was detected by polymerase chain reaction (PCR) on 27% of asymptomatic days and 87% of symptomatic days (Gupta et al., 2004).
   c. Age and sexual activity: Younger age and more frequent sexual activity were associated with higher risk of human immunodeficiency virus 2 (HIV-2) acquisition (Wald et al., 2001).
   d. HIV status: HSV-2 viral shedding rates among human immunodeficiency virus (HIV)-seropositive women was four times greater compared to HSV-2 viral shedding in HIV-seronegative women (13.2% versus 3.6%) (Augenbraun et al., 1995). HSV-2 shedding can occur in 3% of infected adults and is more likely during a first or recurrent genital HSV-2 episode (Wald et al., 2004).

   Health care providers have an obligation to inform their patients about the natural history of disease with potential recurrent episodes and the risk of transmitting HSV during asymptomatic periods. Persons with genital HSV infection should be encouraged to inform their current or prospective sexual partners that they have genital herpes.

Infections by Serological Type

1. HSV-1: Infection typically manifests as oral-labial lesions, but the frequency of HSV-1 genital infections is increasing. Recurrences and subclinical shedding are much less frequent than with genital HSV-2 infection.
2. HSV-2: Infection typically manifests as anogenital lesions. Antibodies are not routinely detected until puberty, when antibody levels correlate with past sexual activity.

PATHOGENESIS

Virus particles can be shed in salivary, cervical, and seminal secretions of infected individuals. The virus gains entry into the body through mucosal surfaces or abraded skin and replicates in the epidermal and dermal cells of a susceptible host. After replication, the virus spreads through contiguous cells to mucocutaneous projections of sensory nerves.

In oral herpes, the virus lodges in the trigeminal ganglion; in genital herpes, the sacral dorsal root (S2 to S4) ganglion is the target site. Centrifugal spread can then occur through peripheral sensory nerves back to the skin surface, so that large areas may be involved.

After resolution of the primary disease, the virus becomes latent. Latency appears to be life long but is interrupted by periods of viral reactivation, leading to silent viral shedding or clinically apparent recurrence. Reactivation of latent virus leads to transport of viral genomes to the skin surface, where replication occurs in the dermis and epidermis. Reactivation can be triggered by a variety of stimuli, such as ultraviolet light, immunosuppression, fever, pneumococcal pneumonia, stress, and local trauma. Frequency and clinical severity of reactivation depend on factors such as the host immunological status and the severity and viral type of the primary infection.

CLINICAL MANIFESTATIONS

Definition of Terms

1. Primary infection: Genital herpes in a patient seronegative for antibody to HSV-1 or HSV-2.
2. First clinical episode: First episode of clinical manifestations due to HSV-1 or HSV-2 infection. This term includes both nonprimary first episodes, (i.e., positive serology), and primary infections.
3. Recurrent clinical episode: Recurrence of genital HSV lesions in a patient with a previously documented symptomatic genital herpes episode.
4. Atypical clinical episode: Episode of clinical manifestations due to HSV-1 or HSV-2 infection that do not include *classic* genital lesions.

Classic Primary Infection

1. Primary genital HSV infection involves both systemic and local symptoms.
2. Incubation: Clinical manifestations begin approximately a week following initial infection.
3. Systemic symptoms occur over the first week of illness in more than half of infected individuals, which may include fever, headache, malaise, and myalgias.
4. Local symptoms include painful lesions (99% of females and 95% of males), dysuria (83% of females and 44% of males), pruritus, vaginal or urethral discharge, and tender inguinal adenopathy.
   a. One third of males develop urethritis whereas 70% to 90% of females develop cervicitis with first episode of infection.
   b. Herpetic lesions can be extensive and can involve the vulva, perineum, vagina, and cervix or, in males, large areas of the penis. Lesions usually begin as small papules or vesicles on an erythematous base that rapidly spread over the genital area. Multiple small pustular lesions coalesce into large areas of ulceration. Pain and irritation from lesions usually peak between days 7 and 11 of disease and heal

over the second week. Crusting and reepithelization occurs in the penile and mons area, but crusting does not occur on mucosal surfaces. Scarring is uncommon. New crops of lesions can form in more than 75% of primary infections. Lesions typically heal by the end of the third week of disease.

5. Central nervous system complaints, such as headache, stiff neck, and mild photophobia, may occur in the first week of illness in almost 70% of females and 40% of males with primary HSV-2 disease.
6. Pharyngeal infection is commonly seen in association with primary genital infection with both HSV-1 and HSV-2.
7. Median duration of viral shedding is 12 days.
8. Complications can include aseptic meningitis and other neurological complications, such as autonomic nervous system dysfunction and transverse myelitis, extragenital lesions located in the buttock, groin, or thighs areas, and disseminated disease.

First Clinical Episode

1. First episodes of genital herpes are more often associated with systemic symptoms, a prolonged duration of lesions and viral shedding, and likely to involve multiple genital and extragenital sites compared to recurrent episodes.
2. Approximately 50% of persons with their first clinical episode of symptomatic genital herpes have serological evidence of prior HSV infection, that is, the first clinical episode is not a result of the primary infection.
3. Prior HSV-1 infection diminishes the severity of first genital herpes episodes.

Recurrent Episodes

1. Clinical manifestations are localized to the genital region and are mild to moderate compared to primary infection.
2. Duration: The duration of the episode usually ranges from 6 to 12 days.
3. Prodromal symptoms: Prodromal symptoms occur in approximately 60% of episodes. Prodromal symptoms vary and can range from mild paresthesias to shooting pains in the buttocks, legs, or hips.
4. Lesions in recurrent episodes are often:
   a. *Unilateral* with a much smaller area of involvement
   b. Associated with *fewer lesions* compared to the primary infection
   c. Occur in predominantly *nonmucosal* skin
5. Clinical episodes can vary considerably in the severity and duration of disease between episodes in the same individual and among different individuals.
6. Symptoms are typically more severe among females.
7. Duration: Lesions typically heal by the second week of disease.
8. Shedding: In untreated patients, the average duration of viral shedding is 4 days.
9. After the first year, recurrences tend to decrease in frequency. Among 59 HSV-1–infected and 191 HSV-2–infected persons, the median annual recurrence rate in the first year following primary infection was one for HSV-1 infection and five for HSV-2 (Benedetti et al., 1999). In the second year, the median was zero recurrences for HSV-1 infection and four recurrences for HSV-2. The annual recurrence rate continued to decline

in subsequent years, even for patients observed for >8 years. However, one third of patients experienced no decrease in recurrences over a 5-year period, and 25% of patients had more recurrences in year 5 than in year 1 (Benedetti et al., 1999).

Atypical Episodes

1. Atypical episodes may have manifestations of either a primary infection or a recurrent episode.
2. Episodes may present with genital pruritus, papules, or fissures, dysuria, urethritis, or cervicitis.

DIFFERENTIAL DIAGNOSIS

Herpes genitalis lesions must be differentiated from early syphilis, chancroid, lymphogranuloma venereum, granuloma inguinale, excoriations, allergic and irritant contact dermatitis, and genital lesions of Behçet syndrome.

DIAGNOSIS

Genital herpes is the most prevalent cause of genital ulcers in the United States. Patients with genital ulcer disease can also be infected with syphilis and/or chancroid. The clinical diagnosis of genital herpes is both insensitive and nonspecific. The classical painful multiple vesicular or ulcerative lesions are absent in many infected persons. Up to 50% of first-episode cases of genital herpes are caused by HSV-1, but recurrences and subclinical shedding are much less frequent for genital HSV-1 infection than genital HSV-2 infection. As the distinction between HSV-1 and HSV-2 influences prognosis and counseling, the clinical diagnosis of genital herpes should be confirmed by laboratory testing.

Laboratory Evaluation

1. Virological tests: Isolation of HSV in cell culture is the preferred virological test in patients who present with genital ulcers or other mucocutaneous lesions. However, sensitivity of culture may be low in recurrent lesions and declines rapidly as lesions begin to heal.
   a. Culture technique: Obtaining the proper specimen and using the appropriate transport medium and conditions is essential for culturing a viable organism.
      • Intact vesicles: If intact vesicles are present, aspirate the vesicle fluid using a fine-gauge needle or, if vesicles are too small to aspirate, gently unroof the vesicle and swab the debris at the vesicle base. Use cotton or Dacron swabs (without a wooden stick) rather than calcium alginate, which inactivates the virus, and place the specimen in viral transport medium.
      • Pustules: If pustules are present, unroof the pustule and wash away purulent material with sterile saline; then swab the base of the lesion.
      • Ruptured vesicle: To culture a ruptured vesicle or ulcer, swab the base of the lesion.
      • Crusted lesion: If a lesion is crusted, wash away necrotic debris with sterile saline, then swab the lesion base. When swabbing the base of a lesion, remember that friction must be used to obtain cells. Avoid contaminating the specimen with alcohol, soap, blood, or stool.

If viral transport medium is not available, substitute sterile distilled water. Leave the swab in the transport medium if transport time is <8 hours. If transport time is longer, swirl the swab vigorously in the medium and remove. If a laboratory courier is used, refrigerate the specimen before pickup.

b. Polymerase chain reaction (PCR) assays: PCR assays for HSV DNA are more sensitive and may be used instead of viral culture; however, PCR tests are not Food and Drug Administration (FDA)-cleared for testing of genital specimens. As with culture, lack of HSV detection does not indicate lack of HSV infection, as viral shedding is intermittent. Both PCR and viral culture should be typed to determine if HSV-1 or HSV-2 is the cause of the infection.

c. Cytological detection: Cytological detection of cellular changes of herpes virus infection is insensitive and nonspecific, both in genital lesions (Tzanck preparation) and cervical Pap smears, and should not be used.

2. Type-specific serological tests: Both type-specific and non–type-specific antibodies to HSV develop during the first several weeks following infection and persist indefinitely. Accurate type-specific assays for HSV antibodies must be based on the HSV-specific glycoprotein G2 for the diagnosis of HSV-2 infection and glycoprotein G1 for diagnosis of HSV-1 infection. Such assays first became commercially available in 1999, but older assays that do not accurately distinguish HSV-1 from HSV-2 antibody, despite claims to the contrary, remain commercially available. Therefore, the type-specific gG-based assays should be specifically requested when serology is performed.

a. Available tests: Currently, the FDA-approved gG-based type-specific assays are moderate complexity, laboratory-based tests, and point-of-care tests that provide results for HSV-2 antibodies from capillary blood or serum. The laboratory gG-based type-specific tests include HerpeSelect 1 ELISA IgG, HerpeSelect 2 ELISA IgG, and HerpeSelect1 and 2 Immunoblot IgG (Focus Diagnostics Inc., Cypress, CA); and CAPTIA HSV-1 IgG Type Specific EIA and CAPTIA HSV-2 IgG Type Specific EIA (Trinity Biotech, Bray, Ireland). The point-of-care tests include the Biokit HSV-2 Rapid Test (Biokit USA, Lexington, MA) and Sure Vue HSV-2 Rapid Test (Fisher Health Care, Houston, TX).

b. Sensitivity and specificity: The sensitivities of these tests for detection of HSV-2 antibody vary from 80% to 98%, and false-negative results may occur, especially at early stages of infection. The specificities of these assays are ≥96%. False-positive results can occur, especially in patients with low likelihood of HSV infection. Repeat or confirmatory testing may be indicated in some settings, especially if recent acquisition of genital herpes is suspected.

c. Meaning of positive test: Most people with HSV-2 antibody by type-specific testing have anogenital HSV infection acquired during adolescence or adulthood, which may be asymptomatic. Most people with HSV-1 antibody have oral HSV infection acquired in childhood, which also may be asymptomatic. However, acquisition of genital HSV-1 appears to be increasing, and genital infection may be asymptomatic. Lack of symptoms in an HSV-1 seropositive person does not distinguish anogenital from orolabial or cutaneous infection. Persons with HSV-1 infection remain at risk for HSV-2 acquisition.

d. Potential uses of type-specific test: Type-specific HSV serological assays may be useful in the following clinical situations:
  • Recurrent or atypical genital symptoms with negative HSV cultures
  • A clinical diagnosis of genital herpes without laboratory confirmation
  • A sex partner with genital herpes
  Some experts believe that HSV serological testing should be included in a comprehensive evaluation for STDs in persons with multiple sexual partners, in persons with HIV infection, and in men who have sex with men (who have a higher risk of HIV acquisition). Screening for HSV-1 or HSV-2 in the general population is not indicated.

3. Additional laboratory workup: Additional evaluation of a genital ulcer should include a serological test for syphilis. In settings where chancroid is prevalent, a *Haemophilus ducreyi* culture should also be performed. Because STD coinfection is frequent among adolescents, evaluation for gonorrhea, chlamydia, trichomonas, and an HIV test should also be performed.

THERAPY

Principles of Genital Herpes Management

Antiviral chemotherapy offers clinical benefits to most symptomatic patients and is the mainstay of management. In addition, counseling regarding the natural history of genital herpes, sexual and perinatal transmission, and methods to reduce transmission is integral to clinical management.

Systemic antiviral drugs partially control the symptoms and signs of herpes episodes when used to treat first clinical episodes and recurrent episodes or when used as daily suppressive therapy. However, these drugs neither eradicate latent virus nor affect the risk, frequency, or severity of recurrences after the drug is discontinued. Randomized trials indicate that three antiviral medications provide clinical benefit for genital herpes—acyclovir, valacyclovir, and famciclovir. Valacyclovir is the valine ester of acyclovir and has enhanced absorption on oral administration. Famciclovir, a prodrug of penciclovir, also has high oral bioavailability. Topical therapy with antiviral drugs for genital HSV offers minimal clinical benefit, and is not recommended (Centers for Disease Control and Prevention, 2006).

First Clinical Episode of Genital Herpes

Many patients with first-episode herpes present with mild clinical manifestations but later develop severe or prolonged symptoms. The Centers for Disease Control and Prevention (CDC) (Centers for Disease Control and Prevention, 2006) recommend that patients with initial genital herpes should receive antiviral therapy.

CDC recommended regimens:

Acyclovir 400 mg orally three times a day for 7 to 10 days, OR
Acyclovir 200 mg orally five times a day for 7 to 10 days, OR
Famciclovir 250 mg orally three times a day for 7 to 10 days,

OR
Valacyclovir 1 g orally twice a day for 7 to 10 days.
Treatment may be extended if healing is incomplete after 10 days of therapy.

Established Herpes Simplex Virus -2 Infection

Most patients with symptomatic, first-episode genital HSV-2 infection subsequently experience recurrent episodes of genital lesions; recurrences are much less frequent following initial genital HSV-1 infection. Intermittent asymptomatic shedding occurs in all patients with genital HSV-2 infection, even in those with long-standing or clinically silent infection. Treatment options should be discussed with all patients, regardless of severity or frequency of recurrent outbreaks. Antiviral therapy for recurrent genital herpes can be administered either episodically to diminish or shorten the duration of lesions, or continuously as suppressive therapy to reduce the frequency of recurrences and possibly decrease the risk of transmission to susceptible partners.

Suppressive Therapy for Recurrent Genital Herpes

Suppressive therapy reduces the frequency of genital herpes recurrences by 70% to 80% among patients who have frequent recurrences (i.e., ≥ 6 recurrences/year), and many patients report no symptomatic outbreaks. Treatment is also effective in patients with less frequent recurrences. Safety and efficacy have been documented among patients receiving daily therapy with acyclovir for as long as 6 years, and with valacyclovir or famciclovir for 1 year. Quality of life is often improved in patients with frequent recurrences who receive suppressive compared with episodic treatment. The frequency of recurrent outbreaks diminishes over time in many patients, and the patient's psychological adjustment to the disease may change. Therefore, the need to continue therapy should be discussed periodically during suppressive treatment (e.g., once a year).

CDC recommended regimens:

Acyclovir 400 mg orally twice a day,
OR
Famciclovir 250 mg orally twice a day,
OR
Valacyclovir 500 mg orally once a day*,
OR
Valacyclovir 1 g orally once a day.
*Valacyclovir 500 mg once a day might be less effective than other valacyclovir or acyclovir dosing regimens in patients who have very frequent recurrences (i.e., ≥ 10 episodes/year).

Overall, valacyclovir and famciclovir are most likely comparable to acyclovir in clinical outcome. Ease of administration and cost also are important considerations for prolonged treatment.

Episodic Therapy for Recurrent Genital Herpes

Effective episodic treatment of recurrent herpes requires initiation of therapy within 1 day of lesion onset, or during the prodrome that precedes some outbreaks. In those with known genital infection, a supply of drug or a prescription can be provided with instructions to self-initiate treatment immediately when symptoms begin.

CDC recommended regimens:

Acyclovir 400 mg orally three times a day for 5 days,
OR
Acyclovir 800 mg orally twice a day for 5 days,
OR
Acyclovir 800 mg orally three times a day for 2 days
OR
Famciclovir 125 mg orally twice a day for 5 days,
OR
Famciclovir 1,000 mg orally twice daily for 1 day,
OR
Valacyclovir 500 mg orally twice a day for 3 days,
OR
Valacyclovir 1 g orally once a day for 5 days.

Severe Disease

Intravenous acyclovir therapy should be provided for patients who have severe disease or complications that necessitate hospitalization, such as disseminated infection, pneumonitis, hepatitis, or complications of the central nervous system (e.g., meningitis or encephalitis). The recommended regimen is acyclovir 5 to 10 mg/kg body weight IV every 8 hours for 2 to 7 days or until clinical improvement is observed, followed by oral antiviral therapy to complete at least 10 days of total therapy (Centers for Disease Control and Prevention, 2006).

Human Immunodeficiency Virus Infection

Immunocompromised patients may have prolonged or severe episodes of genital, perianal, or oral herpes. Lesions caused by HSV are common among HIV-infected patients and may be severe, painful, and atypical. HSV shedding is increased in HIV-infected persons. Although antiretroviral therapy reduces the severity and frequency of symptomatic genital herpes, frequent subclinical shedding still occurs. Subclinical mucosal HSV is associated with higher loads of mucosal HIV. Suppressive or episodic therapy with oral antiviral agents is effective in decreasing the clinical manifestations of HSV among HIV-seropositive persons. HIV-infected persons are likely to be more contagious for HSV; the extent to which suppressive antiviral therapy will decrease HSV transmission from this population is unknown. As HIV-infected persons are evaluated for a variety of chronic infections that may become problematic with increasing immunosuppression, some experts suggest that type-specific serologies should be offered to HIV-infected persons during their initial evaluation, and suppressive antiviral therapy considered.

CDC recommended regimens for daily suppressive therapy in persons infected with HIV:

Acyclovir 400 to 800 mg orally two to three times a day,
OR
Famciclovir 500 mg orally twice a day,
OR
Valacyclovir 500 mg orally twice a day.

Recommended regimens for episodic infection in persons infected with HIV:

Acyclovir 400 mg orally three times a day for 5 to 10 days,

OR
Famciclovir 500 mg orally twice a day for 5 to 10 days,
OR
Valacyclovir 1 g orally twice a day for 5 to 10 days.

In the doses recommended for treatment of genital herpes, acyclovir, valacyclovir, and famciclovir are safe for use in immunocompromised patients. For severe cases, initiating therapy with acyclovir 5 to 10 mg/kg body weight IV every 8 hours may be necessary.

If lesions persist or recur in a patient receiving antiviral treatment, HSV resistance should be suspected and a viral isolate obtained for sensitivity testing. Such patients should be managed in consultation with a specialist, and alternate therapy, such as foscarnet or topical cidofovir gel 1%, should be considered.

Management of Sex Partners

The sex partners of patients who have genital herpes likely benefit from evaluation and counseling. Symptomatic sex partners should be evaluated and treated in the same manner as patients who have genital lesions. Asymptomatic sex partners of patients who have genital herpes should be questioned concerning histories of genital lesions, and offered type-specific serological testing for HSV infection.

PREVENTION

1. Avoidance of intercourse: Sexual transmission of HSV can occur during asymptomatic periods. Persons with active lesions or prodromal symptoms should abstain from intercourse with uninfected partners until the lesions are clearly healed.
2. Condom use: Because viral shedding can occur in the absence of lesions, providers should recommend consistent and correct condoms use to any patient who has had an episode of genital herpes. Male latex condoms may reduce the risk of HSV acquisition and infection. Among 1,843 HSV-2–negative men and women with four or more sexual partners or an STD in the last year, persons reporting more frequent condom use were at lower risk for acquiring HSV-2 than persons who used condoms less frequently (Wald et al., 2005). In a study following 528 monogamous couples discordant for HSV-2 infection, condom use during ≥25% of sex acts was associated with protection against HSV-2 acquisition in for women, but not for men (Wald et al., 2001). Wald also found that the HSV-2 acquisition rate decreased with decreasing sexual activity. Having sex when genital lesions were present increased the risk of HSV-2 acquisition, but the increase did not reach statistical significance (Wald et al., 2001).
3. Use of suppressive therapy: Treatment with valacyclovir 500 mg daily decreases the rate of HSV-2 transmission in discordant, heterosexual couples in which the source partner has a history of genital HSV-2 infection (Corey et al., 2004). HSV-2 discordant couples should be encouraged to consider suppressive antiviral therapy as part of a strategy to prevent transmission, in addition to avoidance of sexual activity during recurrences and consistent condom use. These findings are also likely to apply to persons who have multiple partners, to those who are HSV-2 seropositive without a history of genital herpes, and to men who have sex with men, because the effect of antiviral therapy on viral shedding is unlikely to be related to the behavior of the infected persons.
4. Vaccination: No effective vaccine is yet available for HSV. However, research is continuing in the development of an effective vaccine.

COMPLICATIONS

1. Significant psychological distress: Initially, denial, shock, fear, guilt, feelings of social isolation, and anger are common. Anxiety and depression also occur and may persist in some patients.
2. Local complications: Secondary bacterial infection of lesions, phimosis (males) or labial adhesions (females), urinary retention, constipation, and impotence. Sacral radiculopathy can also occur, causing paresthesias in the lower extremities.
3. Proctitis: Occurs predominately in persons who participate in receptive anal intercourse. Presenting complaints may include rectal bleeding, mucoid discharge, constipation, tenesmus, fever, and, occasionally, impotence.
4. Herpes keratitis: This is predominantly associated with HSV-1 infection.
5. Encephalitis and meningitis: Encephalitis is typically associated with oral HSV-1 infection and aseptic meningitis is typically associated with genital HSV-2 infection.
6. Neonatal herpes: Most mothers of infants who acquire neonatal herpes lack histories of clinically evident genital herpes. The risk for transmission to the neonate from an infected mother is high (30%–50%) among women who acquire genital herpes near the time of delivery and is low (<1%) among women with histories of recurrent herpes at term or who acquire genital HSV during the first half of pregnancy. However, because recurrent genital herpes is much more common than initial HSV infection during pregnancy, the proportion of neonatal HSV infections acquired from mothers with recurrent herpes remains high. Prevention of neonatal herpes depends both on preventing acquisition of genital HSV infection during late pregnancy and avoiding exposure of the infant to herpetic lesions during delivery. Infants exposed to HSV during birth, as documented by virological testing or presumed by observation of lesions, should be followed up carefully in consultation with a specialist.

WEB SITES

For Teenagers and Parents

http://www.ashastd.org. The Herpes Resource Center *(HRC, supported by the American Social Health Association [ASHA]) focuses on increasing education, public awareness, and support to anyone concerned about herpes. The HRC provides accurate information about herpes with informational Web sites, brochures and books, a hotline, a chat room, e-mail responses to questions, and referrals to local Support Groups.* Accessed May 7, 2007.

National Herpes Hotline (supported by ASHA). *Provides accurate information and appropriate referrals to anyone concerned about herpes.* Telephone:1-800-277-8922.

http://www.cdc.gov/std/Herpes/default.htm. Centers for Disease Control and Prevention. *Provides patient HSV information.* Accessed May 7, 2007.

http://www.herpeshelp.com/ (Supported by Glaxo Wellcome). Herpes help informational Web site. Accessed May 7, 2007.

http://www.iwannaknow.org/ (Supported by ASHA). Provides information to teens and parents about teen sexual health and STDs. Accessed May 7, 2007.

www.plannedparenthood.org/. Planned Parenthood HSV informational Web site. Accessed May 7, 2007.

For Health Professionals

http://www.cdc.gov/STD/treatment. Sexually Transmitted Diseases Treatment Guidelines, 2006. Accessed May 7, 2007.

REFERENCES AND ADDITIONAL READINGS

Armstrong GL, Schillinger J, Markowitz L, et al. Incidence of herpes simplex virus type 2 infection in the United States. *Am J Epidemiol* 2001;153:912.

Augenbraun M, Feldman J, Chirgwin K, et al. Increased genital shedding of herpes simplex virus type 2 in HIV-seropositive women. *Ann Intern Med* 1995;123:845.

Benedetti J, Corey L, Ashley R. Recurrence rates in genital herpes after symptomatic first-episode infection. *Ann Intern Med* 1994;121:847.

Benedetti JK, Zeh J, Selke S, et al. Frequency and reactivation of nongenital lesions among patients with genital herpes simplex virus. *Am J Med* 1995;98:237.

Benedetti JK, Zeh J, Corey L. Clinical reactivation of genital herpes simplex virus infection decreases in frequency over time. *Ann Intern Med* 1999;131:14.

Centers for Disease Control and Prevention. Sexually transmitted diseases treatment guidelines 2006. *MMWR* 2006;55 (RR11):16–20.

Chosidow O, Drouault Y, Leconte-Veyriac F, et al. Famciclovir vs. acyclovir in immunocompetent patients with recurrent genital herpes infections: a parallel-groups, randomized, double-blind clinical trial. *Br J Dermatol* 2001;144:818.

Conant MA, Schacker TW, Murphy RL, et al. Valacyclovir versus acyclovir for herpes simplex virus infection in HIV-infected individuals: two randomized trials. *Int J STD AIDS* 2002;13:12.

Corey L, Handsfield HH. Genital herpes and public health: addressing a global problem. *JAMA* 2000;283:791.

Corey L, Wald A. Genital herpes. In: Holmes KK, Sparling PF, Mardh PA, et al., eds. *Sexually transmitted diseases*, 4th ed. New York: McGraw-Hill; 2007.

Corey L, Wald A, Patel R, et al. Once-daily valacyclovir to reduce the risk of transmission of genital herpes. *N Engl J Med* 2004;350:11.

Cowan FM. Testing for type-specific antibody to herpes simplex virus–implications for clinical practice. *J Antimicrob Chemother* 2000;45(Suppl T3):9.

DeJesus E, Wald A, Warren T, et al. Valacyclovir for the suppression of recurrent genital herpes in human. *J Infect Dis* 2003;188:1009.

Druce J, Catton M, Chibo D, et al. Utility of a multiplex PCR assay for detecting herpesvirus DNA in clinical samples. *J Clin Microbiol* 2002;40:1728.

Fleming DT, McQuillan GM, Johnson RE, et al. Herpes simplex virus type 2 in the United States, 1976 to 1994. *N Engl J Med* 1997;337:1105.

Gottlieb SL, Douglas JM Jr, Foster M, et al. Incidence of herpes simplex virus type 2 infection in 5 Sexually Transmitted Disease (STD) clinics and the effect of HIV/STD risk-reduction counseling. *J Infect Dis* 2004;190:1059.

Gupta R, Wald A, Krantz E, et al. Valacyclovir and acyclovir for suppression of shedding of herpes simplex virus in the genital tract. *J Infect Dis* 2004;190:1374.

Haddow LJ, Mindel A. Genital herpes vaccines–cause for cautious optimism. *Sex Health* 2006;3:1.

Laffery WE, Downey L, Celum C, et al. Herpes simplex virus type 1 as a cause of genital herpes: impact on surveillance and prevention. *J Infect Dis* 2000;181:1454.

Langenberg AGM, Corey L, Ashley RL, et al. A prospective study of new infections with herpes simplex virus type 1 and type 2. *N Engl J Med* 1999;341:1432.

Leone PA, Trottier S, Miller JM. Valacyclovir for episodic treatment of genital herpes: a shorter 3-day treatment course compared with 5-day treatment. *Clin Infect Dis* 2002;34:958.

McCormack O, Carboy J, Nguyen L, et al. Clinical inquiries. What is the role of herpes virus serology in sexually transmitted disease screening? *J Fam Pract* 2006;55:451.

Mertz GJ, Benedetti J, Ashley R, et al. Risk factors for the sexual transmission of genital herpes. *Ann Intern Med* 1992;116:197.

Mertz GJ, Schmidt O, Jourden JL, et al. Frequency of acquisition of first-episode genital infection with herpes simplex virus from symptomatic and asymptomatic source contact. *Sex Transm Dis* 1985;12:33.

Miyai T, Turner KR, Kent CK, et al. The psychosocial impact of testing individuals with no history of genital herpes for herpes simplex virus type 2. *Sex Transm Dis* 2004;31:517.

Posavad CM, Wald A, Kuntz S, et al. Frequent reactivation of herpes simplex virus among HIV-1-infected patients treated with highly active antiretroviral therapy. *J Infect Dis* 2004;190:693.

Reeves WC, Corey L, Adams HG, et al. Risk of recurrences after first episodes of genital herpes. Relations to HSV type and antibody response. *N Engl J Med* 1981;305:315.

Romanowski B, Aoki FY, Martel AY, et al., Collaborative Famciclovir HIV Study Group. Efficacy and safety of famciclovir for treating mucocutaneous herpes simplex infection in HIV-infected individuals. *AIDS* 2000;14:1211.

Romanowski B, Marina RB, Roberts JN. Valtrex HS230017 Study Group. Patients' preference of valacyclovir once-daily suppressive therapy versus twice-daily episodic therapy for recurrent genital herpes: a randomized study. *Sex Transm Dis* 2003;30:226.

Sacks SL. Famciclovir suppression of asymptomatic and symptomatic recurrent anogenital herpes simplex virus shedding in women: a randomized, double-blind, double-dummy, placebo-controlled, parallel-group, single-center trial. *J Infect Dis* 2004;189:1341.

Scoular A. Using the evidence base on genital herpes: optimising the use of diagnostic tests and information provision. *Sex Transm Infect* 2002;78:160.

Scoular A, Gillespie G, Carman WF. Polymerase chain reaction for diagnosis of genital herpes in a genitourinary medicine clinic. *Sex Transm Infect* 2002;78:21.

Solomon L, Cannon MJ, Reyes M, et al. Epidemiology of recurrent genital herpes simplex virus types 1 and 2. *Sex Transm Infect* 2003;79:456.

Song B, Dwyer DE, Mindel A. HSV type specific serology in sexual health clinics: use, benefits, and who gets tested. *Sex Transm Infect* 2004;80:113.

Turner KR, Wong EH, Kent CK, et al. Serologic herpes testing in the real world: validation of new type-specific serologic herpes simplex virus tests in a public health laboratory. *Sex Transm Dis* 2002;29:422.

Wald A, Carrell D, Remington M, et al. Two-day regimen of acyclovir for treatment of recurrent genital herpes simplex virus type 2 infection. *Clin Infect Dis* 2002;34:944.

Wald A, Ericsson M, Krantz E, et al. Oral shedding of herpes simples virus type 2. *Sex Transm Infect* 2004;80:272.

Wald A, Huang ML, Carrell D, et al. Polymerase chain reaction for detection of Herpes Simplex Virus (HSV) DNA on mucosal surfaces: comparison with HSV isolation in cell culture. *J Infect Dis* 2003;188:1345.

Wald A, Langenberg AGM, Krantz E, et al. The relationship between condom use and herpes simplex virus acquisition. *Ann Intern Med* 2005;143:707.

Wald A, Langenberg AGM, Link K, et al. Effect of condoms on reducing the transmission of herpes simplex virus type 2 from men to women. *JAMA* 2001;285:3100.

Wald A, Zeh J, Selke S, et al. Virological characteristics of subclinical and symptomatic genital herpes infection. *N Engl J Med* 1995;333:770.

Whittington WL, Celum CL, Cent A, et al. Use of a glycoprotein G-based type-specific assay to detect antibodies to herpes simplex virus type 2 among persons attending sexually transmitted disease clinics. *Sex Transm Dis* 2001;28:99.

Xu F, Sternberg MR, Kottiri BJ, et al. Trends in herpes simplex virus type 1 and type 2 seroprevalence in the United States. *JAMA* 2006;296:964.

Zimet GD, Rosenthal SL, Fortenberry JD, et al. Factors predicting the acceptance of herpes simplex virus type 2 antibody testing among adolescents and young adults. *Sex Transm Dis* 2004;31:665.

CHAPTER 66

Human Papillomavirus Infection and Anogenital Warts

Jessica A. Kahn

HUMAN PAPILLOMAVIRUS

Human papillomavirus (HPV) infection is the most prevalent sexually transmitted infection (STD) in the United States. Most HPV infections are asymptomatic. However, HPV infection may cause anogenital warts, oral warts, recurrent respiratory papillomatosis (RRP), abnormal Pap tests, cervical intraepithelial neoplasia (CIN), and cervical cancer. Other anogenital and oropharyngeal malignancies also are strongly associated with HPV infection. This chapter focuses on the epidemiology of HPV infection and the diagnosis, treatment, and prevention of anogenital warts. Cervical cancer screening and management of abnormal Pap tests are reviewed in Chapter 54.

Human Papillomavirus Genotypes and Clinical Sequelae

Human papillomaviruses are small, nonenveloped, double-stranded DNA viruses of the Papillomaviridae family. More than 130 HPV types have been sequenced and typed, and they are classified as cutaneous or as mucosal (de Villiers et al., 2004). Cutaneous types (e.g., types 1, 2, and 4) cause common skin warts and plantar warts. Mucosal types cause diseases of the anogenital and aerodigestive tracts. Approximately 40 mucosal types have been identified. HPV classification is based on genetic similarities in the viral capsid peptide L1—different types share <90% homology. Genital HPV types are classified as low risk (e.g., 6, 11, 40, 42, 43, 44, 54, 61, 70, 72, 81) and high risk (e.g., 16, 18, 31, 33, 35, 39, 45, 51, 52, 56, 58, 59, 68, 73, 82), depending on their clinical sequelae. Low-risk types (primarily types 6 and 11) cause anogenital warts and are also associated with mild vulvar intraepithelial neoplasia (VIN), vaginal intraepithelial neoplasia (VAIN), CIN, penile intraepithelial neoplasia (PIN), and anal intraepithelial neoplasia (AIN). Vertical transmission of low-risk types from mother to child during delivery rarely may cause RRP in young children. High-risk types (primarily types 16 and 18) may cause mild, moderate, or severe VIN, VAIN, CIN, PIN, and AIN as well as cervical cancer. Persistent infection with high-risk types is a key risk factor for development of CIN and cervical cancer.

The HPV genome is divided into two functional regions. One region encodes for early proteins (E1, E2, E4, E5, E6, and E7). These control viral replication, transcription, and cellular transformation. The E6 and E7 proteins in high-risk HPV types interact with the tumor suppressor gene products p53 and retinoblastoma protein, resulting in cell proliferation and contributing to carcinogenesis. Another region of the genome encodes for the nucleocapsid proteins L1 and L2. When HPV infection occurs, the low-risk types tend to remain extrachromosomal (episomal); in contrast, viral DNA sequences integrate into the host genomes in human cervical carcinomas.

Epidemiology

Prevalence At least 75% of sexually active adult men and women in the United States have been exposed to genital HPV types at some point in their lives. Approximately 20% of adults are currently infected and approximately 5.5 million new infections occur each year. The prevalence of HPV infection peaks during adolescence and young adulthood, and declines with age. Studies have shown that over a 2- to 3-year period, approximately 30% to 40% of college-aged women will acquire HPV infection. In a nationally-representative sample of U.S. women, 20% of 14- to 17-year-olds, 38% of 18- to 21-year-olds, and 42% of 22- to 25-year-olds were HPV-positive. The majority of women with HPV had at least one high-risk type (Kahn et al., 2007). As methods for detection of HPV DNA in men improve, it has become clear that prevalence rates in men are similar to those in women. HPV DNA has been detected from the penile shaft, glans, foreskin, scrotum, and urine in men—sampling additional sites increases detection of HPV DNA.

Prevalence rates of symptomatic anogenital warts vary depending on the population studied. The prevalence rate among U.S. adults is estimated to be 1% to 5%, but prevalence rates up to 40% have been reported in patients presenting to STD clinics. HPV has also been found by polymerase chain reaction (PCR) techniques in 13% to 30% of women who have sex with women (WSW). The prevalence of RRP is approximately 4 cases per 100,000 in children; approximately 7 of 1,000 children born to mothers with genital warts will develop RRP.

Transmission In adolescents, HPV transmission occurs primarily through sexual contact, including genital–genital, oral–genital, and digital–genital contact. Both heterosexual and homosexual transmission occurs. HPV infections as well as high- and low-grade squamous intraepithelial lesions have been detected on Pap tests in WSW who have reported no sexual encounters with men (Marrazzo JM et al., 2001). Adolescents acquire HPV infection rapidly after sexual initiation, often within a few months.

Infants, young children, and preadolescents may acquire HPV infection in several ways—transplacentally through amniotic fluid during gestation, through direct exposure to cervical and genital lesions during birth, through heteroinoculation or autoinoculation after birth, as a result of sexual abuse, and perhaps through fomites. Infection in infants and children presents most commonly as anogenital warts or RRP. Although sexual abuse is less likely than other modes of transmission in children with HPV-associated anogenital warts or RRP, especially in those younger than 4 years, sexual abuse should be carefully considered in all children with these conditions. The likelihood of sexual abuse as the cause for HPV infection increases with age.

Risk Factors The behavioral and biological risk factors for HPV acquisition are as follows:

1. Multiple sexual partners: The number of male sexual partners is strongly linked to HPV infection in women, as is male partners' number of sexual partners.
2. Early age at sexual initiation: The association between early age of first sexual intercourse and HPV infection appears to be mediated primarily by sexual behaviors; that is, those who initiate sexual intercourse at an early age tend to practice sexual behaviors that put them at risk for HPV infection.
3. Nonuse of condoms: In the past, evidence was inconsistent as to whether condom use reduces the risk of HPV acquisition. However, studies have indicated that condom use reduces the risk of genital warts, moderate and severe cervical dysplasia, and invasive cervical cancer. Recent studies have provided more convincing evidence that consistent condom use substantially reduces incident genital HPV infection (Winer et al., 2006).
4. Cigarette smoking: Smoking is linked to HPV acquisition and appears to be a cofactor in cervical carcinogenesis.
5. Immunosuppression: Human immunodeficiency virus (HIV) infection and organ transplantation are important risk factors for HPV acquisition, persistence of infection, progression to cervical cancer and other anogenital cancers, and lack of response to treatment for anogenital warts.
6. Cervical ectopy: Cervical ectopy occurs during puberty when the columnar epithelium that lines the endocervix extends out onto the ectocervix. The process of squamous metaplasia then causes columnar epithelium to differentiate into squamous epithelium. Columnar and metaplastic cells may be particularly vulnerable to infection with STDs such as HPV because their thin epithelium may facilitate HPV infection. In addition, metaplasia is a process of rapid cell proliferation and differentiation, which provides a good environment for HPV replication and protein expression.
7. Oral contraceptive use: It is unclear what impact oral contraceptive pills have on HPV acquisition, as some studies show a protective effect in adolescents (Moscicki et al., 2001; Boardman et al., 2005). However, some studies suggest that oral contraceptive pills may be a cofactor in cervical carcinogenesis.
8. History of genital warts and other STDs, including genital herpes.

Pathophysiology and Natural History of Human Papillomavirus Infection

HPV initially infects the basal layer of epithelial cells through microabrasions in the skin or mucosa. Infection results in proliferation, division, and lateral expansion of infected cells. Subsequently, infected cells migrate to the suprabasal layers, where viral gene expression and thereby viral replication and particle formation occur. As viral particle formation continues in the upper layers of the epidermis or mucosa, viral particles are released to infect adjacent tissue.

Although HPV infection is extremely common in adolescents, infections are usually transient. More than 90% of adolescents with subclinical HPV infection become HPV negative within 9 to 12 months. A recent longitudinal study of sexually active adolescent girls demonstrated that the median time to clearance was 32 weeks for high-risk types and 24 weeks for low-risk types (Brown et al., 2005).

Clinical Manifestations

Types of Anogenital Warts
1. Condylomata acuminata: Cauliflower-shaped growths with a granular surface and finger-like projections. They usually have highly vascular cores that produce punctuated or loop-like patterns unless obscured by overlying keratinized surfaces.
2. Papular warts: Smooth, skin-colored, well-circumscribed papules that are usually 1 to 4 mm in diameter and lack finger-like projections.
3. Keratotic warts: These have a thick, horny (crust-like) layer; they resemble common warts or seborrheic keratoses.
4. Flat-topped papules: These are subclinical lesions that are difficult to detect without techniques such as treatment with a weak acetic acid solution.

Location Typical sites for anogenital warts in women include the cervix, vagina, vulva, urethra, and anus. Typical sites in men include the inner surface of the prepuce, frenulum, corona, penile shaft, glans, scrotum, and anus. Condylomata can be multifocal (one or more lesions at one anatomical site) or multicentric (lesions at multiple separate anatomical sites).

Condylomata acuminata tend to occur on partially keratinized, non–hair-bearing ("moist") skin; keratotic and papular warts tend to occur on fully keratinized (hair-bearing or non–hair-bearing) skin; and flat-topped warts may occur on either skin surface.

Color Pink, red, tan, brown, or gray.

Symptoms Usually asymptomatic but may cause pruritus, burning, pain, urethral or vaginal discharge, urethral bleeding, or postcoital bleeding.

Exacerbating Factors Pregnancy, skin moisture, and/or vaginal or urethral discharge.

Clinical Course Lesions usually appear 2 to 3 months after infection, with a range of approximately 3 weeks to 8 months. However, viral latency may occur and therefore lesions may appear years after infection (Beutner and Ferenczy, 1997). The clinical course of anogenital warts is not well understood. Warts may regress spontaneously, persist, or increase in size or number. They often recur after therapy. However, over a period of months to years most anogenital warts resolve.

Differential Diagnosis

1. Micropapillomatosis labialis of labia minora: Lesions with separate bases that do not converge as do the papillae of condylomata acuminata
2. Pearly penile papules (in males): Parallel rows of small angiofibromas located at the penile corona, which are a normal finding
3. Seborrheic keratoses: Localized hyperpigmented lesions
4. Other benign genital lesions: Skin tags, fibromas, lipomas, hidradenomas, and adenomas
5. Condylomata latum: Owing to secondary syphilis, and diagnosed with dark-field examination and serological testing
6. Molluscum contagiosum: Dome-shaped lesions with central umbilication that are caused by a poxvirus
7. Granuloma inguinale (verrucous type): A rare STD caused by *Calymmatobacterium granulomatis*; Donovan bodies are found in crushed tissue smears
8. High-grade intraepithelial lesions and cancer: Bowen disease, Bowenoid papulosis, dysplastic nevi, VIN, VAIN, PIN, AIN, and squamous cell carcinoma

Diagnosis

Subclinical Human Papillomavirus Infection
The Hybrid Capture II assay is a hybridization and signal amplification technique that detects 13 different high-risk HPV types. PCR-based detection methods are not yet commercially available in the United States. Currently, HPV DNA testing is recommended routinely only in the context of cervical cancer screening in women, as discussed in Chapter 54.

Genital Warts
Genital warts can usually be diagnosed using direct visual inspection with a bright light and, if necessary, magnification. A speculum examination is helpful in women with external genital warts to evaluate for vaginal and cervical warts. An otoscope and small spreader is helpful to inspect the male urinary meatus. Anoscopy should be considered for men and women with recurrent perianal warts and/or a history of anoreceptive intercourse, and urethroscopy should be considered for men with warts at the terminal urethra, and terminal hematuria or an altered urinary stream. Acetowhite testing, HPV DNA testing, and biopsy are not recommended routinely for diagnosis. However, patients with anogenital warts who are not responsive to therapy or have features suggestive of neoplasia (e.g., blue or black discoloration, induration, bleeding, ulceration, increased pigmentation, rapid growth, or fixation to underlying structures) should be referred to a specialist for further evaluation and possible biopsy.

Treatment

General Considerations
The goal of therapy is to eradicate or reduce the size of clinically apparent anogenital warts. However, because anogenital warts may resolve spontaneously and because it is not clear whether treatment of anogenital warts alters the natural history of the infection or decreases future viral transmission, it is reasonable not to begin treatment unless the warts persist or enlarge. Treatment should be guided by the patient's preferences, extent and type of lesion, the provider's experience, and available resources.

General treatment considerations include eliminating or minimizing any predisposing factors and treating co-existing vaginitis and/or cervicitis. Specific treatments for external genital warts can be classified as patient-applied or clinician-applied treatments. Patient-applied therapies require that the patient can adequately visualize the lesions to be treated and can adhere to the specified treatment schedule. There is no definitive evidence that any one treatment is more effective than another. The various treatment strategies, initial treatment success rates, and reported recurrence rates are summarized in Table 66.1, and the instructions for use, and advantages and disadvantages of these strategies are presented in Table 66.2. Clinical trials of treatment strategies vary widely in terms of patient selection, type of wart treated, duration of therapy, length of follow-up, use of concomitant therapies, outcomes assessed, and overall quality. The data in the table should therefore be viewed only as a general guide to treatment efficacy.

Clinicians should be familiar with at least one clinician-applied and one patient-applied therapy. If one treatment strategy fails (e.g., if warts have not improved substantially after three provider-administered treatments or have not completely cleared after six treatments) another may be tried. However, if anogenital warts persist then patients should be referred to a specialist. The use of more than one treatment modality at the same time has not been shown to be effective and may increase the risk of side effects.

Specific Treatment Recommendations and Considerations
1. Patient-applied treatments for external genital warts (Table 66.2): If possible, the provider should apply the first treatment to demonstrate both the application technique and the warts to be treated.
   a. Imiquimod 5% cream
   b. Podophyllotoxin/podofilox 0.5% solution or gel
2. Clinician-applied treatments for external genital warts (Table 66.2):
   a. Podophyllin resin 10% to 25%
   b. Bichloracetic acid (BCA) or trichloroacetic acid (TCA) 80% to 90%
   c. Cryotherapy with liquid nitrogen or cryoprobe
   d. Surgical therapies
3. Treatment of cervical, vaginal, urethral, anal, and oral warts:
   a. Cervical warts: Patients should be referred to a specialist for management of cervical warts, because evaluation for high-grade squamous intraepithelial lesions must be performed before treatment is initiated.

TABLE 66.1

Summary of Data about Clearance and Recurrence Rates Associated with Different Treatment Options for External Genital Warts

Treatment	Clearance Rate (%)	Recurrence Rate (%)
Patient applied		
Imiquimod	27–54	13–19
Podofilox	45–88	4–38
Clinician applied		
Podophyllin resin	23–72	23–65
Trichloroacetic or bichloracetic acid	63–70	
Cryotherapy	27–88	21
Curettage/surgical excision	35–72	19–29
Electrocautery	61–94	22
Laser therapy	23–52	60–77

Data were obtained from randomized controlled trials and well-designed uncontrolled studies. Abstracted from Wiley DJ, Douglas J, Beutner K, et al. External genital warts: diagnosis, treatment, and prevention. *Clin Infect Dis* 2002;35(Suppl 2):S210.

b. Vaginal warts: Cryotherapy with liquid nitrogen (but not a cryoprobe) or TCA/BCA 80% to 90%.

c. Urethral meatus warts: Cryotherapy with liquid nitrogen or podophyllin 10% to 25%. Treated warts must be dry before contact with normal mucosa.

d. Anal warts: Cryotherapy with liquid nitrogen, TCA/BCA 80% to 90%, or surgical removal. Patients with rectal mucosal warts should be referred to a specialist.

e. Oral warts: Cryotherapy with liquid nitrogen or surgical removal.

4. Treatment considerations during pregnancy: Several factors associated with pregnancy, such as hormonal factors and relative immunosuppression, may promote growth of anogenital warts. The only treatments recommended during pregnancy are BCA/TCA, cryotherapy, electrocautery, and surgical excision.

5. Treatment considerations in the setting of immunodeficiency: Adolescents who are immunosuppressed due to HIV infection, organ transplantation, or other conditions may not respond as well as immunocompetent adolescents and may have more frequent recurrences. In addition, squamous cell carcinomas originating in or resembling genital warts occur more frequently among immunocompromised patients. Therefore, evaluation by a specialist should be considered.

Partner Evaluation

It is not clear whether treatment of sexual partners alters the natural history of HPV-related disease. Therefore, although evaluation of sexual partners is not necessary, partner evaluation provides an opportunity for the clinician to screen partners for anogenital warts and other STDs and to educate partners about HPV and genital warts.

Counseling

Providers should educate patients with anogenital warts about HPV infection, its transmission, and its clinical consequences. Key messages are as follows: Genital warts are caused by specific HPV types that are different from the types that cause cervical cancer, genital warts may recur after treatment, it is unclear whether treatment reduces transmission of HPV to partners, condom use may reduce transmission of HPV and acquisition of genital warts, and adolescents with genital warts do not need HPV testing or more frequent Pap testing. They should provide information about available treatment options for genital warts and their prognosis. Web sites that may be helpful are listed in the subsequent text. Providers should also discuss strategies to prevent HPV-related disease and other STDs; for example, abstinence, limiting number of sexual partners, avoiding tobacco, and using condoms consistently. Pap testing should be performed according to published guidelines, but it is not necessary to perform Pap testing more frequently in those with genital warts. Screening for other STDs is indicated in all sexually active adolescents.

Providers should make sure that patients being treated for external genital warts can see their warts, especially those who are using patient-applied therapies. Patients should be advised to examine the areas being treated for signs of inflammation or infection (such as redness, swelling, or discharge) regularly. They should report any signs or symptoms of infection immediately to their provider. General perineal care may promote healing, including sitz baths and keeping the area clean and dry (e.g., with the use of a hair dryer at the lowest setting). During treatment and after visible warts have resolved, follow-up visits are helpful to monitor for complications of therapy, educate adolescents about signs of recurrence, and reiterate prevention messages.

The diagnosis of HPV infection or genital warts may cause anxiety, distress, and fear of social stigmatization in adolescents. Clinicians should provide support and when necessary may refer patients to support groups or for counseling.

Human Papillomavirus Vaccines

Remarkable progress has been made recently in the development of HPV vaccines. HPV vaccines fall into two categories—prophylactic vaccines, which are designed

TABLE 66.2

Recommended Treatment Options for External Genital Warts

Treatment Option	Instructions for Use	Advantages	Disadvantages
Patient applied Imiquimod 5% cream	The cream is provided in individual packets. Apply at bedtime, leave on overnight (6–10 hr), then wash off with soap and water. Use three times per wk for a maximum of 16 wk, until all lesions have disappeared. Wash off before sexual intercourse.	May be applied at home Can be applied to new warts as they appear	Local erythema, erosion, itching, and burning May weaken condoms/diaphragms Takes up to 16 wk to treat warts
Podophyllotoxin/ podofilox 0.5% solution or gel	Using a cotton swab for the solution or a finger for the gel, apply to genital warts twice daily for 3 d, followed by 4 d of no therapy. The cycle can be repeated up to 4 times if needed. Total wart area treated should not exceed 10 cm^2 and total volume of podofilox should not exceed 0.5 mL/d.	Widely available Easy to apply May be applied at home	Local erosion, burning, pain, and itching Not useful for cervical or mucosal lesions or extensive disease
Clinician applied Podophyllin resin 10%–25%	Provider paints the lesions with podophyllin using front or back of a cotton swab, ensures that solution has air-dried before allowing patient to resume a normal position. Treatment repeated weekly if necessary. Patient should wash off podophyllin in 1–4 hr. To avoid toxicity due to systemic absorption, <0.5 mL of podophyllin should be used or an area <10 cm^2 treated per session.	Widely available Easy to apply	Contains mutagenic compounds; therefore, contraindicated during pregnancy, and adolescents receiving it should use effective contraception Possible toxic systemic absorption, associated with bone marrow suppression, hepatocellular dysfunction, neurologic effects, psychosis, nausea, vomiting, diarrhea, and abdominal pain
Trichloroacetic acid (TCA) or bichloracetic acid (BCA) 80%–90%	Provider first applies occlusive ointment to the healthy tissue surrounding lesion, or treats the area with a topical anesthetic (e.g., benzocaine topical solution). The back or front end of a cotton swab is used to apply the solution sparingly until the lesions blanch (frost). The solution should air-dry before the patient resumes a normal position. If necessary, sodium bicarbonate or talc may be applied to remove unreacted acid. Avoid contact with normal skin. Repeat weekly for up to 6 wk until warts have resolved.	Widely available Inexpensive Easy to apply Safe in pregnancy	Pain on application Destroys normal tissue if over-applied

TABLE 66.2

(Continued)

Treatment Option	Instructions for Use	Advantages	Disadvantages
Cryotherapy with liquid nitrogen or cryoprobe	Liquid nitrogen can be used to treat vaginal warts, but use of a cryoprobe is not recommended because of the risk of vaginal perforation or fistula formation. A cotton applicator designed for cryotherapy is placed in liquid nitrogen briefly and then quickly applied with gentle pressure for 2–3 sec to the wart to be treated as well as 2–3 mm of surrounding skin. The surface of the wart should briefly turn white and then return to its normal color. The process can be repeated every 1–2 wk.	Well tolerated Useful for most wart types Safe in pregnancy No anesthesia needed Minimal risk of scarring	Pain, necrosis, blistering Over-application may lead to complications while under-application may lead to poor results
Surgical procedures	These procedures may include excision with a scalpel, curettage, or scissors; electrosurgery; and laser therapy.	Useful for extensive disease or lesions resistant to other modes of therapy Safe in pregnancy Rapid achievement of results	Requires hospital setting, provider expertise, appropriate equipment, and anesthetic Expensive With surgical excision, scarring and bleeding possible Laser is not readily available and intact DNA may be liberated into air with laser vapor

to prevent primary HPV infection by inducing virus-neutralizing antibody, and therapeutic vaccines, which are designed to treat HPV-related diseases. In June, 2006, a prophylactic HPV-6, 11, 16, 18 vaccine (Gardasil, Merck & Co., Inc.) was approved by the U.S. Food and Drug Administration (FDA) for use in girls and women 9 to 26 years of age. The Advisory Committee on Immunization Practices (ACIP) recommended that the vaccine be given routinely to 11- and 12-year-old girls, with catch-up immunization of 13- to 26-year-old girls and women and immunization of 9- and 10-year-old girls at the discretion of the health care provider. An HPV-16 and -18 vaccine (Cervarix), manufactured by GlaxoSmithKline Biologicals, was submitted for regulatory review in Europe and to the FDA in the United States for approval.

These two prophylactic HPV vaccines consist of virus-like particles (VLPs), which are recombinant viral capsids that are identical to HPV virions morphologically, but do not contain viral DNA. Therefore, they cannot replicate and therefore pose no infectious or oncogenic risk. Given that more than 90% of genital warts are caused by HPV-6 and HPV-11 and that approximately 70% of cervical cancer is caused by HPV-16 and HPV-18, these vaccines could have a significant public health impact. Clinical trials have shown that they are highly immunogenic, induce HPV genotype-specific serum antibody responses, are safe, and are well tolerated. Phase III trials suggest that the quadrivalent

HPV vaccine is highly effective in preventing infection and disease caused by the HPV types contained in the vaccines. In an international trial involving over 12,000 women 16 to 26 years of age, vaccine efficacy was 98% (96% confidence interval [CI] 86%–100%) against the combined incidence of HPV 16- or 18-related moderate/severe CIN, adenocarcinoma-in-situ, or invasive cervical cancer in the per-protocol group and 44% (95% CI 26%–58%) in the intention-to-treat group.(FUTURE II Study Group, 2007) Vaccine efficacy in the per-protocol group was 100% (95% CI 94%–100%) for prevention of external anogenital diseases (anogenital warts, VIN, VAIN, or cancer). (Garland et al., 2007). Antibody levels appear to remain high at least 4 years after initial vaccination. Both vaccines are given as three intramuscular injections, Gardasil at 0, 2, and 6 months and Cervarix at 0, 1, and 6 months.

Studies have shown that providers, parents, and adolescents generally find HPV vaccination to be acceptable. When recommending HPV vaccines, providers should address any specific parental or adolescent concerns. Vaccination provides an opportunity for clinicians to reinforce prevention messages that may maximize the effectiveness of HPV vaccines. For example, adolescents must understand that HPV vaccines do not protect against all HPV types or other STDs. They should still postpone sexual initiation, limit number of sexual partners, and use condoms consistently to prevent HPV and other STDs. In addition, physicians should reinforce the importance of continued Pap screening after vaccination. Routine screening is recommended because 30% of cervical cancer is caused by types not contained in the vaccines. In addition, vaccine efficacy may be compromised if women have been infected previously with HPV types contained in the vaccines, if they do not receive all three immunizations, or if immunity wanes over time.

WEB SITES

For Teenagers and Parents

http://www.cdc.gov/std/hpv. CDC Web site that includes fact sheets about HPV for both providers and patients.

http://www.ashastd.org. American Social Health Association site on STDs including excellent information about HPV.

http://www.iwannaknow.org. American Social Health Association site designed specifically for adolescents, which includes information about HPV and other STDs.

http://www.niaid.nih.gov/factsheets/stdhpv.htm. National Institute of Allergy and Infectious Diseases fact sheet on HPV.

www.youngwomenshealth.org. Harvard Medical School site designed for adolescents and young adults, including information on HPV and other STDs.

For Health Professionals

http://www.emedicine.com/derm/topic454.htm. E-medicine chapter on genital warts.

http://www.obgyn.net/femalepatient/default.asp?page= warts_tfp. From "The Female Patient" on management of warts.

http://www.cdc.gov/std/hpv. CDC Web site with excellent fact sheets about HPV for both providers and patients.

http://www.cdc.gov/STD/treatemtent/. CDC Web site including 2006 STD treatment guidelines.

REFERENCES AND ADDITIONAL READINGS

Beutner KR, Ferenczy A. Therapeutic approach to genital warts. *Am J Med* 1997;102:S28.

Beutner KR, Reitano MV, Richwald GA, et al., AMA Expert Panel on External Genital Warts. External genital warts: report of the American Medical Association consensus conference. *Clin Infect Dis* 1998;27:796.

Boardman LA, Stanko C, Weitzen S, et al. Atypical squamous cells of undetermined significance: human papillomavirus testing in adolescents. *Obstet Gynecol* 2005;105:741.

Brown DR, Shew ML, Qadadri B. A longitudinal study of genital human papillomavirus infection in a cohort of closely followed adolescent women. *J Infect Dis* 2005;191:182.

Castellsague X, Bosch FX, Munoz N. Environmental co-factors in HPV carcinogenesis. *Virus Res* 2002;89:191.

Cates W. Estimates of the incidence and prevalence of sexually transmitted diseases in the United States. *Sex Transm Dis* 1999;26(Suppl 4):S2–S7.

Centers for Disease Control and Prevention. Guidelines for treatment of sexually transmitted diseases. *MMWR Morb Mortal Wkly Rep* 2006;55(RR-11):62.

Dempsey AF, Zimet GD, Davis RL, et al. Factors that are associated with parental acceptance of human papillomavirus vaccines: a randomized intervention study of written information about HPV. *Pediatrics* 2006;117:1486.

Garland SM, Hernandez-Avila M, Wheeler CM et al. Quadrivalent vaccine against human papillomavirus to prevent anogenital disease. *NEngl J Med* 2007;356:1928.

Hagensee ME, Cameron JE, Leigh JE, et al. Human papillomavirus infection and disease in HIV-infected individuals. *Am J Med Sci* 2004;328:57.

Harper DM, Franco EL, Wheeler C. Efficacy of a bivalent L1 virus-like particle vaccine in prevention of infection with human papillomavirus types 16 and 18 in young women: a randomised controlled trial. *Lancet* 2004;364:1757.

Ho GYF, Bierman R, Beardsley L, et al. Natural history of cervicovaginal papillomavirus infection in young women. *N Engl J Med* 1998;338:423.

Kahn JA, Bernstein DI. Human papillomavirus vaccines and adolescents. *Curr Opin Obstet Gynecol* 2005;17:476.

Kahn JA, Rosenthal SL, Succop PA, et al. Mediators of the association between age of first sexual intercourse and human papillomavirus infection. *Pediatrics* 2002;109:E5.

Kahn JA, Slap GB, Bernstein DI, et al. Psychological, behavioral, and interpersonal impact of human papillomavirus and Pap test results. *J Womens Health* 2005;14:650.

Kahn JA, Zimet GD, Bernstein DI, et al. Pediatricians' intention to administer human papillomavirus vaccine: the role of practice characteristics, knowledge, and attitudes. *J Adolesc Health* 2005;37:502–510.

Kahn JA, Lan D, Kahn RS. Sociodemographic factors associated with high-risk HPV infection. *Obstetrics and Gynecology* 2007;110:in press.

Koustky LA, Galloway DA, Holmes KK. Epidemiology of genital HPV infection. *Epidemiol Rev* 1988;10:122.

Manhart LE, Koutsky LA. Do condoms prevent genital HPV infection, external genital warts, or cervical neoplasia? A meta-analysis. *Sex Transm Dis* 2002;29:725.

Marrazzo JM, Koutsky LA, Kiviat NB. Papanicolaou test screening and prevalence of genital human papillomavirus among women who have sex with women. *Am J Public Health* 2001;91:947.

Moscicki AB. Cervical cytology testing in teens. *Curr Opin Obstet Gynecol* 2005;17:471.

Moscicki AB, Hills N, Shiboski S, et al. Risks for incident human papillomavirus infection and low-grade squamous intraepithelial lesion development in young females. *JAMA* 2001;285:2995.

Moscicki AB, Shiboski S, Broering J, et al. The natural history of human papillomavirus infection as measured by DNA testing in adolescent and young adult women. *J Pediatr* 1998;132:277.

Sinclair KA, Woods CR, Woods CR, et al. Anogenital and respiratory tract human papillomavirus infections among children: age, gender, and potential transmission through sexual abuse. *Pediatrics* 2005;116:815.

The FUTURE II Study Group. Quadrivalent vaccine against human papillomavirus to prevent high-grade cervical lesions. *N Engl J Med* 2007;356:1915.

Villa LL, Costa RL, Petta CA. Prophylactic quadrivalent human papillomavirus (types 6, 11, 16, and 18) L1 virus-like particle vaccine in young women: a randomised double-blind placebo-controlled multicentre phase II efficacy trial. *Lancet Oncol* 2005;6:271.

de Villiers EM, Fauquet C, Broker TR, et al. Classification of papillomaviruses. *Virology* 2004;324:17.

Wang SS, Hildesheim A. Chapter 5: viral and host factors in human papillomavirus persistence and progression. *J Natl Cancer Inst Monogr* 2003;31:35.

Weaver BA, Feng Q, Holmes KK, et al. Evaluation of genital sites and sampling techniques for detection of human papillomavirus DNA in men. *J Infect Dis* 2004;189:677.

Wiley DJ, Douglas J, Beutner K, et al. External genital warts: diagnosis, treatment, and prevention. *Clin Infect Dis* 2002;35(Suppl 2):S210.

Winer RL, Hughes JP, Feng Q, et al. Condom use and the risk of genital human papillomavirus infection in young women. *New Engl J Med* 2006;354:2645.

CHAPTER 67

Other Sexually Transmitted Diseases Including Genital Ulcers, Pediculosis, Scabies, and Molluscum

Wendi G. Ehrman, M. Susan Jay, and Lawrence S. Neinstein

Chancroid, lymphogranuloma venereum (LGV), and granuloma inguinale constitute the classic minor ulcerative sexually transmitted diseases. All three of these diseases are uncommon but should be considered in the differential diagnosis of genital ulcers. In the United States, the most common causative agent of genital ulcers is the herpes simplex virus (HSV) followed by *Treponema pallidum* or syphilis. Approximately 3% to 10% of these patients will have more than one of these conditions present. In addition, there is an increased risk of human immunodeficiency virus (HIV) infection associated with these ulcerative infections.

CHANCROID

Chancroid is a genital ulcer infection caused by the gram-negative coccobacillus, *Haemophilus ducreyi*. Although uncommon in the United States, it is endemic in some areas of the country. Discrete outbreaks have been associated with poverty, urban prostitution, and illicit drug use. Chancroid is more commonly found in developing countries, with the highest prevalence in southern, central, and eastern Africa. Chancroid is a known risk factor for HIV and an enhancer of disease transmission. In addition, as many as 10% of patients with chancroid acquired in the United States are coinfected with *T. pallidum* or HSV. This number is estimated to be even higher for those case acquired outside the United States.

Epidemiology

1. Incidence: Chancroid was endemic in most parts of the world well into the 20th century. Since then, it has been disappearing in developing countries because of programs targeting increased condom use among commercial sex workers, and improved antibiotics. Despite increased eradication efforts worldwide, there is still an estimated rate of 7 million cases/year. Although outbreaks have occurred sporadically, the incidence of chancroid in the United States has steadily declined from a peak of 5,001 cases in 1988 to 17 cases in 2005. The incidence rate peaked in 1988 at 2.04 per 100,000 and has dropped to <0.01 per 100,000 in 2005. Given that chancroid is difficult to culture, often not considered, and usually diagnosed on the basis of morphological features alone, it is probably significantly under diagnosed.
2. Race: The incidence is increased in African-American and Hispanic patients.
3. Ratio of males-to-females is typically >10:1 in outbreaks.

Clinical Manifestations

1. Incubation period: Three to 10 days
2. Presentation: Chancroid presents as a tender inflammatory papule on the genitalia. It is thought to inoculate through microabrasions on the genital skin, which occur during sexual intercourse. Within 1 to 2 days, the papule becomes pustular, eroded and then ulcerates into an extremely painful, shallow lesion. The characteristic ulcer is soft, friable, and nonindurated with ragged undermined margins, a granulomatous base, and a foul-smelling yellow or gray, necrotic purulent exudate. Multiple lesions may be present, especially in females. Lesions have been known to remain pustular ("dwarf chancroid"), coalesce to form giant or serpiginous ulcers or resemble folliculitis or a pyogenic infection. Within 1 to 23 weeks, painful unilateral inguinal lymphadenitis known as a *bubo*, develops in 40% to 50% of patients. Twenty-five percent of these patients will have progression of the lymphadenitis into a suppurative bubo, which may rupture and ulcerate if not aspirated and drained. If this occurs, the patient can develop autoinoculation with bilateral opposing ulcers, known as *kissing lesions*. Large inguinal abscesses can occur, leading to significant destruction of skin and soft tissue.

   Although males usually present with ulcer or inguinal pain, females may be asymptomatic or develop nontender ulcers along with dysuria, dyspareunia, vaginal discharge, pain with defecation, and rectal bleeding.

Superinfection of ulcers with anaerobes can also occur leading to further ulceration and destruction of genital tissue. Fever and malaise may occur but are rare.

3. Location
   a. In males: Prepuce, coronal sulcus, and frenulum
   b. In females: Vulva, clitoris, cervix, and perianal region
   c. Extragenital sites (rare): Breasts, thighs, fingers, and mouth; has not been shown to spread to distant sites
4. Pregnancy: There have been no reports of adverse effects on pregnancy outcome or on the fetus.
5. HIV-infected patients: Studies on HIV-seropositive males suggest that this group has increased numbers of genital ulcers that may heal slower and require longer courses of therapy.

Differential Diagnosis

Chancroid may be confused with or coexist with herpes genitalis, primary syphilis, LGV traumatic lesions, Behçet syndrome, or fixed drug eruptions. Among adolescents, the most common etiology of genital ulcers would be herpes, followed by nonspecific trauma, syphilis, and chancroid.

1. Herpetic lesions initially present as vesicles, are usually very painful, more superficial, more numerous, and are surrounded by a narrower zone of erythema. Adenopathy is usually bilateral. Constitutional symptoms and lymphadenopathy may occur in first-time infections. Culture or antigen test for HSV should be performed.
2. Syphilitic ulcers are nonpainful and have indurated borders. Dark-field examination and serological examination are needed for confirmation.
3. Lesions associated with LGV are nonpainful and adenopathy develops after the lesions have healed.

Diagnosis

There are currently no easily accessed, highly sensitive tests available to diagnose chancroid. Oftentimes, the diagnosis is difficult because it is based on clinical findings and on the exclusion of HSV, syphilis, LGV, and granuloma inguinale. Accuracy rates from clinical diagnosis alone range from 33% to 80%. The "gold standard" for diagnosis has been culture. However *H. ducreyi* is a fastidious organism that requires special media and specialized laboratory conditions that are not widely available. To assist with diagnosis, all individuals with genital ulcers should receive serological testing for syphilis and if possible, a dark-field examination or direct immunofluorescence for *T. pallidum,* a culture and an antigen test for HSV, in addition to a culture for *H. ducreyi.* Diagnostic options include the following:

1. Microscopy: Direct examination of gram-stained ulcer material or aspirate from an infected lymph node (bubo) may be suggestive if large numbers of gram-negative coccobacilli are seen. Material is collected on a calcium alginate or cotton-tipped swab from the ulcer base and carefully rolled in one direction onto a glass slide for gram staining. The bacteria typically arrange themselves in parallel short chains, described as "schools of fish" and tend to occur close to polymorphonuclear leukocytes. This technique has poor sensitivity and specificity and may be misleading due to the polymicrobial flora often present in genital ulcers. As a result, it should not be used alone for diagnosis.

2. Culture: Culture material may be obtained from genital ulcers or buboes, although intact buboes tend to be sterile. Laboratories should be informed as soon as possible to prepare for the specimens. Compared with newer diagnostic techniques such as multiplex polymerase chain reaction (M-PCR), the sensitivity of culture is 35% to 75% and specificity is 94% to 100%.
3. Immunodiagnostic DNA probes and DNA amplification tests (M-PCR) are being investigated but are not routinely available in the United States. However, testing can be performed by commercial labs that have developed their own polymerase chain reaction (PCR) test. Sensitivity ranges from 56% to 100%.
4. Center for Disease Control and Prevention (CDC) criteria for "probable" chancroid diagnosis are as follows:
   a. One or more painful genital ulcers.
   b. No evidence of *T. pallidum* on dark-field examination of ulcer exudate or by a serological test for syphilis performed at least 7 days after onset of ulcers.
   c. The clinical presentation, appearance of the genital ulcers, and, if present, regional lymphadenopathy are typical for chancroid.
   d. A negative result on HSV test performed on ulcer exudates.
   e. The combination of a painful ulcer with tender inguinal adenopathy is suggestive of chancroid, and when accompanied by suppurative inguinal adenopathy it is almost pathognomonic.

Treatment

1. CDC recommended pharmacotherapy
   a. Azithromycin 1 g orally in a single dose
   b. Ceftriaxone 250 mg intramuscularly (IM) in a single dose
   c. Ciprofloxacin 500 mg orally twice daily for 3 days
      Note: Ciprofloxacin is contraindicated for pregnant and lactating women, children, and adolescents younger than 18 years.
   d. Erythromycin base 500 mg orally three times a day for 7 days.
      Worldwide, several isolates with intermediate resistance to either ciprofloxacin or erythromycin have been reported.
2. Treatment of buboes: Aspiration of fluctuant buboes provides symptomatic relief and can prevent spontaneous rupture. Alternatively, incision and drainage of buboes along with wound packing can avoid the need for frequent reaspirations.
3. HIV and syphilis testing should be performed at the time of diagnosis and repeated in 3 months if initially negative. In addition, patients should be tested for other sexually transmitted diseases such as gonorrhea, chlamydia, and hepatitis B.
4. Follow-up: Follow-up with infected individuals should occur within 3 to 7 days of initiation of therapy and should continue weekly until resolution of signs and symptoms. There should be subjective improvement within 3 days and objective improvement within 7 days. If there is no improvement, the practitioner must consider whether the diagnosis is correct, there is a coinfection with another sexually transmitted disease (STD), the individual is infected with HIV, treatment compliance is poor, or there is resistance to the prescribed antimicrobial. Large ulcers may require more than 2 weeks

to resolve, and fluctuant lymphadenopathy heals even more slowly than ulcers. Healing may also occur more slowly if the ulcers are under the foreskin of an uncircumcised male patient. Adenopathy may progress to fluctuation despite successful therapy and does not represent treatment failure. Patients need to be told that there should be no sexual activity while clinical disease is present.

5. Sexual partners: Treatment should be initiated when sexual contact has occurred within 10 days preceding the onset of symptoms in the infected patient, regardless of whether symptoms are present in the partners.
6. HIV-infected patients: Treatment failures have occurred and these individuals may require longer courses of therapy. The 7-day erythromycin regimen may be better unless very close follow-up is possible.

LYMPHOGRANULOMA VENEREUM

LGV is a systemic, sexually transmitted disease that remains rare in the United States. Although uncommon in most of the industrialized world, LGV is endemic in parts of Africa, India, South America, and the Caribbean. Recent outbreaks of LGV have been reported in the Netherlands and parts of Europe among men who have sex with other men, especially those who were HIV positive. In early 2005, there were already four confirmed cases reported in a similar population in New York City.

Etiology

LGV is caused by the obligate intracellular organism *Chlamydia trachomatis. Chlamydia* has 18 serological variants (serovars) associated with disease. Serovars L_1, L_2, and L_3 are more invasive and cause LGV whereas serovars B and D through K are associated with nongonococcal urethritis and cervicitis.

Epidemiology

1. Frequency: There were 42 known cases in the United States in 2000. This prevalence may be falsely low because of underreporting and misdiagnosis. LGV has not been nationally notifiable since 1995.
2. Age: Peak incidence is from 15 to 40 years of age.
3. Sex: Male to female predominance as high as a 5:1 ratio. A higher prevalence is seen among men who have sex with other men.

Clinical Manifestations

1. Incubation period: Three to 30 days (usually 7 to 12 days)
2. LGV occurs in three separate stages:
   a. Primary stage: The primary lesion of LGV starts out as a small, painless, papule or pustule at the site of inoculation that can erode into an asymptomatic herpetiform ulcer. Although these lesions can be multiple and deeply erosive, they often heal within a week without scarring and may go unnoticed. Primary lesions are typically found on the penis, urethral glans, and scrotum on the male; and on the vulva, vaginal wall, fourchette, and cervix in females. Rectal lesions can occur in both sexes from receptive anal intercourse and can be associated with diarrhea, rectal discharge, and tenesmus. Mucopurulent cervicitis and urethritis may also occur. Females usually have primary involvement of the rectum, vagina, and cervix.
   b. Secondary stage or inguinal stage: This stage typically occurs 2 to 6 weeks after the appearance of the primary lesion and involves painful inflammation and infection of the inguinal and femoral lymph nodes. Inguinal adenopathy is unilateral in 70% of cases. Although most men present during this stage, only 20% to 30% of women develop inguinal adenopathy. The "groove" sign is the result of enlarged inguinal nodes above Poupart ligament and femoral nodes below it and is said to be "pathognomonic" for LGV. Deep pelvic nodes may be involved in females, leading to lower abdominal or back pain. Infected macrophages drain the regional lymph nodes, typically producing unilateral enlargement, infection, and necrotic abscesses. Nodes can become matted and fluctuant. This produces the characteristic bubo. The skin overlying the bubo often becomes attached to the underlying lymph nodes and takes on a characteristic deep reddish blue color ("blue balls"). The buboes may rupture in one third of patients, or develop into hard nonsuppurative masses. Most of these buboes will eventually heal, however, some will develop into sinus tracts. Bubonic relapse can occur in 20% of untreated cases. Constitutional symptoms may occur with the inguinal buboes and be associated with systemic spread of chlamydia leading to arthritis, hepatitis, and pneumonitis. Rarer systemic complications include cardiac involvement, aseptic meningitis, and ocular inflammatory disease.
   c. Tertiary stage or genitoanorectal syndrome: Uncommon but occurs more often in females who were asymptomatic during previous stages of the disease and in homosexual males typically due to receptive anal intercourse. Patients initially develop proctocolitis with symptoms of anal pruritus, rectal discharge, rectal pain, tenesmus, and fever. Later manifestations include perirectal abscesses, rectovaginal and anorectal fistulas, rectal strictures, and rectal stenosis. Chronic inflammation can lead to hyperplasia of intestinal and perirectal lymphatics or "lymphorrhoids." In addition, chronic untreated LGV can lead to a process of repetitive scarring and fistulous tract formation in the genital region. Potential complications from this include elephantiasis of the genitals 1 to 20 years after onset (rare), esthiomene (enlargement, induration, ulceration, and destruction of the vulva), and infertility.

Differential Diagnosis

1. Genital inguinal lesion
   a. Syphilis
   b. Herpes simplex
   c. Chancroid
   d. Granuloma inguinale
   e. Pyogenic infection
   f. Cat-scratch fever
2. Rectal fistulas
   a. Inflammatory bowel disease
   b. Chronic rectal infections: Gonorrhea, amebiasis, tuberculosis
   c. Granuloma inguinale

Diagnosis

The diagnosis of LGV has often been made based on clinical findings, due to lack of available laboratory services for identifying the organism, difficulty in culturing the organism, and the cross-reactivity of serology between several serotypes. For a laboratory diagnosis of LGV, the infective agent must first be identified as *C. trachomatis* and then the LGV serotype of *C. trachomatis* determined. Available laboratory services can be located at www.cdc.gov/std/lgv-labs.htm.

Tests for identification of *C. trachomatis* are as follows:

1. Culture and culture typing: Not a widely available test. *Chlamydia* may be isolated from ulcer material or from a node aspirate. The recovery rate is less than 30% and culture is not highly specific for LGV.
2. NAAT (nucleic acid amplification tests): Not U.S. Food and Drug Administration (FDA) cleared for use with rectal specimens, although some laboratories are able to use this test after meeting Clinical Laboratory Improvement Amendments (CLIA) guidelines. Also not specific for LGV.

Tests for serotyping LGV are as follows:

3. Complement fixation: Titers $\geq 1{:}64$ along with clinical correlation are consistent with a diagnosis of LGV infection. A fourfold increase in titer also supports the diagnosis of LGV. However, titers can also be positive after chlamydial urethritis, psittacosis, or trachoma, although they are rarely higher than 1:16. Disease severity does not correlate with antibody titers.
4. The microimmunofluorescence test is more sensitive and specific than complement fixation but is not routinely available. A high titer (typically >1:128 but can vary by laboratory) is consistent with a diagnosis of LGV. Immunofluorescence techniques are usually applied to lymph node aspirates and may not be applicable in proctitis presentations.
5. Genotyping is not widely available.

Treatment

Owing to the difficulty confirming LGV by diagnostic testing, patients with a clinical syndrome consistent with LGV, including proctocolitis or genital ulcer disease with lymphadenopathy, should be treated for LGV.

1. CDC recommended pharmacotherapy
   a. Doxycycline 100 mg orally twice daily for 21 days
2. CDC alternative regimens
   a. Erythromycin 500 mg orally four times a day for 21 days
   b. Azithromycin 1 g orally weekly for 3 weeks (suggested by some specialists but clinical data lacking)
3. Surgical intervention: Occasionally, aspiration of a fluctuant node or incision and drainage of an abscess is required for prevention of ulcer formation or relief of inguinal pain. The late complications of LGV may necessitate surgical repair after antibiotic treatment is complete.
4. Follow-up: Patients should be monitored clinically until signs and symptoms have resolved.
5. Sex partners: Sexual contacts within 60 days before onset of symptoms should be examined, tested for urethral or cervical chlamydial infection, and treated. In the absence of symptoms, contacts should be treated with azithromycin 1 g oral single dose or doxycycline 100 mg orally twice daily for 7 days.
6. Pregnancy and lactation: Erythromycin should be used to treat pregnant and lactating women. Azithromycin may be an alternative, although published safety and efficacy data are lacking.
7. HIV infection: HIV-infected adolescents should be treated with the same regimens as for noninfected HIV adolescents although prolonged treatment may be necessary.

GRANULOMA INGUINALE

Granuloma inguinale, also known as *Donovanosis*, is a rare STD in the United States but should be considered in the differential diagnosis of chronic progressive genital ulcers. It is endemic in certain tropical, subtropical, and developing areas of the world and is often associated with impoverished communities.

Etiology

Granuloma inguinale is caused by *Calymmatobacterium granulomatis,* a nonmotile, obligate intracellular, encapsulated, gram-negative coccobacillus.

Epidemiology

1. Incidence: Indigenous granuloma inguinale is no longer present in the United States or most other developed countries. Cases that occur in the United States are uncommon and imported. At present this disease is not notifiable in the United States and only eight cases were reported to the CDC in 1997. Granuloma inguinale is considered endemic in Papua, New Guinea, South-East India, South Africa, central Australia, Brazil, and the Caribbean.
2. Sex: Higher prevalence in males.
3. Age: Most cases occurs between the ages of 20 and 40 years.
4. Transmission: Primarily through sexual contact, most commonly from a person with an active infection but possibly also from a person with asymptomatic rectal infection. Transmission may also occur during vaginal childbirth, and young children can acquire infection through infected secretions. Autoinoculation can lead to spread of the disease. Granuloma inguinale is thought to be only mildly contagious, requiring several exposures for clinical disease.

Clinical Manifestations

1. Incubation period: Eight to 80 days
2. Granuloma inguinale has a variety of presentations and atypical lesions, which makes identification a challenge.
   a. Ulcerovegetative or ulcerogranulomatous forms: Most common form; produces large, extensive, nonindurated ulcerations with beefy-red, friable granulation tissue.
   b. Nodular form: Consists of soft red nodules or plaques that erode to form ulcerations.
   c. Hypertrophic or verrucous form: Consists of dry vegetative masses with raised irregular edges that resemble a walnut or condylomata acuminata.

d. Necrotic form: Less common, foul-smelling, deep ulcer that produces rapid and extensive tissue destruction. Unlike most lesions of granuloma inguinale, it is often painful.

e. Sclerotic or cicatricial form: Rare; consists of dry, nonbleeding ulcers that expand into plaques with band-like scarring. Lymphedema can occur due to constriction.

3. True inguinal lymphadenopathy does not occur with granuloma inguinale unless bacterial superinfection develops. However, subcutaneous granulomas near the inguinal nodes (pseudobuboes) can result in inguinal enlargement.

4. Location: Lesions are typically localized without constitutional symptoms. The genital area is involved in 90% of cases and inguinal area in 10%. Extragenital lesions occur in 6% of cases secondary to autoinoculation of primary genital lesions.

   a. Males: Coronal sulcus, prepuce, frenulum, glans penis, and anus. More common in uncircumcised males with poor genital hygiene.

   b. Females: Labia minora and fourchette; can infect the cervix and upper genital tract mimicking cervical cancer.

   c. Extragenital sites: Oropharynx, neck, nose, larynx, and chest.

   d. Hematogenous dissemination is rare and associated with a grave prognosis. Dissemination to the abdominal cavity and organs, lung, bone, and female reproductive organs has occurred and is usually associated with cervical infection related to trauma during pregnancy.

Differential Diagnosis

The disease in its early stages may be confused with syphilis, herpes simplex, chancroid, or carcinoma of the penis if tissue destruction or necrosis is present.

Diagnosis

1. Granuloma inguinale is usually diagnosed by identification of intracytoplasmic inclusion bodies known as *Donovan bodies* within histiocytes of granulation tissue smears or biopsy specimens. Tissue smears are obtained by firmly rolling a cotton swab across the base of a nonbleeding ulcer and then rolling the swab across a slide. "Crush biopsies" are obtained by removing a piece of tissue from the advancing surface of the ulcer and "crushing" or smearing the resultant specimen between two slides. Giemsa or Wright's stain is then used to identify the dark-staining, safety pin–shaped Donovan bodies. Histological examination of biopsy specimens can also be used for diagnosis.

2. PCR tests and serological tests using immunofluorescence have been developed but remain mostly available on a research basis.

   Isolation of *C. granulomatis* is extremely difficult and has not been available although several research labs have reported successful culture of the organism.

3. Lesions should be cultured for *H. ducreyi* to exclude chancroid (pseudogranuloma inguinale). Granuloma

inguinale is frequently misdiagnosed as carcinoma, which can be excluded by histological examination of tissue or by response of the lesion to antibiotics.

Treatment

1. CDC recommended regimens: All treatments should be given for a minimum of 3 weeks and until all lesions have completely healed.

   a. Doxycycline 100 mg orally twice a day for a minimum of 3 weeks or until all lesions healed

2. Alternative regimens

   a. Azithromycin 1 g orally per week for a minimum of 3 weeks

   b. Ciprofloxacin 750 mg orally twice a day for a minimum of 3 weeks (*not used in children younger than 18 years*).

   c. Erythromycin base 500 mg orally four times a day for a minimum of 3 weeks

   d. Trimethoprim-sulfamethoxazole, one double strength tablet orally twice a day for a minimum of 3 weeks or until all lesions healed

3. Resistance: An aminoglycoside such as gentamycin 1 mg/kg IV every 8 hours may be added to any of the regimens if lesions are not responding within the first few days of treatment.

4. Pregnancy: Erythromycin should be used in pregnant and lactating women with consideration for adding a parental aminoglycoside such as gentamycin. Azithromycin is an alternative, although published data is currently not available.

5. HIV: Treatment is the same as in HIV-negative patients although consideration should be given to the addition of an aminoglycoside.

6. Follow-up: Patients should be followed up until complete resolution of clinical signs and symptoms. If therapy is effective, partial healing of the ulcer should be seen within 7 days. Prolonged therapy is required for granulation and reepithelialization of ulcers. Relapses can occur in 6 to 18 months after treatment especially if antibiotics are stopped prematurely. As with other genital ulcer diseases, patients should be tested for other sexually transmitted diseases such as gonorrhea, chlamydia, herpes, syphilis, HIV, and hepatitis B.

7. Sexual partners: Sexual partners should be examined and offered treatment if they had contact with the patient during the 60 days before the onset of symptoms or if they are clinically symptomatic. The value of empirical antibiotic therapy in patients without clinical signs or symptoms is unknown.

PEDICULOSIS AND SCABIES

Scabies and pediculosis are ubiquitous and highly contagious parasitic skin infections that have been present since antiquity and are distributed worldwide. Infections occur both in individuals and in clusters such as school children, homeless people, hospital staff, and immunocompromised persons. Difficulties in management have returned scabies and pediculosis to the limelight.

Pediculosis Pubis

Etiology
Pediculosis pubis is caused by the pubic or crab louse, *Pthirus pubis,* an obligate human parasite. It is a wingless

insect 1 to 3 mm in length with three sets of legs; two that are clawed and one that is shortened and vestigial. The hook-like claws and opposing thumb provide a grasp on the pubic and auxiliary hair. Serrations on its first set of claws also allow it to cling to flat, hairless surfaces. The lice are able to move around the skin surface at approximately 10 cm/day.

Epidemiology

1. Transmission: Pubic lice infestations are most common among adolescents and young adults. Transmission occurs as a result of close bodily contact, chiefly through sexual contact. Condoms do not prevent transmission and frequently infestations coexist with other STDs. Pubic lice can potentially be transmitted by infected clothing, towels, and bedding. Lice have also been found on eyelashes of younger children and may be an indicator for sexual abuse. At present there is no evidence linking ectoparasites to transmission of HIV.
2. Life cycle: The parasite spends its life on skin and feeds on blood. It dies in approximately 24 hours off its human host. The female pubic louse lays approximately three to four eggs/day, which are attached to hair shafts as nits. The nits hatch in 6 to 10 days into nymphs that mature into adult lice within 10 to 14 days. Adult life expectancy is believed to be approximately 1 month.

Clinical Manifestations

1. Symptoms occur 2 weeks or more after contact at which point the infection is usually well established. Pruritus, the main symptom, is related to the louse bite and is probably a hypersensitivity reaction. Secondary infections can occur from scratching. In addition, symptoms occur more rapidly if the patient experienced a prior infestation.
2. Common areas of infection: Pubic hair, hairs of abdomen, chest, thighs, axilla, and perianal area. Occasionally, eyebrows and lashes are involved in young children and beards in males.
3. After prolonged infestation, small blue spots called *maculae caeruleae* may appear on thighs and abdomen. These are uncommon but specific for pubic lice. They represent feeding sites of the louse.
4. Coexisting STDs are common in adolescents infested with pubic lice. One study showed that infested teens were twice as likely to have concurrent chlamydia or gonorrhea than noninfested teens (Pierzchalski et al., 2002).

Diagnosis

Diagnosis of pubic lice is made by direct visualization of lice or nits (eggs) on the hair shafts. Lice appear as tiny, tan to grayish-white oval insects. Nits can be seen as small yellowish-white, glistening oval kernels attached to hair shafts.

Treatment

Pubic lice do not transmit systemic disease. Treatment is mainly for symptomatic relief and prevention of reinfestation and transmission. Topical treatments are more effective when applied to dry hair. Most treatments are toxic to the nervous system of the pubic louse. Embryos may survive initial treatment, requiring a second course of the treatments listed in the subsequent text in 7 to 10 days:

1. CDC recommended regimens
   a. Permethrin 1% creme rinse (Nix) applied to affected area and washed off after 10 minutes. *Treatment of choice because of low toxicity, high cure rate, and possible ovicidal activity.*
   b. Pyrethrins and piperonyl butoxide (nonprescription RID, R & C Lice treatment, Clear, Pronto) applied to the affected area and washed off after 10 minutes.
2. Alternative regimens
   a. Malathion lotion 0.5% (Ovide) applied for 8 to 12 hours then rinsed off in hot water. Reapply in 7 to 9 days if live lice are still present. Used for resistant infestations in adults because of odor and flammability, and toxicity if ingested. Approved for use only in those aged 6 years and older.
   b. Ivermectin at a single dose of 250 µg/kg repeated in 2 weeks (not ovicidal). This drug should not be used on anyone weighing <15 kg, or in pregnant or breast-feeding women. There is some potential for neurotoxicity, so this drug should be used with caution. It may be particularly useful in people who have more than one parasitic infection.
   c. Lindane 1% shampoo applied for no longer than 4 minutes and then thoroughly washed off.
      Note: Not recommended for pregnant or lactating women and children <2 years, anyone with a seizure disorder, or anyone with inflamed or traumatized skin. Should be used only for treatment failures or inability to tolerate other treatment regimens. Has potential for central nervous system toxicity.
3. Clothing or bed linen coming in contact with the patient within the last 2 days should be machine washed at 130°F to 140°F and machine dried (hot cycle for 20 minutes) or dry cleaned. Clothing that cannot be decontaminated as above should be bagged for at least 72 hours. Fumigation is not necessary.
4. Residual nits should be removed with a fine comb. For nits that are difficult to remove, a solution of vinegar and water can be used to loosen them.
5. Sexual contacts within the last month should be treated. Sexual contact should be avoided until both patient and partner are treated and reevaluated for persistence of the infestation.
6. Pregnancy: Use permethrin or pyrethrins with piperonyl butoxide.
7. HIV infection: Use the same therapy as for a noninfected adolescent.
8. Pediculosis of eyelashes: Treat with application of occlusive ophthalmic ointment to the eyelid margins two times a day for 10 days. This smothers the lice and nits. Do not apply lindane or other medications to the eyes. Oral sulfamethoxazole/trimethoprim for 10 days has reportedly been effective but is not FDA approved for this use.

Scabies

Scabies is a highly contagious, ectoparasitic infection. It is one of the most widespread infestations in the world, with approximately 300 million cases of scabies worldwide each year.

Etiology

Scabies is caused by a small mite, *Sarcoptes scabiei* var. *hominis.* The adult mite has a rounded body, has four pairs of legs, and measures 400 µm in length. This parasite is host-specific for humans.

Epidemiology
1. Transmission: The mite is transmitted by prolonged skin-to-skin contact. Sexual transmission is common, as is nonsexual spread in family groups. Transmission can occur before the patient is symptomatic and throughout the infestation as long as it remains untreated. Scabies is frequently found in institutional settings and epidemics are associated with poverty, overcrowding, sexual promiscuity, travel, waning immunity, and other factors.
2. Life cycle: The impregnated female mite burrows into the skin where she lays between 10 and 25 eggs in a 1-cm-long tunnel. Egg-laying is completed in 4 to 5 weeks, and the adult female dies within the burrow. After 3 to 5 days the eggs hatch, and the larvae return to the skin surface to mature in 10 to 17 days. Only 10% of eggs become adults. The average infected host has 3 to 50 adult female mites. Away from the host, human mites have been shown to survive up to 24 to 96 hours.
3. Age: In underdeveloped countries, scabies has the highest prevalence in preschool children and adolescents. In developed nations, the prevalence is similar in all ages.

Clinical Manifestations
1. Incubation: Symptoms occur 3 to 6 weeks after first exposure and 1 to 4 days after reexposure.
2. Lesions: Scabies is an intensely pruritic, papular eruption associated with eczematous lesions and areas of excoriation. Pruritus is often worse at night or after a hot bath and is caused by a cell-mediated immune reaction to the mite and its by-products. The burrows, if seen, appear as short wavy lines a few millimeters to 1 cm in length.
3. Involved areas: Skin lesions are typically seen in between finger webs, on the flexor surfaces of the wrists, in the axillary folds, on the nipples, waist and umbilicus, buttocks, thighs, knees, and ankles. In males, the penis and scrotum are often involved. Scabies usually spares the face, neck, and scalp except in children.
4. Crusted or Norwegian scabies: This is a rare and aggressive form of scabies most often associated with immunodeficient, debilitated, or malnourished patients. Crusted scabies is characterized by a hyperinfestation of the mite with a concomitant inflammatory and hyperkeratotic reaction. The numerous scaling lesions are heavily infested with mites and more contagious than typical scabies. Treatment failures occur frequently and septicemia is a common complication.
5. Differential diagnosis: The lesions can become secondarily infected and eczematized and therefore confused with eczema, atopic or contact dermatitis, or impetigo. Papulovesicular lesions may be confused with papular urticaria, chicken pox, drug eruptions, folliculitis, insect bites, or dermatitis herpetiformis.

Diagnosis
1. Diagnosis is often made on the basis of the body distribution of lesions along with a history of intense itching and similar symptoms in family members or sexual partners. Definitive diagnosis requires microscopic identification of mites, eggs, or feces from skin scrapings of papules or burrows. Burrows are virtually pathognomonic for human scabies but are often difficult to demonstrate.
2. Isolation of mite: Best results are obtained by using a no. 15 scalpel blade to scrape the leading edge of an intact burrow or affected area under fingernails. Visibility of burrows can be enhanced with application of mineral oil, immersion oil, saline, or ink to the skin. Scrapings are transferred to a cover slide under oil or saline and examined under low power for the presence of eggs, feces, or the mite. Alternately, punch or shave biopsies of inflamed lesions may also be used with varying results.

Treatment
1. CDC recommended regimens
   a. Permethrin cream (Elimite) 5% applied to all areas of the body from the neck down and washed off after 8 to 14 hours. Application should include the area beneath the fingernails and skin folds. The cream can be applied at bedtime and removed by bathing the next morning.
   b. Ivermectin 200 µg/kg orally, repeated in 2 weeks. *Note: Ivermectin is not recommended for pregnant or lactating women or children weighing <15 kg. Use may be considered in epidemics, especially if topical scabicides have failed.*
2. Alternative regimens
   a. Lindane (1%) (Kwell) 1 oz of lotion or 30 g of cream applied thinly to all areas of the body from the neck down and washed off thoroughly after 8 hours. Application should include web spaces of digits and under fingernails. Lindane should not be applied immediately after a shower or bath because this may increase unnecessary systemic absorption. *Note: Lindane should not be used by pregnant or lactating women, children <2 years of age, or by those with seizure disorders or with extensive dermatitis. Lindane is not recommended as first-line therapy because of toxicity. It should only be used as an alternative if the patient cannot tolerate other therapies or if other therapies have failed.* Both aplastic anemia and seizures (when used after a bath or by patients with extensive dermatitis) have been reported with use. Lindane resistance has been reported in the United States.
   b. Crotamiton 10% (Eurax) applied for 24 hours once daily for 2 consecutive days followed by bathing 48 hours after the final application. Appears to work better as an antipyretic agent but associated with higher treatment failures, irritation, and allergic reactions. Crotamiton is no longer included by the CDC in their 2006 recommendations.
   c. Other agents used in the past with mixed results include benzyl benzoate, malathion, and sulfur 5% to 10% precipitated in ointment.
3. The patient should not be contagious after 24 hours of treatment.
4. Bedding and clothing worn during the 4 days preceding treatment should be machine washed, machine dried using hot cycle, dry cleaned, or removed from body contact and set aside in a sealed plastic bag for at least 72 hours. Fumigation of living areas is not necessary.
5. Follow-up: Pruritus may persist for up to 2 weeks after treatment. Symptoms persisting longer can be due to a number of factors including resistance to medication, incorrect scabicidal application, poor skin penetration in crusted scabies, reinfection, or other allergies.

Consideration can be given to re-treatment with a different regimen after 1 to 2 weeks, although some specialists recommend this only with the confirmation of live mites.

6. Sex partners and household contacts: Prophylactic treatment is recommend for sex partners, as well as close personal or household contacts within the last month.
7. Pregnant women: Pregnant or lactating women should use permethrin or crotamiton regimens.
8. Oral antipruritics such as hydroxyzine (Atarax), or topical corticosteroids can be used to relieve itching.
9. HIV infection: HIV-infected individuals should use the same treatment as those HIV-negative. Infected individuals are at increased risk for Norwegian scabies, a disseminated infection that should be managed in consultation with a specialist.
10. Crusted scabies: This is a difficult to treat infection that may require combined treatment with Ivermectin and topical scabicides and keratolytic therapy or multiple doses of Ivermectin. Ivermectin is not FDA licensed for this use.

MOLLUSCUM CONTAGIOSUM

Etiology

Molluscum contagiosum is a self-limited, benign, viral skin disease caused by a large DNA poxvirus. It has a worldwide distribution and appears particularly prevalent in warm, humid climates.

Epidemiology

Humans appear to be the only known host of the virus. Transmission occurs by direct person-to-person contact, fomites, or autoinoculation. Transmission has also been associated with swimming pools. Among adolescents, sexual contact is believed to be the most common form of transmission. The incubation period is variable and appears to be from 2 weeks up to 6 months.

Clinical Manifestations

1. Location: The lesions commonly occur on the face, trunk, and extremities. In sexually active adolescents, the lesions are commonly seen on the genital and pubic areas, and inner thighs.
2. Appearance: Lesions are smooth, firm, flesh-colored, dome-shaped papules that can become soft, waxy or pearly gray, and semitranslucent with central umbilication. Immunocompetent hosts typically have less than 20 lesions that grow up to 5 mm in diameter over a period of a couple weeks. HIV-positive and immunocompromised patients may develop hundreds of lesions that may present in clusters. Additionally, HIV-positive patients can present with "giant molluscum" up to 15 mm in diameter that are difficult to eradicate and are easier spread.
3. Symptoms: The lesions are usually asymptomatic; however, approximately 10% of patients will have an encircling eczematoid reaction.

Differential Diagnosis

1. Condylomata acuminata
2. Vulvar syringoma
3. Squamous or basal cell carcinoma
4. Juvenile xanthogranulomas
5. Lichen nitidus

Diagnosis

1. The clinical appearance is usually diagnostic.
2. Wright or Giemsa staining of the caseous material found within the core will reveal intracytoplasmic inclusion bodies known as *molluscum bodies*. Poxvirus can be identified by electron microscopy of these core cells.

Treatment

Owing to the benign nature and self-limiting course of molluscum, nontreatment is an option for nongenital lesions. Individual lesions may resolve in 2 to 6 months but untreated infections can last as long as 5 years. However, autoinoculation can spread the disease and sexually active individuals are at risk of further transmitting the disease. Immunocompromised individuals are also at greater risk of secondary inflammation and bacterial infection. Treatment options include both mechanical and chemical means applied by either the provider or patient:

1. Mechanical ablation: *All are considered safe in pregnancy.*
   a. Curettage or needle extraction of the central molluscum core with/without a local anesthetic such as EMLA. Cauterization of the lesion base with electrodesiccation or application of trichloroacetic acid (TCA) or podophyllin to the base may be of added benefit. Works best when there are only a few lesions.
   b. Cryotherapy through application of liquid nitrogen to the lesions and surrounding area for 5 to 10 seconds. Treatment may need to be repeated in 2- to 4-week intervals. Blistering and scarring are potential side effects.
   c. Electrodesiccation using high frequency electrical current may be used along with a local anesthetic.
   d. Pulse dye laser may be an option for recalcitrant lesions. Laser treatment has been associated with transient hyperpigmentation and development of new lesions after eradication of the old ones.
   e. Duct tape occlusion therapy has been used successfully over a course of months.
2. Chemical cytotoxic agents:
   a. Podophyllin (25%) applied to individual lesions by a health care provider and washed off 1 to 4 hours later. Treatments are given weekly for 4 to 6 weeks and may be associated with significant irritation. Best used when limited number of nonfacial lesions are present. As an alternative, patients can self-apply podofilox twice daily for 3 consecutive days followed by 4 days without treatment, in 4 to 6 cycles. May be associated with pain, irritation, and mild scarring and has a low efficacy and potential toxicity. *Not approved for use in pregnancy.*
   b. TCA (80%–90%) applied by a health care provider to the lesion(s) once a week for 4 to 6 weeks. May result in mild pain, irritation, and scarring. *Safe in pregnancy.*

c. Cantharidin (0.7%–0.9%) carefully applied by a health care provider to lesions, and washed off within 2 to 6 hours. May be repeated in 2 to 4 weeks. Not FDA approved or recommended for face or genitalia use, secondary to significant blistering.

d. Topical 0.5% tretinoin cream or gel applied to lesions daily for 2 to 3 months. Local irritation and dryness are side effects. No controlled clinical trials have been done and it is not recommended in pregnancy.

3. Immunomodulators

Topical 5% imiquimod applied overnight three times per week and washed off in the morning, for 4 to 12 weeks. Currently not FDA approved for this use. May be associated with mild pain and erythema. Not for use in pregnancy.

4. HIV/immunosuppressed patients

Molluscum contagiosum is considered an opportunistic infection in HIV disease and a marker for advanced infection. HIV-infected individuals have high treatment failure rates for almost all standard therapies for molluscum. Imiquimod (5%) may have some benefit, and experimental treatments utilizing the antiviral drug cidofovir (topically or intralesionally) and α-interferon (intralesionally) may be of benefit.

Follow-up

1. Patients should be told to watch for the development of new lesions after several weeks that may have been incubating at the time of the initial treatment.
2. Patients should refrain from sharing clothing or towels with others.
3. Swimming in pools should be discouraged.
4. Partners should be examined and treated for lesions, although the benefits of this are unknown.

WEB SITES

For Teenagers and Parents

http://www.cdc.gov/ncidod/dpd/parasiticpathways/insects.htm. Centers for Disease Control and Prevention (CDC) handouts/information on scabies and public lice.

http://www.ashastd.org. American Social Health Association handout on STDs.

http://www.urologychannel.com/std/index.shtml. Information on sexually transmitted diseases.

For Health Professionals

http://www.cdc.gov/std/lgv. CDC website on diagnosing and testing for LGV.

REFERENCES AND ADDITIONAL READINGS

American Academy of Pediatrics. Summaries of infectious diseases. In: Pickeing LK, ed. *Red book: report of the committee of infectious diseases*, 27th ed. Elk Grove Village, IL: American Academy of Pediatrics; 2006.

Billstein SA. Pubic lice. In: Holmes KK, Sparling PF, Mårdh PA, et al., eds. *Sexually transmitted diseases*, 3rd ed. New York: McGraw-Hill; 1999.

Blank S, Schillinger JA, Harbatkin D. Lymphogranuloma venereum in the industrialized world (comment). *Lancet* 2005;365:1607.

Braue A, Ross G, Varigos G, et al. Epidemiology and impact of childhood molluscum contagiosum: a case seeies and critical review of the literature. *Pediatr Dermatol* 2005;22:287.

Brown TJ, Yen-Moore A, Tyring SK. An overview of sexually transmitted diseases: part I. *J Am Acad Dermatol* 1999;41:4.

Brown TJ, Yen-Moore A, Tyring SK. An overview of sexually transmitted diseases: part II. *J Am Acad Dermatol* 1999;41:5.

Burkhart CG, Burkhart CN, Burkhart KM. An epidemiologic and therapeutic reassessment of scabies. *Cutis* 2000;65:233.

Centers for Disease Control and Prevention. Chancroid–California. *MMWR Morb Mortal Wkly Rep* 1982;31:173.

Centers for Disease Control and Prevention. Lymphogranuloma venereum among men who have sex with men—Netherlands, 2003–2004. *MMWR* 2004;53:985.

Centers for Disease Control and Prevention. Sexually transmitted diseases treatment guidelines 2006. *MMWR* 2006;55 (RR-11).

Centers for Disease Control and Prevention. Other sexually transmitted diseases. In: *Sexually transmitted disease surveillance 2002*. Atlanta, GA: U.S. Department of Health and Human Sevices; 2003:35.

Centers for Disease Control and Prevention. Other sexually transmitted diseases. In: *Sexually transmitted disease surveillance, 2003*. Atlanta, GA: U.S. Department of Health and Human Services; 2004:37.

Chosidow O. Scabies and pediculosis. *Lancet* 2000;355:819.

Clinical Effectiveness Group (Association of Genitourinary Medicine and the Medical Society for the Study of Venereal Diseases). National guideline for the management of scabies. *Sex Transm Infect* 1999;75(Suppl 1):S76.

Dangor Y, Ballard RC, Expostoa F, et al. Accuracy of clinical diagnosis of genital ulcer disease. *Sex Transm Dis* 1990;17:184.

Douglas JM. Molluscum contagiosum. In: Holmes KK, Sparling PF, Mårdh PA, et al., eds. *Sexually transmitted diseases*, 3rd ed. New York: McGraw-Hill; 1999.

Elston DM. Drugs used in the treatment of pediculosis. *J Drugs Dermatol* 2005;2:207.

Flinders DC, De Schweitz P. Pediculosis and scabies. *Am Fam Physician* 2004;69:341.

French P, Ison CA, Macdonald N. Lymphogranuloma venereum in the United Kingdom. *Sex Transm Infect* 2005;81:97.

Hart G. Donovanosis. *Clin Infect Dis* 1997;25:24.

Hurwitz S. *Clinical pediatric dermatology*. Philadelphia: WB Saunders; 1993.

Joseph AK, Rosen T. Laboratory techniques used in the diagnosis of chancroid, granuloma inguinale, and lymphogranuloma venereum. *Dermatol Clin* 1994;12:1.

Kemp DJ, Walton SF, Harumal P, et al. The scourge of scabies. *Biologist* 2002;49:19.

Ko CH, Elston DM. Pediculosis. *J Am Acad Dermatol* 2004;50:1.

Lewis DA. Diagnostic tests for chancroid. *Sex Transm Infect* 2000;76:137.

Lewis DA. Chancroid: clinical manifestations, diagnosis, and management. *Sex Transm Infect* 2003;70:68.

McDonald LL, Stites PC, Buntin DM. Sexually transmitted disease update. *Dermatol Clin* 1997;15:221.

Molino AC, Fleischer AB, Feldman SR. Patient demographics and utilization of health care services for molluscum contagiosum. *Pediatr Dermatol* 2004;21:628.

O'Farrell N. Donovanosis. In: Holmes KK, Sparling PF, Mårdh PA, et al., eds. *Sexually transmitted diseases*, 3rd ed. New York: McGraw-Hill; 1999.

O'Farrell N. Donovanosis: an update. *Int J STD AIDS* 2001;12:423.

O'Farrell N. Donovanosis. *Sex Transm infect* 2002;78:452.

Opaneye AA, Jayaweera DT, Walzman M, et al. Pediculosis pubis: a surrogate marker for sexually transmitted diseases. *J R Soc Health* 1993;113:6.

Orion E, Matz H, Wolf R. Ectoparasitic sexually transmitted diseases: scabies and pediculosis. *Clin Dermatol* 2004;22:513.

Paasch U, Haustein UF. Treatment of endemic scabies with allethrin, permethrin and ivermectin. Evaluation of a treatement strategy. *Hautartz* 2001;52:31.

Patterson K, Olsen B, Thomas C, et al. Development of a rapid immunodiagnostic test for haemophilus ducreyi. *J Clin Microbiol* 2002;40:3694.

Perine PL, Stramm WE. Lymphogranuloma venereum. In: Holmes KK, Sparling PE, Mårdh PA, et al., eds. *Sexually transmitted diseases*, 3rd ed. New York: McGraw-Hill; 1999:423.

Pierzchalski JL, Bretl DA, Matson SC. Phthirus pubis as a predictor for chlamydia infections in adolescents. *Sex Transm Dis* 2002;29:331.

Platts-Mills TAE, Rein M. Scabies. In: Holmes KK, Sparling PF, Mårdh, PA, et al., eds. *Sexually transmitted diseases*, 3rd ed. New York: McGraw-Hill; 1999.

Richens J. Sexually transmitted diseases: microbiology and management. *J Med Microbiol* 2002;51:793.

Roberts LJ, Huffam SE, Walton SF, et al. Crusted scabies: clinical and immunological findings in seventy-eight patients and a review of the literature. *J Infect* 2005;50:375.

Ronald AR, Albritton W. Chancroid and *haemophilus ducreyi*. In: Holmes KK, Sparling PE, Mårdh PA, et al., eds. *Sexually transmitted diseases*, 3rd ed. New York: McGraw-Hill; 1999.

Schachter J, Osoba AO. Lymphogranulom venereum. *Br Med Bull* 1983;39:151.

Sidbury R. What's new in pediatric dermatology: update for the pediatrician. *Curr Opin Pediatr* 2004;16:410.

Smolinski KN, Yan AC. How and when to treat: molluscum contagiosum and warts in children. *Pediatr Ann* 2005;34:211.

Steen R. Eradicating chancroid. *Bull World Health Organ* 2001;79:818.

Thomas A, Platt-Mills E, Rein MF. Scabies. In: Holmes KK, Sparling PF, Mårdh PA, et al., eds. *Sexually transmitted diseases*, 3rd ed. New York: McGraw-Hill; 1999.

Ting PT, Dytoc MT. Therapy of external anogential warts and molluscum contagiosum: a literature review. *Dermatol Ther* 2004;17:68.

Trager J. Sexually transmitted diseases causing genital lesions in adolescents. *Adolesc Med Clin* 2004;15:323.

Tüzün B, Saygin A, Wolf R, et al. Anogenital lesions (viral diseases and ectoparasitic infestations): Unapproved treatments. *Clin Dermatol* 2002;20:668.

Tyring SK. Molluscum contagiosum: the importance of early diagnosis and treatment. *Am J Obstet Gynecol* 2003;189:S12.

Van Dyck E, Piot P. Laboratory techniques in the investigation of chancroid, lymphogranuloma venerum and donovanosis. *Genitourin Med* 1992;68:130.

Veeranna S, Raghu TY. Oral donovanosis. *Int J STD AIDS* 2002;13:855.

Weir E. Lymphogranuloma venereum in the differential diagnosis of proctitis. *CMAJ* 2005;172:185.

Wendel K, Rompalo A. Scabies and pediculosis pubis: an update of treatment regimens and general review. *CID* 2002;35:S146.

Wu JJ, Huang DB, Pang KR, et al. Selected sexually transmitted diseases and their relationship to HIV. *Clin Dermatol* 2004;22:499.

PART XIV

Drug Use and Abuse

CHAPTER 68

Adolescent Substance Use and Abuse

Alain Joffe and Robert E. Morris

Use of alcohol, tobacco, and other illicit drugs (ATOD) by adolescents continues to be a major public health problem. In the short term, drug use is associated with significant adolescent morbidity and mortality. Early use of various substances is a strong predictor of both problem and lifelong use. Most adults with substance use disorders began using drugs as adolescents; hence much of the adult morbidity and mortality attributed to both legal (alcohol and tobacco) and illegal drug use can be traced to behaviors that began during adolescence. Alcohol, tobacco, and marijuana are the three drugs most abused by adolescents, although inhalant use is particularly common among younger adolescents. Other drugs wax and wane in popularity, their use following a predictable pattern. Drug "X" becomes popular, at least in part because it is presumed safe; as its use becomes more widespread, its negative effects become more widely known and its use increasingly perceived as risky. The popularity of drug "X" wanes, to be replaced by use of other presumably safer drugs. Decades later, due to the phenomenon known as *generational forgetting*, drug "X" again becomes popular, as knowledge of its side effects is no longer common knowledge. Recently, abuse of over-the-counter and prescription medications and their ready availability has emerged as a significant problem.

Advances in neuroimaging techniques and research using animal models of human puberty have elucidated the unique vulnerability of the still developing adolescent brain to the effects of alcohol and other drugs; many observed changes in response to drug use may be permanent (Goldstein and Volkow, 2002; Volkow et al., 2003; Chambers et al., 2003). Ongoing research into the brain's reward circuitry (e.g., the ventral tegmental area, the prefrontal cortex, and the nucleus accumbens) continues to demonstrate that in the brain, drugs of abuse share common pathways and exert their effects through similar mechanisms. For example, the active ingredient in marijuana, Δ^9-tetrahydrocannabinol, stimulates the same μ_1 opioid receptor as does heroin. Similarly, when rats that have been chronically exposed to a cannabinoid agonist are given a cannabinoid antagonist to produce an acute withdrawal state, they secrete elevated amounts of corticotropin-releasing factor. This same pattern is seen in withdrawal from other drugs of abuse. Given this growing body of research, drug addiction is best viewed as a chronic disease with relapses being common. However, recent data indicate that treatment of adolescents with drug problems is effective.

EPIDEMIOLOGY

Middle and High School Youth

The best data on adolescent substance abuse come from the *Monitoring the Future (MTF) study*, conducted by the Institute for Social Research at the University of Michigan (www.monitoringthefuture.org). This school-based study began in 1975, surveying a nationally representative sample of 12th graders. Beginning in 1990, data about drug use by 8th and 10th grade students were added. Currently, the sample consists of approximately 50,000 youth. Because the anonymous surveys are conducted in schools, MTF data do not reflect drug use by out-of-school youth (including drop-outs, homeless, and incarcerated youth), whose use is typically higher.

The most important findings from the 2006 MTF survey, focusing especially on the last decade, are as follows:

1. Drug use among 8th graders has decreased by approximately one third since 1996, the peak year in the last decade. Since 1997, the peak year for 10th and 12th graders, drug use is down by 25% and 10%, respectively. For the fifth consecutive year (2002–2006), the proportion of 10th and 12th grade students who use illicit drugs declined (www.monitoringthefuture.org).
2. *Lifetime use*: Use of illicit drugs by 12th graders peaked in 1980 to 1982 and then steadily declined until 1992 when use began to increase again (Fig. 68.1). *Lifetime* use of illicit drugs among 8th grade students peaked in 1996 and has declined since then. *Lifetime* use among 10th and 12th graders peaked in 1997 to 1999, declining since then. In 2006, 20.9% of 8th graders, 36.1% of 10th graders, and 48.2% of 12th graders had ever used an illicit drug.
3. *Annual use (last year)*: Use of any illicit drug peaked in 1996 for 8th graders and in 1997 for 10th and 12th graders, declining in each year thereafter. In 2006, 14.8% of 8th graders, 28.7% of 10th graders, and 36.5% of 12th graders had used an illicit substance in the last year (Figs. 68.2 and 68.3).
4. *Thirty-day use* (i.e., use in the 30 days before the survey) of illicit drugs peaked in 1996 for 8th and 10th graders

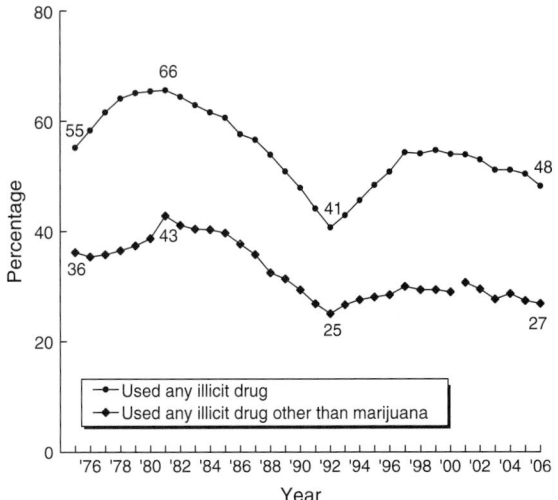

FIGURE 68.1 Trends in lifetime prevalence for an illicit drug use index for 12th graders. (From Johnston LD, O'Malley PM, Bachman JG, et al. *Monitoring the Future national survey results on drug use, 1975–2006: Volume I, Secondary school students*, NIH Publication No. 07–6205. Bethesda, MD: National Institute on Drug Abuse; 2007:229. Available at http://monitoringthefuture.org/pubs/monographs/vol1_2006.pdf.)

and in 1997 for 12th graders and has declined since those peak years. In 2006, 30-day use was 8.1% among 8th graders, 16.8% among 10th graders, and 21.5% among 12th graders.

5. *Daily use*: In 2006, 1% of 8th graders, 3.1% of 10th graders, and 2.8% of 12th graders reported smoking

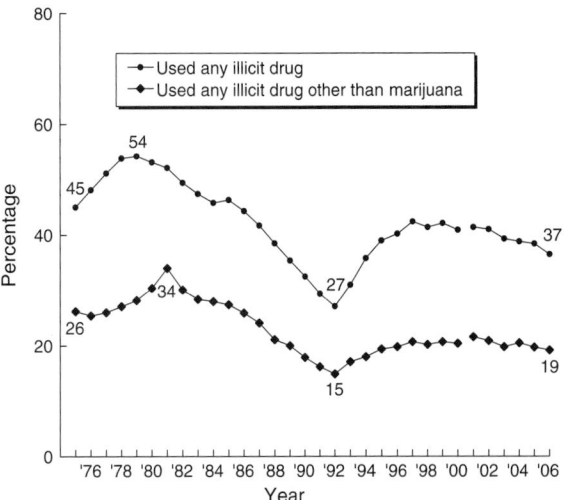

FIGURE 68.2 Trends in annual prevalence of an illicit drug use index for 12th graders. (From Johnston LD, O'Malley PM, Bachman JG, et al. *Monitoring the Future national survey results on drug use, 1975–2006: Volume I, Secondary school students,* NIH Publication No. 07–6205. Bethesda, MD: National Institute on Drug Abuse; 2007:230. Available at http://monitoringthefuture.org/pubs/monographs/vol1_2006.pdf.)

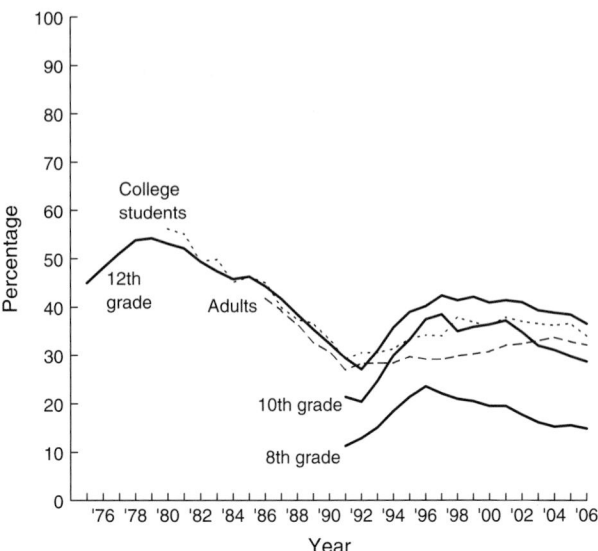

FIGURE 68.3 Trends in annual prevalence of an illicit drug use index across five populations. (From Johnston LD, O'Malley PM, Bachman JG, et al. *Monitoring the Future national survey results on drug use, 1975–2006: Volume I, Secondary school students,* NIH Publication No. 07–6205. Bethesda, MD: National Institute on Drug Abuse; 2007:60. Available at http://monitoringthefuture.org/pubs/monographs/vol1_2006.pdf.)

marijuana or hashish daily; 0.5% of 8th graders, 1.4% of 10th graders, and 3.0% of 12th graders reported drinking alcohol daily. Four percent, 7.6%, and 12.2% of 8th, 10th, and 12th graders, respectively, reported daily cigarette smoking.

6. *Alcohol* continues to be the drug most abused by adolescents. In 2006, approximately 33.6% of 8th graders, 55.8% of 10th graders, and 66.5% of 12th graders had used alcohol in the last year. Binge drinking (defined as five or more drinks in a row) was reported by 10.9% of 8th graders, 21.9% of 10th graders, and 25.4% of 12th graders in the 2 weeks before the survey. Binge-drinking rates have decreased steadily among 8th graders from 1999 to 2005 but there was small increase in 2006; they have remained essentially unchanged since 2002 among 10th and 12th graders, with small nonsignificant decreases occurring from 2004 to 2006. Although males drink more heavily than females, the gap has recently narrowed (Figs. 68.4 and 68.5).

7. *Marijuana*: After alcohol (legal for those aged 21 and older) and tobacco (legal for teenagers aged 18 and older), marijuana is the illicit drug most used by 10th and 12th graders. Among 8th graders, inhalants (17%) and marijuana (16%) are used almost equally. In 2006, 6.5% of 8th graders, 14.2% of 10th graders, and 18.3% of 12th graders reported using marijuana or hashish in the last 30 days (Fig. 68.6A–C).

8. "*Ecstasy*" (methylenedioxymethamphetamine or MDMA) use climbed steeply from 1998 to 2001, then began to decline in 2002 with a small increase 2006; perceived risk of use began increasing in 2001.

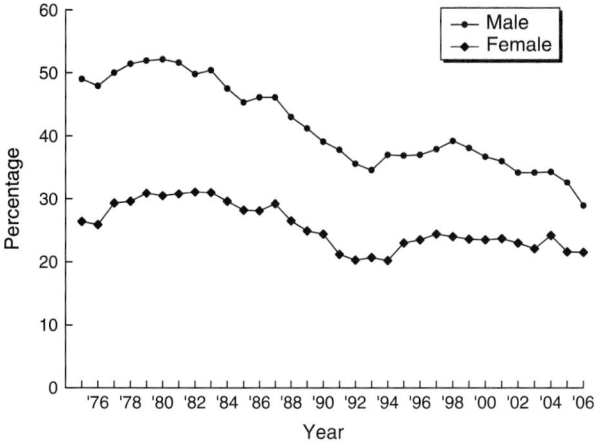

*Due to a coding error, previously released versions of this figure contained values that were slightly off for the measure of five or more drinks in a row for 2005 and 2006. These have been corrected here.

FIGURE 68.4   Trends in 2-week prevalence of heavy drinking (five or more drinks in a row in the last 2 weeks) among 12th graders. (From Johnston LD, O'Malley PM, Bachman JG, et al. *Monitoring the Future national survey results on drug use, 1975–2006: Volume I, Secondary school students,* NIH Publication No. 07–6205, Bethesda, MD: National Institute on Drug Abuse; 2007:247. Available at http://monitoringthefuture.org/pubs/monographs/vol1_2006.pdf.)

9. *Methamphetamine*: Annual use of methamphetamine decreased significantly from 2003 to 2004 among 8th graders but showed a nonsignificant increase in 2005; over the same period, an insignificant decrease was observed among 10th graders. Annual use of methamphetamine decreased significantly among 12th graders from 2004 to 2005 (from 3.4%–2.5%).

10. *Steroid use*: Eighth graders have shown a decline in steroid use since 2000 (but none from 2004–2005); a decline among 10th graders has been occurring since 2002. Twelfth graders demonstrated a significant decline in use from 2004 to 2005 (from 2.5%–1.5% use in the last year).

11. *Rohypnol/GHB*: Use of Rohypnol and GHB among all three grades is low (1.6% or less). Annual use of Rohypnol has shown an upward trend among 8th graders since 2002 but has remained essentially unchanged among 10th and 12th graders since 2002. Annual use of GHB declined among 12th graders from 2004 to 2006 but remained stable among 8th and 10th graders.

12. *Inhalants*: Lifetime use of inhalants showed a significant increase from 2003 to 2004 and a nonsignificant decrease from 2005 to 2006 for 8th graders; annual use of inhalants decreased among 8th graders from 2002 to 2006. From 2003 to 2006, annual use has shown nonsignificant decreases among 10th and 12th graders.

See Figure 68.6A–C and Table 68.1 for detailed information about drug use by adolescents in 2005.

Other surveys that track adolescent substance abuse to varying degrees are the Youth Risk Behavior Surveillance System (YRBSS), also administered in schools, (www.cdc.gov/HealthyYouth/yrbs/index.htm) and the National Survey on Drug Use and Health (NSDUH, www.oas.samhsa.gov/nhsda.htm). The latter survey, administered in the home setting, has the advantage of including out-of-school

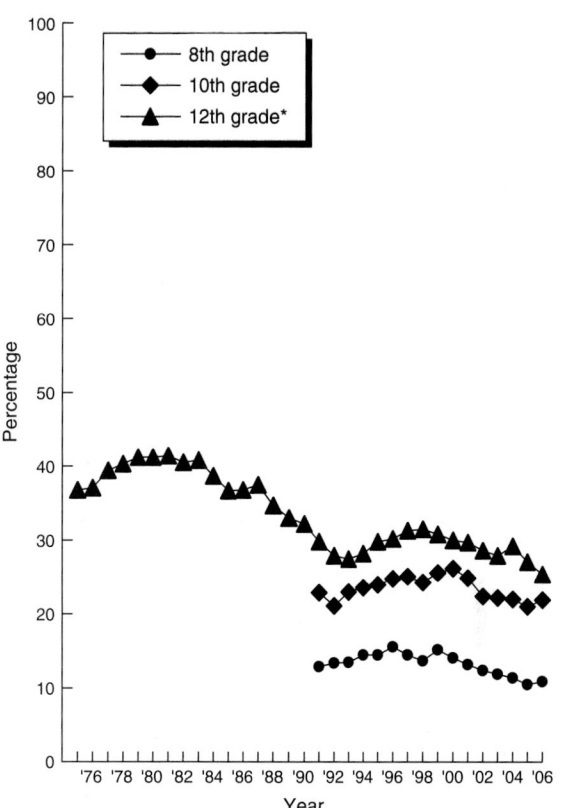

*Due to a coding error, previously released versions of this figure contained values that were slightly off for the measure of five or more drinks in a row for 2005 and 2006. These have been corrected here.

FIGURE 68.5   Trends in 2-week prevalence of heavy drinking (five or more drinks in a row in the last 2 weeks) for 8th, 10th, and 12th graders. (From Johnston LD, O'Malley PM, Bachman JG, et al. *Monitoring the Future national survey results on drug use, 1975–2006: Volume I, Secondary school students,* NIH Publication No. 07–6205. Bethesda, MD: National Institute on Drug Abuse; 2007:241. Available at http://monitoringthefuture.org/pubs/monographs/vol1_2006.pdf.)

youth. However, as parents may be present at home during the survey, results may be subject to underreporting. This may explain why drug use estimates from the MTF surveys consistently yield higher estimates than does the NSDUH. According to the 2000 NSDUH, the average age of new drug users was 16 years for cigarettes, 16.2 for alcohol, 16.6 for marijuana, and 20.4 for cocaine.

Nonmedical Use of Prescription Medications
One worrisome new trend in adolescent drug abuse is nonmedical use of prescription medications (pain relievers, stimulants, tranquilizers, and sedatives). According to the NSDUH, 11.4% of 12- to 17-year-olds surveyed in 2004 had ever abused prescription pain relievers, with 7.4% using them in the last year, and 3% in the last month (http://www.oas.samhsa.gov/NSDUH/2k4nsduh/2k4tabs/Sect1peTabs1to18.pdf). The largest group of new drug users was those who began using prescription pain relievers without a physician's prescription. According to the most recent Partnership for a Drug Free America Tracking Survey, 18% of teenagers have ever used hydrocodone (Vicodin), and

10% have used oxycodone (OxyContin), methylphenidate (Ritalin), or dextroamphetamine/amphetamine (Adderall) without a physician's prescription. Approximately 28% of teens in this survey indicated that these drugs were "very easy" to get, as compared to 48% who felt the same about marijuana and 14% about ecstasy (http://www.drugfree.org/Portal/DrugIssue/Research/PATS_Teens_2004_Report/Teens_Abusing_Rx_and_OTC_Medications). The 2005 MTF data demonstrate that hydrocodone use has declined slightly among 8th, 10th, and 12th graders since 2003. In contrast, annual use of oxycodone from 2002 to 2006 has increased steadily, although nonsignificantly, among 8th graders; remained largely unchanged among 10th graders; and decreased significantly between 2005 and 2006 among 12th graders (from 5.5% to 4.3%).

The European School Survey Project on Alcohol and Other Drugs (ESPAD), conducted in 2003 in 36 European countries and regions among 15- to 16-year-old students

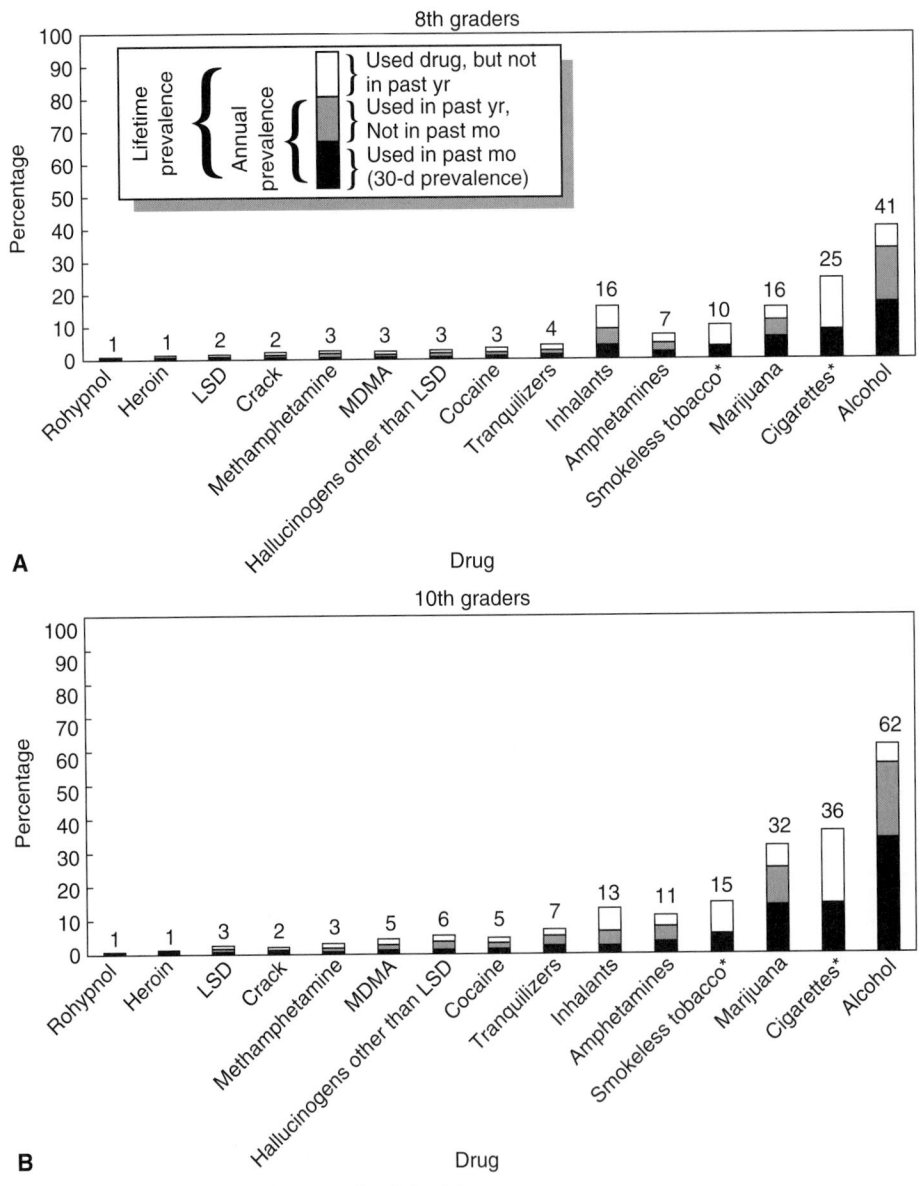

*Annual use not measured for cigarettes and smokeless tobacco.

FIGURE 68.6 **A:** 8th graders; **B:** 10th graders; and **C:** 12th graders. Prevalence and recency of use of various types of drugs for 8th, 10th, and 12th graders, 2006. **B, C:** Annual use not measured for cigarettes and smokeless tobacco. LSD, lysergic acid diethylamide; MDMA, methylenedioxymethamphetamine. (From Johnston LD, O'Malley PM, Bachman JG, et al. *Monitoring the Future national survey results on drug use, 1975–2006: Volume I, Secondary school students,* NIH Publication No. 07–6205. Bethesda, MD: National Institute on Drug Abuse; 2007:136–137. Available at http://monitoringthefuture.org/pubs/monographs/vol1_2006.pdf.)

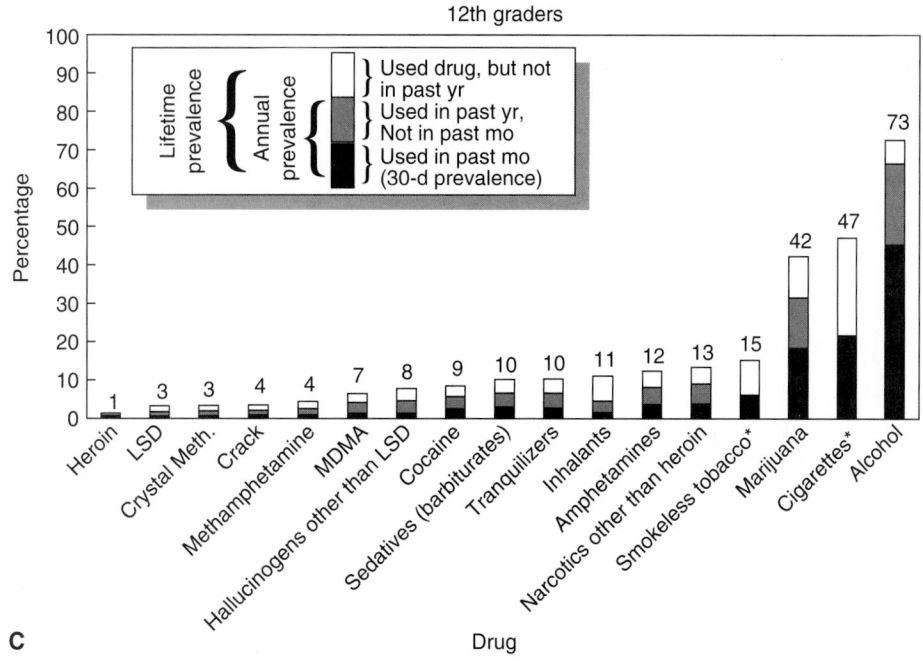

C

Drug

*Annual use not measured for cigarettes and smokeless tobacco.

FIGURE 68.6   *(Continued)*

(mean age 15.8 years), permits comparisons of alcohol use between the United States, where the legal age for alcohol consumption is 21 years, and European countries, most of whom have legal drinking ages below 21. As shown in Figures 68.7 and 68.8, compared to students comprising the 2003 MTF survey cohort, adolescents in most of these countries/regions drink more heavily than do U.S. adolescents and are more likely to be intoxicated (www.udetc.org/documents/CompareDrinkRate.pdf, accessed 12/08/05).

College Students and Their Noncollege Peers

Although most college students and their noncollege peers cannot legally purchase alcohol, the vast majority have used it. Approximately 82% of college students and 79% of noncollege peers have used alcohol in the last year, with 61% of noncollege adolescents and approximately 65% of college students consuming it in the last 30 days. These 30-day use patterns have remained relatively constant over the last decade. Binge drinking among college students (defined as five or more drinks in a row in the prior 2 weeks) has attracted considerable attention. On this measure, college students clearly drink more than their noncollege peers and male college students drink considerably more than female college students. However, the gap between males and females has narrowed somewhat in the last decade (Figs. 68.9 and 68.10).

Binge drinking is especially problematic because of its association with poor academic performance, violence, sexual assault, and unprotected sexual intercourse. According to the Harvard School of Public Health College Alcohol Survey, binge drinking affects not only those who consume alcohol and their partners but other students on campus as well. Nonbinge drinking students on campuses

with medium to high levels of binge drinking are more likely to report having been pushed, hit, assaulted, or having been the victim of a sexual assault/date rape than similar students on campuses with low levels of binge drinking (Wechsler and Nelson, 2001).

Use of illicit drugs in the last 12 months among college and noncollege students reached a low point in 1991 and then began to trend upward, reaching a peak in 2001 (Fig. 68.3). Since then, rates of illicit drug use have remained largely unchanged among college students although increasing somewhat among noncollege students. After alcohol, marijuana is the drug most often used by both college and noncollege students.

Other notable findings regarding drug use in last 12 months are as follows:

1. MDMA ("ecstasy") use grew rapidly in popularity among college students, with peak use occurring in 2001 and declining rapidly after that.
2. Use of narcotics other than heroin has shown a steady upward trend since 1992 and leveling out since 2004.
3. Cocaine use reached a nadir in 1994. Among college students, rates of use plateaued from 2000 to 2002 and then increased in 2003 and 2004 with a slight decrease in 2005 and 2006. Among noncollege students, rates of use increased through 2004 and have remained almost level since that time.
4. In 2006, approximately 7.6% of college students and 9.1% of noncollege students reported nonmedical use of hydrocodone (Vicodin) in the last 12 months. This is a slight decline from 2005 following increases since 2002 when this was first measured. Data from the 2001 Harvard School of Public Health College Alcohol Survey indicate that the prevalence of nonmedical use of prescription opioids and stimulants was 7% and 4.1%, respectively (McCabe et al., 2005a, b).

TABLE 68.1

Prevalence of Use of Various Drugs for 8th, 10th, and 12th Graders, 2006

	Lifetime			Annual			30-Day			Daily		
Grade:	8th	10th	12th	8th	10th	12th	8th	10th	12th	8th	10th	12th
Approximate Weighted n =	*16,500*	*16,200*	*14,200*	*16,500*	*16,200*	*14,200*	*16,500*	*16,200*	*14,200*	*16,500*	*16,200*	*14,200*
Any illicit drug[a]	20.9	36.1	48.2	14.8	28.7	36.5	8.1	16.8	21.5	—	—	—
Any illicit drug other than marijuana[a]	12.2	17.5	26.9	7.7	12.7	19.2	3.8	6.3	9.8	—	—	—
Any illicit drug including inhalants[a,b]	29.2	40.1	51.2	19.7	30.7	38.0	10.9	17.7	22.1	—	—	—
Marijuana/hashish	15.7	31.8	42.3	11.7	25.2	31.5	6.5	14.2	18.3	1.0	2.8	5.0
Inhalants[b]	16.1	13.3	11.1	9.1	6.5	4.5	4.1	2.3	1.5	—	—	0.1
Inhalants, adjusted[b,c]	—	—	11.5	—	—	4.7	—	—	1.7	—	—	—
Amyl/butyl nitrites[d]	—	—	1.2	—	—	0.5	—	—	0.3	—	—	0.2
Hallucinogens	3.4	6.1	8.3	2.1	4.1	4.9	0.9	1.5	1.5	—	—	0.1
Hallucinogens, adjusted[e]	—	—	8.8	—	—	5.3	—	—	1.8	—	—	—
LSD	1.6	2.7	3.3	0.9	1.7	1.7	0.4	0.7	0.6	—	—	0.1
Hallucinogens												
Other than LSD	2.8	5.5	7.8	1.8	3.7	4.6	0.7	1.3	1.3			0.1
PCP[d]	—	—	2.2	—	—	0.7	—	—	0.4	—	—	0.1
MDMA (ecstasy)[f,g]	2.5	4.5	6.5	1.4	2.8	4.1	0.7	1.2	1.3	—	—	*
Cocaine	3.4	4.8	8.5	2.0	3.2	5.7	1.0	1.5	2.5	—	—	0.2
Crack	2.3	2.3	3.5	1.3	1.3	2.1	0.6	0.7	0.9	—	—	0.1
Other cocaine[h]	2.7	4.3	7.9	1.6	2.9	5.2	0.7	1.3	2.4	—	—	0.1
Heroin												
Any use	1.4	1.4	1.4	0.8	0.9	0.8	0.3	0.5	0.4	—	—	*
With a needle[b]	1.0	0.9	0.8	0.5	0.5	0.5	0.2	0.3	0.3	—	—	*
Without a needle[b]	0.9	1.0	1.1	0.5	0.6	0.6	0.2	0.3	0.3	—	—	*
Other narcotics[i]	—	—	13.4	—	—	9.0	—	—	3.8	—	—	0.2
OxyContin[b,j]	—	—	—	2.6	3.8	4.3	—	—	—	—	—	—
Vicodin[b,j]	—	—	—	3.0	7.0	9.7	—	—	—	—	—	—
Amphetamines[i]	7.3	11.2	12.4	4.7	7.9	8.1	2.1	3.5	3.7	—	—	0.3
Ritalin[g,j]	—	—	—	2.6	3.6	4.4	—	—	—	—	—	—
Methamphetamine[g,j]	2.7	3.2	4.4	1.8	1.8	2.5	0.6	0.7	0.9	—	—	*
Crystal methamphetamine (ice)[g]	—	—	3.4	—	—	1.9	—	—	0.7	—	—	*
Sedatives (Barbiturates)[i]	—	—	10.2	—	—	6.6	—	—	3.0	—	—	0.1
Sedatives, adjusted[i,k]	—	—	10.6	—	—	6.8	—	—	3.1	—	—	0.1
Methaqualone[d,i]	—	—	1.2	—	—	0.8	—	—	0.4	—	—	*
Tranquilizers[i]	4.3	7.2	10.3	2.6	5.2	6.6	1.3	2.4	2.7	—	—	0.1
Rohypnol[g,l]	1.0	0.8	—	0.5	0.5	1.1	0.4	0.2	—	—	—	—
GHB[d,j]	—	—	—	0.8	0.7	1.1	—	—	—	—	—	—
Ketamine[b,j]	—	—	—	0.9	1.0	1.4	—	—	—	—	—	—
Alcohol, any use	40.5	61.5	72.7	33.6	55.8	66.5	17.2	33.8	45.3	0.5	1.4	3.0
Been drunk[g]	19.5	41.4	56.4	13.9	34.5	47.9	6.2	18.8	30.0	0.2	0.5	1.6
Flavored alcoholic beverages[d,j]	35.5	58.1	69.9	26.8	48.8	54.7	13.1	24.7	29.3	—	—	1.6
Five or more drinks in a row in last 2 wk[m]	—	—	—	—	—	—	—	—	—	10.9	21.9	25.4
Cigarettes, any use	24.6	36.1	47.1	—	—	—	8.7	14.5	21.6	4.0	7.6	12.2
1/2 pack +/d	—	—	—	—	—	—	—	—	—	1.5	3.3	5.9

TABLE 68.1

(Continued)

	Grade:	Lifetime			Annual			30-Day			Daily		
		8th	10th	12th	8th	10th	12th	8th	10th	12th	8th	10th	12th
Approximate Weighted n =		16,500	16,200	14,200	16,500	16,200	14,200	16,500	16,200	14,200	16,500	16,200	14,200
Bidis[g]		—	—	—	—	—	2.3	—	—	—	—	—	—
Kreteks[g]		—	—	—	—	—	6.2	—	—	—	—	—	—
Smokeless tobacco[d,f]		10.2	15.0	15.2	—	—	—	3.7	5.7	6.1	0.7	1.7	2.2
Steroids[b]		1.6	1.8	2.7	0.9	1.2	1.8	0.5	0.6	1.1	—	—	0.4

[a]For 12th graders only: Use of "any illicit drugs" includes any use of marijuana, LSD, other hallucinogens, crack, other cocaine, or heroin, or any use of other narcotics, amphetamines, barbiturates, or tranquilizers not under a doctor's orders. For 8th and 10th graders only: The use of other narcotics and barbiturates has been excluded, because these younger respondents appear to overreport use (perhaps because they include the use of nonprescription drugs in their answers).

[b]For 12th graders only: Data based on three of six forms; n is one-half of n indicated.

[c]For 12th graders only: Adjusted for underreporting of amyl and butyl nitrites. See text for details. Data for the daily prevalence of use are no longer presented due to low rates of inhalant use and fairly stable rates of nitrite use.

[d]For 12th graders only: Data based on one of six forms; n is one-sixth of n indicated.

[e]Adjusted for underreporting of PCP. See text for details. Data for the daily prevalence of use are no longer presented due to low rates of hallucinogen use and fairly stable rates of PCP use.

[f]For 8th and 10th graders only: Data based on two of four forms; n is one-half of n indicated.

[g]For 12th graders only: Data based on two of six forms; n is two-sixths of n indicated.

[h]For 12th graders only: Data based on four of six forms; n is four-sixths of n indicated.

[i]Only drug use not under a doctor's orders is included here.

[j]For 8th and 10th graders only: Data based on one of four forms; n is one-third of n indicated.

[k]For 12th graders only: "Sedatives, adjusted" data are a combination of barbiturate and methaqualone data. Data based on six forms of barbiturate data adjusted by one form of methaqualone data.

[l]For 8th and 10th graders only: Data based on one of four forms; n is one-sixth of n indicated due to changes in the questionnaire forms.

[m]For 12th graders only: Due to a coding error, previously released versions of this table contained values that were slightly off for the measure of five or more drinks in a row for 2005 and 2006. These have been corrected here.

LSD, lysergic acid diethylamide; PCP, phencyclidine; MDMA, methylenedioxymethamphetamine; GHB, γ-hydroxybutyric acid; —, data not available; *, <.05% but >0%.

From Johnston LD, O'Malley PM, Bachman JG, et al. *Monitoring the Future national survey results on drug use, 1975–2006: Volume I, Secondary school students*, NIH Publication No. 07–6205. Bethesda, MD: National Institute on Drug Abuse;2007:105–106. Available at http://monitoringthefuture.org/pubs/monographs/vol1_2006.pdf.

See Figures 68.3, 68.9, and 68.10 and Tables 84.1 to 84.9 for more detailed data about drug use by college students and noncollege adolescents.

LONG-TERM OUTCOMES OF DRUG USE

Over the last 5 years, a number of studies provide evidence that use of drugs, especially if initiated in early to mid-adolescence, is associated with significant long-term adverse consequences:

1. Marijuana
   a. A retrospective cohort study from Sweden showed that, compared to those who never smoked marijuana those who smoked a total of 11 to 50 times were 2.2 times likely to develop schizophrenia; the risk was 3.1 times for those who smoked more than 50 times. After controlling for use of other drugs, those who smoked marijuana more than 50 times were 8.7 times more likely to develop schizophrenia whereas those who smoked less than 50 times were no longer at increased risk (Zammit et al., 2002).
   b. A longitudinal study from New Zealand showed that, controlling for childhood psychotic symptoms and

other drug use, those who smoked marijuana by age 15 were 7.2 times more likely to develop schizophrenia symptoms at age 26 than controls (Arseneault et al., 2002).
   c. Another longitudinal birth cohort study from New Zealand also demonstrated that cannabis use, especially by age 14 to 15, was significantly related to depression, suicidal ideation and attempts, and participation in violent crimes at age 21, even after controlling for a wide variety of potential confounders (Fergusson et al., 2002).
   d. A study of 1,600 Australian students aged 14 to 15 followed for 7 years demonstrated that weekly use of cannabis among females predicted an almost twofold increase in risk for depression and anxiety at age 21 to 22. In contrast, preexisting depression and anxiety did not predict later cannabis use (Patton et al., 2002).
2. Alcohol
   a. Data from the National Longitudinal Survey of Youth show that binge drinking during adolescence (ages 17–20) is associated with a relative risk of 2.3 for men and 3 for women for binge drinking at age 30 to 31 (McCarty et al., 2004).
   b. A population-based cohort study in England, Scotland, and Wales demonstrated that men who drank

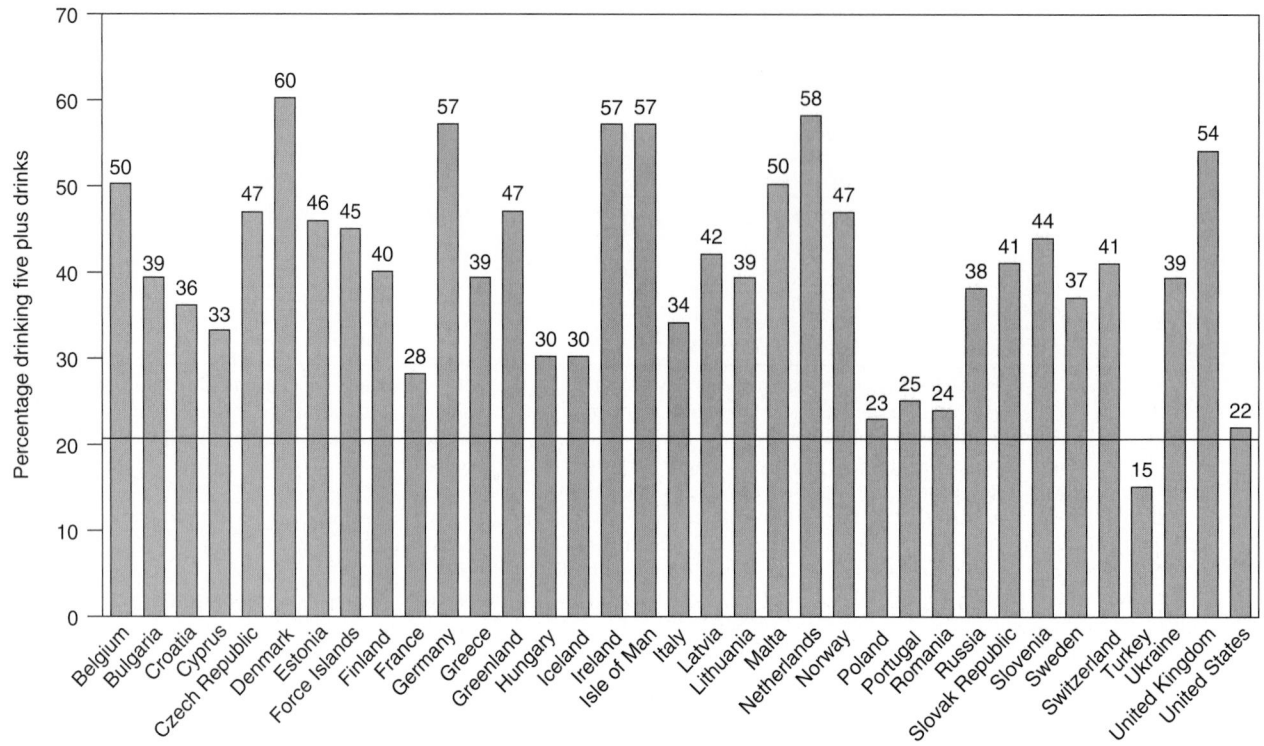

FIGURE 68.7 Prevalence of heavy drinking in the last 30 days: United States and Europe. (From youth drinking rates and problems. A comparison of European Countries and the United States. Office of Juvenile Justice and Delinquency Prevention. Available at www.udetc.org/documents/CompareDrinkRate.pdf [accessed 12/12/05].)

more heavily at age 16 (>7 units/week with 1 unit equal to one small glass of wine) were 1.64 times more likely than light drinkers to binge at age 42. Levels of binge drinking at age 23 increased the odds of binge drinking at 42 (odds ratio 2.10 for men and 1.56 for women) (Jefferis et al., 2005).

c. A cohort study from Australia followed almost 2,000 teenagers from age 14 to age 21, measuring drinking behaviors yearly. Frequent drinking at least once during the 7 years was associated with a twofold increase in the risk for being diagnosed with alcohol dependence at age 20; frequent drinking during more than one period increased the risk threefold. Smoking marijuana weekly or more at one or more times was also associated with an increased risk for being diagnosed as alcohol dependent at age 20 (Bonomo et al., 2004).

RISK AND PROTECTIVE FACTORS FOR DRUG USE

1. Perception of risk

   At a population level, there is a strong link between adolescents' perceptions of the risks of drug use and the prevalence of use. For example, over the last 30 years, the prevalence of marijuana use rose and fell according to how risky its use was perceived to be by adolescents. The percentage of 12th graders who perceived "great risk" in regular marijuana use reached a nadir (~35%) in

1979. In that same year, reported use of marijuana in the last year by 12th graders peaked at approximately 50%. Perceived risk of regular use then began to rise, peaking in 1992. Not surprisingly, use in the last 12 months fell to its lowest level at the same time. Perceived risk then began to fade and use began to rise. In contrast, measures of availability (that a drug is "fairly easy" or "very easy" to get) and disapproval bear little relation to use patterns (Fig. 68.11).

   Similarly, use of ecstasy began climbing steeply in 1998. In 2001, the proportion of 12th graders who perceived great risk in use of this drug increased and in 2002, use began to fall. Over the next 2 years, use continued to decrease as the perception that ecstasy use was risky increased.

2. Race/ethnicity

   One major protective factor associated with drug use is race/ethnicity. Since the MTF survey began in 1975, African-American 12th graders have consistently had lower rates of illicit drug use than white youth, with Hispanic youth having rates in-between those of African-Americans and whites. African-American 8th and 10th graders also have lower rates of illicit drug use than their white classmates although the differences are less pronounced than among 12th graders. In 2004, Hispanic 8th and 10th graders had higher rates of drug use than did whites.

3. Other risk/protective factors

   Adolescent drug use is a complex phenomenon; no single risk factor, when present, predicts with certainty

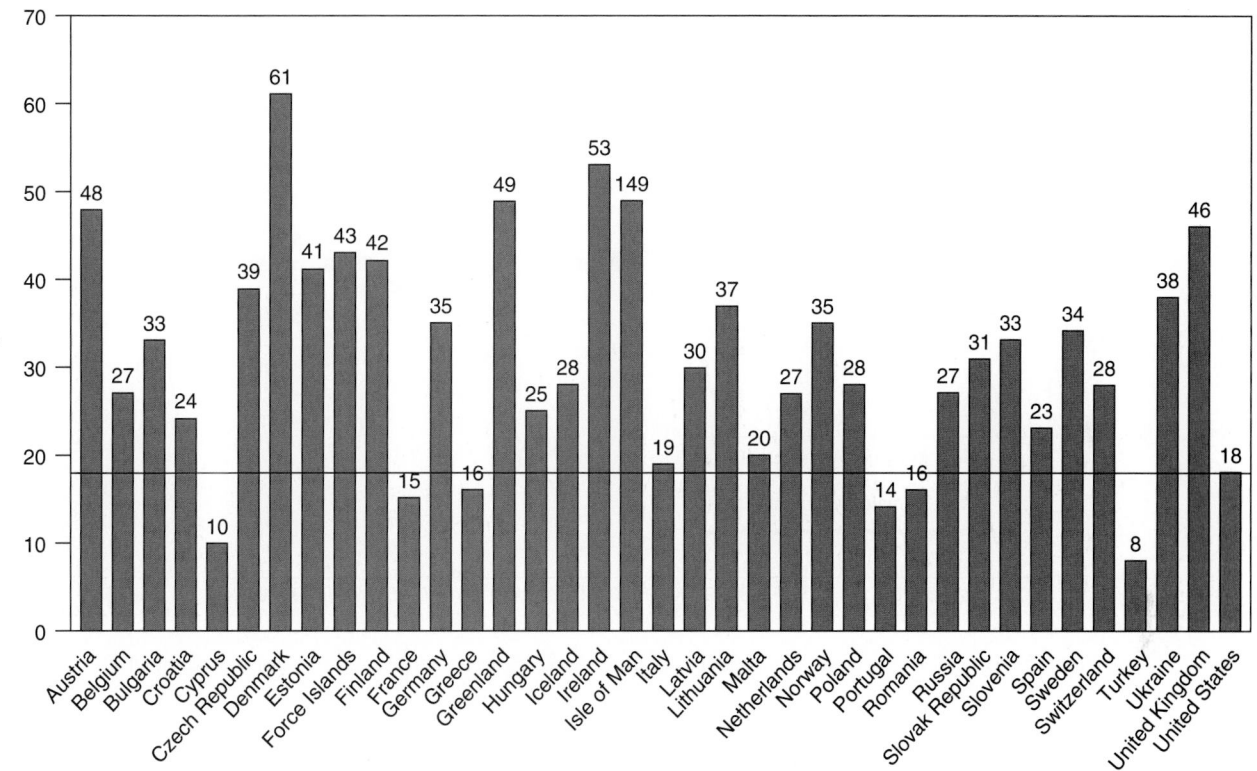

FIGURE 68.8   Prevalence of intoxication in the last 30 days: United States and Europe. (From youth drinking rates and problems. A comparison of European Countries and the United States. Office of Juvenile Justice and Delinquency Prevention. Available at www.udetc.org/documents/CompareDrinkRate.pdf [accessed 12/12/05].)

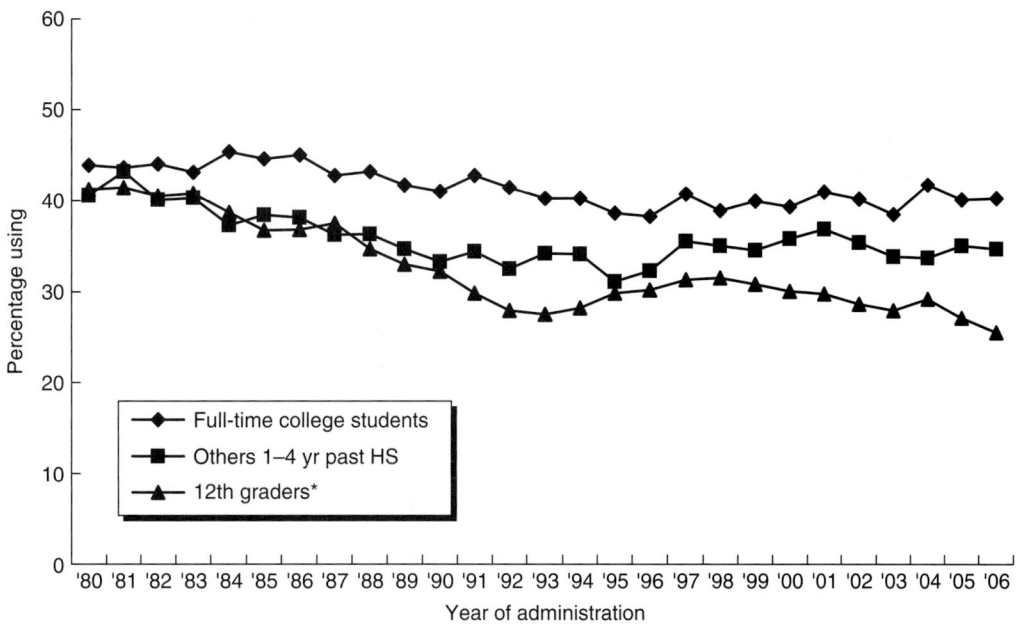

FIGURE 68.9   Alcohol: Trends in 2-week prevalence of five or more drinks in a row among college students versus others, 1 to 4 years beyond high school. (From Johnston LD, O'Malley PM, Bachman JG, et al. *Monitoring the Future national survey results on drug use, 1975–2006: Volume II, College students and adults ages 19–45,* NIH Publication No. 07–6206. Bethesda, MD: National Institute on Drug Abuse; 2007:277. Available at http://www .monitoringthefuture.org/pubs/monographs/vol2_2006.pdf.)

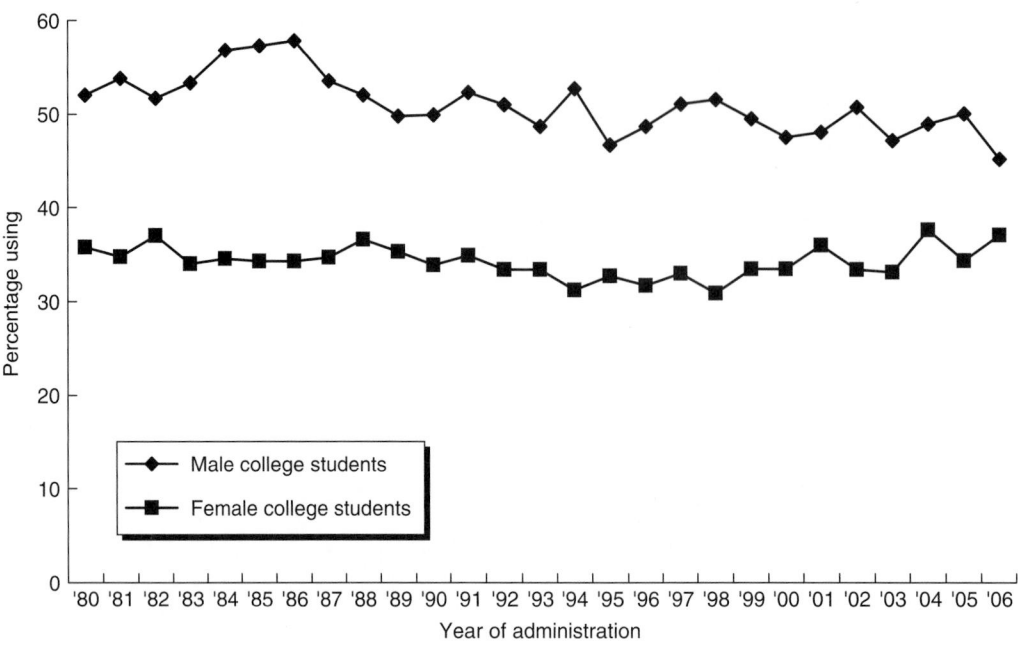

*Due to a coding error, previous versions of this figure contained values (for 12th graders only) that were slightly off for the measure of five or more drinks in a row for 2005. This has been corrected here.

FIGURE 68.10 Alcohol: Trends in 2-week prevalence of five or more drinks in a row among male versus female college students. (From Johnston LD, O'Malley PM, Bachman JG, et al. *Monitoring the Future national survey results on drug use, 1975–2006: Volume II, College students and adults ages 19–45,* NIH Publication No. 07–6206. Bethesda, MD: National Institute on Drug Abuse. Available at http://www.monitoringthefuture.org/pubs/monographs/vol2_2006.pdf.)

FIGURE 68.11 Marijuana: Trends in the perceived availability, perceived risk of regular use, and prevalence of use in last 30 days for 12th graders. (From Johnston LD, O'Malley PM, Bachman JG, et al. *Monitoring the Future national survey results on drug use, 1975–2006: Volume I, Secondary school students,* NIH Publication No. 07–6205. Bethesda, MD: National Institute on Drug Abuse; 2007:379. Available at http://monitoringthefuture.org/pubs/monographs/vol1_2006.pdf.)

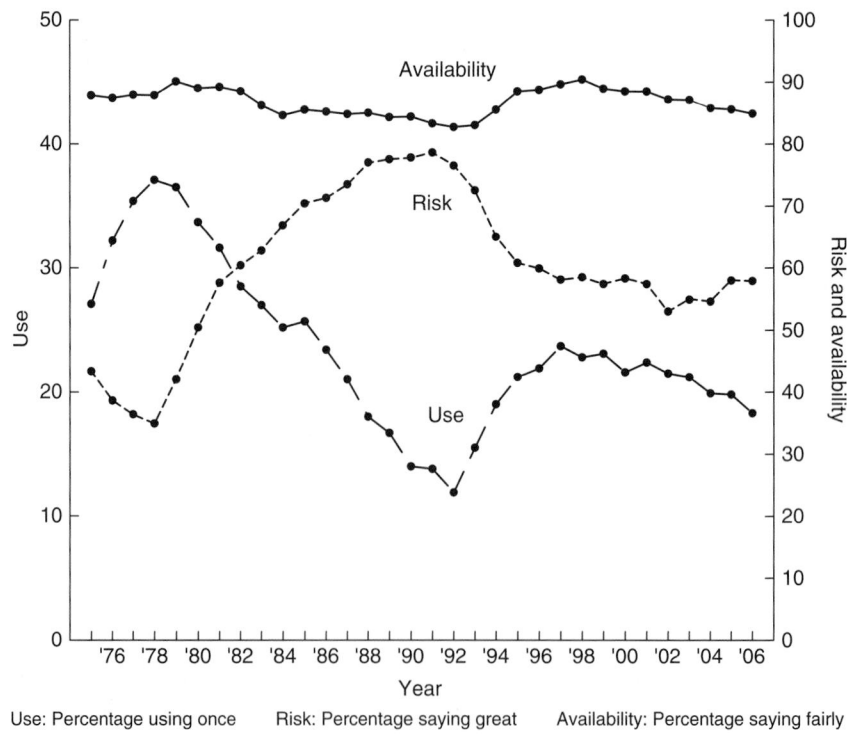

Use: Percentage using once or more in past 30 d (on left-hand scale)

Risk: Percentage saying great risk of harm in regular use (on right-hand scale)

Availability: Percentage saying fairly easy or very easy to get (on right-hand scale)

that an adolescent will use drugs or develop a substance abuse problem, nor does the presence of a single protective factor offer complete reassurance that no use will occur. Rather, drug use or nonuse results from a combination of these factors. Risk and protection can exist at the individual, peer, family, school, and community level or domain (Hawkins et al., 1992). These are outlined in Table 68.2.

ADOLESCENT BRAIN DEVELOPMENT AND SUSCEPTIBILITY TO DRUG USE AND DRUG-ASSOCIATED BRAIN DAMAGE

Use of sophisticated imaging techniques demonstrates that adolescence is a period of significant brain development (Sowell et al., 1999, 2001; Horská et al., 2002). In a longitudinal study of 145 healthy children (56 females, age range 4.2–21.6 years), Giedd et al. (1999) noted the following changes:

1. Linear increases in white matter volume, with greater changes in males than females. The net increase across age 4 to 22 was 12.4%. Increases did not vary by brain region. These changes likely reflect increased myelinization.
2. Gray matter volume changes were nonlinear and varied by lobe. Frontal lobe gray matter increased during early adolescence, reaching peak size at 11 years for females and at 12.1 years for males. Parietal lobe gray matter volume peaked at 10.2 years for females and at 11.8 years for males. Temporal lobe gray matter peaked at 16.5 years for males and at 16.7 years for females. In all three lobes, volumes then decreased. Occipital lobe gray matter continues to increase during adolescence without any leveling off. One explanation for these changes is an initial increase followed by a decrease in the number of synapses in the brain; increased myelinization may also contribute.
3. Observed changes in the frontal cortex are consistent with neuropsychological studies that show that frontal lobes are involved with emotional regulation, planning, organizing, and response inhibition (the latter three constituting "executive functioning").

Studies in rats show that mesolimbic dopamine (DA) synthesis in the nucleus accumbens is lower in preadolescent than adolescent rats, which in turn is lower than in adult rats. Turnover rates for DA are also lower in younger rats as compared with adult rats. Dopaminergic and noradrenergic systems show large increases in neurotransmitter levels and activity during adolescence, particularly in the midbrain and hippocampus. The hippocampus increases significantly in size. The mesolimbic system (which projects from the ventral tegmental area to the nucleus accumbens) may mediate behavioral changes in adolescents and has been shown to play a large role in the reward circuitry of the brain that fuels drug addiction. The hippocampus is intricately involved with new memory formation, a critical process in learning.

Given the significant brain changes that occur during adolescence, including frontal lobe changes linked to impulse control and decision making, and the areas involved in the brain's reward circuitry, it is not surprising that adolescents may be uniquely susceptible to the harmful effects of drug use, including dependence or addiction. Several studies provide clear evidence for this susceptibility; although a few studies have been conducted in humans, for ethical reasons most data derive from studies in rats.

1. Alcohol
   a. Compared with adult rats, adolescent rats are less susceptible to the sedative properties of alcohol and the onset of sedation is slower (Li et al., 2003). This phenomenon may be explained by data showing that cells from adult rats display greater ethanol-induced $GABA_A$ receptor–mediated inhibitory postsynaptic currents than do cells from juvenile or adolescent rats. If this effect were true in humans, then adolescents would be less likely than adults to naturally curtail their intake on the basis of sedation.
   b. In contrast to younger or older rats, adolescent rats displayed a lack of alteration in dopamine and 3,4-dihydroxyphenylacetic acid metabolism with repeated exposure to ethanol. This suggests that adolescents may fail to adapt to repeated alcohol use or may adapt in a way that results in increased reactivity to ethanol (Philpot and Kirstein, 2004).
   c. Adolescent rats are much more vulnerable than adult rats to alcohol-induced learning impairments. Owing to ethical and legal constraints, similar experiments cannot be reproduced in adolescents. However, after ingesting 2 to 3 drinks, young adults in their early twenties display a greater degree of impairment on tasks involving immediate and delayed recall than do young adults in their late twenties who consume the same amount of alcohol (Monti et al., 2005).
   d. After exposure to levels of alcohol consistent with a binge-drinking episode, adolescent rats display greater damage than adult rats to the frontal association cortex and the anterior piriform and perirhinal cortices (which correspond to the orbital-frontal and temporal-cortical areas in humans). Adult rats exposed to binge drinking during adolescence display microglia and long-term changes in serotonergic innervation as compared with control rats (Monti et al., 2005).
   e. Ironically, adolescents display less motor impairment than adults given comparable amounts of ethanol ingestion (White et al., 2002). This is particularly striking given the fact that adolescents have higher peak brain ethanol levels than adults following ethanol administration.
2. Nicotine
   a. Adolescents who smoke cigarettes daily have impairments in working memory compared to nonsmokers, even after controlling for general intelligence, reading achievement, parental education, baseline affective symptoms, and lifetime exposure to alcohol and marijuana. The impairments are more pronounced the younger the age of initiation of smoking is and the severity of impairment at least temporarily increases with smoking cessation. (Jacobsen et al., 2005).
   b. Rats exposed to nicotine in the peri- but not postadolescent period of development become more sensitive to the reinforcing properties of nicotine during adulthood. This is manifested by increased self-administration of nicotine in adulthood and an increase in gene expression of specific subunits

TABLE 68.2

Risk and Protective Factors for Drug Use

Domain	Protective Factors	Risk Factors
Individual	High intelligence	Untreated mental health/behavioral problems (e.g., depression, anxiety, conduct disorder, aggressive behavior, impulsivity)
	Achievement oriented	School problems (including old for grade)
	Positive self-esteem	Genetic vulnerability (family history of alcoholism; "sensation-seeking" personality)
	Optimistic view of future	Early pubertal development
	Good coping skills	Rebelliousness
	Prosocial orientation	Perception that most peers use drugs
	Perception that most peers do not use drugs	Undiagnosed/untreated ADHD
	Treated ADHD	Low religiosity
	High religiosity	Drug use perceived as low risk
	Perception that drug use has risks	After school employment (middle–high income families)
Family	Clear messages about no use	Families expect children will try drugs or expectations about drug use not clear
	Parents model appropriate alcohol/drug use	Familial substance abuse
	Strong family–youth attachment	Alienated from family
	Moderate to high levels of parental monitoring	Permissive parenting
	Supportive parents	Coercive parenting
		Familial conflict
Peers	Peers do not use drugs	Peers use drugs
	Peers have prosocial/conventional values	Peers alienated from community
Schools	Offer opportunities for success and involvement	Poor quality
	Students feel connected to school	Students feel alienated from school
	School personnel perceived as fair and caring	School personnel perceived as uncaring
Community	Good quality with adequate recreational activities	Lack of recreational opportunities
	Strong community institutions	Community institutions lacking
		Lack of community norms about drug use
		Substance abuse common in community
		Drugs easily available
		Socioeconomic deprivation and social disorganization
	Media realistically portrays harms associated with drug use; counter marketing (media used to demonstrate how advertising manipulates youth)	Media portrays drug use as normative and promotes positive expectancies associated with drug use

ADHD, attention-deficit hyperactivity disorder.

of the ligand-gated acetylcholine receptors in the ventral tegmental area of the brain (Adriani et al., 2003).

c. In rats, exposure to nicotine during the periadolescent period (at nicotine levels comparable to that of smokers) is associated with a "profound activation" of midbrain catecholaminergic pathways, followed by a loss of response to an acute nicotine challenge (receptor desensitization). More than 30 days after the last exposure, these rats again showed significant activation of the catecholaminergic pathways with exposure to nicotine. Female rats showed significant late onset cell damage and loss in the hippocampus (Trauth et al., 2001).

3. Marijuana, cocaine, and amphetamines
   a. In both adolescent and adult rats, repeated exposure to the cannabinoid agonist WIN55212.2 (WIN) produced tolerance to its effects. However, adolescent but not adult rats exposed to WIN later displayed long-lasting cross-tolerance to morphine, cocaine, and amphetamines, suggesting a heightened sensitivity to psychoactive substances during a period of brain immaturity (Pistis et al., 2004).
   b. Chronic exposure of periadolescent but not postweanling or adult rats to cocaine and amphetamine results in upregulation of the transcription factor ΔFosB in the nucleus accumbens (Ehrlich et al., 2002).

STAGES OF DRUG USE

It is clinically useful to conceptualize adolescent substance abuse as occurring across a continuum of use. Use generally proceeds from one stage to the next, although some adolescents may skip stages (adapted from MacDonald, 1984).

Stage 0: No drug use. The adolescent is not subject to any health risks posed by his/her own use of illicit substances, although he/she is still subject to risks from use of drugs by friends (e.g., riding with an impaired driver; sexual assault in association with a date rape drug; as a victim in a fight with an intoxicated individual). For clinicians, the primary focus for these adolescents is on safety, praising and normalizing abstinence, and prevention (refusal skills).

Stage 1: Experimentation. Adolescents at this stage may try various drugs, typically out of curiosity or to fit in with friends. The most commonly used drugs are alcohol and tobacco; some may use only marijuana. Once an adolescent crosses from Stage 0 to Stage 1, he/she places himself at risk from the health risks associated with illicit drug use. Even a single episode or very sporadic drug use can involve significant risk—even death—depending on the circumstances of use and the drug(s) used. Some adolescents may move from Stage 1 back to Stage 0, having found the experience unpleasant. For clinicians, the primary focus should be on reviewing risks from drug use, safety, encouraging and normalizing abstinence, and rehearsal of refusal skills.

Stage 2: Learning the mood swing. At this stage, the adolescent will continue to experiment with drugs if available but will not make a concerted effort to obtain the drugs; types of drugs used will increase. Use typically occurs in social settings and positive/pleasurable experiences generally outweigh negative consequences, although the latter may occur. Use typically occurs on the weekends. Significant changes in behavior are not readily apparent although the adolescent may need to change his/her behavior to hide use from parents. For clinicians, the primary focus should be on assessing the adolescent for risk factors associated with progression, reviewing risks, safety, encouraging and normalizing abstinence, and refusal skills.

Stage 3: Seeking/preoccupation with the mood swing. As they progress to this stage, adolescents will actively seek out drug use and begin to organize their lives around assuring a supply of drugs. They will actively seek out settings where drugs are likely to be used and avoid ones where drug use is unlikely. They may buy or even sell drugs to assure a supply. The types of drugs used continue to expand. The social network will largely consist of drug using peers. Straight friends may be dropped. Depending on the types of drugs used and the extent of use, behavioral changes may become apparent. Negative consequences associated with drug use will increase and the adolescent will need to be increasingly vigilant to hide drug use from parents. For clinicians, the focus should be on reviewing risks, safety, assessing for problem use, and challenging the adolescent's perception that he/she controls his/her drug use (abstinence challenges/contracts). Adolescents at this stage need careful follow-up and some will meet the criteria for substance dependence or abuse. Involvement of parents may be necessary despite protestations from the adolescent.

Stage 4: Problem use/dependence. The hallmark of this stage is continued use of drugs despite experiencing significant negative consequences. Adolescents in this stage will often use drugs in order to feel normal. Any adolescent in this stage requires a comprehensive evaluation and will need intensive treatment. Most, if not all, adolescents at this stage will meet criteria for substance dependence or abuse.

PREVENTION

Early efforts at prevention of drug use by adolescents were based on the assumption that use was driven by inadequate knowledge of the harmful effects of drug use. Evaluation of these programs failed to show an effect; indeed, some studies showed an increase in use following presentations on the effects of various drugs. Other efforts relied on the use of authority figures (e.g., police) to deliver antidrug messages. These, too, failed to show an effect (Ennett et al., 1994).

Beginning in the 1980s, prevention efforts became much more sophisticated, recognizing the multiple individual, familial, peer, school, and community factors that bear on use of drugs by adolescents. Given the uptake of drug use by 8th graders (and even earlier for some), these efforts targeted youth before or during junior high school.

1. Life skills approach

Some prevention programs, usually school-based, focus on a "life skills" approach to target numerous risk factors for ATOD use. Such programs generally have the following components (Botvin and Kantor, 2000):

a. ATOD-related information and skills: Information about the short and long-term health risks of ATOD use; providing information about the actual prevalence of ATOD use by adolescents in the community; providing information about the decrease in acceptability of ATOD use among adolescents; refusal skills to resist pressure to use drugs.

b. Personal self-management skills: Improve decision making and problem solving; skills to analyze, interpret, and resist media influences; teaching skills to cope with emotions such as anxiety, frustration, and anger; teaching personal behavior change and self-management skills.

c. Social skills: This component is aimed at improving students' social competence (teaching how to initiate conversations, verbal and nonverbal assertive skills, communicating with others, skills related to male–female relationships).

Such programs require considerable resources to implement. Typically, they use a highly structured curriculum taught over 15 classroom sessions by trained facilitators (not simply classroom teachers). Although some material is didactic, many sessions require role-playing, skills rehearsals, feedback, and homework to practice and reinforce the skills learned in class. In some studies, booster sessions delivered in subsequent years are essential to the program's initial effects at reducing drug use or maintaining the gains as students grow older. Numerous studies have demonstrated that this kind of approach does reduce ATOD use, both in the short and long term. For a comprehensive review of drug prevention programs, see the reviews by Faggiano et al. (2005) and by Skara and Sussman (2003).

2. Risk factor reduction

A second approach is to target the early antecedents of risk factors for substance abuse. For example, Hawkins et al. (1999) found that fifth grade students in high crime areas of Seattle who participated in a program that included training for teachers, parenting classes for parents, and social competence training for students, had lower levels of heavy drinking at 18 years than did control students. In another study, Kellam and Anthony (1998) reported that aggressive/disruptive boys assigned to a 2-year intervention (during grades 1 and 2) aimed at improving behavior in the classroom had lower rates of smoking initiation in early adolescence than did boys in the usual classroom group.

3. Community-based approaches including policy changes and media campaigns

A third approach targets a variety of community approaches including those aimed at policy changes and also media campaigns. These include strict enforcement of laws prohibiting sale of alcohol and tobacco products to minors, counter advertising campaigns, and media criticism. For example, in 1998 the Florida Tobacco Control Program launched a statewide program that included enforcement of regulations against the sale of tobacco to minors and a "truth" counter marketing campaign that sought to counter the tobacco industry's purposeful attempts to market cigarettes to teenagers ("Our brand is truth, their brand is lies"). After 2 years, current cigarette use dropped from 18.5% to 12.1% among middle school students and from 27.4% to 22.6% among high school students. Prevalence of never use increased significantly and prevalence of experimentation decreased significantly. Subsequent analyses showed that the media campaign played a significant role in the program's success (Bauer et al., 2000; Sly et al., 2001; Niederdeppe et al., 2004).

WEB SITES

For Teenagers and Parents

http://www.drugfree.org/. Home page for the Partnership for a Drug Free America. Has comprehensive resources for parents, teenagers, and professionals.

http://camy.org/. Home page of the Center on Alcohol Marketing and Youth. Contains resources to examine and counter the marketing of alcohol to youth.

http://www.freevibe.com/. A youth oriented site developed by the ONDCP.

http://www.nida.nih.gov/students.html. A Web site maintained by NIDA for adolescents, especially for those in grades 5 to 9.

For Health Professionals

http://www.monitoringthefuture.org/. Home page for the MTF survey with links to new press releases and previous research documents.

http://www.cdc.gov/HealthyYouth/yrbs/index.htm. Home page for the CDC's Youth Risk Behavior Surveillance System.

http://www.oas.samhsa.gov/nhsda.htm. Home page for the National Survey on Drug Use and Health.

http://www.samhsa.gov/. Home page for the Substance Abuse and Mental Health Services Administration, where the NSDUH is housed.

http://www.whitehousedrugpolicy.gov/. Office of National Drug Control Policy (ONDCP). Contains much useful information for the discerning reader.

http://www.ncadi.samhsa.gov/research.aspx. A research oriented site maintained by the National Clearinghouse for Alcohol and Drug Information.

http://www.nida.nih.gov/. Home page for the National Institute on Drug Abuse.

http://www.erowid.org/. A Web site that contains extensive information on a wide variety of drugs. Has a search engine to search for information about particular drugs.

http://www.udetc.org/. A good resource for information pertaining to underage drinking.

http://www.hsph.harvard.edu/cas/Home.html. Home page of the Harvard School of Public Health College Alcohol Survey. Contains a page with many links to other alcohol/drug Web sites.

http://www.casacolumbia.org/absolutenm/templates/Home.aspx. Home page of the Center on Addiction and Substance Abuse at Columbia University.

REFERENCES AND ADDITIONAL READINGS

Adriani W, Spijker S, Deroche-Gamonet V, et al. Evidence for enhanced neurobehavioral vulnerability to nicotine during periadolescence in rats. *J Neurosci* 2003;23:4714.

Arseneault L, Cannon M, Poulton R, et al. Cannabis use in adolescence and risk for adult psychosis: longitudinal prospective study. *BMJ* 2002;325:1212.

Bauer UE, Johnson TM, Hopkins RS, et al. Changes in youth cigarette use and intentions following implementation of a tobacco control program. *JAMA* 2000;284:723.

Bonomo YA, Bowes G, Coffey C, et al. Teenage drinking and the onset of alcohol dependence: a cohort study over seven years. *Addiction* 2004;99:1520.

Botvin GJ, Kantor LW. Preventing alcohol and tobacco use through life skills training. *Alcohol Res Health* 2000;24:250.

Chambers RA, Taylor JR, Potenza MN. Developmental neurocircuitry of motivation in adolescence: a critical period of addiction vulnerability. *Am J Psychiatry* 2003;160:1041.

Compton WM, Thomas YF, Conway KP, et al. Developments in the epidemiology of drug use and drug use disorders. *Am J Psychiatry* 2005;162:1494.

Ehrlich ME, Sommer J, Canas E, et al. Periadolescent mice show enhanced ΔFosB upregulation in response to cocaine and amphetamine. *J Neurosci* 2002;22:9155.

Ennett ST, Tobler NS, Ringwalt CL, et al. How effective is drug abuse resistance education? A meta-analysis of project DARE outcome evaluations. *Am J Public Health* 1994;84:1394.

Faggiano F, Vigna-Taglianti FD, Versino E, et al. School-based prevention for illicit drugs' use. *Cochrane Database Syst Rev* 2005;2. Art. No.:CD003020.pub2. DOI: 10.1002/14651858.CD003020.pub2.

Fergusson DM, Horwood LJ, Swain-Campbell N. Cannabis use and psychosocial adjustments in adolescence and young adulthood. *Addiction* 2002;97:1123.

Giedd JN, Blumenthal J, Jeffries NO. Brain development during childhood and adolescence: a longitudinal MRI study. *Nat Neurosci* 1999;2:861.

Goldstein RZ, Volkow ND. Drug addiction and its underlying neurobehavioral basis: neuroimaging evidence for involvement of the frontal cortex. *Am J Psychiatry* 2002;159: 1642.

Hawkins JD, Catalano RF, Kosterman R, et al. Preventing adolescent health-risk behaviors by strengthening protection during childhood. *Arch Pediatr Adolesc Med* 1999;153: 226.

Hawkins JD, Catalano RF, Miller JY. Risk and protective factors for alcohol and other drug problems in adolescence and early adulthood: implications for substance abuse prevention. *Psychol Bull* 1992;112:64.

Horská A, Kaufmann WE, Brant LJ, et al. In vivo quantitative proton MRSI study of brain development from childhood to adolescence. *J Magn Reson Imaging* 2002;15:137.

Jacobsen LK, Krystal JH, Menci WE, et al. Effects of smoking and smoking abstinence on cognition in adolescent tobacco smokers. *Biol Psychiatry* 2005;57:56.

Jefferis BJMH, Power C, Manor O. Adolescent drinking level and adult binge drinking in a national birth cohort. *Addiction* 2005;100:543.

Johnston LD, O'Malley PM, Bachman JG, et al. *Monitoring the Future national survey results on drug use, 1975–2006: Volume I, Secondary school students*, NIH Publication No. 07–6205. Bethesda, MD: National Institute on Drug Abuse; Available at: http://www.monitoringthefuture.org/pubs/monographs/vol1_2006.pdf.

Johnston LD, O'Malley PM, Bachman JG, et al. *Monitoring the Future national survey results on drug use, 1975–2006: Volume II, College students and adults ages 19–45*, NIH Publication No. 07–6206. Bethesda, MD: National Institute on Drug Abuse; 2006. Available at: http://www.monitoringthefuture.org/pubs/monographs/vol2_2006.pdf.

Kellam SG, Anthony JC. Targeting early antecedents to prevent tobacco smoking: findings from an epidemiologically based randomized field trial. *Am J Public Health* 1998;88:193.

Li Q, Wilson WA, Swartzwelder HS. Developmental differences in the sensitivity of hippocampal GABA$_A$ receptor-mediated IPSCS to ethanol. *Alcohol Clin Exp Res* 2003;27:2017.

MacDonald DI. *Drugs, drinking, and adolescents*. Chicago: Year Book Medical; 1984.

McCabe SE, Knight JR, Teter C, et al. Non-medical use of prescription stimulants among US college students: prevalence and correlates from a national survey. *Addiction* 2005a; 99:96.

McCabe SE, Teter CJ, Boyd CJ, et al. Nonmedical use of prescription opioids among U.S. college students: prevalence and correlates from a national survey. *Addict Behav* 2005b;30:789.

McCarty CA, Ebel BE, Garrison MM, et al. Continuity of binge and harmful drinking from late adolescence to early adulthood. *Pediatrics* 2004;114:714.

Monti PM, Miranda R, Nixon K, et al. Adolescence: booze, brains, and behavior. *Alcohol Clin Exp Res* 2005;29:207.

Niederdeppe J, Farrelly MC, Haviland ML. Confirming "truth": more evidence of a successful tobacco countermarketing campaign in Florida. *Am J Public Health* 2004;94:255.

Patton GC, Coffey C, Carlin JB, et al. Cannabis use and mental health in young people: cohort study. *BMJ* 2002;325:1195.

Philpot R, Kirstein C. Developmental differences in the accumbal dopaminergic response to repeated ethanol exposure. *Ann N Y Acad Sci* 2004;1021:422.

Pistis M, Perra S, Pillolla G, et al. Adolescent exposure to cannabinoids induces long-lasting changes in the response to drugs of abuse of rat midbrain dopamine neurons. *Biol Psychiatry* 2004;56:86.

Fonseca FR, Carrera MRA, Navarro M, et al. Activation of corticotropin-releasing factor in the limbic system during cannabinoid withdrawal. *Science* 1997;276:2050.

Skara S, Sussman S. A review of 25 long term adolescent tobacco and other drug use prevention program evaluations. *Prev Med* 2003;37:451.

Sly DF, Hopkins RS, Trapido E, et al. Influence of a counter-advertising media campaign on initiation of smoking: the Florida "truth" campaign. *Am J Public Health* 2001;91:233.

Sowell ER, Thompson PM, Holmes CJ, et al. In vivo evidence for post-adolescent brain maturation in frontal and striatal regions. *Nat Neurosci* 1999;2:859.

Sowell ER, Thompson PM, Tessner KD, et al. Mapping continued brain growth and grey matter density reduction in dorsal frontal cortex: inverse relationships during postadolescent brain maturation. *J Neurosci* 2001;21:8819.

Tanda G, Pontieri FE, Di Chiara G. Cannabinoid and heroin activation of mesolimbic dopamine transmission by a common μ_1 opioid receptor mechanism. *Science* 1997;276:2048.

Trauth JA, Seidler FJ, Ali SF, et al. Adolescent nicotine exposure produces immediate and long-term changes in CAN noradrenergic and dopaminergic function. *Brain Res* 2001;892:269.

Volkow ND, Fowler JS, Wang G-J. The addicted human brain: insights from imaging studies. *J Clin Invest* 2003;111:1451.

Wechsler H, Nelson TF. Binge drinking and the American college student: what's five drinks? *Psychol Addict Behav* 2001;15:287.

White AM, Swartzwelder HS. Hippocampal function during adolescence. A unique target of ethanol effects. *Ann N Y Acad Sci* 2004;1021:206.

White AM, Truesdale MC, Bae JG. Differential effects of ethanol on motor coordination in adolescent and adult rats. *Pharmacol Biochem Behav* 2002;73:673.

Zammit S, Allebeck P, Andreasson S, et al. Self-reported cannabis use as a risk factor for schizophrenia in Swedish conscripts of 1969: historical cohort study. *BMJ* 2002;325: 1199.

Zeigler DW, Wang CC, Yoast RA, et al. The neurocognitive effects of alcohol on adolescents and college students. *Prev Med* 2005;40:23.

CHAPTER 69

Alcohol

Martin M. Anderson and Lawrence S. Neinstein

Alcohol is the most widely used drug in the United States. It is readily available and inexpensive. Alcohol has been used by 76.8% of adolescents by the time they reach 18 years of age. In 2006, 45.3% of high school seniors have used alcohol in the last month and 66.5% used in the last year (Johnston et al., 2007). In 2006, 3.0% of high school seniors used alcohol daily (Johnston et al., 2007). Approximately 25.4% percent of high school seniors reported that they had consumed more than five drinks in a row during the previous 2 weeks; 56.4% of high school seniors have been drunk (Johnston et al., 2007). Table 69.1 depicts trends in prevalence of any use of alcohol among 8th, 10th, and 12th graders between 1991 and 2005 (Johnston et al., 2006).

MORBIDITY AND MORTALITY

An estimated 4.6 million adolescents aged 14 to 17 years have alcohol-related problems.

Motor Vehicle Injuries Motor vehicle accidents caused by driving under the influence of alcohol are the leading cause of death in the 15- to 24-year-old age-group. Annually, approximately 5,000 youth below 21 years of age die from alcohol-related injuries. Alcohol-related motor vehicle accidents account for 1,900 deaths. Alcohol is a factor in 1,500 homicides and 300 suicides (Hingston, 2004). Almost 30% of students (28.5%) nationwide have ridden with a driver who had been drinking, and 9.9% (8.1% female, 11.7% male) have driven a car after drinking (Centers for Disease Control and Prevention, 2006). Forty percent to 50% of young males who drown were drinking when they died. The rate is similar to that for diving accidents (Office of the Inspector General, Report to the Surgeon General, 1992; Chaloupka et al., 2002). A 1985 study of coroner cases of unintentional injury deaths in adolescence showed that approximately 50% had a measurable blood alcohol level (Friedman, 1985). The National Highway Traffic Safety Administration estimates that a legal age of drinking at 21 saves 700 to 1,000 lives per year (NIAAA, 2004/05d). Since 1999 when New Zealand lowered its drinking age to 18, there has been a 12% increase in alcohol-related crashes amongst 18- to 19-year-olds and a 14% increase in 15- to 17-year-olds. For females, the increase was 51% for 18- to 19-year-olds and 24% for 14- to 17-year-olds (www. pire.org; Kypri, 2005).

Other Morbidities Alcohol use is linked to acquisition of sexually transmitted diseases (STDs). Higher alcohol taxes and higher minimum legal drinking ages are associated with lower incidence of STDs among adolescents and young adults (Centers for Disease Control and Prevention, 2000). A 1999 Office of Juvenile Justice and Delinquency Prevention (OJJDP) study estimated that the cost of underage drinking in the United States totals more than $58 billion annually. Alcohol use in adolescents has been associated with several long- and short-term consequences—academic problems, social problems, physical problems, and unwanted, unintended, and unprotected sexual activity. It has been a factor in physical and sexual assaults, suicide, homicide, and alcohol-related unintentional injuries. There is evidence of its role in memory problems and in alterations in brain development (NIAAA, 2004/05b, c).

Alcohol use is not limited to healthy teens. Adolescents with chronic illnesses such as sickle-cell disease or cystic fibrosis engage in risk-taking behaviors such as smoking, sexual activity, and drug and alcohol use. They may use at lower rates than their peers, but should still be screened for health-risk behaviors. Health care providers should not underestimate the effects of alcohol use on adolescents or its consequences.

RISK FACTORS FOR ADOLESCENT ALCOHOL USE

There are many factors that contribute to adolescent alcohol initiation, use, and alcohol-related problem behaviors.

1. Reasons teens give for drinking (Rachal et al., 1975):
   a. Curiosity
   b. Peer conformity
   c. Enjoyment
   d. Escape
   e. Parental encouragement to take first drink to celebrate a special occasion
2. Genetic: The initiation of and use of alcohol are the result of a complex interplay between genes and environment. Several genes have been identified as affecting the risk of alcoholism. A twin study of alcohol use (Rhee et al., 2003) found that alcohol initiation arises from genetic, shared, and nonshared environmental contributions. Problem use has a heritability component

TABLE 69.1

Trends in Prevalence of Any Use of Alcohol for 8th, 10th, and 12th Graders

Grade	1991	1992	1993	1994	1995	1996	1997	1998	1999	2000	2001	2002	2003	2004	2005	2006	2006–2006 Change
8th	70.1	69.3	55.7	55.8	54.5	55.3	53.8	52.5	52.1	51.7	50.5	47.0	45.6	43.9	41.0	40.5	–0.6
10th	83.8	82.3	71.6	71.1	70.5	71.8	72.0	69.8	70.6	71.4	70.1	66.9	66.0	64.2	63.2	61.5	–1.7
12th	88.0	87.5	80.0	80.4	80.7	79.2	81.7	81.4	80.0	80.3	79.7	78.4	76.6	76.8	75.1	72.7	–2.4

Adapted from Johnston LD, O'Malley PM, Bachman JG, et al. *Monitoring the future national survey results on drug use, Overview of key findings.* NIH Publications No. 07-6202, Bethesda, MD: National Institute on Drug Abuse, 2007.

and is influenced by peers more than family. Alcohol use in general is minimally influenced by genetics and is mainly influenced by environment (Rhee et al., 2003).

3. Ethnicity: Asian-Americans and African-Americans are less likely to drink than European Americans (white) or Native Americans. In general, white American adolescents start drinking earlier than nonwhite Americans with the exception of Native Americans (Donovan, 2004). In the 2005 National Youth Risk Behavior Survey, Hispanic high school students and non-Hispanic white students had a higher percent of lifetime use (79.4% and 75.3%) than black students (69%) (Centers for Disease Control and Prevention, 2006). This was also true for current use of alcohol (46.8%, 46.4%, and 31.2% respectively).

4. Family factors: Adolescents' perception of parental approval and parents' use of alcohol are predictive of teens' initiation of alcohol use. If the parents are perceived as being more permissive toward drinking, adolescents are at higher risk of early initiation (Donovan, 2004). Teens with close relationships to their parents are less likely to initiate. Children of alcoholics are 4 to 10 times more likely to become alcoholic as compared with children whose parents were not alcoholic (NIAAA, 2004/05c).

5. Peer factors: Peer involvement in drugs or alcohol, delinquent behaviors, or the perception that there is a high prevalence of alcohol use among peers increases the risk of a teen drinking alcohol.

6. Behavioral risk factors: If teens have tolerant attitudes toward delinquent behavior or approve of alcohol use, they are at higher risk for drinking. Mood disorders, attention-deficit hyperactivity disorder (ADHD), conduct disorder, low school motivation, and low value placed on academic achievement are additional risk factors associated with initiation of alcohol use in adolescence.

7. Risk factor of early initiation: Early onset of alcohol use (before age 14) is often associated with escalated drinking during adolescence and development of alcohol-related problems in adolescents and adults. Approximately one third of adolescents start drinking before 13 years and 10% of 9-year-olds have already started drinking. Youth who start drinking before 13 are 9 times more likely to binge drink than high school students who begin later (NIAAA, 2004/05a).

Factors not predictive of initiation of drinking:

1. Gender: Gender is not predictive of drinking initiation (Donovan, 2004).

2. Social economic status: SES (when family structure is accounted for) does not predict alcohol initiation (Donovan, 2004).

ALCOHOL AND ITS EFFECTS

Physiology and Metabolism Alcohol is a nonionized lipid soluble compound that is completely miscible in water. It is rapidly absorbed from the gastrointestinal (GI) tract and is distributed throughout the total body water. It easily penetrates the central nervous system (CNS) because of its lipid solubility. It is a CNS depressant that also has the ability to increase brain activity in areas that produce endorphins and in those that activate the dopaminergic reward system. The principal ingredient of all alcoholic beverages is ethanol. Most beers and wines contain between 3% and 20% alcohol. A shot of whiskey, a can of beer, and a glass of wine have the same alcohol content. Women, because of their higher percentage of body fat and lower total body water per unit of weight develop higher blood alcohol levels than men with the same alcohol intake.

Intoxication Moderate doses of alcohol in the nontolerant individual induce sedation, euphoria, decreased inhibitions, and impaired coordination. As the dose and corresponding blood alcohol level increase, ataxia, decreased mentation, poor judgment, labile mood, and slurred speech occur. At higher doses, alcohol can induce unconsciousness, anesthesia, respiratory failure, coma, and death (Table 69.2).

Complications Although alcohol can adversely affect many organ systems of the body, adolescent alcohol abusers are usually spared the complications of prolonged alcohol use such as cirrhosis, alcoholic hepatitis, and pancreatitis. Acute withdrawal symptoms such as delirium tremens (DTs) or seizures are also unusual in adolescents. However, Strauss et al. (2000) in a study of obese children and adolescents with elevated liver function test (LFT) values secondary to fatty liver showed a significant *increase in LFTs* with the addition of the alcohol. Acute alcohol intoxication can result in *blackouts* which are caused by acute dysfunction of the hippocampus. Hangovers are a form of *subacute short-term withdrawal*, which are different from acute withdrawals that are mainly found in adults.

Hormonal Changes Human studies as well as studies on animals have identified a variety of potential physiological effects of alcohol in adolescents. Drinking can lower estrogen levels in girls, and testosterone levels in males. In both genders, acute alcohol intake reduces growth hormone levels. Alcohol use in increased amounts can lower bone density in males but not females.

TABLE 69.2

Effects of Alcohol Consumption in the Nontolerant Individual

Blood Alcohol Level (g/100 mL)	Effects
0.02	Reached after approximately one drink; light or moderate drinkers feel some effect—warmth and relaxation
0.04	Most people feel relaxed, talkative, and happy; skin may become flushed
0.05	First sizable changes begin to occur; light-headedness, giddiness, lowered inhibitions, and less control of thoughts may be experienced; both restraint and judgment are lowered; coordination may be slightly altered
0.06	Judgment is somewhat impaired; ability to make rational decisions about personal capabilities is affected (such as being able to drive)
0.08	Definite impairment of muscle coordination and slower reaction time occurs; driving ability becomes suspect; sensory feelings of numbness of the cheeks and lips occur; hands, arms, and legs may tingle and then feel numb (this constitutes legal impairment in Canada and in some U.S. states, e.g., California)
0.10	Clumsiness; speech may become fuzzy; clear deterioration of reaction time and muscle control (this level previously constituted drunkenness in most U.S. states)
0.15	Definite impairment of balance and movement
0.20	Motor and emotional control centers are measurably affected; slurred speech, staggering, loss of balance, and double vision can all be present
0.30	Lack of understanding of what is seen or heard occurs; individuals are confused or stuporous and may lose consciousness
0.40	Usually unconscious; the skin becomes clammy
0.45	Respiration slows and may stop altogether
0.50	Death occurs

From Morrison SF, Rogers PD, Thomas MH. Alcohol and adolescents. *Pediatr Clin North Am* 1995;42:371–387.

Neurotoxicity Alcohol is a neurotoxin. Its full effects on the developing adolescent brain are not yet known. The adolescent brain is continuing to develop. It is a time when the brain's efficiency is enhanced. There is increased myelination and synaptic pruning and development of the hippocampus and prefrontal cortex. The subcortical gray matter and limbic system increase in volume while the prefrontal cortex decreases in volume due to synaptic pruning. These areas of the brain are responsible for planning, integrating information, abstract reasoning, problem solving, and judgment. This is a dynamic developing system that is potentially susceptible to damage due to alcohol.

Research to date demonstrates the following effects:

1. Adolescents are relatively resistant to the sedative effects of alcohol. They show less ataxia, social impairment, and fewer acute withdrawal effects than adults.
2. Imaging studies of teens with significant alcohol use show a reduced volume of the hippocampus and abnormalities of the corpus callosum.
3. Studies show a disruption in learning and memory.
4. Functional magnetic resonance imaging (MRI) shows decreased functional activity of the frontal and parietal areas of the right hemisphere, areas responsible for spatial memory.
5. Neurocognitive testing of long-term users shows decreased visuospatial motor speed, and decreased reading recognition, total reading, and spelling subtests on IQ testing.
6. Increased consumption is associated with decreased memory, abstract thought, and language.

7. Teens with more than 100 drinking episodes showed decreased verbal and nonverbal retention when compared to nondrinking controls.
8. Withdrawal from alcohol also has neurocognitive effects. An increased number of withdrawal episodes is associated with greater decrease in visuospatial function with poor retrieval of verbal and nonverbal information.

These neurocognitive findings could potentially affect the developmental transition from childhood through adolescence to adulthood. Alcohol use is also known to disrupt the sleep–wake cycle resulting in increased sleep latency and increased day-time sleepiness.

Fetal Alcohol Syndrome

Fetal alcohol syndrome is the most common cause of teratogenic mental retardation, and it is also the most preventable. There is no known safe level of alcohol use during pregnancy. Alcohol readily crosses the placenta and can result in the fetal alcohol syndrome, which is characterized by the following:

1. Abnormal facies: Microcephaly; short, upturned nose; thin upper lip; short palpebral fissures; and hypoplastic maxilla
2. Cardiac abnormalities: Especially atrial and ventricular septal defects
3. Renal abnormalities: Deformed kidneys
4. Genital abnormalities: Hypospadias and labial hypoplasia

5. Skeletal abnormalities: Contractures of the extremities; pectus excavatum
6. Hirsutism
7. CNS abnormalities: Electroencephalographic changes, mental retardation
8. Abnormal size: Small for gestational age
9. Behavior: Irritability in infancy; hyperactivity in childhood

PROBLEM DRINKING AMONG ADOLESCENTS

Problem drinking has been defined as having been drunk six or more times in the last year or acknowledging problems in three of the following areas because of drinking:

1. Trouble with a teacher or principal
2. Difficulties with friends
3. Driving after drinking
4. Criticism by dates
5. Trouble with the police

Nationally in the year 2006, 10.9% of 8th graders, 21.9% of 10th graders, and 25.4% of 12th graders were classified as heavy drinkers (five or more drinks in a row during the previous 2 weeks) (Johnston et al., 2007). In addition, 19.5% of 8th graders, 41.4% of 10th graders, and 56.4% of 12th graders said they have been drunk in their life. Daily alcohol use rates are 0.5% in the 8th grade, 1.4% in the 10th grade, and 3.0% in the 12th grade. The percentage of high school students who have a history of being drunk daily in 2006 is 0.2% in 8th grade, 0.5% in 10th grade, and 1.6% in 12th grade.

Adolescents may have little insight into the significance of their excessive alcohol intake. A study of 3,395 Arkansas middle school students showed that 13% (455) were heavy drinkers, but only 16% (65) of these youth acknowledged having an alcohol use problem. These statistics did not include school dropouts, and there is evidence that dropouts use alcohol more heavily than their counterparts who have stayed in school. Problem drinking can seriously interfere with successful completion of the developmental tasks of adolescence, resulting in a maturational arrest.

Harrison and Luxenberg (1995) reported on alcohol and drug use among Minnesota adolescents. They found a continued trend in the proportion of students who reported at least three adverse consequences of alcohol and drug use, including 1% of 6th graders, 7% of 9th graders, and 16% of 12th graders. Alcohol was the primary substance of abuse among students. The most commonly reported consequences included tolerance, blackouts, violence, and school or job absenteeism. The problem users were 2 to 7 times more likely than comparable students with a lesser or no drug history to report parental alcohol or other drug problems, physical abuse, and sexual abuse. They were also 2 to 15 times more likely to have low self-esteem and emotional distress, to exhibit antisocial behavior, and to have made suicide attempts.

Binge drinking adolescents are at higher risk for the harmful effects of acute intoxication. They are also more likely to engage in risk-taking behaviors. They are more likely to carry a gun, use marijuana and cocaine, earn lower grades (D and F), be injured in fights, attempt suicide, and have sex with multiple partners (NIAAA, 2004/05a, d). Alcohol use in college students is discussed in Chapters 68 and 84.

The health care provider must be acutely aware of the differing patterns of use manifested in adolescence so as to be able to formulate accurate diagnostic impressions and thereby use therapeutic interventions with the greatest likelihood of improving outcome. Alcoholism and problem drinking during adolescence may have similar manifestations and consequences. Problem drinking can develop as an attempt to escape the psychic distress resulting from a distinct primary psychiatric disorder such as major depression. It may result in acting out in response to unique psychodynamic circumstances or an evolving personality disorder. In these circumstances, the use will generally subside if the primary disorder is properly identified and treated. If, however, the adolescent does, in fact, have alcoholism, attempts to treat the secondary psychiatric manifestations will do little or nothing to prevent the evolution of this progressive disorder. Because the manifestations of alcoholism in adolescence may be only very subtly distinguished from problem drinking, it is exceedingly important to have a clear understanding of the defining features of the diagnosis of alcoholism.

Characteristics of Alcoholism

Alcoholism is a primary, chronic disease with genetic, psychosocial, and environmental factors influencing its development and manifestations.

1. The disease is often progressive and may be fatal.
2. The individual has impaired control over drinking, progressive preoccupation with alcohol use despite significant adverse consequences, and distortions in thinking, most notably denial.
3. Adverse consequences include impairments in work or school functioning, negative influences on interpersonal relationships, and legal or health-status ramifications.
4. A family history of alcoholism is present in most cases.
5. Research suggests that genetics is a major determinant in the risk of alcoholism. Further recent information shows that the biological features of these genetic determinants create an environment in the dopaminergic mesolimbic reward systems that may predispose a person to progressive use of alcohol and, in addition, may facilitate potent biological reinforcement by substances other than alcohol that also stimulate this region of the brain. Cocaine and amphetamines are two such compounds with a great potential for dependency. Similarly, there appear to be unique elements of the endorphin system in the alcoholic brain that may result in a predisposition to opiate dependency. Although alcoholism is not the only route to dependency on these substances, experimentation with these drugs by an adolescent with suspected alcoholism suggests a more treacherous clinical circumstance and a need for immediate intervention by the health care provider.
6. The biopsychosocial consequences of drug use during adolescence are often the same, whether or not addictions are present. The natural history of the clinical situation and the effectiveness of specific treatments, however, are clearly a function of the specificity of the diagnostic circumstances.
7. Further confounding the diagnostic accuracy is the fact that adolescents who use large amounts of alcohol generally deceive the physicians with whom they come in contact. Because of the teen's (and family's) denial,

the physician often does not recognize the alcohol dependence. The serious medical illnesses and somatic complaints associated with long-term adult drug or alcohol use are generally not available as clues when one is assessing the adolescent. Therefore, the physician is largely dependent on the history in recognizing and diagnosing adolescent alcohol abuse.

DIAGNOSIS

1. Behavioral changes: Certain behavioral changes can arouse the suspicion of alcohol or other drug abuse (but none of them is an absolute indicator of excessive drinking). These include behaviors such as changes in activity; loss of interest in school, play, home, or work; changes in sleeping patterns; changes in eating patterns; and changes in personality. May be reflected in mood changes, fighting with friends and family members, or truancy, manifestations of depression, trouble with the law enforcement system, multiple or frequent accident-related injuries, school failure, and blackouts. Table 69.3 outlines developing signs of alcoholism in teens.
2. Screening instruments: Determining the extent of alcohol abuse and diagnosing alcoholism in the adolescent is crucial. The HEADSS psychosocial profile, as outlined in Chapter 3, is a helpful interview technique for eliciting a history of substance abuse. Several screening devices are also available to help make this diagnosis (see Chapter 73 for details) and include the following:
   a. CAGE (Fig. 69.1)
   b. MAST: The Michigan Alcoholism Screening Test (Fig. 69.2)
   c. CRAFFT: See page 948, Chapter 73.
   d. AUDIT: Alcohol Use Disorders Identification Test

   Fiellin et al. (2000) reviewed performance characteristics of screening methods for alcohol problems through 38 studies conducted between 1966 and 1998. Overall, the AUDIT was most effective in identifying subjects with at-risk, hazardous, or harmful drinking (sensitivity, 51%–97%; specificity, 78%–96%), although the CAGE questions proved better for discovering alcohol abuse and dependence (sensitivity, 43%–94%; specificity, 70%–97%). The authors concluded that these two screening instruments consistently performed better than other methods. However, these tests were not specifically examined in adolescents. CRAFFT has higher sensitivity (76%) and specificity (94%) for two positive responses and has been tested in primary care settings specifically for adolescents (Knight et al., 2002) (see Chapter 73).
3. Family history: A family history of alcoholism or addiction also places the adolescent at high risk for abuse of an addictive substance and subsequent addiction, for the reasons described earlier.

TREATMENT

The American Medical Association Guidelines for Adolescent Preventive Services (GAPS), Bright Futures, and the American Academy of Pediatrics Policy Statement on Substance Abuse all recommend that every adolescent be screened during history taking for alcohol, tobacco, and other drug abuse (ATODA) as part of routine care. If the screen is positive for alcohol, then the clinician must decide what to do next. Research shows that brief interventions in

TABLE 69.3

Developing Signs of Alcoholism in Teenagers

Social/Psychological Signs	Classroom Behavior	Physical Signs
Personality change when drinking	Attendance	A change in tolerance to
Blackouts or temporary amnesia	Misses Monday mornings	alcohol, either an increase or
during and after drinking episodes	Late after lunch	a decrease
Loss of control of drinking	Leaves school early on Fridays	Hangovers
Drinks more than peers and more often	Frequent absences	Marked weight gain or loss
Morning drinking to overcome	General	Repeated minor injuries
hangover effects	Works below expected	Sexual activity beyond standard of
Drinking-related arrests	potential level	peer group
Defensiveness about alcohol usage	Inconsistency in aggressiveness	Characteristics of final
Obsession with consumption of next	and passivity in classroom	phases—obvious and tragic:
drink	participation	Extended binges
Mixing of alcohol with drugs for a	Drinks at school, hides alcohol	Physical tremors
better high	in locker	Hallucinations
Need to drink before going to a party	Boasts about drinking	Deliria
Feeling of remorse about drinking	Alcohol on breath	Convulsions
Occurrence of fights when drinking	Change in peer group affiliation	
Development of elaborate system of	Sleeps during classes	
lies, alibis, and excuses to cover up	General troubles in school	
drinking		

Adapted from the National Council on Alcoholism of San Fernando Valley, California.

1. Have you ever felt you ought to Cut down on your drinking?
2. Have people Annoyed you by criticizing your drinking?
3. Have you ever felt bad or Guilty about your drinking?
4. Have you ever had a drink first thing in the morning to steady your nerves or to get rid of a hangover (Eye opener)?

FIGURE 69.1 CAGE questionnaire for alcoholism. (From Ewing JA. Detecting alcoholism: the CAGE questionnaire. *JAMA* 1985;252:14.)

Circle "Yes" or "No," depending on whether the statement says something true or not true about you. Please answer all questions. The test can be scored to let you know where you lie on a scale from social drinker to addictive drinker. (Underlined answers count for score; in the questionnaire given to the patient, no yes or no answers are underlined.)

1.	Do you feel you are a normal drinker?	Yes	<u>No</u>	2
2.	Have you ever awakened on the morning after some drinking the night before and found you couldn't remember a part of the evening?	<u>Yes</u>	No	2
3.	Do your friends or family ever worry or complain about your drinking?	<u>Yes</u>	No	1
4.	Can you stop drinking without a struggle after one or two drinks?	Yes	<u>No</u>	2
5.	Do you ever feel bad about your drinking?	<u>Yes</u>	No	1
6.	Do friends or relatives think you are a normal drinker?	Yes	<u>No</u>	2
7.	Do you ever try to limit your drinking to certain times of the day or to certain places?	<u>Yes</u>	No	1
8.	Are you always able to stop drinking when you want to?	Yes	<u>No</u>	2
9.	Have you ever attended a meeting of Alcoholics Anonymous (AA)?	<u>Yes</u>	No	5
10.	Have you gotten into fights when drinking?	<u>Yes</u>	No	1
11.	Has your drinking ever created problems with your friends or family?	<u>Yes</u>	No	2
12.	Have your friends or any family member ever gone to anyone for help about your drinking?	<u>Yes</u>	No	2
13.	Have you ever lost friends or spouse because of your drinking?	<u>Yes</u>	No	2
14.	Have you ever gotten into trouble at work or school because of your drinking?	<u>Yes</u>	No	2
15.	Have you ever lost a job because of your drinking?	<u>Yes</u>	No	2
16.	Have you ever neglected your obligations, your family, or your school work for 2 or more days in a row because you were drinking?	<u>Yes</u>	No	2
17.	Do you ever drink before noon?	<u>Yes</u>	No	2
18.	Have you ever been told you have liver trouble?	<u>Yes</u>	No	1
19.	After heavy drinking, have you ever had delirium tremens (DTs) or severe shaking, heard voices, or seen things that were not there?	<u>Yes</u>	No	5
20.	Have you ever gone to anyone for help about your drinking?	<u>Yes</u>	No	5
21.	Have you ever been in a hospital because of your drinking?	<u>Yes</u>	No	5
22.	Have you ever been a patient in a psychiatric hospital or on a psychiatric ward of a general hospital when drinking was part of the problem?	<u>Yes</u>	No	2
23.	Have you ever been seen at a psychiatric or mental health clinic or gone to a doctor, social worker, or clergyman for help with an emotional problem in which drinking played a part?	<u>Yes</u>	No	2
24.	Have you ever been arrested, even for a few hours, because of drunk behavior?	<u>Yes</u>	No	2
25.	Have you ever been arrested for drunk driving or driving after drinking?	<u>Yes</u>	No	2

TOTAL 57

Your score is _____

0–3	Probably not alcoholic
5–10	80% risk of alcoholism
10 or more	Definitely alcoholic

FIGURE 69.2 Michigan Alcoholism Screening Test (MAST) questionnaire on drinking habits. (Adapted from Selzer ML. The michigan alcoholism screening test: the quest for a new diagnostic instrument. *Am J Psychol* 1971;127:89.)

physicians' offices can be effective in assisting patients in changing their behavior.

Components of Successful Treatment of Adolescent Alcohol Abuse and Dependence

See Chapters 72 and 73 for further discussion on alcohol and drug abuse treatment interventions.

1. Accurate diagnosis and assessment: Treatment of any primary psychiatric disturbances that may be identified. If the patient meets criteria for a diagnosis of alcoholism or addiction, then proceed with interventions listed later. If the diagnosis is uncertain, always proceed with these suggestions. Reassessment of psychiatric symptoms should be undertaken after a minimum of 30 days. Very often, prominent psychiatric symptoms remit spontaneously with abstinence.
2. Disease concept of recovery: Viewing alcoholism as a primary progressive disease implies a long-term, ongoing recovery process that requires abstinence and learning to live without alcohol and drugs. The recovery process also helps expose and deal with accumulated feelings of guilt and shame, while rebuilding coping skills and self-esteem.
3. Positive alternatives: Treatment requires that the adolescent learn substitute activities that provide pleasure and reward to replace the "highs" of drug use. These activities should be realistic and attainable.
4. Support systems: Sober peer-support systems are essential for recovery. Alcoholics Anonymous, Cocaine Anonymous, and Narcotics Anonymous provide 12-step programs that are useful for the recovering adolescents.
5. Family involvement: Alcoholism is a family illness. The substance abuse of one member of the family system affects the other members. Dysfunctional coping trends are established. Recovery and treatment should help establish a new, healthier equilibrium. Family members should be encouraged to attend Al-Anon or Alateen, which are 12-step self-help groups for family members.
6. Referrals: The clinician should also be able to provide appropriate referrals for substance abuse services in the community.

RESOURCES

Organizations

Al-Anon/Alateen Family Group Headquarters, Inc., P.O. Box 862 Midtown Station, New York, NY 10018-0862, telephone 1-212-302-7240 or 1-800-344-2666 (U.S.) or 1-800-443-4525 (Canada).

Boys and Girls Clubs of America, National Headquarters. 1275 Peachtree St., NE, Atlanta, GA 30309-3506. Telephone (404) 487–5700.

Friday Night Live, California Friday Night Live Partnership, 2637 W. Burrel, P.O. Box 5091, Visalia, CA 93278-5091, telephone 1-559-733-6496, fax 1-559-737-4231, E-mail: mja@tcoe.k12.ca.us.

National Association for Children of Alcoholics, 11426 Rockville Pike, Suite 100, Rockville, MD 20852, telephone 1-301-468-2600 or 1-800-729-6686.

National Association of Teen Institutes, c/o CADA, 3520 General de Gaulle Dr., Suite 5010, New Orleans, LA 70114. Telephone 1-504-362-4272 or 834–4370.

National Clearinghouse for Alcohol and Drug Information, P.O. Box 2345, Rockville, MD 20852, telephone 1-301-468-2600 or 1-800-729-6686.

National Collaboration for Youth (NCY), The National Assembly of Health and Human Service Organizations, 1319 F Street, NW, Suite 402, Washington, DC 20004, telephone 1-877-693-4248.

National Council on Alcoholism and Drug Dependence, 22 Cortlandt St., Suite 801, New York NY 10007-3128, telephone 1-800-622-2255 or 1-800-475-4673.

National Families in Action, 2957 Clairmont Rd., Suite 150, Atlanta, GA 30329, telephone 1-404-248-9676.

Safe and Drug Free Schools, U.S. Department of Education, 400 Maryland Avenue SW, Washington, DC 20202, telephone 1-202-260-3954.

Publications and Other Resource Materials

Resources for Teens

Contact Substance Abuse and Mental Health Services Administration's (SAMHSA) National Clearinghouse for Alcohol and Drug Information at 1-800-729-6686 or http://www.ncadi.samhsa.gov for the publications and videotapes listed here.

Publications

Alcohol Alert No. 37: Youth Drinking—Risk Factors and Consequences
Alcohol Impairment Chart (for both men and women)
Alcohol, Tobacco, and Other Drugs and the College Experience (ML003)
Alcoholism Tends to Run in Families (PH318)
Children of Alcoholics: Important Facts (NACoA)
Drugs of Abuse: Alcohol
A Guide for Teens: Does Your Friend Have an Alcohol or Other Drug Problem? (PHD688)
How to Cut Down on Your Drinking
Straight Facts about Alcohol
Sex Under the Influence of Alcohol and Other Drugs (ML005)

Resources for Families

Contact SAMHSA's National Clearinghouse for Alcohol and Drug Information at 1-800-729-6686, P.O. Box 2345, Rockville, MD 20847-2345, or http://www.ncadi.samhsa .gov for the publications and videotapes listed here.

Publications

Growing Up Drug Free: A Parent's Guide to Prevention (PHD533)
If Someone Close Has a Problem with Alcohol or Other Drugs (PH317)
TAP 6: Empowering Families, Helping Adolescents: Family-Centered Treatment of Adolescents with Alcohol, Drug Abuse, and Mental Health Problems (BKD81)
Parents, Guardians and Caregivers (MS503)
Alcohol Alert No. 37. Youth Drinking–Risk Factors and Consequences (PH376)
Alcoholism Tends to Run in Families (PH318)
Children of Alcoholics: Important Facts

Videocassettes

Poor Jennifer, She's Always Losing Her Hat (VHS65). Designed to educate adults about the issues faced by children of alcoholics.

Resources for Professionals

Contact SAMHSA's National Clearinghouse for Alcohol and Drug Information at 800-729-6686 or http://www.ncadi .samhsa.gov for the publications and videotapes listed here.

Publications

TIP 3: Screening and Assessment of Alcohol- and Other Drug-Abusing Adolescents (BKD108)

TIP 4: Guidelines for the Treatment of Alcohol- and Other Drug-Abusing Adolescents (BKD109)

TIP 21: Combining Alcohol and Other Drug Abuse Treatment with Diversion for Juveniles in the Justice System (BKD169)

TIP 28: Naltraxone and Alcoholism Treatment (BKD268)

TIP 31: Screening and Assessing Adolescents for Substance Abuse Disorders (BKD306)

TAP 1: Approaches in the Treatment of Adolescents with Emotional and Substance Abuse Problems (PHD580)

The Physician's Guide to Helping Patients with Alcohol Problems. NIAAA, 1995 (PHD360)

Changing Lives: Programs that Make a Difference for Youth at High Risk. Center for Substance Abuse Prevention (CSAP), 1995 (PHD714)

The Young and Restless: Generation X and Alcohol Policy (RPO933)

Children at Risk Because of Parental Substance Abuse. AOS Working Paper. (RPO965)

Prevention Pipeline: Focus on Youth Prevention—Science and Practice in Action (July/August, 1997). *Prevention Pipeline* is an award winning bimonthly magazine developed by the Center for Substance Abuse Prevention.

Videocassettes

Available from SAMHSA, National Clearinghouse for Alcohol and Drug Information

Adolescent Treatment Issues (VHS40). Stresses the importance of understanding the specific treatment needs of adolescents.

Resources for Educators

Contact SAMHSA's National Clearinghouse for Alcohol and Drug Information at 1-800-729-6686 or http://www.ncadi .samhsa.gov/for the resources listed here.

Publications

Alcohol Practices, Policies, and Potentials of American Colleges and Universities: A White Paper (CS01). Exhaustively researched, this resource on alcohol and drinking problems at American colleges and among college students outlines a full range of policy, regulatory, and program responses that some colleges are using to reduce campus drinking problems.

Success Stories from Drug-Free Schools (PHD588). This book salutes the 107 schools honored by the U.S. Department of Education's Drug-Free School Recognition Program. School leaders talk about their achievements, the obstacles they faced, how they overcame them, and what remains to be done.

Getting a Head Start: Teacher's Guide (PHD647). Although these materials were originally designed for Head Start, they are appropriate for early childhood and primary grades to increase awareness of alcohol and drug use.

Strategies for Preventing Alcohol and Other Drug Problems on College Campuses: Faculty Members Handbook (CS04). Faculty members can become involved in efforts to address drinking problems at colleges and universities. This handbook provides resources and tables on recent alcohol and drug use by college students.

Learning to Live Drug Free Curriculum Guides

Schools play a vital role in educating youth about the harmful effects of drugs. This curriculum model provides a framework for prevention education from kindergarten through 12th grade. National Clearinghouse for Alcohol and Drug Information (NCADI) has copied the curricula and grouped them by specific grades: Grades K–3 (RPO894), Grades 4–6 (RPO895), Grades 7–8 (RPO896), and Grades 9–12 (RPO897).

Studies and Reports

Driving After Drug or Alcohol Use: Findings of the 1996 National Household Survey on Drug Abuse

Drinking Under Age 21: Problems and Solutions (RPO961)

The National Household Survey Summary of Findings, 1998

The National Household Survey Population Estimates, 1998

Combating Drunk Driving and Underage Drinking

Monitoring the Future Study, 1975–2004. National Survey Results on Drug Use 1975–2004. Volume I: Secondary Students (NIH Publication #05-5727)

Monitoring the Future Study, 1975–2004. V Survey Results on Drug Use 1975–2004. Volume II: College Students and Adults aged 19–45. (NIH Publication #05-5728)

Prevalence of Youth Substance Abuse: The Impact of Methodological Differences Between Two National Surveys (RPO941)

WEB SITES

For Teenagers and Parents

http://kidshealth.org/teen/. The Nemours Foundation, TeensHealth site has information about alcohol.

http://www.aap.org/. About Alcohol: Ten Tips for Teens.

http://www.al-anon.org. Al-Anon home page.

For Clinicians and Teens

http://ncadi.samhsa.gov/. SAMHSA website.

http://www.nida.nih.gov. National Institute on Drug Abuse (NIDA).

http://www.nofas.org/about/programs.aspx. The National Organization on Fetal Alcohol Syndrome lists several programs to educate the community, youth, and health professionals about the effects of the syndrome and to provide assistance to women in treatment centers. The site includes links to a number of related sites (http://www.nofax.org/resource/links/aspx), as well as to journal articles.

http://www.niaaa.nih.gov/. NIAAA.

For Health Professionals

http://www.cdc.gov/ncbddd/fas/. Web site dedicated to providing information about Fetal Alcohol Syndrome, sponsored by the Centers for Disease Control (CDC). Includes links to CDC activities, publications, fast facts, and current research on the subject. Can also contact by mail at NCBDD, CDC, Mail Stop E-86, 1600 Clifton Rd.,

Atlanta, GA 30333. Phone 1-800-CDC-INFO (232–4636), FAX 404-498-3040, e-mail cdcinfo@cdc.gov.

http://www.healthfinder.gov/orgs/HR0027.htm. SAMHSA's National Clearinghouse for Alcohol and Drug Information—NCADI.

http://www.jointogether.org.

http://www.ncadi.samhsa.gov.

http://www.nida.nih.gov/TB/Clinical/Clinicaltoolbox.html. The NIDA Clinical Toolbox: Science-based materials for drug abuse treatment providers).

http://monitoringthefuture.org/. Monitoring the Future Site with statistics.

http://www.cdc.gov/HealthyYouth.

REFERENCES AND ADDITIONAL READINGS

Abel EL, Hannigan JH. Maternal risk factors in fetal alcohol syndrome: provocative and permissive influences. *Neurotoxicol Teratol* 1995;17:445.

Bauman A, Phongsavan P. Epidemiology of substance use in adolescence: prevalence, trends, and policy implications. *Drug Alcohol Depend* 1999;55:187.

Bertrand J, Floyd RL, Weber MK. Guidelines for identifying and referring persons with fetal alcohol syndrome. *MMWR* 2005;54(RR-11):1.

Blanken AJ. Measuring use of alcohol and other drugs among adolescents. *Public Health Rep* 1993;108:25.

Bobo JK, Husten C. Sociocultural influences on smoking and drinking. *Alcohol Res Health* 2000;24(4):225.

Britto MT, Garrett JM, Dugliss MA, et al. Risky behavior in teens with cystic fibrosis or sickle cell disease: a multicenter study. *Pediatrics* 1998;101:250.

Brown SA, Tapert SF, Granholm E, et al. Neurocognitive functioning of adolescents: effects of protracted alcohol use. *Alcohol Clin Exp Res* 2000;24:164.

Carmichael-Olson H, Feldman JJ, Streissguth AP, et al. Neuropsychological deficits in adolescents with fetal alcohol syndrome: clinical findings. *Alcohol Clin Exp Res* 1998;22:1998.

Centers for Disease Control and Prevention. Alcohol policy and sexually transmitted disease rates–United States, 1981–1995. *MMWR Morb Mortal Wkly Rep* 2000;49:346.

Centers for Disease Control and Prevention. *Fetal alcohol syndrome: guidelines for referral and diagnosis.* Washington, DC: Department of Health and Human Services; July 2004.

Centers for Disease Control and Prevention. Guidelines for identifying and referring persons with fetal alcohol syndrome. Continuing education activity sponsored by CDC. Expiration—October 28, 2007. *MMWR* 2005;54(RR-11):1.

Centers for Disease Control and Prevention. Youth risk behavior surveillance—United States, 2005. *Morb Mortal Wkly Rep Surveill Summ* 2006;55(SS05):1.

Chaloupka FJ, Grossman M, Saffer H. The effects of price on alcohol consumption and alcohol-related problems. *Alcohol Res Health* 2002;26(1):22.

Church MW. The effects of prenatal alcohol exposure on hearing and vestibular function. In: Abel EL, ed. *Fetal alcohol syndrome: from mechanism to prevention.* Boca Raton, FL: CRC Press; 1996:85.

Donovan JE. Adolescent alcohol initiation: a review of psychosocial risk factors. *J Adolesc Health* 2004;35:529–e7.

Donovan JE, Lessor R, Lessor L. Problem drinking in adolescence and young adulthood: a follow-up study. *J Stud Alcohol* 1983;44:109.

Durant RH, Smith JA, Kreiter SR, et al. The relationship between early age onset of initial substance use and engaging in multiple health risk behaviors among young adolescents. *Arch Pediatr Adolesc Med* 1999;153:286.

Ewing JA. Detecting alcoholism: the CAGE questionnaire. *JAMA* 1985;252:14.

Farrow JA, Rees JM, Worthington-Roberts BS. Health, developmental, and nutritional status of adolescent alcohol and marijuana abusers. *Pediatrics* 1987;79:218.

Fiellin DA, Reid MC, O'Connor PG. Screening for alcohol problems in primary care: a systematic review. *Arch Intern Med* 2000;160:1977.

Flanagan P, Kokotailo P. Adolescent pregnancy and substance use. *Clin Perinatol* 1999;26:185.

Frances R, Miller SI. *Clinical textbook of addiction disorders.* New York: The Guildford Press; 1991.

Friedman IM. Alcohol and unnatural deaths in San Francisco youths. *Pediatrics* 1985;76(2):191.

Halpern-Feshler BL, Millstein SG, Ellen JM. Relationship of alcohol use and risky sexual behavior: a review and analysis of findings. *J Adolesc Health* 1996;19:331.

Harrison PA, Luxenberg MG. Comparisons of alcohol and other drug problems among Minnesota adolescents in 1989 and 1992. *Arch Pediatr Adolesc Med* 1995;149:137.

Harwood GA. Alcohol abuse screening in primary care. *Nurse Pract* 2005;30(2):56.

Hingson R, Heeren T, Winter M. Lower legal blood alcohol limits for young drivers. *Public Health Rep* 1994;109:738.

Hingston R, Kenkel D. Social, health, and economic consequences of underage drinking. In: National Research Council and Institute of Medicine. Bonnie, R.J., and O'Connell, M.E., eds. *Reducing Underage Drinking: A Collective Responsibility.* Washington, DC: National Academies Press, 2004;351.

Hingson R, Merrigan D, Heeren T. Effects of Massachusetts raising its legal drinking age from 18 to 20 on deaths from teenage homicide, suicide, and nontraffic accidents. *Pediatr Clin North Am* 1985;32:221.

Johnson MS, Moore M, Mitchell P, et al. Serious and fatal firearm injuries among children and adolescents in Alaska: 1991–1997. *Alaska Med* 2000;42:3.

Johnson VP, Swayze VW, Sato Y, et al. Fetal alcohol syndrome: craniofacial and central nervous system manifestations. *Am J Med Genet* 1996;61:329.

Johnston LD, O'Malley PM, Bachman JG, et al. *Teen drug use down but progress halts among youngest teens.* Ann Arbor, MI: University of Michigan News and Information Services; 2005. December 19, [On-line]. Available: www.monitoringthefuture.org; accessed 6/25/2006

Johnston LD, O'Malley PM, Bachman JG, et al. *Monitoring the future national results on drug use, 1975–2005: volume I, secondary school students.* NIH Publication No. 06–5883 Bethesda, MD: National Institute on Drug Abuse; 2006.

Johnston LD, O'Malley PM, Bachman JG et al. Monitoring the future national results in drug use, overview of key findings. NIH Publications No. 07-6202, Bethesda, MD: National Institute on Drug Abuse, 2007.

Kaemingik K, Paquette A. Effects of prenatal alcohol exposure on neuropsychological functioning. *Dev Neuropsychol* 1999;15:111.

Kandel DB. On processes of peer influences in adolescent drug use: a developmental perspective. *Adv Alcohol Subst Abuse* 1985;4:139.

Knight JR, Sherritt L, Shrier LA, et al. *Validity of the CRAFFT substance abuse screening test among adolescent clinic patients. Arch Pediatr Adolesc Med* 2002;156:607.

Konovalov HV, Lovetsky NS, Bobryshev YV, et al. Disorders of brain development in the progeny of mothers who used alcohol during pregnancy. *Early Hum Dev* 1997;48:153.

Kypri K, Voas RB, Langley JD, et al. Traffic crash injuries among 15 to 19 year olds and minimum purchasing age for alcohol in New Zealand. *Am J Public Health* 2005 Nov 29; published ahead of print as www.ajph.org/cgi/reprint/AJPH .2005.073122v1 (will be printed as *Am J Public Health* 2006; 96(1):1).

Les Dees W, Hiney JK, Srivastava V. Alcohol's effects on female puberty. The role of insulin-like growth factor 1. *Alcohol Health Res World* 1998;22(3):165.

Lewis DD, Woods SE. Fetal alcohol syndrome. *Am Fam Physician* 1994;50:1035.

Lieber CS. Medical disorders of alcoholism. *N Engl J Med* 1995; 333:1058.

Maes HH, Woodard CE, Murrelle L, et al. Tobacco, alcohol, and drug use in eight- to sixteen-year-old twins: the Virginia twin study of adolescent behavioral development. *J Stud Alcohol* 1999;60:293.

Mattson SM, Riley EP, Gramling L, et al. Heavy prenatal alcohol exposure with or without physical features of fetal alcohol syndrome leads to IQ deficits. *J Pediatr* 1997;131:718.

McLennan JD, Shaw E, Shema SJ, et al. Adolescents' insight in heavy drinking. *J Adolesc Health* 1998;22:409.

Meyer R. *Neuropharmacology of ethanol.* Boston: Birkhauser; 1991.

Monforte R, Estruch R, Valls-Sole J, et al. Autonomic and peripheral neuropathies in patients with chronic alcoholism: a dose-related toxic effect of alcohol. *Arch Neurol* 1995;52:45.

Morrison SF, Rogers PD, Thomas MH. Alcohol and adolescents. *Pediatr Clin North Am* 1995;42:371.

National Clearinghouse for Alcohol and Drug Information. *Teens and alcohol don't mix: Alcohol Awareness Month, April* 2000. SAMHSA. Available at http://www.health.org/ seasonal/alcawaremonth/underage.htm#stats.

NIAAA (National Institute on Alcohol Abuse and Alcoholism), U.S. Department of Health and Human Services. Imaging and alcoholism: a window on the brain. *Alcohol Alert* 2000;47:1. Available at http://www.niaaa.nih.gov.

NIAAA (National Institute on Alcohol Abuse and Alcoholism), U.S. Department of Health and Human Services. Alcohol and development in youth—a multidisciplinary overview. The scope of the problem. *Alcohol Res Health* 2004/05a;28(3):111

NIAAA (National Institute on Alcohol Abuse and Alcoholism), U.S. Department of Health and Human Services. Alcohol and development in youth—a multidisciplinary overview. The effects of alcohol on physiological processes and biological development. *Alcohol Res Health* 2004/05b;28(3):125.

NIAAA (National Institute on Alcohol Abuse and Alcoholism), U.S. Department of Health and Human Services. Alcohol and development in youth—a multidisciplinary overview. Genetics, pharmacokinetics, and neurobiology of adolescent alcohol use. *Alcohol Res Health* 2004/05c;28(3):133.

NIAAA (National Institute on Alcohol Abuse and Alcoholism), U.S. Department of Health and Human Services. Alcohol and development in youth—a multidisciplinary overview. Environmental and contextual considerations. *Alcohol Res Health* 2004/05d;28(3):155.

Office of the Inspector General, Report to the Surgeon General. *Youth and alcohol: dangerous and deadly consequences.* Washington, DC: U.S. Department of Education; 1992.

Project CHOICES Research Group. Alcohol-exposed pregnancy: characteristics associated with risk. *Am J Prev Med* 2002; 23:166.

Rachal JV, Williams JR, Brehm ML, et al. *A national study of adolescent drinking behavior, attitudes, and correlates* [conducted by Research Triangle Institute for the National Institute on Alcohol Abuse and Alcoholism]. Washington, DC: U.S. Department of Health, Education, and Welfare; 1975. [Available from National Technical Information Service, Springfield, VA.]

Rhee SH, Hewitt JK, Young SE, et al. Genetic and environmental influences on substance initiation, use, and problem use in adolescents. *Arch Gen Psychiatry* 2003;60:1256.

Robuck TM, Simmons RW, Richardson C, et al. Neuromuscular responses to disturbance of balance in children with prenatal exposure to alcohol. *Alcohol Clin Exp Res* 1998;22:1992.

Selzer ML. The michigan alcoholism screening test: the quest for a new diagnostic instrument. *Am J Psychol* 1971;127:89.

Smith BH, Molina BSG, Pelham WE. The clinically meaningful link between alcohol use and attention deficit hyperactivity disorder. *Alcohol Res Health- Alcohol Comorbid Ment Health Disord* 2002;26(2):122.

Sokol RJ, Delaney-Black V, Nordstrom B. Fetal alcohol spectrum disorder. *JAMA* 2003;290:2996.

Strauss RS, Barlow SE, Dietz WH. Prevalence of abnormal serum aminotransferase values in overweight and obese adolescents. *J Pediatr* 2000;136:727.

Streissguth AP. *Fetal alcohol syndrome: a guide for families and communities.* Baltimore, MD: Paul Brookes Publishing Co; 1997.

Streissguth AP, Barr HM, Kogan J, et al. *Understanding the occurrence of secondary disabilities in clients with Fetal Alcohol Syndrome (FAS) and Fetal Alcohol Effects (FAE): final report.* Seattle, WA: University of Washington Publication Services; 1996.

Sutocky JW, Shultz JM, Kizer KW. Alcohol-related mortality in California, 1980 to 1989. *Am J Public Health* 1993;83:817.

Thomas SE, Kelly SJ, Mattson SN, et al. Comparison of social abilities of children with fetal alcohol syndrome to those of children with similar IQ scores and normal controls. *Alcohol Clin Exp Res* 1998;22:528.

U.S. Preventive Services Task Force. Screening and behavioral counseling interventions in primary care to reduce alcohol misuse: recommendations statement. *Ann Intern Med* 2004;140:554.

U.S. Public Health Service. Alcohol and other drug abuse in adolescents. *Am Fam Physician* 1994;50:1737.

Werenko DD, Olson LM, Fullerton-Gleason L, et al. Child and adolescent suicide deaths in New Mexico, 1990–1994. *Crisis* 2000;21:36.

Wilson DM, Killen JD, Hayward C, et al. Timing and rate of sexual maturation and the onset of cigarette and alcohol use among teenage girls. *Arch Pediatr Adolesc Med* 1994;148: 789.

Windle M, Windle RC. Adolescent tobacco, alcohol, and drug use: current findings. *Adolesc Med* 1999;10:153.

Zeigler DW, Wang CC, Yoast RA, et al. The neurocognitive effects of alcohol on adolescents and college students. *Prev Med* 2005;40:23.

CHAPTER 70

Tobacco

Seth D. Ammerman

"Cigarette smoking is the chief, single avoidable cause of death in our society and the most important public health issue of our time."

—C. Everett Koop, M.D.

This statement made by Dr. Koop when he was United States Surgeon General from 1981 to 1989 remains equally true in the early part of the twenty-first century. The World Health Organization (WHO) estimates that if current smoking patterns continue, tobacco use will cause 10 million deaths each year by 2020. In the United States, approximately 438,000 deaths each year—the equivalent of three 747 fatal airline crashes/day—can be attributed to cigarette smoking. This figure is almost triple the annual number of deaths due to illegal drugs, homicide, alcohol, acquired immunodeficiency syndrome, suicide, and motor vehicle accidents combined (Fig. 70.1). The financial cost for smoking-related health care/year in the United States is approximately $75 billion, or approximately 10% of total medical expenditures, plus an additional $92 billion in productivity losses. Additionally, cigarettes are the leading cause of the approximately 1,000 fire-related deaths and many thousands of fire-related injuries in this country each year, costing approximately $0.5 billion annually just in direct property losses. More than 80% of all cigarette smokers start before the age of 18 years; almost 5% of youth first began smoking by 8 years of age, and another approximately 15% before their 13th birthday. Estimates derived from current smoking rates indicate that approximately 250 million youth worldwide will die prematurely from a tobacco-related disease. Many youth who are daily smokers report that they want to quit smoking. At the same time, a significant number of middle and high school students who have never smoked cigarettes stated that they might try smoking in the next year. Exposure to environmental tobacco smoke (ETS or second-hand smoke) is also a serious problem: In one study >50% of youth were exposed to ETS in the previous week and one third of the youth were exposed to >3 hours of ETS in the previous

week. Therefore, tobacco use should also be considered a pediatric disease. Clinicians can play an important role in preventing cigarette use by their patients and in helping their patients who are already smoking to stop.

PREVALENCE

Use among Adolescents

Tobacco use by adolescents remains a serious problem, with >2,000 American teenagers becoming regular smokers each day. The good news is that usage rates for youth younger than 18 years have been declining in the last decade. The bad news is that the decline in cigarette smoking in young adults (age 18–24 years) has been minimal. The tobacco industry is overtly and heavily targeting the young adult smoker, often sponsoring events in bars and clubs that are popular with young adults. The tobacco industry, to maintain profits, needs ongoing replacement of smokers who have died using their products. Youth are exposed to significant amounts of tobacco advertising on the Internet, and more importantly to tobacco use in movies (see subsequent text on Smoke-Free Movies campaign). Lack of compliance with status laws (i.e., asking for proof of age for those <18 years) also leads to increased smoking among youth.

Prevalence data are gathered from a number of sources; three major sources are the following:

1. National Youth Tobacco Survey (sponsored by the American Legacy Foundation, www.americanlegacy.org, and the Centers for Disease Control and Prevention [CDC] Foundation, www.cdc.gov/tobacco).

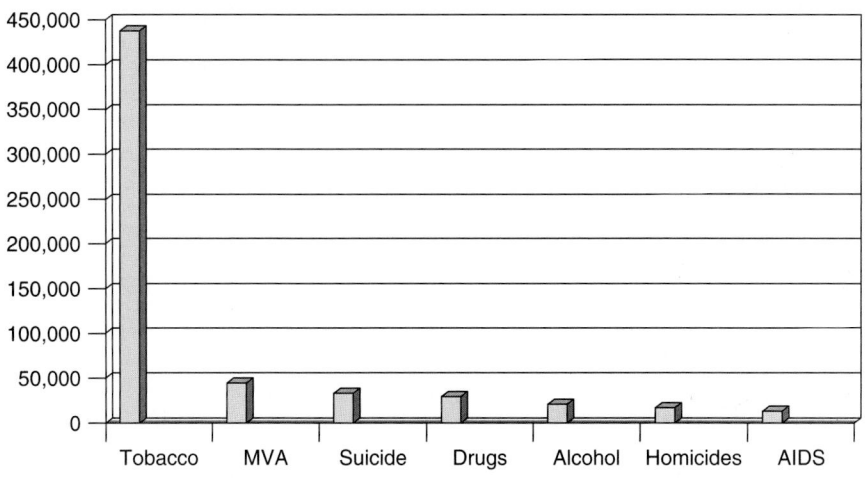

FIGURE 70.1 Deaths in the United States of America, 2004. Tobacco, 438,000; MVA, 43,947; Suicide, 31,647; Drugs, 29,036; Alcohol, 20,398; Homicides, 16,611; AIDS, 12,995. MVA, motor vehicle accident; AIDS, acquired immunodeficiency syndrome. (Adapted from the National Center for Health Statistics, fastats. www.cdc.gov/nchs/fastats/acc-inj.htm; and the *National Vital Statistics Report*, Vol. 54, No.19, June 28, 2006.)

2. Youth Risk Behavior Survey (YRBS) (sponsored by the CDC, http://www.cdc.gov/tobacco; YRBS 2005 and updated data are available at: http://www.cdc.gov/HealthyYouth/yrbs/index.htm).
3. Monitoring the Future (sponsored by the University of Michigan Institute for Social Research, www.monitoringthefuture.org, and the National Institute of Drug Abuse, www.nida.nih.gov).

All three use school-based samples, and the rates of tobacco use shown would likely be greater if high school dropouts had been included in the study samples. A fourth source, which is a home-based survey on alcohol and other drugs, is the National Survey on Drug Use and Health (formerly the National Household Survey on Drug Abuse; sponsored by the Substance Abuse and Mental Health Sciences Administration), and is available at http://oas.samhsa.gov/nsduh.htm.

The 2006 Monitoring the Future data revealed that approximately 8.7% of 8th graders, 14.5% of 10th graders, and 21.6% of 12th graders reported current smoking (i.e., smoking one or more cigarettes during the previous 30 days). Twenty-one percent of 12th grade females and 25% of 12th grade males were current smokers. Furthermore, 4% of 8th graders, 8% of 10th graders, and 12.2% of 12th graders were daily smokers in 2006. Whites have the highest smoking rates, followed by Hispanics, and then African-Americans. Table 70.1 is adapted from the Monitoring the Future study, showing trends in current and daily smoking from 1990 to 2005. For current smokers in both middle and high school, cigarettes are the most commonly used tobacco product, followed by cigars, smokeless tobacco, pipes, bidis, and kreteks. Bidis are small, brown, hand-rolled cigarettes that are made primarily in India and other South Asian countries. They consist of tobacco wrapped in a tendu or temburni leaf (plants native to Asia), and may be secured with a colorful string at one or both ends. They are available in many flavors, such as chocolate, raspberry, and strawberry, making them appealing to adolescent smokers. Kreteks are imported from Indonesia, and typically contain a mixture consisting of tobacco, cloves, and other additives. Both bidis and kreteks deliver more nicotine, carbon monoxide, and tar than conventional cigarettes.

The 2005 YRBS also shows mixed results in high school seniors (Morbidity and Mortality Weekly Report, 2006). Current use of tobacco declined from a high (since 1991) of 36.4% in 1997 to 21.9% in 2003 and increased back to 23% in 2005. Current frequent use (>20 of 30 days in last month) declined from 16.8% in 1999 to 9.7% in 2003 and to 9.4% in 2005. Smoking>10 cigarettes/day declined in high school seniors from 18% in 1991 to 13.7% in 2003 and to 10.7% in 2005.

Table 70.2AA and B shows current use of tobacco products from the 2002 and 2004 National Youth Tobacco Survey. Note that a variety of tobacco products used by adolescents was studied.

Use among College Students and Young Adults

Smoking continues to be a problem for college students and young adults. In 2004, 36% of college students reported having used a tobacco product. There was an equal distribution of use between men and women. Of those who used cigarettes, two third were current smokers and approximately 7% were daily smokers. For both male and female college students, cigarettes are the most commonly used tobacco product, followed by cigars, smokeless tobacco, and pipes. Whites have the highest use of tobacco products, followed by Hispanics, Asians, and African-Americans. College students who use tobacco are more likely to be single, white, and engaged in other risky behaviors involving substance use and sexual activity. They are also more likely to value social life over educational achievement, athletic participation, or religion. Among young adults aged 18 to 24, 26.3% of men and 21.5% of women are current smokers. For more details on tobacco use in college students see Chapter 84.

WHY DO ADOLESCENTS USE TOBACCO?

Adolescent Development

Tobacco use in adolescence can be understood in terms of biopsychosocial development during adolescence. Major developmental tasks during adolescence include establishing independence and autonomy, developing meaningful peer relations, negotiating the changes associated with physical development and puberty, and establishing a coherent self-identity. Cigarette smoking may, for example,

TABLE 70.1

Trends in Prevalence of Use of Cigarettes, for 8th, 10th, and 12th Graders, 1991–2005

	1975	1976	1977	1978	1979	1980	1981	1982	1983	1984	1985	1986	1987	1988	1989	1990
Lifetime																
8th Grade	—	—	—	—	—	—	—	—	—	—	—	—	—	—	—	—
10th Grade	—	—	—	—	—	—	—	—	—	—	—	—	—	—	—	—
12th Grade	73.6	75.4	75.7	75.3	74.0	71.0	71.0	70.1	70.6	69.7	68.8	67.6	67.2	66.4	65.7	64.4
Thirty-day																
8th Grade	—	—	—	—	—	—	—	—	—	—	—	—	—	—	—	—
10th Grade	—	—	—	—	—	—	—	—	—	—	—	—	—	—	—	—
12th Grade	36.7	38.8	38.4	36.7	34.4	30.5	29.4	30.0	30.3	29.3	30.1	29.6	29.4	28.7	28.6	29.4
Daily																
8th Grade	—	—	—	—	—	—	—	—	—	—	—	—	—	—	—	—
10th Grade	—	—	—	—	—	—	—	—	—	—	—	—	—	—	—	—
12th Grade	26.9	28.8	28.8	27.5	25.4	21.3	20.3	21.1	21.2	18.7	19.5	18.7	18.7	18.1	18.9	19.1
1/2 Pack + per day																
8th Grade	—	—	—	—	—	—	—	—	—	—	—	—	—	—	—	—
10th Grade	—	—	—	—	—	—	—	—	—	—	—	—	—	—	—	—
12 th Grade	17.9	19.2	19.4	18.8	16.5	14.3	13.5	14.2	13.8	12.3	12.5	11.4	11.4	10.6	11.2	11.3
Approx, Ns:																
8th Grade	—	—	—	—	—	—	—	—	—	—	—	—	—	—	—	—
10th Grade	—	—	—	—	—	—	—	—	—	—	—	—	—	—	—	—
12th Grade	9,400	15,400	17,100	17,800	15,500	15,900	17,500	17,700	16,300	15,900	16,000	15,200	16,300	16,300	16,700	15,200

	1991	1992	1993	1994	1995	1996	1997	1998	1999	2000	2001	2002	2003	2004	2005	2006	2005–2006 Change
Lifetime																	
8th Grade	44.0	45.2	45.3	46.1	46.4	49.2	47.3	45.7	44.1	40.5	36.6	31.4	28.4	27.9	25.9	24.6	−1.3
10th Grade	55.1	53.5	56.3	56.9	57.6	61.2	60.2	57.7	57.6	55.1	52.8	47.4	43.0	40.7	38.9	36.1	−2.8
12th Grade	63.1	61.8	61.9	62.0	64.2	63.5	65.4	65.3	64.6	62.5	61.0	57.2	53.7	52.8	50.0	47.1	−2.9
Thirty-day																	
8th Grade	14.3	15.5	16.7	18.6	19.1	21.0	19.4	19.1	17.5	14.6	12.2	10.7	10.2	9.2	9.3	8.7	−0.6
10th Grade	20.8	21.5	24.7	25.4	27.9	30.4	29.8	27.6	25.7	23.9	21.3	17.7	16.7	16.0	14.9	14.5	−0.4
12th Grade	28.3	27.8	29.9	31.2	33.5	34.0	36.5	35.1	34.6	31.4	29.5	26.7	24.4	25.0	23.2	21.6	−1.6
Daily																	
8th Grade	7.2	7.0	8.3	8.8	9.3	10.4	9.0	8.8	8.1	7.4	5.5	5.1	4.5	4.4	4.0	4.0	−0.1
10th Grade	12.6	12.3	14.2	14.6	16.3	18.3	18.0	15.8	15.9	14.0	12.2	10.1	8.9	8.3	7.5	7.6	+0
12th Grade	18.5	17.2	19.0	19.4	21.6	22.2	24.6	22.4	23.1	20.6	19.0	16.9	15.8	15.6	13.6	12.2	−1.4
1/2 Pack + per day																	
8th Grade	3.1	2.9	3.5	3.6	3.4	4.3	3.5	3.6	3.3	2.8	2.3	2.1	1.8	1.7	1.7	1.5	−0.1
10th Grade	6.5	6.0	7.0	7.6	8.3	9.4	8.6	7.9	7.6	6.2	5.5	4.4	4.1	3.3	3.1	3.3	+0.2
12th Grade	10.7	10.0	10.9	11.2	12.4	13.0	14.3	12.6	13.2	11.3	10.3	9.1	8.4	8.0	6.9	5.9	−1.0
Approx, Ns:																	
8th Grade	17,500	18,600	18,300	17,300	17,500	17,800	18,600	18,100	16,700	16,700	16,200	15,100	16,500	17,000	16,800	16,500	
10th Grade	14,800	14,800	15,300	15,800	17,000	15,600	15,500	15,000	13,600	14,300	14,000	14,300	15,800	16,400	16,200	16,200	
12th Grade	15,000	15,800	16,300	15,400	15,400	14,300	15,400	15,200	13,600	12,800	12,800	12,900	14,600	14,600	14,700	14,200	

Level of significance of difference between the two most recent classes: s = 0.05, ss = 0.01, sss = 0.001.
'—' indicates data not available.

Any apparent inconsistency between the change estimate and the prevalence of use estimates for the two most recent classes is due to rounding error.

(Johnston LD, O'Malley PM, Bachman JG, et al. *Monitoring the future: decline in teen smoking seems to be nearing its end*. www.monitoringthefuture.org. December 19, 2005.)

TABLE 70.2A

Percentage of Students in Middle School (grades 6–8) Who Were Current Users[a] of Any Tobacco Product, By Product Type, Sex, and Race/Ethnicity—National Youth Tobacco Survey, United States, 2002 and 2004

Characteristic	Any Tobacco[b]		Cigarettes		Cigars		Smokeless Tobacco		Pipes		Bidis		Kreteks	
	%	(95% CI[c])	%	(95% CI)	%	(95% CI)	%	(95% CI)	%	(95% CI)	%	(95% CI)	%	(95% CI)
Middle school, 2004														
Sex														
Male	12.7	(±1.7)	7.7[d]	(±1.3)	6.6	(±1.1)	3.9	(±1.0)	3.3[d]	(±0.8)	2.8	(±0.7)	1.9[d]	(±0.4)
Female	10.7	(±1.8)	8.5	(±1.9)	3.9	(±0.5)	1.9	(±0.5)	1.8	(±0.5)	1.7	(±0.4)	1.2	(±0.4)
Race/Ethnicity														
White, non-Hispanic	11.2	(±1.9)	8.3	(±1.8)	4.4	(±0.8)	3.1	(±0.9)	2.2	(±0.6)	1.8	(±0.5)	1.2	(±0.4)
Black, non-Hispanic	12.3	(±2.5)	7.5	(±1.9)	6.9	(±1.8)	1.8	(±0.8)	2.0[d]	(±0.8)	2.7	(±0.9)	1.6	(±0.6)
Hispanic	14.8	(±1.9)	9.4	(±1.5)	8.0[d]	(±1.2)	3.7	(±0.9)	5.3	(±1.2)	4.3[d]	(±0.8)	3.0	(±0.7)
Asian	3.4[d]	(±1.8)	2.2[d]	(±1.5)	0.7[d]	(±0.6)	1.0	(±0.7)	0.7[d]	(±0.7)	0.5[d]	(±0.6)	0.7[d]	(±0.7)
Total	11.7	(±1.6)	8.1	(±1.5)	5.2	(±0.7)	2.9	(±0.6)	2.6[d]	(±0.6)	2.3	(±0.5)	1.5	(±0.3)
Middle school, 2002														
Sex														
Male	14.7	(±1.6)	9.8	(±1.3)	7.9	(±1.1)	5.3	(±1.3)	5.1	(±0.8)	3.1	(±0.6)	2.7	(±0.6)
Female	11.7	(±1.4)	9.7	(±1.4)	4.1	(±0.7)	1.6	(±0.5)	1.9	(±0.4)	1.7	(±0.4)	1.1	(±0.3)
Race/Ethnicity														
White, non-Hispanic	13.2	(±1.9)	10.1	(±1.6)	5.5	(±1.0)	3.8	(±1.1)	2.8	(±0.6)	1.8	(±0.4)	1.5	(±0.4)
Black, non-Hispanic	13.5	(±2.4)	9.0	(±2.3)	7.3	(±1.7)	2.3	(±0.9)	3.9	(±1.4)	3.1	(±1.0)	2.3	(±0.9)
Hispanic	12.5	(±1.9)	8.7	(±1.5)	6.3	(±1.1)	2.7	(±0.7)	4.3	(±0.9)	2.9	(±0.7)	2.6	(±0.7)
Asian	8.6	(±3.3)	7.4	(±3.3)	5.0	(±2.8)	3.5	(±2.7)	4.6	(±2.7)	3.1	(±2.2)	3.8	(±2.9)
Total	13.3	(±1.4)	9.8	(±1.2)	6.0	(±0.7)	3.5	(±0.7)	3.5	(±0.5)	2.4	(±0.3)	2.0	(±0.4)

[a]Used tobacco on at least 1 day during the 30 days preceding the survey.
[b]Cigarettes, cigars, smokeless tobacco, pipes, bidis (leaf-wrapped, flavored cigarettes from India), or kreteks (clove cigarettes).
[c]Confidence interval.
[d]Significant difference ($p < 0.05$), 2004 versus 2002.
MMWR Morb Mortal Wkly Rep April 1, 2005;54(12):297.

TABLE 70.2B

Percentage of Students in High School (grades 9–12) Who were Current Users[a] of Any Tobacco Product, By Product Type, Sex, and Race/Ethnicity

Characteristic	Any Tobacco[b] %	(95% CI[c])	Cigarettes %	(95% CI)	Cigars %	(95% CI)	Smokeless Tobacco %	(95% CI)	Pipes %	(95% CI)	Bidis %	(95% CI)	Kreteks %	(95% CI)
High school, 2004														
Sex														
Male	31.5	(±3.0)	22.1	(±2.7)	18.4	(±1.8)	10.8	(±2.2)	4.6	(±0.9)	3.6	(±0.7)	3.2	(±0.8)
Female	24.7	(±3.1)	22.4	(±3.1)	7.5	(±1.4)	1.4	(±0.6)	1.6	(±0.6)	1.6	(±0.5)	1.5	(±0.5)
Race/Ethnicity														
White, non-Hispanic	31.5	(±4.1)	25.4	(±3.8)	13.6	(±2.1)	7.5	(±1.6)	2.9	(±0.8)	2.2	(±0.5)	2.3	(±0.7)
Black, non-Hispanic	17.1[d]	(±3.3)	11.4	(±3.1)	10.5	(±2.1)	1.7	(±1.2)	1.8[d]	(±0.8)	2.1	(±0.8)	1.3	(±0.5)
Hispanic	26.2	(±2.9)	21.6	(±3.1)	13.3[d]	(±1.7)	3.5	(±1.1)	5.0	(±1.0)	4.6	(±0.9)	3.3	(±0.7)
Asian	13.1	(±3.3)	11.2	(±2.6)	5.7	(±2.4)	2.1	(±1.7)	2.0	(±1.1)	2.1	(±1.2)	1.4	(±1.0)
Total	28.0	(±2.9)	22.3	(±2.7)	12.8	(±1.5)	6.0	(±1.2)	3.1	(±0.6)	2.6	(±0.5)	2.3	(±0.5)
High school, 2002														
Sex														
Male	32.6	(±2.3)	23.9	(±2.1)	16.9	(±1.4)	10.5	(±2.0)	5.0	(±0.9)	3.7	(±0.8)	3.5	(±0.7)
Female	23.7	(±1.8)	21.0	(±1.9)	6.2	(±0.9)	1.2	(±0.3)	1.4	(±0.4)	1.5	(±0.4)	1.8	(±0.5)
Race/Ethnicity														
White, non-Hispanic	30.9	(±2.0)	25.2	(±1.8)	11.8	(±1.0)	7.3	(±1.4)	2.8	(±0.6)	2.2	(±0.5)	2.7	(±0.6)
Black, non-Hispanic	21.7	(±2.9)	13.8	(±2.8)	12.0	(±1.9)	1.8	(±0.8)	3.7	(±1.2)	3.4	(±1.1)	1.9	(±0.8)
Hispanic	24.1	(±2.7)	19.8	(±2.5)	10.8	(±1.5)	3.3	(±1.1)	4.6	(±1.1)	3.5	(±0.9)	3.0	(±0.8)
Asian	14.6	(±3.8)	12.2	(±3.4)	5.4	(±2.3)	2.1	(±1.5)	2.7	(±1.5)	2.9	(±1.6)	2.1	(±1.7)
Total	28.2	(±1.7)	22.5	(±1.6)	11.6	(±0.9)	5.9	(±1.1)	3.2	(±0.6)	2.6	(±0.5)	2.7	(±0.4)

[a]Used tobacco on at least 1 day during the 30 days preceding the survey.

[b]Cigarettes, cigars, smokeless tobacco, pipes, bidis (leaf-wrapped, flavored cigarettes from India), or kreteks (clove cigarettes).

[c]Confidence interval.

[d]Significant difference ($p < 0.05$), 2004 versus 2002.

National Youth Tobacco Survey, United States, 2002 and 2004.

be viewed as a means of attaining maturity and autonomy, as smoking is a legal adult behavior. Smoking may also be viewed as a social event and a means of fitting in with a peer group. Research has shown that peer influence (e.g., smoking status of best friends) is the most significant and consistent predictor of adolescent smoking. On the other hand, protective factors leading to less smoking among youth include giving clear messages against smoking, involvement in healthy activities such as sports and religious institutions, and limiting exposure to tobacco advertising (including magazines, movies, sporting events, etc.). The price of tobacco products also correlates with adolescent tobacco use: A significant price increase leads to a decrease in adolescent tobacco use.

Psychosocial Factors

Psychosocial factors related to smoking initiation for both genders include low educational aspirations or attainment; low self-esteem or low self-image, or ongoing stress or depression; risk-taking; minimizing perceived hazards of smoking; and favorable attitudes toward smoking or smokers. Other variables associated with adolescent smoking include parental or sibling smoking, perceived support for smoking by parents or peers, having lower socioeconomic status or parental educational attainment, or a history of abuse. There are also gender-specific factors associated with smoking. For example, adolescent girl smokers are more likely to be socially skilled, outgoing, and self-confident. In contrast, adolescent boy smokers may be more insecure in social settings. Teenage girls may use cigarette smoking as a method of weight control and maintenance of a thin appearance. Teenage boys may smoke for a sense of adventure and recreation as well as daring. Youth who identify themselves as gay, lesbian, or bisexual smoke at rates >50% of those of their straight counterparts, and they are four times more likely to use smokeless tobacco products. Preteens and early adolescents may in particular underestimate the addictive nature of cigarettes and may believe that there are many benefits to smoking.

Advertising

Tobacco industry advertising plays an important role in inducing adolescents to smoke. One study found that 86% of 10th graders and 88% of 12th graders who purchase their own cigarettes bought one of the three most heavily advertised brands—Marlboro, Camel, and Newport. In comparison, <50% of adults buy these three brands. Until 1999, when parts of the Master Settlement Agreement between the tobacco companies and the states' attorneys general went into effect, cigarettes were the most heavily advertised product in the outdoor (billboard) media, including the newest and growing form of outdoor advertising—the neighborhood-based bus-stop shelter illuminated billboard. The tobacco industry is now focusing on print media such as magazines with a youth or young-adult focus, electronic media, and movies, so adolescents are constantly exposed to the messages promoted by these advertisers. Studies have shown that >50% of the onset of tobacco use among youth is due to smoking portrayed in the movies. The Smoke-Free Movies campaign has proposed four measures to make sure the U.S. film industry does not act as a marketing arm for the tobacco industry. The American Academy of Pediatrics, the Society for Adolescent Medicine, the WHO, the American Heart Association, the American Medical Association, and the U.S. Public Interest Research Group have endorsed all four measures. They are as follows:

1. *Certify no pay-offs*: Every new smoking movie should run the following affidavit in the closing credits: "No person or entity involved in this motion picture accepted anything from a tobacco company, its agents, or fronts."
2. *Require antismoking ads*: Exhibitors should run effective antitobacco spots before all feature films. Spots should also be added to newly released videos and DVDs of smoking films, regardless of rating; many teens view R-rated movies through these media.
3. *Stop displaying brands*: Use of specific brands gives the appearance of violating agreements against brand placement.
4. *Rate new smoking movies "R"*: All new movies with smoking and tobacco use should receive an R rating from the Motion Picture Association of America (MPAA). Doing so will reduce the amount of smoking in the movies teens see, by >60%. And, because the effect of smoking in the movies depends on the "dose" kids get, an R rating will prevent 535 kids from starting to smoke every day.

Tobacco industry advertisements virtually ignore all health concerns and use themes that appeal to young people. In the messages, use of cigarettes is associated with healthy activities involving adventure and recreation, independence, sexual attractiveness, professional success, confidence in social settings, and weight control and physical appearance. Advertising tobacco in the context of other businesses and services (e.g., household detergents, movies, clothing) helps legitimize tobacco use. The internal documents of tobacco companies demonstrate targeting of youth, women, and minorities. Promotional offerings and "contests," as well as offers of "free" items (e.g., hats, jackets) that are usually redeemable after sending in a specified number of empty cigarette packs, are also inducements to youth to start and continue smoking. Although the Liggett Tobacco Company, in a precedent-setting legal case in March 1997, submitted documents to the Arizona Attorney General admitting that (a) nicotine is addictive, (b) cigarettes cause cancer, and (c) the tobacco industry targets children and teenagers, the tobacco industry continues to promote its deadly products extensively, spending >15 billion/year in the United States alone.

NICOTINE ADDICTION AND HEALTH CONSEQUENCES

Addiction

In addition to being a potent pesticide, nicotine is one of the most addictive substances known. Tobacco use by adolescents, which may have started primarily for psychosocial reasons, may over time become a serious drug addiction. Initial symptoms of nicotine dependence occur, in some teens, within days to weeks of onset of use.

Modes of Action Nicotine seems to function as a positive reinforcer through its actions on nicotinic acetylcholine receptors in the mesocorticolimbic dopamine pathway. Stimulation of brain dopamine systems is of great

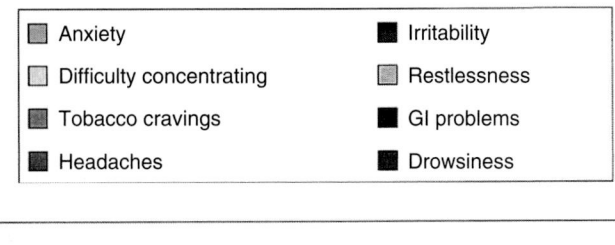

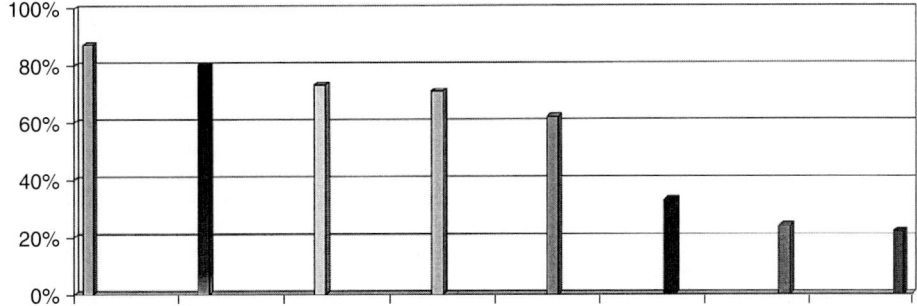

FIGURE 70.2 Nicotine withdrawal symptoms. GI, gastrointestinal. (Adapted from National Center for Chronic Disease Prevention and Health Promotion, Office of Smoking and Health. *The health consequences of smoking: nicotine addiction. A report of the surgeon general.* Washington, DC: U.S. Department of Health and Human Services, Public Health Service, Centers for Disease Control, 1988.)

importance for the rewarding and dependence-producing properties of nicotine. Abstinence from nicotine is associated with depletion of dopamine and other neurotransmitters, which may cause numerous withdrawal symptoms including anxiety, irritability, and cravings (Fig. 70.2). Relapse rates for persons attempting to quit use of nicotine are comparable to those for quitting heroin (Fig. 70.3). There are likely genetic factors (e.g., genetic variants in the dopamine D$_2$ receptor [*DRD2*] gene) in an individual's susceptibility to tobacco addiction as well as to response to the various pharmacological treatments. This is an active area of ongoing research.

Pharmacology
- Each cigarette contains 6 to 11 mg of nicotine, and smokers absorb 1 to 3 mg of nicotine/cigarette.
- Each cigarette contains 10 to 12 doses (puffs) of nicotine; one who smokes half a pack/day therefore inhales approximately 200 doses of the drug daily.
- One pack/day equals 20 to 40 mg of nicotine absorbed/day.
- Each dose of the drug acts on the user within seconds of being inhaled.

Plasma concentrations of nicotine decline in a biphasic manner. Typically the initial half-life is 2 to 3 minutes, and the terminal half-life is 30 to 120 minutes. Most nicotine is metabolized in the liver to cotinine and nicotine-1'-oxide. Cotinine has a plasma half-life that varies from approximately 10 to 40 hours. Nicotine and its metabolites are excreted by the kidneys; approximately 10% to 20% of the nicotine is eliminated unchanged in the urine.

Effects of Other Compounds in Cigarettes

In addition to nicotine, cigarettes contain tar—a toxic compound. Cigarettes usually contain thousands of other chemicals, many poisonous and cancer causing, including ammonia, cadmium, carbon monoxide, cyanide, formaldehyde, nitrosamines, and polynuclear aromatic hydrocarbons. The tobacco industry is actively fighting disclosure of the chemical ingredients in cigarettes, including pesticides and flavor additives, arguing that they are "trade secrets." However, the province of British Columbia, Canada, has mandated the release of all tobacco ingredients, including tobacco, paper, filter, and filter paper (www.healthservices.gov.bc.ca/ttdr).

Systemic Effects of Tobacco

The U.S. Surgeon General's report in 2004 updated the list of diseases related to tobacco use. Use of tobacco products can adversely affect virtually every organ system in the body (www.cdc.gov/tobacco/data_statistics/sgr/sgr_2004/index.htm). Some of these adverse effects include the following:

- Heart and lung disease—ischemic heart disease, and cerebrovascular and peripheral vascular diseases
- Cancers—lung, head and neck, esophageal, gastric, colorectal, bladder, renal, prostate, and cervical cancers
- Diminished bone density
- Pulmonary effects—chronic obstructive pulmonary disease and small airway disease
- Gastrointestinal effects—gastroesophageal reflux and peptic ulcer disease
- Cataracts
- Premature wrinkling of the skin
- Potential adverse effects on immune system
- Pregnancy-related problems including low–birth weight babies and higher rates of spontaneous abortions
- Erectile dysfunction (impotence)

Smokeless Tobacco

Smokeless tobacco users, in addition to suffering from many of the same systemic adverse effects as smokers

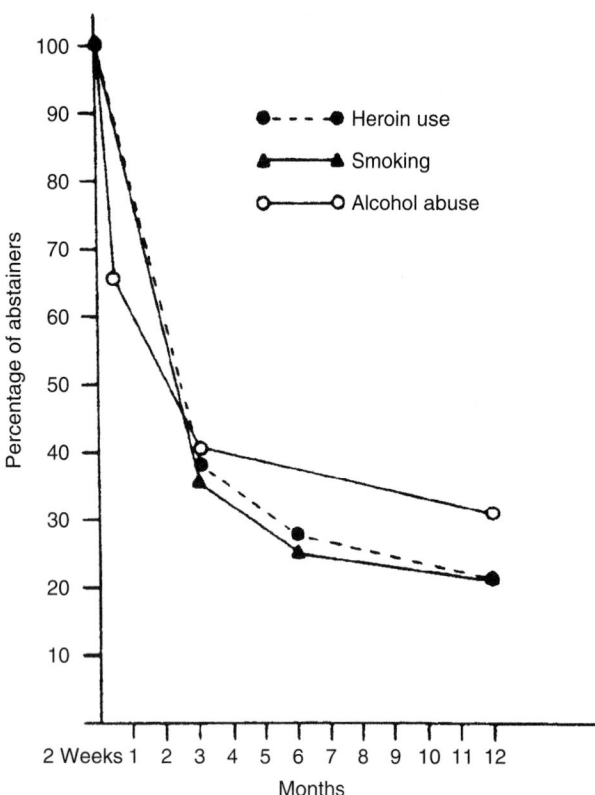

FIGURE 70.3 Relapse over time for heroin use, smoking, and alcohol abuse. (From National Center for Chronic Disease Prevention and Health Promotion, Office of Smoking and Health. *The health consequences of smoking: nicotine addiction. A report of the surgeon general.* Washington, DC: U.S. Department of Health and Human Services, Public Health Service, Centers for Disease Control, 1988.)

due to nicotine, have higher rates of various cancers, including oral, prostate, pancreas, and cervical cancers. Smokeless tobacco use is associated with numerous dental, periodontal, and oral soft tissue problems, including gingival recession, periodontal attachment loss, tooth staining, halitosis, and leukoplakia. Inflammatory bowel disease is more common in smokeless tobacco users.

Environmental Tobacco Smoke

ETS or second-hand smoke has numerous serious adverse health effects. A report by the California Environmental Protection Agency, Air Resources Board, is an excellent resource: "Proposed Identification of Environmental Tobacco Smoke as a Toxic Air Contaminant—June 24, 2005." www .arb.ca.gov/toxics/ets/finalreport/finalreport.htm. Children exposed to ETS may have development of and/or worsening of asthma, higher rates of lower respiratory tract infections (e.g., bronchitis, pneumonia), and higher rates of otitis media. Heart disease, lung cancer, and nasal sinus cancer are also more common with exposure to ETS, as are pulmonary hypertension of the newborn, sudden infant death syndrome (SIDS), and postanesthesia pulmonary complications.

PREVENTION AND TREATMENT

Brief Practitioner Interventions

Research has demonstrated that 3-minute discussions of tobacco use *(brief interventions)* can have a significant impact on smoking prevention or smoking cessation. Busy practitioners can still address the smoking issue in a meaningful way in a short period of time. Dentists and dental hygienists have also been shown to have a positive impact on cessation counseling. There are two types of 3-minute interventions—those directed toward *patients* (Fig. 70.4) and those directed toward *parents* (Fig. 70.5). Strong and direct language is purposefully used, and these kinds of messages have been found to be very helpful. Given the medical problems associated with second-hand smoke, and given that parents are one of the most important role models for adolescents, pediatricians must also provide smoking cessation referrals and/or interventions for the parents. It is much more likely for an adolescent to start smoking, and much more difficult for an adolescent to successfully quit smoking if he or she is living with siblings or parents who smoke. Therefore, siblings and parents need to be encouraged to quit too. Parents should be encouraged to maintain smoke-free homes.

Intensive Smoking Cessation Interventions

More intensive smoking cessation interventions may be more effective in helping addicted smokers quit. These more intensive interventions may involve a medical clinician to discuss health issues and prescribe pharmacotherapy, and a health educator to focus on additional psychosocial or behavioral issues.

Antismoking Messages

The antismoking message should be varied according to the smoking status, age, and developmental stage of the patient. *Prevention* starts with the prenatal visit and continues throughout childhood (as noted earlier, children may start smoking by the age of 8 years) and during the preteen, teen, young adult, and adult years. Anticipatory guidance should always include tobacco-use counseling.

1. Nonsmokers: Nonsmoking should be praised and the behavior normalized. Urge continuation of nonsmoking: "Keep making smart choices."
2. Individuals who are considering starting: For someone who is considering smoking and who lives in an environment with exposure to smokers (e.g., parents, siblings, friends who smoke), offer praise for nonsmoking to date, healthy alternatives to smoking, and role-playing of methods to gracefully bow out of smoking among peers. For example, the teen may refuse opportunities to smoke by saying, "No thanks, I'm not in the mood right now" or "I feel like I'm getting a sore throat and smoking will make it worse" or "I don't want to expose my body to all those nasty chemicals."
3. Patients who smoke: For patients who are smoking, the sooner *treatment* is begun, the more likely successful quitting will occur. The estimates of quitting rates for teen smokers, quitting on their own without help, range from 0% to 11%. For someone who is experimenting with tobacco use, immediate quitting should be encouraged

3-MINUTE CESSATION MESSAGES FOR TEEN PATIENTS

- Nicotine is an addictive drug. Do you want to be chained to a cigarette?

- There are thousands of chemicals in cigarettes. Many of these chemicals are toxic. Some cause cancer. Why pollute your body with these poisons?

- Cigarettes cost a lot of money. Wouldn't it be better to buy a compact disc, or go to a movie?

- Most teens are nonsmokers. Why is that?

- The tobacco companies have admitted that nicotine is addictive. But the tobacco companies think teens are stupid, because they make a lot of money off teen smokers.

- Smoking causes yellow teeth, bad skin and wrinkles, smelly clothes, and bad breath. Do you think that's attractive?

- Why not try to relax in a way that makes your body more fit, like sports, dancing, or exercise?

- Quitting may not be easy, but millions of people have successfully quit smoking. Remember, the average number of quit attempts before successful quitting is 7!

- There are medications to help you during the quit process, if you need them.

- Be smart. Don't let the tobacco companies manipulate you.

FIGURE 70.4 Patient 3-minute pointers. (Adapted from Ammerman SD. Helping kids kick butts. *Contemp Pediatr* 1998;15(2):64.)

3-MINUTE CESSATION MESSAGES FOR PARENTS

- Second-hand smoke is dangerous to your child's health. Please do not smoke around your child.

- If your child is around smokers, he or she will have more respiratory infections and worsening of asthma.

- Smoking during pregnancy is associated with lower birth weights and sudden infant death syndrome (SIDS).

- Cigarettes are expensive: you waste approximately $1,000 a year if you smoke a pack a day. Aren't there better ways to spend that money?

- Your life insurance is much more expensive if you smoke.

- You are more likely to die at a younger age if you smoke; don't you want to see your children grow up, and be around for your grandchildren?

- If you smoke, your children are much more likely to smoke. Do you want your children to smoke?

- Most adults don't smoke. Why do you think you smoke?

- Quitting is easier sometimes if you use medications like the nicotine patch, or Zyban, during your quit attempt.

FIGURE 70.5 Parent 3-minute pointers. (Adapted from Ammerman SD. Helping kids kick butts. *Contemp Pediatr* 1998;15(2):64.)

and a *quit date set*. For someone who is regularly using tobacco, quitting should be encouraged. If the patient wants to quit, the clinician can be more assertive and set a quit date. If the patient does not want to quit, the physician must be less assertive but should raise quitting as an important issue, provide motivational literature, and follow-up at subsequent visits.

United States Public Health Service Clinical Guidelines

The U.S. Public Health Service originally published guidelines that stressed *the five "R's"* for enhancing motivation to quit tobacco use: (a) indicating why quitting is personally *Relevant*; (b) identifying the *Risks* of tobacco use; (c) identifying the medical and psychosocial *Rewards* of quitting; (d) identifying *Roadblocks* to quitting and how to overcome them; and (e) *Repeating* the motivational intervention at every clinic visit.

In 2000, the clinical practice guideline for treating tobacco use and dependence was revised. *The five "A's"—Ask, Advise, Assess, Assist,* and *Arrange*—are used for smoking cessation counseling. There are very few published (and even fewer methodologically sound) studies concerning smoking cessation in teens. Therefore, these treatment guidelines are based primarily on the adult literature.

1. *Ask* systematically about smoking at each visit. A simple and effective way to operationalize this is to add a yes/no question about tobacco exposure and use to the vital sign portion of the chart note (Fig. 70.6A and B). Therefore, when vital signs are taken at every visit, the use of tobacco will be brought up. Using tobacco as a vital sign gives a simple and effective antitobacco use message at the beginning of the visit, helps the health care provider remember to discuss the issue, and helps increase quitting. Smoking status can change quickly in teenagers, and a previous nonsmoker may be smoking by the time of the next visit—or a regular smoker who did not wish to quit in the past may now wish to quit smoking. *Because teens often come in only sporadically for health care, the tobacco issue should be raised at every office visit, no matter what the chief complaint.* In addition to cigarette use, it is important to inquire about the use of other tobacco products. Teens may use cigars, chewing tobacco, snuff, bidis, or kreteks, and they may not realize that these products are harmful. Additionally, adolescents who use tobacco products may also be using alcohol and other drugs. Therefore, an alcohol and other drug use history should be obtained. Concomitant use of tobacco with alcohol or other drugs may make it more difficult for the teen to stop tobacco use without also stopping alcohol or other drug use; this needs to be addressed directly during smoking cessation counseling.

2. Strongly *Advise* all smokers to quit. Advice that is clear and personally relevant is most effective. Physicians are looked on as authoritative figures, even by teens, and giving a consistent cessation message is important. Additionally, be sure that smokers understand that cigarettes labeled "light" or "ultralight" are not safer cigarettes. These cigarettes contain the same amount of nicotine, tar, and many other ingredients as regular cigarettes, but have been used as a marketing ploy by the tobacco industry to encourage smokers to continue smoking.

3. *Assess* patient willingness to make a quit attempt (as noted earlier). A quick and easy method to assess potential success in quitting is to ask the patient two questions, both using a 1 to 10 scale. First, how much *confidence* does the patient have in being able to quit, and second, how much *importance* does the patient attribute to the behavior change. A patient with high self-confidence who feels that this is a highly important behavior change will likely do well, whereas a patient with low self-confidence and not feeling that quitting is very important will likely do poorly. It is usual for patients to be somewhere in the middle on both scales, so both the patient and physician can strategize about doing better on both.

FIGURE 70.6 Tobacco as a vital sign: Teen and parent forms.

A   Tobacco as a Vital Sign

For the Teen

Height _____   Weight _____   P_____   R_____   T _____   BP_____

Ask in a simple straightforward way:

"We now ask teens about tobacco use at each visit. This is confidential. Do you ever use any tobacco products? Are you around tobacco smoke at home or with friends?"

Teen tobacco exposure? Yes_____   No_____   Advice given_____

Teen tobacco use? Yes_____   No_____   Advice given_____

B   Tobacco as a Vital Sign

For the Parent

Height _____   Weight _____   P_____   R_____   T _____   BP_____

Ask in a simple straightforward way:

"We now ask parents about their child's exposure to tobacco at each visit. Is your child ever exposed to tobacco smoke?"

Teen tobacco exposure? Yes_____   No_____   Advice given_____

Teen tobacco use? Yes_____   No_____   Advice given_____

A FIRM QUIT DATE IS AN IMPORTANT STEP IN QUITTING SMOKING

I agree to quit smoking on the following date: _____.

I understand that quitting smoking is the single best thing I can do for my health.

My signature: _____.

My health care professional's signature: _____.

Today's date: _____.

I understand that my health care professional will contact me on or around my quit date

to see how things are going, and to arrange a follow-up visit at the office.

FIGURE 70.7   A firm quit date is an important step in quitting smoking. (Adapted from Ammerman SD. Helping kids kick butts. *Contemp Pediatr* 1998;15(2):64.)

4. *Assist* the patient in stopping smoking.
   a. Motivational steps: *Setting a quit date* has been shown to be an important and effective first step in smoking cessation. An actual calendar date should be chosen and agreed upon by the patient and physician. See Figure 70.7 for an example of a "quit date" form. Once the quit date has been selected (usually 2–4 weeks away), the patient can prepare to become a nonsmoker. Preparation to quit smoking has physical, psychological, and emotional components. For example, in getting ready to quit (before the quit date), the patient should *keep a journal* noting when and why and how much he or she smokes, as well as any routine activities in which smoking plays a part, such as drinking coffee or alcohol. The patient can attempt to *change smoking routines* by keeping cigarettes in a different place, smoking with the other hand, or smoking only in self-designated areas. The patient should occasionally *chew gum or drink a glass of water* instead of smoking a cigarette; he or she will notice that the smoking craving usually subsides within a few minutes. Gum, hard candy, sunflower seeds, or toothpicks can be carried around and used as cigarette substitutes. By the quit date, the patient's *environment should be rid of cigarette cues*. For example, clothes, the living space, and the inside of the car should all be cleaned to get rid of the tobacco smell. Ashtrays and all cigarettes should be got rid of. The patient should make it a point to find nonsmoking spaces to be in and to stay away from places where smoking is permitted (e.g., bars). Patients need to think of themselves as nonsmokers, and they should literally say to themselves that being a nonsmoker is important. Patients should try to remember the benefits of nonsmoking! Writing down the benefits on a 3 × 5 card that the patient can carry around and look at in tempting situations may be helpful. To maintain the quit effort, patients need to know that withdrawal symptoms are common but transient and that pharmacotherapy is available if necessary. *Mild-to-moderate exercise*, such as walking or riding a bicycle, can help attenuate withdrawal symptoms. Suggest that the patient start a *money jar* with the money saved from not buying cigarettes. This will add up quickly, and the patient can reward himself or herself by buying new music, going to the movies, and so on. Psychosocial support has been shown to lead to more successful quit attempts. The patient should *actively elicit support from friends and family*. Going through the process with a "buddy" who is also willing to quit simultaneously can make the whole cessation process easier and should be encouraged. The clinician should provide self-help materials, such as the "quit tips" listed in Table 70.3.
   b. Pharmacotherapy: Pharmacotherapy includes nicotine replacement products (patch, gum, lozenge, inhaler, or nasal spray), and bupropion (Zyban) and varenicline (Chantix). These modalities may be very helpful for addicted smokers. Addiction is usually defined as smoking half a pack of cigarettes or more/day, smoking the first cigarette of the day within 1 hour of awakening, or having had withdrawal symptoms during a previous quit attempt. Nicotine dependence criteria are listed in the American Psychiatric Association's *Diagnostic and Statistical Manual of Mental Disorders, Fourth Edition* (DSM-IV). Withdrawal symptoms and cravings can make quitting very difficult and may be mitigated in large part with use of pharmacotherapy. Prescribing instructions for these medications can be found in Table 70.4. Note that nicotine patches, gum, and lozenges are now over-the-counter medications. Distraction and relaxation techniques should also be encouraged to help patients deal with withdrawal and craving symptoms.

5. Arrange follow-up. Cessation rates have been shown to significantly improve with regular follow-up. For example, we usually call the patient on the quit date to congratulate him or her on the effort, and then talk with or see the patient every 1 or 2 weeks during the first 3 months of the quit attempt—the time of greatest relapse. If a patient is able to quit for 3 straight months, he or she is more likely to successfully quit for good. It is rare for a patient to have a relapse after abstaining from smoking for an entire year.

It is very important for both the pediatrician and the patient to remember that tobacco is an addictive drug and

TABLE 70.3

Guide for Patients: How to Stop Smoking

Quitting smoking is not easy but millions of people have done it and so can you. These tips will help.

Getting ready to quit
- Set a date for quitting. Try to convince a friend to quit with you, so you will have mutual support. Let your family and friends know that you are trying to quit; they can help you through the harder times and give you ongoing encouragement.
- Notice when, where, and how you smoke—list the times when you usually light up—with morning coffee, after a meal, while driving, or whatever your usual smoking occasions are.
- Change your smoking routines. Keep your cigarettes in a different place, do not hold your cigarette in the hand you are used to using, switch brands, and do not carry on any other activity—such as reading, driving, talking on the phone, or watching television—while you smoke.
- Designate one place to smoke—such as the back porch—and do not smoke anywhere else.
- When you want a cigarette, wait a few minutes before you light up. Try doing something else, such as chewing gum or drinking a glass of water, and see if the urge passes.
- Buy only one pack of cigarettes at a time.
- Ask your doctor about medications that ease withdrawal symptoms and reduce cigarette cravings. You may want to have nicotine patches or gum on hand, ready for quit day.

On quitting day
- Get rid of all your cigarettes and put away your ashtrays.
- Change your morning routines, especially where and when you eat breakfast. Try sitting somewhere else, or going out to eat.
- When you get the urge to smoke, do something else instead.
- Carry substitutes to put in your mouth, such as chewing gum, hard candy, or toothpicks.
- Reward yourself at the end of the day. See a movie, or eat a favorite treat.

Staying smoke free
- Do not be upset if you feel sleepy or short tempered. These are symptoms of nicotine withdrawal and they will go away in a few days.
- Exercise regularly. Go for walks, ride a bike, or take part in sports you enjoy.
- Think about the positive aspects of not smoking: Your self-image as someone who has kicked the habit, the health benefit you and your family get from living in a smoke-free environment, and the example you set for others.
- When you feel tense, think about the problem that causes those feelings and try to solve it. Tell yourself that smoking will not make it better.
- Eat regular meals, so you do not have times when you feel hungry and confuse that feeling with the desire to smoke.
- Put the money you would have spent on cigarettes in a money jar every day, and watch it mount up. Plan to buy something special for yourself.
- Let other people know you have stopped smoking. Your friends who still smoke may want to know how you did it.
- If you break down and smoke a cigarette, do not give up. Many former smokers made several attempts to stop before they succeeded. Quit again.

From Ammerman S. Helping kids kick butts. *Contemp Pediatr* 1998;15:71.

that the cessation process is usually difficult. The average number of quit attempts before successful cessation is approximately seven! Therefore, neither the pediatrician nor the patient should get discouraged if the first few quit attempts are unsuccessful. Rather than looking at these unsuccessful quit attempts as failures, the patient should view them as learning experiences. The pediatrician and the patient should discuss what worked and why, and what did not work and why. This helps make the next quit attempt work better. Depression may occur during a quit attempt and the patient should be asked about mood changes. For smokers with numerous unsuccessful quit attempts,

referral to a support group such as Nicotine Anonymous may be helpful.

OFFICE CHANGES

It is important to express a consistent antismoking message to parents and patients throughout the entire medical office. Listed are some simple ways to do this.

1. *Select a smoking cessation coordinator*: This person is in charge of all antismoking efforts and may be anyone who

TABLE 70.4

Pharmacotherapeutic Aids

Type	Indications	Warnings	Adverse Effects	Dosage	Prescribing Instructions	How to Obtain
Patch	Indicated for the relief of nicotine withdrawal symptoms, as part of a comprehensive smoking cessation program	Potential for fetal harm; cardiovascular effects may occur	Local skin reaction, usually mild	Nicoderm CQ and Habitrol: 21 mg (if smoke >10 cigarettes/d; otherwise start with 14 mg) × 6 wk, then 14 mg × 2 wk, then 7 mg × 2 wk; worn 24 hr/d Nicotrol: 15 mg × 6 wk, then 10 mg × 2 wk, then 5 mg × 2 wk, worn either 16 hr while awake, or 24 hr/d	Start the first patch on awakening on quit day Do not smoke while using the patch; if you must smoke, take off the patch Each morning, place a new patch on a relatively hairless spot between the neck and waist Use a different spot each day, to reduce skin irritation	Over the counter
Gum	Appropriate for patients who prefer it, or who have had skin reactions, or failure with the patch	Potential for fetal harm; cardiovascular effects may occur	Mouth soreness, hiccups, dyspepsia, and aching jaws are common, mild, and usually transient	2 mg and 4 mg Use 4 mg if smoking >25 cigarettes/d, use 2 mg if smoking <25 cigarettes/d Preferable to chew at least one piece every 1–2 hr; may chew up to 30 pieces of the 2 mg, or 20 pieces of 4 mg gum/d	Do not smoke while using the gum Chew gum slowly until it tastes minty, peppery, or orange, then park it between the cheek and gum to enhance nicotine absorption Chew slowly and park intermittently for approximately 30 min Reduce number of pieces chewed gradually over time	Over the counter Mint, pepper, or orange flavors
Nasal spray	Same as gum	Not recommended for patients with chronic nasal disorders; keep out of the reach of children	Nasal irritation	1–2 sprays in each nostril/hr, at least 8 times/d, to a maximum of 80 sprays/d; maximum recommended duration of treatment is 3 mo	Use as frequently as needed to counter withdrawal symptoms for approximately 8 wk, then reduce use over the next 4–6 wk	Prescription only
Inhaler	Same as gum	Same as gum	Use with caution in asthma	Up to 20 cartridges/d, up to 6 mo	Insert cartridge into mouthpiece; cartridge lasts approximately 20 min	Prescription only

(continued)

TABLE 70.4

(Continued)

Type	Indications	Warnings	Adverse Effects	Dosage	Prescribing Instructions	How to Obtain
Nicotine lozenge	Same as gum	Same as gum	Same as gum	2 mg or 4 mg Use 4 mg if smoke first cigarette of day within half hr of awakening Otherwise use 2 mg	Do not chew or swallow the lozenge Allow the lozenge to slowly dissolve over 20 or 30 min There may be a warm or tingly sensation in the mouth Intermittently shift the lozenge around in the mouth Reduce number of lozenges used gradually over time	Over the counter
Bupropion	For smokers who have failed to quit using nicotine medications alone	Should not be used in patients already on bupropion, or in patients with anorexia, bulimia, or seizure disorders	Dry mouth, insomnia, headache, rhinitis	150 mg once or twice a d, for up to 6 mo	Start with 150 mg q.o.d for 3 d, increase as needed to a maximum of 300 mg/d Initiate 1 wk q.o.d before quit date, to allow time for blood levels to build up May use in conjunction with nicotine replacement products	Prescription only
Varenicline	For smokers who prefer non-NRT or oral therapy	No studies in patients younger than 18 years, or pregnant women	Nausea, sleep disturbance, constipation, flatulence, vomiting	0.5 mg days 1–3 0.5 mg b.i.d. days 4–7, 1.0 mg b.i.d. day 8—end of treatment May use for up to 6 mo	Initiate 1 wk before quit date, to allow time for blood levels to build up	Prescription only

NRT, nicotine replacement therapy

is interested in the project (e.g., receptionist, nurse, aide, doctor). The immediate goal is to create a smoke-free office.

2. *Select a date to make the office smoke free*: This is the office employees' equivalent of the individual patient's quit date.

3. *Post "no smoking" signs in all office areas*: Prominently display smoking cessation materials and information in your waiting and examination rooms.

4. *Eliminate all tobacco advertising from your waiting room,* either by not subscribing to magazines that carry tobacco advertisements and thereby support the tobacco industry (the Maryland Medicine Society, www.smokefreemd.org, has a list of magazines that do not carry any tobacco ads) or by having the office smoking coordinator write over cigarette ads or place stickers with slogans such as, "Don't fall for this" or "This is a rip-off."

5. *Have prominent office campaigns to publicize the "Great American Smoke-out,"* which is always the Thursday before Thanksgiving, and *"World No-Tobacco Day,"* which is always May 31. These are particularly high-profile public events to encourage smoking cessation.

HEDIS (Health Plan Employer Data and Information Set) Standards and Billing Issues

Smoking prevention and cessation counseling is considered a standard of care, and formal ratings of health plans and individual physicians commonly include these efforts. The National Committee on Quality Assurance (NCQA: www.ncqa.org) issues annual reports on the state of health care quality. Concerning billing issues for follow-up, if smoking cessation per se is not covered, there is almost always a related medical issue that may be billed, such as asthma, bronchitis, cough, pharyngitis, or an upper respiratory infection.

Educational Materials

Educational materials for teens, parents, and physicians are available from a variety of sources either free or for nominal fees. The Web sites listed in this section and at end of the chapter all offer educational materials and provide hypertext links to many other tobacco control groups. These include local chapters of the American Cancer Society (www.cancer.org) and the American Lung Association (www.lungusa.org/tobacco); the American Academy of Pediatrics (www.aap.org); the U.S. Department of Health and Human Services (www.hhs.gov/diseases/index.shtml#smoking); the National Cancer Institute (www.nci.nih.gov); and the Agency for Health Care Policy and Research, now called the *Agency for Health Care Research and Quality* (www.ahcpr.gov), which also provides free smoking cessation guidelines for physicians, and guides for patients. Finally, the federal government's CDC, in conjunction with the Office on Smoking and Health and the National Center for Chronic Disease Prevention and Health Promotion (www.cdc.gov/tobacco), offers educational materials, posters, hypertext links, and other information.

ADVOCACY ISSUES

The most successful tobacco control efforts involve a number of concerted actions. These include the following:

- Increasing the cost of tobacco products through higher taxes on the products
- Litigation against the tobacco industry to hold corporations financially responsible for the disease and death caused by their products
- Ending government subsidies to the tobacco industry (which currently exceed $100 million dollars/year)
- Banning advertising of tobacco products in youth-oriented media (see preceding text concerning the Smoke-Free Movies campaign) and youth-frequented activities such as sporting events
- Enforcing laws that ban minors from buying tobacco products
- Banning cigarette-vending machines
- Promoting adoption of clean indoor air laws and smoke-free facilities such as schools, day care centers, office buildings, restaurants, and bars
- Getting pharmacies to stop selling tobacco products
- Advocating for divestment of tobacco industry stocks by state and local government investment agencies
- Shareholder efforts to change tobacco industry behavior
- Giving the federal government the regulatory oversight of tobacco as a drug

Advocacy organizations such as Action on Smoking and Health (http://www.ash.org), Americans for Nonsmokers' Rights (www.no-smoke.org), and the Campaign for Tobacco-Free Kids (www.tobaccofreekids.org) have many useful fact sheets, educational materials, and up-to-date information on various aspects of the tobacco wars. The American College Health Association published a position statement on tobacco use on college and university campuses; this is available at www.acha.org/info_resources/tobacco_statement.pdf. Smokefree.net (http://www.smokefree.net) is another excellent tobacco advocacy site. It offers daily e-mail updates on a wide variety of tobacco issues, from the latest science to the latest legal battles. In addition, information received from this site can be personalized to one's own areas of interest. Features include tobacco-related news from individual states and a daily document from the tobacco industry files, which were long suppressed by the tobacco industry until 1999. A companion site, www.tobacco.org, features daily updates of "tobacco in the news," as well as related documents and health information. The American Legacy Foundation (www.americanlegacy.org) was founded as part of the master settlement agreement, and particularly involves youth in its tobacco control activities e.g., the Truth counter-advertising campaign. The University of California, San Francisco (www.library.ucsf.edu/tobacco) provides online access to the Tobacco Control Archives Print Collection, tobacco industry Web sites and documents, state-by-state reports on tobacco industry activities, and the "Cigarette Papers."

Internationally, the tobacco industry has not changed its tactics. It has shifted its efforts elsewhere around the globe, and particularly increased them in developing countries, where tobacco control efforts may not be as well established. The tobacco industry continues to aggressively market its damaging and deadly products. To fight this global epidemic of tobacco-related disease, the WHO (http://tobacco.who.int) has developed a treaty on tobacco control, the International Framework Convention on Tobacco Control. The United States has refused to ratify this treaty to date, although >90 other countries have formally adopted the treaty. For more information on this important development, contact the Web site at http://tobacco.who.int.

RESEARCH ISSUES

A number of questions concerning tobacco use prevention and cessation in adolescents are being actively investigated in the research setting, including the following:

1. What are the best methods, and in which settings are programs and clinicians best able to help prevent or delay onset of tobacco use in the pediatric population?
2. How is tobacco addiction in youth similar to, or different from, that of adults?
3. How should successful treatment be defined—for example, is significant decrease in use, as opposed to total quitting, a reasonable treatment outcome for adolescents?
4. How valid is self-reporting of tobacco use, including self-report measures in adolescents?
5. Does biochemical verification (e.g., breath carbon monoxide, salivary or urinary cotinine) significantly increase the validity of self-reporting?
6. How should relapse be defined for adolescents?
7. What are the best methods for recruitment and retention of participants in prevention and cessation studies?
8. What are the reasons for ethnic differences in smoking rates, and what methods are best to prevent smoking as well as target smokers in an ethnically and culturally appropriate manner?

The Society for Research on Nicotine and Tobacco (www.srnt.org) publishes its own research journal *Nicotine and Tobacco Research*. The journal *Tobacco Control* (http://tc.bmjjournals.com) has comprehensive articles on issues related to health, advocacy, and research.

SUMMARY

Tobacco prevention and cessation counseling is one of the most important steps pediatricians can take to improve the short-term and long-term health of patients and their parents. Smoking is a very serious disease with potentially lifelong and life-shortening consequences. Practitioners are in a unique position to help prevent smoking onset or intervene early to stop smoking by adolescents.

WEB SITES

For Teenagers

http://www.thetruth.com. American Legacy Foundation site for adolescents.
http://www.tobaccofreekids.org/youthaction. The Campaign for Tobacco-Free Kids youth component.
http://www.cdc.gov/tobacco/tips4youth.htm. CDC Web site for teens.

For Parents

http://www.cdc.gov/tobacco/smokescreen.htm. CDC education and advocacy sites.
http://www.smokefree.gov. National Cancer Institute Web site for smoking cessation.
http://www.tobaccofreekids.org/. Campaign for Tobacco-Free Kids Web site.

For Clinicians

http://www.americanlegacy.org. American Legacy Foundation Web site.
http://www.tobaccofreekids.org. Campaign for Tobacco-Free Kids Web site.
http://www.cdc.gov/tobacco. CDC Web site on tobacco.
http://www.smokefree.net. A national advocacy Web site.
http://www.surgeongeneral.gov/tobacco/. Surgeon General's Web site for smoking cessation.
http://www.hhs.gov/safety/index.shtml#smoking. Department of Health and Human Services tobacco Web site.
http://www.treatobacco.net/home/home.cfm. A Society for Research on Nicotine and Tobacco related site.
http://www.smokefreemovies.ucsf.edu. Home page for the Smoke-Free Movies campaign.
http://www.tobaccofreeperiodicals.org. Lists magazines that do not accept tobacco advertising.

REFERENCES AND ADDITIONAL READINGS

Abroms L, Simons-Morton B, Haynie DL, et al. Psychosocial predictors of smoking trajectories during middle and high school. *Addiction* 2005;100(6):733.

American Cancer Society. *Cancer prevention and early detection facts and figures*. American Cancer Society, www.cancer.org/docroot/STT/stt/_0.asp. 2006.

American College Health Association. *American College Health Association—National College Health Assessment (ACHA-NCHA) Web Summary*. www.acha.org/projects_programs/ncha_sampledata.cfm. 2005.

American Psychiatric Association. *Diagnostic and statistical manual of mental disorders*, 4th ed. Washington, DC: American Psychiatric Association, 1994.

American Psychiatric Association. Nicotine-related disorders. In: *Diagnostic and statistical manual*, 4th ed. Washington, DC: American Psychiatric Association, 1994.

Ammerman SD. Helping kids kick butts. *Contemp Pediatr* 1998; 15(2):64.

Ammerman SD. Tobacco and pediatrics in the 21st century. *Calif Pediatrician* 1999;Fall/Winter:31.

Ammerman SD, Nolden M. Neighborhood-based tobacco advertising targeting adolescents. *West J Med* 1995;162:514.

Austin SB, Ziyadeh N, Fisher LB, et al. Sexual orientation and tobacco use in a study of US adolescent boys and girls. *Arch Pediatr Adolesc Med* 2004;158:317.

Backinger CL, McDonal P, Ossip-Klein DJ, et al. Improving the future of youth smoking cessation. *Am J Health Behav* 2003; (27 Suppl 2):S170.

Balch GI, Tworek C, Barker DC, et al. Opportunities for youth smoking cessation: findings from a national focus group study. *Nicotine Tob Res* 2004;6(1):9.

Becklake MR, Ghezzo H, Ernst P. Childhood predictors of smoking in adolescence: a follow-up study of Montreal Children. *Can Med Assoc J* 2005;173(4):377.

Biener L, Harris JE, Hamilton W. Impact of the Massachusetts tobacco control program: population-based trend analysis. *BMJ* 2000;321:351.

Biglan A, Ary DV, Smolkwski K, et al. A randomized controlled trial of a community intervention to prevent adolescent tobacco use. *Tob Control* 2000;9:24.

Blum RW, Beuhring T, Rinehart PM. *Protecting teens: beyond race, income, and family structure [Monograph].* Minneapolis, MN: Center for Adolescent Health, University of Minnesota, 2000.

Bolliger CT, Zellweger JP, Danielsson T, et al. Smoking reduction with oral nicotine inhalers: double-blind, randomized clinical trial of efficacy and safety. *BMJ* 2000;321:329.

Braverman MT. Research on resilience and its implication for tobacco prevention. *Nicotine Tob Res* 1999;1:S67.

Bryn Austin S, Ziyadeh N, Fisher LB, et al. Sexual orientation and tobacco use in a cohort study of US adolescent boys and girls. *Arch Pediatr Adolesc Med* 2004;158:317.

Bush T. Preteen attitudes about smoking and parental factors associated with favorable attitudes. *Am J Health Promot* 2005; 19:410.

California Department of Health Services, Cancer Prevention Program. *Does tobacco advertising influence teens to start smoking? Chapter 10: tobacco use in California: a focus on preventing uptake in adolescents.* San Diego: University of California, San Diego, 1993:109.

California Medical Association Foundation. *Pharmacy partnership: prescription for change.* (221 Main Street, 3rd floor, P.O. Box 7690, San Francisco, CA 94120-7690). San Francisco, CA: California Medical Association Foundation, Available at www.RxforChange.org.2002.

Centers for Disease Control and Prevention. Comparison of the cigarette brand preferences of adult and teenaged smokers—United States, 1989, and 10 U.S. communities, 1988 and 1990. *Morb Mortal Wkly Rep CDC Surveill Summ* 1992;41: 169.

Centers for Disease Control and Prevention. Changes in the cigarette brand preferences of adolescent smokers—United States, 1989–1993. *Morb Mortal Wkly Rep CDC Surveill Summ* 1994;43:577.

Centers for Disease Control and Prevention. Strategies for reducing exposure to environmental tobacco smoke, increasing tobacco use cessation, and reducing initiation in communities and health cares systems: a report on recommendations of the Task Force on Community Preventive Services. *MMWR Morb Mortal Wkly Rep* 2000;49(Suppl):RR–12.

Centers for Disease Control and Prevention. Tobacco use among middle and high school students—United States, 1999. *Morb Mortal Wkly Rep CDC Surveill Summ* 2000;49:49.

Centers for Disease Control and Prevention. Youth tobacco surveillance—United States, 1998–1999. *Morb Mortal Wkly Rep CDC Surveill Summ* 2000;49:10.

Centers for Disease Control and Prevention. Cigarette use among high school students—United States, m1991-2003. *Morb Mortal Wkly Rep CDC Surveill Summ* 2004;53:499.

Centers for Disease Control and Prevention. Prevalence of tobacco use among 14 racial/ethnic populations. *Morb Mortal Wkly Rep CDC Surveill Summ* 2004;53;49.

Centers for Disease Control and Prevention. Annual smoking-attributable mortality, years of potential life lost, and productivity losses—United States, 1997–2001. *Morb Mortal Wkly Rep* 2005;54(25):655.

Centers for Disease Control and Prevention. Current smoking among adults—United States, 2003. *Morb Mortal Wkly Rep* 2005;54(20):509.

Centers for Disease Control and Prevention. Use of cigarettes and other tobacco products among students aged 13–15 years–worldwide, 1999–2005. *Morb Mortal Wkly Rep* 2005; 55:553.

Centers for Disease Control and Prevention. Youth risk behavior surveillance—United States, 2005. *Morb Mortal Wkly Rep CDC Surveill Summ* 2006;55(SS05);1.

Colby SM, Monti PM, O'Leary TT, et al. Brief motivational intervention for adolescents in medical settings. *Addict Behav* 2005;30(5):865.

Crosby MH. Religious challenge by shareholder actions: changing the behavior of tobacco companies and their allies. *BMJ* 2000;321:373; *Lancet* 2003;362(9380):281.

Dalton MA, Sargent JD, Beach ML, et al. Effect of viewing smoking in movies on adolescent smoking initiation: a cohort study. *Lancet* 2003;362(9380):281.

Danard RA. The Engle verdicts and tobacco litigation. *BMJ* 2000;321:312.

Davis RM. Moving tobacco control beyond "the tipping point." *BMJ* 2000;321:309.

DiFranza JR, Rigotti NA, McNeill AD, et al. Initial symptoms of nicotine dependence in adolescents. *Tob Control* 2000;9:313.

DiFranza JR, Savageau JA, Rigotti NA, et al. Development of symptoms of tobacco dependence in youths: 30 month follow up data from the DANDY study. *Tob Control* 2002;11:228.

Ellickson PL, Orlando M, Tucker JS, et al. From adolescence to young adulthood: racial/ethnic disparities in smoking. *Am J Public Health* 2004;94:293.

Everett SA, Warren CW, Sharp D, et al. Initiation of cigarette smoking and subsequent smoking behavior among U.S. high school students. *Prev Med* 1999;29:327.

Farkas AJ, Gilpin EA, White MM, et al. Association between household and workplace smoking restrictions and adolescent smoking. *JAMA* 2000;284:717.

Farrelly MC, Davis KC, Haviland ML, et al. Evidence of a dose-response relationship between "truth" antismoking ads and youth smoking prevalence. *Am J Public Health* 2005;95(3):425.

Farrelly MC, Niederdeppe J, Yarsevich J. Youth tobacco prevention mass media campaigns: past, present, and future directions. *Tob Control* 2003;12(suppl 1):i35.

Federal Trade Commission. *Annual report on cigarette sales.* www.ftc.gov/opa/2005/08/cigreport.htm. 2003.

Ferrence R, Ashley MJ. Protecting children from passive smoking. *BMJ* 2000;321:310.

Fiore MC, Bailey WC, Cohen SJ, et al. *Treating tobacco use and dependence: a clinical practice guideline.* AHRQ Publication No. 00–0032. Rockville, MD: U.S. Department of Health and Human Services, 2000.

Francey N, Chapman S. "Operation Berkshire": the international tobacco companies' conspiracy. *BMJ* 2000;321:371.

French SA, Perry CL. Smoking among adolescent girls: prevalence and etiology. *J Am Med Womens Assoc* 1996;51:25.

French SA, Perry CL, Leon GR, et al. Weight concerns, dieting behavior, and smoking initiation among adolescents: a prospective study. *Am J Public Health* 1994;84:1818.

Frieden TR, Blakeman DE. The dirty dozen: 12 myths that undermine tobacco control. *Am J Public Health* 2005;95:1500.

Gansky SA, Ellison JA, Kavanaugh C, et al. Oral screening and brief spit tobacco cessation counseling: a review and findings. *J Dent Educ* 2002;66(9):1088.

Gilpin EA, Pierce JP. Trends in adolescent smoking initiation in the United States: is tobacco marketing an influence? *Tob Control* 1997;6:122.

Gilpin EA, White MM, Farkas AJ, et al. Home smoking restrictions: which smokers have them and how they are associated with smoking behavior. *Nicotine Tob Res* 1999;1: 153.

Glantz S. The truth about big tobacco in its own words. *BMJ* 2000;321:313.

Glantz G, Kacirk K, McCulloch C. Back to the future: smoking in movies in 2002 compared with 1950 levels. *Am J Public Health* 2004;94(2):261.

Glantz SA, Slade J, Bero LA, et al. *The cigarette papers*. Berkeley: University of California Press, 1996.

Godlee F. WHO faces up to its tobacco links. *BMJ* 2000;321:314.

Goodman E, Capitman J. Depressive symptoms and cigarette smoking among teens. *Pediatrics* 2000;106:748.

Gritz ER. Cigarette smoking by adolescent females: implications for health and behavior. *Women Health* 1984;9:103.

Hampl JS, Betts MB. Cigarette use during adolescence: effects on nutritional status. *Nutr Rev* 1999;57:215.

Hastings G, MacFadyen L. A day in the life of an advertising man: review of internal documents from the UK tobacco industry's principal advertising agencies. *BMJ* 2000;321:366.

Heyes E *Tobacco U.S.A.: the industry behind the smoke curtain*. Brookfield, CT: Twenty First Century Books, 1999.

Hoffman D, Hoffman I. The changing cigarette, 1950–1995. *J Toxicol Environ Health* 1997;50:307.

Houston T, Kaufman NJ. Tobacco control in the 21st century: searching for answers in a sea of change. *JAMA* 2000;284:752.

Howell MF, Zakarian JM, Matt GE, et al. Effect of counseling mothers on their children's exposure to environmental tobacco smoke: randomized controlled trial. *BMJ* 2000;321:337.

Hurt RD, Croghan GA, Beede SD, et al. Nicotine patch therapy in 101 adolescent smokers: efficacy, withdrawal symptom relief, and carbon monoxide and plasma cotinine levels. *Arch Pediatr Adolesc Med* 2000;154:31.

Jha P, Chaloupka FJ. *Tobacco control in developing countries*. Oxford: Oxford University Press, 2000.

Johnson JG, Cohen P, Pine DS, et al. Association between cigarette smoking and anxiety disorders during adolescence and early adulthood. *JAMA* 2000;284:2348.

Johnston LD, O'Malley PM, Bachman JG, et al. *Monitoring the future: decline in teen smoking seems to be nearing its end*. www.monitoringthefuture.org. December 19, 2005.

Jordan TR, Price JH, Dake JA, et al. Adolescent exposure to and perceptions of environmental tobacco smoke. *J Sch Health* 2005;75(5):178.

Karp I, O'Loughlin J, Paradis G, et al. Smoking trajectories of adolescent novice smokers in a longitudinal study of tobacco use. *Ann Epidemiol* 2005;15(6):445.

Kessler DA. Nicotine addiction in young people. *N Engl J Med* 1995;333:186.

Killen J, Ammerman S, Rojas N, et al. Do adolescent smokers experience withdrawal when deprived of nicotine? *Exp Clin Psychopharmacol* 2001;9(2):176.

Killen JD, Robinson TN, Ammerman S, et al. Major depression among adolescent smokers undergoing treatment for nicotine dependence. *Addict Behav* 2004;29:1517.

Killen JD, Robinson TN, Ammerman S, et al. Randomized clinical trial of the efficacy of bupropion combined with nicotine patch in the treatment of adolescent smokers. *J Consult Clin Psychol* 2004;72(4):729.

Killen J, Robinson TN, Haydel KF, et al. Prospective study of risk factors for the initiation of cigarette smoking. *J Consult Clin Psychol* 1997;65:1011.

Klein JD, St Clair S. Do candy cigarettes encourage young people to smoke? *BMJ* 2000;321:362.

Klein JD, Graff Havens C, Carlson EJ. Evaluation of an adolescent smoking-cessation media campaign: gottaquit.com. *Pediatr* 2005;116:950.

Klitzner M, Gruenewald PF, Bamberger E. Cigarette advertising and adolescent experimentation with smoking. *Br J Addict* 1991;86:287.

Koop CE. The tobacco scandal: where is the outrage? *Tob Control* 1998;7:393.

Lancaster T, Stead L, Silagy C, et al. Effectiveness of interventions to help people stop smoking: findings from the Cochrane Library. *BMJ* 2000;321:355.

Landrine H, Klonoff EA, Reina-Patton A. Minors' access to tobacco before and after the California STAKE Act. *Tob Control* 2000;9(Suppl II):ii15.

Lasser K, Boyd JW, Woolhandler S, et al. Smoking and mental illness: a population-based prevalence study. *JAMA* 2000;284:2606.

Leatherdale ST, McDonald PW. What smoking cessation approaches will young smokers use? *Addict Behav* 2005;30(8): 1614.

Leistikow BN, Martin DC, Milano CE. Fire injuries, disasters, and costs from cigarettes and cigarette lights: a global overview. *Prev Med* 2000;31:91.

Lerman C, Jepson C, Wileyto EP, et al. Role of functional genetic variation in the dopamine D2 receptor (DRD2) in response to bupropion and nicotine replacement therapy for tobacco dependence: results of two randomized clinical trials. *Neuropsychopharmacoy* 2006;31(1):231.

Levy DT, Cummings KM, Hyland A. A simulation of the effects of youth initiation policies on overall cigarette use. *Am J Public Health* 2000;90:1311.

Levy DT, Cummings KM, Hyland A. Increasing taxes as a strategy to reduce cigarette use and deaths: results of a simulation model. *Prev Med* 2000;31:279.

Luke DA, Stamatakis KA, Brownson RC. State youth-access tobacco control policies and youth smoking behavior in the United States. *Am J Prev Med* 2000;19:180.

McVey D, Stapleton J. Can anti-smoking television advertising affect smoking behavior? Controlled trial of the Health Education Authority for England's anti-smoking TV campaign. *Tob Control* 2000;9:273.

Mermelstein R. Teen smoking cessation. *Tob Control* 2003;12: i25.

Mermelstein R, Colby SM, Patten C, et al. Methodological issues in measuring treatment outcome in adolescent smoking cessation studies. *Nicotine Tob Res* 2002;4:395.

Miller WR, Rollnick S. *Motivational interviewing. Preparing people for change*. New York, NY: The Guilford Press, 2002.

Milton MH, Maule CO, Yee Sl, et al. *Youth tobacco cessation: a guide for making informed decisions*. U.S. Department of Health and Human Services. Centers for Disease Control and Prevention, 2004.

Mitchell P, Chapman S, Smith W. Smoking is a major cause of blindness. *Med J Aust* 1999;171:173.

National Center for Chronic Disease Prevention and Health Promotion, Office of Smoking and Health. Reports of the Surgeon General. *The health consequences of smoking for women, 1980. The health consequences of smoking: nicotine addiction, 1988. Reducing the health consequences of smoking, 1989. Preventing tobacco use among young people, 1994. Tobacco use among U.S. racial/ethnic minority groups, 1998. Reducing tobacco use, 2000. The health consequences of smoking.* Washington, DC: U.S. Dept. of Health and Human Services, Public Health Service, Centers for Disease Control, Available at http://www.cdc.gov/tobacco/sgr/index.htm. 2004.

National Center for Health Statistics. *Health United States, 2000: adolescent health chartbook.* Washington, DC: U.S. Department of Health and Human Services, Centers for Disease Control and Prevention, 2000.

Nichols HB, Harlow BL. Childhood abuse and risk of smoking onset. *J Epidemiol Community Health* 2004;58:402.

Nides M, Oncken C, Gonzales D, et al. Smoking cessation with varenicline, a selective alpha4beta2 nicotinic receptor agonist: results from a 7-week, randomized, placebo and bupropion-controlled trial with 1-year follow-up. *Arch Intern Med* 2006;166(15):1561.

Oncken C, Gonzales D, Nides M, et al. Efficacy and safety of the novel selective nicotinic acetylcholine receptor partial agonist, varenicline, for smoking cessation. *Arch Intern Med* 2006;166(15):1571.

O'Neill HK, Glasgow RE, McCaul KD. Component analysis in smoking prevention research: effects of social consequences information. *Addict Behav* 1983;8:419.

Pechman C, Reibling ET. Anti-smoking advertising campaigns targeting youth: case studies from USA and Canada. *Tob Control* 2000;9(Suppl II):ii–18.

Piasecki M, Newhouse PA, eds. *Nicotine in psychiatry: psychopathology and emerging therapeutics.* Washington, DC: American Psychiatric Press, 2000.

Prabhat J, Chaloupka FJ. The economics of global tobacco control. *BMJ* 2000;321:358.

Pucci LG, Siegel M. Features of sales promotion in cigarette magazine advertisements, 1980–1993: an analysis of youth exposure in the United States. *Tob Control* 1999;8:29.

Quinlan KB, McCaul KD. Matched and mismatched interventions with young adult smokers: testing a stage theory. *Health Psychol* 2000;19:165.

Remafedi G, Carol H. Preventing tobacco use among lesbian, gay, bisexual, and transgender youth. *Nicotine Tob Res* 2005; 7(2):249.

Rigotti NA, Lee JE, Wechsler H. U.S. college students' use of tobacco products: results of a national survey. *JAMA* 2000;284:699.

Rojas N, Killen JD, Haydel KF, et al. Nicotine dependence and withdrawal symptoms in adolescent smokers. *Arch Pediatr Adolesc Med* 1998;152:151.

Sargent JD, Dalton M, Beach M. Exposure to cigarette promotions and smoking uptake in adolescents: evidence of a dose-response relation. *Tob Control* 2000;9:163.

Schroeder SA. What to do with a patient who smokes. *JAMA* 2005;294(4):482.

Simons-Morton B, Haynie DL, Crump AD, et al. Peer and parent influences on smoking and drinking among early adolescents. *Health Educ Behav* 2001;28:95.

Smith TA, House RF, Croghan IT, et al. Nicotine patch therapy in adolescent smokers. *Pediatrics* 1996;98:659.

Sopori ML, Kozak W. Immunomodulatory effects of cigarette smoke. *J Neuroimmunol* 1998;83:148.

Spangler JG. Smoking and hormone-related disorders. *Prim Care* 1999;26:499.

Sussman S, Dent C, Severson H, et al. Self-initiated quitting among adolescent smokers. *Prev Med* 1998;33:2703.

Sussman S, Lichtman K, Ritt A, et al. Effects of thirty-four adolescent tobacco use cessation and prevention trials on regular users of tobacco products. *Subst Use Misuse* 1999;34: 1469.

Sutton CD. A hard road: finding ways to reduce teen tobacco use. *Tob Control* 2000;9:1.

Symm B, Morgan MV, Blackshear Y, et al. Cigar smoking: an ignored public health threat. *J Prim Prev* 2005;26(4):363.

Thun M, Glynn TJ. Improving the treatment of tobacco dependence. *BMJ* 2000;321:311.

Tickle JJ, Sargent JD, Dalton MA, et al. Favourite movie stars, their tobacco use in contemporary movies, and its association with adolescent smoking. *Tob Control* 2001; 10:16.

Tobacco Control Archives. *Library and center for knowledge management.* San Francisco: University of California, Available at www.library.ucsf.edu/tobacco. 2007.

Tuckson RV. Race, sex, economics, and tobacco advertising. *J Natl Med Assoc* 1989;81:1119.

Tyas SL, Pederson LL. Psychosocial factors related to adolescent smoking: a critical review of the literature. *Tob Control* 1998;7:409.

Unger JB, Palmer PH, Dent CW, et al. Ethnic differences in adolescent smoking prevalence in California: are multi-ethnic youth at higher risk? *Tob Control* 2000;9(Suppl II): ii–i9.

Van den bree MB, Whitmer MD, Pickworth WB. Predictors of smoking development in a population-based sample of adolescents: a prospective study. *J Adolesc Health* 2004;35:172.

Wakefield MA, Chaloupka FJ, Kaufman NJ, et al. Effects of restrictions on smoking at home, at school, and in public places on teenage smoking: cross sectional study. *BMJ* 2000;321: 333–337.

Wang MQ, Fitzhugh EC, Westerfield RC, et al. Family and peer influences on smoking behavior among American adolescents: an age trend. *J Adolesc Health* 1995;10:200–203.

Warner KE, Hodgson TA, Carroll CE. Medical costs of smoking in the United States: estimates, their validity, and their implications. *Tob Control* 1999;8:290–300.

Weitzman M, Cook S, Auinger P, et al. Tobacco smoke exposure is associated with the metabolic syndrome in adolescents. *Circulation* 2005;112(6):862.

Wernakulasuriya S. Effectiveness of tobacco counseling in the dental office. *J Dent Educ* 2002;66(9):1079.

World Health Organization. *Why is tobacco a public health priority?* www.who.int/tobacco/health_priority/en/index.html. 2007.

Zhu SH, Anderson CM, Johnson CE, et al. A centralized telephone service for tobacco cessation: the California experience. *Tob Control* 2000;9(Suppl II):ii–48.

Zhu SH, Sun J, Billings SC, et al. Predictors of smoking cessation in US adolescents. *Am J Prev Med* 1999;16(3):202.

CHAPTER 71

Psychoactive Substances of Abuse Used by Adolescents

Sharon Levy and Alan D. Woolf

Misuse of drugs, chemicals, plants and herbs, mushrooms, and other agents continues to be a major cause of mortality and morbidity in adolescents and young adults. According to the 2005 Youth Risk Behavior Survey, nationwide 25.4% of high school students were offered, sold, or given an illegal drug on school property (CDC, 2006). Although overall the proportion of teens who report use of illicit drugs during 2006 has dropped from a peak in the 1990, still almost 50% of high school 12th graders admit to experimenting with an illicit drug, such as cocaine, marijuana, amphetamines, hallucinogens, narcotics, and tranquilizers (Johnston et al., 2007). Furthermore, according to the same survey, the use of prescription medications (including opioid narcotics, benzodiazepines, and stimulants) has risen since the mid to late 1990s, and teenagers report that it is easy to obtain a prescription from a physician (Friedman, 2006). Many teens describe their use of these drugs as for practical effect rather than intoxication, and believe this type of use is "safe" (Friedman, 2006). However, as with all substances of abuse, adolescents are vulnerable to the direct toxic effects of these drugs and chemicals, and also risk long-term addictions, with consequential collateral injury from the effects of their substance abuse on family and social relationships and its detrimental effects on work or school performance. The comorbidities of substance abuse can include lowered self-esteem, lack of motivation, depression, suicidal ideation, and delinquency. Physical trauma can result from motor vehicle accidents and other risk-taking behaviors and poor judgment. Sexual disinhibition and memory loss can result in rape, unplanned pregnancy, and/or sexually transmitted diseases. Some substance-abusing youth will face arrest for infractions of the law, including such offenses as theft, assault, prostitution, or drug possession and/or distribution. The loss of a productive life can follow from the long-term adverse effects of drugs on learning, behavior, personality, vocational choices, and psychosocial adjustment.

In this chapter, we review the clinical toxicology and management of the effects of psychoactive substances of abuse other than alcohol and tobacco. Younger adolescents may experiment first with easily obtained "gateway" drugs such as alcohol, tobacco, marijuana, and over-the-counter cold remedies and inhalants. The complex interplay of genetic, psychological, and family and social factors may underlie whether they later exhibit addictive behaviors and move on to include illicit agents such as the opiates or cocaine. Newer categories of substance abuse include over-the-counter cough and cold and weight loss preparations, herbal remedies and "natural" dietary supplements, and anabolic steroids. The advent of the Internet has provided young people with access to a lot of inaccurate information from the plethora of Web sites portraying substance abuse as a safe and acceptable lifestyle (Boyer et al., 2000). The assessment of such patients by health care providers is complicated by sometimes inaccurate or deliberately misleading histories of substance use, such that the actual substances implicated are unknown. Adolescents may use several drugs and chemicals concurrently, so that the consequent toxic effects may not be those classically associated with one class of substances.

MARIJUANA

Prevalence/Epidemiology

Marijuana is the most widely abused illicit drug in the United States, with >90.8 million adults (42.9%) aged 18 or older admitting marijuana use at least once in their lifetime (SAMHSA, 2005). Among marijuana users, 2.1% reported initiation of its use before age 12 years, 52.7% between ages 12 and 17, and 45.2% at age 18 or older (SAMHSA, 2005). Data from the Monitoring the Future survey suggests that lifetime marijuana use among 12th grade high school students has declined recently from a peak of 49.7% in 1999 to the current prevalence of 42.3% in 2006 (Johnstone et al., 2007). Corresponding figures for lifetime marijuana use in 2006 among 8th graders was 15.7%, and 31.8% for 10th graders. Rates for annual marijuana use in 2006 were 11.7% for 8th graders, 25.2% for 10th graders, and 31.5% for high school seniors (Johnston et al., 2007).

The 2005 Youth Risk Behavior Survey results suggest that the lifetime prevalence of marijuana use among high school students is higher among males (40.9%) than females (35.9%) (CDC, 2006). Lifetime marijuana use was also higher among Hispanic (42.6%) and black (42.6%) students than whites (38%). During the 30 days before the survey, 20.2% of high school students reported that they had used marijuana. Almost one tenth (8.7%) of students nationwide had tried marijuana for the first time before 13 years of age, and 4.5% of students had used marijuana on school property one or more times in the previous 30 days (CDC, 2006).

TABLE 71.1

Common Preparations of Canabis

Canabis Preparations	Description of Preparations
Joint	Chopped up leaves and stems rolled into cigarettes and smoked
Blunt	Cigar sized marijuana cigarette
Pipe	Similar to tobacco pipes, marijuana leaves are placed in the bowl and smoked through a stem
Bong (water pipe)	The bowl of the water pipe is placed below a chamber filled with water, and the marijuana smoke passes through the water, cooling it and removing nonpsychoactive substances, before it is inhaled
Hashish	This preparation is the strongest form of marijuana; it is composed of a pure resin derived from the leaves and flowers of the female plant and is usually pressed into a "brick" and smoked
Cookies/brownies	Marijuana is sometimes baked into cookies or brownies and ingested orally

Because marijuana is so readily available and perhaps not as stigmatized as other substances, it often serves as the introduction of an adolescent to illicit drug use. Marijuana has negative effects on both physical and psychological health and is associated with the development of tolerance, dependence, and a withdrawal syndrome. Regular marijuana use can have adverse effects on learning, with possible psychological and cognitive impairment, and it also affects job performance, driving skills and judgment, social and family relations, and other activities of everyday life. Marijuana use can predict an individual's tendency toward the use and abuse of other substances. One prospective study of 250 addicted individuals, discharged from a detoxification facility, found that continued marijuana use predicted their risk of relapse for cocaine, alcohol, and heroin use (Aharonovich et al., 2005).

Medical Use

There is still significant debate over the medicinal value of marijuana. The active ingredient, delta-9-tetrahydrocannabinol (THC), has been synthesized and is available in capsule form known as *dronabinol* (Marinol). Dronabinol has been considered as a second-line agent for use in the treatment of anorexia associated with weight loss in patients with the acquired immunodeficiency syndrome (AIDS) or for nausea and vomiting associated with chemotherapy. It has also been proposed for the treatment of other conditions such as glaucoma and epilepsy and to help decrease tremors, ataxia, and spasticity in patients with multiple sclerosis.

Preparation and Dose

Marijuana is derived from the resinous oil of the flowering tops and leaves of the plant, *Cannabis sativa*. Although the oil contains >60 cannabinoids the major psychoactive ingredient appears to be THC. The content of THC is highest in the flowering tops and declines in leaves, stems, and seeds. Marijuana joints obtained mainly from the flowering tops and leaves usually have a THC content of 0.5% to 5%, and hashish, which consists of dried cannabis resin and compressed flowers, contains 2% to 20%. Hashish oil may contain 15% to 30% THC.

In the 1960s, the average potency of marijuana was 0.1% to 0.5% THC. Recent analysis shows that today most marijuana averages 4% to 5% THC. Samples of sinsemilla, a marijuana species cultivated to obtain high THC levels, average 7% to 9% but have tested as high as 14%. This increase in potency may be a factor in an increase in reports of side effects.

Routes of Administration and Street Names

Marijuana is usually smoked but may be eaten, brewed in tea, or ingested in pill form. Table 71.1 describes the most common forms and vernacular used by adolescents. Street names include weed, pot, Mary Jane, Acapulco gold, bud, grass, and dope.

Physiology and Metabolism

Two endogenous cannabinoid receptors have been found, CB1 (found mainly in the brain) and CB2 (found only in peripheral tissues, especially in the immune system). Endogenous cannabinoids, anandamide and 2AG, are part of the cannabinoid neurotransmission system in the brain. It appears that cannabinoids may have a natural role in pain modulation, control of movement, cognition, and memory. Marijuana stimulates the dopamine pathway from the ventral tegmental area to the nucleus accumbens. This is believed to be the reward center of the brain. Receptors are most prevalent in the cerebral cortex, hippocampus, basal ganglia, and cerebellum. The location of these receptors helps explain the cognition, motor coordination, memory, and mood changes produced by marijuana.

THC is metabolized primarily in the liver through the cytochrome P-450 system. Peak plasma levels of THC are reached within approximately 10 minutes of smoking marijuana; effects last 2 to 3 hours. Smoked marijuana has 5 to 10 times the bioavailability of the ingested drug. THC is lipid soluble and accumulates in fat stores. Changes in activity or diet that mobilize fat may cause sudden increases in levels of cannabinoids detected in urine. Because marijuana has a long half-life and persists in body tissues, the effects on nerve function may persist after the immediate effects have disappeared.

Cannabinoid metabolites are carried by the enterohepatic circulation to the intestinal lumen and excreted in the feces (65%) or are carried through the renal circulation and excreted in the urine (35%). Carboxy and hydroxy cannabinoids are the major metabolites detected in urine drug screening tests. The cannabinoid metabolites may be

TABLE 71.2

Cannabinoid Physiology

Receptors	Pharmacodynamics	Distribution	Metabolism and Excretion
• CB1–brain • CB2–peripheral tissue	Stimulates the dopamine pathway from the ventral tegmental area to the nucleus accumbens	Lipid soluble; accumulates in fat stores	Cytochrome P-450 system • 65% excreted in feces • 35% in urine

(Pertwee, 1997).

detected for 3 to 10 days in the occasional user and for 1 to 2 months in chronic users (see Table 71.2).

Drug Interactions

Marijuana may enhance sedation when used with alcohol, diazepam, antihistamines, phenothiazines, barbiturates, or narcotics, and it may enhance stimulation when used with cocaine or amphetamines. Marijuana is antagonistic to the effects of phenytoin, propranolol, and insulin.

Effects of Intoxication

1. Low to moderate doses of marijuana: Produce euphoria, time distortion, increased talking, and auditory and visual enhancements or distortions which users find to be pleasant.
2. Acute intoxication: Produces an increased heart rate, erythema of the conjunctivae, dry mouth and throat, dilated pupils, and impaired learning and cognitive functions. As acute effects wear off, marijuana users often have increased appetite and feel sleepy.
3. High doses: High doses of marijuana may produce mood fluctuations, depersonalization, and hallucinations.
4. Toxic reactions: Includes anxiety, panic, organic brain syndrome, psychoses, delusions, hallucinations, and paranoia. Marijuana may produce seizures in epileptic individuals or psychotic episodes in schizophrenic individuals. Marijuana use has also been associated with the precipitation of psychotic episodes in patients not previously diagnosed with schizophrenia. In some cases, these episodes do not resolve with discontinuation of marijuana use.

Adverse Effects

1. Central nervous system: *Acute effects* include the psychological effects described above, many of which are pleasurable, although some may be disturbing and/or disabling.
   a. Psychomotor and reaction times: Marijuana causes a decrease in both psychomotor functions and reaction times, thereby presenting a dangerous risk for the adolescent who drives after getting high (Wilson et al., 1994). Impairments of selective attention, on-task behaviors, and ability to focus and concentrate are notable and possibly related both to frequency and duration of cannabis use (Soliwij et al., 1991; Solowij et al., 1995). Specific functions related to driving skills that are impaired include tracking (the ability to follow a moving object and to control the position of a car in relation to the highway), signal detection (the ability to quickly notice and respond to lights or other unpredictable stimuli), glare recovery time (the ability to see clearly after exposure to bright lights such as headlights). The impairment of these driving skills, in conjunction with marijuana-induced decreased judgment, impaired time and distance estimation, and impaired motor performance, make driving under the influence of marijuana dangerous (DuPont, 1985). There is good evidence that marijuana causes lingering effects on memory and coordination. Striking changes in the ability of pilots to operate a landing simulator persisted 24 hours after exposure to cannabis, during which time the pilots reported no awareness of marijuana after effects (Leirer et al., 1991).
   b. Behavioral problems and neurocognition: Because heavy drug users may already have underlying behavioral problems and may already be depressed, alienated, or bored, it is difficult to distinguish whether marijuana is the cause or the behaviors are preexistent. However, studies have suggested that regular heavy use of marijuana may lead to long-term adverse neurocognitive effects. Pope et al. (1996) studied the neuropsychological residual effects of heavy cannabis use among 65 college students versus 64 control students reporting only "light" use. The results suggested a "drug residue" effect on attention and other executive functions, psychomotor tasks, and short-term memory in heavy users. Pope et al. (1995) also reported that marijuana use may lead to permanent impairment of cognitive function and behavior. Chronic buildup of cannabinoids may affect executive functions such as focus, attention, and ability to filter out irrelevant information or compromise and may impair memory, learning ability, and perception.
   c. Chronic heavy marijuana use may lead to a state of passive withdrawal from usual work and recreational activities known as the *amotivational syndrome*. Schwartz (1987) identified seven components that define this syndrome:
      • Loss of interest, general apathy, and passivity
      • Loss of desire to work consistently and loss of productivity, accompanied by a lack of concern about the poor work performance
      • Loss of energy, and tiredness
      • Moodiness, sullenness, and inability to handle frustration
      • Impairment in concentration and inability to process new material

- Slovenly habits and appearance
- A lifestyle revolving around procurement and use of marijuana and other drugs

2. Pulmonary and cardiovascular: *Marijuana* smoking results in a substantially greater respiratory burden of carbon monoxide and tar than does cigarette smoking (Wu et al., 1988).

  a. Effects on pulmonary function: Heavy marijuana smokers who do not smoke tobacco have functional impairment of airway conductance (Tashkin et al., 1993), and, just as with tobacco, chronic marijuana smoking leads to bronchoconstriction, cellular inflammation and damage, and bronchitis with cough, increased sputum production, and wheezing (Gil et al., 1995; Fligiel et al., 1997). Human studies demonstrate a decrease in forced expiratory volume in 1 second (FEV_1), a decrease in maximal midexpiratory flow rate (MMFR), and an increase in airway resistance. Sherman et al. (1991) found that in contrast to tobacco smokers pulmonary alveolar macrophages of marijuana-only smokers do not produce increased amounts of oxidants, as compared with macrophages of nonsmoking subjects.

  b. Cellular damage: Metaplastic cellular changes have been observed in dogs and humans (Tashkin, 1999). A link between chronic exposure to marijuana smoke and lung cancer in humans has been postulated (Ferguson et al., 1989).

  c. Cardiac effects: Marijuana use leads to an increase in sympathetic tone and a decrease in parasympathetic activity, producing tachycardia, increased myocardial oxygen consumption, and increased cardiac output. In patients with underlying cardiac disease, such effects may induce ischemic chest pain and myocardial infarction (MI) (Mittleman et al., 2001). Vagal stimulation coupled with sympathetic discharge may also produce electrophysiological pathology such as atrial tachyarrhythmias or atrial flutter in some individuals (Fisher et al., 2005).

3. Endocrine and immune function effects: Immune function may be suppressed with heavy doses of THC (Trisler et al., 1994). Chronic administration of high doses of THC in animals lowers testosterone secretion; impairs sperm production, motility, and viability; and alters the menstrual cycle. It is unclear if these effects occur in humans.

Treatment

1. Acute overdose and emergency treatment: Marijuana use in large doses can cause delirium, nausea, vomiting, dizziness, and anxiety in some individuals. It can be contaminated with diarrhea-causing infectious agents such as *Salmonella* species. Marijuana purchased on the street is sometimes mixed with other drugs, which also may cause toxicity. The health care provider should look for symptoms and signs of the toxicities of ethanol, opiates, stimulants, or other substances in addition to marijuana, as the patient may be unaware or choose not to disclose which other chemicals may also be involved in the overdose. Toxicological screening of the blood and urine may be helpful, because THC is distributed into fatty tissues and may subsequently be detectable for days in heavy users.

2. Withdrawal syndrome: A mild withdrawal syndrome from cannabis has been described. Some regular marijuana users develop restlessness, irritability, mild agitation, insomnia, nausea, cramping, and sleep electroencephalographic disturbances on cessation (Crowley et al., 1998).

3. Medical management of addiction: Treatment of marijuana use in the adolescent involves differentiation between experimental or occasional use and the abuse of marijuana. After initially experimenting with marijuana, many adolescents do not use it again or use it very infrequently. However, when counseling families physicians should point out the negative effects of marijuana use in teenagers. Deterioration in school performance, family and social problems, accidents, and legal difficulties suggest the need for intervention and treatment. Frequent marijuana use can interfere with the cognitive, emotional, and social development of adolescents. Research has shown that frequent marijuana use in young girls increases their risk of developing anxiety and depression as compared with peers (Patton et al., 2002). Problems associated with marijuana use accrue slowly and can be quite insidious; many teenagers who meet criteria for marijuana abuse or dependence do not identify marijuana use as connected with other problems in their lives. These teens may be quite ambivalent towards changing their marijuana use. Chapter 73 discusses office-based management in more detail.

COCAINE

Prevalence/Epidemiology

More than 5.9 million Americans aged 12 or older (2.5%) have used cocaine in the last year, with males predominating 2:1 over females as abusers of the drug (SAMHSA, 2005). However, lifetime use of cocaine among U.S. high school students has declined notably since prevalence rates as high as 17.3% were observed in the epidemic of the mid-1980s (Johnston et al., 2005). By 1999 only 4.7% of 8th graders, 7.7% of 10th graders, and 9.8% of high school seniors reported that they had ever used the drug (Johnston et al., 2005). Since then reports of cocaine use have mostly continued to decline. Comparable rates in 2006 were down to 3.4%, 4.8%, and 8.5% respectively (up from 8.0% in 2005). The number of 12th grade students reporting regular cocaine use on an annual basis has remained relatively stable at 5.7%, with 2.5% admitting cocaine use within the preceding 30 days (Johnston et al., 2007).

Lifetime prevalence of crack cocaine use has also declined since rates as high as 5.4% among high school seniors were recorded in 1987. In 2006, the lifetime prevalence of crack cocaine use was reported to be 2.3% among 8th graders, 2.2% among 10th graders, and 3.5% among 12th graders (Johnston et al., 2007). The reader is cautioned that the Monitoring the Future survey data only reflects reports from high school students, and almost certainly underestimates the prevalence of cocaine use among higher risk groups of adolescents, such as school dropouts, delinquents, and homeless youth.

Data from the 2005 Youth Risk Behavior Survey (CDC, 2006) indicated that 7.6% of students had used some form of cocaine during their lifetime. The prevalence of use was higher among Hispanic (12.2%) and white (7.7%)

than black (2.3%) students. Lifetime cocaine use was much higher among white and Hispanic women (7.7% and 9.4%, respectively) than black women (1.2%). This was also true for white and Hispanic males (7.8% and 14.9%, respectively) who reported higher lifetime cocaine use rates than blacks (3.4%).

Medical Use

Cocaine is used medically to provide local anesthesia in surgical repairs. It provides hemostasis in the operative field by the vasoconstriction of mucous membranes, and is often used topically in otolaryngological, plastic surgical, and emergency medical procedures.

Preparation and Dose

1. Cocaine: Cocaine (benzoylmethylecgonine, molecular weight 339.81, $C_{17}H_{21}NO_4$) is a stimulant made from an alkaloid contained in the leaves of the coca bush, *Erythroxylon coca,* first used by the Inca people 3,000 years ago. The cocaine commonly available is actually the hydrochloride salt, which is 89% cocaine by weight. Most cocaine is "cut" by adding an inexpensive substance with similar appearance (white granular or crystalline powder) such as mannitol, lactose, or cornstarch. The "cocaine" sold on the street is actually part cocaine and part an adulterant, and costs $20 to $200/g. Nasal insufflation is often the preferred route of exposure, although local vasoconstriction may delay the onset of effects and prolong the duration of action. Users form the powder into lines approximately $\frac{1}{8}$ in. wide and 2 in. long, each containing approximately 10 to 35 mg cocaine, and then snort the powder through a rolled piece of paper or dollar bill. The cocaine "high" associated with nasal insufflation lasts approximately 60 to 90 minutes.
2. Freebase: Freebase (molecular weight 303.86) refers to cocaine without the hydrochloride. The melting point of freebase is much lower than cocaine hydrochloride, so that it can be smoked without destroying its potency. The old method of making freebase involved mixing cocaine with an alkaline solution and adding a solvent such as ether. The solution would separate into two layers, with the top layer containing freebase cocaine dissolved in the solvent. The solvent would then be evaporated, leaving relatively pure cocaine crystals. This method of preparing freebase is dangerous because of the flammability of the solvents.
3. Crack: Alternatively, "crack" involves converting cocaine hydrochloride to a freebase by an extraction with the use of baking soda, heat, and water. The term *crack* is thought to derive from either the crackling sound the rocks generate as they burn or the shattered appearance of the freebase cocaine when the precipitated layer is dropped to make many small pieces. Because this method is safe, simple, and inexpensive compared with making freebase cocaine with ether, the use of crack spread rapidly in the United States beginning in the mid-1980s. Dealers prefer to sell crack because of its high addiction potential, low cost, and ease of handling. Each vial sold typically contains one or more small, cream-colored chunks resembling rock salt at about $20 to $125/g; a single "rock" can be purchased for as little as $5. It is usually smoked with marijuana in a joint, in a cigarette or cigar, or in a crack pipe. Crack is also sold in larger pieces called "slabs," which resemble a stick of chewing gum. The "high" associated with crack smoking lasts approximately 20 minutes.

Routes of Administration and Street Names

Cocaine is most often insufflated, but may be injected intravenously, ingested orally, or the freebase preparations can be smoked. Inhalation, smoking, and ingestion all result in 20% to 40% absorption. Street names include—coke, Bernice, blow, bump, C, candy, Charlie, flake, nose candy, rock, toot, base, snow, crack, and gold dust. Cocaine may also be used in combination with other drugs, as described in Table 71.3.

TABLE 71.3

Street Names & Colloquial Terms Used for Common Combinations of Cocaine with Other Drugs

Speedball, birdie powder, dynamite, foo-foo stuff, joy powder, junk, lace, leaf	Heroin and cocaine The term was synonymous with intravenous use but now can refer to administration of any opiate with cocaine in close temporal proximity by any route
Primo	Cocaine and marijuana, smoked
Space base	Cocaine and phencyclidine (PCP), smoked
Caviar or champagne	Rock or crack cocaine and marijuana, smoked
Jim Jones	Marijuana cigarette laced with cocaine and dipped in PCP
Snowcap	Cocaine sprinkled on a bowl of marijuana Other names for this combination include banano, blunt, bush, coca puff, hooter, and woolas
Space basing	Rock or crack cocaine with PCP and tobacco
Whacking	Rock or crack cocaine with PCP and tobacco, smoked
Blotter	Cocaine combined with LSD
C and M	Cocaine combined with morphine
Snow seals or turkey	Cocaine and amphetamines

LSD, lysergic acid diethylamide.

TABLE 71.4

Cocaine physiology

Receptors	Pharmacodynamics	Distribution	Metabolism and Excretion
D_1 and D_2 dopamine receptors	• Release of dopamine, epinephrine, norepinephrine, and serotonin • Blockade of neurotransmitter reuptake • Increase sensitivity of postsynaptic receptor sites	Plasma and extracellular fluid	• Hepatic esterases (80%) and plasma cholinesterase to form benzoylecgonine and ecgonine methyl ester • Hepatic-N- demethylation to form norcocaine

Physiology and Metabolism

Cocaine has three different effects on the central nervous system (CNS):

1. Stimulation of D_1 and D_2 presynaptic dopamine receptors, causing the release of dopamine (primarily), serotonin, and norepinephrine into the synaptic cleft
2. Blockade of neurotransmitter reuptake, causing synaptic entrapment and leaving an excess of neurotransmitters in the synapse
3. Increase in the sensitivity of the postsynaptic receptor sites

The dopamine reuptake transporter controls the level of the neurotransmitter in the synapse by carrying dopamine back into nerve terminals. Because cocaine effectively blocks this transporter, dopamine levels remain high in the synapse, affecting adjacent neurons and perpetuating the classic "high" associated with the drug. Because neurotransmitter reuptake is blocked, depletion eventually occurs as entrapped neurotransmitters are broken down by enzymes. This leaves the user feeling dysphoric, with feelings of irritability, restlessness, and depression. This downside can be so intense that it leads to repeated use to overcome the dysphoric feeling. The study of the neurochemical pathways underlying these neuroadaptations is facilitating new approaches to treatment, such as N-methyl-D-aspartate (NMDA) receptor antagonists that block both dopaminergic and reinforcing effects.

Cocaine also blocks neuronal reuptake of norepinephrine and stimulates the release of epinephrine, leading to what has been described as an "adrenergic storm" stimulating the neurological, respiratory, and cardiovascular systems. Cocaine is similar to methamphetamine in that both drugs achieve their reinforcing effects through profound stimulation of the mesolimbic/mesocortical dopaminergic neuronal system, which consists of the ventral tegmental area, nucleus accumbens, ventral pallidum, and medial prefrontal cortex. Repeated exposure results in either sensitization or tolerance depending on dose and pattern of use. Intake of either drug causes neuroadaptation, a process that explains many of the disease aspects of addiction. Sensitization is mediated by the D_1 and D_2 dopamine receptors.

Cocaine is metabolized enzymatically to the inactive metabolite, ecgonine methyl ester, primarily by hepatic esterases and, to a lesser degree, by plasma cholinesterase. Nonenzymatic formation of benzoylecgonine is mediated by hydrolysis. Between 5% and 10% of cocaine is metabolized by cytochrome P-450 mediated N-demethylation into norcocaine, the only active metabolite. Pharmacologically, norcocaine has greater vasoconstrictive and neurological activity than cocaine. Progesterone increases hepatic-N-demethylation, resulting in increased formation of norcocaine. Because of this, women may be more sensitive than men to the cardiotoxic effects of cocaine.

Any medical condition that decreases hepatic perfusion, such as hypotension or low cardiac output, results in increased cocaine levels. Plasma cholinesterase activity is lower in pregnant women, fetuses, infants, and patients with liver disease. Plasma cholinesterase can also be low as a result of genetic or nutritional causes. In these patients, extreme reactions or sudden death can occur after seemingly small doses of cocaine. See Table 71.4 for physiology of cocaine.

Effects of Intoxication

Cocaine has several potent pharmacological actions. It is a *stimulant* of the central and peripheral nervous systems; it has *local anesthetic* activity; and it is a *vasoconstrictor*. The CNS stimulation produces an intense euphoric "rush" (feelings of extreme pleasure, power, strength, and excitement) and "high" (increased alertness, confidence, and a general sense of well-being) upon ingestion when smoked, or injected intravenously. Inhaled cocaine generally produces the high without the rush.

Symptoms of cocaine intoxication include a hyper-alert state, increased talking, restlessness, elevated temperature, anorexia, nausea, vomiting, dry mouth, dilated pupils, sweating, dizziness, hyperreflective reflexes, tachycardia, hypertension, and arrhythmias (see "Adverse Effects" section). People "coming down" from cocaine experience dysphoria, depression, sadness, crying spells, suicidal ideation, apathy, inability to concentrate, delusions, anorexia, insomnia, and paranoia.

Adverse Effects

1. Psychiatric: Toxic psychosis, hallucinations, delirium, formication, body image changes, agitation, anxiety, and irritability.
2. Neurological: Seizures, paresthesias, hyperactive reflexes, tremor, pinprick analgesia, facial grimaces, headache, cerebral hemorrhage, cerebral infractions, cerebral vasculitis, and coma.

3. Skin: Excoriations, rashes, and secondary skin infections.
4. Cardiovascular
   a. Acute: Vasoconstriction, increased myocardial oxygen demand, tachycardia, angina, arrhythmias, chest pain, aortic dissection, hypertension, stroke, MI, and cardiovascular collapse (Mouhaffel et al., 1995; Hollander et al., 1995; Lange et al., 2001). Dysrhythmias and conduction disturbances associated with cocaine use range from sinus tachycardia or bradycardia to bundle branch block or a Brugada pattern, complete heart block, idioventricular rhythms, Torsades de pointes, ventricular tachycardia or fibrillation, or sudden asystole (Lange et al., 2001).
   b. Subacute: In a study of 102 intravenous drug users, an increased rate of bacterial endocarditis was found in those who also routinely used cocaine (Chambers et al., 1987).
   c. Chronic: Accelerated atherosclerosis and thrombosis, endocarditis, myocarditis, cardiomyopathy, coronary artery aneurysms (Willens et al., 1994; Kloner et al., 2003).
5. Gastrointestinal: Acute ischemia, gastropyloric ulcers, perforation of the small and large bowel, colitis, and hepatocellular necrosis.
6. Respiratory: Pneumothorax, pneumomediastinum, pneumopericardium, pulmonary edema, pulmonary hemorrhage, tracheobronchitis, and respiratory failure.
7. Musculoskeletal: Rhabdomyolysis was associated with cocaine use in 39 patients, of whom 13 had associated renal failure (Roth et al., 1988). Six patients in this series, who had associated disseminated intravascular coagulation (DIC), died.
8. Obstetric: Low birth weight, prematurity, microcephaly, and placental abruption.

Acute Overdose and Treatment

Cocaine is short-acting drug; treatment of acute intoxication is not usually necessary. In some patients, acute cocaine use may result in lethal cardiovascular or respiratory collapse. The pathogenesis of these cardiovascular complications has not been fully elucidated, but it may be related to the combination of sympathomimetic and membrane anesthetic effects of cocaine. Treatment of acute overdose is similar to other cardiovascular and respiratory emergencies.

1. Initial management: The primary response in managing cocaine overdose is to support respiratory and cardiovascular functions, monitor vital signs and cardiac rhythm, and establish intravenous access. Cocaine is detectable in urine for up to 72 to 96 hours postexposure; whereas blood levels may fall below detectable thresholds as soon as 60 to 90 minutes after use. A "toxic screen" of the blood and urine may also reveal opiates or other sedative-hypnotics used simultaneously. Electrocardiogram (ECG) monitoring, cardiac isoenzymes, and a chest x-ray are other useful studies in cocaine poisoning. Blood creatine kinase and renal function tests may be necessary in patients suspected of having significant rhabdomyolysis.
2. Removal of residual cocaine: All residual cocaine should be removed from the patient's nostrils. If ingestions are suspected, or if the patient is a "body packer" or "stuffer," then activated charcoal should be administered orally or by gastric tube.

3. Specific interventions
   a. Hypoglycemia: If the patient presents with altered mental status, a blood glucose level should be checked, and hypoglycemia treated if present.
   b. Hyperthermia: Hyperthermia can be treated with antipyretics, a cooling blanket, and iced saline lavage. Muscle paralysis with a nondepolarizing agent may be necessary to reduce muscle contractions contributing to the hyperthermia.
   c. Seizures: Seizures can be treated with benzodiazepines or other standard anticonvulsants.
   d. Arrhythmias: Ventricular dysrhythmias may require an antiarrhythmic agent such as lidocaine; whereas supraventricular arrhythmias may respond to therapy with calcium channel blockers. Cardioversion may be necessary in some patients.
   e. Chest pain: Cocaine-associated chest pain should be treated with nitroglycerin and benzodiazepines. Creatinine kinase (CK and CK-MB fractions) may be elevated after cocaine ingestion even in patients without MI. One prospective study of 302 patients with cocaine-associated chest pain found that those without an evolving clinical picture of ischemia or cardiovascular complications during the initial 9 to 12 hours of observation and monitoring in the emergency department were unlikely to develop life-threatening complications in the subsequent 30-day period (Weber et al., 2003). Thrombolysis should be considered if the symptoms and signs of toxicity, an ECG, and cardiac enzymes are consistent with acute MI.
   f. Hypertensive crisis: Hypertensive crisis can precipitate cerebrovascular hemorrhage and must be treated emergently. Blood pressure elevations may be the result of direct CNS stimulation (treated with benzodiazepines), or peripheral α-agonist effects (treated with either vasodilators [e.g., nifedipine, nitroglycerin, nitroprusside] or an α-adrenergic antagonist such as phentolamine).
   g. Agitation and psychosis: Acutely intoxicated patients should be approached in a subdued manner, with soft voice and slow movements. Agitation and psychosis should be treated with haloperidol or droperidol; chlorpromazine should be avoided because of the possibility of a severe drop in blood pressure, provocation of arrhythmias or seizures, or anticholinergic crisis. Flumazenil should be avoided for fear of unmasking seizure activity.
4. Body stuffer syndrome: Overdose has occurred after leakage or rupture of small bags of cocaine swallowed by an individual while running from law authorities; this type of overdose has been called "body stuffer syndrome" and is associated with hypertension, tachycardia, seizures, and other signs of toxicity (Sporer et al., 1997). People attempting to smuggle cocaine or heroin into the United States from overseas will sometimes swallow 30 to 40 sealed condoms or latex gloves filled with drug and then use purgatives to retrieve the drug after their entry into the country (McCarron et al., 1983). Termed "body packers," these individuals know the catastrophic consequences should one of the bags burst and so they take the time to seal them (unlike the body stuffers, who are much more likely to become symptomatic from hastily wrapped and swallowed drugs). Several cases of acute hepatotoxic effects and hepatocellular necrosis from cocaine use have also been reported (Gourgoutis et al., 1994).

Chronic Use

Cocaine is irritating to the mucosa, skin and airways, and chronic use is associated with erosion of dental enamel, gingival ulceration, keratitis, chronic rhinitis, perforated nasal septum, midline granuloma, altered olfaction, optic neuropathy, osteolytic sinusitis, burns, and skin infarction. People addicted to cocaine also frequently experience anorexia, weight loss sexual dysfunction, and hyperprolactinemia.

Tolerance and Withdrawal

Because of cocaine's powerful euphoric effects and its short half-life, repeated use leads to rapid development of tolerance; addicts can progress from small doses to large daily quantities in a short period. No tolerance to the cardiovascular side effects is developed.

Symptoms of cocaine abstinence or withdrawal include depression, anhedonia, irritability, aches and pains, restless but protracted sleep, tremors, nausea, weakness, intense cravings for more cocaine, slow comprehension, suicidal ideation, lethargy, and hunger. There is currently no widely accepted treatment for cocaine withdrawal. Although many uncontrolled studies have been reported in the literature, and some drugs look promising in early trials, no drug has been proven effective in controlled studies. Relapse rates are very high in cocaine-addicted patients who attempt abstinence.

Cocaethylene

When alcohol is used with cocaine, a third substance, cocaethylene, is formed in the liver (Randall, 1992; Jatlow, 1993; Rose, 1994). The half-life of cocaethylene is 2 hours, compared with 38 minutes for cocaine. Cocaethylene increases the toxicity of cocaine, particularly on the heart. It is also able to block dopamine reuptake, thereby extending the period of intoxication and toxicity. When alcohol is ingested and metabolized along with cocaine, the risk of sudden cardiac death is increased 25 times. In animal models cocaethylene is more likely to cause seizure activity. A recent study (Bolla et al., 2000) showed that neurobehavioral performance was significantly worse in those individuals who combined alcohol and cocaine use, and these effects persisted even after 4 weeks of abstinence.

Betel Nut

Though betel nut is unknown to most Western physicians, it is chewed on a daily basis by 15% of the world's population (600 million people). It is chewed alone or, more commonly, in a "quid." The quid consists of betel nut, catechu gum (produced from the sap of the Malaysian acacia tree), and calcium hydroxide paste (produced by burning limestone, reef coral, or shells) wrapped in betel leaf. This combination is placed in the lateral gingival pocket, and the strongly alkaline saliva-generated calcium hydroxide solution activates enzymes in the catechu gum, releasing eugenol (betel oil) from the betel leaf. Eugenol contains two psychoactive phenols, betel-phenol and chavicol, and an alkaloid stimulant called *cadinene* that has cocaine-like properties. Betel nut releases arecoline, a volatile cholinergic alkaloid and CNS stimulant. Tobacco is frequently added to the quid.

More than 4% of the U.S. population is of Asian or Pacific Island descent, and the use of betel nut (with or without tobacco) is culturally accepted in these communities. Most youth in these communities have experimented with this substance by adolescence. Dependence occurs rapidly, and if the individual leaves the community, transition to tobacco products is common. Knowledge of traditional cultural practices is key to diagnosis.

AMPHETAMINE (AMPHETAMINE, METHAMPHETAMINE, METHYLPHENIDATE, KHAT)

Prevalence/Epidemiology

On the basis of the 2003 National Survey on Drug Use and Health, 20.8 million Americans aged 12 or older (8.8% of the population) had used prescription-type stimulants nonmedically at least once in their lifetime, and an estimated 378,000 persons met the criteria for dependence or abuse within the last year (SAMHSA, 2005). Lifetime use of methamphetamine was reported by 12.3 million; prescription diet pills by 8.7 million; Ritalin or methylphenidate by 4.2 million; and Dexedrine by 2.6 million. Continuing surveillance suggests that methamphetamine use is on the rise. In 2004, the National Survey on Drug Use and Youth estimated that 1.4 million persons aged 12 and older (0.6% of the population) had used methamphetamine within the last year, with 600,000 reporting its use within the last month (SAMHSA, 2005). The average age of first users increased from 18.9 years in 2002, to 20.4 years in 2003, and to 22.1 years in 2004.

The 2006 Monitoring the Future survey of almost 50,000 American high school students (Johnston et al., 2007) documented the continued gradual decline in the lifetime use of amphetamines over the last 10 years from a peak of 13.5% of 8th graders, 17.7% of 10th graders, and 15.3% of 12th graders in 1996 to the current prevalence rates of 7.3%, 11.2% and 12.4% respectively in 2006. Corresponding figures for methamphetamine use among high school students have also dropped to 2.7% of 8th graders, 3.2% of 10th graders, and 4.4% of high school seniors, since lifetime usage rates for this particular drug were first introduced into the survey in 1999 at 4.5%, 7.3%, and 8.2% for the three classes of students, respectively. Separate tallies are also kept for the crystalline form of methamphetamine known as "ice." In 2006, 3.4% of 12th graders reported experimenting with "ice" at least once in their lifetime (Johnston et al., 2007). A second source of information, the 2005 Youth Risk Behavior Survey, reported that 6.2% of students had used methamphetamines one or more times in their lifetime (CDC, 2006).

Such figures should be approached with caution. As suggested with other illicit drugs, the school-based survey likely underestimates use by the total population of adolescents, which includes dropouts, the homeless, working youth, and others. It may also undercount misuse of methylphenidate and other drugs which, although structurally similar to amphetamines, may not be recognized by students as within the amphetamine class of drugs and therefore not reported by them.

Medical Use

Amphetamines have been used as a weight loss aid, although efficacy is questionable. Other uses include treatment of narcolepsy and attention-deficit hyperactivity disorder (ADHD). The recent increase in the diagnosis and medical management of ADHD has increased the availability of amphetamines to adolescents, who may misuse their own prescriptions by taking a higher dose than prescribed, or distribute pills to peers who may misuse them either as study aids or for intoxication. Appropriate treatment of adolescents with ADHD has been shown to decrease the risk of illicit substance use, but must be carefully supervised. Longer-acting medications may have lower addiction potential than short-acting ones.

Preparation and Dose

The term "amphetamine" refers to a class of drugs containing an amphetamine base, available either in prescription form (such as amphetamine, dextroamphetamine, amphetamine sulfate), or illicitly manufactured (mainly in the form of methamphetamine). Amphetamines are CNS stimulants. Methamphetamine has a stronger effect on the CNS than other forms of amphetamine. Methylphenidate is a nonamphetamine stimulant with similar action available in prescription form.

Amphetamine and methamphetamine differ structurally in that a methyl group attaches to the terminal nitrogen to form methamphetamine. Methamphetamine can be produced in clandestine "labs" beginning with ephedrine or pseudoephedrine that can be isolated from over-the-counter cold preparations. Synthesis is relatively easy, and illicit production occurs in home kitchens, workshops, recreational vehicles, and rural cabins. The federal government and some states have enacted laws decreasing the availability of necessary precursor chemicals. Many of these agents can still be obtained in neighboring states or countries.

The methamphetamine produced by ephedrine reduction is a lipid-soluble pure base form that is fairly volatile and can evaporate if left exposed to room air. This product is converted to the water-soluble form, methamphetamine HCl salt. Illicitly synthesized methamphetamine may be contaminated by organic or inorganic impurities. Poisoning from heavy metals (e.g., lead, mercury) or from solvents used in the synthesis process has been reported. Exposures to carcinogenic materials has been noted. Street methamphetamine may be mixed with many drugs, including cocaine. Studies show that 8% to 20% of street-available stimulants contain both drugs. In a report on cocaine intoxication, 7% of patients sought medical help because of the concurrent use of cocaine and amphetamines.

The production process described here results in a high yield of D-methamphetamine, which is cortically more active than the L-isomer (the active ingredient in Vicks Inhaler). Methamphetamine HCl is much more versatile than the hydrochloride salt of cocaine. It has high bioavailability in the salt form by any route of administration, such as snorting, smoking, ingesting by mouth, or passing across other mucous membranes such as the vaginal mucosa. "Ice" consists of pure crystals of D-methamphetamine. There is no difference between smoking street speed and smoking ice.

There are areas in the western and southwestern United States where methamphetamine is the predominant stimulant of abuse. Look-alikes containing combinations of caffeine, ephedrine, and phenylpropanolamine are particularly dangerous. A much larger dose is necessary to achieve the same level of cortical stimulation as achieved with amphetamines. This combination has greater cardiovascular stimulation, so abuse of look-alikes puts the user at great risk for stroke, MI, or hypertensive crisis.

The maximum typically prescribed dose of amphetamine is in the range of 60 to 100 mg, but addicted patients may ingest up to 100 times the daily dose during a binge.

Routes of Administration and Street Names

Prescription amphetamines are typically ingested orally, or through nasal insufflation. Illicit methamphetamine is usually smoked. Either preparation may be ground up, heated, and injected intravenously. Smoking methamphetamine may be more potent and addictive than snorting or ingesting it; smoking produces higher concentrations of drug in the brain for a shorter period. The user places methamphetamine HCl powder, crystals, or ice into a piece of aluminum foil that has been molded into the shape of a bowl, a glass pipe, or a modified light bulb and heats it over the flame of a cigarette lighter or torch; then the volatile methamphetamine fumes are inhaled through a straw or pipe. Street names for amphetamines include A's, meth, speed, crystal, cartwheel, copilots, footballs, magnums, powder, 20–20, whites, white crosses, crank, ice, ups, dexies, bombido, bennies, black beauties, splash, crosses, and crossroads (Table 71.5).

Physiology and Metabolism

Amphetamines are CNS stimulants that work as sympathomimetic drugs. Amphetamines act on the CNS to release neurotransmitters from presynaptic neurons, directly stimulate postsynaptic catecholamine receptors, prevent reuptake of neurotransmitters (dopamine, serotonin, and norepinephrine), and act as a mild monoamine oxidase (MAO) inhibitor. Stimulation of the nucleus accumbens causes the experience of pleasure. Stimulation of the basal ganglia causes repetitive movements that may be seen in amphetamine addicts. Increased serotonin is associated with changes in sleep and appetite patterns, increased body temperature, mood changes, aggressiveness, and psychosis. See Table 71.6 for amphetamine physiology.

Effects of Intoxication

Amphetamines are CNS stimulants. Users experience increased energy, psychological euphoria, and physical well-being. These effects are nearly identical to cocaine use, but last much longer. Smoked methamphetamine results in immediate euphoria that results from rapid absorption in the lungs and deposition in the brain.

Symptoms of amphetamine intoxication include alertness, anxiety, confusion, delirium, dry mouth, tachycardia, hypertension, tachypnea, jaw clenching, bruxism (teeth grinding), reduced appetite, sweating, and psychosis. As with cocaine, depletion of neurotransmitters leads to post

TABLE 71.5

Chemical Names, Brand Names, and Street Names of Amphetamines

Prescription Medications		
Chemical	Brand Name	Street Name
Dextroamphetamine	Dexedrine Adderall	Dexies, hearts, oranges
Amphetamine sulfate	Benzedrine sulfate	Hearts, peaches, footballs
Benzphetamine	Didrex	
Methamphetamine	Desoxyn	Speed, crystal, meth

Illicit Methamphetamine	
Street Name	Description
Ice, crystal	Purified methamphetamine ingested by smoking
Yaba	Methamphetamine and caffeine tablet which may be smoked or ingested orally
Croak	Methamphetamine and crack cocaine

use dysphoria. Deaths related to use of amphetamines have been associated with assaults, suicides, homicides, accidents, driving impairment, and maternal–fetal and infant exposures. Methamphetamine use by pregnant women has been associated with embryopathy and fetal wastage (Stewart et al., 1997).

Adverse Effects

1. Psychiatric: Aggressiveness, confusion, delirium, psychosis.
2. Neurological: Seizures, choreoathetoid movements, cerebrovascular accidents cerebral edema, cerebral vasculitis. One 20-year-old girl suffered hyperreflexia, multiple seizures, and decerebrate posturing after having stuffed bags of methamphetamine into her vagina to avoid their detection. Her serum methamphetamine and amphetamine concentrations were 3,100 ng/mL and 110 ng/mL, respectively (Kashani et al., 2004).
3. Cardiovascular: Tachycardia, hypertension, atrial and ventricular arrhythmias, MI, cardiac ischemia, coronary artery vasospasm, necrotizing angiitis, arterial aneurysms, aortic dissections.
4. Gastrointestinal: Ulcers, ischemic colitis, hepatocellular damage.
5. Musculoskeletal: Muscle contractions, rhabdomyolysis. Intoxicated patients may experience rhabdomyolysis (Richards, 1999) with associated elevated levels of CK and myoglobin, and in some cases may develop secondary acute renal failure.
6. Respiratory: Pneumomediastinum, pneumothorax, pneumo-pericardium; acute noncardiogenic pulmonary edema, pulmonary hypertension.
7. Renal: Acute tubular necrosis.
8. Dental: Chronic gingivitis, numerous dental caries, severe dental abscesses and necrosis known colloquially as "meth mouth."

Overdose and Emergency Treatment

Complications of amphetamine overdose resemble those of cocaine. However, cocaine and the amphetamines are structurally dissimilar. Unlike cocaine, amphetamines do not have anesthetic effects or effects on nerve conduction.

As with cocaine, emergency treatment is directed toward cardiovascular and respiratory stabilization and control of seizures. Because of the ability of methamphetamine to cause significant agitation, patients who present to emergency departments for acute intoxication may require pharmacological intervention. Hyperactive or

TABLE 71.6

Amphetamine Physiology

Receptors	Pharmacodynamics	Distribution	Metabolism
Serotonin binding sites and monoaminergic reuptake sites	• Release of neurotransmitters from the presynaptic neurons • Direct stimulation of postsynaptic catecholamine receptors • Reuptake blockade • Mild monoamine oxidase inhibitor	Crosses into the CNS with CSF levels approximately 80% of plasma levels	• Little metabolism • Renal excretion, enhanced in acidic urine

agitated persons should be treated with droperidol or haloperidol. These are butyrophenones and dopamine-blocking agents that specifically antagonize the central behavioral effects of methamphetamine. Multiple clinical reports attest to the efficacy of droperidol and haloperidol in acute amphetamine toxicity. Patients with acute choreoathetoid syndrome associated with use of amphetamines may show rapid improvement with haloperidol. Diazepam was found to be highly effective in antagonizing the toxic effects of cocaine but not as effective against amphetamines in animal models. A study of 146 patients presenting to an emergency department with agitated, violent, or psychotic reactions due to methamphetamine showed that they responded better to droperidol than to lorazepam, with more rapid and more profound sedation (Richards et al., 1998). Both drugs produced clinically significant reductions in pulse, systolic blood pressure, respiration rate, and temperature over a 60-minute period. Avoid chlorpromazine (Thorazine) because of the possibility of a severe drop in blood pressure, anticholinergic crisis, or seizure activity. Beyond 5 to 10 mg of haloperidol or droperidol, the sedating benefit is minimal and benzodiazepines should be added.

Chronic Use

Chronic use of amphetamines can produce severe psychiatric as well as physical problems, including delusions, hallucinations, and formication, leading individuals to tear and damage their skin. Animal studies have demonstrated that high doses of amphetamines damage neuron cell endings. Some former users seem to have permanent personality changes even after long periods of abstinence from methamphetamine.

Tolerance and Withdrawal

Tolerance does occur with chronic methamphetamine use, and users will frequently escalate their dose or change the route of exposure in order to maintain effect. Symptoms of withdrawal include depression; fatigue; sleep problems; increased appetite, headaches, and drug cravings. These symptoms may begin as soon as the high ends and can last up to 7 to 10 days (McGregor et al., 2005). There is no specific medical treatment for acute amphetamine withdrawal, other than supportive care.

Cathine and Cathinone (Khat)

Cathinone is chemically similar to D-amphetamine, and cathine (D-norisoephedrine) is a milder form of cathinone (Kalix, 1994; Boyer et al., 2000). These compounds are the active ingredients in khat leaves (Catha edulis), which are used as a tea or chewed for their euphoriant and stimulant effects by persons in Africa, the Middle East, and corresponding immigrant and refugee communities in developed nations. The plant grows as a large flowering evergreen shrub or tree. If left unrefrigerated, the cathinone degrades within 48 hours, explaining the preference for fresh leaves. The U.S. Drug Enforcement Agency has classified cathinone as a schedule I narcotic, whereas cathine remains a schedule IV narcotic. Outside the United States, khat is sold by African or Arab sellers and is used within cultural norms with little evidence of abuse. Khat-induced

psychosis is rare but has been described in the literature; it most commonly occurs in the context of nonculturally sanctioned polydrug abuse. Western physicians are frequently unaware of the widespread use and availability of khat in certain African and Arabian communities. Susceptible children and adolescents in these communities are at risk because khat can potentially act as a gateway substance when the protective context of culture and family are absent.

In Russia, methcathinone synthesis from ephedrine in makeshift home laboratories is widespread, and it is one of the most common drugs of abuse, after alcohol and tobacco. When ephedrine is reduced, the hydroxy group is lost and methamphetamine results. When this group is oxidized, methcathinone is produced. Clandestine laboratories producing this substance appeared in the midwestern United States in the 1990s, yet production has been limited and methcathinone has failed to achieve the abuse status of other stimulants. In Russian immigrant and refugee communities, knowledge of and experience with methcathinone may predispose at-risk individuals to seek out methamphetamine or other stimulants. In either population, abuse of khat or methcathinone or a family history of such should be suspected in the substance-abusing adolescent from a representative community.

ECSTASY (METHYLENEDIOXYMETHAMPHETAMINE, [MDMA])

Prevalence/Epidemiology

According to the 2003 National Survey on Drug Use and Health, approximately 2.1 million persons aged 12 and above reported ecstasy use within the last year, with virtually all of them reporting concomitant use of alcohol and 90% reporting use of other illicit drugs also (SAMHSA, 2005). Another survey, the Youth Risk Behavior Survey, reported lifetime ecstasy use rates in 6.3% of students nationwide in 2005 (CDC, 2006). This represented a drop from 11.1% in the 2001 and 2003 surveys. According to the Monitoring the Future survey, reported lifetime use of MDMA by high school students has declined slowly since the drug seemingly peaked in 2001 at rates of 5.2% of 8th graders, 8.0% of 10th graders, and 11.7% of 12th graders to the corresponding current lower rates of 2.5%, 2.8%, and 6.5% in 2006 (Johnston et al., 2007). Still such rates are comparable to the percentage of adolescents reporting use of cocaine and surpass those using crack or lysergic acid diethylamide (LSD). Methylenedioxyamphetamine (MDA) and methylenedioxy-N-ethylamphetamine (MDEA) are synthetic hallucinogens similar to MDMA that were popular in the 1960s. Currently MDMA is much more popular.

Raves and Circuit Parties

Raves are essentially all-night dance parties or mass gatherings of individuals who listen to loud, syncopated, "techno" music being "spun" by a DJ band, often in coordination with laser effects and other visual and auditory stimuli. The music at raves is usually computer generated, without vocals, and noncommercial in nature. Because alcohol is usually not available at raves, there is often no age restriction on admission. Raves are usually held at different venues each time and may not occur as announced, to deter police surveillance. Exact locations may be released only hours before an event takes place. Most attendees are between 15 and 25 years of age, and often they are from middle socioeconomic backgrounds. Circuit parties are large-scale dance parties lasting from one to several days and primarily attended by gay and bisexual men in their thirties and forties. Circuit parties may facilitate the use of drugs such as methamphetamine which, in turn, cause disregard of normal sexual precautions and inhibitions, predisposing the participants to the transmission of diseases such as human immunodeficiency virus (HIV) (Boddiger, 2005).

Although not all attendees use drugs and alcohol is not served, drugs are used liberally and many illicit drugs are available at raves. The term *club drugs* was coined to describe a number of primarily synthetic drugs that are preferred by adolescent and young adult attendees at "raves," nightclubs that stay open all night, and "circuit parties." Drugs used at raves include ecstasy, LSD, ketamine, phencyclidine (PCP), crystal methamphetamine, gamma-hydroxybutyrate (GHB), gamma-butyrolactone (GBL), fentanyl, Rohypnol, cocaine, and marijuana. MDMA started to become more popular in the 1980s, and several features of the drug specifically shaped virtually all aspects of the rave. The intense motor restlessness and stimulation of the "stereotypic behavior" portions of the brain occur as a side effect of MDMA and are relieved by group "movement" (dancing) and "wandering" from one stage area to another. In addition, because of the hallucinogenic properties of MDMA and the predictable occurrence of "seeing tracers," the light show or laser effects are coordinated with the music.

Medical Use

MDMA was first patented in 1912 as an appetite suppressant by a scientist working on the chemical structures found in methamphetamine. However, it was never manufactured and sold commercially, although it did resurface in the 1950s as a potential psychotherapeutic agent for psychoanalysis. However, there are no current medical uses for MDMA.

Preparation and Dose

In the early 1980s MDMA (together with MDA and MDEA) was sold legally, and was in the group of substances called *designer drugs*. "Designer drug" is an imprecise term that describes a synthetic substance closely related to a controlled substance and yet technically legal. Legislation has closed this loophole, but the term "designer drug" persists. "Designer drugs" have included dextromethamphetamine (MDA), MDMA (ecstasy), MDEA, and α-methylfentanyl. In 1985, MDMA was classified as a schedule I drug by the U.S. Food and Drug Administration (FDA) after reports were published of neurotoxicity in laboratory animals, making production and distribution illegal. Most pharmaceutical-grade ecstasy tablets are now produced in Europe and smuggled into the United States. The drug is sold as a tablet or capsule, often with a symbol printed on it. Tablets sold as MDMA may actually contain MDA, MDEA, or something entirely unrelated to the drug such as LSD, caffeine, pseudoephedrine, or dextromethorphan. The typical ecstasy tablet contains 0 to 100 mg of MDMA, although the concentration of MDMA may vary 70-fold or more among tablets sold. Orally ingested doses take approximately 30 minutes for onset of effect and the duration of action is 1 to 2 hours. Many users begin with a low dose (40–70 mg) and gradually add more pills until they experience the desired effect at a common dosage range of 75 to 125 mg, a practice known as "rolling."

Routes of Administration and Street Names

MDMA can be snorted, smoked, or injected, but is usually taken orally. Street names include ecstasy, liquid "X," Adam, "XTC," and MDM. MDEA is referred to as Eve.

Physiology and Metabolism

MDMA causes release of stored serotonin from neuronal vesicles into the synapse. Serotonin binding to post synaptic receptors results in the effects of MDMA. Serotonin is largely broken down in the synapse by MAO, and repeated use of MDMA causes serotonin depletion, after which further doses have little or no effect. MDMA's onset of action is related to the route of administration; for the oral dose, onset usually occurs within 30 to 45 minutes and last 3 to 6 hours. Single doses of MDMA have caused nerve damage in animal studies. See Table 71.7 for MDMA physiology.

Effects of Intoxication

MDMA has both stimulant and hallucinogen effects. Users describe feelings of enhanced well-being and introspection, empathy, love, affection, and increased energy.

Adverse Effects

1. Psychological: Confusion, depression, fatigue, sleep problems, anxiety, paranoia
2. Neurological: Seizures, muscle spasms, bruxism, hyperthermia, sweating, syndrome of inappropriate secretion of antidiuretic hormone (SIADH), blurred vision, faintness, chills, excessive sweating, hyponatremia, serotonin syndrome (with repeated dosing). Water loading, excessive sweating and overheating, and SIADH can contribute to clinically significant hyponatremia or hyponatremic dehydration (Gomez-Balaguer et al., 2000).
3. Musculoskeletal: Muscle rigidity, rhabdomyolysis
4. Cardiovascular: Tachycardia, hypertension, arrhythmias, cardiovascular failure, and asystole. A 27-year-old with no history of cardiac disease claimed that he ingested $\frac{1}{2}$ tablet of MDMA with whiskey at a party. He developed chest pain 3 hours later, which was diagnosed as an acute MI with multiple thrombi visible in the right coronary artery by angiography. His plasma MDMA level was 1,100 ng/mL and his urinary MDMA level was 96,800 ng/mL, with a corresponding urinary MDA level of 13,000 ng/mL, confirming significant exposure (Lai et al., 2003).
5. Gastrointestinal: Nausea, severe hepatic damage. Several cases of severe hepatic damage requiring liver transplantation have been described (Brauer et al., 1997; Andreu et al., 1998; Schwab et al., 1999). In a review by

TABLE 71.7

Methylenedioxymethamphetamine Physiology

Receptors	Pharmacodynamics	Distribution	Metabolism and Excretion
• Serotonin 5-HT$_2$ receptors • Central and peripheral catecholamine receptors	• Release of serotonin into the synapse • Release of endogenous catecholamines • Inhibition of serotonin reuptake • Depletion of serotonin stores occurs with repeated dosing, after which no further effect is achieved by taking more drug	• Few pharmacological studies have been performed in humans • Peak concentrations at 2 hours, half-life 8–9 hours	• Metabolized through cytochrome P-450 isoenzyme CYP2D6 into 3,4-methylenedioxyamphetamine (MDA) • 75% excreted in the urine as parent compound

Andreu et al (1998), MDMA was the second most common cause of liver injury in patients younger than 25 years. It accounted for 20% of the cases in this group of patients—36% if viral hepatitis was excluded. Full recovery occurred in all cases in 3 to 12 months.

Overdose and Emergency Treatment

The most common severe reaction to toxic MDMA ingestion is a syndrome of altered mental status, tachycardia, tachypnea, profuse sweating, and hyperthermia. This syndrome can appear similar to acute amphetamine overdose. The health care provider is cautioned that MDMA may not be detected in routine toxicological screening of the urine for amphetamines (Boyer et al., 2001).

Williams et al. (1998) reported on MDMA users who presented to an emergency room facility. The mean number of tablets taken was two. Approximately 40% had taken MDMA before, and 50% had used another illicit substance, with stimulants and cocaine being most common. The most common features found in those presenting to the emergency room were nonspecific symptoms of feeling unwell or strange; many patients had collapsed or lost consciousness. The most frequent signs were related to sympathetic overactivity and included agitation or disturbed behavior and increased temperature. Serious complications such as delirium, seizures, and profound coma were more frequent with the combination of MDMA and other substances. Teens and young adults who present late at night on weekends and have clinical manifestations of sympathetic overactivity and increased temperature ("Saturday night fever") should be suspected of using stimulants, and MDMA in particular.

The treatment of toxic ingestions of MDMA is supportive and similar to that for amphetamine overdose, including support of airway, breathing, and circulation; assessment and treatment of cardiac arrhythmias; and monitoring of vital signs and level of consciousness. Close monitoring of vital signs, serum electrolytes and fluid balance, and urine output is required because of the possibility of SIADH-induced and/or water loading–induced hyponatremia. Hyperthermia should be treated with cooling blankets and intravenous fluids. Use of muscle relaxants, anticonvulsants, and sedatives may be indicated.

There have been reports of life-threatening toxicity and death associated with ecstasy use. The mechanisms of death appear to be related to fatal hyperthermia, DIC, rhabdomyolysis, renal failure, cardiac arrhythmias and sudden asystole, hyponatremia, and seizures (Henry et al., 1992). Other reports have also included deaths due to serotonin syndrome, DIC and hepatic failure, cerebral infarction, and cerebral hemorrhage. Mueller et al. (1998) report a 20-year-old woman who ingested two ecstasy tablets and within 4 hours presented to the emergency department cyanotic and comatose, with hyperthermia (temperature 107°F) and autonomic instability typically seen in serotonin syndrome. She went on to develop hyperkalemia, multiple seizures, hypotension, and ventricular fibrillation leading to her death 4 hours after presentation. Risky behaviors related to poor judgment induced by MDMA can also lead to accidental deaths (Dowling et al., 1997).

Chronic Use

Research links MDMA to long-term damage to areas of the brain that are critical to thought and memory. In experiments in monkeys, exposure to MDMA for 4 days caused brain damage that was evident 6 years later. Ricaurte et al. (1988) found that both serotonin and 5-hydroxyindoleacetic acid were depleted and serotonergic fibers were damaged in a dose-dependent manner in the brains of monkeys who had been administered MDMA. Curran (2000) reviewed the research on MDMA neurotoxicity in both rodents and nonhuman primates. Her conclusions were that MDMA has been shown to cause serotonergic neuronal toxicity in every animal species tested, although recovery occurred in some. Direct evidence in humans has been more difficult to demonstrate because of the problems with study methods in humans. Bolla et al. (1998) found evidence of verbal and visual memory impairment in previous MDMA users. Parrott (2000a) found that users of ecstasy had impairment of several cognitive functions, including reduced memory for new information, impaired higher executive processing, and heightened impulsivity. Kish (2000) reported that striatal levels of serotonin and hydroxyindoleacetic acid (HIAA) were depleted by 50% to 80% in the brains of chronic users of MDMA. Long-lasting impairment of the 5-hydroxytryptamine (5-HT) system has been found in past users of MDMA, which may be more prominent in females and may be reversible in some patients (Gerra et al., 2000; Reneman et al., 2001).

Withdrawal Syndrome

Ecstasy withdrawal is similar to withdrawal from stimulants; the most common symptoms include depression, anxiety, panic attacks, sleeplessness, paranoia, and delusions. Treatment is supportive. Although depressed effect may persist, there is no role for psychopharmacological management.

OPIOIDS

Prevalence/Epidemiology

Opioids (opium, heroin, meperidine, OxyContin, oxycodone, fentanyl, sufentanil), especially the potent oral analgesics such as hydrocodone (Vicodin), oxycodone (OxyContin), and oxycodone plus acetaminophen (Percocet), continue to be attractive to teenagers. The prevalence of nonmedical oxycodone use increased significantly from 2002 to 2003, with an estimated 11 million Americans aged 12 and older reporting nonmedical oxycodone use at least once in their lifetime (SAMHSA, 2005). The Monitoring the Future survey of high school seniors (which changed its questionnaire in 2002 to include specific examples of these oral opiates) recorded a lifetime prevalence of use rate in 2006 of 13.4% in high school senior and an annual use rate of 9.0% for "other narcotics." In 2006, 3.0% of 8th graders, 7.0% of 10th graders, and 9.7% of 12th graders reported experimenting with Vicodin at least once within the preceding year. Usage rates of OxyContin in the same year were 2.6%, 3.8%, and 4.3%, respectively (Johnston et al., 2007). Heroin use, which had briefly increased in popularity in the late 1990s, has since dropped to lifetime usage rates averaging 1.4% to 1.6% among high school students in the past several years, with prevalence rates of annual use averaging 0.8% to 0.9% among 10th and 12th graders (Johnston et al., 2007). However, the 2005 Youth Risk Behavior Survey reported higher values, with 2.4% of students admitting they had used heroin one or more times during their lifetime (CDC, 2006). The prevalence was higher among Hispanic (3.6%) than white (2.2%) students; and higher among males (3.3%) than females (1.4%).

Medical Use

Opioids have several legitimate medical uses; they are potent antitussives, antidiarrheals, and extremely potent pain relievers. Newer oral medications with extended half-lives are a tremendous asset in the field of pain management. Unfortunately, opioids have a high addiction potential as well, and the development of newer medications has led to increased opioid use and dependence among adolescents. In addition, synthetic narcotics, such as fentanyl, are 80 times more potent than morphine and pose an increased danger of death by overdose.

Preparation and Dose

Opium has been known and used for centuries. The term *opioid* refers to all drugs, natural and synthetic, with morphine-like activity, as well as antagonists that bind to opioid receptors. All opiates are derived from the opium poppy, *Papaver somniferum.* The plant is grown primarily in the Middle East and in the Far East. Crude opium is obtained from the seed pods of the poppy. From this crude opium, morphine, codeine, and heroin are manufactured. The average purity of heroin sold on the street is 38%, up from 18% in 1990. The increased purity allows users to snort or smoke heroin. Over the last 10 years the price of heroin has dropped significantly. The ability to use heroin without needles and the lower prices have made heroin more accessible to adolescents, and the average age at first use dropped from 23 years in 1992 to 19.8 years in 1999.

Synthetic opioid pain relievers such as oxycodone, hydrocodone, and oxymorphone are pharmaceutical products that may be diverted and sold on the street. Many teens believe that these products are safer than drugs manufactured in clandestine laboratories and their popularity has increased dramatically since 2000.

Routes of Administration and Street Names

Opioids can be ingested, insufflated nasally, smoked, or injected intravenously or subcutaneously. Most adolescents first use prescription pain medications either orally or by snorting. OxyContin was developed as a long-acting pain reliever. It is intended to be swallowed whole so as to prolong its analgesic efficacy over 8 to 12 hours. Crushing the tablet destroys this continuous release property and makes the total dose available for a rapid "rush."

The street cost of oxycodone is approximately $1/g. Because of rapid tolerance and the need for increased doses, opioid addiction quickly becomes expensive, and users may begin using heroin which is less expensive. Opioid dependence, regardless of the chosen route of administration, creates intense addictive disease and carries a guarded prognosis. However, newer replacement therapies have been shown to reduce relapse rates substantially (Fudala, 2003), particularly when combined with supportive counseling.

Heroin available on the street is commonly mixed with sugar, talcum powder, Epsom salt, or quinine. This mixture is usually heated into a solution and injected intravenously. Other than leg and arm veins, the veins between the toes, the veins under the tongue, and the dorsal vein of the penis are often used for injection. Heroin is sometimes injected under the skin ("skin popping") or snorted in the same manner as cocaine; the effect is less intense with any of these methods than with intravenous use. The duration of the effects of intravenously injected heroin is 3 to 6 hours.

Street names for heroin include smack, scat, junk, horse, H. Jones, shit, hard stuff, brown, chiva, do-jee, estuffa, hombre, mud, polvo, and stofa. Oxycodone is referred to as OC's, oxy, or percs; hydrocodone is referred to as vics.

Physiology and Metabolism

There are three opioid receptors in humans—μ, κ, and δ; these have been further classified into μ_1 and μ_2; δ_1 and δ_2; and κ_1, κ_2, and κ_3. The μ receptor is the major opioid receptor in the brain and responsible for the majority of neurological effects, including euphoria and pain relief. The κ receptor is found primarily in the brain stem and spinal cord and contributes to pain relief and sedation. The δ receptors are located in the limbic system and are believed to be responsible for affective and emotional changes associated with opioid use.

Morphine is only partially lipid soluble and crosses the blood–brain barrier slowly. By contrast, heroin is very lipid

TABLE 71.8

Opioid Physiology

Receptors	Pharmacodynamics	Distribution	Metabolism and Excretion
μ, κ, and δ Opioid receptors (primarily μ).	Stimulation of opioid receptors produces euphoria, pain relief, and other effects	• Morphine—low lipid solubility, crosses blood–brain barrier slowly • Heroin—high lipid solubility, crosses blood–brain barrier quickly and then is metabolized, creating a "morphine rush"	• Metabolized by the liver (N-demethylation, N-dealkylation, O-dealkylation, conjugation and hydrolysis) • Primarily excreted in the urine (90%)

soluble and crosses the blood–brain barrier quickly, but does not bind to opioid receptors. Heroin is metabolized to morphine within the CNS, which is the active drug. The main effect of heroin is to create a rush of morphine in the CNS. See Table 71.8 for opioid physiology.

Naloxone (Narcan) is a synthetic opioid antagonist. It binds to the opioid receptor with greater affinity than other opioids, and as such it is a useful treatment for overdose. However, naloxone will precipitate sudden withdrawal in patients who have used an opioid. Buprenorphine is a new synthetic opioid partial agonist that has been approved for use as replacement therapy for opioid addiction. It has intermediate avidity for the opioid receptor, between naloxone and other opioids (see Chapter 74 for further information on use of buprenorphine as replacement medication).

Effects of Intoxication

Opioids produce analgesia and, in high doses, euphoria. Symptoms of intoxication include anxiety, slow comprehension, euphoria, floating feeling, flushing, hypotonia, pinpoint pupils, skin picking, sleepiness, poor appetite, and constipation.

Adverse Effects

1. Psychiatric: Sedation, apathy, dysphoria, psychomotor agitation or retardation, impaired judgment, delirium, stupor.
2. Neurological: Diminished reflexes, miosis, pinprick analgesia, ataxia, hypothermia, hypotonia, coma.
3. Cardiovascular: Circulatory collapse, hypotension, hypothermia, peripheral vein thrombosis, phlebitis.
4. Respiratory: Blocked cough reflex, bradypnea, respiratory failure, pulmonary edema.
5. Gastrointestinal: Constipation.
6. Skin: Rashes, allergic reactions, secondary bacterial infections, abscesses, cellulites.
7. Obstetric: Low birth weight, neonatal withdrawal, and respiratory compromise.

Overdose and Emergency Treatment

Opioid overdose results in respiratory depression or failure, and circulatory collapse. Treatment begins with support of respiratory and circulatory function, protection of the airway to prevent aspiration, and treatment of hypoglycemia if present. Patients should receive naloxone (0.4–2 mg) intravenously every 5 minutes until response occurs or up to a maximum of 10 mg. Usually, if there is no response after three intravenous doses, this indicates that the individual has not taken an opioid overdose. Repeated doses may be needed in 2 to 3 hours as the naloxone wears off. Naloxone lasts for approximately 1 or 2 hours, whereas the effects of most opioids last 3 to 6 hours, and that of methadone lasts 24 to 36 hours; necessitating close observation during the treatment for opioid overdose. Resedation and respiratory failure may recur as the effects of naloxone wear off. Naloxone does not reverse hypotension that is caused by opiate-induced histamine release.

Chronic Use

Problems related to chronic use of opioids are primarily related to impurities present in the drugs taken, complications of injection or insufflation, and behaviors associated with addiction, such as prostitution, lying, and stealing. Frequent complications include:

1. Skin: Abscesses and cellulitis caused by injecting infectious organisms directly into the skin.
2. Vascular: Arteritis and thrombosis of the pulmonary vessels, lung abscesses with resulting pulmonary fibrosis and pulmonary hypertension endocarditis, and secondary septic emboli, osteomyelitis, septic arthritis tetanus, HIV, and hepatitis C from injecting infectious organisms directly into a vein.
3. Hepatitis and glomerulonephritis from injecting foreign material (talc, sugar) into a vein.
4. Respiratory: Recurrent aspiration pneumonia from respiratory suppression and blocking of the cough reflex, pulmonary edema, and arrhythmias caused by quinine.
5. Myositis ossificans: Extraosseous metaplasia of muscle caused by needle manipulation.

Tolerance and Withdrawal

Tolerance, dependence, and addiction occur very quickly, and patients must increase dose and frequency constantly to avoid withdrawal symptoms. Opioid withdrawal presents with flu-like symptoms which can be extremely unpleasant, but are not life threatening in otherwise healthy individuals. Symptoms include anxiety, irritability, yawning, restlessness, sleep disturbances, muscle aches, chills and sweating, piloerection, hyperthermia, lacrimation and nasal secretions, abdominal cramps with vomiting and diarrhea, paresthesias, tremors, mydriasis, hypertension, and tachycardia. The Clinical Opiate Withdrawal Scale (COWS) (Table 71.9) was developed to quantify the symptoms of opioid withdrawal and may be useful clinically to help time the induction with buprenorphine (Wesson et al., 2003).

Treatment for opioid withdrawal is supportive, and includes symptomatic treatment of aches and pains with nonsteroidal antiinflammatory medications, abdominal cramping with dicyclomine (Bentyl), and reassurance. Clonidine may also be helpful. Withdrawal can also be managed with buprenorphine (see Chapter 74).

Medical Management of Addiction

Methadone and buprenorphine are two medications that can be used as replacement therapy for opioid-dependent patients. Each of these medications has been shown to reduce the relapse rate in patients seeking treatment (see Chapter 74).

TABLE 71.9

Clinical Opiate Withdrawal Scale (COWS)

Resting pulse rate: (record beats per minute)
Measured after patient has been sitting or lying for 1 minute
0 Pulse rate 80 or below
1 Pulse rate 81–100
2 Pulse rate 101–120
4 Pulse rate greater than 120

Sweating: *Over past $\frac{1}{2}$ hour not accounted for by room temperature or patient activity*
0 No report of chills or flushing
1 Subjective report of chills or flushing
2 Flushed or observable moistness on face
3 Beads of sweat on brow or face
4 Sweat streaming off face

Restlessness: *Observation during assessment*
0 Able to sit still
1 Reports difficulty sitting still, but is able to do so
3 Frequent shifting or extraneous movements of legs/arms
5 Unable to sit still for more than a few seconds

Pupil size:
0 Pupils pinned or normal size for room light
1 Pupils possibly larger than normal for room light
2 Pupils moderately dilated
5 Pupils so dilated that only the rim of the iris is visible

Bone or joint aches: *If patient was having pain previously, only the additional component attributed to opiates withdrawal is scored*
0 Not present
1 Mild diffuse discomfort
2 Patient reports severe diffuse aching of joints/muscles
4 Patient is rubbing joints or muscles and is unable to sit still because of discomfort

Runny nose or tearing: *Not accounted for by cold symptoms or allergies*
0 Not present
1 Nasal stuffiness or unusually moist eyes
2 Nose running or tearing
4 Nose constantly running or tears streaming down cheeks

Gastrointestinal (GI) upset: *Over last $\frac{1}{2}$ hour*
0 No GI Symptoms
1 Stomach cramps
2 Nausea or loose stool
3 Vomiting or diarrhea
5 Multiple episodes of diarrhea or vomiting

Tremor: *observation of outstretched hands*
0 No tremor
1 Tremor can be felt, but not observed
2 Slight tremor observable
4 Gross tremor or muscle twitching

Yawning: *Observation during assessment*
0 No yawning
1 Yawning once or twice during assessment
2 Yawning three or more times during assessment
4 Yawning several times/minute

Anxiety or irritability
0 None
1 Patient reports increasing irritability or anxiousness
2 Patient obviously irritable/anxious
4 Patient so irritable or anxious that participation in the assessment is difficult

Gooseflesh skin
0 Skin is smooth
3 Piloerection of skin can be felt or hairs standing up on arms
5 Prominent piloerection

Total:

Score:
5–12 = mild; 13–24 = moderate; 25–36 = moderately severe; 36+ = severe withdrawal.

NONNARCOTIC CENTRAL NERVOUS SYSTEM DEPRESSANTS

The CNS depressants include the barbiturates such as benzodiazepines; nonbarbiturate hypnotic drugs such as glutethimide (Doriden) and methaqualone (Quaalude), GHB, flunitrazepam (Rohypnol), and major tranquilizers (phenothiazines); and carbamates such as meprobamate (Equanil and Miltown). Physical symptoms of sedative–hypnotic intoxication include slurred speech, incoordination, unsteady gait, nystagmus, decreased reflexes, impaired attention or memory, and stupor or coma; psychiatric symptoms of intoxication include inappropriate behavior, mood lability, impaired judgment, impaired social functioning, and impaired occupational functioning.

Barbiturates

Prevalence/Epidemiology
Nonmedical use of barbiturate tranquilizers continues to be a problem among adolescents. The 2006 Monitoring the Future study recorded an increased in lifetime use of barbiturates among high school seniors from 8.8% in 2003 to 10.2% in 2006, while annual use rates also rose from 6% to 6.6% (Johnston et al., 2007).

Medical Uses
Barbiturates are used as sleep aides, as a sedative–hypnotic anesthesia, as an anticonvulsant, for reduction of intracranial pressure and cerebral ischemia after head trauma, for poststroke management, and for preinduction of anesthesia. Their medical use has decreased over the past decade as they have been replaced by benzodiazepines for several indications.

Preparation and Dose
Barbiturates are sedative/hypnotic drugs derived from barbituric acid. More than 50 types of pills containing barbiturates are available in the United States. The most frequently abused barbiturates are secobarbital and pentobarbital. Many of the illicit pills are made in Mexico and contain varying amounts of secobarbital.

Barbiturates are divided into ultrashort-acting (thiopental [Pentothal] and methohexital [Brevital]), short-acting (secobarbital [Seconal] and pentobarbital [Nembutal]), intermediate-acting (amobarbital [Amytal] and butabarbital [Butisol]), and long-acting types (phenobarbital [Luminal]). Ultrashort-acting barbiturates are often used for anesthesia, whereas short-acting barbiturates are used as sleeping pills. Pentobarbital, for example, has an onset of effect 60 to 90 minutes after ingestion, with peak effects occurring in 1 to 2 hours, whereas phenobarbital has steady-state half-life of approximately 80 to 90 hours in adults. Therapeutic serum concentrations of phenobarbital range from 10 to 25 mcg/mL. Approximately 75% of phenobarbital is hydroxylated in the liver, with 25% excreted unchanged in urine, whereas secobarbital and butabarbital undergo 99% hepatic metabolism with little if any urinary excretion of parent compound.

Routes of Administration and Street Names
Barbiturates are usually taken orally, although some users inject them intravenously.

Street names include reds, red devils, yellow jackets, rainbows, tooies, blue heavens, purple hearts, Mexican reds, nebbies, nimbies, bluebirds, blue devils, blues, yellows, Christmas trees, trees, barbs, beans, goofballs, and stumblers.

Physiology and Metabolism
Barbiturates are γ-aminobutyric acid (GABA) A receptor agonists. GABA is the main inhibitory neurotransmitter of the CNS. Barbiturates bind to a unique location on the GABA receptor (separate from the GABA binding site). Once bound, barbiturates have two functions. First, they enhance binding of GABA to its unique site. Secondly, they open the chloride ion channel of the GABA receptor even in the absence of GABA. These two effects together make barbiturates potent drugs with a narrow window of safety.

By enhancing GABA, barbiturates produce all degrees of CNS depression, from sedation to general anesthesia. The mesencephalic reticular activating system is particularly sensitive to barbiturates.

Barbiturates are metabolized by the liver and enhance liver metabolism, shortening the half-life of other drugs (e.g., anticoagulants, corticosteroids, phenothiazines) and reducing their clinical effectiveness. They can increase the CNS depressant effects of meperidine by increasing its active metabolites. See Table 71.10 for barbiturate physiology.

Effects of Intoxication
Barbiturates are CNS depressants. Low doses result in mild sedation, higher doses result in hypnosis, and still higher doses result in anesthesia and possible death. Symptoms of intoxication include sleepiness, yawning, slowed comprehension, slurred speech, lateral nystagmus, anorexia, dizziness, and orthostatic hypotension. Allergic reactions including bronchospasm, urticaria, dermatitis, fever, and angioneurotic edema can be caused by barbiturates. When barbiturates are used in combination with

TABLE 71.10

Barbiturate Physiology

Receptors	Pharmacodynamics	Distribution	Metabolism and Excretion
GABA A agonists	• Enhance GABA binding • Open the chloride ion channel of the GABA receptor	Barbiturates bind to plasma proteins in varying amounts (50%–97%), and cross into the cerebrospinal fluid and the placenta to varying degrees	• Metabolized in the liver, may enhance metabolism of other compounds • Excreted by the kidney

other depressants such as alcohol or opioids, the effects of both are potentiated and lethal overdoses can occur more easily.

Adverse Effects

1. Fatigue
2. Neurological: Ataxia, slowed comprehension, diplopia, dizziness, dysmetria, hypotonia, poor memory, lateral nystagmus, and slowed speech.
3. Psychiatric: Euphoria or depressed mood, irritability, violent behavior, toxic psychosis.
4. Skin: Cutaneous lesions and bullae.

Overdose and Emergency Treatment

Signs and symptoms of barbiturate overdose include miosis, hypotension, hypothermia, respiratory depression, and decreased gastrointestinal motility. Coma, shock, and death are possible. The presentation is indistinguishable from opiate or other sedative overdose on clinical examination. Urine toxicology can be helpful for diagnosis, but quantitative levels are not predictive of the clinical course.

Treatment of barbiturate overdose is primarily supportive, and aimed at supporting airway, breathing, and circulation. Because of the decreased gastrointestinal motility and delayed gastric emptying drug absorption can continue for a long time after ingestion. Unabsorbed toxins should be removed by gastric lavage followed by activated charcoal for recent ingestion. Absorbed toxins should be removed by alkaline diuresis or dialysis. CNS stimulants should be avoided. Ingestion of >3 g or blood level of >2 mg/dL is the lethal dose for short-acting barbiturates; ingestion of >6 to 9 g or blood level >11 to 12 mg/dL is the lethal dose for long-acting barbiturates.

Tolerance and Withdrawal

Few adolescents use barbiturates with the frequency necessary to develop dependence. However, if dependence is suspected, detoxification must be done under close medical supervision as withdrawal can be life threatening. The severity of the withdrawal syndrome parallels the strength of the drug, the dose used, and the duration of prior abuse. Withdrawal symptoms include anxiety, delirium, hallucinations, irritability, sleep disturbance, seizures, headaches, weakness, hyperactive reflexes, tremor, abdominal cramps, flushing, nausea, sweating, and increased temperature. Orthostatic hypotension may also occur. Barbiturate withdrawal is treated with replacement by phenobarbital followed by a slow taper until the patient is drug free.

Benzodiazepines

Prevalence/Epidemiology

Use of benzodiazepine tranquilizers by teenagers continues to be disturbingly high. The Monitoring the Future study has recently documented a slight drop-off in the lifetime prevalence rates since 2001 to 4.3%, 7.2% of 10th graders, and 10.3% of 12th graders in 2006, although this represents a slight increase since 2005 (Johnston et al., 2007). Annual use rates in 2006 were 2.6%, 5.2% and 6.6% among 8th, 10th, and 12th graders respectively. Rohypnol use has remained relatively constant at approximately 1% of high school 12th grade students, since its availability in the United States for medicinal uses was curtailed in the late 1990s.

Medical Use

Medical use of the benzodiazepines became widespread in the 1970s, and this class of drugs continues to be used clinically as anxiolytic, hypnotic, anticonvulsant, and antispasmodic medication. Benzodiazepines are also used to treat the effects of alcohol withdrawal. Initially benzodiazepines were thought to be free of negative consequences, but it is now known that they carry the risk of dependence, withdrawal, and negative side effects.

Preparation and Dose

Several thousand benzodiazepine formulations have been investigated, but only a handful have found clinical utility. Table 71.11 lists some of the more prominent members of the chemical class, and some of their major uses, although many of these drugs have overlapping clinical indications and may be used for other purposes, such as insomnia, chemical restraint, alcohol withdrawal, and so on.

Long-acting benzodiazepines include diazepam, chlordiazepoxide, clonazepam, flurazepam, and chlorazepate. Typical elimination half-lives for these longer-acting benzodiazepines range from 18 to 100 hours. Short-acting benzodiazepines include oxazepam and lorazepam, with half-lives of approximately 6 hours. Midazolam is an example of an ultra–short-acting benzodiazepine.

Benzodiazepines are sedative-hypnotic medications; many drugs of this class are produced and sold in the United States, and they are readily available on the street. Nearly all the available benzodiazepines have been abused; those that cross the blood–brain barrier more quickly have a higher abuse potential than those that cross more slowly.

Benzodiazepines may be obtained by diverting legitimate prescriptions or by theft from pharmaceutical supplies. Diversion of flunitrazepam tablets across the Mexican border has also been reported. Abuse of benzodiazepines generally occurs within the context of another substance abuse disorder. These drugs are often used to augment the effects of another drug or prevent symptoms of withdrawal (O'brien, 2005). However, benzodiazepines are the drug of choice for a small portion of adolescents with substance abuse problems and sedative-hypnotic dependence has been described.

TABLE 71.11

Major Pharmacological Actions of Various Benzodiazepines

Benzodiazepine	Major Pharmacological Action
Diazepam, chlordiazepoxide, oxazepam, chlorazepate, lorazepam, prazepam, alprazolam, halazepam	Anxiolytic
Flurazepam, temazepam, flunitrazepam, triazolam, midazolam	Sedative–hypnotic
Diazepam, clonazepam	Anticonvulsant
Diazepam	Muscle relaxant

Routes of Administration and Street Names

Benzodiazepines are most often taken orally, although some adolescents may snort them or inject them intravenously. Street names include tranks, downers, blues, yellows, zans, blue footballs, blues, z bars, zan bars, tombstones, totem poles, quad bars, blue magoo, V, and vallies.

Physiology and Metabolism

Benzodiazepines bind to a unique site on the GABA A receptor and enhance the inhibitory effects of GABA. Like barbiturates, benzodiazepines enhance the binding of GABA to its receptor. Unlike barbiturates, however, benzodiazepines do not open the chloride ion channel of the GABA receptor in the absence of GABA. This makes benzodiazepines relatively milder in effect and safer to use than barbiturates. Variability between specific drugs regarding their water solubility and the affinity of the drug for the receptor may be one factor mediating differences among benzodiazepines in the pharmacokinetics of sedation as well as their propensity to cause amnesia.

Benzodiazepines are metabolized by the liver; different drugs in the class have different half-lives based on structural differences. The half-life is often determined by the half-life of active metabolites. Benzodiazepines can be divided into long-acting drugs such as diazepam, chlordiazepoxide, clonazepam, flurazepam, and clorazepate. Diazepam is highly lipophilic and has rapid absorption after ingestion, with an elimination half-life ranging from 18 to 100 hours. It is metabolized in the liver through a two-phased process of demethylation involving the cytochrome P-450 system, followed by glucuronidation. Shorter-acting benzodiazepines include oxazepam and lorazepam, which are metabolized directly in the liver by single-step glucuronidation and have elimination half-lives of approximately 6 hours. Ultra–short-acting agents include triazolam, temazepam, and midazolam. Benzodiazepines can cross the placenta and are excreted in breast milk.

Benzodiazepines and their metabolites may accumulate in the body, resulting in a delayed appearance of adverse reactions and continued clinical effects beyond discontinuation of the drug. Unlike the barbiturates, benzodiazepines do not induce the metabolism of other drugs. See Table 71.12 for benzodiazepine physiology.

Effects of Intoxication

Benzodiazepines are CNS depressants. They produce drowsiness, dizziness, weakness, sedation, and a sense of calmness.

Adverse Effects

1. Psychiatric: Paradoxical aggression, anxiety, delirium, agitation.
2. Neurological: Oversedation, ataxia, memory loss, impaired psychomotor function.
3. Cardiovascular: Mild hypotension.

Overdose and Emergency Treatment

Benzodiazepine overdose typically presents with dizziness, confusion, drowsiness or unresponsiveness, and blurred vision. Some patients may present with anxiety and agitation. Physical examination findings include nystagmus, slurred speech, ataxia, weakness or hypotonia, hypotension, and respiratory depression. Treatment for benzodiazepine overdose is primarily supportive including securing the airway, and cardiovascular and respiratory stabilization. Flumazenil is the first specific benzodiazepine receptor antagonist to become available. To treat severe benzodiazepine overdose, flumazenil is given in incremental doses over a few minutes. If a clinical effect is not seen after five doses have been given, it is unlikely that higher doses will be helpful. Patients who have overdosed on a long-acting benzodiazepine may require redosing to prevent return of symptoms.

In mixed overdoses involving tricyclic antidepressants or other seizure-causing agents, flumazenil is contraindicated. In this setting, it can cause seizure activity by removing any anticonvulsant protection conferred by the benzodiazepine. It is also contraindicated in individuals who are physically dependent on benzodiazepines. This dependence can occur rapidly and use of flumazenil can precipitate a full-blown benzodiazepine withdrawal state (agitation, tremor, flushing).

Chronic Use

Benzodiazepines have a high abuse and dependence potential. Care should be used in prescribing benzodiazepines for management of sleep or anxiety in any patient who has been diagnosed with drug problems. Benzodiazepines are contraindicated in adolescents with alcohol problems, opioid addiction, or on opioid replacement therapy.

Tolerance and Withdrawal

If benzodiazepine dependence is suspected, withdrawal must be carefully supervised. Patients who abruptly stop taking benzodiazepines can develop life-threatening, protracted seizures. Other symptoms of benzodiazepine withdrawal include anxiety, agitation, confusion, sleep disturbance, and flu-like symptoms, including fatigue, headache, muscle pain and weakness, sweating, chills, nausea, vomiting, and diarrhea.

Detoxification from benzodiazepine dependence is done by replacement with long-acting benzodiazepines followed by a taper. The taper can be accomplished either

TABLE 71.12

Benzodiazepine Physiology

Receptors	Pharmacodynamics	Distribution	Metabolism and Excretion
GABA A receptor agonists	Enhance the binding of GABA to the GABA receptor	• Protein bound • Cross into the central nervous system based on their solubility and lipophilicity	• Metabolized in the liver • Many active metabolites, which accounts for wide variation of half-lives

gradually (over 2–3 months) on an outpatient basis by decreasing the dose by one sixth every 10 days or rapidly (over 10–14 days) on an inpatient basis.

"Date Rape" Drugs

Flunitrazepam, GHB, and ketamine are often colorless, tasteless, and odorless. These drugs have the reputation of being the so-called "date rape" drugs because they have been added to beverages and ingested by individuals unknowingly. They can produce both antegrade and retrograde amnesia in the victim, such that they have no memory of events surrounding their use of the drug. In 1996, federal legislation was passed that increased penalties for the use of any controlled substance to aid in sexual assault. Information and educational materials directed toward college students are available from the Rape Treatment Center at Santa Monica—UCLA Medical Center at 1-800-END-RAPE (1-800-363-7273).

Flunitrazepam

Flunitrazepam (Rohypnol), a benzodiazepine, is predominantly a CNS depressant. Use of flunitrazepam began in Europe in the 1970s and appeared in the United States in the early 1990s. Street names include rophies, roofies, roach, and rope. The Monitoring the Future survey included questions on Rohypnol in 1996. In that year, 1.2% of seniors had used Rohypnol at some time; this figure rose to 3% in 1998 before falling to 1.7% in 2001. Although not measured in 12th graders since that time, use in 10th graders has declined from 1.5% in 2001 to 0.8% in 2006 after a peak in 1998 of 2%. Flunitrazepam is rapidly absorbed within 30 minutes of oral ingestion. It is a highly lipophilic drug, readily crossing the blood–brain barrier; consequently CNS depression is rapid in onset. Clinical effects are the same as those of other benzodiazepines, but with an exaggerated amnesia effect. If mixed with alcohol, it can incapacitate victims and prevent them from resisting sexual assault, hence its reputation as a "date rape" drug. Victims may also have impaired memory for the events surrounding the drug's use. This drug can be lethal when combined with alcohol and other depressants. This drug is not approved for use in the United States, and it is illegal to import flunitrazepam into the United States. Occasionally, clonazepam (Klonopin) is sold as "roofies." Flunitrazepam may not be detected in routine laboratory screening for benzodiazepines, but specific testing can detect flunitrazepam in the urine for up to 72 hours after ingestion. Management of patients with suspected overdoses includes decontamination with oral activated charcoal and supportive care.

Gamma-Hydroxybutyrate (Precursors: 1,4 butanediol, Butyrolactone, Gamma-valerolactone)

GHB is a CNS depressant that acts through a metabolite of the inhibitory neurotransmitter GABA and can function as a neurotransmitter itself. GHB triggers the release of an opiate-like substance and can mediate sleep cycles, temperature regulation, memory, and emotional control. In some countries, GHB is used as an anesthetic and for narcolepsy. It is rapidly absorbed after ingestion. Precursors of GHB, such as 1,4 butanediol and butyrolactone, are converted to GHB by the alcohol dehydrogenase enzyme system in the liver (Quang et al., 2002; Quang et al., 2004). Therefore,

sedative effects experienced after these as yet unregulated chemical precursors may be delayed by several hours, until their metabolism is complete.

The illicit use of GHB has grown in the United States, among both body builders and ravers. Body builders claim that it metabolizes fat and builds muscles. Ravers use it as a euphoriant. It has also been mentioned as one of the several "date rape" drugs. It has been sold as a strength enhancer, euphoriant, and aphrodisiac. Some of the common street names include liquid ecstasy, somatomax, scoop, Georgia Home Boy, and grievous bodily harm. The drug comes in both liquid and powder form. Before February 2000, GHB was not illegal to possess, but now it is a schedule I drug. GHB has not been sold over the counter in the United States since 1992. However, products containing precursor chemicals such as gamma butyrolactone (GBL) are used in a number of dietary supplements in health food stores and gymnasiums and are also readily available over the Internet.

Adverse effects include:

1. Cardiorespiratory: Bradycardia, respiratory depression (particularly if used with other depressants), increased or decreased blood pressure
2. Neurological: Hypothermia, dizziness, weakness, ataxia, vertigo, nystagmus, short-term amnesia, coma, tonic-clinic seizures
3. Psychiatric: Confusion, sedation, aggression, impaired judgment, hallucinations
4. Respiratory: Respiratory depression with acidosis
5. Gastrointestinal: Vomiting
6. Endocrine: Mild hyperglycemia
7. Acute respiratory acidosis

Heavy doses can lead to coma and respiratory depression, which can be exacerbated by the use of alcohol. The FDA has issued a warning about GHB because the products have been linked to at least 122 serious illnesses and at least six deaths (O'Connell et al., 2000). The diagnosis of GHB toxicity may be facilitated by the recent finding of an abnormal peak in urinary organic acids (Quang et al., 2005). There is no antidote for GHB overdose; the treatment is supportive care. Withdrawal effects include insomnia, anxiety, tremors, and sweating.

Ketamine

Ketamine ("Special K") is an arylcycloalkylamine chemical congener of PCP; it is similar to PCP pharmacologically, but it has a more rapid onset and is less potent. It is known as a rapid-acting dissociative anesthetic that combines sedative–hypnotic, analgesic, and amnesic effects with the maintenance of pharyngeal reflexes and respiratory function. Like PCP, ketamine is an NMDA receptor antagonist and is used as a human and veterinary anesthetic. Like PCP-induced anesthesia, it occasionally produces unpleasant emergence reactions, anxiety, dysphoria, and hallucinations. Ketamine entered the rave scene in the early 1990s as a substance of abuse and its use has been growing in the United States. Users are attracted to the "dreamy" state of mild hallucinations and "out of body" experiences induced by light ketamine anesthesia. Adverse effects include a cataleptic state, with nystagmus, excessive salivation, involuntary tongue and limb movements, and hypertonus. Laryngospasm, seizures, apnea, and respiratory arrest have all been reported on rare occasions with ketamine-induced anesthesia. Accidents are often of greater threat to the individual than toxicity secondary to the loss of physical control. Ketamine can be used as an alternative to cocaine, and it is often snorted. The drug is also often sold in tablets similar to "ecstasy," and users may take ketamine thinking they are using MDMA. Treatment of ketamine overdose is primarily supportive, with attention to neurological, cardiovascular, and respiratory monitoring. Airway control and ventilatory support may be necessary for some patients. Treatment of agitation related to an emergence reaction entails dim lighting, reduction of extraneous external stimuli, and administration of a benzodiazepine. For idiosyncratic dystonic reactions, intravenous diphenhydramine may be of benefit.

Glutethimide, Meprobamate, Methaqualone

Glutethimide (Doriden), meprobamate (Miltown, Meprosan), and methaqualone (Quaalude) are barbiturates similar in effect and were popularly used in the 1950s and 1960s. They are outmoded drugs and are no longer commercially available in the United States. These drugs are lipophilic, with sedative effects that can last for hours. They have high abuse potential. Tolerance and psychological and physical dependence can all occur. The effects of the drugs include a sense of euphoria, a loss of concern for self, and withdrawal from reality. Heavy use leads to intoxication, with unsteadiness, tremors, loss of memory, irritability, and delirium, and may result in coma and cardiovascular and respiratory failure. Withdrawal from these drugs is dangerous and can result in tremors, insomnia, seizures, coma, and death. Treatment includes oral decontamination with gastric lavage and activated charcoal. Hemoperfusion has been considered in the past for patients with confirmed exposures and life-threatening toxicity.

Baclofen and Muscle Relaxants

Abuse of prescription drugs such as muscle relaxants has become more common among adolescents. Muscle relaxants are diverse in chemical structure and actions; they include such drugs as baclofen, meprobamate, orphenadrine, and methocarbamol. Baclofen (Lioresal) is chemically related to the inhibitory neurotransmitter, GABA, and can induce drowsiness, coma, muscle flaccidity, cardiac dysrhythmias, and respiratory depression or sudden respiratory arrest. Baclofen and other muscle relaxants are not detected in routine toxicological screens of the blood and urine, and should be ordered specifically if an overdose is suspected. Treatment of patients who overdose on muscle relaxants includes oral decontamination with activated charcoal, close monitoring of neurological and cardiovascular status, and supportive care. Intubation and mechanical ventilation may be necessary in cases of severe poisoning. In one retrospective study, 14 teenagers took overdoses of baclofen ranging from 60 to 600 mg at a party. Nine were subsequently admitted to the critical care unit for mechanical ventilation because of respiratory failure. All survived, although the mean length of time on mechanical ventilation was 40 hours (Perry et al., 1998).

INHALANTS

Prevalence/Epidemiology

On the basis of the National Survey on Drug Use and Youth conducted in 2002 and 2003, an annual average of 718,000 (8.6%) of youths aged 12 and 13 years had used an inhalant in their lifetime; and approximately 35% of those had used other illicit drugs (SAMHSA, 2005). The 2006 Monitoring the Future survey of high school students found a lifetime prevalence of inhalant use in 16.1% of 8th graders, 13.3% of 10th graders, and 11.1% of 12th graders in 2006. There has been an upward trend in recent years among 8th graders with a small drop in 2006 (15.2% in 2002, 15.8% in 2003, 17.3% in 2004, 17.1% in 2005 and 16.1% in 2006) (Johnston et al., 2007). This trend may signal resurgence in student acceptance of inhalants as agents for experimentation. The prevalence of inhalant use within the previous year was highest again in 8th graders (9.1%), followed by 10th graders (6.5%) and 12th graders (4.5%). "Fad" use of inhalants is also common, such that misuse of butane lighters or aerosols in food products may gain short-term popularity in a particular school or town based on word-of-mouth reports among teens.

Preparation

Inhalants are attractive to adolescents because of their rapid onset of action, low cost, and easy availability. They are typically used by inhaling from a plastic bag containing the substance ("bagging") or by inhaling a cloth saturated with the substance ("huffing"). The initial effect is stimulation and excitation, which then progresses to a depressant effect on the CNS. Of the myriad products and substances abused, toluene is the most common volatile component. It is present in spray paint, airplane glues, rubber cement, cleaning fluids, inks (magic markers), and lacquer thinner.

Circumstances of Abuse

Inhalants are inexpensive, legal products that do not arouse suspicion in most homes (Table 71.13). When parents report finding fluid saturated cloths, empty spray paint cans or plastic bags in a bedroom, other paraphernalia, or unusual chemicals, they and the physician should suspect inhalant use and ask about it directly. Disinterest in school, declining grades, abandonment of usual friends and activities, secretive or oppositional behaviors, and emotional lability are all the signposts of substance abuse, including inhalant abuse.

Physiology and Metabolism

The effects of inhalants are felt within minutes of inhalation, because of the immediate absorption of the chemicals crossing the large surface area of lung alveoli into the pulmonary circulation. Their lipophilicity facilitates rapid absorption into the brain, and their pharmacology often involves anesthetic effects at the cellular level. Peak effects occur within minutes and excretion is rapid, such that the course of intoxication after one huffing event may last only 15 to 30 minutes.

Effects of Intoxication

Inhalant use results in euphoria, decreased inhibition, and decreased judgment. Symptoms of inhalant use include heavy lidded glazed eyes, slurred speech, lacrimation, rhinorrhea, salivation, and irritation of the mucus membranes.

TABLE 71.13

Classes of Inhalants, Chemical Examples and Toxicity

Class of Inhalant	Product/Chemical Examples	Toxicity
Volatile products	Glues, gasoline, spray paints, butane, paint thinner	Cardiac arrhythmias, respiratory failure, coma, pneumothorax
Gases	Nitrous oxide	Simple asphyxia
Anesthetics	Ether	Coma, respiratory failure
Nitrates	Amyl nitrate, butyl nitrate	Cardiovascular failure, coma methemoglobin

Anesthesia is common with drowsiness, stupor or even obtundation, accompanied by respiratory depression. Users report spinning or floating sensations, with disinhibition, exhilaration, and mild delirium. Feelings of grandiosity and omnipotence impart a sense of control and dominance.

Adverse Effects

Common adverse effects associated with inhalant abuse include gastrointestinal complaints such as anorexia, vomiting, and abdominal pain associated with gastritis. Neurological effects accompanying inhalant abuse include sleepiness, headaches, dizziness, ataxia, incoordination, and diplopia. Users may have a distinctive chemical odor to their breath, hair, or clothing. Disregard of personal hygiene may result in a disheveled appearance. Defatting properties of solvents may lead to perinasal and perioral skin rashes and nosebleeds. Respiratory irritation may cause the user to develop a chronic dry cough, new onset wheezing, and shortness of breath.

Overdose of inhalants can result in life-threatening complications, such as seizures, loss of consciousness, arrhythmias, respiratory failure, or cardiopulmonary arrest (Table 71.14). In addition, specific inhalant groups are associated with unique toxicities.

Death is not an uncommon outcome in adolescent inhalant abuse, either directly due to respiratory or cardiac toxic causes or as a result of trauma from risk-taking behaviors and poor judgment. Sudden sniffing-death syndrome has occurred after inhalation of fluorocarbons or halogenated hydrocarbons. The postulated mechanism involves sensitization of the myocardium by the solvent to the arrhythmogenic effects of epinephrine and increased sympathetic outflow, which occurs during the initial brief excitatory phase of intoxication.

Although tolerance to inhalants may develop, withdrawal symptoms do not usually occur. Inhalants are difficult or impossible to detect in drug samples. Conventional toxicology screening tests give negative results in patients with inhalant abuse.

Chronic Use

Inhalant abuse is notable for escalation in the frequency of use and in binge behaviors, due to the short duration of the "high." Chronic effects of inhalant abuse are characterized by irreversible damage to target organs such as the brain and kidneys. Fatty brain tissues such as myelin and neuronal cell bodies are damaged or destroyed, and white matter degeneration may be evident. One recent study (Rosenberg et al., 2002) compared psychological test scores and magnetic resonance imaging (MRI) studies of 55 solvent abusers to a control group of 61 abusers of other drugs. Solvent abusers had higher rates of MRI abnormalities (44% of the 50 subjects who had an MRI) in subcortical structures including the thalamus, basal ganglia, pons, and cerebellum. Although both groups underperformed on cognitive tests compared to normal populations, solvent abusers did significantly worse than the controls on measures of working memory and executive function (e.g., planning, self-monitoring, ability to focus and concentrate). Mean verbal and performance IQ scores for solvent abusers were 82 and 87, respectively. Such formal psychological testing and imaging studies reveal results typical of a "solvent encephalopathy," consisting of IQ loss, slow mentation, visuospatial dysfunction, faulty memory, poor insight, loss of executive function, cerebral atrophy, and subcortical dementia.

Diagnosis

Many inhalants are so quickly metabolized and/or excreted through pulmonary or other routes that they cannot be detected by the time the patient arrives in the emergency department. Standard toxicological screening tests of the blood or urine do not include such chemicals as hydrocarbons or nitrites. However some products, such as paint thinners or glue, may leave chemical signatures behind. A 14-year-old girl who presented to the emergency department with confusion, hallucinations, and intermittent laughing and crying after inhaling glue several times daily for 5 days consecutively, had elevated

TABLE 71.14

Agent-Specific Toxicities of Inhalant Chemicals

Inhalant Chemical	Agent-Specific Toxicity
Toluene	Renal damage, embryopathy
Amyl and butyl nitrites	Methemoglobinemia, hypotension
Gasoline	Lead poisoning, benzene-induced leukemia
Carbon tetrachloride, trichloroethylene	Hepatitis, cirrhosis
Methylene chloride (Paint thinner)	Carbon monoxide poisoning

urinary hippuric acid levels indicative of heavy toluene exposure (Raikhlin-Eisenkraft et al., 2001).

Treatment

Treatment is supportive, and is aimed at control of arrhythmias, and respiratory and circulatory support. Epinephrine should be avoided because it may provoke cardiac irritability in those patients who have inhaled halogenated hydrocarbons. Intubation and mechanical ventilation may be necessary in severely affected patients who present with respiratory depression and blood gas evidence of hypoxia, hypercarbia, and respiratory acidosis.

Nitrous Oxide

Also known as *laughing gas*, nitrous oxide (N_2O) has long been abused by health care personnel. More recently there has been a resurgence of interest in it among the adolescent population. It is most commonly sold in small balloons or inhaled from whipped-cream cans, in which it is used as a propellant. Occasionally, individual users gain access to a tank of nitrous oxide. Deaths have occurred after prolonged inhalation of 100% N_2O in a closed space.

Nitrites

Amyl, butyl, and isobutyl nitrites are examples of nitrites. They are volatile liquids abused for their vasodilatory action and subjective feeling of light-headedness (known as the "*rush*"). Amyl nitrite requires a prescription and is currently indicated in cyanide poisoning to produce methemoglobin. Butyl and isobutyl nitrite are available over the counter (commonly in "head shops") as a room deodorizer, cologne, or liquid incense.

Individuals abusing nitrites rarely seek medical attention for complications of abuse. The most common side effects are severe headache, dizziness, orthostatic hypotension, and occasionally syncope. These effects are a result of smooth muscle relaxation. Nitrites can be oxidizing agents and as such, can cause methemoglobin formation. However, clinically significant methemoglobinemia is extremely rare as a complication of nitrite abuse.

HALLUCINOGENS

The hallucinogen class of drugs includes LSD, PCP, psilocybin, peyote, mescaline, dimethyltryptamine (DMT), morning glory seeds, serenity-tranquility-peace pill (STP), jimsonweed, dextromethorphan, MDMA, MDA, and MDEA. The term *hallucinogen* ("producer of hallucinations") is actually a misnomer, because prototypical hallucinogens such as LSD, mescaline, and psilocybin at typical dosage levels do not cause hallucinations (sensory perception changes without a corresponding environmental stimulus) but rather illusions (perceptual distortion of a real environmental stimulus) or distortions of perceived reality. True hallucinations do occur with the use of volatile solvents such as gasoline. Set (the user's attitudes and expectations) and setting (the drug-taking environment) greatly influence a user's experience with this class of drugs. With the exception of the hallucinogenic amphetamines, physical withdrawal does not occur. However, long-term recrudescence of fleeting distortions and illusions, termed "flashbacks," are not uncommon, and can occur despite abstinence from further experimentation with the drug.

Overall, the prevalence of hallucinogen use decreased in the late 1970s and early 1980s and then began a slow but definite rise in the late 1980s that continued into the 1990s until about 1997, after which rates have again fallen somewhat. Two trends emerging from the "pop culture" scene are partially responsible for the resurgence of LSD and the emergence of the use of MDMA (ecstasy), a hallucinogenic methamphetamine derivative. "Raves" "house" or "circuit" parties (see pages 916–918) involve alternative forms of rock music played in coordination with colorful, pulsating light effects and augmented by the use of LSD or MDMA. Frequently, the drugs are supplied as part of the admission price or by the organizers of the event. An extremely important fact should be remembered in regard to the current patterns of LSD use. In the 1960s, doses of up to 500 µg were not unusual. The average current dose is in the 20- to 80-µg range. Most users today describe a seemingly mild "trip" with colorful visual "tracers," enhancement of sound, and light sensations. Psychiatric emergency services are not seeing the same level of acuteness as was seen in the 1960s. There is clearly a disregard for and underestimation of the dangers of LSD because of the lower dose. However, even at this lower dosage level, one is at risk for chronic psychiatric problems, acute physical trauma, and other consequences of risk-taking behaviors that might occur under the influence of the drug.

Types of Hallucinogens

Table 71.15 contains the subgrouping of hallucinogens based on distinctive psychoactive effects and structure–activity relationship similarities.

Lysergic Acid Diethylamide

LSD was initially developed as a circulatory stimulant, when it was incidentally found to cause hallucinations. In the 1950s, LSD was marketed under the name Delsyd as a treatment for mental illness; the military also had interest in developing the drug as an agent for "mind control." By the mid-1960s no significant medical benefits of the drug had been found, and development stopped. Nonmedical use of LSD became illegal in 1965 and medical production of the drug ended in 1966.

Prevalence/Epidemiology
The abuse of LSD peaked in the 1960s and then drifted lower during the 1970s and 1980s, reaching a low prevalence rate of use (7.2%) by high school seniors by 1986. Yet the drug then experienced somewhat of a resurgence of popularity among youth in the 1990s. By 1997 the lifetime usage rate of LSD among high school seniors, at 13.6% of students, had surpassed the rate of 11.3% recorded in 1975. However, since that time its popularity has again steadily waned, such that only 3.3% of 12th graders reported that they have ever used with LSD in 2006 (Johnston et al., 2007). Corresponding rates of use in 2006 among 8th and 10th graders were 1.6% and 2.7%, respectively.

TABLE 71.15

Types of Hallucinogens and the Psychoactive Effects They Produce

Category	Psychoactive Effect	Examples
Psychedelics	Prominent hallucinations and synesthesias with mild distortion of time and reality, impaired attention/concentration, mild disruption in ego structure	• Indolealkylamines: LSD, psilocybin, DMT • Phenlyalkylamines: mescaline
Enactogens	Structural similarities to psychedelics (mescaline) and amphetamines; unique psychoactive characteristics include improved communication, empathy with others, and positive mood enhancement	MDMA, MDA, MDEA
Dissociative anesthetics	Causes anesthesia, emergence reactions, and 'out of body' experiences	PCP, ketamine
Other	Mild distortion of time, impaired attention/concentration, mild mood enhancement, euphoria and feelings of well-being	Marijuana

LSD, lysergic acid diethylamide; DMT, dimethyltryptamine; MDMA, methylenedioxymethamphetamine; MDA, methylenedioxyamphetamine; MDEA, methylenedioxy-N-ethylamphetamine; PCP, phencyclidine.

Preparation and Dose

LSD is derived from an alkaloid found in rye fungus. It is made by mixing lysergic acid with diethylamide, freezing the mixture, and then extracting the resulting LSD. The procedure is not easy; therefore, much of the LSD sold on the street is either adulterated or contains no LSD.

LSD is an extremely potent drug with doses measured in micrograms. Low doses of LSD (50–75 μg) produce euphoria whereas higher doses result in typical LSD illusions or "trips." In the 1960s the typical illicit dose of LSD was 100 to 300 μg; currently, the usual dose is 20 to 80 μg.

Routes of Administration and Street Names

The drug is commonly distributed as a soluble powder or liquid. It is usually colorless, odorless, and tasteless in its manufactured state, but it is most often colored when sold. It is sold as cylindrical tablets or gelatin squares or applied to small pieces of paper; these preparations are known on the street, respectively, as microdots, windowpanes, and blotters. LSD is also sold as decals or stickers. The drug is ingested by placing the blotter on the tongue where it is dissolved in saliva and absorbed through the mucus membranes. LSD can also be mixed in with foods or liquids for oral consumption; liquid LSD can be absorbed through

the mucus membranes of the eyes. LSD cannot be smoked as it gets destroyed with heat.

Slang names for LSD include acid, beast, big D, black, blue barrels, blotters, blue cheer, boomers, brown dot, cubes, fry, microdots, orange sunshine, panes, sugar, sunshine, trips, white lightning, window panes, and yellow sunshine.

Physiology and Metabolism

LSD is rapidly absorbed from the gastrointestinal tract, with onset of action in 30 to 40 minutes. It binds to receptors throughout the CNS, including the hippocampus, corpus striatum, cerebral cortex and cerebellum. Its main effects result in the inhibition of release of serotonin, which allows increased firing of sensory neurons, as well as resulting in a nonspecific stress response and resulting autonomic changes. The increased reactivity of sensory neurons results in visual and auditory distortions, which form the basis of hallucinations. See Table 71.16 for hallucinogen physiology.

Effects of Intoxication

LSD intoxication results in euphoria and sensory illusions which may give rise to hallucinations. Symptoms of intoxication include dilated pupils, conjunctival injection,

TABLE 71.16

Hallucinogen Physiology

Receptors	Pharmacodynamics	Distribution	Metabolism and Excretion
Nonspecific intracellular binding throughout the central nervous system	Inhibition of serotonin release, resulting in: • Increased firing of sensory neurons • Nonspecific stress response	Primarily protein bound	Rapidly absorbed through the gastrointestinal (GI) tract • Onset of action is 30–40 minutes • Half-life is 3 hours

hyperthermia, tachycardia, hypertension, flushing, and tremor. The sense of being an observer is frequently reported by LSD users and distinguishes LSD psychosis from schizophrenia.

Adverse Effects
1. Psychiatric: Visual and auditory hallucinations, synesthesias, depersonalization, loss of sense of time, loss of ego boundaries, impairment of attention, motivation and concentration, anxiety, depression, paranoia, confusion, flashbacks.
2. Neurological: Flushing, hyperthermia, piloerection, dizziness, paresthesia, dilated pupils, blurred vision, conjunctival injection, lacrimation, hyperactive reflexes, ataxia and tremor, loss of muscle coordination and pain perception, restlessness and sleep disturbances.
3. Cardiovascular: Hypertension and tachycardia.
4. Gastrointestinal: Anorexia, nausea, dry mouth.

Overdose and Emergency Treatment
LSD overdose may result in grand mal seizures, circulatory collapse, coagulopathies, and coma. Treatment is supportive. LSD can be readily detected in urine by thin layer chromatography or other analytical techniques.

Some LSD users experience "bad trips," which are negative emotional responses triggered both by the circumstances of use as well as feelings within the user. These responses terrify the user and may produce a sense of panic, fragmentation, or fear of "going crazy." LSD users may also experience "flashbacks" or the recurrence of the LSD-induced state after the effects of the drug have worn off. Flashbacks may occur spontaneously for variable lengths of time after original drug ingestion. Concurrent use of selective serotonin reuptake inhibitor agents may induce or worsen the LSD flashback syndrome (Markel et al., 1994), possibly as a result of the similarities in serotonin receptor physiology. Important components of treatment include providing a peaceful, calm environment (darkened lights, few extraneous stimuli), and helping the patient to restore contact with reality. The health care provider should try to calm the user by talking to him or her about familiar things. The patient should be reassured that his or her unusual sensations will cease when the drug wears off. The helping individual should listen carefully to the patient and respond sympathetically. Health care providers should avoid discussing the reasons for use of the drug or personal problems during a bad trip, and medication use should be avoided if possible. It is important to monitor the cycles of lucidity and periods of intense reactions to the drug. If the cycles are frequent, then the individual is probably early in the course of experiencing effects of the drug; if the cycles are less frequent, the drug effects may have peaked.

It is important to remember that one cannot rely on the history when managing alleged use of a hallucinogen. Especially in this class of drugs, adulteration, and misrepresentation of the substance are common. In addition, in the case of a patient with clouded sensorium and fever, even with a history of ingestion of LSD, the differential diagnosis must include CNS infection, endocrine disorder, drug or alcohol withdrawal syndrome, and ingestion of an unknown toxin.

Another dilemma occurs in the situation of the combative patient with a history of hallucinogen use. Although chemical and physical restraints are discouraged, if more passive means of calming the patient have not been effective, restraints must be used to facilitate further clinical evaluation and diagnostic testing. It is essential that every health care provider become adept at using at least one sedative and one major tranquilizer. Lorazepam is probably the best suited of the benzodiazepines because it can be given intramuscularly, intravenously, or orally and is more effective than diazepam as an anticonvulsant. Haloperidol and droperidol are superior to the phenothiazines because they have fewer cardiovascular side effects such as hypotension. Droperidol has come into favor recently because of its more rapid onset of action and shorter half-life and because it is approved for intravenous use. It is also more sedating than haloperidol. A cautionary note is that the major tranquilizers can also lower the seizure threshold.

Chronic Use
Chronic adverse effects may include psychosis, depression, and personality changes. The use of a hallucinogen should be considered in the differential diagnosis of an adolescent who presents with a new onset of psychosis.

Tolerance and Withdrawal
Tolerance to LSD develops rapidly but is short lived. Some daily users of LSD describe the practice of "doubling up" (doubling the previous day's dose when using on consecutive days) to counteract tolerance. No withdrawal syndrome is described, although "flashbacks" are common and can be persistent.

Phencyclidine

Prevalence/Epidemiology
The use of PCP has steadily declined from a high of 12.8% in the late 1970s to a lifetime prevalence use of only 2% to 4% through the 1990s, dropping further to only 2.2% of 12th graders in 2006 (Johnston et al., 2007). Only 0.7% of high school seniors reported using PCP within the previous 12 months in 2006.

Preparation and Dose
PCP (Sernyl) is an arylamine (1-[1-phenyl{cyclohexyl} piperidine]) introduced in the 1950s as a general anesthetic. It is structurally related to ketamine. Clinical trials revealed PCP to be an effective anesthetic, but during surgical recovery the emergence reactions to PCP were frequent and unpleasant, with excessive agitation, excitement, and disorientation. A "drowning swimmer" phenomenon, with feelings of imminent suffocation, was prominent. In 1965, the drug was discontinued as a medicinal product for human use. In the late 1960s, its use increased in San Francisco as an experimental psychedelic drug, called the "*peace pill.*" It was unpopular at that time because of excessive reports of bad trips. However, during the middle and late 1970s its popularity increased tremendously, and it became one of the nation's major drugs of abuse. Until 1978, the drug was still legally manufactured as Semylan for veterinary anesthesia. Dose ranges vary tremendously, from 0.1 to more than 150 mg in one survey. In addition, approximately 20% of drug samples sold as PCP contained no PCP. In terms of potency, <5 mg is considered a low dose, 5 to 10 mg a moderate dose, and >10 mg a high dose.

TABLE 71.17

Phencyclidine Physiology

Receptors	Pharmacodynamics	Distribution	Metabolism and Excretion
Glutamate-*N*-methyl-D-aspartate (NMDA) receptors	• Increases the production of dopamine • Inhibits dopamine reuptake	Metabolites are fat soluble, although not physiologically active	• Metabolized by the liver to monopiperidine conjugate • pH dependent urinary excretion

Routes of Administration and Street Names

PCP may be packaged as a liquid, powder, tablet, leaf mixture, or rock crystal. It can be used intravenously (average dose, 10 mg), intramuscularly, or orally (average dose, 5 mg), or it can be snorted (average dose, 5 mg) or smoked (average dose, 3 mg). Street names for PCP include angel dust, dummy dust, magic dust, peace, peace pill, rocket fuel, whack, zombie weed, and zoom.

Physiology and Metabolism

PCP is the hydrogen chloride salt of PCP. It is a dissociative anesthetic with analgesic, stimulant, depressant, and hallucinogenic properties. The pharmacology of PCP is complex and not fully understood. Its major psychiatric effects are thought to be the result of binding to the glutamate-NMDA receptors, to increase the production of dopamine and inhibit reuptake. The drug acts on the thalamus, midbrain, and sensory cortex to impair proprioception and the brain's ability to organize input. PCP is rapidly inactivated by hepatic metabolism and is excreted in the urine as monopiperidine conjugate. Because PCP is fat soluble, it has the ability to remain in the body for prolonged periods. Its urinary excretion is highly dependent on urine pH, with significantly higher excretion rates at an acidic pH. The half-life of PCP is 3 days. See Table 71.17 for phencyclidine physiology.

Effects of Intoxication

The clinical symptoms of PCP use vary with the dose, the route of administration, and the experience of the user. Intravenous, intramuscular, and oral routes of administration are more difficult to regulate than the smoking of PCP. In addition, inexperienced users have more side effects than experienced users do. PCP usually induces one of several clinical states (see Table 71.18 for PCP intoxication states).

PCP is the only drug of abuse that causes a characteristic *vertical nystagmus*. It can also cause horizontal or rotatory nystagmus. Other symptoms include ataxia, miosis with reactive pupils, hypertension, and increased deep tendon reflexes.

Diagnosis

The diagnosis of PCP use should be suspected in all adolescents with a distorted thought process, especially when there is evidence of analgesia or nystagmus. Any individual with open-eye coma, horizontal and vertical nystagmus, hypertension, and rigidity should be considered to have taken PCP. PCP can be detected in the blood, urine, and gastrointestinal secretions; the best fluid to sample is the urine. A serum concentration of 25 to 100 ng/mL may be found in patients who are in an acute state of confusion; a level of >100 ng/mL may be found in comatose patients. The urinary concentration may vary in different clinical states. Excretion in the urine is highly pH dependent and decreases dramatically as the pH becomes alkaline.

Adverse Effects

Adverse effects associated with PCP use are dose related (Table 71.19).

Overdose and Emergency Treatment

PCP use may result in generalized motor seizures either early in the course of intoxication or delayed in appearance. Hypertension is usually mild, but there was one reported case of hypertensive cerebral hemorrhage in a 13-year-old adolescent (Eastman et al., 1975). Cogen et al (1978) reported rhabdomyolysis in patients with PCP poisoning, due to increased muscular contractions, muscle rigidity, and increased tone. Death can occur and is usually caused by injuries sustained during periods of analgesia and aggression directed at self or others. Death can also occur

TABLE 71.18

Phencyclidine Intoxication States

Acute intoxication	Delusion, disinhibition, dissociation ("out of body" experience)
Acute or prolonged delirium	Disorientation, clouded consciousness, and abnormal cognition
Schizophreniform psychosis	Hallucinations, thought disorder, and delusions
Mania	Hallucinations, elevated mood, elevated self-attitude, feelings of omnipotence
Depressive reactions	Dysphoria, social withdrawal, paranoia, isolation

TABLE 71.19

Adverse Effects of Phencyclidine by Dose

Low dose (<5 mg)	
Blank stare	Behavioral disorders:
Horizontal and vertical nystagmus	• Disorganized thought processes
Ataxia	• Distortion of body image and of objects
Hypertension	• Amnesia
Increased deep tendon reflexes	• Agitated or combative behavior
Decreased proprioception and sensations	• Unresponsive behavior
Miosis or midposition, reactive pupils	• Disinhibition of underlying psychopathology
Diaphoresis	• Schizophrenic reactions
Flushing	• Catalepsy, catatonia
	• Illusions
	• Anxiety, excitement
Moderate dose (5–10 mg)	
Hypertension	Hypersalivation
Vertical and horizontal nystagmus	Mutism
Myoclonus	Amnesia
Midposition pupil size	Anxiety, excitement
Dysarthria	Delusions
Diaphoresis	Behavior:
Fever	• Stupor or extreme agitation
	• Violent or psychotic behavior can occur
High dose (>10 mg)	
Unresponsive, immobile state	Spontaneous nystagmus
Eyes that may remain open during coma	Miosis
Hypertension	Decreased urine output
Arrhythmias	Dysarthria
Increased deep tendon reflexes	Diaphoresis and flushing
Muscle rigidity	Fever
Decerebrate posturing	Amnesia
Convulsions	Mutism
Extremely high dose (>500 mg)	
Prolonged coma	Hypoventilation
Rigidity	Hypertension or hypotension
Extensor (decerebrate) posturing	Prolonged and fluctuating confusional state after
Seizures	recovery from coma

as a result of convulsions and cerebral hemorrhage. One case report described an infant with abnormal behavior and abnormal facies born to a mother who used PCP (Golden et al., 1980).

Reduction of stimuli: When treating patients with PCP overdose, health care providers must use extreme caution. Patients are unpredictable and often have little awareness of the consequences of their behavior. Reducing the levels of light, sound, and other external stimuli can rapidly calm down a PCP user. In an emergency, covering the intoxicated patient with a blanket may be helpful. All hazards should be removed from the environment. Patients should not be touched or cornered. Restraints are not recommended; they may cause the patient to harm himself or herself in an attempt to escape. Health care providers should not attempt to talk to a patient who has recently used PCP.

Supportive care: Treatment for PCP overdose is largely supportive. In addition to basic cardiopulmonary resuscitation, it is essential to check for signs of head, neck, back, and internal injuries, which can occur because of the behavioral effects of the drug. Unconscious victims should be placed on their side so that aspiration does not occur.

Medications: Try to avoid administering other medications, but, if necessary, intravenous diazepam or lorazepam can be used to treat seizures. Severe agitation and psychosis can be treated with haloperidol. Avoid phenothiazines and neuroleptics because of the risk of excessive orthostatic hypotension and the potential for enhancing the cholinergic imbalance. Intravenous diphenhydramine may be used for dystonias.

Recovery: Recovery usually occurs within 24 hours but can take days, depending on the dose and the acidity of the urine. During the recovery phase, an adolescent may require short-term inpatient psychiatric care to deal with paranoia, regressive behavior, and a slow phase of reintegration. With higher doses the coma can last 5 to 6 days and can be followed by a prolonged recovery period marked by behavioral disorders. Cognitive, memory, and speech disorders may last up to 1 year after the last use of PCP. Flashbacks may occur, as with LSD.

Dextromethorphan

Dextromethorphan, the dextro isomer of the codeine analog, levorphanol, has a chemical structure resembling a synthetic opiate, but lacks an opiate's potent analgesic, sedative, or addicting properties. The drug's prominent antitussive properties make it a common ingredient in nonprescription cough and cold syrups, usually in amounts of 10 to 15 mg per teaspoon or per tablespoon. While the use of most hallucinogens is on the decline, the misuse of over-the-counter cold and cough medicines as an inexpensive "high" is one of the fastest growing drugs of abuse. Maximum daily doses range from 30 mg for children to 120 mg for adults. Those engaged in substance abuse may drink 8 to 16 oz of such a cough syrup in an attempt to get high. The volume of cough syrup required to get "high" has led adolescents to order the pure, highly concentrated powder from Internet sources, or to purchase high concentration dextromethorphan-containing tablets such as Coricidin products instead (Kirages et al., 2003). Street language describes the abuse of dextromethorphan as "Robing out," "robo-copping," "triple C," "DXMing," or "Dexing." Dextromethorphan can induce euphoria, and produce dissociative effects.

Physiology and Metabolism Dextromethorphan in high doses binds to opiate sigma receptors, which may account for some of its sedative and psychomimetic properties. The drug is metabolized by O-demethylation to an active metabolite, dextrorphan, which interacts with the same PCP receptor in NMDA neurotransmitter complex. This primary metabolism is under the control of hepatic cytochrome complex, CYP2D6, whose genetic polymorphisms may explain why some users are more susceptible to adverse effects than others (Zawertailo et al., 1998). The dug undergoes secondary conjugation in the liver to inactive glucuronide and sulfate esters, and has an elimination half-life of approximately 3.3 hours.

Intoxication The actions of dextrorphan may explain dextromethorphan's PCP-like symptoms in overdose (Szekely et al., 1991). It can produce somnolence and ataxia, slurred speech, hallucinations, dysphoria, nystagmus, dystonia, tachycardia, and elevated blood pressure. Dextromethorphan also blocks presynaptic serotonin reuptake and has dopaminergic properties. Dextromethorphan may interact with other drugs, including selective serotonin reuptake inhibitors, MAO inhibitors, tricyclic antidepressants, and lithium, to produce movement disorders or the serotonin syndrome of rigidity and hyperthermia. It is also fetotoxic in animal studies.

Treatment Routine toxic screening of the blood for opiates may remain negative despite recent use of dextromethorphan. However in some cases depending on concentration, the test for PCP may be weakly positive in dextromethorphan poisoning. Treatment is supportive; the role of naloxone is not well established although there are case reports of its efficacy (Schneider et al., 1991). Health care providers should note that dextromethorphan poisonings often involve concomitant intoxications with other ingredients in over the counter cold medications such as acetaminophen, antihistamines, pseudoephedrine, and guaifenesin, for which additional medical therapies may be necessary (Schwartz, 2005). Because dextromethorphan is formulated as a hydrobromide salt, an overdose with the drug can also produce toxic effects, such as somnolence, related to bromide poisoning.

Psilocybin

Mushrooms containing psilocybin and psilocin produce effects similar to those of the other hallucinogens. Users reportedly experience euphoria, prominent visual and auditory hallucinations and synesthesias (i.e., perceptual distortions resulting in an apparent ability to visualize sounds or hear colors). The mushrooms are ingested orally, and there is a rapid onset of effects in approximately 15 minutes. The effects peak at 90 minutes, begin to wear off in 2 to 3 hours, and disappear after approximately 5 or 6 hours. The average dose is 4 to 10 mg of psilocybin. Street names for psilocybin mushrooms include "shrooms," mushrooms, Silly Putty, magic Mexican mushrooms, and psychedelic mushrooms. Because many other species can be confused with true *psilocybe* mushrooms, ingestion of misidentified, toxic non-*psilocybe* species can pose a special danger to users.

Jimson Weed

Jimson weed (*Datura stramonium*) is an annual plant found growing wild along roadways and railroad trestles in many parts of the United States, Canada, and the West Indies. Also known as locoweed, thorn apple, devil's apple, angel's trumpet and stink weed, the plant has anticholinergic and mildly hallucinogenic properties. Seed-containing pods ripen in the late summer and autumn. The toxins in the seeds, leaves and roots include tropane belladonna alkaloids such as hyoscyamine, atropine, and scopolamine, with the highest concentrations of these alkaloids present in the seeds. These chemicals act as competitive antagonists to acetylcholine at both central and peripheral parasympathetic receptor sites, with paralysis of parasympathetic innervated organs. Peripheral receptors include exocrine glands controlling sweating, salivation, and smooth and cardiac muscle cells. As tertiary amines, they also cross the blood brain barrier to cause a central anticholinergic syndrome.

Adolescents make tea from the seeds, eat the seeds themselves, or smoke cigarettes made from jimson weed. Pleasurable effects include mild euphoria and hallucinations. However these are more than offset by severe retching, abdominal pain, agitation, headaches, respiratory arrest, and coma. First-time users who experience many of the adverse effects rarely experiment with jimsonweed again. Onset of symptoms is usually within an hour or two; the delayed gastric emptying and slow intestinal motility attributable to anticholinergic effects may prolong the duration of symptoms in untreated patients for as long as several days.

Users may present to the emergency room with the dry mouth, dilated pupils, urinary retention, flushed warm dry skin, tachycardia, and hypo- or hypertension. Decontamination using oral activated charcoal is recommended. Agitated delirium is typical of the central anticholinergic syndrome and will usually resolve upon administration of a benzodiazepine sedative or the cholinergic agent, physostigmine. (Note: Physostigmine should be reserved for only the most severe poisonings and used with precautions such as ECG monitoring, because the administration of cholinergic agents can themselves induce seizures, cholinergic crisis, bradyarrhythmia or asystole). Elevated body temperature remits with the use of fans, cooling blankets, and antipyretics. Repeated retching after jimsonweed use is common and may require treatment with antiemetics; catheterization of the bladder may be necessary to treat urinary retention.

Peyote and Mescaline

Peyote is a cactus (*Lophophora*) that grows in the southwestern United States and in Mexico. The tops of the cactus contain numerous alkaloids, including mescaline (3,4,5-trimethoxyphenethylamine), but they are difficult to find and not readily available to the drug abuse marketplace. Most drugs sold as "mescaline" capsules contain no mescaline, but rather contain LSD, PCP, both LSD and PCP, or something else. Peyote is sold either as buttons derived from the cactus or as capsules containing ground peyote. Street names include big chief, buttons, cactus, mesc, and mescal. The usual human dose ranges from 100 to 500 mg.

Mescaline has its onset of action within 30 minutes to 2 hours after ingestion, and the effects last for 6 to 12 hours. The mescaline high is less intense and less disorienting than LSD and tends to intensify body sense (as opposed to LSD which has a stronger effect on the mind). Mescaline use is frequently accompanied by unpleasant side effects such as nausea and vomiting.

Bad trips are less severe and less frequent with mescaline than with LSD, though tolerance and dependence do occur.

Serenity-Tranquility-Peace Pill

STP (also known as the "*serenity-tranquility-peace pill*") is related to mescaline but approximately 100 times more potent. Its effects are also similar to those of other hallucinogenic drugs, with the exception that with STP the incidence of unpleasant sensations is increased and the effects seem to last longer, up to 72 hours.

Dimethyltryptamine

DMT is a natural constituent of the seeds of several plants found in the West Indies and South America. DMT is usually prepared as an orange liquid in which either tobacco, marijuana, or parsley is soaked and then smoked; it is inactive orally. This drug has effects similar to those of other hallucinogens, except that the "trip" is short, lasting only 1 to 3 hours. DMT is known on the street as the "businessman's special" or "businessman's lunch."

Morning Glory Seeds

The seeds of some members of the bindweed family, including the morning glory (*Rivea corymbosa* and *Ipomoea*), have been used for centuries for their hallucinogenic effects. Morning glory seeds are legally available on seed racks, but, to prevent spoilage, seeds intended for planting are usually coated with dangerous chemicals such as methyl mercury. The active principal ingredient in the seeds is similar to LSD but approximately one tenth as potent. The effects of morning glory seeds are similar to those of LSD; however, there is an increase in side effects such as nausea, dizziness, and diarrhea, and there is an extremely bitter taste.

Nutmeg

Nutmeg is extracted from the dried seed kernels of an evergreen tree found in the South Pacific Islands. This common spice is ubiquitous in household pantries, and outbreaks of its use usually follow media reports of its hallucinogenic properties. However the dried spice quickly loses its potency on the shelf. Fresh nutmeg contains terpene hydrocarbons (e.g., pinene, camphene) as well as eugenol, safrole, borneol, and several hallucinatory allylbenzene derivatives, such as myristicin and elemicin, which can be converted into hallucinogenic amphetamine and mescaline-like congeners. Abuse requires the ingestion of large quantities of freshly ground seed, because the volatile oils, comprising 8% to 15% of a nutmeg by weight, are necessary for its CNS effects. Users typically grind and swallow 3 to 10 or so nutmegs (approximately 20–80 g of powder), containing approximately 3 to 10 g of the myristicin-containing oil (Stein et al., 2001). Effects include delirium, hallucinations, and euphoria, with onset within 30 minutes or so. One 13-year old girl developed visual, auditory, and tactile hallucinations after ingesting 15 to 24 g of nutmeg and smoking marijuana; she recovered after receiving decontamination with oral activated charcoal (Sangalli et al., 2000).

The presence of an extremely potent emetic, geraniol, has discouraged widespread use. The predominant effects of nutmeg overdose are anticholinergic mydriasis, dry mouth, tachycardia, dizziness and repeated vomiting. Some patients may experience anxiety reactions with agitation and restlessness. Others may develop allergic reactions and rashes (Van den Akker et al., 1990). One 18-year-old woman developed severe anxiety, dilated pupils, dry mouth, palpitations, dizziness, tachycardia, and a "trance-like" state, but no hallucinations, 30 minutes after drinking a milk shake containing 50 g of grated nutmeg (Demetriades et al., 2005). She was rehydrated and reassured, and symptoms had resolved 16 hours after the ingestion.

ANABOLIC STEROIDS

Anabolic steroids are synthetic derivatives of testosterone (see also Chapter 18). Abusers of this class of drug exhibit tolerance, withdrawal, and psychological dependence. Treatment may require detoxification and a rehabilitation phase comparable to traditional drug treatment.

The numerous agents fit into two basic categories: the oral agents are 17α-methyl derivatives of testosterone, and the injectable agents are esters of testosterone and 19-nortestosterone. The ideal steroid would have maximal anabolic and minimal androgenic activity and a longer half-life than the parent compound, testosterone. The 17α-alkylated steroids have a half-life of 8 to 10 hours, whereas the injectable forms have half-lives in the range of 21 days. Although these agents have less androgenic activity in lower dosage ranges, this advantage is lost at higher doses. Many abusers use 10 times the usual therapeutic dose and use combinations of oral and injectable agents concurrently in 6- to 12-week cycles ("stacking").

Prevalence and Epidemiology

Use of anabolic steroids by high school students has remained steady, with 1.6% of 8th graders, 1.8% of 10th graders, and 2.7% of 12th graders in 2006 reporting that they have experimented with steroids at least once in their life (Johnston et al., 2007). Annual prevalence of use rates in 2006 slipped to 0.9% in 8th graders (1.7% in 2000), 1.2% of 10th graders (2.2% in 2000) and 1.8% of 12th graders (2.5% in 2004). Whereas it was previously thought that only male athletes used steroids and only for strength training, and that these students did not abuse other drugs, these assumptions were shown to be false by Durant et al. (1993; 1995) to be false. Those students using anabolic steroids were also likely to be engaging in other forms of substance abuse. These researchers analyzed the Centers for Disease Control's Youth Risk Behavior Survey of 12,272 high school students and found that males outnumbered females in steroid use 4:1, but that females also reported steroid use for increasing strength and muscle tone. Adolescent steroid users were more likely than other students to engage in injected drug use and use of other substances such as cocaine, tobacco, amphetamines, and alcohol. In the 2005 Youth Risk Behavior Survey, 4.8% of males in high school and 3.2% of females reported ever having used steroids illegally.

Adverse Effects

1. Psychiatric: Psychosis, mania, mood swings, hyperaggressive behavior, violence. Withdrawal may be associated with depression.
2. Cardiovascular: Decreased high density lipoprotein cholesterol, hypertension, ventricular remodeling, myocardial ischemia, sudden death.
3. Endocrine: Premature epiphyseal closure and shortened stature, female virilization and hypogonadism, testicular atrophy, reduced libido, infertility.
4. Other: Acne, hemolysis, enlarged prostate gland, hepatocellular carcinoma with chronic use.

Treatment of Withdrawal or Dependence

Patients exhibiting psychotic behavior or severe depression require inpatient care. Appropriate pharmacological intervention with antipsychotic, antidepressant, and anxiolytic agents may be indicated, usually for a short period. For the patient meeting DSM-IV criteria (3 of 12 listed) for substance dependence, a traditional drug treatment approach is indicated. Attending 12-step meetings and "working a program" are ideal methods to provide the adolescent with a conceptual framework to work through this problem.

WEB SITES

General

http://www.monitoringthefuture.org/. Monitoring the future is a large epidemiologic survey of the behaviors, attitudes and values of American secondary students, college students and adults.

http://www.nida.nih.gov/MOM/MOMIndex.html. National Institute on Drug Abuse (NIDA), NIH. The Mind Over Matter series is designed to encourage young people in grades 5 through 9 to learn about the effects of drug abuse on the body and the brain. The types of drugs discussed include inhalants, hallucinogens, steroids, opiates, and nicotine. The series also offers a teachers' guide that provides background information and lesson plans.

http://www.nida.nih.gov/DrugAbuse.html. Information from NIDA on many drugs

http://www.nida.nih.gov/DrugsofAbuse.html. Information on side effects of drugs of abuse from NIDA

Specific Substances

Amphetamines/Cocaine
http://www.nida.nih.gov/Infofax/ecstasy.html.
http://www.nida.nih.gov/ResearchReports/Cocaine/Cocaine.html.

Club Drugs
http://www.nida.nih.gov/Infofax/Clubdrugs.html.
http://www.nida.nih.gov/Infofax/RohypnolGHB.html.

Hallucinogens
http://www.nida.nih.gov/MOM/HALL/MOMHALL1.html.
http://ncadi.samhsa.gov/.
http://www.nida.nih.gov/Infofax/lsd.html.
http://www.nida.nih.gov/Infofax/pcp.html.

Opiates
http://www.nida.nih.gov/ResearchReports/Heroin/.

REFERENCES AND ADDITIONAL READINGS

Aharonovich E, Liu X, Samet S, et al. Postdischarge cannabis use and its relationship to cocaine, alcohol, and heroin use: a prospective study. *Am J Psychiatry* 2005;162:1507.

Andreu V, Mas A, Bruguera M, et al. Ecstasy: a common cause of severe acute hepatotoxicity. *J Hepatol* 1998;29:394.

Anonymous. *Drug ID Bible*. Amera-Chem, Inc., Grand Junction, Colorado, 2004.

Bahrke MS, Yesalis CE, Brower KJ. Anabolic-androgenic steroid abuse and performance-enhancing drugs among adolescents. *Child Adolesc Psychol Clin North Am* 1998;7: 821.

Boddiger D. Methamphetamine use linked to rising HIV transmission. *Lancet* 2005;365:1217.

Bolla KI, Funderburk FR, Cadet JL. Differential effects of cocaine and alcohol on neurocognitive performance. *Neurology* 2000;54:2285.

Bolla KI, McCann UD, Ricaurte GA. Memory impairment in abstinent MDMA (Ecstasy) users. *Neurology* 1998;51:1532.

Boyer E, Woolf A. What's new on the street? *Clin Pediatr Emerg Care* 2000;1:180.

Boyer E, Quang L, Woolf A, et al. Dextromethorphan and ecstasy pills. *JAMA* 2001;285:409.

Brauer RB, Heidecke CD, Nathrath W, et al. Liver transplantation for the treatment of fulminant hepatic failure induced by the ingestion of ecstasy. *Transpl Int* 1997;10:229.

Burgess C, O'Donohoe A, Gill M. Agony and ecstasy: a review of MDMA effects and toxicity. *Eur Psychiatry* 2000;15: 287.

Centers for Disease Control and Prevention. Youth Risk Behavior Surveillance—United States, 2005. *MMWR* 2006;55(ss-5): 1. http://www.cdc.gov/mmwr/PDF/SS/SS5505.pdf.

Chambers HF, Morris L, Tauber MG, et al. Cocaine use and the risk for endocarditis in intravenous drug users. *Ann Intern Med* 1987;106:833.

Childers SR, Breivogel CS. Cannabis and endogenous cannabinoid systems. *Drug Alcohol Depend* 1998;51:173.

Cogen FC, Rigg G, Simmons JL, et al. Phencyclidine-associated acute rhabdomyolysis. *Ann Intern Med* 1978;88:210.

Court JM. Cannabis and brain function. *J Paediatr Child Health* 1998;34:1.

Crowley TJ, Macdonald MJ, Whitmore EA, et al. Cannabis dependence, withdrawal, and reinforcing effects among adolescents with conduct symptoms and substance use disorders. *Drug Alcohol Depend* 1998;50:27.

Curran HV. Is MDMA ("Ecstasy") neurotoxic in humans? An overview of evidence and of methodological problems in research. *Neuropsychobiology* 2000;42:34.

Demetriades AK, Wallman PD, McGuiness A, et al. Low cost, high risk: accidental nutmeg intoxication. *Emerg Med J* 2005; 22:223.

Dowling GP, McDonough ET, Bost RO. A report of five deaths associated with the use of MDEA and MDMA. *JAMA* 1997;257:1615.

DuPont RL. Marijuana, alcohol, and adolescence: a malignant synergism. *Semin Adolesc Med* 1985;1(4):311.

Durant RH, Rickert VI, Ashworth CS, et al. Use of multiple drugs among adolescents who use anabolic steroids. *N Engl J Med* 1993;328:922.

Durant RH, Escobedo LG, Heath GW. Anabolic steroid use, strength training, and multiple drug use among adolescents in the United States. *Pediatrics* 1995;96(1 part 1):23.

Eastman JW, Cohen SN. Hypertensive crisis and death associated with phencyclidine. *JAMA* 1975;231:1270.

Ferguson RP, Hasson J, Walker S. Metastatic lung cancer in a young marijuana smoker. *JAMA* 1989;261:41.

Fisher BAC, Ghuran A, Vadamalai V, et al. Cardiovascular complications induced by cannabis smoking: a case report and review of the literature. *Emerg Med J* 2005;22:679.

Fligiel SE, Roth MD, Kleerup EC, et al. Tracheobronchial histopathology in habitual smokers of cocaine, marijuana, and/or tobacco. *Chest* 1997;112:319.

Friedman L, Fleming NF, Roberts DH, eds. *Source book of substance abuse & addiction.* Williams & Wilkins, Baltimore, Md, 1996.

Friedman R. The changing face of teenage drug abuse—the trend toward prescription drugs. *N Eng J Med* 2006;354:14.

Fudala P. Office-based treatment of opiate addiction with a sulingual-tablet formulation of buprenorphine and naloxone. *N Engl J Med* 2003;349:949.

Gerra G, Zaimovic A, Ferri M, et al. Long-lasting effects of (+/−) 3,4-methylenedioxymethamphetamine (ecstasy) on serotonin system function in humans. *Biol Psychiatry* 2000;47:127.

Gil E, Chen B, Kleerup E, et al. Acute and chronic effects of marijuana smoking on pulmonary alveolar permeability. *Life Sci* 1995;56:2193.

Golden NL, Sokol RJ, Rubin L. Angel dust: possible effects on the fetus. *Pediatrics* 1980;65:18.

Gomez-Balaguer M, Pena H, Morillas C, et al. Syndrome of inappropriate antidiuretic hormone secretion and "designer drugs" (ecstasy). *J Pediatr Endocrinol Metab* 2000;13:437.

Gourgoutis G, Das G. Gastrointestinal manifestations of cocaine addiction. *Int J Clin Pharmacol Ther* 1994;32:136.

Henry JA, Jeffreys KJ, Dawling S. Toxicity and deaths from 3,4-methylenedioxymethamphetamine ("ecstasy"). *Lancet* 1992;340:384.

Hollander JE, Burstein JL, Hoffman RS, et al. Cocaine-associated myocardial infarction: clinical safety of thrombolytic therapy. Cocaine Associated Myocardial Infarction (CAMI) Study Group. *Chest* 1995;107:1237.

Jatlow P. Cocaethylene: pharmacologic activity and clinical significance. *Ther Drug Monit* 1993;15:533.

Johnston LD, O'Malley PM, Bachman JG, et al. *Monitoring the future national results on adolescent drug use: Overview of key findings, 2004.* Bethesda Maryland: National Institute on Drug Abuse, 2005. NIH Publication. Available: www.monitoringthefuture.org; accessed 09/23/05.

Johnston LD, O'Malley PMBachman JG, et al. *Teen drug use down but progress halts among youngest teens.* Ann Arbor, MI: University of Michigan News and Information Services, December 19 2005. [On-line]. Available: www.monitoringthefuture.org; accessed 01/19/06 2006.

Johnston LD, O'Malley PM, Bachman JG et al.. *Teen drug use down but progress halts among youngest teens.* Ann Arbor, MI: University of Michigan News and Information Services, December 19, 2005 [On-line]. Available: www.monitoringthefuture.org; accessed 06/23/2006 2006.

Johnston LD, O'Malley PM, Bachman JG, et al. *Monitoring the Future: National results on adolescent drug use: Overview of key findings, 2006.* (NIH Publication No. 07-6202). Bethesda, MD: National Institute on Drug Abuse, 2007:684. NIH Publication No. 06–5883.

Kalix P. Khat, an amphetamine-like stimulant. *J Psychoactive Drugs* 1994;26:69.

Kashani J, Ruha AM. Methamphetamine toxicity secondary to intravaginal body stuffing. *Clin Toxicol* 2004;42:987.

Kirages TJ, Sule HP, Mycyk MB. Severe manifestations of Coricidin® intoxication. *Am J Emerg Med* 2003;21:473.

Kish SJ, Furukawa Y, Ang L, et al. Striatal serotonin is depleted in brain of a human MDMA (Ecstasy) user. *Neurology* 2000;55: 294.

Kloner RA, Rezkalla SH. Cocaine and the heart. *N Engl J Med* 2003;348:487.

Lai TI, Hwang J, Fang C, et al. Methylene 3,4-dioxymethamphetamine-induced acute myocardial infarction. *Ann Emerg Med* 2003;42:759.

Lange RA, Hillis LD. Cardiovascular complications of cocaine use. *N Engl J Med* 2001;345:351.

Leirer VO, Yesavage JA. Marijuana carry-over effects on aircraft pilot performance. *Aviat Space Environ Med* 1991;62:221.

MacKenzie RG, Heischober B. Methamphetamine. *Pediatr Rev* 1997;18:305.

Markel H, Lee A, Holmes RD, et al. LSD flashback syndrome exacerbated by selective serotonin reuptake inhibitor antidepressants in adolescents. *J Pediatr* 1994;125:817.

McCarron MM, Wood D. The cocaine body packer syndrome. *JAMA* 1983;250:1417.

McGee R, Williams S, Poulton R, et al. A longitudinal study of cannabis use and mental health from adolescence to early adulthood. *Addiction* 2000;95:491.

McGregor C, Srisurapanont M, Jittiwutikarn J, et al. The nature, time course, and severity of methamphetamine withdrawal. *Addiction* 2005;100:1320.

McGuire P. Long-term psychiatric and cognitive effects of MDMA use. *Toxicol Lett* 2000;112:153.

Mittleman MA, Lewis RA, Maclure M, et al. Triggering myocardial infarction by marijuana. *Circulation* 2001;103:2805.

Morland J. Toxicity of drug abuse—amphetamine designer drugs (ecstasy): mental effects and consequences of single dose use. *Toxicol Lett* 2000;147:112–113.

Mouhaffel AH, Madu EC, Satmary WA, et al. Cardiovascular complications of cocaine. *Chest* 1995;107:1426.

Mueller PA, Korey WS. Death by 'ecstasy': the serotonin syndrome?. *Ann Emerg Med* 1998;32:377.

National Consensus Development Panel on Effective Medical Treatment of Opiate Addiction. Effective medical treatment of opiate addiction. *JAMA* 1998;280:1936.

O'Brien CP. Benzodiazepine use, abuse and dependence. *J Clin Psychiatry* 2005;66:28.

O'Connell T, Kaye L, Plosay JJ III. Gamma-hydroxybutyrate (GHB): a newer drug of abuse. *Am Fam Physician* 2000;62:2478.

O'Connor PG. Treating opioid dependence: new data and new opportunities. *N Engl J Med* 2000;343:1332.

Parrott AC. Human research on MDMA (3,4-methylenedioxymethamphetamine) neurotoxicity: cognitive and behavioural indices of change. *Neuropsychobiology* 2000a;42:17.

Parrott AC, Sisk E, Turner JJ. Psychobiological problems in heavy "ecstasy" (MDMA) polydrug users. *Drug Alcohol Depend* 2000b;60:105.

Patton G, Coffey C, Carlin J, et al. Cannabis use and mental health in young people: cohort study. *BMJ* 2002;325:1195.

Perry HE, Wright R, Shannon M, et al. Baclofen overdose: drug experimentation in a group of adolescents. *Pediatrics* 1998;101:1045.

Pertwee RG. Pharmacology of cannabinoid CB1 and CB2 receptors. *Pharmacol Ther* 1997;74:129.

Pope HG Jr, Gruber AJ, Yugelun-Todd D. The residual neuropsychological effects of cannabis: the current status of research. *Drug Alcohol Depend* 1995;38:25.

Pope HG, Yurgelun-Todd D. The residual cognitive effects of heavy marijuana use. *JAMA* 1996;275:521.

Porcerelli JH, Sandler BA. Anabolic-androgenic steroid abuse and psychopathology. *Psychol Clin North Am* 1998;21:829.

Quang LS, Shannon MW, Woolf AD, et al. 4-methylpyrazole (4-MP, Fomepizole, Antizol) is an antidote in CD-1 mice for the delayed and additive toxicity from ethanol and 1,4-butanediol (1,4-BD) overdose. *Life Sci* 2002;71(88):771.

Quang LS, Desai MC, Kramer JC, et al. 4-methylpyrazole (4-MP, Fomepizol, Antizol) decreases 1,4-butanediol (1,4-BD) toxicity by blocking its in vivobiotransformation to gamma-hydroxybutyric acid. *Ann NY Acad Sci* 2004;1025:528.

Quang LS, Levy HL, Law T, et al. Use of the urine organic acid analysis to confirm suspected cases of acute gamma-hydroxy-butyrate overdoses: an animal study. *Clin Toxicol* 2005;43:321.

Raikhlin-Eisenkraft B, Hoffer E, Baum Y, et al. Determination of urinary hippuric acid in toluene abuse. *Clin Toxicol* 2001;39:73.

Randall T. Cocaine, alcohol mix in body to form even longer lasting, more lethal drug. *JAMA* 1992;257:1043.

Reneman L, Booij J, de Bruin K, et al. Effects of dose, sex, and long-term abstention from use on toxic effects of MDMA (ecstasy) on brain serotonin neurons. *Lancet* 2001;358:1864.

Ricaurte GA, Fomo LS, Wilson MA, et al. (+) 3,4-methylenedioxymethamphetamine selectively damages central serotonergic neurons in nonhuman primates. *JAMA* 1988;260:51.

Richards JR, Derlet RW, Duncan DR. Chemical restraint for the agitated patient in the emergency department: lorazepam versus droperidol. *JEMS* 1998;16:567.

Richards JR, Johnson EB, Stark RW. Methamphetamine abuse and rhabdomyolysis in the ED: a 5-year study. *Am J Emerg Med* 1999;17:681.

Rochester JA, Kirchner JT. Ecstasy (3,4-methylenedioxy-methamphetamine): history, neurochemistry, and toxicology. *J Am Board Fam Pract* 1999;12:137.

Rose JS. Cocaethylene: a current understanding of the active metabolite of cocaine and ethanol. *Am J Emerg Med* 1994;12:489.

Rosenberg NL, Grigsby J, Dreisbach J, et al. Neuropsychologic impairment and MRI abnormalities associated with chronic solvent abuse. *Clin Toxicol* 2002;40:21.

Roth D, Alarcon FJ, Fernandez JA, et al. Acute rhabdomyolysis associated with cocaine intoxication. *N Engl J Med* 1988;319:673.

Sangalli BC, Chiang W. Toxicology of nutmeg abuse. *Clin Toxicol* 2000;38:671.

Satran A, Bart BA, Henry CR, et al. Increased prevalence of coronary artery aneurysms among cocaine users. *Circulation* 2005;111:2424.

Schneider SM, Michelson EA, Boucek CD, et al. Dextromethorphan poisoning reversed by naloxone. *Am J Emerg Med* 1991;9:237.

Schwab M, Seyringer E, Brauer R, et al. Fatal MDMA intoxication. *Lancet* 1999;353:593.

Schwartz RH. Marijuana: an overview. *Pediatr Clin North Am* 1987;34:305.

Schwartz TH. Adolescent abuse of dextromethorphan. *Clin Pediatr* 2005;44:565.

Sherman MP, Roth MD, Gong H Jr, et al. Marijuana smoking, pulmonary function, and lung macrophage oxidant release. *Pharmacol Biochem Behav* 1991;40:663.

Soliwij N, Michie T, Fox AM. Effects of long-term cannabis use on selective attention: an event-related potential study. [Special issue: Pharmacological chemical, biochemical and behavioral research on cannabis and the cannabinoids.]. *Pharmacol Biochem Behav* 1991;40:683.

Solowij N, Michie PT, Fox AM. Differential impairments of selective attention due to frequency and duration of cannabis use. *Biol Psychiatry* 1995;37:731.

Sporer KA, Firestone J. Clinical course of crack cocaine body stuffers. *Ann Emerg Med* 1997;29:599.

Stein MD. Medical consequences of substance abuse. *Psychol Clin North Am* 1999;22:351.

Stein U, Greyer H, Hentschel H. Nutmeg (myristicin) poisoning—report on a fatal case and a series of cases recorded by a poison information centre. *Forensic Sci Int* 2001;118:87.

Stewart JL, Meeker JE. Fetal and infant deaths associated with maternal methamphetamine abuse. *J Anal Toxicol* 1997; 21:515.

Substance Abuse and Mental Health Services Administration (SAMHSA), Office of Applied Studies, U.S. Department of Health and Human Services. *Highlights of recent reports on substance abuse and mental health, updated on September 22, 2005.* Accessed at www.oas.sanhsa.gov/highlights.htm on September 28, 2005.

Sullivan ML, Martinez CM, Gennis P, et al. The cardiac toxicity of anabolic steroids. *Prog Cardiovasc Dis* 1998;41:1.

Szekely JI, Sharpe LG, Jaffe JH. Induction of phencyclidine-like behavior in rats by dextrorphan but not dextromethorphan. *Pharmacol Biochem Behav* 1991;40:381.

Tashkin DP, Simmons MS, Chang P, et al. Effects of smoked substance abuse on nonspecific airway hyperresponsiveness. *Am Rev Respir Dis* 1993;147:97.

Tashkin E. Effects of marijuana on the lung and its defenses against infection and cancer. *Sch Psychol Int* 1999;20:23.

Trisler K, Specter S. Delta-9-tetrahydrocannabinol treatment results in a suppression of interleukin-2-induced cellular activities in human and murine lymphocytes. *Int J Immunopharmacol* 1994;16:593.

Van den Akker TW, Roesyanto-Mahadi ID, van Toorenenbergen AW, et al. Contact allergy to spices. *Contact Dermatitis* 1990;22:267.

Warner EA. Is your patient using cocaine? Clinical signs that should raise suspicion. *Postgrad Med* 1995;98:173.

Watson SJ, Benson JA Jr, Joy JE. Marijuana and medicine: assessing the science base. A summary of the 1999 Institute of Medicine report. *Arch Gen Psychiatry* 2000;57:547.

Weber JE, Shofer FS, Larkin GL, et al. Validation of a brief observation period for patients with cocaine-associated chest pain. *N Engl J Med* 2003;348:510.

Weir E. Raves: a review of the culture, the drugs and the prevention of harm. *CMAJ* 2000;162:1843.

Wesson DR, Ling W. The Clinical Opiate Withdrawal Scale (COWS). *J Psychoactive Drugs* 2003;35:253.

Willens HJ, Chakko SC, Kessler KM. Cardiovascular manifestations of cocaine abuse: a case of recurrent dilated cardiomyopathy. *Chest* 1994;106:594.

Williams H. "Saturday night fever": ecstasy related problems in a London accident and emergency department. *J Accid Emerg Med* 1998;15:522.

Wilson WH, Ellinwood EH, Mathew RJ, et al. Effects of marijuana on performance of a computerized cognitive-neuromotor test battery. *Psychiatry Res* 1994;51:115.

Wu T, Tashkin DP, Djahed B, et al. Pulmonary hazards of smoking marijuana as compared with tobacco. *N Engl J Med* 1988;318:347.

Zamora-Quezada JC, Dinerman H, Stadecker MJ, et al. Muscle and skin infarction after free-basing cocaine (crack). *Ann Intern Med* 1988;108:564.

Zawertailo LA, Kaplan HL, Busto UE, et al. Psychotropic effects of dextromethorphan are altered by the CYP2D6 polymorphism: a pilot study. *J Clin Psychopharmacol* 1998;18:332.

CHAPTER 72

Laboratory Testing for Psychoactive Substances of Abuse

Sharon Levy and John R. Knight

DRUG TESTING IN THE PRIMARY CARE CLINIC

Drug testing is a complicated procedure that can be controversial and contentious. When done correctly it can be a useful part of a substance use disorder assessment; however, as with any other laboratory test it is best used in conjunction with and not instead of history and physical examination findings. This chapter discusses indications for drug testing, proper specimen collection and validation techniques, interpretation of results, and follow-up.

Indications for Urine Drug Testing in the Primary Care Clinic

Drug use by teens often presents to medical attention with nonspecific signs and symptoms (such as fatigue, excessive moodiness, school failure) and urine drug testing may be a useful assessment tool when parents notice these signs, yet the teenager denies drug use. Health care providers should consider recommending a drug test if a parent has a reasonable basis for suspicion of drug use, such as decrease in school performance, loss of interest in hobbies or extracurricular activities, change in friends, lying or stealing, or is found with drug paraphernalia. However, a drug test may be unnecessary if the teenager is forthcoming regarding his/her drug use history. The health care provider presented with these concerns should interview the patient alone without the parents present at some point during the visit.

In clinical situations in which a drug test is recommended, health care providers and parents should recognize that a single negative drug test result confirms that a patient has not used drugs detectable by the screen in the past 24 to 48 hours (for most substances), but does not rule out a drug use disorder, and, a positive drug test result does not confirm a diagnosis of drug abuse or dependence (Schwartz, 1993). Therefore, although drug testing can provide useful clinical information it must always be considered within the context of the history and physical findings. Health care providers should proceed cautiously when parents request a drug test based on concerns external to the patient (many drugs available in the neighborhood or school, family history of drug problems, and so on). Most experts agree that drug tests are not a

useful screening procedure for general populations as their sensitivity for detecting drug use in unselected populations is low (Hammett-Stabler et al., 2002; Schwartz, 1993).

There is little consensus among physicians regarding the indications for drug testing in adolescents and little consistency in how to proceed when a urine drug test result is positive (Levy et al., 2006). Further evidence-based studies and clinical practice guidelines are needed from health professional organizations (Irwin, 2006).

Consent/Assent

Policy guidelines from the American Academy of Pediatrics state that physicians should obtain assent from competent adolescents before ordering a drug test; parental consent alone is not sufficient (American Academy of Pediatrics, 1996). A health care provider should never order a drug test without explaining the procedure to the patient, as this may decrease trust, impair communication, and make therapeutic alliance between the patient and the health care provider difficult. If a teenager refuses a drug test that is clearly indicated, the health care provider should counsel parents to use appropriate limit setting and consequences. For example, a parent might suspend car privileges or limit socializing with friends until they are reassured that their child is not using drugs. Although drug testing may be an inconvenience to an adolescent, a series of negative drug test results may also present advantages, such as rebuilding trust between parent and child or providing evidence to schools or courts supporting abstinence from drugs.

Confidentiality/Sharing Results

Federal regulations afford information regarding drug use treatment greater confidentiality protection than other information recorded in a medical record. A health care provider should not share drug test results with anyone without the express written consent of the patient (if older than 18 years) or the parent of a minor patient. Drug test results should be omitted from general health summaries or other medical record transmittals as per Health Insurance Portability and Accountability (HIPAA) regulations.

Before ordering a drug test, the health care provider, teenager, and parent(s) should discuss who will receive results. Any patient with a positive drug test result requires further assessment and intervention. Some health care providers require permission to share the interpretation of the drug test result with parents whenever a drug test is ordered because adolescent patients are more likely to comply with follow-up appointments when a parent is involved. However, before sharing a positive drug test result, the health care provider should review the results with the teenager privately, as a drug test may be positive even when a teenager has not used illicit drugs. To avoid false accusation, the health care provider should conduct a private interview with the teenager before interpreting the drug test (see subsequent text).

DRUG TESTING OF TRAUMA VICTIMS IN THE EMERGENCY ROOM DEPARTMENT

The Department of Health and Human Services recommends that all adult trauma patients be screened for drug and alcohol use to determine whether they may have a drug or alcohol disorder (CSAT,1995). Recent research has demonstrated that rates of drug tests positive for cannabis, alcohol, and opiates among 14- to 17-year-old trauma patients was 39% (Ehrlich, 2006). Although drug testing did not alter the acute management of these patients, testing helped to identify drug use by these teenagers and allowed referral for further assessment. On the basis of these data, drug screening should be considered in all adolescent trauma patients after obtaining informed consent. All adolescents who present to an emergency department in an unresponsive condition should have a urine drug screen as part of an evaluation for altered mental status.

TYPES OF DRUG TESTS

Drugs and their metabolites can be detected in several biological matrices, including hair, saliva, breath, blood, and urine (Wolff et al., 1999).

Urine

Urine drug testing has been well studied and standardized. Urine drug concentrations are relatively high and drugs and their metabolites are excreted in the urine for a period of time after acute intoxication, making urine the preferred biological fluid for drug testing in the primary care setting.

There are two principle types of urine drug tests—immunoassays and gas chromatography/mass spectrometry (GC/MS). Immunoassays are relatively nonspecific tests that can detect a variety of drugs. Standard laboratory screening panels are done with immunoassays, as are point of service tests. Immunoassays are quite sensitive and can be used to eliminate samples from further consideration. However, these panels are relatively nonspecific and a number of cross-reacting substances can cause false-positive drug test results (Table 72.1) (Hawks and Chiang, 1986). Therefore, immunoassays are best used as a screen; all positive test results should be confirmed with a second test using a different, more specific testing method such as GC/MS. Requisitions for laboratory tests should include GC/MS confirmation for all positive test results as a separate order. Point of service tests are confirmed by sending the sample to the laboratory for GC/MS. Immunoassay screens should not be repeated for confirmation of an initial positive test result.

Hair/Breath/Saliva/Sweat

1. Hair: Although not a routine method of drug testing, hair testing can provide a longer window of detection (up to 180 days) in patients with long hair and may be useful in some settings. Current drug use can be difficult to distinguish from past use with this testing method. Marijuana use is difficult to confirm by hair testing because of slow deposition into some hair types. Because coarse hair absorbs drugs more readily, the possibility may exist of race/ethnicity inequity in hair testing for drugs (*Med Lett Drugs Ther*, 2002).
2. Breath tests: Breath tests are available for alcohol, and can give a reliable indication of the blood alcohol level at the time of the test (Gullberg, 2003).
3. Saliva tests: Saliva tests are also available for alcohol, and newer tests for a variety of drugs have recently entered the market. Like breath tests, drug levels in saliva reflect blood levels at the time of testing (Drummer, 2005; Verstraete, 2005). Saliva testing has not been nationally standardized and cutoff levels (the threshold level at which a drug test becomes positive) vary from product to product.
4. Sweat tests: Sweat wipes and patches that can be worn for up to 14 days are available, although they are used infrequently because of the high rate of false-positive results from external sources of drugs (Kidwell and Smith, 2001).

PRACTICAL ISSUES IN URINE DRUG TESTING

Test Selection

Substance abuse panels vary and health care providers should be familiar with the panels offered by the laboratories they use. Standard multipanels include the five classes of drugs that are required in federally mandated tests—cannabis, cocaine, amphetamines, phencyclidine (PCP), and opiates (American College of Environmental and Occupational Medicine, 2003). Many laboratories include additional classes of drugs in multiscreen substance abuse panels. Of note, immunoassay screens detect drug classes such as opiates or benzodiazepines, but may not detect every drug in the class. For example, standard opiate screens may not detect synthetic opioids such as oxycodone and hydrocodone (Gourlay et al., 2002). A test for urinary ethyl glucuronide should be ordered to detect alcohol use, as this metabolite has a longer half-life (up to 5 days) and is more sensitive than tests of urinary alcohol (Skipper et al., 2004). Communication and clarification with laboratory staff can reduce interpretation errors.

Specimen Collection

Because of the multitude of methods for falsifying urines, health care providers who choose to order urine drug tests from their offices must be diligent. Most experts recommend either a directly observed urine specimen (the specimen must be directly observed as it passes

TABLE 72.1

Drugs of Abuse, Common Urine Metabolites, Maximum Window of Detection, Molecules that May Cross-react with Screening Panels and Licit Sources of the Drug

Common Name(s)	Urine Metabolite	Maximum Window of Detection	Included in Standard Panels	Substances that Can Cross-react with ELISA Screens[a]	Sources of Clinical False Positives[b]
Alcohol	• Ethanol • Ethylglucuronide	• 24–36 hr • 80 hr	Not part of NIDA-5, but alcohol included on some standard panels		• OTC cough and cold liquid medications • "Nonalcoholic" beer • Foods prepared with uncooked alcohol (such as rum cake)
Marijuana, "weed"	Tetrahydrocannabinol (THC) and other cannabinols	Infrequent users: 3–4 d Daily users: 4–6 wk	Yes	• NSAIDs (ibuprofen, ketoprofen, naproxen) • Promethazine vitamin B supplements	Prescription Marinol use (uncommon in teenagers)
Cocaine	Cocaine, benzoylecgonine	2–3 days	Yes	Amoxicillin	Decocainized teas, commonly in use in South America
Amphetamine	Several members in class	2–4 days	Yes	• Cold medications that contain ephedrine, pseudoephedrine, propylephedrine, phenylephrine, desoxyephedrine • Phenylpropanolamine (present in OTC diet aids)	Prescription use of stimulants (for ADHD or other conditions) including Adderall and Dexedrine

(continued)

TABLE 72.1

(Continued)

Common Name(s)	Urine Metabolite	Maximum Window of Detection	Included in Standard Panels	Substances that Can Cross-react with ELISA Screens[a]	Sources of Clinical False Positives[b]
Methamphetamine	Methamphetamine, p-hydroxymethamphetamine, amphetamine	24–48 hours	Yes, detected on amphetamine panel		• Methamphetamine from OTC medications such as Vicks inhaler[c] • Prescription use of Desoxyn, benzphetamine, dimethylamphetamine, famprofazone, fencamine, furfenorex, selegiline
Ecstasy, 3,4 methylene-dioxymetham-phetamine (MDMA)	MDMA, methylene-dioxyamphetamine (MDA), mono- and dihydroxy derivatives	24–48 hours	No		
Phencyclidine (PCP), "dust"	Glucuronic conjugates of 4-phenyl-4-piperidinocyclo-hexanol and other metabolites	8–10 days	Yes	Dextromethorphan	
Lysergic acid diethylamide (LSD), "acid"	LSD, n-demethylated, deethylated, and hydroxylated metabolites	24 hours	No		

Substance	Metabolites	Detection window	Included in standard panel	Substances causing false-positive results	Comments
Opiates	• Codeine: norcodeine, morphine • Heroin: 6-acetylmorphine, morphine • Morphine: morphine glucuronide, normorphine	2–3 days	Yes, but synthetic opioids are detected only in very high doses	Fluoroquinolone antibiotics	• Consumption of a large quantity of poppy seeds (poppy seeds contain trace amounts of morphine; typical poppy seed consumption produce urine metabolite concentrations under standard thresholds) • Prescription use of opiate medication for pain
Benzodiazepines	Oxazepam common metabolite for several, but not all, benzodiazepines	Up to 2 weeks, but varies for individual drugs	Not part of "NIDA 5", but included in many standard panels		Prescription use of benzodiazepines for anxiety or other conditions
Inhalants	Many in class	<24 hours	No		Inhalants are largely excreted by the lungs although some metabolites may be excreted in the urine; special testing required for detection

ELISA, enzyme-linked immunosorbent assay; NIDA, National Institute on Drug Abuse; OTC, over-the-counter; NSAID, nonsteroidal antiinflammatory drug; ADHD, attention deficit hyperactivity disorder; MDA,;

[a]Gas chromatography/mass spectrometry (GC/MS) confirmation will be negative.
[b]May result in positive drug test results in the absence of illicit drug use.
[c]Vicks inhaler contains the inactive isomer L-methamphetamine, but trace amounts of the D-isomer may be present, resulting in a positive drug test result.

from the urethra into the specimen container) or using the National Institute on Drug Abuse (NIDA) protocol for specimen collection, which is available online (http://www.drugfreeworkplace.com). The Department of Transportation developed this protocol in compliance with the federal mandate to test transit employees, and many commercial laboratories have the necessary facilities and trained staff for specimen collection. The protocol requires the teen (or an accompanying parent) to present photographic identification before donating the sample. The patient then empties his/her pockets, washes his/her hands, and enters a private specimen donation room with all running water shut off. A blue dye is added to the standing water in the toilet. A laboratory staff member checks the temperature of the urine immediately after donation; specimens with a temperature below 90°F or above 100°F are considered substituted or diluted.

Specimen Validation

All drug tests should be ordered with an accompanying specific gravity and urine creatinine level. A negative screen is of absolutely no clinical usefulness in the absence of evidence of adequate urine concentration. Samples with a creatinine <20 mg/dL and a specific gravity of <1.005 are too dilute for proper interpretation and should be repeated with specific instructions regarding water ingestion before specimen donation (American College of Environmental and Occupational Medicine, 2003). In general, patients should be instructed to ingest no more than 20 oz of fluid in the 3 hours preceding donation of a specimen. Although it is impossible to protect against all the possible methods of falsifying urine substances, proper specimen collection and validation significantly decrease the possibility of tampering.

Interpretation

1. Negative test results

   Drug test results have both laboratory and clinical interpretations. The laboratory reading of a drug test result will be negative whenever the drugs in the test panel are not detected in the sample provided. Negative drug test results must be interpreted with caution (Table 72.2). A drug test result will be negative in the context of drug use in the following circumstances:
   - The patient stopped using the substance in question within the window of detection (24–48 hours for most substances). Teens who know they will be drug tested may be able to stop long enough in advance to have a negative result.
   - The patient has diluted the urine sample. Specimens with creatinine levels between 5 and 20 and specific gravity <1.005 are dilute, and should be repeated after limiting fluid ingestion immediately preceding the test. A repeated dilute specimen should be considered clinically positive.
   - The patient has substituted the urine sample. Laboratory specimens with creatinine <5 should be considered substituted (not urine), and the clinical interpretation of the drug test result is positive. Samples may also be substituted with synthetic urine or urine provided by an individual who had not used drugs.
   - The patient has adulterated the urine sample. Bleach, soap, acid, and other chemicals interfere with drug screens and cause false-negative test results. These substances may be detected by laboratory personnel if the sample has an unusual odor or other unusual characteristics. Tests for specific adulterants may be ordered separately (in consultation with laboratory personnel) if adulteration is suspected.
   - The patient has used a drug that is not detected by the panel ordered. Synthetic opioids (such as oxycodone, hydrocodone, and hydromorphone), some benzodiazepines, inhalants, and some hallucinogens are not included on most standard drug testing panels, and the inclusion of alcohol is variable. These drugs must be ordered separately in consultation with the laboratory toxicologist if use is suspected.

2. Positive test results

   The laboratory reading of a drug test result will be positive whenever a molecule in the urine specimen reacts with the test panel, and this also must be interpreted with caution (Table 72.3). A drug test result will be positive in absence of illicit drug use in the following circumstances:
   - A chemical other than an illicit drug has cross-reacted with the drug test panel (Table 72.1). Confirmatory testing with GC/MS will be negative.
   - The patient has consumed the drug in the context of licit use of a prescription or over-the-counter medication, or consumed in a food. A careful patient history, including review of all prescription medications, recently used over-the-counter medications and unusual food consumption may provide an explanation for the positive drug test result if the history is consistent with the result observed.

TABLE 72.2

Interpretation of Negative Urine Drug Test Results

Screen Result	Laboratory Interpretation	Possible Clinical Interpretations	Next Step
Negative	Substance in question not detected in the urine Substance may be either present at a concentration below the sensitivity level set for the test, or not present	• Patient has not used the substance in question within the window of detection (24–48 hours for most substances) • Patient has diluted, substituted or adulterated the urine sample causing a false-negative result	• Adulterated or substituted samples should be considered clinically positive • Dilute samples should be repeated; multiple dilute samples should be considered positive

TABLE 72.3

Interpretation of Positive Urine Drug Test Results

Screen Result	Laboratory Interpretation	Possible Clinical Interpretations	Next Step
Positive	Substance in the urine has reacted with the substrate in the test panel	• True positive—patient has absorbed substance in question • False positive—chemical from an over-the-counter medication, prescribed medication, or food has cross-reacted with substrate in the test panel	• Order GC/MS to confirm result • If GC/MS is positive, discuss with the patient to determine if licit use of prescription or over-the-counter medications, or food consumption would explain a positive test result

GC/MS, gas chromatography/mass spectrometry.

3. Specimens positive for cannabis

Cannabis is lipid soluble and, with chronic use, significant stores can accumulate in fat tissue. Daily users of cannabis can have detectable urine cannabinoid levels for 1 to 2 months after discontinuing use (Schwartz, 1993). The absolute level of urinary cannabinoid excretion varies with urine concentration. Once use is discontinued, however, the ratio of urinary cannabinoids to urinary creatinine will fall over time, and a decreasing ratio supports a history of discontinued use even in a patient with positive urine test results.

Presenting Drug Test Results to Adolescent Patients

All patients with positive, dilute, adulterated, or substituted urine specimens should have a return appointment to interpret drug test results. Teens should be interviewed privately to determine whether an explanation other than illicit drug use might account for the laboratory findings. After the interview, the health care provider should have enough information to determine whether the drug test result is the result of illicit drug use or whether an alternative explanation is realistic.

Some teens will acknowledge drug use when a drug test result is positive, and this may provide an opportunity to have an honest conversation. The health care provider may elicit further drug history in an attempt to clarify diagnoses. If the teenager is willing to abstain from drug use, repeat testing may be useful for monitoring and to help rebuild trust between parent and child. Some teens will deny drug use and insist that the laboratory is in error or offer another inconsistent explanation. The health care provider should avoid arguments, but remain firm in interpretation. Repeat testing and further visits may be required before the teen is ready to give an honest history.

Approach to the Patient Interview When a Drug Test is Positive

Whenever a laboratory drug test result is positive the health care provider should interview the patient privately to determine if an explanation other than illicit drug use might

account for the laboratory findings. The following may serve as an interview guide for these clinical encounters:

• If the test was not done in the office, confirm the date and location, and whether there were problems at the test site.
Did you have a drug test on (date) at (location)?
Were there any problems in the lab when you were there?
• Inform the teen that you have received an unexpected drug test result.
I have the received the results of your drug test and the test was (positive/dilute/adulterated/substituted).
• For positive specimens:
Are you taking any prescription or over-the-counter medications that might account for a positive drug test result?
Did you consume any foods that might have interfered with a drug test?
Determine whether medications or foods listed would account for the positive test result observed. For example, the use of Adderall for attention-deficit hyperactivity disorder (ADHD) would account for a positive amphetamine test result, but not a positive opioid test result.
• For dilute specimens:
Was there anything unusual about that day? Can you explain why your test was so dilute?
Tell the teen that a repeat test will be required and give specific parameters for fluid ingestion (such as no more than 8 oz of fluid in the 2 hours preceding the test). If repeated tests have been dilute inform the teenager that further renal assessment may be required.
• Ask directly about drug use:
Did you use drugs or alcohol before giving a urine test?

Presenting Urine Drug Test Results to Parents

Parental involvement is an important part of intervention for many teens with substance use disorders and disclosing a teen's drug test results to parents may be therapeutically useful, particularly when a teen has not given an honest history. It is, however, important to respect the teen's burgeoning autonomy and, when possible, to protect the therapeutic alliance between the teen and the clinician.

A few guidelines are helpful in deciding what information to share with parents.

Approach to Sharing Urine Drug Test Results with Parents

- Obtain assent or consent (as appropriate) from the teenager to share drug test results *before* ordering the drug test.
- When a drug test result is positive, dilute, adulterated, or substituted always interview the patient privately to interpret drug test results before sharing information with parents.
- Discuss with the teenager exactly which information will be shared with parents. Avoid sharing details that do not impact further assessment or treatment, such as how drugs were obtained or who else used them.
- Offer the teenager the opportunity to speak with parents first (with the clinician present for support and to confirm that information was correctly conveyed).
- If the teenager has not acknowledged the drug use, discuss the teen's alternative explanation for the positive drug test result, but, explain that the explanation offered is inconsistent with laboratory results.

Negative results of drug tests done with proper collection and validation techniques provide good support for a history of no drug use, at least within the window of detection of the substances detected. Health care providers must recognize, however, that even carefully done urine tests have limitations and cannot completely rule out drug use. Parents should understand the limitations of urine drug testing. Continued monitoring by parents, repeat drug testing, or referral to a mental health or substance abuse expert may be indicated if the teenager continues to demonstrate signs and symptoms consistent with drug use, even in the context of a negative drug test result.

WEB SITES

For Teenagers and Parents

http://www.helpguide.org/mental/drug_substance_abuse _addiction_signs_effects_treatment.htm. This site lists signs and symptoms of drug use in adolescents.

For Health Professionals

http://www.drugfreeworkplace.com. This site lists regulations for federally mandated workplace testing programs.
http://www.acoem.org/ This site provides information on medical review officer training.
http://www.hipaa.samhsa.gov/ Part2ComparisonClearedTOC.htm. This site discusses the confidentiality of alcohol and drug abuse patient records and the HIPAA Privacy Rule.

REFERENCES AND ADDITIONAL READINGS

Ahrendt DM, Miller MA. Adolescent substance abuse: a simplified approach to drug testing. *Pediat Ann* 2005;34:956.

American Academy of Pediatrics. Testing for drugs of abuse in children and adolescents. *Pediatrics* 1996;98:305.

American College of Environmental and Occupational Medicine. *Medical review officer drug and alcohol testing comprehensive/fast track course syllabus.* Arlington Heights, IL: American College of Environmental and Occupational Medicine; 2003.

Center for Substance Abuse Treatment. *Treatment Improvement Protocol 16: Alcohol and Other Drug Screening of Hospitalized Trauma Patients.* Available at http://www.ncbi.nlm. nih.gov/books/bv.fcgi?rid=hstat5.chapter.36481.

Drummer O. Review: pharmacokinetics of illicit drugs in oral fluid. *Forensic Sci Int* 2005;150:133.

Ehrlich PF, Brown JK, Drongowski R. Characterization of the drug-positive adolescent trauma population: should we, do we and dose it make a difference if we test?. *J Ped Surg* 2006;41:927.

Gullberg R. Breath alcohol measurement variability associated with different instrumentation and protocols. *Forensic Sci Int* 2003;131:30.

Gourlay G, Heit H, Caplan Y. *Urine drug testing in primary care: dispelling the myths and designing strategies.* San Francisco: California Academy of Family Physicians; 2002.

Hammett-Stabler C, Pesce A, Cannon D. Urine drug screening in the medical setting. *Clin Chim Acta* 2002;315:125.

Hawks RL, Chiang CN, eds. *Urine testing for drugs of abuse.* Rockville, MD: NIDA Research Monograph 73.; 1986.

Irwin CE Jr. To test or not to test: screening for substance use in adolescents. *J Adol Health* 2006;38:329.

Kidwell D, Smith G. Susceptibility of PharmChek drugs of abuse patch to environmental contamination. *Forensic Sci Int* 2001;116:89.

Levy S, Harris SK, Sherritt L, et al. Drug testing of adolescents in general medical clinics, in school and at home: physician attitudes and practices. *J Adol Health* 2006; 38:336.

Med Lett Drugs Ther. Tests for Drugs of Abuse. 2002;44:71.

Schwartz R. Testing for drugs of abuse: controversies and techniques. *Adolesc Med* 1993;4:353.

Skipper GE, Weinmann W, Thierauf A, et al. Ethyl glucuronide: a biomarker to identify alcohol use by health professionals recovering from substance use disorders. *Alcohol Alcohol* 2004;39(5):445.

Verstraete A. Oral fluid testing for driving under the influence of drugs: history, recent progress and remaining challenges. *Forensic Sci Int* 2005;150:143.

Wolff K, Farrell M, Marsden J, et al. A review of biological indicators of illicit drug use, practical considerations and clinical usefulness. *Addiction* 1999;94:1279.

CHAPTER 73

Office-Based Management of Adolescent Substance Use and Abuse

Sharon Levy and John R. Knight

THE ROLE OF PRIMARY CARE PROVIDER

Alcohol and drug use are common among American adolescents; by high school graduation approximately eight of ten American students have tried alcohol, more than half of students have tried an illicit drug, and approximately one third have tried an illicit drug other than marijuana. Almost one third of students try an illicit substance by the end of 8th grade. Alcohol and drug use are related to the four leading causes of death in the adolescent age-group and therefore present a major public health problem. The American Academy of Pediatrics and the Maternal and Child Health Bureau recommend that all adolescents be screened for substance use at each yearly physical examination. Primary care providers should ask every adolescent if they have tried tobacco, alcohol, and other drugs during each yearly health maintenance visit and screen all of those who have used with a validated tool such as the CRAFFT questions (Knight et al., 1999). In most general practices, most teens will report no use or low risk use, and will benefit from praise, encouragement, or brief advice that can be given in a few moments. Those teens who screen positive for high-risk substance use require further assessment and either a brief intervention or referral for more intensive services.

SCREENING

Asking about Drug and Alcohol Use

Large population surveys have demonstrated that all adolescents are at risk of exposure to drugs and alcohol (Centers for Disease Control, 2004). Therefore, every adolescent should be asked yearly about alcohol and drug use, regardless of race, ethnicity, socioeconomic status, religion, or gender.

Health care providers should ask questions regarding substance use in private, after explaining the rules of confidentiality. Adolescents should be afforded confidentiality unless their behavior poses an acute safety concern to themselves or others. Determining whether a specific behavior presents a safety concern is a matter of clinical judgment; the patient's age, other diagnoses, and social situation should be taken into account. Occasional use of alcohol or marijuana can usually be kept confidential. In all cases, adolescents should be assured that if confidentiality is to be broken, the health care provider and patient will review what will be said before speaking with parents, and only diagnostic and planning information will be shared; specific details need not be disclosed.

To avoid miscommunication, questions about substance use should be clear and concise, such as, "Have you ever drunk alcohol? Have you ever smoked marijuana? Have you ever used another drug?" Some health care providers prefer to begin with questions about peers and friends whereas others begin with more direct personal questions.

Substance use may present with nonspecific signs and symptoms, such as change in school performance, loss of interest in hobbies or extracurricular activities, excessive moodiness or irritability, or a change in friends. When a parent reports any of these changes, the health care provider should be particularly alert to the possibility of substance use. In addition, any concerns about use expressed by parents, school officials, coaches, or other adults should be taken seriously. Drug testing may be recommended when parents have reasonable concerns that their child is using drugs and yet the adolescent denies drug use (see Chapter 72).

Screens

All teens who report using alcohol or drugs should receive a structured screening to determine whether their use is of low or high risk. Recent research has demonstrated that reliance on impressions alone may cause even experienced health care providers to underestimate the severity of an adolescent's substance-related problems (Wilson et al., 2004). A number of tools have been created to screen adolescents for alcohol and drug use. These tools fall into two main categories—paper and pencil tools such as the Alcohol Use Disorders Identification Test (AUDIT) (Miles et al., 2001; Reinert and Allen, 2002) and the Problem Oriented Screening Instrument for Teenagers (POSIT) (Knight et al., 1996), and orally administered tools such as the CAGE (see

Chapter 69, Figure 69.1) (Crowe et al., 1997; Ewing, 1984) or CRAFFT (see below) questions (Knight et al., 1999). Written assessments can be self-administered; oral tools are generally administered as part of a routine history. Written tools may screen for a number of disorders simultaneously, but take longer to administer, score, and interpret. Orally administered screens generally require minimal training to use and can be administered very quickly.

The CAGE questions are both valid and reliable for detecting alcohol disorders among adults, but have poor psychometric properties when used with teens and are not recommended for screening adolescents. The CRAFFT questions were developed specifically to screen adolescents for drug and alcohol use disorders simultaneously. Research has demonstrated that CRAFFT is a valid and reliable tool for screening adolescents, with a sensitivity of 76%, specificity of 94%, positive predictive value of 83%, and a negative predictive value of 91% for identifying problem use, abuse, or dependence (Knight et al., 2002b); and its psychometric properties are favorable across age, gender, and race/ethnicity. CRAFFT is a mnemonic acronym created from the first letters of key words in the test's six questions:

During the last 12 months have you ever:

- Ridden in a *CAR* driven by someone, including yourself, who was high or had been using alcohol or drugs?
- Used alcohol or drugs to *RELAX*, feel better about yourself, or fit in?
- Used alcohol or drugs while you are by yourself, *ALONE*?
- *FORGOTTEN* things you did while using alcohol or drugs?
- Had your *FAMILY* or *FRIENDS* tell you that you should cut down on your drinking or drug use?
- Gotten into *TROUBLE* while you were using alcohol or drugs?

Each "yes" response is scored one point. A score of 2 or greater is a positive screen, and indicates that the adolescent is at high risk for having an alcohol- or drug-related disorder.

ASSESSMENT

Interview

All teens who screen positive require further assessment, beginning with a more detailed substance use history. A nonjudgmental, empathetic interviewing style that accepts the patient's point of view encourages more information sharing than an interrogative style. Health care providers should use open-ended questions whenever possible, with an emphasis on the pattern of drug use over time, including whether drug use has increased in quantity or frequency, whether the teen has made attempts at discontinuing drug use and why and whether attempts have been successful. Information about the pattern of drug use and associated problems is more important in making a diagnosis of a substance-related disorder than the absolute quantity or frequency used. A well-conducted history has therapeutic value because it encourages the patient to consider the consequences of drug use that she/he has already experienced.

After interviewing the adolescent about his/her drug of choice, the health care provider should ask about use of other drugs, because use of multiple substances puts an adolescent at higher risk than use of a single substance. This information may also guide treatment planning, particularly if drug testing will be used for monitoring, or if medications are indicated as part of therapeutic management. Table 73.1 lists drugs and classes

---

TABLE 73.1

Guide to Extended Drug History

Drug or Drug Class	Common Street Names[a]
Cocaine	Cocaine or crack
Amphetamines	ADHD medications: Ritalin, Dexedrine, Adderall
	Methamphetamine: meth, crystal meth
Opioids	Pain medications: OxyContin (o.c., oxy), Percocet (percs), Vicodin (vics), codeine, morphine
	Heroin, opium
Benzodiazepines	Klonopin, Valium, Ativan, Xanax, others
Hallucinogens	Cold medications containing dextromethorphan (DXM), often referred to by brand name (Coricidin Cold and Cough [Triple C], Robitussin, NyQuil)
	Psilocybin (mushrooms)
	LSD (acid)
	PCP (dust or angel dust)
Inhalants	Nitrous (often from whipped cream cans or "whippits")
	Lighter fluid
	Paint
	Gasoline
	Markers
	Cleaning fluid
Ecstasy	E
Ketamine	K

ADHD, attention-deficit hyperactivity disorder; LSD, lysergic acid diethylamide; PCP, phencyclidine.
[a]See also Chapter 71.

of drugs that should be included in an extended drug history. For each drug ask the teen:

1. If they have ever used it, and if so whether they are a current user.
2. Whether they have ever tried to quit and why.
3. Whether they have experienced any problems associated with using the drug.

The health care provider should ask about the seven criteria for a diagnosis of drug dependence (Table 73.2) for the drug of choice and each drug the teen has reported using with associated problems.

Physical Examination

A physical examination should be performed as part of a complete assessment. Signs of chronic drug use are rare in teens, but should be noted if present. A list of physical findings associated with acute intoxication, withdrawal, and chronic drug use are presented in Table 73.3.

Laboratory Evaluation

Drug testing may be a useful part of a comprehensive assessment, particularly if symptoms of drug use are present, or parents have specific concerns, yet the teen denies drug use. The use of drug testing as an assessment tool is described in greater detail in Chapter 72.

DIAGNOSIS

Substance Use Disorders

As with many disorders, substance use can be viewed as a spectrum varying from experimentation to drug dependence and addiction. Table 73.2 describes various stages within this spectrum. The Diagnostic and Statistical Manual of Mental Disorders IV (DSM-IV) includes diagnostic criteria for substance abuse and substance dependence disorders. Other designations, while not formal diagnoses, are useful descriptions that can help the health care provider determine the appropriate level of intervention.

Co-occurring Disorders

Many adolescents with substance-related disorders will have symptoms consistent with a co-occurring mental health disorder, and it may be difficult to determine clinically whether the symptoms are solely the result of drug use. In some circumstances, the question of a co-occurring diagnosis cannot be fully resolved until the adolescent has had a period of complete abstinence. However, severe symptoms, symptoms that antedate drug use, or positive family history of a similar disorder all suggest a co-occurring disorder, and warrant concurrent treatment. On the contrary, symptoms beginning after the onset of drug use may resolve completely with abstinence, and patients may be observed and reassessed as necessary. The diagnosis of attention-deficit hyperactivity disorder (ADHD) should not be made unless the adolescent had symptoms before age 10. Dual diagnosis and management is discussed further in Chapter 74.

PRIMARY CARE MANAGEMENT

Most adolescents who use alcohol and drugs can be managed effectively in the primary care setting, and even patients who will ultimately require referral to an addiction or mental health specialist may receive direct benefit, or be more likely to accept treatment recommendations, after a brief office intervention (Borowsky et al., 2003; Fleming et al., 2002; Knight et al., 2000). Research has shown that brief interventions by health care providers, ranging in intensity from a few seconds up to several hours, can significantly reduce drug and alcohol use. In this chapter, we define *brief advice* as an intervention lasting seconds to minutes in which the health care provider gives general information regarding substance use to a patient and *brief intervention* as an individual interactive counseling session focusing on details specific to the patient's substance use.

Abstinence (Positive Reinforcement)

Adolescents who abstain from alcohol and drugs, either primarily or secondarily, should receive praise and encouragement from their health care provider. Statements should be brief yet specific and encourage the adolescent to discuss drug use or ask questions in the future should the need arise. An example is, "It sounds as if you have made some really good decisions about drugs and alcohol. I hope you will come back to me if you ever have questions about drugs, if you are tempted, or even if you try them."

Low Risk (Brief Advice)

Adolescents who have used drugs or alcohol but score 0 or 1 on the CRAFFT questions are "low risk" users, most likely in the experimentation or regular use stage (Knight et al., 2002a,b 2004). These patients may benefit from brief general advice pertinent to the drug they have used. Advice may be targeted at abstinence or risk reduction. Sample statements are listed in Table 73.4. Knowledge of the patient can help the health care provider select the most relevant piece of information to share.

Problem Use and Abuse (Brief Intervention)

Adolescents who have problems associated with drugs may benefit from a brief intervention. It is important for health care providers and parents to realize that behavior change is a process that occurs over time. Prochaska and DiClemente have conceptualized behavior change as occurring in a series of steps, described in Table 73.5. The goal of brief intervention is to encourage the patient to move in the direction of positive behavior change. An intervention that causes an adolescent to move from precontemplation to contemplation should be considered a success, although no observed behavior change will be noted at that time.

Motivational Interviewing

Motivational interviewing (MI) is an empathetic, patient focused, directive counseling style that seeks to create conditions necessary for positive change. It is particularly well suited for brief therapeutic encounters, either as a primary method for assisting patients to change their

TABLE 73.2

Spectrum of Drug Use in Adolescents

Primary abstinence	No history of drug or alcohol use
Experimentation	Initial one or few occasions primarily undertaken to satisfy a curiosity to experience intoxication
Regular use	Regularly recurring drug or alcohol intoxication in social situations without associated problems or consequences
Problematic use	Drug or alcohol use associated with new onset problems with relatively limited consequences such as: Parental punishment School detention or suspension Trouble with the police or risky behavior such as: Driving while intoxicated Overdose or black out
Abuse	Recurrent drug or alcohol use despite problems that interfere with functioning, such as decrease in school performance, decreased performance in sports or hobbies, arrests with legal consequences, or serious medical complications, as defined by DSM-IV criteria (American Psychiatric Association, 1994): A. A maladaptive pattern of substance use leading to clinically significant impairment or distress, as manifested by one (or more) of the following, occurring within a 12-month period: 　1. Recurrent substance use resulting in a failure to fulfill major role obligation at work, school, or home (e.g., repeated absences or poor work performance related to substance use; substance-related absences, suspension, or expulsions from school; neglect of children or household) 　2. Recurrent substance use in situations where it is physically hazardous (e.g., driving an automobile or operating a machine when impaired by substance use) 　3. Recurrent substance-related legal problems (e.g., arrests for substance-related disorderly conduct) 　4. Continued substance use despite having persistent or recurrent social or interpersonal problems caused or exacerbated by the effects of the substance (e.g., arguments with spouse about consequences of intoxication, physical fights) B. The symptoms have never met the criteria for substance dependence for this class of substance
Dependence	Loss of control over a drug or alcohol, as defined by DSM-IV criteria: A. A maladaptive pattern of substance use, leading to clinically significant impairment or distress, as manifested by three (or more) of the following, occurring at any time in the same 12-month period: 　1. Tolerance, as defined by either of the following: 　　a. A need for markedly increased amounts of the substance to achieve intoxication or desired effect 　　b. Markedly diminished effect with continued use of the same amount of the substance 　2. Withdrawal, as manifested by either of the following: 　　a. The characteristic withdrawal syndrome for the substance (refer to Criteria A and B of the criteria sets for withdrawal from the specific substances) 　　b. The same (or a closely related) substance is taken to relieve or avoid withdrawal symptoms 　3. The substance is often taken in larger amounts or over a longer period than was intended 　4. There is a persistent desire or unsuccessful efforts to cut down or control substance use 　5. A great deal of time is spent in activities necessary to obtain the substance (e.g., visiting multiple doctors or driving long distances), use the substance (e.g., chain-smoking), or recover from its effects 　6. Important social, occupational, or recreational activities are given up or reduced because of substance use 　7. The substance use is continued despite knowledge of having a persistent or recurrent physical or psychological problem that is likely to have been caused or exacerbated by the substance (e.g., current cocaine use despite recognition of cocaine-induced depression, or continued drinking despite recognition that an ulcer was made worse by alcohol consumption)
Secondary abstinence	No use and a commitment to abstinence after a period of drug or alcohol use

TABLE 73.3

Physical Signs of Drug Intoxication, Recovery from Intoxication, and Chronic Use[a]

Drug	Acute Intoxication	Recovery from Intoxication/Withdrawal	Chronic Drug Use
Alcohol	Fruity smelling breath, disinhibited or silly, clumsiness, vomiting	Headache, nausea, vomiting, dry mouth	Enlarged liver, increased liver enzymes, hypertension
Marijuana	Erythematous conjunctivae, tachycardia, dry mouth, increased talking, euphoria	Anxiety, nervousness	Chronic cough, wheezing Loss of interest in activities/apathy
Cocaine	Hyperalert state, increased talking, hyperthermia, nausea, dry mouth, dilated pupils, sweating, cardiac arrhythmias	Depression, anhedonia, insomnia, lethargy, mental slowing	Erosion of dental enamel, gingival ulceration, chronic rhinitis, perforated nasal septum, midline granuloma, cardiac arrhythmias, hypertension, paranoia, psychosis
Amphetamines	Similar acute intoxication effects as cocaine	Choreoathetoid movement disorders, skin picking, and ulcerations	
Opioids	Constricted pupils, drowsiness ("nodding"), slowed respirations, bradycardia, slurred speech, slowed comprehension, constipation	Flu-like symptoms, muscle and joint aches, dilated pupils, coryza, lacrimation, sweating, abdominal cramps, nausea, vomiting, diarrhea, hot and cold flashes, piloerection, yawning, tremors, anxiety, irritability	Abscesses, cellulites, phlebitis and scarring (from injection use), chronic constipation, malnutrition
Benzodiazepines	Drowsiness, slowed respirations, slurred speech, slowed comprehension	Seizures (may be life threatening), anxiety, restlessness	Sleep difficulties, anxiety, personality changes
Hallucinogens	Toxic psychosis, paranoia, anxiety, tachycardia, hypertension, dry mouth, nausea, vomiting	Flashbacks, which may occur even after the effects of the drug have worn off, unpredictable or self injurious behavior.	Psychosis, depression, personality changes
Inhalants	Euphoria, slurred speech, ataxia, diplopia, lacrimation, rhinorrhea, salivation, irritation of the mucus membranes, nausea, vomiting, arrhythmias	Headaches, sleepiness, depression	Irritation of mucus membranes, changes in neurological examination
Ecstasy	Euphoria, decreased interpersonal boundaries, tachycardia, hypertension, hyperthermia, sweating, muscle spasms, bruxism, blurred vision, chills, nystagmus	Depression, anxiety, paranoia, dehydration	Cognitive deficits

[a]See also Chapter 71.

TABLE 73.4

Brief Advice Sample Statements

As your doctor, I recommend you stop using
Smoking marijuana damages your lungs and can affect your sports performance
Marijuana directly affects your brain, and can hurt your school performance and your future
Marijuana use can cause life long problems for some people
Alcohol can cause high blood pressure, heart problems, and liver problems.
Alcohol can cause accidents
Drug and alcohol use can lead to sexual assault, sexually transmitted diseases, and unintended pregnancies
Please don't ever get in a car with someone who has been drinking or using drugs
Please don't ever drive a car after using drugs, even if you don't feel high
Make arrangements ahead of time for safe transportation
Marijuana use can slowly get you into trouble—with your parents, at school, or even with the police
Alcohol and marijuana can make you gain weight
Marijuana can be laced with other drugs; you never really know what you are getting

alcohol/drug use, or as a means of encouraging them to accept a referral for more intensive treatment.

MI is based on two important assumptions. The first is that motivation is a product of interpersonal interaction, and not an innate character trait. What a health care provider does or says in counseling sessions can either help or hinder a patient in changing his/her behavior. Confrontation leads to resistance, while empathy and understanding lead to change.

A second assumption is that ambivalence toward change is normal and acceptable. According to this view, adolescents who use alcohol and drugs are in constant conflict, simultaneously experiencing both positive and negative feelings about their use. Their "decisional balance" can be viewed as an old-fashioned pan scale, with the pros and cons of substance use represented by the relative weights on the two sides.

In this model, the counselor is the facilitator while the adolescent presents the arguments for change. The counselor listens carefully for the ambivalence in the patient's own words, and helps the patient to use his or her own negative feelings regarding drug use as the fuel for behavior change by drawing out, repeating, and reinforcing the negative aspects of drug use and positive aspects of change. She/he also looks for opportunities to support self-efficacy, by pointing out strengths, previous successes (no matter how small), and acknowledging the difficulties of making behavioral changes. The counselor avoids resistance by refraining from lecturing or arguing with the patient.

MI techniques: A variety of tools are associated with MI; an exhaustive description is beyond the scope of this chapter (Miller and Rollnick, 2002). Table 73.6 describes several of the most common techniques and gives sample situations in which they may be helpful.

TABLE 73.5

Prochaska and DiClemente Stages of Change Model

Stage	Description
Precontemplation	The patient does not perceive problems related to behavior and has not considered making a change
Contemplation	The patient is considering a behavior change, but is ambivalent
	Perceived benefits of continued behavior are in a dynamic balance with perceived risks
Determination	The patient has decided to make a change and begins to make a specific plan though no change has occurred yet.
Action	The patient is engaged in an action plan and change has occurred.
Maintenance	The behavior change has become internalized
Relapse	The patient has returned to the original behavior

From Prochaska and DiClemente, 1986, 1992.

Written Agreements

When an adolescent does decide to make a behavior change it is useful to make a specific written plan, detailing the change attempted (abstinence, use only on weekends, etc.) and a time frame (usually 30–90 days). This allows both the health care provider and patient to monitor progress, and serves as an excellent starting point at follow-up visits. A sample abstinence contract and controlled use trial (CUT) contract are included in Table 73.7. Sample drinking and driving contracts are available at the Students Against Destructive Decisions (SADD) Web site (http://sadd.org/contract.htm#cf1).

Dependence (Referral)

Most adolescents who meet criteria for substance dependence will need intensive services from an addiction or mental health specialist. Pharmacological treatment may be a useful adjuvant for patients with opioid or alcohol dependence. Intensive therapies are discussed in detail in Chapter 74.

TABLE 73.6

Motivational Interviewing Techniques

Tool	Technique	Situation Example
Open-ended questions	Encourages the patient to explore potential consequences of a behavior	Patients who have not yet begun to think about making a change *"What do you think would happen if you were caught smoking marijuana at school?"*
Reflections	Echo back what the patient has said to emphasize the point	May help "tip the balance" for an ambivalent patient *"You don't use marijuana during lacrosse season because you feel it really slows you down and makes you short of breath"*
"Rolling with resistance"	Acknowledge the patient's point of view, even if not agreeing with it	Redirects the conversation when a patient gets "stuck" or angry *"It is surprising that you were expelled from school for a first drug incident. What do you think you will do about it?"*
Reframing	Point out that the "glass is half full"	Supports self-efficacy while the patient is attempting a behavior change *"So you didn't make your goal completely, but you did cut back your drug use quite a bit. Keep going—that's a great first step."*

THE ROLE OF PARENTS

Parents play a vital role in the prevention and treatment of adolescent substance abuse. Health care providers should encourage the parents of preteens to discuss drugs and alcohol, and to set clear family rules of no use. Health care providers should also encourage parents to set a good example by consuming alcohol only in moderation, never driving after drinking, and avoiding drug use. If parents have had drug or alcohol problems in the past they may decide to share honestly their experiences if their children ask, but do not need to volunteer information.

Some adolescents who are misusing drugs or alcohol will not engage in treatment. In these cases family or parent support counseling may be useful, even if the adolescent refuses to participate. Parents should be advised to set firm limits and avoid enabling substance use. Limit setting refers to consequences designed by the parents, such as the following:

- Limiting privileges to engage in social activities ("grounding")
- Limiting access to entertainment, such as television, computer games
- Limiting car privileges

Ultimately, the adolescent will decide whether to use drugs, but she/he will have to live with the consequences of the decision, including consequences set by parents.

Enabling refers to any activity that intentionally or unintentionally assists the adolescent in obtaining or using

TABLE 73.7

Sample Written Contract

Date: _____

I, _____, agree to not drink alcohol, use drugs, or take anyone else's medication (drink alcohol only _____, not use drugs or take anyone else's medication) for the next _____ days. I also will not provide drugs, alcohol, or prescription medications for anyone else during this time. In addition, I agree to not drive a motor vehicle while under the influence of drugs or alcohol, nor will I ride with a driver who has been drinking or using drugs.

I will come to my follow-up appointment on _____.

Signed _____ Date _____

drugs. Parents may unintentionally enable an adolescent's drug use by providing money, cell phones, E-mail accounts, or a car that teenager uses to obtain drugs. A review of sources of money, communication, and transportation may help parents identify enabling behaviors and eliminate them. If parents are unable to enforce their home rules they may seek assistance from the court system by filing a "Child in Need of Supervision (CHINS)" order with the police department and having a probation officer assigned to assist them.

In all cases, the patient and family should be told that they are welcome to return to the office to discuss drugs and alcohol whenever they are ready. Some patients need more time. A supportive word or two may stay with them, preparing them to ultimately return and engage in treatment.

SUMMARY

Substance use is common among American teenagers. Primary care health supervision visits provide an excellent opportunity for assessment in a one-on-one setting. All teens should be asked confidentially about substance use at each primary care visit. Those who have ever used substances should be screened using the CRAFFT questions. Positive reinforcement for adolescents who have not used substances and brief intervention for those who have but screen negative for high-risk use takes just a few moments but may have significant clinical impact. Teens who screen positive for high-risk use may directly or be more willing to accept a treatment referral after a brief office-based intervention. Primary care visits also provide an opportunity to help parents reduce the likelihood of their child developing a substance use disorder, or to engage parents in the treatment of teens who have developed a substance use disorder.

RESOURCES

American Academy of Pediatrics, Committee on Substance Abuse. Alcohol use and abuse: a pediatric concern. *Pediatrics* 2001;108:185.
American Academy of Pediatrics, Committee on Substance Abuse. *Testing Your Teen for Illicit Drugs: Information for Parents*. Patient education brochure available from the Academy through the AAP Web site (www.aap.org) or by calling (888/227–1770). Accessed 2007.
American Academy of Pediatrics. *Substance abuse: a guide for health professionals*, 2nd ed. Elk Grove Village, IL: American Academy of Pediatrics; 2002.
Kulig JW, Committee on Substance Abuse, American Academy of Pediatrics. Tobacco, alcohol, and other drugs. *Pediatrics* 2005;115(3):816.
Miller WR, Rollnick S. *Motivational interviewing: preparing people for change*, 2nd ed. New York, NY: Guilford Press; 2002.

WEB SITES

http://www.health.org/. National Clearinghouse for Alcohol and Drug Information.
http://www.nida.nih.gov/. National Institute on Drug Abuse.
http://www.niaaa.nih.gov/. National Institute on Alcohol Abuse and Alcoholism.
http://www.samhsa.gov/. Substance Abuse and Mental Health Services Administration.
http://www.saddonline.com/. Students Against Destructive Decisions.

REFERENCES AND ADDITIONAL READINGS

American Psychiatric Association. *Diagnostic and statistical manual of mental disorders*. 4th ed. Washington, DC: American Psychiatric Association; 1994.
Borowsky IW, Mozayeny S, Ireland M. Brief psychosocial screening at health supervision and acute care visits. *Pediatrics* 2003;112(1):129.
Breslin C, Li S, Sdao-Jarvie K, et al. Brief treatment for young substance abusers: a pilot study in an addiction treatment setting. *Psychol Addict Behav* 2002;16(1):10.
Centers for Disease Control. Youth risk behavior surveillance—United States, 2003. *MMWR* 2004;53(SS-5):1.
Crowe RR, Kramer JR, Hesselbrock V, et al. The utility of the brief MAST' and the CAGE' in identifying alcohol problems: results from national high-risk and community samples. *Arch Fam Med* 1997;6(5):477.
Dembo R, Schmeidler J, Brodern P, et al. Examination of the reliability of the Problem Oriented Screening Instrument for Teenagers (POSIT) among arrested youth entering a juvenile assessment center. *Subst Use Misuse* 1996;31(7):785.
Ewing J. Detecting alcoholism: the CAGE questionnaire. *JAMA* 1984;252(14):1906.
Fleming MF, Mundt MP, French MT, et al. Brief physician advice for problem drinkers: long-term efficacy and benefit-cost analysis. *Alcohol Clin Exp Res* 2002;26(1):36.
von Hook S, Harris SK, Brooks T, et al. The "Six T's": barriers to screening teens for substance abuse in primary care. *J Adolesc Health* 2007;40:465.
Knight JR, Goodman E, Pulerwitz T, et al. Reliabilities of short substance abuse screening tests among adolescent medical patients. *Pediatrics* 2000;105(4):948.
Knight JR, Goodman E, Pulerwitz T, et al. Reliability of the Problem Oriented Screening Instrument for Teenagers (POSIT) in an adolescent medical clinic population. *J Adolesc Health*. 2001;29(2):125.
Knight JR, Sherritt L, Gates E, et al. Should the CRAFFT substance abuse screening test be shortened. *J Clin Outcomes Mgmt* 2004;11(1):19.
Knight JR, Sherritt L, Harris SK, et al. Validity of brief alcohol screening tests among adolescents: a comparison of the AUDIT, POSIT, CAGE and CRAFFT. *Alcohol Clin Exp Res* 2002a; 27:67.
Knight JR, Sherritt L, Shrier LA, et al. *Validity of the CRAFFT substance abuse screening test among adolescent clinic patients*. *Arch Pediatr Adolesc Med* 2002b;156:607.
Knight JR, Shrier LA, Bravender TD, et al. A new brief screen for adolescent substance abuse. *Arch Pediatr Adolesc Med* 1999;153:591.

Levy S, Vaugh BL, Angulo M, et al. Buprenorphine replacement therapy for adolescents with opioid dependence: early experience from a children's hospital-based outpatient treatment program. *J Adolesc Health* 2007;40:477.

Miles H, Winstock A, Strang J. Identifying young people who drink too much: the clinical utility of the five-item Alcohol Use Disorders Identification Test (AUDIT). *Drug Alcohol Rev* 2001;20:9.

Miller WR, Rollnick S. *Motivational Interviewing: preparing people for change*, 2nd ed. New York, NY: Guilford Press; 2002.

http://www.powertrain.com *Problem Oriented Screening Instrument for Teenagers (POSIT Version 2)*. Landover, MD: PowerTrain; 1998.

Prochaska J, DiClemente C. Toward a comprehensive model of change. In: Miller WR, Heather N, eds. *Treating addictive behavior: process of change*. New York: Plenum Publishing; 1986:3.

Prochaska JO, DiClemente CC. Stages of change in the modification of problem behaviors. *Prog Behav Modif* 1992;28:183.

Reinert D, Allen J. The Alcohol Use Disorders Identification Test (AUDIT): A review of recent research. *Alcohol Clin Exp Res* 2002;26(2):272.

Schmidt A, Barry KL, Fleming MF. Detection of problem drinkers: the Alcohol Use Disorders Identification Test (AUDIT). *South Med J* 1995;88(1):52.

Stowell RJ, Estroff TW. Psychiatric disorders in substance-abusing adolescent inpatients: a pilot study. *J Am Acad Child Adolesc Psychiatry* 1992;31:1036.

Wilens TE, Biederman J, Abrantes AM, et al. Clinical characteristics of psychiatrically referred adolescent outpatients with substance use disorder. *J Am Acad Child Adolesc Psychiatry* 1997;36(7):941.S.

Wilson CR, Sherritt L, Gates E, et al. Are clinical impressions of adolescent substance use accurate. *Pediatrics* 2004;114: e536.

CHAPTER 74

Intensive Drug Treatment

Brigid L. Vaughan and John R. Knight

PRINCIPLES OF DRUG TREATMENT IN ADOLESCENTS

Primary health care providers, and indeed all health care providers who work with adolescents, have a clear responsibility to screen adolescents for substance use disorders, as described in Chapter 73. Adolescents with low-risk substance use may be amenable to office-based brief interventions. However, adolescents with more severe difficulties, or with substance use disorders, often require more specific or intensive treatment.

The American Academy of Child and Adolescent Psychiatry's (AACAP) Practice Parameter for the Assessment and Treatment of Children and Adolescents with Substance Use Disorders (American Academy of Child and Adolescent Psychiatry, 2005) sets forth evidence-based recommendations regarding the assessment and care of adolescents with substance use disorders (Table 74.1).

A primary requirement in working with adolescents is an explicit review of the limits of confidentiality (American Academy of Child and Adolescent Psychiatry, 2005). Youths are more likely to be honest in discussing their substance use when assured of confidentiality. However, they must also be informed of when and why information will be shared with others, for instance when there is concern of possible harm to the teen or others. Although the adolescent is certainly entitled to confidentiality, the health care provider should not encourage secrets in families. Family involvement is a necessary component in any substance abuse treatment program, but especially with the care of adolescents.

MATCHING PATIENTS TO APPROPRIATE TREATMENT

No single treatment is appropriate for all individuals. Matching of treatment settings, interventions, and services to each patient's problems and needs is critical (Drug Strategies, 2003). Treatment for adolescents must be adolescent-specific, not simply an adult program that tries to accommodate younger patients (American Society of Addiction Medicine, 2001). Adolescents who use substances may have a more rapid progression from casual use to dependence; they are more likely to use multiple substances, and often are at higher risk of co-occurring psychopathology. They must have a comprehensive, multidimensional assessment to adequately formulate an appropriate treatment plan. The American Society of Addiction Medicine (ASAM) and Drug Strategies, a nonprofit research institute, have published documents to help with this process, the *ASAM Patient Placement Criteria for the Treatment of Substance-Related Disorders* (American Society of Addiction Medicine, 2001) and *Treating Teens: A Guide to Adolescent Drug Programs* (Drug Strategies, 2003), respectively. *Treating Teens* includes questions (Table 74.2) to help families and providers in assessing the appropriateness of potential programs.

OVERVIEW OF AVAILABLE TREATMENTS

Inpatient Care

It is important for the health care provider to have a general understanding of the range and types of treatments available, to best counsel patients and families. Treatment should be provided in the least restrictive setting possible (American Academy of Child and Adolescent Psychiatry, 2005). Safety issues, patient or family motivation, medical or psychiatric complications, treatment availability, and failure of treatment in a less-intensive setting, all may lead to the need for an intensive treatment setting.

1. Detoxification: Adolescents usually do not experience physical withdrawal symptoms from the most commonly used substances (e.g., cannabis). However, those who are dependent on alcohol, other sedative-hypnotics, and opioids often experience withdrawal symptoms that require medical management. *Detoxification* is a term used to describe the medical monitoring and treatment of withdrawal symptoms. It can be done on an outpatient basis, but detoxification often requires a 3- to 5-day inpatient medical hospitalization. Detoxification should be considered for all patients who have symptoms of physical dependence on alcohol or benzodiazepines. Opioid withdrawal is not life threatening, as alcohol withdrawal can be, but it is very uncomfortable and can be relieved with detoxification.

2. Psychiatric hospitalization or acute residential treatment: For adolescents whose substance use disorder has caused or has been accompanied by severe

TABLE 74.1

Recommendations for the Assessment and Care of Adolescents with Substance Use Disorders (American Academy of Child and Adolescent Psychiatry, 2005)

The adolescent must be assured of an appropriate level of confidentiality.

Assessment must include developmentally appropriate screening questions regarding the use of alcohol and drugs.

A positive screen necessitates a more formal evaluation.

Toxicology, that is, drug testing, is to be a routine part of assessment and ongoing treatment.

Adolescents who have substance use disorders need specific treatment.

Treatment of substance use disorders should be in the least restrictive setting.

Family therapy and/or substantial family involvement should be included in treatment of adolescents with substance use disorders.

Treatment programs should strive to fully engage adolescents and maximize treatment completion.

Medication to manage craving or withdrawal, or for aversion therapy can be used as indicated.

Treatment of adolescents with substance use disorders must help develop peer support.

Involvement with 12-step groups, like Alcoholics Anonymous (AA) or Narcotics Anonymous (NA), should be encouraged.

Programs should provide comprehensive services, including vocational, recreational, medical services as indicated.

Adolescents with substance use disorders require comprehensive psychiatric assessment, in order to check for comorbid disorders.

Co-occurring psychiatric disorders require treatment.

Programs must provide or arrange for aftercare.

behavioral or even frank psychiatric symptoms, inpatient psychiatric hospitalization or acute residential treatment may be needed (American Academy of Child and Adolescent Psychiatry, 2005). In these settings, patients are stabilized in a safe, structured setting. The initial work of stopping substance use, assessing readiness to change and motivation, and crisis intervention with the teen and family are carried out in these settings over a 1- to 2-week stay. More specific psychiatric assessment and treatment are also initiated when indicated.

Outpatient Care

For medically and behaviorally stable patients, outpatient treatment is the mainstay of substance abuse treatment. This can consist of individual, group, or family therapy,

or any combination of these. Day treatment programs also may be used when an adolescent is transitioning from a more-intensive level of care, or needs greater supervision than provided by outpatient visits. There are multiple treatment modalities that can be used in caring for adolescents with substance use disorders; some of these will be summarized in the subsequent text.

1. Cognitive behavioral therapy: Cognitive behavioral therapy (CBT) is a structured, goal-oriented counseling style (Reinecke et al., 1996) that has been found effective (Azrin et al., 2001; Dennis et al., 2004; Waldron et al., 2001). It is designed to teach patients specific skills that will help them remain abstinent. Cognitive behavioral training teaches patients to identify thoughts and feelings that precede drug use. Once the patient can recognize these situations, she/he can then learn either

TABLE 74.2

Ten Important Questions to Ask of a Treatment Program

1. How does your program address the needs of adolescents?
2. What kind of assessment does the program conduct of the adolescent's problems?
3. How often does the program review and update the treatment plan in light of the adolescent's progress?
4. How is the family involved in the treatment process?
5. How do you engage adolescents so that they stay in treatment?
6. What are the qualifications of program staff and what kind of clinical supervision is provided?
7. Does the program offer separate single sex groups as well as male and female counselors for girls and boys?
8. How does the program follow-up with the adolescent and provide continuing care after treatment is completed?
9. What evidence do you have that your program is effective?
10. What is the cost of the program?

From (Drug Strategies, 2003).

to avoid the situation or to substitute with behaviors other than drug use. CBT is most effective when the patient is willing to practice newly acquired skills. CBT can be used in individual, family, or group therapy settings. It may be used alone or in combination with motivational interviewing, which has been described in Chapter 73.

2. Group therapy: Group treatment for adolescents with substance use disorders is appealing in several ways. Meeting with a group of adolescents who share similar difficulties may be easier for a teen, as she/he will be assured that she/he is not "the only one" with such troubles. Congregating with peers, even if for treatment, coincides with a developmentally normal preference of adolescents. Additionally, in the context of limited resources, being able to provide care for multiple patients simultaneously is cost-effective and allows care for more people. However, studies have yielded mixed reviews (American Academy of Child and Adolescent Psychiatry, 2005). Including youths with more severe conduct disorders in groups may lead to poor outcomes (Dishion et al., 2001). In view of this, careful evaluation of potential group members' appropriateness is warranted.

3. 12-Step fellowships: Another form of peer-based support may be found in 12-step fellowships, namely Alcoholics Anonymous (AA) and/or Narcotics Anonymous (NA). Ideally, adolescents should attend young people's meetings (Jaffe, 2001), or be accompanied to AA/NA meetings by a trusted adult. As is generally recommended for people early in recovery, adolescents would benefit from getting a sponsor. Twelve-step meetings are often an integral part of substance abuse treatment programs (Drug Strategies, 2003). It is imperative that the individual adolescent's developmental level be considered when progressing through the 12 steps (Simkin, 1996).

4. Family therapy: Family therapy has been studied more than any other treatments for adolescent substance use disorders. Limited studies comparing different outpatient studies have found family therapy to be superior (Stanton and Shadish, 1997; Williams and Chang, 2000). There are multiple forms of family therapy that have been studied using randomized clinical studies. These include functional family therapy (Alexander et al., 1990), brief strategic family therapy (Szapocznik et al., 1983, 1988), family systems therapy (Joanning et al., 1992), multidimensional family therapy (MDFT) (Dennis et al., 2002; Liddle et al., 2001), and multisystemic therapy (MST) (Henggeler et al., 1991, 2002).

   MDFT was developed at the University of Miami School of Medicine, and is intended to treat adolescents with substance abuse and behavioral problems. MDFT includes individual and family sessions, with and without the teen, as well as intensive advocacy with social systems, like schools and courts. There are one to four family meetings per week, with frequent interim phone contact. Treatment continues for 4 to 8 months. There are detailed treatment manuals to ensure accurate replication of MDFT; the program has been implemented in 16 other sites in the United States (Drug Strategies, 2003).

   MST is an intensive 4-month program, and was developed to address the needs of adolescents at high risk of incarceration or foster care. Not only are the sessions held in the family's home, but therapists are also always available to assist and provide intervention to families. Parents identify the goals for treatment, and therapists

help them identify the causes and then implement solutions. MST includes comprehensive psychiatric and substance abuse services. The Medical University of South Carolina, where MST was developed, continues to conduct clinical studies of its efficacy and to provide training to outside agencies nation- and worldwide (Drug Strategies, 2003).

5. Drug court: The success of adult drug courts and the increasing prevalence of substance abuse in the adjudicated adolescent population have resulted in the institution of >100 juvenile drug court programs in close to 50 states (American University, 2001). A successful juvenile drug court will use the case management system, which provides a more "user-friendly" interface with the adolescent and family (Drug Strategies, 2003). There should be positive reinforcement for compliance as well as clearly outlined consequences that are swiftly enforced for violation of court-ordered program guidelines. Limited studies indicate that juvenile drug court does reduce recidivism and substance use while the adolescent is participating in the program (Belenko, 2001). Efforts are underway to better utilize juvenile drug courts in delivering research-based treatment interventions to adolescents and families (Belenko and Logan, 2003).

6. Contingency management: Another outpatient treatment model that relies heavily on reinforcement of desirable behaviors is contingency management (Budney et al., 2001). With this treatment model, urine testing is used to detect substance use, and substance abstinence (as detected by a negative drug test result) is reinforced while substance use results in a loss of reinforcement. The reinforcement may be gift certificates, movie tickets, or small amounts of money. Contingency management has been found to be effective in treating adult substance use (Higgins et al., 2002); studies with adolescent patients are promising (Azrin et al., 1994; Corby et al., 2000; Kamon et al., 2005), but additional research is needed (Kaminer, 2000).

Long-term Residential Treatment

For youths who have "failed" outpatient treatment for substance use disorders, longer-term treatment may be in order. As with outpatient treatment, there is a wide range of long-term treatment options. Residential treatment is usually long-term treatment for 6 to 12 months, but may be as brief as 1 month (Drug Strategies, 2003). Residential programs provide a variety of therapeutic sessions daily, including individual, group, and family therapy, as well as an educational component. These programs can accommodate adolescents who may have both psychiatric and substance use disorders. The adolescents who are placed in residential programs have not been able to stop using substances and may well have other concerning behaviors like self-injury or a history of suicide attempts. Some residential programs are "locked" for the most at-risk youths.

1. Therapeutic communities: Therapeutic communities also provide treatment for adolescents with severe substance and behavioral difficulties who have failed less-intensive treatments (Drug Strategies, 2003; Pumariega et al., 2005). These youths are not able to live at home and are not at risk of violent behaviors (Drug Strategies,

2003). This treatment modality is generally of longer duration, 18 to 24 months. Half-way houses, or reentry facilities, provide supervised living for patients recovering from drug dependence (Drug Strategies, 2003). They may serve as a step-down for adolescents who have completed a more-intensive treatment.

2. Therapeutic schools: Therapeutic schools are designed to meet the academic and therapeutic needs of adolescents with a variety of mental health and behavioral problems. Though not designed solely for substance abuse treatment, many schools will have substance abuse services. Therapeutic schools may be residential, include a boarding component, or function solely as a day school with adolescents living at home.

3. Wilderness therapy: For many youths, outpatient treatment is insufficient but inpatient services are too restrictive (Tuma, 1989). For this population, wilderness therapy programs are used at times as an alternative (Russell et al., 1999). Limited studies have been promising (Davis-Berman and Berman, 1989). However, despite the increasing use of wilderness therapy programs they have not been adequately studied (Mulvey et al., 1993); wilderness therapy programs typically serve adolescents having a variety of behavior problems (Drug Strategies, 2003). Adolescents who go for wilderness therapy have generally been resistant to making changes in their behaviors and may have had multiple past treatment experiences (Drug Strategies, 2003; Russell et al., 1999). The treatment involves individual and group therapy, educational curricula, and group living with peers in an unfamiliar environment with application of outdoor-living skills and physical challenges (Russell et al., 1999). The programs are meant to boost responsibility—personal and social—and to encourage emotional growth. Though not specifically designed to treat drug problems, drug use is common among teens in these programs, and most programs will have some specific drug treatment component. Wilderness therapy programs generally last 3 to 8 weeks (Drug Strategies, 2003).

Pharmacotherapy

Developing medication treatments for substance use disorders is an active area of research at this time. This work has even included efforts to develop vaccines to treat drug dependence (Haney and Kosten, 2004; Kosten and Biegel, 2002; Martell et al., 2005; Sofuoglu and Kosten, 2005). However, currently there are few substances of abuse for which there are any corresponding pharmacotherapies (Vocci et al., 2005; Wilkins, 2005). Following is a brief summary of medications currently available to treat problems due to alcohol and opioids.

1. Alcohol: Disulfiram, naltrexone, and acamprosate are the only medications approved for the treatment of alcohol dependence in adults (Mann, 2004); none of them are approved for use in adolescents. Disulfiram was the first medication used for treating alcoholism, and is an aversive therapy that causes an unpleasant reaction if the patient uses alcohol while taking it. The disulfiram–alcohol reaction can result in nausea, vomiting, flushing, headache, diaphoresis, dyspnea, palpitations, chest pain, blurred vision, or confusion (Banys, 1988). Disulfiram is not recommended for use in adolescents. Naltrexone, an opioid antagonist, helps to support abstinence in heavy drinkers by limiting the rewarding effects of alcohol. Acamprosate is the most recent U.S. Food and Drug Administration (FDA)-approved medication for treating alcohol dependence, and acts by alleviating cravings; therefore, is useful as a maintenance medication (Mann, 2004; Schaffer and Naranjo, 1998; Wilkins, 2005). Specific serotoninergic reuptake inhibitors (SSRIs) can be of help to patients with alcohol dependence by treating underlying psychiatric disorders, like depression or anxiety, which may be present (Mann, 2004).

2. Opioids: The treatment of opioid dependence in adults has utilized pharmacotherapy since the mid-1960s when methadone as agonist therapy began (Dole and Nyswander, 1976). The federal government strictly regulates the use of methadone (Rettig and Yarmolinsky, 1995). Patients who have been dependent on heroin for >1 year, and are at least 18-years-old, are eligible for methadone maintenance (Leshner, 2003). This clearly restricts access for adolescents, particularly since they may have a shorter history of opioid dependence.

   Although methadone has been the major medication used for opioid maintenance, newer medications, such as levomethadyl acetate (LAAM) and buprenorphine are similarly effective (Johnson et al., 2000). Concern regarding cardiotoxicity with LAAM has limited its use in treating drug dependence (Joseph, 2005). Buprenorphine is a partial opioid agonist and therefore may have some advantages, including fewer withdrawal symptoms and a lower risk of overdose (O'Connor, 2000). The buprenorphine-naloxone preparation lessens risk of abuse (Fudala et al., 1998; Strain et al., 2000; Weinhold et al., 1992).

TREATMENT OF CO-OCCURRING DISORDERS

Individuals who are struggling with both psychiatric and substance use disorders, have been called *dually diagnosed*; however, more recently they have been thought of as having "co-occurring disorders" because they rarely have difficulties in only two arenas (Drake et al., 2000). Treatment models for patients with co-occurring disorders have included sequential (Weiss and Najavits, 1998), parallel, and integrated care of the psychiatric and substance use disorders (Dennison, 2005). The integrated model for treating co-occurring psychiatric and substance use disorders in adolescents is supported by research (Drug Strategies, 2003; National Institute on Drug Abuse, 1999). Treatment for patients with co-occurring disorders may include psychosocial interventions as well as psychopharmacology.

Mood Disorders

It can be difficult to discern whether a mood disorder preceded or is the result of substance use. Nonetheless depression in adolescents has been correlated with an earlier age at onset of substance use disorders (Deykin et al., 1987). The presence of chronic depression and dysthymia has been found to precede substance use difficulties (Hovens et al., 1994), while major depression has been found to follow it (Bukstein et al., 1992; Hovens et al., 1994). Those participants with primary depression were more likely to be female; additionally, they tended to have a parent with psychiatric difficulties and to have a history of victimization (Deykin et al., 1987). Although studies in adolescents are limited as compared to studies in adults, the use of SSRIs to treat depression in youths with substance use disorders appears to be safe and likely effective (Deas and Thomas, 2001; Lohman, 2002; Riggs, 1997). Bipolar disorder in adolescents may also be associated with substance use disorders, but this has been less well studied (Clark and Neighbors, 1996). Nonetheless, a controlled study by Geller et al. (1998) found that lithium had a good safety profile in treating adolescents with co-occurring bipolar and substance use disorders. Although the study results included greater decline in substance use for teens treated with lithium than those given placebo, pharmacotherapy for the mood disorder did not adequately address the substance use disorder in the absence of specific substance abuse treatment.

Anxiety Disorders

As noted earlier for mood disorders, it can be difficult to determine whether anxiety led to or was caused by substance abuse. Although CBT, often combined with SSRI medication, is an established regimen for treating adolescents with anxiety disorders (March and Wells, 2002), the treatment of teens with anxiety and substance use disorders has not been adequately studied (Riggs, 2003). However, preliminary data suggests that adolescents with substance use disorders and anxiety may be helped by CBT (Najavits, 2003). Additionally, as previously noted, SSRI medications have been found to be safe in adolescents who continue to use alcohol (Lohman, 2002), and so may be used to treat anxiety as well as depression. It is recommended that benzodiazepines not be used to treat co-occurring anxiety in teens with substance use disorders because of their abuse potential (Riggs, 2003).

Attention-Deficit Hyperactivity Disorder

Longitudinal studies have shown that attention-deficit hyperactivity disorder (ADHD) is associated with an increased risk of substance use disorders (Katusic et al., 2003; Molina and Pelham, 2003). Adolescents with ADHD have earlier onset of substance dependence (Biederman et al., 1997). Additionally, a meta-analysis conducted by Wilens et al. (2003) found that stimulant treatment of ADHD is associated with lower risk of substance use disorders. This is especially important because stimulants are the first-line medication for treating ADHD, and are very effective (American Academy of Child and Adolescent Psychiatry, 1997). Health care providers are at times reluctant to prescribe stimulants to patients with ADHD and substance use disorders because the medication can be abused if ground up and used intravenously or intranasally (Wilens, 2004). Longer-acting stimulant medications, particularly osmotic release oral system (OROS) methylphenidate (Concerta), have much less abuse potential (Jaffe, 2002; Wilens, 2004). Nonstimulant medications, like bupropion and atomoxetine, are also effective in treating ADHD (Michelson et al., 2002; Wilens et al., 2001). Bupropion, which does not have a formal indication for treating ADHD, may be helpful for adolescents with comorbid ADHD and depression (Daviss et al., 2001), and so could be considered as an option for teens with co-occurring ADHD and substance use disorders (Riggs, 2003). Additional research is needed in this area.

Acute and Chronic Pain

The topic of pain control in patients with and without history of substance use disorders is quite broad; following is a discussion of salient issues to be considered. The current concerns, in society and the medical community, about undertreatment of pain and opiate abuse/dependence make this a particularly important topic (Ling et al., 2005). Historically, experts in managing pain have underestimated the risk and prevalence of addiction, while substance abuse experts have shown great reluctance to use opioids to treat pain (Passik, 2001). Greater communication and collaboration between professionals is clearly needed in order to adequately treat patients with chronic pain and substance use disorders (Ling et al., 2005).

Pseudoaddiction refers to drug-seeking behavior generated by inadequate pain management (Weissman and Haddox, 1989). The patient's quest for opiate medication is generated by the desire for relief of pain, not by mood-altering effects of the drug (Portenoy et al., 2005; Weissman and Haddox, 1989). Patients with pseudoaddiction may hoard medication, request specific drugs, or escalate medication dose without informing/asking the treating physician (Portenoy et al., 2005). Adequate pain treatment can prevent pseudoaddiction (Ling et al., 2005). If a patient in pain who is complaining of needing more medication becomes involved with illicit drugs or illegal acts (e.g., injecting oral medications, prescription forgery, stealing drugs from others) or exhibits a decline in functioning, then a substance use disorder must be considered (Portenoy et al., 2005).

Patients with a history of past or recent substance abuse or dependence are not immune to pain-related conditions. It has even been suggested that people with opioid dependence are less tolerant to pain (Compton et al., 2000). Patients with both substance use disorders and a pain syndrome, for example, related to cancer or an injury, require comprehensive assessment. This is to include a detailed history of current and past substance use; review of all medical records; permission to contact other current and past health care providers, pharmacies, and family; and urine drug testing as indicated (Portenoy et al., 2005). Ongoing care necessitates continued open communication between all involved providers.

In summary, intensive treatment of substance use disorders in adolescents may occur in a variety of settings and utilize a wide range of services. Common themes, however, include the need for thorough assessment, comprehensive care which involves the family, as well as thoughtful continuing care. The primary care clinician caring for adolescents can serve an important role by educating teens and their families about treatment needs and options, guiding families through various stages of care, and supporting them during difficulties that may arise.

WEB SITES

www.drugstrategies.org. Drug Strategies is a nonprofit research foundation that promotes more effective ways of dealing with the nation's drug and alcohol problems.

Drug Strategies also sponsors www.bubblemonkey.com a confidential Web site dedicated to answering teens' questions about drugs and alcohol.

www.reclaimingfutures.org. This Web site provides information about Reclaiming Futures sites which provide research-based interventions for teens with substance use disorders.

www.dea.gov/pubs/abuse. This site provides text of *Drugs of Abuse,* which provides straightforward information about drugs.

www.buprenorphine.samhsa.gov. This Web site provides information about the use of buprenorphine in treating opioid dependence, as well as a "physician locator" to help patients and families find treatment.

REFERENCES AND ADDITIONAL READINGS

Alexander J, Waldon H, Newberry A, et al. The functional family therapy model. In: Friedman A, Granick S, eds. *Family therapy for adolescent drug abuse.* Lexington, MA: Lexington Books; 1990.

American Academy of Child and Adolescent Psychiatry (AACAP). Practice parameters for the assessment and treatment of children, adolescents, and adults with attention-deficit/hyperactivity disorder. *J Am Acad Child Adolesc Psychiatry* 1997;36:85S.

American Academy of Child and Adolescent Psychiatry (AACAP). Practice parameter for the assessment and treatment of children and adolescents with substance use disorders. *J Am Acad Child Adolesc Psychiatry* 2005;44:609.

American Society of Addiction Medicine (ASAM). *ASAM Patient placement criteria for the treatment of substance-related disorders,* 2001.

American University. Drug court activity update: composite summary information, December 2000. *Drug court clearinghouse and technical assistance project.* Washington, DC: U.S. Department of Justice, Office of Justice Programs; 2001.

Azrin N, Donohue B, Besalel V, et al. Youth drug abuse treatment: a controlled outcome study. *J Child Adolesc Subst Abuse* 1994;3:1.

Azrin N, Donohue B, Teichner G, et al. A controlled evaluation and description of individual-cognitive problem solving and family-behavior therapies in dually-diagnosed youth. *J Child Adolesc Subst Abuse* 2001;11:1.

Banys P. The clinical use of disulfiram (Antabuse): a review. *J Psychoactive Drugs* 1988;20:243.

Belenko S. *Research on drug courts: a critical review 2001 update.* New York: National Center on Addictions and Substance Abuse at Columbia University; 2001.

Belenko S, Logan T. Delivering more effective treatment to adolescents: Improving the juvenile court model. *J Subst Abuse Treat* 2003;25:189.

Biederman J, Wilens T, Mick E. Is ADHD a risk factor for psychoactive substance use disorders. *J Am Acad Child Adolesc Psychiatry* 1997;36:21.

Budney A, Sigmon S, Higgins S. Contingency management: using science to motivate change. In: Coombs R, ed. *Addiction recovery tools: a practical handbook.* Thousand Oaks, CA: Sage; 2001:147.

Bukstein O, Glancy L, Kaminer Y. Patterns of affective commorbidity in a clinical population of dually diagnosed adolescent substance abusers. *J Child Adolesc Psychiatr* 1992; 31:1041.

Clark D, Neighbors B. Adolescent substance abuse and internalizing disorders. In: Jaffe, S, ed. *Child and adolescent psychiatric clinics of North America.* Philadelphia, PA: WB Saunders; 1996:45.

Compton P, Charuvastra V, Kintaudi K. Pain responses in methadone-maintained opioid abusers. *J Pain Symptom Manage* 2000;20:237.

Corby E, Roll J, Ledgerwood D, et al. Contingency management interventions for treating the substance abuse of adolescents: a feasibility study. *Exp Clin Psychopharmacol* 2000; 8:371.

Davis-Berman J, Berman D. The wilderness therapy program: an empirical study of its effects with adolescents in an outpatient setting. *J Contemp Psychother* 1989;19:271.

Daviss W, Bentivoglio P, Racusin R, et al. Bupropion sustained-release in adolescents with comorbid attention-deficit/hyperactivity disorder and depression. *J Am Acad Child Adolesc Psychiatry* 2001;40:307.

Deas D, Thomas S. An overview of controlled studies of adolescent substance abuse treatment. *Am J Addict* 2001;10:178.

Dennis M, Godley S, Diamond G. The Cannabis Youth Treatment (CYT) study: main findings from two randomized trials. *J Subst Abuse Treat* 2004;27:197.

Dennis M, Titus J, Diamond G. The Cannabis Youth Treatment (CYT) experiment: rationale, study design, and analysis plans. *Addiction* 2002;97:16.

Dennison S. Substance use disorders in individuals with co-occurring psychiatric disorders. In: Lowinson, J, Ruiz, P, Millman, R, et al., eds. *Substance abuse: a comprehensive textbook,* 4th ed. New York: Lippincott Williams & Wilkins; 2005: 904.

Deykin E, Buka S, Zeena T. Adolescent depression, alcohol, and drug abuse. *Am J Public Health* 1987;77:178.

Dishion T, Poulin F, Burraston B. Peer group dynamics associated with iatrogenic effects in group interventions with high-risk young adolescents. In: Nangle, D, Erdley C, eds. *The role of friendship in psychological adjustment.* New Directions for Child and Adolescent Development. No. 91. San Francisco: Jossey-Bass; 2001:79.

Dole V, Nyswander M. Methadone maintenance treatment: a ten-year perspective. *J Am Med Assoc* 1976;260:3025.

Drake R, Xie H, McHugo G. Dual diagnosis: fifteen years of progress. *Psychiatr Serv* 2000;51:1126.

Drug Strategies. *Treating teens: a guide to adolescent drug programs. Adolescent Programs and Resources* Washington, DC: Drug Strategies; 2003.

Fudala P, Yu E, MacFadden W. Effects of buprenorphine and naoloxone in morphine-stabilized opioid addicts. *Drug Alcohol Depend* 1998;50:1.

Geller B, Cooper T, Sun K, et al. Double-blind and placebo-controlled study of lithium for adolescent bipolar disorders with secondary substance dependency. *J Child Adolesc Psychiatr* 1998;37:171.

Greydanus DE, Patel DR. The adolescent and substance abuse: current concepts. *Dis Mon* 2005;51:392.

Haney M, Kosten T. Therapeutic vaccines for substance dependence. *Expert Rev Vaccines* 2004;3:11.

Henggeler S, Borduin C, Melton G. Effects of multisystemic therapy on drug use and abuse in serious juvenile offenders: a progress report from two outcome studies. *Fam Dynamics Addict Q* 1991;1:40.

Henggeler S, Clingempeel W, Brondino M, et al. Four-year follow up of multisystemic therapy with substance abusing and substance-dependent juvenile offenders. *J Am Acad Child Adolesc Psychiatry* 2002;41:868.

Higgins S, Alessi S, Dantona R. Voucher-based incentives: a substance abuse treatment innovation. *Addict Behav* 2002; 27:887.

Hovens J, Cantwell D, Kiriakos R. Psychiatric comorbidity in hospitalized adolescent substance abusers. *J Child Adolesc Psychiatr* 1994;33:476.

Jaffe S. *Adolescent substance abuse intervention workbook: taking a first step*. Washington, DC: American Psychiatric Press; 2001.

Jaffe S. Failed attempts at intranasal abuse of Concerta. *J Am Acad Child Adolesc Psychiatry* 2002;41:5.

Joanning H, Quinn W, Thomas F, et al. Treating adolescent drug abuse: a comparison of family system therapy, group therapy and family drug education. *J Marital Fam Ther* 1992;18:345.

Johnson R, Chutuape M, Strain E. A comparison of lev-omethadyl acetate, buprenorphine, and methadone for opi-oid dependence. *N Engl J Med* 2000;343:1290.

Joseph D. *Drugs of abuse*. Washington, DC: Drug Enforcement Administration, US Department of Justice; 2005.

Kaminer Y. Contingency management reinforcement proce-dures for adolescent substance abuse. *J Am Acad Child Adolesc Psychiatry* 2000;39:1324.

Kamon J, Budney A, Stanger C. A contingency management intervention for adolescent marijuana abuse and conduct problems. *J Am Acad Child Adolesc Psychiatry* 2005;44:513.

Katusic S, Barbaresi W, Colligan R. Substance abuse among ADHD cases: a population-based birth cohort study, Paper presented at the *Pediatric academic society annual meeting*. Seattle, WA: May 3–6, 2003.

Kosten T, Biegel D. Therapeutic vaccines for substance dependence. *Expert Rev Vaccines* 2002;1:363.

Leshner A. Accessing opiate dependence treatment medica-tions: buprenorphine products in an office setting. *Drug Alcohol Depend* 2003;70:s103.

Liddle HA. Family-based therapies for adolescent alcohol and drug use. *Addiction* 2004;99(Suppl 2):76.

Liddle H, Dakof G, Parker K, et al. Multidimensional family ther-apy for adolescent substance abuse: results of a randomized clinical trial. *Am J Drug Alcohol Abuse* 2001;27:651.

Ling W, Wesson D, Smith D. Prescription opiate abuse. In: Lowinson J, Ruiz, P, Millman R, et al., eds. *Substance abuse: a comprehensive textbook*, 4th ed. New York: Lippincott Williams & Wilkins; 2005:459.

Lohman M. Perceived motivations for treatment in depressed, substance-dependent adolescents with conduct disorder, Paper presented at the *College on problems of drug depen-dence : 64th annual scientific meeting*. Rockville, MD, 2002.

Mann K. Pharmacotherapy of alcohol dependence: a review of the clinical data. *CNS Drugs* 2004;18:485.

March J, Wells K. Combining medications and psychotherapy. In: Leckman J, Schill L, Charney D, eds. *Pediatric psychophar-macology: principles and practice*. London: Oxford University Press; 2002:426.

Martell B, Mitchell E, Poling J, et al. Vaccine pharmacotherapy for the treatment of cocaine dependence. *Biol Psychiatry* 2005;58:158.

Michelson D, Allen AJ, Busner J, et al. Once-daily atomoxetine treatment for children and adolescents with attention deficit hyperactivity disorder: a randomized, placebo-controlled study. *Am J Psychiatry* 2002;159:1896.

Molina B, Pelham WJ. Childhood predictors of adolescent substance use in a longitudinal study of children with ADHD. *J Abnorm Psychol* 2003;112:497.

Mulvey E, Arthur M, Repucci N. The preventment and treatment of juvenile delinquency: a review of the research. *Clin Psychol Rev* 1993;13:133.

Najavits L. Seeking safety: a new psychotherapy for post-traumatic stress disorder and substance use disorder. In: Ouimette P, Brown P, eds. *Trauma and substance abuse: causes, consequences, and treatment of comorbid disorders*. Washington, DC: American Psychological Association; 2003: 147.

National Institute on Drug Abuse (NIDA). *Principles of drug addiction treatment: a research-based guide, National Institutes of Health Publication No.99–4180*. Rockville, MD: National Institute on Drug Abuse; 1999.

O'Connor P. Treating opioid dependence: new data and new opportunities. *N Engl J Med* 2000;343:1332.

Passik S. Responding rationally to recent report of abuse/diversion of oxycontin. *J Pain Symptom Manage* 2001;21: 359.

Portenoy R, Payne R, Passik S. Acute and chronic pain. In: Lowinson J, Ruiz P, Millman R, et al., eds. *Substance abuse: a comprehensive textbook*, 4th ed. New York: Lippincott Williams & Wilkins; 2005:863.

Pumariega A, Kilgus M, Rodriguez L. Adolescents. In: Lowin-son J, Ruiz P, Millman R, et al., eds. *Substance abuse: a comprehensive textbook*, 4th ed. New York: Lippincott Williams & Wilkins; 2005:1021.

Reinecke M, Dattilio F, Freeman A. *Cognitive therapy with children and adolescents*. New York: Guilford Press; 1996.

Rettig R, Yarmolinsky A. *Federal regulation of methadone treatment*. Washington, DC: Institute of Medicine, National Academy Press; 1995.

Riggs P. Fluoxetine in drug-dependent delinquents with major depression: an open trial. *J Child Adolesc Psychopharmacol* 1997;7:87.

Riggs P. Treating adolescents for substance abuse and comorbid psychiatric disorders. *Sci Pract Perspect* 2003;2:18.

Russell K, Hendee J, Plillips-Miller D. How wilderness therapy works: an examination of the wilderness therapy process to treat adolescents with behavioral problems and addictions, Paper presented at the *Wilderness science in a time of change conference: Wilderness as a place for scientific inquiry*. Missoula, MT, 1999.

Schaffer A, Naranjo C. Recommended drug treatment strategies for the alcoholic patient. *Drugs* 1998;56:571.

Simkin D. Twelve-step treatment from a development perspec-tive. In: Jaffe, S, ed. *Child and adolescent psychiatric clinics of North America: adolescent substance abuse and dual disorders*. Philadelphia, PA: WB Saunders; 1996:165.

Sofuoglu M, Kosten T. Novel approaches to the treatment of cocaine addiction. *CNS Drugs* 2005;19:13.

Stanton M, Shadish W. Outcome, attrition, and family=couples treatment for drug abuse: a meta-analysis and review of the controlled, comparative studies. *Psychol Bull* 1997;122: 170.

Strain E, Stoller K, Walsh S. Effects of buprenorphine versus buprenorphine/naloxone tablets in non-dependent opioid users. *Psychopharmacology* 2000;148:374.

Szapocznik J, Kurtines W, Foote F, et al. Conjoint versus one-person family therapy: some evidence for the effectiveness of conducting family therapy through one person. *J Consult Clin Psychol* 1983;51:889.

Szapocznik J, Perez-Vidal A, Brickman A, et al. Engaging adolescent drug abusers and their families in treatment. *J Consult Clin Psychol* 1988;56:552.

Tuma J. Mental health services for children: state of the art. *Am Psychol* 1989;44:188.

Vocci F, Acri J, Elkashef A. Medication development for addic-tive disorders: the state of the science. *Am J Psychiatry* 2005; 162:1432.

Waldron H, Slesnick N, Brody J, et al. Treatment outcomes for adolescent substance abuse at 4- and 7-month assessments. *J Consult Clin Psychol* 2001;69:802.

Waxmonsky JG, Wilens TE. Pharmacotherapy of adolescent substance use disorders: a review of the literature. *J Child Adolesc Psychopharmacol* 2005;15:810.

Weinhold L, Preston K, Farre M. Buprenorphine alone and in combination with naloxone in non-dependent humans. *Drug Alcohol Depend* 1992;30:263.

Weiss R, Najavits L. Overview of treatment modalities for dual diagnosis patients. In: Kranzler H, Rounsaville B, eds. *Dual diagnosis and treatment: substance abuse and comorbid medical and psychiatric disorders*. New York: Marcel Dekker Inc; 1998:87.

Weissman D, Haddox J. Opioid pseudoaddiction—an iatrogenic syndrome. *Pain* 1989;36:363.

Wilens TE, Spencer TJ, Biederman J, et al. A controlled clinical trial of bupropion for attention deficit hyperactivity disorder in adults. *Am J Psychiatry* 2001;158:282.

Wilens T. Attention-deficit/hyperactivity disorder and the substance use disorders: the nature of the relationship, who is at risk, and treatment issues. *Prim Psychiatry* 2004; 11:63.

Wilens T, Faraone S, Biederman J, et al. Does stimulant therapy of attention deficit hyperactivity disorder beget later substance abuse? A meta-analytic review of the literature. *Pediatrics* 2003;111:179.

Wilkins J. Psychopharmacology for addiction. *Psychiatr Times* 2005;22(2).

Williams R, Chang S. A comprehensive and comparative review of adolescent substance abuse treatment outcome. *Clin Psychol Sci Pr* 2000;7:138.

PART XV

Psychosocial Problems and Concerns

CHAPTER 75

Common Concerns of Adolescents and Their Parents

Mari Radzik, Sara Sherer, and Lawrence S. Neinstein

During the adolescent years, adolescents and their families face a myriad of issues and concerns. As stated earlier in this book, what seems important to the adolescent may not be of concern to his or her parents and vice versa. Often the issues that concern adolescents resolve on their own, may be helped by friends or family, or never come to the attention of a health care provider. In cases where the physician is involved, he or she may be asked to answer questions such as, "Am I normal?", "Is my adolescent normal?", or "What can I do about this problem?" Occasionally, the issue becomes severe enough to create family disruption. In the extreme case, these problems may lead to acting-out behaviors such as truancy, juvenile delinquency, substance abuse, or suicide.

What is normal adolescent behavior? Chapter 2 deals with normal psychosocial development in the adolescent. This chapter emphasizes common psychosocial concerns to which parents and health care providers should be especially sensitive. Unfortunately, there are no clear-cut answers to what is normal adolescent behavior. In an attempt to understand normal behavior and to build an alliance with the adolescent, it is often helpful for the health care provider to remember his or her own adolescence in order to keep things in perspective. Health care providers should consider the following issues when assessing the concerns of the adolescent or his/her family:

1. The severity of the problem: Is this behavior usual for the adolescent or is there a marked change?
2. The chronicity of the problem: Has the problem been present for days, months, or years?
3. Emotional development: Is the adolescent's behavior consistent with his/her developmental stage with respect to independence, body image, peers, school and identity?
4. Daily functioning: Are the problems severe enough to interfere with the daily functioning of the adolescent in areas such as school and social activities?
5. Family functioning: Health care providers must try to understand the adolescent's behavior within the social context of their immediate world, especially their relationship with their caregivers. It is important to develop an understanding of the parenting style. Authoritative parents provide a warm, firm, and involved family climate with consistent and developmentally

appropriate limit setting (Baumrind, 1991). Research has shown that this particular parenting style is associated with increased adolescent competence and psychological well-being (Steinberg, 2000). Therefore, a clear understanding of both the adolescent's acting-out behavior and the nature of his or her relationship with the parent(s) will help the health care provider determine whether an intervention is necessary.

Any concern of an adolescent or parent deserves an assessment. Although some general and routine medical concerns can be handled by discussion and reassurance, other issues such as family conflicts, psychosomatic illnesses, or depression may require several sessions with the adolescent and family. When the problem involves severe or chronic disorders or high-risk violent or self-injurious behavior, then a referral to a health care provider is usually indicated. Indications for considering a referral include the following:

1. Suicidal or self-injurious behavior
2. Mental health disorders such as mood or anxiety disorders
3. Substance abuse
4. Psychotic or other severe psychiatric symptoms
5. Developmental delay or learning disabilities
6. Behavioral problems that have either been present since childhood or have recently become apparent
7. Problems that have persisted despite extensive interventions by the primary caregiver
8. Problems believed to be beyond the skills of the health care provider
9. A problem is present but the health care provider is unsure what it is (e.g., the adolescent with no friends who is socially withdrawn)
10. Severe life stressors or changes in the family such as death, divorce, or suicide of parent or sibling
11. A dramatic change in school behavior and/or performance
12. Runaway behavior
13. Frequent fighting among peers and/or family
14. Acute or chronic illness

Types of behaviors that may indicate common adolescent behavior, a trouble sign, or a problem behavior are shown in Table 75.1.

TABLE 75.1

Common Adolescent Behaviors, Trouble Signs, and Problem Behaviors

Not of Significant Concern	Trouble Sign	Problem Behavior
One or two minor nonviolent violations of the law or school regulations	Repeated violations of the law or school regulations	Any violent act or crime
Sexual activity in the context of a loving relationship	Sexual provocativeness	Sexual promiscuity
Leaving home for a day and in particular running away to a familiar home, once	Running away more than once in 3 months	Running away to the streets
Skipping school or missing a class, once	Skipping school more than once in 3 months	Chronic absenteeism from school
Occasional experimentation with alcohol and drugs	Regular use of drugs and alcohol	Addiction to drugs or drug dealing
Occasional arguing with parents and other adults	Aggressive outbursts	Oppositionalism leading to violence at home or suspension from school

Adapted from Steinberg L, Levine, A. *You and your adolescent: a parents' guide for ages 10–20.* New York: Harper & Row; 1990.

REFERRALS

When the health care provider decides that a referral to a mental health care provider is necessary, several considerations are important. They include:

1. Are the adolescent and parents motivated to seek treatment? Without motivation, compliance is extremely poor.
2. Do the adolescent and family understand the reason for the referral?
3. Is the referral appropriate for the problem? Many options exist for referrals for psychosocial problems, including social workers, family therapists, psychologists, psychiatrists, and vocational counselors. In addition, there are specialized youth programs (Big Brothers/Big Sisters, YMCA), residential programs, and vocational programs (Job Corps) that can provide support.

Several interventions may help in making the referral. They include:

1. The health care provider should reassure the adolescent that the primary health care provider will continue to follow up the adolescent and be involved in his or her care.
2. The health care provider should explain that as part of the total evaluation and treatment of the adolescent's problem, a psychological or psychiatric evaluation is important. It has been shown that screening for mental disorders is not routinely part of the primary care of adolescents (Wren, et al., 2003). Despite this, a routine and practical evaluation for mental disorders is recommended as it will improve the care of the adolescent. If the adolescent and family feel strongly that the problem has an organic etiology, even after a negative medical evaluation, the health care provider can explain that a psychological evaluation is an important part of the diagnostic workup. The health care provider can describe that such a comprehensive assessment is necessary because physical illnesses can lead to psychological problems and that patients with organic disease often have coexistent psychological

disturbances. Psychological support or treatment can often help the adolescent cope with the symptoms.
3. The health care provider should explain his or her concerns to the adolescent and family. As part of this explanation, the health care provider can ask the adolescent whether he or she thinks that "things could be better?" If the adolescent answers "yes", the health care provider can review how counseling may be one way to help the adolescent and the family.
4. The health care provider should reassure the adolescent that often counseling will be arranged for a limited period of time. If the counseling does not work out, the adolescent or family can stop it.
5. The adolescent should be aware that seeing a psychologist or psychiatrist does not mean that they are "crazy". Counseling should be described as an opportunity to help the adolescent feel better, to build coping skills, and to enhance family or interpersonal relations.
6. It is necessary for the health care provider and the parents to distinguish the adolescent from his or her behavior. They must convey acceptance of the adolescent even if they believe the adolescent's behavior to be negative or unhealthy.

CONCERNS OF ADOLESCENTS

Common concerns of adolescents include:

1. Parental conflicts: Rules (e.g., curfew, driving), privacy, expectations, and peer relationships.
2. Peers: Interpersonal concerns regarding friendships, relationships, and sexuality.
3. Identity: Who am I? Concerns surrounding body image, sexual and gender identity, culture, and ethnicity.
4. School: Popularity, academic pressures, teachers, and adjustment to a new school.
5. Sibling/family conflicts: Blended and cross-generational differences.
6. Social situations: Social connectivity, whether isolated or gregarious.
7. Depression: Moderate or severe.

8. Medical concerns: Menstrual disorders, body image issues such as short stature, acne, and weight disorders.
9. Psychosomatic problems: Headaches, stomach pains, and insomnia.
10. Safety concerns: Violence in the environment, community, home, school, and in relationships.
11. Prospects for the future: Economic realities, employment, education, relationship building, and establishing a solid sense of self.

CONCERNS OF PARENTS

Common concerns of parents with regard to their adolescent son or daughter include:

1. Adolescent acting-out behaviors: Mild acting-out behaviors are common in early and middle adolescence. Marked acting-out behaviors however, may be an indication of an emotional or family dysfunction.
2. Risk-taking behaviors: Risk-taking is a common part of the early and middle adolescent process. Life-threatening, risk-taking behavior requires family interventions for the purposes of educating, limit setting, and evaluation of any associated unmet needs of the adolescent and his or her family.
3. Emotional lability: Assessment of the severity, including detailed description of the moods and changes, is required to determine if a mood disorder is the underlying cause.
4. Drug and alcohol use: Evaluation of the type and degree of drug use is required. The use of steroidal drugs for sports performance should also be addressed because the use of anabolic steroid use can be found among athletes (Goldberg, et al., 2000). Furthermore, determination of complimentary and alternative medication use should also be explored.
5. Academic problems: Evaluation of the type and severity of the problem is required. Parents should be encouraged to follow-up with their adolescent's school for any available services that may help him or her. The use of video games and Internet should be monitored as it may often interfere with academic success and expose adolescents to experiences or values that may not be developmentally appropriate (Bremer, 2005; Greenfield, 2004).
6. Sexual activity and identity: Parents should be encouraged to express their concerns. Issues of confidentiality between the adolescent and the health care provider should be explained to the parents. When adolescents know that private and personal information about them will be protected and held in confidence, they are more likely to trust their health care provider and discuss their problems openly. Sexual identity can often be an area of tension in the family, particularly when the adolescent expresses thoughts or behaviors that they may be bisexual, homosexual or transgendered. The parent(s) may reject the adolescent's new sexual identity and may require appropriate resources to help them better understand these issues. Adolescents and their parents should be encouraged to discuss issues of sexuality, sexual identity, and sexual activity whenever possible. Parents often have questions and concerns about limit setting such as, "What is adequate supervision at parties?" "Should I allow my son or daughter to spend time alone in the house or in a room with a girlfriend or boyfriend?" and "What degree and type of sexual activity is normal?" Health care providers should be prepared to help parents explore these issues.
7. Eating disorders: An evaluation of changes in weight, attitudes toward body image, eating habits and behaviors, psychological and emotional health, family functioning, and self-esteem should be undertaken.
8. Safety issues: Violence in the environment or safety while driving (i.e., adolescent or other motorists driving under the influence). The novice adolescent driver is a key stressor for parents and one that brings up many issues of limit setting and sharing of responsibilities.
9. Peer influences: Parents should be aware of the importance of peer influences and should monitor behaviors and activities while understanding that youth need to choose their own friends.
10. Psychosomatic problems: Medical evaluation should include an exploration of any sources of stress that the adolescent may be attempting to cope with psychosomatically.
11. "Wasting time" by the adolescent, especially daydreaming: Parents should be reassured that this is usually a normal part of adolescent development. However, parents should monitor to help redirect youth who may need more direction in their activities.

CONCLUSION

Adolescence is an exciting period of transition and change. It is important to remember the many competencies, strengths, and energy that youth possess. That notwithstanding, health care providers may be confronted by parents and caregivers who struggle with challenging adolescent issues. Parents and caregivers should be encouraged to focus on the positive aspects of adolescence while following up with appropriate resources when needed. Respectful, consistent, and caring parents and caregivers can facilitate a positive transition for their teenager as the move through adolescence toward adulthood.

WEB SITES

http://www.aacap.org/. Questions and answers from the American Academy on Child and Adolescent Psychiatry.
http://www.aamft.org. The American Association of Marriage and Family Therapists Web site.
http://www.adolescenthealth.org. Society of Adolescent Medicine.
http://www.cpc.unc.edu/projects/addhealth. The National Longitudinal Study of Adolescent Health. Beginning in 1994, surveyed key issues of adolescents such as physical health, mental health, and risk behaviors.
http://www.apa.org. The American Psychological Association.
http://www.indiana.edu/%7Ecafs/resources.html. ADOL: Adolescence Directory On-Line is an electronic guide to information on adolescent issues. Service of the Center for Adolescent Studies at Indiana University.
http://www.NationalEatingDisorders.org. National Eating Disorders Association, largest non-profit organization.

http://www.ncfy.com. Supporting Your Adolescent: Tips for Parents, Prepared by the National Clearinghouse on Families & Youth.

http://www.npin.org. The National Parent Information Network.

http://www.pflag.org/. National organization supporting parents of gay, lesbian, bisexual and transgendered persons.

http://www.tnpc.com. Articles on parenting teens from the National Parenting Center, many by Kathleen McCoy and Charles Wibbelsman, M.D., from Teen Body Book.

http://www.4woman.gov/BodyImage. The National Woman's Health Information Center.

REFERENCES AND ADDITIONAL READINGS

Alessi G. The family and parenting in the 21st century. *Adolesc Med* 2000;11:35.

Arnett JJ. Adolescent storm and stress, reconsidered. *Am Psychol* 1999;54:317.

Baumrind D. Parenting style and adolescent development. In: Brook-Gunn J, Lerner R, Peterson AC, eds. *The encyclopedia of adolescence*. New York: Garland; 1991.

Bremer J. The internet and children: advantages and disadvantages. *Adolesc Psychiatr Clin N Am* 2005;14(3):405.

Glascow KL, Dornbusch SM, Troyer L, et al. Parenting styles, adolescents' attributions, and educational outcomes in nine heterogeneous high schools. *Child Dev* 1997;68:507.

Goldberg L, MacKinnon DP, Elliot DL, et al. The adolescents training and learning to avoid steroids program. *Arch Pediatr Adolesc Med* 2000;154:332.

Greenfield PM. Developmental considerations for determining appropriate internet use guidelines for children and adolescents. *Appl Dev Psychol* 2004;25:751.

Steinberg L. We know some things: parent-adolescent relations in retrospect and prospect. *J Res Adolesc* 2000;11(1):1.

Steinberg L, Levine A. *You and your adolescent: a parent's guide for ages 10–20*. New York: Harper & Row; 1990.

Wren FJ, Scholle SH, Heo J, et al. Pediatric mood and anxiety syndromes in primary care: who gets identified? *Int J Psychiatry Med* 2003:33(1):1.

CHAPTER 76

High-Risk and Delinquent Behavior

Robert E. Morris and Ralph J. DiClemente

Changes in society over the last 25 to 30 years have significantly influenced the adolescent years. The educational experience has been prolonged and the job market constricted. Adaptations to intrinsic psychological developmental triggers are now made in an environment of increasing drug use, sexual activity, and media stimulation and weakened family structure. Attempts by adolescents to cope with these pressures often result in social behaviors that are associated with inherent and inconstant degrees of risk to health. The consequences of these health risks may be immediate or long range.

In the United States the following have been estimated:

- Every 37 seconds a teenager becomes pregnant
- About every 1 minute a teen gives birth
- Every 78 seconds a teen attempts suicide
- Every 76 minutes a teen is killed in a car accident
- Every 90 minutes a teen is murdered and another commits suicide

The major causes of death and disability among the approximately 40 million American youth aged 10 to 19 years, who comprise 14% of the U.S. population, have essentially social and behavioral issues at their root—and parenthetically, the majority are preventable!

RISK AND RESILIENCE

The concept of risk has been well established as a characteristic that detrimentally exposes young people to threats to their health and well-being. Related to the concept of risk is the construct of resilience, which has received a great deal of attention through research for many decades. One of the difficulties that persists in understanding this construct is the lack of a unified theoretical framework (Luthar et al., 2000).

A review of the literature on resilience among adolescents suggests that there are two primary operational definitions of this construct (Olsson et al., 2003). First, resilience can be viewed as various psychosocial outcomes characterized by functional behavior patterns among adolescents exposed to risk. Included among such outcomes are mental health functioning, functional capacity, and social competence (Blum, 1998). Absent from this list of psychosocial outcomes defining the construct of resilience is emotional well-being. Rather than conceptualizing emotional well-being as an outcome of the resilient individual facing adverse life events, researchers have suggested that the resilient individual may indeed experience emotional distress; however, what differentiates him/her from the nonresilient individual is his/her ability to function effectively even in the presence of difficult emotions (Luthar, 1991). In other words, emotional difficulty compounds the risk to which an individual is exposed and to which he/she must adapt. Those who are resilient will display good mental health, high functional capacity, and high social competence in adverse circumstances, including those charged with negative emotional stress. In fact, Garmezy (1991) defines resilience as "the capacity to recover and maintain adaptive behavior after insult." This operational definition may be useful in understanding adaptation to adverse events; however, it does not provide much information regarding the mechanism or process by which the impact of a stressful event is modified in such a way as to allow for successful adaptation.

The second way to conceptualize resilience is by investigating the protective mechanisms that contribute to successful adaptation to a stressful event (Olsson et al., 2003). In this view, resilience involves a healthy set of behaviors and coping mechanisms that are integrated into decision making and elicited in response to a threatening situation. The youth responds flexibly and makes positive choices despite impoverished life experiences. Factors associated with resilience as identified in this view include *individual-level factors* such as intelligence (Eccles, 1997), communication skills (Werner, 1995), sociability (Allen, 1998), as well as personal attributes such as self-esteem (Blum, 1998), and tolerance for negative affect (Smith, 1999). Additionally, *family-level factors* are also major contributors to the development of resilience. These include parental warmth, encouragement, and assistance (Smith, 1999; Eccles, 1997), authoritative parenting, that is, acceptance, encouraging psychological autonomy, and behavioral control in a firm but loving manner (Steinberg et al., 1989), as well as cohesion within the family (Maggs et al., 1997). Finally, *social-level factors* include socioeconomic status (Allen, 1998; Maggs et al., 1997), school experiences (Werner, 1995; Rutter, 1987), and supportive communities (Smith, 1999; Werner, 1995).

It is important to note that when considering resilience as a process of interplaying risk and protective factors, the relationship between resilience and adaptability is a multifactorial process. Just as multiple risk factors may have a synergistic effect on one's ability to adapt, protective factors associated with resilience may exert their influence in a similar manner, leading to successful adaptation and coping with a stressful environment.

EPIDEMIOLOGY OF RISK-TAKING BEHAVIOR

Mortality

In 2003, approximately 17,651 adolescents aged 10 to 19 died (Centers for Disease Control and Prevention, 2006). Approximately 75% of deaths occurred from injuries (intentional and unintentional) and 25% from natural causes. The proportion of all deaths from injuries increased with age, from approximately 47% among 10-year-olds to 81% among those 18 years of age. In 2002, motor vehicle- and traffic-related accidents caused 25% of all deaths and 50% of injury-related deaths in 10- to 14-year-olds, 42% of all deaths and 78% of injury-related deaths in 15- to 19-year-olds, and 31% and 75% in 20- to 24-year-olds, respectively. Motor vehicle accidents increase with age, with the greatest increase being between 15 and 16 years of age (see Chapter 5). Many of these events are related to drug or alcohol use. The mortality figures do not reflect the magnitude of morbidity and subsequent disability associated with these leading causes of injury.

Morbidity

It is estimated that 20% of U.S. teenagers have great difficulty making the transition from childhood to adulthood and that this difficulty is often reflected in their risk-taking behaviors. The frequency of these morbidities correlates with the teen's biobehavioral risk profile. The latter is directly dependent on the frequency and number of risky behaviors that the teenager uses to resolve psychological and social developmental needs. Frequent subsequent problems include the following:

1. Pregnancy: In the United States >800,000 pregnancies for females aged 15 to 19 per year are reported with more than 60% of these pregnancies occurring in 18- to 19-year-old females (Henshaw, 2005). From 1990 to 2003, the birth rate for females aged 15 to 19 decreased 33%, from 62 per 1,000 females to 41.6. For 15- to 17-year-olds the birth rate decreased from 38.6 in 1991 to 22.4 in 2003 (Martin et al., 2005). Among all 15- to 19-year-olds in the United States, approximately 10% become pregnant each year, and among those who have had intercourse, approximately 19% become pregnant each year. For younger 10- to 14-year-old females, there are approximately 15,000 pregnancies per year (Abma et al., 2004). Teenage pregnancies are associated with higher rates of complications, particularly low birth weight and infant mortality, and especially when the mother is very young. These complications may be related to the lack of regular prenatal care. Factors increasing pregnancy and parenting risks include poverty, low intellect, lower status of employment and wages, reliance on public assistance, poor literacy and work skills, substance abuse, emotional or sexual abuse, and increased number of children in the family of origin (i.e., many siblings and possibly early pregnancies in the index adolescent's female siblings). Fifty-one percent of adolescents use no contraception during first intercourse, and 20% of adolescent pregnancies occur within 1 month of first intercourse (see Chapter 41).

2. Sexual activity: The 2005 Youth Risk Behavior Survey (YRBS) found that approximately half (46.8%) of all high-school students had had sexual intercourse during their lifetime (CDC, 2006). Female students in grades 11 and 12 (52.1% and 62.4%, respectively) were significantly more likely than female students in grades 9 and 10 (29.3% and 44%, respectively) to have had sexual intercourse. Male students in grades 11 and 12 (50.6% and 63.8%, respectively) were significantly more likely than male students in grades 9 and 10 (39.3% and 41.5%, respectively) to report this behavior. A total of 6.2% of students initiated sexual intercourse before age 13 years (nonabusive) including 8.8% of male and 3.7% of female students. In addition, 14.3% of all students had had sexual intercourse with four or more partners. Approximately 63% of currently sexually active adolescents reported condom use during their last sexual intercourse (CDC, 2006). Sexually transmitted diseases (STDs) are the most commonly reported infectious diseases among sexually active adolescents. Chlamydia and, to a lesser extent, gonorrhea are epidemics in this age-group, with adolescents having the highest prevalence of any age-group nationally, if prevalence is expressed only for those who are sexually active. Although the overall prevalence of human immunodeficiency virus (HIV) infection is relatively low among adolescents, adolescents in some minority and racial groups are disproportionately affected by HIV and acquired immunodeficiency syndrome (AIDS).

3. Substance abuse: In 2005, 43.3% of all high-school students (42.8% of girls and 43.8% of boys) reported alcohol use during the previous 30 days. Binge drinking (consumption of five or more drinks on one occasion) was reported by 23.5% of female students and 27.5% of male students during the same 30-day period. Lifetime use of marijuana, the most commonly reported illicit drug used among high-school students, was reported by 38.4% of high-school students. Current marijuana use was reported by 18.2% of female high-school students and 22.1% of male high-school students. A significant minority of high-school students report lifetime use of other illicit drugs, for example, 6.3% report having used ecstasy, 6.2% report having used methamphetamines, and 7.6% report having used a form of cocaine (CDC, 2006).

4. Runaway behavior: Every year an estimated 500,000 to 1.5 million young people run away or are forced out of their homes. Approximately 200,000 of these are homeless and living on the streets (Administration on Children and Families, 2000). One national study found that an estimated 1,682,900 youth had a runaway or a "throwaway" episode (Hammer et al., 2002). These youth often survive through illegal activities such as survival sex, burglary, or drug dealing (Greene et al., 1999). Approximately 28% of street youth and 10% of shelter youth reported having participated in survival sex. Participation was associated with age, days away from home, victimization, criminal behaviors, substance use, suicide attempts, STDs, and pregnancy (Greene et al., 1999).

5. Suicide: The age-adjusted death rate for suicide, the 11th leading cause of death, has been edging downward during the 1990s. The age-adjusted suicide rate was 10.7 deaths per 100,000 in 2001, compared with 11.5 in 1990 (National Institute of Mental Health, 2004). Suicide is the third leading cause of death among U.S. residents aged 10 to 24 years, accounting for 11.7% of all deaths in this age-group (CDC, 2004). On the otherhand, suicidal ideation or attempting suicide is a powerful indicator of mental and emotional health. In 2002, an estimated 124,409 visits to U.S. emergency departments were made after attempted suicides or other self-harm incidents among persons aged 10 to 24 (CDC, 2004). On the basis of 2005 YRBS data, nationwide, 8.4% of students had actually attempted suicide one or more times during the 12 months preceding the survey (CDC, 2006). Overall, the prevalence of having attempted suicide was higher among female (10.8%) than male (6%) students.

6. Education: Although most adolescents complete high school, those students who drop out of school have fewer opportunities to succeed in the work force or to assume a fully functional place in society. High-school dropouts have lower earnings, experience more unemployment, and are more likely to receive welfare or be in prison. Using the indicator of event dropout rate, which measures the proportion of youth aged 15 through 24 who dropped out of grades 10 to 12 in the 12 months preceding October 2000, and therefore did not successfully complete high school, 5% of young adults enrolled in high school in October 1999 left school without successfully completing a high-school program (National Center for Education Statistics, 2001). The event dropout rate increases with age. The cumulative effect of several hundred thousand adolescents leaving school each year translates into several million young adults out of school and not having a high-school diploma. Socioeconomic status is strongly associated with the decision to stay in school. In 2000, young adults living in families with incomes in the lowest 20% of all family incomes were 6 times as likely as their peers from families in the top 20% of the income distribution to drop out of high school. Students from low-income families had an event dropout rate of 10%, whereas students from middle- and high-income families had event dropout rates of 5.2% and 1.6%, respectively. Members of nonwhite races, with the exception of Asian/Pacific Islander youth, whether as a reflection of socioeconomic status or as an independent variable, are disproportionately represented among dropouts (National Center for Education Statistics, 2001).

7. Crime: In the Youth Health Risk Behavior Surveillance (CDC, 2006), 17% of students had carried a weapon one or more times during the last month (26.9% of males and 6.7% of females). Nationwide, 6.1% of students had carried a gun on >1 occasion in the last 30 days, with the prevalence of having carried a gun higher among male (10.2%) than female (1.6%) students. Almost 41% of males and 25.1% of females reported having been in at least one fight during the previous year. Approximately 5.4% of students reported missing school on 1 or more days during the last month because they felt unsafe at school or when traveling to or from school.

FACTORS INVOLVED IN RISK-TAKING BEHAVIOR

Childhood and adolescence are continuous and contiguous events in the life cycle. The manner in which the developmental challenges of adolescence are expressed is dependent on, if not largely determined by, personality traits and other characteristics established in childhood. The physical, psychological, and social maturational forces of development combine to determine behavior at any moment. During adolescence these behaviors may be perceived by those close to the teenagers as a problem because they may constitute a health risk. Viewed developmentally, however, these behaviors serve a purpose (i.e., that of a developmental task accomplishment). Often the adolescent does not perceive risk-taking behavior as a problem but, rather, as a solution. This paradox helps explain the behavior and also the difficulty of managing youth who engage in high-risk behaviors. *What health professionals see as a problem, youth often see as a solution.* People, in general, do not give up their solutions easily.

General characteristics of risk-taking behaviors in adolescents include the following:

1. Many behaviors that affect health, both positively and negatively, throughout an individual's life, are first tried out during the teenage years (e.g., cigarette smoking, sexual activity, exercise and physical conditioning, dietary changes, study habits).
2. The risk that any behavior has on health may be immediate (e.g., drinking and driving), delayed (e.g., pregnancy and education), or remote (e.g., smoking and lung cancer). *The more immediate the consequence of behavior on health, the greater the likelihood of effecting change through intervention in adolescents.*
3. Consequences of risk behaviors may be universal and invariant (e.g., risk from crack), related to specific factors or cofactors (e.g., environment, gender, situations), or related to the intensity of involvement (e.g., dieting and anorexia nervosa).
4. Factors that significantly influence health-related behaviors are usually acquired or consolidated during adolescence (e.g., values, beliefs, attitudes, motivations, self-concept, general lifestyle).
5. Problem behaviors that contribute to risk tend to occur in combinations or clusters (e.g., smoking, lack of seat belt use, drinking, interpersonal violence, suicidal ideation, school dropout, family discord, and substance use before sexual activity).
6. Risk at any developmental period reflects the number of risk factors present during that period and the cumulative effects of risk factors occurring earlier in life. The effects may be not only cumulative but also compounded and may lead to other risk behaviors (e.g., the effect of long-term alcohol or drug use on driving or suicidal ideation). High-risk adolescents usually have multiple social and psychological handicaps that amplify the severity of the consequences and limit the options for problem solving and task accomplishment.

Biopsychosocial Factors

Many factors have been suggested as contributing to problem behaviors among youth in the United States. Although biological maturational forces have remained relatively constant, the timing of puberty and the social environment in which it occurs have dramatically changed over the last decade. This has put increased pressure on the individual for adaptation to these new norms that define adolescence. These factors include the following:

1. *Menarche occurs earlier (12.5 years), marriage has been delayed (average age, 26 years), and values have changed regarding premarital sexual intercourse.* Incongruence between biological development and psychoemotional preparedness enhances the potential for high-risk behaviors or dysfunctional personal responses to stress, such as early initiation of sexual activity in an attempt to reduce stress.
2. The U.S. population has become more *urbanized*, with lack of purposeful and meaningful work for youth.
3. The American family has *increased mobility*, with a subsequent need for teens to reestablish social relations at a time when social skills are often poorly developed.
4. *Breakdown of the family* results in an increased number of single and working parents, lack of an extended family, and the interposition of the media as an arbiter of family values.
5. The foundation of the adolescent experience, *the educational process, has become more prolonged*, to prepare the individual for a high-tech society. This has resulted in an increased risk for even some mainstream adolescents to drop out.
6. A shift has occurred in *how society views its young*, from being an economic asset to being an economic liability.
7. Western cultures tend to expose rather than protect adolescents from *environmental influences* (e.g., drugs and alcohol, automobiles, violent behaviors).
8. *Change occurs rapidly* during adolescence, and pressures for adaptation are great.
9. Immature processing of emotions: There is the suggestion that young adolescents continue to process emotions and future planning in the amygdala, similar to children, instead of in the frontal lobes. This can lead to physically mature teens' handling information in a manner similar to younger children, which may result in seriously wrong decisions regarding long-term consequences of their behaviors.

Certain youth are predisposed to having difficulty with the transition from childhood to adulthood, including:

1. Youth reared in poverty
2. Youth who have been physically, sexually, or emotionally abused as children
3. Youth living with significant family pathology, parental mental illness, or substance abuse
4. Youth with educational handicaps
5. Youth with a gay or lesbian sexual orientation
6. Youth with a chronic illness

It is important to realize that most of these young people mature successfully through adolescence without apparent long-term problems. The health professional may be on the lookout for problems and offer help when appropriate but should not automatically label these teens as being at high risk.

In summary, high-risk and out-of-control behaviors require prompt evaluation and attention. Associated are a wide spectrum of behaviors, including runaway behavior, truancy, theft, vandalism, substance abuse, sexual promiscuity, and suicide. Loss of parental control must be assessed along with what has been tried to regain control. The health professional must evaluate what are the greatest influences on the teen's present behavior and how those influences are related to developmental needs. Underlying issues often involve autonomy, low self-esteem, frustration, or depression.

INCARCERATED YOUTH AND JUVENILE DELINQUENCY

Definitions

A *juvenile delinquent* is a person younger than 17 or 18 years (depending on the state) who commits any criminal offense as defined by state or local laws. Delinquents are subject to the regulations of the juvenile or family court, with a goal of rehabilitation rather than punishment. For serious offenses including murder, rape, and assault with a deadly weapon, many states have moved jurisdiction from juvenile court to adult criminal court with the possibility of sentencing juveniles to adult prisons where there is little rehabilitation.

A *status offender* is a juvenile younger than 17 or 18 years who commits an offense that would not be illegal for an adult. Examples include disobedience to parents or guardians leading to loss of disciplinary control, truancy, runaway behavior, and curfew violation. Status offenders are often referred to as persons, children, juveniles, or minors in need of supervision (PINS, CHINS, JINS, or MINS, respectively). In some states, juvenile delinquents and status offenders are grouped together. Increasingly, states and local agencies separate the two groups, nonetheless an effective system to deal with status offenders is lacking in most states. Many of these young people are referred to mental health or social service agencies by the court.

Epidemiology

1. Prevalence: Data from the mid-1990s when this data was last collected, showed that >590,000 children are incarcerated each year in public and private juvenile facilities. Another 90,000 are placed in adult jails each year. According to the U.S. Department of Justice, in 1997 and 2003 law enforcement agencies in the United States made an estimated 2.8 and 2.2 million arrests of persons younger than 18 years, respectively. These arrests accounted for 19% and 16% of all reported arrests and 17% and 15% of all violent crimes in 1997 and 2003, respectively (Snyder, 1998, 2005). Of these arrests, 29% involved females compared to 32% in 1997. However, the percentage of arrests for youths younger than 15 years rose from 6% in 1997 to 32% in 2003.

   There was considerable growth in juvenile crime arrests beginning in the late 1980s that peaked in 1994 and dropped every year through 2003 (Snyder, 2005). The violent crime index showed that offenders decreased 48% between 1994 and 2003. Juvenile arrests for murder in 1993 dropped from 3,790 to 1,130 in 2003, a 70% decrease. But, the arrest rate for simple assault increased 102% for males and 269% for females between 1980 and 2003. Arrests for drug abuse increased 19% from 1994 to 2003 with the rate for females increasing much more, to 56% compared to an increase for males at 13% (Snyder, 2005). Table 76.1 compares the types of offenses for

TABLE 76.1

Juveniles in Public or Private Detention, Correctional and Shelter Facilities by Offense, United States, on October 29,1997 and October 22, 2003

Offense	October 29, 1997		October 22, 2003	
	Number	Percentage	Number	Percentage
Total	105,790	100	96,655	100
Violent offenses	35,357	33.4	33,197	34
Murder/manslaughter	1,927	1.8	878	1
Sexual assault	5,690	5.3	7,452	8
Kidnapping	326	0.3	—	—
Robbery	9,451	8.9	6,230	6
Aggravated assault	9,530	9.0	7,495	8
Simple assault	6,630	6.3	8,106	8
Other violent offense	1,903	1.8	3,036	3
Property offenses	31,991	30.2	26,843	28
Household burglary	12,560	11.9	10,399	11
Motor vehicle theft	6,525	6.2	5,572	6
Arson	915	0.9	735	1
Property damage	1,758	1.7	—	—
Theft	7,294	6.9	5,650	6
Other property offense	2,939	2.8	4,487	5
Drug offenses	9,286	8.8	8,002	8
Drug trafficking	3,045	2.9	1,801	2
Drug possession	5,693	5.4	—	—
Other drug offense	548	0.5	6,192	6
Public order offenses	9,718	9.2	9,654	10
Driving under the influence	260	0.2	—	—
Obstruction of justice	1,754	1.7	—	—
Nonviolent sex offense	1,739	1.6	—	—
Weapons offense	4,191	4.0	3,013	3
Other public order offense	1,774	1.7	6,641	7
Probation or parole violation	12,549	11.9	14,135	15
Other delinquent offenses	12	—	—	—
Status offenses	6,877	6.5	4,824	5
Curfew violation	193	0.2	203	0.2
Incorrigibility	2,849	2.7	1,825	2
Running away	1,497	1.4	997	1
Truancy	1,332	1.3	841	0.8
Underage alcohol offense	320	0.3	405	0.4
Other status offense	686	0.6	553	0.5

Adapted from U.S. Department of Justice, Office of Juvenile Justice and Delinquency Prevention. Juvenile offenders in residential placement 1997. Washington, DC. USDOJ, 1999 FS9996 and U.S. Department of Justice, Office of Juvenile Justice and Delinquency Prevention. Juvenile Offenders and Victims: 2006 National Report. Washington, D.C. USDOJ, 2006, NCJ212906.

which juveniles were held in correctional facilities on an index day in 1997 and 2003.

Statistics show that juveniles are more likely to commit crimes in groups and are more likely to be arrested compared to adults. Overall, however, approximately 5% to 10% of the adolescent population accounts for more than 50% of all juvenile crimes and most serious and violent juveniles crimes (Williams, 2006).

As of 2000, there were 73 death row inmates who committed their crime before the age of 18, and 17 had been executed from 1985 through 2000. One of the offenders was 16 at the time of the crime and the remainder were 17 (Sickmund, 2004).

2. Characteristics
   a. Gender: In 2003, males accounted for 71% of juvenile arrests (1,577,300) and 82% of juvenile arrests for violent crimes (75,440) (Snyder, 2005). Female delinquency in the 1950s and 1960s centered mainly on sexual misconduct, acting out, or prostitution. But between 1994 and 2003 arrests of girls for most categories of crime increased more for girls than for boys or decreased at a lower rate in girls compared to boys. For example, during these years simple assault arrests increased 36% for girls but only 1% for boys. Drug abuse violation arrests were up 56% for girls but only 13% for boys. From 1994 to 2003, there were significant

TABLE 76.2

Juveniles in Public or Private Detention, Correctional and Shelter Facilities by Age and Sex, United States on October 29, 1997 and October 22, 2003

| | October 29, 1997 | | | | | | October 22, 2003 | | | | | |
| | Total | | Male | | Female | | Total | | Male | | Female | |
Age (yr)	Number	%	Number	%	Number	%	Number	%	Number	%	Number	%
Total	105,790	100	91,471	100	14,319	100	96,655	100	82,157	100	14,498	100
<13	2,164	2.0	1,782	82.3	382	17.7	1,933	2	1,643	85	290	15
13	4,627	4.3	3,639	78.6	988	21.4	3,866	4	3,054	79	811	21
14	11,584	10.9	9,160	79.1	2,424	20.9	9,666	10	7,636	79	2,030	21
15	21,251	20.0	17,568	82.7	3,683	17.3	18,366	19	14,876	81	3,490	19
16	28,284	26.7	24,455	86.5	3,829	13.5	25,132	26	21,111	84	4,021	16
17	24,754	23.3	22,355	90.3	2,399	9.7	24,166	25	21,024	87	3,142	13
≥18	13,126	12.4	12,512	95.3	614	4.7	13,533	14	14,709	92	1,015	8

Adapted from U.S. Department of Justice, Office of Juvenile Justice and Delinquency Prevention.
Juvenile offenders in residential placement 1997. Washington, D.C. USDOJ, 1999, FS9996 and U.S. Department of Justice, Office of Juvenile Justice and Delinquency Prevention. Juvenile Offenders and Victims: 2006 National Report. Washington, D.C. USDOJ, 2006, NCJ212906.

decreases in arrests of girls for larceny/theft (19% but boy's arrests were down 43%), motor vehicle thefts (reduced 44% for girls and 54% for boys), vandalism (down 11% in girls and 36% in boys), and weapons offenses (down 22% in girls versus 42% for boys) (Snyder, 2005). Table 76.2 compares the gender and ages of juveniles held on an index day in 1997 and 2003.

b. Race: The federal government reported that members of minority races, primarily blacks and Hispanics, accounted for 26% of juvenile arrests in 1997 (Snyder and Sickmund, 1999). In 2003, black youth accounted for 45% of arrests and white youth including Hispanics (reporting parameters changed) accounted for 53% of arrests. This 2003 data can be set against the racial composition of the juvenile population in the United States that was 78% white, 16% black, 4% Asian/Pacific islander, and 1% American Indian (Snyder, 2005). Minorities, especially African-Americans and Hispanics, are disproportionately both the victims and the perpetrators of crime in the United States. Arrests and incarceration is increasing rapidly for Hispanic youth. Black youth accounted for 44% of juvenile arrests for violent crimes in 1997 and for 45% in 2003. In 2003, blacks accounted for 48% of juvenile arrests for murder. In the years preceding 1997, the disproportionate number of minority youth who were incarcerated changed little (63% of all juveniles in residential placement were minorities) (Gallagher, 1999; Sickmund, 2004).

c. Age: Most youths initiate delinquent behavior at the approximate age of 12 or 13 years. Juvenile arrests peak at ages 15 to 16 years and their involvement peaks by age 16 or 17 (Williams, 2006). Eighteen years is the peak age for arrest for violent crimes (homicide, rape, and assault) (Table 76.2).

d. Medical precursors: A number of medical precursors to delinquent and violent behavior have been reported. The contribution of these factors is unknown. It is important to realize that an association may be valid but the incidence is low.

- Head trauma: Head trauma resulting in brain injury is common among delinquent teens. Hyperactivity and impulsivity lead to head injury.
- XYY: Klinefelter syndrome has been associated with offending behaviors such as fire setting in a few boys, but most individuals with this syndrome are not criminal offenders.
- Fetal alcohol syndrome and exposure to illicit drugs: Some individuals with severe prenatal alcohol exposure exhibit difficulty in understanding the consequences of their actions. As a result, they repeatedly engage in behavior that is forbidden and become offenders. Likewise, some adolescents prenatally exposed to cocaine and other psychotropic drugs experience cognitive problems. A better understanding of the long-range effects of prenatal drug exposure will become evident as exposed children mature into their teenage years.
- Lead exposure: Elevated blood lead concentrations have been reported among detained delinquent youths. However, further study is needed to establish a cause and effect association.
- Frontal or temporal lobe epilepsy: This rare form of epilepsy involves complex neurological behavioral and psychiatric symptoms that are usually, but not always, seen in adolescents with *developmental disorders*. Occasionally, there may be explosive or undirected aggression. Nasopharyngeal and/or anterior-temporal leads may be necessary to demonstrate the seizure focus on an electroencephalograph.
- Learning disability and/or attention-deficit disorder: Poor academic performance is found in most delinquent youth. The underlying reasons for this include attention-deficit disorder, other learning disorders, lack of parental supervision, peer pressure, poor schools, and low socioeconomic status.
- Sleep problems: Increased aggression correlates with quantity and quality of sleep among juvenile and young offenders.

e. Social and environmental factors
- Low socioeconomic status
- Lack of employment
- Sense of failure and low self-esteem
- Family conflicts
- Peer-group involvement with delinquent adolescents
- Gang involvement
- Disorganization within the home and/or community environment
- Lack of a sense of belonging
- Lack of appropriate role models
- Lack of at least one caring adult
- Family history of alcoholism, criminal behavior, or psychiatric conditions
- History of physical or sexual abuse (in some cases, physical abuse may cause brain damage)

f. Seriously delinquent adolescents: Those youth with a higher prevalence of violent or sexually assaultive behaviors have a higher prevalence of violent behavior in early childhood, and a history of perinatal trauma, and head and facial trauma. Childhood psychopathology, mostly characterized as conduct disorder, is common.

g. Incarcerated delinquents: Major depression and suicide attempts and frequent risk-taking behaviors are common in this group.

h. Recurrence: A subgroup of adolescents accounts for most juvenile crimes. In one study, 54% of juvenile delinquents were repeaters accounting for 85% of crimes committed, with a subgroup of 6.3% committing 52% of crimes (Wolfgang et al., 1972).

Legal Rights

1. Judicial rights: Adolescent's cases are usually processed through a juvenile court without a jury trial. However, adolescents have the right to legal counsel, the right to notice of charges, the right to remain silent, the right to confront their accuser, and the right to proof of guilt beyond a reasonable doubt. At the end of the proceeding, if the judge believes the youth to be guilty of the offense, he will sustain the petition of delinquency.
2. Treatment rights: In the last 20 years, many laws have been enacted that govern the care of adolescents while in detention. These laws cover specific issues such as staffing requirements and guidelines for the use of psychiatric medications.

Effective Rehabilitation For Delinquent and Violent Youth

Until recently, few interventions to reduce delinquent behavior were rigorously evaluated to determine if they reduced recidivism. Current successful rehabilitation programs address the criminogenic factors of offenders. The major risk factors that correlate with recidivism risk in order of importance are:

1. A history of antisocial behavior and low self control
2. Personnel attitudes, values, beliefs supportive of crime
3. Pro-criminal associates and isolation from anti-criminal others
4. Current dysfunctional family features
5. Callous personality factors
6. Substance abuse

Further information about assessment of risk and case management can be accessed at www.Assessments.com.

The list of most important criminogenic factors varies somewhat from author to author. However, the principle concepts is that attributes related to criminal behavior are targeted by the rehabilitation program and factors such as self esteem that are not related to ongoing delinquent behavior are not stressed.

Effective and cost-efficient programs identify those youth at high risk to re-offend. The programs present their interventions in a responsive manner that meets the learning styles and culture of the youth. Each program must follow ethical guidelines and adhere to program integrity i.e. programs must closely replicate those programs proven to be effective. Some interventions that have been shown to be effective are: Aggression Replacement Training, Multisystemic Treatment, Functional Family Therapy, and Multidimensional Treatment Foster Care. On the other hand, boot camps and scared straight type programs are not effective in reducing recidivism while intensive juvenile probation has a mixed record of success. Considerably more research is needed to develop more effective interventions that address delinquent behavior. In addition researchers must develop collaborative working relationships with legislators who often control the types of rehabilitation available in government funded facilities.

Health Problems

A comprehensive review of mental health and medical issues of institutionalized youth is beyond the scope of this book. The health care provider should know that approximately 1 million adolescents live away from home, and one half of them are in institutions for juvenile offenders. The June 2006 issue of Journal of Adolescent Health and the April 2006 issue of Child and Adolescent Psychiatric Clinics of North America are devoted to health issues of youth in juvenile detention centers.

Between 40% and 80% of these youth have medical problems that may include the following:

1. General medical problems
   a. Unmet nutritional needs that in some cases relate to obesity.
   b. Problems common to adolescents in general: Headaches, chest and abdominal pains, asthma, acne, scoliosis, weight control problems, peptic ulcers, minor trauma, short stature, delayed puberty, gynecological problems, cancers and leukemia, myopia, and hearing loss.
   c. Preexisting conditions that have gone undetected due to poor access to medical care, including hernias, undescended testes, urethral strictures (congenital or acquired), tuberculosis in endemic areas, hepatitis, and congenital heart disease. In addition, decayed and missing teeth are common in most adolescents in juvenile detention facilities (Bolin and Jones, 2006).
2. Problems related to delinquent behaviors and lifestyle
   a. Injuries: Four to eight times more common in institutionalized youth.
   b. Substance abuse and drug withdrawal symptoms affect 70% to 80% of delinquents entering state facilities, especially in short-term detention facilities.
   c. STDs, pregnancy, pelvic inflammatory disease, and occasionally HIV infection. Generally 10% of boys and 20% of girls entering detention will have *Chlamydia* infections.

    d. Retained bullets with increased risk of lead toxicity, especially if the bullet is lodged in healing bone, joints, or lung tissue.

    e. Gunshot wounds and automobile accidents resulting in paraplegia, brain injury, bowel injury, and obstruction.

3. Mental health problems attributable to the social and physical environment: Estimates are that youth in juvenile justice systems have 2 to 4 times the rate of mental health disorders as the general adolescent population. Problems include the following:
    a. Suicide
    b. Institutional violence (gang violence)
    c. Depression
    d. Anxiety

4. Deaths: Gallagher and Dobrin (2006) review death rates for incarcerated youth. Adolescents in juvenile justice facilities have lower risks of death by accident (18.25 deaths per year per 100,000 confined versus 32.79 in general population) and homicide (7.3 versus 9.37). However, those confined have much higher risks of death from suicide (277% higher, 21.9 versus 7.9) and illness (30% higher, 21.9 versus 17). Overall, mortality rates were 7.8% higher in incarcerated youth during their confinement. Higher mortality rates were found in facilities that had a higher percentage of black youth. Accidental deaths were more likely in facilities that had no means of physical security to lock youth inside; however, suicide and illness-related deaths were more likely in larger, highly secure facilities.

Delinquent youth rarely malinger. Many obscure symptoms that result in a confusing clinical picture are either caused by an unusual presentation of a common disease or the presence of an uncommon disease.

Providing medical services to detained youth can be very rewarding. Most institutionalized children have long histories of neglect and abuse. They respond well to kindness and understanding from their care providers. Therefore, medical personnel should remember that they are caregivers and youth advocates rather than correctional staff.

Morris et al. (1995) reviewed the health risk behaviors of youth in juvenile correctional facilities and found that risky behaviors began early and reached a plateau at 15 or 16 years of age. Male and female youths reported comparable rates of drinking, binge drinking, and illicit drug use. By 12 years of age, 62% of those in the study reported a history of sexual intercourse, and 89% were sexually active by age 14. The mean age at onset of sexual intercourse was 12 years. Fighting was common, with 25% reporting fight-related injuries in the last year. Almost one half of the group was in a gang. Suicide had been contemplated by 22%. STDs were common, and fewer than half of the group had used a condom at last intercourse.

In light of these data, incarcerated youth must undergo health and psychiatric screening during intake procedures, and short-term health and mental health care must be available. Guidelines for health care in juvenile detention institutions are available through state boards of correction, from the National Commission on Correctional Health Care (NCCHC) and from the American Correctional Association (ACA).

Clinical health care guidelines for adolescents are available at www.ncchc.org/resources/clinicalguides.html. General health care standards are available at: www.ncchc.org/resources/standards.html and www.aca.org/standards/.

There are many problems facing juvenile correctional facilities, including overcrowding, poorly trained staff, decaying facilities, inadequate medical and psychiatric care, and poor educational resources. These problems tend to persist because of a lack of public scrutiny and disenfranchisement of poor minority youth. For these reasons, a number of states and local jurisdictions are sued each year in order to force improved conditions of confinement.

RUNAWAY BEHAVIOR

Definition

Runaway behavior is defined as an unauthorized absence from home overnight. A *throwaway episode* is defined as a time that a child is asked or told to leave the home by a parent or household adult and, or a time when a child who is away from home is prevented from returning and when no alternative care is offered or provided.

Epidemiology

1. Incidence: In 1999, an estimated 1,682,900 youth had a runaway or "throwaway" episode (Hammer et al., 2002). Approximately 500,000 to 1 million adolescents run away each year (Carper, 1979). In 1997, the federal government reported 136,350 runaways. A Department of Health and Human Services report estimated that in 1983 between 733,000 and 1,300,000 youths in the United States could be classified as either runaways or homeless (Russell, 1995).

2. Age: Most of the runaways/throwaways in the U.S. Department of Justice study were 15 to 17 years of age (68%); however, 28% were 12 to 14 years old and 4% (an estimated 70,000 youth) were between the ages of 7 and 11. Males and females were equally represented among the runaway/throwaway youth (Hammer et al., 2002).

3. Race: Just over half (57%) of the runaway/throwaway youth were white/non-Hispanic. An additional 17% were black/non-Hispanic, 15% were Hispanic, and 11% were of another race/ethnicity (Hammer et al., 2002).

4. Length of time away from home: Nineteen percent of the runaway youth were away for <24 hours, 58% for 24 hours to 1 week, 15% for 1 week to <1 month, 7% for 1 month to <6 months, and <3% did not return (Hammer et al., 2002).

5. Return behavior: Return home on their own, 50%; return home through parental or peer involvement, 30%; return home through police intervention, 14%; never return home, 6%.

6. Distance traveled from home: Just more than one third (38%) traveled <10 mi away, one third (31%) traveled >10 mi but <50 mi, and approximately one fourth (23%) traveled >50 mi from home. No information was available on the remaining 9%. In 83% of the cases, the child did not leave the state. Police were contacted in less than one third of the cases (Hammer et al., 2002).

Types of Runaways

1. Abortive: No actual runaway behavior—just a fantasy.
2. Crisis: A short stay away from home, usually <3 days, secondary to an acute problem.

3. Casual: The streetwise adolescent with frequent runaway episodes.

Reasons for Running Away

Many reasons exist for runaway behavior, including lack of communication with parents, school failure, overly strict or overly permissive parents, discovery of sexual identity discordant with parental values, experimentation, escape from a hopeless situation, being thrown out of the house, revenge, imitation of peers, and the simultaneous crises of adolescence, parental middle-age crisis, and elderly grandparents. Depression is another reason for runaway behavior, 4% of the youth in the Department of Justice study reported previously attempting suicide (Hammer et al., 2002). In this study, 21% of runaway and throwaway youth had been physically or sexually abused at home in the year before leaving home and were afraid of abuse upon return (Hammer et al., 2002).

For those adolescents who become homeless, the situation is aggravated by decreased access to food, shelter, medical services, and social supports. Homeless youth lack a mainstream social network, and create their own social networks within their runaway environment.

An estimated 71% have the potential for being endangered during their runaway/throwaway episode because of substance dependency, use of hard drugs, sexual or physical abuse, presence in a place where criminal activity was occurring, or extremely young age (Hammer et al., 2002). Homeless, runaway, and throwaway youth are at significantly greater risk for health problems including HIV and other STDs, substance abuse, depression and suicide attempts, prostitution, and trauma (Clatts et al., 2005; Greenblatt and Robertson, 1993; Greene et al., 1999; Green et al., 1995; Whitbeck, 2004). Allen et al. (1994) reported HIV prevalence rates of 0% to 7.3% (median, 2.3%) among homeless youth. Rotheram-Borus (1993) reported a suicide attempt in 37% of runaway youth, with 44% of them having made an attempt within the previous month. Girls were significantly more likely than boys to have attempted suicide and to be depressed. Runaways with a history of attempted suicide were significantly more likely to be currently suicidal and depressed.

SUICIDE

This topic is discussed in Chapter 79.

SUBSTANCE ABUSE

This topic is discussed in Chapters 68 to 74.

INTERVENTIONS

For the primary care provider, the contact point with adolescents with high-risk behavior is the presentation of a medical problem. Rather than merely treating the medical problem, the physician needs to gather more background information to elicit the context in which the medical complaint has evolved. A brief psychosocial or lifestyle interview should be conducted. One method is the HEEADSSS Adolescent Risk Profile discussed in Chapter 3.

The HEEADSSS evaluation assesses risk and provides an opportunity to discuss with the adolescent the practices or behaviors that may influence health. The assessment should include the following:

1. Medical evaluation
2. Psychosocial evaluation (HEEADSSS)
3. Family assessment
4. Vocational assessment
5. School assessment

Important considerations include the following:

1. Identifying the youth's needs: Although high-risk youth present with many serious problems that the care provider identifies as paramount in the hierarchy of interventions, the adolescent also has an agenda that must be determined and validated. Failure to meet the young patient's perceived needs often results in his/her failure to "buy into" the professional's plan of care. The adolescent comes to the provider for help, and it is important to provide that help before and during any other interventions that the provider thinks are important.
2. High-risk youth with multiple problems are best dealt with by a *multidisciplinary team* functioning in an interdisciplinary manner. Without available multidisciplinary health professionals, the physician must have a comprehensive listing of local resources. Effective referral, particularly for high-risk youth, is best accomplished through a telephone call to a specific contact person, who should be identified while the adolescent is still in the office.
3. *Basic needs* such as food, shelter, and safety must be addressed before major psychotherapeutic interventions are considered.
4. The approach to the problem should be to draw on the adolescent's own resources or options for change (i.e., to find alternative solutions). Interventions must be both feasible and practical (i.e., within the realm of possibility for that particular teen and capable of serving the appropriate developmental function).
5. *Family involvement*, when indicated, may optimize the intervention strategy, but if such intervention is not done skillfully, the adolescent's problems may simply be compounded. The ability to educate a family for change is inversely proportional to the degree of dysfunction within the family.
6. Risk profiles may be modified by direct or indirect interventions. An example of a direct intervention would be a stop-smoking education program; an indirect method would involve increasing a health-enhancing behavior, such as jogging to discourage smoking.
7. Characteristics intrinsic to health professionals that enhance their ability as vehicles for change include:
   a. Ability to develop trust through establishment of a confidential relationship
   b. Willingness to see the youth's viewpoints as real
   c. Ability to listen
   d. Unconditional positive regard for the adolescent in his or her struggle
   e. Knowledge of self
8. The opportunity to change a system (individual or family) is greatest when the system is unbalanced or in transition. Staff availability during a crisis may be more effective than traditionally scheduled counseling or psychotherapy sessions.

WEB SITES

http://ojjdp.ncjrs.org/. Office of Juvenile Justice and Delinquency Prevention.

http://ncjrs.gov/App/Topics/Topic.aspx?TopicID=122. National Criminal Justice Reference Service.

http://www.childinc.com/runaway.htm. A United Way site on help for those with runaway youth.

http://www.ncjj.org/. National Center for Juvenile Justice.

http://www.njda.com/. National Juvenile Detention Association.

www.ojp.usdoj.gov/bjs/guide.htm. Sourcebook on Criminal Justice Statistics.

http://www.achsa.org/. American Correctional Health Services Association.

http://www.ncchc.org/. National Commission on Correctional Health Care.

http://www.aca.org. American Correctional Association.

REFERENCES AND ADDITIONAL READINGS

Abma JC, Martinez GM, Mosher WD, et al. Teenagers in the United States: sexual activity, contraceptive use, and childbearing, 2002. National center for health statistics. *Vital Health Stat* 2004;23(24):1.

Administration on Children and Families. *Youth programs: runaway and homeless youth program*, 2000. Retrieved November 15, 2005 from the World Wide Web: http://www.acf.hhs.gov/news/facts/youthpr.htm.

Allen JR. Of resilience, vulnerability, and a woman who never lived. *Child Adolesc Psychiatr Clin N Am* 1998;7:53.

Allen DM, Lehman JS, Green TA, et al. HIV infection among homeless adults and runaway youth, United States, 1989–1992. Field services branch. *AIDS* 1994;8:1593.

Bailey S, Doreleijers T, Tarbuck P. Recent developments in mental health screening and assessment in juvenile justice systems. *Child Adolesc Psychiatr Clin N Am* 2006;15(2):391.

Blum RW. Healthy youth development as a model for youth health promotion: a review. *J Adolesc Health* 1998;22:368.

Bolin K, Jones D. Oral health needs of adolescents in a juvenile detention facility. *J Adolesc Health* 2006;38(6):755.

Carper JM. Emergencies in adolescents: runaways and father-daughter incest. *Pediatr Clin North Am* 1979;26:883.

Centers for Disease Control. Surveillance summaries. *MMWR Morb Mortal Wkly Rep* 2000;SS05:1.

Centers for Disease Control and Prevention. Number of deaths and death rates, by age, race, and sex: United States, 2002. Table 3. *Natl Vital Stat Rep* 2004;53(5):21.

Centers for Disease Control and Prevention. Suicide and attempted suicide. *MMWR*, 2004;53(22):471.

Centers for Disease Control and Prevention, Department of Health and Human Services. Youth risk behavior surveillance—United States, 2005. *MMWR Morb Mortal Wkly Rep* 2006;53(SS-5):1.

Centers for Disease Control and Prevention. Deaths final data for 2003. *Natl Vital Stat Rep* 2006;54(13):1.

Clatts MC, Goldsamt L, Yi H, et al. Homelessness and drug abuse among young men who have sex with men in New York city. A preliminary epidemiological trajectory. *J Adolesc* 2005;28(2):201.

Eccles J. The association of school transitions in early adolescence with developmental trajectories through high school. In: Shulenberg J, ed. *Health and risk developmental transitions during adolescence*. New York: Cambridge University Press;1997.

Gallagher CA. Juvenile offenders in residential placement, 1997. *OJJDP fact sheet*, Washington, DC: U.S. Department of Justice, Office of Justice Programs, Office of Juvenile Justice and Delinquency Prevention; 1999: March FS9996.

Gallagher CA, Dobrin A. Deaths in juvenile justice residential facilities. *J Adolesc Health* 2006;38(6):662.

Garmezy N. Resilience in children's adaptation to negative life events and stressful environments. *Pediatr Ann* 1991;20:459.

Golzari M, Hunt SJ, Anoshiravani A. The health status of youth in juvenile detention facilities. *J Adolesc Health* 2006;38(6):776.

Greenblatt M, Robertson M. Lifestyles, adaptive strategies and sexual behaviors of homeless adolescents. *Hosp Community Psychiatry* 1993;44(12):1177.

Greene JM, Ennett ST. Prevalence and correlates of survival sex among runaway and homeless youth. *Am J Public Health* 1999;89(9):1406.

Greene JM, Ennett ST, Ringwalt CL. Prevalence and correlates of survival sex among runaway and homeless youth. *Am J Public Health* 1999;89:1406.

Greene J, Ringwalt C, Kelly J, et al. *Youth with runaway, thrownaway, and homeless experiences: prevalence, drug use and other at-risk behaviors, volumes I, II, III*. Washington, DC: U.S. Department of Health and Human Services, Administration on Children, Youth, and Families; 1995.

Grigorenko EL. Learning disabilities in juvenile offenders. *Child Adolesc Psychiatr Clin N Am* 2006;15(2):353.

Hammer H, Finkelhor DM, Sedkaj AH. Runaway/thrownaway children national estimates and characteristics. *National incidence studies of missing, abducted, runaway, and thrownaway children*. Washington, DC: U.S. Department of Justice, Office of Juvenile Justice and Delinquency Prevention; 2002.

Hayes CD, ed. *Risking the future: adolescent sexuality, pregnancy and child bearing*, vol 1. Washington DC: National Academy Press; 1987.

Henshaw SK. *U.S. teenage pregnancy statistics with comparative statistics for women aged 20–24*. New York: The Alan Gutmacher Institute; 2005.

Luthar SS. Vulnerability and resilience: a study of high risk adolescents. *Child Dev* 1991;62(3):600.

Luthar SS, Cicchetti D, Becker B. The construct of resilience: a critical evaluation and guidelines for future work. *Child Dev* 2000;71(3):5.

Maggs J, Frome P, Eccles J, et al. Psychosocial resources, adolescent risk behaviour and young adult adjustment: is risk taking more dangerous for some than others? *J Adolesc* 1997;20:103.

Martin JA, Hamilton BE, Sutton PD, et al. Births: final data for 2003. *National vital statistics reports*, vol 54 no 2. Hyattsville, MD: National Center for Health Statistics; 2005.

Morris RE, Harrison EA, Knox GW. Health risk behavioral survey from 39 juvenile correctional facilities in the United States. *J Adolesc Health* 1995;17:334.

National Center for Education Statistics. *Dropout rates in the United States: 2000* (Publication No. NCES 2002-114.). Washington, DC: U.S. Department of Education, Office of Educational Research and Improvement; 2001.

National Center for Injury Prevention and Control. *Injury mortality reports and leading causes of death reports*.http://webappa.cdc.gov/sasweb/ncipc/mortrate10.html, accessed 6.30.2006.

National Institute of Mental Health. *Suicide facts and statistics 2004*. Retrieved May 24, 2006 from the World Wide Web: www.nimh.nih.gov/suicide prevention/suifact.cfm.

Olsson CA, Bond L, Burns JM, et al. Adolescent resilience: a concept analysis. *J Adolesc* 2003;26:1.

Ringwalt CL, Greene JM, Robertson M, et al. The prevalence of homelessness among adolescents in the United States. *Am J Public Health* 1998;88:1325.

Rotheram-Borus MJ. Suicidal behavior and risk factors among runaway youths. *Am J Psychiatry* 1993;150:103.

Russell LA. *Homeless youth: child maltreatment and psychological distress*. Dissertation. Los Angeles: University of California, Los Angeles, School of Public Health; 1995.

Rutter M. Psychosocial resilience and protective mechanisms. *Am J Orthopsychiatry* 1987;57:316.

Sickmund M. Juveniles in corrections. *Juvenile offenders and victims. National report series bulletin*, NCJ 202885, Washington, DC: Office of Justice Programs. U.S. Department of Justice Programs. Office of Juvenile Justice and Delinquency Prevention; 2004: June. www.ojp.usdoj.gov/ojjdp.

Smith G. Resilience concepts and findings: implications for family therapy. *J Fam Ther* 1999;21:154.

Snyder HN. Juvenile arrests 1997. *Juvenile justice bulletin*, December; NCJ173938. Washington, DC: U.S. Department of Justice, Office of Justice Programs, Office of Juvenile Justice and Delinquency Prevention; 1998.

Snyder HN, Sickmund M. *Juvenile offenders and victims: 1999 national report*. Pittsburgh: National Center for Juvenile Justice, Office of Juvenile Justice and Delinquency Prevention; 1999.

Snyder HN. Juvenile arrests 2003. *Juvenile justice bulletin* August; NCJ209735. Washington, DC: U.S. Department of Justice, Office of Justice Programs, Office of Juvenile Justice and Delinquency Prevention; 2005: www.ojp.usdoj .gov.

Steinberg L, Elmen JD, Mounts NS. Authoritative parenting, psychosocial maturity, and academic success among adolescents. *Child Dev* 1989;60(6):1424.

Tyler KA, Johnson KA. A longitudinal study of the effects of early abuse on later victimization among high-risk adolescents. *Violence Vict* 2006;21(3):287.

Vermeiren R, Jespers I, Moffitt T. Mental health problems in juvenile justice populations. *Child Adolesc Psychiatr Clin N Am* 2006;15(2):333.

Werner E. Resilience in development. *Curr Dir Psychol Sci* 1995;4:81.

Whitbeck LB. Mental disorder and comorbitity among runaway and homeless adolescents. *J Adolesc Health* 2004;35(2):132.

Williams JH. Addressing incarcerated adolescents' psychological and physical health service needs. *J Adolesc Health* 2006;38(6):638.

Wolfgang ME, Figlio RM, Sellin T. *Delinquency in a birth cohort*. Chicago: University of Chicago Press; 1972.

Woods ER, Lin RG, Middleman A, et al. The association of suicidal attempts with other risk behaviors in adolescents in Massachusetts. *Pediatrics* 1997;99(6):791.

Zerby SA, Thomas CR. Legal issues, rights, and ethics for mental health in juvenile justice. *Child Adolesc Psychiatr Clin N Am* 2006;15(2):373.

CHAPTER 77

Youth Violence

Heather Champion and Robert Sege

Violence is a pervasive problem in American society. Adolescents are particularly likely to be affected by interpersonal violence, as victim, perpetrator, and witness. Despite the welcome decline in the incidence of fatal youth violence since the peak rates of the mid-1990s, recent mortality data still show that homicide and suicide cause more deaths than all natural causes combined among children older than 1 year. Homicide is the second leading cause of death among young people aged 10 to 24 years overall, and is the leading cause of death for African-Americans in this age-group. Violence takes many forms including homicide, physical assault, and other violent crimes, sexual assault, battering in intimate relationships, and suicide. This chapter focuses on interpersonal violence.

Violent behavior is a complex phenomenon that is stimulated by multiple individual, family, community, and societal factors including gender, exposure to violence, and neighborhood disorganization. The most common misconception is that intentional violence is a premeditated event that randomly affects people unknown to the assailant. The opposite is true, with most violent encounters being impulsive acts occurring among friends and acquaintances and within families. Therefore, the distinction between victim and perpetrator is not always apparent. Among males of all ethnic groups, the most common relationship between offender and victim is that of a friend or acquaintance. In approximately 25% of youth homicides, the victim is the initiator of violence. Emergency Department based studies in Boston, Philadelphia, and Washington DC all demonstrated that most violence-related injuries that required medical treatments were the results of arguments between young people who knew each other. For adolescent female victims, the most common perpetrator is a boyfriend, mirroring the situation for female adults, for whom the most common perpetrator is a family member or intimate partner. Ninety percent of female homicide victims are murdered by males.

The consequences of violent behavior are made more lethal by the presence of a firearm, particularly a handgun. Violence results in death, disability, emotional trauma, and tremendous financial cost for our society. Its presence affects all of us, both as citizens and health care providers, and confronts health care providers with particular challenges. This chapter outlines the epidemiology, etiology, risk and protective factors, prevention strategies, and clinical implications of interpersonal violence.

EPIDEMIOLOGY

Homicide

The United States has the highest homicide rate in the world among industrialized countries. The homicide rate for youth aged 18 to 24 years dropped from 25.7 per 100,000 in 1993 to 15.5 per 100,000 in 1999 with a further reduction to 14.72 per 100,000 in 2004 (Table 77.1) (Web-based Injury Statistics Query and Reporting System [WISQARS], www.cdc.gov/ncipc/wisqars). Of particular significance, the homicide rate for African-American males aged 18 to 24 years, the highest risk group for death from homicide, dropped from 191.7 per 100,000 in 1993 to 106.8 per 100,000 in 1999 with a further reduction to 97.01 per 100,000 in 2004. The rate of homicides for juveniles 14–17 also fell from a high of 13.3 per 100,000 in 1993 to 5.1 per 100,000 in 2004.

By 2004, the juvenile arrest rate for homicide fell by 77%, reaching the lowest level since the 1960s. In 2004, juveniles were involved in 5% of murder arrests, involving 1,110 young people, one third the number arrested in 1993. Despite this significant downward trend in homicide rates after 10 years of increasing rates, homicide is the second leading cause of death among 15- to 19-year-olds and the leading cause of death among black youth. The United States is the only industrialized country to have a homicide rate of >5 per 100,000 among young men (age 16–24 years); many countries have a rate <1 per 100,000. In 2004, 5,292 youth aged 10 to 24 were murdered, with 80% being killed with firearms. The Department of Justice reports that youth aged 12 to 17 years were twice as likely as adults to be victims of serious violent crime and 3 times as likely to be victims of simple assault (Snyder and Sickmund, 1999).

Teenage males outnumber females as victims of homicide by a factor of >6:1. Young males are more likely to be victims of violent crimes of all categories, except sexual assault and intimate partner violence. Ninety-four percent of youth younger than 18 years who are convicted of murder are males. Of the 5,292 homicides reported in the 10 to 24 age-group in 2004, 85% (4,518) were males and 15% (774) were females.

Physical Assault and Other Violent Crime

The 2005 Centers for Disease Control's (CDC's) National Youth Risk Behavior Survey (YRBS) has consistently

TABLE 77.1

Adolescent Homicide Rates and Absolute Numbers 1990 to 2004

	Youth Age 14–17 yr; Homicide Rate per 100,000	Youth Age 18–24 yr; Homicide Rate per 100,000	Total Number of Adolescent Homicide Victims Age 18–24 yr	White Males Age 18–24 yr; Rate per 100,000	Black Males Age 18–24 yr; Rate per 100,000	Total Number of Black Male Homicide Victims Age 18–24 yr
1990	11.0	22.2	5,952	17.2	160.1	3,009
1991	12.4	25.0	6,599	18.7	182.7	4,305
1992	12.3	24.7	6,440	19.0	179.9	3,357
1993	13.3	25.7	6,665	18.4	191.7	3,573
1994	12.5	24.8	6,376	19.0	181.9	3,384
1995	11.6	22.2	5,646	18.2	153.4	2,857
1996	9.5	20.4	5,163	15.8	147.0	2,726
1997	7.8	19.5	4,968	15.0	141.6	2,649
1998	6.4	17.4	4,521	14.1	119.7	2,288
1999	6.1	15.5	4,129	12.0	106.8	2,084
2000	5.2	15.5	4,200	12.0	109.5	2,170
2001	5.0	16.3	4,561	13.6	109.4	2,264
2002	5.0	15.8	4,486	12.8	106.5	2,275
2003	4.8	16.1	4,656	13.0	107.3	2,348
2004	5.1	14.72	4,306	12.33	97.01	2,164

Total number of youth homicide victims aged 18–24 yr from 1990–2004:   78,660

Total number of African-American male homicide victims aged 18–24 yr from 1990–2004:   40,553

Data from Centers for Disease Control and Prevention, National Centers for Injury Prevention and Control. Web-based Injury Statistics Query and Reporting System (WISQARS) (2005) (accessed April 25, 2006). Available from: www.cdc.gov/ncipc/wisqars.

found that one third of male high school students (35.9%) had been in one or more physical fights during the previous 12 months. Fights were more common among adolescent boys than adolescent girls (43% versus 28%). Rates were higher among black (43%) and Hispanic (41%) males than whites (33%). Almost 4% of students reported receiving medical attention (which may have been a school nurse) for injuries sustained during a fight.

After a decade long rise in crime from 1983 to 1994, in 2004, the tenth consecutive year of decline, arrests for serious violent crimes (murder, forcible rape, robbery, and aggravated assault) were reduced by 48% (Snyder, 2006). Despite the drop in arrest rates and self-reported rates for homicide, robbery, and rape, arrest rates for aggravated assault remained high at almost 70% above the 1983 level. The arrest rates for simple assault increased from 106% for males and 290% for females from 1980 to 2004.

According to the National Crime Victimization Survey, in 1998 among 12- to 19-year-olds, 1 per 150 was the victim of a robbery, 1 in 13 was the victim of a violent crime, 1 in 16 was the victim of an assault, and 1 in 76 the victim of aggravated assault (Criminal Victimization in the U.S., 2001). Ethnic discrepancies exist for nonlethal violent crime victimization as well. Forty-two per 1,000 Blacks and 32 per 1,000 whites reported experiencing violent crimes in 1999. Native Americans experienced violent crime at more than twice the national average.

Sexual Assault

Female adolescents have the highest risk of any age-group for being subjected to sexual assault. According to a recent CDC study, approximately 9% of women and 1.9% of men report being sexually assaulted before 18 years of age (Tjaden and Thoennes, 2000). The 2005 YRBS found female students (11%) more likely to have been forced to have sexual intercourse compared to male students (4%). Rates of forced sex were higher among black (9%) students than white (7%) students.

Dating Violence

The 2005 YRBS reports that in the 12 months preceding the survey, 9% of students nationwide had been hit, slapped, or physically hurt on purpose by a boyfriend, girlfriend, or date. The prevalence of dating violence was higher among black (12%) students than Hispanic (10%) or white (8%) students. Rates among males and females were comparable within race/ethnicity. Most survey studies conducted in the last decade indicate that males report being victims about as frequently or more than females (Malik et al., 1997), but that females are at increased risk for more severe injuries.

Suicide

In the 12 months preceding the 2005 YRBS, 13% of students nationwide reported a plan to attempt suicide and 8% reported an attempted suicide. Overall, the prevalence of having made a suicide plan was higher among white and Hispanic students than black students (13%, 15%, and 10%, respectively). Completed suicide rates among adolescents are highly correlated with household handgun ownership rates.

RISK FACTORS ASSOCIATED WITH VIOLENCE

Several key risk factors for violence and violence-related injuries have been identified. They are complex, interdependent, and influenced by individual, family, and societal variables and include access to firearms and weapon carrying; gang involvement; exposure to violence at home including violent discipline; domestic violence and child abuse; and exposure to media violence, alcohol, and other drug use.

1. Access to firearms: An estimated 200 million firearms are in civilian hands in the United States, and approximately 60 million of these are handguns. Approximately 43% of homes have one or more handguns; at least 30% of gun owners with children keep one or more loaded guns in the home. Consequently, approximately 9 million adolescents have access to handguns in their own homes. When a teenager fires a gun at home, the most common victim is himself or herself, with the second most common victim being a friend. The victim is essentially never an intruder. When there is a handgun at home, a household member or friend is roughly 43 times more likely to be the victim of the firearm than an intruder. A gun stored in the home is associated with a fivefold increased risk of completed suicide (Kellerman et al., 1992).

   In 2004, 6,540 youths aged 15 to 24 were involved in firearm-related deaths, a decline of over 44% since 1994. Among 15- to 24-year-olds, there were 4,127 homicides using a firearm, 2,104 suicides using a firearm, and 172 accidental firearm deaths (WISQARS). In 2004, 80.6% of homicide victims aged 10 to 24 were killed with a firearm.

2. Weapon carrying: Approximately one fifth of high school students (19%) in the 2005 YRBS reported carrying a weapon (i.e., gun, knife, or club) on at least 1 day in the month before the survey. Several studies, including the YRBS of the CDC, have indicated that surprising numbers of male adolescents carry weapons periodically. Weapon carrying was more commonly reported among boys than girls (30% versus 7%), and 6% of students reported carrying their weapon to school in the last 30 days. The percentage of students carrying weapons decreased between 1991 and 1997 and stabilized between 1997 and 2003 (26%, 18%, and 17%, 19%, respectively).

   Carrying of weapons increases the risk of violent behavior and violence-related injury by providing a false sense of security that contributes to impulsive behavior. The principal effect of having a gun is worsening of the outcomes of violent encounters. Fistfights or assaults result in deaths, retaliation for perceived slights may result in a death, attempted rapes, robberies, and suicidal gestures are completed. *The single most important factor in all kinds of firearm-related injuries is the accessibility to firearms themselves;* recent studies have demonstrated the relationship between firearms ownership rates and overall homicide rate (Miller et al.,

2002). In addition to the substantial risk of homicide associated with firearms availability, access to firearms is also strongly associated with suicide deaths (Miller et al., 2001).

3. Alcohol and other drug use: The role of drug and alcohol use on violent behavior is not clear. Although most violent adolescent offenders use drugs and alcohol, the onset of substance use usually occurs after the onset of violent behavior. In one study, >80% of self-reported violent incidents involved no drugs or alcohol (Huizinga et al., 1995). Risk may be in the social setting of substance use and violence and the co-occurrence of adolescents engaging in multiple risky behaviors. Some violence stems from the need to support drug abuse and from involvement in illicit drug sales.

4. Gang participation: The 1999 National Youth Gang Survey reported >26,000 youth gangs in schools and communities and 840,500 gang members in the United States, a decline of <1% from the peak in 1996. Although gang members represent a relatively small proportion of the adolescent population, they commit most of the serious violence by youth. Children and adolescents who participated in gangs are more likely to promote aggressive attitudes, report victimization experiences, be involved in fights, carry weapons to school, and use drugs or alcohol at school. Nationally, approximately 4% of youth homicides are gang related. However, in inner-city environments, in regions where gangs are prevalent, gang violence may account for as much as 30% to 40% or more of young homicide victims. In 1999, 47% of gang members were Hispanic, 31% black, 13% white, and 7% Asian. Gang members are primarily male (92%). Many young people join gangs out of fear for their safety, or to join a popular group. In those settings, provision of alternative recreation opportunities for youth appears to successfully diverts many of them.

5. Exposure to violence: Exposure to violence includes exposure within one's family including being a victim of and/or witnessing child abuse, witnessing domestic violence; violence in the media, including television and video games; and within one's neighborhood or community. Witnessing violence by children increases the risk that they will react violently later in life. More than half of the 6-year-old inner-city children in a cross-sectional study of exposure to violence had more behavior, emotional, attention, and social problems than those who did not.

6. Violent discipline: The use of violent discipline teaches children that violence is an appropriate means of shaping behavior and solving problems. In addition, children whose parents are unable to set effective limits may develop dysfunctional behavior patterns of interaction, particularly if corporal punishment is used extensively. Dysfunctional interaction may lead to poor performance and social isolation in the early school years and, later, association with peer groups that reward violence and antisocial behavior (Patterson et al., 1989; Tremblay et al., 1994, 2004). Parents appear to use corporal punishment when they have exhausted other means of disciplining their children.

7. Child abuse: Experiencing child abuse as an infant or toddler is a well-documented risk factor for later participation in violent behavior. A longitudinal study designed to examine long-term effects of abuse and neglect found that both physical abuse and neglect (but not sexual abuse) increased the likelihood of

arrest as a juvenile by >50%, arrest as an adult by 38%, and arrest for a violent crime by 38%, compared with a matched comparison group (Widom, 1992). Child abuse prevention is a critical component of violence prevention.

8. Domestic violence: Witnessing violence in the family environment as a young child, in particular spousal battery, has in a number of studies been found to correlate with later violent behavior, both in intimate relationships and in the society at large. Subjecting children to intimate partner violence of parents is a form of emotional abuse of children and in many states may be reported to Child Protective Services.

9. Media violence: More than 3,500 studies now confirm the association between higher levels of viewing violence and increased acceptance of aggressive attitudes and increased aggressive behavior. Children form attitudes about violence at a young age. Children exposed to media violence are more likely to behave aggressively. Watching media violence causes desensitization, particularly among young viewers (Strasburger and Grossman, 2001). The average American child, by the age of 18 years, will have viewed 200,000 acts of violence, including 40,000 murders. Preschoolers watching 2 hours of cartoons daily will be exposed to 10,000 acts of violence annually. These portrayals help form early values and perceptions. Pediatricians may effectively counsel parents concerning media exposure (Sege and Dietz, 1994), by suggesting that children younger than 2 years do not watch television and that older children be limited to 2 hours/day of total screen time. With the advent of V-Chips and television rating systems, more information is now available to parents regarding the content of television and other media.

RESILIENCE

Protective Factors

Protective factors are individual or environmental factors that buffer or moderate the risk of violence. The Surgeon General's Report on Youth Violence reviews several proposed individual-level protective factors including an intolerant attitude toward deviance (including violent behavior), high IQ, female gender, positive social orientation, perceived sanctions for transgression; family-level factors including a warm, supportive relationship with parents or other adults, and parental monitoring or supervision of activities; and school- or community-level protective factors including commitment to school, involvement in school activities, and having friends who behave conventionally. Only two of these factors have been shown to buffer the risk of youth violence—an intolerant attitude toward deviance and a commitment to school.

Recent studies using the National Longitudinal Survey of Youth have demonstrated the importance of protective factors, including community, family, and individual factors. At the community level, youth reported less violence involvement if they felt connected to school, to adults outside their families, and if they felt safe in their neighborhoods. Lower levels of violence were reported by teens who felt connected to their families, shared activities with their parents, and felt that they could talk about their problems with their parents. Interestingly, religiosity was a protective factor for girls, but not for boys. At all levels of risk, the effects of these protective factors—which the authors describe as "connectedness"—strongly reduce the likelihood of violence (Resnick et al., 2004).

A cross-sectional study in Vermont demonstrated an inverse relationship between the number of protective factors and health risk behaviors, including violence (Murphey et al., 2004). School-based programs that increase social connection reduce the incidence of violence and are more effective than traditional risk-based programs. In the office setting, parents and providers both have strong preferences for asset- or strength-based counseling and assessment (Sege et al., 2006). The American Academy of Pediatrics has just released a new violence-prevention program, Connected Kids: Safe, Strong Secure, which is primarily based on the promotion of resilience.

Other Factors: Schools

The U.S. Department of Education reported 188,000 fights or physical attacks not involving weapons, 11,000 fights involving weapons, and 4,000 incidents of sexual assault in schools during the 1996 to 1997 school year. Nevertheless, school remains by far the safest place for children. Vital statistics estimate that fewer than 1% of child and adolescent homicides occur in school (WISQARS), and the overwhelming proportion of assaults that do occur in school are relatively minor in severity. For perspective, about twice the number of Americans are killed by lightning each year as are killed on school campuses.

School is a critical environment for young people to learn socially appropriate and constructive behaviors and methods of addressing conflict. Adolescents who fail at school, or leave for any reason, are at vastly increased risk for violence-related injury compared with teens who attend school. Homicide is, in the scope of violent events, relatively rare, and other violent encounters such as fights and robberies are much more common. Young people who emerge as bullies, develop uncontrolled rage, engage in threatening language or behavior, carry weapons, or engage in frequent fighting or other antisocial activity must be identified, preferably helped, to reduce their antisocial behaviors, and if necessary, placed in settings where they are not a threat to other young people. When young people do engage in a violent act, it is unusual for them to have been no preceding signs. All of the events that have involved multiple homicides on campuses and in communities by youth have one thing in common—the young perpetrators had easy access to firearms, on some occasions, automatic firearms.

ASSESSMENT OF RISK

To implement interventions which decrease the risk of violence, it is recommended that health care providers assess the risk of the youth's involvement with violence, including taking a thorough history of the teen's involvement with violence as an aggressor, a victim, a witness to violence in the community, a nonviolent problem solver, or a participant in gender role–related violence. In assessing risk, as with other situations, one must be cognizant of the developmental stage of the youth, and the clustering of risk factors. For example, among males there is a strong

TABLE 77.2

FISTS

FISTS: *F*ighting-*I*njuries-*S*ex-*T*hreats–*S*elf-defense
This mnemonic provides the basis for assessment of an adolescent's risk for involvement in violence

Fighting
How many fights have you been in during the past year?
When was your last fight?

Injuries
Have you ever been injured in a fight?
Have you ever injured someone else in a fight?

Sex
Are you scared of disagreeing with your partner?
Does your partner criticize or humiliate you in front of others?
Are you scared by your partner's violent or threatening behaviors?
Has your partner ever forced you to do something sexual you didn't want to do?
Every family argues. What are fights like in your family or with people you're dating? Do they ever become physical?
Do you think that couples can stay in love when one partner makes the other afraid?

Threats
Has someone carrying a weapon ever threatened you? What happened?
Has anything changed since then to make you feel safer?

Self-defense
What do you do if someone tries to pick a fight with you?
Have you ever carried a weapon in self-defense?

Asking about weapons in the context of self-defense facilitates a more candid response. In all cases, carrying a
 firearm indicates high risk. Carrying a knife is not as clearly identified with violent behavior. For example, a small
 pocketknife may or may not be considered high risk.

The FISTS mnemonic is adapted with permission from the Association of American Medical Colleges. Alpert EJ, Bradshaw YS, Sege
RD. Interpersonal violence and the education of physicians. *J Acad Med* 1997;72:S46.

association between cigarette smoking and weapons carry-ing. Complete assessment should include focused attention on connectedness of the teen to school and community. The mnemonic device FISTS (*F*ighting-*I*njuries-*S*ex-*T*hreats-*S*elf-defense) can be used as a guide in the collection of a violence-related medical history (Table 77.2).

Youth at low risk do not report recent fights, are in school, and do not report use of illicit drugs or alcohol. Moderate-risk youth may report one to two fights in the last year, or associated risk factors on the FISTS screen or occasional drug or alcohol use. High-risk individuals are not in school, or they report two or more fights in the last year. Moderate-risk and high-risk individuals may need further counseling or referral.

PREVENTION AND INTERVENTION

Recently, there has been a proliferation of violence-prevention programs. Programs tend to be funded for relatively short periods and limited in scope, so longitudinal effects on participants and broader societal measures of violent incidents are not valid measures. Promising approaches begin as early in life as possible, are sustained over time, and enhance nurturing and nonviolent parenting methods. Resources for successful prevention programs

are included in the Internet resources at the end of this chapter.

Primary Prevention Interventions

Primary prevention strategies are either directed at the entire population or focused on selected populations at greatest risk. Any serious strategy of violence preven-tion must include efforts directed at young children, during which time basic values and approaches to frus-tration and conflict are learned. Particular issues to be addressed include familial violence, corporal punish-ment, child abuse, and early exposure to media violence, which are known to correlate with later violent behav-ior of children and adolescents. Recent research has suggested that effective primary prevention programs will be directed toward the promotion of resilience, as well as risk reduction. Effective strategies include the following:

1. Identification of young, stressed, and particularly so-cially isolated parents, and providing them with home visitation and early intervention parenting training pro-grams.
2. Increasing financial stability of impoverished families at risk, particularly families headed by single parents.

3. Identification and referral of pregnant and parenting teenagers and their partners to teen parenting and support groups.
4. Preschool programs that address intellectual, emotional, and social needs of young children and encourage the development of nonviolent conflict-resolution skills.
5. Reduction of early childhood exposure to media violence, including cartoon violence.
6. Engaging teens, particularly young teens, in supervised recreational activities.
7. Improving the quality of the school environment, and development of stable after-school programs with extensive activities for youths.
8. Provision of safe, supervised routes ("safe corridors") to and from school for youths in troubled neighborhoods.
9. Increased access to after-school programs.
10. Prevention of school truancy and dropout.
11. Employment programs for teenagers, including those who are out of school, or after-school and vacation employment for teens in school.

In addition, curricula for conflict resolution have been developed for use in secondary schools. Specific curricula approaches that appear to be effective are as follows:

1. Alternative solution generation
2. Self-esteem enhancement
3. Peer negotiation skills
4. Problem-solving skills training
5. Anger management

Effective primary prevention programs must be developmentally appropriate and comprehensive in approach (particularly those involving teenagers) and must include multiple components, reinforcing nonviolent behaviors in various contexts such as the family, school, peer groups, and the media. These approaches attempt to provide access to ongoing relationships with nonviolent, caring adult mentors, particularly for those teens from stressed or single-parent families. By reducing risk factors, children and adolescents are empowered to resist effects of detrimental life circumstances.

While many of these programs are community based, office-based counseling may also be effective. The American Academy of Pediatrics (AAP) Connected Kids program offers clinical resources and public education materials to support violence prevention in the primary care setting.

Firearms Fundamental to a public health approach to prevention is a change in environmental risk factors. Access to firearms is the principal environmental risk factor for *lethal* violence. Removal of firearms from the environment of adolescents through legislation, strict enforcement of existing laws, and removal of firearms from the home environment is essential in the prevention of the grave consequences of violent behavior. It should be recognized that a serious consideration of the adolescent emotional developmental characteristics must lead one to the conclusion that educational interventions alone are unlikely to be successful with many children and adolescents (American Academy of Pediatrics, Committee on Injury and Poison Prevention, 2000).
Recommendations include the following:

1. Removal of firearms: Parents of adolescents and children should be encouraged to remove firearms from their homes. This is consistent with the recommendations of the American Academy of Pediatrics, Center to Prevent Handgun Violence (1994). Attempts at interventions short of removal have not been shown to reduce mortality. Parents who keep loaded firearms at home should be informed that this is extremely dangerous for their children, and they may be held legally culpable for any adverse consequences. Parents must be made aware that if they keep a gun at home, the most likely victim is their teenage son/daughter and that firearms at home are far more likely to be used to shoot a friend or a family member than an intruder. Additionally, parents may enquire about the presence of loaded firearms in the homes of their children's friends and require that they be eliminated before children can play in the area.
2. Locked containers: If parents are unwilling to remove firearms from the home, they should be advised to separate ammunition from the weapons and keep both in separate securely locked containers. Trigger locks should be placed on all firearms. It must be emphasized, however, that although this may reduce impulsive access to firearms in the home, teenagers have manual dexterity equal to that of adults and these measures may have a limited impact on the adolescent's ability to obtain and use a firearm if he or she is determined to do so. Weapons should therefore always be stored unloaded, with the ammunition locked separately.
3. Safety classes: Because accidental discharges make up few firearm injuries, safety classes in use of firearms have never been shown to reduce the risk associated with firearm ownership. In contrast, several studies have shown that gun safety classes do not overcome the natural curiosity of children.
4. Strict laws: Most states have laws that make it an offense for a minor to be in possession of a firearm under most circumstances.
5. Handgun regulations: American Academy of Pediatrics, Center to Prevent Handgun Violence (1994) and many other medical and health organizations recommend that private, unlicensed ownership of handguns be banned. Regulations may, over time, reduce the number of handguns in circulation. Preliminary studies in California indicate that most firearms used in homicides were purchased within 2 years of use in a crime. Reductions in sales may have a more rapid impact on reducing public access than is generally thought.

Secondary Prevention Interventions

Although the causes of juvenile violence are not completely understood and programs designed to prevent delinquency have not been thoroughly evaluated, successful approaches to intervention appear to have the following characteristics:

1. They are appropriately supportive of children and adolescents and their families.
2. They are intensive (i.e., they involve the commitment of considerable time, personnel, and effort).
3. They are broad based; that is, they intervene in a number of systems, including family, school, and peer, in which the child or adolescent is involved and use multiple services including educational, health, and social as appropriate for the individual child or adolescent.

Secondary interventions may be directed at teens who have been identified after their risk behaviors have become apparent. These interventions support adolescents identified as at risk in making a successful transition through school and into employment; they help nurture relationships with supportive adults (Elliot, 1994). They may include the following:

1. Enhancement of the school environment with smaller-size classes and supervised after-school activities
2. Supporting successful transition to adult roles through access to job training, apprenticeship, and job placement
3. Providing caring, nonviolent adult mentors
4. Integrating adolescents into activities with nondisturbed peers
5. Intensive individual or family psychotherapy

Children and youth hospitalized for violence-related injuries are at particular risk. Hospital based psychoeducational approaches to risk reduction have not been as effective as once hoped; it appears that long-term improvement in outcome depends on linkages with community resources. Several cities have adopted promising programs that link injured youths with community-based service organizations that offer ongoing programs that positively engage these patients, and, when needed, provide concrete services and support (Marcelle and Melzer-Lange, 2001).

Tertiary Intervention

Tertiary intervention takes place after a teen has become embroiled in violent activities and may occur largely through the juvenile justice system. When the juvenile justice system was created approximately 100 years ago, it was intended to be a "kind and just parent," acknowledging that children were inherently different from adults, less culpable for their acts, more amenable to rehabilitation, and that a community-based, comprehensive approach was the most effective way to achieve rehabilitation. By 1915, almost all states had a juvenile court and the model spread internationally. The original goals of the juvenile court were to shield children from adults, protect the privacy of children, and allow adolescents to enter the workforce without a police record. During the 1990s, despite the fact that crime rates had been dropping significantly, these goals were rapidly eroded. Many states passed legislation making sentences more punitive, facilitating transfers of juveniles to adult court, and corroding protections of confidentiality. In effect, these measures blur the distinctions between adult and juvenile offenders (National Academy Press, Juvenile Crime, Juvenile Justice. (2001) Commission on Behavioral and Social Sciences and Education. National Research Council, Commission on Behavioral and Social Sciences and Education, 1993). These policies rely less and less on rehabilitation and increasingly attempt to manage juveniles through the adult criminal justice system. More than 90% of children involved in the juvenile justice system are nonviolent offenders, with most offences involving property or substance offenses such as theft, burglary, and drugs. On any given day, >90,000 children are in juvenile detention or correctional facilities; in addition, more than an estimated 9,000 adolescents younger than 18 years are in adult jails (Snyder and Sickmund, 1999). This is a cause for concern, because children held in adult jails are 8 times more likely than those held in juvenile facilities to commit suicide, 5 times more likely to be sexually assaulted, and twice as likely to be beaten by prison staff (Forst et al., 1989).

The effectiveness of punishment on antisocial behavior is of significant debate, and there is no clear evidence that punishment either improves behaviors or reduces the recidivism rate. Research that exists tends to indicate that incarceration efforts of the judicial system tend to actually worsen the outcomes for young people. Evidence for the effectiveness of incarceration in reducing later illegal activity does not exist. Incarcerated adolescents have a 50% to 70% chance of being arrested within 2 years of release. Juvenile justice policies are frequently not designed based on prevention research but in a legislative response to particular aberrant and well-publicized events. For example, boot camps have been widely adopted as a model for treatment of incarcerated teens, with no evidence of effectiveness at all; in fact, studies indicate that teens who have participated in boot camps have a 75% recidivism rate, even worse than incarceration. In addition, recent investigations into some of the 50 boot camps operating around the country have revealed widespread abuse and neglect (Children's Defense Fund, 2001).

The disproportionate incarceration of minority adolescents, particularly Latino and African-American teens, has been a source of grave concern for many years. Research indicates that this overrepresentation is a product of actions occurring through the entire juvenile justice system, from the decision to make the initial arrest, the decision to hold a youth in detention, the decision to refer a case to juvenile court, the prosecutor's decision to prosecute a case, to the actual judicial decision, and the subsequent penalty (Building Blocks for Youth, 2000). At every step of the process, minority adolescents are more likely to be treated in a way that inflates the charges and magnifies their chances of incarceration, including the incarceration of minority adolescents as adults, than are white teens for the same offenses (Males and Macallair, 2000). Minority adolescents are 8.3 times more likely than their white counterparts to be sentenced by an adult court to imprisonment in a California Youth Authority facility. The juvenile justice system has a budget of approximately $10 billion nationally; most is used for incarceration.

Family-focused, community-based, supervised programs involving offending teens have markedly lower recidivism rates. There is much room for continued research and modification of public policy regarding our approach as a society to young people who are apprehended for illegal activities (Mendel, 2000). Parenthetically, health care for teens in juvenile confinement is a serious concern because incarcerated teens have a greater than average number of health problems that may worsen during confinement, and only 1% of eligible juvenile justice facilities have been accredited as meeting existing voluntary standards for providing health care.

WEB SITES

http://www.aap.org/vipp.
http://www.cjcj.org/. Justice Policy Institute.
http://www.colorado.edu/cspv/. Center for the Study and Prevention of Violence.
http://www.buildingblocksforyouth.org. Building Blocks for Youth.
http://www.aypf.org. American Youth Policy Forum.

Federal Resource Sites

http://www.albany.edu/sourcebook/toc.html. Source book on juvenile crime statistics.

http://www.cdc.gov/HealthyYouth/YRBS. Center for Disease Control and Prevention, National Center for Chronic Disease Prevention and Health Promotion, Youth Risk Behavior Surveillance.

http://www.cdc.gov/ncipc/factsheets/yvoverview.htm. Center for Disease Control and Prevention, Factsheet on youth violence.

http://www.cdc.gov/ncipc/wisqars/. Center for Disease Control and Prevention, National Center for Injury Prevention and Control, Web-based Injury Statistics Query and Reporting System (WISQARS).

http://www.juvenilenet.org. The Corrections Connection Network, Juvenile Info Network.

http://www.ojp.usdoj.gov/bjs/welcome.html. Department of Justice, Bureau of Justice Statistics.

http://www.ojjdp.ncjrs.org. Office of Juvenile Justice and Delinquency Prevention.

http://www.safeyouth.org. National Youth Violence Prevention Resource Center.

http://www.surgeongeneral.gov/library/youthviolence. Youth Violence: A report of the Surgeon General.

REFERENCES AND ADDITIONAL READINGS

American Academy of Pediatrics, Center to Prevent Handgun Violence. *Steps to prevent firearm injury*. Elk Grove, IL: The Academy of Pediatrics; 1994.

American Academy of Pediatrics, Committee on Communications. Media violence. *Pediatrics* 1995;95:949.

American Medical Association. Adolescents as victims of family violence. *JAMA* 1993;270:1850.

American Psychological Association. *Violence and youth: psychology's response*. Washington, DC: American Psychological Association; 1993.

American Academy of Pediatrics, Committee on Injury and Poison Prevention. Firearm-related injuries affecting the pediatric population. *Pediatrics* 2000;105:888.

American Academy of Pediatrics, Committee on Communications. Children, adolescents, and television (RE0043). *Pediatrics* 2001;107(2):423.

Amnest J, Mercy J, Gibson D, et al. National estimates of nonfatal firearm related injuries: beyond the tip of the iceberg. *JAMA* 1995;273:1749.

Anderson RN, Smith BL. Deaths: leading causes for 2001. *Natl Vital Stat Rep* 2003;52(9):1.

Autphenne V, Gluckin A, Iverson E. *Teen relationship abuse, regional needs assessment*, Children's Hospital Los Angeles, Division of Adolescent Medicine; 1998.

Building Blocks for Youth. *And justice for some*. Available at www.buildingblocksforyouth.org, 2000.

Bureau of Justice Statistics. *Violent crime in the United States, 1990*. Washington, DC: U.S. Department of Justice; 1991.

Bureau of Justice Statistics. *Homicide trends in the U.S.: Intimate Homicide 1998–2001*. Washington, DC: U.S. Department of Justice. Available at www.ojp.usdoj.gov/bjs/homicide/intimates.htm, 2001.

Centers for Disease Control and Prevention. Weapon carrying among high school students—United States, 1990. *MMWR Morb Mortal Wkly Rep* 1991;40:681.

Centers for Disease Control and Prevention. Violence-related attitudes and behaviors of high school students—New York city, 1992. *JAMA* 1993;270:2032.

Centers for Disease Control and Prevention. Rates of homicide, suicide, and firearm-related death among children in 26 industrialized countries. *MMWR Morb Mortal Wkly Rep* 1997; 46:101.

Centers for Disease Control and Prevention. *Deaths: Final Data for 1998 MMWR Natl Vital Stat Rep*. 2000;48(11).

Centers for Disease Control and Prevention. Surveillance for Fatal and Nonfatal Injuries—United States, 2001. *MMWR* 2004;53(SS-7).1–57

Centers for Disease Control and Prevention, National Center for Injury Prevention and Control. Web-based Injury Statistics Query and Reporting System (WISQARS) [online]. (2005) [cited 2006 Apr 25].~ Available from URL: www.cdc.gov/ncipc/wisqars.

Centers for Disease Control and Prevention. Youth risk behavior surveillance—United States, 2005. *MMWR* 2006;55 (SS-5):1. Available at: http://www.cdc.gov/HealthyYouth/yrbs/index.htm, accessed June 13, 2006.

Centerwall BS. Homicide and the prevalence of handguns: Canada and the United States, 1976 to 1980. *Am J Epidemiol* 1991;134:1245.

Children's Defense Fund. *Yearbook 2000, the state of America's children*. Washington, DC: CDF Publication; 2001.

Clancy TV, Misick LN, Covington D, et al. The financial impact of intentional violence on community hospitals. *J Trauma* 1994;37:1.

Coben JH, Weiss HB, Dearwater SR. A primer on school violence prevention. *J Sch Health* 1994;64:309.

Cotten NU, Resnick J, Browne DC, et al. Aggression and fighting behavior among African-American adolescents: individual and family factors. *Am J Public Health* 1994;84:618.

Criminal Victimization in the U.S.. 1999, Bureau of Justice Statistics, U.S. Department of Justice. http://www.ojp.usdoj.gov/bjs/cvict.htm, 2001.

Department of Health and Human Services (US). Youth Violence: A report of the Surgeon General [online] 2001.

Dolins JC, Christoffel KK. Reducing violent injuries: priorities for pediatrician advocacy. *Pediatrics* 1994;94:638.

DuRant RH, Cadenhead C, Pendergrast RA, et al. Factors associated with the use of violence among urban black adolescents. *Am J Public Health* 1994;84:612.

Elliot D. *Youth violence: an overview, 1994*. Colorado: Center for the Study and Prevention of Violence; 1994. Available at www.colorado.edu/cspv.

Eron LD. Media violence. *Pediatr Ann* 1995;24:84.

Fingerhut LA, Ingram DD, Feldman JJ. Firearm homicide among black teenage males in metropolitan counties. Comparison of death rates in two periods, 1983 through 1985 and 1987 through 1989. *JAMA* 1992;267:3054.

Fingerhut L, Kleinman J. International and interstate comparisons of homicide among young males. *JAMA* 1990;263:3292.

Forst M, Fagan J, Vivona T. Youth in prisons and training schools: perceptions and consequences of the treatment/custody dichotomy. *Juv Fam Ct J* 1989;40:1.

Garbarino J, Dubrow N, Kostelny K, et al. *Children in danger: coping with the consequences of community violence*. San Francisco: Jossey Bass Publishers; 1992.

Garrett D. Violent behaviors among African-American adolescents. *Adolescence* 1995;30:209.

Golding AM. Leading article—understanding and preventing violence: a review. *Public Health* 1995;109:91.

Goodwillie S. *Voices from the future, our children tell us about violence in America. Children's express.* New York: Crown Publishers; 1993.

Groves BM, Zuckerman B, Marans S. Silent victims. Children who witness violence. *JAMA* 1993;269:262.

Hammond WR, Yung B. Psychology's role in the public health response to assaultive violence among young African-American men. *Am Psychol* 1993;48:142.

Harms PD, Snyder HN. *Trends in the murder of juveniles: 1980–2000.* Washington, DC: Office of Juvenile Justice and Delinquency Prevention; 2004.

Hausman AJ, Spivak H, Prothrow-Stith D. Adolescents' knowledge and attitudes about and experience with violence. *J Adolesc Health* 1994;15:400.

Huizinga D, Loeber R, Thornberry TP. *Recent findings from the program of research on the causes and correlates of delinquency.* (U.S. Department of Justice, Office of Justice Programs, Office of Juvenile Justice and Delinquency Prevention, NCJ 159042). Washington, DC: U.S. Government Printing Office; 1995.

Jaffe PG. *Children of battered women.* Newbury Park: Sage Publications Inc; 1990.

Johnson EM, Belfer ML. Substance abuse and violence: cause and consequence. *J Health Care Poor Underserved* 1995;6:113.

Kellam SG, Prinz R, Sheley J. *Preventing school violence: plenary papers of the 1999 conference on criminal justice research and evaluation-enhancing policy and practice through research, May 2000.*, National Institute of Justice. U.S. Department of Justice; 2000.

Kellerman AL, Rivarra FP, Somes G, et al. Suicide in the home in relation to gun ownership. *N Engl J Med* 1992;327:467.

Males M, Macallair D. *The color of justice: an analysis of juvenile adult court transfers in California,* Center of Juvenile and Criminal Justice, 2000. www.buildingblocksforyouth.org.

Malik S, Sorenson S, Aneshensel C. Community and dating violence among adolescents: perpetuation and victimization. *J Adolesc Health* 1997;21:291.

Marcelle DR, Melzer-Lange MD. Project UJIMA: working together to make things right. *Wis Med J* 2001;100(2):22.

Mendel R. *Less hype, more help: reducing juvenile crime, what works and what doesn't.* American Youth Policy Forum; 2000. Available at www.aypf.org. American Youth Policy Forum.

Miller M, Azrael D, Hemenway D. Firearm availability and unintentional firearm deaths. *Accid Anal Prev* 2001;33:477.

Miller M, Azrael D, Hemenway D. Rates of household firearm ownership and homicide across US regions and states, 1988–1997. *Am J Public Health* 2002;92(12):1988.

Moffitt T. *Partner violence among young adults.* Presentation to the National Institute of Justice; 1997.

Mondragon D. Clinical assessment of gang violence risk through history and physical exam. *J Health Care Poor Underserved* 1995;6:209.

Murphey DA, Lamonda KH, Carney JK, et al. Relationships of a brief measure of youth assets to health-promoting and risk behaviors. *J Adolesc Health* 2004;34(3):184.

National Research Council, Commission on Behavioral and Social Sciences and Education. *Commission on Behavioral and Social Sciences and Education.* National Academy Press, Juvenile Crime, Juvenile Justice..(2001).

National Research Council. *Understanding and preventing violence.* Washington, DC: National Academy Press; 1993.

O'Donnell L, Cohen S, Hausman A. Forum on youth violence in minority communities. Evaluation of community-based violence prevention programs. *Public Health Rep* 1991;106:276.

Panel on High-Risk Youth, National Research Council. *Losing generations: Adolescent in high-risk settings.* Washington, DC: National Academy Press; 1993.

Patterson GR, DeBaryshe D, Ramsey E. A developmental perspective on antisocial behavior. *Am Psychol* 1989;44:331.

Prothrow-Stith D. *Violence prevention, curriculum for adolescents. Teenage health teaching modules.* Newton, MA: Education Development Center; 1987.

Prothrow-Stith D. *Deadly consequences.* New York: Harper-Collins; 1991.

Prothrow-Stith DB. The epidemic of youth violence in America: using public health prevention strategies to prevent violence. *J Health Care Poor Underserved* 1995;6:95.

Rachuba L, Stanton B, Howard D. Violent crime in the United States: an epidemiologic profile. *Arch Pediatr Adolesc Med* 1995;149:953.

Resnick M, Ireland M, Borowsky I. Youth violence perpetration: what protects? What predicts. *J Adolesc Health* 2004;35:424–e1.

Rivara FP, Farrington DP. Prevention of violence: role of the pediatrician. *Arch Pediatr Adolesc Med* 1995;149:421.

Rodriguez MA, Brindis CD. Violence and latino youth: prevention and methodological issues. *Public Health Rep* 1995;110:260.

Ropp L, Visintainer P, Uman J, et al. Death in the city: an American childhood tragedy. *JAMA* 1992;267:2905.

Rosenberg ML. Academic medical centers have a major role in preventing violence. *Acad Med* 1993;68:268.

Sege R, Dietz W. Television viewing and violence in children: the pediatrician as agent for change. *Pediatrics* 1994;94:600.

Sege RD, Flanigan E, Levin-Goodman R, et al. American academy of pediatrics' connected kids program case study. *Am J Prev Med* 2005;29(5 Suppl 2):215.

Sege RD, Hatmaker-Flanigan E, De Vos E, et al. Anticipatory guidance and violence prevention: results from family and pediatrician focus groups. *Pediatrics* 2006;117(2):455.

Sege RD, Hoffman JS. Training health professionals in youth violence prevention overview of extant efforts. *Am J Prev Med* 2005;29(5 Suppl 2):175.

Sege RD, Licenziato VG, Webb S. Bringing violence prevention into the clinic the Massachusetts medical society violence prevention project. *Am J Prev Med* 2005;29(5 Suppl 2):230.

Seltzer F. Trend in mortality from violent deaths: unintentional injuries, United States, 1960–1991. *Stat Bull Metrop Insur Co* 1995;76:19.

Sheley J. *Controlling violence: what schools are doing—preventing school violence: plenary papers of the 1999 conference on criminal justice research and evaluation.* Washington, DC: National Institute of Justice; 2000: Available at www.ojp.usdoj.gov/nij.

Sheley JF, McGee ZT, Wright JD. Gun-related violence in and around inner-city schools. *Am J Dis Child* 1992;146:677.

Singer MI, Anglin TM, Song LY, et al. Adolescents' exposure to violence and associated symptoms of psychological trauma. *JAMA* 1995;273:477.

Slaby RG, Stringham P. Prevention of peer and community violence: the pediatrician's role. *Pediatrics* 1994;94:608.

Sloan JH, Kellermann AL, Reay DT, et al. Handgun regulations, crime, assaults, and homicide: a tale of two cities. *N Engl J Med* 1988;319:1256.

Snyder HN. *Juvenile arrests 2004.* Washington, DC: U.S. Department of Justice, Juvenile Justice Bulletin, Office of Juvenile Justice and Delinquency Prevention; 2006. Available at www.ncjrs.org. Dec.

Snyder HN, Sickmund M. *Juvenile offenders and victims; 1999 national report*. Washington, DC: U.S. Department of Justice, Office of Juvenile Justice and Delinquency Prevention; 1999. September

Strasburger VC, Grossman D. How many more Columbines? What can pediatricians do about school and media violence. *Pediatr Ann* 2001;30:87.

Tjaden P, Thoennes N. *Full report of the prevalence, incidence, and consequences of violence against women*. Washington, DC: U.S. Department of Justice; 2000.November, Available at www.ojp.usdoj.gov/nij.

Tomes H. Research and policy directions in violence: a developmental perspective. *J Health Care Poor Underserved* 1995;6:146.

Tremblay RE, Pihl RO, Vitaro F, et al. Predicting early onset of male antisocial behavior from preschool behavior. *Arch Gen Psychiatry* 1994;51:732.

Tremblay RE, Nagin DS, Seguin JR, et al. Physical aggression during early childhood: trajectories and predictors. *Pediatrics* 2004;115:e43.

U.S. Advisory Board on Child Abuse and Neglect. *A nation's shame: fatal child abuse and neglect in the United States*. Washington, DC: U.S. Congress; April 1995.

U.S. Department of Justice. *Crime in the United States, uniform crime reports*. Washington, DC: Federal Bureau of Investigation; 1992; August 30.

Waller JA, Skelly JM, Davis JH. Characteristics, costs, and effects of violence in Vermont. *J Trauma* 1994;37:921.

Webster DW, Wilson ME. Gun violence among youth and the pediatrician's role in primary prevention. *Pediatrics* 1994; 94:617.

Weil DS, Hemenway D. Loaded guns in the home: analysis of a national random sample of gun owners. *JAMA* 1992;267:3033.

White MP. A comprehensive approach to violence prevention. *J Health Care Poor Underserved* 1995;6:254.

Widom C. *The cycle of violence*. Washington, DC: National Institute of Justice, U.S. Department of Justice, 1992.October.

Wilson-Brewer R, Spivak H. Violence prevention in schools and other community settings: the pediatrician as initiator, educator, collaborator, and advocate. *Pediatrics* 1994;94:623.

CHAPTER 78

Adolescent Depression and Anxiety Disorders

Stan Kutcher and Sonia Chehil

Depression and anxiety disorders are common psychiatric disorders during adolescence. According to the World Health Organization, these disorders contribute the largest single burden of disease in young people (World Health Organization, 2003). Depression and anxiety disorders may occur concurrently or separately. Individually, each disorder is often accompanied by symptoms of the other and both are often preceded by impairing anxiety symptoms that start in childhood. Childhood anxiety is in fact one of the best predictors of depression later in life. Early diagnosis and effective interventions can enhance the short- and long-term functioning and prevent or significantly modify the characteristic lifelong chronic nature of these illnesses.

DEPRESSION

Depression, as a clinical entity, is the prolonged presence of persistent low mood, negative cognition, and withdrawn behavior that leads to significant functional difficulties in many aspects of life (social, interpersonal, family, educational, and vocational). It must be differentiated from the usual, expected, and relatively transient mood difficulties that most individuals experience in the course of their daily living, which in popular parlance is also called *depression*, as well as from a state of "demoralization," which is a more prolonged mood disturbance, usually resulting from ongoing negative life experiences. The importance of differentiating "normal" transient low mood states and demoralization phenomenon from clinical depression in adolescents may be difficult. Mood states during the teen years may fluctuate rapidly and may be expressed in a variety of different affective, cognitive, and behavioral dimensions, some of which, if not critically considered, may be mistaken for symptoms of a clinical depression. For example, the teen who emphatically states, "I am so depressed that I can not stand it"; or the teen who thinks "now that my boyfriend has left me I can't go on with life"; or the teen who locks himself in his room for a couple of days because he was removed from the basketball team, may not be depressed at all, but just be demonstrating the expected enhanced emotionality of the adolescent years. Careful diagnostic assessment is necessary to avoid overdiagnosis and subsequent exposure to unnecessary treatment or underdiagnosis and subsequent denial of needed treatment.

In the clinical situation, it may take two or more visits and an independent perspective (such as that of the parents) before the clinician is able to determine the presence or absence of a depressive syndrome with a high degree of certainty (Table 78.1).

Epidemiology

1. Self-reported symptoms of depression are very common in normal adolescent populations. In studies of adolescents in the United States, up to 50% of teens report feeling depressed within the 6-month period before the questioning with significant numbers (up to approximately 20%) reporting suicidal ideation. When Diagnostic and Statistical Manual of Mental Disorders (DSM) criteria are applied, studies show that approximately 5% to 8% of teens will qualify for the diagnosis of major depressive disorder (MDD) (perhaps slightly fewer if strict functional disability criteria are stringently applied).
2. In the 2005 Youth Risk Behavior Surveillance (Centers for Disease Control and Prevention, 2006), 28.5% of high school students reported feeling sad or hopeless almost everyday for over 2 weeks in a row during the last year. This rate was 36.7% in females and 20.5% in males. Rates were highest in Hispanic high school students—36.7% compared to black (28.4%) and white (25.8%).
3. Rates by age: The rates range from approximately 1% prepubertally to near adult rates (8%–10%) by the end of the teen years.
4. Gender: Girls are approximately twice as likely to demonstrate clinical depression as boys.

These data illustrate the importance of differentiating depressive symptoms from clinical depression (Kessler et al., 2001; Birmaher et al., 1996a,b).

Suicide

Trends in suicide rates across the lifespan tend to parallel those of depression with low suicide rates reported prepubertally followed by a rapid rise in suicide rates over the adolescent years, peaking in early adulthood and remaining relatively level until the geriatric phase of the life cycle. In the United States, adolescent suicide is consistently amongst the top three causes of mortality in this age-group. It is highly correlated with unidentified

TABLE 78.1

Distinguishing Clinical Depression from Common "Similar" Conditions

Condition	Description
Depression (symptoms)	Usually transient mood, behavioral, and somatic symptoms. Often associated with negative life events. Does not cause significant functional impairment. This is not a psychiatric disorder, does not require medical intervention.
Demoralization	Mood, behavioral, and somatic symptoms may be relatively long standing but clearly related to external situation and would resolve if the situation resolves, does not cause significant functional impairment. May be secondary to effects of another mental disorder (such as the demoralization experienced by teenagers with ADHD who have difficulties with schoolwork and who may fail subjects as a result). This is not a psychiatric disorder and does not require medical intervention although if secondary to another mental disorder should be addressed within the context of the treatment of the other illness.
Depression (as a clinical syndrome)	Includes the DSM diagnostic categories of MDD and dysthymic disorder. Meets severity and duration criteria for one of the DSM categories and must include significant functional impairment. This is a psychiatric disorder and medical treatment is indicated—either pharmacological or psychological or both.

ADHD, attention-deficit hyperactivity disorder; DSM, Diagnostic and Statistical Manual of Mental Disorders; MDD, major depressive disorder.

and untreated depression. Although suicide rates in adolescents have increased over the period 1950 to 1990, the last decade has seen a significant decrease in suicide rates in the United States. Although the reasons for this are not clear and the cause is likely to be multifactorial, there is a strong association between this decrease in suicide and an increase in the use of selective serotonin reuptake inhibitors (SSRIs) in the treatment of adolescent depression (Simon et al., 2006; Olfson et al., 2003; American Academy of Pediatrics, Committee on Adolescence, 2000). See Tables 79.3 and 79.4 for suicide rates in high school students from the Youth Risk Behavior Survey. Any adolescent complaining of suicidal intent or who has made a suicide attempt must be evaluated carefully for the presence of a depressive disorder (DD).

Risk Factors for Adolescent Depression

A multitude of "risk factors" have been identified for adolescent depression. However, it has been difficult to separate risk factors which are *highly predictive (causal) from associated factors.*

- Highly predictive risk factors: Their presence usually foreshadows the onset of adolescent depression in the future.
- Associated risk factors: Factors that often occur concurrently with adolescent depression but are not necessarily predictive of future onset of adolescent depression.

Highly Predictive Risk Factors
1. Maternal history of MDD
2. Previous episode of MDD

Associated Risk Factors
1. Family conflict with poor affective involvement and significant communication difficulties
2. Exposure to significant negative life events

In "real life" cases it may be difficult to determine the nature of the risk factors identified.

For example, a depressed teen may have a depressed parent and also live in a family where conflict and poor affective support exist. It is hard to determine if the causal factor is the genetic risk passed on through the depressed parent or the environment which itself may be the result of parental depression, or both.

In addition, studies are just now beginning to help differentiate *proximal versus distal risk factors.*

- Proximal risk factors: Those occurring immediately or shortly before the onset of the event—in this case an episode of depression.
- Distal risk factors: Those occurring at some point in time before the onset of the event—in this case depression.

Proximal Risk Factors
1. Anxiety disorder such as panic disorder (PD), social anxiety disorder (SAD), and so on
2. Medical condition such as diabetes or cancer

If the clinician is aware that the teenager has a positive family history of MDD or bipolar disorder, "preventive counseling" in the prepubertal period may help the parent and teen identify significant mood disturbances should they arise. If such mood disturbances are identified, the parent and teen will to be better prepared to seek clinical attention early.

Distal Risk Factors
1. Family history of MDD or bipolar disorder (especially the female children of a mother who has had a clear episode of MDD)
2. Early prolonged abuse (sexual or physical)
3. Early death of a parent

Negative Life Events
Negative life events are commonly but often mistakenly considered to be causal risk factors for adolescent depression.

These events include but are not limited to breakup of a romantic relationship, school problems, geographic moves, or family difficulties. The reality is that these life events are so common among adolescents that if they were causal, every teenager would be clinically depressed. These events however may lead to distress, depressive symptoms, and even demoralization but are not likely to be single substantive causal factors for MDD. Another difficulty in exploring the impact of negative life events on MDD is understanding the timing of the onset of depression in adolescents. Typically, DDs are not known to have a sudden onset; instead, they have a gradual and insidious onset. In fact, the onset is often so gradual, that the associated dysfunction can be overlooked. It is not uncommon for the gradual onset of the DD (and not yet identified) to lead to significant life events such as interpersonal problems, family difficulties, romantic breakups, and a variety of school difficulties. Following these events, the depression may become more clearly manifest. Therefore, events which may be identified as "causal" for a depressive episode may actually be the result of the episode itself.

Diagnosis

The diagnosis of depression is made using DSM-IV-TR criteria (American Psychiatric Association, 2000) or the International Classification of Diseases (ICD) criteria (World Health Organization, 1992). In the United States, the DSM criteria are most commonly used. The DSM classifies three types of DDs:

1. MDD
2. Dysthymic disorder
3. Depressive disorder not otherwise specified (DD-NOS)

There is good consensus about the diagnostic categories of MDD and Dysthymic disorder. There is less consensus about the category of DD-NOS. In the opinion of the authors of this chapter, the DD-NOS diagnosis should not be used to justify medical interventions in this age-group.

DSM Criteria for MDD
In order to meet DSM criteria for MDD, the young person must have experienced one or more major depressive episodes (MDEs) without ever having experienced a manic, mixed, or hypomanic episode.

Diagnostic Criteria for a Major Depressive Episode (Adapted from DSM-IV-TR)
For at least 2 consecutive weeks the adolescent has experienced five (or more) of the following symptoms which represent a change from previous functioning; one of the symptoms must be either depressed or irritable mood or markedly diminished interest or pleasure.

1. Depressed or irritable mood most of the day, nearly every day.
2. Markedly diminished interest or pleasure in all or almost all activities nearly every day.
3. Significant weight loss when not dieting or a weight gain of >5% of body weight in a month *or* a decrease/increase in appetite nearly every day.
4. Insomnia or hypersomnia nearly every day.
5. Psychomotor agitation or retardation nearly every day (this symptom *must* be noticeable to others and not merely subjective feelings).

6. Fatigue or loss of energy nearly every day.
7. Feeling of worthlessness or excessive/inappropriate guilt nearly every day (this does *not* include self-reproach or guilt about being sick).
8. Diminished ability to think or concentrate, or indecisiveness nearly every day.
9. Recurrent thoughts of death, recurrent suicidal ideation, a suicide attempt, or a specific plan for committing suicide.

In addition to the symptom complex described earlier, the following *must* also be present:

- The symptoms cause *clinically significant* distress or *impairment* in social, occupational, or other important areas of functioning.
- The symptoms are not due to the direct physiological effects of a substance (e.g., a drug of abuse, a medication) or a general medical condition (e.g., hypothyroidism).
- The symptoms are not better accounted for by bereavement.

If *all* of the aforementioned conditions are not met, then the adolescent does not meet the diagnosis for a MDE.

Some youth may experience long-standing and persistent depressive symptoms that are not demoralizing and cause functional difficulties. These youth may be demonstrating DD which is a chronic mood disturbance characterized by depressive symptoms that are present most days for at least a period of 1 year.

Diagnosis of Dysthymic Disorder (Adapted from DSM-IV-TR)
1. Depressed or irritable mood for most of the day, for most days for at least 1 year.
2. Two or more of the following must be present:
   a. Poor appetite or overeating
   b. Insomnia or hypersomnia
   c. Low energy or fatigue
   d. Low self-esteem
   e. Poor concentration or difficulty making decisions
   f. Feelings of hopelessness

In neither MDD nor Dysthymic disorder can the symptoms be part of a schizophrenic, schizoaffective, bipolar, or delusional illness. The two DDs described here may have a seasonal component. It is important to note that should there be a seasonal component present this does not affect diagnosis or treatment of the disorder.

Identifying the Depressed Adolescent

Underrecognition of clinical depression in teens is common in primary care (Asarnow et al., 2002; Rushton et al., 2002). This may be in part due to the different clinical presentation of depression in teens as compared to adults (youth may present with marked irritability rather than sad or depressed mood) and may be compounded by the hesitance of teens to self disclose symptoms of depression if not asked directly about these symptoms during a clinical assessment.

Screening Tests
It is reasonable for clinicians to screen for depression, because it is one of the most common medical disorders that begin in the teenage years. Screening tests include the Kutcher Adolescent Depression Scale, the KADS-11

(an 11-item version of the KADS self-report questionnaire), the Beck Depression Inventory (Beck and Steer, 1987), the Reynolds Adolescent Depression Scale (RADS) (Reynolds, 1987), and the Mood and Feelings Questionnaire (Thapar and McGuffin, 1998). Most of these take longer to administer than the six-item KADS and their sensitivities and specificities range from 0.70 to 0.90 and 0.39 to 0.90, respectively.

Some general health screening tools for adolescents have been studied in primary care. These include the Patient Health Questionnaire for Adolescents (Johnston et al., 2002) and the Safe Times Questionnaire (Schubiner et al., 1994). Screening tools in the primary care setting is strongly recommended, as the evidence suggests that sole reliance on a teenager's reporting of depression as a chief complaint may miss a significant number of depressed youth (Zuckerbrot and Jensen, 2006).

1. *The KADS* (six-item version) (Fig. 78.1) has been validated as a screening tool for depression in adolescents (LeBlanc et al., 2002; Brooks, 2004; Brooks et al., 2003). One study found that in a population of students in the 7th to 12th grade, the brief instrument was as good as the Beck Depression Inventory and better than the 16-item KADS in its overall diagnostic ability, with sensitivity of 92% and a specificity of 71% at a cutoff score of 6 (LeBlanc et al., 2002). A distinct advantage of the six-item KADS is its brevity and the ability to combine it with other brief tools in the screening of mental illnesses. It is a brief self-report questionnaire, which the teenager can fill out while waiting for an appointment. It can also be used to screen large numbers of adolescents (such as a secondary school population) if a public health framework is being considered. A score of 6 or higher (or a score of 2 or higher on question six) should lead to a careful clinical assessment directed at determining the presence or absence of a depressive syndrome (clinical depression).

2. *An 11-item version of the KADS self-report questionnaire (KADS-11)* is ideal for assessment and monitoring purposes in clinical settings (Fig. 78.2). The items on the KADS-11 are worded using standard and colloquial terminology, and responses are scored on a simple 4-point scale. Once the youth has completed the KADS-11, clinicians can review and discuss the individual items of the KADS with the teen and an informant (usually a parent or guardian, if available), in order to gain a more comprehensive understanding of the teen's difficulties and to rule in or rule out a definitive diagnosis of depression.

Although not a screening tool, *The Chehil and Kutcher Clinical Assessment of Adolescent Depression* (CAAD, See Fig. 78.3) is designed to accompany the 11-item version of the KADS. Additional items found in the CAAD that are not present in the KADS-11 include assessment of current substance use and an overall rating of symptoms, function and safety.

Scores on the 11 items in the KADS are reviewed for both the following:
a. Frequency scale: Rated on a four-point frequency scale from "hardly ever" to "all of the time."
b. Severity scale: Clinicians ask the teen and the informant to rate the severity of each symptom on a four-point scale (0–3) where
   • "0" represents the absence of the symptom
   • "1" is used to denote a symptom that is present but is experienced as mild and tolerable by the patient and is not associated with impairment

• "2" is used to denote a symptom that is present, is moderate in severity, is experienced as problematic by the patient but does not significantly impair the patient's functioning
• "3" is used to denote a symptom that is present and severe, difficult to tolerate, and associated with significant impairment

On the basis of the information obtained from the teen and the informant, the clinician also provides a "composite" rating for each symptom using the same four-point scale. The CAAD can be used effectively by the clinician to conduct a detailed clinical interview needed to arrive at a diagnosis of MDD.

3. *The RADS* is an instrument used primarily on adolescents 13 to 18 years of age. It is a self-report, 30-item tool to screen for identification of depression and evaluation of treatment in adolescents. Internal consistency reliability has ranged from 0.92 to 0.96 and concurrent validity from 0.70 to 0.89 (Weber, 2000).

4. *Children's Depression Inventory (CDI)*. The CDI, developed from the Beck Depression Inventory, is a self-rated instrument and represents five factors common to children and adolescents. It has been utilized in studies that have included various developmental ages and diverse ethnic populations. The construct validity of this test has been questioned in a study by Myers et al. (2002). They reported an internal consistency reliability of 0.59 to 0.88, a poor discriminate validity, and a high false-negative rate in adolescents.

BIPOLAR DISORDER (MANIC DEPRESSION)

If MDD occurs together with mania the diagnosis is bipolar disorder. This illness usually has its onset approximately 10 to 15 years postpuberty and is a chronic psychiatric disorder characterized by periods of depressed mood (which meet the criteria of MDD described earlier) and periods of significantly elevated mood (mania). Mania is characterized by intense energy, hyperactivity, elation, grandiosity, sleeplessness, racing thoughts, pressured speech, excessive risk-taking behaviors, excessive impulsive behaviors (such as spending sprees without the means to pay), and hypersexuality. In most teens with bipolar disorder, a "classic" MDE may be the first presentation of the illness; the initial diagnosis of MDD is revised after the first clear manic episode has been experienced. In some teenagers, an antidepressant medication can precipitate the development of a manic episode. While the following clinical points may be of help in identification of individuals at higher risk of bipolar disorder, at the present time we have no effective way of accurately predicting which teen presenting with MDD will go on to develop a bipolar disorder. The clinical points listed in the next section may be of help in identifying teens at higher risk of bipolar disorder.

Clinical Risk Factors for Bipolar Disorder in a Clinically Depressed Teenager

• Rapid onset of MDD
• Psychotic symptoms occurring together with MDD
• Family history of bipolar disorder

6-ITEM Kutcher Adolescent Depression Scale: KADS-6

NAME: _____ CHART NUMBER: _____

DATE: _____ ASSESSMENT COMPLETED BY: _____

OVER THE LAST WEEK, HOW HAVE YOU BEEN "ON AVERAGE" OR "USUALLY" REGARDING THE FOLLOWING ITEMS:

1. **Low mood, sadness, feeling blah or down, depressed, just can't be bothered.**

    ☐   ☐   ☐   ☐
    0 - Hardly Ever   1 - Much of The Time   2 - Most of The Time   3 - All of The Time

2. **Feelings of worthlessness, hopelessness, letting people down, not being a good person.**

    ☐   ☐   ☐   ☐
    0 - Hardly Ever   1 - Much of The Time   2 - Most of The Time   3 - All of The Time

3. **Feeling tired, feeling fatigued, low in energy, hard to get motivated, have to push to get things done, want to rest or lie down a lot.**

    ☐   ☐   ☐   ☐
    0 - Hardly Ever   1 - Much of The Time   2 - Most of The Time   3 - All of The Time

4. **Feeling that life is not very much fun, not feeling good when usually (before getting sick) would feel good, not getting as much pleasure from fun things as usual (before getting sick).**

    ☐   ☐   ☐   ☐
    0 - Hardly Ever   1 - Much of The Time   2 - Most of The Time   3 - All of The Time

5. **Feeling worried, nervous, panicky, tense, keyed up, anxious.**

    ☐   ☐   ☐   ☐
    0 - Hardly Ever   1 - Much of The Time   2 - Most of The Time   3 - All of The Time

6. **Thoughts, plans or actions about suicide or self-harm.**

    ☐   ☐   ☐   ☐
    0 - Hardly Ever   1 - Much of The Time   2 - Most of The Time   3 - All of The Time

TOTAL SCORE: [   ]

1

© Dr Stan Kutcher, 2006

FIGURE 78.1 Six-Item Kutcher Adolescent Depression Scale. (The Six-Item KADS is under copyright to Dr. Stan Kutcher. Use is with written permission only. Individuals wishing to use the six-item KADS can contact Dr. Kutcher at skutcher@dal.ca for permission.)

6-ITEM Kutcher Adolescent Depression Scale: KADS-6

OVERVIEW

The Kutcher Adolescent Depression Scale (KADS) is a **self-report** scale specifically designed to diagnose and assess the severity of adolescent depression, and versions include a 16-item, an 11 item and an abbreviated 6-item scale.

SCORING INSTRUCTIONS

TOTAL SCORE	SCORE INTERPRETATION
0 – 5	Probably not depressed
6 and ABOVE	Possible depression; more thorough assessment needed

REFERENCE

LeBlanc JC, Almudevar A, Brooks SJ, Kutcher S: Screening for Adolescent Depression: Comparison of the Kutcher Adolescent Depression Scale with the Beck Depression Inventory, Journal of Child and Adolescent Psychopharmacology, 2002 Summer; 12(2):113-26.

Self-report instruments commonly used to assess depression in adolescents have limited or unknown reliability and validity in this age group. We describe a new self-report scale, the Kutcher Adolescent Depression Scale (KADS), designed specifically to diagnose and assess the severity of adolescent depression. This report compares the diagnostic validity of the full 16-item instrument, brief versions of it, and the Beck Depression Inventory (BDI) against the criteria for major depressive episode (MDE) from the Mini International Neuropsychiatric Interview (MINI). Some 309 of 1,712 grade 7 to grade 12 students who completed the BDI had scores that exceeded 15. All were invited for further assessment, of whom 161 agreed to assessment by the KADS, the BDI again, and a MINI diagnostic interview for MDE. Receiver operating characteristic (ROC) curve analysis was used to determine which KADS items best identified subjects experiencing an MDE. *Further ROC curve analyses established that the overall diagnostic ability of a six-item subscale of the KADS was at least as good as that of the BDI and was better than that of the full-length KADS. Used with a cutoff score of 6, the six-item KADS achieved sensitivity and specificity rates of 92% and 71%, respectively—a combination not achieved by other self-report instruments. The six-item KADS may prove to be an efficient and effective means of ruling out MDE in adolescents.*

2

© Dr Stan Kutcher, 2006

FIGURE 78.1   *(Continued)*

11-ITEM Kutcher Adolescent Depression Scale: KADS-11

NAME: _____   CHART NUMBER: _____

DATE: _____ ASSESSMENT COMPLETED BY: _____

OVER THE LAST WEEK, HOW HAVE YOU BEEN "ON AVERAGE" OR "USUALLY" REGARDING THE FOLLOWING ITEMS:

1. **Low mood, sadness, feeling blah or down, depressed, just can't be bothered.**

   ☐ 0 - Hardly Ever   ☐ 1 - Much of The Time   ☐ 2 - Most of The Time   ☐ 3 - All of The Time

2. **Irritable, losing your temper easily, feeling pissed off, loosing it.**

   ☐ 0 - Hardly Ever   ☐ 1 - Much of The Time   ☐ 2 - Most of The Time   ☐ 3 - All of The Time

3. **Sleep Difficulties - different from your usual (over the years before you got sick): trouble falling asleep, lying awake in bed.**

   ☐ 0 - Hardly Ever   ☐ 1 - Much of The Time   ☐ 2 - Most of The Time   ☐ 3 - All of The Time

4. **Feeling Decreased Interest In: hanging out with friends; being with your best friend; being with your partner / boyfriend / girlfriend; going out of the house; doing school work or work; doing hobbies or sports or recreation.**

   ☐ 0 - Hardly Ever   ☐ 1 - Much of The Time   ☐ 2 - Most of The Time   ☐ 3 - All of The Time

5. **Feelings of worthlessness, hopelessness, letting people down, not being a good person.**

   ☐ 0 - Hardly Ever   ☐ 1 - Much of The Time   ☐ 2 - Most of The Time   ☐ 3 - All of The Time

1

Dr. Stan Kutcher, 2006

FIGURE 78.2 11-Item Kutcher Adolescent Depression Scale. (The 11-Item KADS is under copyright to Dr. Stan Kutcher. Use is with written permission only. Individuals wishing to use the 11-item KADS can contact Dr. Kutcher at skutcher@dal.ca for permission.)

6. **Feeling tired, feeling fatigued, low in energy, hard to get motivated, have to push to get things done, want to rest or lie down a lot.**

☐ 0 - Hardly Ever   ☐ 1 - Much of The Time   ☐ 2 - Most of The Time   ☐ 3 - All of The Time

7. **Trouble concentrating, can't keep your mind on schoolwork or work, daydreaming when you should be working, hard to focus when reading, getting "bored" with work or school.**

☐ 0 - Hardly Ever   ☐ 1 - Much of The Time   ☐ 2 - Most of The Time   ☐ 3 - All of The Time

8. **Feeling that life is not very much fun, not feeling good when usually (before getting sick) would feel good, not getting as much pleasure from fun things as usual (before getting sick).**

☐ 0 - Hardly Ever   ☐ 1 - Much of The Time   ☐ 2 - Most of The Time   ☐ 3 - All of The Time

9. **Feeling worried, nervous, panicky, tense, keyed up, anxious.**

☐ 0 - Hardly Ever   ☐ 1 - Much of The Time   ☐ 2 - Most of The Time   ☐ 3 - All of The Time

10. **Physical feelings of worry like: headaches, butterflies, nausea, tingling, restlessness, diarrhea, shakes or tremors.**

☐ 0 - Hardly Ever   ☐ 1 - Much of The Time   ☐ 2 - Most of The Time   ☐ 3 - All of The Time

11. **Thoughts, plans or actions about suicide or self-harm.**

☐ 0 - No thoughts or plans or actions   ☐ 1 - Occasional thoughts, no plans or actions   ☐ 2 - Frequent thoughts, no plans or actions   ☐ 3 - Plans and/or actions that have hurt

TOTAL SCORE: ☐

2

Dr. Stan Kutcher, 2006

FIGURE 78.2 *(Continued)*

11-ITEM Kutcher Adolescent Depression Scale: KADS-11

OVERVIEW

The Kutcher Adolescent Depression Scale (KADS) is a **self-report** scale specifically designed to diagnose and assess the severity of adolescent depression, and versions include a 16-item, a 11-item, and an abbreviated 6-item scale.

SCORING INTERPRETATION

There are no validated diagnostic categories associated with particular ranges of scores. All scores should be assessed relative to an individual patient's baseline score (higher scores indicating worsening depression, lower scores suggesting possible improvement).

REFERENCE

LeBlanc JC, Almudevar A, Brooks SJ, Kutcher S: Screening for Adolescent Depression: Comparison of the Kutcher Adolescent Depression Scale with the Beck Depression Inventory, Journal of Child and Adolescent Psychopharmacology, 2002 Summer; 12(2):113-26.

Self-report instruments commonly used to assess depression in adolescents have limited or unknown reliability and validity in this age group. We describe a new self-report scale, the Kutcher Adolescent Depression Scale (KADS), designed specifically to diagnose and assess the severity of adolescent depression. This report compares the diagnostic validity of the full 16-item instrument, brief versions of it, and the Beck Depression Inventory (BDI) against the criteria for major depressive episode (MDE) from the Mini International Neuropsychiatric Interview (MINI). Some 309 of 1,712 grade 7 to grade 12 students who completed the BDI had scores that exceeded 15. All were invited for further assessment, of whom 161 agreed to assessment by the KADS, the BDI again, and a MINI diagnostic interview for MDE. Receiver operating characteristic (ROC) curve analysis was used to determine which KADS items best identified subjectsexperiencing an MDE. *Further ROC curve analyses established that the overall diagnostic ability of a six-item subscale of the KADS was at least as good as that of the BDI and was better than that of the full-length KADS. Used with a cutoff score of 6, the six-item KADS achieved sensitivity and specificity rates of 92% and 71%, respectively—a combination not achieved by other self-report instruments. The six-item KADS may prove to be an efficient and effective means of ruling out MDE in adolescents.*

3

Dr. Stan Kutcher, 2006

FIGURE 78.2   *(Continued)*

NAME: _____   INFORMANT: _____

Chehil & Kutcher CLINICAL ASSESSMENT OF ADOLESCENT DEPRESSION (CAAD)

Record the frequency of occurrence OVER THE PAST ONE WEEK for each symptom below then rate the symptom on a 4 point scale (0–3) in the *symptom* column. Document relevant clinical information in the *Clinician Review* column (i.e. course, aggravating/mitigating factors, impact on home/school/recreational functioning, etc.) and rate the symptom from 0–3 based on the composite information obtained.

Symptom Rating: 0 = Does not bother the adolescent
1 = Mild distress and no significant impairment in home, school, or social function
2 = Moderate distress and some impairment in home, school, or social function
3 = Severe distress and significant impairment in home, school, or social function

SYMPTOM: Low mood, sadness, blah, down, depressed, just can't be bothered.			
Over the past week I have experienced this: ☐ Hardly ever ☐ Much of the time ☐ Most of the time ☐ All of the time	Patient Symptom Rating (0–3)	Informant Symptom Rating (0–3)	Clinician Composite Symptom Rating (0–3)

Notes:

SYMPTOM: Irritable, losing temper easily, feeling pissed off, loosing it.			
Over the past week I have experienced this: ☐ Hardly ever ☐ Much of the time ☐ Most of the time ☐ All of the time	Patient Symptom Rating (0–3)	Informant Symptom Rating (0–3)	Clinician Composite Symptom Rating (0–3)

Notes:

1

FIGURE 78.3   Chehil and Kutcher Clinical Assessment of Adolescent Depression. (The Clinical Assessment of Adolescent Depression is under copyright to Dr. Sonia Chehil and Dr. Stan Kutcher. Use is with written permission only. Individuals wishing to use the CAAD can contact Dr. Chehil at schehil@dal.ca or Dr. Kutcher at skutcher@dal.ca for permission.)

SYMPTOM: Sleep Difficulties—different from usual (over the years before getting sick): trouble falling asleep, lying awake in bed.			
Over the past week I have experienced this: ☐ Hardly ever ☐ Much of the time ☐ Most of the time ☐ All of the time	Patient Symptom Rating (0–3)	Informant Symptom Rating (0–3)	Clinician Composite Symptom Rating (0–3)

Notes:

SYMPTOM: Decreased Interest In: being with friends / best friend / partner / boy or girl friend; going out; school work; work; hobbies; sports; recreation.			
Over the past week I have experienced this: ☐ Hardly ever ☐ Much of the time ☐ Most of the time ☐ All of the time	Patient Symptom Rating (0–3)	Informant Symptom Rating (0–3)	Clinician Composite Symptom Rating (0–3)

Notes:

SYMPTOM: Sense of worthlessness, hopelessness, letting people down, not being a good person.			
Over the past week I have experienced this: ☐ Hardly ever ☐ Much of the time ☐ Most of the time ☐ All of the time	Patient Symptom Rating (0–3)	Informant Symptom Rating (0–3)	Clinician Composite Symptom Rating (0–3)

Notes:

2

FIGURE 78.3 *(Continued)*

SYMPTOM: Tired, fatigued, low in energy, hard to get motivated, have to push to get things done, want to rest or lie down a lot.			
Over the past week I have experienced this: ☐ Hardly ever ☐ Much of the time ☐ Most of the time ☐ All of the time	Patient Symptom Rating (0–3)	Informant Symptom Rating (0–3)	Clinician Composite Symptom Rating (0–3)

Notes:

SYMPTOM: Trouble concentrating, can't keep mind on school/work, daydreaming, hard to focus when reading, getting "bored" with work or school.			
Over the past week I have experienced this: ☐ Hardly ever ☐ Much of the time ☐ Most of the time ☐ All of the time	Patient Symptom Rating (0–3)	Informant Symptom Rating (0–3)	Clinician Composite Symptom Rating (0–3)

Notes:

SYMPTOM: Life is not very much fun, not able to enjoy things once enjoyed, not getting as much pleasure from fun things as before getting sick.			
Over the past week I have experienced this: ☐ Hardly ever ☐ Much of the time ☐ Most of the time ☐ All of the time	Patient Symptom Rating (0–3)	Informant Symptom Rating (0–3)	Clinician Composite Symptom Rating (0–3)

Notes:

3

FIGURE 78.3   *(Continued)*

SYMPTOM: Worried, nervous, panicky, tense, keyed up, anxious.			
Over the past week I have experienced this: ☐ Hardly ever ☐ Much of the time ☐ Most of the time ☐ All of the time	Patient Symptom Rating (0–3)	Informant Symptom Rating (0–3)	Clinician Composite Symptom Rating (0–3)
Notes:			

SYMPTOM: Physical expression of worry: headaches, butterflies, knots in the stomach, nausea, tingling, restlessness, diarrhea, shakiness.			
Over the past week I have experienced this: ☐ Hardly ever ☐ Much of the time ☐ Most of the time ☐ All of the time	Patient Symptom Rating (0–3)	Informant Symptom Rating (0–3)	Clinician Composite Symptom Rating (0–3)
Notes:			

SYMPTOM: Thoughts, plans or actions about suicide or self-harm.

Over the past week I have experienced this:

☐ No thoughts or plans or actions
☐ Occasional thoughts, no plans or actions
☐ Frequent thoughts, no plans or actions
☐ Plans and/or actions that have hurt

Patient Symptom Rating (0–3)

Clinician Composite Symptom Rating (0–3)

☑ RISK FACTOR	YES	NO
☐ Suicidal Ideation		
☐ Suicidal Intent		
☐ Suicidal Plan		
☐ Access to lethal means		
☐ Past Suicide Behavior		
☐ Problems Seem Unsolvable		
☐ Hopelessness/worthlessness		
☐ Anger/impulsivity		

Notes:

4

FIGURE 78.3 *(Continued)*

Substance Use: NO ☐ YES ☐ list: _____

Current Substance Use:	Patient Symptom Rating (0–3)	Informant Symptom Rating (0–3)	Clinician Composite Symptom Rating (0–3)
☐ None in the last 1 month ☐ 1 substance once weekly or less ☐ 1 substance 2–3x /week or 2 substances 1–2x /week ☐ 1 substance 4x / week or 2 substances 2–3 /week or polysubstance use (>3 substances)	☐	☐	☐

Notes:
_____
_____

OVERALL RATING	PATIENT RATING				INFORMANT RATING				CLINICIAN RATING			
SYMPTOMS	0	1	2	3	0	1	2	3	0	1	2	3
SIDE EFFECTS	0	1	2	3	0	1	2	3	0	1	2	3
SCHOOL/WORK FUNCTION	0	1	2	3	0	1	2	3	0	1	2	3
FAMILY FUNCTION	0	1	2	3	0	1	2	3	0	1	2	3
PEER FUNCTION	0	1	2	3	0	1	2	3	0	1	2	3
RECREATION FUNCTION	0	1	2	3	0	1	2	3	0	1	2	3
SAFETY	0	1	2	3	0	1	2	3	0	1	2	3
OVERALL:	0	1	2	3	0	1	2	3	0	1	2	3

NOTES: _____
_____
_____
_____
_____
_____
_____
_____
_____
_____
_____
_____
_____
_____
_____
_____

PLAN: _____
_____
_____
_____
_____

REFERRAL/DISPOSITION: _____

F/U CLINICIAN: _____ DATE/TIME: _____

ASSESSMENT COMPLETED BY: _____ DATE: _____

Signature: _____

© Dr Sonia Chehil & Dr Stan Kutcher

FIGURE 78.3 (*Continued*)

A diagnosis of bipolar disorder is not to be made lightly. Concerns have been raised with recent increases in the use of a variety of thymoleptic medications (e.g., lithium, valproate) and antipsychotics (e.g., olanzapine, risperidone) to treat "bipolar spectrum" disorders in this age-group. Such interventions are not benign and carry risks of significant side effects. The use of these compounds by health care professionals in teens who demonstrate mood lability or persistent behavioral disturbances, but who do not meet rigorous DSM diagnostic criteria for bipolar disorder, is not encouraged. These interventions should be reserved for use in those disorders where these medications have been clearly demonstrated to be effective.

ANXIETY DISORDERS

Anxiety symptoms which are mild, transient, and not associated with significant impairment are common in the adolescent population. However, many young people experience symptoms of anxiety that are severe and significantly affect their ability to function at school, in recreational activities, at home, in their relationships, or with their peers. As with clinical depression, teens who have anxiety disorders must experience certain clearly demarcated symptoms for a specified amount of time, which are associated with impaired function or significant distress. The diagnosis of an anxiety disorder is made using the DSM-IV-TR (American Psychiatric Association, 2000) or the ICD criteria (World Health Organization, 1992). There are a number of different yet related anxiety disorders which commonly occur during the adolescent years. These anxiety disorders include generalized anxiety disorder (GAD), social anxiety disorder (SAD) (also known as *social phobia*), panic disorder (PD), and obsessive compulsive disorder (OCD). Post-traumatic stress disorder (PTSD) may also occur in teenagers given the proper confluence of circumstance and constitution. Coexisting depressive symptoms are common and many teens may fulfill criteria for both depressive as well as anxiety disorders. In terms of the anxiety disorders themselves, these also often co-occur.

Generalized Anxiety Disorder

GAD is characterized by uncontrollable, excessive, and unrelenting worry that is inappropriate and not restricted to particular events or situations but rather involves many "usual" things such as safety of self and others, being on time, school work, performance, or illness. The worrying leads to significant emotional distress and functional impairment. Adolescents with GAD often also experience irritability, difficulty concentrating, and restlessness as well as many physical symptoms of anxiety such as recurrent headaches, stomach upset, muscle tension, fatigue, and sleep disturbance. Teens with GAD may experience social exclusion or bullying.

Panic Disorder

The onset of PD often occurs in mid- to late adolescence and is characterized by recurrent, unexpected, rapid onset, time limited, intense episodes of severe anxiety (panic attacks) occurring in a crescendo–decrescendo pattern usually peaking within 10 minutes and lasting 30 to 45 minutes.

Panic attacks are associated with autonomic hyperarousal, respiratory and cardiac distress, and cognitions of dread and fear. Adolescents with PD also experience anticipatory anxiety (the teen fears having an attack) between panic attacks as well as phobic avoidance (the teen avoids locations in which panic attacks occurred). Severe cases of PD can lead to agoraphobia.

Social Anxiety Disorder

SAD is characterized by excessive fears of social situations (e.g., public speaking, going to a party, standing up in class, changing in the locker room) in which the teen thinks that they are the subject of negative scrutiny by others. They feel embarrassed and anxious and may even experience panic attacks when faced with the dreaded social situation. They avoid or tolerate (with extreme difficulty) the feared situations and as a result experience social, interpersonal, and academic/vocational impairment. SAD in teens may be associated with school refusal or avoidance.

Obsessive Compulsive Disorder

OCD is characterized by the presence of recurrent, intrusive, unwanted thoughts or images that the teen knows are not true (e.g., "my hands are covered with deadly germs") called *obsessions* and/or repetitive physical or mental rituals (e.g., counting, ordering, washing) called *compulsions*. These symptoms create significant emotional distress and lead to functional impairment.

Post-Traumatic Stress Disorder

PTSD may occur in young people who are exposed to severe stressors that violate their personal safety (such as assault or rape) or in those who have witnessed or experienced a horrific event (traffic accident death, murder) or natural disaster (hurricane, earthquake). In addition to functional impairment, PTSD symptoms include reexperiencing the event (e.g., through dreams, flashbacks, vivid memories), persistent avoidance of situations or persons associated with the event, or increased hyperarousal. PTSD must be distinguished from the acute stress reaction which is a normal response to severe stressors and resolves over a period of a few months without clinical intervention.

Epidemiology of Anxiety Disorders

Anxiety disorders are very common in adolescents. At any one time up to one third of youth in the community may suffer from one of the anxiety disorders (Costello et al., 2005). Retrospective reports of adults with anxiety disorders suggest that the onset of anxiety disorders generally begin in childhood or adolescence. The incidence of anxiety disorders is greater in girls than boys, and girls tend to have an earlier age at onset than boys.

Risk Factors for Adolescent Anxiety Disorders

Like DD, anxiety disorders tend to run in families. A family history of parental anxiety or mood disorder has been shown to be a risk factor for an adolescent anxiety disorder. Other risk factors for the development of anxiety disorders include female gender, inhibited or anxious temperament, anxiety sensitivity, increased startle reflex, and increased autonomic reactivity (Merikangas, 2005; Costello et al., 2005).

LABORATORY EVALUATION FOR DEPRESSION AND ANXIETY

There are no diagnostic or laboratory tests that can be used to establish a diagnosis of depression or anxiety. Both depression and anxiety disorders are "clinical diagnosis" requiring the clinician to rely on current and longitudinal symptoms elucidated from the patient and informants where appropriate. All teens suspected of having one of these disorders should have a careful medical history and physical examination to rule out the presence of an underlying or contributing medical disorder. "Screening" tests for medical conditions which may present with depressive or anxiety symptoms such as thyroid stimulating hormone for hypothyroidism or thyroxine for hyperthyroidism are not cost-effective given their low positive predictive value in this population. If there is evidence from the history or physical examination to suggest the presence of a particular medical condition, the appropriate laboratory investigations should be carried out to confirm or reject the diagnostic possibility. Once a diagnosis of a DD or anxiety disorder is confirmed, a pregnancy test in adolescent females may be indicated if medication treatment is being considered.

MANAGEMENT

Baseline Evaluation

Once the diagnosis has been made, a proper baseline evaluation of the depressed or anxious adolescent must be conducted. This includes a measure of symptom severity and a measure of functional impairment. In addition, a baseline evaluation of somatic symptoms and psychoeducation should be conducted.

Symptom Severity
Symptom severity is best measured using an observer rated tool. For the depressed teen, the CAAD (Fig. 78.3) provides a useful clinical tool for measuring the severity of depressed symptoms in a teenager. It can also be repeatedly applied over the course of treatment to measure treatment response. Similar tools for anxiety disorders include the Screen for Child Anxiety Related Emotional Disorders (SCARED) or the Pediatric Anxiety Rating Scale (Birmaher et al., 1999; Research Units on Pediatric Psychopharmacology Study Group, 2002).

Functional Impairment
A simple, clinically meaningful, and easily applied measure of overall functional impairment is a four-point scale to ascertain the composite level of impairment as a summary of difficulties experienced in each of the following domains—family functioning, school functioning, work functioning, peer functioning, and recreational functioning. For

each functional domain the following scoring system is suggested:

- 0: No problems in functioning in any domain.
- 1: Some problems in functioning in one or more domains (such as grades slipping at school, noticeable decrease in usual social activity; more family disagreements; more time spent watching television instead of outdoor activities).
- 2: Significant problems in functioning in one or more domains (such as clear evidence of decreased grades at school; avoidance of social interactions; increased family conflicts; lack of interest in usual recreational activities).
- 3: Significant problems in functioning in one or more domains and at least one domain with severe problems (such as not attending school; refusal to socialize with most friends; anger outbursts at family members; refusal to participate in usual recreational activities).

It is not unusual for adolescents with DDs or anxiety disorders to experience markedly poor functioning in one or two domains and moderately impaired functioning in others. In such situations, the domain(s) with the most impairment should be identified for particular attention.

A clinically useful tool that can be routinely used to measure a depressed or anxious teen's functioning at baseline and during treatment is the Clinical Measurement of Functioning in Adolescent Depression and Anxiety Disorders (Table 78.2).

Evaluation of Somatic Symptom Side Effects
Somatic symptoms should be systematically assessed at baseline and at appropriate intervals during treatment. Such an assessment will provide the clinician and the patient with useful information about which physical complaints are actually treatment emergent side effects and which are more likely to be somatic manifestations of the depressive syndrome or the anxiety disorder.

A simple but clinically useful side-effect tool such as the one found in Table 78.3 can be used at baseline and repeated at each clinic visit. A four-point scoring system as described in the subsequent text can be used to evaluate each somatic complaint:

- 0: Not present
- 1: Present but mild, tolerable, no impairment

TABLE 78.2

Clinical Measurement of Functioning in Adolescent Depression and Anxiety Disorders

Domain of Functioning	Score (0–3)[a]	Comments
Family		
School		
Work		
Peer		
Recreation		
Overall		

[a]See scoring scale in text.

TABLE 78.3

Somatic Side Effects Evaluation Scale

Item	Score (0–3)[a]	Item	Score (0–3)
Dry mouth		Headaches	
Drowsiness		Insomnia	
Loss appetite		Nausea	
Agitation		Tremor	
Anxiety/nervousness		Sweating	
Diarrhea		Sexual problems	

Suicidal ideation_____ Suicidal intent_____ Suicide plans_____

[a]See scoring scale in text.

- 2: Present but moderate, some difficulty tolerating, some impairment may be evident
- 3: Present and severe, difficult to tolerate, impairment evident

Psychoeducation

Educating the teenager and the parents or guardians about the disorder and its treatment is a necessary part of the baseline evaluation. After an informed discussion, the treatment for the depression and the relevant anxiety disorder should be determined by consensus with all interested parties. Ongoing individual and family support will be needed. The adolescent and parents will benefit from practical advice on how to approach common problems. Clinician intervention with the school system is often indicated, especially if grades are a problem or behavioral difficulties have been identified by school officials.

An appropriate period of psychoeducation before starting treatment is time well spent in the care of the depressed or anxious teenager. When properly conducted, it may serve to help establish a positive therapeutic relationship that will underlie whatever interventions are to follow. There is no rush to begin treatment (either medication or psychotherapy), as the only indication for emergency intervention is risk of self-harm or suicide (in which case hospitalization is required). A week to 10 days from time of diagnosis to the initiation of treatment will provide an opportunity for the teen and parents to read about the disorder and its treatments and to raise any issues that may come up. In addition to direct discussions, the clinician should have available scientifically valid literature on the topics and should direct the patient and family to appropriate Web sites for their own research.

Evidence-Based Treatments for Adolescent Depression and Anxiety Disorders

Current scientific evidence supports only a few interventions as having therapeutic efficacy for adolescent depression and anxiety disorders—SSRI medications (particularly fluoxetine and possibly sertraline or citalopram), psychological treatments (cognitive behavioral therapy [CBT], and interpersonal therapy [IPT]) (Harrington et al., 1998; Mufson et al., 2004; Ryan, 2005; AACAP, 2002; Waslick, 2005).

For adolescent depression, the best available scientific evidence favors fluoxetine (March et al., 2004) as the single best intervention and fluoxetine combined with CBT as the best intervention overall (March et al., 2004). Regardless of the intervention chosen, clinicians should be aware that the placebo response rates in the treatment of adolescent depression range from approximately 35% to 50%. The placebo response rate in the treatment of adolescent anxiety disorders appears to be lower than that seen in depression. Recent research suggests that the previous enthusiasm for the effectiveness of specific psychotherapies (CBT and IPT) in adolescent depression may have been overrated (National Institutes of Mental Health Meeting, 2006).

Both SSRIs and CBT have individually been found to be effective strategies in the treatment of a variety of anxiety disorders including GAD, SAD, and OCD. Unfortunately, there are no comparative studies addressing whether CBT or SSRI treatment alone is superior or whether combining the two treatment options has any added benefit for most of the anxiety disorders with the exception of OCD. The evidence for the treatment of OCD has shown that the combination of fluvoxamine with CBT or fluoxetine and CBT is superior to either alone. In general, the benefits of CBT for anxiety disorders are better than those found in the treatment of depression.

For adolescents with mild symptoms of depression and minimal functional impairment, a period of watchful monitoring following psychoeducation may be considered. A similar approach can be used with any of the anxiety disorders. This should include regular telephone contact, frequent face to face visits, and supportive problem-based counseling. Continuous evaluation of suicidality is required. If this does not lead to substantial symptom resolution over a period of 4 to 6 weeks, more intensive medical or psychological intervention is indicated.

For adolescents presenting with moderate to severe depressive symptoms accompanied by functional impairment, the initiation of medication or psychological treatments is indicated. This recommendation is similar for teenagers presenting with anxiety disorders. In some cases, the primary care clinician may not be trained to carry out CBT. If this is the case and referral for this intervention is not timely or possible, the use of cognitive therapy techniques (such as challenging dysfunctional thoughts and "all or none" reasoning) can be applied as part of ongoing support while medications are being prescribed. In all cases, ongoing monitoring of suicidality is required. Both at baseline and throughout treatment, the clinician should also address the issue of drug or alcohol use, abuse or dependence, as both depression and anxiety disorders increase the risk of substance abuse in young people.

If a depressed adolescent presents with psychotic symptoms or the clinician is concerned that there may be a psychotic disorder or bipolar illness underlying the depressive presentation, referral to an appropriate mental health professional for a thorough diagnostic assessment and perhaps hospitalization may be necessary. Suicidal intent or suicidal actions require a hospital admission to maintain safety and to provide immediate stabilization and proper evaluation.

Medication

While the recent controversies about SSRI medications causing suicide have been played out in the popular press, multiple independent investigations of the data by qualified groups and individuals have sufficiently addressed this issue and shown that SSRI use has not been associated with an increased risk of completed suicide. On the contrary, by playing a significant role in the treatment of teen depression, SSRI treatment may be protective and lead to a reduction in teen suicide. Recent prospective data (March et al., 2004) shows that the initiation of treatment with fluoxetine alone significantly decreases suicidality. Further, a health plan record analysis of SSRI use demonstrated a highly significant decrease in suicidality following the initiation of SSRI treatment in adolescents compared with the period before SSRI treatment (Simon et al., 2006). However, compared to placebo, SSRIs are associated with an increase in suicidal ideation and self-harm behaviors (but not completed suicide) (Cheung et al., 2005, 2006). As a result, the U.S. Food and Drug Administration (FDA) has issued a "black box" warning to advise consumers that these medications can cause these behaviors.

This data notwithstanding, prescribing clinicians require a good understanding of the pharmacokinetics and pharmacodynamics of these medications. This includes understanding the various physical and behavioral side effects that can be experienced as a result of the medication treatment. The most concerning of these behavioral side effects is enhanced suicidality (suicidal thinking) and possibly self-harm behaviors which can occur soon after the initiation of antidepressant treatment. Other behavioral adverse effects such as impulsivity, hostility, and restlessness can also be experienced by some patients. It is essential that the clinician inform the patient and family about the possibility of adverse effects, provide appropriate monitoring, and work out a contingency plan with the patient and family should the patient experience these adverse effects (Kutcher et al., 2004).

Individual Medication Categories
Selective Serotonin Reuptake Inhibitors
The SSRI medications, particularly fluoxetine, sertraline, and citalopram, have the best overall evidence supporting their use in the treatment of adolescent depression and anxiety disorders (Cheung et al., 2005; Wagner, 2005; Ryan, 2005). These medications work by blocking the reuptake of serotonin in presynaptic neurons. Doses for older adolescents parallel those of adults, whereas younger adolescents are generally started at lower doses and titrated upward more slowly. The advantages of the SSRIs are as follows:

- Minimal binding to histamine 1 (H_1), so less sedation and weight gain
- Minimal binding to α_1 receptors, so less orthostatic hypotension
- Less binding to muscarinic cholinergic receptors, so less dry mouth, blurred vision, and constipation
- Do not potentiate effects of alcohol or sedative-hypnotic agents
- Once-daily dosing

Overall these medications are well tolerated and safe, with a much lower risk in overdose situations. However, there are also some disadvantages to consider:

- Inhibition of cytochrome P-450 enzyme system, which can lead to possible drug–drug interactions
- Sexual dysfunction including impotency and loss of libido can occur, which can reduce compliance
- Possible gastrointestinal side effects
- Disinhibition

- Induction or exacerbation of suicidality
- Precipitation of a hypomanic-manic episode

Given the available evidence, it is not possible to recommend the use of venlafaxine, nefazodone, monoamine oxidase inhibitors, or any tricyclic antidepressant (TCA) in adolescents. Randomized controlled trials (RCTs) of venlafaxine and TCAs have not shown these compounds to be significantly better than placebo in treating depressed adolescents younger than 18 or 19 years. While there is evidence for efficacy in adults, the number of individuals aged 18 to 25 in these studies is very small and therefore it is difficult to assess efficacy and safety in the young adult population. The FDA data base on child and adolescent pharmacotherapy identified that venlafaxine was the antidepressant most likely to be associated with suicidality in this age-group. The TCAs are known to have more cardiotoxic side effects than the SSRIs. Both these medications lack substantive evidence of efficacy, and the increased risk of use suggests that neither venlafaxine nor a TCA should be used in this population. Similarly, no RCT evidence for the efficacy, safety, and tolerability of Monoamine-oxidase inhibitor (MAOIs) exists in the teen population. The expected risk-benefit ratio of these compounds does not support their use in adolescent depression. Finally, nefazodone has not been demonstrated to be more effective than placebo treatment in this age-group. Bupropion may be considered as a second-line medication as there is theoretical rationale and some clinical evidence that this medication may be useful in teenagers with MDD who have comorbid attention-deficit hyperactivity disorder (ADHD).

Bupropion (Wellbutrin)
Mechanism of action: Bupropion is a dopamine reuptake inhibitor with some norepinephrine reuptake inhibition as well. It has stimulant–like properties, is well tolerated and may be particularly beneficial for patients with depression and significant psychomotor retardation. Bupropion is available in both regular-release as well as sustained release formulations. Only the sustained release formulation should be used for young people.

Advantages

- Minimal affinity for H_1, α_1, and muscarinic receptors
- Low risk in overdose situations
- Does not potentiate effects of alcohol or sedative-hypnotic agents
- No significant cytochrome P-450 drug–drug interactions
- Least likely to cause sexual dysfunction

Disadvantages of regular release bupropion

- Short half-life requires multiple dosing
- Higher risk of seizures with doses >450 mg
- Can have dose-dependent increase in blood pressure

Benzodiazepines
Although not well studied, clinical experience and some open label studies suggest that low doses of the benzodiazepine clonazepam (0.25–1 mg b.i.d.) may be of value in some of the anxiety disorders (such as PD). Some adolescents may experience a paradoxical response to a benzodiazepine characterized by agitation, insomnia, and disinhibition. If a benzodiazepine is to be used in teens, the clinician must look out for the occurrence of this paradoxical response and must inform the patient and caregivers that this might occur. Rapid onset, short-acting benzodiazepines should be avoided. Long-term use of benzodiazepines is

TABLE 78.4

Examples of Selective Serotonin Reuptake Inhibitor Dosing in Adolescent Depression and Anxiety Disorders

Medication	Generic Name	Starting Dose	Increments (mg)	Effective Dose (mg)	Maximum Dose (mg)
Fluoxetine	Prozac	5–10 mg q.d./o.d.	10–20	20	60
Citalopram	Celexa	10 mg q.d./o.d.	10	20	60

generally not recommended and rapid discontinuation should be avoided whenever possible.

Antipsychotic Medications and Mood Stabilizers
Antipsychotic medications or mood stabilizers should not be used as first-line treatments for either depression or anxiety disorders. They may have some utility in highly specific and limited circumstances, for example, with psychotic depression or for treatment-resistant OCD where they can be used to augment antidepressants. Such augmentation strategies should be preceded by appropriate subspecialist consultation.

Prescribing Advice

Comfort with prescribing and monitoring antidepressant medications stem from knowledge and familiarity. An effective strategy to use in clinical practice is to choose a couple of antidepressant medications with demonstrated safety and efficacy in teens and use these compounds preferentially (Ambrosini et al., 1995). In this way, the clinician will become familiar with the range of effects that these compounds exhibit at different doses and in different individuals. Continued use of a small number of different medications will enable the clinician to build up an expertise with these medicines over time. Furthermore, given the available evidence pertaining to treatment effects of the SSRI compounds, the knowledge of two of these medications will be sufficient. On the basis of available literature, in order of preference, fluoxetine, citalopram, and sertraline would be reasonable SSRIs to choose. Table 78.4 provides a dosing guide using two of these SSRIs as an example for clinicians. Table 78.5 lists common SSRI medications and other antidepressant medications, including doses and side effects. Teens with anxiety disorders may be sensitive to the side effects of the SSRIs, particularly the activation side effects which generally occur early on in treatment.

Initiation
1. Lower initiation dose: Some clinicians choose to use lower initiation doses for teens with anxiety disorders. In addition, some clinicians may add a low dose of clonazepam (0.25 mg b.i.d.) for a week or two when beginning SSRI treatment to cover anxiety symptoms until the SSRIs are titrated to a therapeutic dose and their antianxiety properties begin to take effect. When initiating treatment with an SSRI in an adolescent, always start at a low dose (ideally at half the manufacturer's recommended initiation or lower) and increase gradually over a 1- to 2-week period to the initial target dose (see fluoxetine initiation and titration example in Table 78.6). It is a good idea to call the pharmacy used by the patient, to find out what the lowest available dose of the medication is. Sometimes starting with a liquid formulation may be reasonable if the dose available in tablets or capsules is higher than needed.

2. Expected time to improvement: In adolescent depression, significant symptom improvement may require 6 to 8 weeks following achievement of the initial target dose (e.g., 20 mg of fluoxetine daily) while remission may not be evidenced for 8 to 12 weeks. Similar time courses can be expected in the anxiety disorders apart from OCD in which significant symptom improvement may not become evident for 10 to 12 weeks (see Table 78.6 for fluoxetine initiation and dose titration). Care must be taken to ensure that the proper dose of medication is maintained for an appropriate length of time. Rapid dose increases are not likely to lead to faster or better improvement. This may in fact lead to more side effects. Ongoing psychoeducation, psychotherapy, or face to face counseling as described earlier is an important component of medication treatment.

3. Stopping treatment: With the exception of fluoxetine, which has a very long half-life, antidepressant medications should not be stopped abruptly. Sudden discontinuation may lead to a withdrawal syndrome. Symptoms of antidepressant withdrawal are outlined in Table 78.7. Given the demonstrated therapeutic benefits of these medications and the importance of monitoring for adverse effects the treatment and monitoring model discussed in the following text is suggested (Kutcher et al., 2004).

Patient Treatment and Monitoring Model

The model described in the subsequent text identifies the primary care practitioner as providing most of the care with ongoing consultation from the psychiatric specialist.

Patient Evaluation

1. Ensure that the adolescent has a DD or one of the anxiety disorders using DSM-IV criteria. Remember that DDs and anxiety disorders may be comorbid with each other. Clinicians should always assess substance (including alcohol) use, abuse, and dependence. The 11-item KADS in conjunction with the CAAD can provide a useful guide to the clinical assessment of adolescent depression.

2. Conduct a thorough psychiatric assessment addressing carefully other disorders which may present with depressive symptoms (such as a schizophrenia prodrome). Remember that the presence of depressive symptoms does not equal a clinical depression. Similarly, anxiety symptoms in the absence of an anxiety disorder should not lead to medical treatment.

3. Take a careful family history focusing on mood disorders and bipolar disorder. When obtaining the patient's present and past psychiatric history, complete a careful search for bipolar symptoms and substance abuse. Always inquire about a family history of anxiety disorders. Many of these anxiety disorders (in particular, PD) have strong genetic components.

TABLE 78.5

Common Selective Serotonin Reuptake Inhibitor Medications and Other Antidepressants Medications Doses and Side Effects[a]

Medication	Dose Range	Usual Dose	Typical Dosing	Half-life (hr)	Anticho-linergic (%)	Sedation (%)	Insomnia (%)	Weight Gain	Dizziness (%)	Adverse Effects
SSRIs										
Tier one: SSRIs with evidence-based use in adolescents										
Fluoxetine (Prozac)	20–80 mg/d	20 mg/d	Once a day	48–216	10	12	17	±	6	Nausea, anxiety, insomnia, diarrhea, anorexia, dry mouth
Sertraline (Zoloft)	50–200 mg/d	50–100 mg/d	Once a day	26–104	16	13	16	±	12	Nausea, headache, diarrhea, sexual dysfunction (most common of all SSRIs), insomnia, dry mouth
Citalopram (Celexa)	20–60 mg/d	20–40 mg/d	Once a day	35	—	—	—	—	—	Nausea, dry mouth, somnolence, insomnia, sweating, tremor, diarrhea, sexual dysfunction, dyspepsia, asthenia, anxiety, anorexia
SSRIs not recommended for use in adolescents (without evidence-based use in adolescents)										
Paroxetine (Paxil)	10–50 mg/d	20 mg/d	Once a day	10–24	18	23	13	±	13	Nausea, sedation, headache, dry mouth, fatigue, insomnia
Fluvoxamine (Luvox)	50–300 mg/d	100 mg/d	1–2 times/d	13.6–15.6	14	22	21	1%	11	Nausea, sedation, fatigue, headache, dry mouth, insomnia

(continued)

TABLE 78.5

(Continued)

Medication	Dose Range	Usual Dose	Typical Dosing	Half-life (hr)	Anticho-linergic (%)	Sedation (%)	Insomnia (%)	Weight Gain	Dizziness (%)	Adverse Effects
Other common antidepressant medications										
Tier two: Use in adolescents										
Bupropion (Wellbutrin)	200–450 mg/d	300 mg/d	t.i.d.	8–24	27	20	19	±	22	Agitation, dry mouth, constipation, headache, Nausea, insomnia, dizziness
Bupropion sustained release	200–450 mg/d	300 mg/d	b.i.d.	—	—	—	—	—	—	—
Other common antidepressants not recommended for use in adolescents (without evidence-based use in adolescents)										
Nefazodone (Serzone)	200–600 mg/d	300–400 mg/d	1–2 times/d	2–4	25	25	11	±	17	Nausea, somnolence, dry mouth, dizziness, constipation, asthenia, blurred vision
Trazodone (Desyrel)	150–600 mg/d	100–300 mg/d	b.i.d.–t.i.d.	4–9	18	29	5	±	22	Drowsiness, dizziness, nervousness, dry mouth, Fatigue, nausea, headache, insomnia
Venlafaxine (Effexor)	75–375 mg/d	75–150 mg/d	b.i.d.–t.i.d.	5–11	22	23	18	±	21	Nausea, headache, somnolence, insomnia, dizziness, dry mouth, Nervousness, constipation
Venlafaxine extended release	75–225 mg/d	75–150 mg/d	Once a day							

SSRIs, selective serotonin reuptake inhibitors.

[a] In the author's opinion, the risk : benefit ratio based on the currently available evidence does not support the use of tricyclics, MAOI's or venlafaxine in the treatment of adolescent depression.

TABLE 78.6

Fluoxetine (Prozac) Initiation and Dose Titration in Adolescent Depression and Anxiety Disorders

Day	Dose (mg)	Monitoring of Response
0	0	Patient assessment and baseline measurement of symptoms, function, and side effects
1	5	Check for side effects (by phone if not possible in person)
3	10	Check for side effects (by phone if not possible in person)
7	20	Check for side effects: If 10 mg is well tolerated increase dose to 20 mg
14–54	20	Check for side effects and monitor symptoms and function
54–75[a]	20	Check for side effects and monitor symptoms and function
		Decide on next steps regarding treatment depending on outcome

[a]In adolescent obsessive compulsive disorder (OCD) this period should be lengthened for 14–21 more days because a longer period of time is needed to determine therapeutic response at a fixed dose in this disorder.

4. Determine the presence or absence of symptoms and the degree of functional impairment that the symptoms are causing. Measure the symptoms and the concurrent functional impairment appropriately. The CAAD can be used at baseline and for appropriate monitoring periods for depression. The SCARED (see preceding text) may be used for anxiety disorders.

5. Provide the patient and parent(s)/guardian(s) comprehensive information about the disorder and the various treatment options. Selected literature should be available in your office to share with the patient and parent(s)/guardian(s). Information sheets that provide appropriate Web sites can be given to the patient(s) for review. This type of information can be helpful to the patient and parents in their decision about medication. Refer patient and parent(s) to the Web sites identified at the end of the chapter.

6. Provide the patient and parent(s)/guardian(s) with all the information about somatic and behavioral side effects of the medication and the expected length of time to symptomatic improvement. Remember that in adolescent depression the time to improve might be longer than that of adults. Six to 8 weeks of medication treatment at an appropriate dose accompanied by supportive or cognitive based counseling is necessary for depression and most of the anxiety disorders. A longer period is needed for OCD. Providing this information in written form may be helpful.

7. Treat judiciously following a proper risk-benefit evaluation. A period of active monitoring in mild to moderately depressed or anxious adolescents is reasonable. This will allow the patient and parent(s)/guardian(s) time to digest the information provided and to weigh the pros and cons of different treatment options.

8. Provide opportunity for open dialogue and discussion regarding treatment options with the adolescent and family or other caregivers. Come to a joint decision about the most appropriate treatment.

If Medication Treatment is to be Initiated

1. Appropriately measure all somatic and behavioral "side effects" before initiating the intervention. Use a clinically useful scale (Table 78.3) at baseline. If the patient has a history of self-harm behaviors and exhibits significant restlessness and agitation, closer monitoring when starting an SSRI medication is indicated.

2. Check for symptoms of panic and impulsivity. The presence of these may suggest an enhanced sensitivity to the adverse behavioral effects of SSRIs. In cases of severe anxiety, short-term treatment with a benzodiazepine such as clonazepam may be indicated.

3. Begin treatment with a small test dose (ideally at half the dose recommended by the manufacturer for initiation) and increase gradually over a 1- to 2-week period to the initial target dose.

4. Carefully monitor for behavioral and somatic adverse affects during this initiation phase. Provide telephone contact opportunities. Address treatment emergent side effects as they arise. Use the telephone for patient contact between scheduled office visits.

5. Once initial therapeutic dose is reached, wait 6 to 8 weeks before increasing the dose further (10–12 weeks for OCD). During this time, provide appropriate psychotherapeutic interventions or ongoing counseling using face to face sessions weekly and establish telephone contact as necessary.

6. Conduct the appropriate laboratory investigations, not as a shotgun screening but when concerned about ongoing medical conditions. All female patients should have a pregnancy test.

7. If significant improvement is not obtained after 6 to 8 weeks of appropriate intervention (10–12 weeks for OCD) consultation with a psychiatric specialist is indicated.

8. If the intervention demonstrates only partial improvement, the treatment plan should be carefully reviewed, the diagnosis reconsidered, and treatment adherence addressed. If adverse effects are not significant, an increase in dose could be implemented at this time. If this strategy is not successful, switching to another antidepressant from the same class can be considered. In addition, a psychiatric consultation should be sought.

TABLE 78.7

Symptoms of Antidepressant Withdrawal Syndrome

Dizziness	Headaches
Weakness	Anxiety/nervousness
Nausea	Difficulty sleeping
Tremor	"Electricity sensations"

9. The role of the primary care clinician, even if the patient has been referred to a specialist, should be continued throughout. Communication between clinicians is important and shared management of the depressed adolescent may be the most appropriate method of providing care.

Monitoring Throughout the Course of Treatment
1. Monitor for suicide risk.
2. Focus on enhancing the developments of a trusting and supportive relationship with the patient and family.
3. Measure objectively and subjectively the course of symptoms, side effects, and functioning.

Other Interventions

Anecdotal evidence and some limited research suggest that light therapy may be a potentially useful adjunct to other interventions for adolescent depression occurring in the winter months. Electroconvulsive therapy (ECT) may be indicated in very specific circumstances (psychotic depression) and should be provided by experts only under highly controlled conditions. There is no rationale for using ECT in the treatment of anxiety disorders. Transcranial magnetic stimulation and other biological treatments have not been well studied in this population.

CONCLUSIONS

Adolescent depression and anxiety disorders are significant public health problems. Adolescent depression can cause a high degree of morbidity and significant mortality usually due to suicide. Adolescent anxiety disorders can be significantly disabling and may be associated with substance abuse and other chronic life difficulties. Effective treatments are available and when properly administered can be helpful in the primary care setting. Evidence-based interventions should be used to guide treatment. Ongoing careful monitoring of therapeutic effectiveness and the presence of adverse events within the context of a supportive and trusting relationship is the cornerstone of effective treatment.

Primary care clinicians are in a unique position to develop and implement a treatment plan for the depressed teenager. Clinicians treating depressed adolescents will need to be well versed in the effective medication options available. To date, the SSRIs (specifically fluoxetine, citalopram, and sertraline) are the only class of antidepressant medications that have been shown to be safe and effective in treating depression in adolescents. In addition, fluvoxamine has proven effect in OCD. Careful monitoring of medication treatment and the judicious application of psychotherapeutic strategies is necessary.

WEB SITES

For Teenagers and Parents

http://www.aacap.org/about/glossary/depress.htm. American Academy of Child and Adolescent Psychiatry.
http://www.nmha.org/infotr/factsheets/24.cfm. National Mental Health Association fact sheet and other information on adolescent depression.

http://www.nlm.nih.gov/medlineplus/depression.html. National Library of Medicine information regarding adolescent depression.
http://www.nimh.nih.gov/HealthInformation/anxietymenu .cfm. National Institutes of Mental Health information on anxiety disorders.
http://www.samhsa.gov/. US Department of Health and Human Services, Substance Abuse and Mental Health Services Administration information on adolescent anxiety disorders.
http://www.dbsalliance.org/. US Department of Veterans Affairs, National Center for PTSD information on PTSD in children and adolescents.

REFERENCES AND SUGGESTED READINGS

AACAP. Practice parameters for the assessment and treatment of children and adolescents with depressive disorders. *J Am Acad Child Adolesc Psychiatry* 2002;37(10 Suppl):63S.

Ambrosini PJ, Emslie GJ, Greenhill LL, et al. Controversies and opinions: selecting a sequence of antidepressants for treatment depression in youth. *J Child Adolesc Psychopharmacol* 1995;5(4):233.

American Academy of Pediatrics, Committee on Adolescence. Suicide and suicide attempts in adolescents. *Pediatrics* 2000; 105:871.

American Psychiatric Association. *Diagnostic and statistical manual of mental disorders*, 4th ed (Text Revision) DSM-IV-TR. Washington, DC: American Psychiatry Association; 2000.

Asarnow JR, Jaycox LH, Anderson M. Depression among youth in primary care models for delivering mental health services. *Child Adolesc Psychiatr Clin N Am* 2002;11:477.

Beck AT, Steer RA. *Manual for the beck depression inventory*. San Antonio, TX: The Psychological Corporation; 1987.

Birmaher B, Brent D, Chiapetta L, et al. Psychometric properties of the Screen for Child Anxiety Related Emotional Disorders (SCARED): A replication study. *J Am Acad Child Adolesc Psychiatry* 1999;38:1230.

Birmaher B, Ryan ND, Williamson DE, et al. Childhood and adolescent depression: a review of the past 10 years. Part I. *J Am Acad Child Adolesc Psychiatry* 1996a;35:1427.

Birmaher B, Ryan ND, Williamson DE, et al. Childhood and adolescent depression: a review of the past 10 years. Part II. *J Am Acad Child Adolesc Psychiatry* 1996b;35:1575.

Brooks S. The Kutcher Adolescent Depression Scale (KADS). *Child Adolesc Psychopharmacol News* 2004;9(5).

Brooks S, Krulewicz S, Kutcher S. The kutcher adolescent depression scale: assessment of its evaluative properties over the course of an 8-week pediatric pharmacotherapy trial. *J Child Adolesc Psychopharmacol* 2003;23:239.

Centers for Disease Control and Prevention. Youth risk behavior surveillance—United States, 2005. *Morb Mortal Wkly Rep CDC Surveill Summ* 2006;55(SS05):1.

Cheung Am, Emslie G, Mayes T. Review and safety and efficacy of antidepressants in youth with depression. *J Child Psychol Psychiatry* 2005;46(7):735.

Cheung A, Emslie G, Mayes T. The use of antidepressants to treat depression in children and adolescents. *Can Med Assoc J* 2006;174:193.

Costello EJ, Egger HL, Angold A. The developmental epidemiology of anxiety disorders: phenomenology, prevalence, and comorbidity. *Child Adolesc Psychiatr Clin N Am* 2005;14:631.

Hammad TA. *Results of the analysis of suicidality in pediatric trials of newer antidepressants.* Presentation at the Food and Drug Administration, Psychopharmacologic Drugs Advisory Committee and the Pediatric Advisory Committee. 13 September, 2004.

Harrington R, Whittaker J, Shoebridge P, et al. Systematic review of efficacy of cognitive behaviour therapies in childhood and adolescent depressive disorder. *BMJ* 1998;316 (7144):1559.

Hazell P, O'Connell D, Healthcote D, et al. Tricyclic drugs for depression in children and adolescents. *Cochrane Database Syst Rev* 2002;2:CD002317.

Johnston JG, Harris ES, Spitzer Rl, et al. The patient health questionnaire for adolescents: validation of an instrument for the assessment of mental disorders among adolescent primary care patients. *J Adolesc Health* 2002;30: 196.

Kessler RC, Avenevoli S, Ries Merikangas K, et al. Mood disorders in children and adolescents: an epidemiologic perspective. *Biol Psychiatry* 2001;15:1002.

Kutcher S, Gardiner D, Virani A. A clinical Approach to Treating Major Depressive Disorder with SSRIs in Adolescents: 12 Steps to Careful Monitoring. *Child and Adolescent Psychopharmacology News.* 2004;9(5):1.

LeBlanc JC, Almudevar A, Brooks S, et al. Screening for adolescent depression: comparison of the kutcher adolescent depression scale with the beck depression inventory. *J Child Adolesc Psychopharmacol* 2002;12:113.

March JU, Silva S, Petrycki S, et al. Treatment for Adolescents with Depression Study (TADS) Team. Fluoxetine, cognitive-behavioural therapy, and their combination for adolescents with depression: Treatment for Adolescents with Depression Study (TADS) randomized controlled trial. *JAMA* 2004;292(7):807.

Merikangas KR. Vulnerability factors for anxiety disorders in children and adolescents. *Child Adolesc Psychiatr Clin N Am* 2005;14:649.

Mufson L, Dorta KP, Wickramaratne P, et al. A randomized effectiveness trial of interpersonal psychotherapy for depressed adolescents. *Arch Gen Psychiatry* 2004;61(6):577.

Myers K, Winters N C. Ten-year review of rating scales, VII: scales assessing functional impairment. *Journal Of The American Academy Of Child Adolescent Psychiatry.* 2002;41(6):634.

National Institutes of Mental Health Meeting. *Treating children and adolescents with depression: what we know and what else we need to know through research.* Washington, February 6 and 7, 2006.

Olfson M, Shaffer D, Marcus S. Relationship between antidepressant medication treatment and suicide in adolescents. *Arch Gen Psychiatry* 2003;609:978.

Research Units on Pediatric Psychopharmacology Study Group. The pediatric anxiety rating scale (PARS): development and psychometric properties. *J Am Acad Child Adolesc Psychiatry* 2002;41:1061.

Reynolds WM. *Reynolds adolescent depression scale.* Odessa, FL: Psychol Assess Resour; 1987.

Rushton J, Bruckman D, Kelleher K. Primary care referral of children with psychosocial problems. *Arch Pediatr Adolesc Med* 2002;156:592.

Ryan ND. Treatment of depression in children and adolescents. *Lancet* 2005;366:933.

Schubiner H, Tzelpis A, Podany E. The clinical utility of the Safe Times Questionnaire. *J Adolesc Health.* 1994 Jul;15(5):374–82.

Schubiner H, Tzelpis A, Podany E. The clinical utility of the safe times questionnaire. *J Adolesc Health Care* 1994;15:374.

Shaffer D, Craft L. Methods of adolescent suicide prevention. *J Clin Psychiatry* 1999;60(2 Suppl):70.

Simon GE, Savarino J, Operskalski B, et al. Suicide risk during antidepressant treatment. *Am J Psychiatry* 2006;163:41.

Thapar A, McGuffin P. Validity of the shortened mood and feelings questionnaire in a community sample of children and adolescents: a preliminary research note. *Psychiatry Res* 1998;81:259.

US Food and Drug Administration. Antidepressant use in children, adolescents and adults. http://www.fda.gov/cder.drug .antidepressants/default.htm. Accessed Nov. 25, 2005.

Vitiello B, Calderoni D, Mazzone L. Pharmacologic treatment of children and adolescents with major depressive disorder. In Vitiello B, Masi G, Maarazziti D. *Handbook of child and adolescent psychopharmacology.* Abingdon, UK: Informa Healthcare; 2006:53.

Wagner KD. Pharmacotherapy for major depression in children and adolescents. *Prog Neuropsychopharmacol Biol Psychiatry* 2005;29:819.

Waslick B. Psychopharmacology interventions for pediatric anxiety disorders: a research update. *Child Adolesc Psychiatr Clin N Am* 2005;15:51.

Weber S. Factor structure of the Reynolds Adolescent Depression Scale in a sample of a school-based adolescents. *J Nurs. Meas.* 2000 Summer;8(1):23–40.

Whittington C, Kendall T, Fongay P. Selective serotonin reuptake inhibitors in childhood depression: systematic review of published versus unpublished data. *Lancet* 2004;363:1341.

World Health Organisation, *International statistical classification and related health problems: ICD-10.* Geneva, 1992–1994.

World Health Organization. *Caring for children and adolescents with mental disorders: Setting WHO Directions.* Geneva: WHO; 2003.

Zuckerbrot RA, Jensen PS. Improving recognition of adolescent depression in primary care. *Arch Pediatr Adolesc Med* 2006; 160:694.

CHAPTER 79

Suicide

Sara Sherer

Suicide in adolescents is especially tragic because of the many years of life lost. Adolescent suicide is often precipitated by a stressor that once relieved, greatly reduces the suicidal tendency. Despite the fact that suicide is rare before puberty, it is a significant contributor to adolescent mortality worldwide. More teenagers and young adults die of suicide than from cancer, heart disease, acquired immunodeficiency syndrome, birth defects, stroke, pneumonia and influenza, and chronic lung disease combined. Suicide is the third leading cause of death in adolescence after unintentional injuries and homicide.

Adolescent suicide rates have varied dramatically over the last 50 years. From 1950 to 1990, the suicide rate for adolescents 15- to 24-years-old increased threefold. This increase has been attributed to greater access to firearms and an increase in substance use and abuse. Since 1990, adolescent suicide rates have decreased. A substantial national campaign to reduce the availability of firearms has contributed to a significant reduction in suicide by firearm. In addition, the increase use of antidepressant medications (selective serotonin reuptake inhibitors) is also thought to contribute to the decrease in teen suicide rates.

Although accurate data on attempted suicides are not available, researchers estimate that there are a minimum of 8 to 25 attempted suicides to one completed suicide. Six times as many male youth die by suicide, but girls attempt suicide more often. Tracking youth at high risk for suicide is a complex task. The Center for Disease Control and Prevention (CDC) has collected data on nonlethal suicide behaviors since the early 1990 using the Youth Risk Behavior Surveillance (YRBS). Recent YRBS data does not show a parallel decline in suicide attempts to the decline observed for completed suicides. However, the 2005 YRBS data does show a significant linear decline since 1991 in those high schools students seriously considering suicide in the last 12 months and also those teens who had made a suicide plan in the last 12 months. More studies are necessary to fully understand the relationship between nonlethal suicide behaviors and death by suicide.

Suicidal behaviors may be conceptualized as the adolescent's ultimate, yet inadequate coping behavior. For the adolescent, a suicide attempt may represent an attempt to escape pain or to obtain relief. For the family, suicide imposes grief at the loss, rage at the act of suicide, and guilt for having failed to prevent an untimely death. For the health care professional, a suicide attempt presents a crisis that he or she may feel totally inadequate to handle if lacking prior training.

This chapter discusses adolescent suicide and suicide attempts, including epidemiology, risk profile, etiology, warning signs, evaluation, and treatment.

EPIDEMIOLOGY

1. Suicide rates: Efforts to estimate attempted and completed suicides are confounded by the fact that many suicide attempts are recorded as accidents. In 2003, 11.9% of all deaths in the 15- to 24-year-old age-group were attributed to suicide (CDC, http://www.cdc.gov/ncipc/wisqars/). The CDC reported 4,316 suicides among 15- to 24-year-olds in the United States in 2004. Thirty-seven percent were 15- to 19-year-old adolescents and 63% were 20- to 24-year-old young adults. In that same year, 283 adolescents 10- to 14-years-old died by suicide. Suicide was also the third leading cause of death for adolescents 10- to 14-years-old (after unintentional injuries and malignant neoplasias).

   Since 1950, suicide rates have increased 3 to 4 times for 15- to 24-year-old males. The suicide rate has also increased by approximately 10% for females in the same age-group. Since 1990, suicide rates declined by 28% in 15- to 19-year-old group (from 11.4 to 8.2 per 100,000) and by 17% in 20- to 24-year-olds (from 15.1 to 12.47 per 100,000). However, suicide rates are still higher than what they were in the 1950s.
   a. Suicide rates for adolescent males in the United States are shown in Table 79.1.
   b. Suicide rates for adolescent females in the United States are shown in Table 79.2.
   c. Trends in suicide rates from 1950 to 2004 in the 15 to 24 years age-group are shown in Figure 79.1.
2. Suicide attempts: Table 79.3 and 79.4 review the results of the 2005 YRBS. The YRBS showed that it is not uncommon for adolescents to consider suicide. It reported that 28.5% of students felt so sad or hopeless almost every day for >2 consecutive weeks that they stopped doing their usual activities. Female and Hispanic teens were more likely to feel sad or hopeless. Overall, 16.9% of students had seriously considered attempting suicide during the 12 months before the

TABLE 79.1

Adolescent Male Suicide Rates in the United States

Year	Suicide Rate in 15- to 19-Year-Olds (per 100,000)	Suicide Rate in 20- to 24-Year-Olds (per 100,000)
1950	3.5	9.3
1960	5.6	11.5
1970	8.8	19.3
1980	13.8	26.8
1990	18.1	25.7
2000	13.0	21.4
2001	12.9	20.5
2002	12.2	20.8
2003	11.62	20.25
2004	12.65	20.85

From US Department of Health and Human Services. Center for Disease Control and Prevention. National Center for Health Statistics. Health, United States, 2004 With Chartbook on trends in Health of Americans. Hyattsville, Maryland: 2004 and National Center for Injury Prevention and control: at http://www.cdc .gov/nchs/data/hus/hus04.pdf.

TABLE 79.2

Adolescent Female Suicide Rates in the United States

Year	Suicide Rate in 15- to 19-Year-Olds (per 100,000)	Suicide Rate in 20- to 24-Year-Olds (per 100,000)
1950	1.8	3.3
1960	1.6	2.9
1970	2.9	5.7
1980	3.0	5.5
1990	3.7	4.1
2000	2.7	3.2
2001	2.7	3.1
2002	2.4	3.5
2003	2.66	3.39
2004	3.52	3.59

From US Department of Health and Human Services. Center for Disease Control and Prevention. National Center for Health Statistics. Health, United States, 2004 With Chartbook on trends in Health of Americans. Hyattsville, Maryland: 2004 and National Center for Injury Prevention and control: at http://www.cdc .gov/nchs/data/hus/hus04.pdf.

survey, 13% had a specific suicide plan, and 8.4% had attempted suicide during the preceding 12 months. Youth not attending high school are at higher risk for suicide than those attending school and as such the YRBS probably underestimated the prevalence of nonlethal suicidal behaviors because it is a survey of high school students. Chapter 84 reviews suicide rates in college students.

3. Ratios of suicide attempts to completed suicide range from 8:1 to 200:1 depending on the study. In 2004 there were 4,316 suicides, approximating anywhere from 32,000 to 800,000 suicide attempts per year. Preventing and accurately assessing for suicide attempts is essential because about one third of all adolescent suicides are committed by youth who were previously known to attempt suicide.

4. Gender: Males outnumber females (6:1) in completed suicides, whereas females outnumber males (4:1) with respect to suicidal ideation and attempts. The gender difference in the rate of completed suicides is attributed to the suicide method. Males tend to use firearms, a method that is more fatal and prevents high rates of rescue. Females most often ingest poisons, which in the United States results in better rescue opportunities. In 2003, among all age-groups nationwide, white males accounted for 72.5% of all suicides and both white males and females accounted for >90% of all suicides.

5. Race: As in previous years, the 2004 suicide rate among Native American male adolescents (30.90 per 100,000) was significantly higher than the overall suicide rate and the rates reported for non-Hispanic white males (18.95 per 100,000), African-American males (12.2 per 100,000), and Latino males (13.45 per 100,000). From 1980 to the early 1990s, suicidal behaviors among all adolescents increased. However, rates for African-American adolescents increased at a higher rate, having more than doubled during that time and therefore dramatically shrinking the gap between the races. Since the early 1990s, adolescent suicide rates have been falling, but the suicide rate

for African-American youth between 10 and 19 years of age fell by only 26.5%, demonstrating a higher vulnerability in this group. Hispanic adolescents report more suicide attempts than any other ethnic group. In the 2005 YRBS, 11.3% of the Latino high school students reported a suicide attempt compared to 7.6% African-American and 7.3% white students. Latino females were 2.5 times more likely to report a suicide attempt than Latino males.

6. Age: Suicide is uncommon in adolescents younger than 14 years. There is a dramatic rise in the rates of suicide thereafter. The largest increase in suicide rates since 1970 has been in 15- to 19-year-old males.

7. Psychiatric comorbidity: Rich et al. (1986) summarized their study results by concluding that "psychiatric illness is a necessary (but insufficient) condition for suicide." A review of the literature indicates that a history of a suicide attempt and a history or diagnosis of a mental or addictive disorder is associated with 90% of suicides. The most common psychiatric illnesses are mood disorders, alcohol and substance use disorders, conduct disorders, and anxiety disorders. Sixty percent of youth who complete suicide suffered from depression. Suffering from a depressive disorder and the expression of hopelessness is also associated with suicidal ideation and attempts. Other factors contributing to suicide attempts include impulsive, aggressive, and antisocial behaviors.

8. Method used for completed suicides
   a. Firearms and explosives: Firearms are the most common method used in adolescent suicide. This is the case for both males and females. The use of firearms is more common in male suicides. However, firearm suicides have increased significantly in female adolescents. In 2004, firearms accounted for 49% of adolescent suicides. The CDC attributes almost all of the increase in the suicide rates since the 1980s to firearm-related suicides.

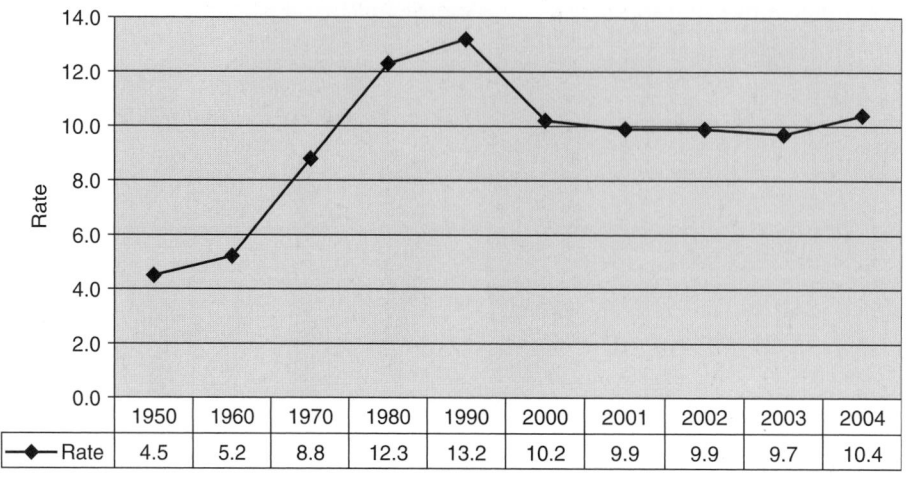

FIGURE 79.1   Suicide rates for adolescents 15 to 24 years of age, 1950 to 2004. (Adapted from U.S. Department of Health and Human Services.Center for Disease Control and Prevention. National Center for Health Statistics. *Health, United States, 2006 with chartbook on trends in health of Americans.* Hyattsville: 2006.)

b. Suffocation: Among adolescents 10 to 14 years old, suffocation (especially hanging) has replaced firearms as the most common method used in suicides. In 2004, suffocation accounted for 35% of suicides in 15- to 24-years-olds.

c. Poisoning: In 2004, poison was used in 8.4% of adolescent suicides.

d. Other: A small percentage of suicides are accomplished through gas poisoning, cutting and piercing with a sharp instrument, or jumping from high places.

9. Marital status: In the general population, suicide rates are lower for married individuals. In contrast, married adolescents between 15 and 19 years of age have a 1.5 to 1.7 times higher suicide rate compared to unmarried individuals.

10. Season: Suicide rates increase in the spring and fall.

11. Geography: Suicide rates are highest in the western United States and Alaska and lowest in the southern, north-central, northwestern, and midwestern states. The lowest rates for both African-American and

TABLE 79.3

Behaviors Related to Attempted Suicide Among High School Students During 12 Months Preceding Survey, 2005

Category	Seriously Considered Attempting Suicide (%)	Made a Suicide Plan (%)	Attempted Suicide (%)	Suicide Attempt Required Medical Attention (%)
Sex				
Female	21.8	16.2	10.85	2.9
Male	12.0	9.9	6.0	1.8
Grade				
9	17.9	13.9	10.4	3.0
10	17.3	14.1	9.1	2.3
11	16.8	12.9	7.8	2.2
12	14.8	10.5	5.4	1.6
Race or ethnicity				
White	16.9	12.5	7.3	2.1
African-American	12.2	9.6	7.6	2.0
Hispanic	17.9	14.5	11.3	3.2
Total	16.9	13.0	8.4	2.3

From Centers for Disease Control and Prevention. Youth risk behaviors surveillance—United States, 2005, *Surveillance Summaries*, June 9, 2006. MMWR 2006;55 (No. SS-5).

TABLE 79.4

Trends in Behaviors Related to Suicide Among High School Students During 12 Months Preceding Survey, 2005

Category	Seriously Considered Attempting Suicide[a] (%)	Made a Suicide Plan[a] (%)	Attempted Suicide[b] (%)	Suicide Attempt Required Medical Attention[b] (%)
1991	29.0	18.6	7.3	1.7
1993	24.1	19.0	8.6	2.7
1995	24.1	17.7	8.7	2.8
1997	20.5	15.7	8.7	2.6
1999	19.3	14.5	8.3	2.6
2001	19.0	14.8	8.8	2.6
2003	16.9	16.5	8.5	2.9
2005	16.9	13.0	8.4	2.3

[a]Significant linear decrease in rates between 1991 and 2005.
[b]No significant change between 1991 and 2005.
From Centers for Disease Control and Prevention. Youth risk behaviors surveillance—United States, 2003, *Surveillance Summaries,* May 21, 2004. MMWR 2004; 53 (No. SS-2):[45–47].

white suicides are in the northeast and the deep south.

12. Suicide at college: Suicide is the third leading cause of death on college campuses. Most studies indicate that suicide rates in college students are no higher than that in the general population for the same age-group. College students who commit suicide tend to be depressed, quiet, and socially isolated, whereas young adults in the noncollege population tend to abuse substances and demonstrate impulsive and risk-taking behaviors. Approximately 10% of college students contemplate suicide each year; 5% to 6% make a plan and approximately 1.5% attempt (see Chapter 84 for more information on suicide in college students).

RISK FACTORS

To date, there are no assessment tools to help identify adolescents who will attempt suicide. Risk factors for suicide frequently occur in combination with each other. Certain risk factors should increase the health care provider's index of suspicion for a potentially suicidal adolescent. A risk assessment identifies both risk factors and protective factors and can help differentiate the risk factors that can be modified from ones that cannot. The following text outlines risk factors for suicide:

1. A history of co-occurring mental disorder and substance abuse disorder: More than 90% of teen suicide victims have a mental disorder such as depression and/or a history of alcohol or drug abuse. Studies report that the rate of substance abuse disorders is 7.5 to 9 times higher in adolescents who complete suicide compared to their nonsuicidal peers. Psychological autopsies reveal that most teens who complete suicide suffered from depression and experienced higher levels of hopelessness, helplessness, or low self-esteem than their nonsuicidal peers. There appears to be a strong association between adolescent suicide behavior and substance abuse. Adolescents who abuse psychoactive substances experience greater psychological distress and appear to be at higher risk for suicidal behavior.

2. Prior suicide attempts: A previous suicide attempt is one of the strongest predictors of both future attempts and death by suicide. Approximately one third of teenage suicide victims have made a previous suicide attempt. A male teen who has attempted suicide in the past is >30 times more likely to complete a suicide than a male who has never attempted before. A female teen with a history of a suicide attempt presents with 3 times the risk of suicide. This relationship is the strongest among adolescents suffering from mood disorders. It is important to assess the adolescent's intention to repeat, the agent used in a past attempt (jumping and shooting are of higher risk than ingestion or cutting), and the location and likelihood of rescue (the risk is higher among adolescents who have attempted suicide in a remote site or who have taken steps to eliminate or reduce the probability of discovery).

3. History of suicide in the family: A history of suicide attempt(s) or completed suicides among first- or second-degree relatives substantially increases the likelihood of attempted and completed suicides in the adolescent. This relationship exists even when studies control for parental psychopathology.

4. History of prior physical and sexual abuse: Adolescents who had been physically or sexually abused are significantly more likely to experience suicidal thoughts and behaviors than those adolescents who have not been exposed to this type of abuse. Some studies report up to a 5 times greater risk of suicide in adolescents with a prior history of physical abuse and a threefold increase of suicidal behaviors in teens with a history of sexual abuse. Runway and homeless youth, who often report escaping abuse and neglect, are especially vulnerable.

5. Family history of mental and substance abuse disorders: The parents of suicidal adolescents consistently show higher rates of mood disorders, substance abuse, and aggressive and suicidal behaviors. Environmental

and genetic mechanisms may contribute to this relationship.

6. History of a broken family or family discord including low levels of communication with parents: Parent–child conflict and lack of family support increases the likelihood of suicidal behaviors. Other family influences include a history of violence, family disruption due to death, divorce, moving, and rapid sociocultural changes. This relationship is strongest among younger adolescents.

7. Stressful life event or loss: Psychosocial problems and stressors are often cited by adolescents as reasons for attempting suicide. It is important to recognize that the degree of stress the adolescent experiences is subjective and reflects a personal level of vulnerability (such as experiencing a loss of a significant person or relationship, a conflict with parents or peers, problems at school, or the risk of incarceration). Suicidal behaviors resulting from stressful life events are more common in adolescents than in adults.

8. Gay and bisexual adolescents: Gay and bisexual youth are confronted by challenges in domains such as identity development, family and community values that stigmatize homosexuality, and a climate of homophobic attitudes. Research shows that gay and bisexual adolescents experience higher rates of depression and gay males are 4 times more likely than their heterosexual peers to attempt suicide.

9. Easy access to firearms: In 2004, almost half of 15- to 24-year-olds who completed suicide used a firearm. The most common location for teen suicides by firearms is in their homes. The risk is directly related to the accessibility and the number of guns in the home. The presence of firearms in the home is associated with a 31.3 to 107.9 times increase in adolescent suicide even in the absence of clear psychiatric illness. Some researchers claim that suicides by firearms tend to be more impulsive and spontaneous.

10. Suicide contagion: Suicide clusters and imitating suicide has been reported throughout human history. They account for 1% to 5% of all teen suicides in the United States. Although rare, they are observed on high school and college campuses, among religious sects, in prisons, and among marine troops. They often follow highly publicized suicides of teenagers and popular young adults. They can be provoked by membership in the same educational or social groups and shared environmental stressors. It is not necessary for the decedents to know each other or to have direct contact.

Research in chronic illness in adolescents and young adults show a significant association between chronic illness, emotional distress, and suicidality that persists even after adjusting for depressive illness and alcohol use. The association is especially significant for adolescent females. The findings support the need to screen for suicidality in general medical settings, especially in adolescents presenting with a range of physical health problems and in those with chronic illness.

THE ADOLESCENT SUICIDE ATTEMPT

Although each suicidal adolescent is different, many exhibit a behavioral pattern that can be broken down into the following four components:

1. Long-standing history of difficulties: Suicide is a disease of deficiency, a deficiency of early social connections that a developing teen uses later as the basis for conflict resolution and problem-solving skills. Many adolescents who attempt suicide exhibit a long history of deficiency that creates an underlying vulnerability. These problems include parents or relatives who have attempted suicide, one or both natural parents absent from the home, unwanted stepparents, divorce in the family, history of family conflicts, parents with alcohol problems, history of foster placements, or marked residential mobility.

2. Escalation phase: For many adolescents who have attempted suicide, the vulnerability created during childhood increases during adolescence. This period of escalating difficulties is characterized by frequent family conflicts as the family fails to deal adequately with the adolescent developmental process. The adolescent often begins to feel isolated from his or her family and other social structures. Significant physical or mental illness in the family and loss of the family unit may also exacerbate the adolescent's vulnerability.

3. Progressive social isolation: Failure of available adaptive techniques for coping with old and new problems often leaves the suicidal adolescent feeling progressively more socially isolated. This is often associated with a significant breakdown of communication with parents. The adolescent seems to have lost or never developed the capability to appropriately express his or her feelings. Although these adolescents are often depressed, one must remember that child and adolescent depression may not mirror the typical adult behaviors of depressed affect. In fact, adolescent depression may manifest itself through oppositional or evasive behaviors such as reduced school attendance and performance, substance abuse, delinquency, runaway behavior, early onset of sexual activity, or sexual promiscuity.

4. Final stage: The suicide attempt is often preceded by a precipitating event that caps this long process of increasing despair. Precipitating events often include a family conflict, loss of a girlfriend or boyfriend, school problems, pregnancy, or loss or death of a friend or relative.

Warning Signs

Several signs should alert family, friends, and health care providers to the potential for suicide. These prodromal signs include sadness, hopelessness, emptiness, lack of energy, insomnia, eating problems, loss of interest in social life and school, boredom, loneliness, irritability, truancy, substance abuse, or a change in social behavior. Other signs include atypical accident proneness, giving away prized possessions, and statements such as, "My family (or the world) would be better off without me."

ASSESSMENT OF THE SUICIDAL ADOLESCENT

Interview and History

All adolescents identified to be at risk of suicide need help. Most suicidal adolescents are not likely to initiate help-seeking behaviors. The adolescents who seek help should be interviewed alone as long as they can provide a clear history. The clinician should involve parents or guardians at some point during the assessment. Asking adolescents about suicide or using a screening tool will not cause them to attempt suicide. In fact, asking an adolescent about suicidal feelings can come as a great relief and can provide an opportunity for the adolescent to get help.

The interview with the adolescent should consist of open-ended nonjudgmental questions. For instance, "When you feel sad or depressed do you ever feel like there is no hope?" If the answer is yes, the clinician should follow-up with more direct, close-ended questions like, "Have you ever felt so sad or depressed that you thought about killing yourself?" If the response is yes, the clinician should follow-up with questions to assess suicide risk. Any adolescent with a well-thought-out plan that includes intent, plan for place and time, and access to lethal means should be considered to be at high risk. Even adolescents presenting with low or medium risk must be screened to assess past and present suicide-related factors. On the basis of the screening, the degree of protection and intervention necessary can then be determined.

The following issues need to be assessed:

1. All suicidal adolescents
   a. Sex and age of adolescent
   b. History of mental disorders including history of substance abuse
   c. Description of current depressive symptoms
   d. History of accidents or prior self-destructive behavior
   e. History of suicide attempts, mental disorders, or substance abuse in family members
   f. History of family, school, or peer problems
   g. History of incest or abuse (physical, sexual, or emotional)
   h. Sexual orientation
   i. Recent experience of loss
   j. Prior use of coping strategies
   k. Available support systems including reaction by parents and others: Do the parents take the attempt seriously and are they supportive of seeking help? What family or peer support system will the adolescent be returning to at home?
2. Adolescents who present with suicidal ideation
   a. Suicidal ideations (type and frequency)
   b. Plan and motivation
   c. Access to methods (especially firearms)
   d. History or evidence of prior suicide attempts
   e. History of depression
   f. History of substance use
   g. Life stressor (e.g., school difficulties, relationship issues, job loss) that precipitated the thoughts
   h. Access to firearms and other weapons
   i. Access to potentially harmful medications
3. Adolescent who has attempted suicide
   a. Medical therapy: The first priority is to treat any life-threatening medical complication of the suicide attempt.
   b. Physical protection: The suicidal adolescent should be provided with immediate physical protection so that a reattempt does not occur. Depending on the degree of risk and the resources available, an adolescent should be hospitalized or sent home with family members who know how to ensure the youth's safety and are aware of the help resources that are available to the family.

c. Psychological evaluation: As soon as the medical evaluation and treatment are completed, an initial evaluation should be performed. This evaluation should attempt to assess the following:
   - Method: Lethality and access to means
   - Timing: Sudden impulse versus a well planned attempt
   - Intent: Strength of intention to die
   - Desire to repeat
   - Circumstances surrounding the attempt: Possibility of rescue versus an attempt carried out in isolation
   - Life stressor (e.g., school difficulties, relationship issues, job loss) that precipitated the attempt
   - Access to firearms and other weapons
   - Access to potentially harmful medications

Mental Status

Evaluating the adolescent's mental status includes the following:

1. Level of depression, level of hopelessness, helplessness, and self-esteem
2. Feelings of expendability (e.g., the adolescent feels not important to the family and that to some extent the family would be "better off" without the adolescent)
3. Openness to further interventions
4. Level of panic and disorganization
5. Attitude about death
6. A suicide scale such as the Child-Adolescent Suicide Potential Index or voluntary school screening instruments such as the Columbia Suicide Screen can also be administered. These scales and screening instruments must be followed by a clinical interview conducted by a mental health professional. Furthermore, they cannot substitute for a thorough suicide assessment, which will help determine if further evaluation and treatment are needed. Following the clinical interview, the parents or guardians of the minor adolescent must be informed about treatment recommendations. In addition, appropriate referral information must be provided to the patient and family.

Disposition

The disposition of the suicidal adolescent often depends on the resources available to the patient, family, and health care provider. Although a consultation with a mental health provider is recommended for all suicide assessments, this service is not always available. The following is intended as guiding principles to help determine the most appropriate arrangement for the suicidal adolescent:

1. Indications for inpatient hospitalization
   a. Medical complications
   b. Patient is psychotic
   c. Attempt was near-lethal, premeditated, or involved use of a lethal method with clear intent to die
   d. An uncommunicative adolescent who cannot establish a trusting relationship with the evaluator, someone who communicates ambivalence regarding the will to live, or someone who has a persistent intent to die
   e. History of a psychiatric disorder(s) or substance abuse (especially with current intoxication)

f. Current agitation, poor judgment, or refusal of help
g. Lack of family support

High-risk adolescents (presenting with a strong wish to die and a persistent plan to hurt themselves) must remain in a safe and protected environment. Patient and parental consent is highly recommended. However, if the adolescent refuses voluntary admission, procedures for involuntary hospitalization should be initiated. Discharge should be considered once the suicide risk has declined and the youth and family are able to utilize appropriate resources. Following discharge, the adolescent and the family should receive intense outpatient mental health services to manage the psychological needs of the adolescent.

2. Indications for outpatient management
   a. Outpatient management should only be considered if the adolescent has demonstrated a low suicide risk (no current wish to die and no current plan to hurt oneself; close outpatient follow-up) and if the adolescent has a supportive home environment where appropriate supervision can be established.
   b. Adolescent no longer feels actively suicidal and does not wish to die.
   c. No history of a serious suicide attempt (plan, method, and intent have low lethality).
   d. No evidence of long-standing psychiatric disorder, especially severe depression or substance abuse.
   e. Adolescent has a supportive family willing to help, and communication at home is appropriate. An adult at home is capable of securing the environment and accessing additional services as determined.
   f. Appropriate medical and psychosocial follow-up has been arranged.

Follow-up

Every suicidal adolescent should have conscientious follow-up care by a psychiatrist, psychologist, or other qualified mental health provider. The adolescent and family should be provided with these services when a decision is made to either not hospitalize the adolescent or discharge the adolescent from the hospital. The collaborative care between a medical physician and the mental health providers is an essential component to follow-up. Initially, weekly or more frequent mental health visits should be scheduled. During this period, the adolescent's problems can be explored, with careful attention given to the areas of school, social and family problems, and existing support mechanisms.

The outpatient management of an at-risk adolescent is characterized by close follow-up with an appropriate mental health provider. Often a no-suicide contract is established. A no-suicide contract is an agreement in which the adolescent promises not to harm or kill himself or herself. No-suicide contracts can be written or verbal. The no-suicide contract is a tool used to document the adolescent's and family's responsibilities, expectations, and desire for change. Although it is common practice to develop and sign a no-suicide contract in the outpatient setting, the health care provider should be aware that a signed contract does not eliminate suicide risk. This tool should be used as an adjunct to an ongoing comprehensive evaluation and treatment plan. These contracts do not provide legal protection and should be viewed as a tool to assess the degree to which the adolescent feels capable to keep oneself safe. If the attempt to develop a no-suicide contract reveals suicidal ideations, or the suicide potential is judged to be high, voluntary or involuntary hospitalization should be reconsidered. If the adolescent is at risk of suicide, the appropriate persons should be notified.

Suicidal ideation, gestures, or attempts must be taken seriously, even if one suspects that these behaviors are a "manipulative attempt" to get attention. The clinician should attend to these behaviors in a supportive and professional manner.

RECOMMENDATIONS FOR PRIMARY CARE PHYSICIANS

Adapted from a policy statement by the American Academy of Pediatrics (April, 2000).

1. Know the risk factors associated with adolescent suicide. Be prepared to serve as a resource to adolescents, parents, and other members of the community.
2. Routinely ask questions about depression and suicide.
3. Ask specific questions about the availability of firearms. Advise parents of suicidal teens to remove firearms and other potential methods from the home.
4. Recognize the medical and psychiatric needs of the suicidal adolescent, and work closely with health care professionals and family members to best manage the suicidal adolescent.
5. Physicians should become familiar with local, state, and national resources concerned with youth suicide. Working relations should be established with colleagues specializing in adolescent suicide to manage the care and follow-up of adolescents at risk of suicide.

SUICIDE PREVENTION

In 1999, David Satcher, the Surgeon General, hosted a press conference where he unveiled a blueprint to prevent suicide in the United States. The document entitled *The Surgeon General's Call to Action to Prevent Suicide* outlined more than a dozen steps that individuals, communities, organizations, and policy makers can take to prevent suicide. The call for action resulted in a task force established by the Department of Health and Human Services (DHHS). In 2001, the DHHS published the National Strategy for Suicide Prevention (NSSP): Goals and Objectives for Action. The document identified multiple goals and objectives in the areas of awareness, intervention, and methodology of suicide prevention. The NSSP represents the first U.S. attempt at suicide prevention through a coordinated approach. Information about NSSP is available at the DHHS Web site www.mentalhealth.samhsa.gov/suicideprevention/strategy.asp.

WEB SITES

http://www.suicidology.org Provides information on current research, prevention, and help for the suicidal person. A list of crisis centers and support groups is also included.

http://www.afsp.org The American Foundation for Suicide Prevention provides research, education, and current statistics regarding suicide.

http://www.suicidehotlines.com Suicide Crisis Center provides a state-by-state listing of suicide-prevention resources.

http://www.aap.org/pubed/ZZZ7FR2VR7C.htm?&sub_cat=1 Information on suicide from the American Academy of Pediatrics and fact sheets for parents and caregivers on teen depression and preventing youth suicide.

http://www.safeyouth.org/scripts/index.asp National Youth Violence Prevention Resource Center includes hot topics on youth suicide.

http://www.aacap.org/publications/factsfam/suicide.htm The American Academy of Child and Adolescent Psychiatry Web site includes facts for families, including information on teen suicide, depression, and other related topics.

http://www.cdc.gov/nchs/hus.htm Center for Disease Control and Prevention (CDC), the National Center for Health Statistics.

http://www.spanusa.org Suicide Prevention Advocacy Network.

http://www.suicidology.org American Association of Suicidology or call-1-800-273-TALK.

http://www.teenscreen.org/index.htm Columbia University Teen Screen program.

REFERENCES AND ADDITIONAL READINGS

American Academy of Child and Adolescent Psychiatry. Practice parameter for the assessment and treatment of children and adolescents with suicidal behavior. *J Am Acad Child Psychiatry* 2001;40(Suppl 7):24S.

American Academy of Pediatrics, Committee on Adolescents. Suicide and suicide attempts in adolescents. *Pediatrics* 2000; 105:871.

Anderson RN, Smith BL. Deaths: leading causes for 2002. *National vital statistics reports*, Vol. 53 No. 17 Hyattsville, MD: National Center for health Statistics, 2005.

Bagley C, Tremblay P. Elevated rates of suicidal behavior in gay, lesbian, and bisexual youth. *Crisis: J Crisis Interv Suicide* 2000;21(3):111.

Beautrais AL. Gender issues in youth suicidal behaviour. *Emerg Med (Fremantle)* 2002;14(1):35.

Beautrais AL. Risk factors for suicide and attempted suicide among young people. *Aust N Z J Psychiatry* 2000;34(3):420.

Berman AL, Jobes DA. *Adolescent suicide: assessment and intervention*. Washington, DC: American Psychological Association, 1991.

Brent DA, Baugher M, Bridge J, et al. Age-and sex-related risk factors for adolescent suicide. *J Am Acad Child Adolesc Psychiatry* 1999;38:1497.

Brent DA. Assessment and treatment of the youthful suicidal patient. *Ann N Y Acad Sci* 2001;932:106.

Canetto SS. Meanings of gender and suicidal behavior during adolescence. *Suicide Life Threat Behav* 1997;27(4):339.

Cantor CH, Baume PJ. Access to methods of suicide: what impact? *Aust N Z J Psychiatry* 1998;32(1):8.

Cavaiola AA, Lavender A. Suicidal behavior in chemically dependent adolescents. *Adolescence* 1999;34:735.

Cavanagh JT, Carson AJ, Sharpe M, et al. Psychological autopsy studies of suicide: a systematic review. *Psychol Med* 2003;33(3):395.

Craney JL, Geller B. A prepubertal and early adolescent bipolar disorder-I phenotype: review of phenomenology and longitudinal course. *Bipolar Disord* 2003;5(4):243.

Centers for Disease Control and Prevention. Methods of suicide among persons aged 10–19 years, United States, 1992–2001. *MMWR* 2004;53:471.

Centers for Disease Control and Prevention. *Surveillance Summaries. MMWR* 2004;53(SS-2).

Center for Disease Control and Prevention. *WISQARS*. National Center for Health Statistics (NCHS) National Vital Statistics System, 2005.

Centers for Disease Control and Prevention. Youth risk behavior surveillance—United States, 2005. *MMWR CDC Surveill Summ* 2006;55(SS05):1.

Douglas J, Brewer M. American psychiatric association practice guideline for assessing and treating patients with suicidal behaviors. *Psychiatr Ann* 2004;34(5):373.

Druss B, Pincus H. Suicidal ideation and suicide attempts in general medical illnesses. *Arch Intern Med* 2000;160:1522.

Esposito-Smythers C, Spirito A. Adolescent substance use and suicidal behavior: a review with implications for treatment research. *Alcohol Clin Exp Res* 2004;28(Suppl 5):77S.

Evans E, Hawton K, Rodham K. Factors associated with suicidal phenomena in adolescents: a systematic review of population-based studies. *Clin Psychol Rev* 2004;24(8):957.

Evans E, Hawton K, Rodham K. Suicidal phenomena and abuse in adolescents: a review of epidemiological studies. *Child Abuse Negl* 2005;29(1):45.

Fergusson DM, Horwood LJ, Beautrais AL. Is sexual orientation related to mental health problems and suicidality in young people? *Arch Gen Psychiatry* 1999;56:876.

Frankenfield D, Keyl PM, Gielen A, et al. Adolescent patients—healthy or hurting? Missed opportunities to screen for suicide risk in the primary care setting. *Arch Pediatr Adolesc Med* 2000;154:162.

Galloucis M, Francek H. The Juvenile Suicide Assessment: an instrument for the assessment and management of suicide risk with incarcerated juveniles. *Int J Emerg Ment Health* 2002;4(3):181.

Gary FA, Yarandi HN, Scruggs FC. Suicide among African Americans: reflections and a call to action. *Issues Ment Health Nurs* 2003;24(3):353.

Gould MS Suicide Contagion. *Research article—American Foundation for Suicide Prevention*. http://www.afsp.org/research/articles/gould.html.

Gould MS, Greenberg T, Velting DM, et al. Youth suicide risk and preventive interventions: a review of the past 10 years. *J Am Acad Child Adolesc Psychiatry* 2003;42(4):386.

Gould MS, Marrocco FA, Kleinman M, et al. Evaluating iatrogenic risk of youth suicide screening programs: a randomized controlled trial. *JAMA* 2005;293(13):1635.

Haliburn J. Reasons for adolescent suicide attempts. *J Am Acad Child Adolesc Psychiatry* 2000;39:13.

Handwerk ML, Larzelere RE, Friman PC, et al. The relationship between lethality of attempted suicide and prior suicide communications in a sample of residential youth. *J Adolesc* 1998;21:407.

Hart TA, Heimberg RG. Presenting problems among treatment-seeking gay, lesbian, and bisexual youth. *J Clin Psychol* 2001; 57(5):615.

Hawton K, James A. Suicide and deliberate self harm in young people. *BMJ* 2005;330(7496):891.

James A, Lai FH, Dahl C. Attention deficit hyperactivity disorder and suicide: a review of possible associations. *Acta Psychiatr Scand* 2004;110(6):408.

Kennedy SP, Baraff LB, Suddath R, et al. Emergency department management of suicidal adolescents. *Ann Emerg Med* 2004;43(4):452.

Koplin B. Agathen J Suicidality in children and adolescents: a review. *Curr Opin Pediatr* 2002;14(6):713.

Kulkin HS, Chauvin EA, Percle GA. Suicide among gay and lesbian adolescents and young adults: a review of the literature. *J Homosex* 2000;40(1):1.

Lebson M. Suicide among homosexual youth. *J Homosex* 2002; 42(4):107.

Links PS, Gould B, Ratnayake R. Assessing suicidal youth with antisocial, borderline, or narcissistic personality disorder. *Can J Psychiatry* 2003;48(5):301.

Londino DL, Mabe PA, Josephson AM. Child and adolescent psychiatric emergencies: family psychodynamic issues. *Child Adolesc Psychiatr Clin N Am* 2003;12(4):629.

Malone KM, Oquendo MA, Haas GL, et al. Protective factors against suicidal acts in major depression: reasons for living. *Am J Psychiatry* 2000;157:1084.

McBride HE, Siegel LS. Learning disabilities and adolescent suicide. *J Learn Disabil* 1997;30:652.

McKeown RE, Garrison CZ, Cuffe SP. Incidence and predictors of suicidal behaviors in a longitudinal sample of young adolescents. *J Am Acad Child Adolesc Psychiatry* 1998;37:612.

McQuillan CT, Rodriguez J. Adolescent suicide: a review of the literature. *Bol Asoc Med P R* 2000;92(1–3):30.

Miller AL. Dialectical behavior therapy: a new treatment approach for suicidal adolescents. *Am J Psychother* 1999;53(3): 413.

Miller AL, Glinski J. Youth suicidal behavior: assessment and intervention. *J Clin Psychol* 2000;56(9):1131.

Mino A, Bousquet A, Broers B. Substance abuse and drug-related death, suicidal ideation, and suicide: a review. *Crisis* 1999;20:28.

Moscicki EK. Identification of suicide risk factors using epidemiologic studies. *Psychiatr Clin North Am* 1997;20(3):499.

Moskos MA, Achilles J, Gray D. Adolescent suicide myths in the United States. *Crisis: J Crisis Interv Suicide* 2004;25(4): 176.

National Center for Health Statistics. *Health, United States, 2004 With Chartbook on Trends in Health of Americans.* Hyattsville, MD: 2004. Accessed at http://www.cdc.gov/nchs/data/hus/hus04.pdf

Pelkonen M, Marttunen M. Child and adolescent suicide: epidemiology, risk factors, and approaches to prevention. *Paediatr Drugs* 2003;5(4):243.

Pfeffer C, Normandin L, Kakuma T. Suicidal children grow up: suicidal behavior and psychiatric disorders among relatives. *J Am Acad Child Adolesc Psychiatry* 1994;33:8.

Pfeffer CR. Childhood suicidal behavior. A developmental perspective. *Psychiatr Clin North Am* 1997;20(3):551.

Pfeffer CR. Diagnosis of childhood and adolescent suicidal behavior: unmet needs for suicide prevention. *Biol Psychiatry* 2001;49(12):1055.

Pfeffer CR, Jiang H, Kakuma T. Child-Adolescent Suicidal Potential Index (CASPI): a screen for risk for early onset suicidal behavior. *Psychol Assess* 2000;12(3):304.

Poland S, Lieberman R. Questions and answers: suicide interventions in the schools. *NASP Communique* 2004;31:7.

Pumariega AJ, Rothe E. Cultural considerations in child and adolescent psychiatric emergencies and crises. *Child Adolesc Psychiatr Clin N Am* 2003;12(4):723.

Remafedi G. Sexual orientation and youth suicide. *JAMA* 1999;282:1291.

Rich CL, Young D, Fowler RC. San Diego suicide study. I. Young vs. old subjects. *Arch Gen Psychiatry* 1986;43:577.

Rosenberg ML, Mercy JA, Potter LB. Firearms and suicide [Editorial]. *N Engl J Med* 1999;341:1609.

Rosewater KM, Burr BH. Epidemiology, risk factors, intervention, and prevention of adolescent suicide. *Curr Opin Pediatr* 1998;10(4):338.

Rowan AB. Adolescent substance abuse and suicide. *Depress Anxiety* 2001;14(3):186.

Safer DJ. Self-reported suicide attempts by adolescents. *Ann Clin Psychiatry* 1997;9(4):263.

Safer DJ. Adolescent/adult differences in suicidal behavior and outcome. *Ann Clin Psychiatry* 1997;9(1):61.

Sanchez LE, Le LT. Suicide in mood disorders. *Depress Anxiety* 2001;14(3):177.

Shaffer D, Pfeffer CR. Practice parameter for the assessment and treatment of children and adolescents with suicidal behavior. *J Am Acad Child Adolesc Psychiatry* 2001;40(7):24S.

Shaffer D, Scott M, Wilcox H, et al. The Columbia suicide screen: validity and reliability of a screen for youth suicide and depression. *J Am Acad Child Adolesc Psychiatry* 2004;43:71.

Shenassa ED, Rogers ML, Spalding KL, et al. Safer storage of firearms at home and risk of suicide: a study of protective factors in a nationally representative sample. *J Epidemiol Community Health* 2004;58(10):841.

Spirito A, Overholser J. The suicidal child: assessment and management of adolescents after a suicide attempt. *Child Adolesc Psychiatr Clin N Am* 2003;12(4):649.

Suicide Prevention Resource Center. *Promoting mental health and preventing suicide in college and university settings.* Newton, MA: Education Development Center, Inc, 2004.

Suris JC, Parera N, Puig C. Chronic illness and emotional distress in adolescence. *J Adolesc Health Care* 1996;19(2):153.

U.S. Department of Health and Human Services. *National strategy for suicide prevention; Goals and objectives for action.* Rockville, MD: U.S. Department of Health and Human Services, 2001.

U.S. Preventive Services Task Force Screening for suicide risk: recommendation and rationale. *Ann Intern Med* 2004;140:820.

U.S. Public Health Service. *The surgeon general's call to action to prevent suicide.* Washington, DC: U.S. Public Health Service, 1999.

Van Heeringen C. Suicide in adolescents. *Int Clin Psychopharmacol* 2001;16(Suppl 2):S1.

Welch SS. A review of the literature on the epidemiology of parasuicide in the general population. *Psychiatr Serv* 2001; 52(3):368.

Wilcox HC, Conner KR, Caine ED. Association of alcohol and drug use disorders and completed suicide: an empirical review of cohort studies. *Drug Alcohol Depend* 2004;76 (Suppl):S11.

Willis LA, Coombs DW, Drentea P. et al Uncovering the mystery: factors of African American suicide. *Suicide Life Threat Behav* 2003;33(4):412.

CHAPTER 80

School Problems and Attention-Deficit Hyperactivity Disorder

Peter R. Loewenson, Howard Schubiner, Arthur L. Robin, and Lawrence S. Neinstein

School problems, including school phobia, truancy, dropout, academic performance problems, attention-deficit hyperactivity disorder (ADHD), and learning disabilities, represent common concerns for adolescents and their families. The adolescent's primary care clinician can play a critical role in the evaluation and management of such problems in the following manner:

1. Evaluating the adolescent for biomedical disorders such as hearing and vision dysfunction, ADHD, learning disorders, sleep disorders, thyroid disorders, subtle cognitive impairments, and seizure disorders
2. Screening the adolescent for emotional disorders such as depression, anxiety, and family conflict and initiating referrals as necessary
3. Assessing the impact of chronic illness (or its treatment) on the adolescent and his or her family
4. Assessing the impact of family, school, or community factors on academic performance
5. Initiating and coordinating appropriate referrals for the psychological and psychometric testing necessary to determine the presence of learning disabilities, ADHD, and related problems
6. Demystifying learning disabilities, ADHD, and related problems, educating the adolescent and the family about such disabilities, and encouraging the adolescent to develop appropriate attitudes for coping effectively with these disabilities
7. Educating the patient and the family about the legal obligations of public schools to meet the educational needs of youngsters with disabilities
8. Cooperating with public schools in determining the eligibility for special education services, and providing physician certification when required
9. Contributing to the development and coordination of an overall school-based intervention plan and serving as an advocate for the adolescent
10. Providing short-term counseling for milder school- and home-related problems and anticipatory guidance to prevent the development of additional complications (e.g., adjustment reactions and parent–teen conflict)
11. Providing medical therapy for anxiety and affective disorders, as well as for ADHD
12. Serving as care coordinator with whom the adolescent can periodically "check in" to monitor the overall progress of comprehensive medical, educational, and psychological services

SCHOOL PHOBIA/AVOIDANCE

School phobia or school avoidance is a persistent and irrational fear of going to school. The problem usually arises either because the adolescent cannot cope with the pressures and challenges at school or as a result of other stresses, usually related to family or peers. Common stress factors include the following:

1. Fear of undressing in a group
2. Fear of confrontations with teachers or students
3. Fear of poor grades
4. Fear of being picked first or last for a team or school project
5. Fears related to participation in athletics
6. Family dysfunction
7. Fear of being criticized by peers (openly or otherwise)
8. Fears related to poverty or financial circumstances
9. Fears related to sexual expression or sexual orientation
10. Fear of inadequate vocational or academic preparation
11. Fear of individuating or separating from parents

The health care provider must explore with the adolescent his or her fears and reasons for disliking school. A gentle and accepting approach is critical as most adolescents with this disorder are embarrassed or afraid to disclose the nature of their fears or phobia. Depending on the home situation, the practitioner may recommend more parental involvement and an immediate return to school, or in overrestrictive families the health care provider may wish to lessen parental involvement by working out a contract regarding school attendance between the health care provider and the adolescent. Psychological referral may be advisable, depending on the severity and type of underlying problem (e.g., family dysfunction or clinical phobia). Because anxiety disorders such as social phobia or generalized anxiety disorder are a common cause of school phobia, medications for anxiety disorders can be useful as part of the overall management plan. The serotonin selective reuptake inhibitors (SSRIs) have been shown to be useful for these disorders and are generally very well tolerated. Paroxetine (Paxil, usual doses of 10–40 mg every day), fluoxetine (Prozac, usual doses of 10–40 mg every day), and sertraline (Zoloft, usual doses of 50–150 mg every day) have been most often used. The adolescent must be monitored closely for new or worsening symptoms and for emergence of suicidal thinking after starting an SSRI. Buspirone (BuSpar, usual doses of 10–20 mg three times a day) may also be effective.

SCHOOL TRUANCY AND DROPOUT

Although the adolescent with school phobia has some fear of attending school, the adolescent who is truant or who drops out of school is making a conscious decision to miss school. It is clear that school failure is one of the common precursors to truancy and school dropout. And most importantly, school failure or school dropout often precedes high-risk social behaviors such as involvement in gangs and violence, running away, sexual promiscuity, and excessive drug or alcohol use. Therefore, an educational history that investigates potential causes of poor academic performance is important. School dropout is a major problem, particularly among lower socioeconomic classes, and can reach as high as 50% in certain school districts, particularly among male students. Data from college admissions reveal a significant gender difference, with males accounting for only 43% of students at colleges and universities at all levels. In addition to the risk behaviors seen in dropouts, they have higher rates of unemployment and lower incomes than those of high-school graduates.

As mentioned, one of the primary causes of truancy and dropout is poor academic performance and its antecedents. In addition, truancy and dropout may be caused or exacerbated by substance abuse, pregnancy, marriage, or the need to work to support family members.

It is critical to address the primary causes of truancy and dropout. For those at risk for dropping out (e.g., those with early school failure, truancy, high-risk behaviors, poor "fit" within a school system), it will be necessary to work with the adolescent and the family to identify any primary learning disabilities, ADHD, or related conditions, and then to establish appropriate goals for academic achievement and define an appropriate placement. In addition, the health care provider will need to assess the motivation of the adolescent and family for academic performance, their short- and long-term goals, conflicts at home or at school, relationships with peers and teachers, and medical causes of academic difficulties. This information is necessary to develop a plan to improve performance or resolve barriers to continuing involvement in school. A behavioral plan of rewards and consequences is often needed to reestablish parental control and motivate the adolescent to attend school and complete homework. The adolescent should be involved in the development of this type of plan to attempt to optimize compliance. It is critical to identify and support the academic or extracurricular strengths of an adolescent. Educational options may include work-study programs, vocational programs, independent study programs, early graduation, or adult education programs. Follow-up is essential to determine if the initial plan is working and what further steps need to be taken.

It should be kept in mind that some of the world's most accomplished and well known people had difficulties in traditional school settings, so there may be room for optimism (particularly for those who have above-average intelligence). However, the fact remains that most school dropouts have a tough road ahead of them in our present economic milieu.

ACADEMIC PERFORMANCE PROBLEMS

Adolescents who are having difficulty with academic performance constitute a significant group of patients seen in the outpatient setting. During middle school and high school, there is increased dependence on reading, and an increased need to organize materials, develop appropriate study habits, and use abstract thought processes. Therefore, it is not uncommon for academic problems to arise during these years and in fact may be the presenting issue for an office visit. In addition, there will be a number of students who have never done well in school and now that they are adolescents, may have poor academic performance that becomes complicated by other health risk behaviors. An interview with a parent or guardian is crucial in uncovering academic performance problems, because the adolescent may be less concerned with a drop in grades.

Poor academic performance can be due to a wide variety of causes related to the individual adolescent, or to school, family, or community factors. However, it is also common to have multiple factors that coexist and thereby make the evaluation and management more complex. The specific causes of poor academic performance are not always clear. For example, it is commonly believed that substance abuse and membership in a gang are likely causes of school failure. However, academic failure may actually precede some of these health risk behaviors, as students gravitate toward other youth who are also failing at school. Motivation toward academic performance is a critical factor that often requires intensive interventions.

Defining and Identifying the Problem

The identification of academic performance problems is a critical step in the evaluation of every adolescent (see Chapter 4). This is particularly crucial because school performance may be an important marker of other health risk behaviors. Therefore, the adolescent's health care provider should inquire about grades and absences at all routine office visits.

If a potential problem is identified, it is important to clearly define the problem.

1. What is the specific problem?
   a. Has there been a drop in grades, behavior problems, inconsistent performance, emotional issues, or under-achievement for the presumed level of intelligence?
2. Who "owns" the problem?
   a. Does the adolescent have concerns about his or her progress?
   b. Are parents concerned with "average" work because it may not be sufficient for matriculation into certain elite colleges?
   c. Have the teachers identified particular issues that should be resolved?

It is necessary to obtain information from the patient, the family, and the school to understand the nature of the problem and to begin an evaluation.

Causes of Poor Academic Performance

1. Biomedical causes
   a. Hearing or vision problems: Such problems are unlikely to be the primary cause for an adolescent but may contribute to the overall picture.
   b. Mental impairment or low intellectual ability: Subtle forms of mental impairment may not have been picked up earlier. For example, patients with fragile X syndrome (or female carriers of this syndrome), Klinefelter syndrome, Turner syndrome, XXX chromosome syndrome (females only), tuberous sclerosis, neurofibromatosis, or the fetal alcohol syndrome may not have been formerly diagnosed. Some teenagers may not have severe cognitive impairments, but they may score in the borderline range of intellectual ability (an intelligence quotient [IQ] of 70–79). Youngsters with borderline intellectual ability often cannot meet the demands of a regular education curriculum and are considered slow learners. They typically need additional help, but may not qualify for special education services.
   c. Chronic illness: Patients with severe asthma, cystic fibrosis, diabetes mellitus, sickle cell anemia, juvenile rheumatoid arthritis, epilepsy, congenital heart diseases, or other disorders may have had sufficient absences to cause academic problems. In addition, the side effects of medications may impair cognitive function. Chronic infections, such as sinusitis, or obstructive sleep apnea, may also adversely affect school performance.
   d. Neurological disorders: Certain seizure disorders such as simple generalized or partial complex seizures may be subtle enough to be missed. Borderline forms of cerebral palsy may also present difficulties in early diagnosis. Rarely, progressive neurological diseases such as Wilson disease or subacute sclerosing panencephalitis may present as cognitive impairment. Antiepileptic medications may also cause mild cognitive impairments.
   e. Sleep disorders: It is increasingly recognized that some adolescents suffer from undiagnosed obstructive sleep apnea, central hypoventilation syndrome, or have poor sleep hygiene, any of which may have adverse effects on learning.
2. ADHD: Some adolescents may not have been diagnosed as a child, whereas others may have been diagnosed but never treated. In particular, females with attention-deficit disorder without hyperactivity are often not diagnosed in elementary school.
3. Learning disabilities: Specific learning disabilities are common (occurring in approximately 3%–5% of students); usually related to specific problems in reading, spelling, mathematics, or written expression.
4. Psychological and behavioral causes: An adolescent's school performance may be affected by depression, substance abuse, anxiety disorders, conduct disorder, or physical, sexual, or emotional abuse.
5. Family issues: Various family problems may affect academic performance, including parental depression, drug or alcohol abuse, and divorce; conflict within the family (parent–teen or parent–parent); or mismatches between parent–adolescent–school expectations for achievement.
6. School and peer relationships: Adolescents who have poor peer relationships or interact with a peer group that does not value academic achievement may present with academic problems. The school may not be able to meet the needs of certain students (e.g., the bright and bored, those with special needs, those who learn in different ways, or those who do not value the educational experience).
7. Cultural or environmental factors: Adolescents who did not have an opportunity to achieve adequately, who received poor teaching, or had cultural or economic disadvantages that interfere with appropriate education may also present with academic performance problems. Children from ethnic or cultural backgrounds that are different from the prevailing school norm, or in which English is not the primary language may also experience difficulty with a standard curriculum. The practitioner should attempt to distinguish such cultural or environmental factors from all of the other previously mentioned causes of academic performance problems.

Evaluation

History
The history is the most important and often the most challenging part of the evaluation. It is necessary to develop rapport with the adolescent to let him or her know that your interest is to help him achieve his educational goals, rather than to "take the side of the parents or the school."

1. Interview with the parents
   a. Developmental history
      - Prenatal history (use of drugs, alcohol, medications)
      - Perinatal history (prematurity, birth history, sepsis, asphyxia)
      - Developmental milestones (for delays in language acquisition, communications skills, and other discrete areas)
      - Speech, vision, or hearing problems
   b. Medical history
      - Chronic illnesses such as asthma, otitis media
      - Neurological disorders such as head injuries, neurological symptoms
      - Hospitalizations
      - Family history of neurological or psychological disorders, ADHD, or learning disabilities (a family history of resistance to thyroid hormone is strongly associated with ADHD)
   c. Behavioral history
      - Peer and family relationships
      - Suspected drug or alcohol use
      - Psychological symptoms
      - Antisocial behaviors
      - Symptoms of ADHD (inattention, impulsivity, restlessness)
   d. School history (attempt to get similar information from the school)
      - History of prior problems
      - Behaviors reported in school
      - Specific problems (i.e., which classes, which hours, which teachers, missing assignments, missing homework, poor test scores)
      - Motivation and goals
      - Grades, attendance, suspensions

- Parents' educational level and their expectations for their adolescent
- Prior attempts to improve the situation
- Prior educational or IQ testing

2. Interview with the adolescent
   a. School history
      - The perspective of the adolescent on the problem or lack thereof
      - Assessment of motivation and goals
      - Likes and dislikes about school
      - Specific problem areas in school: This area is important to assess both for motivation and for specific deficits that may be indicative of a learning disorder or ADHD. Ask about difficulties in specific classes (to screen for learning disorders in math, reading, language skills), difficulties with specific teachers unrelated to course content, capability and willingness to do homework, difficulty with tests (what kind of tests pose particular problems), overall workload, and difficulty of the assignments.
      - Factors that prevent academic achievement
      - Future plans for employment
      - Specific strengths: This is a critical area to identify. If an adolescent has one strong area (e.g., art, music, computers, sports), you can often build self-esteem by encouraging development in that area while using it as a "hook" to keep the adolescent motivated to stay in school.
   b. Medical and behavioral history
      - Psychological symptoms (particularly anxiety and depression)
      - Symptoms of acute or chronic illness
      - Drug and alcohol use
      - Peer support and influences
      - Family conflicts or problems with parents
3. School records or telephone interviews with teachers are helpful to obtain the school's perspective and to identify the interventions that have been attempted.

Physical Examination

1. Height, weight, body mass index (BMI), and blood pressure.
2. General inspection
   a. For nutritional status
   b. For minor anomalies (e.g., short palpebral fissures, epicanthal folds, thin upper lip of fetal alcohol syndrome; clinodactyly, wide-set eyes, epicanthal folds of XXX syndrome)
3. Ears, nose, and throat; neck: For otitis, tonsillar, or thyroid enlargement
4. Genital: For sexual maturity rating, testicular size (large testes in fragile X syndrome, small testes in Klinefelter syndrome)
5. Neurological: Neurological examination is indicated when a neurological problem is suspected. This may include testing of cranial nerves, muscle strength and tone, gait, coordination, involuntary movements (particularly looking for tics) and reflexes, and sensory examination. Some recommend testing for "soft" neurological signs. These may include reflex asymmetry, strabismus, hyperkineses, coordination difficulties, poor fine visual-motor coordination, confused laterality, choreiform movements, overflow and mirror movements, and extinction to double simultaneous tactile stimulation. Five percent of healthy children display one or two "soft" signs.

Testing

1. Audiometric testing.
2. Visual acuity testing.
3. Cognitive ability testing: General intellectual ability test such as the Wechsler Intelligence Scale for Children-IV for up to age 16 years and the Wechsler Adult Intelligence Scale, third edition, for those older than 16 years. The Woodcock-Johnson III Tests for Cognitive Abilities are sometimes used by schools as well.
4. Achievement testing: Such as Woodcock-Johnson III Test of Achievement, Wechsler Individual Achievement Test II, Kaufman Test of Educational Achievement.
5. Learning disability analysis: Compare IQ and achievement test results, looking for significant discrepancies between average IQ and below-average achievement (usually discrepancies of at least two standard deviations). Occasionally, further educational testing of specific reading, mathematics, writing, and language skills must be done after determining that there is a significant discrepancy.
6. Neuropsychological testing: Testing is indicated if there is either an unusual pattern of functioning on IQ or achievement tests that defy a traditional learning disability explanation or if there are indications of neurological problems.
7. ADHD screening: See next section on ADHD.
8. Psychopathology screening: May ask parent or youth to complete a standardized self-report that broadly screens for psychopathology such as the Child Behavior Checklist (CBCL) or the Behavior Assessment System for Children (BASC-2). T scores higher than 70 would suggest the need for a follow-up clinical interview.
9. Family problems screening: May ask the adolescent or parent to complete a self-report screening of family conflict such as the Conflict Behavior Questionnaire.
10. Adolescents with low or borderline IQ scores should be screened for chromosomal anomalies, such as the Fragile X syndrome.

ATTENTION-DEFICIT HYPERACTIVITY DISORDER

ADHD is a developmental disorder affecting approximately 4% to 12% of children and adolescents, characterized by developmentally inappropriate degrees of inattention, impulsivity, and hyperactivity. It arises in early childhood, is relatively chronic and pervasive in nature, and is not accounted for on the basis of gross neurological, sensory, language, or motor impairment, mental retardation, or severe emotional disturbance. As a result of these core symptoms, adolescents with ADHD have difficulty getting their schoolwork done, organizing their personal lives, resolving disputes, communicating with their parents, following rules established by adult authority figures, and maintaining good peer relationships. Eventually, such cumulative life failure may thwart them from accomplishing the developmental tasks of adolescence, including independence seeking, identity formation, mature same- and opposite-sex interpersonal relationships, and vocational planning. As a result, many such adolescents develop low self-esteem and depressed affect.

Contemporary follow-up studies have suggested that ADHD is truly a life span disorder; 60% to 80% of ADHD children continue to manifest the full clinical syndrome in adolescence, and >50% continue to manifest the full clinical syndrome in adulthood. In adolescence, paying attention and controlling impulses remain the greatest problems, whereas motoric hyperactivity usually diminishes and/or transforms into mental restlessness. Those adolescents with ADHD alone (i.e., without oppositional-defiant disorder or conduct disorder) may exhibit comorbid difficulties such as learning disorders, low self-esteem, depression, or other emotional problems (see subsequent text), whereas those with ADHD plus oppositional-defiant disorder, conduct disorder, or bipolar disorder are more likely to develop problems with truancy, dropout, substance abuse, and severe family conflict.

Epidemiology

1. Prevalence: Four percent to 12% of school-aged children are estimated to have ADHD by combining recent community prevalence studies.
2. Sex: Male to female ratio is approximately 3:1 in community samples.
3. Age: The problem typically starts in early grade school, with an increased prevalence of school- and home-based problems in adolescence. Because the transitions to middle and high school entail increased organizational demands, many brighter youngsters or less hyperactive youngsters with ADHD may first become educationally impaired by attention problems in adolescence, resulting in diagnosis and treatment. For 50% to 60% of adolescents with ADHD, there will be residual impairments into adulthood.

Etiology

Although the exact cause of ADHD remains unknown, mounting evidence from neurochemical, brain imaging, genetic, and family studies converge to suggest that in most cases, ADHD is an inherited condition with a biochemical basis. Considerable evidence implicates the neurotransmitters dopamine and norepinephrine in the pathophysiology of ADHD. Brain imaging studies have shown differences between individuals with ADHD and controls in the structure of the basal ganglia and the right frontal anterior lobes and these small differences in brain volumes are present in children and adolescents with ADHD who have never been treated with stimulant medications. Family genetic studies show clustering of ADHD, as well as anxiety, affective disorders, and substance use disorders. In short, ADHD is a biologically disabling condition that cannot be "cured." The goal of treatment is to maximize function and the quality of the adolescent's daily life and to facilitate completion of the developmental tasks of adolescence through flexible combinations of medical, psychosocial, and educational interventions.

Diagnostic Criteria

The *Diagnostic and Statistical Manual of Mental Disorders, fourth edition* (*DSM-IV-TR*) includes a list of nine inattention criteria and a list of nine hyperactivity/impulsivity criteria. Subtypes of ADHD are based on various combinations of these lists (1a and 1b), together with criteria 2 to 5.

1. Either inattention (a) or hyperactivity/impulsivity (b)
   a. Inattention: At least six of the following symptoms of inattention have persisted for at least 6 months to a degree that is maladaptive and inconsistent with developmental level
      - Often fails to give close attention to details or makes careless mistakes in schoolwork, work, or other activities
      - Often has difficulty sustaining attention in tasks or play activities
      - Often does not seem to listen when spoken to directly
      - Often does not follow through on instructions and fails to finish schoolwork, chores, or duties in the workplace (not due to oppositional behavior or failure to understand instructions)
      - Often has difficulty organizing tasks and activities
      - Often avoids, dislikes, or is reluctant to engage in tasks that require sustained mental effort (such as schoolwork or homework)
      - Often loses things necessary for tasks or activities (e.g., toys, school assignments, pencils, book, tools)
      - Is often easily distracted by extraneous stimuli
      - Is often forgetful in daily activities
   b. Hyperactivity/impulsivity: At least six of the following symptoms of hyperactivity/impulsivity have persisted for at least 6 months to a degree that is maladaptive and inconsistent with developmental level
      - Hyperactivity
        – Often fidgets with hands or feet or squirms in seat
        – Often leaves seat in classroom or in other situations in which remaining seated is expected
        – Often runs about or climbs excessively in situations in which it is inappropriate (in adolescents or adults, may be limited to subjective feelings of restlessness)
        – Often has difficulty playing or engaging in leisure activities quietly
        – Is often "on the go" or often acts as if "driven by a motor"
        – Often talks excessively
      - Impulsivity
        – Often blurts out answers before questions have been completed
        – Often has difficulty awaiting turn
        – Often interrupts or intrudes on others (e.g., butts into conversations or games)
2. Some symptoms that caused impairment were present since 7 years of age.
3. Some impairment caused by the symptoms is present in two or more settings (e.g., at school, work, or at home).
4. There must be clear evidence of clinically significant impairment in social, academic, or occupational functioning.
5. The symptoms do not occur exclusively during the course of a pervasive developmental disorder, schizophrenia, or other psychotic disorder and are not better accounted for by another mental disorder (e.g., mood disorder, anxiety disorder, dissociative disorder, or personality disorder).
6. DSM-IV subtypes
   a. 314.01. ADHD, combined type: If both criteria 1a and 1b are met for the past 6 months.

b. 314.00. ADHD, predominantly inattentive type: If criterion 1a is met but criterion 1b is not met for the past 6 months.
c. 314.01. ADHD, predominantly hyperactive/impulsive type: If criterion 1b is met but criterion 1a is not met for the past 6 months.
d. 314.09. ADHD, not otherwise specified: If prominent symptoms of inattention or hyperactivity/impulsivity are present that do not meet criteria for ADHD.

Although the DSM-IV criteria capture the core ADHD symptoms of inattention, impulsivity, and restlessness, contemporary conceptualizations of ADHD have placed these symptoms within the broader context of executive functions of the brain. Executive functions of the brain are higher order self-regulatory functions, often likened to the conductor of an orchestra. Just as the conductor directs the orchestra, telling various instruments when to start, stop, and how to interpret the music, the executive functions of the brain direct the individual to behave in a self-controlled, task-oriented manner. These executive functions include organizing and activating to work, sustaining concentration and attention, sustaining energy and controlling emotions, and utilizing working memory and recall (Brown, 1996). In ADHD executive functions are ineffective, as if the conductor of the orchestra were not doing a good job.

Although used for purposes of standardization, there are a number of problems with the DSM-IV approach to diagnosis: (a) The DSM-IV is developmentally insensitive in that the same number of symptoms are required for a positive diagnosis at all ages; research has suggested that fewer symptoms should be required in older adolescents (five out of nine) and adults (four out of nine); (b) the DSM-IV assumes that ADHD is a categorical diagnosis (e.g., you either have it or you do not); research clearly indicates that inattention and behavioral inhibition are dimensional, not categorical, and adolescents may have different degrees of difficulties in these areas; the practitioner is referred to the *Diagnostic and Statistical Manual for Primary Care (DSM-PC)—Child and Adolescent Version* for an approach to addressing this problem; and (c) the DSM-IV item set was developed with school-age boys in mind and does not adequately capture the phenomenology of ADHD in adolescents, particularly adolescent girls; readers interested in a detailed discussion of ADHD in middle- and high-school girls should consult *Understanding Girls with ADHD* (Nadeau et al., 1999).

Associated Features or Comorbidity

Psychosocial and/or psychiatric comorbidity is common in ADHD

1. Oppositional-defiant disorder: A pattern of negativistic, hostile, and defiant behavior lasting at least 6 months, involving loss of temper, frequent arguments with adults, refusing to comply with requests, deliberately annoying others, being angry and vindictive, and blaming others for one's mistakes. Thirty-five percent of children with ADHD have oppositional-defiant disorder.
2. Conduct disorder: A repetitive pattern of antisocial behavior violating others' basic rights or societal norms, involving physical aggression, threats, use of weapons, cruelty to people or animals, destruction of property, deceitfulness and theft, repeated running away from home, frequent truancy, or sexual assault. Approximately 26% of children with ADHD have conduct disorder. There is sometimes a progression from oppositional-defiant disorder to conduct disorder, and persistent conduct disorder is termed *antisocial personality disorder* in adulthood.
3. Learning disabilities or academic achievement problems: A significant discrepancy between average to above-average intellectual ability and below-average academic achievement in reading, math, spelling, handwriting, or language may reflect a processing deficit. At least 20% to 30% of children with ADHD have learning disabilities in at least one area. Although most adolescents with ADHD do not have learning disabilities, they do consistently show academic achievement problems, with scores on Standardized Achievement Tests lower than those of matched controls, and a greater likelihood of grade retentions, school dropout, or expulsions.
4. Depressive and anxiety disorders: Many adolescents with ADHD are somewhat depressed because of their school and home problems. As a result, their self-esteem suffers. A coexisting depressive disorder is present in 18% of children with ADHD, which further impairs functioning. Anxiety disorders are present in 26% of children with ADHD.
5. Substance abuse: Adolescents with ADHD show more cigarette and alcohol use than matched controls, with these findings accounted for primarily by the subgroup with comorbidity for conduct disorder. A substance use disorder is more likely to be diagnosed in adolescents with ADHD, and is also diagnosed at an earlier age. Some have attributed this to the use of methylphenidate, labeling it "a gateway drug." Effective treatment with stimulant medication, however, has been clearly shown to reduce the risk of subsequent substance use disorder in individuals with ADHD. Marijuana is a commonly used illicit drug among adolescents with ADHD.
6. Driving behavior: Adolescents with ADHD show less sound driving skills or habits than matched control groups, with greater likelihood of accidents, more bodily injuries associated with crashes, and more traffic citations, particularly for speeding. The subgroup with comorbid oppositional-defiant disorder or conduct disorder is at the highest risk for such deficient driving skills or habits. Medical treatment for ADHD has been shown to improve driving performance in adolescents.
7. Family relationships: Adolescents with ADHD and their parents display more negative, controlling interactions, fewer positive, facilitative interactions, and more conflicts than matched controls. Mothers of adolescents with ADHD report more personal psychological distress than mothers of matched controls. The adolescents themselves underestimate the degree of family conflict, compared with their mothers.
8. High-risk sexual behaviors: Adolescents with ADHD have an earlier age at first sexual intercourse, more sexual partners, less use of birth control, more sexually transmitted diseases, and more teen pregnancies that their non-ADHD peers.
9. Sleep disorders: Sleep disturbances are more common in children with ADHD. Because insomnia is a common side effect of stimulant therapy, it is important to thoroughly assess sleep before and after starting stimulant medication.

Making a Diagnosis of Attention-Deficit Hyperactivity Disorder: Clinical Guidelines

In May 2000, the American Academy of Pediatrics (AAP) published evidence-based clinical guidelines for primary care evaluation and diagnosis of ADHD (Table 80.1). These guidelines were developed in conjunction with the National Initiative for Children's Healthcare Quality (NICHQ). The AAP and NICHQ released a toolkit for implementing these guidelines in 2002. "Caring for Children with ADHD: A Resource Toolkit for Clinicians" may be purchased from the AAP and may also be downloaded from the NICHQ Web site at http://www.nichq.org/NICHQ/Topics/ChronicConditions/ADHD/.

1. Inclusion criteria: Does the adolescent meet the DSM-IV inclusion criteria for ADHD? Because of performance inconsistency, information from parents, adolescents, and teachers is required to answer this question. Interview the parents and the adolescent with reference to the DSM-IV criteria. Some health care providers prefer to rely upon an in-depth clinical interview performed by an experienced psychologist. There has been some concern that the DSM-IV criteria lack developmental perspective, that is, they remain the same over the spectrum of childhood and adolescence. Symptoms of inattention tend to remain stable across this developmental spectrum, but symptoms of hyperactivity/impulsiveness may diminish significantly. The DSM-PC can provide a developmental perspective on normal behavioral differences across the age spectrum.

2. Differential diagnosis: If the adolescent meets the DSM-IV inclusion criteria, can alternative syndromes that resemble ADHD be ruled out? Refer the adolescent for psychological testing to explore learning disabilities, and conduct (or refer for) a thorough interview to address other psychiatric syndromes. Inquire about the major life stressors in the adolescent's history, and examine the temporal relationship between the ADHD symptoms and the major life stressors. For example, poor concentration is a frequent clinical feature of major depression.

3. Rating scales: A number of questionnaires and rating scales have been developed to assess behavioral characteristics. There are both ADHD-specific and global ("broadband") scales available. The AAP guidelines consider the ADHD-specific scales an option in clinical assessment, with several caveats. These scales may not function as well in a primary care clinic as in the ideal conditions of the study setting (e.g., comparison of apparently healthy children in referral sites). The questions in the rating scales are subjective; bias may be introduced and a false sense of validity may result. The use of broadband scales in the evaluation of ADHD is discouraged by the AAP guidelines. These global scales, however, are helpful in screening for coexisting conditions. The practitioner should use at least one psychometrically sound parent, teacher, and adolescent self-report rating scale.

Three examples of ADHD-specific rating scales include the following:
a. NICHQ Vanderbilt Parent and Teacher Scales: These scales are included in the AAP toolkit, and may be copied for use in the office or clinic. Each of the 18 DSM-IV behavior descriptions is addressed, and scoring is based on number of behaviors endorsed on a four-point scale. Screening questions for comorbid conditions, for example, conduct disorder, oppositional-defiant disorder, and anxiety/depression are also included. One advantage of this scale is that impairment measures are included for assessing the degree of impairment in the home setting, in academic performance, and in classroom behaviors. These are normed scales for children 5 to 11 years of age.
b. Conners Rating Scales-Revised (CRS-R): There are short and long versions of each of the parent, teacher, and adolescent self-report scales. All DSM-IV symptom subscales are included, and scoring is based on conversion of raw scores into T scores. Conners forms have been in use for 20 years, and are normed forms for adolescents up to age 17 (available from Multi-Health Systems, http://www.mhs.com/).

TABLE 80.1

American Academy of Pediatrics Clinical Guidelines for Attention-Deficit Hyperactivity Disorder Diagnosis and Evaluation

In a child 6- to 12-years-old who presents with inattention, hyperactivity, impulsivity, academic underachievement, or behavior problems primary care clinicians should initiate an evaluation for ADHD

The diagnosis of ADHD requires that a child meet DSM-IV criteria

The assessment of ADHD requires evidence directly obtained from parents or caregivers regarding the core symptoms of ADHD in various settings, age at onset, duration of symptoms, and degree of functional impairment

The assessment of ADHD requires evidence directly obtained from the classroom teacher (or other school professional) regarding the core symptoms of ADHD, duration of symptoms, degree of functional impairment, and associated conditions

Evaluation of the child with ADHD should include assessment for associated (coexisting) conditions

Other diagnostic tests are not routinely indicated to establish the diagnosis of ADHD but may be used for the assessment of other coexisting conditions (e.g., learning disabilities and mental retardation)

ADHD, attention-deficit hyperactivity disorder; DSM-IV, *Diagnostic and Statistical Manual of Mental Disorders, fourth edition.*

c. Brown Attention-Deficit Disorder (ADD) Scale for Adolescents. The Brown ADD Scale for Adolescents (Brown, 1996) is a psychometrically sound adolescent self-report measure which can be administered either as a semistructured interview or as a written rating scale. It consists of 40 items rated on a four-point Likert scale yielding total summary scores and five subscale scores for the following executive functions—organizing and activating to work, sustaining attention and concentration, sustaining energy and effort, managing affective interference, and utilizing working memory and accessing recall.

4. Integration of information from ratings and interview: Make a diagnosis and clearly present it to the family and the adolescent.

LEARNING DISABILITIES

Public schools define learning disabilities in accordance with the Individuals with Disabilities Education Act (IDEA), the recertified version of PL 94–142. Specific learning disabilities consist of disorders in one or more of the basic psychological processes involved in understanding or in using language, spoken or written, which may manifest itself in an imperfect ability to listen, think, speak, read, write, spell, or do mathematical calculations. The term includes such conditions as perceptual handicaps, brain injury, minimal brain dysfunction, dyslexia, and developmental aphasia. The term does not include learning problems that are primarily the result of visual, hearing, or motor disabilities; mental retardation; emotional disturbance; or environmental, cultural, or economic disadvantage.

An information processing model can help us understand how an individual adolescent's learning disability in reading, writing, mathematics, or language is a complex interplay of the following four stages of cognitive processing:

1. Input: Input disabilities include visual perception problems, auditory perception problems, and sensory integration problems.
2. Integration: Integrative disabilities involve understanding information, sequencing, abstracting, and organizing.
3. Memory: Memory difficulties may involve short- or long-term memory.
4. Output: Output disabilities may involve language or writing problems and motor disabilities.

Educators commonly summarize such information processing disabilities in terms of reading, mathematics, writing, and language disorders. They commonly interpret the presence of a significant discrepancy between actual and expected achievement for a given adolescent's intellectual ability as evidence of a learning disability. Practically, a discrepancy of two standard deviations between scores on an IQ test and scores on an achievement test is often presumptive evidence of a learning disability. For example, an individual with a full-scale IQ score of 100 and a reading achievement test score of 78 would qualify (assuming these tests have a mean of 100 with a standard deviation of 10). Learning disabilities are also often suspected when a significant discrepancy exists between the verbal and performance scores on IQ testing.

In recent years educators have increasingly recognized the limitations of a discrepancy model for operationalizing learning disabilities. A new model, "Response to Intervention," is evolving through educational practice and research. When a student exhibits difficulty with a basic learning process such as reading, the educator locates an evidence-based intervention and applies that intervention to remediate the student's difficulty. If the intervention is successful, it is continued in regular education and no learning disability is diagnosed. If the intervention is not successful, the student is considered to have a learning disability, and special education services are provided. The emphasis within this model is the prevention of later learning problems through the early identification and remediation of deficits using evidence-based interventions. The 2004 recertification of the Individuals with Disability Act authorized the public schools to switch from a discrepancy model to a response-to-intervention model for learning disabilities. To date, most applications of the response-to-intervention model have been in elementary schools, but the practitioner should be aware that this evolving model will increasingly be applied in middle- and high-school environments.

Reading Disorders

Reading involves (a) decoding (the act of transcribing a printed word back into speech) and (b) comprehension (the act of interpreting the message or meaning of the text). With dyslexia, the most common reading disorder, the adolescent's decoding skills are impaired, but comprehension is intact. Common clinical indicators of decoding difficulties include guessing at words, having trouble with sound-letter combinations, and making spelling errors involving mispronunciations of words. In addition, dyslexic teens may have trouble sequencing speech into words, syllables, and phonemes, and rearranging sounds into spoken words. If decoding is intact, but comprehension is impaired, this relatively rare reading disability is called *hyperlexia*. The hyperlexic adolescent can read any text but not understand what has been read; they often also have oral language disabilities.

Math Disorders

The terms *dyscalculia* and *acalculia* are often applied to the disorders in teenagers with impairment in the ability to do arithmetic computations or develop number and spatial concepts, resulting in math achievement far below than that expected for grade and intellectual level. Such youngsters have trouble learning to use number words and facts and have difficulty applying math to common life problems. One subgroup of dyscalculic adolescents also has pervasive learning disorders in reading and spelling. There is a second group, however, with low math achievement and poor spatial skills, which have average to superior reading achievement and verbal abilities. This subset has been described as having a nonverbal learning disability. IQ testing reveals that these adolescents consistently show high verbal and low performance ability; neuropsychological testing confirms that their verbal abilities are intact, but their spatial abilities are deficient.

Writing Disorder

The term *writing disorder* refers to difficulty with spelling and other linguistic aspects of writing, such as composing and punctuating sentences and organizing cohesive paragraphs; it does not refer to difficulties with handwriting. Because writing disorders often coexist with reading disorders, dyslexic adolescents should also always be evaluated for a possible writing disorder. The adolescent with a writing disorder is capable of formulating complex thoughts but because of difficulties with spelling is unable to express them in writing at the level expected for his or her intellectual ability. Paragraphs will be poorly organized; sentences will be short with abrupt endings; and expository writing will read more like a list of answers to test questions than a fluent essay. Writing disorders become particularly debilitating in high school and college, when there are increased demands for written expression.

Management of Learning and Achievement Problems

Legal Responsibilities of the Public Schools Children with disabilities are guaranteed a free and appropriate education by the following three federal laws:

1. IDEA: This basic special education act outlines that schools are obligated to conduct multidisciplinary evaluations for adolescents suspected of having a disability, and if the disability is confirmed, provide special education interventions. These interventions are encoded in an Individualized Education Program written at a team meeting that includes the parents. This law outlines specific types of disabilities such as learning disabilities, emotional impairment, mental impairment, and other health impairments. Since 1997, the other health impairment category has been revised to cover children with both ADHD and educational handicaps. IDEA has a funding stream associated with it at the local, state, and federal levels.
2. Section 504 of the Rehabilitation Act of 1973: Section 504 is a civil rights law that outlaws discrimination against individuals with a disability in federally funded programs in education and at the workplace. Schools are required to make reasonable accommodations to educate individuals with disabilities. ADHD has been interpreted as an educational disability under Section 504. Children suspected of having a disability must be evaluated and, if confirmed, reasonable accommodations are typically made first in regular education. Section 504 has no funding stream associated with it.
3. Americans with Disabilities Act: This law basically extends the protections of Section 504 to college students, adults, and the private sector, and therefore may apply to older adolescents who are working.

Also, specific state laws and local policies within school districts elaborate on the federal laws. Most state education departments provide free manuals to professionals and parents explaining special education procedures. Primary care clinicians should become familiar with these laws, inform parents about them, and encourage parents of adolescents suspected of having disabling conditions to make *written* requests for school-based evaluations and interventions. Although an exhaustive account of educational interventions is not possible in this chapter, a summary of the most common accommodations helpful to adolescents with ADHD and learning disabilities follows in the subsequent sections.

ACCOMMODATIONS

Failure to complete or hand-in assignments on time is a major deficit of ADHD and learning disabled teens. Some common accommodations for adolescents with ADHD include the following:

1. Modifying lesson presentation: This will make it easier for the inattentive youngster to remain on task and complete assignments. It often involves breaking lessons into short segments, frequently monitoring on-task behavior, redirecting the adolescent to the task if the adolescent's attention wanders, and providing frequent positive feedback for successful task completion. When a paper is due in 1 month, for example, the teacher might construct intermediate steps to monitor the adolescent: (a) hand in a reference list, (b) hand in notes, and (c) hand in a first draft.
2. Adjusting testing procedures: Adjusting testing procedures by permitting extended time to complete examinations, providing a quiet environment, or administering oral tests.
3. Organizational assistance: This may take the form of note-taking training, assignment sheets, a second set of textbooks at home, checks to make sure students have the materials they need to complete assignments, and monitoring of hand-in assignments.
4. Computers: Students with writing disorders often benefit from an early emphasis on computers, using word processors in school to complete examinations and home assignments.
5. Weekly home or school progress reports: Coordination of weekly home or school progress reports, with home-based incentives for positive teacher ratings, motivates task completion, and cements teacher–parent communication.

Special Education

A continuum of alternative placements for students certified as learning disabled or otherwise health impaired includes resource rooms, separate self-contained rooms, separate schools, residential placements, and even homebound instruction. Placement is usually in the least restrictive environment to best prepare the disabled individual to live in a society with nondisabled individuals. Instructional procedures for reading, mathematics, and writing disabilities rely heavily on contemporary cognitive and developmental psychology and emphasize selecting alternative teaching methods that help the learner bypass his or her area of disability.

MANAGEMENT OF ATTENTION-DEFICIT HYPERACTIVITY DISORDER

Management of ADHD requires a comprehensive plan that includes the adolescent in the decision-making process. A treatment plan that allows the adolescent to participate in setting goals and developing strategies is more likely to succeed. Many adolescents with ADHD have had significant conflicts with their parents, and often the treatment plan includes negotiation of those conflicts to help the parents and adolescent work toward common goals. As described

TABLE 80.2

American Academy of Pediatrics Clinical Guidelines for Attention-Deficit Hyperactivity Disorder Treatment

Primary care clinicians should establish a treatment program that recognizes ADHD as a chronic condition

The treating clinician, parents, and child, in collaboration with school personnel, should specify appropriate target outcomes to guide management

The clinician should recommend stimulant medication and/or behavior therapy as appropriate to improve target outcomes in children with ADHD

When the selected management for a child with ADHD has not met target outcomes, clinicians should evaluate the original diagnosis, use of all appropriate treatments, adherence to the treatment plan, and presence of coexisting conditions

The clinician should periodically provide a systematic follow-up for the child with ADHD; monitoring should be directed to target outcomes and adverse effects, with information gathered from parents, teachers, and the child

ADHD, attention-deficit hyperactivity disorder.

earlier in this chapter, many adolescents with ADHD have comorbid conditions, which should be considered in the treatment plan.

The principles of management of ADHD include education, medication, home interventions, counseling, school interventions (see previous discussion), and advocacy. In 2001, the AAP published evidence-based guidelines for ADHD treatment, emphasizing the importance of viewing this as a chronic condition (Table 80.2).

Education

Education about ADHD should be provided for the adolescent, for the parents and family, for the school, and sometimes even for the friends of the adolescent. A wide array of useful pamphlets, books, and videos are available from the ADD Warehouse (800-233-9273, http://addwarehouse.com). In addition, the AAP has published *ADHD: A Complete and Authoritative Guide*, which many families might find helpful. However, it is critical to take some time to explain in person some of the basics to ensure that the teen has a clear understanding of the condition. This begins with the process of informing the adolescent and the parents of the diagnosis. It is common for adolescents to have some resistance to this diagnosis, as it may be regarded as a "psychological problem" that makes them feel different from their peers. It is important to explain the diagnosis fully and carefully to the adolescent and the parents. Blame for the condition can be deflected by describing the genetic origin and neurochemical nature of the disorder, which may make ADHD seem more acceptable to the family and adolescent.

Adolescents must know that there is hope for improved functional and academic performance. This is important, because adolescents with ADHD often have low self-esteem due to their poor grades, frequently hearing "they could do better if they only tried," and seeing reports of "not living up to potential." If health care providers take a small amount of time at each visit to offer some education about ADHD to the adolescent, they will find that the adolescent is more likely to accept the diagnosis and begin to understand why he or she may act in certain ways. This is the first step in the development of insight, which can play a crucial role in allowing the adolescent to consciously alter his or her behaviors. A useful analogy in explaining ADHD is that of poor eyesight. Poor eyesight is hereditary and not someone's "fault." It causes one to have difficulty

"focusing" and therefore may cause problems in school and in overall functioning. Simple interventions, such as wearing glasses, can help one see clearly and improve academic and overall performance. ADHD is an inherited "biochemical" condition that causes difficulty in focusing and organizing. Medical and behavioral interventions can help the person function better. If adolescents understand this line of reasoning, they will have an easier time in accepting the diagnosis and therapy. In addition, they may be less likely to feel some of the stigma that may be attached to the diagnosis.

Medication

Medication (Table 80.3) should not generally be the only treatment received by the adolescent, but it is frequently the cornerstone of treatment for ADHD, because when it is successful, it appears to correct the underlying disorder in the brain. Because 75% to 90% of adolescents respond to medical therapy, a medication trial should be undertaken for almost all adolescents diagnosed with ADHD. Results from the large Multimodal Treatment Trial of ADHD (MTA) show that medication therapy was the single most effective intervention, and that intensive and closely monitored medical therapy was more effective than the usual provision of stimulant medications in the community (The MTA Cooperative Group, 1999).

Stimulants The stimulants are considered first-line agents because they are the most effective of the available medication options and have an excellent record of safety. They have been shown to be effective in improving the core symptoms of ADHD. Recent studies have also shown that social interactions, academic productivity, and normal reaction times (potentially important in preventing motor vehicle accidents) are also improved.

Immediate-release methylphenidate (Ritalin, Methylin, Focalin) has been the most commonly prescribed stimulant for ADHD. However, the development and acceptance of longer-acting stimulants has led to increased flexibility in providing individual patients with a medication regimen that meets their needs. Shorter-acting medications have the potential for the following disadvantages: (a) need for more frequent and "during school" doses and (b) increased likelihood of "wearing off" and "rebound" symptoms, such as irritability and fatigue. It should be recognized that

TABLE 80.3

Stimulant Medications

Generic Name	Trade Name	Available Doses	Length of Action (hr)	Dose Range
Methylphenidate	Ritalin	5, 10, 20 mg	3–5	5–30 mg b.i.d.–t.i.d.
	Methylin	5, 10, 20 mg; 2.5, 5 mg chewable; 5 and 10 mg/5 mL	3–5	5–30 mg b.i.d.–t.i.d.
	Focalin	2.5, 5, 10 mg	3–5	2.5–10 mg b.i.d.
Intermediate-release methylphenidate	Ritalin-SR	20 mg	4–8	20 mg q.d.–b.i.d.
	Metadate-ER, Methylin-ER	10, 20 mg	4–8	10–20 mg q.d.–b.i.d.
Extended-release methylphenidate	Concerta	18, 27, 36, 54 mg	8–12	18–72 mg q.d.
	Metadate-CD	10, 20, 30, 40, 50, 60 mg	8–12	20–60 mg q.d.
	Focalin XR	5, 10, 20 mg	8–12	5–20 mg q.d.
	Ritalin-LA	20, 30, 40 mg	8–12	20–60 mg q.d.
Methylphenidate patch	Daytrana	10, 15, 20, 30 mg	Up to 12	10–30 mg q.d.
Dextroamphetamine tablets	Dexedrine	5 mg	3–4	5–20 mg b.i.d.–t.i.d.
Dextroamphetamine Spansules	Dexedrine, Dextrostat	5, 10, 15 mg	6–8	5–30 mg q.d.–b.i.d.
Amphetamine and dextroamphetamine	Adderall	5, 7.5, 10, 12.5, 15, 20, 30 mg	4–8	5–30 mg b.i.d.–t.i.d.
	Adderall XR	5, 10, 15, 20, 25, 30 mg	10–12	20–60 mg q.d.

ADHD affects the whole fabric of an adolescent's life including their sports performance, relationships with friends and family, risk for injury (from their potential inattentive or impulsive actions while bicycling, skateboarding, rollerblading, boating, or driving), and decisions about lifestyle risks (e.g., impulsive use of drugs or alcohol). Therefore, as they mature, it makes sense to negotiate a treatment plan that considers coverage by medication throughout the day and on weekends. This is particularly important for those adolescents who experience irritability when the dose "wears off." Therefore, many patients with ADHD benefit from using one of the longer-acting medications, such as dextroamphetamine spansule capsules (Dexedrine), combination dextroamphetamine and amphetamine (Adderall or Adderall XR), or methylphenidate in a timed-release preparation (Concerta, Metadate-ER and Metadate-CD, Methylin-ER, Focalin XR, or Ritalin-LA). Tolerance to stimulants rarely develops after the first month or two on medication, and drug "holidays" are not usually required (with the exception of those few adolescents who show decreases in their growth velocity).

Side Effects of Stimulants

Serious side effects (and relative contraindications to use) include the following:

1. Elevated blood pressure
2. Arrhythmias (particularly when used in association with alcohol, caffeine, or sympathomimetics such as decongestants)
3. Development of psychosis

Concerns about cardiovascular risks associated with the use of stimulant medications prompted the requirement of a "black-box warning." Significantly increased risks have not been subsequently confirmed, nevertheless, careful screening of patients, including a family history, is essential to rule out the presence of cardiovascular disease or risk factors. Routine electrocardiogram (ECG) screening is not currently recommended.

There has been much debate about the development of tics in patients treated for ADHD (especially with stimulants). In children and adolescents with Tourette syndrome, 50% to 75% may also have ADHD; it is possible that the Tourette syndrome may become apparent after ADHD treatment has begun. Tics are not uncommon in childhood and adolescence, and are a relative, not absolute, contraindication for stimulant use. Of children and adolescents with ADHD who also have tics, approximately one third experience worsening of their tics on stimulant medication, one third notice no change, and one third experience improvement in their tics. Patients with comorbid ADHD and Tourette syndrome may respond well to a combination of a stimulant and an α_2-agonist, for example, clonidine or guanfacine.

Minor side effects of stimulants include the following:

1. Weight loss (usually mild)
2. Headaches
3. Abdominal pain
4. Dizziness
5. Dry eyes or mouth
6. Nausea
7. Irritability
8. Insomnia (sleep onset): This may occur if the medication is taken too late in the evening, although many patients seem to have an easier time falling asleep while taking stimulants.

When a dosage trial is undertaken, persistent symptoms of nervousness or jitteriness and feeling "spaced out" or "overfocused" are indications that the dose is too high. Suppression of growth is rarely a problem in adolescents (particularly those receiving lower doses) but should be monitored. It has been shown that ultimate height is not compromised. Some patients develop rebound (periods of irritability or increased ADHD symptoms) when the dose of stimulant is wearing off. This is particularly common with short-acting stimulants. These patients should be given doses at shorter intervals or be switched to a longer-acting preparation.

There has been controversy around a possible association between stimulant use, particularly methylphenidate, and substance abuse. Routine use of methylphenidate as a prescribed therapy has been decried as a "gateway drug" to subsequent abuse of other substances. There is considerable evidence now that the opposite is true. Untreated ADHD is a risk factor for later substance abuse, and treatment of ADHD with stimulants appears to reduce later substance use by as much as 50%. Still, diversion of stimulants is a legitimate concern and adolescents for whom stimulants are prescribed should be warned of the legal and ethical consequences of providing these agents to other adolescents.

Immediate-Release Methylphenidate
Short-acting methylphenidate is no longer recommended as first-line treatment for ADHD. The usual role of short-acting methylphenidate is as an adjunct to longer-acting medications (see subsequent text). If short-acting methylphenidate is used as primary therapy, it should be started at low doses before titrating up to the optimal dose. The dose range is usually 5 to 30 mg/dose, given at intervals of approximately 4 hours (two to three times daily), up to a maximum of 60 mg/day. A typical titration method is to start with 5 mg and increase by 5-mg doses at weekly intervals to 20-mg doses, checking weekly by telephone for positive effects and side effects. The onset of action is approximately 30 minutes. Doses are usually given in the morning, at lunchtime, and after school. A new preparation, the D-isomer of methylphenidate (Focalin), may have fewer side effects and requires approximately half of the usual dose to be effective.

Intermediate-Release Methylphenidate (Ritalin-SR, Metadate-ER, Methylin-ER)
Sustained-release methylphenidate can be useful, because its duration of action is approximately 4 to 8 hours and can be given once or twice daily. Ritalin-SR, however, only comes in a 20-mg preparation and is often not as effective as the short-acting tablet. Therefore, it is not commonly used as a single agent. However, it can be helpful for patients who require lower stimulant doses or those who experience too many "ups and downs" with the short-acting methylphenidate. A good strategy in these situations is to use both short-acting and intermediate-release methylphenidate together as one would use regular and long-acting insulin. A common regimen for this would be sustained-release 20-mg plus 10- to 20-mg short-acting methylphenidate three times a day. Metadate-ER and Methylin-ER are extended-release preparations, and may be given 20 to 40 mg daily, or in varied doses such as 40 mg in the morning and 20 mg in the early afternoon.

Timed-Release Methylphenidate Capsule (Concerta, Metadate-CD, Focalin XR, Ritalin-LA), and the Methylphenidate Patch (Daytrana Patch)
Concerta consists of methylphenidate packaged using a medication delivery system similar to that used in the long-acting medications for hypertension and diabetes mellitus. The capsule contains an outer coating of methylphenidate that is released quickly and a minute hole in the capsule that allows the active ingredient to be released at a constant rate for up to 12 hours. Preliminary studies show good efficacy in the treatment of ADHD and most patients do not need a dose during school hours. Concerta is available in 18-, 27-, 36-, and 54-mg capsules, with most patients requiring 36 to 72 mg/dose.

Metadate-CD consists of beads of methylphenidate with two different release patterns; 30% of the beads are immediately released and absorbed, while the other 70% are released slowly over 8 to 12 hours. Doses of 20 to 60 mg/day in the morning are usually required.

Focalin XR provides an extended-release form of d-methylphenidate. It comes in doses of 5, 10, and 20 mg and appears to be effective up to 12 hours.

Ritalin-LA consists of methylphenidate beads in a 1:1 ratio of immediate and slow release forms. Half of the dose is released immediately and the rest is released approximately 4 hours later to provide 8 hours of medication effect. Morning doses of 20 to 60 mg are used.

A methylphenidate sustained action transdermal system (Daytrana) is now available. For adolescents who are willing to wear a patch, it offers steady-state dosing and variable duration of action. The effects continue for 2 to 3 hours after removing the patch. Skin reactions may occur but are usually mild. It is very difficult to elute the methylphenidate from the patch for purposes of abuse.

Dextroamphetamine (Dexedrine Spansules)
Dextroamphetamine is an effective long-acting preparation and is also tolerated quite well. It comes in 5-, 10-, and 15-mg spansules. The duration of action is usually approximately 8 hours, so it is generally given before school and after school. The usual doses are 10 to 20 mg twice daily, with some patients requiring doses up to 30 mg twice daily. Short-acting dextroamphetamine in seldom used in ADHD.

Combination Dextroamphetamine and Amphetamine (Adderall and Adderall XR)
Adderall is another stimulant for the health care provider to consider. There is good evidence of its effectiveness and it is very well tolerated. Long-acting Adderall XR is effective for 10 to 12 hours with a single morning dose of 10 to 40 mg. Shorter-acting Adderall can be used as an adjunct to Adderall XR. Some adolescents will have better results with short-acting Adderall dosed before and after school. Commonly used doses are 10 to 20 mg two or three times a day, with some patients requiring up to 30 or 40 mg/dose.

Pemoline (Cylert), a long-acting stimulant rarely used because of its potentially fatal hepatotoxicity, is no longer available in the United States.

Atomoxetine Atomoxetine (Strattera) is a selective norepinephrine reuptake inhibitor, the only nonstimulant medication approved by the U.S. Food and Drug Administration (FDA) for the treatment of ADHD, and is the only medication approved for the treatment of ADHD in adults.

It is available as 10-, 18-, 25-, 40-, 60-, 80-, and 100-mg tablets and is given in a single daily dose. The starting dose is 0.5 mg/kg body weight, which may be increased to 1.2 mg/kg/day after 3 to 7 days. The maximum daily dose is 1.4 mg/kg/day or 100 mg/day, whichever is lower. Common side effects include stomach upset, decreased appetite, nausea or vomiting, fatigue, dizziness, mild increase in pulse and blood pressure, and growth delay. There have been several reports of (apparently reversible) severe liver injury associated with atomoxetine use. A recent analysis showed an increased risk of suicidal thinking in children and adolescents during the first few months of treatment with atomoxetine, leading to a black-box FDA warning for this medication. However, the absolute risk of suicidal thinking is quite low.

Tricyclic Antidepressants Tricyclic antidepressants have been generally considered second-line agents in the medical treatment of ADHD, but some health care providers now prefer atomoxetine as a second-line medication because of tricyclic side effects. They may be the medication of choice for patients who do not tolerate stimulants (generally each of the stimulants should be tried before making this determination), for those who have coexistent enuresis, or in whom a tic disorder has developed. Imipramine (Tofranil) and desipramine (Norpramin) have been used successfully. A trial of 4 to 6 weeks at adequate doses should be attempted (blood levels are useful to confirm this because children often metabolize tricyclic medications faster than adults), and careful monitoring is important, including heart rate, blood pressure, complete blood count, and serum levels. ECG monitoring should be done initially and periodically to look for cardiac toxicity (heart rate >130 bpm, PR interval >0.20 seconds, QRS duration >0.12 seconds, QT interval >0.45 seconds). Relative contraindications include a history of cardiac arrhythmias, heart disease, syncope, or family history of sudden death. Side effects include drowsiness, dry mouth, constipation, nausea, sweating, tremor, and postural hypotension. Rarely, neurological side effects such as seizures, an acute organic brain syndrome, and hypomania can occur. Rare instances of sudden death have been reported in children and adolescents. The daily dose of imipramine and desipramine is approximately 3 to 5 mg/kg of body weight. Toxicity is more likely to occur at the higher dose ranges.

Bupropion The antidepressant bupropion (Wellbutrin) has been shown to be effective for inattention and impulsivity in children and may be beneficial in some adolescents with ADHD, especially those with comorbid depression or anxiety. Bupropion (sold as Zyban) is also approved for use in nicotine addiction, and may be helpful in adolescents with ADHD and substance abuse, especially those desiring smoking cessation. It is available in sustained-release (Wellbutrin SR) and extended-release (Wellbutrin XL) formulations. The immediate-release preparation may have a higher incidence of side effects in adolescents. The usual doses are 100 to 150 mg twice daily for Wellbutrin SR and 150 to 300 mg daily for Wellbutrin XL. It is contraindicated in patients with seizures or eating disorders; common side effects include nausea, anorexia, agitation, restlessness, drowsiness, and headaches.

Clonidine Clonidine (Catapres) is a central-acting α_2-agonist that has been shown to have limited effectiveness in the treatment of ADHD. However, it can be useful in patients with comorbid conditions, such as sleep disturbances, tic disorders, or severe aggressiveness (associated with oppositional-defiant disorder or conduct disorder). Clonidine comes in tablets of 0.1, 0.2, and 0.3 mg, as well as skin patches of similar strengths. The tablets are taken 2 to 4 times a day (or at night only for insomnia) starting with 0.05 mg, and then increasing by 0.05 mg/day every 7 days. The maximum daily dose is 0.3 mg/day. The patch is effective for 3 to 7 days. Some experts recommend obtaining a baseline ECG and blood glucose before starting clonidine. Compliance must be carefully monitored since missed doses or abrupt discontinuation of clonidine can precipitate hypertensive crisis, even in those with no history of hypertension. A long-acting α_2-agonist, guanfacine (Tenex), can be used in place of clonidine.

Behavioral or Psychological Interventions

In the large MTA study, a comprehensive behavioral intervention alone was compared with medication alone, a combination of behavioral intervention and medication, and standard community care (The MTA Cooperative Group, 1999). Medication was generally found to be more effective in reducing ADHD symptoms than behavioral intervention, and there were few differences between the combined treatment and medication alone in effectively managing ADHD symptoms. However, when it came to other domains of functioning, such as oppositional/aggressive symptoms, internalizing symptoms, teacher-rated social skills, parent–child relationships, and reading achievement, there was evidence that the combined treatment was superior to community care whereas medication alone was not. Behavioral interventions, when combined with medication, add an important dimension to the positive outcomes on the variables other than ADHD symptoms. In interpreting these results, the health care provider must keep in mind that the study was limited to school-age children, not adolescents.

The MTA study suggests the need to include behavioral interventions to have an impact on various issues other than ADHD symptoms (such as conduct disorder, oppositional-defiant disorder, poor self-esteem, family conflict, depression, anxiety disorders, and the use or abuse of alcohol and other drugs) that require attention. If the initial evaluation reveals a significant substance use disorder, the health care provider should refer the adolescent for a substance abuse workup or treatment before undertaking any additional intervention. The presence of oppositional behavior, family conflict, peer relationship difficulties, depression, or anxiety is an indication to refer the family for behavioral or psychological interventions. The most common behavioral or psychological interventions include family therapy, individual therapy, and social skills training. It is often useful for families with adolescents who are newly diagnosed with ADHD to have a burst of 10 to 15 sessions of behavioral or psychological intervention, followed by less frequent checkups. If new problems surface during a follow-up checkup, another burst of therapy may be scheduled. Individual therapy is usually helpful in building self-esteem and reducing anxiety but does not reliably result in behavioral changes in the classroom or at home.

Behavioral family system therapy is the treatment of choice for the home-based problems and conflicts between teenagers with ADHD and their parents. Early in treatment, the therapist divides the family issues into two categories: (a) nonnegotiable issues (basic rules for living in a family, such as no violence, drugs, or alcohol) and (b) negotiable issues (all other independence-related conflicts that may be subject to negotiation and compromise). Strategic structural intervention techniques are used to reinforce parental authority around the nonnegotiable issues (i.e., the therapist teaches the parents how to establish and consistently follow behavioral contracts for these basic rules). External authorities such as the juvenile justice system or mental health inpatient system are used to back up parents when they no longer have the ability to exert any control over the adolescents.

In the case of issues that can be negotiated between parents and adolescents, problem-solving communication training is used to teach parents and adolescents to work out mutually acceptable compromise solutions. The therapist instructs, models, and coaches the family to learn and practice the steps of problem solving: (a) clearly define the problem in a nonaccusatory manner; (b) brainstorm a list of alternative solutions; (c) systematically evaluate the positive or negative impacts of each solution, culminating in a mutually acceptable compromise solution; and (d) plan the details for implementing the solution. The family resolves a number of significant conflicts with the therapist present as a coach and then is given successively more complex assignments to apply problem-solving skills at home in weekly family meetings. As the family begins to practice problem-solving skills in the sessions and at home, the therapist targets negative communication patterns, again coaching families to replace accusatory, defensive language with more productive, goal-oriented language.

As part of an overall family intervention, it is also useful to teach parents the effective use of behavior modification techniques. A manual has been written to guide the health care provider in teaching parents contingency management techniques and integrating these techniques with problem-solving communication training (Barkley et al., 1999). These techniques are crucial for parents of adolescents with ADHD to help them teach their children to stay motivated to complete homework assignments and household chores. Setting up explicit rewards for appropriate activities and punishments for proscribed activities is a cornerstone of behavioral management. Health care providers can help parents with home interventions by offering advice on how to carry out simple behavioral contracts. Two clinical trials have now demonstrated the effectiveness of behavioral family systems therapy for reducing conflict between parents and their adolescents with ADHD (Barkley et al., 1992, 2001).

SUMMARY

In summary, health care providers can best help adolescents with ADHD and learning disabilities by encouraging them, believing that they can succeed, helping them to understand their disorder and how it affects them, mediating conflict between them and their parents, finding the optimal medication regimen (if appropriate), and helping them obtain the services they require through their school system and within their community.

WEB SITES

For Teenagers and Parents

http://www.chadd.org. Official Web site for the support group, Children and Adults with ADHD.

http://www.help4adhd.org/. National Resource Center on ADHD, funded cooperatively by the Centers for Disease Control and CHADD.

http://www.nimh.nih.gov/publicat/adhd.cfm. National Institutes of Health information on ADHD.

http://www.addvance.com. Commercial Web site, with link specifically for girls and women with ADHD.

http://www.add.org. National Attention Deficit Disorder Association (ADDA).

http://www.LDAAmerica.org. Learning Disabilities On Line.

http://www.wrightslaw.com. Commercial site for special education law and advocacy.

http://www.ideapractices.org. Information about the Individuals with Disabilities Act.

http://www.ldanatl.org. Learning Disabilities Association of America.

http://www.ed.gov/about/offices/list/osers/codi.html. Clearinghouse on Disability Information, Office of Special Education and Rehabilitative Services, U.S. Department of Education. Specializes in questions about funding, federal legislation, and federal programs that serve persons with disabilities at national, state, and local levels.

http://www.interdys.org. The International Dyslexia Association.

http://www.nichcy.org. National Dissemination Center for Children and Youth with Disabilities.

http://www.ncld.org. National Center for Learning Disabilities.

For Health Professionals

www.nichq.org/nichq/topics/chronicconditions/ADHD/ADHDhomepage.htm. National Initiative for Children's Healthcare Quality (NICHQ) Web site, with link to the ADHD Toolkit.

REFERENCES AND ADDITIONAL READINGS

Achenbach T. Subtyping ADHD: a request for suggestions about relating empirically based assessment to DSM-IV. *ADHD Rep* 1996;4(4):5.

Ahmann PA, Waltonen SJ, Olson KA, et al. Placebo controlled evaluation of ritalin side effects. *Pediatrics* 1993;91:1101.

Ambalavanan G, Holten KB. How should we evaluate and treat ADHD in children and adolescents. *J Fam Pract* 2005;54 (12):1058.

Ambrosini PJ, Bianchi MD, Rabinovich H, et al. Antidepressant treatments in children and adolescents. 11. Anxiety, physical, and behavioral disorders. *J Am Acad Child Adolesc Psychiatry* 1993;32:483.

American Academy of Pediatrics. *Diagnostic and statistical manual for primary care (DSM-PC)*, Child and adolescent version. Elk Grove, IL: American Academy of Pediatrics; 1996.

American Academy of Pediatrics. Clinical practice guideline: diagnosis and evaluation of the child with attention-deficit/ hyperactivity disorder. *Pediatrics* 2000;105:1158.

American Academy of Pediatrics. Clinical practice guideline: treatment of the school-aged child with attention-deficit/hyperactivity disorder. *Pediatrics* 2001;108:1033.

American Psychiatric Association. *The diagnostic and statistical manual of mental disorders, text revision*, 4th ed. Washington, DC: American Psychiatric Association; 2000.

Barkley R. *ADHD and the nature of self-control*. New York: Guilford Press; 1997.

Barkley R. *Attention deficit hyperactivity disorder: a handbook for diagnosis and treatment*. New York: Guilford Press; 1998.

Barkley RA, Edwards G, Laneri M, et al. The efficacy of problem-solving communication training alone, behavior management training alone, and their combination for parent-adolescent conflict in teenagers with ADHD and ODD. *J Consult Clin Psychol* 2001;69:926.

Barkley R, Edwards G, Robin AL. *Defiant teens: a clinician's manual for assessment and family intervention*. New York: Guilford Press; 1999.

Barkley RA, Guevremont DG, Anastopoulous AD, et al. A comparison of three family therapy programs for treating family conflict in adolescents with attention-deficit hyperactivity disorder. *J Consult Clin Psychol* 1992;60:450.

Biederman J, Wilens T, Mick E, et al. Pharmacotherapy of attention-deficit/hyperactivity disorder reduces risk for substance use disorder. *Pediatrics* 1999;104(2):e20.

Brown TE. *Brown attention-deficit disorder scales manual*. San Antonio: The Psychological Corporation; 1996.

Brown RT, Amler RW, Freeman WS, et al. American Academy of Pediatrics Committee on Quality Improvement. American Academy of Pediatrics Subcommittee on Attention-Deficit/Hyperactivity Disorder. Treatment of attention-deficit/hyperactivity disorder: overview of the evidence. *Pediatrics* 2005;115(6):e749.

Castellanos FX, Lee PP, Sharp W, et al. Developmental trajectories of brain volume abnormalities in children and adolescents with attention deficit/hyperactivity disorder. *JAMA* 2002;288:1740.

Christman AK, Fermo JD, Markowitz JS. Atomoxetine, a novel treatment for attention-deficit-hyperactivity disorder. *Pharmacotherapy* 2004;24:1020.

DePaul GJ, Stoner G. *ADHD in the schools: assessment and intervention strategies*. New York: Guilford Press; 1994.

DeVries BB, Halley DJ, Oostra BA, et al. The fragile X syndrome. *J Med Genet* 1998;35(7):579.

Dworkin PH. School failure. *Pediatr Rev* 1989;10:301.

Faigel HC, Sznajderman S, Tishby O, et al. Attention deficit disorder during adolescence: a review. *J Adolesc Health* 1995;16:174.

Fischer M, Barkley RA, Fletcher K, et al. The adolescent outcome of hyperactive children: predictors of psychiatric, academic, social, and emotional adjustment. *J Am Acad Child Adolesc Psychiatry* 1993;32:324.

Gadow KD, Sverd J. Attention deficit hyperactivity disorder, chronic tic disorder, and methylphenidate. *Adv Neurol* 2006;99:197.

Gadow KD, Sverd J, Sprafkin J, et al. Efficacy of methylphenidate for attention-deficit hyperactivity disorder in children with tic disorder. *Arch Gen Psychiatry* 1995;52:444.

Goyette CH, Conners CK, Ulrich RE, et al. Attention-deficit/hyperactivity disorder in children and adolescents: interventions for a complex costly clinical conundrum. *Pediatr Clin North Am* 2003;50:1049.

Illingworth R. Early failure of the famous. *Pediatrician* 1986;13:70.

Levy HB, Harper CR, Weinberg WA. A practical approach to children failing in school. *Pediatr Clin North Am* 1992;39:895.

Lipkin PH, Goldstein IJ, Adesman AR. Tics and dyskinesias associated with stimulant treatment in attention-deficit hyperactivity disorder. *Arch Pediatr Adolesc Med* 1994;148:859.

The MTA Cooperative Group. A 14-month randomized clinical trial of treatment strategies for attention deficit/hyperactivity disorder. *Arch Gen Psychiatry* 1999;56:1088.

Nadeau KG, Littman EB, Quinn PO. *Understanding girls with AD/HD*. Silver Spring, MD: Advantage Press; 1999.

Palmer FB, Capute AJ. Mental retardation. *Pediatr Rev* 1994;15:473.

Palumbo D, Lynch PA. Psychological testing in adolescent medicine. *Adolesc Med Clin* 2006;17(1):147.

Prince JB. Pharmacotherapy of attention-deficit hyperactivity disorder in children and adolescents: update on new stimulant preparations, atomoxetine, and novel treatments. *Child Adolesc Psychiatr Clin N Am* 2006;15(1):13.

Rappley MD. Attention deficit-hyperactivity disorder. *N Engl J Med* 2005;352:165.

Reiff MI, Stein MT. Attention-deficit/hyperactivity disorder evaluation and diagnosis, a practical approach in office practice. *Pediatr Clin North Am* 2003;50:1019.

Robin AL. Training families with ADHD adolescents. In: Barkley R, ed. *Attention deficit hyperactivity disorder: a handbook for diagnosis and treatment*, 2nd ed. New York: Guilford Press; 1998a:413.

Robin AL. *ADHD in adolescents: diagnosis and treatment*. New York: Guilford Press; 1998b.

Robin AL, Foster SL. *Negotiating parent-adolescent conflict: a behavioral family systems perspective*. New York: Guilford Press; 1989.

Rourke BP. *Nonverbal learning disabilities*. New York: Guilford Press; 1989.

Rubenstein JS, Hastings EM. School refusal in adolescence: understanding the symptom. *Adolescence* 1980;15:775.

Schubiner H, Robin AL. Attention-deficit/hyperactivity disorder in adolescence. *Adolesc Health Update* 1998;10(2):1.

Spencer T, Biederman J, Wilens T. Tricyclic antidepressant treatment of children with ADHD and tic disorders. *J Am Acad Child Adolesc Psychiatry* 1994;33:8.

Steingard R, Biederman J, Spencer T, et al. Comparison of clonidine response in the treatment of attention deficit hyperactivity disorder with and without comorbid tic disorders. *J Am Acad Child Adolesc Psychiatry* 1993;32:350.

Swank LK. Specific developmental disorders. *Child Adolesc Psychiatr Clin N Am* 1999;8:89.

U. S. Food and Drug Administration, Center for Drug Evaluation and Research. (September 29, 2005). *FDA Alert [9/05]: Suicidal Thinking in Children and Adolescents* (Alert posted on the World Wide Web). Washington, DC. Retrieved November 1, 2005 from the World Wide Web:. http://www.fda.gov/cder/drug/infosheets/hcp/atomoxetinehcp.htm

Wilens TE, Biederman J, Spencer T. Clonidine for sleep disturbances with attention-deficit hyperactivity disorder. *J Am Acad Child Adolesc Psychiatry* 1994;33:424.

Wilens TE, Faraone SV, Biederman J, et al. Does stimulant therapy of attention-deficit/hyperactivity disorder beget later substance abuse? a meta-analytic review of the literature. *Pediatrics* 2003;111:179.

Wolraich ML, Wibbelsman CJ, Brown TE, et al. Attention-deficit/hyperactivity disorder among adolescents: a review of the diagnosis, treatment, and clinical implications. *Pediatrics* 2005;115(6):1734.

CHAPTER 81

Sexual Assault and Victimization

Vaughn I. Rickert, Owen Ryan, and Mariam R. Chacko

SEXUAL ASSAULT

Sexual assault and victimization among adolescents and young adults has been referred to as a hidden epidemic because of the high rates of occurrence and its infrequent disclosure (Rickert et al., 2004). In fact, female adolescents aged 16 to 19 years and young adults 20 to 24 years of age, are 4 times more likely to be sexually assaulted than women in all other age-groups (Golding et al., 1997). Since prevalence estimates of sexual victimization have been largely geared toward women and those in heterosexual relationships, prevalence of victimization among adolescents and young adults in same gender relationships is yet to be determined. Regardless, in most instances among adolescents and young adults, the perpetrator of sexual victimization is a date or an acquaintance rather than a stranger.

Sexual assault and victimization is one of the most devastating encounters a person can experience and can dramatically change the victim's view of self and the world. The victim is the object of a hostile, dehumanizing attack that can have long-lasting effects on concepts of self-worth and identity. This is particularly true for the adolescent who is learning to manage feelings of sexual arousal, developing new forms of intimacy and autonomy, experiencing intimate interpersonal relationships, and building skills to control the consequences of sexual behavior. Sexual victimization or attempted assault as a first or early sexual experience may cause confusion between intercourse and violence and can jeopardize the person's sexual health.

The disclosure of sexual assault and victimization requires prompt medical and psychological intervention, but is rarely forthcoming. When forensic evidence is required, as in the case of sexual assault, only those primary care providers who are willing to devote the time and support needed should examine the sexual assault victim. Equally as important is a clinician's familiarity with the proper protocol for intervention including clinical, legal, and psychosocial techniques.

Provider-initiated screening to detect sexual victimization represents an important public health strategy to overcome the difficulty that some victims face when disclosing these violent events (Irwin and Rickert, 2005). Currently, fewer than half of providers routinely screen their adult patients for intimate partner violence; the prevalence or acceptability of screening practices among adolescents and young adults is unknown.

The terms used to describe the range of victimizations included in sexual assault are sometimes used interchangeably and yet not often particularly clear. Some of these terms have legal ramifications and reporting requirements that greatly impact prevalence and incidence rates. Following is a list of terms and definitions that will help provide a solid understanding of terminology used in the rest of this chapter. If a work is cited that has used a different definition, that definition is provided.

Sexual assault: Any act, either physical or verbal, of a sexual nature committed against another person that is accompanied by actual or threatened physical force. Sexual assault is an umbrella term that contains several different aspects of sexual violence and victimization.

Rape: Rape is a legal term with a definition that varies widely from state to state. In general, this term implies unlawful nonconsensual sexual activity carried out forcibly or under threat of injury against the will of the victim. Nonconsensual sex can be divided into two categories—those perpetrated by a stranger and those perpetrated by an acquaintance. *Stranger rape* applies to the former whereas the term *acquaintance rape* refers to the latter. *Date rape*, nonconsensual sex that occurs between two people in a romantic relationship, is a subset of acquaintance rape.

Sexual abuse: Usually refers to the sexual victimization of a minor. In certain contexts, the term can include consensual sex between minors or a minor and an adult (*statutory rape*, see "Legal Issues" section). Occasionally, the terms *incest* and *intrafamilial sex* become confused with sexual abuse. We define *incest* as sexual intercourse between closely related persons while *intrafamilial* sex consists of intercourse in a caregiving situation—both are forms of abuse. Sexual abuse, as with rape, is also primarily a legal term.

Epidemiology of Sexual Assault

The Bureau of Justice Statistic's (BJS) 2004 National Crime Victimization Survey (NCVS) reports that although aggregate numbers for violent crime reached their lowest point since 1973, aggregate numbers for rape and sexual assault rose by 6%. To understand the trend more precisely, however, it is necessary to consider these crimes separately. When rape (defined as forced penetration perpetrated on either a man or a woman) is considered by itself, there is a decrease of 28% in reported cases since 2001. Alternately, the more expansive category of sexual assault has seen consistent increases during the same time—a trend masked by the overall drop in reported rape cases. The disparity in these two trends emphasizes the need to consider sexual assault more broadly. According to NCVS, of the 203,680 rape and sexual assault cases where a female was the victim, only 34% of perpetrators were identified as strangers. Amongst the 6,200 male rape and sexual assault victims, a stranger perpetrated 50% of the attacks. Therefore, in a large majority of sexual assault cases, the victim knew the perpetrator.

Several studies have highlighted a significant period of vulnerability for adolescent females. The vast majority of assaults occur between the ages of 12 and 24 years with the largest number occurring between the ages of 16 and 24 years. Reporting of rape and sexual assault has remained inconsistent since 1993 with a high of approximately 50% reported in 2002 and a low of 30% throughout the 1990s. Currently, the reporting rate rests between 35% and 40%. However, providers must understand that prevalence estimates, especially trend analyses, are not without problems. Depending on the survey, different definitions are employed. For example, the BJS surveys exclude rape and sexual assault that result in homicide and the FBI's Uniform Crime Reporting (UCR) Program identifies rape as "carnal knowledge of a female forcibly and against her will." Additionally, surveys that rely on police reports are often skewed by socioeconomic status. Therefore, prevalence estimates must be cautiously compared. Stratification of sexual assault estimates by demographic characteristics can be difficult to generalize and inappropriately interpreted.

1. Risk factors
   a. Females: Age 16 to 19 years and 20 to 24 years
   b. A history of abuse (sexual or other) as a child or adolescent
   c. For females with younger age at menarche, greater number of dating and/or sexual partners, and a sexually active peer group
   d. For males, homelessness and disability (physical, cognitive, psychiatric)
   e. Alcohol use by perpetrator or victim, especially in a dating situation
   f. Dating relationships that include verbal or physical abuse
2. Incidence
   a. In the 2005 Centers for Disease Control and Prevention (CDC, 2006) National Health Risk Behavior Surveillance report on adolescents, 7.5% of youth, 10.8% of females, and 4.2% of males reported that they had been forced to have sexual intercourse.
   b. A recent study reported that 1 in 12 children and youth (82 per 1,000) aged 2 to 17 years had experienced one or more sexual victimization during their lifetime; 32 per 1,000 had experienced a sexual assault; and 22 per 1,000 had experienced a completed or attempted rape (Finkelhor et al., 2005).
   c. Adults are responsible for a few victimizations (15% of general sexual victimizations and 29% of sexual assault) confirming that a vast majority of victimizations are perpetrated by peer acquaintances (Finkelhor et al., 2005).

d. A 2000 survey by the National Center for Juvenile Justice found that two thirds of sexual assault victimizations reported to the police involved juvenile victims.
e. In the U.S. Department of Justice's (DOJ) "Full Report of the Prevalence, Incidence and Consequences of Violence Against Women," 17.6% of surveyed women stated they had been the victim of a completed or attempted rape at some time in their lives. Of those with a history of rape, 21.6% were younger than 12 years when they were first raped, 32.4% were aged 12 to 17. Therefore 9% of women in the overall population reported being a victim of sexual assault before the age of 18 years.
f. Adolescents $\leq$18 years who experience sexual victimization are twice as likely to experience a future assault during their college years.
g. Approximately 60% of sexual assaults occur at home or at the home of an acquaintance.
h. The incidence of reported rapes is higher during the summer months and on weekends, and approximately two thirds of sexual assaults occur between 6 p.m. and 6 a.m. Sexual assaults are least frequent in December (FBI, 1999). The National Center for Juvenile Justice study found that there was increased vulnerability for adolescents and young adults immediately after school (3 p.m.) and later at night (between 11 p.m. and midnight).
i. Forceful verbal resistance, physical resistance, and fleeing were all associated with rape avoidance, whereas nonforceful verbal resistance and no resistance were associated with being raped. Injury rates were no higher in women who used forceful resistance.
j. Use of date rape drugs such as gamma hydroxybutyrate (GHB) acid and flunitrazepam (Rohypnol) are of concern, but limited data are available as to the prevalence of their use. Unfortunately, testing for these agents is compromised by time and drug test facilities (Weir, 2001).
3. Sequelae
   Most of the sexual violence that clinicians will encounter when treating adolescents and young women is that which has been perpetrated by an acquaintance or, in fact, a date. As a result, spontaneous disclosure of the victimization is not likely—either because the young person does not perceive this as a sexual assault, they are embarrassed, or they believe it is their own fault. Clinicians need to be aware of the sequelae that result from sexual victimization of adolescents to more appropriately identify youth in need of services.

   Some of the reactions of adolescent victims are similar to those of adults, but there are important differences stemming from the developmental tasks facing adolescents. The major developmental tasks of adolescents include individuation and emancipation, intimacy, identity formation, and mastery, all of which may be affected by the experience of sexual victimization. Such an event often disrupts the adolescent's sense of equilibrium and growing identity. The assault itself and the reactions of family members may inhibit the growing need for independence and autonomy. Adolescent victims must deal with the realization that the events may not be under their control, a fact that may delay successful emancipation. Identity formation issues often cause adolescent victims to question their sense of self and sexuality. In the aftermath, an adolescent may act in an unexpected bizarre or inappropriate manner; for example, he or she may be aggressive or withdrawn, resent peer and parental attention, or act as if nothing happened.

Much of the specialized research in the study of sexual assault has focused solely on stranger rape, and, while these are important findings, they do not address the vast majority of sexual victimizations that occur in this population. The information provided in the following text has been broadened to include findings from research aimed to identify sequelae of sexual violence in general.

Adolescents who have been victimized experience significantly higher levels of depression and anxiety. Male and female high school–aged victims report decreased life satisfaction coupled with suicidal ideation and attempts. An adolescent's sexual health is greatly impacted by victimization. Typically, sexually victimized youth engage in higher risk sexual behaviors, have poorer attitudes and beliefs regarding sex, and demonstrate a greater prevalence of consequences from sexual activity, that is, unintended pregnancies and sexually transmitted diseases (STDs).

Several common responses to victimization among adolescents include the following:
a. Phobias
b. Somatic reactions
c. Self-blame
d. Loss of appetite
e. Sleep disturbance
f. Somatic responses

Sequelae particular to date rape may include self-blame, decreased self-esteem, and a difficult time maintaining relationships. Somatic responses can manifest as chronic pelvic pain or recurrent abdominal pain. In the most general case, the first 2 months postvictimization is a time of particular vulnerability for severe depression. Signs of post-traumatic stress disorder are not uncommon within the first year (Rickert et al., 2003).

Data suggest a link between sexual victimization, alcohol, and illicit drug use. These adolescents or young adults can be 2 or even 3 times as likely to begin using illicit drugs, smoke, or regularly consume alcohol as compared to their nonvictimized peers (Diaz et al., 2002).

SEXUAL ABUSE

1. Incidence
   In 2005, the National Child Abuse and Neglect Data System (NCANDS) published the findings of its 2003 survey. Their data is derived from substantiated claims of abuse filed by state child welfare agencies. In 2003, sexual abuse accounted for 10% of all victimizations of children, totaling 45,634 cases—4 of which resulted in the death of the child. Unlike other types of child victimization that have seen recent declines, child sexual abuse has remained constant at 1.2 children per every 1,000. The most recent National Incidence Survey (NIS) found that girls were 3 times as likely as boys to be sexually abused, and that vulnerability to sexual abuse remained consistent after age 3.

   The NCANDS statistics confirm that adolescents and young adults are most vulnerable to sexual abuse at the hands of those closest to them. Sixty-nine percent of perpetrators were a parent, a relative, or a partner to the parent—the largest percentages falling in the first two categories. It has also been shown that sexual abuse cases are less likely to receive services from child welfare agencies than any other type of abuse. Reasons for this disparity were not explored.

   Only 8.5% of sexual abuse case reporting came from medical professionals, just slightly higher than the 7.9% reported by parents. This figure underscores the acute need for trained medical professionals who feel comfortable and are skilled at screening for victimization.

2. Situations that should alert the provider to suspect abuse:
   a. STD infection (including gonorrhea, syphilis, herpes, *Trichomonas* infection, and condylomata) in a prepubertal adolescent or any adolescent with no history of sexual intercourse.
   b. Recurrent somatic complaints, particularly involving the gastrointestinal, genitourinary, or pelvic areas.
   c. Behavioral indicators include:
      • Significant change in mood, onset of withdrawal from usual family, school, and social activities
      • Patterns of disordered eating
      • Running away from home
      • Suicidal and self-injurious gestures
      • Rapid escalation of alcohol and/or drug abuse
      • Onset of promiscuous sexual activity
      • Early adolescent pregnancy
      • Onset of sexual activity before age 13 years
      • Sexualized play in the prepubescent child

3. Sequelae
   The occurrence of sexual abuse during childhood has been linked to a variety of psychological and emotional problems during adolescence, with some continuing into adulthood. The relationship between severity of abuse, frequency of abuse, and subsequent mental health disorders remains elusive. Some data suggest a strong and positive relationship between severity of abuse and subsequent symptom expression, while other studies do not. Regardless, sequelae include depression, suicidal ideation and attempts, substance abuse, post-traumatic stress disorder, eating disorders, and precocious sexual behaviors (e.g., earlier age at first coitus and greater number of lifetime partners). In addition, childhood sexual abuse for females has been linked to acquaintance and date rape as an adolescent or young adult. Therefore, victims of child sexual abuse are likely to present with a number of immediate psychological and emotional sequelae and have subsequent symptoms during the recovery process.

UNDERSERVED POPULATIONS

Male Adolescents

Male adolescents who have been sexually abused are often overlooked and underserved. Most studies of victimization are weighted toward younger children or females. However, male sexual abuse is not uncommon and is significantly underreported. Since most perpetrators of sexual violence against adolescent males are male themselves, these victims may remain silent due to the homosexual aspect of an assault. In addition, practitioners may fail to recognize and pursue this possibility because of their lack of awareness of this problem.

Gay, Lesbian, and Bisexual

A small amount of research has been conducted on violence in same sex relationships. Of these, there is an even smaller amount that is applicable or can be generalized toward gay and lesbian adolescents (or those with same gender sexual partners). Critics maintain that studies of gay and lesbian populations either tend not to use standardized measures or provide obscure data regarding victim/perpetrator relationship.

A recent study attempted to map out victimization of gay, lesbian, and bisexual men and women across their lifetime (Balsam et al., 2005). The results identified a dramatically increased risk of child sexual abuse and adolescent victimization amongst gay, lesbian, and bisexual persons. Over the lifetime, gay and bisexual men were 5 times more likely to be sexually assaulted than heterosexual men; lesbian and bisexual women were twice as likely as heterosexual women.

As a comparison group, the researchers used heterosexual siblings of the sexual minority participants. They were able to identify that even within family groups, sexual orientation was a significant predictor of sexual victimization either by persons within the family or outside of it.

Research such as this can easily become tied up in misdirected debates of causality (e.g., did the childhood victimization result in homosexuality or bisexuality?) and thereby make claims of particular vulnerability difficult. With little doubt, although, it can be asserted that there is a great disparity in regard to sexual victimization between sexual orientations.

Transgendered Adolescents

There is limited research identifying the particular vulnerabilities of transgendered adolescents and young adults in regard to sexual victimization. This is an area of acute concern considering the data showing increased sexual health risks amongst transgendered men and women.

Developmentally Delayed Children

The NCANDS (2005) found that children with disabilities accounted for 6.5% of all victims. Disabilities included mental retardation, emotional disturbance, visual impairment, learning disability, physical disability, behavioral problems, or another medical problem. It is important for the clinician to remember that these data reflect substantiated cases of abuse; children with such conditions are undercounted as not every child receives a clinical diagnostic assessment by child protective service. Specific data for teens with disabilities are not available.

Earlier studies conducted among developmentally delayed populations suggest that most victims were women (72%). However, these studies included developmentally delayed individuals who had little difficulty with verbal communication. As expected, most of the perpetrators were men (88%) and included other individuals with mental retardation, paid staff, family members, and others. Most sexual abuse occurred in the victim's residence, and in 92% of cases the victim knew the abuser (Furey, 1994).

Homeless/Street Youth

Studies have found that homeless and street youth are particularly vulnerable to victimization and violence. One study noted that 85% of surveyed homeless youth had experienced violence, 34% of whom were sexually assaulted. The numbers highlight that not only are homeless youth more prone to sexual violence but youth who have been sexually victimized are prone to homelessness as well—15% of youth living on the street were victimized before their homelessness (Kipke et al., 1997).

DISCLOSURE AND REPORTING

Screening

Disclosure of sexual assault as well as sexual victimization is rarely spontaneous and often deeply impacted by the adolescent's or young adult's beliefs surrounding their own victimization. Such sensitive information is more often revealed weeks or months after the assault rather than within a timeline in which emergency room care could be beneficial (Rickert et al., 2004). This lapse leaves primary care providers with an obligation to inquire about past and present sexual victimization in as sensitive a manner as possible.

1. Screening measures: There are currently several useful screening measures that can be easily employed by a clinician and take <15 minutes.
   a. Home, Education, Activities Drugs, Depression, Suicidal ideation, Sex, Safety (HEADSSS) inventory: As listed in Chapter 3, the HEADSSS inventory is a helpful device to collect important psychosocial information. Other screening tools for adolescents and young adults include:
   b. Conflict in Adolescent Relationship Inventory (Wolfe et al., 2001)
   c. Sexual Experience Survey (Koss and Oros, 1982)
   d. Date and Family Violence and Abuse Scale (Symons et al., 1994)
   e. Sexual Aggression Questionnaire (Muehlenhard and Linton, 1987)
   In addition, information pamphlets designed to help patients self-screen for dating violence or to increase awareness of sexual health issues can also be helpful. Some clinicians also find *anticipatory guidance,* a conversation centering on sexual health risk factors and warning signs for violence in partners, more helpful in completely serving the adolescent's needs.
2. Screening process: Regardless of what sources are used, screening is a very delicate process. It is as important to elicit information of possible victimization as it is to create a supportive environment for the adolescent patient.
   a. Barriers: The main barriers for not disclosing information are mistrust of adults and professionals, a fear of the consequences of disclosure for their family and offender, and ignorance of the existence of protective agencies.
   b. Environments: Environments that allow adolescents to talk and have their concerns valued, can do much to overcome these obstacles.

Within the patient/clinician conversation, adolescents should be provided *accurate information* about the help they can receive from their social network, protective agencies, rape crisis centers, and hotlines. It is recommended that the screening take place in *a private, quiet space* where only the provider and the adolescent or young adult are present. An example of an icebreaker that prepares the patient for some of the questions they will be asked is,

> Because I want to help my patients, I ask everyone about topics that may be very sensitive or may make you uncomfortable. Sadly, some young adults come to my office having been hurt by people around them. It is important that I know those things to be able to help them out.

The concept of *limited confidentiality* should be introduced to the patient in a manner that conveys the legal obligations of the clinician, should any disclosure occur. Some providers choose to use a direct but nonthreatening statement similar to,

> Generally, what you say in here stays in here, but there are some exceptions. If I feel that you may hurt yourself or someone else, or that you have been abused by someone, I will need to talk to others to help make sure you get all the care you need.

Consistently asking patients about sexual history, even if negative answers were received in prior instances, can allow for this part of the examination to become more routine.

a. Sexual history: Once these preliminary steps have been taken, a provider can begin to collect a sexual history that includes sexual partners and experience, any unwanted touch, or previous victimization. The incidence rate amongst young women makes this step in their care especially necessary.
b. Examination: If the patient discloses that injuries were sustained, a thorough examination, consented to by the patient and described in detail in the section "Physical Examination", will be required. This consent must not be general. The adolescent will need to know and consent to the specific purpose and procedures involved in the examination, including the stages of a rape kit.

It should be noted that for those adolescents who have experienced a recent victimization or are seeking treatment because of assault, it may be important to have *a family member or friend present* for the examination. Additionally, the provider can help the victim regain a sense of control over his or her body by encouraging them to make as many decisions during their examination as possible. It is crucial that the victim be informed that he or she is in control of what will be done and that, at any point, they can refuse examination, treatment, or stop the examination. For further clinical interventions in sexual violence refer to the section "General Forensic Background".

Reporting

The following professional guidelines have been endorsed by several prominent organizations regarding the screening and reporting of sexual victimization among adolescents and young adults (Society for Adolescent Medicine, 2004).

1. Sexual activity and sexual abuse are not synonymous. It should not be assumed that adolescents who are sexually active are, by definition, being abused. Many adolescents have consensual sexual relationships.
2. It is critical that adolescents who are sexually active received appropriate confidential health care and counseling.
3. Open and confidential communication between the health professional and the adolescent patient, together with careful clinical assessment, can identify most sexual abuse cases.
4. Physicians and other health professionals must know their state laws and report cases of sexual abuse to the proper authority, in accordance with those laws, after discussion with the adolescent and parent as appropriate.
5. Federal and state laws should support physicians and other health care professionals and their role in providing confidential health care to their adolescent patients.
6. Federal and state laws should affirm the authority of physicians and other health care professionals to exercise appropriate clinical judgment in reporting cases of sexual activity.

Their position stresses the power of health care workers involved in primary care to clinically assess for sexual abuse or victimization. It equally emphasizes how state and federal laws that require health care providers to report particular sexual activity to adults responsible for the child's care impede this power.

LEGAL ISSUES RELATED TO REPORTING OF SEXUAL ASSAULT AND VICTIMIZATION

All 50 states require reporting of sexual abuse (also referred to as sexual assault) of minors; but there are a variety of ways in which states approach these issues under their mandatory child abuse reporting laws. Many states laws include a definition of sexual abuse, sexual intercourse, and other sexual acts that involve minors under a specific age (Society for Adolescent Medicine, 2004). Some states include only abuse that is perpetrated by parents, guardians, custodians, or caretakers, while others include acts of unrelated third parties. There are also state statutes for the screening and reporting of domestic violence, partner abuse, and violent injuries that may apply to adolescents and young adults. The child abuse and other reporting laws however, do not always encompass all aspects of assault and victimization and therefore some issues, such as victimization that occurs between adolescent and young adult dating partners, may fall outside the purview of mandatory reporting.

Every state has mandatory reporting of a reasonable suspicion of child abuse, including sexual abuse, to a designated authority. Mandated reporters of child abuse include virtually all medical and health professionals involved in the care of adolescents. The abuse does not need to be proved before being reported. An area of concern is that confidentiality is broken when abuse is reported, whether the teen or family does or does not want the incident reported. Society has determined that the public's right to protect a victim of child abuse supersedes a patient's right of privacy. This leads to more reporting of suspected abuse, but less protection of physician–patient confidentiality. In the role of mandated reporters, health care professionals are generally afforded legal immunity for making reports of suspected abuse. Failure to report can result in civil liability or criminal penalties.

In recent years, there has been an increased effort at the federal level and in many states to increase the reporting by health care providers of sexual activity involving minors under child abuse reporting laws. In addition, an area of potential confusion and controversy is the reporting of "statutory rape." Although this term does not appear in most states' laws, it is generally used to refer to sexual intercourse that is illegal even if it is consensual; and can refer either to sexual contact between two minors or between a minor and an adult. Policy makers at the federal and state levels have attempted to increase the enforcement of statutory rape laws, partially in response to suggested links between teenage pregnancy and "statutory rape."

Many states have attempted to increase the reporting of sexually active minors under child abuse reporting laws, either through legislative and policy changes or enforcement of existing laws. These efforts have focused particular attention on younger adolescents who are sexually active. An area of particular confusion and controversy is the reporting of statutory rape—defined as consenting sexual contact between two minors or one minor and an adult. At least one state has attached legislative riders to state appropriations measures for programs that provide family planning services, imposing specific conditions on service contracts for these programs (Title V, X, XX, and Medicaid). In that state, according to health department regulations, these funds will only be distributed to recipients who show good faith efforts to comply with all child abuse reporting guidelines and requirements. Health departments conduct random monitoring of records of minors on an annual basis. The impact of implementing these measures is yet unknown. However, based on experience, many providers sense that law enforcement officials do not process most of these reports.

In summary, there are a variety of considerations that can have a bearing on when sexual activity, especially in a young adolescent, must be reported. These include use of coercion or pressure, force or the threat of force, or a wide age difference between partners even if the adolescent and parent(s) consider the current relationship consensual and nonabusive. Owing to the variations in reporting laws among states, it is essential that health care providers consult their local legal and medical authorities regarding laws for their state and be aware of their institution policies as it relates to the screening and reporting of child abuse, sexual abuse, sexual victimization, and violence.

EVALUATION OF SEXUAL ABUSE AND ASSAULT IN ADOLESCENTS: MEDICAL AND FORENSIC ASPECTS

Medical Evaluation

The following pages are meant as a guide for clinicians performing medical examinations on sexually victimized adolescents and young adults. It is important to understand that a large majority of these individuals will present with conditions that do not lend themselves to examination. Victimizations of coercion or date rape can often involve "forced consent," leaving the victim with more palpable psychological scars than physical.

Owing to the burden of incidence on young women, the information provided is skewed toward the perspective of a female victim. Following the information on forensic examination and treatment, there is a special note on STD prevalence in sexual victimization and a smaller piece on the legal processes involved in prosecution.

General Forensic Background

Facilitating an Appropriate Medical Examination
Medical and mental health providers who suspect that their patient has experienced sexual victimization during the course of their clinical practice need to facilitate an appropriate medical examination based on established procedures. Clearly, the earlier an examination is performed the more likely the evidence of trauma will be noted. Because this is an extremely vulnerable situation for the victim, only practitioners with the time, sensitivity, and training required to conduct a full examination should do so.

Physicians and nurses have an obligation to provide care to victims, which involves being both a "medical detective" (being able to provide a legal defense in all cases including those in which a *rape kit* may or may not have been done) and a supportive care provider. Therefore, these individuals must be trained and comfortable in examining the sexually abused or assaulted adolescent. The training includes the ability to complete a *rape kit*, and to have knowledge of internal and external genital and anal anatomy in females and males. It also includes the ability to be vigilant in the documentation of a detailed history of acute and chronic traumatic injuries. To the experienced examiner, what might otherwise seem like subtle findings can actually be determinants of previous trauma to the genital area.

Facilitating Appropriate Forensic Procedures
The *rape kit* enables collection of evidence such as semen, clothing, and debris for forensic examination. In some jurisdictions, the cutoff period for collecting evidence for the *rape kit* has been extended beyond the standard 72 hours of a sexual abuse or assault incident, since sperm has been identified in the cervix up to a week later even after showering and bathing. In addition, the availability of deoxyribonucleic acid (DNA) amplification technology now used to identify assailants more accurately allows for collecting evidence beyond the 72-hour period (American Academy of Pediatrics, 2001; U.S. Department of Justice, Office on Violence Against Women, 2004). Individual jurisdictions determine the maximum time interval (36 hours to 1 week) in which evidence may be collected. Changing clothes, showering, brushing teeth can also change the yield of the forensic examination.

In the event that the adolescent declines a forensic examination, a speculum examination should not be undertaken to obtain STD tests until after 96 hours. This allows the victim the time to change her mind and permit a forensic examination within the designated time. A speculum examination conducted before forensic work will call into question the accuracy of evidence that may later be collected.

Magnification Aids and Photography

Magnification aids and photography are not absolutely necessary but can be useful in the evaluation and documentation of genital trauma. Photographs can provide an accurate record of significant genital injuries and fresh trauma (bloody tears and complete clefts). They can also be available at a later date for a second opinion. However, photographs and magnification may not be as helpful in documenting subtle findings such as erythema, swelling, or small labial tears. Providers have typically used the colposcope because it has excellent magnification, light, and a built-in 35-mm camera with approximately 12 in. between the examiner and the body. An alternative to the colposcope is the medscope, an adapted dental camera that takes digital prints. It has greater depth of field, can be used to document injuries elsewhere on the body, and

is easy to operate, portable, and less cumbersome than the colposcope. Images are taken using the foot, freeing the hands to conduct the examination and reducing the risk of contaminating the evidence. Since the medscope does not have definite magnification ranges like the colposcope, the digital prints cannot be enlarged or reprinted like 35-mm prints (U.S. Department of Justice, Office of Justice Programs, Office for Victims of Crime Bulletin, 2001).

A clear protocol for the secure filing of print and digital photographs for forensic evidence will reassure a fearful adolescent about the security of the photographs.

Interpretation of Findings

A classification system has been developed by Adams (2004) to assist clinicians in the interpretation of physical

TABLE 81.1

Findings Diagnostic of Trauma and/or Sexual Contact[a]

1. Moderate specificity for abuse
   a. Acute lacerations or extensive bruising of labia, perihymenal tissues, penis, scrotum, or perineum (may be from unwitnessed accidental trauma).
   b. Scar of posterior fourchette (discrete, pale, off the midline). Scars are very difficult to assess unless acute injury at same location was documented.
   c. Fresh laceration of the posterior fourchette, not involving the hymen (must be differentiated from dehisced labial adhesion or failure of midline fusion, or may be caused by accidental injury).
   d. Perianal scar. Discrete, pale, off the midline (rare, difficult to assess unless acute injury at the same location was previously documented; may be due to other medical conditions such as Crohn disease, or previous medical procedures).
2. High specificity for abuse (diagnostic of blunt force penetrating trauma)
   a. Laceration (tear, partial or complete) of the hymen, acute.
   b. Ecchymosis (bruising) on the hymen.
   c. Perianal lacerations extending deep to the external anal sphincter (not to be confused with partial failure of midline fusion).
   d. Hymenal transection (healed). An area where the hymen has been torn through, to or nearly to the base, so there appears to be virtually no hymenal tissue remaining at that location, confirmed using additional examination techniques such as a swab, prone knee-chest position, Foley catheter, water to float the edge of the hymen. This finding has also been referred to as a *complete cleft* in sexually active adolescents and young women.
3. Presence of infection confirms mucosal contact with infected genital secretions; contact most likely to have been sexual in nature
   a. Positive confirmed culture for gonorrhea, from genital area, anus, and throat, in a child outside the neonatal period.
   b. Confirmed diagnosis of syphilis, if perinatal transmission is ruled out.
   c. *Trichomonas vaginalis* infection in a child older than 1 year, with organisms identified (by an experienced technician or clinician) in vaginal secretions by wet mount examination or by culture.
   d. Positive culture from genital or anal tissues for *Chlamydia*. If child is older than 3 years at time of diagnosis, and specimen was tested using cell culture or comparable method approved by the Centers for Disease Control and Prevention. Positive serology for HIV, if neonatal transmission and transmission from blood products has been ruled out.
4. Diagnostic of sexual contact
   a. Pregnancy.
   b. Sperm identified in specimens taken directly from a child's body.

HIV, human immunodeficiency virus.
[a]Findings which in the absence of a clear, timely, plausible history of accidental injury or nonsexual transmission should be reported to child protective services.
Adapted from Adam J, Medical evaluation of suspected sexual abuse. *J Pediatr Adolesc Gynecol* 2004;17:191 (with permission).

and laboratory findings and to provide an opinion as to the likelihood of sexual abuse or assault in children and adolescents (Table 81.1).

Conducting the Medical History

- If a rape kit is being completed, consent needs to be obtained from the adolescent for the forensic examination, treatment, collection of evidence, and release of medical records.
- A brief description of the incident including body parts touched, orifices penetrated, the geographic location of the assault, identity of the assailant or alleged perpetrator (if known), whether a condom was used, whether any bleeding was noted from contact sites at the time of the abuse or assault, and method by which the assailant left the scene.
- Whether a weapon was used and any injuries sustained at the time of attack.
- Whether any illicit drugs or alcohol were used to render the victim helpless.
- Date of last menses and use of sanitary pads and/or tampons.
- Date and time of last voluntary coitus, other recent sexual experiences.
- History of previous STDs.
- History of prior pregnancy.
- Use of contraception.
- Any significant actions after alleged assault, such as showering or douching, rinsing of mouth, and brushing of teeth.

Physical Examination

- Before examining the patient, the medical provider should provide a step-by-step explanation of what he or she will be doing and why.
- Reassure the patient that he or she will be in control.
- Keep personal contact with the patient, both through verbal and eye contact.
- Proceed slowly, allowing the patient to relax.
- During the examination, comment on unremarkable or normal findings. Frequently, the patient feels abnormal as a result of the attack and wonders whether his or her body is still the same. It is crucial to convey a sense of normalcy where appropriate. When physical findings are remarkable and injury is present, the medical provider should stress that these injuries are not the patient's fault.
- The examination must include a thorough physical examination for bruises and healing abrasions followed by a genital examination for evidence of trauma and collection of specimens for STD.

General Physical Findings

- General appearance, emotional state, and behavior should be recorded.
- Condition of patient's clothing should be observed and documented.
- All areas of the body should be explored for signs of trauma. Look closely at the neck and upper arms, where bruises resulting from forced restraint are apt to appear.
- Examine the throat.
- Check for abdominal crepitus; this may signify vaginal or rectal laceration with intra-abdominal bleeding.

Gender-Specific Considerations
Females
- The proportion of adolescent females with genital injuries from nonconsensual intercourse is significantly higher than those from consensual intercourse (Adams, 2004).
- Straddle injuries or injuries from sharp objects to the genital area are extremely rare.
- Complete hymenal clefts are not commonly associated with tampon use but may occur during painful insertion (Emans et al., 1994). It would seem prudent for physicians to interpret such data in the court in the context of a specific case with adequate and detailed history (Goodyear-Smith, 1998).
- Estrogen affects the adolescent hymen by making it elastic and thereby permitting penile penetration without tearing. Therefore, while posterior hymenal notches or clefts strongly suggest trauma to the area, absence of hymenal notches or clefts should not exclude the possibility of vaginal penetration.
- Even when penile–vaginal penetration is certain, definitive findings may not be present (Kellogg, 2004).

Males
- Evidence of trauma has been found in only approximately 20% to 37% of adolescent male sexual abuse or assault victims.
- Most genital injuries from sexual abuse and assault involve the rectum and the penis. The perineum, scrotum, or testes follow far behind (Doan, 1983).
- Rectal lacerations from sexual abuse or assault tend to be located at the 1, 5, 7, and 11 o'clock positions (Kadish et al., 1998).

Genital, Pelvic, and Rectal Examination
- Position: An examination on an adolescent female is performed in the lithotomy position. Young and petite adolescent females and males can be examined in the knee-chest position for easier visualization of the anogenital area. The anal area in the larger and older male adolescent should be visualized with the adolescent lying in the lateral position and with one or both knees flexed.
- External genitalia: Note and record signs of blood secretions and sites of bruising, hematoma, ecchymoses, abrasions, lacerations and redness, and swelling in the external genitalia, including the hymen. Application of toluidine blue will make local injuries in the female (the fossa navicularis, posterior fourchette, and hymenal membrane) more apparent.
- Hymen: The hymen can be observed by using a cotton applicator swab moistened with water. Gently stretch the hymen all around to clearly define any partial or complete fresh hymenal tears, and the amount of hymenal tissue present, especially at the 6 o'clock position of the posterior rim where acute hymenal tears are more likely to be found (Slaughter 1997). Spread apart any areas that appear to be notches or clefts with the swab to define the depth of the notch or cleft. An alternative method to detect hymenal damage is by using a Foley catheter balloon technique. The provider inserts the balloon in the distal vaginal vault and expands the estrogenized hymen to full capacity so that injuries along the edge of the hymen can be visualized. This technique also allows for improved photodocumentation (Jones

et al., 2003; Danielson and Holmes, 2004). Remember that the absence of notches does not rule out previous penetration; therefore, the term "*intact*" hymen should be avoided.

- Anus: When anal penetration is reported in females or males, the perianal and anal area needs to be inspected carefully for scars, fissures, sphincter tears, evidence of chronic fissuring, distortion of the anus, skin tags, and localized venous engorgement. Recurrent anal penetration must be suspected when the skin around the anal opening is smooth and thickened and the external sphincter has lost its tone and it does not contract readily. Loss of tone is assessed by presence of a relaxed external anal sphincter almost to the point of gaping, along with loss of puckering of the mucous membrane. Location of anal findings using the face of a clock must be documented.
- Internal examination: An internal pelvic and rectal examination must be performed if there is pain, bleeding, a history of vaginal or rectal penetration, or signs of injury. This should be performed after a thorough examination of the entire body. A primary responsibility of the physician is to avoid further trauma to the patient in performing this part of the examination. A warm water-lubricated speculum should be used for the vaginal examination. In the young peripubertal adolescent, a small-sized metal speculum is preferred for easier insertion and visualization. General anesthesia may be indicated. Injuries such as ecchymoses and tears to the vagina and cervix must be noted. An anoscopy or a proctoscopy is recommended when internal trauma and pathology (warts) is suspected. Internal trauma should be suspected when rectal bleeding, fever, or signs of an acute abdomen are present.

Collection of Specimens

- Treatment for any and all significant trauma, including soft tissue injury as well as injury to the genital area should precede collection of medicolegal information.
- When the kit is opened, the examiner should familiarize himself/herself with the contents of the rape kit and all hospital laboratory tests should be set up on the counter.
- The provider first sees an instruction sheet, a consent form, and numerous sexual assault forensic examination forms. The sexual assault forensic examination forms include history, physical and genital examination records, a checklist of evidence items, follow-up plans, body diagrams for documentation of injuries, and police department documents (receipt of information and authorization for examination and payment). Finally, the rape kit also contains a paper sheet, envelopes, slides, and swabs.
- Collection of legally mandated tests for the rape kit has to be synchronized with the general physical examination, pelvic examination, and hospital laboratory tests. For example, all tests for the rape kit or the hospital laboratory that are needed from the genital area should be obtained during the pelvic examination and blood tests for the rape kit and the hospital laboratory should be done upon completion of the examination. Remember patient permission is required for photographs of areas of trauma.
- Legally mandated tests for evidence collection may include foreign hair collection, clothing, blood from

victim for typing, filter paper disk with saliva from victim, and swabs from perianal, anal verge, and rectal canal for presence of acid phosphatase. Appropriate specimens for DNA testing should be obtained. The "chain of evidence" must be maintained when collecting forensic specimens by strictly following rape kit protocols or evidence will not be of value in criminal prosecution.
- The Wood's lamp has been shown to be unreliable in screening for the presence of semen, but may be helpful in identifying foreign debris (Santucci et al., 1999).
- Evidence for the kit is collected and handed over to a police officer according to legal procedure with associated specimen analysis cost covered by the police.

Hospital Laboratory Tests
- Cultures: *Gonorrhea* cultures should be obtained from the endocervix, rectum, and pharynx. *Chlamydia* cultures should be obtained from the endocervix and rectum. Noncultural techniques (i.e., U.S. Food and Drug Administration [FDA]-approved nucleic acid amplification tests) should not be used because they have inadequate specificity for criminal prosecution (Centers for Disease Control and Prevention, 2002).
- Gram stain of any urethral or anal discharge should be obtained. A Gram stain from the cervix or vagina is not useful.
- If genital ulcers or vesicles suspicious for *herpes genitalis* are present, a viral culture from the lesions should be sent for *herpes simplex* virus.
- Wet mount of vaginal secretions should be prepared and examined for evidence of *Trichomonas* and bacterial vaginosis. If sperm are identified, the laboratory technician validates these findings with the examiner and/or a senior pathologist.
- Serum sample for reactive protein reagin (RPR) or Venereal Disease Research Laboratory (VDRL) test should be obtained as a baseline test and repeated within 6 to 8 weeks for syphilis.
- Serum sample for hepatitis B surface antigen and antibody should be obtained.
- Discuss possible testing for human immunodeficiency virus (HIV) and provide appropriate pretest counseling. If testing is desired, a serum sample should be obtained and repeated at 6 weeks, 3 months, and 6 months.

Treatment

- Patient instructions for managing any injuries, including those to the genital area should be provided, that is, cleaning area with an antibacterial agent, application of local antibiotic ointment, and sitz baths.
- Clinicians need to be sensitive to the likelihood of gastrointestinal side effects from multiple oral medications dispensed or prescribed following a sexual assault evaluation. In this event, treatment should begin with emergency contraception and intramuscular medication for gonorrhea. Medications for other common STDs can begin after the emergency contraception regimen is completed.
- Tetanus toxoid 0.5 mL intramuscularly (plus tetanus immune globulin if dirty wound) is indicated for severe or penetrating trauma.

- STD prophylaxis: Many specialists recommend routine preventive therapy after a sexual assault. Prophylactic treatment for chlamydia, gonorrhea, *Trichomonas* infections, and bacterial vaginosis may be provided. Recommended regimens include: Ceftriaxone 125 mg IM in a single dose PLUS metronidzole 2 g orally in a single dose PLUS azithromycin 1 g orally in a single dose OR doxycycline 100 mg orally twice a day for 7 days.
- Hepatitis B infection: Empiric treatment for hepatitis B with hepatitis B immune globulin (HBIG) following sexual assault is controversial. Its efficacy in adolescents who are already immunized against hepatitis B infection is unknown. The Centers for Disease Control and Prevention (CDC) recommends postexposure hepatitis B vaccine without HBIG as adequate protection against hepatitis B infection.
- HIV postexposure prophylaxis (PEP): It is difficult to discuss PEP issues in the acutely traumatized victim. See Chapter 31 for more information and Web sites on PEP.
  - First assess the risk for HIV infection in assailant and evaluate circumstances of assault that may affect risk for HIV transmission. PEP is best reserved for individuals at higher risk, that is, those who had penetration by an assailant known to be HIV positive or at high risk for HIV infection (men who have sex with men, injection drug users, men with recent incarceration).
  - Consult a specialist in HIV treatment in your local area if PEP is considered.
  - If the victim is eligible for PEP, discuss antiretroviral prophylaxis including toxicity and unknown efficacy.
  - If the victim accepts PEP, provide prescription for 7 days of medication and follow-up in 7 days to assess tolerance to medication.
- Prevention of pregnancy: Emergency contraception may be provided without speculum examination. If the adolescent has not been using prescription methods of contraception, pregnancy prophylaxis should be discussed, that is, emergency contraception within 5 days of an incident. Although Plan B may be taken as a single dose medication, most other approved regimens require two doses. When these are prescribed, it is recommended that the adolescent receive her first dose with an antiemetic in the emergency room and the second dose 12 hours later. However, some hospitals and physicians do not prescribe emergency contraception on religious and ethical grounds. Therefore, if emergency contraception is indicated, it is very important that the provider refer the adolescent to a hospital that does dispense or prescribe emergency contraception.
- Sleep aids: These can be prescribed if indicated but should be given in small quantities.
- Medical follow-up: An appointment with a health care provider should be scheduled as indicated or within 14 to 21 days after the assault, especially in adolescents who have suffered penetration and penetrative injuries. A third visit may be scheduled at 8 to 12 weeks to repeat initial serological studies including tests for syphilis, hepatitis B, or HIV infection. The adolescent should be followed up and evaluated for psychological symptoms (i.e., post-traumatic stress disorder, depression, and/or anxiety). Health care providers should determine the appropriate supports and treatment required.
- Psychological supports: Advocates, law enforcement representatives, and other responders can coordinate with the health care provider to discuss a range of issues before discharge from the emergency center. In many cities, rape crisis centers will send a supportive individual to the emergency department, if notified. The adolescent victim should ideally see a social worker or counselor trained in this area of work, before and after the medicolegal evaluation.

Areas to explore with the adolescent during the initial examination and follow-up are the following:
- Feelings during the assault.
- Feelings and worries regarding the rape, medical examination, and the legal process.
- Concerns regarding physical health, emotional reactions, sexuality, and unusual behaviors.
- Feelings regarding the perpetrator, family, peers, school, and job.
- Willingness to receive crisis intervention services (from professionals, paraprofessional, peers, religious, and other possible resources).
- Issues around her safety should be reviewed and she should be released to a caring friend or family member. Eligibility for protection orders and/or enhanced security measures should be assessed. Telephone numbers of rape hotlines or crisis centers should be provided as well.
- A follow-up appointment should be scheduled with a counselor.
- Written materials: Written materials regarding victims' rights, the rape experience, reporting rape, feelings about rape, and special reactions (the teenage victim, male victim, and the disabled victim) should be given to the victim before leaving the hospital. Providers can obtain this information from Web sites and their local District Attorney's Office. In addition, most states and urban centers have resources and organizations dedicated to providing support for sexual assault victims. Web site resources including pamphlets for victims and their families are listed at the end of this chapter.

Sexually Transmitted Disease Transmission in Sexual Victimization of Adolescents

It is difficult to estimate the risk a sexually abused or assaulted adolescent has of acquiring an STD due to empirical treatment of syphilis, gonorrhea, and chlamydia at the time of sexual assault examinations. A major confounding factor is a report of prior consensual sexual activity by an adolescent at the time of the medical examination. As it stands now, the only determination regarding frequency and incidence that can be made is that bacterial STDs are more commonly isolated than viral STDs.

Factors that should be considered when determining STD risk include the duration between the genital examination and the reported event and pubertal development of a female adolescent. Adult male sex offenders may be at higher risk for STDs than males in the general population based on a history of multiple consensual and nonconsensual sexual encounters with both males and females. Moreover, males from correctional facilities are at higher risk for STDs and HIV infection (Beck–Sague et al., 1999).

When an infection has been determined, the possibility of nonsexual transmission, especially in a young adolescent, should be considered. Unlike for young children (below 3 years of age), nonsexual transmission of STDs through perinatal means is highly unlikely in adolescents. Transmission through fomites is also unlikely. In one controlled experiment, *Trichomonas vaginalis* was reported to survive in young girls who were bathing in tanks in India for religious rituals. This manner of transmission is highly unlikely in adolescents in the United States (Chacko, 2004).

Published studies on STD infection among sexually abused or assaulted adolescents have been predominantly determined from female samples. *Neisseria gonorrhoeae* has been isolated in 0% to 26.3% of cases, *T. vaginalis* in 0% to 19% of cases, *Chlamydia trachomatis* in 4% to 17% of cases, *Treponema pallidum* or syphilis in 0% to 5.6% of cases, and human papillomavirus (HPV) in 0.6% to 2.3% of cases. Of note, empirical treatment for *T. vaginalis* was not standard care at the time of sexual assault evaluations about a decade ago. Under these circumstances, trichomoniasis has been detected in 14.7% of victims in the emergency room visit, and an additional 13.8% at their 2-week follow-up; suggesting that this infection resulted directly from the incident (Reynolds et al., 2000). The literature on STDs in sexually abused or assaulted adolescent males is sparse. One study reported no STDs in any of the 80 males (including adolescents) evaluated for sexual abuse (Seigel et al., 1995). There is a limited number of reports of the occurrence of HIV infection in sexually assaulted adolescents, either male of female.

Little is also known about the infectivity of an STD organism after a single contact. In an adolescent who denies any prior sexual activity, the chance of isolating an STD on the day of an assault is low. It is also possible that such a positive test result would represent bacteria or virus present in the semen of the perpetrator. Emergence of an infection depends on the incubation period and varies depending on the specific organism. The incubation period and/or manifestation of symptoms of common STDs is approximately 1 to 14 days for *N. gonorrhoeae* urethritis in males and up to 10 days for cervicitis in females; 7 to 21 days for *C. trachomatis* in males and females; 10 to 90 days for *T. pallidum* (an average of 2–3 weeks for primary and 4–10 weeks for secondary lesions); 5 to 28 days for *T. vaginalis*; 2 days for *herpes simplex virus* lesions; and 4 to 6 weeks for HPV.

The anatomical site may also influence the likelihood of acquiring an STD in adolescent females. For example, because of the ability of *N. gonorrhoeae* and *C. trachomatis* to infect columnar epithelium of the cervix, penile–vaginal penetration may make acquisition of these STDs more likely as compared to penile-anal or oral penetration. In one case series, 4.6% of pubertal girls had *N. gonorrhoeae*—all were isolated from the cervix. Two had concurrent rectal gonorrhea and one had pharyngeal gonorrhea (Seigel et al., 1995). *C. trachomatis* was isolated from the cervix in pubertal girls (Seigel et al., 1995). The less mature lining of the vaginal mucosa in a young premenstrual adolescent allows for easier occurrence of vaginitis by organisms like *N. gonorrhoeae* and *C. trachomatis*. Unlike bacterial STDs, HIV is more likely to be transmitted through anal intercourse.

The Investigative Process and Legal Outcomes

The effort to prosecute sexual assault perpetrators has its own requirements. A single, dedicated individual who can ensure an unbroken chain of evidence during the forensic examination and is able to follow through with detailed, immediate documentation is essential for providing factual testimony in court (U.S. Department of

Justice, Office on Violence Against Women, 2004). In some areas, sexual assault nurse examiner (SANE) programs provide prompt access to emergency medical care by providing a dedicated examination room, a specially trained forensic examiner who is competent in collection of evidence for the investigation, expert witnesses, and a collaborative team approach. In large metropolitan areas, a community-based victim advocate can assist and counsel the victim and family (U.S. Department of Justice, Office of Justice Programs, Office for Victims of Crime Bulletin, 2001). In small towns and rural areas, such assistance is rarely available and is provided by the local law enforcement officer. Together, these factors can lead to successful prosecution.

Following the medical evaluation, the investigative process involves the following:

- An interview of the victim by the police department if this had not occurred, so that charges can be filed. The police cannot investigate and pursue prosecution unless the victim is willing to talk to them.
- Detaining the alleged perpetrator and evidence for an arrest reviewed. Following an arrest, the alleged perpetrator may be eligible to post bail. At this time, the victim may decide to drop charges and data suggest that charges were dropped in approximately half of cases where an arrest had been made (Gray–Eurom et al., 2002).
- The prosecuting attorney will review the case. Since sexual assault is an offense against the state, the victim is a witness to the state and the state is the prosecuting party. The prosecuting attorney makes all decisions in regard to legal proceedings.
- If the case goes forward, the prosecuting attorney will contact the victim to determine (a) whether the victim is willing to participate, (b) to evaluate the victim as a potential witness, and (c) to assess whether guilt can be proved beyond a reasonable doubt. Therefore, the ability of the victim to provide a detailed description of the event is vital.
- The decision whether to prosecute is ongoing and is determined by several factors. Data suggest successful prosecution has been found to be significantly associated with victims who are <18-years-old, with the presence of genital trauma, and with the use of a weapon by the assailant (Gray–Eurom et al., 2002). Among sexually abused children, the conviction of the alleged perpetrators occurred in victims with normal or nonspecific findings of sexual abuse and in those who were older and reported penetration, pain, and blood when the event occurred (Adams et al., 1994). De Jong and Rose (1991) reported that the highest rate of felony convictions (83%) was in adolescent victims 12 years of age and older based on both the victim's description of the event and presence of physical findings. Therefore, the decision to proceed with criminal charges is often based on either physical evidence, the minor's ability to describe the abuse in detail, or both.

Testifying

- Usually the provider first learns of a case going to court when he or she is subpoenaed or when the medical record is subpoenaed.
- The provider needs to present the medical facts much like an expert witness. These skills are usually acquired through training and experience. A verbal explanation to acknowledge that the lack of physical evidence is

not inconsistent with sexual penetration in child sexual abuse cases may be necessary.

- Pretrial preparation is strongly encouraged and begins with the provider communicating with the prosecuting attorney after receipt of the subpoena. Some institutions prefer that the provider first seek guidance from an in-house attorney before contacting the prosecutor.
- The provider should be prepared to discuss his or her educational background, qualifications, and clinical experience. It will be necessary to listen carefully and be guided by questions posed. Use of medical jargon should be avoided and terms and concepts should be explained in a straightforward and simple manner. Finally, the provider should avoid getting emotional and argumentative especially during cross-examination.

WEB SITES

http://nccanch.acf.hhs.gov/. National Clearing House on Child Abuse and Neglect.

http://www.cdc.gov/ncipc/factsheets/svfacts.htm. CDC Sexual Violence Fact Sheet.

http://www.ncjrs.org/pdffiles1/ovw/206554.pdf. A National Protocol on the Sexual Assault Medical Forensic Examinations, Adults/Adolescents, 2004.

http://www. usdoj.gov. U.S. Department of Justice, Office for Victims of Crime.

http://www.dhhs.gov. U.S. Department of Health and Human Services.

http://www.acf.dhhs.gov. The Administration for Children, Youth, and Their Families.

http://www.ndacan.cornell.edu/. National Data Archive on Child Abuse and Neglect.

http://www.childrensdefense.org. Children's Defense Fund.

http://www.cwla.org. Child Welfare League of America.

http://www.atsa.com. Association for the treatment of Sexual Abusers.

http://www.faithtrustinstitute.org/. The Faith Trust Institute.

http://www.youthlaw.org. National Center for Youth Law.

http://www.nsvrc.org. National Sexual Violence Resource Center.

http://www.menagainstsexualviolence.org/. Men Against Sexual Violence.

http://www.ncdsv.org/. National Center on Domestic and Sexual Violence.

http://www.usdoj.gov/ovw/. U.S. Department of Justice, Violence Against Women Office.

http://www.rainn.org/. Rape Abuse and Incest National Network.

http://www.4woman.gov/faq/sexualassault.htm. Department of Health and Human Services Sexual Assault fact sheet.

REFERENCES AND ADDITIONAL READINGS

Adams JA. Medical evaluation of suspected child sexual abuse. *J Pediatr Adolesc Gynecol* 2004;17:191.

Adams JA, Botash AS, Kellogg N. Differences in hymenal morphology between adolescent girls with and without a history of consensual sexual intercourse. *Arch Pediatr Adolesc Med* 2004;158:280.

Adam JA, Girardin RN, Faugno D. Adolescent sexual assault: documentation of acute injuries using photo-colposcopy. *J Pediatr Adolesc Gynecol* 2001;14:175.

Adams JA, Harper K, Knudson S, et al. Examination findings in legally confirmed child sexual abuse: it's normal to be normal. *Pediatrics* 1994;94:310.

American Academy of Pediatrics, Committee on Adolescence. Care of the adolescent sexual assault victim. *Pediatrics* 2001; 107:1476.

American College of Emergency Physicians. Management of the patient with the complaint of sexual assault. *Ann Emerg Med* 1995;25:728.

Anderson SC, Griffith S, Bach CM, et al. *Sexual abuse of adolescent males: an overview.* Paper presented at the *Third international congress on child abuse and neglect*; Amsterdam, The Netherlands; April 1981.

Anderson J, Martin J, Mullen P, et al. Prevalence of childhood sexual abuse experiences in a community sample of women. *Am Acad Child Adolesc Psychiatry* 1993;32:5.

Balsam KF, Rothblum ED, Beauchaine TP. Victimization over the life span: a comparison of lesbian, gay, bisexual, and heterosexual siblings. *J Consult Clin Psychol* 2005;3:477.

Bechtel K, Podrazik M. Evaluation of the adolescent rape victim. *Pediatr Clin North Am* 1999;46:809.

Beck—Sague CM. Sexual assault and STD. In: Holmes KK, Sparling PF, Mardh P-A, et al., eds. *Sexually transmitted diseases*, 3rd ed. San Francisco: McGraw-Hill, Health Professionals Division;1999:1433.

Browne A, Finkelhor D. Impact of child sexual abuse: a review of the research. *Psychol Bull* 1986;99:66.

Bureau of Justice Statistics. *Sexual Assault of Young Children as Reported to Law Enforcement: Victim, Incident, and Offender Characteristics.* US Department of Justice. July 2000.

Catalano S. *Criminal Victimization,2004.* Bureau of Justice Statistics—US Department of Justice; 2005.

Centers for Disease Control and Prevention. Youth risk behavior surveillance, June 9, 2006. *MMWR Morb Mortal Wkly Rep* 2005;55(SS-5).

Centers for Disease Control and Prevention. Sexually transmitted diseases and guidelines 2006. *MMWR* 2006;55 (RR-11):80.

Chacko MR, Staat M, Woods C. Genital infections in childhood and adolescence. In Feigin RD, Cherry JD, Demmler GJ, eds. *Textbook of pediatric infectious diseases*, 5th ed, Vol 1. Philadelphia, Pennsylvania: Saunders, an Imprint of Elsevier Science; 2003:562.

Chacko MR, Wiemann CM, Smith PB. Chlamydia and gonorrhea screening in asymptomatic young women. *J Pediat Adolesc Gynecol* 2004;17:169.

Committee on Adolescent Health Care. Adolescent acquaintance rape. ACOG Committee opinion. *Int J Gynaecol Obstet* 1993;42:209.

Cunningham RM, Stiffman AR, Dore P, et al. The association of physical and sexual abuse with HIV risk behaviors in adolescence and young adulthood: implications for public health. *Child Abuse Negl* 1994;18:233.

Danielson CK, Holmes MM. Adolescent sexual assault: an update of the literature. *Curr Opin Obstet Gynecol* 2004;16:383.

Deisher RW, Bidwell RJ. Sexual abuse of male adolescents. *Semin Adolesc Med* 1987;3:47.

De Jong AR, Emmett GA, Hervada AA. Epidemiologic factors in sexual abuse of boys. *Am J Dis Child* 1982;136:990.

De Jong AR, Rose M. Legal proof of child sexual abuse in the absence of physical evidence. *Pediatrics* 1991;88:506.

Dewdney D. Treatment of physically abused adolescents. *Semin Adolesc Med* 1987;3:55.

Diaz A, Simatov E, Rickert VI. Effect of abuse on health: results of a national survey. *Arch Pediatr Adolesc Med* 2002;156:811.

Doan LA, Levy RC. Male Sexual Assault. *J Emerg Med.* 1983;1:45.

Dunn SF, Gilchrist VJ. Sexual assault. *Prim Care* 1993;20:359.

Emans SJ, Woods ER, Allred EN, et al. Hymenal findings in adolescent women: impact of tampon use and consensual sexual activity. *J Pediatr* 1994;125:153.

Farber ED, Joseph JA. The maltreated adolescent: patterns of physical abuse. *Child Abuse Negl* 1985;9:201.

Federal Bureau of Investigation. *Crime in the United States, 2004, Uniform Crime Reports.* U.S. Department of Justice; 1999: Available at www.fbi.gov/ucr.

Ferris LE, Sandercock J. The sensitivity of forensic tests for rape. *Med Law* 1998;17:333.

Finkelhor D. *Sexually victimized children.* New York: Free Press; 1979.

Finkelhor D. Risk factors in the sexual victimization of children. *Child Abuse Negl* 1980;4:265.

Finkelhor D. *Child sexual abuse: new theory and research.* New York: Free Press; 1984.

Finkelhor D. *Current information on the scope and nature of child sexual abuse.* Future Child 1994;4(2):31.

Finkelhor D, Browne A. The traumatic impact of child sexual abuse: a conceptualization. *Am J Orthopsychiatry* 1985;55:530.

Finkelhor D, Ormrod R, Turner H. The victimization of children and youth: a comprehensive, national survey. *Child Maltreat* 2005;10(1):5.

Furey EM. Sexual abuse of adults with mental retardation: who and where. *Ment Retard* 1994;32:173.

Gagnon J. Female child victims of sex offenses. *Soc Probl* 1965;13:176.

Gans JE, Blyth DA, Elster AB, et al. *Americas Adolescents: how healthy are they?* Chicago: American Medical Association; 1990.

Glaser JB, Hammerschlag MR, McCormack WM. Sexually transmitted diseases in victims of sexual assault. *N Engl J Med* 1986;315:625.

Golding JM. Sexual assault history and physical health in randomly selected Los Angeles women. *Health Psychol* 1994;13:130.

Golding JM, Cooper ML, George LK. Sexual assault history and health perceptions: seven general population studies. *Health Psychol* 1997;16:4.

Goodyear-Smith FA, Laidlaw TM. Can tampon use cause hymen changes in girls who have not had sexual intercourse? A review of the literature. *Forensic Sci Int* 1998;94:147.

Greenfeld L. *Sex offenses and offenders: an analysis of data on rape and sexual assault.* Washington, DC: Bureau of Justice Statistics; February 1997.

Greydanus DE, Shaw RD, Kennedy EL. Examination of sexually abused adolescents. *Semin Adolesc Med* 1987;3:59.

Gray—Eurom K, Seaberg DC, Wears RL. The prosecution of sexual assault cases: correlation with forensic evidence. *Ann Emerg Med* 2002;39:61.

Guidelines for the interview and examination of alleged rape victims. A conjoint effort of the Committee on Evolving Trends in Society Affecting Life and the Advisory Panels of Obstetrics and Gynecology, Pathology, and Psychiatry of the Scientific Board of the California Medical Association. *West J Med* 1975;123:420.

Hampton HL. Care of the woman who has been raped. *N Engl J Med* 1995;332:234.

Hanson KA, Gidycz CA. Evaluation of a sexual assault prevention program. *J Consult Clin Psychol* 1993;61:1046.

Hickson FC, Davies PM, Hunt AJ, et al. Gay men as victims of nonconsensual sex. *Arch Sex Behav* 1994;23:281.

Holmes M. Sexually transmitted infections in female rape victims. *AIDS Patient Care STDs* 1999;13:703.

Irwin KL, Edlin BR, Wong L. Urban rape survivors: characteristics and prevalence of human immunodeficiency virus and other sexually transmitted infections. Multicenter crack cocaine and HIV infection study team. *Obstet Gynecol* 1995;85:330.

Irwin CE, Rickert VI. Coercive sexual experiences during adolescence and young adulthood: a public health problem. *J Adolesc Health* 2005;36:359.

Jones JS, Dunnuck C, Rossman L, et al. Adolescent foley catheter technique for visualizing hymenal injuries in adolescent sexual assault. *Acad Emerg Med* 2003;10:1001.

Jones JS, Rossman L, Wynn BN, et al. Comparative analysis of adult versus adolescent sexual assault: epidemiology and patterns of anogenital injury. *Acad Emerg Med* 2003;10:872.

Kadish HA, Schunk JE, Britton H. Pediatric male rectal and genital trauma: accidental and nonaccidental injuries. *Pediatr Emerg Care* 1998;14:95.

Kellogg ND. Genital anatomy in pregnant adolescents: "normal" does not mean "nothing happened". *Pediatrics* 2004;113:e67.

Kellogg N. American academy of pediatrics committee on child abuse and neglect. The evaluation of sexual abuse in children. *Pediatrics* 2005;116:506.

Kellogg ND, Huston RL. Unwanted sexual experiences in adolescents: patterns of disclosure. *Clin Pediatr* 1995;34:306.

Kipke M, Simon T, Montgomery S, et al. Homeless youth and their exposure to and involvement in violence while living on the streets. *J Adolesc Health* 1997;20:360.

Kormos KC, Brooks CI. Acquaintance rape: attributions of victim blame by college students and prison inmates as a function of relationship status of victim and assailant. *Psychol Rep* 1994;74:545.

Koss MP, Oros CJ. Sexual experiences survey: a research instrument investigating sexual aggression and victimization. *J Consult Clin Psychol* 1982;50(3):455.

Lakey JE. The profile and treatment of male adolescent sex offenders. *Adolescence* 1994;29:755.

Linden JA. Sexual assault. *Emerg Med Clin North Am* 1999;17:685.

Lindon J, Nourse CA. A multi-dimensional model of groupwork for adolescent girls who have been sexually abused. *Child Abuse Negl* 1994;18:341.

Mann EB. Self-reported stresses of adolescent rape victims. *J Adolesc Health Care* 1981;2:29.

Martin CA, Warfield MC, Braen GR. Physician's management of the psychological aspects of rape. *JAMA* 1983;249:501.

McCormack A, Janus M, Burgess AW. Runaway youths and sexual victimization: gender differences in an adolescent population. *Child Abuse Negl* 1986;10:387.

Muehlenhard CL, Linton MA. Date rape and sexual aggression in dating situations: Incidence and risk factors. *J Couns Psychol* 1987;34:186.

Munt LC. Sexual abuse of children and adolescents. *J Curr Adolesc Med* 1980;2:30.

Neinstein LS, Goldenring J. Nonsexual transmission of sexually transmitted diseases: an infrequent occurrence. *Pediatrics* 1984;74:67.

Peipert JF, Domagalski LIZ. Epidemiology of adolescent sexual assault. *Obstet Gynecol* 1994;84:867.

Rabkin JG. The epidemiology of forcible rape. *Am J Orthopsychiatry* 1979;49:634.

Ramos B, Carlson BE, McNutt LA, et al. Lifetime abuse, mental health, and African American women. *J Fam Violence* 2004;19:3.

Reynolds MW, Peipert JF, Collins B. Epidemiologic issues of sexually transmitted diseases in sexual assault victims. *Obstet Gynecol Surv* 2000;55:51.

Rickert VI, Edwards S, Harrykissoon SD, et al. Violence in the lives of young women: clinical care and management. *Curr Womens Health Rep* 2001;1:94.

Rickert VI, Vaughan R, Wiemann C. Violence against young women: implications for clinicians. *Contemp Ob Gyn* 2003; 48:30.

Rickert VI, Wiemann C. Date rape among adolescents and young adults. *J Pediatr Adolesc Gynecol* 1998;11:167.

Rickert VI, Wiemann C. Date rape: office-based solutions. *Contemp Ob Gyn* 1998;43:133.

Rickert VI, Wiemann CM, Vaughan RD, et al. Rates and risk factors for sexual violence among an ethnically diverse sample of adolescents. *Arch Pediatr Adolesc Med* 2004;158: 1132.

Rickert VI, Wiemann CM, Vaughan RD. Disclosure of date/ acquaintance rape: who reports and when. *J Pediatr Adolesc Gynecol* 2005;18:17.

Rimza ME, Niggeman MS. Medical evaluation of sexually abused children: a review of 311 cases. *Pediatrics* 1982;69:8.

Rosenberg MS. Rape crisis syndrome. *Med Aspects Hum Sex* 1986;20:65.

Rubinstein M, Yeager CA, Goodstein C. Sexually assaultive male juveniles: a follow-up. *Am J Psychiatry* 1993;150:262.

Runtz M, Brierz J. Adolescent "acting out" and childhood history of child abuse. *J Interpers Violence* 1986;1:326.

Santucci KA, Nelson DG, McQuillen KK, et al. Wood's lamp utility in the identification of semen. *Pediatrics* 1999;104:1342.

Schaaf KK, McCanne TR. Relationship of childhood sexual, physical, and combined sexual and physical abuse to adult victimization and posttraumatic stress disorder. *Child Abuse Negl* 1998;22:1119.

Schor DP. Sex and sexual abuse in developmentally disabled adolescents. *Semin Adolesc Med* 1987;3:1.

Schwartz RH, Milteer R, LeBeau MA. Drug-facilitated sexual assault ('date rape'). *South Med J* 2000;93:558.

Seigel RM, Schubert CJ, Myers PA, et al. The prevalence of sexually transmitted diseases in children and adolescents evaluated for sexual abuse in cincinnati: rationale for limited STD testing in prepubertal girls. *Pediatrics* 1995;96: 1090.

Shaw JA, Campo-Bowen AE, Applegate B, et al. Young boys who commit serious sexual offenses: demographics, psychometrics, and phenomenology. *Bull Am Acad Psychiatry Law* 1993;21:399.

Shearer SL, Herbert CA. Long-term effects of unresolved sexual trauma. *Am Fam Physician* 1987;36:169.

Silber TJ. Ethical issues in the treatment of the sexually abused adolescent: a clinician's perspective. *Semin Adolesc Med* 1987;3:39.

Slaughter L, Brown CRV, Crowley S, et al. Patterns of genital injury in female sexual assault victims. *Am J Obstet Gynecol* 1997;176:609.

Society for Adolescent Medicine. Protecting adolescents: ensuring access to care and reporting of sexual activity and abuse. *J Adolesc Health* 2004;35:420.

Stevenson J. The treatment of the long-term sequelae of child abuse. *J Child Psychol Psychiatry* 1999;40:89.

Struckman-Johnson C, Struckman-Johnson D. Men pressured and forced into sexual experience. *Arch Sex Behav* 1994; 23:93.

Summit R. Beyond belief: the reluctant discovery of incest. In: Kirkpatrick M, ed. *Women's sexual experience*. New York: Plenum Publishing; 1982.

Symons PY, Groer MW, Kepler-Youngblood P. Prevalence and predictors of adolescent dating violence. *J Child Adolesc Psychiatr Nurs* 1994;7:14.

Tipton AC. Child sexual abuse: physical examination techniques and interpretation of findings. *Adolesc Pediatr Gynecol* 1989;2:10.

Tjaden P, Thoennes N. *Full report of the prevalence, incidence, and consequences of violence against women*, U.S. Department of Justice; 2000: November Available at www.ojp.usdoj.gov/nij.

Tomlinson DR, Harrison J. The management of adult male victims of sexual assault in the GUM clinic: a practical guide. *Int J STD AIDS* 1998;9:720.

U.S. Department of Justice, Office on Violence Against Women. A national protocol on the sexual assault medical forensic examinations, adults/adolescents, 2004. Available at www.ncjrs .org/pdffiles1/ovw/206554.pdf.

U.S. Department of Justice, Office of Justice Programs, Office for Victims of Crime Bulletin. Sexual Assault Nurse Examiner (SANE) Programs: Improving the Community Response to Sexual Assault Victims, 2001. Available at www.usdoj.gov/ ovw/publication.

U.S. Department of Health and Human Services Administration on Children Youth and Families. (2005). *Child maltreatment* 2003. Washington, DC: U.S. Government Printing Office.

Walsh WA, Wolak J. Nonforcible Internet-related sex crimes with adolescent victims: prosecution issues and outcomes. *Child Maltreat* 2005;10:260.

Watkins B, Bentovim A. The sexual abuse of male children and adolescents: a review of current research. *J Child Psychol Psychiatry* 1992;33:197.

Weir W. Drug-facilitated date rape. *Can Med Assoc J* 2001;165:80.

Wiebe ER, Comay SE, McGregor M, et al. Offering HIV prophylaxis to people who have been sexually assaulted: 16 months' experience in a sexual assault service. *Can Med Assoc J* 2000;162:641.

Wolfe DA, Scott K, Reitzel-Jaffe D, et al. Development and validation of the conflict in adolescent dating relationships inventory. *Psychol Assess* 2001;13(2):277.

Zoucha-Jansen JM, Coyne A. The effects of resistance strategies on rape. *Am J Public Health* 1993;83:1633.

CHAPTER 82

Chronic Illness in the Adolescent

Susan M. Coupey

With the extraordinary technological advances in medicine that have occurred in the last few decades, the prevalence of chronic conditions in adolescents has increased dramatically. Many more children with conditions such as congenital heart disease, renal failure, cystic fibrosis, and even congenital human immunodeficiency virus (HIV) infection, survive into their teens and beyond (Table 82.1). Despite the availability of excellent biomedical treatment for most common chronic diseases, optimal management of illness in adolescents is not limited to biomedical prescription alone. Developmental, psychosocial, and family factors all feature prominently in the ongoing care of adolescents with chronic diseases. Chronic conditions, by definition, have no cure and therefore must be endured and managed on a daily basis. Having such a condition is a continuing source of stress for the adolescent and his or her family and can contribute to maladaptive coping and dysfunction. On the other hand, the experience of successfully managing a chronic illness also may foster accelerated maturation and coping skills in adolescents and their families. Helping adolescents manage the chronic illness well and reach their full developmental potential can be very rewarding for the clinician. This chapter emphasizes developmental and behavioral issues in management of chronically ill or hospitalized adolescents. It is beyond the scope of this book to discuss medical management of all the specific chronic conditions that can affect adolescents. The references at the end of this chapter address a number of the major chronic illnesses in this age-group.

DEFINITION AND PREVALENCE

Stein et al. (1993; 1997) developed a noncategorical, or generic, approach to defining and measuring chronic health conditions in children, rather than using a list of diagnoses. Three definitional concepts provide the framework, all of which must be present for a child or adolescent to be classified as having a chronic health condition:

1. Disorder on a biological, psychological, or cognitive basis
2. Duration or expected duration of at least 12 months
3. Consequences of the disorder:

a. Functional limitations compared with healthy peers in the same age-group
b. Reliance on compensatory mechanisms or assistance, such as medications, special diet, medical technology, assisting device, or personal assistance
c. Need for medical care or related services, psychological services, or educational services over and above the usual for the child's age

Applying this definition and using data from the 1994 National Health Interview Survey Disability Supplement for Children aged 0 through 17 years, Stein and Silver (1999) estimated that 10.3 million children (14.8%) had chronic conditions. In 2001, the Maternal and Child Health Bureau of the National Institutes of Health (NIH) conducted the National Survey of Children with Special Health Care Needs

TABLE 82.1

Prevalence of Selected Chronic Conditions in Adolescents Aged 10–17 Years

Condition	Cases per 1,000 U.S. Adolescents
Impairments	
Musculoskeletal impairments	20.9
Speech defects	18.9
Deafness and hearing loss	17.0
Blindness and visual impairments	16.0
Diseases	
Asthma	46.8
Heart disease	17.4
Arthritis	8.7
Epilepsy and seizures	3.3
Diabetes mellitus	1.5
Sickle cell disease	0.9

From Westbrook LE, Stein RE. Epidemiology of chronic health conditions in adolescents. *Adolesc Med* 1994;5:197–209, with permission. Based on Newacheck PW, McManus MA, Fox HB. Prevalence and impact of chronic illness among adolescents. *Am J Dis Child* 1991;145:1367–1373.

using a different but similar definition of "children with special health care needs," namely:

> "...those who have or are at increased risk for a chronic physical, developmental, behavioral, or emotional condition and who also require health and related services of a type or amount beyond that required by children generally."

The 2001 survey found that 12.8% of children younger than 18 years or approximately 9.4 million children in the United States had special health care needs. Both sets of analyses found that children with chronic health conditions or special health care needs were disproportionately older and male. The 2001 survey found that among adolescents aged 12 through 17, 15.8% have special health care needs. Asthma and other chronic respiratory tract conditions and musculoskeletal disorders account for most of the physical disabilities. Mental health disorders, including developmental, behavioral, and emotional problems, also are a leading cause of disability in this age-group.

INTERACTION OF ADOLESCENT DEVELOPMENT AND CHRONIC ILLNESS

Early adolescence is a period of accelerated physical growth and pubertal development, and in middle and later adolescence, acceleration in cognitive and psychosocial development predominates. The interaction of chronic illness with these different developmental streams is complex and bidirectional; the illness may affect the development and/or the development may affect the illness. For example, some chronic diseases such as cystic fibrosis or sickle cell disease can cause delayed puberty, but for other chronic diseases such as diabetes mellitus, normal puberty can cause exacerbation of the disease. Similarly, disabling chronic conditions that impede peer interaction such as spina bifida can delay psychosocial development; conversely, normal psychosocial development that includes increasing independence from parents with experimentation and risk taking can lead to poor medication adherence and exacerbation of illnesses such as asthma or chronic renal failure.

Specific psychosocial areas, notably achieving independence and family relationships, have been found to be most vulnerable to dysfunction in adolescents with chronic health conditions. Wolman et al. (1994) examined emotional health in adolescents with and without a chronic illness. They found that although adolescents with chronic conditions do less well than adolescents without chronic conditions, the illness is not the most influential factor in emotional well-being. Family connectedness is of fundamental importance for adolescents' emotional well-being. Bennett (1994) reviewed 60 studies of depressive symptoms among children and adolescents with chronic medical problems. Although the findings indicate that children and adolescents with a chronic medical problem are at slightly elevated risk of having depressive symptoms, most were not clinically depressed. Mintzer et al. (2005) looked at post-traumatic stress disorder (PTSD) in >100 adolescents who had an organ transplantation (kidney, liver, or heart) a mean of 7 years previously and found that, although the majority (70%) had no symptoms, 16%

met criteria for a diagnosis of PTSD. The type of transplant did not predict PTSD but adolescents with acute onset of organ failure precipitating the need for transplant were more likely to have PTSD than those having transplantations resulting from chronic or congenital conditions. Most studies indicate that the presence of a chronic physical illness, even with its attendant problems and stresses, does not necessarily lead to emotional dysfunction. Adolescents with a chronic condition, who are also disabled, however, are at increased risk for psychosocial and emotional dysfunction.

Another approach put forward by Rutter (1985) and reiterated by Patterson and Blum (1996) is to evaluate the total burden of risk and protective factors borne by each adolescent and to view chronic physical illness as one of several important risk factors for psychosocial and emotional dysfunction. Risk factors other than chronic illness include the following:

- Male sex
- Psychiatric illness and/or criminality in a parent
- Severe family discord
- Low socioeconomic status

Protective factors include the following:

- Positive temperament
- Above-average intelligence
- Social competence
- A supportive relationship with at least one parent
- Family closeness
- Adequate rule setting

Using this approach, clinicians can target adolescents with multiple risk factors, in addition to the chronic illness, for enhanced intervention to prevent dysfunction.

Specific Developmental Risks

Independence–Dependence The medical requirements of managing a chronic illness and/or the perception of vulnerability of the ill adolescent can impede the movement toward independence that usually occurs during early and middle adolescence. Because chronic illness may prolong dependence on parents and others, including physicians, the adolescent may become compliant and child-like or noncompliant and rebellious.

Body Image As stressed in earlier chapters, adolescents are highly concerned with and are self-conscious about their developing bodies. Delayed puberty or visible markers of the illness may interfere with the development of a healthy body image. This abnormal body image may lead to the following:

- Lowered self-image and self-esteem
- Segregation from peers
- Increased absences from school and other activities
- Increased anxieties over sexuality, sexual attractiveness, sexual function, and sexual relations
- Disordered eating or eating disorders
- Depression, anger, or both

Peer Group Chronic illness may limit teenagers' activities, not only because of physical, mental, or sensory disabilities but also even without overt disability, because of illness-related fatigue, frequent medical appointments, and hospitalizations. Chronically ill adolescents may be rejected by peers or have fantasies of such rejection. These problems may lead to fear of peer involvement and social isolation.

Identity The adolescent with a chronic illness often has difficulties consolidating a mature identity. Concerns about future vocation, financial resources, separation from parents, marriage, and reproduction may all lead to identity problems.

Modifying Factors

Age at Onset The stage of development during which the chronic illness appears may have considerable bearing on the psychological impact of the illness on the adolescent.

1. Preadolescence: Chronic illness or disability that originates at birth or in early childhood may lead early on to altered parental expectations. Lowered parentally perceived potential of the developing adolescent may foster reduced self-expectations in the teen. These misconceptions have major implications for the setting and achievement of future goals for the adolescent.
2. Early adolescence: Because the early adolescent has yet to separate from his or her parents, there may be little struggle for independence or the parents may become overprotective and resist normal and reasonable independence overtures by their child. Chronic illness diagnosed in early adolescence may be particularly likely to provoke deep concerns about body integrity and body image. Such concerns can set the stage for dysfunctional coping, and if not resolved, eating disorders may develop later on. Gross et al. (2000) assessed the prevalence of eating disorder symptoms in a sample of young women with physical disabilities and found that 8% had a sufficient number of symptoms to suggest clinical disorder. Neumark-Sztainer et al. (1998) in a survey of a representative population of high school students in Connecticut, found that prevalence rates of disordered eating (using laxatives, diet pills, or vomiting to control weight) were twice as likely to be reported by boys with chronic illness than healthy boys and 1.6 times more likely to be reported by girls with chronic illness than healthy girls. Eating disorders are also reported with some frequency in adolescents with diabetes mellitus and inflammatory bowel disease, diseases that often have their onset in early adolescence.
3. Middle adolescence: This age may be the most devastating time for a chronic illness to strike. During this phase, the adolescent is intensely involved with separation, peers, and sexual development. A chronic illness may thwart the adolescent's progress in these areas, in addition to conflicting with the high energy levels and feelings of omnipotence typical of middle adolescence. Poor adherence to medical therapy is a frequent problem during this period, as is depression, sexual acting out, and substance use.
4. Late adolescence: Chronic illness with an onset in late adolescence usually causes less upheaval. At this stage, the teenager should have already gained self-confidence and a secure identity. Concerns are focused on how the disease may disrupt vocational and educational plans, as well as future serious relationships, parenthood, and the prospects for living independently.

Nature of the Illness Perrin et al. (1993) list 12 dimensions, other than age at onset, for describing chronic illness that potentially may have an impact on the adolescent's adjustment:

1. Duration	7. Cognition
2. Limitation of age-appropriate activities	8. Emotional/social
	9. Sensory functioning
3. Visibility	10. Communication
4. Expected survival	11. Course
5. Mobility	12. Uncertainty
6. Physiological functioning	

For example, a highly visible disease such as psoriasis may cause more emotional disruption than a life-threatening malignancy such as Hodgkin disease. However, as is true for all of these dimensions, there is a complex relationship between visible deformities and adjustment. Sheerin et al. (1995) evaluated psychosocial adjustment in children with facial port-wine stains compared with adjustment in children with prominent ears. The children with disfiguring facial birthmarks were found to be as well as or better adjusted than nondisfigured peers, whereas those with prominent ears were less well adjusted. To explain this counterintuitive finding, the authors suggest that having a clearly abnormal disfigurement, such as a port-wine stain, elicits uniformity of both opinion and support from family, whereas having a "deformity" such as prominent ears, which is merely an exaggeration of normal, is not as likely to elicit support and may explain the poorer mental health in that marginally disfigured group.

An exacerbating and remitting course of illness with the accompanying uncertainty and lack of control over when the symptoms will strike, seems to be more likely to be associated with emotional problems. In reviewing studies among children and adolescents with chronic medical problems, Bennett (1994) found that certain disorders with these characteristics (i.e., asthma, recurrent abdominal pain, and sickle cell anemia) are associated with a greater risk for depression than other disorders that are more predictable (i.e., cancer, cystic fibrosis, and diabetes mellitus). Ireys et al. (1994) studied young adults (mean age, 21.9 years) with chronic illness and found that hearing and speech problems, unpredictability of symptoms, and restricted activity days were illness characteristics that had significant adverse effects on mental health status. Diseases that interfere with cognition, sensory function, or communication are particularly likely to be associated with poor adjustment. Howe et al. (1993) found that adolescents with brain-based conditions had more behavioral problems, less autonomous functioning, and poorer school achievement than those without brain dysfunction.

COPING WITH CHRONIC ILLNESS

To cope with difficulties and frustrations of chronic illness, the adolescent usually adopts one or more of the following coping mechanisms:

- Insightful acceptance: Unusual in adolescents, particularly during early and middle adolescence.
- Denial: A common coping strategy used by adolescents. Some forms of denial may be adaptive and helpful, but more often, this strategy leads to poor adherence

behaviors such as missed appointments and forgotten medications.

- Regression: Also common in chronically ill adolescents. With regression, the teenager becomes abnormally dependent on parents and other adults and exhibits inappropriate child-like behavior.
- Projection: This coping mechanism allows feelings of rage, frustration, or guilt to be transferred onto parents or health care providers. Projection is often observed on adolescent inpatient units, where anger is transferred to members of the staff.
- Displacement: A similar coping mechanism to projection, but the anger is usually transferred to an object or an activity. Displacement is observed frequently on adolescent units and is typified by behavior such as throwing of objects.
- Acting out: Similar to displacement but less constructive. In frustration, the adolescent exhibits out-of-control behavior, necessitating disciplinary management.
- Compensation: A highly useful coping strategy in which the patient alters usual activities in response to the restrictions of the disease. For example, an adolescent who formerly achieved self-esteem through dancing switches to performing music for fulfillment.
- Intellectualization: This coping mechanism separates the realities of the disease from the emotional impact. Teenagers who become highly involved in the technical aspects of their disease use intellectualization. Although intellectualization can be positive, there needs to be some period during which the adolescent acknowledges his or her emotional concerns.

Over time, the adolescent with a chronic illness or disability likely uses many of the listed coping mechanisms, often using different mechanisms to cope with different situations. Most adolescents who come from psychologically healthy and supportive families can cope amazingly well with a multitude of stressors and are even able to use these situations as emotional growth experiences. It is not uncommon to observe regressed behavior in an adolescent during a period of acute distress, with a rapid regaining of maturational status almost immediately afterward (e.g., when a bone marrow aspiration needle is removed).

With maturation and experience in dealing with chronic illness and its treatment, many adolescents are able to use cognitive reframing of situations to render them less threatening and stressful. Such adolescents also develop an array of coping strategies that have worked for them and learn to reuse those successful strategies instead of continuing to try unsuccessful ones. Exposure to multiple stresses of a similar nature permits stress inoculation and the ability to respond more rapidly and often more appropriately to familiar challenges.

For those adolescents who cannot consistently meet the challenges of chronic illness, breakdown of coping may be manifested behaviorally by poor adherence to treatment recommendations, increased risk-taking behaviors, or overall withdrawal from developmental tasks as a manifestation of depression.

RISK BEHAVIORS

Risk taking, particularly in the areas of sexuality and substance use, contributes substantially to morbidity in healthy adolescents. When this behavior interacts with chronic illness, however, negative health consequences are often exacerbated. It is ironic that risk taking among chronically ill teenagers is probably directly related to improved management, which most often results in normal or near-normal growth, pubertal development, and fertility; better nutritional status; normal energy levels; and age-appropriate opportunities for social interaction that can, and often do, include risk-taking behaviors.

Sexuality

For adolescents with a chronic illness, the health risks of sexual activity may be exacerbated by the illness itself, the medications used to treat it, or by a maladaptive emotional response to illness. However, studies show that many adolescents with chronic illness and disability are sexually active and most have concerns about their sexual attractiveness, normalcy of their reproductive system and sexual response, fertility, safety of contraception use, and genetic aspects of their disease.

1. Prevalence of sexual activity: Table 82.2 shows prevalence of sexual activity among chronically ill adolescents.

TABLE 82.2

Prevalence of Sexual Activity among Chronically Ill Adolescents

Study Population	Sample Size	Age Range (yr)	Sexually Active (%)
School-based, Minnesota, various diseases[a]			
Males—visible conditions	148	13–18	49
Females—visible conditions	308	13–18	42
Inner-city, New York, various diseases[b]	217	14–17	33
Tertiary care centers, North Carolina, sickle cell disease[c]	205	12–19	51
Tertiary care centers, North Carolina, cystic fibrosis[c]	116	12–19	28

[a]Suris J, Resnick MD, Cassuto N, et al. Sexual behavior of adolescents with chronic disease and disability. *J Adolesc Health* 1996;19:124–131.

[b]Alderman EM, Lauby JL, Coupey SM. Problem behaviors in inner-city adolescents with chronic illness. *J Dev Behav Pediatr* 1995;16:339–344.

[c]Britto MT, Garrett JM, Dugliss MAJ, et al. Risky behavior in teens with cystic fibrosis or sickle cell disease: a multicenter study. *Pediatrics* 1998;101:250–256.

Suris et al. (1996) conducted a statewide survey of Minnesota high school students and showed that for both boys and girls, there was no difference in age at first intercourse between those with chronic illness and those without, and no effect of visibility of illness on age at first intercourse. Cheng and Udry (2002) in an analysis of physically disabled adolescents (mainly with musculoskeletal disorders) interviewed in the National Longitudinal Study of Adolescent Health found that by age 16, physically disabled teens were at least as sexually active as their nondisabled peers with 39% and 42% of severely disabled boys and girls, respectively, reporting sexual intercourse versus 37% and 34% of nondisabled boys and girls, respectively. In a study of inner-city adolescents with various chronic diseases (e.g., asthma, diabetes mellitus, cancer, sickle cell disease, and others) and their healthy friends aged 14 through 17 years, Alderman and Lauby (1995) found that approximately one third of both the chronically ill group and the healthy group were sexually active, with a mean age at first intercourse in the 13th year. However, these investigators also found that the interaction between gender and sexual debut was significantly different; boys without chronic illness initiated intercourse at a younger age (12.9 years) than boys with illness (13.4 years), and the reverse was true for girls, those with chronic illness initiated intercourse at a younger age (13.8 years) than their healthy friends (15.3 years). Britto et al. (1998) surveyed adolescents with cystic fibrosis and sickle cell disease from five pediatric tertiary care centers in North Carolina and compared their sexual behavior with that of controls matched for age, race, and gender. Fewer teens with cystic fibrosis (28%) and sickle cell disease (51%) than matched controls (46% and 76%, respectively) reported sexual activity. Also, the age at first intercourse for girls was older in those with chronic illness compared with matched controls, 15.7 versus 14.6 years and 14.8 versus 13.9 years for those with cystic fibrosis and sickle cell disease, respectively. The same was true for boys, only the ages at first intercourse were approximately 1 year younger in all groups.

As the study by Britto et al. shows, sexual debut may be delayed in adolescents with illnesses that delay puberty such as cystic fibrosis and sickle cell disease. Onset of sexual activity may also be delayed for adolescents with mobility limitations and brain-based conditions that result in fewer opportunities for peer interaction. Sexual assault is also a salient issue, particularly for cognitively impaired adolescent girls who are uniquely vulnerable to exploitation.

2. Fertility: Some chronic conditions are associated with impaired fertility related to the disease itself or to the treatment. For example, males with cystic fibrosis are infertile, but females are fertile and many have children. In a large study of survivors of childhood cancer, Byrne et al. (1987) demonstrated that compared with sibling controls, radiation therapy below the diaphragm had the greatest adverse effect on fertility in females. It is important to remember, however, that most chronic illnesses do not impair fertility, and particularly for sexually active girls, effective contraception is extremely important. Girls with chronic illness should be counseled about the necessity of carefully planning pregnancies to minimize teratogenicity from medications and treatments and to ensure the best outcome for mother and fetus. Chapter 42 reviews contraceptive options in teens

with various chronic illnesses and Table 82.3 outlines contraceptive options for selected chronic diseases.

3. Sexually transmitted diseases: Girls who are immunosuppressed either due to the disease (e.g., HIV) or the treatment (e.g., organ transplant, lupus) are at risk for a prolonged and more complicated course if infected with a sexually transmitted disease. These girls should receive detailed instruction and frequent reinforcement regarding barrier contraceptive use. Genital infection with human papillomavirus (HPV) is particularly virulent in girls who are immunocompromised, and they are at increased risk of developing cervical cancer. In the future, with widespread use of HPV vaccines, this risk may be considerably mitigated.

Substance Use

Substance use by adolescents with chronic illness can contribute significantly to morbidity and mortality. Alcohol, illicit drugs, or over-the-counter herbal preparations may interact with prescribed medications to cause deleterious effects. Certain specific chronic conditions, notably heart disease, put affected adolescents at particular risk of death from even one-time use of stimulants such as cocaine, amphetamines, or "Ecstasy" (methylenedioxymethamphetamine [MDMA]).

Prevalence of Substance Use Westbrook et al. (1991) compared substance use in three different groups of adolescents, aged 13 to 19 years. The groups included 34 patients with idiopathic epilepsy, 32 with various chronic diseases other than epilepsy, and 50 with no chronic illness. Fewer adolescents with epilepsy were daily smokers (9%) than adolescents who had other chronic diseases (19%) or were healthy (30%). Approximately 15% of the teens in each group reported drinking alcohol once a week or more, and 20% in each group reported that they used marijuana, with less than half using it once a week or more. The study by Britto et al. (1998) in North Carolina also found that fewer teens with cystic fibrosis versus matched controls smoked regularly (2.6% versus 29.6%), were binge drinkers (18.0% versus 35.3%), or tried marijuana (9.7% versus 29.4%), respectively. Tyc et al. (2006) reviewed smoking rates in children and adolescents with chronic illness. They reported that some of these adolescents had smoking rates at least comparable to those of their healthy peers. The article also reviewed suggested interventions for smoking cessation in youth with a chronic illness. Although the proportion of adolescents with chronic illness using substances may be less than that of their healthy peers, the absolute numbers are still quite high, and the risk for health complications are greater. Screening by history for substance use, and anticipatory guidance and counseling regarding specific substances and their effect on the adolescent's illness are mandatory.

MANAGEMENT OF CHRONIC ILLNESS IN THE ADOLESCENT

General Principles

Optimal care of the adolescent's medical condition is of primary importance. However, high-quality treatment often

TABLE 82.3

Choice of Contraceptives for Girls with Selected Chronic Conditions

Condition	Special Considerations	Suggested Contraceptives
Diabetes mellitus	Low-dose OCPs do not affect glucose tolerance. Estrogen-dominant pills promote a favorable lipid profile. Obesity is often a problem in type 2 diabetes.	Second- or third-generation combination OCPs, patch, or ring plus male latex condom. Avoid DMPA in girls with type 2 diabetes.
Heart disease	OCPs, patch, and ring contraindicated with pulmonary vascular disease, thromboembolic disease, and cerebrovascular disease.	Progestin-only injectable or implantable methods plus male latex condom. Consider progestin-releasing IUD (Mirena). May use OCPs if no contraindications.
Immunosuppression	STDs, especially viral pathogens such as HPV, are more virulent and hard to treat.	Male latex condoms preferred. Consider female condom. May use hormonal methods as well if no contraindications.
Mental retardation	Compliance is an issue unless parent will administer pills. Barrier methods difficult to use.	Long-acting injectable or implantable methods are preferred.
Seizure disorder	OCPs, patch, and ring have lowered efficacy with some seizure medications but not with valproic acid.	DMPA or combination OCPs plus male latex condom. Progestin-only OCPs are contraindicated.
Sickle cell disease	Hormonal methods reduce frequency of vasoocclusive crises. OCPs, patch, and ring contraindicated with history of stroke.	DMPA with male latex condoms is preferred. OCPs, patch, or ring may be used if no contraindications.
Spina bifida	May have latex allergy. OCPs have lowered efficacy with some seizure medications. OCPs, patch, and ring may have higher thrombosis risk in immobilized patients. DMPA may exacerbate osteopenia in immobilized patients.	Polyurethane condoms (male or female) plus hormonal methods if no contraindications. DMPA is not advised for those who are wheelchair bound. Consider progestin-releasing IUD (Mirena–reduced uterine bleeding, no osteopenia).

OCP, oral contraceptive pill; DMPA, depot medroxyprogesterone acetate; IUD, intrauterine device; HPV, human papillomavirus; STD, sexually transmitted disease.

cannot be achieved without consideration and exploration of the adolescent's mental health, developmental progress, and family relationships. Simply prescribing treatment is not enough. The adolescent must cooperate with the health care team, believe that adhering to a complex regimen is better than the alternative, and have family support and assistance in carrying out the treatment plan. Helpful principles for management include the following:

1. Educate: Inform the adolescent about the nature of the disease and the limitations of treatment. The educational process should be directed at both patient and family and should use language that is easy to understand. For illnesses diagnosed early in life, update adolescents as they become more cognitively mature and capable of understanding their condition better.
2. Respond to emotion: Listen carefully, give permission, and allow time for the adolescent and the family to express feelings, fears, and hopes.
3. Involve the family: Family support and guidance are crucial. Help families to allow their adolescents increased autonomy and independence over time. Families must be coached to avoid the "overs"—overprotection, overanxiety, and overattention.
4. Involve the patient: The more an adolescent is involved with his or her own care, the greater the

chance for improved compliance and a greater sense of self-determination.
5. Use a multidisciplinary team: Many health care professionals are usually necessary to optimally manage adolescents with chronic illness, including physicians, psychologists, social workers, nurses, occupational therapists, physical therapists, and nutritionists. Respect for the skills of these individuals, as well as communication in interdisciplinary conferences, can improve the care of the adolescent.
6. Provide continuity of care: The chronically ill adolescent needs an advocate whom he or she can trust. At least one member of the health care team, preferably a primary care clinician, should maintain an ongoing relationship with the patient and family. This clinician's role is to coordinate care among various specialty disciplines, monitor adolescent development, provide support and anticipatory guidance, and treat intercurrent illnesses.
7. Provide comprehensive ambulatory services: Such services would include psychological, educational, speech and hearing, social work, and other special services. It may be difficult for families to obtain insurance reimbursement for such necessary services, although they are cost-effective. Liptak et al. (1998) showed that

comprehensive ambulatory service decreased number of inpatient hospitalizations, length of stay, hospital costs, and readmissions for chronically ill children.

8. Referral to peer and disease support groups: Participation in such groups allows for increased expression of concerns and anxieties by both patients and families and sharing of information among families with similar problems. A number of support group agencies are listed at the end of this chapter.

9. Consider self-help techniques: Training the adolescent in various cognitive-behavioral techniques to manage stress and pain can enhance feelings of self-control and reduce disease- and treatment-related stress. Examples of these strategies include hypnosis, relaxation and distraction techniques, guided imagery, and thought stopping.

10. Limit setting: If compliance or behavior is a problem, limits must be set and the entire health care team and the parents must agree and enforce the limits. Avoidance of splitting and pitting one member of the team against another is crucial.

11. Inpatient care: When necessary, inpatient hospital care is best handled in an environment conducive to the developmental needs of the adolescent.

HEALTH CARE TRANSITION FROM PEDIATRIC TO ADULT SERVICES FOR YOUNG ADULTS WITH CHRONIC ILLNESS

Approximately half a million youth with special health care needs will turn 18 each year in the United States and most will need to be transitioned into the adult health care system. An appropriately timed transition to adult-oriented health care allows youth to optimize their independence and to more successfully assume adult roles and functioning. Indeed, the Healthy People 2010 initiative has established a goal that "All youth with special health care needs will receive the services necessary to make transitions to all aspects of adult life, including adult health care, work, and independence." A joint consensus statement issued in 2002 by leading pediatric and adult health care societies recommends that a written health care transition plan for adolescents with special health care needs be created by age 14 and that affordable, continuous health insurance coverage be ensured throughout adolescence and adulthood. However, there are several barriers to effecting a successful health care transition for chronically ill youth and their families. Such barriers include the following:

- Lack of adequately trained or accessible adult-oriented physicians to manage chronic childhood conditions such as congenital heart disease or cystic fibrosis
- Loss of health insurance coverage when the young adult is no longer covered on the parents' policy
- Reluctance of patients, families, and pediatric subspecialists to terminate a long-standing relationship

The Society for Adolescent Medicine in its 2003 position paper outlined several principles of successful transition services. Such services should have the following features:

- Be appropriate for both chronological age and developmental attainment

- Address common concerns of young people such as growth and development, sexuality, mental health disorders, and substance use
- Facilitate self-reliance and autonomy, and increase personal responsibility
- Be flexible enough to meet the needs of a wide range of young people
- Have a designated professional who, along with the patient and family, takes responsibility for the process

Scal and Ireland (2005) evaluated the adequacy of transition services in an analysis of parent reports from the 2001 National Survey of Children with Special Health Care Needs. These investigators found that overall, 50% of youth and parents had discussed transition issues with the adolescent's doctor but only one in six (16%) had developed a plan. The strongest predictors of the adequacy of health care transition services were a high-quality parent–provider interaction, a greater number of needed services, female gender, and older age. This study provides us with a first look at how we are doing as a nation in providing optimal care for our adolescents and young adults with chronic illness and indicates that we have much room left for improvement.

RESOURCES

http://www.pacer.org/links/national/disability.htm. PACER Center (Parent Advocacy Coalition for Educational Rights): This site has up-to-date links and addresses for more than 160 specific disability resources including organizations and associations such as Autism Society of America, National Fragile X Foundation, American Diabetes Association, Cystic Fibrosis Foundation, March of Dimes Birth Defects Foundation, Candlelighters Childhood Cancer Foundation, and many others. Resources are listed for 14 different categories of disability including: Attention Deficit Disorder, Autism Spectrum Disorders, Cognitive and Developmental Disabilities, Deaf Blind, Deaf and Hard of Hearing, Emotional and Behavioral Disorders, Genetic Disorders, Health Impairments, Learning Disabilities, Neurological Disorders, Physical Disabilities, Speech or Language Impairments, Traumatic Brain Injury, and Visually Impaired.

WEB SITES

http://www.nichcy.org. National Dissemination Center for Children with Disabilities. Information on disabilities in children and youth, special education, and research.
http://www.depts.washington.edu/healthtr/. Adolescent Health Transition Project at the Center on Human Development and Disability at the University of Washington, Seattle. This site contains extensive high quality information for health care providers and educators, parents and families, and teens and young adults.
http://www.hrtw.org. Healthy and Ready to Work National Center. This Center is part of the Division of Services for Children with Special Health Care Needs of the MCHB. It is filled with information for professionals, parents, and youth.
http://www.youngwomenshealth.org. This site is sponsored by the Children's Hospital Boston. There is

excellent information for girls, parents, and professionals on contraception and sexual health as well as on chronic gynecologic conditions including reproductive consequences for cancer survivors, poly cystic ovary syndrome, endometriosis, congenital anomalies of the female genital tract, and ovarian failure.

REFERENCES AND ADDITIONAL READINGS

Alderman EM. Reproductive health for girls with chronic illness. In: SM Coupey, ed. *Primary care of adolescent girls.* Philadelphia: Hanley & Belfus, 2000:127–135.

Alderman EM, Lauby JL, Coupey SM. Problem behaviors in inner-city adolescents with chronic illness. *J Dev Behav Pediatr* 1995;16:339.

American Academy of Pediatrics, American Academy of Family Physicians, American College of Physicians, American Society of Internal Medicine. A consensus statement on health care transitions for young adults with special health care needs. *Pediatrics* 2002;110:1304.

American Academy of Pediatrics, Committee on Children With Disabilities. General principles in the care of children and adolescents with genetic disorders and other chronic health conditions. *Pediatrics* 1997;99:643.

Bennett DS. Depression among children with chronic medical problems: a meta-analysis. *J Pediatr Psychol* 1994;19:149.

Blum RW. Sexual health contraceptive needs of adolescents with chronic conditions. *Arch Pediatr Adolesc Med* 1997; 151:290.

Britto MT, Garrett JM, Dugliss MAJ, et al. Risky behavior in teens with cystic fibrosis or sickle cell disease: a multicenter study. *Pediatrics* 1998;101:250.

Byrne J, Mulvihill JJ, Myers MH, et al. Effects of treatment on fertility in long-term survivors of childhood or adolescent cancer. *N Engl J Med.* 1987;317:1315.

Cheng MM, Udry JR. Sexual behaviors of physically disabled adolescents in the United States. *J Adolesc Health* 2002;31:48.

Desguin BW, Holt IJ, McCarthy SM. Comprehensive care of the child with a chronic condition. II. Primary care management. *Curr Probl Pediatr* 1994;24:230.

Freed GL, Hudson EJ. Transitioning children with chronic diseases to adult care: current knowledge, practices, and directions. *J Pediatr* 2006;148:824.

Garwick AE, Millar HEC. *Promoting resilience in youth with chronic conditions and their families.* Rockville, MD: U.S. Department of Health and Human Services, Maternal and Child Health Bureau, Health Resources and Service Administration, Public Health Service, April 1996.

Hauser ST, DiPlacido J, Jacobson AM, et al. Family coping with an adolescent's chronic illness: an approach and three studies. *J Adolesc* 1993;16:305.

Holden EW, Chmielewski D, Nelson CC, et al. Controlling for general and disease specific effects in child and family adjustment to chronic childhood illness. *J Pediatr Psychol* 1997;22:15.

Howe GW, Feinstein C, Reiss D, et al. Adolescent Adjustment to chronic physical disorders. I. Comparing neurological and non-neurological conditions. *J Child Psychol Psychiatry.* 1993;34:1153.

Ireys HT, Werthamer-Larsson LA, Kolodner KB, et al. Mental health of young adults with chronic illness: the mediating effect of perceived impact. *J Pediatr Psychol* 1994;19:205.

Kyngas HA, Kroll T, Duffy ME. Compliance in adolescents with chronic diseases: a review. *J Adolesc Health* 2000;26:379.

Liptak GS, Burns CM, Davidson PW, et al. Effects of providing comprehensive ambulatory services to children with chronic conditions. *Arch Pediatr Adolesc Med* 1998;152:1003.

Maternal and Child Health Bureau. *Achieving success for all children and youth with special health care needs: a 10-year action plan to accompany Healthy People 2010.* Rockville, MD: Maternal and Child Health Bureau, 2001.

McPherson M, Arango P, Fox H, et al. A new definition of children with special health care needs. *Pediatrics* 1998; 102:137.

Mintzer LL, Stuber ML, Seacord D, et al. Traumatic stress symptoms in adolescent organ transplant recipients. *Pediatrics* 2005;115:1640.

National Survey of Children with Special Health Care Needs Chartbook 2001. *Prevalence of children with special health care needs.* http://mchb.hrsa.gov/chscn/pages/prevalence.htm. 2001.

Neal W, Coupey SM. Biopsychosocial aspects of chronic illness. *Adolesc Med* 1996;7:427.

Neumark-Sztainer D, Story M, Falkner NH, et al. Disordered eating among adolescents with chronic illness and disability. *Arch Pediatr Adolesc Med* 1998;152:871.

Newacheck PW, Strickland B, Shonkoff JP, et al. An epidemiologic profile of children with special health care needs. *Pediatrics* 1998;102:117.

Patterson J, Blum RW. Risk and resilience among children and youth with disabilities. *Arch Pediatr Adolesc Med* 1996;150: 692.

Perrin EC, Newacheck P, Pless IB, et al. Issues involved in the definition of chronic health conditions. *Pediatrics.* 1993;91:787.

Rosen DS, Blum RW, Britto M, et al. Transition to adult health care for adolescents and young adults with chronic conditions: position paper of the Society for Adolescent Medicine. *J Adolesc Health* 2003;33:309.

Rutter M. Resilience in the face of adversity: protective factors and resistance to psychiatric disorder. *Br J Psychiatry* 1985;147:598.

Saetermoe CL, Farruggia SP, Lopez C. Differential parental communication with adolescents who are disabled and their healthy siblings. *J Adolesc Health* 1999;24:427.

Scal P, Ireland M. Addressing transition to adult health care for adolescents with special health care needs. *Pediatrics* 2005;115:1607.

Sheerin D, MacLeod M, Kusumakar V. Psychosocial adjustment in children with port-wine stains and prominent ears. *J Am Acad Child Adolesc Psychiatry* 1995;34:1637.

Stein RE, Bauman LJ, Westbrook LE, et al. Framework for identifying children who have chronic conditions: the case for a new definition. *J Pediatr* 1993;122:342.

Stein RE, Silver EJ. Operationalizing a conceptually based noncategorical definition: a first look at U.S. children with chronic conditions. *Arch Pediatr Adolesc Med* 1999;153:68.

Stein RE, Westbrook LE, Bauman LJ. The questionnaire for identifying children with chronic conditions: a measure based on a noncategorical approach. *Pediatrics* 1997;99:513.

Stuber ML. Psychiatric sequelae in seriously ill children and their families. *Psychiatr Clin North Am* 1996;19:481.

Suris J, Resnick MD, Cassuto N, et al. Sexual behavior of adolescents with chronic disease and disability. *J Adolesc Health* 1996;19:124.

Tyc VL, Throckmorton-Belzer L. Smoking rates and the state of smoking interventions for children and adolescents with chronic illness. *Pediatrics* 2006;118:471.

Valencia LS, Cromer BA. Sexual activity and other high risk behaviors in adolescents with chronic illness: a review. *J Pediatr Adolesc Gynecol* 2000;13:53.

Westbrook LE, Stein RE. Epidemiology of chronic health conditions in adolescents. *Adolesc Med* 1994;5:197.

Wolman C, Resnick MD, Harris LJ, et al. Emotional well-being among adolescents with and without chronic conditions. *J Adolesc Health* 1994;15:199.

References for Specific Conditions

Asthma

Angsten JM. Use of complementary and alternative medicine in the treatment of asthma. *Adolesc Med* 2000;11:535.

CDC. Self-reported asthma among high school students—United States, 2003. *MMWR* 2005;54:765.

Howenstine MS, Eigen H. Medical care of the adolescent with asthma. *Adolesc Med* 2000;11:501.

Morikawa A, Mochizuki H, Shigeta M, et al. Age-related changes in bronchial hyperreactivity during the adolescent period. *J Asthma* 1994;31:445.

Reznik M, Sharif I, Ozuah PO. Classifying asthma severity: prospective symptom diary or retrospective symptom recall? *J Adolesc Health* 2005;36:537.

Rodriguez MA, Winkleby MA, Ahn D, et al. Identification of population subgroups of children and adolescents with high asthma prevalence. *Arch Pediatr Adolesc Med* 2002;156:269.

Vila G, Nollet-Clemencon C, Vera M, et al. Prevalence of DSM-IV disorders in children and adolescents with asthma versus diabetes. *Can J Psychiatry* 1999;44:562.

Zbikowski SM, Klesges RC, Robinson LA. Risk factors for smoking among adolescents with asthma. *J Adolesc Health* 2002;30:279.

Cancer

American Academy of Pediatrics. Guidelines for pediatric cancer centers. *Pediatrics* 2004;113:1833.

Bahadur G, Whelan J, Ralph D. Gaining consent to freeze spermatozoa from adolescents with cancer: legal, ethical, and practical aspects. *Hum Reprod* 2001;16:188.

Bassal M, Mertens AC, Taylor L, et al. Risk of selected subsequent carcinomas in survivors of childhood cancer: a report from the childhood cancer survivor study. *J Clin Oncol* 2006;24:476.

Bleyer WA. Cancer in older adolescents and young adults: epidemiology, diagnosis, treatment, survival, and importance of clinical trials. *Med Pediatr Oncol* 2002;38:1.

Grant J, Cranston A, Horsman J, et al. Health status and health-related quality of life in adolescent survivors of cancer in childhood. *J Adolesc Health* 2006;38:504.

Green DM, Zevon MA, Reese PA, et al. Factors that influence the further survival of patients who survive for five years after the diagnosis of cancer in childhood or adolescence. *Med Pediatr Oncol* 1994;22:91.

Grundy R, Gosden RG, Hewitt M, et al. Fertility preservation for children treated for cancer: scientific advances and research dilemmas. *Arch Dis Child* 2001;84:355.

Hudson MM, Mertens AC, Yasui Y, et al. Health status of adult long-term survivors of childhood cancer. *JAMA* 2003; 290:1583.

Kazak AE. Evidence-based interventions for survivors of childhood cancer and their families. *J Pediatr Psychol* 2005; 30:29.

Klopfenstein KJ. Adolescents, cancer, and hospice. *Adolesc Med* 1999;10:437.

Nicholson HS, Byrne J. Fertility and pregnancy after treatment for cancer during childhood or adolescence. *Cancer* 1993;71:3392.

Sarafoglou K, Boulad F, Gillio A, et al. Gonadal function after bone marrow transplantation for acute leukemia during childhood. *J Pediatr* 1997;130:210.

Shankar S, Robison L, Jenney MEM, et al. Health-related quality of life in young survivors of childhood cancer using the Minneapolis-Manchester quality of life—youth form. *Pediatrics* 2005;115:435.

Von Essen L, Enskar K, Kreuger A, et al. Self-esteem, depression, and anxiety among Swedish children and adolescents on and of cancer treatment. *Acta Pediatr* 2000;89:229.

Wu X, Chen VW, Steele B, et al. Cancer incidence in adolescents and young adults in the United States, 1992–1997. *J Adolesc Health* 2003;32:405.

Cystic Fibrosis

Bartholomew LK, Parcel GS, Swank PR, et al. Measuring self-efficacy expectations for the self-management of cystic fibrosis. *Chest* 1993;103:1524.

Birnkrant DJ, Hen J, Stern RC. The adolescent with cystic fibrosis. *Adolesc Med* 1994;5:249.

Britto MT, Garrett JM, Konrad TR, et al. Comparison of physical activity in adolescents with cystic fibrosis versus age-matched controls. *Pediatr Pulmonol* 2000;30:86.

Graetz BW, Shute RH, Sawyer MG. An Australian study of adolescents with cystic fibrosis: perceived supportive and nonsupportive behaviors from families and friends and psychological adjustment. *J Adolesc Health* 2000;26:64.

Nasr SZ. Cystic fibrosis in adolescents and young adults. *Adolesc Med* 2000;11:589.

Sawyer SM, Rosier MJ, Phelan PD, et al. The self-image of adolescents with cystic fibrosis. *J Adolesc Health* 1995;16:204.

Thompson RJ, Gustafson KE, George LK, et al. Change over a 12-month period in the psychological adjustment of children and adolescents with cystic fibrosis. *J Pediatr Psychol* 1994; 19:189.

Zindani GN, Streetman DD, Streetman DS. Adherence to treatment in children and adolescent patients with cystic fibrosis. *J Adolesc Health* 2006;38:13.

Diabetes Mellitus

Daviss WB, Coon H, Whitehead P, et al. Predicting diabetic control form competence, adherence, adjustment, and psychopathology. *J Am Acad Child Adolesc Psychiatry* 1995;34:1629.

Draznin MB, Patel DR. Diabetes mellitus and sports. *Adolesc Med* 1998;9:457.

Farrell SP, Hains AA, Davies WH, et al. The impact of cognitive distortions, stress, and adherence on metabolic control in youths with type 1 diabetes. *J Adolesc Health* 2004;34:461.

Fagot-Campagna A, Pettitt DJ, Engelgau MM, et al. Type 2 diabetes among North American children and adolescents: an epidemiologic review and a public health perspective. *J Pediatr* 2000;136:664.

Hoare P, Mann H. Self-esteem and behavioral adjustment in children with epilepsy and children with diabetes. *J Psychosom Res* 1994;38:859.

Jacobson AM, Hauser ST, Lavori P, et al. Family environment and glycemic control: a four-year prospective study of children and adolescents with insulin-dependent diabetes mellitus. *Psychosom Med* 1994;56:401.

Lawrence JM, Standiford DA, Loots B, et al. Prevalence and correlates of depressed mood among youth with diabetes: the SEARCH for diabetes in youth study. *Pediatrics* 2006;117:1348.

Mellin AE, Neumark-Sztainer D, Patterson J. Unhealthy weight management behavior among adolescent girls with type 1 diabetes mellitus: the role of familial eating patterns and weight-related concerns. *J Adolesc Health* 2004;35:278.

Pettitt DD, Jones KL, Arslanian SA. Type 2 diabetes mellitus in minority children and adolescents: and emerging problem. *Endocrinol Metab Clin North Am* 1999;28:709.

Pollock M, Kovacs M, Charron-Prochownik D. Eating disorders and maladaptive dietary/insulin management among youths with childhood-onset insulin-dependent diabetes mellitus. *J Am Acad Child Adolesc Psychiatry* 1995;34:291.

Sperling MA. Diabetes in adolescence. *Adolesc Med* 1994;5:87.

Svoren BM, Butler D, Levine B, et al. Reducing acute adverse outcomes in youths with type 1 diabetes: a randomized controlled trial. *Pediatrics* 2003;112:914.

Weissberg-Benchell J, Glasgow AM, Tynan WD, et al. Adolescent diabetes management and mismanagement. *Diabetes Care* 1995;18:77.

Disabled Adolescent

Apple DF Jr, Anson CA, Hunter JD, et al. Spinal cord injury in youth. *Clin Pediatr* 1995;34:90.

Balogh R, Bretherton K, Whibley S, et al. Sexual abuse in children and adolescents with intellectual disability. *J Intellect Disabil Res* 2001;45:194.

Clark MW. The physically challenged athlete. *Adolesc Med* 1998; 9:491.

Greydanus DE, Rimsza ME, Newhouse PA. Adolescent sexuality and disability. *Adolesc Med* 2002;13:223.

Hallum A. Disability and the transition to adulthood: issues for the disabled child, the family, and the pediatrician. *Curr Probl Pediatr* 1995;25:12.

Langley JD, Stanton WR, McGee RO, et al. Disability in late adolescence. I. Introduction, methods, and overview. *Disabil Rehabil* 1995;17:35.

Saetermoe CL, Farruggia SP, Lopez C. Differential parental communication with adolescents who are disabled and their healthy siblings. *J Adolesc Health* 1999;24:427.

Taniguchi MH, Schlosser GA. Adolescent spinal cord injury: considerations for post-acute management. *Adolesc Med* 1994;5:327.

Epilepsy

Hoare P, Mann H. Self-esteem and behavioral adjustment in children with epilepsy and children with diabetes. *J Psychosom Res* 1994;38:859.

Raty LKA, Larsson BMW, Soderfeldt BA, et al. Health-related quality of life in youth: a comparison between adolescents and young adults with uncomplicated epilepsy and healthy controls. *J Adolesc Health* 2003;33:252.

Westbrook LE, Silver EJ, Coupey SM, et al. Social characteristics of adolescents with idiopathic epilepsy: a comparison to chronically ill and non-chronically ill peers. *J Epilepsy* 1991; 4:87.

Heart Disease

Cetta F, Graham LC, Lichtenberg RC. Piercing and tattooing in patients with congenital heart disease: patient and physician perspectives. *J Adolesc Health* 1999;24:160.

Doroshow RW. The adolescent with simple or corrected congenital heart disease. *Adolesc Med* 2001;12:1.

Gillum RF. Epidemiology of congenital heart disease in the United States. *Am Heart J* 1994;127:919.

Mendelson MA. Gynecologic and obstetric issues in the adolescent with heart disease. *Adolesc Med* 2001;12:163.

Inflammatory Bowel Disease

Engstrom I. Inflammatory bowel disease in children and adolescents: mental health and family functioning. *J Pediatr Gastroenterol Nutr* 1999;28:S28.

Griffiths AM. Inflammatory bowel disease. *Adolesc Med* 1995;6:351.

Lindberg E, Lindquist B, Holmquist L, et al. Inflammatory bowel disease in children and adolescents in Sweden, 1984–1995. *J Pediatr Gastroenterol Nutr* 2000;30:259.

Renal Disease

Cameron JS. Lupus nephritis in childhood and adolescence. *Pediatr Nephrol* 1994;8:230.

Furth SL, Hwang W, Yang C, et al. Relation between pediatric experience and treatment recommendations for children and adolescents with kidney failure. *JAMA* 2001;285:1027.

Hogg RJ, Furth S, Lemley KV, et al. National kidney foundation's kidney disease outcomes quality initiative clinical practice guidelines for chronic kidney disease in children and adolescents: evaluation, classification, and stratification. *Pediatrics* 2003;111:1416.

Manifica S, Dazord A, Cochat P, et al. Quality of life of children and adolescents after kidney or liver transplantation: child, parents and caregiver's point of view. *Pediatr Transplant* 2003;7:228.

Watson AR, Shooter M. Transitioning adolescents from pediatric to adult dialysis units. *Adv Perit Dial* 1996;12:176.

Rheumatological Conditions

Adam V, St-Pierre Y, Fautrel B, et al. What is the impact of adolescent arthritis and rheumatism? Evidence from a national sample of Canadians. *J Rheumatol* 2005;32:354.

Bentas W, Karch H, Huppertz HI. Lyme arthritis in children and adolescents: outcome 12 months after initiation of antibiotic therapy. *J Rheumatol* 2000;27:2025.

Britto MT, Rosenthal SL, Taylor J, et al. Improving rheumatologists' screening for alcohol use and sexual activity. *Arch Pediatr Adolesc Med* 2000;154:478.

Cuneo KM, Schiaffino KM. Adolescent self-perceptions of adjustment to childhood arthritis: the influence of disease activity, family resources, and parent adjustment. *J Adolesc Health* 2002;31:363.

Hollister JR. Medical treatment of adolescents with rheumatic disease. *Adolesc Med* 1998;9:163.

Sathananthan R, David J. The adolescent with rheumatic disease. *Arch Dis Child* 1997;77:355.

Shaller J. Diagnosis and management of rheumatic diseases in adolescence. *Adolesc Med* 1998;9:1.

Silva CA, Hallak J, Pasqualotto FF, et al. Gonadal function in male adolescents and young males with juvenile onset systemic lupus erythematosus. *J Rheumatol* 2002;29:2000.

White PH. Psychosocial aspects of rheumatic disease in childhood and adolescence. *Adolesc Med* 1998;9:171.

White PH. Transition to adulthood. *Curr Opin Rheumatol* 1999; 11:408.

Sickle Cell Anemia

Athale UH, Chintu C. The effect of sickle cell anaemia on adolescents and their growth and development: lessons from the sickle cell anaemia clinic. *J Trop Pediatr* 1994;40:246.

Britto MT, Garrett JM, Dugliss MA, et al. Preventive services received by adolescents with cystic fibrosis and sickle cell disease. *Arch Pediatr Adolesc Med* 1999;153:27.

Kell RS, Kliewer W, Erickson MT. Psychological adjustment of adolescents with sickle cell disease: relations with demographic, medical, and family competence variables. *J Pediatr Psychol* 1998;23:301.

Lemanek KL, Steiner SM, Grossman NJ. Too little, too late: primary vs. secondary interventions for adolescents with sickle cell disease. *Adolesc Med* 1999;10:385.

Mantadakis E, Cavender D, Joe RN. Prevalence of priapism in children and adolescents with sickle cell anemia. *J Pediatr Hem Oncol* 1999;21:518.

Ohene-Frempong K, Weiner SJ, Sleeper LA, et al. Cerebrovascular accidents in sickle cell disease: rates and risk factors. *Blood* 1998;91:288.

Platt OS, Brambilla DJ, Rosse WF, et al. Mortality in sickle cell disease—life expectancy and risk factors for early death. *N Engl J Med* 1994;330:1639.

Yang YM, Cepeda M, Price C, et al. Depression in children and adolescents with sickle-cell disease. *Arch Pediatr Adolesc Med* 1994;148:457.

Spina Bifida

Appleton PL, Minchom PE, Ellis NC, et al. The self-concept of young people with spina bifida: a population-based study. *Dev Med Child Neurol* 1994;36:198.

Ammerman RT, Kane VR, Slomka GT, et al. Psychiatric symptomatology and family functioning in children and adolescents with spina bifida. *J Clin Psychol Med Settings* 1998; 5:449.

Blum RW, Resnick M, Nelson R, et al. Family and peer issues among adolescents with spina bifida and cerebral palsy. *Pediatrics* 1991;88:280.

Coakley RM, Holmbeck GN, Friedman D, et al. A longitudinal study of pubertal timing, parent-child conflict, and cohesion in families of young adolescents with spina bifida. *J Pediatr Psychol* 2002;27:461.

Gross SM, Ireys HT, Kinsman SL. Young women with physical disabilities: risk factors for symptoms of eating disorders. *J Dev Behav Pediatr* 2000;21:87.

McDonnell GV, McCann JP. Issues of medical management in adults with spina bifida. *Childs Nerv Syst* 2000;16:222.

Sandler AD, Worley G, Leroy EC, et al. Sexual knowledge and experience among young men with spina bifida. *Eur J Pediatr Surg* 1994;4(Suppl 1):36.

Silber TJ, Sheer C. Eating disorders in adolescent girls with spina bifida. *J Adolescent Health* 1996;18:139.

Wolman C, Basco DE. Factors influencing self-esteem and self-consciousness in adolescents with spina bifida. *J Adolesc Health* 1994;15:543.

CHAPTER 83

Complementary and Alternative Medicine in Adolescents

Cora Collette Breuner and Michael Cirigliano

Complementary and alternative medicine (CAM), also known as *integrative, non-allopathic, unconventional, holistic,* or *natural therapy,* encompasses a whole spectrum of healing resources, modalities, and practices other than those intrinsic to the conventional, traditional health systems in a particular society.

One study reported that in 1990 more than one third of Americans used "unconventional" therapies (Eisenberg, 1997). This number increased by 38% between 1990 and 1997. Expenditures for visits to alternative medicine providers were estimated at $21.2 billion and more than half was paid from out of pocket. Approximately one in five people taking prescription medicines were also taking herbs or high-dose vitamin supplements.

CAM use in children and adolescents is more common in certain geographic areas of North America and in young people with chronic illnesses. Importantly, homeless youth have a 70% utilization rate for CAM. In order of prevalence, the therapies most frequently used were chiropractic, homeopathy, naturopathy, and acupuncture. Parents who use CAM for their children and adolescents are older and have a higher level of maternal education. Medical conditions most frequently treated with CAM include respiratory (including ears, nose, and throat), musculoskeletal, skin, gastrointestinal (GI), allergies, chronic conditions such as cystic fibrosis, cancer, arthritis, and illnesses that require surgery.

IMPORTANT ISSUES FOR THE HEALTH CARE PROVIDER

Knowledge/Open Discussion

It is imperative that the adolescent or their parents inform their health care provider regarding CAM use in order to appropriately answer questions that are brought to them. If the provider is open to the discussion of CAM, the teen or parent is less likely to rely on erroneous and false information gleaned from friends, family, and the Internet. Clearly, if health care providers embrace this approach, rather than having a negative or critical attitude, patients will benefit and receive accurate information.

Medicolegal Issues

The combination of lack of sufficient medical research and the desire of the patient to utilize alternative treatments may present an ethical dilemma for the health care provider. There is genuine concern for patient safety, as well as the potential for medicolegal issues. According to Cohen and Kemper (2005), important questions for patients, families, and health care providers who elect to use CAM include:

- Will effective care be utilized when the patient's condition is life threatening?
- Will using CAM treatments prevent the use of conventional treatment?
- What is known about the safety and/or efficacy of the treatment?
- Has the patient consented to the use of CAM?
- Will this proposed CAM therapy be acceptable to another clinician?
- Does this treatment have some support in the medical literature?

In many instances, it is not the health care provider who wishes to use such a treatment but the patient. The health care provider must then decide what to recommend. The health care provider should provide advice that is based on the best available evidence and is congruent with the patient's personal needs and the clinician's best judgment.

Adequate Medical History

Health care providers need to ask adolescents about their use of any form of CAM during every office visit, given that adolescents use CAM (including taking herbal products or supplements). Many herbal treatments have the potential to interact with standard pharmaceutical agents. Screening for CAM use may prevent a significant drug–herb interaction or treatment complication. It also allows the health care provider to assess whether all treatments are actually necessary. Young people may not report CAM use because they believe that their health care provider will not approve or that their health care provider will have insufficient information about CAM modalities. Health care providers involved in adolescent health care should be knowledgeable regarding the use of CAM including side effects, toxicity, and potential interactions. Health care providers should also inform adolescents that just because something is natural, does not guarantee its safety.

HERBAL THERAPIES

Consumer use of herbal therapies has increased over the last several years. Sales of herbal therapies have increased yearly by approximately 5% to 6% until recently when sales have stabilized. Despite concerns among the medical community, consumer use remains popular and is rarely discussed with the health care provider. Given the overwhelming popularity of herbal therapies, health care providers should be encouraged to follow basic clinical guidelines to ensure patient safety (Table 83.1).

Regulation

The Dietary Supplement Health and Education Act (DSHEA) of 1994 defines herbal therapies as supplements. As such, herbal therapies are not tested according to the same scientific standards as conventional drugs. Packaging or marketing information does not need to be approved by the U.S. Food and Drug Administration (FDA) before a product reaches the market. The herbal therapy need only describe how the "structure and function" of the human body is affected and cannot be marketed for the diagnosis, treatment, cure or prevention of disease. No protection is offered against misleading or fraudulent claims. The American Academy of Pediatrics (AAP) Committee on Children with Disabilities has issued guidelines for discussing CAM use (specifically herbal therapies) with families (http://www.aap.org/healthtopics/complementarymedicine.cfm).

Accurate Clinical Research Data

Clinical data is often lacking for many herbal therapies. Because herbal therapies are considered dietary supplements and not drugs, premarket testing and studies on safety and efficacy are not required. More recently, studies of herbal therapies using sound investigational methodology are being published in peer-reviewed journals. This will undoubtedly assist in making informed decisions regarding the use of herbal therapies.

Herb–Drug Interactions

Clinicians should be aware of various herb–drug interactions (Table 83.2). One of the most significant such interactions is by agents that cause antiplatelet activity. Recent evidence shows serious interactions with St. John's wort and cyclosporine, oral contraceptives, and antiretroviral agents including indinavir. A number of herbal therapies when combined with warfarin (Coumadin) or nonsteroidal antiinflammatory drugs have led to bleeding complications. Preoperative counseling on the risks of these herbal therapies should be provided to patients undergoing surgery. To ensure safety, discontinuation of these herbs at least 2 weeks before surgery should occur, until more data is available. At a minimum, frequent measurements of the prothrombin time and/or the international normalized ratio may be necessary to avoid complications.

Herb Toxicity

Herbal therapies have been known to cause toxicity to various organ systems (Table 83.3) including:

1. Liver: The organ that appears to be the most common target of serious herbal toxicity is the liver. Two common types of liver insults are hepatitis and venoocclusive disease. Chaparral has been implicated in acute hepatitis causing subacute hepatocellular necrosis leading to cholestatic hepatitis and eventually liver failure requiring transplantation. Additionally, germander has been thought to be involved in causing hepatotoxicity and fatality. Several Chinese herbal therapies have been found to cause liver toxicity including *Jin Bu Huan*, which contains the alkaloid levo-tetrahydropalmatine. This herbal therapy contains structural similarities to hepatotoxic pyrrolizidine alkaloids previously documented to cause liver damage. Clinically, exposure to this compound may lead to hepatomegaly and ascites caused by hepatic

TABLE 83.1

Guidelines for Use of Herbal Therapies in the Clinical Setting

All patients should be asked about use of alternative/complementary treatments during routine office visits and initial visits

Care should be exercised when combining herbal therapies with standard pharmaceuticals

Because herbal contaminants have been documented in a number of products due to poor manufacturing and lack of standardization, use of herbal therapies by reputable manufacturers is advised

Larger than recommended doses of herbal therapies should be discouraged

Until safety data exist, herbal therapies should not be used in pregnancy or lactation

Long-term use of herbal therapies should be done only under the supervision of a knowledgeable health care provider

Herbal therapies with known toxicity and side effects should not be used in children and adolescents

Use of herbal stimulants and performance enhancers in the adolescent population should be discouraged

All proven treatment options should be discussed with patients and their families before entertaining any form of complementary therapies

From *The review of natural products*. St. Louis, MO: Facts and Comparisons, 1999, with permission.

TABLE 83.2

Selected Drug–Herb Interactions Important in Adolescent Health

Herbal Product	Drug or Drug Class	Potential Interaction
Green tea	Warfarin	Decreased anticoagulant activity due to vitamin K content
Kava	Alprazolam	Additive or synergistic effects
St. John's wort	Cyclosporine Digoxin OCP Protease inhibitors TCAs Theophylline	Significant metabolism through P-450 system may lead to decreased serum drug levels
	Warfarin Iron SSRIs	May lead to decreased absorption or iron May lead to increased side effects as well as the serotonin syndrome
	Benzodiazepam	May reduce the effectiveness in reducing anxiety and may increase the risk of side effects such as drowsiness
	Photosensitizing drugs (e.g. lansoprazole, omeprazole, piroxicam, and sulfonamide antibiotics)	Increased risk of sun sensitivity
Valerian	Barbiturates Benzodiazepines	Possible synergistic effects Increased sedation and increased side effects
Yohimbe	TCAs	Hypertension
Panax ginseng Garlic Feverfew Ginkgo	Anticoagulants	Inhibition of platelet aggregation through inhibition of thromboxane synthetase, arachidonic acid production, inhibition of epinephrine, platelet thromboxane synthetase aggregation inhibition of platelet-activating factor
Panax ginseng	Oral hypoglycemics	Enhanced effects
Echinacea	Immunosuppressants	Interference with immunosuppression

OCP, oral contraceptive pill; SSRI, selective serotonin reuptake inhibitor; TCA, tricyclic antidepressant.
Adapted from Drug-herb interactions. In: *The review of natural products*. St. Louis, MO: Facts and Comparisons, 1999, with permission.

central vein dilation and fibrosis. In utero exposure has been linked with hepatic venoocclusive disease and death in the newborn.

2. Cardiotoxicity: Cardiotoxicity has been associated with ingestion of herbal therapies containing aconite alkaloids. These therapies are thought to activate sodium channels and have widespread effects on the excitable membranes of cardiac, neural, and muscle tissue. Enhancement of transmembrane inward currents induces automaticity. Fatal arrhythmias have been described in case reports.

Herbal therapies possess the potential for harm, although the widespread use to date has not led to large numbers of complications. This may be in part due to underreporting of herbal acute drug reactions and toxicities. Herbal therapies have the potential to add a great deal to the existing treatment options available to patients. Further study and long-term trials are needed to assess safety and efficacy.

Dosing Issues and Active Compounds

In traditional medicine, clinicians have become accustomed to using pharmaceutical agents that by definition possess the same strength and high quality. This is not always the case with herbal medicines. Because herbs represent complex entities containing hundreds of constituents, it is difficult to find one particular component representing the active agent. In many cases, particular herbal treatments have been evaluated with a focus on individual extracts and chemical entities such as *Ginkgo biloba* extract (EGb 761). Patients should be counseled on the use of a specific extract in an herbal product that has been clinically studied. If manufacturers have not produced an herbal product using a particular extract, this product should not be recommended.

Whether there is benefit to standardizing an herbal therapy to one identifiable component is a matter of current debate. According to some, the worthy goal of standardization—to achieve a consistent level of the main

TABLE 83.3

Examples of Herbal Therapies Associated with Adverse Effects

Name	Responsible Ingredient	Adverse Effect
Aconite (*Aconitum napellus*)	Contains toxic alkaloids (aconitine)	Heart failure
Aristolochia species	Aristolochic acid is nephrotoxic and mutagenic	Renal failure
Celandine (*Chelidonium majus*)	Toxic alkaloids	Hemolytic anemia, hepatitis
Chamomile (*Chamomilla recutita*)	Sesquiterpene lactone	Potent skin sensitizer
Chaparral (*Larrea tridentata*)	Nordihydroguaiaretic acid	Hepatitis, renal carcinoma
Chaste tree (*Vitex agnus-castus*)	Estrogen-like substances	Hormonal effects
Comfrey (*Symphytum officinale*)	Pyrrolizidine alkaloids	Hepatitis
Ephedra species	Ephedrine	Heart problems, circulatory problems, death
Goldenseal (*Hydrastis canadensis*)	Isoquinoline alkaloids	Uterine contractions
Kelp (*Fucus pyriferus*)	Iodine	Hyperthyroidism
Licorice (*Glycyrrhiza glabra*)	Glycyrrhizin	Mineralocorticoid effects
Mistletoe (*Viscum album*)	Viscotoxins, lectins	Local irritation, allergic reactions
Senna (*Cassia senna*)	Anthranoid derivatives	Suspected mutagenicity

From Ernst E, Pittler MH. Herbal Medicine. *Medical Clinics of North America* 2002; 86(1): 149–161.

therapeutically effective active plant constituent—remains remote. Efforts to achieve this will require characterization, bioactivity assessment, and correlation with clinical end points. The standardization of phytomedicines serves as a precaution for the quality of medicinal plant extracts.

The dosage and length of treatment of various herbal therapies also remains controversial.

Long-term Use

Use of herbal therapies for extended periods of time presents a dilemma for the practicing clinician. Most studies involving herbal therapies do not evaluate long-term effects. Herbal therapies containing tannins have documented an increase risk of certain oropharyngeal cancers with long-term exposure. Additionally, several other herbals have been thought to possess components that may be carcinogenic over time. Herbal therapies should only be used on a time- limited basis until more data is available regarding long-term safety. Adolescents wishing to remain on herbal therapies should be monitored periodically for signs of toxicity and potential adverse effects. Ultimately, adolescents should be informed that the long-term effects of most herbal therapies are unknown. As such, close follow-up is recommended.

Contamination

A lack of quality control and regulation has resulted in contamination and misidentification of plant species (Table 83.4). Herbal therapies may be contaminated with heavy metals or bacteria/fungal organisms when being manufactured or stored. In one study, blood lead levels were significantly higher in children consuming Chinese herbal therapies compared to those who were not. Furthermore, fungal contamination has been noted to be

a problem. In one report from Croatia, 62 samples of medicinal plant material and 11 samples of herbal tea were found to be contaminated with fungal elements. Patients and families should be advised to use products from reputable manufacturers, which use higher regulatory standards (e.g., European agencies such as German Commission E) to ensure the safe manufacturing of herbal therapies.

Use in Pregnancy and Lactation

Women contemplating pregnancy, currently pregnant, or nursing should not use herbal therapies, given the lack of evidence on safety.

Consultation

Adolescents and their families who wish to use herbal therapies may seek the advice of a naturopath, herbalist, or traditional Chinese medicine practitioner. Information

TABLE 83.4

Documented Contaminants/Adulterants Found in Herbal Therapies: Not All Inclusive

Aluminum	Indomethacin
Arsenic	Lead
Aspirin	Mercury
Cadmium	Theophylline
Caffeine	Thiazide diuretics
Corticosteroids	Zinc
Diazepam	

From *Am J Med* 1998;104:175, with permission.

on these practitioners is available through their respective licensing organizations.

Common Herbal Therapies in the Adolescent Population

Among adolescents, it is quite common to find the use of herbal therapies for a number of conditions—weight loss, depression and anxiety, upper respiratory tract infections, and the enhancement of athletic performance. A brief review on commonly used herbal therapies is outlined in the following text.

PSYCHOACTIVE HERBAL THERAPIES

St. John's Wort

Uses Historically, St. John's wort has been used for depression and wound healing.

Mechanism of Action The two active ingredients are hypericin and hyperforin, which inhibit the reuptake of serotonin, norepinephrine, and dopamine. Various studies have noted monoamine oxidase inhibition in vitro along with modulation of melatonin secretion.

Clinical Studies Several studies comparing St. John's wort to tricyclic antidepressants (TCAs) in patients with mild depression, have found that St. John's wort was superior to placebo and as effective as low-dose TCAs. More recently, several studies comparing St. John's wort to selective serotonin reuptake inhibitors (SSRIs) found comparable efficacy using high doses of St. John's wort and low doses of SSRIs. This has not been confirmed in the treatment of major depression.

Side Effects St. John's wort has been noted to have a low incidence of side effects including GI symptoms, dizziness, and confusion. Phototoxicity may occur with ingestion of high doses. Although this is rare, it resolves with the discontinuation of the herb.

Drug Interactions St. John's wort has been shown to induce the cytochrome P-450 metabolic pathway. Studies have shown a significant interaction with St. John's wort and cyclosporine, oral anticoagulants, oral contraceptives, and certain antiretroviral agents including indinavir. The concomitant use of St. John's wort with standard antidepressants is also contraindicated because of the risk of serotonin syndrome.

Kava

Uses Historically, kava was an important cultural entity in the South Pacific, particularly in the Fiji Islands where it is used as a ceremonial drink. It was also used for its calming effects. More recently, it has been used as a natural alternative to sedatives and anxiolytics.

Mechanism of Action It is thought to work by inhibiting γ-aminobutyric acid (GABA) receptor binding.

Clinical Studies In a number of small studies, kava was found to reduce the scores on anxiety scales when compared with the scores of those taking a placebo. Kava was effective as a standard anxiolytic.

Side Effects Heavy kava drinkers acquire yellowing and flaking of the skin, known as *kava dermopathy*. This resolves with discontinuation of the herb. There is a potential risk of severe liver injury associated with the use of kava-containing dietary supplements. There are several reports of extrapyramidal-like dystonic reactions with kava use.

Drug Interactions Combined use of sedatives and alcohol should be avoided as it has been reported to cause oversedation.

Valerian Root

Uses Valerian root has been used for centuries as a sedative agent and sleep aid. Recently, it has been used as an aid for insomnia and jet lag. It is also used for migraine headaches, fatigue, and intestinal cramps.

Mechanism of Action Valerian root has effects on GABA receptors, leading to its sedative effects.

Clinical Studies Several human trials confirm a mild sedative effect. Few studies exist regarding the anxiolytic effects of valerian root in vivo.

Side Effects Headache, excitability, uneasiness, and cardiac disturbances.

Drug Interactions Care should be exercised when combining valerian root with other sedative agents and alcohol.

Chamomile

Uses Historically, chamomile has been used for GI discomfort, peptic ulcer disease, pediatric colic, and mild anxiety.

Mechanism of Action Chamomile may act by binding to central benzodiazepine receptors.

Clinical Studies Several small trials on humans have noted chamomile to have hypnotic–sedative properties. However, none of these trials have been randomized or controlled.

Side Effects The FDA regards chamomile as safe when used as a spice, seasoning, or flavoring agent. Although several cases of significant allergic reactions to chamomile have been reported, no significant toxicity has been reported.

Drug Interactions No drug–herb interactions have been noted.

HERBS FOR WEIGHT LOSS

Ma Huang (Ephedra)

Uses Ephedra, also known by its Chinese name Ma Huang, is a naturally occurring substance derived from plants. Its principal active ingredient is ephedrine. Ephedra products have been used to aid weight loss, enhance sports performance, and increase energy. In 2004, the FDA banned the sale of dietary supplements containing ephedra owing to reported serious adverse effects.

Mechanism of Action Ephedra acts by increasing the levels of norepinephrine, epinephrine, and dopamine, and by stimulating both α and β adrenoreceptors. This leads to anorectic and thermogenic effects by increasing metabolism. The addition of caffeine to ephedra appears to blunt the negative feedback control on the release of norepinephrine. The combination of adrenergic and dopaminergic effects leads to heightened alertness, decreased fatigue, and a lessened desire for sleep. At higher doses, the release of norepinephrine causes anxiety, restlessness, and insomnia.

Clinical Studies In a meta-analysis of 52 controlled trials and 65 case reports, ephedrine and ephedra were shown to promote modest short-term weight loss (≈ 0.9 kg/month compared to placebo) (Shekelle, 2003).

Side Effects It is well known that Ma Huang has the potential to cause serious side effects that have led to a number of reported deaths. On the basis of known side effects and minimal benefit, this product should not be recommended for use. The combination of caffeine and ephedra has an increased risk of psychiatric symptoms, such as euphoria, neurotic behavior, agitation, depressed mood, giddiness, irritability, and anxiety. Other side effects may include increased blood pressure, palpitations, tachycardia, chest pain, coronary vasospasm, and even cardiomyopathy. The structural similarity of ephedrine to amphetamine raises concern about possible abuse.

Guaraná (*Paullinia cupana, P. crysan, P. sorbilis*)

Uses Guaraná is a small shrub native to Venezuela and northern Brazil, known for the high stimulant content of the fruit. Guaraná contains a caffeine-like product guaranine, along with theobromine, theophylline, xanthine, and other xanthine derivatives and acts as a stimulant. A number of energy drinks containing guaraná are available.

Mechanism of Action The applicable part of guaraná is the seed. Guaraná contains 3.6% to 5.8% caffeine (compared to 1%–2% in coffee). Caffeine is responsible for the pharmacological effects of guaraná.

Clinical Studies One study of overweight adults reported that the combination of yerba mate (leaves of *Ilex paraguayensis*), guaraná (seeds of *Paullinia cupana*), and damiana significantly delayed gastric emptying, causing prolonged perceived gastric fullness with an associated weight loss over 45 days (Andersen, 2001).

Side Effects Similar to those of ephedra and caffeine.

Hydroxycitric Acid (Garcinia Cambogia)

Uses Garcinia is marketed as an herbal weight-loss product.

Mechanism of Action It is thought that hydroxycitric acid can increase fat oxidation by inhibiting citrate lyase, an enzyme that plays a crucial role in energy metabolism during de novo lipogenesis.

Clinical Studies Several clinical trials have shown no benefit of this herbal compared to placebo.

Side Effects Minor side effects have been reported. Higher doses have caused abdominal pain and vomiting.

Hoodia Gordonii

Uses Hoodia gordonii looks like a cactus, but it is a succulent from the Kalahari Desert in southern Africa. Bushmen from the area have been using hoodia for centuries to help ward off hunger during long trips in the desert.

Mechanism of Action A steroidal glycoside termed *P57AS3* (P57) has been isolated from hoodia gordonii and may increase the content of adenosine triphosphate (ATP) causing a decrease in hunger.

Clinical Studies Preliminary data suggests that overweight men who consume P57 have significantly lower calorie intake than those taking a placebo.

Side Effects None reported.

HERBAL THERAPIES FOR SPORTS ENHANCEMENT

Ginseng (Panax Ginseng)

Uses Ginseng has been used for >2,000 years to strengthen both mental and physical capacity. Recently, ginseng has become popular as an "adaptogenic" (stress-protective) agent.

Mechanism of Action Ginseng is thought to have effects on nitric oxide synthesis in endothelial tissue of lung, heart, and kidney. In addition, effects on serotonin and dopamine may also be responsible for its actions. Other effects may be related to activity on the hypothalamic–pituitary–adrenal system.

Clinical Studies To date, seven trials investigating ginseng's effects on physical performance in young, active volunteers during cycle ergometer exercises have been reported. Four studies found no significant difference between ginseng and placebo, whereas three studies found a significant decrease in heart rate and increase in maximal oxygen uptake with ginseng.

Side Effects Adverse effects may include nervousness, insomnia, and GI disturbance associated with prolonged use. Because of the estrogen-like effect, ginseng has been reported to cause mastalgia and vaginal bleeding in women.

Drug Interactions Ginseng may interact with oral anticoagulants, antiplatelet agents, corticosteroids, and hypoglycemic agents.

MISCELLANEOUS HERBAL THERAPIES

Echinacea

Uses Echinacea (E. angustifola, E. pallida, E. purpurea) has been used for centuries by Native Americans for aches and colds. It has also been used as a topical analgesic for snake bites, stings, and burns. It has become extremely popular as a natural immune booster.

Mechanism of Action Echinacea works by protecting the integrity of the hyaluronic acid matrix and by stimulating the alternate complement pathway. It also promotes nonspecific T-cell activation by binding to T cells and increasing interferon production. The polysaccharides arabinogalactan and echinacin are the active ingredients of Echinacea and are felt to have immune-modulating effects on the body. Other ingredients include glycosides, alkaloids, alkylamides, polyacetylenes, and fatty acids that are believed to inhibit viral replication, improve the motility of polymorphonuclear cells, and enhance phagocytosis. Echinacea may also enhance natural killer cell activity.

Clinical Studies In a Cochrane review, Echinacea preparations were found to be better than placebo for the treatment of upper respiratory symptoms, but no better than placebo for the prevention of the common cold (Linde, 2006).

Side Effects Adverse effects are usually mild and may include skin rash, GI upset, and diarrhea. Patients with progressive systemic diseases such as multiple sclerosis, tuberculosis, systemic lupus erythematosus, autoimmune diseases, and human immunodeficiency virus infection should not use Echinacea because of its possible effects on the immune system.

Drug Interactions Echinacea should not be used in patients who are immunosuppressed or in those who are on immunosuppressant medications.

Feverfew

Uses Feverfew has become a very popular herbal therapy for the prevention and treatment of migraine headaches. Historically, it has been used for URI, melancholy, and GI distress.

Mechanism of Action Feverfew is thought to inhibit prostaglandin, thromboxane, and leukotriene synthesis. It also reduces serotonin release from thrombocytes and polymorphonuclear leukocytes. The mechanism of action for preventing migraine headaches is unknown.

Clinical Studies Two randomized trials have shown benefit of feverfew use for the prevention of migraines. However, these studies did not address acute treatment of migraines.

Side Effects Adverse effects include occasional mouth ulcerations, contact dermatitis, dizziness, diarrhea, and heartburn.

Drug Interactions Feverfew may interact with anticoagulants and antiplatelet agents because of its platelet aggregation inhibition.

Garlic

Uses Garlic has long been used as a medicinal agent to increase physical strength and as a topical antiseptic. In recent years, it has been used as a natural cholesterol-lowering agent.

Mechanism of Action Garlic causes a reduction in cholesterol synthesis by reducing the hepatic activity of β-hydroxy-β-methylglutaryl-CoA (HMG-CoA) reductase, an enzyme essential to cholesterol biosynthesis.

Clinical Studies A number of small studies have noted a modest reduction in the total cholesterol level when compared to placebo. Other studies have found no reduction in cholesterol. The negative findings may be due to the preparation lacking the active ingredients in fresh garlic.

Side Effects Garlic is generally considered safe although, may cause some GI distress including gas symptoms and skin irritation.

Drug Interactions Garlic has some antiplatelet activity and therefore should not be used in patients on anticoagulant medication.

Adverse events associated with kava and all other herbal therapies should be reported as soon as possible to FDA's MedWatch program by calling their toll-free number (1-800-332-1088) or through the Internet (http://www.fda.gov/medwatch).

ACUPUNCTURE

Overview

Acupuncture is widely used in children and adults. In 1991, an estimated $14 billion out-of-pocket expenses were used for acupuncture therapy. Data from family practice physicians and internists have shown that it is one of the most frequently recommended CAM therapies.

Theory

Originating in China >2,000 years ago, acupuncture is an ancient Chinese therapeutic treatment based on the premise that energy (Qi,Chi) flows through the body along channels known as *meridians*, connected by acupuncture points. The flow of Qi is manipulated by insertion of fine needles at acupuncture points along the involved meridians. Since the 1600s, acupuncture has been practiced in European cultures. In 1916, Sir William Osler recommended acupuncture for the treatment of pain. There has been increased use of acupuncture in the United States during the 20th century due in part to the writings of a New York Times editor whose postoperative pain was managed with this treatment.

In assessing a patient, an acupuncturist takes a history and then performs an examination, which includes the determination of the shape, color, and coating of the tongue and the force, flow, and character of the radial pulse. The specific treatment is based on the diagnosis and may include solid sterile needle placement, moxibustion (the practice of burning dried herbs over the acupuncture needles), acupressure, or cupping.

The flow of Qi through acupuncture points is difficult to translate into typical Western biomedical theory. There is segmental inhibition of pain impulses at the local site of needle stimulation that is carried in the slower unmyelinated C fibers and sensory A-δ fibers. Opioid peptides and other neurotransmitters are released, and naloxone has been shown to reverse the analgesic effects of acupuncture. Acupuncture may also stimulate the hypothalamus and pituitary glands and may modify neurotransmitter secretion.

Evidence of Health Benefits

- Dental pain
- Postoperative nausea and vomiting
- Chemotherapy nausea and vomiting

Possible Health Benefits

- Migraine/tension headaches
- Back pain
- Dysmenorrhea
- Acute and chronic pain
- Substance abuse

Complications

- Pneumothorax, angina, septic sacroiliitis, and epidural and temporomandibular abscess

YOGA

Yoga is widely known for helping to build strength and flexibility through a combination of meditation, controlled breathing, and stretches. Research has explored yoga's potential value as an adjunct treatment for such health problems as anxiety, hypertension, heart disease, depression, low-back pain, headaches, and cancer. More studies are needed to evaluate the efficacy of this intervention.

MASSAGE

Overview

Consumers in the United States spend two to four billion dollars annually on 75 million visits to massage therapists.

More than 150,000 trained massage therapists practice in the United States.

Theory

Massage therapy is thought to release muscle tension, remove toxic metabolites, and facilitate oxygen transport to cells and tissues. Of the five forms of massage therapy, the most common is traditional European or Swedish. Swedish massage is performed on a special massage table or chair. The focus is to relax the muscles and improve circulation. Deep-muscle or deep-tissue massage technique is commonly used in sports. Structural massage and movement integration also called *bodywork* utilizes deep-tissue massage to correct posture problems and movement imbalances. Chinese healers may perform acupressure and shiatsu, known as the *Oriental method*. Reflexology is an energy form of massage where the focus is primarily on the hands, feet and ears.

Evidence of Health Benefits

- Preterm infants have shortened hospital stays
- Improved glucose control in type 1 and 2 diabetes mellitus
- Decreased pain in juvenile rheumatoid arthritis

Possible Health Benefits

- Less need for topical steroids in atopic dermatitis
- Improved pulmonary function in patients with cystic fibrosis
- Decreased anxiety in eating disorders
- Improved mood in depression
- Improved control in asthma

Complications

- None reported

CHIROPRACTIC

Overview

Doctors of Chiropractic (DCs) are the most frequently visited CAM providers. Chiropractors treat many conditions including low-back pain, cervical pain, headache, otitis media, dysmenorrhea, and carpal tunnel syndrome. In one study, 70% of the visits to a chiropractor were for back and neck problems. In 1993, 20 million children and adolescents in the United States were seen by chiropractors for respiratory problems (including asthma); ear, nose, and throat problems; colic; enuresis; allergies and general preventative care.

Theory

Chiropractic, founded by Daniel David Palmer, is based on the theory that all disease can be traced to malpositioned bones in the spinal column called *subluxations*, which lead to the entrapment of spinal nerves. Subluxations produce symptoms of disease because optimal functioning of tissues and organs are not allowed. Physical adjustment of the spine restores proper alignment of the spine by relieving nerve entrapments. For example, many DCs believe that improper eustachian tube drainage associated with acute or chronic otitis media is caused by atlantooccipital joint misalignment.

There are two theories underlying the practice of chiropractic medicine. The International Chiropractic Association (ICA) focuses on the use of chiropractic adjustments for health promotion. Vertebral subluxations are thought to disrupt spinal nerves, which can result in a variety of problems with function. By correcting the subluxations, the bodies' self-healing powers may lead to optimal health. This organization is known for its advancement of pediatric chiropractic care and its opposition to mandatory immunizations and comprises 5% to10% of all DCs in the United States. The American Chiropractic Association (ACA) uses a wide range of diagnostic tools including laboratory tests and advanced imaging (magnetic resonance imaging and computed tomography). They also support nutritional supplements and herbal remedies as treatment options.

Evidence of Health Benefits

• Decreased pain in acute low-back pain

Possible Health Benefits

• Improvement in symptoms of acute otitis media

Not effective

• Asthma

Complications

• Stroke, myelopathies, and radiculopathies after cervical manipulation
• Adverse outcomes are most likely to occur with bleeding dyscrasia, when improper diagnosis is made in the presence of a herniated disc or when an improper manipulative method is utilized

HOMEOPATHIC MEDICINE

Overview

Homeopathy is a medical discipline first promoted in the late 18th century by Samuel Hahnemann (1755–1843). In 1990, there were approximately 5 million visits to homeopathic providers in the United States. Homeopathic medicine sales increased from $100 million in 1988 to $250 million in 1996. In some European countries, up to 40% of physicians use homeopathy in their practice.

Theory

Three concepts embody the philosophy of homeopathic medicine: (a) finding the similum or similar substance, (b) treating the totality of symptoms, and (c) using the minimum dose through potentization.

The "principle of similars" is that highly dilute preparations of substances causing specific symptoms in healthy volunteers are reported to stimulate healing in ill patients who have similar symptoms.

The preparation of homeopathic remedies requires serial dilution and succussion (shaking). A "30C potency" is a remedy that has been diluted by a factor of 1:100 thirty successive times. There are several theories for the mechanism of action of these highly dilute substances. The "memory of water" theory is basic to homeopathy, and holds that water is capable of containing "memory" of particles dissolved in it. This memory allows water to retain the properties of the original solute even when there is no solute left in the solution. In other words, the curative power of the remedy is engrafted into the water molecules and the water retains a "memory" of these changes.

Homeopathy is one of the most controversial of the CAM therapies. Many health care providers remain suspicious that infinitesimally diluted substances retain their biological effects. As a result, many question the effectiveness of this intervention. Others believe that homeopathic remedies are a permissible approach for many medical problems.

Research Evidence

Anecdotal support of the efficacy of homeopathy has been replaced with more scientific evidence. In a meta-analysis of 32 trials in adults, individualized homeopathy was significantly more effective than placebo in treating symptomatic seasonal allergies and postoperative ileus among other complaints. However, when the analysis was restricted to the methodologically sound trials, no significant effect was seen. A second meta-analysis of 110 trials of homeopathy and 110 matched conventional medicine trials for respiratory tract infections, gynecological problems, and musculoskeletal disorders demonstrated weak evidence for specific effects of homeopathic remedies.

Possible Health Benefits

• Recurrent upper respiratory tract infections
• Otitis media
• Attention-deficit disorder

Complications

• Aggravation of symptoms
• Contamination of remedy

In conclusion, clinicians need to understand and appreciate the variety of health care options available to adolescents and their families. Open, honest, and nonjudgmental discussions with adolescents using or planning to use CAM will bring about a safe and rational use of these treatments for which there is evidence of efficacy, and enable adolescents to make informed choices. Improved communication can be addressed by following the recommendations outlined in Table 83.5. Health care providers need to inquire regularly about CAM use because such insight will help clinicians provide better care to adolescents.

TABLE 83.5

Talking with Your Patients about Complementary and Alternative Medicine

Be open-minded. Most patients are reluctant to share information about their use of CAM therapies because they are concerned their physicians will disapprove. By remaining open-minded, you can learn a lot about your patients' use of unconventional therapies. These strategies will help foster open communication.

Ask the question. I recommend asking every patient about his or her use of alternative therapies during routine history taking. One approach is simply to inquire, "Are you doing anything else for this condition?" It's an open-ended question that gives the patient the opportunity to tell you about his or her use of other health care providers or therapies. Another approach is to ask, "Are you taking any over-the-counter remedies such as vitamins or herbs?"

Avoid using the words "alternative therapy," at least initially. This will help you to avoid appearing judgmental or biased.

Don't dismiss any therapy as a placebo. If a patient tells you about a therapy that you are unaware of, make a note of it in the patient's record and schedule a follow-up visit after you have learned more—when you'll be in a better position to negotiate the patient's care. If you determine the therapy might be harmful, you'll have to ask the patient to stop using it. If it isn't harmful and the patient feels better using it, you may want to consider incorporating the therapy into your care plan.

Discuss providers as well as therapies. Another way to help your patients negotiate the maze of alternative therapies is by stressing that they see appropriately trained and licensed providers and knowing whom to refer to in your area. Encourage your patients to ask alternative providers about their background and training and the treatment modalities they use. By doing so, your patients will be better equipped to make educated decisions about their health care.

Discuss CAM therapies with your patients at every visit. Charting the details of their use will remind you to raise the issue. It may also help alert you to potential complications before they occur.

CAM, complementary and alternative medicine.
Breuner CC. Complementary medicine in pediatrics: a review of acupuncture, homeopathy, massage and chiropractic therapies. *Current Probs in Pediatric and Adolescent Health Care.* 2002;32(10):347–384.

WEB SITES

General

http://www.nccam.nih.gov. National Center for Complementary and Alternative Medicine.
http://www.amfoundation.org. Alternative Medicine Foundation.

Herbal Medicine

http://www.herbmed.org. HerbMed database.
http://www.herbs.org. Herb Research Foundation.
http://www.herbalgram.org. American Botanical Council.
http://www.naturaldatabase.com. Natural Medicines Comprehensive Database.

Mind Body Medicine

http://www.umassmed.edu/cfm/clinical.cfm. The Stress Reduction Clinic at the University of Massachusetts.
http://www.holisticmedicine.org. The American Holistic Medical Association.
http://www.ahha.org. The American Holistic Health Association.
http://www.nicabm.com. The National Institute for Clinical Applications of Behavioral Medicine.
http://www.cmbm.org. The Center for Mind Body Medicine.

Yoga

http://www.americanyogaassociation.org/.

Acupuncture

http://www.aaom.org. American Association of Oriental Medicine.
http://www.acuall.org. Acupuncture and Oriental Medical Alliance.
http://www.medicalacupuncture.org. American Academy of Medical Acupuncture.

Chiropractic

http://www.amerchiro.org. American Chiropractic Association.
http://www.chiropractic.org. International Chiropractors Association.

Homeopathy

http://www.homeopathic.org. National Center for Homeopathy.

Massage

http://www.amtamassage.org. American Massage Therapy Association.

http://www.ncbtmb.com. National Certification Board for Massage Therapy and Bodywork.

REFERENCES AND ADDITIONAL READINGS

Abuaisha BB, Costanzi JB, Boulton AJ. Acupuncture for the treatment of chronic painful peripheral neuropathy. *Diabetes Res Clin Pract* 1998;39:115.

Adoga GI. The mechanism of the hypolipidemic effect of garlic oil extract in rats fed on high sucrose and alcohol diets. *Biochem Biophys Res Commun* 1987;142:1046.

Almeida JC, Grimsley EW. Coma from the health food store: interaction between kava and alprazolam. *Ann Intern Med* 1996;125:940.

American Academy of Pediatrics, Committee on Children with Disabilities. Counseling families who choose complementary and alternative medicine for their child with chronic illness or disability. *Reaffirmed in Pediatrics*. 2005;115:1438.

Andersen T, Fogh J. Weight loss and delayed gastric emptying following a South American herbal preparation in overweight patients. *J Hum Nutr Diet* 2001;14(3):243.

Angell M, Kassirer JP. Alternative medicine—the risks of untested and unregulated remedies. *N Engl J Med* 1998; 339(12):839.

Arnold LE. Alternative treatments for adults with attention-deficit hyperactivity disorder (ADHD). *Ann N Y Acad Sci* 2001;931:310.

Assendeff W, Bouter L, Knipschild P. Complications of spinal manipulation: a comprehensive review of the literature. *J Fam Pract* 1996;42:475.

Awang DVC, Kindack DG. Herbal medicine: *Echinacea*. *Can Pharm J* 1991;124:512.

Baischer W. Acupuncture in migraine. Long-term outcome and predicting factors. *Headache* 1995;35:472.

Balon J, Aker PD, Crowther ER, et al. A comparison of active and simulated chiropractic manipulation as adjunctive treatment for childhood asthma. *N Eng J Med* 1998;339(15):1013.

Barnett ED, Levatin JL, Chapman EH, et al. Challenges of evaluating homeopathic treatment of acute otitis media. *Pediatr Infect Dis J* 2000;19:273.

Barron RL, Vanscoy GJ. Natural products and the athlete: facts and folklore. *Ann Pharmacother* 1993;27:607.

Batchelor WB, Heathcote J, Wanlesa IR. Chaparral induced hepatic injury. *Am J Gastroenterol* 1996;90:831.

Bent S, Ko R. Commonly used herbal medicines the Unites States: a review. *Am J Med* 2004;116:478.

Bergmann T, Peterson D, Lawrence D. *Chiropractic technique: principles and procedures*. New York, NY: Churchill Livingstone, 1993:747.

Berkowitz CD. Homeopathy: keeping an open mind. *Lancet* 1994;344:701.

Berthold HK, Sudhop T, von Bergmann K. Effect of a garlic oil preparation on serum lipoproteins and cholesterol metabolism: a randomized controlled trial. *JAMA* 1998;279: 1900.

Blumenthal M. Herb sales down 3% in mass market retail stores—sales in natural food stores still growing, but at lower rate. *HerbalGram* 2000;49:68.

Blumenthal M, Busse W, Goldberg A, et al. *The complete German Commission E monographs: therapeutic guide to herbal medicines*. Austin, TX: American Botanical Council, 2000.

Braun CA, Bearinger LH, Halcon LL, et al. Adolescent use of complementary therapies. *J Adolesc Health* 2005;37(1):76.

Brevoort P. The booming U.S. botanical market: a new overview. *HerbalGram* 1998;44:33.

Breuner CC. Complementary medicine in pediatrics: a review of acupuncture, homeopathy, massage and chiropractic therapies. *Curr Probl Pediatr Adolesc Health Care* 2002;32(10):347.

Breuner CC, Barry P, Kemper KJ. Alternative medicine use by homeless youth. *Arch Pediatr Adolesc Med* 1998;152(11):1071.

Brewington V, Smith M, Lipton D. Acupuncture and detoxification treatment: an analysis of controlled research. *J Subst Abuse Treat* 1994;11:289.

Brumbaugh AG. Acupuncture new perspectives in chemical dependency treatment. *J Subst Abuse Treat* 1993;10:35.

Bullock ML. Controlled trial of acupuncture for severe recidivist alcoholism. *Lancet* 1989;1(8652):1435.

Canadian Pediatric Society. Children and natural health products; what every clinician should know. *Paediatr Child Health* 2005;10(4):227.

Carey TS, Garrett J, Jackman A, et al. The outcomes and costs of care for acute low back pain among patients seen by primary care practitioners, chiropractors, and orthopedic surgeons. The North Carolina back pain project. *N Engl J Med* 1995;333(14):913.

Cirigliano MD, Sun A. Advising patients about herbal therapies. *JAMA* 1998;280:1565.

Cohen MH, Kemper KJ. Complementary therapies in pediatrics: a legal perspective. *Pediatrics* 2005;115(3):774.

Cohen MH, Hrbek A, Davis RB, et al. Emerging credentialing practices, malpractice liability policies and guidelines governing complementary and alternative medical practices and dietary supplement recommendations. *Arch Intern Med* 2005;165:289.

Colson CRD, Debroe ME. Kidney injury from alternative medicine. *Adv Chronic Kidney Dis* 2005;12(3):261.

Committee on the Use of Complementary and Alternative Medicine by the American Public, Board on Health promotion and Disease Prevention, Institute of Medicine of the National Academies. *Complementary and alternative medicine in the United States*. Washington, DC: The National Academies Press, 2005.

Coulter ID. Patients using chiropractors in North America: who are they, and why are they in chiropractic care?. *Spine* 2002;27(3):291.

Day AS, Whitten KE, Bohane TD. Use of complementary and alternative medicines by children and adolescents with inflammatory bowel disease. *J Paediatr Child Health* 2004;40: 681.

DeLange deKlerk ESM, Blommers J, Kuik DJ, et al. Effect of homeopathic remedies medicines on daily burdens of symptoms in children with recurrent upper respiratory infections. *Brit Med J* 1994;309.

Diehl DL, Kaplan G, Coulter I, et al. Use of acupuncture by American physicians. *J Altern Complement Med* 1997;3:119.

Durant CL, Verhoef MJ. Chiropractic treatment of patients under 18 years of age. Fact. *Focus Altern Complement Ther* 1998; 2(4):198.

Eisenberg DM. Advising patients who seek alternative medical therapies. *Ann Intern Med* 1997;127(1):61.

Eisenberg DM, Davis RB, Ettner SL, et al. Trends in alternative medicine use in the United States, 1990–1997. *JAMA* 1998; 280:1569.

Eisenberg DM, Kessler RC, Foster C, et al. Unconventional medicine in the United States. *N Engl J Med* 1993;328:246.

Ernst, E. Adverse effects of spinal manipulation. In: Jonas WB, Levin JS, eds. *Essentials of complementary and alternative medicine.* Philadelphia: Lippincott Williams & Wilkins, 1999: 176.

Ernst E. Prospective studies of the safety of acupuncture: a systematic review. *Am J Med* 2001;110(6):481.

Ernst E, Kaptchuck TJ. Homeopathy revisited. *Arch Int Neurol* 1996;156:2162.

Ernst E, Pittler MH. Herbal Medicine. *Med Clin North Am* 2002; 86(1):149.

Fearon J. A reflective overview of complementary therapies for children 1995–2005. *Complement Ther Clin Pract* 2005; 11(1):32.

Field T. Massage and relaxation therapies' effects on depressed adolescent mothers. *Adolescence* 1996;31(124):903.

Field T, Morrow C, Valdeon C, et al. Massage reduces anxiety in child and adolescent psychiatric patients. *Am Acad Child Adolesc Psychiatry* 1992;31:125.

Field T, Quintino O, Hernandez-Reif M, et al. Adolescents with attention deficit hyperactivity disorder benefit from massage therapy. *Adolescence* 1998;333:103.

Field T, Schanberg S, Kuhn C, et al. Bulimic adolescents benefit from massage therapy. *Adolescence* 1998;33:555.

Firenzuoli F, Gori L. Garcinia cambogia for weight loss. *JAMA* 1999;282:234.

Fugh-Berman A. Herb-drug interactions. *Lancet* 2000;355:134.

Gardiner P, Kemper KJ. Herbs in pediatric and adolescent medicine. *Pediatr Rev* 2000;21(2):44.

Gillis CN. Panax ginseng pharmacology: a nitric oxide link? *Biochem Pharmacol* 1997;54:1.

Goldberg H. Feverfew for prevention of migraine. *Altern Med Alert* 1999;2(4):41.

Goldhaber-Fiebert S, Kemper K. *Echinacea.* The Longwood Herbal Task Force, 1999.

Halt M. Moulds and mycotoxins in herb tea and medicinal plants. *Eur J Epidemiol* 1998;14:269.

Heymsfield SB, Allison DB, Vasselli JR, et al. Garcinia cambogia (hydroxycitric acid) as a potential antiobesity agent: a randomized controlled trial. *JAMA* 1998;280:1596.

Hobbs C. *Echinacea,* a literature review: botany, history, chemistry, pharmacology, toxicology, and clinical uses. *HerbalGram* 1994;30:33.

Hondras MA, Linde K, Jones AP. Manual therapy for asthma. *Cochrane Database Syst Rev* 2005;3.

Hopkins MP, Androff L, Benninghoff AS. Ginseng face cream and unexplained vaginal bleeding. *Am J Obstet Gynecol* 1988; 159:1121.

Hypericum depression trial study group. Effect of Hypericum perforatum (St. John's wort) in major depressive disorder: a randomized controlled trial. *JAMA* 2002;287:1807.

Izzo AA, Ernst E. Interactions between herbal medicines and prescribed drugs: a systematic review. *Drugs* 2001;61:2163.

Jussofie A, Schmiz A, Hiemke C. Kavapyrone-enriched extract from Piper methysticum as modulator of the GABA binding site in different regions of rat brain. *Psychopharmacology* 1994;116:469.

Kaptchuk T. *The web that has no weaver.* New York: Congdon and Weed, 1983.

Kaptchuk TJ, Eisenberg DM. Chiropractic: origins, controversies and contributions. *Arch Inter Med* 1998;158:2215.

Katz M, Saibil F. Herbal hepatitis: subacute hepatic necrosis secondary to chaparral leaf. *J Clin Gastroenterol* 1990;12:831.

Kaufman DW, Kelly JP, Rosenberg L, et al. Recent patterns of medication use in the ambulatory adult population of the United States. *JAMA* 2002;287:337.

Kelly JP, Kaufman DW, Kelley K, et al. Recent trends in use of herbal and other natural products. *Arch Intern Med* 2005; 165:281.

Kinzler E. Effect of a special kava extract in patients with anxiety, tension, and excitation states of nonpsychotic genesis. *Arzneimittelforsch* 1991;41:584.

Kriketos AD, Thompson HR, Greene H, et al. Hydroxycitric acid does not affect energy expenditure and substrate oxidation in adult males in a post absorptive state. *Int J Obes Relat Metab Discord* 1999;23:867.

Lamont J. Homeopathic treatment of attention deficit disorder. *Br Homoeopath J* 1997;86:196.

Lee KP, Carlini WG, McCormick GF, et al. Neurologic complications following chiropractic manipulation: a survey of California neurologists. *Neurology* 1995;45:1213.

Lee ACC, Li DH, Kemper KJ. Chiropractic care for children. *Arch Pediatr Adolesc Med* 2000;154:401.

Lindahl O, Lindwell L. Double-blind study of a valerian preparation. *Pharmacol Biochem Behav* 1989;32:1065.

Linde K, Barrett B, Wolkart K, Bauer R, Melchart D. Echinacea for preventing and treating the common cold. *Cochrane Database Syst Rev.* 2006; Jan 25:(1):CD000530.

Linde K, Clausius N, Ramirez G, et al. Are the clinical effects of homeopathy placebo effects; a meta analysis of placebo-controlled trials? *Lancet* 1997;350:834.

Linde K, Melchart D. Randomized controlled trials of individualized homeopathy: a state-of-the-art review. *J Altern Complement Med* 1998;4(4):371.

Linde K, Ramirez G, Mulrow CD, et al. St. John's wort for depression: an overview and meta-analysis of randomized clinical trials. *Br Med J* 1996;313:238.

Linde K, Streng A, Jurgens S, et al. Acupuncture for patients with migraine. *JAMA* 2005;293:2118.

Losier A, Taylor B, Fernandez CV. Use of alternative therapies by patients presenting to a pediatric emergency department. *J Emerg Med* 2005;28(3):267.

Lyon MR, Cline JC, Totosy de Zepetnek J, et al. Effect of the herbal extract combination Panax quinquefolium and Ginkgo biloba on attention-deficit hyperactivity disorder: a pilot study. *J Psychiatry Neurosci* 2001;26(3):221.

Martinet A, Hostettmann, Schutz Y. Thermogenic effects of commercially available plant preparations aimed at treating human obesity. *Phytomedicine* 2000;6(4):231.

Matthews MK. Association of Ginkgo biloba with intracerebral hemorrhage. *Neurology* 1998;50:1933.

Miller FG, Emanuel EJ, Rosenstein DL, et al. Ethical issues concerning research in complementary and alternative medicine. *JAMA* 2004;291:599.

Morris CA, Avorn J. Internet marketing of herbal products. *JAMA* 2003;290:1505.

Mostefa-Kara N, Pauwela A, Pines E, et al. Fatal hepatitis after herbal tea. *Lancet* 1992;340:674.

Newall C, Anderson L, Phillipson J. *Herbal medicines: a guide for healthcare professionals.* London: Pharmaceutical Press, 1996.

NIH Consensus Conference. Acupuncture. *JAMA.* 1998;280:1518.

O'Hara M, Kiefer D, Farrell K, et al. A review of 12 commonly used medicinal herbs. *Arch Fam Med* 1998;7:523.

Ohye H, Fukata S, Kanoh M, et al. Thyrotoxicosis caused by weight-reducing herbal medicines. *Arch Intern Med* 2005; 165:831.

Ondrizck RR. An alternative medicine study of herbal effects on the penetration of zona-free hamster oocytes and the integrity of sperm deoxyribonucleic acid. *Fertil Steril* 1999; 71(3):517.

Palmer BV, Montgomery ACV, Monteriro JCMP. Ginseng and mastalgia. *Br Med J* 1996;313:253.

Pepper K, Trautwein W. The effect of aconitine on the membrane current in cardiac muscle. *Pfluggers Arch* 1967;296:328.

Pillans PI. Toxicity of herbal products. *N Z Med J* 1995;108:469.

Piscitelli SC, Burstein AH, Chai HD, et al. Indinavir concentrations and St. John's wort. *Lancet* 2000;355:134.

Rose KD, Croissant PD, Parliament CF, et al. Spontaneous spinal epidural hematoma with associated platelet dysfunction from excessive garlic ingestion: a case report. *Neurosurgery* 1990;26:880.

Rotblatt M, Ziment I. *Evidence based herbal medicine.* Philadelphia: Hanley & Belfus, 2002.

Roulet M, Laurini R, Rivier L, et al. Hepatic veno-occlusive disease in a newborn infant of a women drinking herbal tea. *J Pediatr* 1988;112:433.

Rusy LM, Weisman SJ. Complementary therapies for acute pediatric pain management. *Pediatr Clin North Am* 2000;47(3):589.

Saper RB, Kales SN, Paquin J, et al. Heavy metal content of ayruvedic medicine products. *JAMA* 2004;292:2868.

Sawni-Sikand A, Schubiner H, Thomas RL. Use of complementary/alternative therapies among children in primary care pediatrics. *Ambul Pediatr* 2002;2(2):99.

Schoneberger D. Influence of the immunostimulating effects of the pressed juice of *Echinaceae* purpurae on the duration and intensity of the common cold: results of a double-blind clinical trial. *Forum Immunol* 1992;2:18.

Schulz V, Hansel R, Tyler VE. *Rational phytotherapy: a physicians' guide to herbal medicine.* Berlin: Springer-Verlag, 2004.

Shekelle PG, Hardy ML, Morton SC, et al. Efficacy and safety of ephedra and ephedrine for weight loss and athletic performance: a meta-analysis. *JAMA* 2003;289:1537.

Shelton RC, Keller MB, Gekenberg A, et al. Effectiveness of St. John's wort in major depression, a randomized control trial. *JAMA* 2001;285:1807.

Shang A, Huwiler-Muntener KH, Juni P, et al. Are the clinical effects of homeopathy placebo effects? Comparative study of placebo controlled trials of homeopathy and allopathy. *Lancet* 2005;366:726.

Sorrentino M. Garlic: is the "stinking rose" good for the cholesterol count? *Altern Med Alert* 1998;1(9):97.

Spigelblatt L, Laine-Ammara G, Pless IB, et al. The use of alternative medicine by children. *Pediatrics* 1994;94:811.

Stewart JH. Hypnosis in contemporary medicine. *Mayo Clin Proc* 2005;80:511.

Sticher O. Quality of ginkgo preparations. *Planta Med* 1993;59.

Stux G, Pomeranz B. *Basics of Acupuncture.* Germany: Springer-Verlag, 1998.

Tai Y, But P, Young K, et al. Cardiotoxicity after accidental herb-induced aconite poisoning. *Lancet* 1992;340:1254.

Taylor JA, Weber W, Standish L, et al. Efficacy and safety of *Echinacea* in treating upper respiratory tract infections in children: a randomized controlled trial. *JAMA* 2003;290(21): 2824.

Telles S, Joshi M, Dash M, et al. An evaluation of the ability to voluntarily reduce the heart rate after a month of yoga practice. *Integr Physiol Behav Sci* 2004;39(2):119.

Trigazis L, Tennankore D, Vohra S, et al. The use of herbal remedies by adolescents with eating disorders. *Int J Eat Disord* 2004;35(2):223.

Turner RB, Bauer R, Woelkart K, et al. An evaluation of *Echinacea angustifolia* in experimental rhinovirus infections. *N Engl J Med* 2005;353(4):337.

Udani JK, Ofman JJ. *Echinacea* for the common cold. *Altern Med Alert* 1998;1(2):16.

Wilson K, Klein J. Adolescents' use of complementary and alternative medicine. *Ambul Pediatr* 2002;2:99.

Wong AHC, Smith M, Boon HS. Herbal remedies in psychiatric practice. *Arch Gen Psychiatry* 1998;55:1033.

Woolf GM, Petrovic LM, Rojter SE, et al. Acute hepatitis associated with the Chinese herbal product Jin Bu Huan. *Ann Intern Med* 1994;121:729.

Yussman S, Auginger P, Weitzman M, et al. Complementary and alternative medicine use in children and adolescents. *J Adolesc Health* 2002;30:105.

Yussman S, Wilson K, Graff C, et al. Herbal products and their association with substance abuse in adolescents. *J Adolesc Health* 2002;30:122.

CHAPTER 84

Overview of Health Issues for College Students

Lawrence S. Neinstein, Paula L. Swinford, and James A. H. Farrow

More than 17.6 million students were enrolled in 2006 in the nation's 4,392 colleges and universities with an anticipated 19.5 million by 2014. Almost two thirds (63%) of these students are in the 14- to 24-year-old age-group. College students of traditional age (18–24 years) compromise a unique population with specific health-related assets and vulnerabilities, whereas the college campus is a unique health environment that creates both risks and opportunities (Keeling, 2002). This makes colleges and universities, collectively referred to as Institutions of Higher Education (IHEs), critical settings for preventing or reducing health-risk behaviors and enhancing well-being among many young adults.

College health has as its mission the enhancement of the health of college students in support of advancing student academic success and the learning environment. IHEs provide a variety of services including the provision of health care to approximately 10 million adolescents, young adults, and adults in the United States. Nationally, there are approximately 1,600 colleges or universities that provide some level of services to advance the health of students (Patrick, 1988). Most common are medical or clinical services directed by a physician, nurse, nurse practitioner, or administrator. More than 150 of these institutions maintain an ambulatory health care center accredited by either the Accreditation Association for Ambulatory Health Care (AAAHC) or the Joint Commission on Accreditation of Healthcare Organizations (JCAHO). However, what specific services are offered varies widely in the United States, ranging from part-time nurses providing triage and referral to comprehensive ambulatory health care centers, and even public health, counseling, education, prevention services, and sometimes disability and recreational services. There are approximately 10 million students making as many as 30 million visits to these services per year at an approximate cost of $1.4 billion dollars. Approximately 5% to 25% of these visits were made to counseling services.

While it is beyond the scope of this book to offer a comprehensive review of the history and scope of college health, this chapter provides an overview of the following:

- The philosophy of a model college health program
- Demographics of the student population
- Demographics of IHEs in the United States

- Statistics regarding morbidity, mortality, and the health status in this student population
- Information for providers when their patients start attending college
- Information for parents when their children start attending college
- Web-based resources for college students, parents, and health care professionals

Issues of college health may also be important to pediatricians and other health care professionals serving adolescents and young adults, for the following reasons:

1. Health care providers often perform precollege examinations or provide care during college years.
2. Health care providers may communicate with college health professionals regarding health care needs of a student while at school.
3. Employment and career opportunities exist in the college setting.
4. Opportunities for collaboration often exist between professionals in adolescent health and college health.
5. Collaboration among insurance providers, local health care providers, health care providers in the college health program, and the university health care systems or medical schools can benefit all parties and especially students.
6. College health professionals may be a source of ongoing referrals to other health care professionals of patients needing hospitalization or secondary and tertiary care consultations.
7. Significant opportunities exist for both teaching and research.

THE PHILOSOPHY OF A MODEL COLLEGE HEALTH PROGRAM

Services that support and enhance the health of college students developed in colleges and universities over the last 150 years for numerous reasons such as the following (Swinford, 2002):

- A call from faculty to create a support system to maintain the student's health for academic studies

- The public health and communicable disease concerns of a compact campus community, particularly before the advent of vaccines and antibiotics
- The specialized medical needs of a predominantly adolescent and young adult population that may differ from health care provided in the surrounding community
- The confidentiality needs of young adults as they establish a new relationship with parents and their health care providers
- The need for access to care and treatment for the many uninsured individuals in the college student population

A college health program is more than just the provision of quality medical services on campus. At its best, college health embraces a model that encompasses a variety of services focused on students' physical, emotional, and social health in the context of their cultural and academic influences. The "college health program" model is defined as a coordinated and planned set of policies, procedures, activities, programs, and services to enhance, protect, promote and improve the health and well-being of students, faculty, and staff of colleges, universities, and other IHEs (AAHE, 2006). This model includes significant interactions with the campus community and uses the best methods of health promotion and prevention including primary, secondary, and tertiary prevention. In addition, college health programs are usually staffed by a multidisciplinary team that includes members from various professional disciplines including medical, nursing, counseling, health promotion, and ancillary services staff. The Carnegie Foundation outlined college health as:

> "The caring intersection between health and education. It is a community with a shared vision and common cause... college health is developmentally appropriate, educationally effective, medically expert, accessible, and convenient."
>
> (Boyer, 1987)

Similar to the best of adolescent health care, health care for college students involves treating medical conditions while assessing, intervening, and preventing the student's behavioral and health risks. College health services also seek to reduce risk and reinforce behaviors that create health for the individual and for the community. The best practices in college health continually assess the student population on the particular campus to track their health status and identify service needs. Then the health center can provide a portfolio of services that include high-quality medical care, attention to psychosocial and developmental needs, primary prevention within the campus community, reduction of risk, and promotion of health at the individual and campus level. This may involve assessing health status and promoting health in students, who may never visit the health center, through, for example, population-based primary prevention programs such as mandatory prematriculation alcohol education. This may also involve campus outreach vaccination programs. Campus involvement often overlaps academic life, and student affairs programs such as residential life and orientation. The best practice of college health seeks such educational opportunities and promotes learning not just during the clinical visit or counseling appointment but throughout the campus culture.

Depending on the population's needs and the campus resources, a college health program may include the following (ACHA, 1999):

1. Providing primary care, including medical and counseling services that are more accessible than community services and are specifically designed for students
2. Providing services based on informative data regarding the health status and risk behaviors of the population and the change in response to that information
3. Providing of health services that are caring and student centered
4. Engaging health care professionals and campus partners in a multidisciplinary team approach
5. Participating in campus life and advancing the academic mission and student learning mission of the institution
6. Working with student affairs partners within a student development framework
7. Preventing of illness, injury, and disease and reducing risk behaviors and promoting health-enhancing behaviors as a primary mission parallel to screening, treatment, and cure of illness, injury, and disease
8. Welcoming the diversity of the student population by building cultural competency skills for the staff
9. Encouraging of student participation as advisors to development and review of services
10. Teaching students to become wise health care consumers, knowledgeable about accessing services in the health care delivery system
11. Using prepayment to help maximize access to preventive services and treatment care without financial barriers

The American College Health Association (ACHA)'s *Guidelines for a College Health Program* states that: "Current sociological trends, high-risk identification, public health issues, health care finance reform, and changes in preventive medicine have broad institutional implications. College health programs have a unique opportunity to help meet those new challenges."

ENROLLMENT

There are almost 4,400 IHEs in the United States, with approximately 17.6 million students in Fall 2006, likely rising to approximately 18.8 million by the year 2010 and 19.5 million by 2014 (Hussar, 2005; National Center for Education Statistics, 2003). Data and extensive tables are available from the National Center for Education Statistics at http://nces.edu.gov/programs/digest as well as the almanac issues of the Chronicle of High Education.

Gender

Approximately 42% are male and 58% female.

Full Time Versus Part Time

Approximately 62% are full time and 38% part-time.

Age Distribution (Fall, 2005)

(Digest of Education Statistics, NCES 2007)

Age	Millions Actual 2005 Projected 2006	Percent Actual 2005 Projected 2006
14–17 years	0.176	1.0
	0.181	1.0
18–19 years	3.660	20.9
	3.700	21.0
20–21 years	3.728	21.3
	3.780	21.4
22–24 years	3.047	17.4
	3.049	17.3
25–29 years	2.456	14.0
	2.538	14.4
30–34 years	1.312	7.5
	1.294	7.3
>35 years	3.108	17.8
	3.105	17.6

Overall, 60.6% of enrolled students are 24 years or younger.

Digest of Education Statistics, 2006, National Center for Education Statistics, U.S. Department of Education, http://nces.ed.gov/programs/digest.

College Enrollment by Racial Group (1995–2005)

(The Chronicle of Higher Education, Almanac Issue 2007–2008)

	1995 (%)	2005 (%)
White	72.2	65.7
Black	10.3	12.6
Hispanic	7.6	10.8
Asian or Pacific Islander	5.5	6.5
American Indian/Alaska native	0.9	1.0
Non-resident alien	3.2	3.3

Total high school graduates enrolled in college by race: (61.6%)

Race	2001	1978
White	64.2%	50.5%
Black	54.6%	46.4%
Hispanic	51.5%	41.5%

Types of Universities (2005–2006)

(National Center for Education Statistics, 2006, N = 4,276 universities and colleges)

Four year (60% with majority being private)	
Public 4-year institutions	640
Private 4-year institutions	1,942
Two year (40% with majority being public)	
Public 2-year institutions	1,053
Private 2-year institutions	641

Number of Colleges by Enrollment, Fall 2005

	All	Public	Private
Under 200	483	14	469
200–499	616	52	564
500–999	605	91	514
1,000 to 2,499	916	328	588
2,500 to 4,999	657	382	275
5,000 to 9,999	484	384	100
10,000 to 19,999	311	263	48
20,000 to 29,999	126	113	13
30,000 or more	55	48	7

Level of Student

Approximately 86% of enrolled students in 2004 were undergraduate students

Undergraduate: 14,780,630/17,272,044 = 85.6%
Postbaccalaureate: 2,491,414/17,272,044 = 14.4%
    First-professional: 334,529 (1.9%)
    Graduate: 2,156,885 (12.5%)
    (Chronicle of Higher Education, 2006)

Changing Student Profile

1. The enrollment of students aged 25 years and above increased from 4.9 million in 1987 to 6.89 million in 2005; and increase of 41%. Although the proportion of students aged 25 years and above increased from 38% in 1987 to 43.8% in 1995, this percentage dropped in 2005 back down to 39.3% (The Chronicle of Higher Education, Almanac of Higher Education 2007–8).
2. Women played a major role in the increase of enrollment between 1982 and 2005. The enrollment of women in college increased from 6.4 million in 1982 to over 10 million in 2005, representing an average annual growth rate of more than 2.5%, for a 57.5% increase over the period (The Chronicle of Higher Education, Almanac of Higher Education 2007–8).
3. After several years of stagnation, the number of international college students coming to the United States was up again from 1998 onward, with an increase of almost 14% between 2000 and 2003. The number of international students has increased from approximately 179,000 in 1976 to 407,000 in 1990 and to 584,000 in 2005. Almost two thirds of the international students are from Asia.
4. Approximately 25% of students do not have health insurance coverage and it is estimated that another 18% to 24% have inadequate insurance. Nationally, noninsurance rates rise rapidly with level of students from approximately 12% as freshman to almost 30% as seniors.
5. Increasing numbers of undergraduate college students are on financial aid with the percentage of any aid rising from 58.7% in 1992–1993 to 72.5% in 1999–2000 to 76.1% in 2003–2004 (Digest of Education Statistics, 2006, National Center for Education Statistics, U.S. Department of Education, http://nces.ed.gov/programs/digest).
6. Enrollment as a percentage of all 18- to 24-year-olds has increased between 1990 and 2001 from 35.2% to 39.3% for white, non-Hispanics; from 25.3% to 31.3% for African-Americans; and from 15.8% to 21.7% for Hispanic students (National Center for Education Statistics, 2005).
7. Projections of future enrollment
   a. Between 2004 and 2014 enrollment is expected to go up from 17.6 million to 19.5 million in colleges and universities.

b. By age: The above increase is expected to be 16% for students 18 to 24 years old and 5% for students who are 35 years and older.

c. By sex: The above increase is expected to be 12% for men and 21% for women.

d. By attendance status: The above increase is expected to be 20% for full-time students and 14% for part-time students.

e. By level: The increase is expected to be 16% for undergraduates, 21% for graduates, and 32% for first-professional students.

f. By public versus private institutions: The increase is expected to be 17% in public institutions and 19% in private institutions.

By far the majority (80%) of college students attend campuses that have some organized arrangement for advancing their health (Patrick, 1988). Nationally, there are approximately 1,500 to 1,650 college health centers. There are approximately 10 million students making as many as 30 million visits per year at an approximate cost of $1.4 billion. In addition, approximately 5% to 25% of these students use the counseling center.

MORBIDITY AND MORTALITY

Availability of data regarding morbidity and mortality in college students is less than that in other populations. Although an age-group is easily identified in most data sets, current college enrollment is rarely collected as part of standard demographic data. Given this, in recent decades the college student population has attracted specific focus. There was overall data collected from the youth risk behavior surveillance: National College Health Risk Behavior Survey (NCHRBS)—United States, 1995. While this was over 10 years ago, currently yearly health status data is available from the ACHA as the American College Health Association-National College Health Assessment Survey, the ACHA-NCHA (since 1999). National data are also available specifically on drug use from several studies, including Monitoring the Future Study (since 1975), Core Alcohol and Drug Survey (since 1989), the College Alcohol Study (Wechsler, 1997; 1999; 2002), and the Cooperative Institutional Research Program (CIRP) Freshman Survey.

Some overall trends found in the CIRP Freshman Survey have included the following:

- Tobacco use: Down since 1966 (15%), to 1987 (7.2%), and 2006 (5.3%)
- Alcohol use: Beer use down since 1987(65.4%) to 2006 (42.3%) and "wine and other liquor" down since 1987 (67.8%) to 2006 (48.6%)
- Mental health: Feeling "Overwhelmed" has been up since 1987 (18.6%) to 2006 (28.7%). However, this is lower than the 30.7% listing this in 1999. "Feeling depressed" has been down since 1987 (9%) to 2006 (7.3%).

2006 Spring ACHA-NCHA

Acknowledging the need for college student population health status data, the ACHA began conducting national surveys in the spring of 2000. The 2006 ACHA-NCHA data set (results available at www.acha.org) includes 117 IHEs (113, 4-year and 4, 2-year institutions) that chose randomly selected students (N = 94, 806). While the students are selected on a randomized manner, the IHEs were not chosen on a random basis. In terms of student enrollment, 24 had more than 20,000 students; 37 had between 10,000 and 19,999; 26 had between 5,000 and 9,999; 14 had between 2,500 and 4,999; and 16 had less than 2,500. The sample of students was 61% female and 82% undergraduate. The ethnicity of the students was 73% white, 5% African-American, 6% Hispanic, 12% Asian, and 4% other. Almost 88% of the students reported having some kind of health care insurance. Thirteen percent of the students sample had a monthly unpaid credit card balance of $1,000 or more. This data is available at ¡http://www.acha.org/projects_programs/assessment.cfm¿. The ACHA-NCHA data throughout the rest of this chapter is from the aforementioned Web site or from the ACHA-NCHA's Reference Group Data Report (Spring, 2006).

The ACHA-NCHA suggests the following:

- Many college students were involved in activities that placed them at increased risks.
- Heavy drinking episodes: More than one third (37%) of college students reported at least one event of consuming five or more alcoholic drinks at a setting, during the 2-week period preceding the survey.
- Many college students fail to protect themselves against sexually transmitted diseases (STDs) and pregnancy. Of the students who are sexually active, a little more than half (52%) used a condom the last time they had vaginal intercourse.
- Approximately 60% of students failed to engage in vigorous or moderate physical activity at recommended levels 3 or more times/week.

INJURIES

Unintentional Injuries

2006 ACHA-NCHA data (within the last school year)

- 5.9% rarely or never used a seat belt (of drivers).
- 67.5% rarely or never wore bicycle helmets (of riders).
- 84.6% rarely or never wore helmets when inline skating (of skaters).
- 22.4% rarely or never wore motorcycle helmet (of riders).
- 5% drove a car after having five or more drinks in last 30 days (of drivers).

Intentional Injuries

2006 ACHA-NCHA data (within the last school year)

- 6.2% were involved in fights (11.3% in males and 3% in females).
- 1.4% experienced sexual penetration against their will (1.8% females and 0.7% males) while 2.7% experienced attempted sexual penetration against their will.
- 8.4% experienced sexual touching against their will (10.7% females and 4.2% males).

Suicide

2006 ACHA-NCHA data

Suicidal ideation and attempt (within the last school year)

	Suicidal Ideation	Suicide Attempt
Total	9.3%	1.3%
Female	9.8%	1.3%
Male	8.4%	1.2%

Although lower than the high school adolescent population, in which almost 12% of female adolescents and 5.6% of boys have attempted suicide, the rates are still significant. Of the group, 43.8% reported feeling so depressed it was difficult to function in the last year.

ALCOHOL, TOBACCO, AND OTHER DRUG USE

Monitoring the Future data for college students is available in the figures and tables in this chapter and further information is available in Volume II of the National Survey Results on Drug Use, 1975–2006, Monitoring the Future (Johnston et al., 2005, www.monitoringthefuture.org). This data examines both young adult high school graduates aged 19 to 32 as well as college students. See Tables 84.1 to 84.5 for lifetime, annual, 30 day, and 30-day daily prevalence use of drugs among college students compared to their age-matched peers not in college. Tables 84.6 to 84.9 give the trends in these prevalence rates from 1980 to 2006. Figure 84.1 shows trends in annual prevalence of any illicit drug, Figure 84.2 shows trends in 2-week prevalence of five or more drinks in a row, and Figure 84.3 shows trends in daily cigarette usage. Starting in 1980, the 2006 survey marks the 26th year of following up drug use in the college population. Trends noticed in this report include the following:

- Overall, use of illicit drugs fell among American college students and young adults between late 1970s and early 1990s. These declines seemed most correlated with perceived risk and not availability of the drug. However, there have been increases in the usage rates since 1994 for many drugs among high school seniors and college students.
- In 2006, the rank order for annual prevalence of using any illicit drug was 12th graders (36.5%), college students (33.9%), 19- to 28-year-olds (32.1%), 10th graders (28.7%), and 8th graders (14.8%). In general, the trends for most illicit drugs use in college students paralleled noncollege peers in the 1980s. However, in the 1990s the trends diverge; college students showed less increase than their age-mates not in college. In 2006, for most categories of drugs, college students showed rates of use that are similar to those of their age peers. Annual prevalence for any illicit drug is 33.9% among college students versus 32.1% among noncollege age-mates. For any illicit drug other than marijuana this difference is 18.1% versus 18.4%. For a few drugs, college students show higher rates of use than their age-mates including Ritalin, marijuana and hallucinogens. While college-bound seniors have below-average rates of use in high school for all of the illicit drugs, these students' eventual use of some illicit drugs becomes equal or exceeds those not attending college. This has become known as the "*catching up*" or "*college effect*." This influence has been correlated to leaving the parental home after graduation (more likely in college students) or getting married (less likely in college students).
- *Smoking:* In the first half of the 1990s, smoking rose among college students and their same-age peers, although the increases were not as steep for either group as they were among high school seniors. However, in 1998 and 1999, while smoking was declining among secondary school students in all grades, smoking increased significantly

for college students. Between 1990 and 1999, the 30-day prevalence of cigarette smoking in college students rose from 22% to 31% and daily smoking rose from 12% to 19%. The year 2000 shows, for the first time in several years, a decline in college student smoking. This is likely reflective of the decline in younger students as they work their way into college. In 2006, out of all the substances studied, cigarette smoking showed the greatest absolute difference between age-matched college students and non–college students (9.2% daily smoking prevalence versus 18.6% for same aged high school graduates not in college). Among college students, females had a slightly higher probability of being a daily smoker from 1980 through 1994, with a reversal of this from 1994 to 2001. Since 2001, there is little consistent gender difference in smoking among college students.
- *Alcohol use:* Alcohol has been tried by 86.6% of college students. In 2006, the lifetime and annual use of alcohol among college students was not significantly different from age-matched peers not in college. In 2006, 30-day use was higher (65%) in college students than non–college age-matched peers (61%) but daily drinking in college students was lower (4.8%) than their non–college peer group (5.7%). However, college students have the highest rate of occasions of heavy drinking (five or more drinks in a row in the last 2 weeks). In 2006, this was 11% for 8th graders, 22% for 10th graders, 25.1% for 12th graders, 40.2% (45.2% in males) for college students, and 34.7% for age-matched peers not in college. Episodes of heavy drinking have declined far less among college students than high school seniors and noncollege age-mates. Between 1981 and 1992, heavy drinking dropped by 11 percentage points among noncollege 19- to 22-year-olds, but only by 2 percentage points among college students. Therefore, college students stand out as having high rates of binge (or party) drinking. Because college-bound seniors in high school are consistently less likely to report occasions of heavy drinking compared to non–college-bound students, it appears that the higher rates of heavy drinking episodes in college indicate a college-related increase in binge drinking or what is being called the "*college effect*." Among college students and young adults in general, there are substantial gender differences in alcohol use. College males drink the most with 50% of college males reporting five or more drinks in a row over prior 2 weeks compared to 34.4% of college females. Over the years of this survey, alcohol use did not increase as other illicit drug use decreased and in fact the opposite appeared true. This supports the notion that alcohol use moves much more in parallel with other illicit drugs, rather than in the opposite direction.
- *Marijuana use:* The annual prevalence of marijuana use among college students decreased markedly from 1981 through 1991, from 51% to 27%. In the 1990s, there was an increase in marijuana use in college students that followed the increase in high school students as these students replaced their peers in college. This was a reversal of the way the epidemic started in the 1960s when drug usage started on college campuses and spread downward to high school students and then to junior high school students. Daily marijuana use rose substantially among college students between 1992 and 2003 but appears to have decreased since.
- *Lysergic acid diethylamide (LSD):* During the early 1980s, one of the largest proportional declines in college

TABLE 84.1

Lifetime Prevalence of Use for Various Types of Drugs, 2006: Full-Time College Students versus Others Among Respondents 1 to 4 Years Beyond High School (Entries are percentages)

	Total		Males		Females	
	Full-Time College	Others	Full-Time College	Others	Full-Time College	Others
Any illicit drug[a]	50.6	61.0	55.0	58.0	47.8	63.3
Any illicit drug[a]						
Other than marijuana	26.3	35.5	29.2	33.9	24.4	36.7
Marijuana	46.9	57.8	52.8	55.0	43.1	59.8
Inhalants[b]	7.4	11.9	8.5	12.6	6.6	11.4
Hallucinogens	10.6	14.9	15.5	17.0	7.5	13.4
LSD	3.5	6.8	4.7	7.9	2.8	6.1
Hallucinogens						
Other than LSD	10.1	13.6	15.3	15.7	6.8	12.0
Cocaine	7.7	17.1	10.5	18.3	6.0	16.2
Crack[c]	2.3	6.2	2.7	6.5	2.0	6.0
Other cocaine[d]	6.2	17.1	8.8	18.1	4.7	16.4
MDMA (Ecstasy)[b]	6.9	12.3	7.0	11.3	6.8	13.0
Heroin	0.7	2.0	1.1	2.5	0.4	1.7
With a needle[e]	0.3	0.6	0.8	1.0	*	0.3
Without a needle[e]	0.8	1.9	0.8	3.3	0.8	0.8
Other narcotics[f]	14.6	19.7	18.5	19.2	12.1	20.0
Amphetamines, adjusted[f,g]	10.7	17.5	11.9	15.2	9.9	19.2
Methamphetamine[e]	2.9	10.5	4.0	11.3	2.2	10.0
Ice[e]	1.7	8.1	3.3	6.8	0.7	8.9
Sedatives (Barbiturates)[f]	6.3	11.1	8.5	11.3	4.9	10.9
Tranquilizers[f]	10.0	16.1	12.4	15.1	8.4	16.8
Alcohol	84.7	83.8	83.0	83.8	85.7	83.8
Been drunk[b]	73.1	76.4	72.1	79.4	73.7	74.2
Flavored alcoholic beverage[h]	80.9	79.5	78.7	75.5	82.4	82.2
Cigarettes	NA	NA	NA	NA	NA	NA
Steroids[e]	1.9	1.3	3.9	3.0	0.7	*
Approximate weighted n =	1,280	870	500	370	780	500

LSD, lysergic acid diethylamide; MDMA, methylenedioxymethamphetamine

"*" indicates a percentage of <0.05%.

[a]Use of "any illicit drug" includes any use of marijuana, hallucinogens, cocaine, heroin or other narcotics, amphetamines, sedatives (barbiturates), or tranquilizers not under a doctor's orders.

[b]This drug was asked about in three of the six questionnaire forms. Total n in 2006 for college students is approximately 640.

[c]This drug was asked about in five of the six questionnaire forms. Total n in 2006 for college students is approximately 1,060.

[d]This drug was asked about in four of the six questionnaire forms. Total n in 2006 for college students is approximately 850.

[e]This drug was asked about in two of the six questionnaire forms. Total n in 2006 for college students is approximately 430.

[f]Only drug use that was not under a doctor's orders is included here.

[g]On the basis of the data from the revised question, which attempts to exclude inappropriate reporting of nonprescription amphetamines.

[h]This drug was asked about in one of the six questionnaire forms. Total n in 2006 for college students is approximately 210.

From Johnston LD, O'Malley PM, Bachman JG, et al. (2007). *Monitoring the Future national survey results on drug use, 1975–2006: Volume II, College students and adults ages 19–45* (NIH Publication No. 07-6206). Bethesda, MD: National Institute on Drug Abuse;2007:234. Available at: http://www.monitoringthefuture.org/pubs/monographs/vol2_2006.pdf.

TABLE 84.2

Annual Prevalence of Use for Various Types of Drugs, 2006: Full-Time College Students versus Others Among Respondents 1 to 4 Years Beyond High School (Entries are percentages)

	Total		Males		Females	
	Full-Time College	Others	Full-Time College	Others	Full-Time College	Others
Any illicit drug[a]	33.9	39.7	39.2	39.3	30.6	39.9
Any illicit drug[a]						
Other than marijuana	18.1	23.0	22.6	23.6	15.2	22.5
Marijuana	30.2	35.2	35.8	34.9	26.6	35.3
Inhalants[b]	1.5	3.5	1.6	3.8	1.4	3.3
Hallucinogens	5.6	5.7	10.1	7.1	2.7	4.6
LSD	1.4	2.5	1.9	3.6	1.0	1.6
Hallucinogens						
Other than LSD	5.4	4.8	9.7	6.1	2.7	3.7
Cocaine	5.1	9.9	7.3	12.9	3.7	7.6
Crack[c]	1.0	2.1	1.0	2.3	1.0	2.0
Other cocaine[d]	3.8	9.8	5.9	14.1	2.6	6.7
MDMA (Ecstasy)[b]	2.6	5.2	3.8	4.7	1.9	5.6
Heroin	0.3	1.0	0.5	1.3	0.2	0.7
With a needle[e]	0.3	0.5	0.8	0.7	*	0.3
Without a needle[e]	0.3	1.2	0.6	2.1	0.2	0.6
Other narcotics[f]	8.8	11.9	12.8	13.3	6.3	10.9
OxyContin[e]	3.0	3.6	5.4	4.8	1.5	2.8
Vicodin[e]	7.6	11.1	12.3	12.4	4.6	10.2
Amphetamines, adjusted[f,g]	6.0	8.6	7.2	7.9	5.3	9.0
Ritalin[e,f]	3.9	3.0	5.0	4.5	3.1	1.9
Methamphetamine[e]	1.2	4.7	1.2	5.8	1.2	3.8
Ice[e]	0.6	3.3	0.9	2.4	0.4	4.0
Sedatives (Barbiturates)[f]	3.4	6.3	4.7	6.1	2.6	6.4
Tranquilizers[f]	5.8	8.5	8.0	8.9	4.4	8.1
Rohypnol[e]	0.2	0.7	0.3	1.5	0.2	0.2
GHB[e]	*	0.4	*	0.8	*	0.2
Ketamine[e]	0.9	1.3	1.5	0.8	0.5	1.6
Alcohol	82.1	78.9	80.5	80.0	83.0	78.0
Been drunk[b]	66.2	63.6	66.5	68.0	66.0	60.4
Flavored alcoholic beverage[h]	63.5	59.0	59.7	54.2	66.0	62.2
Cigarettes	30.9	44.6	34.1	45.9	28.8	43.6
Steroids[e]	0.8	0.7	2.0	1.6	*	*
Approximate weighted n =	1,280	870	500	370	780	500

LSD, lysergic acid diethylamide; MDMA, methylenedioxymethamphetamine; GHB, gamma hydroxybutyrate.

"*" indicates a percentage of <0.05%.

[a]Use of "any illicit drug" includes any use of marijuana, hallucinogens, cocaine, heroin or other narcotics, amphetamines, sedatives (barbiturates), or tranquilizers not under a doctor's orders.

[b]This drug was asked about in three of the six questionnaire forms. Total n in 2006 for college students is approximately 640.

[c]This drug was asked about in five of the six questionnaire forms. Total n in 2006 for college students is approximately 1,060.

[d]This drug was asked about in four of the six questionnaire forms. Total n in 2006 for college students is approximately 850.

[e]This drug was asked about in two of the six questionnaire forms. Total n in 2006 for college students is approximately 430.

[f]Only drug use that was not under a doctor's orders is included here.

[g]On the basis of the data from the revised question, which attempts to exclude inappropriate reporting of nonprescription amphetamines.

[h]This drug was asked about in one of the six questionnaire forms. Total n in 2006 for college students is approximately 210.

From Johnston LD, O'Malley PM, Bachman JG, et al. (2007). *Monitoring the Future national survey results on drug use, 1975–2006: Volume II, College students and adults ages 19–45* (NIH Publication No. 07-6206). Bethesda, MD: National Institute on Drug Abuse;2007:235. Available at: http://www.monitoringthefuture.org/pubs/monographs/vol2_2006.pdf.

TABLE 84.3

Thirty-Day Prevalence of Use for Various Types of Drugs, 2006: Full-Time College Students versus Others Among Respondents 1 to 4 Years Beyond High School (Entries are percentages)

	Total		Males		Females	
	Full-Time College	*Others*	*Full-Time College*	*Others*	*Full-Time College*	*Others*
Any illicit drug[a]	19.2	21.8	23.4	21.5	16.6	22.0
Any illicit drug[a]						
Other than marijuana	8.2	10.6	10.3	11.3	6.9	10.1
Marijuana	16.7	18.6	21.3	18.9	13.8	18.3
Inhalants[b]	0.4	0.6	0.7	0.9	0.3	0.5
Hallucinogens	0.9	1.2	1.5	1.2	0.5	1.3
LSD	0.3	0.4	0.4	0.5	0.2	0.4
Hallucinogens						
Other than LSD	0.7	1.0	1.2	1.0	0.4	0.9
Cocaine	1.8	3.2	3.2	3.5	1.0	3.0
Crack[c]	*	0.5	0.1	0.4	*	0.6
Other cocaine[d]	1.3	3.2	2.3	3.7	0.7	2.8
MDMA (Ecstasy)[b]	0.6	1.1	0.7	1.3	0.6	0.9
Heroin	0.2	0.4	0.4	0.6	0.0	0.2
Other Narcotics[e]	3.1	4.8	4.3	5.6	2.3	4.3
Amphetamines, adjusted[e,f]	2.5	3.0	2.1	3.2	2.7	2.9
Ice[g]	*	1.5	*	2.0	*	1.1
Sedatives (Barbiturates)[e]	1.3	2.6	1.3	2.2	1.2	2.8
Tranquilizers[e]	2.1	3.7	2.9	4.9	1.6	2.9
Alcohol	65.4	61.0	65.7	64.9	65.2	58.1
Been drunk[b]	47.6	40.2	52.2	46.9	44.7	35.2
Flavored alcoholic beverage[h]	26.2	30.5	19.7	34.2	30.6	28.1
Cigarettes	19.2	35.7	20.9	38.3	18.1	33.8
Approximate weighted n =	1,280	870	500	370	780	500

LSD, lysergic acid diethylamide; MDMA, methylenedioxymethamphetamine.

"*" indicates a percentage of <0.05%.

[a]Use of "any illicit drug" includes any use of marijuana, hallucinogens, cocaine, heroin or other narcotics, amphetamines, sedatives (barbiturates), or tranquilizers not under a doctor's orders.

[b]This drug was asked about in three of the six questionnaire forms. Total n in 2006 for college students is approximately 640.

[c]This drug was asked about in five of the six questionnaire forms. Total n in 2006 for college students is approximately 1,060.

[d]This drug was asked about in four of the six questionnaire forms. Total n in 2006 for college students is approximately 850.

[e]Only drug use that was not under a doctor's orders is included here.

[f]On the basis of the data from the revised question, which attempts to exclude inappropriate reporting of nonprescription amphetamines.

[g]This drug was asked about in two of the six questionnaire forms. Total n in 2006 for college students is approximately 430.

[h]This drug was asked about in one of the six questionnaire forms. Total n in 2006 for college students is approximately 210.

From Johnston LD, O'Malley PM, Bachman JG, et al. (2007). *Monitoring the Future national survey results on drug use, 1975–2006: Volume II, College students and adults ages 19–45* (NIH Publication No. 07-6206). Bethesda, MD: National Institute on Drug Abuse;2007:236. Available at: http://www.monitoringthefuture.org/pubs/monographs/vol2_2006.pdf.

students was for use of LSD with annual prevalence rates falling from 6.3% in 1982 to 2.2% in 1985. However, usage increased after 1985, reaching 6.9% in 1995. After peaking in 1995, use among college students and young adults declined through 2005 (0.7%) but increased in 2006 to 1.4%. However, there is some evidence that at the same time there may have been some displacement of LSD usage to ecstasy (methylenedioxymethamphetamine [MDMA]) as well as tranquilizer usage.

- *MDMA (ecstasy):* MDMA (ecstasy) had a substantial increase in annual use in college students starting in 1995

(3.6%) to 2001 (9.2%). However, 2002 (6.8%) marked the beginning of a decline with the annual prevalence rate at 2.6% in 2006.

- *Amphetamines:* Between 1982 and 1992 amphetamine annual use declined among college students from 21% to 3.6%. However, annual use increased among college students to 7.2% in 2001 and has decreased since then to 6.0% in 2006. The annual use prevalence is 8.6% for age-matched peers not in college. The perceived risk dropped in 1993 and this may account for the increase in usage in the 1990s.

TABLE 84.4

Thirty-Day Prevalence of Daily Use for Various Types of Drugs, 2006: Full-Time College Students versus Others Among Respondents 1 to 4 Years Beyond High School (Entries are percentages)

	Total		Males		Females	
	Full-Time College	Others	Full-Time College	Others	Full-Time College	Others
Marijuana[a]	4.3	6.7	5.5	8.0	3.6	5.7
Cocaine[a]	0.1	0.2	0.2	0.2	*	0.3
Amphetamines, adjusted[a,b,c]	0.4	0.1	0.3	*	0.4	0.2
Alcohol						
Daily[a]	4.8	5.7	7.3	7.5	3.2	4.3
Five or more drinks in a row in past 2 wk	40.2	34.7	45.2	41.1	37.1	29.8
Cigarettes						
Daily	9.2	25.8	9.9	27.2	8.7	24.8
Half-pack or more per day	4.9	17.0	6.9	17.6	3.6	16.5
Approximate weighted n =	1,280	870	500	370	780	500

"*" indicates a percentage of <0.05%.

[a]Daily use is defined as use on 20 or more occasions in the past 30 days except for cigarettes, for which actual daily use is measured, and for five or more drinks, for which the prevalence of having five or more drinks in a row in the last two weeks is measured.

[b]Only drug use that was not under a doctor's orders is included here.

[c]On the basis of data from the revised question, which attempts to exclude inappropriate reporting of nonprescription amphetamines.

From Johnston LD, O'Malley PM, Bachman JG, et al. (2007). *Monitoring the Future national survey results on drug use, 1975–2006: Volume II, College students and adults ages 19–45* (NIH Publication No. 07-6206). Bethesda, MD: National Institute on Drug Abuse;2007:237. Available at: http://www.monitoringthefuture.org/pubs/monographs/vol2_2006.pdf.

TABLE 84.5

Lifetime, Annual, and 30-Day Prevalence of an Illicit Drug Use Index, 2005: Full-Time College Students versus Others among Respondents 1 to 4 Years beyond High School

	Total		Males		Females	
	Full-Time College	Others	Full-Time College	Others	Full-Time College	Others
	Lifetime					
Any illicit drug[a]	52.3	61.6	54.2	62.1	51.3	61.3
Any illicit drug other than marijuana	26.5	35.2	29.0	36.5	25.1	34.1
	Past 12 Months					
Any illicit drug	36.6	39.6	40.7	40.8	34.2	38.7
Any illicit drug other than marijuana	18.5	23.4	21.1	24.0	16.9	23.0
	Past 30 Days					
Any illicit drug	19.5	23.9	22.9	27.0	17.5	21.7
Any illicit drug other than marijuana	8.2	11.0	10.3	11.0	7.0	11.0
Approximate weighted N =	1,360	850	500	360	860	490

Entries are percentages

[a]Use of "any illicit drug" includes any use of marijuana, hallucinogens, cocaine, heroin or other narcotics, amphetamines, sedatives (barbiturates), or tranquilizers not under a doctor's orders.

From Johnston LD, O'Malley PM, Bachman JG, et al. *Monitoring the future volume II of the national survey results on drug use, 1975–2005*, Bethesda, MD: National Institute on Drug Abuse, www.monitoringthefuture.org. 2006.

TABLE 84.6

Trends in Lifetime Prevalence of Various Types of Drugs Among College Students 1 to 4 Years Beyond High School

Percentage who used in lifetime

	1980	1981	1982	1983	1984	1985	1986	1987	1988	1989	1990	1991	1992	1993	1994	1995	1996	1997	1998	1999	2000	2001	2002	2003	2004	2005	2006	'05–'06 change
Approximate weighted n	1,040	1,130	1,150	1,170	1,110	1,080	1,190	1,220	1,310	1,300	1,400	1,410	1,490	1,490	1,410	1,450	1,450	1,480	1,440	1,440	1,350	1,340	1,260	1,270	1,400	1,360	1,280	
Any illicit drug[a]	69.4	66.8	64.6	66.9	62.7	65.2	61.8	60.0	58.4	55.6	54.0	50.4	48.8	45.9	45.5	45.5	47.4	49.0	52.9	53.2	53.7	53.6	51.8	53.9	52.2	52.3	50.6	−1.8
Any illicit drug[a] Other than marijuana	42.2	41.3	39.6	41.7	38.6	40.0	37.5	35.7	33.4	30.5	28.4	25.8	26.1	24.3	22.0	24.5	22.7	24.4	24.8	25.5	25.8	26.3	26.9	27.6	28.0	26.5	26.3	−0.3
Marijuana	65.0	63.3	60.5	63.1	59.0	60.6	57.9	55.8	54.3	51.3	49.1	46.3	44.1	42.0	42.2	41.7	45.1	46.1	49.9	50.8	51.2	51.0	49.5	50.7	49.1	49.1	46.9	−2.2
Inhalants[b]	10.2	8.8	10.6	11.0	10.4	10.6	11.0	13.2	12.6	15.0	13.9	14.4	14.2	14.8	12.0	13.8	11.4	12.4	12.8	12.4	12.9	9.6	7.7	9.7	8.5	7.1	7.4	+0.3
Hallucinogens[c]	15.0	12.0	15.0	12.2	12.9	11.4	11.2	10.9	10.2	10.7	11.2	11.3	12.0	11.8	10.0	13.0	12.6	13.8	15.2	14.8	14.4	14.8	13.6	14.5	12.0	11.0	10.6	−0.5
LSD	10.3	8.5	11.5	8.8	9.4	7.4	7.7	8.0	7.5	7.8	9.1	9.6	10.6	10.6	9.2	11.5	10.8	11.7	13.1	12.7	11.8	12.2	8.6	8.7	5.6	3.7	3.5	−0.2
Hallucinogens Other than LSD[c]	11.6	9.0	10.6	8.3	9.2	8.1	7.8	6.8	6.2	6.2	6.0	6.0	5.7	5.4	4.4	6.5	6.5	7.5	8.7	8.8	8.2	10.7	11.0	12.8	10.1	10.6	10.1	−0.5
MDMA (Ecstasy)[d]	NA	NA	NA	NA	NA	NA	NA	NA	NA	3.8	3.9	2.0	2.9	2.3	2.1	3.1	4.3	4.6	6.8	8.4	13.1	14.7	12.7	12.9	10.2	8.3	6.9	−1.3
Cocaine	22.0	21.5	22.4	23.1	21.7	22.9	23.3	20.6	15.8	14.6	11.4	9.4	7.9	6.3	5.0	5.5	5.0	5.6	8.1	8.4	9.1	8.6	8.2	9.2	9.5	8.8	7.7	−1.1
Crack[e]	NA	NA	NA	NA	NA	NA	NA	3.3	3.4	2.4	1.4	1.5	1.7	1.3	1.0	1.8	1.2	1.4	2.2	2.4	2.5	2.0	1.9	3.1	2.0	1.7	2.3	+0.6
Other cocaine[f]	NA	NA	NA	NA	NA	NA	NA	18.1	14.2	16.0	10.2	9.0	7.6	6.3	4.6	5.2	4.6	5.0	7.4	7.8	8.1	8.3	8.6	8.5	9.3	8.1	6.2	−1.9
Heroin	0.9	0.6	0.3	0.5	0.4	0.4	0.6	0.3	0.7	0.3	0.3	0.5	0.5	0.6	0.1	0.6	0.7	0.9	1.7	0.9	1.7	1.2	1.0	1.0	0.9	0.5	0.7	+0.2
Other narcotics[g,h]	8.9	8.3	8.1	8.4	8.9	6.3	8.8	7.6	6.3	7.6	6.8	7.3	7.3	6.2	5.1	7.2	5.7	8.2	8.7	8.7	8.9	11.0	12.2	14.2	13.8	14.4	14.6	+0.2
Amphetamines, adjusted[g,i]	29.5	29.4	30.1	27.8	27.8	25.4	22.3	19.8	17.7	14.6	13.2	13.0	10.5	10.1	9.2	10.7	9.5	10.6	10.6	11.9	12.3	12.4	11.9	12.3	12.7	12.3	10.7	−1.6
Methamphetamine[j]	NA	NA	NA	NA	NA	NA	NA	NA	NA	NA	NA	NA	NA	NA	NA	NA	NA	NA	NA	7.1	5.1	5.3	5.0	5.8	5.2	4.1	2.9	−1.2
Crystal meth. (Ice)[j]	NA	NA	NA	NA	NA	NA	NA	NA	NA	NA	1.0	1.3	0.6	1.6	1.3	1.0	0.8	1.6	2.2	2.8	1.3	2.3	2.0	2.9	2.2	2.4	1.7	−0.7

(continued)

TABLE 84.6

(Continued)

Sedatives

Drug																												s
(Barbiturates)[g]	8.1	7.8	8.2	6.6	6.4	4.9	5.4	3.5	3.6	3.2	3.8	3.5	3.8	3.5	3.2	4.0	4.6	5.2	5.7	6.7	6.9	6.0	5.9	5.7	7.2	8.5	6.3	−2.2 s
Sedatives, adjusted[g,k]	13.7	14.2	14.1	12.2	10.8	9.3	8.0	6.1	4.7	4.1	NA	NA	NA	NA	NA	NA	NA	NA	NA	NA	NA	NA	NA	NA	NA	NA	NA	—
Methaqualone[g]	10.3	11.4	11.1	9.2	9.0	7.2	5.8	4.1	2.2	2.4	NA	NA	NA	NA	NA	NA	NA	NA	NA	NA	NA	NA	NA	NA	NA	NA	NA	—
Tranquilizers[c,g]	15.2	11.4	11.7	10.8	10.8	9.8	10.7	8.7	8.0	8.0	7.1	6.8	6.9	6.3	4.4	5.4	5.4	6.9	7.7	8.2	8.8	9.7	10.7	11.0	10.6	11.9	10.0	−1.9
Any Rx drug[l]	35.9	34.2	34.9	33.7	32.3	29.8	28.5	26.3	24.2	22.0	20.5	20.3	18.4	17.0	15.1	17.6	15.5	18.4	17.7	19.3	19.8	21.1	20.7	22.8	22.9	22.9	22.2	−0.7
Alcohol[m]	94.3	95.2	95.2	95.0	94.2	95.3	94.9	94.1	94.9	93.7	93.1	93.6	91.8	89.3	88.2	88.5	88.4	87.3	88.5	88.0	86.6	86.1	86.0	86.2	84.6	86.6	84.7	−2.0
Been drunk[n]	NA	NA	NA	NA	NA	NA	NA	NA	NA	NA	NA	79.6	76.8	76.4	74.4	76.6	76.2	77.0	76.8	75.1	74.7	76.1	75.1	74.9	73.4	72.9	73.1	+0.2
Flavored alcoholic beverage[o]	NA	NA	NA	NA	NA	NA	NA	NA	NA	NA	NA	NA	NA	NA	NA	NA	NA	NA	NA	NA	NA	NA	NA	NA	79.0	84.5	80.9	−3.6
Cigarettes	NA	NA	NA	NA	NA	NA	NA	NA	NA	NA	NA	NA	NA	NA	NA	NA	NA	NA	NA	NA	NA	NA	NA	NA	NA	NA	NA	NA
Steroids[p]	NA	NA	NA	NA	NA	NA	NA	NA	NA	NA	1.5	1.4	1.7	1.9	0.5	0.8	0.6	1.6	0.9	1.3	0.6	1.5	1.2	1.2	1.6	1.0	1.9	+0.9

LSD, lysergic acid diethylamide; MDMA, methylenedioxymethamphetamine.

Level of significance of difference between the two most recent years: s = 0.05, ss = 0.01, sss = 0.001. Any apparent inconsistency between the change estimate and the prevalence estimates for the two most recent years is due to rounding.

"NA" indicates data not available.

a"Any illicit drug" includes use of marijuana, hallucinogens, cocaine, heroin or other narcotics, amphetamines, sedatives (barbiturates), methaqualone (until 1990), or tranquilizers not under a doctor's orders.

bThis drug was asked about in four of the five questionnaire forms in 1980–1989; in five of the six questionnaire forms in 1990–1998, and in three of the six forms in 1999–2006. Total n in 2006 is approximately 650.

cIn 2001 the question text was changed on half the questionnaire forms. "Other psychedelics" was changed to "other hallucinogens," and "shrooms" was added to the list of examples. For tranquilizers, "Miltown" was replaced with "Xanax" in the list of examples. Beginning in 2002 the remaining forms were changed to the new wording.

dThis drug was asked about in two of the five questionnaire forms in 1989, in two of the six questionnaire forms in 1990–2001, and in three of the six questionnaire forms in 2002–2006. Total n in 2006 is approximately 650.

eThis drug was asked about in two of the five questionnaire forms in 1987–1989, in all six questionnaire forms in 1990–2001, and in five of the six questionnaire forms in 2002–2006. Total n in 2006 is approximately 1,070.

fThis drug was asked about in one of the five questionnaire forms in 1987–1989 and in four of six questionnaire forms in 1990–2006. Total n in 2006 is approximately 850.

gOnly drug use that was not under a doctor's orders is included here.

hIn 2002 the question text was changed on hall of the questionnaire forms. The list of examples of narcotics other than heroin was updated: Talwin, laudanum, and paregoric—all of which had negligible rates of use by 2001—were replaced by Vicodin, OxyContin, and Percocef. The 2002 data presented here are based on the changed forms only; n is one half on n indicated. In 2003 the remaining forms were changed to the new wording. The data are based on all forms in 2003 and beyond.

iOn the basis of the data from the revised question, which attempts to exclude inappropriate reporting of nonprescription amphetamines.

jThis drug was asked about in the two of the six questionnaire forms. Total n in 2006 is approximately 430.

k"Sedatives, adjusted" data are a combination of barbiturate and methaqualone data.

lUse of "Any Rx Drug" includes any use of amphetamines, sedatives (barbiturates), tranquilizers, and/or narcotics other than heroin not under a doctor's orders.

mIn 1993 and 1994, the question text was changed slightly in three of the six questionnaire forms to indicate that a "drink" meant "more than just a few sips." Because this revision resulted in rather little change in reported prevalence in the surveys of high school graduates, the data for all forms combined are used in order to provide the most reliable estimate of change. After 1994 the new question text was used in all six of the questionnaire forms.

nThis drug was asked about in three of the six questionnaire forms. Total n in 2006 is approximately 640.

oThis drug was asked about in one of the six questionnaire forms. Total n in 2006 is approximately 220.

pThis drug was asked about in one of the five questinnaire forms in 1989 and in two of the six questionnaire forms in 1990–2006. Total n in 2006 is approximately 430.

qDaily use is defined as use on 20 or more occasions in the past 30 days except for cigarettes, for which actual daily use is measured, and for five or more drinks, for which the prevalence of having five or more drinks in a row in the last 2 weeks is measured.

rRevised questions about amphetamine use were introduced in 1982 to more completely exclude inappropriate reporting of nonprescription amphetamines. The data in italics are therefore not strictly comparable to the other data.

From Johnston LD, O'Malley PM, Bachman JG, et al. (2007). Monitoring the Future national survey results on drug use, 1975–2006: Volume II. College students and adults ages 19–45 (NIH Publication No. 07-6206). Bethesda, MD: National Institute on Drug Abuse;2007:249–251. Available at: http://www.monitoringthefuture.org/pubs/monographs/vol2.2006.pdf.

TABLE 84.7

Trends in Annual Prevalence of Various Types of Drugs Among College Students 1 to 4 Years Beyond High School

Percentage who used in past year

	1980	1981	1982	1983	1984	1985	1986	1987	1988	1989	1990	1991	1992	1993	1994	1995	1996	1997	1998	1999	2000	2001	2002	2003	2004	2005	2006	'05–'06 change
Approximate weighted n	1040	1130	1150	1170	1110	1080	1190	1220	1310	1300	1400	1410	1490	1490	1410	1450	1450	1480	1440	1440	1350	1340	1260	1270	1400	1360	1280	
Any illicit drug[a]	56.2	55.0	49.5	49.8	45.1	46.3	45.0	40.1	37.4	36.7	33.3	29.2	30.6	30.6	31.4	33.5	34.2	34.1	37.8	36.9	36.1	37.9	37.0	36.5	36.2	36.6	33.9	−2.6
Any illicit drug[a] Other than marijuana	32.3	31.7	29.9	29.9	27.2	26.7	25.0	21.3	19.2	16.4	15.2	13.2	13.1	12.5	12.2	15.9	12.8	15.8	14.0	15.4	15.6	16.4	16.6	17.9	18.6	18.5	18.1	−0.4
Marijuana	51.2	51.3	44.7	45.2	40.7	41.7	40.9	37.0	34.6	33.6	29.4	26.5	27.7	27.9	29.3	31.2	33.1	31.6	35.9	35.2	34.0	35.6	34.7	33.7	33.3	33.3	30.2	−3.2
Inhalants[b]	3.0	2.5	2.8	2.4	3.1	3.9	3.7	4.1	3.7	3.9	3.5	3.1	3.0	3.8	3.0	3.9	3.6	4.1	3.0	3.2	2.9	2.8	2.0	1.8	2.7	1.8	1.5	−0.4
Hallucinogens[c]	8.5	7.0	8.7	6.5	6.2	5.0	6.0	5.9	5.3	5.1	5.4	6.3	6.8	6.0	6.2	8.2	6.9	7.7	7.2	7.8	6.7	7.5	6.3	7.4	5.9	5.0	5.6	+0.5
LSD	6.0	4.6	6.3	4.3	3.7	2.2	3.9	4.0	3.6	3.4	4.3	5.1	5.7	5.1	5.2	6.9	5.2	5.0	4.4	5.4	4.3	4.0	2.1	1.4	1.2	0.7	1.4	+0.7
Hallucinogens Other than LSD[c]	5.2	4.7	3.9	4.1	3.9	3.8	NA	3.1	3.4	3.1	3.0	3.1	2.6	2.7	2.8	4.0	4.1	4.9	4.4	4.5	4.4	5.5	5.8	7.1	5.6	5.0	5.4	+0.5
MDMA (Esctasy)[d]	NA	NA	NA	NA	NA	NA	NA	NA	NA	2.3	2.3	0.9	2.0	0.8	0.5	2.4	2.8	2.4	3.9	5.5	9.1	9.2	6.8	4.4	2.2	2.9	2.6	−0.3
Cocaine	16.8	16.0	17.2	17.3	16.3	17.3	17.1	13.7	10.0	8.2	5.6	3.6	3.0	2.7	2.0	3.6	2.9	3.4	4.6	4.6	4.8	4.7	4.8	5.4	6.6	5.7	5.1	−0.6
Crack[e]	NA	NA	NA	NA	NA	NA	1.3	2.0	1.4	1.5	0.6	0.5	0.4	0.6	0.5	1.1	0.6	0.4	1.0	0.9	0.9	0.4	0.4	1.3	1.3	0.8	1.0	+0.2
Other cocaine[f]	NA	NA	NA	NA	NA	NA	NA	10.7	10.6	9.3	5.1	3.2	2.4	2.5	1.8	3.3	2.3	3.0	4.2	4.2	4.1	4.1	5.0	5.1	6.3	5.0	3.8	−1.2
Heroin	0.4	0.2	0.1	*	0.1	0.2	0.1	0.2	0.2	0.1	0.1	0.1	0.1	0.1	0.1	0.3	0.4	0.3	0.6	0.2	0.5	0.5	0.1	0.2	0.4	0.3	0.3	−0.1
Other narcotics[g,h]	5.1	4.3	3.8	3.8	3.8	2.4	4.0	3.1	3.1	3.2	2.9	2.7	2.7	2.5	2.4	3.8	3.1	4.2	4.2	4.3	5.7	7.4	7.4	8.7	8.2	8.4	8.8	+0.4
OxyContin[j]	NA	NA	NA	NA	NA	NA	NA	NA	NA	NA	NA	NA	NA	NA	NA	NA	NA	NA	NA	NA	NA	NA	1.5	2.2	2.5	2.1	3.0	+0.9
Vicodin[j]	NA	NA	NA	NA	NA	NA	NA	NA	NA	NA	NA	NA	NA	NA	NA	NA	NA	NA	NA	NA	NA	NA	6.9	7.5	7.4	9.6	7.6	−2.1
Amphetamines[g]	22.4	22.2	NA	NA	NA	NA	NA	NA	NA	NA	NA	NA	NA	NA	NA	NA	NA	NA	NA	NA	NA	NA	NA	NA	NA	NA	NA	—
Amphetamines, adjusted[g,i]	NA	NA	21.1	17.3	15.7	11.9	10.3	7.2	6.2	4.6	4.5	3.9	3.6	4.2	4.2	5.4	4.2	5.7	5.1	5.8	6.6	7.2	7.0	7.1	7.0	6.7	6.0	−0.7
Ritalin[g,j]	NA	NA	NA	NA	NA	NA	NA	NA	NA	NA	NA	NA	NA	NA	NA	NA	NA	NA	NA	NA	NA	NA	5.7	4.7	4.7	4.2	3.9	−0.4
Methamphetamine[j]	NA	NA	NA	NA	NA	NA	NA	NA	NA	NA	NA	NA	NA	NA	NA	NA	NA	NA	NA	3.3	1.6	2.4	1.2	2.6	2.9	1.7	1.2	−0.5
Crystal meth.(Ice)[j]	NA	NA	NA	NA	NA	NA	NA	NA	NA	NA	0.1	0.1	0.2	0.7	0.8	1.1	0.4	0.8	1.0	0.5	0.5	0.6	0.8	0.9	1.1	1.4	0.6	−0.7

(continued)

TABLE 84.7

(Continued)

																														Change
Sedatives																														
(Barbiturates)[g]	2.9	2.8	3.2	2.2	1.9	1.3	2.0	1.2	1.1	1.0	1.4	1.2	1.5	1.4	1.2	2.0	2.3	3.0	3.2	2.5	3.7	3.2	3.7	3.8	3.7	4.1	4.2	3.9	3.4	−0.5
Sedatives, adjusted[g,k]	8.3	8.0	8.0	4.5	3.5	2.5	2.6	1.7	1.5	1.0	NA	NA	NA	NA	NA	NA	NA	NA	NA	NA	NA	NA	NA	NA	NA	NA	NA	NA	NA	—
Methaqualone[g]	7.2	6.5	6.6	3.1	2.5	1.4	1.2	0.8	0.5	0.2	NA	NA	NA	NA	NA	NA	NA	NA	NA	NA	NA	NA	NA	NA	NA	NA	NA	NA	NA	—
Tranquilizers[c-g]	6.9	4.8	4.7	4.6	3.5	3.6	4.4	3.8	3.1	2.6	3.0	2.4	2.4	2.9	1.8	2.9	2.8	3.8	3.8	3.9	4.2	5.1	6.7	6.9	6.7	6.9	6.4	6.4	5.8	−0.6
Any Rx drug[l]	26.0	24.8	23.9	21.2	18.6	15.0	14.4	11.1	10.2	9.0	9.0	8.0	7.0	7.3	7.7	9.6	8.3	9.6	11.0	10.5	11.5	12.7	13.7	14.8	14.7	15.0	14.7	15.0	14.6	−0.4
Rohypnol[j]	NA	NA	NA	NA	NA	NA	NA	NA	NA	NA	NA	NA	NA	NA	NA	NA	NA	NA	0.7	0.3	0.4	0.7	0.6	0.3	0.4	0.3	0.7	0.1	0.2	+0.1
GHB[j]	NA	NA	NA	NA	NA	NA	NA	NA	NA	NA	NA	NA	NA	NA	NA	NA	NA	NA	NA	NA	NA	0.6	0.7	0.6	0.6	0.3	0.7	0.4	*	−0.4
Ketamine[j]	NA	NA	NA	NA	NA	NA	NA	NA	NA	NA	NA	NA	NA	NA	NA	NA	NA	NA	NA	NA	NA	1.0	1.3	1.0	1.5	0.9	1.5	0.5	0.9	+0.3
Alcohol[m]	90.5	92.5	92.2	91.6	90.0	92.0	91.5	90.9	89.6	89.6	89.0	88.3	85.1	86.9	82.7	83.2	83.0	82.4	83.6	84.6	83.2	83.6	83.0	82.9	81.7	81.2	83.0	83.0	82.1	−1.0
Been drunk[n]	NA	NA	NA	NA	NA	NA	NA	NA	NA	NA	NA	69.1	65.6	67.3	63.1	62.1	64.2	66.8	67.0	65.4	64.7	66.0	68.8	66.0	64.7	67.1	66.2	64.2	66.2	+2.0
Flavored alcoholic beverage[g]	NA	NA	NA	NA	NA	NA	NA	NA	NA	NA	NA	NA	NA	NA	NA	NA	NA	NA	NA	NA	NA	NA	NA	NA	63.2	63.2	67.0	67.0	63.5	−3.6
Cigarettes	36.2	37.6	34.3	36.1	33.2	35.0	35.3	38.0	36.6	34.2	35.5	35.6	37.6	37.3	38.8	39.3	41.4	43.6	44.5	44.3	41.3	39.0	38.3	35.2	36.7	36.0	36.0	36.0	30.9	−5.1 ss
Steroids[p]	NA	NA	NA	NA	NA	NA	NA	NA	NA	0.4	0.5	0.6	0.2	0.2	0.9	0.4	0.2	0.7	0.6	0.9	0.1	0.2	0.5	0.3	0.6	0.3	0.5	0.6	0.8	+0.2

LSD, lysergic acid diethylamide; MDMA, methylenedioxymethamphetamine; GHB, gamma hydroxybutyrate

Level of significance of difference between the two most recent years: s = 0.05, ss = 0.01, sss = 0.001. Any apparent inconsistency between the change estimate and the prevalence estimates for the two most recent years is due to rounding.

"NA" indicates data not available.

[a] "Any illicit drug" includes use of marijuana, hallucinogens, cocaine, heroin or other narcotics, amphetamines, sedatives (barbiturates), methaqualone (until 1990), or tranquilizers not under a doctor's orders.

[b] This drug was asked about in four of the five questionnaire forms in 1980–1989, in five of the six forms in 1990–1998, and in three of the six forms in 1999–2006. Total n in 2006 is approximately 650.

[c] In 2001 the question text was changed on half the questionnaire forms. "Other psychedelics" was changed to "other hallucinogens," and "shrooms" was added to the list of examples. For tranquilizers, "Miltown" was replaced with "Xanax" in the list of examples. Beginning in 2002 the remaining forms were changed to the new wording.

[d] This drug was asked about in two of the five questionnaire forms in 1989, in two of the six questionnaire forms in 1990–2001, and in three of the six questionnaire forms in 2002–2006. Total n in 2006 is approximately 650.

[e] This drug was asked about in two of the five questionnaire forms in 1987–1989, in all six questionnaire forms in 1990–2001, and in five of the six questionnaire forms in 2002–2006. Total n in 2006 is approximately 1,070.

[f] This drug was asked about in one of the five questionnaire forms in 1987–1989 and in four of six questionnaire forms in 1990–2006. Total n in 2006 is approximately 850.

[g] Only drug use that was not under a doctor's orders is included here.

[h] In 2002 the question text was changed on hall of the questionnaire forms. The list of examples of narcotics other than heroin was updated: Talwin, laudanum, and paregoric—all of which had negligible rates of use by 2001—were replaced by Vicodin, OxyContin, and Percocef. The 2002 data presented here are based on the changed forms only; n is one half on n indicated. In 2003 the remaining forms were changed to the new wording. The data are based on all forms in 2003 and beyond.

[i] On the basis of the data from the revised question, which attempts to exclude inappropriate reporting of nonprescription amphetamines.

[j] This drug was asked about in the two of the six questionnaire forms. Total n in 2006 is approximately 430.

[k] "Sedatives, adjusted" data are a combination of barbiturate and methaqualone data.

[l] Use of "Any Rx Drug" includes any use of amphetamines, sedatives (barbiturates), tranquilizers, and/or narcotics other than heroin not under a doctor's orders.

[m] In 1993 and 1994, the question text was changed slightly in three of the six questionnaire forms to indicate that a "drink" meant "more than just a few sips." Because this revision resulted in rather little change in reported prevalence in the surveys of high school graduates, the data for all forms combined are used in order to provide the most reliable estimate of change. After 1994 the new question text was used in all six of the questionnaire forms.

[n] This drug was asked about in three of the six questionnaire forms. Total n in 2006 is approximately 640.

[o] This drug was asked about in one of the five questionnaire forms. Total n in 2006 is approximately 220.

[p] This drug was asked about in one of the five questionnaire forms in 1989 and in two of the six questionnaire forms in 1990–2006. Total n in 2006 is approximately 430.

[q] Daily use is defined as use on 20 or more occasions in the past 30 days except for cigarettes, for which actual daily use is measured, and for five or more drinks, for which the prevalence of having five or more drinks in a row in the last 2 weeks is measured.

[r] Revised questions about amphetamine use were introduced in 1982 to more completely exclude inappropriate reporting of nonprescription amphetamines. The data in italics are therefore not strictly comparable to the other data.

From Johnston LD, O'Malley PM, Bachman JG, et al. (2007). Monitoring the Future national survey results on drug use, 1975–2006: Volume II, College students and adults ages 19–45 (NIH Publication No. 07-6206). Bethesda, MD: National Institute on Drug Abuse;2007:252–253. Available at: http://www.monitoringthefuture.org/pubs/monographs/vol2.2006.pdf.

TABLE 84.8

Trends in 30-Day Prevalence of Various Types of Drugs Among College Students 1 to 4 Years Beyond High School

	1980	1981	1982	1983	1984	1985	1986	1987	1988	1989	1990	1991	1992	1993	1994	1995	1996	1997	1998	1999	2000	2001	2002	2003	2004	2005	2006	'05-'06 change
									Percentage who used in last 30 days																			
Approximate weighted n	1040	1130	1150	1170	1110	1080	1190	1220	1310	1300	1400	1410	1490	1490	1410	1450	1450	1480	1440	1440	1350	1340	1260	1270	1400	1360	1280	
Any illicit drug[a]	38.4	37.6	31.3	29.3	27.0	26.1	25.9	22.4	18.5	18.2	15.2	15.2	16.1	15.1	16.0	19.1	17.6	19.2	19.7	21.6	21.5	21.9	21.5	21.4	21.2	19.5	19.2	-0.3
Any illicit drug[a] Other than marijuana	20.7	18.6	17.1	13.9	13.8	11.8	11.6	8.8	8.5	6.9	4.4	4.3	4.6	5.4	4.6	6.3	4.5	6.8	6.1	6.4	6.9	7.5	7.8	8.2	9.1	8.2	8.2	0.0
Marijuana	34.0	33.2	26.8	26.2	23.0	23.6	22.3	20.3	16.8	16.3	14.0	14.1	14.6	14.2	15.1	18.6	17.5	17.7	18.6	20.7	20.0	20.2	19.7	19.3	18.9	17.1	16.7	-0.4
Inhalants[b]	1.5	0.9	0.8	0.7	0.7	1.0	1.1	0.9	1.3	0.8	1.0	0.9	1.1	1.3	0.6	1.6	0.8	0.7	0.6	1.5	0.9	0.4	0.7	0.4	0.4	0.3	0.4	+0.1
Hallucinogens[c]	2.7	2.3	2.6	1.8	1.8	1.3	2.2	2.0	1.7	2.3	1.4	1.2	2.3	2.5	2.1	3.3	1.9	2.1	2.1	2.0	1.4	1.8	1.2	1.8	1.3	1.2	0.9	-0.3
LSD	1.4	1.4	1.7	0.9	0.8	0.7	1.4	1.4	1.1	1.4	1.1	0.8	1.8	1.6	1.8	2.5	0.9	1.1	1.5	1.2	0.9	1.0	0.2	0.2	0.2	0.1	0.3	+0.2
Hallucinogens Other than LSD[c]	1.9	1.2	1.4	1.0	1.2	0.7	1.2	0.8	0.8	1.1	0.8	0.6	0.7	1.1	0.8	1.6	1.2	1.2	0.7	1.2	0.8	0.8	1.1	1.7	1.2	1.1	0.7	-0.3
MDMA (Ecstasy)[d]	NA	NA	NA	NA	NA	NA	NA	NA	NA	0.3	0.6	0.2	0.4	0.3	0.2	0.7	0.7	0.8	0.8	2.1	2.5	1.5	0.7	1.0	0.7	0.8	0.6	-0.2
Cocaine	6.9	7.3	7.9	6.5	7.6	6.9	7.0	4.6	4.2	2.8	1.2	1.0	1.0	0.7	0.6	0.7	0.8	1.6	1.6	1.2	1.4	1.9	1.6	1.9	2.4	1.8	1.8	0.0
Crack[e]	NA	NA	NA	NA	NA	NA	NA	0.4	0.5	0.2	0.1	0.3	0.1	0.1	0.1	0.1	0.1	0.2	0.2	0.3	0.3	0.1	0.3	0.4	0.4	0.1	*	-0.1
Other cocaine[f]	NA	NA	NA	NA	NA	NA	NA	3.5	3.2	3.2	1.0	1.0	0.9	0.6	0.3	0.8	0.6	1.3	1.5	1.0	0.9	1.5	1.4	1.9	2.2	1.8	1.3	-0.5
Heroin	0.3	*	*	*	*	*	*	0.1	0.1	0.1	*	0.1	*	*	*	0.1	*	0.2	0.1	0.1	0.2	0.1	*	*	0.1	0.1	0.2	+0.1
Other narcotics[g,h]	1.8	1.1	0.9	1.1	1.4	0.7	0.6	0.8	0.8	0.7	0.5	0.6	1.0	0.7	0.4	1.2	0.7	1.3	1.1	1.0	1.7	1.7	3.2	2.3	3.0	3.1	3.1	0.0
Amphetamines[g]	13.4	12.3	NA	NA	NA	NA	NA	NA	NA	NA	NA	NA	NA	NA	NA	NA	NA	NA	NA	NA	NA	NA	NA	NA	NA	NA	NA	—
Amphetamines, adjusted[g,i]	NA	NA	9.9	7.0	5.5	4.2	3.7	2.3	1.8	1.3	1.4	1.0	1.1	1.5	1.5	2.2	0.9	2.1	1.7	2.3	2.9	3.3	3.0	3.1	3.2	2.9	2.5	-0.4
Methamphetamine[j]	NA	NA	NA	NA	NA	NA	NA	NA	NA	NA	NA	NA	NA	NA	NA	NA	NA	NA	NA	1.2	0.2	0.5	0.2	0.6	0.2	0.1	0.2	+0.1
Crystal Meth. (Ice)[j]	NA	NA	NA	NA	NA	NA	NA	NA	NA	*	*	*	*	0.3	0.5	0.3	0.1	0.2	0.3	*	*	0.1	*	0.3	0.1	0.2	*	-0.2

(continued)

T A B L E 8 4 . 8

(Continued)

Sedatives																												Change
(Barbiturates)[g]	0.9	0.8	1.0	0.5	0.7	0.4	0.6	0.5	0.5	0.2	0.2	0.3	0.2	0.4	0.4	0.7	0.4	0.5	0.8	1.2	1.1	1.1	1.1	1.5	1.7	1.7	1.5	1.3	1.3	0.0
Sedatives, adjusted[g,k]	3.8	3.4	2.5	1.1	1.0	0.7	0.6	0.6	0.6	0.2	0.2	NA	NA	NA	NA	NA	NA	NA	NA	NA	NA	NA	NA	NA	NA	NA	NA	NA	NA	NA
Methaqualone[g]	3.1	3.0	1.9	1.4	1.2	1.1	0.7	0.5	0.4	0.4	0.3	0.2	0.1	NA	NA	NA	NA	NA	NA	NA	NA	NA	NA	NA	NA	NA	NA	NA	NA	−0.1
Tranquilizers[c,g]	2.0	1.4	1.4	1.2	1.1	1.4	1.9	1.0	1.1	0.8	0.5	0.6	0.6	0.4	0.4	0.5	0.7	1.2	1.3	1.1	2.0	1.5	3.0	2.8	2.7	2.2	2.1	—	—	0.0
Any Rx drug[l]	15.6	13.3	11.4	8.4	7.1	5.7	5.5	3.9	3.5	2.6	2.5	2.2	2.3	2.6	2.2	3.3	2.3	4.1	3.9	4.3	5.6	5.4	6.4	6.6	6.9	6.5	6.5	—	—	−2.5
Alcohol[m]	81.8	81.9	82.8	80.3	79.1	80.3	79.7	78.4	77.0	76.2	74.5	74.7	71.4	70.1	67.8	67.5	67.0	65.8	68.1	69.6	67.4	67.0	68.9	66.2	67.7	67.9	65.4	—	—	+4.5
Been drunk[n]	NA	NA	NA	NA	NA	NA	NA	NA	NA	NA	NA	45.0	45.0	43.8	42.8	37.9	40.3	46.4	44.3	44.6	43.9	44.7	44.4	40.4	47.4	43.1	47.6	—	—	−4.7
Flavored alcoholic beverage[o]	NA	NA	NA	NA	NA	NA	NA	NA	NA	NA	NA	NA	NA	NA	NA	NA	NA	NA	NA	NA	NA	NA	NA	NA	34.0	30.9	26.2	—	—	—
Cigarettes	25.8	25.9	24.4	24.7	21.5	22.4	22.4	24.0	22.6	21.1	21.5	23.2	23.5	24.5	23.5	26.8	27.9	28.3	30.0	30.6	28.2	25.7	26.7	22.5	24.3	23.8	19.2	—	—	−4.6ss
Steroids[p]	NA	NA	NA	NA	NA	NA	NA	NA	NA	*	0.2	0.3	0.2	0.2	0.2	0.1	*	0.2	0.2	0.4	*	0.3	*	0.1	*	*	*	—	—	0.0

LSD, lysergic acid diethylamide; MDMA, methylenedioxymethamphetamine.

Level of significance of difference between the two most recent years: s = 0.05, ss = 0.01, sss = 0.001. Any apparent inconsistency between the change estimate and the prevalence estimates for the two most recent years is due to rounding.

"*" indicates a percentage of <0.05%

"NA" indicates data not available.

a"Any illicit drug" includes use of marijuana, hallucinogens, cocaine, heroin or other narcotics, amphetamines, sedatives (barbiturates), methaqualone (until 1990), or tranquilizers not under a doctor's orders.

b This drug was asked about in four of the five questionnaire forms in 1980–1989, in five of the six forms in 1990–1998, and in three of the six forms in 1999–2006. Total n in 2006 is approximately 650.

c In 2001 the question text was changed on half the questionnaire forms. "Other psychedelics" was changed to "other hallucinogens," and "shrooms" was added to the list of examples. For tranquilizers, "Miltown" was replaced with "Xanax" in the list of examples. Beginning in 2002 the remaining forms were changed to the new wording.

d This drug was asked about in two of the five questionnaire forms in 1989, in two of the six questionnaire forms in 1990–2001, and in three of the six questionnaire forms in 2002–2006. Total n in 2006 is approximately 650.

e This drug was asked about in two of the five questionnaire forms in 1990–2001, in all six questionnaire forms in 2002–2006. Total n in 2006 is approximately 1,070.

f This drug was asked about in one of the five questionnaire forms in 1987–1989 and in four of six questionnaire forms in 1990–2006. Total n in 2006 is approximately 850.

g Only drug use that was not under a doctor's orders is included here.

h In 2002 the question text was changed on half of the questionnaire forms. The list of examples of narcotics other than heroin was updated: Talwin, laudanum, and paregoric—all of which had negligible rates of use by 2001—were replaced by Vicodin, OxyContin, and Percocet. The 2002 data presented here are based on the changed forms only; n is one half on n indicated. In 2003 the remaining forms were changed to the new wording. The data are based on all forms in 2003 and beyond.

i On the basis of the data from the revised question, which attempts to exclude inappropriate reporting of nonprescription amphetamines.

j This drug was asked about in the two of the six questionnaire forms. Total n in 2006 is approximately 430.

k"Sedatives, adjusted" data are a combination of barbiturate and methaqualone data.

l Use of "Any Rx Drug" includes any use of amphetamines, sedatives (barbiturates), tranquilizers, and/or narcotics other than heroin not under a doctor's orders.

m In 1993 and 1994, the question text was changed slightly in three of the six questionnaire forms to indicate that a "drink" meant "more than just a few sips." Because this revision resulted in rather little change in reported prevalence in the surveys of high school graduates, the data for all forms combined are used in order to provide the most reliable estimate of change. After 1994 the new question text was used in all six of the questionnaire forms.

n This drug was asked about in three of the six questionnaire forms. Total n in 2006 is approximately 640.

o This drug was asked about in one of the six questionnaire forms. Total n in 2006 is approximately 220.

p This drug was asked about in one of the five questionnaire forms in 1989 and in two of the six questionnaire forms in 1990–2006. Total n in 2006 is approximately 430.

q Daily use is defined as use on 20 or more occasions in the past 30 days except for cigarettes, for which actual daily use is measured, and for five or more drinks, for which the prevalence of having five or more drinks in a row in the last 2 weeks is measured.

r Revised questions about amphetamine use were introduced in 1982 to more completely exclude inappropriate reporting of nonprescription amphetamines. The data in italics are therefore not strictly comparable to the other data.

From Johnston LD, O'Malley PM, Bachman JG, et al. (2007). Monitoring the Future national survey results on drug use, 1975–2006: Volume II, College students and adults ages 19–45 (NIH Publication No. 07-6206). Bethesda, MD: National Institute on Drug Abuse;2007:254–255. Available at: http://www.monitoringthefuture.org/pubs/monographs/vol2_2006.pdf.

TABLE 84.9

Trends in Thirty-Day Prevalence of Daily Use of Various Types of Drugs Among College Students 1 to 4 Years Beyond High School, 2006

Percentage who used daily in last 30 days

	1980	1981	1982	1983	1984	1985	1986	1987	1988	1989	1990	1991	1992	1993	1994	1995	1996	1997	1998	1999	2000	2001	2002	2003	2004	2005	2006	'05–'06 change
Approximate weighted n	1,040	1,130	1,150	1,170	1,110	1,080	1,190	1,220	1,310	1,300	1,400	1,410	1,490	1,490	1,410	1,450	1,450	1,480	1,440	1,440	1,350	1,340	1,260	1,270	1,400	1,360	1,280	
Marijuana[q]	7.2	5.6	4.2	3.8	3.6	3.1	2.1	2.3	1.8	2.6	1.7	1.8	1.6	1.9	1.8	3.7	2.8	3.7	4.0	4.0	4.6	4.5	4.1	4.7	4.5	4.0	4.3	+0.3
Cocaine[q]	0.2	*	0.3	0.1	0.4	0.1	0.1	0.1	0.1	*	*	*	*	*	0.1	*	*	*	*	*	*	*	*	*	*	0.1	0.1	0.0
Amphetamines[g,q]	0.5	0.4	NA	NA	NA	NA	NA	NA	NA	NA	NA	NA	NA	NA	NA	NA	NA	NA	NA	NA	NA	NA	NA	NA	NA	NA	NA	—
Amphetamines, adjusted[g,i,q]	NA	NA	0.3	0.2	0.2	*	0.1	0.1	*	*	*	0.1	*	0.1	0.1	0.1	*	0.2	0.1	0.1	0.1	0.2	0.1	0.3	0.2	0.2	0.4	+0.1
Alcohol[m]																												
Daily[q]	6.5	5.5	6.1	6.6	6.6	5.0	4.6	6.0	4.9	4.0	3.8	4.1	3.7	3.9	3.7	3.0	3.2	4.5	3.9	4.5	3.6	4.7	5.0	4.3	3.7	4.6	4.8	+0.2
Been drunk[n,q]	NA	NA	NA	NA	NA	NA	NA	NA	NA	NA	NA	0.5	0.2	0.3	0.8	0.5	0.1	1.3	0.8	1.0	0.7	0.5	0.8	1.1	0.8	0.5	0.6	0.0
Five or more drinks in a row in last 2 wk	43.9	43.6	44.0	43.1	45.4	44.6	45.0	42.8	43.2	41.7	41.0	42.8	41.4	40.2	40.2	38.6	38.3	40.7	38.9	40.0	39.3	40.9	40.1	38.5	41.7	40.1	40.2	+0.1
Cigarettes																												
Daily	18.3	17.1	16.2	15.3	14.7	14.2	12.7	13.9	12.4	12.2	12.1	13.8	14.1	15.2	13.2	15.8	15.9	15.2	18.0	19.3	17.8	15.0	15.9	13.8	13.8	12.4	9.2	−3.2 ss
Half-pack or More per day	12.7	11.9	10.5	9.6	10.2	9.4	8.3	8.2	7.3	6.7	8.2	8.0	8.9	8.9	8.0	10.2	8.5	9.1	11.3	11.0	10.1	7.8	7.9	7.6	6.8	6.7	4.9	−1.8 s

Level off significance of difference between the two most recent years: s = 0.05, ss = 0.01, sss = 0.001. Any apparent inconsistency between the change estimate and the prevalence estimates for the two most recent years is due to rounding.

"*" indicates a percentage of <0.05%.

"NA" indicates data not available.

[g]Only drug use that was not under a doctor's orders is included here.

[i]On the basis of the data from the revised question, which attempts to exclude inappropriate reporting of nonprescription amphetamines.

[m]In 1993 and 1994, the question text was changed slightly in three of the six questionnaire forms to indicate that a "drink" meant "more than just a few sips." Because this revision resulted in rather little change in reported prevalence in the surveys of high school graduates, the data for all forms combined are used in order to provide the most reliable estimate of change. After 1994 the new question text was used in all six of the questionnaire forms.

[n]This drug was asked about in three of the six questionnaire forms. Total n in 2006 is approximately 640.

[q]Daily use is defined as use on 20 or more occasions in the past 30 days except for cigarettes, for which actual daily use is measured, and for five or more drinks, for which the prevalence of having five or more drinks in a row in the last 2 weeks is measured.

From Johnston LD, O'Malley PM, Bachman JG, et al. (2007). *Monitoring the Future national survey results on drug use, 1975–2006: Volume II, College students and adults ages 19–45* (NIH Publication No. 07-6206). Bethesda, MD: National Institute on Drug Abuse;2007:256–257. Available at: http://www.monitoringthefuture.org/pubs/monographs/vol2.2006.pdf.

FIGURE 84.1 Any illicit drug: Trends in annual prevalence among college students vs. others. (From Johnston LD, O'Malley PM, Bachman JG, et al. (2007). *Monitoring the Future national survey results on drug use, 1975–2006: Volume II, College students and adults ages 19–45* (NIH Publication No. 07–6206). Bethesda, MD: National Institute on Drug Abuse;2007:258. Available at: http://www.monitoringthefuture .org/pubs/monographs/vol2_2006 .pdf.)

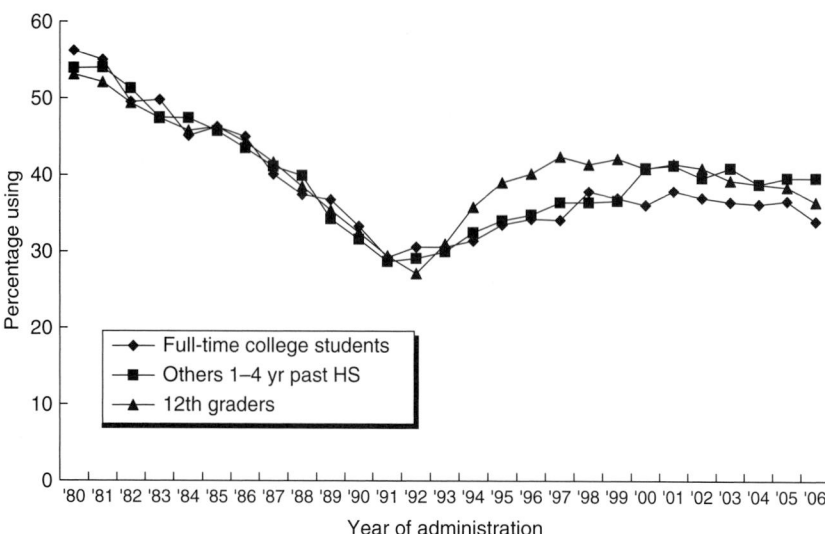

- *Cocaine:* Use of cocaine in college students dropped dramatically from 1983 to 1994 (17.3% annual use to 2%), however this has increased to 5.1% in 2006.
- *Other drugs:* Among college students, the annual prevalence of Vicodin use increased from 6.9% in 2002 to 7.6% in 2006, Rohypnol use decreased from 0.7% to 0.2%, GHB use decreased and ketamine use also decreased from 1.3% to 0.9%. Ritalin usage decreased slightly in annual use from 5.7% in 2002 to 3.9% in 2006. Tranquilizers also followed a similar pattern as cocaine usage with annual prevalences falling from 6.9% in 1980 to 1.8% in 1994 and then reversing to 6.9% in 2003. The rates from 2003–2006 have decreased to 5.8%. Overall, LSD use has fallen precipitously since 2001 while narcotics other than heroin and tranquilizers have become much more important drugs of illicit use.

Tobacco

2006 ACHA-NCHA "Number of days of any cigarette use in last 30 days"

	≥10 Days	1–9 Days
Total	8.4%	9.3%
Female	7.8%	8.7%
Male	9.2%	10.2%

Interestingly, the students' perception of tobacco use rates of students was much higher. Reported actual daily use of cigarettes for all students within the last 30 days was 4.3%, which compares with how often students perceived the typical student on campus used cigarettes within the same time. The perceived daily use of cigarettes by all students was 32.1%.

Alcohol

2006 ACHA-NCHA "How many days did you consume any alcohol in last 30 days?"

	≥10 Days	1–9 Days
Total	15.6%	54%
Female	13%	55.9%
Male	20%	51.1%

Interestingly, the students' perception of alcohol use rates of students was much higher. For all students, 17.2% reported actually never drank alcohol within the last 30 days, which compares with how often students perceived the typical student on campus used alcohol within the same time. The perception was only 3.6% of all students never drank alcohol within the last 30 days.

High-risk drinking (five or more drinks at a sitting in last 2 weeks)

Frequency	Total	Female	Male
None	62.9%	68%	54%
1–2 times	21.4%	21%	25%
3–5 times	11.3%	9%	15%
≥6 times	3.4%	1%	6%

Consequences of Drinking in Last School Year for Those Who Drink Alcohol
- 18.2% had an injury to self.
- 4.1% injured another person.
- 35.7% did something they later regretted.
- 1.3% were involved in forced sexual activity by someone else.
- 13.9% were involved in unprotected sexual activity.

College Students: Who Drinks? Evidence suggests that the highest number of high-risk drinkers (defined as having five or more drinks at a sitting for men and four or more drinks at a sitting for women) are in fraternities and sororities (Fig. 84.4).

Marijuana Use

2006 ACHA-NCHA "How many days did you use marijuana in last 30 days?"

	≥10 Days	1–9 Days
Total	4.5%	10%
Female	3%	9%
Male	6%	11%

Interestingly, the students' perception of marijuana use rates of students was much higher. Reported actual daily

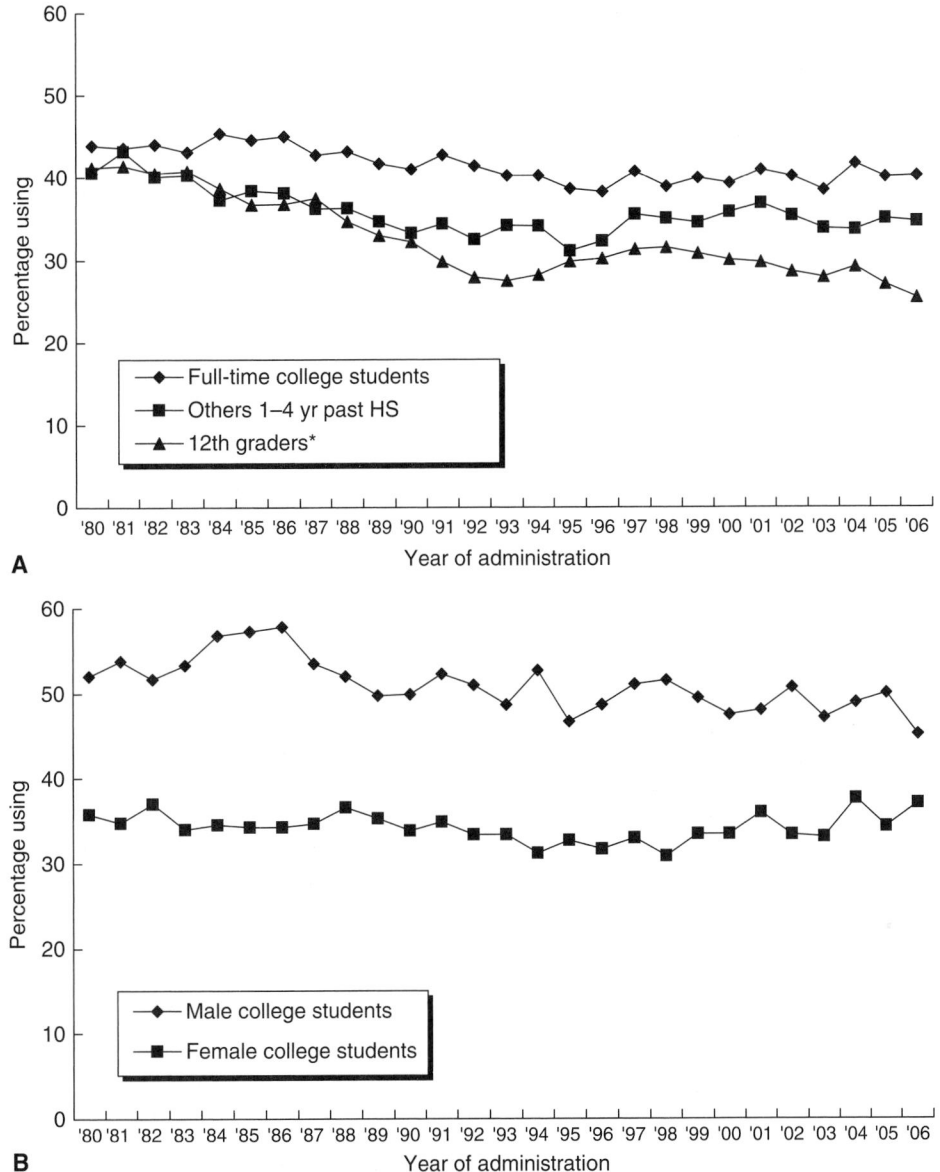

FIGURE 84.2 **A:** Alcohol: Trends in 2-week prevalence of five or more drinks in a row among college students versus others. **B:** Alcohol: Trends in 2-week prevalence of five or more drinks in a row among male versus female college students. (From Johnston LD, O'Malley PM, Bachman JG, et al. (2006). *Monitoring the Future national survey results on drug use, 1975–2006. Volume II, College students and adults ages 19–45* (NIH Publication No. 07-6206). Bethesda, MD: National Institute on Drug Abuse;2007:274. Available at: http://www.monitoringthefuture.org/pubs/monographs/vol2_2006.pdf.)

use of marijuana for all students within the last 30 days was 1.2%, which compares with how often students perceived the typical student on campus used marijuana within the same time. The perceived daily use of marijuana by all students was 18.5%.

SEXUALITY

Sexually Transmitted Diseases

College populations are generally unidentifiable in overall reports on STDs. There are no random frequency studies

that have been performed in this population. In general, national STD studies focus on adolescents and homeless and incarcerated youth. College students often do not recognize the risks and availability of treatment for most STDs.

Chlamydia

Although there are no randomized frequency studies on college campuses, the overall prevalence appears to be falling. One college reported a rate of >9% in 1990, falling to just >3% by 1994.

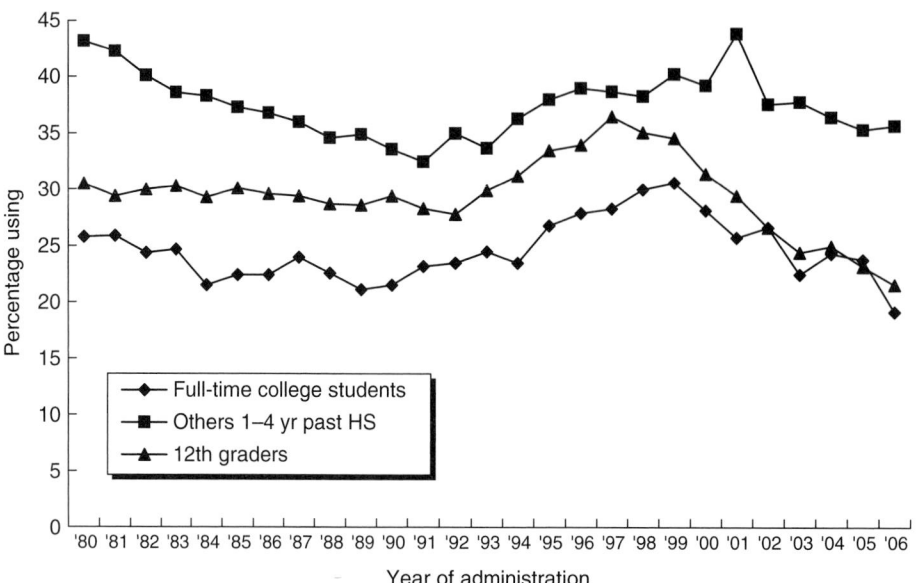

FIGURE 84.3   Cigarettes: Trends in 30-day prevalence of daily use among college students versus others. (From Johnston LD, O'Malley PM, Bachman JG, et al. (2007). *Monitoring the Future national survey results on drug use, 1975–2006: Volume II, College students and adults ages 19–45* (NIH Publication No. 07-6206). Bethesda, MD: National Institute on Drug Abuse;2007:278. Available at: http://www.monitoringthefuture.org/pubs/monographs/vol2_2006.pdf.)

Sexual Behaviors

2006 ACHA-NCHA Prevalence of intercourse

	Ever Had Vaginal Intercourse	Ever Had Anal Intercourse	Ever Had Oral Intercourse
Total	68.6%	25.1%	72.1%
Female	69%	23%	72%
Male	68%	29%	73%

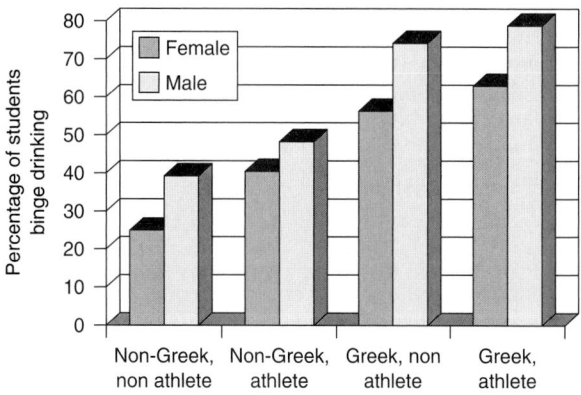

FIGURE 84.4   College students—who drinks? (From Wechsler H, Davenport AE, Dowdall GW, et al. Binge drinking, tobacco, and illicit drug use and involvement in college athletics: a survey of students at 140 American colleges. *J Am Coll Health* 1997;45:195, with permission.)

Prevalence condom use at last sexual intercourse (excluded if "never did this activity")

	During Vaginal Intercourse	During Anal Intercourse	During Oral Intercourse
Total	52.1%	27.7%	3.8%

Number of partners (vaginal, oral, anal intercourse) within the last school year

	None	One	Two or Three	Four or More
Total	29.2%	46.5%	16.7%	7.6%
Female	29%	49%	16%	5%
Male	30%	43%	17%	11%

Emergency Contraception Use and Unintended Pregnancies—Last Year

- 11.2% of sexually active college students reported using (or reported their partner used) emergency contraception ("morning after pill") within the last school year (male, 9.7%; female, 12.7%)
- 2.1% of college students who had vaginal intercourse within the last school year reported experiencing an unintentional pregnancy or their partner pregnant within the last school year (male, 2.2%; female, 2%)

DIETARY, PHYSICAL ACTIVITY AND SLEEP BEHAVIORS

Dietary Behaviors

2006 ACHA-NCHA "In the last 30 days, to lose weight you . . ."

	Dieted	Exercised	Purged	Used Diet Pills
Total	34.5%	55.2%	2.5%	3.6%
Females	42.4%	62.7%	3.6%	4.6%
Males	22.1%	43.7%	0.7%	1.9%

Physical Activity Behaviors

2006 ACHA-NCHA "In the last week, participated in exercise for at least 20 minutes . . ."

	None	1 or 2 Days	3 to 5 Days	6 or 7 Days
Total	24.4%	31.4%	35.6%	8.6%
Females	25.7%	31.2%	35%	8%
Males	22.1%	31.7%	36.6%	9.6%

Sleep Behaviors

2006 ACHA-NCHA "In the last week, getting enough sleep to feel rested in the morning . . ."

	None	1 or 2 Days	3 to 5 Days	6 or 7 Days
Total	10.4%	28%	47.7%	13.9%
Females	10.8%	28.3%	47.1%	13.8%
Males	9.4%	27.4%	49.1%	14.1%

Body Mass Index

2006 ACHA-NCHA Data Estimated body mass index (BMI) incorporates reported gender, height, and weight (Table 84.10).

PREVENTATIVE HEALTH CARE, PROBLEMS, AND HEALTH INFORMATION

Preventative Health Care Practices

2006 ACHA-NCHA Preventive health care practices among college students:

Hepatitis B vaccination	73.4%
Meningococcal vaccination	57.1%
Chicken pox vaccination	50%
Flu immunization last year	26%
Dental examination last year	77.2%
Testicular self-examination last month	38.8%
Breast self-examination last month	39.4%
Gynecological examination last year	59.2%
Cholesterol check in last 5 years	45.1%

Health Problems

2006 ACHA-NCHA Within the last school year, college students reported experiencing:

Back pain	46.6%
Allergy problems	45.5%
Sinus infection	28.8%
Depression	17.8%
Strep throat	13.2%
Anxiety disorder	12.4%
Asthma	11.2%
Ear infection	9.3%
Seasonal affective disorder	8.1%
Bronchitis	7.8%
Carpal tunnel	6.8%
Fracture	4.7%
High blood pressure	4.5%
Substance abuse	3.4%
High cholesterol	4%
Chronic fatigue	3.4%
Bulimia	2.3%
Genital warts	2.2%
Monoucelosis	2.2%
Anorexia	1.9%
Endometriosis	1%
Genital herpes	1%
Diabetes	0.9%
Chlamydia	0.8%
Hepatitis B or C	0.4%
Pelvic inflammatory disease	0.3%
Human immunodeficiency virus	0.3%
Tuberculosis	0.2%
Gonorrhea	0.2%

Health Information

2006 ACHA-NCHA Health information believability and sources

	Believe	Use as Source of Information
Medical staff	90.1%	59.7%
Health educators	89.2%	51.6%

TABLE 84.10

Weight Classification (BMI in kg/m^2) for Males and Females

	<18.5 Underweight	18.5–24.9 Healthy Weight	25–29.9 Overweight	30–34.9 Class I Obesity	35–39.9 Class II Obesity	≥40 Class III Obesity
Total	4.5%	64.1%	21.9%	6.2%	2.1%	1.2%
Females	5.6%	67.6%	17.8%	5.5%	2%	1.4%
Males	2.6%	58.2%	28.8%	7.4%	2.1%	0.8%

	Believe	Use as Source of Information
Parents	64.3%	73.2%
Faculty/coursework	66.3%	37.8%
Leaflets/pamphlets	60.8%	51.1%
Campus newspaper	47%	26.7%
Peer educators	46.1%	18.4%
Resident assistant/advisors	36%	16.9%
Friends	24.4%	60.6%
Magazines	22%	52.5%
Religious center	24.2%	9.9%
Internet	23%	72.4%
Television	12.6%	43.2%

It appears that medical staff members and health educators have high believability among students but are used only by approximately 50% of students for their health information. At the same time, 61% of students use friends for their health information but only 24% believe them. Television and the Internet are also ranked low on believability but are sources of health information for approximately half of students.

IMPEDIMENTS TO ACADEMIC SUCCESS

2006 ACHA-NCHA Data: *Within the last school year students reported the following factors affecting their individual academic performance, that is, received an incomplete, dropped a course; received a lower grade in a class, on an examination, or on an important project:*

Stress	32%
Cold/flu/sore throat	26%
Sleep difficulties	23.9%
Concern for a troubled friend or family	18%
Depression/anxiety disorder/seasonal affective disorder	15.7%
Relationship difficulty	15.6%
Internet use/computer games	15.4%
Death of a friend/family member	8.5%
Sinus or ear infection/bronchitis/step throat	8.3%
Alcohol use	7.3%
Allergies	4.2%
Injury	3.3%
Learning disability	3.2%
Chronic pain	2.9%
Chronic illness	2.7%
Drug use	2.3%
Mononucleosis	1.5%
Eating disorder/problem	1.3%
Pregnancy (yours or partner's)	0.9%
Assault (sexual)	0.8%
Assault (physical)	0.6%
Sexually transmitted disease	0.4%

With more than 87.3% of students having some type of medical access insurance and the quality and convenience of health care on campus, it appears that of the top ten impediments to academic success only two are biomedical, while psychosocial issues, such as depression, relationships, and stress carry the greatest impact on student learning. Alcohol use, ranked at number ten, creates high-risk situations for both the individual student and the institution. Other issues, such as sexual assault, are not as prevalent but have devastating consequences. This is the first data of its type and illuminates the relationship between health and learning.

TYPES OF HEALTH PROBLEMS

Students presented to health centers with the following:

1. Acute medical problems: Primary care including minor infections (Epstein-Barr virus infections, genitourinary tract infections, upper respiratory tract infections, and acute gastroenteritis), musculoskeletal injuries, minor trauma, and skin problems. Occasionally, some of the infections become life threatening, such as meningitis and tuberculosis. Reproductive issues are common, including the diagnosis and treatment of STDs, contraception, emergency contraception, routine gynecology, men's health care, and unintended pregnancies.
2. Chronic medical problems: Many college undergraduate and older graduate students receive care at the health center for chronic medical conditions, including asthma, diabetes, seizure disorders, thyroid disorders, hypertension, hyperlipidemia, eating disorders, and malignancies. In addition, the incidence rates of certain malignancies such as Hodgkin disease, melanoma, testicular neoplasms, leukemia, and primary bone cancer in this age-group are increased compared with those of other age-groups.
3. Mental health issues: Many college students are under increased stress and the following are frequent on college campuses—stress-related symptoms, eating disorders, anxiety, depression, suicidality, chronic fatigue, and other disorders affecting academic performance such as attention-deficit disorder.
4. Substance abuse: Diagnosis and treatment
5. Screening for STDs
6. Immunization requirements
7. Screening for tuberculosis
8. Routine screening for other health risks including smoking and hyperlipidemia
9. Behavioral health issues such as unsafe sexual behaviors, high-risk alcohol use, and tobacco use.

Trends

Some trends that appear to be occurring among college students include (data may not be available) the following:

- More students are entering college with chronic disease such as asthma, diabetes, physical disabilities, and treated mental health disorders.
- More students are traveling abroad.
- More students are interested in herbal and complementary medicine interventions.
- Few universities have overnight infirmaries. Most IHEs can no longer justify the cost, risk, and resources associated with overnight infirmaries and so students attend to each other in their place of residence, are

hospitalized in local facilities, or go to the residence of a parent or guardian for care.

Challenges

With the many changes in the health care field, there are numerous challenges facing both student affairs and health care professionals in the college health setting of the 21st century. Some of these include the following:

1. Stability of finances: In a 1991 survey of 400 colleges the source of funds was as follows:
   a. 85% funding prepaid (46% general fees and 39% a designated health fee)
   b. 5% service fees
   c. 10% grants and donations
   However, as funding becomes tighter in higher education, college health programs will need to continue to explore alternative, cost-effective funding mechanisms. Many college health clinics have formed fund-raising and development programs of their own and participate in funded research.
2. Continued national accreditation of ambulatory care services.
3. Continued integration into campus and academic life.
4. Improved information technology: Students comprise one of the largest groups with high-speed access to Internet information. They are also a group that expects communication through this modality. College health programs will need to adapt to these changes and use this technology for communication regarding appointments, laboratory results, medical care, and prevention services. In a review of electronic communication by college health centers with students, Neinstein (2000) found that 64% of health centers used electronic communication with patients and 27% used e-mail to give out medical advice. Other uses included giving out laboratory test results, making appointments, and communicating insurance issues. Many health centers now use an electronic health record.
5. Improved facilities: Many student health center buildings are old, outdated, and need replacement. This, along with other student services, often has a lower priority to academic buildings in IHEs.
6. Strong supplemental insurance policies: Another critical issue among college students is coverage for health care, particularly beyond what a college health program can cover. Approximately 20% to 33% of the 19- to 24-year-old age-group are uninsured or underinsured. In addition, coverage may not extend outside the local area. It is critical that college health programs explore adequate coverage opportunities for students and that students and their parents strongly consider insurance options during college years. Important questions to explore include the following:
   a. What are the deductibles and co-payments and what is the maximum lifetime coverage?
   b. What coverage is provided when the student is out of school during winter and summer breaks?
   c. Does the coverage include common items such as contraception, acne treatment, immunizations, mental health, smoking cessation, and substance abuse?

THE PRECOLLEGE VISIT

Information for Providers to Consider When Sending Their Patients Off to College

The precollege visit marks the beginning of the transition for the adolescent from health care that has largely been supervised by the parent to health care that is a personal responsibility. There are various concepts of what might be included in this visit. Stashwick (1997) describes a comprehensive visit as that intended to update the medical history, perform a complete physical examination, screen for health-risk behaviors, update immunizations, and provide counseling and education. Time constraints and prematriculation health requirements of the university may alter the nature and focus of this visit.

Prematriculation Requirements Most universities require certain immunizations and tuberculosis screening, and others will have a health form that must be completed before the student arrives on the campus. The parental expectations for this visit then will be to have these prematriculation requirements met so the college-bound student may register for classes.

Health History Health-risk behaviors are important to consider before the adolescent leaves for college. Screening questions should cover the following:

- Eating disorders
- Tobacco use
- Alcohol and other potential substances of abuse including anabolic steroids
- Sexual behaviors
- Emotions that indicate depression or risk of suicide
- History of emotional, physical, or sexual abuse
- Learning or school problems especially prior evaluation and treatment of attention-deficit disorder
- Risk factors for tuberculosis

Given the time constraints of the visit, the provider may elect to do the screening history by a questionnaire. The major drawback to this approach is that the adolescent will most likely be accompanied by a parent, and given the sensitivity of the questions that need to be asked, the adolescent may not feel comfortable responding openly. Alternative approaches include having the adolescent complete the questionnaire in an examination room or having the provider ask the questions directly once the parent has left the room.

An example of comprehensive screening questions on these topics can be found in the NCHA survey, which is posted on the ACHA Web site (at www.acha.org). Table 84.11 gives examples of a simplified version of these questions. Another potential source for screening questions is the National Health and Nutrition Examination Survey created by the National Center for Health Statistics and available at the Centers for Disease Control and Prevention (CDC) Web site (at www.cdc.gov). Figure 84.5 is a screening form given to students at the University of Southern California on the first visit.

Examination If a complete physical examination had been performed in the last 3 years, the assessment during the precollege visit may be limited to determination of the

TABLE 84.11

Examples of Screening Questions

Eating disorders:
- Do you worry about gaining weight? Do you feel that food controls your life?
- Do you do any of the following (select all that apply)?
  1. Exercise to lose weight
  2. Diet to lose weight
  3. Vomit or take laxatives to lose weight
  4. Take diet pills to lose weight
  5. None of the above
- Have you ever been told that you had anorexia nervosa or bulimia? Tobacco use:
- Have you ever used any tobacco products (cigarettes, cigars, smokeless tobacco)?

Alcohol and other abusable substances:
- Do you drink alcohol (beer, wine, liquor)?
- Do you use marijuana (pot, hash, hash oil)?
- Do you use cocaine (crack, rock, freebase)?
- Do you use amphetamines (diet pills, speed, meth, crank)?
- Do you use steroids for body building or to improve athletic performance?
- Do you use other drugs such as Rohypnol (roofies), GHB or liquid X?

Sexual behaviors:
- Have you ever been sexually active?
- Are you currently sexually active?
- Have you ever been diagnosed with a sexually transmitted infection (STD) such as chlamydia, gonorrhea, syphilis, pelvic inflammatory disease, genital warts (human papillomavirus), herpes, hepatitis B, or HIV?
- Do you practice safe sex (use a condom or dental dam)?
- Do you use a method of contraception?
- Have you unintentionally become pregnant or gotten someone else pregnant?
- Have you been tested for HIV?

Mental heatlh
- Do you have any mental health disorders?
- Do you feel depressed, sad, or lonely?
- Have you ever seriously considered or attempted suicide?
- Do you have difficulty controlling your temper?

Emotional, physical, or sexual abuse:
- Have you been or are you in a relationship that is emotionally, physically, or sexually abusive?

Learning problems
- Have you been told you had a learning disorder or attention deficit disorder?

Risk for tuberculosis infection:
- Have you ever had a positive skin test for tuberculosis?
- Were you born in a country other than the United States? If yes, where?
- Have you ever injected street drugs?
- Have you tested positive for HIV?
- Have you ever resided in, volunteered in, or worked in a prison, nursing home, hospital, residential facility for patients with acquired immunodeficiency syndrome, homeless shelter, or a refugee camp?
- Have you ever been on steriods (prednisone, cortisone) for at least a month?

GHB, gamma-hydroxybutyrate; HIV, human immunodeficiency virus.

height, weight, and blood pressure, as well as performance of a focused physical examination based on problems uncovered in the screening history. For the sexually active female, a pelvic examination with Papanicolaou (Pap) smear and testing for STDs is indicated. If the college-bound student presents for a preparticipation sports physical, a more comprehensive physical assessment is necessary and the reader is referred to excellent summaries on this topic (Smith, 1997).

The Body Mass Index The BMI is helpful in assessing whether the adolescent is underweight or overweight. A simplified calculation of BMI, along with its classification has been published by the National Heart, Lung, and Blood Institute Obesity Education Initiative. To estimate BMI, multiply the adolescent's weight (in pounds) by 703 and divide by the height (in inches) squared. This approximate BMI can then be classified as in Table 84.12. Underweight individuals may have anorexia nervosa and further

University of Southern California   **Patient History Form**
University Park Health Center
849 W. 34th Street, Los Angeles, CA 90089-0311

Date: _____

Name: _____   USC 10-Digit I.D. #: _____

Local telephone: _____   Date of birth: _____ / _____ / _____
                                                                        MM / DD / YY

It is the philosophy of the staff of the University Park Health Center to provide you with the best care possible. To accomplish this, it is important for us to review significant health issues that might impact your health. Our health screening form is given to all students on their first visit to the health center. You may leave any question blank if you choose. **This history form is a confidential document that will be kept in your medical record in the University Park Health Center. No information may be released without your written consent, unless required by law.**

Allergies (list all)

Allergy	Type of reaction

Serious Illnesses or Injuries (not including hospitalizations)

Year	Reason

Current Prescribed Medications (list all prescribed medications)

Medication	Dosage if known

Current Herbal/Vitamins or Non-Prescribed Medications

Medication	Dosage if known

Hospitalizations / Surgery (list all)

Year	Reason

Immunizations

1. Have you been immunized for hepatitis B?   ❑ Yes ❑ No ❑ Unsure
2. When was your last PPD (tuberculosis skin test)? _____
3. Have you received a tetanus shot within the last 10 years?   ❑ Yes ❑ No ❑ Unsure

Health habits

1. Have you ever used tobacco regularly?   ❑ Yes ❑ No
2. Do you currently smoke cigarettes?   ❑ Yes ❑ No
   If yes, how often? _____ Do you want to quit? ❑ Yes ❑ No
3. Do you consume caffeine containing products?   ❑ Yes ❑ No
   If yes, what type? _____ how often? _____
4. Do you exercise regularly?   ❑ Yes ❑ No
   If yes, what type? _____

Family history Have any close relatives (parents, siblings) ever had any of the following? (check all that apply)

❑ Alcoholism   ❑ Hereditary disease
❑ Allergies   ❑ High blood pressure
❑ Blood or clotting disorders   ❑ High cholesterol
❑ Cancer   ❑ Stroke
❑ Depression / psychiatric illness ❑ Tuberculosis
❑ Diabetes   ❑ Other serious illness
❑ Heart disease

Explain any item checked: _____
_____

List any close relatives (parents, siblings) who have died:

Age	Relationship	Cause of Death

(Office use): *Reviewed by* _____ _____ _____ _____
                              Initials/Date *Initials/Date* *Initials/Date* *Initials/Date*

continued on back . . . .

FIGURE 84.5 Patient history screening form. (From USC University Park Health Center. www.usc.edu/uphc, with permission.)

Name: _____   USC 10-Digit I.D. #: _____

Personal History (Have you had or do you now have any of the following? If yes, note date of occurrence if known.)

Head / Neurologic	Yes	No	Heart / Circulation / Chest	Yes	No	Chronic diseases	Yes	No
Frequent headaches/migraines	❑	❑	Severe chest pain or pressure	❑	❑	Diabetes mellitus	❑	❑
Dizziness or fainting	❑	❑	Heart disease or murmur	❑	❑	Asthma	❑	❑
Loss of consciousness	❑	❑	Rapid or irregular pulse	❑	❑	High blood pressure	❑	❑
Head injuries	❑	❑	Blood clots or vein problems	❑	❑	Arthritis	❑	❑
						Sickle cell disease	❑	❑
Eyes			**Respiratory**			Seizures or epilepsy	❑	❑
Vision or eye problems	❑	❑	Chronic cough (over 1 month)	❑	❑	Thyroid disease	❑	❑
Glasses or contact lenses	❑	❑	Pneumonia	❑	❑	Elevated cholesterol	❑	❑
			Tuberculosis or positive PPD	❑	❑			
Ears / Nose / Throat			Shortness of breath	❑	❑	**Genitourinary**		
Allergies or hay fever	❑	❑				Urinary or kidney problems	❑	❑
Ear or hearing problems	❑	❑	**Gastrointestinal**					
Frequent sinusitis	❑	❑	Adominal pain (severe / recurrent)	❑	❑	**Additional medical history**		
Dental problems or TMJ	❑	❑	Ulcer	❑	❑	Cancer	❑	❑
			Bowel movement problems	❑	❑	Unusual fatigue (over 1 month)	❑	❑
Skin			Blood in stool	❑	❑	Recent gain or loss of weight		
Severe acne or skin disorder	❑	❑	Hepatitis	❑	❑	(over 10 pounds)	❑	❑
New or changing moles	❑	❑	Hernia	❑	❑			
						Eating disorder	❑	❑
Blood disorder			**Musculoskeletal**					
Anemia	❑	❑	Swollen or painful joints			**Other:**		
Bleeding disorder	❑	❑	or extremities	❑	❑	_____		
Enlargement of glands or			Chronic or severe back					
lymph nodes			problems	❑	❑	_____		
	❑	❑						

Explain all "Yes" answers above: _____

_____

WOMEN'S HEALTH (women answer only)

1. Age when you had your first period? _____   Are your periods regular?   ❑ Yes ❑ No
   Periods come every: ___ days. Periods last: ___ days. Last period began:_____
2. Have you had any pain or abnormal bleeding with your periods?   ❑ Yes ❑ No
3. Do you have significant problems with premenstrual syndrome (PMS)?   ❑ Yes ❑ No
   If yes, symptoms: _____
4. Have you ever had a pelvic examination ?   ❑ Yes ❑ No
5. Date of your last pap smear or pelvic exam? _____ Was it normal?   ❑ Yes ❑ No
6. Do you check your breasts monthly for lumps or discharge?   ❑ Yes ❑ No
7. Have you ever been pregnant? If yes, when? _____   ❑ Yes ❑ No
   How many: live births?_____ miscarriages?___ terminations?___
8. Have you had any pregnancy complications?   ❑ Yes ❑ No
   If yes, explain: _____

9. Have you ever had:
   gynecological problems without surgery (e.g. cyst, fibroid)   ❑ Yes ❑ No
   abnormal pap smear   ❑ Yes ❑ No
   breast lumps or discharge   ❑ Yes ❑ No
   vaginal infections or abnormal discharge   ❑ Yes ❑ No
   pain or bleeding with intercourse   ❑ Yes ❑ No

MEN'S HEALTH (men answer only)
1. Do you have any penile discharge or change in urination?   ❑ Yes ❑ No
2. Have you ever had undescended testicles, testicular problems or cancer?   ❑ Yes ❑ No
3. Have you ever had prostate problems?   ❑ Yes ❑ No
5. Do you regularly examine your testicles for swellings or lumps?   ❑ Yes ❑ No
6. Would you like information on how to examine your testicles?   ❑ Yes ❑ No

continued on next page . . . .

FIGURE 84.5 *(Continued)*

Name: _____ USC 10-Digit I.D. #: _____

CONFIDENTIAL (men and women answer) This information will not be released to anyone without your written consent. Answers to the following questions help your clinician provide appropriate care for you. Leave questions blank if you are uncomfortable answering them. Please feel free to discuss any concerns with your clinician.

1. Have you ever been sexually active (i.e. any genital contact with another person)? ❑ Yes ❑ No
2. Are you currently sexually active? ❑ Yes ❑ No
3. Have your sexual partners been: ❑ Men ❑ Women ❑ Both
4. Do you have any concerns/questions regarding

   sexual functioning or orgasm? ❑ Yes ❑ No
   sexual orientation? ❑ Yes ❑ No
   gender identity? ❑ Yes ❑ No
   your own sexuality? ❑ Yes ❑ No

5. Have you ever had any of the following sexually transmitted diseases (STD's):
   chlamydia ❑ Yes ❑ No
   pelvic inflammatory disease ❑ Yes ❑ No
   genital warts / HPV ❑ Yes ❑ No
   herpes ❑ Yes ❑ No

   other ❑ Yes ❑ No

6. Does your current partner display any symptoms of an STD? ❑ Yes ❑ No ❑ Not sure
7. Have you practiced safe sex (use condom, dental dam, etc):
   with your current partner ❑ Yes ❑ No ❑ Sometimes
   with past partners ❑ Yes ❑ No ❑ Sometimes
   during last sexual contact ❑ Yes ❑ No ❑ Sometimes
8. Are you presently using a method of birth control? ❑ Yes ❑ No ❑ N/A
   If yes, what type? _____
   Are you in need of a contraceptive method? ❑ Yes ❑ No
9. Are you aware that emergency contraception ("morning-after pill")
   is available for women? ❑ Yes ❑ No
10. Do you have any questions or concerns regarding any of the following?

    family alcoholism or drug abuse ❑ Yes ❑ No
    your appearance or weight? ❑ Yes ❑ No
    rape, sexual abuse, or unwanted sexual activity ❑ Yes ❑ No
    physical abuse ❑ Yes ❑ No
    dating or domestic violence ❑ Yes ❑ No
    death of a loved one within the past 12 months ❑ Yes ❑ No
    termination of a pregnancy (you or your partner) ❑ Yes ❑ No

11. Have you felt sad, lonely or depressed for over two consecutive weeks? ❑ Yes ❑ No
12. Do you have any mental health condition? ❑ Yes ❑ No

    If yes, please indicate what kind of condition: _____

    Present or past medications for this condition: _____

13. How many days per week do you drink alcohol? (circle one) 0 1 2 3 4 5 6 7

    When you drink alcohol, how many standard drinks do you have? _____

14. Within the last year, have you experienced any problems or
    injuries as a result of drinking? ❑ Yes ❑ No
15. Have you used any recreational drugs such as: ecstasy, narcotics, stimulants,
    cocaine, LSD, or other street drugs? ❑ Yes ❑ No
16. Do you use marijuana? ❑ Yes ❑ No
17. Do you frequently use tranquilizers or sleeping pills? ❑ Yes ❑ No

3 of 4

FIGURE 84.5 (*Continued*)

TABLE 84.12

Classification for Body Mass Index

Classification	Body Mass Index
Underweight	≥ 18.5 kg/m^2
Normal weight	18.5–24.9 kg/m^2
Overweight	25–29.9 kg/m^2
Obesity (class 1)	30–34.9 kg/m^2
Obesity (class 2)	35–39.9 kg/m^2
Extreme obesity (class 3)	≥ 40 kg/m^2

From National Heart, Lung, and Blood Institute. *Obesity Education Initiative. The practical guide to identification, evaluation and treatment of overweight and obesity in adults.* National Heart, Lung, and Blood Institute. Available at www.nhlbi.nih.gov/guidelines/obesity/ob_home.htm, with permission.

screening should be performed. Weight-loss counseling should be provided for those individuals whose BMI is ≥ 25 kg/m^2 as well as screening for hyperlipidemia and type 2 diabetes.

Blood Pressure Screening Blood pressure standards based on gender and percentile of height have been developed for the older adolescent. Blood pressure readings above the 95th percentile should be considered indicative of hypertension and should be investigated for an organic cause. Blood pressure readings between the 90th and 95th percentile indicate the need for careful monitoring over the next few months (Table 84.13).

Diagnostic Testing Diagnostic testing during the precollege visit is limited.

1. Cholesterol: The Expert Panel on Blood Cholesterol Levels of Children and Adolescents recommends that adolescents whose parents have a serum cholesterol of >240 mg/dL and adolescents older than 19 years should be screened for total blood cholesterol level (nonfasting) at least once. If the parental cholesterol level is unknown or if the adolescent has other risk factors for future cardiovascular disease (e.g., smoking, hypertension, obesity, diabetes mellitus, excessive consumption of dietary saturated fats, and cholesterol), then ordering a screening serum cholesterol level (nonfasting) is also reasonable.
2. STD screening: Screening tests for chlamydia, gonorrhea, syphilis, and/or human immunodeficiency virus (HIV) should be based on risk factors. A Pap smear (preferably liquid-based) should be obtained annually for all sexually active females.
3. Tuberculosis screening: A skin test for tuberculosis should be placed only if there are risk factors for tuberculosis exposure (CDC, 2000). The major risk factor for exposure to tuberculosis in the college-bound population is birth in a tuberculosis-endemic country. The ACHA guidelines indicate that students should undergo tuberculin skin testing if they have arrived within the last 5 years from countries *except* those on the following list:
   a. American region:
      - Canada
      - Jamaica
      - Saint Kitts and Nevis
      - Saint Lucia
      - United States of America
      - Virgin Islands (United States)
   b. European region:
      - Belgium
      - Denmark
      - Finland
      - France
      - Germany
      - Greece
      - Iceland
      - Ireland
      - Italy
      - Liechtenstein
      - Luxembourg
      - Malta
      - Monaco
      - Netherlands
      - Norway
      - San Marino
      - Sweden
      - Switzerland
      - United Kingdom
   c. Western Pacific region:
      - American Samoa
      - Australia
      - New Zealand

   Other risk factors for tuberculosis that would prompt a skin test include HIV infection, injection drug use, and clinical conditions such as diabetes, chronic renal failure, cancer, low body weight, gastrectomy, chronic malabsorption syndromes, prolonged corticosteroid therapy, or other immunosuppressive disorders. Also at risk are those who have lived in, worked in, or volunteered in high-risk congregate settings such as prisons, nursing homes, hospitals, residential facilities for patients with acquired immunodeficiency syndrome, or homeless shelters. Guidelines for interpretation of the skin test result can be found in the CDC's core curriculum on tuberculosis, which is available at state health departments or at the CDC Web site (at www.cdc.gov). Individuals with positive skin test results should have a chest radiograph. If the chest radiograph is negative and there are no contraindications to preventive therapy, isoniazid should be prescribed daily for 9 months.
4. Immunizations: Most colleges and universities mandate proof of certain immunizations before arrival on campus. Although the ACHA, 2000 report gives guidelines for institutional prematriculation immunizations, the institution may vary these requirements as mandated by state law or otherwise. Therefore, to minimize disruption in the enrollment process, the health history form provided to the college-bound student by the college or university should be consulted. If proof of immunization cannot be obtained, then titers demonstrating immunity may often be substituted. An alternative is to reimmunize. Many colleges now require or strongly recommend immunization against varicella and hepatitis B. These inoculations may be begun at the precollege visit and either completed before leaving for college or after arriving on campus.

TABLE 84.13

A: Blood Pressure Levels for the 90th and 95th Percentiles of Blood Pressure for Girls Aged 16 and 17 Years by Percentiles of Height

Age (yr)	Height Percentiles	Systolic BP (mm Hg)							Diastolic BP (mm Hg)						
		5%	10%	25%	50%	75%	90%	95%	5%	10%	25%	50%	75%	90%	95%
16	90th	122	122	123	125	126	127	128	79	79	79	80	81	82	82
	95th	125	126	127	128	130	131	132	83	83	83	84	85	86	86
17	90th	122	123	124	125	126	128	128	79	79	79	80	81	82	82
	95th	126	126	127	129	130	131	132	83	83	83	84	85	86	86

B: Blood Pressure Levels for the 90th and 95th Percentiles of Blood Pressure for Boys Aged 16 and 17 Years by Percentiles of Height

Age (yr)	Height Percentiles	Systolic BP (mm Hg)							Diastolic BP (mm Hg)						
		5%	10%	25%	50%	75%	90%	95%	5%	10%	25%	50%	75%	90%	95%
16	90th	125	126	128	130	132	133	134	79	79	80	81	82	82	83
	95th	129	130	132	134	136	137	138	83	83	84	85	86	87	87
17	90th	128	129	131	133	134	136	136	81	81	82	83	84	85	85
	95th	132	133	135	136	138	140	140	85	85	86	85	88	89	89

BP, blood pressure.
From National High Blood Pressure Education Program, update on the Task Force. *On blood pressure in children and adolescents.* National Institutes of Health; September 1996. NIH publication no. 96–3790.

Meningococcal vaccination: The 2005 recommendation by the CDC's Advisory Committee on Immunization Practices (ACIP) is to:

a. Immunize adolescents aged 11 to 12 years (during the pre-adolescent visit) or
b. Immunize adolescents aged 15 years (high school entry) or
c. Immunize incoming college freshmen living in dormitories.

The older groups would be phased out when younger groups are immunized.

College freshmen living in dormitories or residence halls are at modestly increased risk of meningococcal disease (4.6 per 100,000) relative to other persons their age who are not attending college (1.4 per 100,000). Vaccination with the meningococcal polysaccharide vaccine will decrease the risk for meningococcal disease in these individuals but efficacy is less than 100% against serogroups C, Y, W-135, and A. It will confer no protection against serogroup B disease, and should an outbreak of meningococcal disease occur on campus even those who have been vaccinated should seek medical attention. There are two vaccines available, a quadrivalent polysaccharide vaccine and a quadrivalent conjugate vaccine. The conjugate vaccine has the potential for higher antibody levels, longer protection, and potential elimination of the carrier state.

Pertussis vaccination: In recent years, pertussis (whooping cough) has increased approximately 400% in adolescents and adults. It appears to account for 20% to 30% of cough lasting more than 2 weeks in adolescents and adults. It also appears that adolescents and young adults are a significant source vector (76% of cases) leading to the rising infection rates in infants. Recent ACIP recommendations include

a. Tdap should replace Td for all 11- and 12-year-olds and those aged 13 to 18 years who have not yet received a Td booster should receive Tdap in place of Td.
b. Adults who have not received a Td immunization during the last 10 years should receive a single dose of Tdap vaccine. In addition, those not previously given Tdap vaccine may be given Tdap vaccine at shorter intervals (<10 years) following last Td immunization in settings of wound management and increased risk (including pertussis outbreaks) and contact with infants.
c. In addition, women are encouraged to receive Tdap vaccine before conception.

Tdap and conjugate meningococcal vaccine should be given simultaneously.

It would therefore appear that college students may be a prime group to get revaccinated with Tdap. This could prevent significant morbidity during college semesters and also prevent significant infections in at-risk infants. This would also be important in the urgent care setting in college health centers.

Health Guidance

The remainder of the precollege visit should be devoted to the provision of health guidance information. Selected information, based on responses to the screening questionnaire, may be discussed during the office visit and additional information may be given out as handouts or brochures. The American Academy of Pediatrics publishes a brochure entitled "Health Care for College Students," which covers recommendations for sleep, nutrition, exercise, responsible sexual activity including abstinence, responsible drinking including abstinence, common health problems, mental health, and safety on campus. The ACHA publishes a multitude of brochures on many of these topics as well. The Healthy Student, A Parent's Guide to Preparing Teens for the College Years is available from the Society for Adolescent Medicine (http://www.adolescenthealth.org/The_Healthy_Student.pdf).

For the adolescent with chronic medical conditions, an attempt should be made to arrange for transition of care, either to the health care providers in the college health service or to community providers near the college or university. The parent should sign a release of information (for the minor child) and a copy of the medical record, or an introductory letter summarizing the medical history should be sent to the new provider.

Information for Parents to Consider When Sending Their Children Off to College

Available College Health Center Services and Costs The college-bound student and parents should ask for information about the college health service. Services provided by the college health service are often found on the college's Web site. Campus health services vary from large multispecialty centers providing all outpatient primary care, specialty, and diagnostic services to those that provide only rudimentary first aid. In general, however, college health services provide high-quality, low-cost accessible primary care and health education services. Parents and students should determine what services are available and what the student health fee (if any) covers.

After-hours Care Information about provision of after-hours care and emergency services, pharmacy services, and the location of the referral hospital should be obtained and the information kept in an accessible location.

Health Insurance Most colleges have no facilities such as infirmaries for overnight stays. Parents should ensure that the college-bound student has adequate health insurance to cover hospitalization and emergency, specialty, and diagnostic health services. It is estimated that currently 25% to 30% of college students are uninsured. An unexpected medical bill can interrupt or terminate a college career, and it is strongly recommended that students not go without adequate health insurance. Many campuses sponsor a group health insurance plan for students at reasonable rates. Parents should check the following:

1. Benefits: It is wise to explore the benefits of any and all plans to determine prescription drug policies, whether there are in-network providers in the college area, and the basics about out-of-network coverage, particularly as it concerns access to emergency care and hospitalization.
2. Insurance card: The student should be advised to carry a copy of his or her health insurance card *at all times* and have the name and phone number of the primary care provider.

Consent and Confidentiality

1. Minor consent: If the college-bound student will be an unemancipated minor child on arrival on campus, the parent should sign a generic "consent for treatment" and forward this to the college health service. Many institutions provide this statement on their prematriculation health history form. The parent should be aware that certain disorders or conditions may be treated without parental consent, even if the student is an unemancipated minor. These may include diagnosis and treatment of STDs, contraception, pregnancy, and family planning; mental health or emotional disturbance; and/or substance abuse.
2. Alcohol use: As of 1998, federal law permits, but does not require, colleges and universities to notify parents any time a student younger than 21 years violates drug or alcohol laws. Many institutions have since adopted a policy of mandatory parental notification if a student is found to be involved in risky or illegal behavior such as underage drinking, public drunkenness, drugs, or criminal activity. Because colleges and universities vary in their approach to this issue, the parent should become familiar with the policies on their child's campus.
3. Confidentiality: Once the student is of age 18 years, he or she is considered an adult. At this point, the college health service will adopt a policy of strict confidentiality regarding medical records and medical information. Medical information will not be released to anyone (even the parent who is paying the tuition and fees) without the student's written consent or a court order. This new approach to confidentiality often causes anguish and frustration on the part of the parent but is essential if the student is to engage openly in a professional relationship with the health care provider. Furthermore, confidentiality is essential if the college health service is to assist the student in assuming increasing responsibility for personal health care. Counseling services on campus will adopt the same policy of strict confidentiality.

Personal Health Information The parent should ensure that the student is knowledgeable about his or her personal health information.

1. Medications: The student should have a list of all medications, dosages, and frequency of dosing and should be aware of why the medication was prescribed.
2. Allergies: The student should be aware of all allergies to medications, foods, and others, and should have some knowledge of the type of reaction (e.g., hives, rash, trouble breathing, and shock).
3. Family medical history: The student should be aware of important family medical history and should keep this current.
4. Prior health problems and records: If the student has a prior history of a chronic or significant medical or psychiatric condition, make sure a copy of these records is sent to the student health service or counseling service.
5. Precollege examination and immunizations: This can be an important opportunity/time to review health history including reproductive health and mental health issues with a student's primary care physician. It is also a time to bring immunizations up to date. This information is discussed previously in this chapter.

First Aid Supplies Every student should have basic health care supplies and equipment to deal with minor illnesses and injuries.

1. First aid kit
   a. Bandages
   b. Antibiotic ointment
   c. Elastic wrap such as an Ace wrap

d. Liquid soap
e. 2 × 2 Gauze pads
f. Acetaminophen
g. Ibuprofen
h. Pepto-Bismol
i. Cough and cold medicine
j. Sore throat lozenges or throat spray
k. Allergy medicine
2. Electronic thermometer
3. Ice pack or chemical cold pack

Guidance Regarding Transition Parents should be aware that entering college marks a transition for the student that reaches far beyond merely leaving home. Parents will no longer be personally responsible for attending to the health care needs of their son or daughter. Rather, the student begins the process of learning self-care and good health practices. Parents can assist with this process by "letting go" and allowing students to engage in their own decision making. The campus health service will assist with this transition, by one-on-one counseling and education within the clinic and through programmed health promotion activities on campus. Through these combined efforts, the student will transition toward a state of optimal health, physically, emotionally, socially, intellectually, and spiritually.

WEB SITES

Health Resources

http://www.columbia.edu/cu/healthwise/alice.html. Go Ask Alice includes health question and answers from Columbia University.
http://www.health.gov/healthypeople/. Healthy people 2010 home page.

Organizations

http://www.nces.ep.gov. National Center Education Statistics.
http://www.acha.org/. American College Health Association home page, includes position papers.
http://www.chronicle.com/ Chronicle of Higher Education.
http://www.acpa.org/. American College Personnel Association - College Student Educators International.
http://www.nacubo.org/. National Association of College and University Business Officers.
http://www.naspa.org/. National Association of Student Personnel Administrators.
http://www.aaahc.org/. Accreditation Association for Ambulatory Health Care.
http://www.jcaho.org/. Joint Commission on Accreditation of Healthcare Organizations, home page.
http://www.edc.org/hec/. The U.S. Department of Education established the center to provide nationwide support for campus alcohol and other drug-prevention efforts.

REFERENCES AND ADDITIONAL READINGS

Advisory Committee on Immunization Practices. Meningococcal disease and college students: recommendations of the Advisory Committee on Immunization Practices (ACIP), *MMWR* 2000;49(RR-11-20).
American Association for Health Education, National Commission for Health Education Credentialing, Inc., & Society for Public Health Education. *A competency-based framework for health educators.* Allentown, PA, 2006.
American College Health Association. *Guidelines for a college health program.* Baltimore, 2001.
American College Health Association. *Recommendations for institutional prematriculation immunizations.* American College Health Association. 2005. Available at www.acha.org.
American College of Health Association. The American College Health Association National College Health Assessment (ACHA-NCHA), Spring 2003 Reference Group report. *J Am Coll Health* 2005:53;199.
Boyer EL. *College: the undergraduate experience in America.* New York: Harper & Row, 1987.
Centers for Disease Control and Prevention. *Core curriculum on tuberculosis: what the clinician should know?* 4th ed. Atlanta, GA: Centers for Disease Control and Prevention, 2000. Available at state health departments or at www.cdc.gov/nchstp/tb/pubs/corecurr/.
Christmas WA. The evolution of Medical Services for Students at College and Universities in the United States. *J Am Coll health.* 1995;43:241.
Chronicle of Higher Education. Almanac issue 2007–2008, http://chronicle.com/free/almanac/2007.
DeArmond M. *College health 2000,* American College Health Association, 1987.
DeArmond MM. The future of college health. *J Am Coll Health* 1995;43:258.
DeArmond MM, Bridwell MW, Cox JW, et al. College health toward the year 2000. *J Am Coll Health* 1991;39:249.
Digest of Education Statistics, 2006, National Center for Education Statistics. U.S. Department of Education, http://nces.ed.gov/programs/digest.
Elster AB, Kuznets NJ, eds. *AMA Guidelines for Adolescent Preventive Services (GAPS): recommendations and rationale.* Baltimore: Williams & Wilkins, 1994.
Goldstein MA. Preparing adolescent patients for college. *Curr Opin Pediatr* 2002;14:384.
Greydanus DE, Rimsza ME, Matytsina L. Contraception for college students. *Pediatr Clin North Am* 2005;52:135.
Hussar WJ. *Projections of Education Statistics to 2014 (NCES 2005–074).* U.S. Department of Education, National Center for Education Statistics. Washington, DC: U.S. Government Printing Office, 2005.
Jackson M, Weinstein H. The importance of healthy communities of higher education. *J Am Coll Health* 1997;45:237.
Johnston LD, O'Malley PM, Bachman JG, et al. *Monitoring Future national survey results on drug use, 1975–2006, Volume I, Secondary school students.* NIH Publication No. 07-6205. Bethesda, MD: National Institute on Drug Abuse; Available at: http://www.monitoringthefuture.org/pubs/monographs/vol1_2006.pdf.
Johnston LD, O'Malley PM, Bachman JG, et al. *Monitoring the Future national survey results on drug use, 1975–2006, Volume II: College students and adults ages 19–45 NIH Publication No. 07-6206.* Bethesda, MD: National Institute on Drug Abuse. Available at: http://www.monitoringthefuture.org/pubs/monographs/vol2_2006.pdf.
Keeling RP. Why college health matters [Editorial]? *J Am Coll Health* 2002;50:261.
Lyznicki JM, Nielsen NH, Schneider JF. Cardiovascular screening of student athletes. *Am Fam Physician* 2000;62:765.

National Association of Student Personnel Administrators and American College Health Association. *Principles of good practice for student affairs: statement and inventories.* National Association of Student Personnel Administrators and American College Health Association, May 1998.

National Center for Education Statistics. http://www.nces.ed.gov. 2005.

National Heart, Lung, and Blood Institute. *Obesity Education Initiative. The practical guide to identification, evaluation and treatment of overweight and obesity in adults.* Available at www.nhlbi.nih.gov/guidelines/obesity/ob_home.htm. Accessed 2007

Packwood W. *College student personnel services.* Charles C. Thomas Publisher, 1977:298–365.

Patrick K. Student health: medical care within institutions of higher education. *JAMA* 1988;260:3301.

Prouty AM, Protinsky HO, Canady D. College women: eating behaviors and help-seeking preferences. *Adolescence* 2002;37:353.

Pryor JH, Hurtado S, Saenz VB, et al. *The American Freshman: Forty Year Trends.* Los Angeles: Higher Education Research Institute, UCLA 2007.

Rimsza ME. Sexually transmitted infections: new guidelines for an old problem on the college campus. *Pediatr Clin North Am* 2005;52:217.

Rimsza EM, Kirk GM. Common medical problems of the college student. *Pediatr Clin North Am* 2005;52:9.

Smith DM. American Academy of Family Physicians, Preparticipation Physical Evaluation Task Force. *Preparticipation physical evaluation,* 2nd ed. Minneapolis: Physician and Sportsmedicine, 1997.

Stashwick CA. The pre-college visit: make the most of it. *Intern Med* 1997;14:89.

Swinford PL. Advancing the health of students: a rationale for college health programs. *J Am Coll Health* 2002;50:309.

Wechsler H, Davenport AE, Dowdall GW, et al. Binge drinking, tobacco, and illicit drug use and involvement in college athletics: a survey of students at 140 American colleges. *J Am Coll Health* 1997;45:195.

Wechsler H. Molnar BE. Davenport AE. Baer JS. College alcohol use: a full or empty glass?. *J Am College Health.* 1999;47(6):247.

Wechsler H. Lee JE. Kuo M. Seibring M. Nelson TF. Lee H. Trends in college binge drinking during a period of increased prevention efforts. Findings from 4 Harvard School of Public Health College Alcohol Study surveys: 1993–2001. *J Am College Health.* 2002;50(5):203.

Working Group Report from the National High Blood Pressure Education Program, Update on the Task Force (1987). *On blood pressure in children and adolescents.* National Institutes of Health; September 1996. NIH publication no. 96–3790.

Appendices

Reference Materials on Adolescence

Lawrence S. Neinstein

GENERAL ADOLESCENT MEDICINE

American Academy of Pediatrics. *Guidelines for health supervision III*. Elk Grove Village: American Academy of Pediatrics, 2002.

Aten CB, Gotlieb EM, eds. *Caring for adolescent patients*, 2nd ed. Elk Grove Village: American Academy of Pediatrics, 2006.

Braithwaite RL, Taylor SE, eds. *Health issues in the black community*. San Francisco: Jossey-Bass, 2001.

Coupey SM. *Primary care of adolescent girls*. Philadelphia: Hanley & Belfus, 2000.

Elster AB, Kuznets NJ. *AMA guidelines for adolescent preventive services [GAPS]: recommendations and rationale*. Chicago: American Medical Association, 1995.

Friedman SB, Fisher M, Schonberg K. *Comprehensive adolescent health care*, 2nd ed. St. Louis: Mosby, 1998.

Gallagher R, Heald F, Carrell D. *Medical care of the adolescent*. New York: Appleton-Century-Crofts, 1976.

Goldstein MA. *Boys into men: staying healthy through the teen years*. Westport: Greenwood Press, 2000.

Greydanus DE, Patel DR, Pratt HD. *Essential adolescent medicine*. New York: McGraw-Hill, 2006.

Hofmann AD, Greydanus DE, eds. *Adolescent medicine*, 3rd ed. Stamford: Appleton & Lange, 1997.

Holmes KI, Mardh PA, Sparling PF, et al. eds. *Sexually transmitted diseases*, 3rd ed. New York: McGraw-Hill, 1999.

Irwin C. *Principles of adolescent medicine*. New York: Elsevier Science, 2000.

Jacobson MS, ed. *Adolescent nutritional disorders: prevention and treatment*. New York: New York Academy of Sciences, 1997.

Kaufman M. *Easy for you to say: questions and answers for teens living with chronic illness or disability*. Buffalo: Firefly Books, 2005.

Koss-Chioino JD, Vargas LA. *Working with Latino youth: culture, development, and context*. San Francisco: Jossey-Bass, 1999.

McAnarney ER, Kriepe RE, Orr PP, et al. eds. *Textbook of adolescent medicine*. Philadelphia: WB Saunders, 1992.

McDonald RE, Avery DR, eds. *Dentistry for the child and adolescent*, 7th ed. Harcourt Health Sciences, 1999.

Moore S. *Youth, AIDS, and sexually transmitted diseases (adolescence and society)*. London, New York: Routledge, 1996.

Neinstein LS. *Adolescent health care: a practical guide*. Philadelphia: Lippincott Williams & Wilkins, 2008.

Prescott HM. *A doctor of their own: the history of adolescent medicine*. Cambridge: Harvard University Press, 1998.

Rickert VI, ed. *Adolescent nutrition: assessment and management*. New York: Chapman & Hall, 1996.

Ryan C, Futterman D. *Lesbian & gay youth: care and counseling*. New York: Columbia University Press, 1998.

Shannon JB. *Adolescent health sourcebook*, 2nd ed. Detroit: Omnigraphics, 2006.

Sorenson RC. *Adolescent sexuality in contemporary America*. New York: World Publishing, 1973.

Stanitski CL. *Pediatric and adolescent sports medicine*. Boston: Little, Brown and Company, 1994.

Tanner IM. *Growth at adolescence*. London: Blackwell Science, 1962.

U.S. Congress, Office of Technology Assessment, *Adolescent Health—Volume I: Summary and Policy Options, OTA-H-468* (Washington, DC: U.S. Government Printing Office, 1991).

U.S. Congress, Office of Technology Assessment, *Adolescent Health—Volume II: Background and the Effectiveness of Selected Prevention and Treatment Services, OTA-H-466* (Washington, DC: U.S. Government Printing Office, 1991).

World Health Organization. *The health of young people: a challenge and a promise*. Geneva: World Health Organization, 1993.

PSYCHOSOCIAL CONCERNS

Adams G, ed. *Adolescent development: the essential readings*. Malden: Blackwell Science, 2000.

Aguilera DC. *Crisis intervention: theory and methodology*. St. Louis: Mosby–Year Book, 1998.

Allmond BW, Tanner LJ, Gofman HF. *The family is the patient: Using family interviews in children's medical care*, 2nd ed. Baltimore: Lippincott Williams & Wilkins, 1999.

Bauman L. *The ten most troublesome teen-age problems and how to solve them*. Secaucus: Carol, 1997.

Barrett PM, Ollendick TH. *Handbook of interventions that work with children and adolescents: prevention and treatment*. Hoboken: John Wiley and Sons, 2004.

Berman AL, Jobes DA. *Adolescent suicide: assessment and intervention*. Washington, DC: American Psychological Association, 2006.

Blos P. *The adolescent passage: developmental issues*. New York: International Universities Press, 1979.

Bonino S, Cattelino E, Ciairano S. *Adolescents and risk: behaviors, functions, and protective factors*. New York: Springer-Verlag New York, 2005.

Brach H. *The golden cage: the enigma of anorexia nervosa*. New York: Vintage Books, 1979.

Bruch H. *Eating disorders: anorexia nervosa, obesity, and the person within*. New York: Basic Books, 1973.

Brumbert JJ. *Fasting girls: the history of anorexia nervosa*. New York: Vintage Books, 2000.

Caissy GA. *Early adolescence: understanding the 10- to 15-year-old*. New York: Insight Books, 1994.

Carnegie Council on Adolescent Development. *Great transitions: preparing adolescents for a new century/concluding report, Carnegie council on adolescent development*. New York: Carnegie Corporation of New York, 1995.

Cheng K, Myers K. *Child and adolescent psychiatry: the essentials*. Philadelphia: Lippincott Williams & Wilkins, 2005.

Costin C. *The eating disorder sourcebook: a comprehensive guide to the causes, treatments, and prevention of eating disorders*, 3rd ed. New York: McGraw-Hill, 2007.

D'Onofrio A. *Adolescent self-injury: a comprehensive guide for counselors and health care professionals*. New York: Springer-Verlag New York, 2007.

Elkind D. *A sympathetic understanding of the child: birth to sixteen*, 3rd ed. Boston: Allyn & Bacon, 1994.

Elkind D. *All grown up and no place to go: teenagers in crisis*. Reading: Addison Wesley, 1998.

Erikson E. *Identity, youth, and crises*. New York: WW Norton, 1968.

Fishman HC. *Treating troubled adolescents: a family therapy approach*. New York: Basic Books, 1988.

Forgatch M, Patterson G. *Parents and adolescents: living together. II*, 2nd ed.Champaign: Research Press, 2005.

Freeman A, Reinecke M, eds. *Personality disorders in children and adolescents*. Hoboken John Wiley and Sons, 2007.

Fritz GK. *Child and adolescent mental health consultation in hospitals, schools, and courts*. Washington, DC: American Psychiatric Press, 1993.

Gallagher J, Harris HI. *Emotional problems of adolescents*. New York: Oxford University Press, 1976.

Goreczny AJ, Hersen M. *Handbook of pediatric and adolescent health psychology*. Boston: Allyn & Bacon, 1999.

Green WH. *Child and adolescent clinical psychopharmacology*. Philadelphia: Lippincott Williams & Wilkins, 2007.

Holinger PC. *Suicide and homicide among adolescents*. New York: Guilford Press, 1994.

Hughes JN, La Greca AM, Conoley JC. *Handbook of psychological services for children and adolescents*. New York: Oxford University Press, 2000.

Jaffe M. *Adolescence*. New York: John Wiley and Sons, 1998.

Jessor R, ed. *New perspectives on adolescent risk behavior*. Cambridge, New York: Cambridge University Press, 1998.

Jessor R, Jessor SC. *Problem behavior and psychosocial development: a longitudinal study of youth*. New York: Academic Press, 1977.

Kasper S, den Boer JA, Ad Sitsen JM. *Handbook of depression and anxiety*, 2nd ed. New York: Marcel Dekker Inc, 2003.

King RA, Apter A. *Suicide in children and adolescents*. New York: Cambridge University Press, 2003.

Lask B, Bryant-Waugh R. *Eating disorders in childhood and adolescence*. New York: Taylor and Francis, 2007.

Le Grange D. *Treating bulimia in adolescents: a family-based approach*. New York: Guilford Press, 2007.

Lerner RM, Lerner JV, eds. *Theoretical foundations and biological bases of development in adolescence*. New York: Garland, 1999.

Mattis SG, Ollendick TH. *Panic disorder and anxiety in adolescence*. Malden: Blackwell Science, 2002.

Minuchin S, Rosman BL, Baker L. *Psychosomatic families: anorexia nervosa in context*. Cambridge: Harvard University Press, 1978.

Offer D, Ostroy E, Howard KI, eds. *Patterns of adolescent self-imaging*. San Francisco: Jossey-Bass, 1984.

Offer D, Sabshin M, Offer J. *The psychological world of the teenager: a study of normal adolescent boys*. New York: Basic Books, 1969.

Patterson G, Forgatch M. *Parents and adolescents: living together. I. The basics*. Champaign, Illinois, Research Press, 2005.

Reynolds WM, Johnston HE. *Handbook of depression in children and adolescents*. New York: Plenum Publishing, 1994.

Rice FP. *Child and adolescent development*. Upper Saddle River: Prentice Hall, 1997.

Robin AL. *ADHD in adolescents: diagnosis and treatment*. New York: Guilford Press, 1998.

Santrock JW. *Adolescence*, 11th ed. Boston: McGraw-Hill, 2007.

Scales P. *Developmental assets: a synthesis of the scientific research on adolescent development*. Minneapolis: Search Institute, 1999.

Shaffer DR. *Developmental psychology: childhood and adolescence*, 7th ed. Belmont: Wadsworth/Thomson, 2007.

Sorenson RC. *Adolescent sexuality in contemporary America*. New York: World Publishing, 1973.

Spruijt-Metz D. *Adolescence, affect, and health*. Hove, East Sussex, UK: Psychology Press, 1999.

Steinberg L. *Adolescence*, 7th ed. Boston: McGraw-Hill, 2005.

Stubbe D. *Child and adolescent psychiatry: a practical guide*. Philadelphia: Lippincott Williams & Wilkins, 2007.

Weiss SI. *Coping with the beauty myth: a guide for real girls*. New York: Rosen, 2000.

Wiener JM, Dulcan MK, eds. *Textbook of child and adolescent psychiatry*, 3rd ed. Washington, DC: American Academy of Child and Adolescent Psychiatry and American Psychiatric Press, 2004.

Wodarski JS, Wodarski LA, Dulmus CN. *Adolescent depression and suicide: a comprehensive empirical intervention for prevention and treatment*. Springfield: Charles C Thomas Publisher, 2003.

Wolfe DA. *Adolescent risk behaviors: why teens experiment and strategies to keep them safe New Haven*. Yale University Press, 2006.

Wolfe DA, Mash EJ. *Behavioral and emotional disorders in adolescents: nature, assessment, and treatment*. New York: Guilford Press, 2006.

Wolman BB. *Adolescence: biological and psychosocial perspectives*. Westport: Greenwood Press, 1998.

ADOLESCENT GYNECOLOGY

Carpenter SEK, Rock JA, eds. *Pediatric and adolescent gynecology*. Philadelphia: Lippincott Williams & Wilkins, 2000.

Curtis MG, Overhold S, Hopkins MP, eds. *Glass' office gynecology*. Philadelphia: Lippincott Williams & Wilkins, 2006.

Emans SJH, Laufer MR, Goldstein DP. *Pediatric and adolescent gynecology*, 5th ed. Philadelphia: Lippincott Williams & Wilkins, 2005.

Garden AS, ed. *Paediatric and adolescent gynaecology*. London, New York: Arnold, Oxford University Press, 1998.

Goldfarb AF. *Clinical problems in pediatric and adolescent gynecology*. Philadelphia: Current Medicine, 1998.

Hatcher RA, Trussel J, Nelson AL, et al. *Contraceptive technology*, 19th ed. Atlanta, Contraceptive Technology Communications, 2008.

Mishell DR, ed. *Reproductive endocrinology*. Philadelphia: Current Medicine, 1999.

Sanfilippo JS, Muram D, Lee PA, et al. eds. *Pediatric and adolescent gynecology*, 2nd ed. Philadelphia: WB Saunders, 2001.

Womens Health Care Physicians. *Health care for adolescents*. Washington, DC American College of Obstetricians and Gynecologists, 2003.

BOOKS FOR TEENS AND PARENTS

Anderson A. *Making weight: men's conflicts with food, weight, shape and appearance*. Carlsbad: Gurze Books, 2000.

Beecher M. *Parents on the run: a common sense book for today's parents*. New York: Calahad Books, 1974.

Bennett D, Rowe L. *What to do when your children turn into teenagers*. New York: Doubleday Division of Random House, 2003.

Blume J. *Letters to Judy: what your kids wish they could tell you*. New York: Putnam's Sons, 1986.

Canfield J, Hansen MV, Kirberger K. *Chicken soup for the teenage soul: 101 stories of life, love and learning*. Deerfield Beach: Health Communications Inc, 1997.

Cole B. *Hair in funny places: a book about puberty*. New York: Hyperion Books for Children, 2000.

Collins L. *Eating with your anorexic: how my child recovered through family-based treatment and yours can too*. New York: McGraw-Hill, 2005.

Columbia University Health Education Program. *The "Go Ask Alice" book of answers: a guide to good physical, sexual and emotional health*. New York: Henry Holt & Co, 1998.

Coombs HS. *Teenage survival manual: how to reach 20 in one piece (and enjoy every step of the journey)*, 5th ed. new millennium ed. San Francisco: Halo Books, 1998.

Cordes H. *Girl power in the mirror: a book about girls, their bodies and themselves*. Minneapolis: Lerner, 2000.

Crompton V, Kessner EZ. *Saving beauty from the beast: how to protect your daughter from an unhealthy relationship*. Boston: Little, Brown and Company, 2003.

De Prisco J, Riera M. *Field guide to the American teenager: a parent's companion*. Cambridge: Perseus Publishing, 2000.

Dinkmeyer D, McKay GD. *The STEP approach to parenting your teenager*. Circle Pines: American Guidance Service, 1998.

Elkind D. *Understanding your child from birth to sixteen*. Boston: Allyn and Bacon, 1999.

Fairchild B, Hayward N. *Now that you know: a parent's guide to understanding their gay and lesbian children*. New York: Harcourt Brace, 1998.

Forgatch M, Patterson G. *Parents and adolescents: living together. II.*, 2nd ed.Champaign: Research Press, 2005.

Freeman CG. *Living with a work in progress: a parent's guide to surviving adolescence*. Columbus: National Middle School Association, 1996.

Gaffney CR. *Dr. Gaffney's coaching guide for better parents and stronger kids*. Wilsonville: BookPartners, 1997.

Ginsburg KR. *A parent's guide to building resilience in children and teens: giving your child roots and wings*. Elk Grove Village: American Academy of Pediatrics, 2006.

Ginsburg K, Jones M, Jablow MM. *Less stress, more success: a new approach to guiding your teen through college admissions and beyond*. Elk Grove Graphics: American Academy of Pediatrics, 2006.

Ginott HG. *Between parent and teenager*. New York: Macmillan, 1969.

Gordon S. *When living hurts*. New York: Union of American Hebrew Congregations, 1994.

Gordon S, Gordon J. *Raising a child responsibly in a sexually permissive world*. Holbrook: Adams Media, 2000.

Gravelle K. *What's going on down there?: answers to questions boys find hard to ask*. New York: Walker and Co, 1998.

Haffner D. *Beyond the big talk: every parent's guide to raising sexually healthy teens–from middle school to high school, and beyond*. New York: Newmarket Press, 2001.

Haffner D. *From diapers to dating: a parent's guide to raising sexually healthy children*, 2nd ed. New York: Newmarket Press, 2004.

Harris SO. *When growing up hurts too much: a parent's guide to knowing when and how to choose a therapist with your teenager*. Lexington: Lexington Books, 1990.

Harris RH, Emberley M. *It's perfectly normal: changing bodies, growing up, sex, and sexual health*. Cambridge: Candlewick Publishers, 2004.

Kaufman M, ed. *Mothering teens: understanding the adolescent years*. Charlottetown: Genergy Books, 1997.

Kimball G. *The teen trip: the complete resource guide*. Chicago: Equality Press, 1997.

Madaras L. *My body, my self for boys*. New York: New Market Press, 1995.

Madaras L. *The what's happening to my body? book for boys: the new growing-up guide for parents and sons*, 3rd ed. New York: Newmarket Press, 2001.

Madaras L. *The "what's happening to my body" book for girls: the new growing-up guide for parents and daughters*, 3rd ed. New York: Newmarket Press, 2001.

McCoy K. *Understanding your teenager's depression: issues, insights, and practical guidance for parents*. New York: Berkley Publishing Group, 1994.

McCoy K. *Growing and changing*. New York: Berkley Publishing Group, 2003.

McCoy K, Wibbelsman C. *Crisis-proof your teenager*. New York: Bantam Books, 1991.

McCoy K, Wibbelsman C. *Life happens: a teenager's guide to friends, failure, sexuality, love, rejection, addiction, peer pressure, families, loss, depression, change, and other challenges of living.* New York: Berkley Publishing Group, 1996.

McCoy K, Wibbelsman C. *The teenage body book.* New York: Perigee, 1999.

McGraw J. *Life strategies for teens.* New York: Fireside, 2000.

Middleman AB, Pfeifer KG. *American Medical Association boys' guide to becoming a teen.* San Francisco: Jossey-Bass, 2006.

Ng G. *Everything you need to know about self-mutilation: a helping book for teens who hurt themselves.* New York: Rosen, 1998.

Panzarine S. *A parent's guide to the teen years: Raising your 11 to 14 year old in the age of chat rooms and navel rings.* New York: Facts On File, 2000.

Patterson G, Forgatch M. *Parents and adolescents: living together. The basics.* Champaign, Illinois, Research Press, 2005.

Patterson GR, Forgatch MS. *Parents and adolescents living together: Part 2: family problem solving.* 2nd Edition. Champaign Illinois: Research Press, 2005.

Pollack W. *Real boys: rescuing our sons from the myths of boyhood.* New York: Henry Holt & Company, 1999.

Ponton L. *The sex lives of teenagers.* New York: Dutton, 2000.

Pruitt D. *Your adolescent: emotional, behavioral, and cognitive development from early adolescence through the teen years.* New York: NY Collins Publishing, 2000.

Richardson J, Schuster MA. *Everything you never wanted your kids to know about sex, (but were afraid they'd ask): the secrets to surviving your child's sexual development from birth to the teens.* New York: Crown Publishers, 2003.

Siegel M. *Surviving an eating disorder: strategies for family and friends.* New York: HarperPerennial, 1997.

Slap GB, Jablow MM. *Teenage health care.* New York: Pocket Books, 1994.

Steinberg L. *The ten basic principles of good parenting.* New York: Simon & Schuster, 2004.

Steinberg LD, Levine A. *You and your adolescent: a parent's guide for ages 10 to 20.* New York: Harper & Row, 1997.

Weisman B, Weisman M. *What we told our kids about sex.* San Diego: Harcourt Brace Jovanovich, 1987.

Weston C. *Girl talk: all the stuff your sister never told you.* New York: Harper Perennial, HarperCollins, 1997.

Wolf AE. *"Get out of my life, but first could you drive me and Cheryl to the mall?": a parent's guide to the new teenager.* New York: Farrar, Straus and Giroux, 2002.

JOURNALS

Adolescence

Libra Publishers, 391 Willets Road, Roslyn Heights, NY 11577 (Quarterly journal of current research in areas of social work and psychology.)

Adolescent Medicine Clinics

Elsevier Science Publishing Co, 6277 Sea Harbor Drive Orlando, FL 32887–4800655. *Adolescent Medicine Clinics* is the journal of the AAP Section on Adolescent Health. The hardcover journal is published 3 times annually.

Archives of Pediatrics and Adolescent Medicine

American Medical Association P.O. Box 10946 Chicago, IL 60610-0946

Current Problems in Pediatric and Adolescent Health Care

Mosby, A Division of Elsevier Science Publishing Co, 6277 Sea Harbor Drive Orlando, FL 32887–4800655

Jounral of Adolescent and Pediatric Gynecology

Elsevier Science Publishing Co, 6277 Sea Harbor Drive Orlando, FL 32887–4800655 (Official quarterly publication of the North American Society for Pediatric and Adolescent Gynecology.)

Journal of Adolescent Health

Elsevier Science Publishing Co, 6277 Sea Harbor Drive Orlando, FL 32887–4800655 (Official quarterly publication of the North American Society for Pediatric and Adolescent Gynecology.)

Journal of Adolescent Research

Sage Publications, Inc., 2455 Teller Road, Newbury Park, CA 91320, 805-499-0721 (Official publication of the Society for Research on Adolescence.)

Journal of American College Health

Heldref Publications, 4000 Albemarle Street, NW, Washington, DC 20016 (Journal dedicated to the exchange of information related to health care issues in community colleges, colleges, and universities.)

Journal of Youth and Adolescence

Plenum Publishing Corp., 233 Spring Street, New York, NY 10013 (Multidisciplinary quarterly research journal.

Other Resources and Services

Lawrence S. Neinstein

GENERAL RESOURCES AND SERVICES

The Center for Early Adolescence, School of Medicine, University of North Carolina at Chapel Hill, D-2 Carr Mill Town Center, Carrboro, NC 27510; 919-966-1148. (Offers bibliographies and booklets on many areas concerning young adolescents, such as community services, parenting, and sexuality.)

Available from the center:
   Understanding Early Adolescence: A Framework, by
       J. P. Hill
   Understanding Families With Young Adolescents, by
       L. D. Steinberg
   *Schools for Young Adolescents: Adapting the Early
       Childhood Model,* by S. Feeney
Resource Lists
   "Adolescent Literature"
   "Community Resources"
   "Early Adolescence"
   "Educating Young Adolescents"
   "Parenting"
   "Religion"
   "Sex Education"

ABORTION SERVICES

Check telephone listings under
   Clergy counseling service
   National Abortion Federation Hotline: 800-772-9100
   National Organization for Women
   Planned Parenthood

COUNSELING SERVICES

Check telephone listings under
   Family Services Association
   County department of health
   Counseling clinics
   Mental health clinics
   United Fund

HOTLINE SERVICES

Adolescent Crisis Intervention and Counseling (the "nine" line): 800-999-9999 (24 hours, 7 days)
AIDS
   Centers for Disease Control and Prevention (CDC)
       Acquired Immunodeficiency Syndrome (AIDS)
           Hotline: 800-342-2347 (24 hours, 7 days)
       Spanish: 800-344-7432 (8 a.m. to 2 a.m., Eastern
           time, 7 days)
       TTY: 888-232-6348 (Monday through Friday, 10 a.m.
           to 10 p.m., Eastern time)
   Teens AIDS: 800-440-8336 (staffed by teens for teens;
       Fridays and Saturdays, 6 p.m. to midnight, Eastern
       time)
   Teens TAP (Teaching AIDS Prevention), an AIDS infor-
       mation line for teens (not a crisis line): 800-234-8336
       (Monday through Friday, 4 p.m. to 8 p.m., Central
       Standard time)
Gay and Lesbian Youth Hotline (not a crisis line): 800-773-
   5540 (Thursday through Saturday, 12 p.m. to 8 p.m.,
   Eastern time)
Hit Home, a national youth crisis line for suicide, abuse,
   pregnancy, depression, counseling, and intervention:
   800 442–4673 (24 hours, 7 days)
National Child Abuse Hotline, for suspected child abuse
   reports and for referrals: 800-422-4453 (800 4-A-CHILD)
   (24 hours, 7 days)
National Domestic Violence/Child Abuse/Sexual Abuse:
   800-799-SAFE/800-799-7233/800-787-3224 TDD, 800-942-
   6908 Spanish Speaking 24-hour-a-day 7 days a week
   hotline, Provides crisis intervention and referrals to
   local services and shelters for victims of partner or
   spousal abuse.
National Herpes Hotline: 919-361-8488 (Monday through
   Friday 9 a.m. to 7 p.m., Eastern time)
National Runaway Switchboard Hotline (for youth or
   parents:1 800 RUNAWAY (800) 786–2929) (24 hours)
National Youth Crisis Hotline: 1-**800-442-HOPE (4673)** Provides counseling and referrals to local drug treatment
   centers, shelters, and counseling services. Responds
   to youth dealing with pregnancy, molestation, suicide,
   and child abuse. Operates 24 hours, 7 days a week.
Rape Hotline 1800 656-HOPE

STD Hotline: 800-227-8922 (Monday through Friday, 8 a.m. to 11 p.m., Eastern time)

Check local operator or directory for hotlines listed under
Crisis counseling
Counseling
Drug abuse
Rape
Runaways
Suicide

Information also available from

National Clearinghouse for Mental Health Information, P. O. Box 2345, Rockville, MD 20847-2345, (800) 729–6686

See also "Adolescent Clinics" section later in this appendix.

ALCOHOL AND DRUG PROBLEMS

Books

Bukstein OG. *Adolescent substance abuse: assessment, treatment, and prevention.* New York: John Wiley and Sons, 1995.

Carroll CR, Durrant LH. *Drugs in modern society.* Boston: McGraw-Hill, 2000.

Dayton T. *Trauma and addiction: ending the cycle of pain through emotional literacy.* Deerfield Beach: Health Communication, 2000.

Dodgen CE, Shea MW. *Substance use disorders: assessment and treatment.* San Diego: Academic Press, 2000.

Erlich LB. *A textbook of forensic addiction, medicine, and psychiatry.* Springfield: Charles C Thomas Publisher, 2001.

Falkowski C. *Dangerous drugs: an easy-to-use reference for parents and professionals.* Center City: Hazelden, 2000.

Frances RJ, Miller SI. *Clinical textbook of addictive disorders.* New York: Guilford Press, 1998.

Gold MS. *Smoking and illicit drug use.* New York: Haworth Medical Press, 1998.

Hardiman M. *Overcoming addiction: a common sense approach.* Freedom: Crossing Press, 2000.

Henderson EC. *Understanding addiction.* Jackson: University Press of Mississippi, 2000.

Kandel DB. *Stages and pathways of drug involvement: examining the gateway hypothesis.* New York: Cambridge University Press, 2001.

Ladewig D. *Basic and clinical science of substance related disorders.* New York: Basel, 1999.

Lawton SA. *Drug information for teens : health tips about the physical and mental effects of substance abuse.* Detroit: Omnigraphics, 2006.

Liddle HA, Rowe CL. *Adolescent substance abuse : research and clinical advances.* New York: Cambridge University Press, 2006.

Lowinson JH. *Substance abuse: a comprehensive textbook.* Philadelphia: Lippincott Williams & Wilkins, 2005.

McCrady BS, Epstein EE. *Addictions: a comprehensive guidebook.* New York: Oxford University Press, 1999.

McNeece AC, DiNitto DM. *Chemical dependency: a systems approach.* Boston: Allyn and Bacon, 1998.

Maisto SA, Galizio M, Connors GJ. *Drug use and abuse.* Fort Worth: Harcourt Brace College Publishers, 1999.

Margolis RD. *Treating patients with alcohol and other drug problems: an integrated approach.* Washington, DC: American Psychological Association, 1998.

Milkman HB, Sunderwirth SG. *Craving for ecstasy: how our passions become addictions and what we can do about them.* San Francisco: Jossey-Bass, 1998.

Miller NS. *The principles and practice of addictions in psychiatry.* Philadelphia: WB Saunders, 1997.

Niesink RJM. *Drugs of abuse and addiction: neurobehavioral toxicology.* Boca Raton: CRC Press, 1999.

Orcutt JD, Rudy DR. *Drugs, alcohol, and social problems.* Lanham: Rowman and Littlefield, 2003.

Ott PJ, Tarter RE, Ammerman RT. *Sourcebook on substance abuse: etiology, epidemiology, assessment, and treatment.* Boston: Allyn and Bacon, 1999.

Rogers PD, Werner MJ. *Substance abuse.* Philadelphia: WB Saunders, 1995.

Rotgers F. *Main title: treating alcohol problems.* Hoboken: Wiley-Liss, 2006.

Schuckit MA. *Drug and alcohol abuse: a clinical guide to diagnosis and treatment.* New York: Springer-Verlag New York, 2006.

Schaler JA. *Addiction is a choice.* Chicago: Open Court, 2000.

Senay EC. *Substance abuse disorders in clinical practice.* New York: WW Norton, 1998.

Sheen B. *Teen alcoholism.* San Diego: Lucent Books, 2004.

Smith DE, Seymour RB. *Clinician's guide to substance abuse.* New York: McGraw-Hill, Health Professions Division, 2001.

Sullivan E, Fleming M. *A guide to substance abuse services for primary care clinicians.* Rockville: U.S. Department of Health and Human Services; Public Health Service; Substance Abuse and Mental Health Services Administration, 1997.

Winters KC, ed. *Adolescent substance abuse: new frontiers in assessment.* New York: The Haworth Press, 2006.

Yoshida R, ed. *Trends in alcohol abuse and alcoholism research.* Hauppauge: Nova Science Publishers, 2006.

Organizations

Al-Anon Family Group Headquarters
1600 Corporate Landing Parkway, Virginia Beach, VA 23454-5617; (888) 4AL-ANON

Alcohol and Drug Helpline
800-821-4357 (Provides referrals to local facilities where adolescents and adults can seek help for alcohol and drug problems.)

Alcohol Hotline
800-252-6465 (800-ALCOHOL)

Alcoholics Anonymous
PO Box 459, Grand Central Station, New York, NY 10163; 212-870-3400; or check local office

American Council on Alcoholism
800-527-5344 (Provides treatment referrals, counseling, and advice for alcoholics and their families and friends.)

Boys Clubs of America
1275 Peachtree Street, N.E., Atlanta, GA 30309-3506, (404) 487–5700

Cocaine Anonymous World Services
National Referral Information line (not a hotline): 800-347-8998
World Service Office: 310-559-5833
National Cocaine Hotline: 800-262-2463 (800-COCAINE)

Narcotics Anonymous
PO Box 9999, Van Nuys, CA 91409; 818-773-9999; Fax: 818-700-0700

National Clearinghouse for Alcohol Information
PO Box 2345, Rockville, MD 20847-2345; 800-729-6686

National Clearinghouse for Alcohol and Drug Information
PO Box 2345, Rockville, MD 20847-2345; 800-729-6686

National Council on Alcoholism
22 Cortlandt Street, Suite 801, New York, NY 10007-3128;
(800) 475-HOPE

National Council on Alcoholism and Drug Dependence, Inc
800-622-2255 (Provides information and referrals to local counseling.)

National Federation of Parents for Drug-Free Youth
11159-B South Town Square St. Louis, MO 63123(314)
845-1933

National Institute on Drug Abuse
6001 Executive Boulevard, Bethesda, MD 20892-9561;
301-443-1124

Parent Resources Institute for Drug Education
40 Hurt Plaza, Suite 210 Atlanta, GA 30303(404) 577-4500

SEXUALITY

Books

The Alan Guttmacher Institute (AGI). *Sex and America's teenagers*. New York: Alan Guttmacher Institute, 1994.

Bell R. *Changing bodies, changing lives: a book for teens on sex and relationships*. New York: Times Books, 1998.

Carrera MA. *Adolescent sexuality and pregnancy prevention*. New York: Bernice and Milton Stern National Training Center for Adolescent Sexuality and Family Life Education, The Children's Aid Society, 1996.

Cocca C. *Adolescent sexuality: a historical handbook and guide*. Westport: Praeger, 2006.

Columbia University Health Education Program. *The "Go Ask Alice" book of answers: a guide to good physical, sexual and emotional health*. New York: Henry Holt & Co, 1998.

Gordon S. *Seduction lines heard around the world and answers you can give*. Buffalo: Prometheus Books, 1987.

Gordon S, Gordon J. *Raising a child responsibly in a sexually permissive world*. Holbrook: Adams Media, 2000.

Haffner D. *Beyond the big talk : every parent's guide to raising sexually healthy teens–from middle school to high school, and beyond*. New York: Newmarket Press, 2001.

Haffner D. *From diapers to dating : a parent's guide to raising sexually healthy children*, 2nd ed. New York: Newmarket Press, 2004.

Harris RH, Emberley M. *It's perfectly normal: changing bodies, growing up, sex, and sexual health*. Cambridge: Candlewick Publishers, 2004.

Hyde M, Forsyth EH. *Safe sex 101: an overview for teens*. Minneapolis: Twenty-First Century Books, 2006.

McCoy K. *Growing and changing*. New York: Berkley Publishing Group, 2003.

McCoy K, Wibbelsman C. *The teenage body book*. New York: Perigee, 1999.

Nardo D. *Teen sexuality*. San Diego: Lucent Books, 1997.

Park JM, Card JJ, Muller KL. *Just the facts: what science has found out about teenage sexuality and pregnancy in the U.S.* San Jose: Sociometrics Corporation, 1998.

Rekers GA. *Handbook of child and adolescent sexual problems*. New York: Lexington Books, 1995.

Reisser PC. *Parents' guide to teen health: raising physically and emotionally healthy teens*. Wheaton: Tyndale House Publishers, 2001.

Sawyer K. *Sex and the teenager: choices and decisions*. Notre Dame: Ave Maria Press, 1999.

Organizations

AIDS Information Line, CDC, National Human Immunodeficiency Virus (HIV) and AIDS Hotline
800-232-4636

American Social Health Association
PO Box 13827, Research Triangle Park, NC 27709; 919-361-8400

Center for Population Options
140016th Street, N.W. Suite 100, Washington, DC 200036;
202-667-1142

International Planned Parenthood Federation, Western Hemisphere Regional Office
120 Wall Street, 9th floor, New York, NY 10005-3092;
212-248-6400

National Family Planning and Reproductive Health Association
1627 K Street, NW, 12th floor, Washington, DC 20006;
202-293-3114

National Sex and Drug Forums
330 Ellis Street, San Francisco, CA 94102

Planned Parenthood-World Population
434 West 33rd Street, New York, New York 10001; 212-541-7800

Sex Information and Education Council of the United States (SIECUS) (main office)
130 West 42nd Street, suite 350, New York, NY 10036-7802; 212-819-9770

Society for Adolescent Medicine (SAM)
1916 Copper Oaks Circle, Blue Springs, MO 64015; 816-224-8010

Sex Education Resources

Manuals Contact the following organizations for up-to-date educational manuals:

Planned Parenthood, national and local
Family Planning Federation
Local school district
National Clearinghouse for Family Planning Information, Rockville, MD
U.S. Department of Health and Human Services (U.S. Government Printing Office)

Other Resources
Odin Books
1110 West West Broadway, Vancouver, BC; 800-223-6346 (Education resource lists available on education curricula and reference lists on topics such as self-esteem, attention-deficit disorder, depression, child abuse, eating disorders, and teen pregnancy.)

ETR Associates
4 Carbonero Way, Scotts Valley, CA 95066 ; 1-800-321-4407 (Many pamphlets and books on AIDS, family life, sexual abuse, sexuality, drug abuse prevention, and reproductive health.)

POPLINE (POPulation information onLINE)

Johns Hopkins University, Population Information Program, 111 Market Place, suite 310, Baltimore, MD 21202-4024; 410-659-6300

Online service: National Library of Medicine, Bethesda, MD; 800-638-8480 (for user ID and password) (Citations and abstracts to the worldwide literature on population and family planning.)

Planned Parenthood Federation of America

434 W 33rd Street,, New York, NY 10001; 800 829–7732 (Many pamphlets, books, and videotapes on reproductive health care; also available is *Current Literature in Family Planning,* a monthly review of literature in family planning.)

Teenage Pregnancy

Books

Alan Guttmacher Institute.

Disparities in rates of unintended pregnancy in the United States, 1994 and 2001 perspectives on sexual and reproductive health article. June 2006.

In the know: questions about pregnancy, contraception and abortion frequently asked questions. May 2006.

Assessing costs and benefits of sexual and reproductive health interventions: detailed data and analysis on the benefits of investing in sexual and reproductive health care. December 2004.

U.S. teenage pregnancy statistics: overall trends, trends by race and ethnicity and state-by-state information state-level data on teenage pregnancy. February 2004.

Unintended pregnancy in the United States most current data (update in progress). January 1998.

Contraception counts: ranking state efforts state and congressional district fact sheets on meeting women's needs for contraception. February 1996.

Sex and America's teenagers. New York: Alan Guttmacher Institute, 1994.

Battle SE. *The black adolescent parent.* New York: Haworth Press, 1987.

Becker E, Rankin E, Rickel AU. *High-risk sexual behavior: interventions with vulnerable populations.* New York: Plenum Publishing, 1998.

Breedlove GK, Schorfheide A. *Adolescent pregnancy.* White Plains: March of Dimes, 2001.

Cherry AL, Dillon ME, Rugh D. *Teenage pregnancy: a global view.* Westport: Greenwood Press, 2001.

Cothran H. *Teen pregnancy and parenting.* San Diego: Greenhaven Press, 2001.

Dudley W. *Pregnancy.* San Diego: Greenhaven Press, 2001.

Furstenberg FL, Brooks-Gunn J, Morgan SP. *Adolescent mothers in later life.* New York: Cambridge University Press, 1987.

Hardy JB, ed. *Adolescent pregnancy in an urban environment: issues, programs, and evaluation.* Washington, DC: Urban Institute Press, 1991.

Humenick SS, Wilkerson NN, Paul NW. *Adolescent pregnancy: nursing perspectives on prevention.* White Plains: March of Dimes Birth Defects Foundation, 1991.

Lawson A, Rhode DL. *The politics of pregnancy: adolescent sexuality and public policy.* New Haven: Yale University Press, 1993.

Lerman E, Moffett J. *Teen moms: the pain and the promise.* Buena Park: Morning Glory Press, 1997.

Luker K. *Dubious conceptions: the politics of teenage pregnancy.* Cambridge: Harvard University Press, 1996.

Mayden B, Castro W, Annitto M. *First talk: a teen pregnancy prevention dialogue among Latinos.* Washington, DC: CWLA Press, 1999.

Merrick E. *Reconceiving black adolescent pregnancy.* Boulder: Westview Press, 2000.

Robinson BE. *Teenage fathers.* Lexington: Lexington Books, 1988.

U.S. Department of Education. *Compendium of school-based and school-linked programs for pregnant and parenting adolescents.* Washington, DC: National Institute on Early Childhood Development and Education, Office of Educational Research and Improvement, U.S. Department of Education, 1999.

Zabin LS. *Adolescent sexual behavior and childbearing.* Newbury Park: Sage Publications Inc, 1993.

Zollar AC. *Adolescent pregnancy and parenthood: an annotated guide.* New York: Garland, 1990.

Adolescent Clinics

Alabama

Adolescent Health Clinic

Department of Pediatrics

University of Alabama

1600 7th Avenue South

Birmingham, AL

35233; 205-939-9231

Arizona

Adolescent Clinic

Department of Pediatrics

University of Arizona

1501 North Campbell Avenue

Tucson, AZ 85724-5073

520-694-7432

Adolescent and Young Adult Clinic

Phoenix Indian Medical Center (serves only Native Americans)

Primary Care Medical Center

4212 North 16th Street

Phoenix, AZ 85016

602-263-1200

California

UCLA Adolescent Medicine Clinic

UCLA

200 Medical Plaza, suite 265

Los Angeles, CA 90095

310-825-5744

Other UCLA sites include:

UCLA Adolescent Medicine Clinic

UCLA

11318 National Boulevard

Los Angeles, CA 90064

310-391-7043

UCLA Adolescent Medicine Clinic

UCLA

15200 Sunset Boulevard, #107

Pacific Palisades, CA 90272

310-459-7736

Adolescent Clinic
  Children's Health Clinic
  4460 East Huntington Boulevard
  Fresno, CA 93702
  559-459-5664
Youth and Young Adult Clinic
  Packard Children's Hospital, Stanford University
  Division of Adolescent Medicine
  730 Welch Road, #325
  Palo Alto, CA 94304
  650-736-7642
Adolescent Clinic
  University of California Medical Center
  400 Parnassus Avenue, 2nd floor
  San Francisco, CA 94143
  415-353-2002
Adolescent Clinic
  University of California San Francisco
  3333 California Street, suite 245
  San Francisco, CA 94118
  415-476-2184
Adolescent Clinic
  Harbor-University of California at Los Angeles Medical
    Center
  1000 West Carson Street
  Torrance, CA 90509
  310-222-2321
Adolescent Clinic
  University of California at San Diego Medical Center
  4168 Front Street
  San Diego, CA 92103
  619-543-7872
Adolescent Clinic
  Stanford University
  730 Welch Road, suite 325
  Palo Alto, CA 94304
  650-736-7642
Adolescent Clinic
  Children's Hospital Los Angeles
  5000 Sunset Boulevard, 4th floor
  Los Angeles, CA 90027
  323-669-2153
Adolescent Clinic
  Oakland Children's Hospital
  747 52nd Street
  Oakland, CA 94609
  510-428-3387
Adolescent Clinic
  San Francisco General Hospital
  1001 Potrero Avenue, 6 ms
  San Francisco, CA 94110
  415-206-8376

Colorado

Adolescent Clinic
  The Children's Hospital
  1056 East 19th Avenue, B025
  Denver, CO 80218
  303-861-6133
Eating Disorder Program
  The Children's Hospital
  1056 East 19th Avenue, B025
  Denver, CO 80218
  303-861-6133

Connecticut

Adolescent Clinic
  Yale New Haven Hospital
  20 York Street
  Primary Care Center/Adolescent Clinic
  New Haven, CT 06510-3202
  203-688-2471
Adolescent Clinic
  Bridgeport Hospital
  267 Grant Street
  Bridgeport, CT 06610
  203-384-3064
  Department of Child and Adolescent
    Psychiatry
  Mt. Sinai Hospital
  675 Tower Avenue, #301
  Hartford, CT 06112
  860-714-2747
Adolescent Medicine
  Fair Haven Clinic
  274 Grand Avenue
  New Haven, CT 06513
  203-777-7411
Adolescent Medicine
  St. Francis Hospital
  1000 Asylum Avenue
  Hartford, CT 06105
  860-714-4332

District of Columbia

Adolescent Clinic
  Walter Reed Army Medical Center
  Georgia Avenue and 16th Street
  Washington, DC 20307-5001
  202-782-6101
Adolescent Clinic
  Walter Reed Army Medical Center
  8901 Wisconsin Avenue
  Bethesda, MD 20889
  301-295-4902
Adolescent Clinic
  Children's National Medical Center
  111 Michigan Avenue, NW
  Washington, DC 20010
  202-884-2178
Adolescent Clinic
  Howard University Hospital
  2041 Georgia Avenue, NW
  Washington, DC 20060
  202-865-1304
Pediatrics
  Georgetown University
  Children's Medical Center
  3800 Reservoir Road, NW
  Washington, DC 20007
  202-444-5437

Hawaii

Adolescent and Young Adult Clinic
  Tripler Army Medical Center
  1 Jarrett White Road
  Tripler AMC, HI 96859
  808-433-4165

Adolescent Clinic
  Kapiolani Children's Medical Center
  1319 Punahou Street
  Honolulu, HI
  808-983-8394

Illinois
Adolescent Clinic
  Rush Presbyterian Hospital
  1645 West Jackson Boulevard, #315
  Chicago, IL 60612-3227
  312-942-2777
Adolescent Clinic
  Cook County Hospital
  1901 W. Harrison
  Chicago, IL 60612
  312-864-3585
Adolescent Clinic
  Department of Pediatrics
  Loyola University
  2160 South First Avenue
  Maywood, IL 60153
  708-327-9119

Indiana
Adolescent Clinic
  Riley Outpatient Parking Garage
  575 North West Drive, #070
  Indianapolis, IN 46202
  317-274-8812
Wishard Hospital Adolescent Community Clinics
  Wishard Primary Care
  1002 Wishard Boulevard, 2nd floor
  Indianapolis, IN 46202
  317-692-2363
Blackburn Health Center
  2700 Martin Luther King Drive
  Indianapolis, IN 46208
  317-931-4300
Cottage Corners Health Center
  1434 South Shelby Street
  Indianapolis, IN 46203
  317-655-3200
Grassy Creek Health Center
  9443 East 38th Street
  Indianapolis, IN 46236
  317-890-2100
North Arlington Health Center
  2505 North Arlington Avenue
  Indianapolis, IN 46218
  317-554-5200
Bellflower Clinic
  1101 West 10th Street
  Indianapolis, IN 46202
  317-221-8300
Methodist Hospital Adolescent Clinics
  1701 Senate Blvd.
  Indianapolis, IN 46202
  317-962-8067

Iowa
Adolescent Clinic
  University of Iowa Hospitals and Clinics
  200 Hawkins Drive
  Iowa City, IA 52242
  319-356-2229

Kansas
Adolescent Clinic
  University of Kansas Medical Center
  3901 Rainbow Boulevard
  Kansas City, KS 66160
  913-588-5908

Kentucky
Adolescent Clinic
  Kosair Children's Hospital
  231 East Chestnut Street
  Louisville, KY 40202
  502-629-7700

Louisiana
Adolescent Medicine
  Department of Pediatrics
  SL 37, Tulane Medical Center
  1415 Tulane Avenue
  New Orleans, LA 70112
  504-988-5795

Maine
Teen and Young Adult Clinic at the Family Practice Clinic
  895 Union Street, suite 12
  Bangor, ME 04401
  207-973-7979
Adolescent Clinic
  University of Maryland Hospital
  120 Penn Street
  Baltimore, MD 21201
  410-328-6495

Massachusetts
Adolescent Clinic
  New England Medical Center
  750 Washington Street
  PO Box 351
  Boston, MA 02111
  617-636-1332
Adolescent Clinic
  Boston Medical Center
  1 Boston Medical Center Place
  Boston, MA 02118
  617-638-8000
Adolescent/Young Adult Practice
  Children's Hospital
  333 Longwood Avenue, 5th floor
  Boston, MA 02115
  617-355-7181
Adolescent Clinic
  Milford-Whitinsville Regional Hospital
  Vittori Marsell Young Women's Health
  14 Prospect
  Milford, MA 01757
  508-482-5444
Pediatric Clinic
  University of Massachusetts Memorial Health Center
  Benedict Building, 2nd floor
  55 Lake Avenue North
  Worcester, MA 01655
  508-856-5624
Adolescent Clinic
  Family Health and Social Services (Community Health Center)

26 Queen Street
Worcester, MA 01610
508-860-7700

Michigan

Teenage and Young Adult Health Program
University of Michigan
Briarwood Health Specialists
325 Briarwood Circle, Building 5
Ann Arbor, MI 48108
734-647-9000
www.med.umich.edu/ahp
Adolescent Medicine Clinic
Children's Hospital of Michigan
3901 Beaubien Boulevard
Detroit, MI 48201
313-745-4045
Adolescent Clinic
Hurley Children's Clinic
806 Tuuri Place
Flint, MI 48503
810-257-9773
Adolescent Medicine Program
Department of Pediatrics/Human Development
Michigan State University, College of Human Medicine
B-240 Life Sciences Bldg.
East Lansing, MI 48824-1317
517-353-5042
Adolescent Clinic
University Hospital University of Michigan
4260 Plymouth Road
Ann Arbor, MI 48109
734-647-5680
Internal Medicine Program
University Hospital University of Michigan
1500 East Medical Center Drive
Ann Arbor, MI 48109
734-936-5582

Minnesota

Adolescent Health
University of Minnesota Hospital and Clinic
McNamara Center, 200 Oak Street, SE, suite 260
Minneapolis, MN 55455
612-626-2820

Mississippi

Teen Medicine Center
University of Mississippi Medical Center
Department of Pediatrics
2500 North State Street
Jackson, MS 39216
601-984-2925

Missouri

Adolescent Clinic
Children's Mercy Hospital
4605 Paseo
Kansas City, MO 64110
816-234-3050

Nebraska

Youth Village
Children's Memorial Hospital

8200 Dodge Street
Omaha, NE 68114
402-955-5400
Omaha Children's Clinic
12802 Augusta Avenue
Omaha, NE 68144
402-330-5690

Nevada

Adolescent Medicine
University of Nevada School of Medicine
Department of Pediatrics
2040 West Charleston Boulevard, #402
Las Vegas, NV 81902
702-671-2231
Teen Clinic
Washoe County District Health Department
PO Box 11130
Reno, NV 89520
775-328-2400

New Hampshire

Pediatric and Adolescent Clinic
Dartmouth–Hitchcock Medical Center
1 Medical Center Drive
Lebanon, NH 03756
603-653-9663

New Jersey

Adolescent Clinic
Monmouth Medical Center
270 Broadway
Long Branch, NJ 07740
732-923-6702
Adolescent Clinic
University Medical Group
(University of Medicine and Dentistry of NJ–Robert
Wood Johnson Medical School)
89 French Street
New Brunswick, NJ 08903
732-235-7896
Adolescent Clinic
Morristown Memorial Hospital
Children's Medical Center
100 Madison Avenue, Box-54
Morristown, NJ 07962
973-971-6475
www.TeenHealthFx.com.

New Mexico

Adolescent Clinic
University of New Mexico
Health Sciences Center & University Hospital
ACC 3rd floor
815 Camino De Salud
Albuquerque, NM 87131
505-272-5551

New York

Adolescent Clinic
North Shore University Hospital
410 Lakeville Road
New High, NY 11021
516-465-3270

Jordan Health Center Teen Center
82 Holland Street
Rochester, NY 14605
585-423-2846
Threshold Center for Alternative Youth Services
80 St. Paul Street, 4th floor
Rochester, NY 14604
585-454-7530
Adolescent Clinic
Mount Sinai Medical Center
312 East 94th Street
Manhattan, NY 10128
212-423-3000
Adolescent Clinic
The Door
555 Broome Street
New York, NY 10013
212-941-9090
Adolescent Clinic
Children's Hospital
601 Elmwood Avenue
Box 690
Rochester, NY 14642
585-275-2964
Adolescent Oncology
Roswell Park Cancer Institute
Carlton and Elm Street
Buffalo, NY 14263
877-275-7724
Montefiore Hospital and Medical Center
Division of Adolescent Medicine
111 East 210th Street
The Bronx, NY 10467
718-920-4321
Schneider Children's Hospital of Long Island
Division of Adolescent Medicine
410 Lakeview Road, #108
New Hyde Park, NY 11040
516-465-3270
Brookdale Hospital and Medical Center
Division of Adolescent Medicine
1380 Linden Boulevard
Brooklyn, NY 11212
718-240-5055
Adolescent Clinic
Coney Island Hospital
2601 Ocean Parkway
Brooklyn, NY 11235
718-616-3991
Adolescent Clinic
North Shore University Hospital
410 Lakeview Road
New High Park, NY 11040
516-465-3270

North Carolina
Pediatric Ambulatory Care Center
University of North Carolina
CB No. 7735
Mason Farm Road
Chapel Hill, NC 27599-7735
919-966-2491
Duke Medical Center
Department of Pediatrics
4020 North Roxbro Road

Durham, NC 27704
919-620-5374

Ohio
Teen Health Center
Children's Hospital Medical Center
Division of Adolescent Medicine
3333 Burnet Avenue
Cincinnati, OH 45229
513-636-4200
Adolescent Clinic
Children's Hospital
899 E. Broad Street
Columbus, OH 43205
614-722-2450
Lakewood Hospital Teen Health Center
15644 Madison Avenue, #108
Lakewood, OH 44107
216-391-8336
No Listing
Pediatric Clinic
Metro Health Center
2500 Metro Health Drive, 1st floor
Cleveland, OH 44109
216-778-2222
Pediatric and Adolescent Clinic
University Internal & Pediatric Clinic
234 Goodman Street
Cincinnati, OH 45219
513-584-1000

Oklahoma
Adolescent Medicine
Children's Hospital of Oklahoma
940 N.E. 13th Street
room 4419
Oklahoma City, OK 73104
405-271-6208

Oregon
Adolescent and Young Adult Clinic
Doernbecher Children's Hospital
Oregon Health Sciences University
3181 SW Sam Jackson Park Road
Portland, OR 97201-3098
503-418-5700
Outside In Health Clinic (serves homeless and high risk youth)
1132 S.W. 13th Avenue
Portland, OR 97205
503-223-4121

Pennsylvania
Adolescent Health Center
Children's Hospital of Pittsburgh
3420 Fifth Avenue
Pittsburgh, PA 15213
412-692-6677
Adolescent Clinic
Children's Hospital
350 Market Street
Philadelphia, PA 19104
215-590-3537

Rhode Island

Adolescent Medicine
  Rhode Island Hospital
  Department of Pediatrics
  APC-585-A, 593 Eddy Street
  Providence, RI 02902
  401-444-4712

Texas

The Center for Adolescent Health
  People's Community Clinic
  2909 N I H 35
  Austin, TX 78722
  512-478-4939
Adolescent Clinic
  Children's Hospital
  1935 Motor Street
  Dallas, TX 75235
  214-648-3563
Adolescent Medicine
  Kids Place
  6410 Fannin Boulevard, #500
  Houston, TX 77030
  832-325-7111
Adolescent and Sports Medicine
  Texas Children's Hospital
  6601 Fannin Street, 11th Floor
  mc-cc610.01
  Houston, TX 77030
  832-822-4887
Adolescent Clinic
  University of Texas
  301 University Boulevard
  Galveston, TX 77555-0764
  409-772-3630
Eating Disorders Program
  (Eating disorders evaluations and treatment only).
  The Menninger Clinic
  2801 Gessner Drive
  Houston, Texas 77080
  785-350-5000

Utah

Pediatric Clinic
  University of Utah Hospital
  50 North Medical Drive
  Salt Lake City, UT 84132
  801-581-2321

Virginia

Adolescent Health
  Medical College of Virginia
  1001 E. Marshall Street
  Richmond, VA 23219
  804-828-9449
Pediatric Endocrinology and Adolescent Medicine
  Children's Hospital of the King's Daughters
  601 Children's Lane
  Norfolk, VA 23507
  757-668-7816

Washington

Adolescent Clinic
  University of Washington

Division of Adolescent Medicine
  CH Regional
  4800 Sandpoint Way N.E.
  MS # M2-4
  Seattle, WA 98105
  206-987-2028
The Adolescent Center
  13451 SE 36th Street
  Bellevue, WA 98006
  425-562-1352
The Kent Teen Clinic
  613 West Gowe Street
  Kent, WA 98032
  206-296-7450
The Teen Pregnancy and Parenting Clinic
  125 16th Avenue E.
  MS (CWB-F112)
  Seattle, WA 98112
  206-326-2656
The Renton Teen Clinic
  275 Bronson Way NE, (RNT)
  Renton, WA 98056-4099
  425-254-2710

West Virginia

Pediatrics
  West Virginia University
  Department of Pediatrics
  PO Box 9214
  Morgantown, WV 26506-9214
  304-293-1225

Wisconsin

Pediatric and Teen Clinic
  University of Wisconsin Hospital and Clinics
  2880 University Avenue
  Madison, WI 53705
  608-263-9000
Adolescent Clinic
  Children's Hospital
  1020 North 12th Street
  Milwaukee, WI 53233
  414-277-8900
Pediatrics and Adolescent Clinic
  Marshfield Clinic
  1000 North Oak Avenue
  Marshfield, WI 54449
  800-335-5251
Pediatric and Adolescent Department
  Beaumont Clinic LTD
  P.O. Box 19070
  Green Bay, WI 54307-9070
  920-496-4700

Canada

Adolescent Clinic
  British Columbia Children's Hospital
  4480 Oak Street
  Vancouver, BC 6H3V4
  604-875-2130
Adolescent Clinic
  St. Justine Hospital
  3175 Chemin Cote Ste.-Catherine
  Montreal, Quebec H3T1C5
  514-345-4722

Adolescent/Teen Clinic
    Hospital for Sick Children
    555 University Avenue
    Toronto, Ontario M5G1X8
    416-813-5804
Child and Adolescent Services
    Allan Memorial Institute
    Royal Victoria Hospital
    3666 McTavish Street
    Montreal, Quebec H3A1Y2
    514-843-1619

Sleep Disorder Resources

Arizona
Banner Regional Sleep Disorder Program
    Good Samaritan Medical Center
    1111 East McDowell Road
    Phoenix, AZ 85006
    602-239-2000

California
North Valley Sleep Disorders Center
    11550 Indian Hills Road, suite 291
    Mission Hills, CA 91345
    818-361-0996
Sleep Disorders Center
    University of California
    Irvine Medical Center
    101 The City Drive, Route 23
    Orange, CA 92868
    714-456-5105
Stanford Sleep Disorders Clinic
    401 Quarry Road, suite 3301-A
    Stanford, CA 94305
    650-725-5917
UCLA Sleep Disorders Center
    University of California
    Los Angeles, 24–221 CHS
    Box 957069
    Los Angeles, CA 90095-7069
    310-206-8005

Florida
Sleep Disorders Clinic
    Mount Sinai Medical Center
    4701 N. Meridian Avenue
    Miami Beach, FL 33140
    305-674-2613

Illinois
Sleep Disorders Center
    Northwest Memorial Hospital
    201 East Huron
    Galter 7th floor
    Chicago, IL 60611
    312-926-2650
Sleep Disorders Center
    Rush Medical Center
    710 S. Paulin Street, Suite 600S
    Chicago, IL 60612
    312-942-5440
Sleep Disorders Center
    University of Chicago (TS-301)

5815 South Maryland MC 9091
Chicago, IL 60637
773-702-1782

Louisiana
Tulane Sleep Disorders Center
    1415 Tulane Avenue
    Box HC17
    New Orleans, LA 70112
    504-988-1657

Maryland
The Johns Hopkins Sleep Disorders Center
    Asthma and Allergy Building
    room 4B-50
    5501 Hopkins Bay View Circle
    Baltimore, MD 21224
    410-550-0571

Massachusetts
Center for Pediatric Sleep Disorders
    The Children's Hospital
    300 Longwood Avenue
    Honeywell 2
    Boston, MA 02115
    617-355-6000/6663/6242
Sleep Clinic
    Brigham and Women's Hospital
    Sleep HealthCenter
    1505 Commonwealth Avenus
    Brighton, MA 02135
    617-783-1441
Sleep Disorders Clinic
    Tufts-Newton Wellesley Hospital
    2014 Washington Street
    Newton, MA 02462
    617-243-6624
Sleep Disorder Center
    University of Massachusetts Memorial
    119 Belmont Street
    Worcester, MA 01605
    508-334-8191

Michigan
Sleep Disorders Clinic
    Clara Ford Pavilion
    2799 West Grand Boulevard
    Detroit, MI 48202
    313-916-5176

Minnesota
Minnesota Regional Sleep Disorders Center
    Hennepin County Medical Center
    #867B, 701 Park Avenue South
    South Minneapolis, MN 55415
    612-873-6201

New Hampshire
Sleep Disorders Center
    Dartmouth–Hitchcock Medical Center
    1 Medical Center Drive
    Lebanon, NH 03756
    603-650-7534

New York

Sleep Disorders Center
   University Hospital
   240 Middle Country Road
   Smithtown, NY 11787
   631-444-2500
Sleep-Wake Disorders Center
   Montefiore Medical Center
   3411 Wayne Avenue
   The Bronx, NY 10467
   718-920-4841

Oklahoma

Sleep Disorders Center
   Presbyterian Hospital and Medical Center
   700 NE 13th Street
   Oklahoma City, OK 73104
   405-271-6312

Pennsylvania

Sleep Evaluation Center
   Western Psychiatric Institute and Clinic
   3811 O'Hara Street
   Pittsburgh, PA 15213-2593
   412-624-2000
Sleep Research and Treatment Center
   Milton S. Hershey Medical Center
   500 University Drive
   Hershey, PA 17033
   717-531-8520

Tennessee

Sleep Disorders Center
   Baptist Memorial Hospital
   1500 W. Popular
   Collierville, TN 38017
   901-861-9001
Sleep Disorders Clinic
   Vanderbilt University Medical Center
   Marriott Hotel
   2525 W End Street
   Nashville, Tenn. 37232
   615-343-5888

Texas

Sleep Disorders and Research Medicine
   Baylor College of Medicine & VA Medical Center
   2002 Holcombe Boulevard, room 6C344
   Houston, TX 77030
   713-794-7563

Organizations Involved In Adolescent Health

Healthfinder.gov. This site has links with most health organizations including nonprofit organizations. http://www.healthfinder.gov/.
American Academy of Child and Adolescent Psychiatry
   3615 Wisconsin Avenue, NW
   Washington, DC 20016
   202-966-7300
   www.aacap.org/
American Academy of Family Physicians (AAFP)
   11400 Tomahawk Creek Parkway

   Leawood, KS 66211-2672
   913-906-6000
   www.aafp.org/
American Academy of Pediatrics
   141 Northwest Point Boulevard
   Elk Grove Village, IL 60007-1098
   847-434-4000
   www.aap.org/
American College Health Association
   PO Box 28937
   Baltimore, MD 21240-8937
   410-859-1500
   www.acha.org
American College of Obstetricians and Gynecologists
   Division of Program Services, Department of Adolescent Health Care
   409 12th Street, SW., PO Box 96920
   Washington, DC 20090-6920
   202-638-5577
   www.acog.org/
American College of Physicians
   190 N. Independence Mall West
   Philadelphia, PA 19106-1572
   215-351-2600; 800-523-1546 ext. 1546
   www.acponline.org/
American College of Preventive Medicine
   1307 New York Avenue, N.W., Suite 200
   Washington, DC 20005
   202-466-2044
   www.acpm.org/
American Dietetic Association
   120 South Riverside Plaza, Suite 200
   Chicago, IL 60606-6995
   800-877-1600
   www.eatright.org/
American Medical Association (AMA)
   Department of Adolescent Health
   515 North State Street
   Chicago, IL 60610
   800-621-8335
   www.ama-assn.org/
American Osteopathic Association
   142 East Ontario Street
   Chicago, IL 60611
   800-621-1773
   www.osteopathic.org
American Psychiatric Association
   1000 Wilson Boulevard, Suite 1825
   Arlington, VA 22209-3901
   703-907-7300
   www.psych.org/
American Psychological Association
   750 First Street, N.E.
   Washington, DC 20002-4242
   800-374-2721
   www.apa.org/
American Public Health Association
   800 I. Street NW
   Washington, DC 20001-3710
   202-777-APHA
   www.apha.org/
American School Health Association
   PO Box 708
   Kent, OH 44240
   330-678-1601
   www.ashaweb.org/

American Society for Adolescent Psychiatry
PO Box 570218
Dallas, TX 75357-0218
972-686-6166
www.adolpsych.org/
Association of State and Territorial Health Officials
1275 K. Street N.W. Suite 800
Washington, D.C. 20005-4006
(202) 371–9090
www.astho.org/state.html
Canadian Paediatric Society
2305 St. Laurent Blvd.
Ottawa, Ontario, K1G 4J8, Canada
(613) 526–9397
http://www.cps.ca/english/index.htm
Centers for Disease Control and Prevention (CDC)
1600 Clifton Road
Atlanta, GA 30333
404-639-3311
www.cdc.gov/

Healthy Teen Network

The Healthy Teen Network, Inc., formerly the National Organization on Adolescent Pregnancy, Parenting, and Prevention, Inc. (NOAPPP), is an interdisciplinary 501(c) (3) membership association for leaders in the field of adolescent reproductive health and parenting. The organization and its members are dedicated to educating providers, organizations, teens and their parents, policymakers, and the public about critical issues that impact reproductive information and services to teens, teen parents, and their children.
509 2nd Street NE
Washington, DC, 20002
(202) 547–8814
www.healthyteennetwork.org

International Association for Adolescent Health
PO Box 2137
Christchurch, New Zealand
www.iaah.org
Maternal and Child Health Bureau
Health Resources and Services Administration
U.S. Public Health Service, Department of Health and Human Services
5600 Fishers Lane, room 1805
Rockville, MD 20857
301-443-2170
National Association of Social Workers
750 First Street NE, suite 700
Washington, DC 20002-4241
202-408-8600
800-638-8799
www.naswdc.org/
National Alliance for Hispanic Health
1501 16th Street NW
Washington, DC 20036-1401
202-387-5000
www.hispanichealth.org/
National Institute on Alcohol Abuse and Alcoholism
Prevention Research Branch
5635 Fishers Lane, MSC-9304
Bethesda, MD 20892-9304
301-443-1677
www.niaaa.nih.gov/

National Institute on Drug Abuse
6001 Executive Boulevard
Bethesda, MD 20892-9561
301-443-1124
www.nida.nih.gov/
National Medical Association (NMA)
1012 Tenth Street, NW
Washington, DC 20001
202-347-1895
www.nmanet.org/
National Mental Health Association (NMHA)
2000 N Beaurregard Street, 6th Floor
Alexandria, VA 22311
703-684-7722
www.nmha.org/
Office of Disease Prevention and Health Promotion
U.S. Public Health Service
Department of Health and Human Services
1101 Wootton Parkway, Suite LL100
Rockville, MD 20852
240-453-8280
http://odphp.osophs.dhhs.gov/
Planned Parenthood Federation of America
www.plannedparenthood.org
The Robert Wood Johnson Foundation
College Road East/Route 1
PO Box 2316
Princeton, NJ 08543
888-631-9989
www.rwjf.org/index.jsp
Sexuality Information and Education Council of the United States
130 West 42nd Street, suite 350
New York, NY 10036
212-819-9770
www.siecus.org/
Society for Adolescent Medicine (SAM)
1916 Copper Oaks Circle
Blue Springs, MO 64015
816-224-8010
www.adolescenthealth.org/
Society for Research in Adolescence
3131 S. State Street, Suite 302
Ann Arbor, MI 48104-1623
socresadol@umich.edu
734-998-6567
www.s-r-a.org/
William T Grant Foundation
570 Lexington Avenue, 18th floor
New York, NY 10022
212-752-0071
http://williamtgrantfoundation.org
World Health Organization
Avenue Appia 20
1211 Geneva 27
Switzerland
(+41 22) 791 21 11
www.who.int/en/

Sports Medicine Organizations

Academy for Sports Dentistry
University of Iowa Hospitals and Clinics,
Department of Otolaryngology
Iowa City, IA 52242
www.sportsdentistry-asd.com

American Academy of Orthopaedic Surgeons
 6300 North River Road
 Rosemont, IL 60018-4262
 847-823-7186
 www.aaos.org/
American Academy of Pediatrics
 141 Northwest Point Blvd.
 Elk Grove Village, IL 60007-1098
 847-434-4000
 www.app.org
American College Health Association
 PO Box 28937
 Baltimore, MD 21240-8937
 410-859-1500
 www.acha.org
American College of Sports Medicine
 401 W. Michigan Street
 Indianapolis, IN 46202-3233
 317-637-9200 ext. 138
 www.acsm.org/
American Council on Exercise
 4851 Paramount Drive
 San Diego, CA 92123
 858-279-8227
 www.acefitness.org/
American Heart Association
 7272 Greenville Avenue
 Dallas, TX 75231-4596
 800-242-8721
 www.americanheart.org/
American Medical Association (AMA)
 Department of Adolescent Health
 515 North State Street
 Chicago, IL 60610
 800-621-8335
 www.ama-assn.org/
American Medical Society for Sports Medicine
 11639 Earnshaw
 Overland Park, KS 66210
 913-327-1415
 www.amssm.org/contactus.htm
National Athletic Trainers Association
 2952 Stemmons Freeway
 Dallas, TX 75247
 214-637-6282
 www.nata.org/
National Collegiate Athletic Association
 700 W. Washington Street
 Indianapolis, IN 46206-6222
 317-917-6222
 www.ncaa.rg/
President's Council on Physical Fitness and Sports
 200 Independence Avenue, S.W., Room 738-H
 Washington, DC 20001-004
 202-690-9000
 www.fitness.gov/

Statistical Resources

See Chapter 5 for further listing of statistical web-based
 resources.

Alan Guttmacher Institute
 120 Wall Street, 21st Floor
 New York, NY 10005
 212-248-1111

www.guttmacher.org
 (Contraceptive data, pregnancy rates, and marital and
 fertility patterns.)
CDC
 Health, United States, 2006: Available at: http://www.cdc
 .gov/nchs/hus.htm
 Reproductive Health Division
 1600 Clifton Road, NE
 Atlanta, GA 30333
 404-639-3311
 www.cdc.gov/reproductivehealth/index.htm
National Institutes of Health
 National Institute of Child Health and Human Develop-
 ment
 Center for Population Research
 9000 Rockville Pike
 Bethesda, MD 20892
 301-496-4000
 www.nih.gov/
Center for Population Research
 www.nichd.nih.gov/about/cpr/
Healthfinder
 www.healthfinder.gov/
Population Studies Center
 www.psc.isr.umich.edu/
Monitoring the Future Web site on Drug Usage
 www.monitoringthefuture.org/
National Cancer Institute, Surveillance Epidemiology and
 End Results, http://seer.cancer.gov/publicdata/
National Center for Educational Statistics (trend informa-
 tion)
 http:/nces.ed.gov
National Center for Injury Prevention and Control (NCIPC)
 (http://www.cdc.gov/ncipc/wisqars/default.htm)
National Center for Health Statistics
 3700 East-West Highway
 Hyattsville, MD 20782-2003
 301-458-4000
 www.cdc.gov/nchs
National Institutes of Health
 Demographic and Behavioral Sciences Branch
The National Survey of Family Growth (*http://www.cdc.gov/
 nchs/nsfg.htm*)
National Vital Statistics System—http://www.cdc.gov/nchs/
 nvss.htm
Statistical Abstract of the United States
 www.census.gov/prod/www/statistical-abstract-
 us.html
 U.S. Census Bureau—www.census.gov/compendia/
 statab/).
Youth Risk Behavior Survey (YRBSS): (http://www.cdc.gov/
 HealthyYouth/yrbs/index.htm) The Youth Risk Behav-
 ior

WEB SITES

The world wide web has exploded as a source of
health information including a wealth of information about
adolescent medicine and general medical topics. This
section reviews the following:

1. How to subscribe to SAM and College listserv groups
2. Tips on health Web searching
3. Best sites for browsing
4. Best sites to get statistical and other information

How to subscribe to the SAM and College listserv groups

An electronic mailing list (listserv) is a group of individuals interested in an area, who can post questions and comments and receive responses to these questions, as well as in all the posts that are listed. This is a wonderful format for communicating information and asking questions—clinical, educational, research, or administrative. However, when you are on a listserv, you may receive several to 50 or more e-mails per day depending on the volume of posts to a particular listserv. It is recommended that users learn how to use the "delete" button quickly.

SAM ListServ (SAM-L)

The Society for Adolescent Medicine maintains its own listserv. Through this listserv, SAM members and other health care professionals interested in adolescent medicine and adolescent's health issues can share ideas. If an individual who is not a SAM member wants to join the listserv, he/she should first contact the SAM office at sam@adolescenthealth.org or 816.224.8010 and provide brief work contact information.

To subscribe to this free communication mode, you perform the following steps:

- Send a message to sam-L@adolescenthealth.org. The message should only say *subscribe SAM-L "your name"* (e.g., subscribe SAM-L "Mary Jones").
- When you want to post to the Listserv, e-mail to sam-l@adolescenthealth.org (this is an "L," not the number 1 after "sam").
- When you receive a Listserv message and you want to provide an answer and/or share your thoughts with the sender, do *not* click on the Reply button; if you do, everyone on the Listserv message will receive your reply. Instead, note the sender's e-mail address, and send a new message using that address only.
- To unsubscribe, one needs to contact the SAM office at sam@adolescenthealth.org or 816.224.8010 asking to be removed from the system.

College Health ListServ

SHS Listserv: The Student Health Service discussion group (SHS) is the major forum and information source for college health professionals, students involved in health promotion, and any other interested parties. The subscription base is more than 1,200 college health professionals. Instructions:

1. Send an e-mail to: listserv@listserv.utk.edu
2. Under the SUBJECT, type Subscription
3. In the MESSAGE, type SUB SHS (Your Name).

You will then receive confirmation of the subscription and a formal electronic welcome with instructions from the group. You may cancel the subscription at any time.

The College Health Promotion List

The College Health Promotion List (Hlthprom) provides a forum for the exchange of information among professionals providing health promotion and prevention services at colleges/universities. Discussions might address such topics as sexuality, STDs, HIV/AIDS, alcohol, tobacco, and drugs use, nutrition, peer education, and administration.

To join HLTHPROM, fill in the form on this page: https://lists.wisc.edu/read/all_forums/subscribe?name=hlthprom

The Clinical Medicine List

The Clinical Medicine List (Clinmed) provides a forum for clinical medicine providers in the college health field. It is maintained at the University of Colorado-Boulder.
Instructions:

1. Send an email to: listproc@lists.colorado.edu
2. Leave the subject line blank
3. In the message, type: subscribe clinmed (your name)

You will then receive confirmation of the subscription and a formal electronic welcome with instructions from the group. You may cancel the subscription at any time.

The SHSaAMc ListServ

For directors of student health services at academic medical centers. Instructions:

1. Send an email to Majordomo@list.pitt.edu
2. Type in the body of the email message:
       Subscribe SHSAAMc@list.pitt.edu

After you are subscribed, you may then send emails to the list address: SHSAAMc@list.pitt.edu. Only list subscribers will be able to post to this list.

College Mental Health List

For discussion of issues among professionals providing mental health services at colleges/universities.
Instructions:

1. Send a message to: listserver@relay.doit.wisc.edu
2. Leave the subject link blank
3. In the message, type: subscribe univn [your name]

Insert your real name and do not include the brackets.
You will then receive confirmation of the subscription and a formal electronic welcome with instructions from the group. You may cancel the subscription at any time.

The College Nutrition ListServ

For college health nutritionists and registered dietitians and anyone working in college health with an interest in nutrition.
Instructions:

1. To subscribe, unsubscribe, or change settings, visit the ADACOMM Web page at https://mailman.csupomona.edu/mailman/listinfo/adacomm
2. For questions, contact the mailing list owner at jv-grizzell@csupomona.edu

Students in Student Health List

The Students in Student Health List (StudHeal) provides a forum for the exchange of information among students involved in student health issues. Discussions might address such topics as programming, SHACs, peer education groups, and involvement in ACHA. Subscriptions are free. The list is operated by Arizona State University.
Instructions:

1. Send an e-mail to: listserv@asuvm.inre.asu.edu
2. Leave the subject line blank
3. In the message, type: subscribe studheal (your name)

You will then receive confirmation of the subscription and a formal electronic welcome with instructions from the group. You may cancel the subscription at anytime.

LGBT-Health
A forum to discuss and work on lesbian, gay, bisexual, and transgender health issues in the college setting primarily, but not limited to college life.
Instructions:

1. Send an email to listserv@usm.maine.edu
2. Leave the subject line blank
3. In the message, type: subscribe lgbt-Health

Tips on Health Web Searching

One can gain a wealth of information and data quickly utilizing a concise approach to searching the Web.

Web Searching
Some of the best Web search tools include www.google.com and www.yahoo.com.Google.com uses an approach that combines finding the keywords and the utilization pattern of the Web sites by users. In practice, this means that in most cases, the most useful sites are found early in the search. In addition to putting down the keyword, it is useful to add a second keyword that may help refine the search. For example, you can search on gonorrhea. In fact, with the Google searcher, the top two sites are a CDC and an NIH site on gonorrhea. If you want CDC information, you could narrow this search by placing both *gonorrhea* and *CDC* in the search area. With a Web search tool, you are likely to find hundreds of "hits." Each hit is usually titled, has a brief description, and has the Web address. These can be very helpful to glance at quickly to help you narrow which "hits" to explore. In health sites, the addresses often lead to either government sites, academic centers, commercial health sites, commercial product sites (pharmaceutical companies and others), and private health care provider sites. Looking at the address can help you determine if you want to explore that site or not. There are some important questions to ask yourself about each site:

- Is the advice provided by qualified trained medical professionals?
- How old is the information? Often a site can look great, but the information was last updated 3 or 4 years ago.
- Who pays for the site? Is this a commercial for-profit site?
- Do you need to register or provide personal information? Make sure you read the privacy information before giving out such information.
- Where do these links go to (as outlined previously).

Health Portals
There are also some specific health finders and portals that can help in finding health information. These include the following:

- www.healthfinder.gov. Health searching tool from the NIH.
- www.healthatoz.com/. Commercial health searching tool.
- www.nlm.nih.gov/medlineplus. National Library of Medicines database of medical journal abstracts and resources such as clearinghouses, libraries, and medical dictionaries.
- www.nlm.nih.gov/. National Library of Medicines regular search of Library of Congress.

- http://loc.gov/. National Library of Congress.
- www.emedicine.com. Medical textbook online.
- www.cdc.gov. A wealth of information from the CDC that includes searchable health information, fact sheets, *Morbidity Mortality Weekly Reports*, supplements, statistics, travelers health updates, and much more.

Patient-oriented Overall Health Sites
- www.intelihealth.com. Site from Aetna Healthcare and Harvard University Medical Schools featuring information on common health problems.
- www.mayohealth.org. Other site of basic information that's written for the public from Mayo Clinic.
- www.kidshealth.org. Portal for extensive health information for teens and parents.
- www.webmd.com/. Commercial site of health information.
- www.noah-health.org. Comprehensive health information on many topics. Available in Spanish.
- www.goaskalice.columbia.edu/about.html. College student-oriented site on many topics with questions and answers.
- www.talkingwithkids.org. Site from Kaiser Family Foundation to facilitate communication between parents and teens.
- http://familydoctor.org. From the American Academy of Family Physicians, this site offers patient education documents for common medical concerns and conditions. All of the information within familydoctor.org has been written and reviewed by physicians and patient education professionals at the American Academy of Family Physicians.
- http://cpmcnet.columbia.edu/texts/guide/. This resource is the online version of the third Revised Edition, 1995 of this standard consumer health text.
- http://www.merckhomeedition.com/home.html. The online interactive edition of "The Merck Manual of Medical Information—Home Edition," a comprehensive consumer text.
- http://www.vh.org/commonproblems/commonproblems.html. The Virtual Hospital is a digital health sciences library created in 1992 at the University of Iowa to help meet the information needs of health care providers and patients. The site contains hundreds of books and brochures.

Best Sites for Browsing

In addition to the sites already listed, there are many other excellent sites for browsing. Many of these are listed in individual chapters of this book. Some highlights include the following:

Reproductive Health
- www.agi-usa.org. Alan Guttmacher Institute with a wealth of information on reproductive health and statistics.
- www.reproline.jhu.edu/. Reproductive Health Online affiliated with Johns Hopkins University, promoting information on reproductive health issues.
- www.teenpregnancy.org/. Information from the National Campaign to Prevent Teen Pregnancy, with information and data on teenage pregnancy.
- www.iwannaknow.org. Teen awareness site on STDs from the American Social Health Association.

- www.teenwire.com. Teen health and awareness site from Planned Parenthood.
- www.engenderhealth.org/wh/fp/index.html. Web site from AVSC, an overview of information about contraceptive devices.
- www.cdc.gov/nchstp/dstd. The CDC home page on STD information and guidelines.
- www.4woman.org/faq/adoles.htm. National Women's Health Information Center.

Clinical Guidelines

- www.acc.org/clinical/topic/topic.htm. Clinical guidelines from the American College of Cardiology and the American Heart Association.
- http://www.guideline.gov/. National Guideline Clearinghouse. Database of clinical criteria from numerous health organizations.
- http://www.ahrq.gov/clinic/cpgonline.htm. Agency for Healthcare Research and Quality—Clinical Guidelines Online.

Health Prevention and Promotion

- www.health.gov/healthypeople/. The Department of Health and Human Services Web sites on goals for the health of the United States in 2010.
- http://familydoctor.org/healthfacts/. AAFP, patient handouts.
- http://nccam.nih.gov. National Center for Complementary and Alternative Medicine disseminates information to practitioners and public.

Best Sites to get Statistical and Other Information:

See chapter 5 and statistical resources above.

INDEX

Page numbers followed by *f* in italics indicate figures; those followed by *t* indicate tabular material.

Urinalysis, 45*t*
  Chlamydia trachomatis and, 812
  cystitis, 379
  enuresis, 388–389
  hematuria, 398
  laboratory test, 63
  pelvic inflammatory disease and, 821
  proteinuria, 395–396
Urinary tract infection, 380*f*, 397
Urine drug testing, practical issues, 942, 946–948
Urticaria, 318, 321–322
U.S. Census Bureau, 81, 82*t*
U.S. Preventive Services Task Force (USPSTF), preventive care, 44, 45*t*, 49
Uterine defects, 706
Uterine bleeding, dysfunctional, 687–690
Uterine neoplasms, 708
Uterine synechiae, 694–695
Uterovaginal agenesis, 707
Uterus
  amenorrhea and, 692, 694, 695
  congenital absence of, 692, 694, 695
  congenital anomalies, 706
  neoplasms, 708
  palpation, 669

V
Vaccinations, (see immunizations)70– 77, 451
Vagal nerve stimulation (VNS), epilepsy, 341
Vagina
  discharge, 729–731
  normal, 723
Vaginal-abdominal examination, 669
Vaginal contraceptive rings, 612–613
Vaginal defects, 706–707
Vaginal spermicides, 637–638
Vaginitis, 378*t*, 668, 777–778
  bacterial vaginosis, 728–729
  causes of vaginal discharge, 729–731
  Trichomoniasis vaginalis, 726–728
  vulvovaginal candidiasis (VVC), 724–726
Vaginosis, pubertal females, 724
Valacyclovir, 838, 839
Valerian root, 1069*t*, 1071
Valproic acid
  headaches, 353
  seizure treatment, 335, 338*t*
  side effects, 336, 341
  teen pregnancy, 575
Valvular aortic stenosis, 223*t*, 224–225
Valvular heart disease, contraceptive methods, 591*t*
Valvular pulmonary stenosis, 223*t*, 224
Vanishing testis syndrome, 145
Varicella, 76–77, 451
Varicocele, 405*f*, 407–408
Vascular headaches, 346, 347
Vasopressin, enuresis, 387, 390–391
VDRL, for syphilus, 826, 828–829
Vegans, guidelines, 121
Vegetarian diets, guidelines, 121
Vehicular accidents, 878, 889*f*
Venereal disease, consent, 125, 130–131

Venereal Disease Research Laboratory (VDRL), test for syphilus, 826, 828, 829
Venereal warts, 319
Venlafaxine, 1014*t*
  premenstrual syndrome, 682*t*
Ventricular septal defect, 223*t*, 224
Verrucae, 319–320
Vertebral osteomyelitis, 262
Vertigo, 361–363
Very low-density lipoprotein, 188–190
Victimization
  homicide rates, 89*f*
  sexual assault and, 1042–1043
Vigabatrin, hormonal contraceptives, 601, 602*t*
Violence
  assessment of risk, 987–988
  epidemiology, 984–986
  fighting-injuries-sex-threats–self-defense (FISTS), 988*t*
  homicide, 984, 985*t*
  objectives, 83*t*
  prevention and intervention, 988–990
  resilence, 987
  risk factors, 986–987
  screening, 53*f*, 57*f*
Violent discipline, 986
Viral pneumonia, 419
Virilization, 746–752
  diagnosis, 748–751
Vision, screening, 45*t*, 63
Vitamins
  hyperlipidemia, 200
  premenstrual syndrome and , 679, 681
  requirements, 120
  vegetarians, 121
Vitamin therapy
  hyperlipidemia, 200
  premenstrual syndrome, 679, 681
Vitex agnus-castus, premenstrual syndrome, 681
Vitiligo, 320
Von Willebrand disease, 689
Vulvodynia, 730
Vulvovaginal candidiasis, vaginitis, 724–726, 730*t*
Vulvovaginitis
  prepubertal females, 723
  pubertal females, 724

W
Waist-hip ratio (WHR), nutrition, 117–118
Walking pneumonia, 418–419
Warfarin
  hormonal contraceptives, 602*t*
  teen pregnancy, 576
Warts, 319–320. *See also* Human papillomavirus (HPV)
  anogenital, 843
  flat, 319
  genital, 779–780, 842–848
  plantar, 319
  venereal, 319
  Verruca vulgaris, 319
Weapons, 53*f*, 57*f*
  violence, 986, 989

Web-based Injury Statistics Query and Reporting System (WISQARS), mortality, 82
Weight, 53*f*, 57*f*
  amenorrhea, 693, 697
  athlete nutrition, 122
  changes with contraceptive use, 609, 654, 658
  herbs, 1072
  hypertension, 214
  nutrition, 116
  puberty, 15–16
Weight-for-age
  boys, 20*f*
  girls, 18*f*
Weight-for-height percentile
  obesity, 467
  polycystic ovary disease and, 702
  puberty and, 10, 12*f*
  reduction, 214
  sports examination, 265, 267
Withdrawal syndromes
  amphetamines, 918
  anabolic steroids, 937
  barbiturates, 925
  benzodiazepines, 926–927
  cocaine, 915
  ecstasy, 921
  hallucinogens, 932
  marijuana, 911
  nicotine, 895
  opioids, 922–923
  recovery from, for drugs, 953*t*
Wolff–Parkinson–White syndrome, 359*t*, 363
Wolfram syndrome, diabetes, 171
World Health Organization (WHO), contraception, 589, 590*t*, 651*t*, 652*t*
Writing disorder, 1034–1035

X
X chromosomal abnormality, amenorrhea and, 691–692

Y
Yoga, 1074
Yohimbe, 1069*t*
Youth Risk Behavior Survey (YRBS), morbidity, 85, 86*t*, 539*t*, 540*f*, 541*f*, 542*f*
Yuzpe regimen, emergency contraception, 641–646

Z
Zalcitabine, 455
Zanamivir, influenza, 423
Zidovudine, 446–447, 455
Zinc
  requirements, 120
  risk of deficiency, 122
Zolmitriptan, migraine headaches, 352–353
Zonisamide, seizure treatment, 336, 339*t*